INTEGRATIVE MEDICINE

Fourth Edition

David Rakel, MD

Professor and Chair
Department of Family and Community Medicine
University of New Mexico School of Medicine
Albuquerque, New Mexico

ELSEVIER

ELSEVIER

1600 John F. Kennedy Blvd.
Ste 1800
Philadelphia, PA 19103-2899

Notices

Knowledge and best practice in this field are constantly changing. As new research and experience broaden our understanding, changes in research methods, professional practices, or medical treatment may become necessary.

Practitioners and researchers must always rely on their own experience and knowledge in evaluating and using any information, methods, compounds, or experiments described herein. In using such information or methods they should be mindful of their own safety and the safety of others, including parties for whom they have a professional responsibility.

With respect to any drug or pharmaceutical products identified, readers are advised to check the most current information provided (i) on procedures featured or (ii) by the manufacturer of each product to be administered, to verify the recommended dose or formula, the method and duration of administration, and contraindications. It is the responsibility of practitioners, relying on their own experience and knowledge of their patients, to make diagnoses, to determine dosages and the best treatment for each individual patient, and to take all appropriate safety precautions.

To the fullest extent of the law, neither the Publisher nor the authors, contributors, or editors, assume any liability for any injury and/or damage to persons or property as a matter of products liability, negligence or otherwise, or from any use or operation of any methods, products, instructions, or ideas contained in the material herein.

Previous editions © 2012, 2007, 2003

Library of Congress Cataloging-in-Publication Data

Names: Rakel, David, editor.
Title: Integrative medicine / [edited by] David Rakel.
Other titles: Integrative medicine (Rakel)
Description: Fourth edition. | Philadelphia: Elsevier, 2017. | Includes
    bibliographical references and index.
Identifiers: LCCN 2017000204 | ISBN 9780323358682 (hardcover: alk. paper)
Subjects: | MESH: Integrative Medicine--methods | Complementary
    Therapies--methods | Preventive Medicine--methods | Primary Health
    Care--methods
Classification: LCC R733 | NLM WB 113 | DDC 616--dc23 LC record available at
    https://lccn.loc.gov/2017000204

Senior Content Strategist: Sarah Barth
Senior Content Development Specialist: Joan Ryan
Publishing Services Manager: Catherine Jackson
Project Manager: Kate Mannix
Design Direction: Patrick Ferguson
Illustrations Manager: Amy Faith Heyden

Printed in the United States

Last digit is the print number: 9 8 7 6 5 4

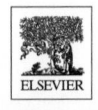

Working together
to grow libraries in
developing countries

www.elsevier.com • www.bookaid.org

For the students, residents, fellows, friends, and colleagues
at the University of Wisconsin School of Medicine and Public Health.
Thank you for your support and guidance over the past 16 years.

CONTRIBUTORS

Robert Abel, Jr., MD
Delaware Ophthalmology Consultants
Wilmington, Delaware;
Former Clinical Professor of Ophthalmology
Thomas Jefferson University School of Medicine
Philadelphia, Pennsylvania

Ather Ali, ND, MPH, MHS
Assistant Professor of Pediatrics and Medicine
Director
Yale Adult and Pediatric Integrative Medicine Clinic;
Medical Director, Integrative Medicine
Smilow Cancer Hospital at Yale-New Haven
Yale University School of Medicine
New Haven, Connecticut

Judith Balk, MD, MPH
Associate Professor
Obstetrics and Gynecology
Allegheny Health Network, Temple University
Pittsburgh, Pennsylvania

Bruce Barrett, MD, PhD
Professor
Department of Family Medicine and Community Health
University of Wisconsin School of Medicine and Public
    Health
Madison, Wisconsin

David K. Becker, MD
HS Clinical Professor
Department of Pediatrics
Osher Center for Integrative Medicine
University of California, San Francisco School of Medicine
San Francisco, California

Paul E. Bergquist, MD
Physician Member
American Institute of Homeopathy;
Family Practice Physican
Family Practice and Complementary Medicine
Vernon Memorial Hospital and Clinics
Viroqua, Wisconsin

Apple A. Bodemer, MD
Assistant Professor
Department of Dermatology
University of Wisconsin
Madison, Wisconsin

Robert Alan Bonakdar, MD
Director of Pain Management
Scripps Center for Integrative Medicine
Health Sciences Assistant Clinical Professor (Nonsalaried)
Department of Family Medicine and Public Health
University of California, San Diego School of Medicine
La Jolla, California

Samudragupta Bora, PhD
Postdoctoral Fellow
Pediatric Newborn Medicine
Brigham and Women's Hospital;
Postdoctoral Fellow
Pediatrics
Harvard Medical School
Boston, Massachusetts

Suhani Bora, MD
Research Fellow
Department of Pediatric Newborn Medicine
Brigham and Women's Hospital
Harvard Medical School
Boston, Massachusetts

Amy C. Brown, PhD
Department of Complementary and Alternative Medicine
John A. Burns School of Medicine
University of Hawaii
Honolulu, Hawaii

Remy R. Coeytaux, MD, PhD
Associate Professor
Department of Community and Family Medicine
Duke Clinical Research Institute
Durham, North Carolina

Stephen Dahmer, MD
Assistant Clinical Professor of Family Medicine and
    Community Health
Icahn School of Medicine at Mount Sinai
New York, New York

Douglas E. Dandurand, PhD, MDiv, MA, MAS
Spiritual Facilitator
Minnesota Personalized Medicine
Minneapolis, Minnesota

Alan M. Dattner, MD
CEO and Founder
HolisticDermatology.com
New York, New York

Brian Degenhardt, DO
Associate Research Professor
Kirksville College of Osteopathic Medicine
A. T. Still University;
Director
A. T. Still Research Institute
Kirksville, Missouri;
Co-Medical Director
Ridgway Integrative Medicine
Ridgway, Colorado

Gautam J. Desai, DO, FACOFP
Professor, Division of Primary Care
Kansas City University
Kansas City, Missouri

Stephen Devries, MD, FACC, FAHA
Executive Director
Gaples Institute for Integrative Cardiology;
Associate Professor
Division of Cardiology
Northwestern Feinberg School of Medicine
Chicago, Illinois

Dennis J. Dowling, DO
Private Practice
Osteopathic Manipulative Medicine Associates
Syosset, New York;
Director of Osteopathic Manipulative Medicine
Clinical Skills Testing Center
National Board of Osteopathic Medical Examiners
Conshohocken, Pennsylvania;
Director of Osteopathic Manipulative Services
Physical Medicine and Rehabilitation
Nassau University Medical Center
East Meadow, New York

Jeanne A. Drisko, MD
Director and Professor
KU Integrative Medicine
University of Kansas Medical Center
Kansas City, Kansas

Jeffery Dusek, PhD
Research Director
Integrative Health and Medicine Research Center
Allina Center for Healthcare Innovation
The Penny George Institute for Health and Healing
Minneapolis, Minnesota

Connie J. Earl, DO, ABIHM
Director of Integrative Medicine
West County Health Centers
Forestville, California;
Assistant Professor of Family Medicine
University of California San Francisco–Santa Rosa
    Family Medicine Residency
Santa Rosa, California

Robert Z. Edwards, MD
Family Physician
GHC of South Central Wisconsin
DeForest, Wisconsin

Joseph Eichenseher, MD, MAT
Access Community Health Center;
Clinical Assistant Professor
University of Wisconsin
Madison, Wisconsin

Ann C. Figurski, DO
Osteopathic Family Medicine Physician
Clinical Instructor
Department of Family Medicine and Community
    Health
University of Wisconsin
Madison, Wisconsin

Amanda C. Filippelli, MSN, MPH, RN, APRN
Pediatric Nurse Practitioner
Pulmonary Department
Connecticut Children's Medical Center
Hartford, Connecticut

Luke Fortney, MD, FAAFP
Family and Integrative Medicine
Sauk Prairie Healthcare
Spring Green, Wisconsin

Alan R. Gaby, MD
Past President of the American Holistic Medical
    Association
Author of the textbook *Nutritional Medicine*
Former Professor of Nutrition and Clinical Faculty
Bastyr University
Kenmore, Washington

Louise Gagné, MD
Clinical Assistant Professor
Community Health and Epidemiology
University of Saskatchewan
Saskatoon, Saskatchewan, Canada

Paula Gardiner, MD, MPH
Assistant Professor
Family Medicine
Boston Universtiy Medical School
Boston, Massachusetts

Tracy Gaudet, MD
Executive Director
National Office of Patient Centered Care and Cultural
    Transformation
Washington, DC

Jeffrey Geller, MD
Director of Integrative Medicine and Group Visits
Family Practice
Greater Lawrence Family Health Center;
    Director of HIP Fellowship
Integrative Medicine
Lawrence Family Practice Residency
Lawrence, Massachusetts

Katherine Gergen-Barnett, MD
Assistant Professor
Department of Family Medicine
Boston University School of Medicine
Boston, Massachusetts

Andrea Gordon, MD
Director of Integrative Medicine
Tufts University Family Medicine Program
Cambridge Health Alliance
Malden, Massachusetts;
Associate Professor
Tufts University School of Medicine
Boston, Massachusetts

Russell H. Greenfield, MD
Director
Greenfield Integrative Healthcare, PLLC
Charlotte, North Carolina;
    Clinical Professor of Medicine
University of North Carolina–Chapel Hill School of
    Medicine
Chapel Hill, North Carolina

Hana Grobel, MD
Integrative Family Physician
San Mateo, California

Thomas G. Guilliams, PhD
Adjunct Assistant Professor
University of Wisconsin School of Pharmacy
Madison, Wisconsin;
Vice President–Scientific Affairs
Ortho Molecular Products Inc.
Stevens Point, Wisconsin

Steven Gurgevich, PhD
Clinical Assistant Professor of Medicine
Arizona Center for Intergrative Medicine
University of Arizona College of Medicine;
Faculty, Fellow, and Approved Consultant
The American Society of Clinical Hypnosis;
Private Practice
Behavioral Medicine, Ltd.
Tucson, Arizona

Fasih A. Hameed, MD, ABIHM
Director of Integrative Services
Petaluma Health Center
Petaluma, California
Assistant Clinical Professor
University of California, San Francisco-Santa Rosa
    Family Medicine Residency
Santa Rosa, California;

Adrienne Hampton, MD
Department of Family Medicine
University of Wisconsin
Madison, Wisconsin

Patrick J. Hanaway, MD
Medical Director
Center for Functional Medicine
Cleveland Clinic
Cleveland, Ohio

Joshua Harbaugh, OMSIV
Kansas City University of Medicine and Biosciences
Kansas City, Missouri

John W. Harrington, MD
Division Director
General Academic Pediatrics
Children's Hospital of The King's Daughters;
Professor of Pediatrics
Eastern Virginia Medical School
Norfolk, Virginia

James Harvie, PEng
Executive Director
Institute for a Sustainable Future
Duluth, Minnesota

Supriya Hayer, MD
Research Specialist
Department of Family Medicine
University of Wisconsin School of Medicine and
    Community Health
Madison, Wisconsin

Michael Hernke, PhD
Lecturer
University of Wisconsin School of Business
Madison, Wisconsin

Michael J. Hewitt, PhD
Research Director for Exercise Science
Department of Exercise Physiology
Canyon Ranch Health Resort
Tucson, Arizona

Randy J. Horwitz, MD, PhD
Medical Director
Arizona Center for Integrative Medicine;
Associate Professor of Medicine
University of Arizona College of Medicine
Tucson, Arizona

Mark Houston, MD, MS, MSc
Associate Clinical Professor of Medicine
Medicine
Vanderbilt University School of Medicine
Nashville, Tennessee
Instructor in Medicine
Physical Medicine
Georgetown Medical School
Washington, DC

Corene Humphreys, ND
Director
Nutritional Medicine Ltd.
Medical Research Consultant
Auckland, New Zealand

Alexandra Ilkevitch, MD
Clinical Instructor
Department of Orthopedics and Rehabilitation
University of Wisconsin School of Medicine and Public
  Health
Madison, Wisconsin

Robert S. Ivker, DO
Co-founder and Former President
American Board of Integrative Holistic Medicine;
Medical Director
Fully Alive Medicine
Boulder, Colorado

Bradly Jacobs, MD, MPH, ABOIM
CEO and Executive Medical Director
BlueWave Medicine
Sausalito, California

Sarah James, DO
Department of Family Medicine
University of Wisconsin School of Medicine and
  Community Health
Madison, Wisconsin

Hwee Soo Jeong, MD
Associate Professor of Family and Integrative Medicine
Dongguk University College of Medicine
Gyeongju, Korea

Julia Jernberg, MD
Clinical Assistant Professor of Medicine
Department of Internal Medicine
Section of Geriatrics, General Medicine, and Palliative
  Medicine
University of Arizona College of Medicine
Tucson, Arizona;
Clinical Assistant Professor of Medicine
Department of Internal Medicine
University of Wisconsin Hospitals and Clinics
Madison, Wisconsin

Wayne Jonas, MD
Professor of Family Medicine
Georgetown University
Washington, DC;
Adjunct Professor
Uniformed Services University of Health Sciences
President and Chief Executive Officer
Samueli Institute
Alexandria, Virginia

Scott Karpowicz, MD
Lead Preceptor
Contra Costa Family Medicine Residency
Staff Physician
Department of Family Medicine
Contra Costa Regional Medical Center
Martinez, California

Amanda J. Kaufman, MD, ABIHM
Private Practice
Integrative Healthcare Providers
Ann Arbor, Michigan

David J. Kearney, MD
Professor of Medicine
University of Washington School of Medicine
Director, MBR Program
VA Puget Sound Health Care System
Seattle, Washington

Kathi J. Kemper, MD, MPH
Director
Center for Integrative Health and Wellness
Professor
Pediatrics
Ohio State University
Columbus, Ohio

David Kiefer, MD
Clinical Assistant Professor
Department of Family Medicine and Community
  Health
University of Wisconsin School of Medicine and Public
  Health
Madison, Wisconsin

Marcia Klein-Patel, MD, PhD
Assistant Professor
Temple University School of Medicine
Allegheny Health Network
Philadelphia, Pennsylvania

Benjamin Kligler, MD
Professor of Family Medicine and Community Health
Icahn School of Medicine at Mount Sinai
New York, New York

Mikhail Kogan, MD
Medical Director
GW Center for Integrative Medicine;
Assistant Professor
Department of Medicine
Associate Director, Geriatrics Fellowship
George Washington University
Washington, DC

Wendy Kohatsu, MD
Director, Integrative Medicine Fellowship
Santa Rosa Family Medicine Residency;
Culinary Medicine Chef
Santa Rosa, California;
Assistant Clinical Professor
Family and Community Medicine
Univeristy of California San Francisco
San Francisco, California

Greta J. Kuphal, MD
Clinical Assistant Professor
University of Wisconsin Integrative Medicine
Department of Family Medicine
University of Wisconsin School of Medicine and Public
    Health
Madison, Wisconsin

Jost Langhorst, MD
Director, Center for Integrative Gastroenterology
University of Duisburg-Essen
Essen, Germany

Taryn Lawler, DO
University of Wisconsin-Madison
Department of Family Medicine and Community Health
Academic Integrative Medicine Fellow
Madison, Wisconsin

Richard T. Lee, MD
Associate Professor
Department of Medicine
Case Western Reserve University School of Medicine;
Medical Director, Supportive and Integrative Oncology
    Program
University Hospitals Seidman Cancer Center
Cleveland, Ohio

Roberta Lee, MD, CaC
Primary Care
Southern Arizona Veteran's Administration
    Healthcare System;
Assistant Professor of Clinical Medicine
University of Arizona
Tucson, Arizona

Russell Lemmon, DO
Department of Family Medicine and Community
    Health
University of Wisconsin
Madison, Wisconsin

David M. Lessens, MD, MPH
Integrative & Family Medicine
Alaska Native Medical Center
Anchorage, Alaska

Sanford H. Levy, MD, FACP, ABIHM
Clinical Associate Professor of Medicine
State University of New York at Buffalo Medical School
Buffalo, New York

Edward (Lev) Linkner, MD
Founding Member
American Board of Integrative Holistic Medicine
Clinical Associate Professor
Department of Family Medicine
University of Michigan Medical School;
    Faculty, Department of Family Practice
St. Joseph Mercy Hospital;
Private Practice
Ann Arbor, Michigan

Natalia O. Litbarg, MD
Assistant Professor of Medicine/Nephrology
University of Illinois at Chicago;
Jesse Brown VA Medical Center
Chicago, Illinois

Yue Man Onna Lo, MD, ABIHM
Board Certified Family Medicine Physician
Private Practice
Albany, California

Amy B. Locke, MD, FAAFP, ABIHM
Associate Professor
Department of Family and Preventative Medicine
Office of Wellness and Integrative Health
University of Utah
Salt Lake City, Utah;
Adjunct Assistant Professor
Department of Family Medicine
University of Michigan
Ann Arbor, Michigan

Abigail Love, MD, MPH
Director of Maternity Services
Department of Family Medicine
Cambridge Health Alliance
Cambridge, Massachusetts;
Clinical Instructor, Part-time
Department of Population Medicine
Harvard Medical School
Boston, Massachusetts

Tieraona Low Dog, MD
Education and Fellowship Director
Academy of Integrative Health and Medicine
San Diego, California

Junelle H. Lupiani, RD
Registered Dietician and Nutrition Expert
Miraval Spa and Resorts
Tucson, Arizona

Victoria Maizes, MD
Executive Director
Arizona Center for Integrative Medicine
Professor of Clinical Medicine, Family Medicine, and
    Public Health
University of Arizona
Tucson, Arizona

D. Jill Mallory, MD
Integrative Family Physician
Wildwood Family Clinic
Madison, Wisconsin

John Douglas Mann, MD
Professor of Neurology
Neurology
University of North Carolina
Chapel Hill, North Carolina

Lucille R. Marchand, MD, BSN
Professor
Stuart J. Farber, MD, and Annalu Farber Endowed
    Faculty Fellow in Palliative Care Education
Department of Family Medicine
Section Chief of Palliative Care
Director, Palliative Care Program
University of Wisconsin Medical Center
University of Washington School of Medicine
Seattle, Washington

John D. Mark, MD
Clinical Professor of Pediatrics
Pediatric Pulmonary Medicine
Stanford University School of Medicine
Palo Alto, California

Michelle E. Martinez, MPH
MBSR Program Administrator
VA Puget Sound Health Care System
Seattle, Washington

Richard McKinney, MD
Clinical Professor
Family and Community Medicine
Osher Center for Integrative Medicine
University of California San Francisco;
San Francisco, California

Michelle J. Mertz, MD
Resident Physician
Family Medicine
Santa Rosa Family Medicine Residency
Santa Rosa, California

Aaron J. Michelfelder, MD
Chair, Department of Family Medicine
Co-Director, Institute for Transformative
    Interprofessional Education (I-TIE)
Professor of Family Medicine, Bioethics and Health
    Policy, and Medical Education
Loyola University Chicago Stritch School of Medicine
Maywood, Illinois

Vincent J. Minichiello, MD
Department of Family Medicine and Community Health
University of Wisconsin School of Medicine and Public
    Health
Madison, Wisconsin

Matthew Moher, MD
Hospitalist Medicine
Royal Jubilee Hospital
Victoria, British Columbia, Canada

Daniel Muller, MD, PhD
Rheumatologist
University of Colorado Health
Fort Collins, Colorado

Gerard E. Mullin, MD
Associate Professor of Medicine
Johns Hopkins University School of Medicine
Baltimore, Maryland

Sarah A. Murphy, MD
Private Practice;
Assistant Professor
University of Alaska Anchorage
WWAMI Medical School
Anchorage, Alaska

Harmon Myers, DO†
Preceptor
Program in Integrative Medicine
University of Arizona College of Medicine
Tucson, Arizona

Rubin Naiman, PhD
Clinical Assistant Professor of Medicine
Arizona Centrer for Integrative Medicine
University of Arizona
Tucson, Arizona

Kaushal Nanavati, MD, FAAFP, ABIHM
Director, Integrative Medicine
Upstate Cancer Center;
Assistant Professor of Family Medicine
Upstate Medical University
Syracuse, New York

James P. Nicolai, MD
Family Physician
Hospice and Palliative Medicine
Casa De La Luz Hospice
Tucson, Arizona

Bobby Nourani, DO
Clinical Assistant Professor
Department of Family Medicine and Community
    Health
University of Wisconsin School of Medicine and Public
    Health
Madison, Wisconsin

Brian Olshansky, MD
Professor Emeritus
Department of Internal Medicine
University of Iowa Hospitals and Clinics
Iowa City, Iowa;
Electrophysiologist
Mercy North Iowa
Mason City, Iowa

Sunil T. Pai, MD
House of Sanjevani
Integrative Medicine Health and Lifestyle Center
Albuquerque, New Mexico

Alyssa M. Parian, MD
Assistant Professor of Medicine
Division of Gastroenterology and Hepatology
Johns Hopkins School of Medicine
Baltimore, Maryland

Adam I. Perlman, MD, MPH
Executive Director
Duke Integrative Medicine
Duke University Health System;
Associate Professor
Department of Medicine
Duke School of Medicine;
Durham, North Carolina

Surya Pierce, MD
Assistant Professor
University of New Mexico Center for Life;
Department of Internal Medicine
University of New Mexico School of Medicine
Albuquerque, New Mexico

Gregory A. Plotnikoff, MD, MTS
Senior Consultant
Minnesota Personalized Medicine
Minneapolis, Minnesota

Rian Podein, MD
Department of Family Medicine and Community
    Health
University of Wisconsin
Madison, Wisconsin

David Rabago, MD
Associate Professor
Department of Family Medicine and Community
    Health
University of Wisconsin School of Medicine and
    Community Health
Madison, Wisconsin

David Rakel, MD
Professor and Chair
Department of Family and Community Medicine
University of New Mexico School of Medicine
Albuquerque, New Mexico

Jacqueline Redmer, MD, MPH
Northlakes Community Clinic
Family Medicine/Integrative Medicine
Iron River, Wisconsin;
Honorary Fellow
University of Wisconsin Department of Family Medicine
University of Wisconsin Madison
Madison, Wisconsin

Eric Reed, BA
Upstate Medical University
Syracuse, New York

Robert Rhode, PhD
Clinical Psychologist and Adjunct Lecturer
Department of Psychiatry
Arizona Health Sciences Center
Tucson, Arizona

J. Adam Rindfleisch, MPhil, MD
Integrative Health Medical Director
Associate Professor
Department of Family Medicine and Community
    Health
University of Wisconsin School of Medicine and Public
    Health
Madison, Wisconsin

Melinda Ring, MD
Executive Director
Osher Center for Integrative Medicine
Drs. Pat and Carl Greer Distinguished Physician in
    Integrative Medicine
Clinical Associate Professor of Medicine
Clinical Associate Professor of Medicine and Medical
    Social Sciences
Northwestern University Feinberg School of Medicine
Chicago, Illinois

Eric J. Roseen, DC
Department of Family Medicine
Boston Medical Center
Boston, Massachusetts

Lisa Rosenberger, ND, Lac
Adjunct Clinical Professor of Acupuncture
University of Bridgeport Acupuncture Institute
Bridgeport, Connecticut;
Naturopathic Physician
East West Integrative Health Clinic, LLC
Branford, Connecticut

Maret Rossi
Research Assistant
Blue Wave Medicine
Sausalito, California

Martin L. Rossman, MD
Clinical Faculty
Department of Ambulatory and Community Medicine
University of California San Francisco
San Francisco, California;
Director, Marin Integrative Medicine and Medical
    Acupuncture
Founder, The Healing Mind, Inc.
Greenbrae, California;
Co-Founder, Academy for Guided Imagery
Malibu, California

Pooja Saigal, MD
Professional Staff Physician
Family Medicine
NorthShore University Health System
Glenview, Illinois;
Clinical Educator
Family Medicine
University of Chicago
Hyde Park, Illinois

Bonnie R. Sakallaris, PhD, RN
Samueli Institute
Alexandria, Virginia

Anju Sawni, MD, FAAP, FSAHM
Director of Adolescent Medicine
Hurley Children's Hospital/Hurley Medical Center;
Assistant Professor
Department of Pediatrics and Human Medicine
Michigan State University College of Human Medicine
Flint, Michigan

Craig Schneider, MD
Director of Integrative Medicine
Department of Family Medicine
Maine Medical Center
Portland, Maine;
Clinical Assistant Professor
Tufts University School of Medicine
Boston, Massachusetts

Howard Schubiner, MD
Director, Mind Body Medicine Center
Department of Internal Medicine
Providence Hospital/Ascension Health
Southfield, Michigan;
Clinical Professor
Michigan State University
Detroit, Michigan

Nancy J. Selfridge, MD
Professor and Chair
Department of Clinical Medicine
Ross University School of Medicine
Dominica, West Indies

Tanmeet Sethi, MD
Faculty Physician
Director of Integrative Medicine Curriculum
Swedish Cherry Hill Family Medicine Residency
Swedish Medical Center;
Clinical Assistant Professor
University of Washington Medical School
Seattle, Washington

Adam D. Simmons, MD
Director, Parkinson's Disease Center
Hospital for Special Care
New Britain, Connecticut;
Assistant Professor of Neurology
Yale School of Medicine
New Haven, Connecticut

Tracy L. Simpson, PhD
Associate Professor
Psychiatry and Behavorial Sciences
University of Washington School of Medicine;
Clinical Investigator
VA Puget Sound Health Care System
Seattle, Washington

Coleen Smith, DO
Founder
Johnson City Osteopathic Medicine
Johnson City, Tennessee

Myles Spar, MD, MPH
Integrative Internal Medicine
West Hollywood, California;
Clinical Faculty
University of California, Los Angeles School of
  Medicine
Los Angeles, California

Srivani Sridhar, MD
Integrative Family Physician
Family Medicine
Swedish American Medical Group
Rockford, Illinois

Tina M. St. John, MD
Owner and Principal
St. John Health Communications and Consulting
Vancouver, Washington;
Editor-in-Chief
The Carlat Primary Care Report
Newburyport, Massachusetts

James A. Stewart, MD, FACP
Chief, Hematology/Oncology
Baystate Medical Center
Springfield, Massachusetts;
Professor of Medicine
Tufts University School of Medicine
Boston, Massachusetts

Larry Stoler, PhD, MSSA
Clinical Psychologist
Budding Spring Healing
Wilmette, Illinois

Nancy L. Sudak, MD, ABIHM
Director of Integrative Health
Essentia Health
Duluth, Minnesota

Jonathan Takahashi, MD, MPH
Academic Integrative Medicine Fellow
Department of Family Medicine
University of Wisconsin School of Medicine and Public
  Health
Madison, Wisconsin

Leslie Mendoza Temple, MD, ABOIM
Clinical Assistant Professor
Department of Family Medicine
University of Chicago Pritzker School of Medicine,
Chicago, Illinois;
Medical Director
Integrative Medicine Program
NorthShore University HealthSystem
Glenview, Illinois

Malynn L. Utzinger, MD, MA
Director of Integrative Practices
Promega Corporation;
Co-Executive Director
Usona Institute
Madison, Wisconsin

Donald Warne, MD, MPH
Chair
Department of Public Health
Mary J. Berg Distinguished Professor of Women's
    Health College of Health Professions
North Dakota State University
Fargo, North Dakota

Allan Warshowsky, MD, FACOG, ABIHM
Private Practice
Rye, New York

Michael J. Weber, MD
Clinical Assistant Professor
Department of Family Medicine and Community
    Health
University of Wisconsin School of Medicine and
    Community Health
Madison, Wisconsin

Andrew Weil, MD
Director
Arizona Center for Integrative Medicine
Clinical Professor of Medicine
Professor of Public Health
University of Arizona
Tucson, Arizona

Joy A. Weydert, MD
Associate Professor of Pediatrics and Integrative
    Medicine
Department of Pediatrics
University of Kansas Medical Center,
Kansas City, Kansas

Myrtle Wilhite, MD, MS
Medical Director
A Woman's Touch Sexuality Resource Center
Madison, Wisconsin

Theodore Wissink, MD
Integrative Medicine and Family Medicine
Department of Family Medicine
Main Medical Center
Portland, Maine;
Assistant Clinical Professor
Tufts University
Boston, Massachusetts

Andrew J. Wolf, MEd
Exercise Physiologist
Miraval Spa and Resorts
Tucson, Arizona

Rev. Daniel Wolpert, MDiv, MA
Executive Director
Minnesota Institute of Contemplation and Healing
Crookston, Minnesota;
Spiritual Director
The Penny George Institute for Health and Healing
Minneapolis, Minnesota

Jimmy Wu, MD, MPH
Community Preceptor/Clinical Instructor
Santa Rosa–University of California, San Francisco
    Family Medicine Program;
Red Clinician Lead
Vista Family Health Center
Santa Rosa, California

Aleksandra Zgierska, MD, PhD
Assistant Professor
Department of Family Medicine
University of Wisconsin School of Medicine and
    Community Health
Madison, Wisconsin

FOREWORD

After the publication of the first edition of *Integrative Medicine* in 2003, this text, now in its fourth edition, has become the go-to textbook for clinicians wanting evidence-informed guidance to make the best integrative therapeutic choices.

In medical education it is important that our tools adapt to the changing needs of clinicians in their chosen environments. *Integrative Medicine* does just that.

More than 140 integrative medicine experts have contributed 118 chapters to this volume. As the focus of our national medical system shifts from volume to value, we need reliable information on value-based care. Integrative medicine uses evidence within the context of an individual's life to select the best methods of treatment to achieve a healthy outcome. In general, it prefers safer, less invasive, less costly therapies over more aggressive ones, as dictated by the circumstances of illness.

As with previous editions, the text is divided into three parts. The first presents the philosophy and foundational principles of integrative medicine. The second focuses on integrative approaches to specific conditions, and the third covers "tools for your practice," with practical advice on how to best select and implement specific treatments and interventions.

Each chapter in the second part of the book has a *Therapeutic Review* summary that weighs the evidence for benefit versus the evidence for harm. Each method is rated with a visual icon to give you a time-efficient way to assess it. Each chapter also includes highlighted clinical pearls that the author feels are most important, as well as a *Prevention Prescription* of recommendations based on the best research to prevent a condition from occurring or reoccurring.

Fifteen new chapters have been added to the updated 103 chapters from the third edition. The growth of the field of integrative medicine has allowed for the recruitment of many new gifted authors (35%) who have given their time to keep the information fresh and useful to busy clinicians.

Some of these new chapters include guidance on posttraumatic stress disorder, adrenal fatigue, MTHFR mutation, food allergy and intolerance, the FODMaPs diet, chelation therapy, integrative medicine for the underserved, and the whole-health process of care.

As we work together to create a true health care system, Rakel's *Integrative Medicine* uses the best available data to empower us to be of service to others in achieving healthy outcomes. I highly recommend it.

Andrew Weil, MD
Director, Arizona Center for Integrative Medicine
Clinical Professor of Medicine
Professor of Public Health
University of Arizona
Tucson, Arizona
July, 2016

PREFACE

As the field of integrative medicine continues its health mission, the larger medical culture of which it is a part is adopting and implementing its therapeutic strategies. Reducing cost and improving quality with better outcomes can be achieved with an integrative approach where professionals combine their expertise in service of facilitating health within the complexity of people's lives. This text is a tool to guide this important process.

The fourth edition includes expertise from 148 authors, 35% of whom are new. They have contributed to 118 chapters, including 15 new chapters on hot topics such as posttraumatic stress disorder, adrenal fatigue, the FODMaPs diet, integrative medicine for the underserved, chelation therapy, and MTHFR mutation, to name a few.

New to this edition is the inclusion of three to four multiple choice questions that follow each chapter on ExpertConsult.com. These were included to prepare the reader for taking and passing the board exam in integrative medicine. The answer includes a short explanation that provides insight and further education on clinical topics.

As with previous editions, the text is divided into three parts. Part 1, Integrative Medicine, is an overview of the field and the foundations from which it is delivered. Part 2, Integrative Approach to Disease, is the core of the text and discusses integrative approaches to treating disorders that range from insomnia to diabetes to the most common types of cancer. Part 3, Tools for Your Practice, includes practical, how-to information on the most clinically useful integrative therapeutic interventions.

We strive to make extracting the information you need as efficient as possible. Each disease-focused chapter concludes with a Therapeutic Review that summarizes an integrative approach. After each recommendation, there is an evidence versus harm icon that provides the busy clinician a quick assessment of the balance of the level of evidence for benefit with the level of potential harm. Each chapter also has a Prevention Prescription that lists those interventions that have been found to be most useful in preventing the specific disease and its recurrence. Clinical pearls are highlighted in note boxes throughout the text.

The science and research of our work is often linear. We have a cause, a result, and a treatment. But how we apply it is circular. It intertwines within the context of someone's life, artfully prescribed based on insight gained from listening to someone's story. I hope the information within these pages empowers you to use the best science to serve your patients. We likely will never master this craft, but we can strive together to improve our understanding how to reproduce health, healing, and resiliency within circular and dynamic ecosystems. Thank you for engaging in this important work.

David Rakel, MD

ACKNOWLEDGMENTS

It has taken the expertise of a talented group of professionals to complete this fourth edition. I am very grateful to Joan Ryan for her persistence in managing the content and gracefully supporting the authors in completing the many manuscripts. Kate Mannix took it from there to produce and edit the final drafts and Sarah Barth and Kate Dimock oversaw the big picture towards completion. This Elsevier team has been a joy to work with and their investment has supported a high quality text that has been checked and double-checked for accuracy.

As I transition from the University of Wisconsin in Madison to The University of New Mexico in Albuquerque, I would also like to acknowledge the students, residents, faculty, and staff to whom this book is dedicated. I am also grateful to my long-time colleague Adam Rindfleisch for his support over the years and for continuing to lead the Integrative Medicine program at the University of Wisconsin. I am grateful to my practice partners, Greta Kuphal, Michael Weber, and Samantha Sharp, for their back up when other, nonclinical tasks required attention, and to Bruce Barrett for his friendship, education, and research collaboration. I'm also grateful to Char Luchterhand, Mike Johnson, Jackie Kuta-Bangsberg, and Katharine Bonus for their support for our UW Integrative Medicine program over the years.

I have also been honored to be part of a national educational initiative with the Pacific Institute of Research and Evaluation (PIRE) and the Office of Patient Centered Care and Cultural Transformation within the Veteran's Health Administration. I am grateful to have been able to learn from a variety of gifted and passionate people to work towards a more personalized, proactive, and patient-driven VA health system. I am grateful to Tracy Gaudet, David Rychener, Bernie Murphy, Kathy Atwood, Russ Greenfield, Marite Hagman, David Kiefer, Kelly Peyton-Howard, Janet Vertrees, and Christine Milovani. Their work is, in part, summarized in Chapter 4, The Whole Health Process.

I would not have the energy to do this work if it were not for those that give me energy: my wife, Denise, and three children, Justin, Sarah (and our future son-in-law Adam), and Lucas.

As always, I am grateful to the 148 authors that contributed their time and expertise to help us all do our job a little better.

CONTENTS

■ PART I
INTEGRATIVE MEDICINE

1 PHILOSOPHY OF INTEGRATIVE MEDICINE, 2
David Rakel, MD • Andrew Weil, MD

2 CREATING OPTIMAL HEALING
ENVIRONMENTS, 12
David Rakel, MD • Bonnie R. Sakallaris, PhD, RN •
Wayne Jonas, MD

3 THE HEALING ENCOUNTER, 20
David Rakel, MD • Luke Fortney, MD, FAAFP

4 THE WHOLE HEALTH PROCESS, 27
David Rakel, MD • J. Adam Rindfleisch, MPhil, MD •
Tracy Gaudet, MD

■ PART II
INTEGRATIVE APPROACH TO DISEASE

SECTION I
AFFECTIVE DISORDERS, 35

5 DEPRESSION, 36
Craig Schneider, MD • Theodore Wissink, MD

6 ANXIETY, 46
Roberta Lee, MD, CaC

7 ATTENTION DEFICIT DISORDER, 53
Anju Sawni, MD, FAAP, FSAHM • Kathi J. Kemper, MD, MPH

8 AUTISM SPECTRUM DISORDER, 64
John W. Harrington, MD • Samudragupta Bora, PhD

9 INSOMNIA, 74
Rubin Naiman, PhD

10 POSTTRAUMATIC STRESS DISORDER (PTSD), 86
David J. Kearney, MD • Michelle E. Martinez, MPH •
Tracy L. Simpson, PhD

SECTION II
NEUROLOGY, 94

11 ALZHEIMER DISEASE, 95
Mikhail Kogan, MD • Hwee Soo Jeong, MD

12 HEADACHE, 108
Remy R. Coeytaux, MD, PhD • John Douglas Mann, MD

13 PERIPHERAL NEUROPATHY, 120
Sunil T. Pai, MD

14 MULTIPLE SCLEROSIS, 133
Bradly Jacobs, MD, MPH, ABOIM • Surya Pierce, MD

15 PARKINSON'S DISEASE, 143
Adam D. Simmons, MD

SECTION III
INFECTIOUS DISEASE, 152

16 OTITIS MEDIA, 153
David K. Becker, MD

17 CHRONIC SINUSITIS, 157
Robert S. Ivker, DO

18 VIRAL UPPER RESPIRATORY INFECTION, 170
Bruce Barrett, MD, PhD

19 HIV DISEASE AND AIDS, 180
Stephen Dahmer, MD • Benjamin Kligler, MD

20 HERPES SIMPLEX VIRUS, 191
Maret Rossi • Bradly Jacobs, MD, MPH, ABOIM

21 CHRONIC HEPATITIS, 198
Tina M. St. John, MD

22 URINARY TRACT INFECTION (UTI), 211
Amy B. Locke, MD, FAAFP, ABIHM

23 LYME DISEASE, 218
Ather Ali, ND, MPH, MHS

SECTION IV
CARDIOVASCULAR DISEASE, 229

24 HYPERTENSION, 230
Gregory A. Plotnikoff, MD, MTS • Jeffery Dusek, PhD

25 HEART FAILURE, 242
Russell H. Greenfield, MD

26 CORONARY ARTERY DISEASE, 253
Stephen Devries, MD, FACC, FAHA

27 DYSLIPIDEMIA, 264
Mark Houston, MD, MS, MSc

28 ARRHYTHMIAS, 276
Brian Olshansky, MD

SECTION V
ALLERGY/INTOLERANCE, 287

29 ASTHMA, 288
John D. Mark, MD

30 THE ALLERGIC PATIENT, 300
Randy J. Horwitz, MD, PhD

31 FOOD ALLERGY AND INTOLERANCE, 310
Alan R. Gaby, MD

SECTION VI
METABOLIC/ENDOCRINE DISORDERS, 319

32 INSULIN RESISTANCE AND THE METABOLIC SYNDROME, 320
Edward (Lev) Linker, MD • Corene Humphreys, ND

33 DIABETES MELLITUS, 334
Matthew Moher, MD

34 HYPOTHYROIDISM, 347
Leslie Mendoza Temple, MD, ABOIM • Pooja Saigal, MD

35 POLYCYSTIC OVARIAN SYNDROME, 361
Melinda Ring, MD

36 OSTEOPOROSIS, 370
Louise Gagné, MD • Victoria Maizes, MD

37 AN INTEGRATIVE APPROACH TO OBESITY, 382
James P. Nicolai, MD • Junelle H. Lupiani, RD • Andrew J. Wolf, MEd

38 MTHFR, HOMOCYSTEINE AND NUTRIENT NEEDS, 395
Thomas G. Guilliams, PhD

39 ADRENAL FATIGUE, 404
Jacqueline Redmer, MD, MPH

SECTION VII
NEPHROLOGY, 410

40 CHRONIC KIDNEY DISEASE, 411
Natalia O. Litbarg, MD

SECTION VIII
GASTROINTESTINAL DISORDERS, 422

41 IRRITABLE BOWEL SYNDROME, 423
Patrick J. Hanaway, MD

42 GASTROESOPHAGEAL REFLUX DISEASE, 433
David Kiefer, MD

43 PEPTIC ULCER DISEASE, 439
Joseph Eichenseher, MD, MAT

44 CHOLELITHIASIS, 450
Ann C. Figurski, DO

45 RECURRING ABDOMINAL PAIN IN PEDIATRICS, 457
Joy A. Weydert, MD

46 CONSTIPATION, 466
Tanmeet Sethi, MD

SECTION IX
AUTOIMMUNE DISORDERS, 474

47 FIBROMYALGIA, 475
Nancy J. Selfridge, MD

48 CHRONIC FATIGUE SYNDROME, 484
Sanford H. Levy, MD, FACP, ABIHM

49 RHEUMATOID ARTHRITIS, 493
Daniel Muller, MD, PhD

50 INFLAMMATORY BOWEL DISEASE, 501
Alyssa M. Parian, MD • Gerard E. Mullin, MD • Jost Langhorst, MD • Amy C. Brown, PhD

SECTION X
OBSTETRICS/GYNECOLOGY, 517

51 PRECONCEPTION COUNSELING AND FERTILITY, 518
Victoria Maizes, MD

52 LABOR PAIN MANAGEMENT, 526
Michelle J. Mertz, MD • Connie J. Earl, DO, ABIHM

53 POSTDATES PREGNANCY, 535
D. Jill Mallory, MD

54 NAUSEA AND VOMITING IN PREGNANCY, 542
Andrea Gordon, MD • Abigail Love, MD, MPH

55 MANAGING MENOPAUSAL SYMPTOMS, 550
Marcia Klein-Patel, MD, PhD • Katherine Gergen-Barnett, MD • Judith Balk, MD, MPH

56 PREMENSTRUAL SYNDROME, 560
Tieraona Low Dog, MD

57 DYSMENORRHEA, 569
Greta J. Kuphal, MD

58 UTERINE FIBROIDS (LEIOMYOMATA), 578
Allan Warshowsky, MD, FACOG, ABIHM

59 VAGINAL DRYNESS, 592
Myrtle Wilhite, MD, MS

SECTION XI
UROLOGY, 600

60 BENIGN PROSTATIC HYPERPLASIA, 601
David Rakel, MD

61 UROLITHIASIS (KIDNEY AND BLADDER STONES), 608
Jimmy Wu, MD, MPH

62 CHRONIC PROSTATITIS/CHRONIC PELVIC PAIN SYNDROME, 616
Myles Spar, MD, MPH

63 ERECTILE DYSFUNCTION, 623
Luke Fortney, MD, FAAFP

64 TESTOSTERONE DEFICIENCY, 630
Robert Z. Edwards, MD

SECTION **XII**
MUSCULOSKELETAL, 638

65 OSTEOARTHRITIS, 639
Adam I. Perlman, MD, MPH • Lisa Rosenberger, ND, LAc •
Ather Ali, ND, MPH, MHS

66 MYOFASCIAL PAIN SYNDROME, 651
Robert Alan Bonakdar, MD

67 CHRONIC LOW BACK PAIN, 662
Russell Lemmon, DO • Eric J. Roseen, DC

68 NECK PAIN, 676
Alexandra Ilkevitch, MD • Taryn Lawler, DO •
J. Adam Rindfleisch, MPhil, MD

69 GOUT, 689
Fasih A. Hameed, MD, ABIHM

70 CARPAL TUNNEL SYNDROME, 697
Gautam J. Desai, DO, FACOFP • Dennis J. Dowling, DO •
Joshua W. Harbaugh, OMSIV

71 EPICONDYLOSIS, 707
David Rabago, MD • Sarah James, DO •
Aleksandra Zgierska, MD, PhD

SECTION **XIII**
DERMATOLOGY, 715

72 ATOPIC DERMATITIS, 716
Amanda J. Kaufman, MD, ABIHM

73 PSORIASIS, 726
Apple A. Bodemer, MD

74 URTICARIA, 739
Apple A. Bodemer, MD

75 APHTHOUS STOMATITIS, 747
David Rakel, MD

76 SEBORRHEIC DERMATITIS, 753
Alan M. Dattner, MD

77 ACNE VULGARIS AND ACNE ROSACEA, 759
Hana Grobel, MD • Sarah A. Murphy, MD

SECTION **XIV**
CANCER, 771

78 BREAST CANCER, 772
Lucille R. Marchand, MD, BSN • James A. Stewart, MD, FACP

79 LUNG CANCER, 785
Kaushal B. Nanavati, MD, FAAFP, ABIHM • Eric Reed, BA

80 PROSTATE CANCER, 790
Richard T. Lee, MD

81 COLORECTAL CANCER, 800
Srivani Sridhar, MD

82 PALLIATIVE AND END-OF-LIFE CARE, 806
Lucille R. Marchand, MD, BSN

SECTION **XV**
SUBSTANCE ABUSE, 817

83 ALCOHOLISM AND SUBSTANCE ABUSE, 818
Donald Warne, MD, MPH

SECTION **XVI**
OPHTHALMOLOGY, 829

84 CATARACTS, 830
Robert Abel, Jr., MD

85 AGE-RELATED MACULAR DEGENERATION, 838
Robert Abel, Jr., MD

■ **PART III**
TOOLS FOR YOUR PRACTICE

SECTION **IA**
LIFESTYLE: NUTRITION, 848

86 THE ELIMINATION DIET, 849
Suhani Bora, MD • J. Adam Rindfleisch, MPhil, MD

87 GLYCEMIC INDEX AND GLYCEMIC LOAD, 863
Yue Man Onna Lo, MD, ABIHM

88 ANTIINFLAMMATORY DIET, 869
Wendy Kohatsu, MD • Scott Karpowicz, MD

89 THE DASH DIET, 878
David M. Lessens, MD, MPH • David Rakel, MD

90 THE FODMAP DIET, 882
David Rakel, MD

SECTION **IB**
LIFESTYLE: EXERCISE, 886

91 WRITING AN EXERCISE PRESCRIPTION, 887
Michael J. Hewitt, PhD

92 THERAPEUTIC BREATHING, 895
Vincent J. Minichiello, MD

93 LOW BACK PAIN EXERCISES, 901
Brian Degenhardt, DO • Coleen Smith, DO

SECTION II
MIND-BODY, 908

94 RELAXATION TECHNIQUES, 909
Vincent J. Minichiello, MD

95 SELF-HYPNOSIS TECHNIQUES, 914
Steven Gurgevich, PhD

96 ENHANCING HEART RATE VARIABILITY, 922
Malynn L. Utzinger, MD, MA

97 GUIDED IMAGERY AND INTERACTIVE GUIDED IMAGERY, 930
Martin L. Rossman, MD

98 JOURNALING FOR HEALTH, 937
Adrienne Hampton, MD • David Rakel, MD

99 FORGIVENESS, 940
J. Adam Rindfleisch, MPhil, MD

100 RECOMMENDING MEDITATION, 945
Luke Fortney, MD, FAAFP

101 MOTIVATIONAL INTERVIEWING, 954
Robert Rhode, PhD

102 EMOTIONAL AWARENESS FOR PAIN, 963
Howard Schubiner, MD

103 ENERGY PSYCHOLOGY, 971
Larry Stoler, PhD, MSSA

SECTION III
BIOCHEMICAL, 978

104 PRESCRIBING BOTANICALS, 979
Paula Gardiner, MD, MPH • Amanda C. Filippelli, MSN, MPH, RN, APRN • Tieraona Low Dog, MD

105 PRESCRIBING PROBIOTICS, 986
Jonathan Takahashi, MD, MPH • J. Adam Rindfleisch, MPhil, MD

106 DETOXIFICATION, 996
Luke Fortney, MD, FAAFP • Rian Podein, MD • Michael Hernke, PhD

107 CHELATION THERAPY 1004
Jeanne A. Drisko, MD

108 INTEGRATIVE STRATEGIES FOR PLANETARY HEALTH 1016
Nancy L. Sudak, MD, ABIHM • James Harvie, PEng

SECTION IV
BIOMECHANICAL, 1027

109 STRAIN/COUNTERSTRAIN, 1028
Harmon Myers, DO • Julia Jernberg, MD

110 ACUPUNCTURE FOR HEADACHE, 1038
Aaron J. Michelfelder, MD

111 ACUPUNCTURE FOR NAUSEA AND VOMITING, 1044
Aaron J. Michelfelder, MD

112 PROLOTHERAPY FOR CHRONIC MUSCULOSKELETAL PAIN, 1047
David Rabago, MD • Bobby Nourani, DO • Michael J. Weber, MD

113 NASAL IRRIGATION FOR UPPER RESPIRATORY CONDITIONS, 1054
David Rabago, MD • Supriya Hayer, MD • Aleksandra Zgierska, MD, PhD

SECTION V
BIOENERGETICS, 1057

114 INTEGRATING SPIRITUAL ASSESSMENT AND CARE, 1058
Gregory A. Plotnikoff, MD, MTS • Daniel Wolpert, MDiv, MA • Douglas E. Dandurand, PhD, MDiv, MA, MAS

115 THERAPEUTIC HOMEOPATHY, 1064
Paul E. Bergquist, MD

116 BIOFIELD THERAPIES, 1073
J. Adam Rindfleisch, MPhil, MD

SECTION VI
OTHER, 1081

117 CREATING A GREENER CLINIC: THE IMPACT OF GLOBAL WARMING ON HEALTH 1082
Rian Podein, MD • Michael Hernke, PhD

118 INTEGRATIVE MEDICINE FOR THE UNDERSERVED, 1088
Richard McKinney, MD • Jeffrey Geller, MD

USING THE EVIDENCE-VERSUS-HARM GRADING ICONS

In the busy practice of medicine, being able to access information quickly and efficiently is important for obtaining the highest quality data in the shortest period of time in the effort to enhance care.

The Strength of Recommendation Taxonomy (SORT)[1] rating for evidence has been an excellent step in this direction. The A, B, and C ratings give us a quick and simple way to judge the quality of evidence for a particular intervention. There are limitations to making decisions based only on the evidence of benefit. One limitation is the absence of the potential harm of the evidence. Even if the evidence may be grade A, the potential harm of that intervention may negate its effect.

An example is the Randomized Aldactone Evaluation Study (RALES) published in the *New England Journal of Medicine* in 1999.[2] This study showed that spironolactone significantly improved outcomes in patients with severe heart failure. A follow-up article published in the same journal in 2004[3] showed that after the publication of this study, the number of prescriptions written for spironolactone significantly increased in Ontario, Canada, from 34 per 1000 patients in 1994 to 149 per 1000 patients in 2001. Thus the Canadian physicians were practicing evidence-based medicine, and their prescribing habits resonated with this. The follow-up study also noted that despite this evidence-based practice, there was a significant increase in the number of hospital admission and in the death rate related to hyperkalemia when spironolactone and ACE inhibitors were used together. In fact, when the investigators took into account the number of deaths related to hyperkalemia, there was no decrease in the number of admissions or the death rate for congestive heart failure patients after the publication of RALES. The initial benefit of improving outcomes in congestive heart failure with spironolactone seen in the original study was not evident in the application of the evidence in the clinical setting. The potential harm of the evidence was not taken into account, and this drug may have caused more harm than good.

Adding a rating for potential harm will enhance the rating of the evidence for the clinician but is by no means a final guiding rule. Decision making goes beyond the evidence and the harm and is grounded in the much broader insights obtained through relationship-centered care. It is only a tool that we hope will make the clinician's life a little easier in recommending specific therapeutic interventions.

GRADING THE EVIDENCE

The authors of this text used the SORT criteria for grading the evidence for the therapies that are recommended in the Therapeutic Review sections of the chapters. A simplified summary follows:

Grade A	Based on consistent, good-quality, patient-oriented evidence (e.g., systematic review or meta-analysis showing benefit, Cochrane Review with clear recommendation, high-quality patient-oriented randomized controlled trial). Example: Acupuncture for nausea and vomiting.
Grade B	Based on inconsistent or limited-quality patient-oriented evidence. Example: Ginger for osteoarthritis.
Grade C	Based on consensus, usual practice, opinion, disease-oriented evidence (e.g., study showing a reduction in blood sugar but no studies in humans to show a benefit to those with diabetes).

GRADING THE POTENTIAL HARM

Unlike grading for evidence, there is no unified, acceptable grading system for harm. In grading the three levels of harm, we used the following grading scale:

Grade 3 (most harm)	This therapy has the potential to result in death or permanent disability. Example: Major surgery under general anesthesia or carcinogenic effects of the botanical *Aristolochia* (birthwort).
Grade 2 (moderate harm)	This therapy has the potential to cause reversible side effects or interact in a negative way with other therapies. Example: Pharmaceutical or neutraceutical side effects.
Grade 1 (least harm)	This therapy poses little, if any, risk of harm. Examples: Eating more vegetables, increasing exercise, elimination diets, encouraging social connection.

The resulting icons incorporate a weighing of the evidence versus the potential harm. If the evidence is strong (A) with the least potential harm (1), the arrow will point up. If the evidence is weak (C) with the most potential harm (3), the arrow will point down.

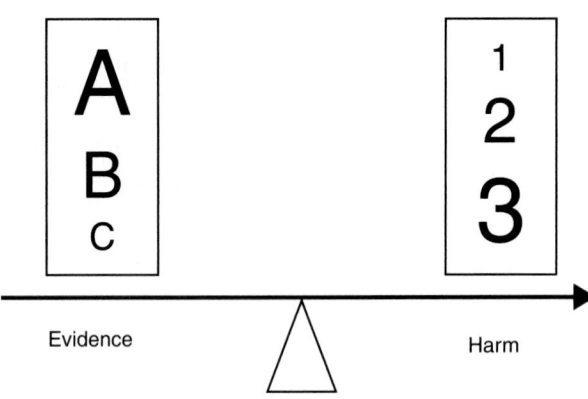

Examples:

Clinical Recommendation
- Exercise for diabetes management (A,1)

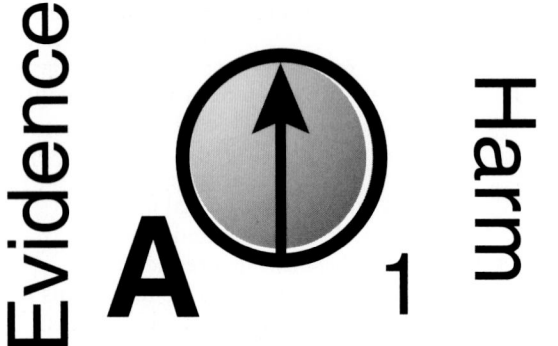

- Hypnosis for irritable bowel syndrome (B,1)

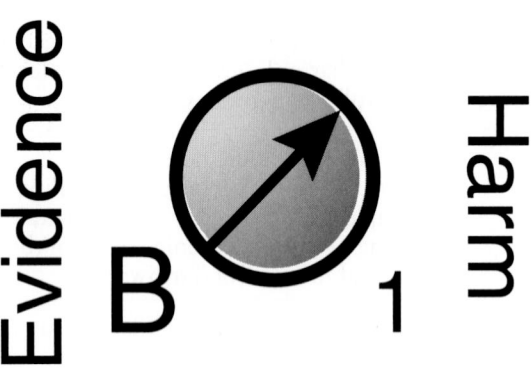

- Zinc supplementation for infectious diarrhea (B,2)

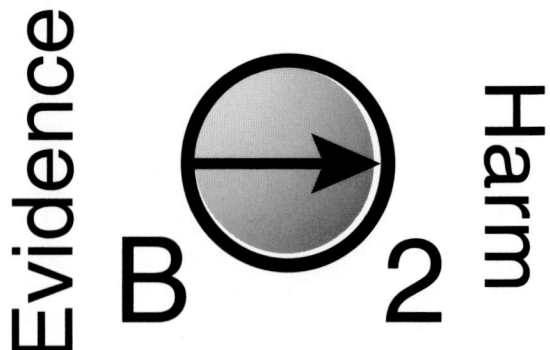

- Astragalus root for infectious hepatitis (C,2)

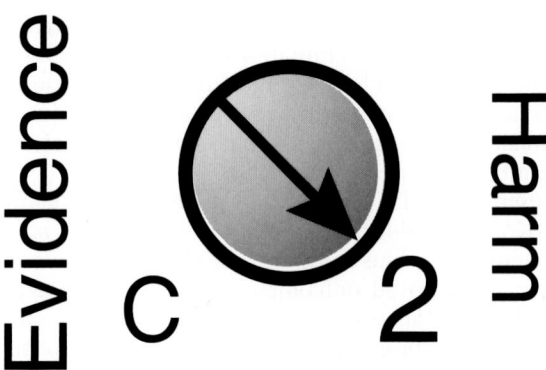

- *Aristolochia* (birthwort) to support immunity (C,3)

Rating Options	Arrow	Icon
(A,1)	↑	A ⬆ 1
(A,2) (B,1)	↗	A ⬈ 2 B ⬈ 1
(A,3) (B,2) (C,1)	→	A → 3 B → 2 c → 1
(B,3) (C,2)	↘	B ↘ 2 c ↘ 2
(C,3)	↓	c ↓ 3

STRENGTHS OF EVIDENCE-VERSUS-HARM GRADING

- Gives quick access to the balance of available evidence and potential harm for a given therapy.
- Works best for therapeutic interventions for chronic disease compared with acute or emergency treatments.
- Gives more credibility to therapies that have little potential harm. For example, we know that encouraging social support, reducing stress, and enhancing spiritual connection are beneficial for quality of life and health, but the evidence may not be strong. The potential harm will always be low, giving the benefit a more positive outlook.
- Helps us honor our primary goal, which is to "first, do no harm." This rating scale allows us to include this important fact in medical decision making. This is very important, seeing that adverse drug reactions from medical therapy have been found to be the sixth leading cause of hospital deaths in the United States.[4]

LIMITATIONS OF EVIDENCE-VERSUS-HARM GRADING

- Is used only for those therapies proved to have a positive benefit. There may be good evidence showing that a therapy does not work. If this was the case, the therapy was not included in the Therapeutic Review.
- Does not reward the potentially life-saving interventions that are risky and have little available evidence showing benefit. For example, there has not been a meta-analysis showing that emergency repair of a dissecting aortic aneurysm has therapeutic benefit. The potential harm of this therapy is high (Grade 3). On the evidence-versus-harm scale, this therapy would have an arrow pointing toward the negative side, but without the therapy the patient would likely die.
- Those therapies that have the most potential for economic gain often have the most evidence. For example,

there are more resources to do high-quality research for a potentially profitable pharmaceutical that can be patented than for a whole food or plant that cannot. Therapies such as pharmaceuticals will have a higher quality of evidence in general when compared with botanicals, mind-body therapy, and spiritual connection.
- This rating scale can be reductionistic. It is much easier to complete high-quality research based on our scientific model on a physical process, drug, or supplement. It is harder to show an enhanced quality of life or a reduction in suffering from reducing social isolation, for example.

SUMMARY

This model includes potential harm along with the strength of the evidence. The arrows will give a quick reference for potential benefit when the evidence and harm are weighted against each other. For example, strong (heavy) evidence with little (light) potential harm will result in an arrow pointing up. This will be most helpful for recommendations for chronic disease. Unlike acute life-threatening conditions that often need more aggressive intervention with higher potential risk, chronic disease is often managed using lifestyle choices that will be supported by this model.

REFERENCES

1. Ebell MH, Siwek J, Weiss BD: Strength of recommendation taxonomy (SORT): a patient-centered approach to grading evidence in the medical literature, *Am Fam Physician* 69:548–556, 2004.
2. Pitt B, Zannad F, Remme WJ, et al.: The effect of spironolactone on morbidity and mortality in patients with severe heart failure. Randomized Aldactone Evaluation Study Investigators, *N Engl J Med* 341:709–717, 1999.
3. Juurlink DN, Mamdani MM, Lee DS: Rates of hyperkalemia after publication of the randomized aldactone evaluation study, *N Engl J Med* 351:543–551, 2004.
4. Lazarou J, Pomeranz BH, Corey PN: Incidence of adverse drug reactions in hospitalized patients, *JAMA* 279:1200–1205, 1998.

PART I

INTEGRATIVE MEDICINE

CHAPTER 1

PHILOSOPHY OF INTEGRATIVE MEDICINE

David Rakel, MD • Andrew Weil, MD

A BRIEF HISTORY OF INTEGRATIVE MEDICINE

When religion was strong and medicine weak, men mistook magic for medicine;

Now, when science is strong and religion weak, men mistake medicine for magic.

THOMAS SZASZ, THE SECOND SIN

The philosophy of integrative medicine is not new. It has been talked about for ages across many disciplines. It has simply been overlooked as the pendulum of accepted medical care swings from one extreme to the other. We are currently experiencing the beginning of a shift toward recognizing the benefits of combining the external, physical, and technological successes of curing with the internal, nonphysical exploration of healing.

Long before magnetic resonance imaging and computed tomographic scanners existed, Aristotle (384–322 BC) was simply able to experience, observe, and reflect on the human condition. He was one of the first holistic physicians who believed that every person was a combination of both physical and spiritual properties with no separation between mind and body. It was not until the 1600s that a spiritual mathematician became worried that prevailing scientific materialistic thought would reduce the conscious mind to something that could be manipulated and controlled. René Descartes (1596–1650), respecting the great unknown, did his best to separate the mind from the body to protect the spirit from science. He believed that the mind and spirit should be the focus of the church thus leaving science to dissect the physical body. This philosophy led to the "Cartesian split" of mind–body duality.

Shortly afterward, John Locke (1632–1704) and David Hume (1711–1776) influenced the reductionist movement that shaped our science and medical system. The idea was that if we could reduce the natural phenomena to greater simplicity, we could understand the larger whole. So, to learn about a clock, all we need to do is study its parts. Reductionism facilitated great discoveries that helped humans gain control over their environment. Despite this progress, clinicians had few tools to treat disease effectively. In the early 20th century, applied science started to transform medicine through the development of medical technologies. In 1910, the Flexner report[1] was written, and it had a significant impact on the development of allopathic academic institutions. They came to emphasize the triad that prevails today: research, education, and clinical practice. Reductionism and the scientific method produced the knowledge that encouraged the growth of these institutions.

The scientific model led to greater understanding of the pathophysiological basis of disease and the development of tools to help combat its influence. Subspecialization of medical care facilitated the application of the new information. We now have practitioners who focus on the pieces and a society that appreciates their abilities to fix problems. Unfortunately, this approach does not work well for chronic disease that involves more than just a single organ. In fact, all body organs are interconnected, so simply repairing a part without addressing the underlying causes provides only temporary relief and a false sense of security. This, in part, resulted in a very expensive health care system in America with poor health outcomes.[2]

More Technology, Less Communication

The tremendous success of medical science in the 20th century was not without cost. Total health care expenditures reached $2.9 trillion in 2013, an amount that was 17.4% of the gross domestic product (GDP), and translated to $9255 per U.S. resident. The health care market grows when more attention is focused on single diseases that can be treated with drugs or procedures. In 10 years (2003–2013), drug spending in the United States rose 66.4% from $180 billion to $271 billion.[3] Financial rewards increase when we have more subtypes of disease to which treatments can be matched. The system encourages patients to believe that tools are the answer to their physical woes and discourages them from paying attention to the interplay of the mind, community, and spirit. Technology is the golden calf in this scenario. We have become dependent on it, and overuse has widened the barrier of communication between the patient and provider. The old tools of the trade—rapport, gestalt, intuition, and laying on of hands—were used less and less as powerful drugs and high-tech interventions became available.

To help curtail costs, managed care and capitation were born. These new models reduced excessive costs and further eroded the patient-provider relationship by placing increased time demands on physicians that did not involve patient care. Physician and patient unrest followed. Physicians are unhappy, in part, because of the loss of autonomy in practicing medicine. Patients are unhappy, in part, because they believe they are not receiving the attention they need. Most upset are patients with chronic medical conditions whose diseases do not respond well to the treatments of specialized medicine. This comes at a time when the incidence of chronic and degenerative diseases is at an all-time high. Diseases such as heart disease, diabetes, irritable bowel syndrome, chronic fatigue, and chronic pain syndromes are quite common. They require evaluation and treatment of much more than any one organ. The public has started to realize the limitations of Western medicine and wants more attention paid to health and healing of the whole person, especially when someone has no "part" to be fixed.

Public Interest Influences Change

The deterioration of the patient-provider relationship, the overuse of technology, and the inability of the medical system to treat chronic disease adequately has contributed to rising interest in complementary and alternative medicine (CAM). The public has sent this message with their feet and their pocketbooks. In fact, more visits were made to CAM providers in the early 1990s than to all primary care medical physicians, and patients paid for these visits out of pocket, with an estimated expenditure of $13 billion.[4] This trend continued throughout the 1990s; 42% of the public used alternative therapies, and expenditures increased to $27 billion from 1990 to 1997.[5] Patients are also demanding less aggressive forms of therapy, and they are especially leery of the toxicity of pharmaceutical drugs. Adverse drug reactions had become the sixth leading cause of death in hospitalized patients,[6] and in 1994, botanicals were the largest growth area in retail pharmacy.[7] Research shows that people find complementary approaches to be more aligned with "their own values, beliefs, and philosophical orientations toward health and life."[8] The public, before the medical establishment, realized that health and healing involved more than pills and surgery. Less invasive, more traditional treatments such as nutrition, botanicals, manipulation, meditation, massage, and others that were neglected during the explosion of medical science and technology are now being rediscovered with great enthusiasm (Fig. 1.1).

Medicine Gets the Message

The popularity of CAM therapies created a need for research in these areas. In 1993, an Office of Alternative Medicine was started within the National Institutes of Health (NIH). The initial budget was $2 million, a fraction of the $80 billion budget of the NIH. The office was later upgraded to the National Center for Complementary and Alternative Medicine (NCCAM), and in 2014, the name was changed to the National Center for Complementary and Integrative Health (NCCIH). The amount of money available for scholarly research kept pace with this growth. By 2010, the NCCAM budget grew to $127 million.[9] Unfortunately, with a shrinking NIH budget, the NCCIH budget dropped in 2013 to $120.6 million and rose only to $124.5 million in 2015, still lower than in the previous decade.[10] Despite the challenges in research funding, there was still the opportunity to explore ways in which these areas of medicine could enhance health care delivery. At first, researchers tried to use traditional methods to learn

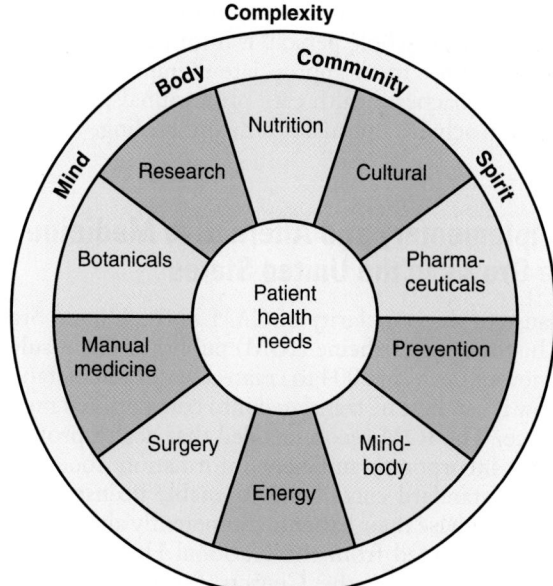

FIG. 1.1 ■ Integrative medicine pie chart.

about CAM therapies. These methods were sufficient for studying some areas such as botanicals. The limitations of the reductionist model became apparent, however, when it was applied to more dynamic systems of healing such as homeopathy, traditional Chinese medicine, and energy medicine. New methods were required to understand the multiple influences involved. Outcome studies with attention to quality of life were initiated. Research grants in "frontier medicine" were created to help learn about fields such as energy medicine, homeopathy, magnet therapy, and therapeutic prayer. Interest grew in learning how to combine the successes of the scientific model with the potential of CAM to improve the delivery of health care.

Academic Centers Respond

In 1997, one of the authors of this chapter, Andrew Weil, started the first fellowship program in integrative medicine at the University of Arizona. This 2-year clinical and research fellowship was created to train physicians in the science of health and healing and to teach more about therapies that were not part of Western medical practice. Since then, other fellowship programs have been created, as well as projects to incorporate integrative medicine into 4-year family medicine and pediatric residency training models. NIH-sponsored R25 grants have been awarded to medical schools across the country to bring these concepts into medical school curriculums. The Academic Consortium for Integrative Health and Medicine (ACIHM) now comprises more than 62 medical schools (40%) across the United States and Canada, and it brings academic leaders together to transform health care through rigorous scientific studies, new models of clinical care, and innovative educational programs that integrate biomedicine, the complexity of humans, the intrinsic nature of healing, and the rich diversity of therapeutic systems.[11]

Integrative medicine reaffirms the importance of the relationship between the practitioner and patient, focuses on the whole person, is informed by evidence, and makes use of all appropriate therapeutic and lifestyle approaches, health care professionals, and disciplines to achieve optimal health and healing.

Complementary and Alternative Medicine Use Grows in the United States

Because of the popularity of CAM in the United States, the Institute of Medicine (IOM) published the results of a review of CAM in 2004 to create a better understanding of how it can best be translated into conventional medical practice. The IOM recommended that health profession schools incorporate sufficient information about CAM into the standard curriculum to enable licensed professionals to advise their patients competently about CAM.[12]

Data collected from the National Health Interview Survey in 2002 by the Centers for Disease Control and Prevention's National Center for Health Statistics showed that 62% of U.S. adults used CAM within 12 months of being interviewed. When prayer was excluded as a CAM therapy, the percentage dropped to 36%.[13] This survey was repeated in 2007, during which the use of CAM rose slightly from 36% to 38.3%. The 2007 survey included children, in whom it showed 11.8% use of CAM therapy, most commonly for back/neck pain (6.7%) and colds (6.6%) (Fig. 1.2). The 10 most commonly used CAM therapies can be reviewed in Fig. 1.3. The use of natural products was the most common at 17.7%. Pain conditions were the most common reason for CAM therapy in adults, and low back pain accounted for the highest percentage of CAM use at 17.1% (Fig. 1.4).[14] A review also showed an increase in the use of CAM in those who did not have access to conventional medical care, thus showing the

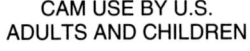

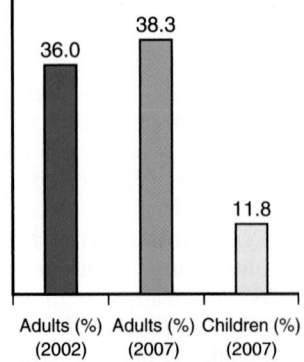

CAM USE BY U.S.
ADULTS AND CHILDREN

FIG. 1.2 ■ Adults and children who have used complementary and alternative medicine (CAM): United States, 2007. (From Barnes PM, Blook B, Nahin R. *Complementary and alternative medicine use among adults and children: United States, 2007.* National Health Statistics Report No. 12. Hyattsville, MD: National Center for Health Statistics; 2008.)

importance of CAM as an option for the uninsured.[15] These data suggest that people value other ways of treating illness and that they want to be empowered to be active participants in their care. They also feel that CAM offers them more opportunity to tell their story and explore a more holistic view of their problem.[16]

Avoiding Complementary and Alternative Medicine Labels

With the growth of good scientific research regarding many CAM therapies, we are realizing that the labels once used to classify these therapies are no longer needed (Fig. 1.5). The use of the terms *complementary* and *alternative* serve only to detract from a therapy by making it sound second class. Therapies that are often labeled under the heading of CAM include nutrition and spirituality. Many would argue that a lack of attention to these important influences on health has resulted in epidemics of obesity, diabetes, and substance abuse. Stress, which many CAM-labeled mind–body therapies address, was found to be the second leading risk factor for heart disease after smoking in one of the largest studies ever completed across multiple cultures.[17] CAM therapies are hardly of lesser significance than conventional therapies.

Labeling therapies as CAM also avoids the deeper issues that need to be addressed in health care delivery and promotes further fragmentation of care. Simply adding CAM therapies without changing our health care model is like increasing the number of specialists with no primary care infrastructure, an approach that increases cost and reduces the quality of care.[18] Having multiple providers treating the patient in many different ways prevents what is needed most in the restructuring of health delivery: a medical home that is founded in relationship-centered care.

The term *integrative medicine* stressed on the importance of using evidence to understand how best to integrate CAM therapies into our health care model and allowed us to better understand how they can be used to facilitate health and healing. This evolving understanding helped influence positive change in our health care system.

Signs of this evolution away from CAM are the name changes of many of the educational and research organizations supporting its mission. A general theme is a transition from integrative medicine to integrative health that supports the importance of the process of achieving health outcomes (Table 1.1).

Changing the Medical Culture

In 2001, the IOM published a report on the overall state of U.S. health care. The IOM concluded that the U.S. health care system was so flawed it could not be fixed and an overhaul was required.[19] In 2006, a report from the American College of Physicians (ACP) stated that "Primary care, the backbone of the nation's health care system, is at grave risk of collapse due to a dysfunctional financing and delivery system. Immediate and comprehensive reforms are required to replace systems that undermine and undervalue the relationship between patients and their personal physician."[20]

This crisis has led to proposals for a restructuring of health care that resonate with the philosophy of integrative medicine. The family medicine community has joined the IOM and the ACP in creating their own proposal for a new model of care that promotes a relationship-centered medical home for the establishment of excellence

in health creation in the outpatient setting. Principles of the medical home include the following[21]:

1. Access to care based on an ongoing relationship with a personal primary care clinician who is able to provide first contact and continuous and comprehensive care
2. Care provided by a physician-led team of professionals within the practice who collectively take responsibility for the ongoing needs of patients

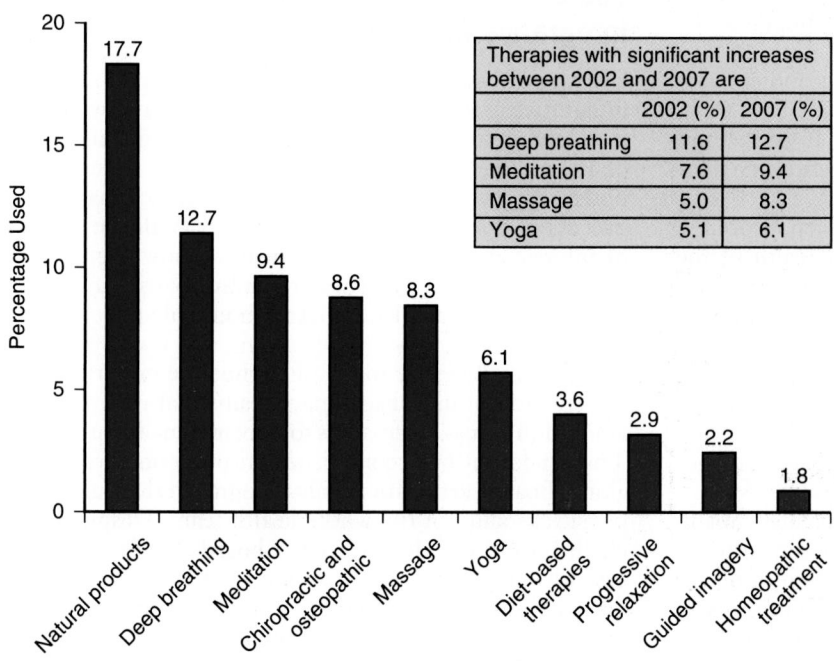

FIG. 1.3 ■ The 10 most commonly used complementary and alternative medicine (CAM) therapies among adults and a list of the most significant increases in therapies from 2002–2007. (From Barnes PM, Blook B, Nahin R. *Complementary and alternative medicine use among adults and children: United States, 2007.* National Health Statistics Report No. 12. Hyattsville, MD: National Center for Health Statistics; 2008.)

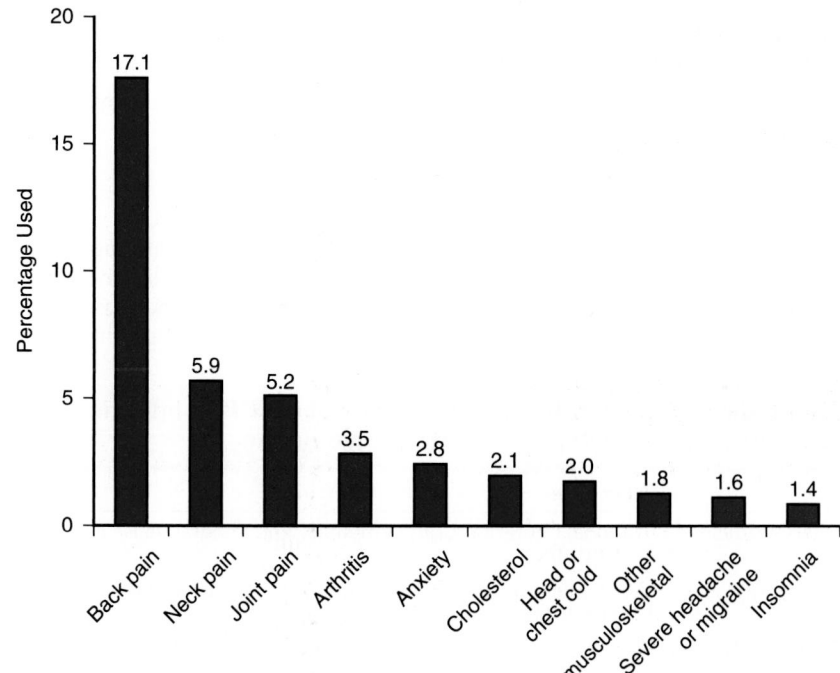

FIG. 1.4 ■ Diseases and conditions for which complementary and alternative medicine (CAM) is most frequently used in adults. (From Barnes PM, Blook B, Nahin R. *Complementary and alternative medicine use among adults and children: United States, 2007.* National Health Statistics Report No. 12. Hyattsville, MD: National Center for Health Statistics; 2008.)

3. Care based on a whole-person orientation in which the practice team takes responsibility for either providing care that encompasses all patient needs or arranging for the care to be done by other qualified professionals
4. Care coordinated or integrated across all elements of the complex health care system and the patient's community
5. Care facilitated by the use of office practice systems such as registries, information technology, health information exchange, and other systems to ensure that patients receive the indicated care when and where they need and want it in a culturally and linguistically appropriate manner
6. A reimbursement structure that supports and encourages this model of care

A similar set of goals was stated by the IOM in their proposal for a new health system for the twenty-first century (Table 1.2).

In 2009, the Bravewell Collaborative sponsored a summit on Integrative Medicine and the Health of the Public at the IOM in Washington, D.C. The goal of this conference was to share the science in the field and the potential for ways in which it can improve the health care of the nation. It succeeded in opening up dialogue among clinicians, administrators, and politicians to bring awareness of how the field could bring balance to a health care system that is weighted heavily toward disease management. A report of the meeting is available online.[22]

The field of integrative medicine was created not to fragment the medical culture further by devising another silo of care but to encourage the incorporation of health and healing into the larger medical model. The culture of health care delivery is changing to adopt this philosophy,

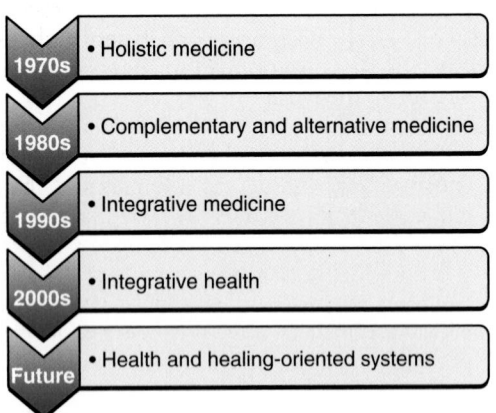

FIG. 1.5 ■ Evolution of titles in the field.

and the integration of nontraditional healing modalities will make this goal more successful.

> It is important to see the benefits and limitations of our current allopathic system and realize that science alone will not meet all the complex needs of our patients.[23]

The Creation of Board Certification In Integrative Medicine

Creating a board certification process for physicians in integrative medicine was not without controversy. There were competing incentives. The underlying philosophy of integrative medicine was not to create a new field, potentially fragmenting care further, but to enhance the process of the medical delivery model. With the growth of interest in integrative medicine, acknowledgment of competency in the field was required, particularly with training programs arising that were not adequate in time and scope.

Another challenge for the field was the importance of the creation of interdisciplinary teams that required collaboration across professions to improve health outcomes. This could not be accomplished through one profession alone. Board certification only recognized the training of physicians and not the whole health team. Despite these challenges, it was decided that a board certification process was needed to recognize the time and commitment invested in learning a body of knowledge for physicians that supported competence in the field.

In 2013, The American Board of Integrative Medicine (ABIOM) was formed through the American Board of Physician Specialties (ABPS). The first diplomats were awarded board certification in 2014. Although grandfathering was allowed initially, fellowship training in integrative medicine will be required after 2016 to sit for the board exam. The requirements for fellowship training programs to meet eligibility are currently being defined and will be available through the ABPS website[24] (see Key Web Resources).

INTEGRATIVE MEDICINE

Integrative medicine is healing-oriented and emphasizes the centrality of the physician-patient relationship. It focuses on the least invasive, least toxic, and least costly methods to help facilitate health by integrating both

TABLE 1.1	Name Changes of Integrative Medicine Organizations as Examples of a Shift in Intention From the Tools of Integrative Medicine to the Process of Integrative Health	
Old Name	**New Name**
National Center for Complementary and Alternative Medicine (NCCAM)	National Center for Complementary and Integrative Health (NCCIH)
The Consortium of Academic Health Centers for Integrative Medicine (CAHCIM)	Academic Consortium for Integrative Medicine and Health (ACIMH)
The American Board of Integrative and Holistic Medicine (ABIHM)	Academy of Integrative Health and Medicine (AIHM)

TABLE 1.2 Simple Rules for the Twenty-First Century Health Care System

Old Rule	New Rule
Care is based primarily on visits.	Care is based on continuous healing relationships.
Professional autonomy drives variability.	Care is customized according to the patient's needs and values.
Professionals control care.	The patient is the source of control.
Information is a record.	Knowledge is shared, and information flows freely.
Decision making is based on training and experience.	Decision making is evidence based.
"Do no harm" is an individual responsibility.	Safety is a system priority.
Secrecy is necessary.	Transparency is necessary.
The system reacts to needs.	Needs are anticipated.
Cost reduction is sought.	Waste is continuously decreased.
Preference is given to professional roles rather than the system.	Cooperation among clinicians is a priority.

From Institute of Medicine, Committee on Quality of Health Care in America. *Crossing the quality chasm: a new health system for the 21st century.* Washington, D.C.: National Academy Press; 2001.

TABLE 1.3 Defining Integrative Medicine

- Emphasizes relationship-centered care
- Integrates conventional and complementary methods for treatment and prevention
- Involves removing barriers that may activate the body's innate healing response
- Uses natural, less invasive interventions before costly, invasive ones when possible
- Engages mind, body, spirit, and community to facilitate healing
- Maintains that healing is always possible, even when curing is not

allopathic and complementary therapies. These therapies are recommended based on an understanding of the physical, emotional, psychological, and spiritual aspects of the individual (Table 1.3).

> The goal of integrative medicine is to facilitate health within complex systems, from the individual to the communities and environment in which all things live.

Health and Healing-Oriented Medicine

"Health" comes from the Old English word *Hal*, which means wholeness, soundness, or spiritual wellness. Health is defined by the World Health Organization (WHO) as "a state of complete physical, mental, and social well-being and not merely the absence of disease or infirmity."[25] Cure, on the other hand, refers to doing something (e.g., giving drugs or performing surgery) that alleviates a troublesome condition or disease. Healing does not equal curing. We can cure a condition such as hypertension with a pharmaceutical product without healing the patient. Healing would facilitate changes that reduce stress, improve diet, promote exercise, and increase the person's sense of community. In doing this,

we help improve the balance of health of the body that may result in the ability to discontinue a pharmaceutical agent and thereby reduce the need for the cure.

An example of this can be seen in Fig. 1.6. Here we have two trees, A and B. Tree A is obviously in a better state of health than tree B. This is likely because of its ability to be in balance with its environment. If a branch breaks on tree A, we can feel comfortable that if we mend the branch, it will likely heal well, or even heal itself. If a branch breaks on tree B and we mend it, the branch is not going to heal because the tree is not in a state of health. The point here is that our focus in medicine has been on fixing the branch while neglecting the health of the tree. If we give more attention to helping tree B find health either by removing barriers that are blocking its own ability to heal or by improving areas of deficiency, the branch will heal itself—we will not need to spend as much time and money fixing the parts.

Integrative medicine is about changing the focus in medicine to one of health and healing rather than disease. This involves understanding the influences of the mind, spirit, and community, as well as the body. It entails developing insight into the patient's culture, beliefs, and lifestyle that will help the clinician understand how best to trigger the necessary changes in behavior that will result in improved health and thus bring more value to health care delivery.

> Cure and fix when able, but if we ignore healing, the cure will likely not last or will give way to another disease that may not have a cure.

Increasing Value Through Integrative Medicine

You get what you pay for. In the past, the economics of health care delivery rewarded treating disease. When this is what is rewarded, health systems need more disease to sustain themselves financially. Here lie the crossroads.

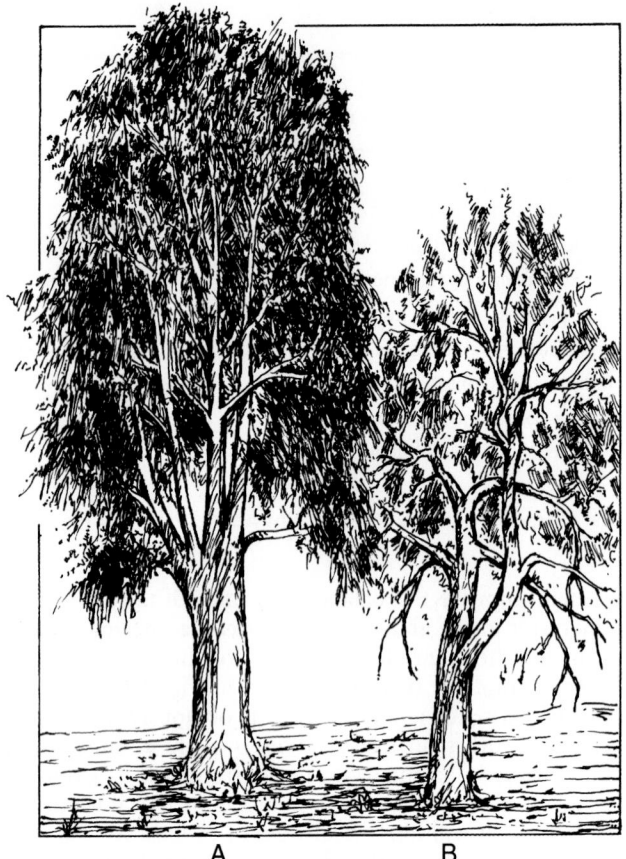

FIG. 1.6 ■ Healthy *(A)* and sickly *(B)* trees. It is important to see the benefits and limitations of our current allopathic system and to realize that science alone will not meet all the complex needs of our patients.[23]

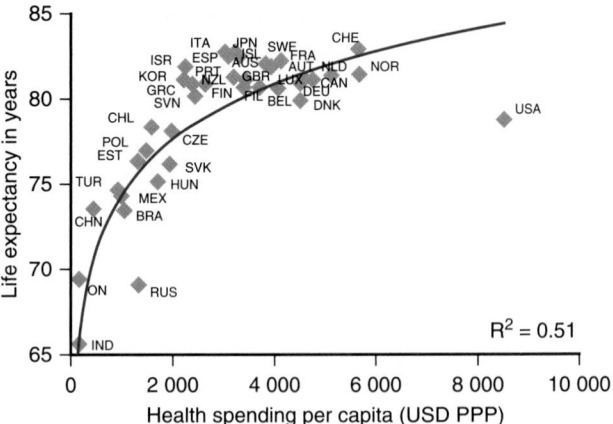

FIG. 1.7 ■ Data points comparing Organizations for Economic Co-operation and Development (OECD) countries with high- and low-income U.S. states in relation to average life expectancy in years and health care expenditures by percentage of the gross domestic product (GDP). (From Fuchs VR. Critiquing US health care. *JAMA.* 2014;312:2095–2096.)

If we are to truly shift health care delivery to health, we have to start financially rewarding health outcomes.

If the United States spent as much of their GDP as the second most expensive country after the United States, there would be an extra trillion dollars available for the United States to support health outcomes. The state with the lowest health care costs (Colorado) still outspends all of the Organisation for Economic Co-operation and Development (OECD) countries, most of which offer universal health care coverage. Those states with the lowest incomes have similar spending with worse than average life expectancy (Fig. 1.7).[26]

Achieving high value for patients and incentivizing practitioners to foster health will become the overarching goal of health reimbursement in the future. In fact, Sylvia Burwell, the U.S. Secretary of Health and Human Services, has stated that *"Our goal is to have 85% of all Medicare fee-for-service payments tied to quality or value by 2016 and 90% by 2018."*[27] Value is defined by the health outcomes achieved per dollar spent. It depends on results, not just inputs, and should be measured by the ways we can improve the quality of patients' lives, not by the number of patients seen in a day. This will require a reimbursement model that rewards team-based care that transcends the one-on-one office visit and allows multiple avenues for patient communication and education among an interdisciplinary team of professionals. This is more

complicated than attaching a payment to a procedure or diagnostic code. To understand how to promote health, the interprofessional team must address all aspects of what it means to be human, both physical and nonphysical.

Integrative medicine can increase value and lower costs through two of its foundational values: (1) by shifting the emphasis of health care to health promotion, disease prevention, and enhanced resiliency through attention to lifestyle behaviors; and (2) by bringing low-tech, less expensive interventions into the mainstream that preserve or improve health outcomes. This approach requires that these professionals have time to recognize the complexity of someone's life, and it cannot be done without a sound commitment to the practitioner-patient relationship.

Relationship-Centered Care

It is much more important to know what sort of patient has a disease than what sort of disease a patient has.
                                                                    SIR WILLIAM OSLER

Observing practitioners of various trades, such as biomedicine, manual medicine, Chinese medicine, and herbal medicine, helps us realize that some practitioners have better results with their chosen trade. Those with more success are able to develop a rapport, understanding, and empathy that help them facilitate healing with their therapy. The relationship fosters healing not only by allowing the practitioner to gain insight into the patient's situation but also by building the patient's trust and confidence in the provider. This trust acts as a tool to activate the patient's natural healing response and supports whatever technique the provider uses, whether it is acupuncture, botanicals, pharmaceuticals, or surgery.

The evidence behind the benefits of relationship-centered care is solid, particularly with regard to reducing health care costs. This approach to care has been found to reduce expenditures on diagnostic tests,[28] reduce hospital admissions,[29] and lower total health care costs.[30,31]

Developing a holistic understanding and relationship with patients allows the practitioner to guide them toward health more efficiently. The integrative clinician can point the way toward health while realizing that the patient will have to do the work to get there. This attitude does a great deal to remove pressure and guilt from providers who have been trained to think of themselves as failures when they cannot fix problems. In fact, relationship-centered care is a necessity when dealing with the many chronic conditions that do not have simple cures. Success is now defined as helping the patient find an inner peace that results in a better quality of life, whether the problem can be fixed or not (see Chapter 3).

Prevention

Integrative medicine encourages more time and effort on disease prevention instead of waiting to treat disease once it manifests. Chronic disease now accounts for much of our health care costs and also causes significant morbidity and mortality. The incidences of heart disease, diabetes, and cancer could be significantly reduced through better lifestyle choices. Instead, these diseases are occurring in epidemic proportions. The system needs a reallocation of resources. Unfortunately, this is a large ship to turn. In the meantime, integrative practitioners can use their broad understanding of the patient to make recommendations that will lead to disease prevention and slow or reverse disease progression.

Integration

Integrative medicine involves using the best possible treatments from both CAM and allopathic medicine based on the patient's individual needs and condition. This selection should be based on good science and neither rejects conventional medicine nor uncritically accepts alternative practices. It integrates successes from both worlds and is tailored to the patient's needs using the safest, least invasive, most cost-effective approach while incorporating a holistic understanding of the individual.

CAM is not synonymous with integrative medicine. CAM is a collection of therapies, many of which have a similar holistic philosophy. Unfortunately, the Western system views these therapies as tools that are simply added on to the current model, one that attempts to understand healing by studying tools in the toolbox. David Reilly said it well in an editorial in *Clinical Evidence:* "We are the artists hoping to emulate Michelangelo's David only by studying the chisels that made it. Meantime, our statue is alive and struggling to get out of the stone."[32]

Integration involves a larger mission that calls for a restoration of the focus on health and healing based on the provider–patient relationship.

REDUCING SUFFERING

The secret of the care of the patient is in caring for the patient.

FRANCIS PEABODY, MD

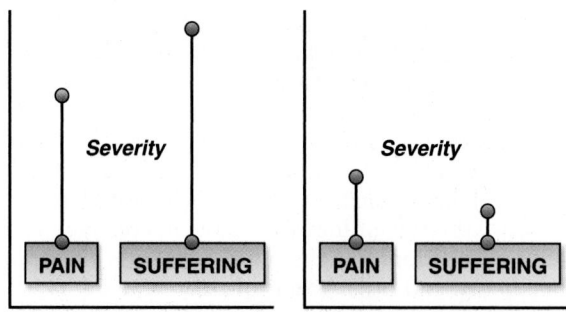

FIG. 1.8 ■ Suffering's effect on the same source of pain. Treating suffering will help reduce the severity of pain and improve the quality of life and should be at the core of our work in integrative medicine.

Good caring and a weak medicine can give a better outcome than poor caring and a strong medicine.

UNKNOWN

At the core of the delivery of health and healing is our ability to relieve suffering. This is not something that we learn in a book, but it requires that we explore our own suffering before we can understand how to help others with theirs. We are our own first patient, and part of our continuing education requires a recurring exploration of our inner self, so we can understand what it means to be truly present without judgment.

The integrative medicine practitioner is not afraid to turn toward suffering in the care of another. As each addresses what is real, the authenticity of the truth draws both toward healing.

In learning this, it is helpful to understand how suffering influences the severity of pain and our quality of life. Pain and suffering are intricately connected but are not the same. Pain is a normal bodily reaction; suffering is not. Pain helps protect us from further harm; suffering is an opportunity to learn. Suffering influences how our body perceives pain—"the more I suffer, the more pain I experience" (Fig. 1.8). Our job is to reduce suffering so we can distil the pain to the most physiological reason for its presence. In treating someone's suffering, we can often make pain more tolerable. In recognizing the severity of suffering, we can often avoid long-term medications that are used to suppress the symptom. It is often through our listening and our presence that we are best able to treat suffering. When no "right" answer or "drug cure" exists, it is our human compassion, connection, and unconditional positive regard that always works, even when our tools do not. This is the most important part of our work and is the reason that we heal in the process of helping others do the same.

THE FUTURE

Although the information age will continue to increase the amount of data on the variety of therapies available, it will only complicate how we apply them. Informed patients will be looking for competent providers who can help them navigate the myriad therapeutic options, particularly for those conditions for which conventional approaches are not effective. These patients will demand scientifically trained providers who are knowledgeable about the body's innate healing mechanisms and who understand the role of lifestyle factors in creating health, including nutrition and the appropriate use of supplements, herbs, and other forms of treatment from osteopathic manipulation to Chinese and Ayurvedic practices. They will be seeking providers who can understand their unique interplay of mind, body, and spirit to help them better understand what is needed to create their own balance of health. This will require a restructuring of medical training that will involve more research and education on how the body heals and how the process can be facilitated.

Health-focused teams will be created within delivery models that assess the health needs of the population being served. Based on this need, the optimal team of professionals will be recruited to work together to improve health outcomes. This requires a common vision in which everyone works together toward each community's unique health needs.

CONCLUSION

The philosophy of health based on a balance of mind, body, and spirit is not new or unique to integrative medicine. This understanding has been around since the time of Aristotle. What we call it is not important, but the underlying concepts are. It is time that the pendulum swings back to the middle, where technology is used in the context of healing and physicians acknowledge the complexity of the mind and body as a whole. Integrative medicine can provide the balance needed to create the best possible medicine for both the physician and patient. We will know that we are near this balance when we can drop the term integrative. The integrative medicine of today will then simply be the good medicine of the future.

THERAPEUTIC REVIEW

INTEGRATIVE MEDICINE

- Emphasizes relationship-centered care
- Develops an understanding of the patient's culture and beliefs to help facilitate the healing response
- Focuses on the unique characteristics of the individual person based on the interaction of the mind, body, spirit, and community
- Regards the patient as an active partner who takes personal responsibility for health
- Focuses on prevention and maintenance of health with attention to lifestyle choices, including nutrition, exercise, stress management, and emotional well-being
- Encourages providers to explore their own balance of health that will allow them better to facilitate this change in their patients
- Requires providers to act as educators, role models, and mentors to their patients
- Uses natural, less invasive interventions before costly, invasive ones when possible
- Recognizes that we are part of a larger ecosystem that requires our efforts in sustaining its health so we can continue to be a part of it

- Uses an evidence-based approach from multiple sources of information to integrate the best therapy for the patient, be it conventional or complementary
- Searches for and removes barriers that may be blocking the body's innate healing response
- Sees compassion as always helpful, even when other therapies are not
- Focuses on the research and understanding of the process of health and healing (salutogenesis) and how to reproduce it
- Accepts that health and healing are unique to the individual and may differ for two people with the same disease
- Works collaboratively with the patient and a team of interdisciplinary providers to improve the delivery of care
- Maintains that healing is always possible, even when curing is not
- Agrees that the job of the physician is to cure sometimes, heal often, support always–*Hippocrates*

Key Web Resources

Academic Consortium for Integrative Medicine and Health (ACIMH): This organization strives to advance the principles and practices of integrative health care within academic institutions. Its members include more than 62 academic health centers in North America.

https://www.imconsortium.org/index.cfm

National Center for Complementary and Integrative Health (NCCIH): This branch of the National Institutes of Health focuses on complementary and integrative health research. It includes literature reviews and education on CAM modalities and integrative practice.

https://nccih.nih.gov/

Academy of Integrative Health and Medicine: The Academy is the evolution of the American Board of Integrative Holistic Medicine that offered board certification prior to the establishment of the American Board of Integrative Medicine. The Academy is an interprofessional organization that focuses on education and fellowship training.

https://aihm.org/

Key Web Resources—cont'd

The American Board of Integrative Medicine through the American Board of Physician Specialties: Provides information for physicians interested in becoming board certified in integrative medicine.

http://www.abpsus.org/integrative-medicine

University of Arizona Center for Integrative Medicine: This center offers education and fellowship training in integrative medicine for physicians, family nurse practitioners, and physician's assistants.

http://integrativemedicine.arizona.edu/

University of Wisconsin Integrative Medicine Program: This program offers patient handouts and educational material for integrative approaches to common medical conditions. It focuses on bringing integrative medicine into primary care delivery models.

http://fammed.wisc.edu/integrative

The Institute for Functional Medicine: An interprofessional organization that focuses on underlying causes of disease that uses a systems-oriented approach through a therapeutic patient partnership.

https://www.functionalmedicine.org/

REFERENCES

References are available online at ExpertConsult.com.

CHAPTER 2

CREATING OPTIMAL HEALING ENVIRONMENTS

David Rakel, MD • Bonnie R. Sakallaris, PhD, RN • Wayne Jonas, MD

Many health practitioners who go into primary care want to both treat and heal, to care for the whole person, to be patient advocates, to apply the best science, and to serve the suffering. In short, we seek to be healers.

However, we often find in medical school and in our practice that the skills needed to be healers and the environment needed to execute those skills are not taught, available, or funded. We know, for example, the factors that increase the risk of disease, but we wait until illness arrives. We understand that relationships, a positive attitude, and behavioral skills form the foundation for compliance and self-care, prevention, and well-being, but we find ourselves without the time to develop them. We see the search for meaning in patients' eyes when they suffer from a serious illness, and yet our science cannot help them find the coherence they seek. For optimal healing to take place, we need to be proactive in creating an environment where these things can happen—to give patients realistic hope.

Every medical recommendation is done in a dynamic environment of care delivery. This environment consists of both physical and nonphysical elements. It often includes a synergy among factors that can either promote or hinder the healing process. Our goal in this chapter is to describe the foundational characteristics of an optimal healing environment (OHE) so that any therapy that is prescribed within this space (shown as a container in Fig. 2.1) will be more successful.

THE OPTIMAL HEALING ENVIRONMENT

We define an OHE as an environment in which the social, psychological, spiritual, physical, and behavioral components of health care are oriented toward support and stimulation of innate healing capacities and the achievement of wholeness. This definition is an expansion of Engel's biopsychosocial model, which created a foundation for understanding the dynamic influences of health.[1] An OHE consists of people in relationships, their health-creating behaviors, and the surrounding physical environment.[2] The Samueli Institute has been a leader in researching and implementing a framework to optimize the potential for healing.[2,3] To enhance clinical delivery, this framework is organized into four environments as shown in Fig. 2.2: internal, interpersonal, behavioral, and external. Each of these environments has two essential constructs that work synergistically to support and stimulate health as shown in Table 2.1.

Internal

- Healing intention
- Personal wholeness

The internal environment recognizes that each person has a unique interaction of mind, body, and spirit that can be directed and supported towards healing. The internal environment is vital to healing because our thoughts, emotions, and spirit have a direct effect on our bodies, our choices, and our relationships. This process is fostered by inner beliefs and expectations that healing and wellness can and will occur.[3] Such belief requires self-reflection, in which each individual becomes aware of his or her own internal wholeness, trusting its healing potential.

It is difficult to connect truly with intention until we have explored our own inner nature.

Patient care starts with us and our preparation to be healers through practices that foster cohesion of body, mind, and spirit. As this connection grows, our ability to sit fully with another suffering human will be enhanced, and appreciation in our work will grow. This growth brings forward foundations in healing that include personal wholeness, positive expectation, hope, faith, and compassion.[4]

Interpersonal

- Healing relationships
- Healing organizations

The interpersonal environment stresses the importance of personal, family, professional, and organizational therapeutic relationships that support and encourage healing. Healing relationships are the connections between persons who hold an intention for healing to occur. The attribute that distinguishes a healing relationship from other positive relationships is the intentional and covenantal nature of the connection, which involves positive emotional engagement with mutual benefit.[3] This relationship includes the art of the clinician, who intentionally learns about the patient in the context of life to recruit the innate ability present in each person for healing[5,6] (see Chapter 3, The Healing Encounter). Healing organizations are as important, as they provide the structures, processes, and resources to stimulate and support healing through intention, relationships, person-centered strategic planning, and shared decision-making.

Through the intent of healing relationship, unhealthy emotions are released and optimism and positive expectations are born. This can be the fulcrum that shifts behavior.

Optimal Healing Environments

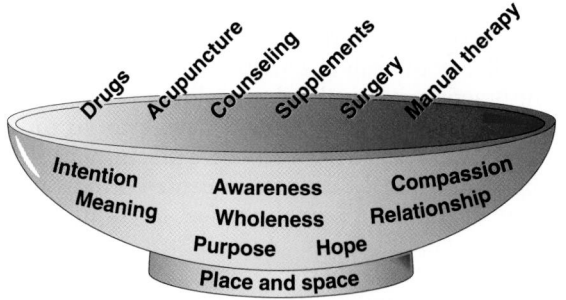

FIG. 2.1 ■ Schematic showing that the therapy we prescribe comes from within a container of influences that can enhance its effectiveness.

Behavioral

- Healthy lifestyles
- Integrative care

Healthy lifestyles and behaviors involve actions that promote health, prevent or even treat disease, and enhance self-healing mechanisms.[7,8] These actions should be directed by the patient but supported by the most appropriate professional in an integrative care team to help the individual succeed in achieving their health goals (see Chapter 4, The Whole Health Process). These behaviors, when motivated by personal meaning, are the main drivers of health outcomes.[9-13] Empowering the individual to best care for himself or herself so both the provider and the patient are active participants in the healing process is a key factor. Some would say that all

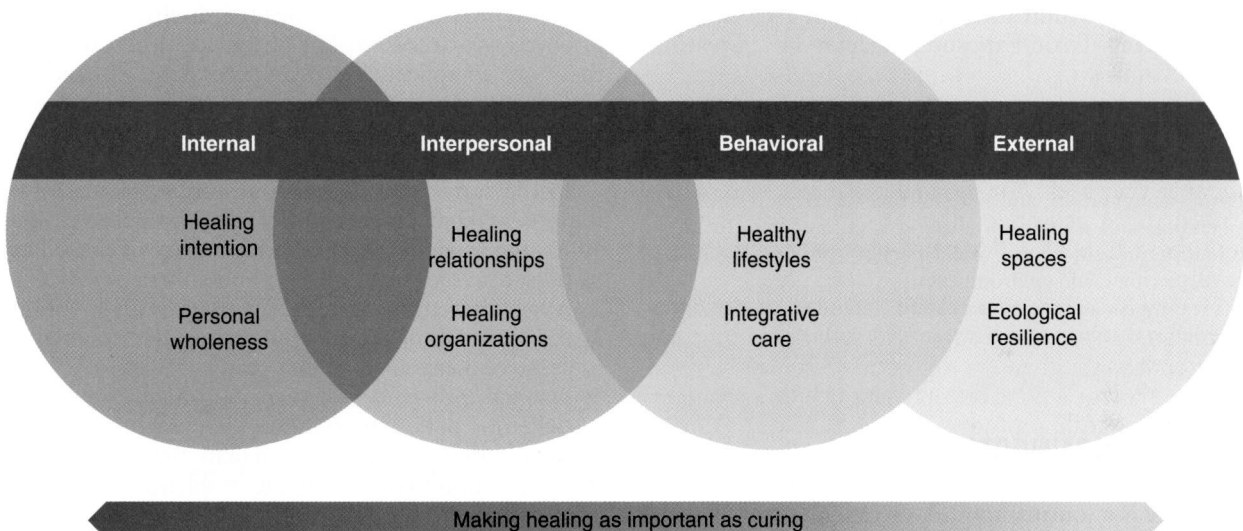

FIG. 2.2 ■ Optimal healing environments. (Copyright© 2015 Samueli Institute, Alexandria, Virginia.)

TABLE 2.1	**Optimal Healing Environments**					
Inner Environment to the Outer Environment						
Healing intention	Personal wholeness	Healing relationships	Healing organizations	Healthy lifestyles	Integrative collaborative medicine	Healing spaces
Expectation	Mind	Compassion	Leadership	Diet	Person oriented	Nature
Hope	Body	Empathy	Mission	Movement	Conventional	Light
Understanding	Spirit	Social support	Culture	Relaxation	Complementary	Color
Belief	Family Community	Communication	Teamwork	Addictions	Culturally appropriate	Architecture
Enhanced awareness expectancy	Enhanced personal integration	Enhanced caring communication	Enhanced delivery process	Enhanced healthy habits	Enhanced medical care	Enhanced healing structure

Modified from Jones WB, Chez RA: Toward optimal healing environments in health care, *J Altern Complement Med.* 10(suppl 1):51-56, 2004.

healing is self-healing, and we, as integrative medicine practitioners, are at our best when we are able to facilitate individuals to care for themselves most successfully. The integrative care team should have this principle as their collective goal. These behaviors can have epigenetic influences on the expression of a healthy phenotype.[14,15]

External

- Healing spaces
- Ecological resilience

The external environment consists of using and sustaining a physical place that supports the health of living beings and the global environment in which all things live. Nature, color, light, fresh air, music, fine arts, and architecture should be used to create influences that support the health and well-being of those who enter the space. This healing space is not only aesthetically pleasing but supports the engagement of its occupants to explore the internal, interpersonal, and behavioral process described above. The importance of ecological resilience is vital, as our health is impeded if we are not able to live within a healthy ecosystem (see Chapter 108, Reducing Toxic Exposure; Chapter 117, Creating a Green Clinic).

Healing can be defined as the dynamic process of recovery, repair, reintegration, and renewal that increases resilience, coherence, and wholeness. Healing is an emergent, transformative process of the whole person—physical, mental, social, spiritual, and environmental.

Healing is a unique personal and communal process and experience that may or may not involve curing.[16]

SPIRITUAL CONNECTION

Spirituality is a journey toward, or experience of, a connection that gives life meaning. This journey is unique to each individual and often drives action. Motivation for changing behaviors often comes from an individual's connection to meaning. As Viktor Frankl writes, *"Those who have a 'why' to live, can bear with almost any 'how'."* It is unfortunate that the importance of this connection rarely enters consciousness until it is threatened by a heart attack or the diagnosis of cancer. Creating awareness between the chasm of our behaviors and what gives life meaning is the key ingredient in the success of motivational interviewing (see Chapter 101, Motivational Interviewing Techniques). The spiritual process of connecting to meaning and purpose empowers the OHE to be effective and sustainable.

CREATING AN OPTIMAL HEALING ENVIRONMENT IN THE CLINICAL SETTING

How can we bring the components of an OHE into a busy practice? Although transforming a practice into a

healing environment may seem like a daunting task, or one with little practical value, experience and evidence indicate that attention to simple and inexpensive details often gradually moves the focus of care from cure alone to one filled with healing activity.[17]

The practitioner can develop healing-oriented sessions within the clinical space without having to go through major renovations. The primary care practitioner already has the foundational relationship-centered tools needed to create an OHE. The nonphysical intention is much more important than the physical space. Healing can occur anywhere, whether it is in an $8 million healing center or in an underfunded inner city clinic for the homeless (Table 2.2).

FOUNDATIONS OF A HEALING ENCOUNTER

To understand the intrinsic value of a therapeutic modality, the scientific model requires that we isolate it from the environment in which it is prescribed. The investigation is also blinded so that the belief systems of the patient and the prescriber do not influence the results. This model is important for research but unrealistic when we look at the more complicated environment in which health care is delivered. In fact, the environment in which the prescribed therapy is given may be more effective than the therapy itself.[18]

In the early 1990s, Frank and Frank[19] described four ingredients that are present in a healing encounter:

1. An emotionally charged relationship with a helping person
2. A healing setting (an expected place to go for healing)
3. An explanation for the symptoms that resulted in a sense of control and understanding
4. A ritual, procedure, or plan that involves active participation of both parties that each believes will restore the person to a state of health (a mutual belief followed by an action to overcome the problem)

When one of the chapter authors, David Rakel, was in practice in rural Idaho, he believed that a selective serotonin reuptake inhibitor was the most successful drug he prescribed. In retrospect, however, the fulfillment of these four criteria may have played a major role in patient improvement. If we look at an example of what happens before we prescribe medication to someone who is depressed, we can better understand this concept.

A depressed gentleman whose life is in chaos comes to see you, his physician, with whom he has a relationship based on trust and a holistic understanding of who he is. The patient has come to a healing setting (medical clinic), where he has the expectation that he will receive help. You give him a logical explanation for his symptoms ("a reduction in the level of serotonin") that offers a sense of control and understanding. Both you and the patient agree on a prescribed therapy that you believe will restore health. You then write down the "answer" on a prescription pad and hand it to him, which then completes the healing ceremony.

When this ritual was performed in a study of St. John's wort, sertraline (Zoloft), and placebo for major depression, it was not the plant or the pill that had the greatest

TABLE 2.2 Optimal Healing Environment

Description of Sample Case Study

OHE Ingredients	OHE Present	OHE Absent
General case description	Mike is a 42-year-old man with low back pain for 8 weeks. He has no history of acute injury, no radicular symptoms, and no improvement despite chiropractic manipulation and over-the-counter NSAIDs.	Mike is a 42-year-old man with low back pain for 8 weeks. He has no history of acute injury, no radicular symptoms, and no improvement despite chiropractic manipulation and over-the-counter NSAIDs.
Relationship-centered care	Mike goes to see Dr. Smith because he knows and trusts her. She helped him through his divorce several years ago.	Mike has no primary care provider. He goes to a local health care clinic close to his home and sees whichever physician is available at the time he visits.
Healing space	Mike likes Dr. Smith's office. It is warm and welcoming and makes him feel at ease, safe, and comfortable.	The clinic is cold and uninviting. You can hear traffic noises from the busy street as you hear the paging system overhead telling the physician that the patient is ready in Room 3.
Self-care	Dr. Smith seems to "walk the talk." Mike sees her jogging around town at lunch, and she never seems stressed out like so many other physicians.	Dr. Jones seems rushed and stressed by the demands of all the patients backed up in the waiting room. She appears to be overweight, pale, and fatigued.
Intention and awareness	What Mike likes best about his physician is that she seems totally present when she sees him. He feels like he is the most important thing on her mind during his visits.	Mike feels sorry for the overworked physician and wants to give her information in an efficient manner so that she can do her job quickly. She remains standing, offers little eye contact, and seems distracted by the many demands on her time. Mike feels disconnected.
Holism	Dr. Smith does a full physical examination that shows muscle spasm in the right quadratus lumborum muscle group but no other concerning signs. Mike feels comfortable telling Dr. Smith about the loss of his job a few months back. She educates him about how the body can sympathize and experience symptoms when the mind is under stress.	Dr. Jones focuses on Mike's back pain and asks directed questions related to his discomfort. Time does not allow for questions beyond Mike's physical symptoms. The examination shows muscle spasm in the right quadratus lumborum muscle group, but no other concerning signs are noted.
Collaborative care	Dr. Smith refers Mike for counseling to develop further insight into how his life situation can influence his health. He will also see an acupuncturist to help reduce the severity of his pain.	Dr. Jones is concerned about the length of Mike's symptoms without resolution. She orders an MRI scan and refers Mike to an orthopedic surgeon for further evaluation. She educates Mike about the potential benefits of an epidural block.
Lifestyle	Dr. Smith sees that Mike has gained 18 lb in the last year and discusses the need for him to start a gradual exercise program and work on getting back to his ideal body weight. She also recommends a book that discusses the relationship between back pain and stress.	Mike is given a prescription for hydrocodone and a patient education handout on low back pain exercises. He is told that if nothing helps, he may be a candidate for long-term opioid pain management.
Spiritual connection	Dr. Smith knows that Mike has a love of photography and the outdoors. Many of his photographs can be found around town in local shops. She encourages Mike to take this opportunity to direct his career to fulfill those things that he loves to do.	Mike leaves hopeful that the medication will reduce his pain and discomfort.

Compare and Contrast	OHE Present	OHE Absent
Outcome	Dr. Smith encourages the development of personal insight into how Mike's life situation is influencing his health. She understands what Mike can do to help this situation resolve.	Dr. Jones focuses on symptom resolution.
Goal	The initial goal is symptom resolution.	The initial goal is symptom suppression.
Symptom management	Dr. Smith recruits internal resources to facilitate health and healing.	With Dr. Jones' approach, the lack of a holistic view and of relationship-centered care results in a focus on the physical symptom without encouraging the patient's insight.
Use of resources	The use of resources is reduced.	The use of resources increases.
Cost	The long-term cost is low.	The long-term cost is high.
Side effects	Most side effects are potentially positive (e.g., joy in a new hobby, insight into behavior, increased well-being, and reduced risk factors).	Most side effects are potentially negative (e.g., nausea from hydrocodone, potential drug addiction, and possible surgery).

MRI, magnetic resonance imaging; NSAIDs, nonsteroidal antiinflammatory drugs; OHE, optimal healing environment.

effect, but the ritual (placebo) 8 weeks after initiating therapy.[20] A meta-analysis and review of data submitted to the U.S. Food and Drug Administration for drug treatment of depression also found little difference between the medication and the placebo for mild to moderate depression; both had beneficial effects[21,22] (see Chapter 3, The Healing Encounter).

During the early development of family medicine, this process was known as the "art of medicine" and was held to be an important feature of the specialty. With the rise and dominance of pharmaceuticals and evidence-based medicine, it became known as the placebo effect and was not supported in medical care. Subsequently, accumulating evidence on the importance of the healing context and encounter resulted in a re-interpretation of this effect as the creation of an OHE.[5] It is important to be aware of these key healing elements so they can be systematically brought into clinical practice.

A Case of Low Back Pain

The case of Mike, a 42-year-old man with low back pain discussed in Table 2.2, illustrates how treatment may progress in the presence or absence of an OHE. This case touches on the complexity of applying the best evidence within the context of each human being's unique life, culture, and belief system. Actively recruiting the ingredients of an OHE can dramatically influence the outcomes achieved with the therapy prescribed.

Acupuncture Versus Epidural Steroids

Acupuncture and epidural steroids have been studied for the treatment of low back pain. Both involve sticking an object through the skin and both include a therapeutic ritual between clinician and patient. As with all therapies, each may be perceived differently by the patient based on their culture and belief system. If we look at the evidence regarding acupuncture, it appears to work better than no treatment but not significantly better than sham acupuncture for low back pain.[23] If we look at the evidence for epidural steroids, they work better than no treatment, but adding a steroid does not seem to result in better outcomes compared to injecting xylocaine alone.[24] Acupuncture's effect may last longer, up to 2 years,[25] whereas epidural steroids have only short-term benefits.[26] Acupuncture is less expensive and less invasive than epidural steroids and likely explains why acupuncture but not epidural steroids was approved by the United Kingdom's National Institute for Health and Care Excellence (NICE) guidelines for treating low back pain.[27]

Specific and Nonspecific Variables

Evidence suggests that the specific effect of acupuncture may be slightly better than the specific effects of epidural steroids, with lower cost and less potential for harm. The OHE is used to enhance the effect size of a therapy through nonspecific variables that include meaning and context (MAC). Examples of the importance of meaning and context include the choice

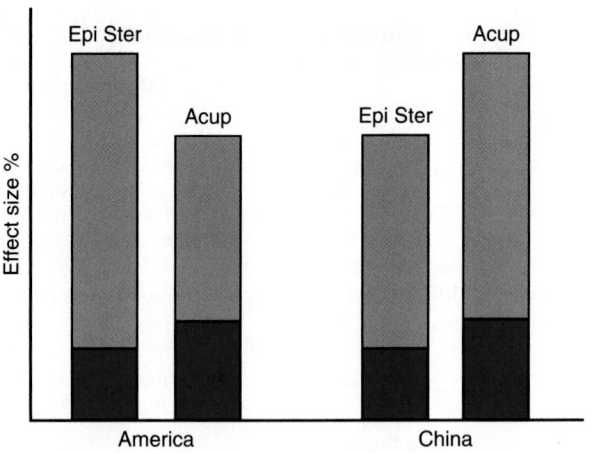

FIG. 2.3 ■ Acupuncture vs epidural steroids. Epi Ster, epidural steroids; MAC, meaning and context; OHE, optimal healing environment.

of words used by a clinician while administering a therapy and the matching of a therapy to the culture that has influenced the patients' beliefs. Both of these actions can enhance the OHE by creating positive expectations.

In a study evaluating areas of the brain affected by the administration of acupuncture needles, there was a significant difference if the needles were simply placed without words compared to being placed by a therapist who created positive therapeutic expectations. The former action merely activated the sensory cortical areas of the brain, while the latter stimulated both the sensory and the limbic centers.[28] Using encouraging words ("This acupuncture meridian will help calm your pain") to create positive expectations can have dramatic effects on the therapeutic outcome, adding to the specific effects.[29] An OHE stacks the deck towards a more robust healing response.

Moerman looked at the healing of ulcers in dozens of placebo-controlled studies from multiple countries. The healing effects of the therapeutic ritual (placebo group) ranged from 0% to 100%, with wide variation from country to country. Patients in Germany experienced large effects, while those in the Netherlands experienced small effects.[30] What was effective in one country was not effective in another. This "country of origin" effect shows that the outcomes are affected in part by the context of the patient and the culture they grew up in. These are just a few of many examples of the power that the OHE can add to the specific effects of any therapy. Fig. 2.3 shows the hypothetical power of these multiple effects, which honors the power of meaning and context supported by the OHE. Even though the evidence indicates that acupuncture is more effective than epidural regarding specific effects, the context and culture in which the treatment is given can determine how well it works. The reason the data in Fig. 2.3 is so variable is that there are many important nonspecific effects that can influence outcomes. These factors are summarized in Table 2.3.

TABLE 2.3	Techniques to Maximize Healing Through an OHE

Have a skilled clinician in communication create positive expectation towards healing.[34,35]

Listen and provide empathy and understanding.[34,51]

Match the therapy to the patient's culture and belief system.[30,52]

Provide an explanation for a problem that increases the sense of control and understanding.[53]

Create positive expectations of the therapy being prescribed.[54]

Deliver the therapy with confidence from a credible source.[55]

Provide therapy in a therapeutic setting that includes elements of nature.[56]

Research the treatment so the prescriber has belief in the therapy being recommended.[57]

Touch the patient.[58,59]

Use the newest therapy.[60,61]

Use a name brand well-known by the culture with more information on the label.[62]

Charge a higher price but not too high.[62,63]

Cut or stick the skin when it is believed to be important.[60]

Create a therapeutic ritual using a tool such as a knife, pin, pill, laser, or light.[62,64]

Write down a plan that both the clinician and patient agree will facilitate health (therapeutic contract).[19]

From Jonas WB: Reframing placebo in research and practice, *Philosophical Transactions of the Royal Society of London. Series B, Biological Sciences* 366(1572):1896-1904, 2011.

The Practitioner's Influence on Healing

Psychotherapy is a good area to explore the ways in which therapeutic interaction influences healing because it employs few external physical tools such as drugs and surgery. When researchers looked at factors that influence positive health change in psychotherapy, the factor within the therapist's control that influenced healing the most (30%) was the establishment of a therapeutic relationship in which the patient felt a sense of trust and rapport.[31] A study on the "most effective" psychotherapists found that those patients receiving counseling from therapists most talented in developing trusting relationships were much more likely to respond positively to medications than were those patients seeing less effective therapists.[32] In fact, when psychiatrists who were rated "high" in relationship and rapport treated depressed patients using a placebo, they had better outcomes than did psychiatrists who were rated lower and who used active drugs.[33] Thus, the practitioner, rather than the pill, had the largest impact on the outcome.

The quality of the clinician-patient interaction influences outcomes. Studies of practitioners' effects on the severity and duration of the common cold and irritable bowel syndrome showed significant enhancement of the therapeutic effect when the treatment was given through an "enhanced" or "augmented" clinical visit in which the

Contributions to the Healing Process

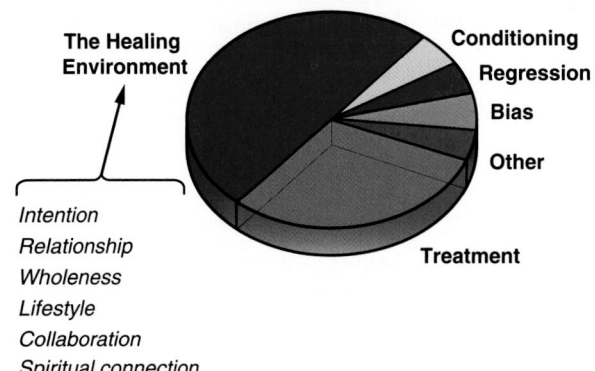

FIG. 2.4 ■ Influences on the healing process.

clinician took time to create a connection that was perceived as empathetic.[34,35]

In treating one of the most common conditions encountered in primary care—diabetes—high ratings of physician empathy by diabetic patients correlated with better outcomes in diabetes management.[36] Nonspecific healing influences found within the clinical encounter should be the foundational intent of interdisciplinary teams focusing on health outcomes of populations (Fig. 2.4).[37]

Creating an OHE will bring more joy to your work. It will allow you to connect with those key elements that attracted you to health care, and in doing so, you will find more meaning and purpose.

Health Teams

New models of care are being designed to improve value and access and reduce cost in the United States. The practitioners of integrative medicine will be leaders in this movement because its philosophy places health creation as its highest priority. Both integrative and conventional medicine will require the assembly of teams of professionals based on the health needs of the community they serve. However, these teams are not simply a potpourri of professionals working independently in proximity. For example, if 30% of a community suffers from obesity, metabolic syndrome, and diabetes, the strategic medical home base will recruit professionals best suited to address this need. This team may include nutritionists, exercise physiologists, spiritual guides, psychologists, health coaches, and physicians. These team members need adequate communication so that the services of each are used to maximize the benefit to the patient. When professionals from varied disciplines come together, shared knowledge allows for insight from different perspectives that can stimulate an "ah ha!" moment in which new ideas allow them to transcend old models of care. When this happens, an interdisciplinary team becomes a transdisciplinary team, and new models of delivery are defined.[38] Multifaceted team-based interventions in primary care are more effective in influencing positive lifestyle behaviors than is isolated specialty care (Table 2.4).[39-41]

TABLE 2.4	**Defining Disciplinary Teams**
Multidisciplinary team	**Additive.** "Comprising more than two professionals from different health care disciplines who work with the same patient, set of patients, or clinical condition, but provide care independently of each other" (interdisciplinary team building). For example, a patient may have visits with both a primary care practitioner (PCP) and a physical therapist (PT). Although the PCP may view clinical notes or a report from the PT, the two disciplines usually do not interact.
Interdisciplinary team	**Interactive.** "Dedicated to the ongoing and integrated care of one patient, set of patients, or clinical condition" (interdisciplinary team building). Team members develop collegial relationships with shared goals and joint decision making. They interact, support, as well as question each other's opinions and negotiate to develop health strategies based on the needs of the individual.
Transdisciplinary team	**Holistic.** Professionals learn from each other and in the process transcend traditional disciplinary boundaries that may result in the emergence of new knowledge. Often, the greater the difference between professions (epistemologic distance; e.g., engineering and humanities), the more likely insight will develop toward the creation of a new way to solve a problem.

From Rakel DP, Jonas W: The patient-centered medical home. In Rakel R, Rakel D, editors: *Textbook of Family Medicine.* 8th ed, Philadelphia, 2011, Saunders; data from Choi BC, Pak AW: Multidisciplinarity, interdisciplinarity, and transdisciplinarity in health research, services, education and policy: 3. Discipline, inter-discipline distance, and selection of discipline, *Clin Invest Med* 31:E41-E48, 2008.

Environment's Influence on Genetic Expression

The goal of an integrative medicine health-oriented team is to work together to create OHEs. Environments can have an influence on the genome of the organisms that live within them. The scientific evidence for this epigenetic influence is exploding and gives power and hope to the individual to make positive lifestyle choices by attending to and changing their environment (Fig. 2.5).

Animal studies showed that genetically identical agouti mice that were bred to develop obesity and diabetes could have this expression suppressed when the mothers were fed methyl-donating foods (genistein) before they gave birth.[42] An Amish community was assessed to see whether carriers of the *FTO* obesity gene would become overweight, and it was found that carriers who averaged 18,000 steps in 1 day remained at a normal weight. Their lifestyle habits trumped their genetic risk.[15]

Telomeres are the protective DNA-protein complexes at the end of the chromosomes that promote stability. Loss in their length has been associated with increased

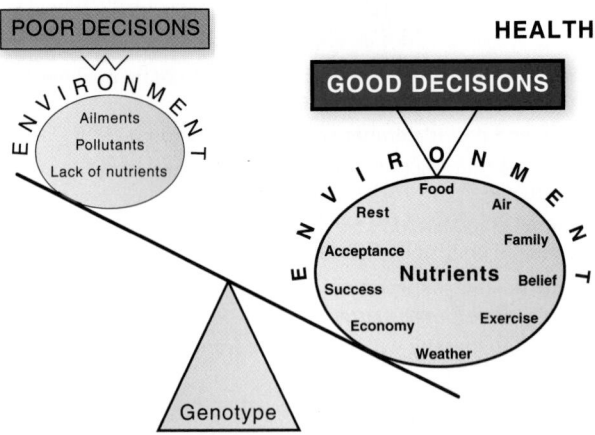

FIG. 2.5 ■ Depicted is a balance representing the person's unique genetic constitution and the direction into which his or her decisions will poise the organism's well-being, determined by the presence of nutrients, ailments, or pollutants. A nutrient can be understood as any element that nourishes the body and mind.

risk of disease and premature mortality. Telomere shortening is counteracted by the enzyme telomerase, and more of this enzyme is beneficial. Ornish et al.[14,43,44] investigated telomerase levels in 30 men with prostate cancer. After 3 months of healthy lifestyle changes including moderate exercise, a low-fat, plant-based diet, and social support, the telomerase levels rose[43] and oncogene expression was inhibited.[44] Exercise alone can increase telomerase activity[45] and brain volume.[46] Stress can decrease telomerase levels,[47] whereas practicing the relaxation response can have a positive influence on genetic expression[48] and reduce the expression of genes that promote inflammation.[49] Although these behaviors are powerful, they are not the sole dictator of outcomes. The body–mind is complex and mysterious. The clinician should be careful not to instill guilt regarding lifestyle habits when cancer or heart disease is diagnosed. Instead, the clinician should reassure the patient that, even when disease progresses, improved well being and function are more likely if he or she continues or adopts healthy behaviors while incorporating interventions that will have the most benefit.

THE VALUE OF CREATING OPTIMAL HEALING ENVIRONMENTS

Business Case for Optimal Healing Environments

Most health care leaders agree that healing is at the core of their mission. The reality of current incentives and cost-containment initiatives has caused many practices to set aside healing practices in favor of direct revenue-producing activities. The Samueli Institute studied three financially-thriving organizations who committed additional time and resources to create an OHE. Each of the organizations reported a cost per patient day or encounter that is higher than the average. However, the costs are minimal when compared to overall budgets. They found that creating an OHE provided market differentiation, improved community engagement, and promoted positive staff and physician engagement and positive patient experience scores.[50] In addition, the organizations studied realized efficiencies related to the emphasis on person-centered and team-based care. When patients are involved in decisions and in the plan of care, wait times and frustration points are minimized. Integrating multiple disciplines into care provides checks and balances and communication patterns that reduce errors.

Health as a Continuum

The continuum of health starts with ourselves, is supported by others, is influenced by lifestyle choices, and is shaped by our inner and outer environments. This continuum recognizes the importance of the interconnectedness of all things. Health is not found in isolated parts but throughout the whole. Being an integrative medicine practitioner means recognizing the dynamic and complex ecosystem in which we live and working to support its health. In doing so, we occasionally pause to witness the mystery of how nature continuously strives for balance despite the odds we have created against it.

I would rather live in a world where my life is surrounded by mystery than live in a world so small that my mind could comprehend it.

HARRY EMERSON FOSDICK

Several years ago, a primary care clinic in England introduced a spiritual healer into its practice. This was done quietly, without advertisement. Patients who had refractory, chronic illnesses, were high-frequency health care users, and were taking multiple drugs were offered 12 sessions with the healer. Health care use costs, symptoms, and well-being were measured before and after the study period. Almost all patients got better: health care visits decreased; patients improved in their energy and well-being; and although the diseases were not actually cured, suffering was relieved.

Costs were reduced by $2000 per patient per year. Most interesting, however, was the change this approach had on the physicians in the practice. When the investigators examined what the healer did during sessions, the procedures were simple. The healer spent a long time listening intently to the patients and hearing what their concerns were about the illness, linking it up with family events, and challenging patients to perceive their connectivity beyond themselves, to imagine a future that was better and improved. The healer then spent time doing some bioenergy work, holding her hands over the patient in the traditional laying-on-of-hands manner. The physicians in the clinic soon realized that many of these same behaviors were similar to things they had been taught to value in medical school but had not often been able to incorporate into their own practice. These physicians then found themselves spending a few more moments with patients and asking them about social and family issues that earlier they would have glossed over or ignored. They provided and received feedback about the meaning of a person's illness and listened and responded in a warmer fashion.

In other words, the physicians realized that they, too, could become healers in the classic sense of the term.[61]

Key Web Resources

The Samueli Institute Study of Optimal Healing Environments http://www.samueliinstitute.org/research-areas/optimal-healing-environments/ohe-framework	The Samueli Institute has sponsored research on the development of optimal healing environments and provides resources and papers on the topic through this website.
The National Institute of Building Sciences https://www.wbdg.org/resources/therapeutic.php	Reviews key factors for producing therapeutic environments within building structures.
Planetree http://planetree.org/	The Planetree organization focuses on incorporating optimal healing environments into health systems through patient-centered care.

REFERENCES

References are available online at ExpertConsult.com.

CHAPTER 3

THE HEALING ENCOUNTER

David Rakel, MD • Luke Fortney, MD, FAAFP

To find health should be the object of the doctor. Anyone can find disease.

T. STILL, MD

To write prescriptions is easy, but to come to an understanding of people is hard.

FRANZ KAFKA

What kind of doctor do I need to be for this patient today?
MICHAEL BALINT

Medical encounters in the recent past have been dominated by the 15-minute "problem-focused" office visit that only addresses symptoms and disease. While this *pathogenesis*-focused encounter addresses the creation of disease, the healing encounter has a different goal of *salutogenesis*, which focuses on health and prevention.[1] Here the clinician's intent is to develop an understanding of what the person needs to self-heal and be well. This chapter focuses on how the clinician can most efficiently *allow* this process to unfold. At its deepest level, this healing process is not one-sided, but allows both the patient and the clinician to be transformed by the process together. The result can be the most rewarding aspect of the medical profession.

> *Salutogenesis* means "the creation of health," which is the opposite of *pathogenesis* (the creation of suffering and disease). The goal of the healing encounter is to facilitate health and well-being that transcends the physical alone and results in less suffering, greater understanding, and improved quality of life.

PRACTITIONER VERSUS PILL

The mind often attributes healing to external influences outside of ourselves, such as from drugs, herbs, an acupuncture needle, etc. These specific variables are often the most thoroughly studied and are thought to contribute the most benefit, partly because they are physical treatments that can be easily quantified. The gold standard in medical research, the double-blind placebo-controlled trial, focuses on removing nonspecific variables that can often be more powerful than the pill or procedure being studied. These nonspecific variables include aspects of care that are difficult to quantify and include trust, empathy, a sense of control, and compassion, which are key ingredients of the healing encounter. These nonspecific variables are important to healing. For

example, they have been found to enhance the effects of acupuncture for irritable bowel syndrome,[2] shorten the duration of the common cold,[3] trump antidepressants for mild to moderate depression,[4-6] and improve clinical outcomes in patients with diabetes,[7] among others. The nonspecific effects that have been most thoroughly studied in influencing healing in the clinical encounter can be summarized through the *PEECE mnemonic*: P, positive prognosis; E, empathy; E, empowerment; C, connection; and E, education.[8] Many of these healing influences can be cultivated through the practice of mindful awareness.

MINDFULNESS IN YOUR PRACTICE

Mindfulness is a way of being in the present moment, on purpose, non-judgmentally.

JON KABAT-ZINN[9]

When we sit with a patient, the mind will naturally wander and be distracted. Without intentional redirection of the attention back to the patient, however, we may lose the opportunity to understand the person sitting across from us. When we are not present and anchored in the moment, we can slip into seeing patients not as who they truly are but as we prematurely judge them to be. Medical training conditions us to label patients with disease. As we become more adept at recognizing the disease states within people, however, our perception of each other can shift and only recognize the label rather than the individual.

> The previous edition of the International Classification of Disease code book (ICD-9) had approximately 13,000 diagnostic codes. The 10th edition (ICD-10) has more than 68,000.

In an observational study from 1973, eight *sane* people presented to eight different psychiatric hospitals in California with the complaint of, "*I am hearing thuds.*" After being admitted, these people behaved in a normal and healthy way. The researchers wanted to see what diagnoses they would be given and how long they would remain in the hospital. All eight were given the diagnosis of schizophrenia in remission, and the average length of stay was 19 days. One of the eight participants was in the hospital for 52 days.[10] The doctors and nurses were not able to see the *sane* patients for who they really were because of their disease-focused conditioned thinking. Recognizing

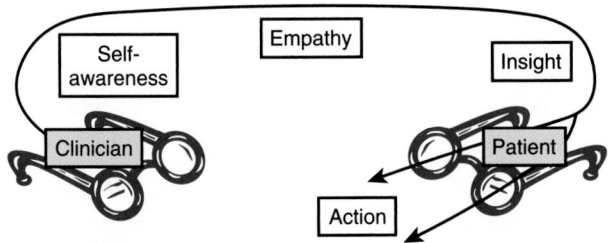

FIG. 3.1 ■ Seeing From the Patient's Perspective.

disease patterns is an important part of a clinician's everyday work. If we are not aware and do not recognize the habitual nature of these snap judgments, however, we risk being stuck in these conditioned perspectives and may not recognize arising moments and situations when it is appropriate to step out of these perspectives. The people who questioned the appropriateness of the eight *sane* patients' admissions to the psychiatric hospital were not the doctors or nurses but their fellow inpatients—those with whom the sane people developed relationships through meals, group therapy, and daily activities. Through close relationships, the other inpatients were able to see the individuals as they truly were.

Self-Reflection

The healing encounter requires that the practitioner be aware of and recognize his/her own mind states, which may or may not be helpful in any given moment. Noticing personal bias can help minimize unconscious snap-judgments and projections. The mindful clinician will be better equipped to meet patients where they are by recognizing their true needs. In being aware and present in the moment, we can be more successful in helping others if we are able to recognize our own beliefs and then do our best to also see the world through the lens of our patient from his/her life perspective (Fig. 3.1). For example, primary care clinicians trained in mindfulness report improved mood and sense of personal well-being, which, in turn, can have a positive impact on patient care.[11,12] A study of psychotherapists in training found that the patients under the care of those therapists who practiced mindfulness had better outcomes and greater symptom reduction than the patients of therapists who did not practice mindfulness. This study indicates that the personal practice of clinicians may influence the outcomes of patients in their care.[12]

To be of service to a person in need is difficult if the clinician is suffering more than the patient. As the saying goes, "you can't give what you don't have."

There is nothing like a difficult patient to show us ourselves.

WILLIAM CARLOS WILLIAMS

Most people do not listen with the intent to understand; they listen with the intent to reply. They're either speaking or preparing to speak. They're filtering everything through their own paradigms, reading their autobiography into other people's lives.

STEPHEN COVEY

Empathy

Empathy is defined as a cognitive attribute that involves an understanding of experiences, concerns, and perspectives of another person, combined with the capacity to communicate this understanding.[13] Empathy is a foundational ingredient of the healing encounter. It asks that we initially set aside what we know, feel what patients are communicating, and then communicate this back to them so they know they were heard. Patients often do not remember what you tell them, but they remember how you made them feel. We perceive first through empathy, and *then* we proceed in taking action based on the information obtained through mindful listening combined with medical knowledge and training. Unfortunately, it is not surprising that empathy declines significantly through medical school and residency as learners focus solely on increasing their technical-medical knowledge at the expense of emotional health and personal awareness.[14] The combination of empathetic insight with knowledge best serves the authentic needs of the patient to experience healing—both are important and necessary.

Compassion Training

The challenge with empathy is that when you feel someone's suffering day in and day out, it can lead to negative feelings, withdrawal, nonsocial behavior, and even burnout. This process is known as *empathic distress*.[1,15] A helpful remedy for this is compassion training. In a study where groups were shown videos of human suffering, one group was first given empathy training and then compassion training. The other group was taught a memory exercise at both time points. The researchers evaluated positive and negative effects after each training program. The memory group had a gradual decline in positive effect. The group taught empathy had more negative emotions; however, negative effect went down and positive effect went up after being taught compassion. Functional MRI analysis showed that the compassion training activated the same areas of the brain that are associated with reward, affiliation, and love.[16]

Why is compassion training a remedy for empathic distress? Compassion comes from "compati" (to feel pity), "com" (come together), and "pati" (to suffer). In short, it means that when one person suffers, we all suffer together. This social integration activates areas of the brain (ventromedial prefrontal cortex and ventral striatum) that are associated with enhanced well-being and love, even when experiencing suffering in another. Compassion training encourages us to love one another as part of an interconnected whole, and this gives us resiliency to be with one another during difficult times (see Table 3.1, which summarizes a type of compassion training used in this study).

Insight and Intuition

Insight requires empathy and is the process by which information is gained that allows clinicians to understand how best to serve the health needs of the patient. Intuition is a unique human ability that is both subtle and

TABLE 3.1 Compassion Training

Start with yourself	May I be filled with loving kindness May I be well May I be peaceful and at ease May I be happy
Then to your loved ones	May you be filled with loving kindness May you be well May you be peaceful and at ease May you be happy
Then to a neutral person you do not know	May you be…
Then to someone who is challenging or difficult for you	May you be…
Then to all living beings	May all beings be filled with loving kindness May all be well May all be peaceful and at ease May all be happy

Start by taking a few calming breaths and then focus your attention to each of the five groups in the order shown. This short practice, if done regularly, can have neuroplastic effects that build therapeutic resiliency, which can protect against burnout.
(This practice is adapted from the book *Loving-Kindness* by Sharon Salzberg. Boston. Shambhala Publishing; 2002).

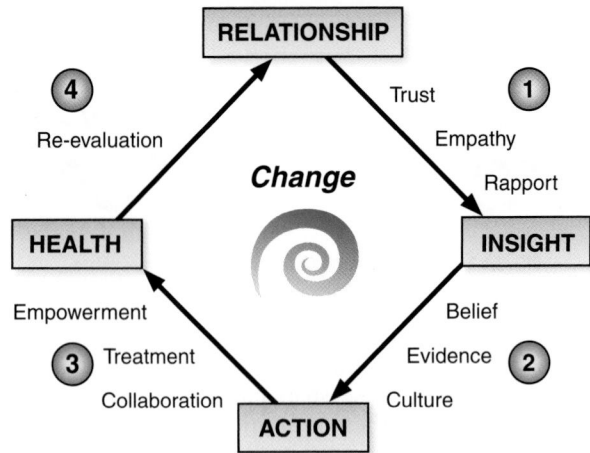

FIG. 3.2 ■ **The Dynamic Process of Facilitating Health and Healing.** (From Rakel DP. The healing power of relationship-centered care. In: Rakel DP, Faass N, eds. *Complementary medicine in clinical practice.* Boston: Jones & Bartlett; 2006).

complex. It is a process of perception, of incorporating a variety of different unrelated bits of information (both conscious and unconscious), and arriving at a logical conclusion. The more information we have to work with, the more accurate the intuition. If a patient is seen only as a disease or a dysfunctional organ system, the clinician will often start with what he or she already knows from medical training, and the additional information obtained through listening and feeling will not be incorporated into the patient's care. This is why ongoing face-to-face, relationship-centered care is so important: it can enhance the accuracy of our intuition and insight. A clinician who has an established therapeutic relationship with a patient is more likely to have accurate insight and intuition based on the many bits of information (analytical and emotional) assimilated over time. This ongoing therapeutic relationship is why a strong primary care infrastructure results in a 15-fold return on investment in medical spending.[17] Insight obtained in this way results in action that guides the patient most efficiently to health (Fig. 3.2).

Functional magnetic resonance imaging research has shown a strong coupling between speakers' and listeners' brains that vanishes when communication is poor. With good communication, the listener can anticipate what is going to be communicated before speech is produced, thus leading to greater understanding of the information conveyed.[18]

Action

The Buddhist tradition has a saying, "action without wisdom is dangerous, and wisdom without action is useless."

The healing encounter requires a collaborative action that both the clinician and patient believe will bring health. If we do not bring a mindful approach to listening *before* moving into action, we may not serve the true needs of the patient and may even cause harm. When we recommend a therapy that the patient does not follow through with, the clinician may blame the patient for being noncompliant. In actuality, the clinician should assume partial responsibility for not making the effort to fully understand the patient's concerns and make recommendations that would better match the patient's needs. Nonadherence is really a situation where two people are miscommunicating and working toward different goals. The healing encounter involves a process that must unfold before action can be of service and the patient's goals can be met. To simplify, we summarize this process into the three Ps of a healing encounter: *Pause, Presence,* and *Proceed.*

THE 3 PS: PAUSE, PRESENCE, AND PROCEED

Pause

Before entering the clinical examination room, take a moment to pause, take a deep breath, and allow yourself to direct your full attention to the patient in the room. Use the threshold of the exam room doorway to remind you to drop into the sensations of your own breathing so that you may be more present with the patient. A threshold is a metaphor for a transition to a new understanding or awareness that the clinician and patient find together. Taking advantage of the opportunity to pause, drop in, and be present can help us center and be more attentive to the patient.*

---

*For more information on this topic, go to http://www.fammed.wisc.edu/mindfulness/pip.

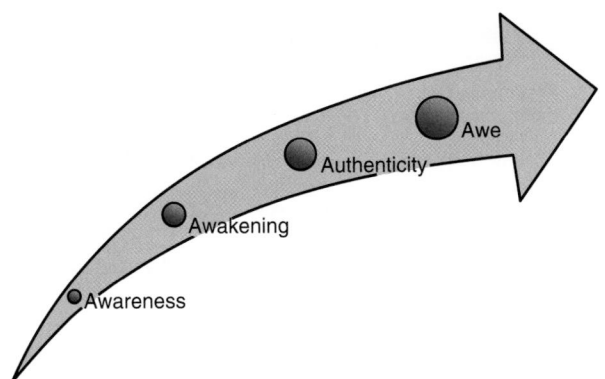

FIG. 3.3 ■ **The Four As of the Healing Encounter.**

Presence

Intentionally directing the attention to the physical sensations of breathing or feeling the feet making contact with the floor helps ground and center the mind. Taking two to three deep breaths into the lower abdomen just beneath the umbilicus is a good start (see Chapter 92). In martial arts, this area is called the *hara*, and bringing awareness to this area of the body allows the settled mind to respond more appropriately to the changing needs of each moment. According to some Eastern practices, life energy flows from the hara (see Chapter 116). A suggestion to "practice in your practice" involves using your computer log-in as an opportunity to drop in and check in with your own body as you prepare to work with a patient. When the mind and body show up in the same place at the same time, the clinician is better equipped to engage with the patient. The computerized or paper chart need not be a barrier between patient and provider.

Being present and alert moment by moment can awaken us to mystery and awe in an authentic way (Fig. 3.3). When we pause and become present with what is really happening, we are more likely to recognize what is beautiful in each moment, such as in seeing a flower or a living cell. The same is true with suffering; even though suffering is associated with pain and discomfort, the more we explore and lean into it, the more we come to understand and learn from it. The mindful encounter brings two people together in the fullness of life including suffering, joy, peace, unrest, creativity, and frustration. The mindful clinician is able to remain present with a wide range of emotions and experiences without being overwhelmed by or overidentifying with suffering.

Patients are able to feel whether you are truly present and listening. If they sense that you are compassionate and attentive, they will feel more comfortable and will often share important information and amazing stories. Creating this space results in more meaningful conversation that engenders understanding. In telling their stories, patients are able to reflect on the cause of their symptoms. This insight can be empowering and help motivate the patient to make changes. The clinician's empathy can provide comfort and reduce the feeling of isolation that patients with chronic illness often have. Ultimately, mindful listening may be our most effective therapeutic

tool.[19] As the saying goes, "you were given two ears and one mouth to be used in that proportion."

Proceed

In pausing, being present, and listening to the patient, insight arises. This insight allows a plan to be created that both the clinician and patient believe will be of benefit. The plan should increase the sense of control that patients feel in taking action that helps them move from disease to wellness. The health plan should recognize both physical and nonphysical factors that the patient can use to manage symptoms and prevent illness in the future. Helpful questions that can bring an understanding to this process are reviewed in Box 3.1.

The health plan may have one recommendation or several, based on the needs of the patient. For example, if a patient has had recurring headaches and diarrhea ever since his or her divorce, the health plan may only involve one recommendation, such as working toward self-care and forgiveness (see Chapter 99). If another patient wants to prevent a recurrence of breast cancer, however, the health plan may include recommendations on stress reduction, nutrition, spiritual connection, improving sleep, and the use of medications and supplements.

Before computerized medical records, the "answer" to the patient's problem was often conveyed as a quick fix on the prescription pad. The practice of integrative medicine recognizes that health be defined by much more than a medication. Instead, the power of the ritual process around the actual prescription should be cultivated. This ritual transfers knowledge and a sense of control that gives confidence that something may help the patient transcend suffering. The clinician's recommendations, based on the insight that arises from the healing encounter, should be summarized in writing and given to the patient at the conclusion of the visit.

Healing is not something easily reproduced or taught. Often, the best we can do is create an environment where it can unfold, grow, and teach us.

FIVE QUESTIONS TO CONSIDER BEFORE PRESCRIBING A THERAPY

The integrative medicine practitioner uses relationship-centered care to develop insight into the most effective therapy for the patient's needs. Before prescribing a specific therapy, the practitioner should consider the following five questions:

1. **Does the therapy result in symptom resolution or symptom suppression?** Our initial goal should always be the resolution of the symptom to enable us to use fewer external influences to maintain health. This often requires that we explore the mind and spiritual aspects of a symptom. A physical symptom can also be seen as our body asking for some type of change. If we simply suppress the symptom without understanding what it may need to go away, it will likely recur or arise in another part of the body. A good example of this is the use of proton pump inhibitors (omeprazole [Prilosec], lansoprazole [Prevacid], and rabeprazole [Aciphex]) for epigastric pain. These are excellent medications to help suppress symptoms or heal ulcers. If we over-rely on this pharmacotherapy, however, it may prevent us from exploring the symptom further. It may also keep us from listening to the patient's story, in which the use of metaphor may give us further insight into the mind-body influences on health. For example, a person with epigastric pain may say that his or her job is "eating me up inside." If we do not deal with this stress, the body will not truly heal even though the symptom may be suppressed through use of a medication. Ultimately, this can lead to long-term use of a medication that may result in a change of the natural environment of the body. Long-term acid suppression is now known to be associated with increased risk of pneumonia[20]; malabsorption of B vitamins, calcium, magnesium, and iron[21]; a higher prevalence of *Clostridium difficile* colitis[22]; and increased risk of myocardial infarction[23] and fractures of the hip[24,25] and spine.[26]

To foster symptom resolution, we need to explore both the external and internal reasons for its expression (Fig. 3.4). An external therapy (medications, acupuncture, surgery, or manual therapies) will not have lasting benefit unless it is coupled with an internal exploration and understanding of why the symptom is there in the first place (e.g., emotions, stress, meaning, and purpose). The physical and nonphysical are inseparable, and if we do not address both, it will be difficult for the symptom to fully resolve. However, when a condition has been fully evaluated and we have explored all aspects of it but find no resolution, it is appropriate to consider suppression of the symptom with medication and procedures to reduce suffering and improve quality of life.

2. **What is the evidence?** The scientific model allows us to understand which therapies have the most intrinsic value. Once we have reviewed the evidence, we can combine it with the "art of medicine" to stack the deck further in favor of a positive response. Unfortunately, the amount of evidence we have to rely on is limited. Out of 2404 treatments reviewed in medical care, 15% were found to be beneficial and 47% to have not been adequately tested.[27]

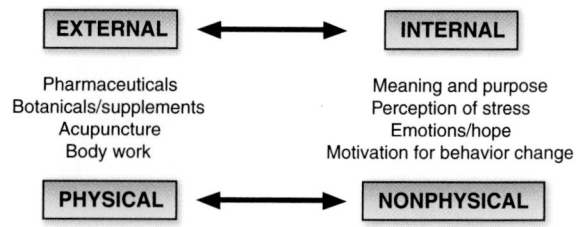

FIG. 3.4 ■ Dynamic Interplay Between the Physical and Nonphysical Influences on Health and Disease.

It is expensive and time and labor intensive to conduct meaningful research, and the therapies that have the best quality of evidence are often those therapies that have the greatest potential for economic gain. Unfortunately, little economic incentive exists to promote therapies that result in healing in our current health care model. You will not see representatives from the wood and paper industry promoting the use of pencils and paper to support the health benefits of journaling on asthma and rheumatoid arthritis despite the evidence showing benefit.[28] The responsibility falls to the academic institutions and the government to provide funding to research all potential therapies despite their lack of economic rewards.

3. **What is the potential harm?** It can be dangerous if we look only at the evidence for the benefits of any given therapy without also considering the evidence for potential harm. For example, in the 1950s, evidence showed that diethylstilbestrol prevented miscarriages; however, the potential harm to the unborn fetus was not taken into consideration until after many lives were affected. In addition, evidence initially indicated that flecainide improved arrhythmias observed on electrocardiography in cases of supraventricular tachycardia; however, subsequent research demonstrated that flecainide can also increase mortality.[29] The integrative medicine practitioner first considers the least harmful, least invasive therapies before moving on to more invasive therapies. As a result, it is imperative that we continue to research not only the potential benefits but also the potential harms of the therapies we prescribe. Because of the potential risks associated with many extrinsic medical therapies (e.g., medications and surgeries), we should first encourage healthy lifestyle changes with the least risk (e.g., nutrition, stress-reduction, exercise, spiritual connection, etc.). This can lead to fewer high-risk interventions, thereby resulting in overall harm reduction. For this reason, this text includes an icon that weighs the evidence of benefit against the evidence of harm to help guide the clinician.

4. **What is the cost?**

One of the first duties of the physician is to educate the masses not to take medicine.

SIR WILLIAM OSLER

Complementary therapies are generally low tech and low cost and reduce the need for more expensive interventions. Users of CAM report that their use of prescription drugs and conventional therapies decreases.[33] When CAM was combined with biomedicine, one study showed a reduction of pharmaceutical use by 51.8%, a decrease in outpatient surgeries and procedures use by 43.2%, and a reduction of hospital admissions by 43%.[34]

Incorporating mind-body stress reduction techniques into the treatment of 4452 subjects enrolled in the Relaxation Response Resiliency Program compared to a cohort of controls that did not receive this training showed that the program participants had a 43% reduction in billable medical encounters, reducing costs by $2360 per patient per year.[35]

Another study randomized participants to three groups: a wait list control, an 8-week exercise program, or an 8-week mindfulness program to see if this training would reduce the incidence and cost of upper respiratory illness. The cost of care related to upper respiratory illness per group member was $214 for the wait list control, $136 for the exercise program, and $65 for the mindfulness meditation program.[36] In addition, as far back as the 1980s, Dean Ornish et al.[37] showed how coronary heart disease can be reversed by incorporating lifestyle changes, including nutrition, exercise, stress management, group psychosocial support, and smoking cessation.

Much of the economic incentive for physicians in the United States is fixated on acute care management and driven by relative unit value (RVU), with little incentive for lifestyle education and prevention that would reduce the need for expensive medications and procedures. These studies are examples of how an integrative approach can result not only in self-healing but also in economic savings in morbidity, mortality, and the money needed to treat them. The implementation of lifestyle modification and prevention medicine has the potential for tremendous cost savings and improved quality of care.

5. **Does the therapy match the patient's culture and belief system?** In our conventional medical system, we have traditionally pulled patients into our paradigm of thought and have told them what they need. This method is often necessary for acute illness; however, we will be more effective if we offer treatment plans that better match patients' belief systems for chronic conditions that have no "easy" answer (see Chapter 4). In this way, we can activate the internal healing response, a process that we know as the placebo effect. Instead of brushing this off as a nuisance, the talented clinician will use it to enhance healing. Being able to integrate various methods of healing from different cultures can enable the clinician to better match the therapy to the individual. The art of medicine may lie in the clinician's ability to activate this response without deception. We should give patients what they need before we give them what we know.

STEPS TO ENHANCE THE HEALING ENCOUNTER

Creating Salutogenesis-Oriented Sessions

A healing encounter can be created in a brief 5-minute interaction or during an hour-long discussion. To serve the complexity of health and healing most effectively, however, practitioners need to protect time in their schedules to create the space for a healing ritual (i.e., the salutogenesis-oriented session, SOS).[38] Any health care clinic can create an SOS that stacks the deck in favor of the healing encounter. The following subsections describe key ingredients that will help create a healing environment for this approach to unfold and be sustainable.

Protect Time in Your Schedule

Reserve time in your weekly work schedule for SOS appointments. Some practitioners may schedule these as they would a yearly physical; others may protect a half-day a week focused only on these sessions. Many integrative medicine consultative clinics work in this way. Each session should be scheduled for at least 40 minutes, and patients should be encouraged to arrive 15 minutes before their appointments to allow as much face-to-face time as possible with the clinician.

Create Space

Consider redecorating an existing examination room to give the feeling that you are in a special and comforting place. Incorporate soft colors and fabric, and limit sterile and cold medical equipment when possible. If you are unable to do this, simply introduce an element of nature, such as a flower, plant, or water fountain.

Create Patient Expectations

Let the patient know that these sessions are intended to allow time for exploring deeper issues that may help facilitate salutogenesis. A typical scenario for creating expectation may be something like the following:

> *"We have ruled out a physical cause for your headaches, and no evidence indicates a tumor. We do not have time scheduled today, but I would like you to come back on a Wednesday morning when I have set aside time for a session that will allow us more time to explore other aspects of life that can have a significant impact on your physical health and symptoms. I want to understand more clearly what may be going on in your life that may be influencing the amount of pain, fatigue, and sleep problems you have been experiencing. Often, in these sessions, we find common underlying causes that may help us get at the root of many of your symptoms."*

Offer Support

Relationship-centered care is based on trust and support. An SOS can result in the emergence of past traumas or events that must be supported and processed further. Often, we may need to collaborate with a psychologist to help understand how we can help patients heal from these events. We should not create an environment in which this information comes out and then not offer support and guidance on how to process it. This represents abandonment and can turn an SOS into a pathogenesis-oriented session. Interprofessional collaborative care allows healing to occur within a team that can support it.

Code Appropriately

We need to make sure that our time is appropriately coded so these sessions can be incorporated into clinical care as an important factor. The hope is that the medical system will eventually recognize the cost-saving potential of an SOS. As we explore the root of how the body self-heals, we may need fewer costly interventions. As the cost of disease-focused care escalates, this approach will gain more acceptance.

You need 45 minutes of face-to-face time to bill a "99204" (new patient) or 40 minutes for a "99215" (established patient). Be sure to document the amount of time spent and include that "greater than 50% of time was spent counseling and/or coordinating care." This needs to be included if you are billing based on time spent with the patient. If you document only total time and not the percentage of time spent counseling and coordinating care, then you must document the required components of the history, examination, and medical decision making per usual.

For integrative medicine consultations, the code is "99244" for a 60-minute and "99245" for an 80-minute consult appointment. Be sure to document the practitioner who referred the patient for consultation.

CONCLUSION

Pausing to be present before proceeding with an action plan for health is a simple task that, if practiced, can help two people efficiently find a healing path within a dynamic and complex setting. Ideally, the visit itself is therapeutic, even before something is prescribed. Communication between clinician and patient gives the patient perspective and support that encourages both parties to pause, learn from symptoms, and proceed toward a better place together.

> *The meeting of two personalities is like the contact of two chemical substances; if there is any reaction, both are transformed.*
>
> CARL JUNG

THERAPEUTIC REVIEW

- Self-reflect to learn of your own implicit biases so these unconscious beliefs become conscious and do not interfere with your goal of facilitating health in another.
- Pause before crossing the threshold of the clinic room to clear your own clutter so the clinical stool becomes your meditation cushion where you focus on one thing well, the person in front of you.
- Practice compassion, realizing that in serving others you serve yourself.
- Be fully present and mindfully aware, creating insight into the individual's authentic needs.
- Proceed towards action that you both agree will bring focus to a healing path.

Key Web Resources

University of Wisconsin Integrative Medicine Program. This website includes instructions, exercises, videos, and audio files to help the clinician bring mindfulness into the clinical encounter. It complements this chapter.	http://www.fammed.wisc.edu/mindfulness
Foundation for Active Compassion. Offers guidance on practicing compassion to foster healing for others and ourselves.	http://foundationforactivecompassion.org/
The University of Rochester Mindful Practice Training Program. Offers training for clinicians in mindfulness to increase self-awareness and resiliency towards improved patient care and outcomes.	https://www.urmc.rochester.edu/family-medicine/mindful-practice.aspx

REFERENCES

References are available online at ExpertConsult.com.

CHAPTER 4

THE WHOLE HEALTH PROCESS

David Rakel, MD • J. Adam Rindfleisch, MPhil, MD • Tracy Gaudet, MD

We can't solve problems by using the same kind of thinking we used when we created them.
ALBERT EINSTEIN

VALUE OVER VOLUME

As health care spending in the US surpasses three trillion dollars a year, there is a push to shift the focus of health care delivery away from volume and toward increased value by improving quality at less cost. This "Value over Volume" approach is quickly changing reimbursement models and encouraging health care systems to create new models of care.[1]

This evolution honors the advances achieved using the biomedical model while at the same time enhancing it with a much needed transition away from a reactive, disease-centric approach toward one that prioritizes improving health outcomes. New approaches place greater importance on patient engagement, highlight health promotion, and place care within the context of each individual.

One of the most important ways to enhance value is to strategically tailor health care resources according to the context of each person's life. Ongoing, relationship-centered care allows the clinician to understand what sort of person has a disease (to paraphrase Osler) instead of simply focusing on what disease the person has. This context helps explain why there is a predicted 15-fold return on investment when health systems have a strong primary care foundation.[2]

PATIENT-DEFINED GOALS

To improve health outcomes, goals that drive clinical care must arise from the individual or community that is served. This structure requires that we work beyond the traditional biomedical model that has been directed by physician-dominated dialogue.

Research on contextual errors has shown that even when clinicians are told by a patient that "I can't afford my asthma medication," 50% of physicians will prescribe it anyway.[3,4] Often the clinician will "do the right thing" according to the evidence protocol for a condition that is concrete instead of working the evidence into the context of someone's real life, which is more complex than general guidelines can accommodate (Table 4.1).

A better balance is needed to combine the scientific, biomedical model by artfully adapting it to be as relevant and useful as possible to the person being treated.[5] Doing so will ensure patient adherence to a plan of care that emphasizes what is needed most to change behavior over time. Ideally, this approach recruits the self-healing mechanisms possessed by all living beings. When the self-healing potential is tapped, there will be less need for costly and potentially harmful interventions, be they pharmaceuticals, surgery, or acupuncture needles. How is this value most efficiently obtained? We start by asking each patient to explore what matters to them most and then to define his or her own health goals.

Organizing resources around patients' self-defined health goals is the most efficient way to motivate sustainable behavior change. These goals are those most relevant within the context of people's lives, so they are much more likely to foster patient engagement and adherence to the plan of care. This approach shifts our focus from asking, "what's the matter with you" to "what matters to you."

INNOVATIVE HEALTH SYSTEMS

After more than 50 years of treatment by the Indian Health Services, more than 60,000 Alaska Native and American Indians living in Southcentral Alaska became the owners of their own health care system, the Southcentral Alaska Foundation. Known as the Nuka System of Care,[6] the system focuses on establishing long-term, trusting, accountable relationships built upon a shared-decision model where the patient's health goals are primary.[7,8] After implementation in 1999, urgent care and emergency department use decreased by 40%, specialist use decreased by 50%, and hospitalization days decreased by 30%.[9] Blood sugar and blood pressure control improved,[10] and customer satisfaction data showed that 91% of customer-owners rated their care as "favorable."[7] In this model, patients and their families are the principal drivers of health, which has reduced dependence on the health system (Fig. 4.1).

The Nuka strategy resulted in significant improvements in the health of a population that was at high risk for disease. A similar high-risk population is American Veterans. A conventional biomedical model that places the patient in a passive role as they receive treatments for symptoms and disease states does not serve Veterans (or other Americans) well. Such a model risks the potential harm of polypharmacy while not recruiting the person's active participation in their health.[11] In 2012, The Office of Patient-Centered Care and Cultural Transformation (OPCCCT) was created to bring needed change to

TABLE 4.1	**Patient-Defined Goals**
Volume (Biomedical Model)	**Value (Health Outcomes Model)**
Concrete	Context
Reductionistic	Holistic
Data and science	Poetry and the arts
More things	Less things
Projection of science's "truth"	Internal motivation for change
Requires compliance	Self-sustaining

TABLE 4.2	**Models of Care**
Traditional Medical Assessment	**Whole Health Process**
Chief complaint	Engage patient's meaning
History of present illness	Personalized health assessment
Family and social history	Patient-defined goals
Physical exam	Professional expertise and alignment
Diagnostic tests and imaging	Interdisciplinary team support
Assessment with appropriate coding	Personalized health plan
Therapeutic plan	Tracking outcomes and goal achievement

Both these models are valuable, but the Whole Health Process will add more value.

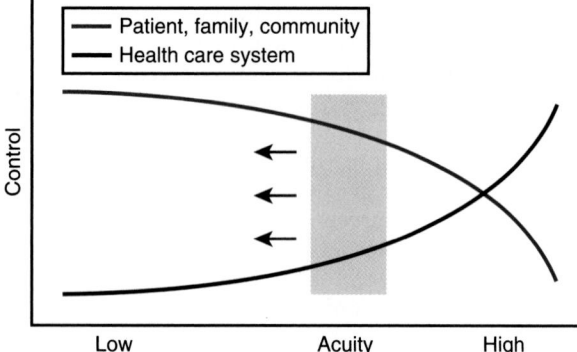

FIG. 4.1 ■ The Alaska Native Health Care model moved the column to the left, reducing dependence on high-cost medical interventions by increasing the control of the patient, their family, and community. This change resulted in better health and fewer acute health care needs. (From Rakel DP, Jonas WB: The patient-centered medical home. In Rakel RE, Rakel DP, editors: *Textbook of family medicine,* ed 9, Philadelphia, 2016, Elsevier, pp 17-24.)[24]

the largest health care system in the US, The Veterans Health Administration (VHA). Directed by one of the coauthors, Tracy Gaudet, the OPCCCT is leading the charge towards a shift in health care delivery. The VHA has declared that its primary strategic priority is "to provide personalized, proactive, patient-driven health care to Veterans, and engages and inspires Veterans to their highest possible level of health and well-being."[12] This model moves beyond the traditional health assessment, as is highlighted in Table 4.2.

THE CIRCLE OF HEALTH

The diagram "Components of Proactive Health and Well-Being," known more informally as the "Circle of Health," is featured in Fig. 4.2. This elegant framework focuses attention on "Me," the individual, who is placed at the center. Moving outward from the center, "mindful awareness"—paying attention to one's thoughts and patterns—is the next circle. Next is the light blue circle, which encompasses eight smaller circles, the "Circles of Proactive Self-Care." Here, after we see that the central focus is on the individual and on what a person can do for self-care, does the diagram then draw in the navy blue "Professional Care" circle, which incorporates prevention, conventional

therapy, and complementary approaches—all the aspects of care that involve other people besides oneself. The outermost circle, "Community," encompasses the entire circle, emphasizing that while self-care is fundamental, no one has to seek health alone. The person at the center of the circle is the captain of a team of people who all value that person's well-being at many different levels.

Personalized, Proactive, Patient-Driven Care

A personalized process recognizes that every human being has a unique story that puts any therapy into the context of their lives. For example, 20 people with hypertension may have 20 different therapeutic plans to lower blood pressure. One person may need to change diet, while another may need to address stress. A personalized health plan is more likely to promote long-term health, as each individual's main health needs are explored.

A proactive approach encourages recognition of health risks and seeks to proactively minimize them. It supports each human being's powerful, innate self-healing process, attempting to mobilize it rather than just suppress symptoms.

Patient-driven care requires that the locus of control be given to each individual. Clinicians assist patients with recruiting the most appropriate professionals needed for their individual success. All healing is self-healing, and the Whole Health process empowers people to find their particular paths to self healing. They are placed in charge of their own health destiny.

THREE QUESTIONS

The Whole Health process can be challenging to incorporate, as it suggests a shift in focus that is unfamiliar to both clinicians and patients. Several key questions can be asked to initiate the Whole Health encounter, but the first question below is perhaps the most important and

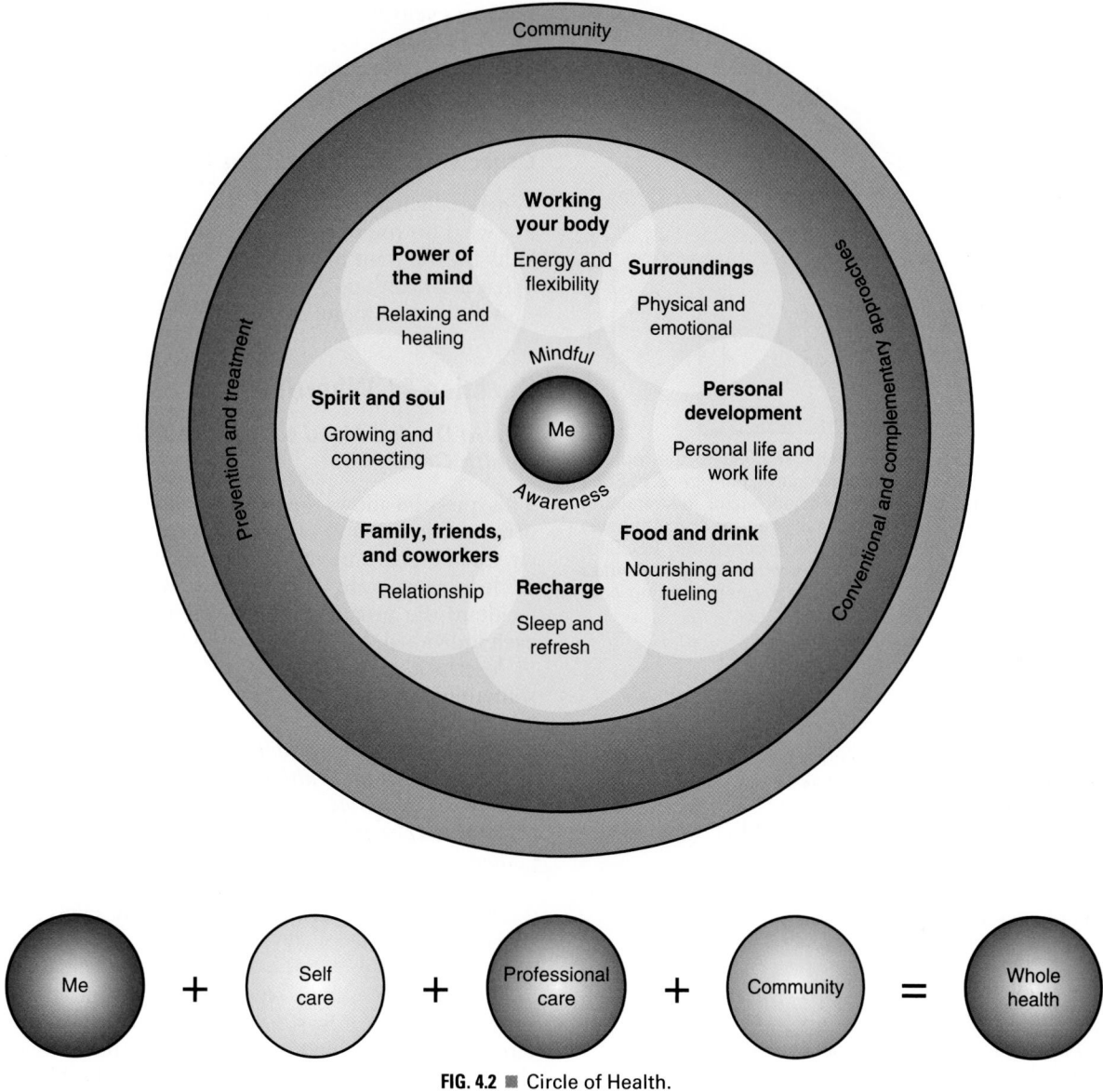

FIG. 4.2 ■ Circle of Health.

the most challenging. If framed correctly, it can connect people to their personal meaning, getting to the heart of a personalized, proactive, and patient-driven approach. The first question is at the center of the Fig. 4.2, the mindful awareness of ME.

Question #1, What?

What Gives Your Life Meaning?

This question can be asked in a number of different ways, but the goal of the question is to connect the individual to what is most important. Without this connection, even a health goal that is defined by the individual will most likely be unsustainable. This deeper exploration helps to discover the underlying motivational driver that can allow for sustainable healthy behaviors.[13,14] For example, a smoker whose clinician informs them of the evidence linking smoking to increased risk of cancer, heart disease,

and death is much less likely to change their behavior than the person who wants to stop smoking because the daughter they love recently developed asthma. The hemoglobin (Hgb) A1c test may just be an abstract idea, while the fear of losing one's eyesight or requiring dialysis may be much more real. Eliciting emotional reasons for change is much more effective than recruiting cognitive reasoning.

Experience in asking this question has provided valuable lessons. Many people initially may not understand the question or may say, "I don't know, you're the doctor, you tell me." Providing context before asking the question can help with comprehension. Consider the following script:

In our clinic we are shifting focus from what is wrong with you to a process that helps us understand what you want your health for. This way we can use the resources of the health system to help you live your fullest life. Achieving

What matters to you?

vs.

Diabetes mgmt.

FIG. 4.3 ■ Aligning our work with what matters to the individual empowers them to be a proactive participant in care. Such patient involvement is the most important factor in sustaining healthy outcomes. Treating one disease at a time (e.g., diabetes management) is disconnected from the larger whole. T.S. Eliot describes the bottom graphic well in his introduction to *Dante's Inferno*: "The definition of hell is a place where nothing connects with nothing."

health is much more about what you do than what you take. I want to know what matters most to you, because this will help us both know where to invest our time and energy to help you get where you want to go.

If the response is, *"I want to be healthy,"* explore further, as in the following sample dialog:

"If you were healthy, what would your life look like?"
"I would be able to travel and spend time with my wife and kids."
"What will you need to be able to travel and connect to your wife and kids?"
"I need to get this arthritis pain under better control."
"That's a great health goal! I am going to put down in your chart that your health goal is that you want to travel and spend time with your wife and kids."

The process of asking this question is as important as the answer. The focus of the office visit changes from a superficial conversation to a place of deeper meaning that is rewarding and energizing for both the clinician and the patient. Such interaction enhances the therapeutic relationship while directing care towards value because the action that follows the question will have significant downstream health effects. This first question invites the patient to begin exploring what is most meaningful to them and is a powerful first domino that drives positive health outcomes (Fig. 4.3). Surprisingly, the data show that such interaction does not require more time and, more importantly, changes the type of conversation we are having with our patients.[4] It is important to recognize that this question is deep, and to truly explore it will take time and iterations. Typically, people begin to reflect on such matters when they are in health crisis, facing cancer or recovering from a heart attack. To explore this issue before

such an event is a great opportunity but also a significant shift. This exploration can be further supported by self-reflection tools or group approaches outside of the clinical encounter.

Other Versions of Question 1 Include

What really matters to you?
For what do you want your health?
Why do you want to be healthy or improve your health?
What is a health goal that will help you connect to what is most meaningful in your life?

Question #2, Where?

Where Do You Need to Start to Achieve Your Health Goal?

This question allows the patient to self-reflect and to prioritize which area of self-care depicted by the light blue circles in Fig. 4.2 are of highest priority. Each of the eight circles incorporate the foundational ingredients that facilitate the proactive, self-healing mechanisms within each individual.

A script that one may use to ask question #2 could go something like this:

These eight circles include key ingredients that are important in the health of any human being. What they all have in common is that they are linked to self-care. That is, they are things that you can work on yourself, though we will be sure to talk about who can support you with them along the way. Point to one or two areas that you feel you need to work on most to achieve your health goal.

Ideally, the savvy information technology (IT) team of the health system would populate each of the circles with available community resources relevant to the patient's health goal. For example, the "Food and Drink" circle would include resources on how to access a nutrition consultant, healthy cooking classes, or mindful eating classes.

To continue the previous scenario:

The patient whose health goal is to travel and spend time with his wife and kids points to "Working Your Body" and "Personal Development" as the two areas that he feels need the most attention. He wants to move his body more since he feels his arthritis is leading to a sedentary lifestyle. He also wants to make sure he can afford the travel that he is looking forward to with his loved ones, so he wants to add money to his retirement plan at work. For that reason, he wants to get a promotion.

Question #3, Who?

Who Do You Need to Support You in Achieving Your Health Goal?

This question recruits the most appropriate professionals, family members, friends, or community resources needed to support achievement of the health goal. The Whole Health process identifies the interdisciplinary team that will offer support and guidance with the next steps of the process. This team is linked to the outer two rings in the Circle of Health (see Fig. 4.2). The Whole Health approach stresses the importance of creating a team that will help the individual succeed in achieving his or her goals.

A script for question #3 could go something like this:

Now we need to recruit services or individuals to help you achieve your health goal. Who do you feel will be most important in helping you be successful?

To use the military metaphor, we ask the Veteran **what** is their mission for health, **where** do they need the most support, and **who** do we need to recruit to ensure a successful outcome?

In the case of the man whose health goal is to travel and spend time with his wife and kids, we recruit an acupuncturist to help improve the pain and function of his knees. We refer him to physical therapy to increase his strength and improve his mobility. Finally, we recommend that he connect to human resources at work to improve his chances of getting a better-paying job that was posted recently. This Whole Health process is directed and organized by his primary health care team in the patient-centered medical home, but he, the patient, has been consistently directing the process.

Case Scenario: Mt. Kilimanjaro

A 48-year-old female veteran named Betty visited her physician every 3 to 4 months to monitor her type II diabetes. She would often feel frustrated because she never felt good enough. She would hear that she needed to lose more weight and improve her nutrition to get her Hgb A1C and low-density lipoprotein (LDL) cholesterol under better control. She soon became frustrated with how many medicines she was asked to take.

After a period of self-reflection, she realized that she wanted the resources of the VA medical system to help her achieve what she wanted to work towards. She had a personal goal of climbing to the top of Mt. Kilimanjaro by her 50th birthday. So the next time she visited her doctor, she told him of this goal. He was resistant initially, but was eventually swayed to refocus attention not just on her Hgb A1C levels but towards helping her achieve her health goal, that which connected her to meaning.

Betty's health care team now consisted of the professionals she needed to help her achieve her goal, including a nutritionist, physical therapist, and a health psychologist; her primary care physician organized her care. In her 50th year, she made it to the top of Mt. Kilimanjaro. Betty was happy to have reached her health goal, and Betty's team shared in the joy of her success. Everyone was energized, as the focus of work was on connecting to meaning, not only for the patient but for that of the whole medical team. Not surprisingly, Betty's Hgb A1C and LDL cholesterol improved as a side effect.

DEVELOPING THE PERSONAL HEALTH PLAN

Whole Health has been introduced to dozens of VA facilities since 2013. Different facilities have experimented with innovative approaches to making care more personalized, proactive, and patient driven. One of the questions that frequently comes up is, "But how do I apply this model to the real world of practice? I have time constraints, I have to be sure I always ask about things like tobacco use and safety at home. How can I possibly fit more in?" Many clinicians find it helpful to keep a few key pointers in mind as they begin to do Personal Health Planning under the Whole Health model.

No clinician writes the health plan alone. We have been indoctrinated with the idea that care happens in a one-to-one interaction, with the clinician—often a physician—taking responsibility for the plan. This approach can be effective on its own but is enhanced by a team approach. There are clinics in which the entire team collaborates on health planning, from the receptionist who provides the intake forms (the VA has created a "Personal Health Inventory," see the following Key Web Resources) to the nurse who reviews the inventory with them and the psychologist and social workers who are integrated into the team to help with various aspects of follow up and support. Health coaches can also be invaluable to the process.

Much of the foundation for the personalized health plan can be done outside of the clinic, allowing more time and support to reflect on one's life. The VA has created a 9-week Whole Health program in which facilitators are trained to lead the group and guide Veterans through the Circle of Health. Through this process, the Veteran creates the foundation of their overarching personal health plan, and interactions with their providers in the clinical setting can be much more streamlined.

Health plans take many forms. A health plan may be as simple as a one-item recommendation. "Bob, it sounds like you are up for switching over to sparkling water between now and our next visit, what do you think?" If this is all Bob is up for, it is best not to hit him with more than he can handle. Another person may be just the opposite. Some people love to have multiple items on a to-do-list to follow. Remember, though, that they should be coauthors of that list!

Health plans are built on continuity and follow up. No one expects you to cover every issue during a single visit. Everyone who interacts with the person can help with the plan, tweaking it as appropriate. Focusing on question one helps to clear the clutter of the crowded problem list, allowing the team to focus on what matters most. A useful question may be, *if we focused on one thing that would help all your other problems get better as a side effect, what would that one thing be?*

Believe it or not, this approach saves time. People who adopt it find that not only does their work feel much more gratifying, but they are also more efficient. Time and energy are saved by asking someone what they think is going to help them the most. The question "What are you willing to do today to make your health better?" can write the health plan itself.

You, as the clinician, also have a place at the center. One of the most powerful ways to understand this process is to apply it to your own life. Clinician self-care matters. You may find that you learn a great deal by applying this entire process to your own individualized care needs. For what do *you* want your health? And you might just find that this process gives you a kick-start that reconnects you to meaning in your work.

FOUR-STEP PROCESS FOR HEALTH PLANNING

Largely due to the efforts of the VA facilities in the Boston area, a pragmatic process for health planning has been developed.[15] This process involves four steps, which may not all happen at once:

1. Assessment. Gathering information—and doing it in a different way—is critical. Yes, if the patient is being seen for a specific concern, you should have that in mind. Rarely, someone will not want you to use this approach; fair enough—respecting their choice is a way to personalize care. However, if they are willing, asking the three questions listed above can be an excellent way of doing an assessment.

2. Shared goal setting. In health professions training, we learn about how to interview people. One of the issues that arises during such training is agenda setting. Remember, *you do not give up your own priorities for the visit.* Rather, you weave them into the overall process. For our example patient previously, the clinician may have the goal of bringing down the patient's heart disease risk. The items noted in the health plan, such as a potential reduction in financial stress by attaining a better-paying job, are useful for this process.

3. Health planning. Health planning is the step in which the clinician and patient work together to talk about what they will do. Patients often have great ideas already—just ask. Clinicians should bring up their own ideas as well. Remember, for a plan to be successful, you have to have their buy-in. Now is the time for you to decide whether you do have their buy-in and how to increase it.

4. Skill-building and support. Health planning does not end when the patient leaves the room. It is incumbent upon the health care team to provide guidance to the person seeking care. What skills do they need to have? Does someone teach them a mind–body approach? Do they need help signing up to do volunteer work? Is there a meditation practice you would like them to try? Providing the information and connections they need is important. As is the case with any clinical visit, you also need be very clear in stating what steps will follow. When will they see you again? When will they

follow up with other members of the team? The quest for health is lifelong, and you can show them possible routes that they can follow along the way.

THE VALUE OF THE WHOLE HEALTH PROCESS

The Whole Health process incorporates key ingredients that promote sustainable health outcomes, as shown in Figs. 4.2 and 4.3. Patients sit in the driver's seat and clarify, with support, which areas are most important to them. This process is not only empowering but also activates their innate capacity to heal, tapping into the wisdom within each of us.

The value of this approach has become increasingly clear through recent research. For example, many people choose "Power of the Mind" as an area of focus on the Circle of Health because of the high levels of perceived stress in their lives. Self-care in this area can result in significant cost savings. In a 2015 study, 4452 subjects were taught mind–body skills to reduce stress and build resiliency. After following this cohort for 4.2 years, those who completed the training had a 43% overall reduction in the use of health-related care than did the 13,149 controls. Clinical encounters decreased by 41.9%, lab encounters dropped by 43.5%, and procedures were decreased by 21.4%.[16] In another study investigating the incidence and cost of treatment for upper respiratory illness, those who were taught mindfulness had a 70% lower cost ($65 per meditator vs $214 per control) than did untreated controls.[17]

The Diabetes Prevention Trial confirmed the value of healthy lifestyle choices, noting they were not only more effective clinically in reducing the incidence of progression to diabetes when compared to metformin[18] but were also more cost effective.[19] Avoiding smoking, moving the body, improving nutrition, maintaining a healthy body weight, and limiting excessive alcohol use dramatically improved the cost effectiveness. Practicing these lifestyle behaviors was shown to decrease the incidence of coronary events by 83% in 84,129 women followed in the Nurse's Health Study[20,21] and by 79% in 20,721 Swedish men followed for 11 years.[22] These key determinants of health were also associated with living 14 years longer in 20,244 people followed in the EPIC–Norfolk Study.[23] The Whole Health approach allows us to link meaning to action so that those we serve are more likely to incorporate these powerful behaviors into their own lives.

What one does is much more effective than what one takes. Value is added when we are able to encourage and support personalized, proactive, patient-driven care. The Whole Health approach is a powerful and innovative way to achieve value by valuing what matters to the people who seek our care.

Key Web Resources

The Veterans Administration Office of Patient-Centered Care and Cultural Transformation http://www.va.gov/PATIENTCENTEREDCARE/about.asp	Provides information on incorporating this Whole Health Concept within the VA Medical System Includes resources and strategies on a personalized, proactive, patient-centered approach
The Veterans Administration www.va.gov/patientcenteredcare/multimedia-and-resources.asp	Videos from the VA's patient-centered care that explores the Whole Health process
Whole Health Video http://bcove.me/7si4hxcv	A VA-sponsored video that conveys the vision of the Whole Health Process of Care
Personal Health Planning Video http://bcove.me/35dbfmed	A VA-sponsored video that summarizes the process of Personal Health Planning

REFERENCES

References are available online at ExpertConsult.com.

PART **II**

INTEGRATIVE APPROACH TO DISEASE

PART OUTLINE

SECTION I AFFECTIVE DISORDERS

SECTION II NEUROLOGY

SECTION III INFECTIOUS DISEASE

SECTION IV CARDIOVASCULAR DISEASE

SECTION V ALLERGY/INTOLERANCE

SECTION VI METABOLIC/ENDOCRINE DISORDERS

SECTION VII NEPHROLOGY

SECTION VIII GASTROINTESTINAL DISORDERS

SECTION IX AUTOIMMUNE DISORDERS

SECTION X OBSTETRICS/GYNECOLOGY

SECTION XI UROLOGY

SECTION XII MUSCULOSKELETAL

SECTION XIII DERMATOLOGY

SECTION XIV CANCER

SECTION XV SUBSTANCE ABUSE

SECTION XVI OPHTHALMOLOGY

SECTION I

AFFECTIVE DISORDERS

SECTION OUTLINE

5 DEPRESSION

6 ANXIETY

7 ATTENTION DEFICIT DISORDER

8 AUTISM SPECTRUM DISORDER

9 INSOMNIA

10 POSTTRAUMATIC STRESS DISORDER (PTSD)

CHAPTER 5

DEPRESSION

Craig Schneider, MD • Theodore Wissink, MD

Centers for Disease Control and Prevention surveys indicate that nearly 1 in 10 residents of the United States who is 18 years old or older has a depressive disorder.[1] Annual prevalence rates in patients with chronic disease are about 25%.[2] In fact, depression is one of the chronic conditions for which alternative therapies are most frequently used.[3] This statistic is not surprising considering that pharmaceutical antidepressant medications are not as effective as once believed for many patients with less severe forms of depression.[4] Many people seen in primary care settings fall under the DSM-5 category "persistent depressive disorder." The Patient Health Questionnaire-2 (PHQ-2) can be used for screening,[5] and the longer Patient Health Questionnaire (PHQ-9) (see Key Web Resources, later) can be used both for diagnosis and tracking of depression treatment outcomes in the primary care setting.[6] Clinicians should discuss the spectrum of treatment options including antidepressant medications and/or psychotherapy and integrative medicine treatments.[7]

PATHOPHYSIOLOGY

The pathophysiology of depression is not fully understood. The stress–diathesis model of illness emphasizes that significant emotional, social, and environmental antecedents such as the loss of a family member or a romantic or professional disappointment, as well as genetic and acquired vulnerabilities, are clearly involved. Significant stressors appear to be more frequently involved with initial episodes. In recurrent depression, vulnerability appears to increase as episodes become less and less related to stress and more autonomous in a process known as kindling.[8,9] With repeated episodes of illness (kindling), central nervous system dysfunction increases, as manifested by hypercortisolemia, decreased slow-wave (restful) sleep, and increased rapid eye movement (arousing) sleep and disruption of neuroplasticity.[10] Inflammation is now considered another important mediator. High levels of inflammatory biomarkers are found in depressed patients and improve as symptoms resolve.[11] The biochemical impact of depression may be stored in neurons through changes in the activity of gene transcription factors and neuronal growth factors.[12] A common final pathway is the biochemical imbalance of biogenic amines or neurotransmitters (e.g., serotonin, norepinephrine, gamma-aminobutyric acid [GABA], and dopamine) and their relationships with their respective receptors in the brain. Potential effects on neurotransmitters include impaired synthesis, increased breakdown, and increased pump uptake, with consequent alterations in neurotransmitter levels. This increasingly sophisticated understanding of the underpinnings of depression may one day lead to improved treatment, but for now pharmaceutical approaches to treating depression involve correction of altered neurotransmitter levels and of neurotransmitter receptor interactions.

INTEGRATIVE THERAPY

Exercise as Medicine

More than 1000 trials have examined the relationship between exercise and depression, and most have demonstrated an inverse relationship between them.[13,14] Physical activity may also prevent the initial onset of depression.[15,16]

Regularly performed exercise is as effective an antidepressant as psychotherapy or pharmaceutical approaches.[13,17–21] Well-designed studies also support that exercise combined with pharmacologic treatment is superior to either alone, but exercise appears to be superior in maintaining therapeutic benefit and preventing recurrence of depression.[22–26] Evidence provides some support for the use of exercise. A recent Cochrane review (updated from 2009) included 32 studies (n=1858) involving exercise for the treatment of researcher-defined depression. From these studies, 28 randomized controlled trials (RCTs) (n=1101) were included in a meta-analysis revealing a moderate to large effect in favor of exercise over standard treatment or control. However, only four trials (n=326) with adequate allocation concealment, blinding, and ITT analysis were found, resulting in a more modest effect size in favor of exercise. Pooled data from seven trials (n=373) with long-term follow-up data also found a small clinical effect in favor of exercise.[28] The additional benefits that may be attained by patients who exercise, including increased self-esteem, increased level of fitness, and reduced risk of relapse, make exercise an ideal intervention for patients suffering from depression.

Both aerobic and anaerobic activities are effective.[19,23,33,34] Regardless of the type of exercise, the total energy expenditure appears more important than the number of times a week a person exercises, and high-energy exercises are superior to low-energy exercises.

Exercise to Prevent Pregnancy-Related Depression

According to recommendations from both the American College of Obstetricians and Gynecologists and the Royal College of Obstetricians and Gynaecologists, pregnant women without medical contraindications should engage in regular aerobic and strength-conditioning exercise during the perinatal period.[29] A study of prenatal aerobic exercise in women without depression has shown that exercise or physical activity was associated with fewer depressive symptoms in pregnancy.[30] Few controlled studies have evaluated the effectiveness of exercise as a treatment for postpartum depression. Two RCTs comparing a 12-week intervention of exercise to a control situation in postnatal depression symptoms demonstrated a significantly greater reduction in these symptoms with exercise as compared to controls.[31,32] Based on this small number of studies, we recommend the following for the general health of perinatal patients: 30 minutes of exercise per day, most days of the week, in the absence of either medical or obstetric complications and after consultation with a physician.

Exactly why exercise relieves or prevents depression is not understood. Although exercise may increase levels of serotonin, norepinephrine, and endorphins, its benefits have been reported even when naloxone is administered to block endorphins. Exercise may also increase nerve cell growth in the area of brain that modulates mood, similar to pharmaceuticals.[35,36]

Exercise is inexpensive, has proven benefits beyond the treatment of depression, has a low occurrence of side effects, and is available to everyone. The appropriate exercise prescription depends on the specific patient's health, motivation, level of fitness, and interests (see Chapter 91, Writing an Exercise Prescription). For more seriously depressed patients and those with significant psychomotor retardation, the exercise regimen should be started as adjunct therapy.

> Write an exercise prescription for all patients; tailor the type of exercise to something the patient enjoys, whether aerobic or anaerobic.

NUTRITION
Caffeine and Simple Sugars

Cross-national epidemiologic studies suggest a correlation between sugar intake and rates of major depressive disorders.[37] Examination of the diets of people suffering from depression reveals increased consumption of sucrose compared with the general population.[38] A small cohort trial found that eliminating refined sucrose and caffeine from the diets of people experiencing unexplained depression resulted in improvements by 1 week, and symptoms worsened when patients were challenged with these substances but not with placebo.[39] However, protective effects in women of drinking 2 to 5 cups of coffee daily have been demonstrated,[40] and an inverse relationship appears to exist between daily tea drinking and depression.[41] At this point, no clear cause and effect has been demonstrated.

Dietary Patterns

Prospective data suggest a protective effect of a whole foods traditional diet (vegetables, fruit, beef, lamb, fish, and whole grains) or Mediterranean-style diet (omega-3 fatty acids [from fish], monounsaturated fatty acids [from olive oil], and natural folate and other B vitamins [from legumes, fruit and nuts, and vegetables]) versus a Western-style diet (high levels of energy, saturated fats, and refined sugar, as well as fried and highly processed foods)[42] across a number of populations (British, Australian, Spanish, Korean) after adjusting for potential confounders.[43–46] At this point, no

large, high-quality clinical trials have been published supporting the use of diet for treating depression (although one is underway),[47] but the evolving understanding of the underpinnings of depression, including inflammation, suggest a rationale for dietary manipulation in treatment.

Alcohol

A systematic review confirmed that alcohol-related problems are more common in depressed individuals than in the general population and are associated with worse outcomes.[48] Although consumption of alcohol transiently increases the turnover of serotonin, the long-term result is diminished levels of serotonin and catecholamines.[49] Elimination of alcohol intake appeared to reduce depressive symptoms in a number of studies.[42] Because of the safety, potential health benefits in other areas, and low cost of this intervention, limiting alcohol consumption is warranted.

> Recommend that patients adhere to a traditional or Mediterranean dietary pattern and limit sugar and alcohol consumption.

Omega-3 Fatty Acids

Epidemiologic data suggest that a deficiency of omega-3 fatty acids or an imbalance in the ratio of omega-6 and omega-3 fatty acids correlates positively with increased rates of depression.[50] Because dietary polyunsaturated fatty acids and cholesterol are the major determinants of membrane fluidity in synaptic membranes involved in the synthesis, binding, and uptake of neurotransmitters, it is hypothesized that alterations may lead to abnormalities contributing to increased rates of depression.[51] Although the current evidence does not support using omega-3 fatty acids as monotherapy to treat depression,[52] small, well-designed studies support the use of omega-3 fatty acids as adjuncts to conventional antidepressant therapy.[53,54] Preliminary evidence also suggests that children with depression and women with depression during pregnancy may benefit from supplementation with omega-3 fatty acids.[55,56]

A recent meta-analysis suggests omega-3 supplements containing 60% or more eicosapentaenoic acid (EPA), with a ceiling of 2000 mg of EPA in excess of docosahexaenoic acid (DHA), appears to be most effective.[57] Consumption of two or three servings each week of smaller cold-water fish (herring, mackerel, wild salmon, sardine) may be comparable. One caveat to consider is the issue of heavy metal and pesticide contamination of available seafood and supplemental fatty acids. Larger fish and some farmed fish may bioconcentrate toxins, including mercury and polychlorinated biphenyls. Vegetarian alternatives to consider include flaxseed oil or ground flaxseed meal (2 tablespoons daily) and a small handful of walnuts each day, but these substances have not been studied with respect to depression (see Chapter 88, The Antiinflammatory Diet).

> The role of docosahexaenoic acid is generally more structural (important for brain and retina development), while that of eicosapentaenoic acid is generally more functional (improves communication across cell membranes).

DIETARY SUPPLEMENTS
Vitamin D

Epidemiological evidence shows that Vitamin D deficiency is associated with an 8% to 14% increase in depression.[58–60] However, causality and efficacy of supplementation remain controversial awaiting confirmation by systematic review and meta-analysis. These reviews have produced conflicting results but include studies with many different designs and flaws (e.g., ineffective interventions that failed to increase or actually decreased 25OHD [25-hydroxy vitamin D] levels or failed to measure a baseline 25OHD level). A recent meta-analysis that included only studies without such flaws found a statically significant effect of vitamin D supplementation on depression scores, comparable to the magnitude of the effect of typical antidepressant medications.[61] These results are promising, but clearly, more studies are needed to make a more definitive statement on the effectiveness of Vitamin D supplementation on depression.

B Vitamins

Folic acid and vitamin B_{12} are intimately linked with the synthesis of S-adenosylmethionine (SAMe), and each functions as a methyl donor, carrying and donating methyl groups to a variety of brain chemicals, including neurotransmitters. Although large-scale clinical studies are lacking, a trial of a B-complex vitamin is advisable, particularly for older patients, in whom B_{12} deficiency is common, and for persons with suboptimal diets. Vitamin B_6 is essential in the manufacture of serotonin, and vitamin B_6 levels have been found to be low in many depressed patients, particularly in premenopausal women taking oral contraceptive pills or replacement estrogen.[25,50,62]

DOSAGE

One B-complex vitamin daily. A B-50 has approximately 50 mcg or mg of most of the B vitamins, and a B-100 has about 100 mcg or mg. Both are safe. The one B-vitamin that can be neurotoxic at doses > 200 mg daily is B6 (pyridoxine).

Folic Acid

Up to one-third of depressed adults have borderline or low folate levels. A subgroup of depressed patients with folate deficiency and impaired methylation and monoamine neurotransmitter metabolism has been identified.[63] In fact, depression is the most common symptom of folate deficiency.[64] Patients with low levels of folate also appear to respond more poorly to therapy with selective serotonin reuptake inhibitors (SSRIs).[67] Limited evidence from a Cochrane Review suggests that the addition of folate to conventional antidepressant therapy is beneficial.[65] More recent trials have used L-methylfolate, the active and more bioavailable form of folic acid.[66]

Folate may also have other health benefits (e.g., prevention of neural tube defects and reduction of elevated homocysteine). Supplementation with vitamin B_{12} concomitantly makes sense to avoid masking a deficiency (see Chapter 38, MTHFR Mutation).

DOSAGE

400 mcg to 1 mg daily (although doses of 5 to 20 mg daily have been used in studies). Consider L-methylfolate 7.5 to 15 mg, which may be better tolerated.

PRECAUTIONS

High doses of folic acid have been reported to cause altered sleep patterns, vivid dreaming, irritability, exacerbation of seizure frequency, gastrointestinal disturbances, and a bitter taste in the mouth, and concerns have emerged about possible increased risk of some cancers.

S-Adenosylmethionine

SAMe (Fig. 5.1) is the major methyl donor in the body and is involved in the metabolism of norepinephrine, dopamine, and serotonin. Its synthesis is impaired in depression, and supplementation results in increased brain monoamine levels, enhanced binding of neurotransmitters to receptors, and increased brain cell-membrane fluidity. Although larger trials are warranted, multiple open and RCTs suggest that SAMe is an effective natural antidepressant. An RCT comparing SAMe (1600 mg orally, daily) with imipramine (150 mg orally, daily) over 6 weeks demonstrated equivalent efficacy and superior tolerability of SAMe.[67] Another small, double-blind, placebo-controlled trial of SSRI nonresponders with major depression compared adjunctive SAMe (800 mg orally, twice daily) with placebo and found SAMe significantly more likely to lead to remission.[68] A more recent RCT from 2014 compared SAMe, escitalopram, and placebo and showed similar significant improvement in depression for all three treatments after 12 weeks.[69] An agency for Healthcare Research and Quality evidence report and technology assessment in 2002 found SAMe to be superior to placebo and comparable to conventional antidepressants, based on available evidence. SAMe is generally well-tolerated and has a more rapid onset of action than that of standard pharmaceutical antidepressants.[70] Because of this characteristic, some clinicians start SAMe

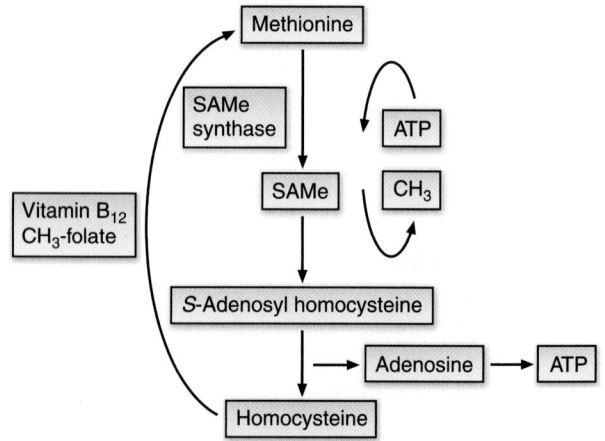

FIG. 5.1 ■ **S-Adenosylmethionine (SAMe) metabolism.** SAMe may cause hypomania or mania in patients with bipolar disease and should be avoided in this population. *ATP*, adenosine triphosphate; *CH₃*, methyl group.

concurrently with another dietary supplement or pharmaceutical approach to therapy of depression that has been more thoroughly studied and then taper the dose of SAMe to zero as the other antidepressant begins to take effect. The most stable and bioavailable oral form appears to be 1,4-butane-disulfonate (Actimet), which is stable for up to 2 years at room temperature. SAMe does not have known cardiac, anticholinergic, or orthostatic effects. Larger clinical trials comparing SAMe with placebo and standard of care will help elucidate its role in treating depression.

DOSAGE

Initial treatment of depression may require 1600 mg daily given in two equal doses. We recommend starting with 200 mg once or twice daily followed by slow titration up over 2 weeks to minimize gastrointestinal side effects.

PRECAUTIONS

High dosages can cause nausea, vomiting, flatulence, and diarrhea. Avoid giving the second dose close to bedtime because it can cause insomnia.

Hydroxytryptophan

Hydroxytryptophan (5-HTP) is the intermediate in the metabolism of tryptophan to serotonin. Open trials and RCTs have suggested that 5-HTP is as effective as standard antidepressants.[71,72] A Cochrane Review found only 2 of 108 trials of sufficient quality for inclusion, but in these trials, 5-HTP was superior to placebo.[73] Tryptophan itself appeared promising as a treatment for insomnia and depression but was removed from the market (although it is available again) when a contaminated batch was linked to an outbreak of eosinophilia myalgia syndrome in people with abnormal activation of the kynurenin pathway. Although 5-HTP is not metabolized along this pathway, case reports link 5-HTP to an illness resembling eosinophilia myalgia syndrome. The suspected culprit is a family of contaminants known as peak X that is commonly found in commercially available 5-HTP.[74] Because uncertainty surrounding 5-HTP remains, it seems advisable to avoid recommending its use pending further information. Case reports of seizures in Down syndrome and dermatomyositis in conjunction with the use of carbidopa have appeared in the literature. Use with other serotonin agonists is not recommended, to avoid serotonin syndrome.

DOSAGE

5-HTP 50-200 mg three times daily. We recommend starting with 50 mg and titrating up over a few weeks if needed.

BOTANICALS
St. John's Wort (Hypericum perforatum)

The exact mechanism of action of St. John's wort (SJW) remains unknown, but this botanical affects serotonin,

dopamine, norepinephrine, and GABA reuptake inhibition and also in vitro monoamine oxidase inhibition and L-glutamate.[67] SJW also appears to inhibit interleukin-6 and increase cortisol production, which may result in an additional indirect antidepressant effect.[75] Clinical effects are probably the result of a combined contribution of multiple mechanisms, each individually too weak to account for the action.[76] SJW has been a licensed prescription medication in Germany since 1984, and nearly twice the number of prescriptions are written for it as for all other antidepressants in that country. Two large US trials found that SJW was not effective for treating severe major depression.[77] The most recent Cochrane Reviews examined the findings of 29 trials (nearly 5500 patients) comparing SJW with placebo or standard antidepressants and concluded that available evidence suggests that SJW is superior to placebo and is as effective as conventional antidepressants and better tolerated.[78] Large-scale postmarketing surveillance studies of SJW extracts (14,245 patients) recorded rates of adverse effects 10-fold lower than for conventional antidepressants.[79]

Indication

SWJ is indicated for mild to moderate depression.

DOSAGE

300 mg three times daily has been used most frequently in clinical trials. 450 mg twice daily has also been used. Choose a product standardized to a minimum of 2% to 5% hyperforin or 0.3% hypericin such as those used in clinical trials. Examples include Lichtwer LI 160 found in Kira and WS5572, containing a minimum level of 3% hyperforin found in Perika (Schwabe, Nature's Way). Once clinical improvement has been obtained, consider twice-daily dosing. Up to 2 months may be required before full effects are noted.

PRECAUTIONS

Although side effects are fewer than with current pharmacologic antidepressants, they can include gastrointestinal upset, allergic reaction, fatigue, dry mouth, restlessness, constipation, sexual side effects, and possibly increased risk of cataracts.

St. John's wort can activate the cytochrome P-450 3A4 detoxification system in the liver, as well as p-glycoprotein, and thereby reduce the serum levels of drugs metabolized by this pathway. Caution should be used in patients receiving antiretroviral, warfarin, cyclosporine, and oral contraceptive therapy.

Saffron

In addition to its well-known culinary uses, saffron has long been used in traditional Persian medicine to treat mood disorders.

Small, controlled trials now suggest that a specific saffron extract can improve symptoms of depression as effectively as imipramine (100 mg daily) and fluoxetine (20 mg daily) in patients with mild to moderate depression after 6 weeks of treatment and is well-tolerated.[80,81]

DOSAGE

30 mg daily (Novin Zaferan Co., Iran)

Safety

Saffron has "Generally Recognized as Safe (GRAS)" status in the US

MIND–BODY THERAPY

Antidepressants and psychotherapy are first-line treatments for depression according to the American Psychiatric Association (APA); even so, only 60% of those treated will have a clinically significant response, and many others may have residual symptoms.[82] Many psychotherapies can be considered mind–body approaches. One-fourth of patients with depression have tried some type of mind–body therapy,[83,84] and two-thirds of those found it beneficial.[84]

Depression-specific psychotherapies are designed to provide acute, time-limited interventions. They are present-oriented and pragmatic, focusing on depression and issues considered relevant to both its onset and its perpetuation.[85] Primary care physicians can provide limited, supportive psychotherapy at frequent visits necessary to monitor the effectiveness of medications.[86] In fact, generic counseling appears to be preferred by patients over antidepressant drugs and is as effective, although slower in onset, for treating mild to moderate depressive illness.[87] Cognitive therapy in which the physician or therapist assists the patient in replacing negative patterns of thinking with a more positive and realistic approach is the most-studied psychotherapeutic approach to major depression. Multiple studies have demonstrated the equivalency of this modality to rigorous antidepressant medication regimens.[85]

Mind–body therapies encourage an active process through which the patient learns from their symptoms versus taking a medication or supplement during which the individual is a passive recipient.

There is an ever-growing diversity of psychotherapeutic approaches including "third wave cognitive behavioral therapies" (e.g., mindfulness-based cognitive therapy, compassionate mind training, acceptance and commitment therapy) and psychodynamic therapies, as well as integrative approaches that combine aspects of various models. However, evidence is lacking as to which psychotherapeutic approach is most effective.[87A]

Mindfulness-Based Cognitive Therapy

Based upon the work of Jon Kabat Zinn's "Mindfulness Based Stress Reduction," MBCT focuses on allowing distressing emotions, thoughts, and sensations to come and go, without grasping onto the need to suppress, fight, or escape them.[88] This specific method has been successful for treating depression in a variety of patient populations.[89] Several initial studies also demonstrate that MBCT can decrease the recurrence of depression.[90–92] MBCT appears to be particularly effective in patients who have had three or more relapses and may be equal to medication in preventing relapse in this difficult-to-treat population.

Other Mind–Body Therapies

Yoga

Yoga is rooted in Indian philosophy and has become a popular route in Western culture towards improving physical and mental well-being. Yoga is most often associated with physical postures, breath control, and meditation. Different yoga schools have emerged that put varying degrees of focus on the physical and meditation practices. A recent systematic review located 12 RCTs (pooled n = 619) studying the effect of yoga on the severity of depression. Moderate evidence indicated a beneficial short-term effect of yoga compared to usual care, and limited evidence indicated such a benefit compared to relaxation and aerobic exercise.[93] Aside from the physiological benefits of yoga, the mindfulness component may also provide a form of focus that may quell rumination (which is common in depression).

At this point, distinguishing between the different types of yoga is not possible, although initial studies using Hatha and Vinyasa yoga both appeared promising.[94,95]

Tai Chi

Tai chi combines martial arts and meditative movements that promote balance and healing of the mind and body. Tai chi involves a series of slowly performed, dance-like postures that flow into one another. As it comprises concentration, balance, muscle relaxation, and relaxed breathing, tai chi shows potential for becoming widely integrated into the prevention and rehabilitation of a number of medical and psychological conditions. One recent meta-analysis was performed on three RCTs that used depression as an outcome measure and demonstrated that tai chi interventions have beneficial effects for various populations on a range of psychological well-being measures including depression, anxiety, general stress management, and exercise self-efficacy.[96] The authors concluded that despite these positive outcomes, the studies had significant methodological limitations, and more RCTs with rigorous research design are needed to establish the efficacy of tai chi in improving psychological well-being and its potential to be used in interventions for populations with various clinical conditions.

OTHER TRADITIONAL HEALING TECHNIQUES

Although well-designed clinical studies investigating the role of hypnosis and imagery in the treatment of depression are limited, centuries of experience in traditional healing systems (e.g., Ayurvedic, Tibetan) support this kind of therapeutic approach. In our experience, these mind–body techniques are often extremely useful therapeutic adjuncts that appear to enhance the efficacy of other treatments. Emerging data suggest that relaxation therapy appears promising.[97] Some evidence has also shown the effectiveness and durability of prayer as an adjunct to other therapy for depression.[98,99] We recommend that interested patients explore one of these approaches (see Chapter 94, Relaxation Techniques).

ACUPUNCTURE

Acupuncture has been used for centuries in Asia for the treatment of virtually all known disease states. The exact mechanism of action is unknown, but human and animal studies have demonstrated that the stimulation of certain acupuncture points can alter neurotransmitter levels.[100] The United Nations World Health Organization recognized acupuncture as effective in treating mild to moderate depression. Published data suggest that acupuncture, including manual-, electrical-, and laser-based modalities, is a generally beneficial, well-tolerated, and safe monotherapy for depression. However, acupuncture augmentation in antidepressant partial responders and nonresponders is not as well studied as monotherapy.[101] A recent review of the current literature (January 2000 through April 2013) for acupuncture in cancer-related psychological symptoms showed positive results for acupuncture for the treatment of depression, anxiety, sleep disturbance, and for improving quality of life, with most results showing statistical significance. However, only a handful of acupuncture studies were specifically designed to evaluate depression, sleep disturbance, and quality of life as primary outcomes. Published studies in cancer patients and survivors show that acupuncture treatment is not only safe but also more acceptable, with fewer side effects than standard of care pharmacological treatments like antidepressants.[102] However, there are several limitations of these studies (small sample sizes, imprecise enrollment criteria, problems with randomization and blinding, brief duration of study, and lack of follow-up); thus evidence supporting acupuncture for depression remains inconclusive pending further study. The Cochrane Reviews investigators concluded that evidence was insufficient to recommend acupuncture for depression.[103,104]

PHOTOTHERAPY

Phototherapy is commonly used for patients with seasonal affective disorder and appears to be useful as an adjunctive modality with pharmacotherapy in both unipolar and bipolar depression.[105] The effect of phototherapy is thought to involve manipulation of the sleep-wake cycle and biological rhythms. Two meta-analyses supported at least modest benefit of bright light phototherapy when compared with placebo for nonseasonal depression.[106,107] In small studies, it appears to be an effective adjunct for adolescents, adults, and the elderly.[108–110] The APA guidelines for the treatment of major depressive disorder consider bright light therapy a low-risk and low-cost option.[111] Consider recommending 30 to 60 minutes of bright, white light (full-spectrum, 10,000 Lux) daily from special bulbs, lamps, or light boxes.

PHARMACEUTICALS

Antidepressants are believed to work by inhibiting the degradation and reuptake of neurotransmitters important in regulating psychological and neurovegetative function (serotonin, norepinephrine, dopamine), thus increasing neurotransmitter availability at the synaptic level. Newer theories suggest that pharmaceuticals may also mediate intracellular signaling systems that affect neurotrophic factors vital to the functioning of neuronal systems involved in mood regulation. Attempts to determine the most cost-effective approach to treating depression are limited by the quality of these evaluations, but SSRIs and newer antidepressants such as venlafaxine, mirtazapine, and nefazodone consistently are superior to tricyclic antidepressants (TCAs).[112] Systematic reviews suggest that escitalopram and sertraline may offer the best combination of efficacy and tolerability.[113,114] Studies of antidepressant medications increasingly are questioned because of the potential bias owing to unblinding, given that side effects of the drugs (as opposed to inert placebos) may reveal the identity of the true medication to participants or investigators. Trials using an "active" placebo that mimics some of the side effects of antidepressants to counteract this potential bias suggest that differences between antidepressants and active placebos are small.[115]

Selective Serotonin Reuptake Inhibitors and Mixed Reuptake Blockers

The APA continues to recommend the use of an SSRI as first-line treatment for all levels of depression: mild, moderate, and severe.[116] Recommendations for secondary steps include switching or augmenting current therapy (pharmacotherapy or psychotherapy) and depend on the initial treatment choice. *Maintenance therapy* is defined as continuation of the initial treatment to prevent recurrence of depression. For acute treatment of major depressive disorder (MDD), approximately 60% of patients respond to second-generation antidepressants[117] with a 40% relapse rate after 1 year.[118] A relatively recent meta-analysis of second-generation antidepressants summarized 4 comparative trials and 23 placebo-controlled trials and found that second-generation antidepressants were generally comparable to each other.[119] Safety in overdose and side effect profiles for SSRIs and mixed reuptake blockers are greatly improved over those of cyclic antidepressants and monoamine oxidase inhibitors. Even so, one-half of all patients discontinue their medication in the first 4 months after treatment initiation, and two-thirds of these patients report a side effect as the reason for stopping treatment.[120] In addition, meta-analyses of antidepressant medications have reported only modest benefits over placebo treatments.[121]

Be aware that concern is emerging over the long-term effects of SSRIs, including uncommon but serious neurologic sequelae of seizures and extrapyramidal symptoms,[122] as well as worsening of long-term outcomes despite effective short-term control.[123] The Food and Drug Administration (FDA) has mandated a black box warning on SSRIs regarding the risk of increasing suicidality in children and adolescents. This risk appears to occur within the first 2 weeks of initiating therapy, and whether this risk exists for adults is unclear.[120] Some work suggests that adults treated with antidepressant drugs, including SSRIs, are no more likely to attempt or complete suicide than those not treated with an antidepressant.[124]

DOSAGE

See Table 5.1.

PRECAUTIONS

Nausea, cramping, agitation, insomnia, headache, decreased libido, delayed ejaculation, erectile dysfunction, and anorgasmia have been reported in patients taking SSRIs.[120] Gastrointestinal side effects are more pronounced with sertraline but may be minimized by taking the drug with food and water. Fluoxetine

TABLE 5.1 **Drug and Supplement Dosages Used in Depression Treatment**

Drug/supplement	Initial dose (mg/day[†])	Range (mg/day[†])	Frequency
Vitamin B complex 100	1 tablet	—	Daily
Folic acid or L-methylfolate	400 mcg	400–800 mcg	Daily
Fish oil	1000	1000–6000	Daily
SAMe (1,4-butane-disulfonate)	200	200–800	bid
Hydroxytryptophan (enteric coated)	100	100–200	tid
St. John's wort (standardized to 5% hyperforin)*	300	900–1200	tid
Saffron	30 mg		bid
Selective Serotonin Reuptake Inhibitors and Mixed Reuptake Blockers			
Fluoxetine	20	20–60	Daily (AM)[‡]
Sertraline	50	50–200	Daily
Paroxetine	20	20–60	Daily (AM)
Paroxetine, extended release	12.5	25–75	Daily
Citalopram	20	20–60	Daily
Escitalopram	10	10–20	Daily
Serotonin Norepinephrine Reuptake Inhibitors			
Venlafaxine, immediate release	37.5	75–375	bid
Venlafaxine, extended release	37.5	75–375	Daily (at bedtime)
Desvenlafaxine	50	50	
Duloxetine	60	60–120	Divided daily–bid
Dopamine Norepinephrine Reuptake Inhibitor			
Bupropion, immediate release	150	300–450	tid[∥]
Bupropion, sustained release	150	300–400	bid
Bupropion, extended release	150	300–450	Daily
Serotonin Modulators			
Nefazodone	50	200–300	bid
Trazodone	150	150–400	bid–tid
Norepinephrine Serotonin Modulator, Alpha 2 Antagonist			
Mirtazapine	15	15–45	Daily (at bedtime)

bid, twice daily; SAMe, *S*-adenosylmethionine; tid, three times daily.
*Cytochrome P-450 3A4 and drug pump P-glycoprotein induction by St. John's wort requires that care be taken when prescribing this botanical in the setting of other drugs metabolized along these pathways. Perhaps the most clinically relevant interactions occur with cyclosporine (lowering serum cyclosporine concentration) and with other antidepressants, particularly the selective serotonin reuptake inhibitors (SSRIs; serotonin syndrome), antiretroviral therapy (reducing the concentration of protease inhibitors in patients infected with human immunodeficiency virus), and warfarin-type anticoagulants (increasing anticoagulation). Concern exists that St. John's wort may interfere with the efficacy of oral contraceptives. Avoid the use of St. John's wort concurrently with SSRIs; also avoid its use in pregnancy and lactation. High doses may predispose patients to photodermatitis.
†Unless otherwise indicated.
‡Maximum range, 20 to 80 mg.
§Doses greater than 100 mg should be divided dose, with the greater dose given at bedtime.
∥Initial dose: 100 mg bid for 3 days; then 100 mg tid.

is generally the most activating. Paroxetine has mild anticholinergic properties, including nausea and possibly weight gain. Venlafaxine has side effects similar to those of the other SSRIs but may cause serious hypertension over time. Although venlafaxine and paroxetine may have an increased risk of nausea, this can be reduced by using the extended-release forms.[120] Citalopram and escitalopram have the fewest side effects and the least impact on the cytochrome P-450 enzyme system. Duloxetine appears to play a role in mediating chronic pain and appears effective in older patients.[125] Rare side effects of SSRIs may include increased risk of gastrointestinal bleeding when these drugs are used with nonsteroidal antiinflammatory drugs, but more research is needed.[120] Other rare side effects include cardiac conduction abnormalities with venlafaxine and liver enzyme abnormalities with duloxetine.[120]

Tricyclic Antidepressants

TCAs have significant side effects (anticholinergic effects, weight gain, and cardiac dysrhythmias) and can be lethal in overdoses as small as an average 10-day supply.

Heterocyclic Serotonin Modulator and Dopamine Norepinephrine Reuptake Inhibitor Antidepressants

Heterocyclic antidepressants are much safer than TCAs in overdose, and they have side effect profiles that make them useful in specific clinical circumstances. Several studies have demonstrated that heterocyclic antidepressants are equally effective as SSRIs.[126] Amoxapine is useful in treating psychotic depression. Trazodone is highly sedating and is useful in low doses (25 to 50 mg nightly) when taken in combination with SSRIs to induce sleep. Bupropion is highly stimulating and may be a good option for patients wishing to discontinue smoking tobacco; it also has decreased fatigue and somnolence, but it is associated with seizures in underweight people. Nefazodone has anxiolytic properties and may be useful in patients who develop anxiety and insomnia while taking SSRIs. Nefazodone and bupropion also tend to have fewer sexual side effects compared with the SSRIs and serotonin norepinephrine reuptake inhibitors. Nefazodone and bupropion have the least likelihood of causing weight gain compared with SSRIs, whereas mirtazapine increases appetite and tends to cause weight gain. Mirtazapine also increases fatigue and somnolence, which may be desirable in some cases.[120]

Rare side effects that need further investigation in heterocyclic antidepressants include the following: seizures and atopic reactions with bupropion; thrombocytopenia, neutropenia, and bone marrow suppression with mirtazapine; and hepatotoxicity, cardiac conduction problems, and priapism with trazodone.

ELECTROCONVULSIVE THERAPY

Electroconvulsive therapy (ECT) reportedly is effective in achieving remission in 70% to 90% of patients with depression within 7 to 14 days in clinical trials (although it is less effective in community settings).[127] Generally, ECT is reserved for suicidal, psychotic, or catatonic patients; it is also helpful in patients refractory to other treatment modalities. ECT should be used with caution in patients with recent myocardial infarction, cardiac arrhythmia, or intracranial space-occupying lesions. Transient postictal confusion and anterograde and retrograde memory impairment are expected.[111]

DOSAGE

ECT, which requires referral to an experienced treatment center, generally involves sessions three times a week for up to 4 weeks, until symptoms abate.

THERAPIES TO CONSIDER FOR DEPRESSION

Estrogen Replacement Therapy

No abnormality of ovarian hormones has been identified that distinguishes women with depression from those without depression during the menopause transition.[128] However, estrogen replacement was demonstrated to reduce symptoms in perimenopausal and postmenopausal women with depression in some small studies, and discontinuation of hormone replacement therapy (HRT) appears to be associated with the rapid recurrence of depression in some women with a history of depression.[129] An RCT comparing HRT (estradiol valerate 2 mg, dienogest 2 mg) with placebo suggests that in women with mild to moderate depression in the setting of postmenopausal syndrome, HRT clearly and clinically relevantly reduced symptom severity by the Hamilton Rating Scale for Depression (HAM-D) at 24 weeks.[130] Studies assessing the relationship between hormone status and depression are inconsistent, and this topic remains an active area of research. Practitioners should consider recommending HRT after weighing the risks and benefits.

Transcranial Magnetic Stimulation

Transcranial magnetic stimulation uses a magnetic coil close to the scalp to generate rapidly alternating magnetic fields to produce electrical stimulation of superficial cortical neurons. It requires no general anesthesia and has minimal side effects. This technique was cleared by the FDA in 2008 for use in patients with major depressive disorder who have not responded adequately to at least one antidepressant trial. Meta-analysis suggests that TMS may be as effective as electrical conductive therapy (ECT) for nonpsychotic depression.[131]

Aromatherapy

Aromatherapy, which is the use of essential oils most often topically combined with MT or as inhaled vapors, has roots in ancient healing traditions. Several small studies demonstrate the impact of aroma on mood. One small open pilot trial found that adjunctive aromatherapy allowed for reductions in the dose of antidepressants compared with usual therapy. This nonrandomized trial included patients using various types and doses of antidepressants.[132] Short-term but not persistent benefits were found for aromatherapy MT with citrus oil in patients with cancer who were dealing with depression.[133] Aromatherapy may be promising as a gentle adjunctive therapy, but larger, well-designed trials are necessary before conclusions can be drawn.

Music Therapy

In music therapy, patients actively perform or listen to music to promote health and healing. Numerous trials of music therapy, largely in an older population, suggest potential antidepressant benefits when this modality is added to usual care, and a dose effect exists with increased response as treatment continues.[134-136] Most trials are small and lack blinding to intervention and appropriate control for attention of professionals. In addition, concurrent interventions that are not music specific (e.g., guided imagery and relaxation) make conclusions difficult to draw. A Cochrane Review identified only five trials meeting inclusion criteria and concluded that although music therapy is well tolerated by people with depression and appears to be associated with improvements in mood, the small number and low quality of studies preclude clear determination of effectiveness until better studies are conducted.[137] Although proof of benefits will require more thorough study, music therapy may be a useful intervention, especially for the elderly, in whom avoiding polypharmacy is of great importance.

Sleep Deprivation Therapy

Sleep deprivation therapy (SDT) is defined as maintaining wakefulness in patients all or part of the night. Multiple studies have suggested a rapid antidepressant effect of sleep deprivation therapy, but unfortunately, the effect tends to be limited, often followed by full or partial relapse after recovery sleep or even small naps. Some trials have suggested a more durable effect may be achieved through the addition of phototherapy or sleep-phase advancement.[138] One limitation of these studies is the inability for blinding, but chronobiology remains an active area of depression research.

NOVEL TREATMENTS HAVING PRELIMINARY STUDIES
Psilocybin

A small pilot study investigated the effect of psilocybin on 12 patients with advanced-stage cancer and a diagnosis of adjustment disorder with anxiety and generalized anxiety disorder. Using a crossover design, the patients were treated with psilocybin and niacin placebo (to cause flushing) several weeks apart. Psilocybin did not cause any clinically significant adverse effects. It caused a significant decrease in anxiety, as assessed by the State-Trait Anxiety Inventory at 1 and 3 months after treatment, and improved mood, as measured by the Beck Depression Inventory after 6 months.[139]

Botox

The theory that treatment of frown lines with botulinum toxin might improve the mood of depressed patients might seem farfetched. Wollmer and colleagues[140] studied the effect of injecting botulinum toxin into 3 sites in the glabella region of 15 depressed patients who were stable on up to 2 antidepressant treatments. The treatment was the same as that used in the cosmetic treatment of frown lines, and 15 participants received a placebo of saline injections at the same sites. There was a significant decrease in depression scores from 2 weeks to the end of the trial at 4 months for the active treatment relative to placebo. Similar results were seen on the Beck Depression Inventory and the Clinical Global Impressions Scale.[140]

PREVENTION PRESCRIPTION

The following steps are recommended for prevention of depressive symptoms:

- Remove exacerbating factors.
- Review current medications and supplements that could be contributing to depression, and consider decreasing dosages or discontinuing drugs that are suspect if they are not vital to the patient's well-being.
- Recommend a whole foods/low–processed foods diet such as the Mediterranean or antiinflammatory style eating plan, low in refined sugar (sucrose), , and alcohol. Encourage a diet rich in omega-3 fatty acids. Recommend two or three servings of cold-water fish (salmon, herring, mackerel, sardines) each week and 2 tablespoons of ground flaxseed or flaxseed oil daily.
- Consider recommending vitamin D_3 1000 units daily.
- Consider recommending a B-complex vitamin daily.
- Prescribe physical activity. Encourage daily aerobic (e.g., walking, jogging, cycling) or anaerobic (weight-lifting) exercise. Explore options, and help patients select activities they feel are enjoyable. Emphasize starting slowly and setting realistic short-term goals. Gradually increase to an ideal exercise prescription (see Chapter 91, Writing an Exercise Prescription).
- Foster an increase in a sense of community and investment in meaningful relationships to reduce social isolation.

THERAPEUTIC REVIEW

LIFESTYLE

- Suggest regular practice of aerobic or anaerobic exercises most days of the week.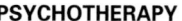
- Encourage activities that will increase social connection and enhance meaningful relationships.

NUTRITION

- Eliminate simple sugars from the diet.
- Consume a Mediterranean-style or whole foods (low–processed foods) diet.

DIETARY SUPPLEMENTS AND BOTANICALS

- Vitamins: Augment conventional antidepressant medication with vitamin B complex and 400 mcg to 1 mg of additional folic acid (L-methylfolate) daily.
- St. John's wort: Take 900 mg daily in three equal doses. Choose a product standardized to a minimum of 2% to 5% hyperforin or 0.3% hypericin. Examples include Kira, or Perika. If no improvement is seen after 4 to 6 weeks, consider switching to SAMe or a pharmaceutical antidepressant. Concurrent psychotherapy is recommended, if this approach is acceptable to the patient.
- S-Adenosylmethionine (SAMe): Start at 200 mg once or twice daily to minimize gastrointestinal side effects; then titrate upward to effect over 1 to 2 weeks. Initial treatment of depression may require 1600 mg daily given in two equal doses, followed by a maintenance dose of 200 mg twice daily. If recommending a pharmaceutical antidepressant, consider using SAMe initially (because of its rapid onset of action) along with it to minimize the latency period. SAMe may be withdrawn after 4 to 6 weeks.
- If SAMe is given without a pharmaceutical antidepressant, consider switching to another agent if no resolution of symptoms is noted after 2 weeks. Choose a product containing 1,4-butane-disulfonate (Actimet), which is stable for up to 2 years at room temperature. Concurrent psychotherapy is recommended, if this approach is acceptable to the patient.
- Fish oil: Take 1 g daily. If this dose is not effective, consider titrating up to 6 g of omega-3 fatty acids. In the case of an intake higher than 3 g per day, caution must be used because antiplatelet effects

are more likely. Choose a product with at least 60% EPA that also includes DHA and that has been tested for pesticides and heavy metal residues and keep refrigerated.

PSYCHOTHERAPY

The combination of supportive psychotherapy with antidepressant supplements or pharmacotherapy is generally recommended. Primary care physicians can provide limited psychotherapy at frequent visits to monitor lifestyle modifications, dietary supplements, or drug therapy. Alternatively, referral for cognitive or interpersonal therapy is recommended.

PHARMACEUTICALS

If no improvement is obtained with the use of lifestyle modification measures and dietary supplements (or if the patient has severe depression), discontinue the supplements, and start a pharmaceutical antidepressant. All currently approved antidepressant drugs are equally effective and have similar latency periods.[47] Choice of a selective serotonin reuptake inhibitor, mixed reuptake blocker, or heterocyclic antidepressant should be guided by matching the most appropriate side effect profile to each patient's symptoms. Continue treatment for at least 6 months after improvement, and consider full-dosage maintenance if the patient has a history of recurrent depression ([moderate to severe depression] or [mild depression]). If only a partial response has occurred at 6 weeks, either change the class of antidepressant medication or continue the antidepressant and consider adding lithium carbonate, 300 mg three times a day (necessitates experience in monitoring serum levels), or liothyronine sodium (Cytomel), 25 to 50 mcg.

PHOTOTHERAPY

Suggest phototherapy with 30 to 60 minutes of bright, white (full-spectrum, 10,000 Lux) light daily from special bulbs, lamps, or light boxes.*

REFERRAL

Consider referral to a psychiatrist if the patient remains refractory to treatment, is suicidal or psychotic, or requires psychiatric hospitalization or electroconvulsive therapy or transcranial magnetic stimulation.

---

*Information and therapeutic lights are widely available, including from the following manufacturers: BioBrite, Inc., 1-800-621-LITE (1-800-621-5483), www.biobrite.com; and SunBox Company, 1-800-548-3968, www.sunboxco.com

Key Web Resources

American Psychiatric Association. http://www.psychiatryonline.com/pracGuide/pracGuideTopic_7.aspx http://www.psychiatry.org/dsm5	American Psychiatric Association Guidelines for Treatment of Major Depression
http://www.phqscreeners.com/overview.aspx	The PHQ-2 is a useful tool for screening. The PHQ-9 questionnaire is a useful tool to diagnose and monitor depression treatment.
http://www.consumerlab.com	Independent testing of dietary supplements
http://naturaldatabase.therapeuticresearch.com	Evidence-based resources on dietary supplements

REFERENCES

References are available online at ExpertConsult.com.

CHAPTER 6

ANXIETY

Roberta Lee, MD, CaC

Anxiety disorders are some of the most commonly encountered medical conditions in primary care. According to the National Institute of Mental Health, the 1-year prevalence rate of anxiety disorders is 18.1% of the US population, a total of 40 million individuals. Underdiagnosis is common, with the average patient with an anxiety disorder consulting 10 health care professionals before receiving a definitive diagnosis.[1,2] Furthermore, patients with a diagnosis of anxiety use primary care services at significantly higher rates than other patients.[3] In the past, underdiagnosis was more common with patients receiving elaborate medical workups despite a definitive diagnosis remaining elusive in many cases. These patients became categorized as the "worried well." Nevertheless, because anxiety can be masked in numerous psychosomatic ways, practitioners must maintain a high index of suspicion for this disorder.

Anxiety disorders encompass a wide variety of subtypes, the most common being generalized anxiety disorder (GAD), obsessive-compulsive disorder (OCD), panic disorder, phobias, and posttraumatic stress disorder (PTSD). All are marked by irrational, involuntary thoughts. One of the most defining diagnostic elements of anxiety disorders is the disruption of daily life by overt distress. Frequently, patients have a significant reduction in the ability to carry out routine tasks, whether social, personal, or professional, with the prevalence of GAD as high as 8% to 10% in primary care practice.[4] This chapter provides an integrative approach to the management of GAD, as defined in the fifth edition of the *Diagnostic and Statistical Manual of Mental Disorders* (DSM-5).[4]

DEFINITION AND DIAGNOSTIC CRITERIA

GAD involves unremitting, excessive worry involving a variety of issues. These concerns may be related to family, health, money, or work. Once the initial concern subsides, another quickly takes its place. The practitioner observes the development of pervasive and repetitive concerns over time. Additionally, the distress seems out of proportion to actual life circumstances.

To meet the DSM-5 criteria for GAD, intense worrying must occur on majority of days during a period of at least 6 continuous months.[4] In addition, three of the following signs and symptoms must be present: easy fatigability, difficulty concentrating, irritability, muscle tension, restlessness, and sleep disturbance. Patients usually present with physical complaints and fail to recognize stress as the causative factor. The most frequent signs and symptoms are diaphoresis, headache, and trembling.[5] GAD is also associated with psychological manifestations. Patients often report impaired memory or a diminished ability to concentrate or take directions and frequently make statements such as "I can't seem to stop thinking of..."

COMORBID CONDITIONS

Approximately 40% of individuals with GAD have no comorbid conditions, but many develop other disorders as time evolves.[5] In fact, concurrent or coexistent organic or psychiatric disease is the rule rather than the exception in patients with GAD.[6] For example, panic disorder is common among persons who have irritable bowel syndrome, with a shared brain-gut mechanism incorporating a link with serotonin hypothesized.[7] Psychiatric overlap is common. Anxiety disorders and depression frequently coincide and either may trigger the other. In cases of coexisting depression, particularly of significant severity, the treatment of depression is the primary objective. Subsequent visits may reveal whether the anxiety is relieved simply by addressing underlying depression. Many individuals coping with anxiety use alcohol or drugs to mask their distress, with approximately 30% of individuals with panic disorder reported to abuse alcohol, and use of drugs occurs in 17%.[1]

PATHOPHYSIOLOGY

The pathophysiology of GAD is multifactorial and remains incompletely understood. Studies in animals and humans have attempted to identify body structures and systems involved in the pathogenesis of anxiety. One such structure is thought to be the amygdala, a small structure deep inside the brain that communicates with the autonomic nervous system to relay perceived danger to other centers of the brain which, in turn, readies the body to respond to perceived danger. Furthermore, the memory of these dangers stored in the amygdala appears to be indelible, thus creating a pathophysiologic phenomenon that may contribute to the pathogenesis of GAD.

> Although the pathophysiology of generalized anxiety disorder is multifactorial, the amygdala in the brain appears to be a focus for stressful memories that stimulate the autonomic nervous system when the body and mind perceive danger.

Other contributing factors may lie in the realm of cognitive phenomena. Current research is evaluating the association between exposure to stress early in life and subsequent development of GAD.[7]

In PTSD, a subtype of anxiety, studies have identified low cortisol levels (and high levels of corticotropin-releasing factor) and an overabundance of norepinephrine and epinephrine as contributing factors.[8]

Finally, genetic factors are also thought to contribute to GAD, with previous studies reporting genetic concordance with certain genetic loci that produce functional serotonin polymorphisms.[9]

Ruling out Organic Disease

The symptoms of anxiety disorders can resemble those of a variety of medical conditions, and a full medical workup is required for accurate diagnosis (Table 6.1).

INTEGRATIVE THERAPY

Exercise

Numerous studies have assessed the effects of both short-term and long-term exercise on anxiety. The bulk of these studies have measured the effects of exercise according

TABLE 6.1 Medical Conditions Often Associated With Symptoms of Anxiety

System	Specific Disorder
Cardiovascular	Acute myocardial infarction Angina pectoris Arrhythmias Congestive heart failure Hypertension Ischemic heart disease Mitral valve prolapse
Endocrine	Carcinoid syndrome Cushing's disease Hyperthyroidism Hypothyroidism Hypoglycemia Parathyroid disease Pheochromocytoma Porphyria Electrolyte imbalance
Gastrointestinal	Irritable bowel syndrome
Gynecologic	Menopause Premenstrual syndrome
Hematologic	Anemia Chronic immune diseases
Neurologic	Brain tumor Delirium Encephalopathy Epilepsy Parkinson disease Seizure disorder Vertigo Transient ischemic attack
Respiratory	Asthma Chronic obstructive pulmonary disease Pulmonary embolism Dyspnea Pulmonary edema

to the presence of signs and symptoms of elevated anxiety rather than by using a diagnostic system such as the DSM.[10] Nonetheless, the results of the majority of studies have generally indicated a reduction in symptoms with increased physical activity.

Aerobic exercise programs appear to produce a larger effect than obtained with weight training and flexibility regimens, although all forms of exercise appear to be effective in improving mood.[10,11] The length of physical activity also appears to be important. In one study, programs exceeding 12 minutes for a minimum of 10 weeks were required to achieve significant anxiety reduction,[12] with the beneficial effect of exercise reportedly maximal at 40 minutes per session.[10] Furthermore, the benefits appear to be long-lasting. In one study assessing the long-term effects of aerobic exercise, initially recorded psychological benefits were maintained in participants evaluated at 1-year follow-up. Participants reported their exercise routines were either the same as those in the original study design or less intensive at 12-month follow-up.[13]

The exact mechanisms underlying the improvement of mood with exercise are not completely understood. However, increased physical activity has been correlated with changes in brain levels of monoamines, namely norepinephrine, dopamine, and serotonin, which may account for improved mood.[14] The endorphin hypothesis is another explanation for the beneficial effects of exercise on mood. Many studies have demonstrated significant endorphin secretion with increased exercise, with beneficial effects on state of mind. However, blockade of endorphin elevation with antagonists, such as naloxone, during exercise has not been shown to decrease mental health benefits.[14] A number of investigators have argued that the latter findings are explained by flaws in methodologic design.

Both length of exercise session and physical activity program duration appears to be important in maximizing the beneficial effect of exercise on anxiety reduction.

Regardless of the underlying mechanisms, the involvement of individual patients in active recovery may confer a sense of independence leading to increased self-confidence. In turn, patient ability to cope with challenging life events is increased. This process is consistent with the integrative philosophy of healing. Furthermore, the paucity of side effects, low cost, and general availability of exercise make it a crucial component of integrative management.

The level of exertion and specific exercise prescription should be determined according to patient level of fitness, interest in specific physical activities, and health concerns (see Chapter 91).

Nutrition

Caffeine

On average, U.S. residents consume 1 or 2 cups of coffee per day, which represents approximately 150 to 300 mg of caffeine. Although the majority of individuals are able to handle this amount with no effect on mood, some experience increased anxiety. People who are prone to feeling stress have reported that they experience increased anxiety from small amounts of caffeine. With long-term use, caffeine has been linked with anxiety and depression. Discontinuation of caffeine intake may be warranted in patients with anxiety.[15]

Alcohol

With long-term use, alcohol has been found to diminish levels of serotonin and catecholamine. Discontinuation of alcohol consumption may therefore be warranted in cases of anxiety.[16]

Omega-3 Fatty Acids

Epidemiologic data indicate that omega-3 fatty acid deficiency or imbalance between the ratio of dietary omega-6 and omega-3 fatty acids are associated with increased anxiety and depression. Animal studies have demonstrated that levels of polyunsaturated fats and cholesterol metabolism influence neuronal tissue synthesis, membrane fluidity, and serotonin metabolism.[17] Primarily indirect evidence, particularly in depression, suggests that correction of the ratio of omega-6 to omega-3 consumption may improve mood. Given the evidence concerning neuronal tissue synthesis and serotonin metabolism, increased supplementation with omega-3 fatty acids may be beneficial in patients with depression.[18] Recommending consumption of cold water fish (sardines, mackerel, tuna, salmon, herring) at least two or three times a week, flaxseed oil (1000 to 2000 mg/day), or freshly ground flaxseed (2 tablespoons daily), may also be appropriate in such patients (see Chapter 88).

Supplements

B Vitamins

Nutrient deficiencies may alter brain function and therefore lead to anxiety. Deficiency of certain vitamins, including the B vitamins, has been linked with mood disorders. The B vitamins, including B_6 (pyridoxine) and B_{12}, are linked with the synthesis of S-adenosylmethionine (SAMe), which carries and donates methyl molecules to many chemicals in the brain including neurotransmitters. Vitamin B_6 is essential for the production of serotonin and has been linked with improvement in various mood disorders including anxiety when administered as a supplement.[19] Although large-scale clinical studies are lacking, a trial of a B-complex supplement appears warranted, particularly in older individuals or those taking medications that may deplete B vitamins, for example, oral contraceptives or replacement estrogen (Premarin).[20]

DOSAGE

Vitamin B_6 is administered as a B-complex vitamin supplement.

Folic Acid

Studies have shown that folic acid supplementation has benefit in individuals with depression (see section on folic acid use in Chapter 5). Patients with low levels of folic acid reportedly respond less well to selective serotonin reuptake inhibitors (SSRIs).[21] Serum vitamin B_{12} levels should be checked in patients receiving folic acid supplementation, particularly if megaloblastic anemia is noted in laboratory tests because vitamin B_{12} deficiency can be masked by folic acid supplementation.

DOSAGE

The recommended dose of folic acid for supplementation is 400 to 1000 mcg per day.

PRECAUTIONS

High doses of folic acid have been reported to cause altered sleep patterns, exacerbation of seizure frequency, gastrointestinal disturbances, and a bitter taste in the mouth.

5-Hydroxytryptophan

5-Hydroxytryptophan (5-HTP) is an amino acid precursor used in the formation of serotonin. 5-HTP has been used as an oral supplement alternative to boost serotonin.[22] It has been shown in studies to improve depression, but only preliminary evidence is available suggesting that 5-HTP also may improve anxiety. L-Tryptophan, another amino acid found to improve mood, is converted to 5-HTP and then to serotonin. 5-HTP readily crosses the blood–brain barrier. The metabolism of 5-HTP by monoamine oxidase and aldehyde dehydrogenase forms 5-indoleacetic acid, which is excreted in the urine.

DOSAGE

For anxiety or depression, the dose is 150 to 800 mg daily.

PRECAUTIONS

Anyone using conventional medications for depression or anxiety, particularly those agents that boost serotonin, should discuss the use of 5-HTP with his or her health care practitioner before initiating supplementation to avoid excessively elevated levels of serotonin. 5-HTP can cause gastrointestinal side effects such as nausea, belching, and heartburn.

Caution. Some concern exists that 5-HTP, like L-tryptophan, can cause a condition known as eosinophilia myalgia syndrome. The suspected culprit is a group of contaminants identified from the peak X family. However, current evidence is insufficient to suggest that this element is consistently responsible. Case reports have been sporadic.[23,24]

Pharmaceuticals

Conventional options for initial therapy in GAD are based on various factors and drug side effect profiles. Depression frequently coexists with GAD, so antidepressants are often considered. Several of the SSRIs can be considered (paroxetine, sertraline, citalopram, escitalopram, fluoxetine, fluvoxamine) for the treatment of GAD, although some agents have been approved for panic disorder, social phobia, and PTSD. Because less cardiotoxicity is associated with SSRIs than with tricyclic antidepressants, an SSRI may be a better choice for

TABLE 6.2 Supplement and Drug Recommendations for Treatment of Anxiety

Drug/Supplement	Initial Dose (Range)	Frequency
Vitamin B complex 100	1 tablet	Daily
Folic acid	400–800 mcg	Daily
Kava	50–70 mg (of kava lactones)	tid
Valerian root	150–300 mg every AM and 300–600 mg at bedtime	
5-Hydroxytryptophan	150–300 mg	Daily
Selective Serotonin Reuptake Inhibitors and Mixed Reuptake Blockers		
Fluoxetine (Prozac)	10–20 mg (10–80)	Daily
Fluvoxamine (Luvox)	50 mg (50–300)	Daily
Paroxetine (Paxil)	10 mg (10–60)	Daily
Sertraline (Zoloft)	50 mg (50–200)	Daily
Escitalopram (Lexapro)	10 mg (10–20 mg)	Daily
Citalopram (Celexa)	20 mg (20–40 mg)	Daily
Others		
Venlafaxine (Effexor)	75 mg (37.5–75 mg)	bid
Nefazodone (Serzone)	200 mg (100–300 mg)	bid
Bupropion (Wellbutrin)	100 mg (50–125 mg)	bid
Duloxetine (Cymbalta)	60 mg (30–120 mg)	Daily
Azapirones		
Buspirone (BuSpar)	5 mg (15–30 mg)	bid

bid, Twice daily; tid, three times daily.

patients with heart disease. Other conventional options for treatment of GAD involve the use of multiple receptor agents. Serotonin norepinephrine reuptake inhibitors (e.g., venlafaxine (Effexor) and duloxetine (Cymbalta)) are also approved for GAD. The use of tricyclic antidepressants has always been a consideration, but the difficulty in using these medications is that they can have anticholinergic and cardiovascular side effects, as well as a more pronounced sedative effect. Most experts recommend a trial of at least 4 to 6 weeks to determine efficacy.

For short-term treatment of GAD, the use of anxiolytics, especially benzodiazepines, has always been a consideration. However, the risk of abuse and habituation has made most primary care practitioners cautious about prescribing these medications. The nonbenzodiazepine anxiolytic buspirone (BuSpar) may be a conventional alternative lacking the problematic issue of drug dependence and excessive sedation.

DOSAGE
See Table 6.2.

Botanicals

Kava (Piper methysticum)

In the field of botanical pharmaceuticals, kava has become known as a botanical option for the treatment of GAD in the United States and Europe. It is derived from the pulverized lateral roots of a subspecies of pepper plant, *Piper methysticum*, and is indigenous to many Pacific Island cultures. In Europe, kava is recognized by health authorities as a relatively safe remedy for anxiety.[24] A recent metaanalysis of six of the eleven published randomized clinical trials evaluated the efficacy of kava in GAD,[25] with kava found to be superior to placebo in the symptomatic treatment of GAD.

The constituents of kava considered to be most pharmacologically active are lactones, which have a chemical structure similar to that of myristicin, found in nutmeg.[26] Kava lactone structures are lipophilic and are present in the highest concentration in the lateral roots. Of the 15 isolated kava lactone structures, 6 are concentrated maximally in the root and vary depending on the variety of *Piper methysticum*.[27] The mechanism of action of kava in GAD has yet to be completely elucidated, although the action appears to be similar to that of benzodiazepines. However, conflicting results have been reported in studies in rats and cats.

Benzodiazepines exert their actions by binding to the gamma-aminobutyric acid (GABA) site and benzodiazepine receptors in the brain. Animal studies analyzing the anxiolytic activity of kava, however, have demonstrated mixed and minor effects at both sites. Other studies indicate that kava constituents produce anxiolytic effects by altering the limbic system, particularly at the amygdala and hippocampus.[28] Other documented uses of kava have been as a muscle relaxant, an anticonvulsant, an anesthetic, and an antiinflammatory agent.

Indication. Mild to moderate GAD.

DOSAGE
Kava is taken for anxiety at a dose of 50 to 70 mg (purified extract, kava lactones) three times daily.

PRECAUTIONS
Anecdotal reports have noted excessive sedation when kava is combined with other sedative medications.[29] Extrapyramidal side effects were reported in four patients using two different preparations of kava. Thus, kava should be avoided in patients with Parkinson syndrome.[30] The effects were reported to diminish once the extract was discontinued. A yellow, ichthyosiform condition of the skin, known as kava dermopathy, has been observed in patients with heavy kava consumption. This condition is reversible with discontinuation of kava.[31] The overdose potential of kava appears to be low. In many cases, skin rash, ataxia, redness of the eyes, visual accommodation difficulties, and yellowing of the skin have been reported in studies from Australia and the Pacific region after ingestion of up to 13 liters per day, equivalent to 300 to 400 g of dried root per week. This amount of kava represents a dose 100 times that of the recommended therapeutic dose.[32]

Caution. There are insufficient data to determine the teratogenicity of kava. For this reason, it is wise to avoid the use of kava during pregnancy. Kava is present in the milk of lactating mothers and its use is therefore discouraged during breast-feeding.[33] The use of kava with other sedative medications should be avoided.

Kava has been reported to cause idiopathic hepatotoxic hepatitis. To date, all case reports (a total of 31) have been in patients from Europe who used concentrated extracts manufactured in Germany or Switzerland. The exact cause of the observed effects are currently under investigation. Kava should not be used in individuals who have liver problems, nor should it be used concomitantly in patients who are taking multiple medications that are metabolized by the liver or in individuals who drink alcohol on a daily basis.[34] Liver tests should be routinely performed in individuals who use kava on a daily basis, and patients should be counseled regarding the signs and symptoms of hepatotoxicity (jaundice, malaise, and nausea). Furthermore, daily use of kava should be discontinued after approximately 4 months.

Valerian (Valeriana officinalis)

Valerian represents a botanical alternative for the treatment of GAD. The clinical efficacy of valerian has predominantly been evaluated in the treatment of treating sleep disturbances, with fewer clinical studies assessing its use in anxiety available and mixed reports regarding efficacy. Nevertheless, valerian has been used in Europe for more than a thousand years as a tranquilizer and calmative.[35] The use of valerian in combination with either passionflower (*Passiflora incarnata*) or St. John's wort (*Hypericum perforatum*) for anxiety has been studied in small clinical trials. One study evaluated valerian root in combination with passionflower (100 mg of valerian root with 6.5 mg of passionflower extract) compared with chlorpromazine hydrochloride (Thorazine, 40 mg daily) over a period of 16 weeks. In this study, 20 patients were randomly assigned to the two treatment groups after being identified as suffering from irritation, unrest, depression, or insomnia. Electroencephalographic changes in both groups consistent with relaxation were comparable, with the use of two psychological scales demonstrating scores consistent with reduced anxiety.[36] A further study evaluated anxiety in 100 anxious individuals receiving either a combination of 50 mg of valerian root plus 90 to 100 mg of standardized St. John's wort for 14 days or 2 mg of diazepam (Valium) twice daily in the first week and up to 2 capsules twice daily in the second week. The results of this study demonstrated reduced anxiety in the phytomedicine treatment group compared to healthy individuals. Patients in the diazepam treatment group continued to have significant anxiety scores after treatment.[37]

Indication. Mild to moderate anxiety.

Contrary to common belief, valerian is not suitable for short-term treatment of anxiety or insomnia, with several weeks required to observe a beneficial effect.

Mind-Body Therapy

Psychotherapy

Psychotherapy has been shown to be effective as a therapeutic option in the treatment of GAD with or without medical intervention. Two clinically proven forms are frequently used: behavioral therapy and cognitive-behavioral therapy. Behavioral therapy focuses on changing specific unwanted actions by using several techniques to stop the undesired behavior. In addition, both behavioral therapy and cognitive-behavioral therapy help patients to understand and change their thinking patterns so that they can react differently to their anxiety.

Relaxation Techniques

Relaxation training, stress reduction techniques, and breath work are of proven benefit. In fact, imaginal exposure is used as a tactic for repeated exposure to induce anxiety (in a gradual way). Patients learn to cope with and manage their anxiety through repeated exposure rather than to eliminate it. Relaxation training paired with interceptive therapy is often useful. Patients who admit to their anxiety are often willing to confront and learn to cope despite an inability to relax completely. Depending on patient preference, patients should choose a relaxation technique that reinforces a sense of calm. Therapies that can be used for this purpose are massage, sound therapy, aromatherapy, guided interactive imagery, and hypnosis. Because many patients have somatic sensations that accompany their anxiety, a complementary therapy that imparts a "remembrance" of a deeply relaxed state (see Chapter 94) should also be used to reinforce on a more somatic-kinesthetic level.

Therapies to Consider

Traditional medical systems, such as acupuncture and Ayurvedic medicine, may provide other options for the treatment of anxiety.[40-42] Several small trials assessing relaxation in an anxious state have reported reduction of anxiety in psychologically normal patient populations through the use of auricular acupuncture.[41,42] Although the mechanisms underlying the efficacy of these treatment are not well elucidated, such systems may have beneficial effects on autonomic nervous system balance.

PREVENTION PRESCRIPTION

- Maximize nutrition to include foods rich in omega 3-fatty acids, B vitamins, and folic acid.
- Follow a regular exercise routine (even walking with tracking using a pedometer).
- Institute a daily mind-body exercise program to enhance the relaxation response.
- Keep a journal to develop a "feeling inventory" and enhance self-awareness.
- Limit the use of personal digital assistants, cellphones, and BlackBerry devices. Do not access these devices during meals and special times with family and friends. Turn to "off" at 10 p.m. and "on" at 6 to 7 a.m. Do not recharge these devices next to your bed!
- Get enough sleep to feel refreshed.

THERAPEUTIC REVIEW

The following four steps are recommended for initial management of patients with generalized anxiety disorder (GAD).
1. Remove exacerbating factors. Review current medications and supplements that could contribute to anxiety (particularly botanical supplements, such as ephedra, and over-the-counter stimulant preparation). Supplements that are unnecessary should be discontinued.
2. Screen for diseases that mimic anxiety. Screening should be performed for underlying medical conditions that produce anxiety, such as hyperthyroidism or withdrawal syndrome.
3. Improve nutrition. Nutritional support is recommended, such as with omega-3 fatty acid supplementation (two to three servings of cold water fish per week, or flaxseed oil 2 tablespoons a day or 1000 mg of flaxseed oil in a capsule). In addition, caffeine and alcohol consumption should be avoided. **A**①₁
4. Institute physical activity. Physical activity (aerobic or anaerobic) at least 5 days out of 7 should be encouraged. To ensure long-term compliance, an activity that is enjoyable to the patient is important. Furthermore, adherence to a regular exercise regimen and setting realistic short-term goals may require emphasis. Increases in exercise level and intensity should be gradual (see Chapter 91). **A**①₁

SUPPLEMENTS
- Vitamin B6 included in a vitamin B 100 complex preparation with the addition of folic acid (400 mcg daily) should be considered. **A**②₂
- Folic acid
- 5-Hydroxytryptophan (150 to 300 mg daily) may be considered as a serotonin boosting alternative; however, close monitoring should be undertaken to screen for eosinophilia myalgia syndrome. **B**②₂ **C**⊕₃

BOTANICALS
- Kava can be administered at 50 to 70 mg three times a day (purified kava lactones). Choose a standardized product with either 30% or 50%–55% kava lactone concentration.
- If no improvement is observed after 4 to 6 weeks, consider valerian, a valerian combination, or a pharmaceutical anxiolytic (use for at least 6 weeks before evaluating efficacy). **B**⊕₂
- Concurrent psychotherapy is highly recommended if this approach is acceptable to the patient.

MIND-BODY THERAPY
- Psychotherapy: The combination of psychotherapy in conjunction with supplements, botanicals, or a pharmaceutical anxiolytic or antidepressant is highly recommended, particularly in GAD. An integrative therapeutic approach is associated with higher success rates in cases of severe anxiety. Often, psychotherapy can provide the patient with skills for coping with anxiety, as opposed to extinguishing the symptoms. Primary care physicians are able to monitor lifestyle modification, dietary and supplement interventions, and drug therapy. However, referral to a psychotherapist is advised. **A**①₁
- Relaxation training: Patients are educated in relaxation techniques, allowing control of anxiety symptoms when required. **B**②₁

TRADITIONAL MEDICAL SYSTEMS
- Use of traditional medicine systems (TMSs) is problematic as TMSs have historically been used to provide primary care for a variety of medical ailments (including anxiety). In allopathic medicine, TMSs are generally used as an adjunctive modality. However, the use of a TMS (e.g., Chinese medicine or Ayurvedic medicine) may represent an appropriate primary therapeutic option in patients with strong feelings regarding the use of singular botanical preparations (predominantly as being insufficient for treatment) or whose medical conditions appear mild, as long as the well-being of the patient is not in jeopardy. **C**⊖₁

PHARMACEUTICALS
- The use of a pharmaceutical anxiolytic or antidepressant should be considered if no improvement is obtained with lifestyle measures, dietary measures, or supplement interventions in conjunction with botanical supplements. Depending on the severity of the anxiety and the degree of lifestyle impairment, a conventional prescriptive option with dietary and lifestyle interventions in combination with complementary therapy (e.g., acupuncture, mind-body therapy) may be used to induce a sense of relaxation before reduction of the prescriptive treatment (often a couple of months later). Depending on the severity of the disorder, botanical supplements (e.g., kava) may also be useful. **A**②₂
- Different clinical responses may be obtained with various anxiolytics (and selective serotonin reuptake inhibitors). Optimal management may require a change of medication according to patient symptoms. For long-term therapy, the use of benzodiazepines should be limited due to the risk of tolerance and dependence.
- Referral to a psychiatrist should be considered if the patient remains refractory to treatment, is suicidal or psychotic, or requires psychiatric stabilization in a hospital unit.

Key Web Resources

Benson-Henry Institute for Mind Body Medicine. http://www.massgeneral.org/bhi/.	The Institute was founded in 1988 as a nonprofit scientific and educational organization building on the work of Herbert Benson at Harvard Medical School on the relaxation response. The website covers research, education, training programs, clinical programs, books, videotapes, audiotapes, and more.
Mind and Life Institute. www.MindandLife.org.	The Institute is dedicated to creating dialogue and collaboration in research at the highest possible level between modern science and the great living contemplative traditions, especially Buddhism. The website provides information regarding conferences and events, research initiatives, publications, and the work of the Dalai Lama.
Mindfulness-Based Stress Reduction (MBSR). www.umass-med.edu/cfm.	The Center for Mindfulness at the University of Massachusetts sponsors the MBSR program. The website covers clinical care, education, research, training, a bibliography, and more.
Shambhala. www.shambhala.org/.	This worldwide network of meditation centers was founded by Chogyam Trungpa Rinpoche, a Tibetan Buddhist master of the Shambhala and Buddhist teachings. The website is an international guide to Shambhala centers and their activities, books and recordings, and essays on mindfulness meditation.
Transcendental Meditation (TM) Program. www.tm.org/.	The official U.S. website of the TM program. The website provides a description of the program, scientific research on TM, news articles and books, places to study, and an explanation of the uses of TM in enhancing function and the treatment of a variety of conditions.
Wildmind Buddhist Meditation. www.wildmind.org/.	This website provides a wealth of information on Buddhist practices, including guided meditations in RealAudio format and online meditation courses led by an experienced instructor.

REFERENCES

References are available online at ExpertConsult.com.

CHAPTER 7

ATTENTION DEFICIT DISORDER

Anju Sawni, MD, FAAP, FSAHM • Kathi J. Kemper, MD, MPH

DEFINITIONS, EPIDEMIOLOGY, AND PATHOPHYSIOLOGY

Attention-deficit/hyperactivity disorder (ADHD) is one of the most commonly diagnosed and costly neurodevelopmental disorders affecting school-aged children in the United States. ADHD is characterized by symptoms of developmentally inappropriate levels of inattention and/or hyperactivity-impulsivity for which there is no other explanation. ADHD may also lead to significant impairment of academic or work performance. ADHD is a lifelong condition with 60% to 80% of children reported to have ADHD symptoms that persist into adulthood,[1,2] with the prevalence of ADHD in adults estimated at 4.4%.[3]

Current data indicate ADHD is diagnosed in 3%–11% of children between 4 and 17 years of age (depending on age, gender, and community), with rates increasing in the past 10 years from 3%–5% per year.[3] ADHD is diagnosed more commonly in boys than girls (3:1 ratio), with a peak age of diagnosis between 8 and 10 years. Drugs used to treat ADHD, such as methylphenidate (Concerta), atomoxetine (Strattera), and a combination of amphetamine and dextroamphetamine (Adderall), are three of the top five (ranked by spending) treatments for children younger than 18 years in the United States. Unlike acute bacterial infection, ADHD is a chronic condition requiring ongoing management.

The classic presentation of ADHD is that of an energetic boy who is easily distracted, talks a lot, interrupts others, acts as if driven by a motor, fidgets and squirms, has a messy room, acts impulsively, has trouble following rules, and often breaks or loses things, and often admonished to sit still, pay attention, and clean up his room. The quiet girl who daydreams and is inattentive in class represents a second presentation of ADHD (ADHD without hyperactivity). The diagnosis is based on the most recent edition of the *Diagnostic and Statistical Manual* (DSM-5),[4] characterized by an age of onset less than 12 years and consistent perceptions of a particular pattern of behavior, such as the following:

- Persistence of symptoms (at least 6 months).
- Pervasive (present in at least two settings) patterns of inattention and/or hyperactivity-impulsivity (at least six symptoms up to the age 17 and five symptoms at age 17 and older).
- Symptoms are inappropriate for developmental level and disrupt age-appropriate academic, social, or occupational functioning.

Knowledge of normal child development is essential in making a diagnosis of ADHD, as normal behavior for a 2 year old includes impulsivity and a short attention span that would be abnormal in an 8 year old.

The majority of clinicians use behavioral checklists, such as the Vanderbilt Parent and Teacher Rating Scales, to diagnose ADHD and monitor treatment progress. No laboratory or imaging modalities have demonstrated utility in confirming the diagnosis of ADHD, although clinicians often use laboratory or neuropsychological tests to rule out contributory problems, such as hearing or vision problems, anemia, hypothyroidism, absence seizures, reading or math learning disabilities, and short-term memory impairment.

Common comorbidities include oppositional defiant disorder (ODD) and conduct disorders (CD) (30% to 50%), mood or anxiety disorders (15% to 30%), learning disabilities (20% to 25%), sleep problems (25% to 50%), and tic disorders such as Tourette syndrome (10% to 60%).[2,5,6] Strengths often include creativity, imagination, sociability, flexible attention, interest in the environment, energy, vitality, enthusiasm, adaptability, confidence, exuberance, spontaneity, and desire to please others.[7] A strengths-based, specific behavioral goal-oriented approach is popular in the management of ADHD.

Consequences of persistent, poorly treated ADHD include: an increased risk of injuries; increased cost of medical care; an increased risk of addiction to tobacco, alcohol, and illicit drugs; an increased risk of incarceration; and a diminished ability to maintain employment or relationships.[8,9]

Although a single pathophysiological mechanism underlying ADHD has yet to be described, genetic associations, multiple environmental agents, and psychosocial characteristics (e.g., poverty, stressed parents and households, families with mental health or substance abuse challenges, difficulty setting limits, disorganized routines) affect the risk of developing or being labeled with ADHD. Genes found to be significantly associated with ADHD include *DRD4, DRD5, DAT, DBH, 5-HTT, HTR1B,* and *SNAP-25.* Other risk factors for ADHD include male gender, maternal tobacco use during pregnancy or early childhood, intrauterine growth retardation, excessive exposure to television, and exposure to certain pesticides.[10–12] Of the 358 industrial chemicals, pesticides, and pollutants found in studies of the umbilical cord blood of infants in the United States, more than 200 are known to be toxic to the brain. Multiple brain regions, including the prefrontal cortex, frontostriatal networks, and cerebellum, and neurotransmitters, particularly dopamine and norepinephrine, appear to be involved in ADHD deficits.[13–16]

In summary, ADHD is a common clinical diagnosis in both children and increasingly in adults, and has multiple genetic, environmental, and psychosocial effects on several neurotransmitter systems and regions of the brain.

INTEGRATIVE THERAPY

Integrative therapy focuses on the goals of the patient and family in the context of values, culture, and community. Goals for treating ADHD may include improvements in the ability to focus or pay attention and in following directions, greater persistence in the presence of difficulty, improved ability to delay gratification, more consistent anticipation of consequences, improving grades, better organizational skills, better short-term memory, greater neatness, less procrastination, improved social relationships, greater obedience, better sleep, and fewer injuries, among other goals. Each of these goals requires a complex interaction of specific skills and resources.

Requirements for learning to manage attention are as follows:
1. *Motivation* (it is easier to pay attention to things that interest us)
2. The ability to *perceive* sensory data, such as sounds (as words) and symbols (written words or gestures), accurately and to *process* these data into meaningful information
3. *Tuning out of irrelevant* sensory information (e.g., ignoring music or conversation in the background while reading a book) while being *flexibly responsive* to changing priorities (a fire by a smoke detector, a cry for help, or ringing telephone)
4. *Monitoring* of one's own attention ("Oh, was I listening to the music instead of focusing on the words? How many times have I read this sentence?")
5. *Redirection* of attention (let us get back to the book)
In addition to managing attention, learning to *follow directions* also requires certain abilities:
1. Understanding the meaning of the request
2. Recognizing the tools and skills needed to complete it
3. Assessing the availability of these tools and skills
4. Using available resources and asking for help when needed
5. Monitoring performance

The choice of specific therapies depends, to some extent, on individual-specific goals; however, general mental and physical health can always be supported by appropriate attention to the fundamentals: *healthy habits in a healthy habitat.* Four fundamental healthy habits have been identified: exercise, balanced with optimal sleep; nutrition and avoidance of toxins in the diet; management of stress and emotions; and establishment of healthy communication and supportive, rewarding social relationships.[17] A healthy habitat includes both the physical and psychosocial environment (Fig. 7.1).

LIFESTYLE

Exercise

A minimum of 30 to 60 minutes of aerobic activity daily is necessary for general physical and mental health.[18] A study conducted in 2009 of children with developmental coordination disorder found that regularly playing table tennis was beneficial for both coordination and ability to sustain focus.[19] Exercise outdoors in nature is even

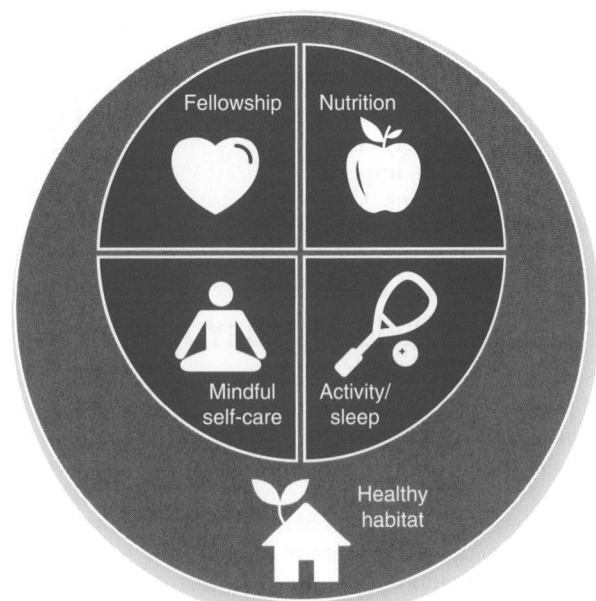

FIG. 7.1 ■ Healthy habits in a healthy habitat.

better than exercise in a gym or urban setting.[20] Exercise increases brain-derived neurotrophic factor levels and enhances neurogenesis, thereby promoting overall cognitive function, including attention and memory, which are both required for academic achievement.[21,22] Cerebellar dysfunction has been implicated in ADHD.[23] This has led to growing interest in activities that build balance and coordination such as yoga, juggling, cross-midline exercises, the Interactive Metronome method, and Brain Gym. Quiet, mindful exercises, such as tai chi and yoga, encourage focus on body movements and can thereby improve ability to focus and allow individuals to be more deliberate and less impulsive.[24] Martial arts training promotes discipline. Dr. David Katz of Yale University in Connecticut recommends the ABCs: Activity Bursts in the Classroom (or Corporation).[25]

> A minimum of 30 to 60 minutes of aerobic activity daily is necessary for general physical and mental health.

Safety

Impulsive, distracted people are prone to injuries. Encourage appropriate use of bike and ski helmets in addition to protective padding for skateboarding. Encourage enrollment in organized sports or lessons with small classes with close supervision and low student-teacher ratios (karate, tae kwon do, tai chi, or yoga) to help develop body awareness and self-discipline. Counsel the patient to avoid overuse injuries.

Sleep

Sleep deprivation impairs focus, organizational skills, diligence, and self-discipline during boring tasks. Inadequate sleep and poor sleep quality impair attention and judgment, increase fidgeting, lower performance, and lead to more mistakes, automobile collisions, and injuries. Although many patients with ADHD report sleep problems, even before starting treatment, stimulant medications may contribute to insomnia. Improved sleep may lead to improvements in daytime focus on behavior. Clinicians should routinely inquire about sleep and recommend sleep hygiene measures (e.g., cool, quiet, dark room; comfortable bedding; avoidance of television in the bedroom or exercise late in the day; routine bedtime) to promote optimal sleep. Even a brief behavioral intervention to improve sleep hygiene may improve quality of life and overall functioning in addition to sleep quality.[26]

Nutrition

Despite weighing less than 5% of total body weight, the brain uses approximately 20% of the body's energy supply. To function well, the brain requires a steady supply of high-quality fuel (Table 7.1). Accordingly, regular meals supplying optimal amounts of essential fatty acids for cell membranes, amino acids for the production of neurotransmitters, vitamin and mineral cofactors for neurotransmitter production and metabolism, and a steady supply of glucose are required to meet whole-body energy needs. Optimally, nutrients are ingested in the diet; however, supplements may be required in patients with a poor diet. Children with ADHD are at increased risk of deficiencies of several essential nutrients, including vitamin D, iron, magnesium, and zinc.[27]

Omega-3 Fatty Acids

Low levels of omega-3 fatty acids are associated with ADHD and behavioral problems in both adults and children.[28,29] Supplementation with fish oils (which are rich sources of omega-3 fatty acids) can alleviate ADHD symptoms and decrease depression, anger, anxiety, impulsivity, and aggression, in addition to improving academic achievement.[30-36] Although flaxseed, walnuts, and green leafy vegetables contain the omega-3 fatty acid *linolenic acid*, humans convert only 5% to 10% of linolenic acid to useful *eicosapentaenoic acid* (EPA) and *docosahexaenoic acid* (DHA). Patients should be encouraged to eat either sardines, salmon, or mackerel twice weekly, consume 1 to 2 tablespoons of flaxseeds daily, or consider a supplement containing between 500 and 2000 mg of combined EPA and DHA.

Amino Acids

The results of two small studies indicate *carnitine* supplements may help improve attention and behavior in children and adults with ADHD, particularly the inattentive type.[37,38] Additional studies are required to determine optimal dosing, frequency, and duration, particularly for patients with varying intake of foods rich in amino acids.

Minerals

Iron deficiency interferes with memory, concentration, behavior, and both physical and mental performance.

TABLE 7.1 Dietary Essentials for Optimal Attention

Dietary Essentials	Foods Sources
Amino acids	Soy, tofu, beans, lentils Seeds and nuts Milk, cheese, eggs Fish, fowl, meat
Essential fatty acids (omega-3 fatty acids: EPA, DHA, and linolenic acid)	Fish (tuna, salmon, sardines, and mackerel) Flax seeds, walnuts Dark green leafy vegetables Animals raised on eaten omega-3–rich diets (e.g., eggs from chickens fed flaxseed; pasture-raised and grass finished beef; lamb; bison; wild game)
B vitamins, including folate and B12	Beans, lentils, nuts and seeds Leafy green vegetables, asparagus Oranges and other citrus fruits and juices Whole grains Yeast (e.g., brewer's), dairy, eggs, meat, poultry, fish, and shellfish
Minerals: iron, magnesium, zinc	Peas, beans, lentils, peanuts, peanut butter Leafy green vegetables: spinach, kale Avocado Raisins Whole grains, brown rice, wheat bran and germ Nuts: almonds, cashews Dairy, eggs Meat, fish, poultry, oysters

DHA, docosahexaenoic acid; EPA, eicosapentaenoic acid.

Correcting iron deficiencies (indicated by low ferritin levels) has been shown to have utility in improving attention and restlessness.[39-44] *Magnesium* supplements have benefit in children with ADHD who are excitable, easily stressed, or worriers, as well as those who also suffer from constipation.[45] *Zinc* supplements has been shown to improve behavior in individuals deficient in zinc.[46,47] The best dietary sources of essential minerals are considered to be plants and animals raised on mineral-rich soils.

Vitamins

The B vitamins function as essential cofactors in the production of neurotransmitters. Many children who avoid leafy green vegetables consume insufficient amounts of folate. Those who are strict vegans may benefit from vitamin B_{12} supplements. For picky eaters or those who eat poor-quality diets, multivitamin and mineral supplementation may be beneficial; however, megadoses have not been shown to have efficacy and are associated with side effects.[48]

Water

Dehydration may impair attention and mood.[49] In a small study of first graders, ingestion of water prior to a test led to increased attention and greater happiness.[50]

Sugar

At least a dozen double-blind studies have demonstrated that sugar does not cause hyperactivity. However, eating simple sugars can cause blood sugar swings that impair mental and emotional stability. Calories should be consumed in the form of complex carbohydrates, such as whole grains, rather than simple sugars.[51] Furthermore, many sweet, processed food products also contain artificial colors and preservatives that may contribute to behavior problems.

Feingold Diet, Artificial Colors, Flavors, and Preservatives

The Feingold diet does not exclude sugar but does eliminate salicylates (at least initially before slowly reintroducing fruits containing them), several synthetic food additives, and certain synthetic sweeteners:
- Artificial colors (petroleum-based certified FD&C and D&C colors)
- Artificial flavors
- BHA, BHT, TBHQ (preservatives)
- The artificial sweeteners Aspartame (now called Truvia), Neotame, and Alitame

Artificial food colors significantly worsen hyperactivity in many cases.[52] The Center for Science in the Public Interest (CSPI) has called on the U.S. Food and Drug Administration (FDA) to ban dyes linked to hyperactivity and behavior problems. The colorings the CSPI would like to see banned are as follows:
- Blues 1 and 2
- Green 3
- Orange 8
- Reds 3 and 40
- Yellows 5 and 6

In studies of children with ADHD who received the Feingold diet, 73% had improved behavior.[53,54] Studies involving more than 1800 children have reported significant improvements in hyperactive behavior in participants consuming a diet free of benzoate preservatives and artificial colors and flavors.[55,56] Some families find diets free of artificial colors, flavors, and preservatives difficult to follow. When families focus on healthy foods, use supplements wisely, and avoid exposure to artificial ingredients and environmental toxins, they often see remarkable improvements in mood, attention, and behavior, with a proportion of patients able to reduce reliance on stimulant medications.

Coffee and Other Caffeine-Containing Foods

Caffeine has demonstrated greater efficacy in improving attention than placebos but has not been shown to be as potent as prescription medications.[57-60] Some families find caffeine a useful substitute for stimulant medications. In addition to caffeine, green tea contains the amino acid theanine, which leads to a feeling of calm that can counteract the jitteriness a proportion of individuals experience with coffee.[61] Coffee and tea contain variable amounts of caffeine depending on growing conditions and preparation techniques. Side effects of caffeine include insomnia, jitteriness, anxiety, palpitations, panic attacks, and dehydration. Coffee can be addictive, and withdrawal symptoms include headaches and feeling irritable, sleepy, depressed, anxious, or fatigued. Withdrawal symptoms can occur with as little as 1 to 2 cups daily. Caffeinated sodas and energy drinks often contain artificial flavors, colors, and preservatives and are considered less appropriate choices than coffee or tea. Caffeine should not be used as a substitute for regular high-quality sleep.

Food Sensitivities

Approximately 6% to 10% of children have allergies or sensitivities to foods. In addition to classic allergies, a significant proportion of individuals are lactose intolerant and approximately 1% of individuals are sensitive to gluten. The most common food sensitivities are to wheat, corn, soy, milk products, eggs, tree nuts, shellfish, citrus, and peanuts. If sensitivities are suspected, families should be encouraged to keep a careful *food diary*. Blood testing, skin testing, biopsies (for gluten sensitivity), and elimination diets may be useful in some cases. However, allergy test results may be negative even in affected individuals because many reactions are not true allergies. Some studies have posited that the use of few foods or oligoantigenic diets may improve symptoms in more than half of children with ADHD.[62] An elimination diet typically removes all foods and artificial ingredients that commonly cause problems for at least 2 weeks before slowly reintroducing specific foods one at a time every 3 to 4 days while monitoring symptoms. Nutritional counseling to avoid deficiencies should be recommended if families pursue this option.

Organic or Not?

Products that contain the highest levels of pesticide contamination include apples, bell peppers, celery, cherries, imported grapes, nectarines, peaches, pears, potatoes, raspberries, spinach, and strawberries. Organic crops contain lower levels of pesticides and other agrochemical residues than nonorganic crops.[63] Children who regularly eat organic produce have lower levels of toxic pesticide chemicals than children who eat nonorganic produce.[64] As historical farming practices waned, mineral levels in fruits, vegetables, meat, and milk fell by up to 76% between 1940 and 1991.[65] Organic crops contain significantly more minerals and antioxidants than crops raised with petroleum-derived (so-called conventional) fertilizers.[66,67] Milk from cows that graze on grass (botanically diverse pasture) has higher levels of the essential omega-3 fatty acids than milk from cows fed grains such as corn.[60,68]

Mind-Body Therapies

Know Thy Self

Several studies have reported that children with ADHD tend to have deficits in central executive function and short-term working memory.[69,70] Accordingly, training in cognitive function and short-term memory may be useful for patients with ADHD.[71] A meta-analysis of 16 randomized controlled trials of cognitive training for children and adolescents with ADHD demonstrated significant improvements in working memory but not necessarily in other symptoms.[72]

Managing Stress and Emotional Self-Regulation

Learning to manage stress is an important lifelong skill. Major pediatric stressors include physical or sexual abuse; divorce; moving; parental loss of a job or house; serious health challenges; war; neighborhood violence; exposure to domestic violence; parental addiction, incarceration, deployment, or depression; and loss of a loved one. Stress interferes with concentration and self-discipline. Numerous successful strategies for managing stress are available and may be common sense or require training and practice or professional counseling.

Common Sense Stress Management

Common sense strategies include preventive strategies, such as practicing gratitude (counting blessings), and in-the-moment strategies, such as taking a deep breath and counting to 10 before reacting impulsively. Learning to understand one's own triggers, strengths, and weaknesses is also helpful in proactively planning how to manage stressful situations, such as tests, conflicts, running late, or losing something. Rehearsing an anticipated event can help decrease the stress of the actual experience (Table 7.2). For example, at a calm time, a parent and child may imagine how to handle a situation in which a teacher asks the child to hand in homework and the child

TABLE 7.2 Stress Management Strategies

Common Sense

Gratitude. Develop the habit of listing three things you are grateful for before meals or bed.

Count on it. Count to 10 before reacting.

Identify your early warning signs: tight muscles, faster breathing, red face, clenched hands, and tight jaw.

Know yourself. Plan activities based on whether you are a morning person or a night owl and a visual or auditory learner.

Plan ahead. Being organized and consistent reduces stress.

Reflect. Develop the daily practice of reflecting on what went well and what could be improved.

Rehearse. Anticipate difficult situations and rehearse or role play before the situation.

Formal Practices, Often Learned with a Teacher or Trainer

Sitting meditation (concentration or mindfulness types)

Moving meditation (e.g., yoga, tai chi, qi gong)

Other Practices, Often Best Learned with Professional Coaching

Biofeedback

Autogenic training, guided imagery

is unable to find it in his backpack. What can he do to *prevent* this from happening? If it does happen, how can he *handle* it in a way that is respectful to him, his teacher, his classmates, and his parents? Learning how to anticipate and manage problems proactively is a critical skill that requires practice and effective coaching. *Timing* in training and problem-solving is important, too. Night owls may wish to save perplexing problems until later in the day, whereas morning people (larks) may wish to get up earlier to tackle challenging tasks. *Reflecting* on the day's events after the heat of the moment can also help children learn to identify negative patterns and create opportunities for meeting challenges.

Meditation

Meditation improves attention, stability, creativity, and mental clarity and reduces errors, aggressiveness, anxiety, and depression, particularly in the presence of stress or distractions. Meditation leads to calm coherence with more focused electroencephalographic (EEG) patterns.[73,74] Regular meditation practice changes cortical blood flow and increases the size of areas dealing with attention, focus, planning, emotional self-regulation, and mood.[75-80]

Just as many forms of sport improve physical fitness, many kinds of meditation improve attention and reduce stress reactivity. Just as some kinds of sports involve rackets, bats, or balls, meditation can be performed with eyes open or closed, while sitting still or moving, in silence or not, while visualizing or not, and alone or in groups. *Concentration-based* meditation practices involve focusing on a word, sound, object, idea, emotion (e.g., gratitude), or movement. When other thoughts, sensations, or emotions arise, they are gently placed aside and the mind returns to its object of concentration. Students who practice concentration-types of meditation reportedly have fewer problems with absenteeism and suspension for behavioral problems,[81] less distractibility and better creativity,[82] and better cognitive function and grades.[83,84] *Mindfulness* meditation is the moment-to-moment practice of nonjudgmental awareness of sensations, thoughts, emotions, and experiences; when the mind wanders to past or future concerns, it is also gently returned to the present. Studies in school settings have demonstrated that mindfulness-based meditation training can improve attention, emotions, and behavior, with students having fewer fights and improved grades.[85-91] For hyperactive patients, types of meditation that involve movement, such as yoga, tai chi, or qi gong, may be more appropriate than sitting meditation.[24,92] Regular practice reduces test anxiety and improves academic achievement, with those who practice the most reaping the greatest rewards.[93,94]

> Regular meditation practice changes cortical blood flow and increases the size of cortical regions dealing with attention, focus, planning, emotional self-regulation, and mood.

The need for formal training and the intensity, duration, and frequency of practice vary. Some clinicians undertake specific training and certification to provide specific kinds of meditation training (e.g., mindfulness-based stress reduction, mindfulness-based cognitive-behavioral therapy, or dialectical behavior therapy). Nevertheless, it is prudent to ask about a provider's training and experience in case of the absence of consistent state or national certification for mind-body training. As with other clinicians, look for those who are welcoming, warm, empathetic, and show genuine interest in people, not just in their favorite techniques. The most effective teachers and trainers offer steadfast acceptance and positive regard. They also create an atmosphere of safety and trust while fostering independence and acknowledging the strengths and capacities of students.

Just as national guidelines recommend 30 to 60 minutes daily of physical exercise to maintain physical health, recommendations for meditation practice typically range from just a few minutes for young children to 10 minutes twice daily for school-age children to 40 to 60 minutes daily for older adolescents and adults.

Biofeedback

EEG biofeedback (neurofeedback) has been shown to significantly improve behavior, attention, and intelligence quotient (IQ) scores.[95-104] In fact, neurofeedback can be as effective as standard therapies, even for children with Asperger's syndrome and those with mental retardation.[100,105–109] The majority of studies provided at least 20 to 40 EEG biofeedback training sessions with a professional trainer. EEG biofeedback training develops a particular skill. Unlike medications, whose effects stop when the pills stop, EEG biofeedback training benefits can be expected to persist if the skill is mastered and practice continues.

Typical costs range from $75 to $200 per session; however, insurance reimbursement for neurofeedback varies. The majority of professionals who offer EEG biofeedback are psychologists, therefore, their professional services may be covered by insurance. Despite promising preliminary evidence, neurofeedback remains controversial.[110]

> Neurofeedback shows promising results as an active treatment where the child learns skills rather than relying on medications or supplements that are passive and whose effects disappear on treatment cessation.

Professional Counseling

The results of large studies indicate that, at least in the short term, the most effective treatment for children with ADHD is an integrated strategy including both behavioral therapy and stimulant medication.[2,111,112] Cognitive-behavioral therapy can be particularly useful in helping patients learn to question assumptions and thoughts underlying negative emotions. Given all the negative feedback patients with ADHD commonly receive regarding their behavior and academic performance, it is not surprising that they frequently internalize many of these messages and develop low self-esteem. Negative self-labels are occasionally projected onto others, thus leading to blaming and oppositional behavior. By recognizing, questioning, and transforming negative self-talk, one can build confidence, self-esteem, and problem-solving capacities. Professional counseling may also be helpful for those who have comorbidities, such as anxiety, depression, ODD, or CD, or for chaotic families where parents may not be effective role models. Psychological or neuropsychological testing has utility in identifying children with specific learning disabilities, thus allowing specific educational accommodations in school. For adults with ADHD, "metacognitive" therapy can help teach skills, such as time management, organization, and planning. This type of training promotes significant improvements in daily life skills and job performance.[113] Although professional counseling takes more time to be effective compared to medication, the skills learned in behavioral therapy can provide long-term and lasting benefits.[114]

Social Relationships

Effective communication is key to developing positive social relationships. Most children want to win the approval of their parents and teachers, and receiving frequent criticism, punishment, and negative feedback can be very disheartening. Parents are also often frustrated, confused, discouraged, angry, feel helpless, or consider themselves ineffective parents. This can generate a cycle of maladaptive patterns with high levels of criticism, negative expectations, and negative emotions. Helping families break this cycle can be one of the most beneficial treatments for ADHD. Several common sense steps to do so are summarized in *Transforming the Difficult Child: The Nurtured Heart Approach* by Howard Glasser and Jennifer Easley.[115]

1. Take a strengths-based approach to communication. Recognize the child's strengths and where possible, reframe negative labels or challenges as positive opportunities or gifts (Table 7.3).
2. Identify clear, specific rules with achievable, measurable behaviors and clear time-linked consequences. In behavioral pediatrics, this is referred to as a SMART plan: Specific, Measurable, Achievable, Relevant, and

TABLE 7.3 Reframing Labels

Negative Label	Reframed as a Positive
Hyper	Exuberant, vigorous
Distractible	Aware of details that others miss
Spacey	Rich inner life
Driven by a motor	Energetic
Off task	Creative
Impulsive	Eager, enthusiastic, willing
Inattentive	Listening to a different drummer
Poor concentration	Flexibly aware of changes in the environment
Accident-prone	Fearless

Timely. For example, "start to get ready for bed by brushing your teeth at 8 pm" is more specific, measurable, and timely than "go to bed soon." "Spend 15 minutes studying spelling words before 4 pm" is more timely than, "you'll have to work harder on homework."

3. Frame rules in positive terms. For example, "please play with your toys in your bedroom," is more positive than "don't leave your toys in the kitchen."
4. Make accommodations for learning challenges. If it's easier for the child to pay attention when sitting in front of the classroom, ask for those seating arrangements. If the child cannot remember to bring books home, ask for a second set of books for home. If the child has learning problems, ask for educational accommodations such as more time for tests. If he or she forgets his or her assignments, ask that the teacher communicate them directly to the parent. Recognize that children with ADHD are generally trying their best and make accommodations to help them succeed.[116] These can be part of a standard 504 educational plan.
5. Break it down. Rather than asking a young child to "set the table" or "put plates, silverware, glasses, and napkins out," start with just one request, such as "put a plate at each person's place at the kitchen table." When that task is done, give positive feedback and then say, "Thank you! That's so helpful. Now put out the forks." As the child's memory and capacity improve, you can increase the number of steps or the complexity of the request.
6. Anticipate that the child will test the rules. Testing rules and limits is how children establish a sense of cause and effect, trust, and reliability. This is normal and can be expected. For example, if you ask a child who dislikes peas to "eat his peas," he may well leave a few (or many) on the plate to find out exactly what you mean. Or he may bargain ("what if I eat all the carrots and leave some peas?"), rationalize ("I shouldn't have to eat peas since I had a salad") compare ("Suzy didn't eat all of HER peas"), distract ("look at Dad" while feeding peas to the dog), or sabotage (roughly reaching for something and spilling the plate on the floor). It may be helpful to practice or rehearse a few of these scenarios in clinic in a playful way to help families anticipate how to handle these common situations when they arise in the heat of the moment.
7. Give positive feedback frequently and negative feedback neutrally. This practice will help counter the pattern of criticism and sense of failure that are all too common among families confronted with ADHD. "Catch them being good" is a cornerstone of behavioral pediatrics. It is easy to pick on the faults, failures, and lapses. This is not to say that problems should be ignored, but instead make sure there is a balance of at least three praises for every one correction. Help parents rehearse corrective language, too. "We all make mistakes. How do you imagine handling it next time Johnny forgets his homework?"

The benefits of nurturing behavioral strategies can be more profound and long-lasting than medications. For example, when the Tolson School in Tucson began applying this approach, they found a sharp decline in discipline problems, improved test scores, and a decrease in the number of students requiring special education (from 31 students to 7 students), with just 2 out of 519 students requiring medications for ADHD.[116]

Social support is useful for most families managing chronic conditions such as ADHD. National support groups usually have local chapters with ongoing support and local resources. See Key Web Resources for the URL of key social support groups that include *All Kinds of Minds (AKOM)*, *The National Federation of Families of Children's Mental Health*, *Learning Disabilities Association of America (LDA)*, and *Mental Health America*.

Alliance With Schools

Clinicians should help teachers and school administrators recognize the child's unique gifts and challenges. Families should schedule regular meetings with their child's teachers to monitor progress and advocate for seating arrangements that put the child near the front of the classroom. Encourage families to advocate for the child to receive the public services to which he or she is legally entitled. According to the 1999 addendum to the U.S. Individuals with Disability Education Act (IDEA), children and youth whose disabilities adversely affect their educational performance should receive special services or accommodations that address their problem (i.e., ADHD) and its effects. Section 504 of the U.S. Vocational Rehabilitation Act prohibits discrimination against any person with a disability. Under Section 504, students may receive services such as a smaller class sizes, tutoring, modification of homework assignments, help with organizing, and other assistance.

If the patient has not received sufficient services or accommodation within 6 months of asking the teacher or principal, write to the school district's director or chairperson for special educational services. The letter should specifically request an evaluation for specific learning disabilities and a functional assessment to determine how the disabilities are affecting the child's classroom performance. These evaluations are required to develop an Individual Educational Plan (IEP) or a 504 Accommodation Plan. Middle school and high school students diagnosed with ADHD are also entitled to these evaluations and, if appropriate, an IEP or accommodation plan. With an IEP, the child may qualify for extra help, special classes, extra time for tests or projects, an extra set of books for home study, permission to take notes on a computer keyboard rather than by hand, extra breaks in the day, fewer classes, and other accommodations, such as support teachers and administrators who offer creative, effective strategies to promote children's strengths.

Encourage parents to try other activities that explore the child's interests, talents, and possible lifelong passions or vocations. When choosing activities, consider the adult-child ratio. Music, art, tutoring, and individual language lessons may offer more individual attention than soccer leagues. Look for consistency. A class that meets every Tuesday is easier to schedule and attend than a sports team that has inconsistent practice and game schedules requiring frequent changes in the family driving routine.

Environment

Increasing time in nature may help soothe irritable children and adults, allow room for exploratory and creative play, and build on innate strengths and skills. Encourage families to reduce electronic screen time to less than 2 hours daily. Ask, advise, and assist families in reducing or eliminating exposure to tobacco smoke and help adults learn to be better role models when managing stress (i.e., not using alcohol or drugs). Remind families to use proper safety equipment (e.g., seat belts, helmets). Reduce the use of pesticides at home and in schools. Consider using music as a way of reinforcing positive behavior, a learning strategy (songs with rhymes to assist in memorization), and a way to influence the environment subtly to cue wake up times and bedtimes. Encourage families to use calendars and posted schedules to promote structure and predictability for the day, week, and month (Table 7.4).

BIOCHEMICAL THERAPIES

Botanicals & Dietary Supplements

Melatonin

Melatonin does not improve daytime symptoms of ADHD but can help improve sleep, particularly for shift workers and those with delayed sleep phase syndrome.[117-120] The typical adult dose of melatonin is 0.3 to 5 mg taken 1 hour before the desired bedtime. However, melatonin is not a substitute for a healthy sleep routine. One study followed children with ADHD who had started taking melatonin as part of a clinical trial on sleep. At nearly 4 years later, more than two thirds of children were still using melatonin as they reported it helpful with no serious side effects.[121]

Calming Herbs

Historically, certain varieties of herbs have been used to promote calm and decrease agitation; however, none can replace a healthy lifestyle. Calming herbs, such as chamomile, hops, kava, lavender, lemon balm, passionflower, and valerian, may promote sleep but are not usually helpful for calming daytime hyperactivity, inattentiveness, or impulsivity.[122]

Other Herbs

Coffee and tea containing caffeine are natural stimulants. Green tea also contains theanine, which can be calming and thereby offset some of the unpleasant side effects of caffeine.[123-125] Caffeine helps enhance attention and promotes positive cognitive performance in both children and adults.[126-129] To minimize the risk of insomnia due to caffeine, caffeinated beverages should not be consumed within 6 hours of the planned bedtime. No controlled trials have demonstrated significant benefits for other commonly used stimulant herbs, such as ginseng, for ADHD. A pilot study from Italy indicated that ginkgo may help improve ADD symptoms.[130] A Canadian product (AD-fX) that combines ginseng and ginkgo benefitted patients with ADHD or dyslexia in one manufacturer-sponsored study.[131] Similarly, pycnogenol or European pine bark extract was significantly better than placebo in improving concentration and decreasing hyperactivity in children in several European studies funded in part by pycnogenol producers.[132-134] Neither evening primrose oil (which contains gamma-linoleic acid, GLA) nor St. John's wort supplements have greater efficacy than placebo in treating ADHD. Variations in the quality of herbal products and the paucity of research studies indicate further studies and product standardization are required before the routine administration of these products (Table 7.5).

Pharmaceuticals

In the United States, stimulant medications combined with behavioral therapy comprise the first-line treatment for young individuals with ADHD, although the long-term effectiveness of this therapeutic regime remains unclear.[2,112,135,136] The British National Institute for

---

TABLE 7.4   Environmental Dos and Don'ts

Do

Spend more time in nature.

Be more mindful of use of music to calm, focus, and reinforce behavior.

Use clocks, calendars, and lists to organize time.

Post schedules, chore charts, and other tools to organize activities and expectations.

Use proper safety equipment (e.g., bike helmets and seat belts).

Don't

Spend more than 2 hours in front of electronic devices daily.

Spend time around tobacco smoke.

Model the use of alcohol or drugs as skillful stress management strategies.

TABLE 7.5   Herbs as Additional Therapy

Calming Herbs

Tea: chamomile, hops, lemon balm, passionflower

Valerian: tincture, glycerite, or capsule

Aromatherapy: chamomile, lavender

Avoid kava because of concerns about hepatotoxicity

Stimulant Herbs

Coffee

Tea: black and green

Ginseng or ginseng/ginkgo combination

Other Herbs

Pycnogenol (pine bark extract, also known as OPC): benefits shown in small, industry-funded studies

Evening primrose oil: ineffective in a randomized controlled trial

St. John's wort: ineffective in a randomized controlled trial

Health and Clinical Excellence (NICE) guidelines for treating ADHD recommend stimulant medications as a first-line therapy for adults with ADHD, but only for children with severe symptoms and not mild or moderate ADHD.[137] Initially, stimulants (which are classified as controlled substances) benefit approximately two thirds of patients. Stimulant medications typically do not improve oppositional or defiant behaviors, or overall quality of life; however, their adverse effects on appetite, sleep, and growth require ongoing monitoring. Research conducted by scientists without conflicts of interest (unlike previous studies in which investigators occasionally received payments from pharmaceutical companies) have reported that stimulants have limited additional efficacy compared to placebo.[138]

> The National Institute of Clinical Excellence (NICE) recommends stimulant medications only for children with severe symptoms and not those with mild to moderate ADHD.

Stimulant medications include short-acting (3 to 6 hours), medium-acting (4 to 8 hours), and long-acting (more than 8 hours) methylphenidates (Ritalin, Methylin, Metadate, Concerta, and Quillivant), dexmethylphenidate (Focalin), methylphenidate transdermal patches (Daytrana), and amphetamines (Adderall, Dexedrine, and Vyvanse). As with coffee, the effects of the majority of stimulants are observed after approximately 20 minutes (Table 7.6).

Nonstimulant medications used to treat ADHD include atomoxetine (Strattera), clonidine (Catapres, extended-release Kapvay), guanfacine (Tenex and extended-release Intuniv), bupropion (Wellbutrin), and other antihypertensives and antidepressants. Atomoxetine is the most commonly prescribed nonstimulant medication for ADHD and has been shown to be significantly superior to placebo in improving the ability to focus, to be organized, and to regulate attention and emotions, in addition to enhancing short-term memory in adults.[139] Atomoxetine has also been shown to be beneficial in children with ADHD; however, side effects such as sleepiness and decreased appetite have limited its wider use.[140] In addition to having limited efficacy in a proportion of patients, stimulant medications have several limitations:

1. *Side effects.* The most common side effects of stimulant medications are decreased appetite, poor growth, and insomnia. Less common side effects include nausea, headaches, stomachaches, sweating, jitteriness, tics, dizziness, a racing heart, and, paradoxically, drowsiness. Of greater concern, stimulant use may be linked to psychosis, hallucinations, heart arrhythmias, and sudden death.[141,142]

2. *Failure to work when not taken.* Medications do not represent a cure for ADHD. Medications will not work when a dose is missed or if patients stop taking their medication. More than half of patients with ADHD stop taking stimulant medication without being advised to do so by their physician.[143,144]

3. *Reliance on medications.* Patients may rely on these agents instead of making healthy changes in lifestyle and environment.

4. *Long-term costs.* Continuous dependence on medications is costly for individuals and society. An estimated 3.5% of U.S. children received stimulant medication in 2008, up from 2.4% in 1996. Over the period of 1996 to 2008, stimulant use increased consistently at an overall annual growth rate of 3.4%.[145] In terms of the overall costs of medications, of the top five drugs prescribed for children, three were medications for ADHD.

5. *Long-term effects.* The effects of long-term medication use or of the concurrent use of multiple medications are unknown. Although stimulant medications have been used for decades, no long-term studies have eval-

TABLE 7.6 Short-, Medium-, and Long-Acting Stimulant Medications for Attention Deficit Hyperactivity Disorder

Short (3–6 hours)	Medium (4–8 hours)	Long (>8 hours)
Ritalin (methylphenidate) 5, 10, 20 mg bid or tid	Ritalin LA (methylphenidate long acting) 10, 20, 30, 40, 60 mg daily	Concerta (methylphenidate) 18, 27, 36, 54 mg daily
Methylin (methylphenidate) 2.5, 5, 10 mg, or 5, 10 mg/5 mL bid or tid		Focalin XR (dexmethylphenidate extended release) 5, 10, 15, 20, 25, 30, 35, 40 mg daily
Focalin (dexmethylphenidate) 2.5, 5, 10 mg bid	Metadate CD (methylphenidate extended release) 10, 20, 30, 40, 50, 60 mg daily	Daytrana (methylphenidate patch) 10, 15, 20, 30 mg daily
	Metadate ER (methylphenidate extended release) 20 mg daily to bid	Adderall XR (amphetamine/dexamphetamine extended release) 5, 10, 15, 20, 25, 30 mg daily
Adderall (amphetamine/ dexamphetamine) 5, 7.5, 10, 12.5, 15, 20, 30 mg daily to bid		Quillivant XR (methylphenidate–liquid) 5 mg/mL
		Vyvanse (lisdexamfetamine) 10, 20, 30, 40, 50, 60, 70 mg daily

bid, twice daily; tid, three times daily.

uated the developmental impact of using these medications daily for 30 years. Short-term use has been evaluated for one drug at a time; however, the impact of taking multiple medications simultaneously remains unknown.

Misuse, diversion, and abuse. As the number of prescriptions for stimulant medications has grown, so has the number of reports that these drugs are being diverted or sold to people who do not have ADHD. A 2009 study reported a 76% increase in the number of calls to Poison Control Centers related to adolescent abuse of prescription ADHD medications.[146]

Given these concerns regarding stimulant medications, many pediatricians do not provide prescriptions for stimulant medications without first conducting *N*-of-1 trials to determine the short-term benefits and risks for individual patients. Such trials can be repeated annually to assess the ongoing need for such medications.

Therapies to Consider

Massage, Chiropractic, Acupuncture, and Osteopathy

Scientific studies support the regular use of massage for improving ADHD symptoms.[147-149] Massage affects blood flow and neurotransmitters involved in focus and clarity.[150,151] Massage also reduces stress, improves mood, decreases pain, and alleviates anxiety, all of which can improve concentration, deliberation, and self-discipline.[152-154] Even a 15-minute chair massage has been shown to improve speed and accuracy on standard tests.[155] Additional studies are required to determine the best type of massage, the duration and frequency of treatments, and whether massage provided by friends or family members has similar effectiveness to care provided by a licensed professional.

Aside from case reports, there are few studies evaluating the effectiveness of chiropractic adjustments in improving ADHD symptoms. There are insufficient studies to recommend chiropractic as a front-line treatment for ADHD.[156] There is also insufficient data to recommend acupuncture as a proven strategy to address ADHD.[157] The results of one small study in 2014 indicated osteopathic manipulative therapy may improve some test scores in children with ADHD compared to standard treatment.[158]

Massage is safe when common sense precautions are used, such as avoiding massage over rashes, infections, bruises, or burns. Do not force massage therapy on patients who have suffered physical or sexual abuse or who are particularly shy. The wishes of adolescents for privacy should also be respected. In the United States, massage therapists are licensed or certified as health professionals in 40 states and licensed by cities or counties elsewhere. Licensed professionals in the United States can be found through the American Massage Therapy Association's Locator Service.

PREVENTION PRESCRIPTION

- Advise pregnant women to stop smoking and avoid drinking alcohol.
- Advise parents not to smoke around their children and to limit exposure to television and pesticides.
- Encourage families to live a healthy lifestyle focusing on the following: a whole foods diet that limits intake of artificial colors, flavors, sweeteners, and preservatives and foods that cause

sensitivity reactions and that avoids deficiencies of essential omega-3 fatty acids, amino acids, vitamins, and minerals; daily physical activity, preferably outdoors in natural surroundings; adequate sleep; effective stress and emotional self-management; strength-based communication skills and participation in supportive community networks; and a safe, structured, well-organized environment.

THERAPEUTIC REVIEW

ACCURATE DIAGNOSIS

Use standard rating scales, such as the Vanderbilt Parent and Teacher Rating Scales, to assess ADHD symptoms and response to interventions.

Rule out medical and neuropsychological conditions that impair attention and self-discipline, such as hypothyroidism and vision, hearing, and specific learning deficits. Consider requesting a neuropsychological examination to assess IQ and learning difficulties.

ENCOURAGING HEALTHY HABITS IN A HEALTHY HABITAT

Dietary

Assess diet and correct nutritional deficiencies with an improved diet or dietary supplements.

Encourage patients to maintain a steady blood glucose level by eating regular meals with low glycemic index foods. Foods containing artificial colors, sweet-

eners, flavors, and preservatives should be avoided, as should foods with heavy contamination with pesticides.

Instruct patients to avoid dehydration.

Consider recommending coffee or tea as mild dietary stimulants and monitoring for insomnia and other common side effects.

Sleep and Activity

Promote adequate sleep with sleep hygiene. Consider melatonin (0.3 to 3 mg an hour before bed) or sedative herbal remedies (a cup of chamomile tea or lavender aromatherapy) as a first-line approach to improving sleep.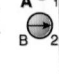

Encourage vigorous daily activity, at least 30 minutes daily of activity vigorous enough to break a sweat or make it difficult to talk and move at the same time.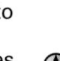

Stress Management and Emotional Self-Management Skills

Assess stress management and emotional self-management skills.

Counsel families regarding stress management.

Consider referral for meditation training, including moving meditation practices such as yoga and tai chi. Consider referral for effective counseling and cognitive-behavioral therapy.

Social Support

Refer families to support networks of other families such as Children and Adults with Attention Deficit Hyperactivity Disorder (CHADD).

Encourage positive family communication, focusing on goals rather than problems. Help families view overall long-term goals in terms of short-term achievable objectives and learn to make specific, measurable, achievable, relevant, time-specific (SMART) plans, including ways to celebrate success.

Consider referring families for additional support for parenting, strengths-based communication, and discipline skills, as well as time management and organizational skill development.

Healthy Environment

Advocate for appropriate testing and learning accommodations at school.

Referral for Additional Professional Assistance

Consider referral to a psychologist for neurofeedback.

Consider a referral for massage therapy.

Pharmaceutical Management

Remember that 65% of individuals do respond to stimulant medication, at least initially.

Consider recommending an *N*-of-1 trial of a stimulant medication, comparing a low dose (e.g., 2.5 to 5 mg methylphenidate twice daily) and a middle dose (5 to 10 mg twice daily) with placebo for 1 week each.

If patients report improvement, consider switching to a longer-acting medication to reduce the number of pills or doses required daily.

Monitor and Support Families With Regular Follow-up Every 3 to 4 Months

---

Key Web Resources

Rating Scales

Vanderbilt Teacher Rating

Vanderbilt Parent Rating Scale

http://www.brightfutures.org/mentalhealth/pdf/professionals/bridges/adhd.pdf

http://www.vanderbiltchildrens.org/uploads/documents/DIAGNOSTIC_PARENT_RATING_SCALE(1).pdf

Activity

U.S. Centers for Disease Control & Prevention

ABC for Fitness. Activity bursts in the classroom

http://www.cdc.gov/healthyyouth/physicalactivity/

http://www.davidkatzmd.com/abcforfitness.aspx

Diet

Feingold diet

Nutrition information from the Center for Science in the Public Interest

Food pesticide levels from Environmental Working Group

www.feingold.org.

http://www.cspinet.org/

http://www.foodnews.org/

Support Groups

All Kinds of Minds (AKOM)

Children and Adults with Attention Deficit Hyperactivity Disorder (CHADD)

The National Federation for Families of Children's Mental Health

Learning Disabilities Association of America (LDA)

Mental Health America

www.allkindsofminds.org

www.chadd.org

www.ffcmh.org

https://ldaamerica.org/

www.nmha.org

Environment

Collaborative on Health and the Environment

National Environmental Education Foundation's Children and Nature Initiative

http://healthandenvironment.org/

http://www.neefusa.org/health/children_nature.htm

Biofeedback

Association for Applied Psychophysiology and Biofeedback

www.aapb.org

Massage

American Massage Therapy Association

www.amtamassage.org

REFERENCES

References are available online at ExpertConsult.com.

CHAPTER 8

AUTISM SPECTRUM DISORDER

John W. Harrington, MD • Samudragupta Bora, PhD

Autism spectrum disorder (ASD) and autism are now used interchangeably in research literature; however, ASD emphasizes that this disorder is based on a continuum of neurodevelopmental problems characterized by deficits in social communication and interactions in addition to restrictive and repetitive patterns of behaviors, interests, and activities.[1] Recently published data from the Centers for Disease Control and Prevention (CDC) demonstrate that autism continues to increase in prevalence, with 1 in 68 children now affected. Because boys are more commonly affected than girls, at a ratio of 4:1, this translates to 1:42 boys and 1:189 girls diagnosed with an ASD by age 8 in the United States of America.[2] Recent estimates from the United States and the United Kingdom suggest that the average lifetime costs associated with ASD are remarkably high ($1.4 million–$2.4 million in 2011), not accounting for the hidden costs to families.[3] With approximately 1%–2% of the population being affected by ASD, clinicians, public health, and research experts agree that understanding of the factors underlying the increased prevalence of ASD is an urgent matter. Three major hypotheses still prevail to some extent: a true increase in prevalence; heightened awareness and therefore earlier diagnosis; and the criteria used to define autism are too subjective, leading to "diagnostic substitution" with other disorders. This final hypothesis was possibly ameliorated with the release of the *Diagnostic and Statistical Manual of Mental Disorders*, Fifth Edition (DSM-5) in May of 2013.[4] The DSM-5 merges communication and social interaction behaviors into one symptom category and increases the importance of repetitive and restrictive behavior regarding the requirements for a diagnosis of an ASD (Table 8.1). In addition, unlike the DSM-IV, the DSM-5 allows the diagnosis of co-occurring diagnoses, such as attention-deficit/hyperactivity disorder (ADHD), with ASD. The impact of these changes on the diagnostic criteria for ASD has not been fully realized, making it difficult to predict the potential effect on the incidence of ASD over time. Some experts believe the new criteria will exert a downward pressure on the prevalence of ASD[5]; however, new prevalence data from the CDC monitoring networks, which review data from both schools and clinicians, may provide better information regarding the true incidence of ASD and is expected to be reported again in 2016.

PREVALENCE, CHARACTERISTICS, AND GUIDELINES FOR COMPLEMENTARY AND ALTERNATIVE MEDICINE THERAPIES IN AUTISM

More than 3000 patients in the autism treatment network completed a complementary and alternative medicine (CAM) usage survey, with 28% of patients reported to use CAM and 17% using special diets overall.[6] Rates of CAM usage were higher in children with more severe ASD, those diagnosed at an earlier age, and those with seizures or gastrointestinal symptoms.[6] In a separate study by Akins et al., no significant difference in CAM use was observed between ASD and developmental disability.[7] However, a higher level of parental education was associated with increased CAM usage, and families who used > 20 hours per week of conventional services were more likely to use CAM. Clinicians should be aware that families who use CAM are likely to use more than one CAM treatment, and children using CAM should be monitored for possible treatment interactions.[8] Interestingly, CAM treatments are viewed as safe by parents because they are perceived as natural.[9] Unfortunately, while the search for a consistent etiology or cure for autism continues, therapies that extend beyond educational and behavioral interventions are readily contemplated by parents hoping to help their child with autism. In addition, because many comorbidities are associated with ASD, children are often referred to CAM for the treatment of ADHD, oppositional defiant disorder, repetitive and restricted behaviors, depression, and anxiety.

It is important for parents and practitioners to have a framework from which to work from when considering and discussing the safety of CAM therapies. Following is a table that highlights the guidelines parents should review (Table 8.2). Table 8.3 provides an ethics and advice table first produced by Cohen et al.[10] that may inform practitioners and health care providers when counseling parents regarding the use of a CAM therapy.

PATHOPHYSIOLOGY

Genetic/Environmental/Epigenetics

Many genetic disorders and syndromes have been shown to have strong associations with autism, including Angelman, Down, Fragile X, and Williams syndromes in addition to tuberous sclerosis and neurofibromatosis.[11] In addition, increasingly refined genetic techniques, such as comparative genomic hybridization microarrays, whole genome linkage, and gene association studies, have allowed researchers to identify numerous chromosomal regions with specific single nucleotide polymorphisms or copy number variants that may be associated with autism.[12] However, even with these developments in genetic testing, the likelihood that a primary care provider will be able to test and uncover a significant genetic finding reportedly remains less than 20%.[13] The vast majority

TABLE 8.1 Comparison of Changes Between the DSM-IV and DSM-5 for ASD

DSM-IV for Autism	DSM-5 Changes for ASD
1. Rett disorder	1. Rett disorder is removed as it is considered a genetic disease
2. Pervasive developmental disorder-not otherwise specified, Asperger disorder, and childhood disintegrative disorder	2. These three disorders will now officially be termed autism spectrum disorder
3. Unusual sensory behaviors not part of the criteria	3. Unusual sensory behaviors will be added to the criteria
4. 3 symptom categories (impairment in social interaction, impairment in communication, and repetitive and restrictive behaviors)	4. Two symptom categories (deficits in social communication and social interaction combined, repetitive and restrictive behaviors) but more criteria required per category

ASD, autism spectrum disorder; DSM-IV, Diagnostic and Statistical Manual of Mental Disorders, 4th edition; DSM-5, Diagnostic and Statistical Manual of Mental Disorders, 5th edition.

TABLE 8.2 Guidelines for Parents Interested in Starting CAM Therapies

1. Research the medication or therapy and try and find out safety and efficacy
2. Isolate the behavior you hope to improve in your child
3. Start only one new treatment at a time
4. Understand that all children with autism will improve in their development over time
5. Children may naturally have good and bad weeks regardless of treatment
6. Observe other confounding factors that may affect outcome (life transitions, new infant, vacation, etc.)
7. Assess poor sleep and improve sleep hygiene before CAM trial if possible

CAM, complementary and alternative medicine.
Reproduced from Harrington JW, Allen K. The clinician's guide to autism. *Pediatr Rev.* 2014;35(2):62-78; quiz 78.

TABLE 8.3 Ethical 2 by 2 Table

Safe	Effective	
	Yes	No
Yes	Use/recommend	Tolerate
No	Monitor closely	Advise against

Reproduced from Cohen MH, Kemper KJ, Stevens L, Hashimoto D, Gilmour J. Pediatric use of complementary therapies: ethical and policy choices. *Pediatrics.* 2005;116(4):e568-575.

of cases of ASD are presumed to be caused by an underlying genetic predisposition and interplay between the genetic code and environmental factors, referred to as the *epigenetics of autism*.[14,15] One of the largest, longitudinal, population-based studies to date, involving 1.6 million families, revealed that genetic and environmental factors contribute equally to the development of ASD, with the relative risk of autism directly correlated with increasing genetic relatedness.[16] There are currently multiple studies being conducted evaluating these environmental risks: the Study to Explore Early Development (SEED),[17] the Childhood Autism Risk Factors from Genetics and Environment (CHARGE) study,[18] the Early Autism Risk Longitudinal Investigation (EARLI),[19] and the Early Markers for Autism study (EMA).[20] Results from these studies have demonstrated factors that increase the risk of autism include prematurity, twins or multiple pregnancies, advanced maternal and paternal age at conception

and that folic acid supplementation in mothers may have a protective affect against having a child with autism.[18,19]

> The vast majority of ASD is presumed to be caused by an underlying genetic predisposition and the interplay between the genetic code with environmental factors, referred to as the *epigenetics of autism*.

Unfortunately, without a consistent genetic or biologic marker for autism, common procedures and practices, such as vaccines, were wrongly considered to have a causal link with autism. Several hundred studies have since proven that autism and vaccines have only a temporal association with no causal link with autism demonstrated. The recent outbreak of measles at Disneyland in 2015, affecting predominately unvaccinated or undervaccinated children, clearly highlights the problems that can be wrought in public health when parents neglect the immunization of their child and clinicians, along with media, fail to practice according to evidenced-based guidelines.

Neuroimaging Findings

Autism remains a disorder defined by its clinical presentation. However, there is growing information from postmortem and neuroimaging studies highlighting the role of brain abnormalities in the pathogenesis of ASD, although a clear description of the phenotypic neuropathology remains lacking. Alterations in brain structural development, primarily in the frontal and temporal lobes, cerebellum, amygdala, and hippocampus, have consistently been reported. A recent meta-analysis of 16 whole-brain voxel-based morphometric studies, pooling data from 277 ASD patients and 307 healthy controls, found alterations in the lateral occipital lobe, pericentral region, medial temporal lobe, basal ganglia, and the insula/parietal operculum in ASD patients.[21] Similarly, a separate meta-analysis of 20 studies, comprising 497 patients with ASD and 471 healthy controls, confirmed alterations of brain structures related to social cognition in patients with autism.[22] Although no statistically significant difference in global gray matter volumes between ASD patients and controls was observed in this meta-analysis, regional alterations with markedly lower gray matter volumes were observed in the amygdala-hippocampus complex and the precuneus. Altered development and functioning of brain areas involved in face processing, verbal and nonverbal communication, and social interaction have been consistently reported by previous studies, although the nature of these alterations has yet to be elucidated. The discrepancies in the findings of these studies may be attributable to various factors, including small sample size, methodological differences in data acquisition and analysis across neuroimaging studies, effects of medication status, and heterogeneity among ASD patients in terms of etiology and symptom manifestation. Consistent with reported neuroimaging findings, postmortem studies of ASD patients have demonstrated focal cortical dysplasia and reduced gamma-aminobutyric acid-B ($GABA_B$) receptors in the cingulate cortex and fusiform gyrus, providing additional evidence indicating neuroanatomical alterations are associated with autism.[23,24] Finally, in addition to alterations in specific brain structures, abnormal brain size and volume has been observed in autism. Despite inconsistent findings between studies, a meta-analysis published in 2005 including all published studies at that time using a range of methodologies to estimate brain size from birth to age 65 years demonstrated early brain overgrowth during infancy and toddler years in children with ASD, followed by age-related decline in brain size.[25]

While the pathophysiology of ASD remains unknown, in addition to neuroanatomical abnormalities, studies have demonstrated metabolic abnormalities, including neurotransmitter, hormonal, and immune imbalance, in patients with autism. These changes will be briefly discussed in the following sections.

INTEGRATIVE THERAPY

Intensive Behavioral Therapy

Early diagnosis is the most important aspect of interventional therapy because every published study has demonstrated that earlier interventions in patients with autism are associated with improved outcomes. Intensive behavioral therapy, referred to as applied behavioral analysis or ABA, represents the only conventional therapy proven through evidence-based methods to marginally treat the core disorder of ASD.[26,27] ABA is a behavioral treatment approach designed to increase socially appropriate behavior and decrease the severity and/or emergence of challenging behaviors.[28] ABA focuses on teaching specific behaviors in a systematic manner in the context of repeated trials. ABA has utility in improving communication, social relatedness, and decreasing repetitive behaviors.[29] The ABA framework is used in other treatment modalities, such as Pivotal Response Training, Treatment and Education of Autistic and Related Communication Handicapped Children (TEACCH), and Developmental, Individual-Difference, Relationship based model (DIR)/Floortime[30-32] (see Key Web Resources). Many children with autism also receive conventional services, such as speech and language therapy, to address expressive and receptive language deficits and occupational therapy to address sensory integration issues commonly seen in autism. The use of additional or CAM therapies

is common in autism and requires an understanding of their genesis.

Understanding the Theoretical Gastrointestinal Link to Autism

Due to the frequency of gastrointestinal problems in autism, it is important for clinicians involved in the treatment of ASD to understand theories related to immune function and gut-brain theory, intestinal permeability, and dysbiosis.[33,34] The reported prevalence of gastrointestinal problems in children with autism ranges from 9%–91%, with abdominal pain and discomfort, constipation, diarrhea, and chronic diarrhea the most common complaints.[35-43] Because two-thirds of the human immune system is composed of gastrointestinal mucosal cells, this further implies immune dysfunction is associated with the documented inflammation in gastrointestinal biopsies from children with autism.[36] There have also been multiple reports of altered immune function in terms of cytokine function, T-cell abnormalities, and an augmented immune response in patients with autism.[44,45] Familial histories of autoimmune disorders have been reported in patients with autism,[46] along with maternal increases in autoantibodies directed at central nervous system proteins (an extension of the gut-brain theory) of their child with autism.[47-49]

Leaky Gut

Altered intestinal permeability ("leaky gut"), possibly in response to allergy or inflammatory response, may play a pathogenic role in autism. There have been several studies reporting impaired intestinal barrier function in autism.[50] In addition, Altieri et al. reported elevated levels of a bacterial product (p-cresol) in the urine of young children with autism versus controls.[51] Other studies have also shown that children with autism have higher concentrations of *Clostridia*, *Bacteroidetes*, and *Firmicutes* than controls.[52,53] This dysbiosis, or abnormalities of gastrointestinal microflora, is thought to be interrelated with intestinal permeability.[54] Nutritional factors may be inhibited from effective transport through the gastrointestinal tract and, in addition, interstitial permeability may allow active neuropeptides to move from the gastrointestinal tract into the bloodstream, have an end-organ effect on the brain, and contribute to the core symptoms of autism and possibly anxiety.[43,55]

Dietary/Lifestyle Treatments

Probiotics. The theoretical pathogenic model of ASD described previously endorses the use of probiotics to aid digestion and improve immune function. Probiotics have been found to influence the composition of microbiota, potentially improving intestinal barrier function and mucosal immune responses in children with autism. The restoration of the gut microbiota to normal levels using probiotics may have utility in reducing inflammation, restoring epithelial barrier function, and improving behavioral symptoms in children with ASD.[56] A recent study of plasma myeloperoxidase (MPO) levels in children with autism found probiotics decreased MPO levels and may affect the overall absorption properties of the gastrointestinal tract.[57] Unfortunately, no studies have conclusively demonstrated the benefits or dose response of probiotics that would allow practitioners to make standard recommendations for their use.[58] However, the use of probiotics has not been shown to have harmful effects, other than occasional diarrhea, and therefore are likely be well-tolerated if parents agree with their use.[59] The most commonly used probiotics are *Lactobacillus rhamnosus GG* and *Saccharomyces boulardii*. These probiotics are provided at many concentrations that range between 1 and 10 billion cells per oral daily dose.[60]

Gluten-Free, Casein-Free Diet. One of the most popular dietary treatments tried by parents is the combination of a gluten-free/casein-free diet (GFCF). The premise of this diet is centered on the theory of the "leaky gut," as previously described, whereby increased intestinal permeability allows gluten and casein peptides to leak from the gut and promote opioid activity resulting in ASD behaviors.[61] Interestingly, there does not appear to be an increased rate of celiac disease in patients with autism, nor has any consistent increase in opioids been observed in the urine of children with autism.[62,63] The most recent systematic review of studies including children with autism using the GFCF diet published between 1970 and 2013 concluded that there was no convincing evidence of benefit.[64] Although previous studies have reported mixed results, there is consensus that the potential risks related to maintaining a GFCF diet include low intake of calcium, vitamin D, and amino acids in addition to decreased bone density.[64] There were additional concerns regarding rice milk, almond milk, and potato milk as poor sources of protein. Previous studies have also reported high dropout rates and a significant proportion of participants being unable to maintain the diet, highlighting the difficulty in adhering to such a strict diet in children who already have restrictive dietary behaviors. At the population level, the GFCF diet may not have a beneficial effect; however, the majority of previously reported studies were not adequately powered to detect significant benefit effects on gastrointestinal disease between subgroups of children. If parents do wish to try their child or family on the GFCF diet, we suggest the following: consultation with a dietician to limit the risks of decreased protein and calcium intake; listing of current dietary and behavioral problems they wish to monitor; and setting a clear start and stop date, usually 60–90 days, to help verify any observed changes.

Exercise. Exercise has been found to be beneficial for several psychiatric and developmental disorders.[65] The mechanisms underlying the beneficial effects of exercise in reducing hyperactive and repetitive behaviors by children with autism may be through stimulation of the release of neurotransmitters such as acetylcholine and beta-endorphins.[66] In a systematic review published in 2010, the vast majority of previously reported studies of antecedent aerobic exercise (6–20 minutes) found a decrease in self-stimulatory behaviors and an improvement in academic performance.[67] Although a proportion of these studies had significant limitations, exercise is cheap, safe, and easy to adhere to for children, with benefits that include improved sport skills, improved physical fitness, and increased control of obesity. Aerobic activities that may be performed in groups but do not require strict rules, such as running, swimming, and treadmill or biking exercise, are generally recommended.

PHARMACEUTICALS

It must be stressed that there are currently no medications known to treat the core symptoms of autism. Children with autism generally have other common medical problems, such as sleep disorders, constipation, and food limitations, which may be treated with conventional or, in some cases, complementary therapies. However, pharmaceutical treatments based on previous studies should be considered as adjuncts to robust behavioral or counseling programs in patients with emotional and behavioral disturbances that commonly co-occur with autism, such as anxiety, ADHD, compulsions and repetitive behaviors, depression, irritability, and aggression.

Stimulants

When using an inclusive definition of all types of ADHD (inattention, hyperactivity, and combined), ADHD may be apparent in up to one-half of patients with autism.[68] Occasionally, children are diagnosed and treated for ADHD before a diagnosis of autism is made.[69] Some studies have even suggested that ADHD may be part of a continuum with autism.[70] Regardless, it is important to understand that the very few randomized, double-blind, placebo-controlled studies that have been published limits the evidence supporting the treatment of inattentiveness and hyperactivity with stimulants (methylphenidate and amphetamines).[71] Anecdotally, children with autism tend to be more sensitive to stimulants and may have an increased incidence of common adverse effects, such as increased irritability, heightened emotionality, decreased appetite, and insomnia.[1,71] As a result of these side effects, the mantra for most pharmaceutical medications, particularly in autism, is "start low, and go slow."[1,58] Therefore, a half tablet of a 5 mg short-acting methylphenidate is typically trialed initially. When using amphetamine, which tends to be twice as potent as methylphenidate, one should consider a half tablet of a 2.5 mg amphetamine drug. If the stimulant does not prove helpful or has side effects that make continuing the stimulant difficult (tics or hyperemotionality), an alpha agonist, such as guanfacine or clonidine, should be used either alone or as an adjunctive therapy; however, there have been very few clinical trials to validate the efficacy of this treatment approach.[72] Once no side effects are noted with a short-acting alpha agonist, the use of a long-acting guanfacine (such as Intuniv) at 1 to 2 mg daily is recommended.

When considering a nonstimulant medication for inattentiveness and hyperactivity, recent studies have demonstrated the efficacy of the norepinephrine reuptake inhibitors Atomoxetine or Strattera in decreasing hyperactivity and stereotypic behaviors.[73,74] These medication are titrated at an initial dose of 0.4 mg/kg for several days and can be increased to approximately 1.2 mg/kg daily as a single dose. The norepinephrine reuptake inhibitors appear to have significantly less side effects than stimulants. The benefits of norepinephrine reuptake inhibitors may take six to eight weeks to be fully realized, and this should be explained to the parent and child.

Antipsychotics

The antipsychotics risperidone and aripiprazole are the only medicines with FDA approval for use in autism for irritability and explosive behaviors.[75] Risperidone continues to be used as the first-line medication and its use has significantly increased over the last several years in children with autism.[76] Common side effects with risperidone include rapid weight gain precipitated by a voracious appetite, drowsiness, and hypertriglyceridemia with early signs of diabetes.[75,76] In addition, patients should be monitored for extrapyramidal symptoms (EPS), including tremors, dyskinesia, and rigidity. Liquid preparations (1 mg/mL) should be used with caution as parents have been known to accidentally overdose children via decimal point confusion (5.0 mL versus 0.5 mL).[77]

Aripiprazole may also be used for managing severe irritability and aggression in ASD. Aripiprazole has a similar side effect profile to risperidone (increased appetite, weight gain, drowsiness, and EPS) despite initially being marketed as causing fewer side effects.[76] Aripiprazole, as with other antipsychotics, requires blood monitoring for neutropenia, electrocardiography if prolonged QT syndrome is suspected, and monitoring for suicidal ideation.[78] Generally, liquid aripiprazole (1 mg/mL) is initially administered at 1 mL two times a day and increased by 1–2 mL per week to a total of 5 mL or 5 mg two times per day.

Serotonin Reuptake Inhibitors and Selective Serotonin Reuptake Inhibitors

SRI and SSRI may be used to treat anxiety, phobias, and compulsions in children, adolescents, and adults with autism; however, the results of previous studies of the efficacy of these treatment have been mixed.[79] Citalopram, escitalopram, and fluoxetine have been the most commonly studied drugs in randomized controlled trials.[80] Fluoxetine is preferred in children and adolescent groups using a liquid preparation (4 mg/mL) for titration, because low doses tend to be tolerated better for anxiety and compulsions than the higher doses used for depression.[81] Fluoxetine administration should be initiated at 1 mL/4 mg/week and titrated up by 1 mL/4 mg/week until effect or to 5 mL/20 mg because doses above 20 mg are associated with increased side effects.[82] The main side effects of SRI and SSRIs are agitation, increased energy, and poor sleep.[82] Overall, the side effect profile and limited efficacy in children have led the Cochrane Database report to support only

very limited use of these medications in children with autism.[80]

Newer Pharmacological Agents

Many pilot or trial studies of nonconventional pharmacological agents have recently been reported in children with autism aimed at manipulating specific receptor-associated channels and neurotransmitters in the brain related or sensitive to glutamate, glutamine, glycine, Gamma-amino-butyric acid (GABA), N-methyl D-aspartic acid (NMDA), nicotinic, or opioids. There is hope that these pharmacological agents may target the core symptoms of autism, with N-acetylcysteine (NAC), memantine, D-cycloserine, naltrexone, and oxytocin demonstrating utility in improving comorbid symptoms or as potential subgroup treatments for core symptoms. All of these therapies are currently in the research phase and require validation by further clinical trials before their use in children with ASD is fully endorsed.

NAC is a glutamate modulator administered orally at 900 mg 1–3 times a day. NAC has demonstrated benefit in decreasing irritability either alone or in conjunction with risperidone.[83-85]

Memantine was originally developed to treat Alzheimer's disease. A connection between Alzheimer's and autism was hypothesized several years ago following results from Fragile X studies.[86] Memantine modulates glutamate neurotransmission and is administered at 10–20 mg doses daily. In a systematic review, memantine therapy was associated with improvements in the core symptoms of autism in eight of nine studies, including one double-blind, placebo-controlled study.[87]

D-Cycloserine acts on the NMDA receptor, which is thought to have effects on improving sociability.[88] Two recent studies have been done by the same authors, using a randomized, double-blind trial and assessing dosage of 50 mg of D-cycloserine daily versus weekly, which show improvements in both the Social Responsiveness Scale and the Aberrant Behavior Checklist.[89,90]

Naltrexone, an opioid antagonist, has been trialed in children with autism in several studies to determine its utility in treating the core symptoms of autism. A recent systematic review of previous literature concluded that naltrexone provided some improvement in hyperactivity and restlessness but had no discernible effect on the core symptoms of autism.[91] Reported dosages were between 0.5 mg/kg and 2.0 mg/kg, with an onset of action of 30 minutes and peak effect at 6–12 hours. The most common side effect of naltrexone therapy was weight loss.[91]

Oxytocin is a naturally occurring peptide in the brain that increases socialization and promotes parental nurturing and social bonds. It has been developed into an intranasal medicine and trialed in autism in the hope that it will improve social cognition and reciprocity.[92] Currently, there are numerous studies underway (ClinicalTrials.gov); however, early results are mixed with some studies reporting modest improvements in social engagements and others reporting nonmeasurable affects.[93] The dosage of intranasal oxytocin is 0.4 IU/kg/dose and appears to be safe in short trials.[92,93]

Older Unproven or Disproven Pharmacological Treatments and Agents

The use of antifungal medications (fluconazole or nystatin) and/or antibiotics as a treatment for autism remains popular and based on the unproven hypothesis that there is an overgrowth of yeast and/or intestinal microbes in the gastrointestinal systems of children with autism. There is currently no evidence to support the efficacy or safety of any antifungal agents or bacterial treatments, and there have been no studies of the effectiveness of antiviral therapies.[94] A trial of the use of minocycline to modulate neurotrophic growth factors demonstrated no effect on the clinical symptoms of regressive autism.[95]

Chelation

Chelation is a process of administering a medication to remove heavy metals from the blood. The most commonly used medications are ethylene diamine tetra-acetic acid (EDTA), 2,3-dimercaptosuccinic acid (DMSA), and 2,3-dimercaptopropane-1-sulfonate (DMPS). Chelation has been used in children with autism based on the theory that ASD is caused by heavy metal poisoning, specifically with mercury. Mercury and other heavy metals are thought to accumulate due to increased exposure or an inability to clear toxins due to metabolic dysfunction, or a combination of both. Chelation is occasionally referred to under the larger umbrella of detoxification, where patients initially have their gastrointestinal tract prepared by removing dysbiotic flora and the addition of essential nutrients before the initiation of a course of chelation. This theory also relies on monitoring urine after chelation to determine treatment response. This process was utilized in two related studies published involving 65 children with autism and chelation that reported treatment responses in 49 children with elevated urinary excretion of heavy metals.[96,97] These 49 children were randomly assigned to receive 6 more rounds of DMSA or placebo treatment. Although a small but significant difference in language, cognition, and sociability was reported by this study, the side effect profile of the chelating agents was considered to be unacceptably high and is likely to prevent further studies due to substantial renal and hepatic toxicity and a reported death due to hypocalcemia.[98,99]

> Although slight improvements in autism symptoms have been reported with chelation therapy, the side effects, including hepatotoxicity and one reported death, outweigh any minimal potential benefits.

Secretin

Secretin is a gastrointestinal hormone that inhibits intestinal motility and the release of gastric acid, and stimulates the secretion of pancreatic fluid. There are anecdotal reports that secretin has benefit in children with autism and gastrointestinal problems. These reports culminated in a special feature on *60 Minutes*, a CBS news program, where a small study of injectable secretin was followed and debunked on an episode aired on February 20, 1994, and recounted in Paul Offit's novel.[100] Since that time, more than 900 children with autism have been evaluated in double-blind, placebo-controlled trials, with no behavioral benefit of secretin observed.[94]

Immunotherapy

Immunotherapy for children with autism is based on the hypothesis that early fetal brain development is sensitive to the prenatal immune response.[101] Although this hypothesis concerning an epigenetic immune phenomenon has been supported by recent studies of biological markers,[102,103] the successful development of therapeutic treatments with intravenous immunoglobulin (IVIG) or oral immunoglobulin is not currently supported by published data.[104,105]

There does not appear to be any ongoing clinical trials or any FDA-approved clinical use of an immunomodulatory treatment for autism. The potential adverse effects of IVIG and other immune therapies include transmission of blood-borne pathogens and transfusion reactions.

SUPPLEMENTS

Folic Acid

Folic acid may be considered in patients with autism for several reasons. There were initial concerns that children and mothers with methylenetetrahydrofolate reductase (MTHFR) deficiency were at risk of autism or having a child with autism[106] (see Chapter 38). Open trials of folinic acid and B12 supplementation in children with autism have reported improvements in language both expressive and receptive.[107] In recent studies, the risk of women near conception having a child with autism was significantly reduced by supplementation with folic acid at levels above the recommended requirements (600–800 mcg rather than 400 mcg).[18]

Methyl B12 Injections

Methyl B12 is a vital cofactor for the regeneration of methionine from homocysteine by providing methyl groups for the transmethylation and transsulfuration metabolic pathways. Methyl B12 deficiency causes reduced synthesis of transsulfuration pathway products, specifically glutathione and cysteine, which are important antioxidants responsible for controlling macromolecular damage produced by oxidative stress.[108] However, there is currently only one reported double-blind, placebo-controlled, randomized crossover trial using subcutaneous injection of methyl B12 at 65–75 mcg/kg every 2–3 days.[109] The results were mixed with no statistical significance observed in behaviors between the two groups, but a subgroup of approximately a third of all patients had some improvements in language and social interaction.

Although injections were well tolerated in this study, methyl B12 injections do not appear to be a viable option for many families of children with autism due to the frequency of visits required and as yet unproven benefits.

Amino Acid Therapy

Glutamine, taurine, and carnosine are all amino acids that have been hypothesized to have a neuroprotective effect in children with autism. It is thought that the metabolism of these amino acids, as well as many others, is impaired in children with autism and supplementations may have a positive neurological effect. Previous studies of amino acid therapy have proven inconclusive, with no current therapy presently having sufficient evidence to be recommended.

Dimethylglycine and Trimethylglycine

Dimethylglycine (DMG) and trimethylglycine (TMG) are both derivatives of the amino acid glycine and have been posited to reduce lactic acid, enhance oxygen use, and reduce seizure activity during times of stress.[110] The use of DMG and TMG is based on the theory that metabolic derangements contribute to the development of autism. There has been very little research on the use of DMG and TMG, with only 2 studies reporting essentially no benefits of the use of DMG in patients with autism.[110,111]

Vitamin B6 and Magnesium

Vitamin B6 (Pyridoxine) and magnesium represent some of the oldest therapies used for children with mental health disorders and have subsequently been trialed for children with autism.[112] A systematic review of more than 25 studies reported the evidence for treatment with B6 and magnesium to be inconclusive and equivocal.[112] The main concern with vitamin B6 and magnesium therapy is that high dose of vitamin B6 (>100 mg/day) may cause neuropathy and magnesium may cause diarrhea.

Melatonin

Melatonin is a hormone produced by the pineal gland in response to decreasing levels of light and is involved in the regulation of sleep by inducing drowsiness. Melatonin is synthesized from serotonin, and abnormalities in these pathways have been reported in children with autism.[113] Sleep problems have been reported in children with autism 50%–80% of the time.[114] Several studies have demonstrated abnormally low levels of melatonin in children with autism and other developmental disabilities.[115] Therapy with melatonin at doses ranging from 1–10 mg at bedtime have been shown to improve the overall amount of sleep and shorten sleep latency in the majority of studies involving children with autism.[116,117] Melatonin is available in many different preparations and dosages. The 3-mg pills are preferred because this dose tends to work well as an initial dose and allows easy titration to 6 and 9 mg. For children with autism that are unable to swallow pills, melatonin is available in a 1 mg/mL solution, which can be initiated at doses of 1 mL to 3 mL at one to two hours before bedtime.

Omega-3 Fatty Acids

Omega-3 fatty acids (FA) are essential for brain function and development. Omega-3 FA are nutrients that primarily function at the cell membrane and aid in synaptic plasticity and neuroprotection.[118] The two omega-3 FA of primary interest for the treatment of autism are eicosapentaenoic acid (EPA) and docosahexaenoic acid (DHA). Low levels of omega-3 FA have been reported in children with autism.[119] The use of omega-3 FA in children with autism has become ubiquitous in primary care practices despite surprisingly little evidence regarding their efficacy in the treatment of the core symptoms of ASD.[94] However, that practitioners may be using omega-3 FA to treat comorbidities, such as ADHD and depression, where omega-3 FA have also been posited to have utility despite a current lack of evidence.[120,121] The initial dose of omega-3 FA is typically approximately 600 mg (equal amounts of DHA and EPA) daily as a trial dose for treatment before titration up to 2 g. Doses can be reduced in patients that develop diarrhea while receiving higher doses.

Multivitamins and Minerals

Studies of multivitamin and mineral supplementation, along with specific vitamin and mineral therapies, have reported mixed results.[94] Previous multivitamin and mineral studies have had significant methodological flaws that have made the interpretation of their results difficult. Previous literature supports supplementation with vitamins A, C, and D3 for the prevention of nutritional deficiencies, such as scurvy and rickets, that may occur in children with autism due to restricted diets or stressed maternal environments.[122,123] Several important metal minerals have also been linked to the expression of autism, including iron, zinc, and copper.[124,125] These metals are critical in synaptic transmission and deficiencies in these metals may have significant cognitive, behavioral, and neurodegenerative consequences.[126,127] The strongest research to date indicate both low maternal iron stores and low infant or child stores of iron are potential risk factors for the development of autism. Further, there is good evidence to indicate that deficiencies in either prenatal mothers or infants and children should be treated with iron supplementation.[128,129]

> The most important mineral deficiency to screen for and treat in individuals with autism is iron.

BOTANICALS AND HERBAL

There is a lack of studies of botanicals and herbal remedies for the treatment of children with ASD.

MIND-BODY MEDICINE

Biofeedback and Neurofeedback

Biofeedback and neurofeedback therapies were initially considered as a treatment for autism because it was noted that children with autism had abnormal electroencephalogram (EEG) patterns compared to controls.[130-132] Teaching participants with ASD to regulate these patterns reportedly improves social interactions, verbal and nonverbal communication skills, and executive function.[133-135] The underlying mechanism remains unknown; however, current research is focusing on mechanisms responsible for a proportion of children with autism responding better than others and the utility of this method in improving cognitive flexibility.[136]

Music Therapy

Music therapy for children with ASD refers to musical experiences and the relationships that develop through music that enable communication and expression and help to improve the core symptoms of autism such as joint attention, communication, expression, and engagement.[137] Music therapies involve structured and unstructured individual and group sessions with and without a leader that include playing and/or listening to music. A recent Cochrane database review concluded that music therapy has benefits for children with autism in the areas of social interaction, verbal communication, initiating behaviors, and social-emotional reciprocity.[138] Additional studies with larger sample sizes and longitudinal followup are required to determine if the effects of music therapy are reproducible and enduring.

Yoga

Yoga involves breathing, positioning, and relaxation exercises that can easily be taught to children with autism. Unfortunately, very few studies evaluating the utility of yoga as a therapy for autism have been reported. In one study, yoga was combined with dance and was found to result in significant changes in the behavioral and cognitive areas of the Behavioral Assessment System for Children (BASC).[139] A separate study of a 16-week program in school reported significant improvements in maladaptive behaviors of children with autism compared to controls.[140]

Body-Based Practices, Energy Medicine

Acupuncture

Acupuncture involves the systemic insertion of needles or pressure to specific points on the body and is widely used in traditional Chinese medicine. Previous studies have reported that acupuncture increases levels of beta-endorphins, serotonin, and noradrenaline, which may reduce the symptoms of depression or anxiety.[141] The majority of studies of acupuncture in children with autism has been performed in China and are thus difficult to review. A systematic review published in 2011 by Lee et al. concluded that acupuncture is safe but with conflicting results across the 11 studies they were able to review.[142] A more recent review by Yang et al. evaluating all uses of acupuncture in children found unclear benefits of acupuncture in children with autism.[143]

Auditory Integrative Training

Auditory integration training was developed as a technique for improving abnormal sound sensitivity in children and individuals with behavioral disorders, specifically ASD. Sound therapies that use these principals include the Tomatis Method and Samonas Therapy. Studies of this therapy with controls, such as waiting lists, usual therapy, and sham placebo, found no benefits and no evidence to support the use of auditory integrative training in children with autism.[144] Accordingly, auditory integration training and sound therapies are not currently recommended or supported by research literature.

Transcranial Magnetic Stimulation

Transcranial magnetic stimulation (TMS) or neuromodulation is an energy-based therapy that has been posited to work through electromagnetic induction, thereby modifying neuroexcitability. TMS uses noninvasive focal cortical stimulation, involving small, variable intracranial electrical currents generated by a rapidly fluctuating extracranial magnetic field.[145] This is a new field of research in autism with very few randomized control trials reported; however, preliminary work is intriguing. The use of low frequency TMS has been shown to include improvements in EEG indices that correspond to attention and information processing, and improvements in repetitive behaviors.[146] In addition, the use of high frequency stimulation has been shown to improve self-reported social relating and social anxiety.[147]

Hippotherapy

Hippotherapy (therapeutic horseback riding) for children with ASD is based upon the hypothesis that riding a horse stimulates multiple areas of functioning for children, including cognitive, social, and gross motor functioning.[148] Several very small and nonrandomized trials have reported improvements in parent-reported emotional and social functioning, improvements in adaptive behaviors, and dose–response benefits.[149-151] Despite the potential benefits, the cost and risk of injury associated with hippotherapy should be considered before recommending this therapy. The use of a helmet and appropriately trained supervision should also be strongly advised.

Massage and Qigong

Qigong is a Chinese movement therapy that, along with massage therapy alone, has gained increasing popularity with the recognition and addition of sensory abnormalities to the diagnostic criteria of ASD in the DSM-5. Abnormalities in tactile sensation may delay early self-regulation milestones and social development in young children with ASD. Parents are best positioned to promote more tactile stimulation through therapeutic massage protocols that may improve developmental outcomes.[152] Several small studies have reported the benefits of qigong in improving parental perceptions and decreasing parental stress, with children benefiting from decreases in tactile impairment and improved self-regulation.[152] Qigong represents an extremely low risk therapy with potential benefits.

Other

Hyperbaric Oxygen Therapy

Hyperbaric oxygen therapy (HBOT) has been posited to enhance oxygen delivery to potentially damaged areas of the brain, reduce swelling, and promote brain recovery in children with autism.[153] A multicenter, randomized control trial published in 2009 including 62 children with autism between the ages of 2 and 7 years reported potential benefits with the use of low pressure and low oxygen levels.[154] The results of this study included improvements in overall function, receptive language, social interaction, eye contact, and sensory/cognitive awareness.[154] Unfortunately, this study was limited by a short follow up and a period of strong placebo effect. The results of this study have never been reproduced but retain strong support in the autism community.[155] The reported side effects of HBOT include ear barotrauma, reversible myopia, pulmonary barotrauma, pulmonary oxygen toxicity, and seizures.[156,157] However, these side effects are typically seen at higher atmospheric pressures rather than the lower pressures used in the previous studies. Overall, the number of dives required for HBOT (40 dives in total) and high cost ($100-$200/dive) may make this therapy prohibitive for many families. Accordingly, it may be difficult to recommend such an expensive and unproven therapy in most cases of autism.

Therapies to Consider

There is a lack of studies on healing touch therapy, reiki, and prayer, as well as evidence to support their use in children with autism; however, all are safe and seem reasonable to recommend.

There is also a lack of studies on the potential efficacy of craniosacral manipulation/therapy, chiropractic, and homeopathy in children with autism; however, such therapies may compete with other validated therapies for limited time and resources and may therefore be difficult to support.

PREVENTION PRESCRIPTION

No definitive strategies exist for the prevention of autism. The results of recent epigenetic studies suggest the following:

- Women of childbearing age should receive folic acid supplementation at > 400 mcg to 600 mcg–800 mcg daily and iron supplements to maintain normal hemoglobin and ferritin levels.
- Births should be spaced by at least 2 years if possible, and mothers should be encouraged to have children before the age of 35.
- Avoid pesticide exposure where possible.

- Supplementation of the child's daily intake with a multivitamin is advisable; however, megadoses of any individual vitamin or mineral may confer little to no benefit.
- The avoidance of immunizations will put the child and other children who cannot be immunized at risk of vaccine-preventable diseases.
- Prevent exposure of pregnant women and infants to any toxic household cleaning products or insecticides.

THERAPEUTIC REVIEW

NUTRITION

A 60-day trial of a gluten-free/casein-free diet (GF/CF; strongly consider consultation with a nutritionist or dietician). B₂

EXERCISE

Aerobic exercise, 20 minutes daily. C₁

SUPPLEMENTS

- Folic acid (>400 mcg daily) in children and preconception females. B₁
- Probiotics containing lactobacilli, bacteroidetes, and saccharomyces (1–10 billion cells daily). C₁
- Omega 3 fatty acids (EPA + DHA; 500–2000 mg). B₁
- Iron (3–6 mg/kg daily if deficient and 1–3 mg/kg for supplementation) in children and preconception females. B₁

- Melatonin (1–9 mg taken one or two hours before bedtime). B₁

MIND-BODY

- Intensive behavioral therapy (ABA, TEACCH, DIR/Floortime, see web resources for more information). B₁
- Music therapy. C₁

PHARMACEUTICALS

- Oxytocin (0.4 IU/kg/dose) 1–2 doses daily. C₁
- Memantine (10–20 mg daily). C₁
- Methyl B12 injections (65–75 mcg/kg every 2–3 days). C₁

OTHERS

- Qigong/massage. C₁
- Transcranial magnetic stimulation (TMS). C₁
- Hippotherapy (horseback riding). C₁
- Hyperbaric oxygen therapy (HBOT).  C₂

Key Web Resources

Research Autism has updated data on recent research studies of many of the complementary and alternative therapies discussed in a searchable database.	http://www.researchautism.net/interventions
Much of the epigenetic and environmental research is being performed through the MIND (Medical Investigation of Neurodevelopmental Disorders) Institute at the University of California, Davis.	http://www.ucdmc.ucdavis.edu/mindinstitute/
Autism Science Foundation has evidence-based information.	http://www.autismsciencefoundation.org/
Interactive Autism Network (IAN) is housed from the Kennedy Krieger Institute and allows families to register for research.	http://www.IANresearch.org/
Intensive Behavioral Therapy Resources Applied Behavioral Analysis	http://www.centerforautism.com/aba-therapy.aspx
TEACCH stands for *Treatment and Education of Autistic and related Communication Handicapped Children.*	http://teacch.com/about-us/what-is-teacch
DIR/Floortime. DIR stands for *Developmental, Individual Difference, Relationship-Based* and uses a developmental intervention approach integrating psychodynamic and cognitive learning principles.	http://www.interactingwithautism.com/section/treating/floort

REFERENCES

References are available online at ExpertConsult.com.

CHAPTER 9

INSOMNIA

Rubin Naiman, PhD

Insomnia is prevalent, associated with a broad range of illnesses, and presents a significant medical, social, and economic burden. Largely undiagnosed and untreated despite the existence of effective interventions, insomnia has been described as "unremitting, disabling, costly, pervasive, and pernicious."[1] Because it is strongly linked to lifestyle and mind-body dynamics and is resistant to conventional medical treatment, insomnia deserves much greater consideration from integrative medicine researchers and practitioners. In fact, a National Health Interview Survey reported that 1.6 million adults already use complementary and alternative medicine (CAM) to treat insomnia.[2]

The National Institutes of Health reports that 60 million adults in the United States struggle with insomnia annually.[3] Depending on definition, the prevalence of insomnia among adults ranges from 10% to 30% and increases with age and in female gender, as well as with a broad range of medical and psychiatric comorbidities.[4]

Patients with insomnia are at increased risk for comorbid medical disorders, including chronic pain, cardiovascular disease, cancer, neurological and gastrointestinal disorders,[5,6] obesity,[7] and diabetes.[8-10] Sleep loss has been associated with insulin dysregulation,[9,10] disruptions of cortisol rhythms,[11,12] and immune function and inflammatory markers.[13-16]

Psychiatric illness, especially depression or anxiety,[17] is the most common comorbidity linked to insomnia.[18,19] Approximately 40% of adults with insomnia have a psychiatric illness, most commonly depression.[18,19] Persistent insomnia significantly increases the risk of clinical depression, anxiety disorders, and substance abuse.[20,21] The traditional presumption that insomnia is secondary to psychiatric illness has been challenged by several findings that suggest insomnia more often precedes, and is likely a significant risk factor for, mood disorders.[22-25]

Although psychiatric illness,[18] medical disorders,[26] and shift work[27] significantly increase the risk for insomnia, they are not causal but precipitating factors in patients already predisposed to the disorder.[28] Primary sleep and circadian rhythm disorders, such as restless legs syndrome,[29] periodic limb movement disorders, delayed sleep phase, and sleep-related breathing disorders, are also frequently associated with insomnia.[30]

Insomnia is associated with significant impairment in quality of life,[31-33] increased risk of accidents,[34] and decrements in work productivity.[35] The economic burden of insomnia in the United States has been estimated to be as high as $63.2 billion annually.[36]

Although conventional sleep medicine has clearly made advances in understanding and evaluating sleep and sleep disorders, one can argue that it lags in terms of developing effective treatment and prevention strategies for insomnia. Despite their serious limitations, hypnotic agents remain the primary focus of conventional insomnia treatment. Advances in cognitive-behavioral therapy for insomnia (CBT-I) challenge the conventional emphasis on medication and are associated with a chasm between conventional and behavioral sleep medicine. Among the most significant limitations of conventional approaches to insomnia is a widespread tendency to "treat the chart" that offers remarkably limited regard for subjective experiences of the patient.

An integrative medicine approach to understanding and managing insomnia (1) restores the place of subjectivity, as is evident in CBT-I; (2) emphasizes the promotion of sleep health, as opposed to symptom suppression; (3) acknowledges the important social and relational context of sleep; (4) underscores the critical role of natural rhythms in life and health; and (5) strongly emphasizes the role of lifestyle. An integrative approach to insomnia also calls for personalization of treatment based on a thorough evaluation.

DEFINITIONS

Insomnia disorder refers to difficulties with initiating or maintaining sleep, as well as nonrestorative sleep that is associated with excessive sleepiness or fatigue and with functional decrements for at least 4 weeks. Primary insomnia is not attributable to medical or psychiatric causes, whereas secondary insomnia has historically been viewed as a symptom of a primary disorder that would resolve with treatment.[28] A National Institutes of Health (NIH) State of the Science Conference[5] recommended that secondary insomnia be considered *comorbid insomnia* to encourage its direct treatment. Insomnia is frequently comorbid with other conditions, most commonly primary sleep disorders (Box 9.1), chronic pain syndromes, and psychiatric disorders, especially depression and substance abuse.

ETIOLOGY

The etiology of insomnia is commonly understood in terms of a "Three P" model,[37,38] including predisposing, precipitating, and perpetuating factors. Predisposing factors comprise a broad range of biomedical, psychological, and lifestyle factors that increase the risk of developing insomnia. These include (1) dependence on substances such as alcohol, caffeine, nicotine, and other drugs; (2) the long-term use of stimulant, sedating, or circadian

BOX 9.1   Comorbid Primary Sleep Disorders

- Restless legs syndrome (RLS)
- Periodic limb movements in sleep (PLMS)
- Gastroesophageal reflux disease (GERD)
- Sleep-phase disorders
- Narcolepsy
- Obstructive sleep apnea (OSA)
- Nocturia

BOX 9.2   Medications That Can Interfere With Deep or Rapid Eye Movement Sleep

- Alcohol
- Antiarrhythmics
- Anticonvulsants
- Antihistamines
- Appetite suppressants
- Benzodiazepines
- Bronchodilators
- Caffeine
- Carbidopa/levodopa
- Corticosteroids
- Diuretics
- Decongestants
- Estrogen
- Lipophilic beta blockers
- Monoamine oxidase inhibitors
- Nicotine
- Pseudoephedrine
- Selective serotonin reuptake inhibitors
- Sedatives
- Statins
- Sympathomimetics
- Tetrahydrozoline
- Thyroid hormones
- Tricyclic antidepressants

rhythm–disrupting medications; (3) illnesses associated with nocturnal pain or discomfort; (4) primary sleep disorders, such as restless legs syndrome, periodic limb movements in sleep, gastroesophageal reflux disease, and obstructive sleep apnea; and (5) circadian rhythm disorders associated with shift work, jet lag, and advanced or delayed sleep-phase syndromes.

Precipitating factors in insomnia commonly include stress associated with family, occupation, or health challenges. These factors are usually negative challenges, such as divorce, death of a loved one, or illness, but they can also involve stress associated with positive events, such as the birth of a child or retirement.[37,38]

Perpetuating factors in insomnia refer to behaviors intended to manage or compensate for sleeplessness that inadvertently exacerbate the condition. Examples include (1) excessive waking time spent in bed; (2) an irregular sleep–wake schedule including napping and dozing; (3) excessive use of caffeine, alcohol, and other drugs; and (4) anxiety associated with attempts at controlling sleep, as well as the daytime consequences of sleeplessness. Dependence, habituation, and rebound effects associated with sedative-hypnotics can also perpetuate insomnia.

The common practice of spending excessive time in bed to compensate for lost sleep results in conditioned insomnia, a negative association of the bed with wakefulness that significantly perpetuates the problem.

Conditioned insomnia is measured in terms of *sleep efficiency*, the ratio of total time spent asleep to the amount of time spent in bed. A sleep efficiency below 85% is considered problematic.[37,38]

Additional biomedical factors that can predispose to, precipitate, or perpetuate insomnia include iatrogenic influences of extended hospitalizations, as well as a broad range of medications that interfere with sleep, such as analgesics, benzodiazepines, antidepressants, and anticholinergic medications. Beta blockers, calcium channel blockers, diuretics, and other medications may also suppress melatonin (MT) and interfere with sleep. Box 9.2 provides a more extensive listing of medications that can interfere with sleep.

Exposure to ordinary room light before bedtime suppresses MT onset and duration in humans,[39] potentially disrupting sleep and circadian rhythms. Other environmental factors, including sound, temperature, and air and bedding quality, can also predispose one to precipitate or perpetuate insomnia, although these factors have not received the attention they warrant.

PATHOPHYSIOLOGY

The most compelling pathophysiological model for insomnia suggests a strong association with chronic cognitive-emotional hyperarousal, which may be a premorbid characteristic of the disorder.[40-42] Compared with controls, patients with insomnia have elevated heart rates,[43,44] increased body and brain metabolic rates,[45,46] elevated core body temperature,[47] increased beta and gamma electroencephalography, and neuroendocrine dysregulation including elevated nighttime cortisol and decreased serum MT.[48-51] Insomnia has also been linked to nocturnal sympathetic activation and overactivation of the hypothalamic-pituitary-adrenal axis.[52,53]

Chronic cognitive-emotional hyperarousal associated with elevated metabolic rate, sympathetic overactivation, and chronic inflammation is a common substrate of insomnia.

Insomnia appears to be bidirectionally associated with chronic inflammation. A single night of sleep deprivation in human subjects can alter cellular immune responses[54] and increase levels of inflammatory markers.[55-58] Inflammatory conditions have been shown to disrupt sleep by increasing pain, anxiety, and depression.[59,60] Chronic inflammation is fundamentally a process of immune system overactivation, which can be understood as yet another expression of hyperarousal.

Sleepiness and sleep propensity appear to be strongly influenced by circadian core body temperature rhythms. Specific types of insomnia have been linked to specific patterns of disrupted temperature rhythms. Sleep onset difficulties have been associated with a delayed circadian temperature rhythm, early morning awakenings with an advanced circadian temperature rhythm, sleep maintenance insomnia with a nocturnally elevated core body temperature, and mixed insomnia with a 24-hour elevation of core body temperature, consistent with the hyperarousal model.[61]

Hyperarousal can be further elucidated by the widely accepted dual-process model of sleep regulation,[62] which views sleep in terms of a dynamic interaction between homeostatic and circadian processes. As the homeostatic sleep drive gradually increases through the waking day, the circadian pacemaker exerts an equal but opposite force to maintain alertness. The potential for sleep normally occurs with the nightly, rhythmic release of circadian alertness.

As a consequence of their 24-hour hyperarousal, insomnia patients are generally less sleepy during the day than normal sleepers. However, they may be significantly more fatigued (a construct independent of sleepiness)[63,64]—a condition strongly associated with major depression.[65] Theoretically, fatigue, which draws one toward rest, and hyperarousal, which encourages activity, can result in a state of chronic isometric tension that characterizes the insomnia–depression complex. Suspended in a limbic zone between fatigue and hyperarousal, neither a healthy descent into sleep nor a passionate ascension into waking are possible.[66]

Modern lifestyles are associated with the widespread suppression of rapid eye movement (REM) sleep and dreaming. Excessive alcohol consumption, most sleep medications, and many psychiatric medications suppress REM sleep. Sleep maintenance insomnia, early morning awakenings (including those caused by an alarm clock), obstructive sleep apnea, and short sleeping can further limit REM sleep and dreaming.[67]

Human and animal studies confirm that the selective deprivation of REM sleep results in its rebound in the form of a reduced REM latency and disrupted deep sleep. This same pattern characterizes the sleep of depressed patients.[68] The classic psychodynamic notion that depression is "a loss of one's dreams" appears to have a literal underpinning.

> Hyperarousal may be understood as circadian alertness (wakefulness) that has gone awry and overrides both normal sleep drive and the excessive daytime sleepiness one would expect with chronic insomnia.

Evaluating Insomnia

The scope of an insomnia evaluation should be comprehensive, including any and all biomedical, psychological, and environmental factors potentially affecting sleep. Box 9.3 provides a list of essential clinical interview and history topics.

> Subjective measures, including the clinical interview and history, are the most critical components of the evaluation of insomnia.

BOX 9.3	Clinical Interview and History

1. The presenting complaint
2. The sleep–wake routine
3. Daytime functioning and symptoms
4. Sleep conditions and routines
5. Previous treatment effects
6. Other sleep disorder symptoms
7. Comorbid medical conditions
8. Psychiatric conditions and stressors
9. Medication and substance use
10. Relevant family history

Adapted from Mai E, Buysse DJ. Insomnia: prevalence, impact, pathogenesis, differential diagnosis, and evaluation. *Sleep Med Clin.* 2008;3:167-174.

The adage that as important as knowing which disease the patient has is knowing which patient has the disease is most pertinent here. It is critical to elicit each patient's personal sleep *and dream* story. Evidence from a study of bad dreams and nightmares suggests that patients may respond to these dreams with sleep avoidant behaviors.[68] Eliciting the patient's basic posture toward sleep and dreams is a critical component of the insomnia evaluation. In addition to providing essential diagnostic information, doing so can engage the patient more deeply, strengthen the therapeutic alliance, and improve treatment adherence. The patient's story should be complemented with information gathered through personalized sleep logs or diaries, which should be recorded over a period of 1–2 weeks. Sleep logs and diaries (see Key Web Resources) provide data about sleep patterns, habits, and daytime effects as well as related cognitive, affective, and behavior patterns. Interviewing available bed partners may also be helpful to corroborate information about snoring and movement disorders.

Self-Report Scales

Self-report scales can be useful for the assessment of sleepiness, fatigue, and hyperarousal. Empirically supported tools include the Pittsburgh Insomnia Rating Scale,[69] the Athens Insomnia Scale,[70] and the Bergen Insomnia Scale.[71] The Epworth Sleepiness Scale[72] is a brief, public domain questionnaire that provides an effective measure of current sleepiness (see Key Web Resources). Although the Epworth Sleepiness Scale is helpful as a screening device, it does not provide useful discriminative information for insomnia; however, it may have value in screening for comorbid sleep apnea, narcolepsy, or other sleep disorders. Also in popular use, the Stanford Sleepiness Scale[73] offers sensitivity to patterns of daytime wakefulness. Finally, the Insomnia Severity Index[74] is a self-report scale that assesses insomnia type, severity, and impact on daily life.

Objective Measures (Fig. 9.1)

Polysomnography (PSG), as its name implies, measures multiple sleep parameters including indices of respiration,

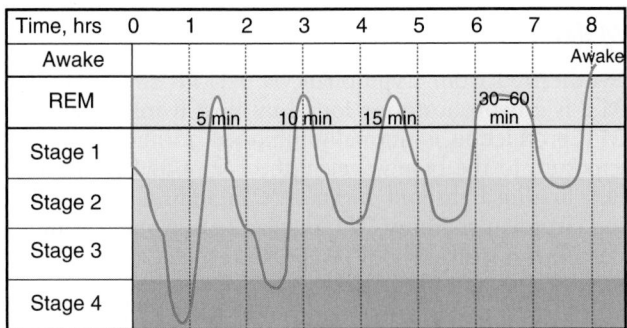

FIG. 9.1 ■ Stages of Sleep.

electroencephalography, and movement and muscle tone. Widely considered the gold standard of sleep evaluation, PSG is not, however, routinely indicated for insomnia because it provides little information useful for diagnosis or treatment.

PSG may be necessary to rule out periodic limb movements in sleep, obstructive sleep apnea, or other conditions underlying persistent insomnia.[75] With advances in remote monitoring technologies, home-based PSG is increasingly being used. Other home use devices, such as actigraphy, allow for longitudinal studies that can reveal useful information about circadian rhythms and other sleep parameters.[5]

INTEGRATIVE THERAPY

"The best cure for insomnia," said W.C. Fields, "is sleep." A common temptation among both patients and practitioners is to oversimplify the causes and treatment of insomnia. As suggested earlier, treatment of insomnia calls for lifestyle change. Promoting general health with proper nutrition, exercise, and psychological well-being provides an essential backdrop to the comprehensive integrative treatment of insomnia. There are no magic bullets. Treatment typically entails multicomponent interventions that address all three P factors contributing to the noise of hyperarousal, including comorbid medical and psychiatric conditions. Ongoing monitoring and evaluation using subjective reports and objective measures should be an integral part of treatment.

> If there is a secret to a good night's sleep, it is a good day's waking.

From the patient's perspective, interventions for insomnia can be classified in terms of two basic approaches: *taking something to sleep* and *letting go of something to sleep*. Patients who struggle with insomnia are inclined to consume sleeping medication, alcohol, warm milk, herbal teas, MT, botanicals, nutraceuticals, a wide range of comfort foods, and more. The fundamental belief underlying this approach is that insomnia results from *insufficient sleepiness* that can be ramped up with sleep-promoting ingestibles.

Sleep Promotion: Principles of Taking Something to Sleep

Both conventional and CAM approaches offer a wide array of options for *taking something to sleep* when indicated by psychological or medical crises. Short-term use of safe alternatives minimize the risk of dependence and the erosion of sleep self-efficacy. With the possible exception of MT, which regulates circadian rhythms, both conventional and alternative sleep aids do little to address the underlying "noise" of hyperarousal.

> Most chronic insomnia results not from insufficient sleepiness, but from excessive wakefulness. *Letting go of something to sleep* refers to an approach concerned with reducing the noise of this excessive wakefulness.

Pharmaceuticals and Substances

Epidemiological studies suggest that alcohol, cannabis, OTC antihistamines, and prescription sedative-hypnotics are the most common treatments used by insomnia patients. Data suggesting that sedative-hypnotics can be effective in ameliorating insomnia raise serious questions about pharmaceutical industry influence and bias. At best, positive outcomes are negligible, and harmful side effects are substantial.[76]

Box 9.4 provides a list of the most common U.S. Food and Drug Administration–approved and off-label medications used to treat insomnia. Long-term use of most of these medications is associated with serious side effects (Box 9.5). Additional studies have raised concerns that the hypnotic agents may increase the risk of cancer.[77,78] Other findings revealed a 10%–15% increase in mortality among occasional users of sleeping pills and a 25% increase in mortality among nightly users of these drugs.[79]

> In the end, most sleep medications do little more than temporarily suppressing the neurophysiological symptoms of hyperarousal—and they do so with risk.

Despite these concerns, an unprecedented surge in the use of sleep medications has been underway since 2000.[80] This trend is certainly a factor in the rising tide of psychiatric polypharmacy.[81]

Supplements

Numerous botanical sleep aids have been in use around the globe for centuries. In contrast to conventional sleep medications, CAM sleep aids, including botanical medicines as well as nutraceuticals, generally provide less of a knockout and more of a gentle assist to sleep with significantly fewer adverse effects. Although L-tryptophan and 5-hydroxytryptophan (5-HTP), precursors to serotonin and MT, are widely used, reports about the effectiveness

BOX 9.4	Common Medications for Insomnia

OVER-THE-COUNTER AGENTS
- Diphenhydramine
- Doxylamine
- Benzodiazepines
- Estazolam
- Flurazepam
- Quazepam
- Temazepam
- Triazolam

NONBENZODIAZEPINE HYPNOTICS
- Eszopiclone
- Zaleplon
- Zolpidem
- Melatonin receptor agonists
- Ramelteon

ANTIDEPRESSANTS (TRICYCLIC OR TETRACYCLIC ANTIDEPRESSANTS)
- Amitriptyline
- Doxepin
- Trazodone
- Mirtazapine

OTHER AGENTS
- Clonidine
- Gabapentin
- Quetiapine
- Sodium oxybate (gamma-hydroxybutyric acid sodium salt [GHB])

BOX 9.5	Common Side Effects of Sedative-Hypnotics

- Dependence
- Tolerance
- Damaged sleep architecture
- Diminished deep sleep
- Rapid eye movement suppression
- Parasomnias
- Anterograde amnesia
- Morning hangover
- Undermined self-efficacy
- Rebound insomnia with discontinuation
- Increased risk of falls
- Cognitive impairment
- Symptom suppression
- Increased mortality

of these agents in treating insomnia are mixed. Kava has empirical support for use in treating insomnia; however, controversial findings have raised serious questions about its safety.[82] More rigorous research into such alternatives has been hindered by limited financial incentives, conventional sleep medicine biases, and the natural complexity of many botanicals. Of the many alternatives to conventional sleep medications available, MT, valerian, hops, l-theanine, and lemon balm have been reviewed in greater detail, are in common use, and are generally regarded as safe.

Melatonin

Synthesized from tryptophan via 5-HTP and serotonin, MT is a neurohormone found in most living organisms. MT production is normally inhibited during the day by exposure to the blue wavelength of light and is disinhibited by dim light and darkness.[83] In addition to regulating circadian rhythms; MT mediates sleep and dreaming; decreases nocturnal body temperature; and has antiinflammatory, immune-modulating, and free-radical scavenging effects.[84] The suppression of endogenous MT through overexposure to light at night,[85-87] in advancing age,[88] and by common substances and medications (e.g., caffeine, nicotine, alcohol, beta blockers, diuretics, calcium channel blockers, and over-the-counter analgesics[89]) may be a factor in the development of insomnia, depression, and cancer. A growing number of animal, human, and population studies suggest that MT may have oncostatic properties.[90,91] Other findings suggest that high doses of MT may actually disrupt sleep.[92] Anecdotal reports suggest that MT may heighten awareness of dreams. Doses as high as 50 mg can dramatically increase REM sleep and dreams. Certain psychoactive drugs, including cannabis and lysergic acid diethylamide (LSD), increase MT synthesis and may emulate MT activity in the waking state as a "waking dream."[93] Although an Agency for Healthcare Research and Quality report suggested that MT had limited effectiveness in treating insomnia,[94] a more recent meta-analysis of the effects of exogenous MT confirmed its beneficial effects on sleep-onset latency, total sleep time, and sleep efficiency.[95]

Preparations. MT is available in oral, sublingual, and transdermal immediate or sustained-release formulations. Sublingual MT can avoid first-pass liver metabolism, thereby resulting in more reliable serum levels. Given its short half-life (approximately 0.5–2 hours), sustained-release formulations administered at or near bedtime are more likely to maintain effective levels throughout the sleep period, while immediate-release sublingual formulations administered at awakening may be more effective in treating sleep maintenance insomnia and early morning awakenings.

DOSAGE

The recommended dose of MT is 0.3–0.5 mg for adults.[95] A sustained-release formulation more closely approximates the natural pattern of release. Although anecdotal data suggests higher doses may be effective for some, they can also disrupt sleep.

PRECAUTIONS

MT generally has a good safety profile; however, it is contraindicated in pregnancy, and concerns about it exacerbating autoimmune illness have been raised. One meta-analysis found adverse effects to be uncommon and more likely with high doses.[96,97]

Valerian Root (Valeriana officinalis)

Valerian is a sedating botanical with purported anxiolytic and hypnotic properties. In contrast to prescription sedative-hypnotics, valerian does not impair psychomotor or cognitive performance.[98,99] One review concluded that valerian was safe but did not have significant effects on sleep.[100] A second study concluded that valerian appeared effective for mild to moderate insomnia.[101] Valerian is nonaddictive, resulting in no withdrawal symptoms on discontinuation. Valerian may sometimes require weeks of nightly use before producing an effect.[102]

Preparation. Valerian is available as whole powdered root and an aqueous or ethanolic extract standardized to 0.8% valerenic acids. High-quality products have an unpleasant odor, which confirms potency.

DOSAGE

For adults: 300–900 mg standardized extract of 0.8% valerenic acid or as a tea of 2–3 g of dried root steeped for 10–15 minutes and taken 30–120 minutes before bedtime for 2–4 weeks to assess effectiveness

PRECAUTIONS

Valerian has a good safety profile.[100] Possible herb-drug interactions can increase sedation or alter drug metabolism. Caution should be exercised during pregnancy or in patients with a history of liver disease.

Hops (Humulus lupulus)

Hops refers to the flower clusters atop the *Humulus lupulus*. Best known for its use in beer, hops has also been used in traditional preparations to treat a broad range of conditions, including insomnia. The German Commission E Monographs listed hops as an approved remedy for insomnia.[102] More recent findings have shown a modest hypnotic effect of a valerian-hops combination in treating adult insomnia.[103] Hops are believed to have antispasmodic properties that can help reduce muscle tension and promote relaxation.[104] Additional evidence suggests that hops may be beneficial in alleviating hot flashes and other menopausal symptoms.[105]

DOSAGE

Prescribe 5:1 ethanolic extract, one-half to one dropper full, 30–60 minutes before bedtime.

PRECAUTIONS

Although no evidence indicates toxicity at medicinal dosages, avoiding the use of hops in pregnancy may be advisable.

L-theanine

L-theanine is a unique amino acid commonly found in green and black tea. Although human research is limited, animal studies and anecdotal experience suggest that l-theanine may be useful in managing anxiety, hypertension, the stimulant effects of caffeine, and sleeplessness.[106]

DOSAGE

There is limited data supporting l-theanine dosages for insomnia. Typical recommendations range from 50 to 400 mg taken 30–60 minutes before bedtime.

PRECAUTIONS

Although theanine is generally regarded as safe by the FDA, it is not recommended for pregnant or lactating women. Theanine can have an antihypertensive effect, so it should be used with caution when combined with antihypertensive medications. Avoid supplements that contain extracts of D-theanine.

Lemon Balm (*Melissa officinalis*)

Lemon balm leaves have been used medicinally for centuries to address insomnia. Available in capsules, teas, and essential oil, lemon balm is frequently combined with other sedating botanicals or nutraceuticals, such as valerian, hops, or l-theanine, to promote sleep. Lemon balm has an uplifting lemon-like fragrance and can be an effective aromatherapy agent.[107]

DOSAGE

Capsules of dried leaf: 300–500 mg, or as a tincture: 60 drops

PRECAUTIONS

Lemon balm should not be used by pregnant or lactating women.

Cannabis

The recent legalization of recreational and medical marijuana use in many states has sparked interest in cannabis as a potential sleep aid. Tetrahydrocannabinol (THC) has been shown to cause a 400-fold increase in endogenous MT.[108] Existing research suggests that cannabis does impact sleep, including REM sleep, but there are striking contradictions and inconsistencies in these findings. Older research relied on marijuana that was relatively weak in potency compared to the array of high potency hybrid products available today. Because rigorous, well-controlled studies are still lacking, the impact of cannabis on sleep likely depends on the specific kind utilized, the characteristics of the user, and the setting in which it is used.[109]

Numerous additional botanical and nutraceuticals supplements are available to promote sleep. Proprietary blends that include a number of ingredients run the risk of providing too little of any one of them. It goes without saying that healthy nutrition is essential for sleep and a range of nutrient deficiencies can contribute to insomnia. The role of vitamin D in promoting healthy sleep, for example, is now receiving substantial attention.[110,111]

Although it is beyond the scope of this chapter, a number of aromatherapeutic agents have also shown promise in promoting healthy sleep. Most notably, the effects of jasmine were found to be comparable to a benzodiazepine in a recent trial.[112]

MIND-BODY THERAPY

The Noise Reduction Approach for Insomnia

The breadth of an integrative approach to insomnia treatment can overwhelm patients. Too often, the misguided temptation is to reduce sophisticated integrative strategies that support a shift in consciousness and lifestyle to a simple sleep hygiene checklist. The Noise Reduction Approach for Insomnia (NRAI)[113] provides a comprehensive and face valid framework for patients by organizing complex and numerous etiological and therapeutic recommendations into an understandable and manageable system. More specifically, the NRAI uses a *body*, *mind*, and *bed* framework in which body refers to biomedical factors, mind refers to psychological factors, and bed refers to sleep environmental factors.

The NRAI conceptualizes healthy sleep in terms of a *sleepiness-to-noise ratio* in which *sleepiness* refers to the propensity to sleep and *noise* refers to any kind of stimulation that interferes with sleep. Noise is used to denote the subjective experience of hyperarousal. Both sleepiness and noise can derive from body, mind, or bed factors. Although insomnia can result from insufficient sleepiness caused by daytime sleep or dozing, inadequate activity, sedating medications, and circadian rhythm disorders, it usually results from excessive noise.

Noise resulting from body, mind, or bed factors is cumulative. For example, the stimulating effects of ordinary work stress, two cups of coffee, or minor reflux alone may not interfere with sleep; however, their cumulative effect may well reach a threshold that does. Insomnia occurs when an individual's noise level exceeds their sleepiness, whereas sleep occurs when noise levels fall below the threshold of sleepiness. Because the propensity to sleep is our natural default, the NRAI is less concerned with promoting sleepiness and more concerned with the identification and management of factors that produce noise.

Reducing Body Noise

The essential focus of body noise reduction is decreasing physiological manifestations of hyperarousal. In addition to the importance of promoting basic health through exercise, nutrition, and stress management, reducing body noise involves attending to a range of biomedical and lifestyle factors that commonly disrupt sleep. Box 9.6 summarizes the major components of body noise reduction.

Simultaneously addressing all comorbid disorders is essential. This is especially true for depression, primary sleep disorders, and disorders characterized by pain and discomfort. The reasonable assumption is that doing so may have a synergistic effect. For example, reducing pain will obviously improve sleep, but improving deep and REM sleep can raise pain thresholds by 60% and 200%, respectively.[114]

Managing the sleep-disruptive side effects of medications and substances (see Box 9.2), as well as managing caffeine and alcohol, is essential to reducing body

---

> **BOX 9.6** **Reducing Body Noise**
>
> - Manage all comorbid conditions, especially other sleep disorders, depression, and chronic pain.
> - Manage the sleep side effects of medications.
> - Manage alcohol and caffeine use.
> - Manage symptoms of women's health issues (e.g., premenstrual dysphoric disorder, menopause).

---

noise. Although individual variations exist, the half-life of caffeine is approximately 5 hours and can range from 2 hours for tobacco smokers to more than 10 hours for women who are pregnant or using oral contraceptives. Consuming two 8-ounce cups of drip coffee within an hour of morning awakening will leave approximately 35 mg of caffeine, the amount found in a cola drink, in one's system near bedtime. "Energy drinks," which contain 2–500 mg of caffeine per serving, have soared in popularity. Because the depressant effects of alcohol can facilitate sleep onset, it is widely used as a sleep aid. Insomnia increases the risk of relapse in patients recovering from alcoholism.[115] Alcohol, especially if consumed without food or near bedtime, commonly compromises sleep quality and results in subsequent arousals.

Common women's health concerns, including premenstrual syndrome and premenstrual dysphoric disorder,[116] pregnancy,[117] and menopause,[118] are strongly linked to insomnia. These conditions and any associated insomnia are most effectively addressed independently. Additionally, MT may be helpful in managing premenstrual syndrome and premenstrual dysphoric disorder,[119,120] possibly through regulating rhythmic features of the disorder. Menopausal symptoms, particularly hot flashes, are commonly blamed for repeated awakenings. Disrupted sleep, however, is not a likely consequence of menopause.[121]

> Menopause neither causes nor exacerbates sleep problems for most women.

Reducing Mind Noise

The basic goal of mind noise reduction is decreasing psychological and behavioral expressions of hyperarousal. This is largely achieved through CBT-I (cognitive-behavioral therapy for insomnia). CBT-I combines cognitive restructuring, which addresses insomnia-related dysfunctional thoughts and beliefs, with behavioral interventions including sleep hygiene education, stimulus control therapy (SCT), sleep restriction therapy (SRT), and relaxation practices. CBT-I also addresses common maladaptive coping reactions to insomnia that function as perpetuating factors. In addition to the treatment of individuals, CBT-I can be used in group settings, as well as through automated and web-based formats. Box 9.7 provides a list of mind noise reduction therapies. This list primarily contains CBT-I components, but it is expanded to include dream health, which is not typically addressed in conventional treatment.

BOX 9.7	**Mind Noise Reduction (Cognitive-Behavioral Therapy for Insomnia)**

- Sleep hygiene education
- Cognitive restructuring
- Stimulus control therapy
- Sleep restriction therapy
- Relaxation practices
- Restoring dream health

BOX 9.8	**Dysfunctional Thoughts About Sleep**

- I should sleep at least 8 hours every night.
- I should fall asleep quickly.
- I should always sleep through the night.
- I can and must get myself to sleep.
- I should just rest in bed if I cannot sleep.
- I will have a terrible day if I do not sleep well.

BOX 9.9	**Stimulus Control Therapy Instructions**

1. Get into bed with the intention to sleep only when sleepy.
2. Use the bed and bedroom only for sleep and sexual activity.
3. Do not watch the clock.
4. If awake after approximately 15 minutes, leave the bedroom, engage in restful activity, and return to bed when sleepy. Repeat as needed.
5. Keep a fixed morning rising time irrespective of the amount of sleep obtained.
6. Avoid napping until nighttime sleep is normal.

Compelling evidence indicates the effectiveness of CBT-I for primary insomnia,[5,122,123] and support for CBT-I in comorbid insomnia is growing.[22] CBT-I has been shown to be at least as effective as prescription medications in the short-term treatment of chronic insomnia, with beneficial effects extending well beyond the completion of treatment and no evidence of adverse effects.[124] Patients with insomnia who were treated with CBT-I experienced greater increases in deep sleep and decreases in wake time than those treated with zopiclone (Canadian hypnotic with similar action to eszopiclone). These benefits were still present at a 6-month follow-up in contrast to patients treated with zopiclone who showed no ongoing benefits of treatment.[125] CBT-I alone was also found to be no less effective than CBT-I paired with zolpidem.[126] CBT-I has also been shown to enhance depression outcomes for patients with comorbid insomnia.[127]

Sleep Hygiene. *Sleep hygiene* refers to a list of basic behavioral and environmental recommendations that promote healthy sleep. These can include most of the suggestions reviewed earlier, such as managing substances, regulating one's sleep–wake schedule, obtaining adequate exercise, and creating an environment conducive to sleep. Sleep hygiene has not been demonstrated effective as a stand-alone intervention, although most sleep specialists believe that it can be an effective aid to a multicomponent treatment approach.[128]

Cognitive Restructuring. Cognitive restructuring techniques systematically review, reconsider, and replace thoughts and beliefs that trigger sleep-disruptive anxiety and rumination. Box 9.8 provides examples of common dysfunctional thoughts about sleep. These thoughts are dysfunctional because they distort the truth, set up unrealistic expectations, and inevitably trigger anxiety. For example, the belief that "I can and must get myself to sleep" is nearly ubiquitous among patients with insomnia. Because it implies that falling asleep is under one's conscious control, this belief leads to excessive sleep effort, which then backfires by increasing arousal. Similarly, the common belief that "I should always sleep through the night" sets the stage for a reflexive reaction of frustration, disappointment, and even self-recrimination with wakefulness after sleep onset. In reality, what wakes one up is not necessarily what keeps one awake. Frequently, our strong reaction to the awakening, which is based on a dysfunctional belief, is the real problem. Similar cycles of disappointment, frustration, arousal, and anxiety can ensue from comparable dysfunctional thoughts and beliefs, and their effects can be cumulative.

Stimulus Control and Sleep Restriction Therapies. Both SCT and SRT are effective behavioral interventions for managing conditioned insomnia and reducing sleep efficiency.[129,130] Both approaches systematically minimize the amount of waking time spent in bed in an effort to increase sleep efficiency. SCT does so through self-monitoring and staying out of bed when sleepless. Box 9.9 provides basic SCT instructions.

SRT requires patients to limit the amount of time in bed to their average total sleep time established at baseline. Time in bed is then gradually increased as sleep efficiency improves. The administration of SRT is challenging to both patients and clinicians and should be used only by professionals trained in this intervention. Both SCT and SRT may be contraindicated in patients with sleep apnea, mania, epilepsy, and parasomnias and those at risk of falling.

Relaxation Practices. Relaxation practices, which have been included under the rubric of CBT-I, are useful in reducing sympathetic tone, decreasing mind noise, and familiarizing patients with the waking state of rest that serves as a transition to sleep. A myriad of effective techniques are available and should be matched to patients' interests and personalities. Breathing exercises are among the easiest and most portable practices.[131] Early research combining mindfulness meditation and CBT-I showed a reduction in sleep-related arousals[132] (see Chapter 94).

Restoring Dream Health. In contrast to conventional approaches, integrative therapies for insomnia are concerned with the restoration of dream health. From antiquity through recent times, dreams have been revered as rich sources of psychological insight, healing, and spirituality. Healthy REM sleep and dreaming are critical to the consolidation of procedural memory, as well as to the processing of emotion.[133]

BOX 9.10	Promoting Healthy Dreaming

- Identify and manage dream thieves
- Arise slowly in the morning to enhance recall
- Journal or talk about dreams
- Join a dream circle or support group
- Note dreamlike aspects of waking life

Trying to promote healthy sleep without considering dreams is like trying to promote healthy nutrition without regard for the taste of food.

Given the frequency of bad dreams and the common belief that high-quality sleep is devoid of dreaming, it is not surprising when patients with insomnia state that they would prefer not to dream at all. Dream avoidance, evident in Hamlet's classic remark, "To sleep, perchance to dream...," is clearly seen in patients with frequent nightmares and can result in sleep avoidance and arousals.[68]

Box 9.10 offers recommendations for promoting healthy dreaming. Simply asking patients whether they have dream recall can be an essential first step in sensitizing them to the importance of dreaming. In addition to avoiding dream thieves—REM-suppressant drugs, substances, and activities—it may be useful to intentionally recall and attend to one's dreams.[134] Because we usually awaken from dreams, arising slowly in the morning with a receptive attitude can improve recall. Bridging dream experiences to waking life through journaling, discussion, and noting the "waking dream," dreamlike aspects of ordinary waking life, can also be helpful.

Reducing Bed Noise

Although the sleep environment can have a critical impact on sleep, it has not yet received the attention it warrants. Recognizing the bedroom as not only a physical location, but also a temporal and psychological space, the goals of bed noise reduction include the following: (1) minimizing the toxic burden of the physical environment, (2) regulating circadian rhythms through entrainment with light and darkness, and (3) creating a sense of sanctuary that is free of ordinary waking life stimulation.

A Healthy Sleep Environment. Sensitivities or allergies to bedroom irritants or toxins can be pronounced or subtle. Awareness is increasing, as reflected in the growth of the natural mattress industry, of the importance of an environmentally friendly and toxin-free bedroom. In addition to recommendations to keep the bedroom quiet and cool (68°F or lower), compelling arguments have been made on behalf of "green" (organic) beds and bedding as well as clean bedroom air.[134,135] Box 9.11 lists common sources of bedroom toxicity that should be evaluated and addressed to improve sleep. Bedroom air quality can be improved with high-efficiency particulate air (HEPA) filtration systems as well as with varieties of ordinary houseplants. Because electromagnetic fields can suppress endogenous MT,[136] it is advisable to clear them from the sleep area.

BOX 9.11	Common Sources of Bedroom Toxicity

- Pesticide-laden fabrics in bed and bedding
- Synthetic materials in mattresses and pillows
- Outgassing from furnishings, floors, walls, or carpeting
- Polluted indoor air
- Electromagnetic fields

BOX 9.12	Regulating Circadian Rhythms

- Use phototherapy, with timed exposure to light and darkness.
- Maintain a regular sleep-wake pattern.
- Simulate dusk by dimming the lights or using blue blocker technology 1–2 hours before sleep.
- Supplement with melatonin.
- Sleep in total darkness.

Regulation of Circadian Rhythms. Time can be conceptualized in two distinct ways. Ordinary waking life is structured by linear or clock time. However, human biology, including sleep–wake cycles, operates on cyclic time, most evident in circadian rhythms. Nature's darkness may invite us to sleep, whereas culture, with its vast array of evening distractions, encourages us to stay awake.[70]

Sleep disorders, in part, are chronic skirmishes between nature and culture—between linear and cyclic time.

Zeitgebers (from the German, "time giver") refer to environmental and behavioral factors that regulate circadian rhythms. These include temporal patterns of feeding, activity or exercise, socialization, and, most importantly, the timing of exposure to light and darkness. Bright light signals the start of morning, whereas dim light or darkness conveys a sense of night to the brain's circadian pacemaker. Sleep-phase disorders, most commonly advanced or delayed sleep-phase syndromes, are common predisposing factors in insomnia. These disorders can be effectively treated by systematically manipulating exposure to light and darkness to restructure the position of the patient's sleep phase within their circadian cycles.

Regulating circadian rhythms (Box 9.12) is a critical component of treating insomnia. Maintaining a regular sleep–wake pattern 7 days per week is essential in promoting a healthy sleep rhythm. Bright light exposure for approximately 30–45 minutes shortly after morning arising is a most potent Zeitgeber[137] as well as a potential antidepressant.[138] When natural light is not an option, light boxes that provide comparable lux levels are commercially available. Exposure to higher lux levels of natural light throughout the waking day may also reduce daytime sleepiness.[139]

Given the relentless demands of daily living, dusk simulation practices—dimming lights for 2 to 3 hours before

| BOX 9.13 | Creating a Sense of Sanctuary |

- Establish the bedroom as a stress-free and work-free zone.
- Limit exposure to stressful imagery from books, television, and radio.
- Conceal ready access to clocks.
- Establish a sense of personal safety.
- Maintain peace with your sleep partner.

bedtime—are particularly challenging. Dim light diminishes the blue wavelength of light prominent in natural daylight, artificial lighting, and computer and television screens. The blue wavelength of light has been shown to signal the brain to suppress MT production, thus delaying the start of the sleep phase.[140] Newer blue light filtration technology in the form of goggles and light bulbs can provide illumination without suppressing MT (see Key Web Resources) and can minimize the negative impact of reading or watching television.

Because even small amounts of light can trickle across closed eyelids and suppress MT, sleeping in total darkness or with a sleep mask is ideal.

Creating a Sense of Sanctuary. For many who struggle with insomnia, the bedroom is a place of work, entertainment, and other activities that may be antagonistic to sleep. Reimagining the bedroom as a sanctuary (Box 9.13), a place of retreat from the world of waking, is helpful. To do so, the bedroom should be a work-free, stress-free, and clock-free zone. Exposure to stressful imagery from reading material, television, or radio should be avoided. Clock watching is a common compulsion among patients with insomnia and serves only to exacerbate sleeplessness by tethering them to the waking world of linear time. Establishing a deep sense of personal or psychological safety in the bedroom is also important. For some patients, this may mean installing a security system, whereas for others it may mean keeping a religious icon on the bed stand.

The percentage of couples sleeping apart, largely as a result of sleep disorders, has increased dramatically and now stands at 23%.[141] Sleeping apart is associated with negative effects on the relationship.[142] Addressing sleep symptoms (e.g., snoring or periodic limb movements in sleep) that may provoke one's sleep partner is essential. Differing sleep environment preferences can also be negotiated. Creating a sense of sanctuary in the bedroom encourages an essential shift from waking to *night consciousness*.[70]

Fundamentally, insomnia is associated with inadvertently smuggling waking consciousness into the world of night and sleep.

Behavioral Sleep Medicine Specialists

Although some components of CBT-I can be implemented by patients on their own, this complex therapy generally requires specialized training. The stepped care model for CBT-I recommends a hierarchy of five increasing levels of interventions associated with clinician expertise and patient needs (Fig. 9.2). Behavioral sleep medicine specialists, formally trained and certified in the use of CBT-I, are a small but steadily growing and key professional resource in this model (see Key Web Resources).

A Basic Primary Care Intervention

Due to the shortage of behavioral sleep medicine specialists, practical implementation of CBT-I has been lagging. Today, the majority of insomnia patients rarely, if ever, see a behavioral sleep medicine specialist. Given that primary care is the front-line contact for most insomnia patients, providers need to be educated in their diagnosis and treatment. New research suggests that insomnia patients may be effectively treated by primary care providers with a brief, single-session of sleep restriction therapy.[143]

PREVENTION PRESCRIPTION

Preventing insomnia by intentionally maintaining healthy sleep is considerably less daunting than treating it.

- Recognize the value and joy of sleep.
- Attend to and journal dreams.
- Engage in relaxation practices daily.
- Perform adequate regular exercise.
- Obtain daily exposure to morning light.
- Limit the use of stimulants and sedatives.
- Maintain a regular sleep–wake schedule.
- Dim lights or use blue blocker tools 1–2 hours before sleep.
- Sleep in total darkness or use a sleep mask.
- Sleep in a cool environment
- Consider low-dose melatonin replacement therapy.

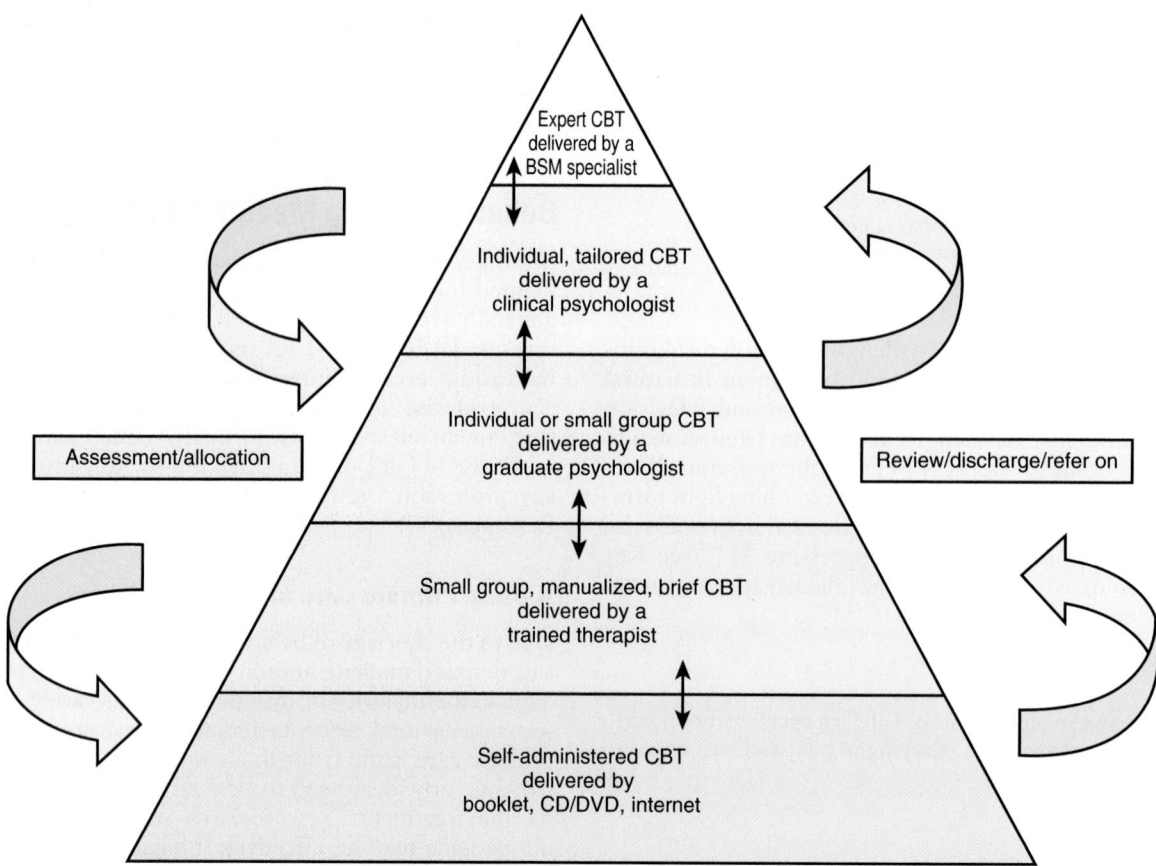

FIG. 9.2 ■ A Stepped Care Model for Cognitive-Behavioral Therapy for Insomnia (CBT-I). This evidence-based model for CBT illustrates how patients may be allocated to resources. *Arrows* represent referral movements. BSM, behavioral sleep medicine. (From Espie CA. "Stepped care": a health technology solution for delivering cognitive behavioral therapy as a first line insomnia treatment. *Sleep.* 2009;32:1549-1558).

THERAPEUTIC REVIEW

REDUCE BODY NOISE

- Directly address all comorbid conditions, especially primary sleep disorders, depression, chronic pain, and women's health issues. Evaluate and manage sleep side effects of all medications (see Box 9.2). Evaluate and manage alcohol, caffeine, and other stimulant use.
- Melatonin: 0.3–0.5 mg at bedtime, especially if the patient may have an associated circadian rhythm disorder
- Avoid sedative-hypnotics , and use complementary and alternative medicine sleep aids as needed, preferably on a short-term (2- to 4-week) basis. Consider one or a combination of the following:
  - Valerian, for adults: 300 to 900 mg standardized extract of 0.8% valerenic acid or as a tea of 2–3 g of dried root steeped for 10–15 minutes and taken 30–120 minutes before bedtime for 2–4 weeks to assess effectiveness
  - Hops: in a 5:1 ethanolic extract, ½; to one dropper full, 30–60 minutes before bedtime
  - L-theanine: 50–400 mg taken 30–60 minutes before bedtime.
  - Lemon balm: 300–500 mg or 60 drops of tincture; can be used in blends with valerian, l-theanine, or other soporifics.

REDUCE MIND NOISE

- Encourage patients to select and engage in a daily relaxation practice. The 4-7-8 relaxing breath exercise (Box 9.14) is an easy and effective option.

- Use stimulus control therapy for sleep efficiency lower than 85%.
- Consider sleep restriction therapy as a standalone intervention in lieu of sedative-hypnotics.
- Evaluate and discuss basic dysfunctional beliefs and thoughts about sleep. Refer the patient to a behavioral sleep medicine specialist for more elaborate cognitive restructuring therapy as needed.
- Encourage dream recall by limiting "dream thieves," and promote daily dream journaling and participation in dream support groups. Refer patients with chronic nightmares to a behavioral sleep specialist for image rehearsal therapy.

REDUCE BED NOISE

- Recommend reduction of bedroom toxicity from beds, bedding, and furnishings, as well as air filtration with high-efficiency particulate air (HEPA) filters or houseplants. Encourage evaluation of and protection from electromagnetic fields.
- Urge the patient to maintain a regular sleep–wake schedule, including on weekends. The patient should simulate dusk by dimming lights or using blue blocker technology (see Key Web Resources) 1–2 hours before sleep, and sleep in total darkness. Exposure to morning light is important.
- Encourage patients to create a sense of sanctuary by establishing the bedroom as a stress-free and work-free zone, limiting exposure to stressful imagery and clocks, ensuring a sense of personal safety, and maintaining peace with bed partners.

BOX 9.14	4-7-8 Relaxing Breath Exercise

1. Place the tip of your tongue against the ridge behind your front teeth and exhale completely through your mouth.
2. Inhale through your nose for a count of 4.
3. Hold your breath for a count of 7.
4. Exhale through your mouth with a swooshing sound to the count of 8.
5. Repeat this cycle three more times for a total of four breaths.

The ratio of 4:7:8 is key, not the actual time spent on each breath cycle. Practice at least twice daily, beginning with no more than four breath cycles at one time for the first month and increasing to eight breath cycles afterward if desired. This exercise can be used to increase presleep relaxation and to facilitate sleep onset in bed.

Key Web Resources

American Academy of Sleep Medicine. This website provides professional information and resources for sleep medicine.	http://www.aasmnet.org/
Society of Behavioral Sleep Medicine. This official website includes links to lists of certified behavioral sleep medicine specialists.	http://www.behavioralsleep.org/
Epworth Sleepiness Scale. This official website provides an overview of and access to the Epworth Sleepiness Scale.	http://epworthsleepinessscale.com/
Fatigue Severity Scale. This Medscape website provides information about fatigue and the Fatigue Severity Scale.	http://www.medscape.org/viewarticle/472869
Sleep diary forms. These documents assist patients in collecting and monitoring data essential for initial and ongoing evaluation.	http://www.sleepeducation.org/docs/default-document-library/sleep-diary.pdf
The Dark Side of Sleeping Pills. Dr. Daniel Kripke's complementary e-book discusses the risks of sedative-hypnotics.	http://www.darksideofsleepingpills.com/all.html
Low Blue Lights. This commercial website provides information, research, and products related to blue light filtering technology.	https://www.lowbluelights.com/index.asp
SHUTi (Sleep Health Using the Internet). This is an automated web-based program of cognitive-behavioral therapy for insomnia that was developed by the University of Virginia.	http://www.myshuti.com/
Dr. R. Naiman. This website promotes the development of integrative sleep medicine.	http://www.drnaiman.com/

REFERENCES

References are available online at ExpertConsult.com.

CHAPTER 10

POSTTRAUMATIC STRESS DISORDER (PTSD)

David J. Kearney, MD • Michelle E. Martinez, MPH • Tracy L. Simpson, PhD

DEFINITION AND DIAGNOSTIC CRITERIA

Posttraumatic stress disorder (PTSD) is a common consequence of trauma that, without treatment, can persist for decades.[1] The lifetime risk of developing PTSD is estimated to be 6.8%, with women more likely to be affected than men.[2] The clinical hallmarks of PTSD include recurrent, intrusive recollections or reexperiencing of a traumatic event, avoidance of external or internal trauma reminders, negative changes in cognitions and mood, and changes in arousal and reactivity.[3] PTSD has been shown to have a greater impact on quality of life than major depression and obsessive-compulsive disorder, and it is estimated that the typical person with PTSD experiences active symptoms for at least two decades over their lifespan.[1] PTSD is also significantly associated with an increased lifetime risk of suicide, with a stronger association with suicidality than any other anxiety disorder.[4] PTSD often results in severe reductions in quality of life, including disruptions in interpersonal relationships and ability to work in addition to increased risk of mood and substance/alcohol use disorders.[5,6] PTSD is also associated with an increased risk of developing physical conditions, including arthritis, coronary artery disease, metabolic syndrome, chronic pain syndromes, and asthma, after adjusting for other risk factors.[7,8]

A number of different types of treatments for PTSD have been evaluated, including pharmacological, traditional cognitive-behavioral (CBT) interventions, and complementary and alternative (CAM) interventions. In this chapter, we provide a brief overview of these treatments, with particular emphasis on various CAM approaches for PTSD. Where possible, we have used comprehensive systematic reviews and meta-analyses as guides, with greater weighting given to the results of randomized clinical trials (RCTs) than open trials or case studies. We begin by describing the least invasive approaches before providing an overview of psychotherapeutic approaches and conclude with an overview of current psychopharmacology literature.

INTEGRATIVE THERAPY

Exercise

Previous studies have demonstrated that exercise is effective in reducing anxiety and reactivity,[9] which are prominent components of PTSD symptoms. Three PTSD studies were identified in a review of research exploring the anxiety-reducing effect of exercise on a range of anxiety disorders.[9] Each of these studies used aerobic exercises (rather than weight lifting or circuit training) as the intervention, and the length and frequency of exercise varied between the studies. In a pre–post open trial involving a sample of adolescent females, an exercise routine of 40-minute sessions three times a week for 8 weeks led to a reduction in PTSD symptoms, depression, and anxiety.[10] A separate open trial of adolescent females reported the efficacy of 5 weeks of 3 weekly sessions of aerobic exercise in treating PTSD. Heart rates were measured at the conclusion of the 12th minute of moderate-intensity exercise to ensure rates had decreased to between 60%–90% of the maximum calculated heart rate. The intervention resulted in significant reductions in PTSD symptoms at posttreatment for 90% of participants, and general anxiety was significantly reduced in >50% of participants.[11] Significant reductions in the symptoms of PTSD, anxiety, and depression were observed posttreatment in an open trial of adults who participated in a program involving twelve 40-minute sessions of exercise that maintained 60%–80% of their calculated maximum heart rate.[12] In all three studies, symptom improvement was maintained at 1-month followup.[9] Although these findings provide encouraging preliminary evidence, future studies in this area should use larger sample sizes and appropriate control groups to strengthen the evidence base for aerobic exercise as a treatment option for PTSD.

> Encouraging exercise may have utility in reducing PTSD symptoms, anxiety, and depression. Exercise is also posited to lead to reductions in coping-oriented alcohol use without patients making specific efforts to cut back on alcohol consumption.

There is preliminary evidence that exercise may be associated with a decreased risk of symptoms that commonly co-occur with PTSD, including suicidal ideation and use of alcohol as a coping strategy. For example, veterans in inpatient PTSD treatment who reported engaging in relatively more exercise were found to be at decreased risk of suicide and depression, and to have improved sleep patterns.[13] In a separate correlational study, vigorous-intensity exercise (≥6 resting metabolic equivalents) was found to be inversely correlated with alcohol use as a coping strategy among individuals who had experienced trauma, indicating that encouraging exercise may lead to reductions in coping-oriented alcohol use without any special efforts to cut back on alcohol consumption.[14]

MIND-BODY

In the interest of providing patients with increased options for treatment, there has been increasing interest in CAM modalities for the treatment of PTSD. Further, the Institute of Medicine (IOM) has called for more research in these areas.[15] The following overview of the literature pertaining to CAM and mind-body interventions for PTSD is an extension of the comprehensive systematic review published by Helané Wahbeh et al. in 2014.[16] We have provided summaries of their findings along with information about relevant studies that have been published since 2013 when their literature search concluded.

Meditation

Meditation can be considered a broad term that encompasses a wide variety of practices involving attention and mental focus.[17,18] Mindfulness practice may involve techniques that run counter to tendencies to suppress or avoid painful emotions and thoughts, as is characteristic of PTSD. A small body of literature suggests that meditation may have benefit in cases of PTSD. In their systematic review of CAM for PTSD, Wahbeh et al. reported on 9 studies of meditation (5 RCTs and 4 pre–post studies).[16] Of note, all pre–post studies showed positive outcomes and the majority of RCTs (which were of variable quality) reported favorable outcomes for meditation compared to waitlist controls.[16] Because there are a wide variety of techniques for practicing meditation, which differ according to how mental focus is cultivated,[18] we review specific meditation practices that have been postulated to be effective in the treatment of PTSD in this section.[18] These include mindfulness meditation, mantra repetition meditation, and compassion-based meditation.[18]

> Mindfulness practice may involve techniques that run counter to tendencies to suppress or avoid painful emotions and thoughts, as is characteristic of PTSD.

Mindfulness Meditation

Mindfulness is defined as "the awareness that emerges by way of paying attention on purpose, in the present moment, and nonjudgmentally to the unfolding of experience moment by moment."[19] In mindfulness-based interventions, individuals are taught to pay attention to experiences with an attitude of curiosity, openness, acceptance, and kindness. In this way, mindfulness practice runs counter to tendencies to suppress or avoid painful emotions and thoughts, as is characteristic of PTSD.[20]

Mindfulness practice is postulated to represent a form of exposure therapy.[21]

Two of the most widely available clinical programs for teaching mindfulness meditation are an 8-week class series called Mindfulness-Based Stress Reduction (MBSR) and Mindfulness-Based Cognitive Therapy (MBCT). A well-designed RCT (n = 116) compared MBSR to an active control condition and found that patients randomized to MBSR had greater improvements in PTSD symptom severity, depression, and quality of life at 2-month followup.[22] In addition, a significantly greater proportion of patients randomized to MBSR experienced clinically significant improvements in PTSD symptoms compared to the control condition (49% vs. 28%; $P = 0.03$).[22] These findings corroborate the results of two before-and-after studies of MBSR in individuals with a high prevalence of PTSD, which both reported significant improvements in symptoms of PTSD, depression, and quality of life over time.[23,24] A separate small trial comparing MBCT to usual care for veterans with PTSD reported greater PTSD symptom reductions after MBCT.[25] Other studies of mindfulness-based interventions have indicated the benefit of a telehealth mindfulness intervention[26] and a mindfulness-based stretching and deep breathing exercise program[27] in improving PTSD symptoms. Further definitive trials of mindfulness-based intervention for PTSD are required and are currently ongoing.

Mantra Meditation

A mantra is a sacred word or phrase that is repeated silently over the course of the day as a means of training attention with the intent of bringing about a sense of peace and relaxation.[18] As noted in the review by Wahbeh et al.,[16] both a before-and-after study[28] and an RCT (compared with a waitlist control)[29] evaluating mantram repetition reported that participation in the intervention was associated with significant reductions in PTSD. More recent research on a mantram repetition program (not included in the Wahbeh review)[16] include an RCT (n = 146) comparing this intervention (6-week duration, 90 min per week) to usual care for military veterans with PTSD and observed an associated with significantly greater reductions in PTSD symptoms and depression than treatment as usual alone.[30] In this study, reductions in PTSD symptoms were mediated by enhanced existential spiritual wellbeing[31] and mindfulness.[32] Transcendental meditation (TM) is another type of mantra meditation practice in which one's attention is placed on a mantra as an object of attention. TM is generally practiced with eyes closed for 15–20 minutes, twice per day. The evidence supporting the use of TM for PTSD is limited. However, a small RCT comparing TM to psychotherapy among Vietnam veterans[33] and a before-and-after study involving Operation Iraqi Freedom/Operation Enduring Freedom veterans[34] (included in the Wahbeh review)[16] both found that TM was associated with reductions in PTSD. A moderate-sized RCT comparing TM to no intervention among Congolese refugees.[35] TM is hypothesized to reduce hyperarousal by effects on the autonomic nervous system.[18]

Loving-Kindness/Compassion Meditation

Loving-kindness and compassion meditation practices are intended to enhance one's capacity for kindness and compassion to self and others. Self-compassion is associated with healthy psychological functioning and negatively associated with self-criticism, rumination, thought suppression, and depression,[36] which are phenomena frequently associated with PTSD.[37] Loving-kindness and compassion practices are theorized to represent an innovative approach to address emotional numbing, which is common in chronic PTSD. In loving-kindness meditation, individuals silently repeat a series of phrases that invoke the desire for safety, happiness, health, and ease or peace for self and others. Two studies evaluating this approach were not included in the Wahbeh review. A before-and-after study of veterans with PTSD (n = 42) reported improvements in symptoms of PTSD and depression, as well as increases in self-compassion and pleasant emotions over time.[38,39] Another self-compassion intervention, "Compassionate mind training," appeared promising for people with a history of trauma in a small open trial[40] (see Chapter 100).

Relaxation Exercises

There is little evidence to support relaxation training as an effective treatment modality for PTSD. Relaxation, which typically involves teaching patients various scripted exercises, has been studied primarily as a control condition in trials of PTSD treatment. In the systematic review by Wahbeh et al., four trials that assessed relaxation techniques for PTSD (two randomized controlled trials, one before-and-after, and one crossover) were described.[16] The studies were all limited by significant methodological shortcomings and reported mixed or negative results (see Chapter 94).

Visualization and Guided Imagery

Visualization or imagery-based therapies for PTSD have predominantly focused on addressing chronic nightmares, as opposed to the full range of symptoms. These therapies include imaginal confrontation with nightmare contents (ICNC), imagery rescripting and rehearsal (IRR), imagery rehearsal therapy (IRT), and imagery rescripting and exposure therapy (IRET). In a meta-analytic review of 20 studies of treatments incorporating IRR or ICNC for PTSD nightmares, in addition to sleep quality, depression, anxiety, and PTSD severity, both IRR and ICNC were found to be effective. However, the quality of this evidence has been called into question. In a review of 16 trials that used a range of imagery rehearsal approaches for PTSD, Harb et al. found that most had low methodological quality due to a lack of details regarding treatment delivery (which inhibits replication of the treatment in a future trial) and poor descriptions of sample populations.[41] Research investigating the impact of visualization on the full range of PTSD symptoms (rather than nightmares alone) is also lacking. A recent randomized controlled trial described in the Wahbeh review[16] incorporated guided imagery into its treatment arm; however, this was coupled with healing touch, which

limited the ability of the study to determine which treatment was responsible for the improvements observed.[42] Currently, the evidence base for visualization treatments is too underdeveloped to determine its clinical value as a PTSD treatment method, although it may have utility as a supplement to an evidence-based approach due to its apparent safety (see Chapter 97).

Yoga

Yoga is a practice that typically includes physical postures, breathing exercises, and meditation, with the relative emphasis on each of these components varying according to the style of yoga practiced.[43] Yoga also involves paying attention to emotional and physical stimuli. In this way, yoga can be considered a form of mindfulness practice.[43,44] Yoga has been hypothesized to influence pathways that may favorably impact PTSD, including upregulation of the parasympathetic nervous system, downregulation of the sympathetic nervous system, and decreased basal cortisol and catecholamine levels.[44] In addition, practicing yoga may represent a form of behavioral activation[43] and may encourage grounding in the body, both of which may counter PTSD-related avoidance and hyperarousal symptoms.

There is growing evidence indicating a beneficial effect of yoga for PTSD, with four of five comparative trials reporting benefit. A nonrandomized trial (n = 183; included in the Wahbeh review)[16] compared a yoga breath intervention for tsunami survivors to a yoga breath intervention plus exposure therapy or a waitlist control. A similar level of symptom reduction was observed with the two interventions such that exposure therapy component did not confer additional benefit; however, both active interventions were found to be superior to the waitlist control.[45] In a recent, well-designed RCT (n = 60; published since the Wahbeh review)[16] that compared a 10-week duration (one hour per week) yoga intervention to an active control (supportive health education), yoga was associated with significantly greater improvements in PTSD symptoms compared to the active control and was well tolerated.[46] Two smaller randomized trials (n = 38 and n = 22; not included in the Wahbeh review)[16] reported conflicting results regarding PTSD outcomes as compared to control groups that did not receive treatment.[44,47] Larger randomized controlled trials are required to clarify the effectiveness of yoga practice in reducing PTSD symptoms and improving quality of life; however, the current small body of evidence indicates the benefit of yoga in treating PTSD symptoms.[48]

Emotional Freedom Technique and Thought Field Therapy

Thought field therapy (TFT) and emotional freedom technique (EFT) are similar methods that use a combination of exposure through visualization and acupoint tapping to address emotional disturbances. In these treatments, PTSD is conceptualized as an emotional disturbance resulting from conflicts in the body's energy field (also known as the meridian system) or thought fields.[49]

EFT or TFT involves eliciting the imagery, narrative, and physiological arousal associated with a traumatic memory while tapping on the ends of one's energy meridians located at certain points on the body in a specific sequence. This process is theorized to release energy blockages that create the negative emotions associated with the disturbing memory.

There is some preliminary evidence that TFT and EFT may be effective treatments for PTSD. An open trial of participants receiving TFT found that posttreatment total scores and symptom subgroupings of the DSM criteria for PTSD dropped significantly from pretreatment scores.[50] In a small RCT (n = 46), individuals with PTSD were assigned to EFT or eye movement desensitization and reprocessing (EMDR) and assessed 3 months later. Results showed similar therapeutic gains for both interventions.[49] A more recent before-and-after study provided male veterans and their spouses with a multimodal intervention that involved EFT and other energy/psychology methods that was associated with significant decreases in PTSD symptoms, which were maintained through followup.[51] Finally, a more recent randomized controlled trial compared 6-hour-long sessions of EFT and standard care to a waitlist group (standard care only) and observed significant decreases in psychological distress and PTSD symptom levels in EFT subjects, with 90% of those receiving EFT no longer meeting PTSD criteria at the end of the study (compared to 4% in the standard care/waitlist group).[52] Though these studies are encouraging, validation by further studies is required due to high drop-out rates[49] and a lack of control arms in open trials[50,51] (see Chapter 103).

Hypnotherapy

As a treatment for PTSD, hypnosis provides guided, controlled access to traumatic memories that may be kept out of normal consciousness.[53] Hypnotherapists can help patients access and experience traumatic memories and then assist in reshaping these experiences. More specific forms of hypnotherapy can also be employed. For example, hypnotherapeutic olfactory conditioning may be used to treat resistant olfactory-induced flashbacks.[54]

Wahbeh et al. reviewed two RCTs comparing hypnosis to an active control arm.[16] In a study using cognitive behavioral therapy as the active control, hypnotherapy was found to be associated with comparable outcomes to CBT at 3-year followup.[55] The other study focused on PTSD-related insomnia and used Zolpidem as a pharmaceutical active control.[56] The hypnotherapy group had significantly better outcomes compared to patients treated with Zolpidem with regard to improved insomnia and other symptoms; however, Zolpidem was not expected to improve PTSD symptoms unrelated to sleep.

Abreactive Ego State Therapy

Abreactive ego state therapy (AEST) is a form of hypnosis based on the psychodynamic view of personality being comprised of several "ego states." In the framework of AEST, it is believed that the underlying pathology of PTSD results from memory encodings specific to the traumatic event and tied to particular ego states, which are treatable through hypnosis-guided emotional catharsis. Abreactive hypnosis activates expression of the trauma-related ego state to release affect through subcortical processes. Therapists provide support, encouragement, and foster adaptive communication among patient ego states, thereby altering attitudes and emotional reactions related to trauma at subcortical (subconscious) levels.[57]

Ego state therapy has been internationally embraced for a range of trauma disorders, but it is not as commonly used in the United States. However, there is preliminary evidence that supports it as a treatment for PTSD. Barabasz et al. conducted two recent studies of AEST for PTSD (neither of which were included in the Wahbeh review)[16] comparing a single five- to six-hour session of AEST with a 3-phase active placebo involving an informational video about PTSD and an introduction to the "counting method."[58-60] Both treatment arms led to significant improvements in common measures of PTSD symptoms at posttreatment; however, the effect sizes within the placebo group were markedly smaller than those in the AEST group. Additionally, improvements following AEST continued through follow-up measures, whereas the therapeutic impact observed in the placebo groups had disappeared by the first follow-up visit. This was true for both studies. Although these results are encouraging, further high-quality studies are required.

Psychotherapy

Psychotherapies for PTSD and other psychiatric disorders emphasize the reduction of painful thoughts and feelings and seek to achieve this through a variety of means, including skill building to cope more effectively with trauma cues and stressors, desensitization and habituation through repeated or prolonged exposure to imaginal and in vivo trauma cues, and restructuring maladaptive thoughts and beliefs pertaining to traumatic events. Stress inoculation treatment (SIT), prolonged exposure (PE), eye movement desensitization and reprocessing (EMDR), and cognitive processing therapy (CPT) all have been evaluated in multiple RCTs and are considered empirically supported treatments for PTSD (EST).[61]

Psychotherapies for PTSD can generally be categorized as trauma-focused therapies and nontrauma-focused therapies.

Trauma-focused therapies are forms of cognitive behavioral therapy that address memories, thoughts, emotions, and beliefs associated with the traumatic event(s), and include cognitive processing therapy (CPT), prolonged exposure therapy (PE), and eye movement desensitization and reprocessing therapy (EMDR).

Nontrauma-focused interventions emphasize the development of skills (e.g., stress management, relaxation, or problem-solving) and provide instructions regarding the application of these skills in daily life, such as reminders of the trauma, relationship difficulties, and daily stressors. In contrast to trauma-focused therapies, nontrauma-focused approaches do not directly attempt to address trauma-related beliefs, emotions, or memories. Present centered therapy (PCT) is a nontrauma-focused intervention that facilitates the use of patients' own coping strategies and has recently been found to have results that are only marginally inferior to trauma-focused CBT and superior with regard to treatment retention.[62,63]

Narrative exposure therapies, which involve individuals constructing a story of their lives that they then tell another person either directly or through an interpreter, have been found to be effective in reducing PTSD and trauma symptoms among refugees, particularly when administered by counselors who themselves are refugees.[64]

The literature base regarding psychological interventions for children and adolescents with PTSD is far more limited than for adults. To date, CBT has most consistently been found to be effective at reducing PTSD symptoms,[65] with trauma-focused variants possibly the most efficacious.[66] EMDR has not been found to outperform conventional treatment in children with regard to overall PTSD symptoms, and narrative therapy has been shown to be associated with short-term but not longer-term gains.[65]

There is even more limited research on psychological approaches for preventing PTSD. Early efforts evaluating single-session critical incident debriefing strategies were found to not be helpful and to actually be harmful such that those who underwent them were over two and a half times more likely to meet diagnostic criteria for PTSD at follow-up than those in the no-treatment control conditions.[67] More recently, a meta-analysis of multiple session interventions for preventing PTSD also failed to find these approaches helpful and noted a trend toward increased PTSD symptoms at follow-up in patients who received active interventions compared to formal intervention.[68] In contrast, brief trauma-focused CBT has been found to be helpful in reducing acute traumatic stress symptoms in a number of studies. Acute traumatic stress is defined as meeting the diagnostic criteria for PTSD when less than 1 month has elapsed posttrauma.[69]

> Cognitive behavior therapy is recommended for the treatment of children and adolescents with PTSD because CBT has the most substantial evidence base for reducing PTSD symptoms in this population.

ACUPUNCTURE

There is growing evidence that acupuncture may be an effective treatment for PTSD, particularly as a supplement to other forms of treatment. Three RCTs have provided evidence that acupuncture or acupoint stimulation significantly improves PTSD symptoms compared to control conditions, two of which were included in the Wahbeh review.[16] In the first, acupuncture and CBT were compared to waitlist control, with both found to be significantly more effective than the control and similar to each other.[70] The other found that a combination of acupoint stimulation and CBT was more effective than CBT alone.[71] In a more recent study, 55 service members

were randomized to acupuncture (eight 60-minute sessions of acupuncture twice weekly) or treatment as usual. Patients in the acupuncture group reported significant improvements in PTSD severity as well as depression, pain, and physical and mental health functioning compared to the treatment as usual group.[72] A meta-analysis of two RCTs compared acupuncture plus moxibustion to SSRIs and concluded the results favored acupuncture plus moxibustion for PTSD symptoms, depression, and anxiety.[73]

> Acupuncture is a reasonable treatment approach for patients with PTSD who do not wish to pursue traditional psychotherapeutic options.

Although these outcomes are encouraging, additional placebo or sham-controlled trials are warranted. Side effects of acupuncture are uncommon but include dizziness, nausea and vomiting, pain, fainting, and infection of needle insertion points. Acupuncture may be appropriate for patients whose preference is to not engage in more conventional therapies.

REPETITIVE TRANSCRANIAL MAGNETIC STIMULATION

Repetitive transcranial magnetic stimulation (rTMS) is a multisession treatment that uses magnetic fields to stimulate nerve cells associated with mood control and depression, reaching no more than 5–6 cm into the right dorsolateral prefrontal cortex of the brain. rTMS is a noninvasive procedure, and side effects are rare but may include seizures (rTMS is not recommended for patients with epilepsy), pain at the stimulation site, muscle twitching during treatment, posttreatment headache, and toothache. It is primarily used to treat medication-resistant major depression; however, there is emerging evidence of its efficacy in treating PTSD. A systematic review[16] and meta-analysis[74] of three RCT trials applying rTMS to subjects with PTSD have indicated significant differences favoring rTMS for improvement in PTSD symptoms, overall anxiety, and depressive symptoms. Additional studies are required. Also, rTMS is not widely available, which currently limits its utility in clinical practice.

PHARMACOTHERAPIES

The U.S. Food and Drug Administration (FDA) has approved the use of the selective serotonin reuptake inhibitor (SSRI) antidepressant medications, sertraline and paroxetine, based on a series of positive RCTs favoring these medications.[75-78] Although a recent large meta-analysis of medications for PTSD supported the use of paroxetine in adults, sertraline was not found to consistently outperform placebo treatments.[79] This meta-analysis also found that two additional SSRIs, fluoxetine and venlafaxine, outperformed placebo on both clinician and self-rated symptoms of PTSD.[79]

Because SSRIs typically have limited effects on PTSD, with significant symptom reduction observed in approximately 60% of patients and full remission in only 30%, the use of the atypical antipsychotic medications, such as risperidone and olanzapine, has also been evaluated in adults.[80] A recent meta-analysis of the use of atypical antipsychotics for PTSD based on eight RCTs found that they both outperformed placebo and, importantly, were well-tolerated.[81]

Other types of medications have also been subjected to double-blind tests of efficacy for the treatment of PTSD among adults, including prazosin, an alpha-1 adrenergic receptor antagonist, and nabilone, a synthetic cannabinoid. Prazosin has been found to ameliorate PTSD-related nightmares and sleep disturbance and improve overall clinical status in several trials.[82-85] In a small crossover double-blind trial of nabilone, the active medication was found to reduce nightmares and improve global functioning relative to placebo;[86] however, further studies of nabilone are required before its adoption into clinical practice.

Pharmacotherapies have only recently begun to be evaluated among children and young adults, with the majority of available information based on small open trials.[87] Thus far, double-blind RCTs involving children and youth have not found sertraline to outperform placebo.[88,89] Small open label-trial studies involving children and/or young adults indicate the noradrenergic agent, guanfacine, along with propranolol, respiridone, and the mood stabilizer carbamazepine may be worthy of further study.[90]

Pharmacological approaches have also been evaluated for the prevention of PTSD following exposure to trauma in adults. Pharmacological agents have been studied due to their potential to inhibit the formation of trauma memories. A recent Cochrane review of nine relevant RCTs concluded that there is moderate quality evidence (based on four trials) supporting the use of hydrocortisone (relative risk, 0.17), but no support for propranolol, escitalopram, temazepam, or gabapentin (the final three medications have only been tested in one RCT each), in preventing PTSD. Although results regarding the efficacy of hydrocortisone in preventing PTSD in adults are promising, the authors concluded that there is not sufficient evidence to endorse hydrocortisone use in routine clinical practice.[91]

Therapies to Consider

Biofeedback

Biofeedback uses electronic instruments to provide immediate information to patients so that they can learn to control physiological functions. For PTSD, biofeedback attempts to teach patients techniques for detecting and controlling physiological changes associated with increased arousal, which in turn is theorized to lead to reductions in symptoms.[92,93] Heart rate variability (HRV), a marker of parasympathetic nervous system function, is typically the physiological parameter monitored. Patients are trained to control their breathing pattern in order to increase HRV. However, literature regarding biofeedback for PTSD remains very limited. There have been four trials conducted of biofeedback for PTSD (two RCTs, one nonrandomized controlled trial, and one before-and-after study),[16] with the controlled trials reporting mixed results.[92-94] Further research on biofeedback for PTSD is warranted (see Chapter 96).

Natural Products

The clinical efficacy of natural products for PTSD is not well-studied. Wahbeh et al.[16] reviewed a small double-blind crossover trial (n = 13) that compared the efficacy of inositol, a carbohydrate chemical compound found in fruits such as cantaloupe and oranges, to placebo in reducing PTSD core symptoms.[95] Although depression was lowered in the inositol group, core symptoms of intrusion and avoidance were unaffected. A separate study compared ginkgo biloba to placebo and reported significant improvements in PTSD in the ginkgo biloba group.[96]

PREVENTION PRESCRIPTION

PTSD prevention is a complex topic and, as noted in the psychotherapy section, is not without pitfalls (e.g., critical incident debriefing strategies and multiple session interventions have been shown to increase the risk of developing PTSD rather than prevent PTSD, whereas brief trauma-focused CBT has been shown to reduce the risk of developing PTSD; see psychotherapy section previously). From a societal perspective, attempts to reduce trauma exposure (e.g., through public safety laws) may be expected to reduce the risk of PTSD. For example, lower speed limits and the required use of seatbelts have reduced the incidence of severe traffic accidents and injuries. However, exposure to potentially life-threatening traumatic events (e.g., natural disasters, interpersonal violence, motor vehicle accidents) remains common over the course of an individual's life. Although the majority of individuals recover from traumatic events without lasting adverse psychological consequences, a small proportion will develop PTSD. Below are factors that may serve to prevent trauma exposure, minimize the negative psychological effects of trauma, or bolster natural recovery:

- Physical fitness and safety: Participating in regular aerobic exercise and avoiding unsafe, high-risk behaviors.
- Social support[97,98]: Social support reduces the likelihood of developing PTSD. Maintenance of social support networks provides an avenue for individuals who have sustained trauma to share their experience, which appears to play a role in natural recovery.

PREVENTION PRESCRIPTION—cont'd

- Adjusting negative cognitive biases: A negative attributional style, a tendency to ruminate and appraise situations negatively, and fear of one's own emotions increases vulnerability to PTSD. Conversely, learning to view things in a less negative way and to become emotionally aware and accepting may protect against PTSD.[99]
- Cognitive flexibility: The ability to "reframe, redefine, re-story" and to use alternative thinking to identify benefits and solve problems is a characteristic of resilient individuals.[100] Participation in programs or approaches that develop these abilities, such as psychotherapy, may help to foster resilience and mitigate the effects of trauma.
- Experiencing positive emotions and accepting/tolerating negative emotions: People who are realistically optimistic, laugh often (and can laugh at themselves), hopeful, and have positive self-image are more resilient,[100] whereas those who fear and avoid their emotions are at increased risk of PTSD. Participation in programs or activities that build emotional awareness and acceptance (e.g., meditation practices or

psychotherapy) may help with emotional clarity and regulation.
- Spirituality and "meaning making"[98,100]: Having a sense of meaning and purpose in life enhances resilience and reduces the risk of developing PTSD after trauma. For many individuals, the ability to find meaning in difficult experiences is assisted by faith or spirituality; however, it can also be supported by any value system that provides a moral compass and sense of altruism.

For people whose risk of traumatic exposure is especially high due to occupation or environment (e.g., military personnel, first responders, firefighters, female college students, etc.), resiliency programs may be offered to help bolster the qualities and capacities listed previously. For example, mindfulness-based mind fitness (MMFT)[101] and stress resilience in virtual environments (STRIVE)[102] have been used to promote predeployment resiliency in the military as a way of preventing the development of combat-related PTSD. Further, mindfulness-based resilience training (MBRT)[103] has received initial support as a method of building resiliency among police officers.

THERAPEUTIC REVIEW

A broad range of approaches have been studied for PTSD including exercise, CAM interventions, and psychotherapy. We briefly summarize the findings pertaining to different modalities that have some evidence for successfully treating PTSD, noting strengths and limitations of the extant literatures.

EXERCISE

- Uncontrolled trials and correlational studies indicate regular aerobic exercise (up to 60%–90% of maximal heart rate) is associated with improvements in PTSD symptoms, anxiety, and depression.

MIND BODY

- Meditation
  - Mindfulness-based stress reduction (MBSR)
  - Mindfulness-based cognitive therapy (MBCT)
  - Mantram repetition
  - Loving-kindness meditation
- Yoga
  - Hatha yoga
- Tapping: thought field therapy and emotional freedom technique
- Hypnotherapy
- Abreactive ego state therapy (AEST)

- Psychotherapy
  - Stress inoculation treatment (SIT)
  - Prolonged exposure (PE)
  - Eye movement desensitization and reprocessing (EMDR)
  - Cognitive processing therapy (CPT)

ACUPUNCTURE

- Eight 60-min sessions of acupuncture twice weekly are associated with improvements in PTSD severity in addition to depression, pain, and physical and mental health functioning.[72]

PHARMACOTHERAPIES

Selective serotonin reuptake inhibitor (SSRIs) and serotonin norepinephrine reuptake inhibitors (SNRIs) with the best evidence for benefit in treating PTSD include:
- Paroxetine 20–60 mg daily
- Fluoxetine 10–60 mg daily
- Venlafaxine 37.5–300 mg daily
Alpha-1 adrenergic receptor agonists have been found to reduce nightmares and sleep disturbance but may cause hypotension.
- Prazosin 1 mg at bedtime. Titrate to a maximum of 15 mg at bedtime until nightmares are controlled.[84]

Key Web Resources

Website/Purpose	URL
Overview of psychotherapy treatment for PTSD from Psych Central	http://psychcentral.com/lib/treatment-of-ptsd/
American Psychological Association: "PTSD treatments grow in evidence, effectiveness"	http://www.apa.org/monitor/jan08/ptsd.aspx
National Institute of Mental Health: Posttraumatic stress disorder information	http://www.nimh.nih.gov/health/publications/post-traumatic-stress-disorder-ptsd/index.shtml
Innovative resources and online continuing education (PTSD) from the Zur Institute	http://www.zurinstitute.com/ptsd_resources.html
PTSD patient information from the BMJ Group (.pdf)	http://bestpractice.bmj.com/best-practice/pdf/patient-summaries/532670.pdf
From the VA National Center for PTSD	
Evidence-based treatments for PTSD (.pdf)	http://www.ptsd.va.gov/Public/understanding_TX/CourseList/Course_NCPTSD_Treatment_1435/assets/00015006.PDF
PTSD screening and referral source for health care providers	http://www.ptsd.va.gov/professional/provider-type/doctors/screening-and-referral.asp
Sexual trauma information for women's health care providers	http://www.ptsd.va.gov/professional/treatment/women/ptsd-womens-providers.asp
PTSD assessment overview	http://www.ptsd.va.gov/professional/assessment/overview/index.asp
Continuing PTSD education for mental health providers	http://www.ptsd.va.gov/professional/continuing_ed/index.asp

REFERENCES

References are available online at ExpertConsult.com.

SECTION II

NEUROLOGY

SECTION OUTLINE

11 ALZHEIMER DISEASE

12 HEADACHE

13 PERIPHERAL NEUROPATHY

14 MULTIPLE SCLEROSIS

15 PARKINSON'S DISEASE

CHAPTER 11

ALZHEIMER DISEASE

Mikhail Kogan, MD • Hwee Soo Jeong, MD

Alzheimer disease (AD) presents as a progressive cognitive decline affecting an individual's memory, language, and social functioning. Later stages lead to complete dependency for basic activities of daily life and premature death.

An estimated 44 million people have AD worldwide, including more than 5 million people in the United States alone. Approximately 500,000 people die of AD every year in the United States. AD is the most common form of dementia comprising 70%–90% of all cases. The annual cost of dementia care in the United States is thought to be between $150 and $215 billion. In 2010, Alzheimer's Disease International estimated the global cost of dementia care, including informal care from family and caregivers, at $600 billion. Care costs in Europe and North America accounted for 70% of this burden.[1,2]

For decades, dementia has been one of the most expensive diseases in the United States in terms of total costs to the economy; the annual cost of formal dementia care exceeds the direct health care expenditures for heart disease or cancer.[3] It is projected that by 2040, nearly 10 million Americans will have dementia, including 50% of those aged more than 80.

PATHOPHYSIOLOGY

Scientists have long understood that AD is caused by brain lesions known as *plaques*—beta-amyloid clusters that build up between nerve cells. As plaques accumulate, they block cell-to-cell signaling and trigger an inflammatory response from the brain's immune system that kills nerve cells. Twisted strands of dead nerve cells, known as *tangles*, also provide stimuli for inflammation. Inflammation is clearly an important contributor to the pathological process of AD. A seminal paper entitled, "Inflammation and Alzheimer's Disease," describes a complex web of interacting inflammatory mediators in the periphery and in the AD brain.[4] High plasma levels of C-reactive protein (CRP) in mid-life and elevated interleukin-6 in old age are strong predictors of AD risk.[5-7] Neurons contain large amounts of metabolically active mitochondria, and synaptic activity depends on good mitochondrial function. A recent theory proposes that accumulation of beta-amyloid damage may cause mitochondrial dysfunction and memory loss in AD[8,9] (see Table 11.1 and Table 11.2 for a summary of risk factors).

Methylation and Homocysteine

One of the key steps of methylation is the final step of the folate cycle that is regulated by methylenetetrahydrofolate reductase (*MTHFR*). MTHFR single nucleotide polymorphisms (SNPs) (mostly C677T and A1298C) slow down conversion of folic acid or dietary folate into 5-methyltetrahydrofolate (5MTHF), a step regulating the homocysteine cycle, glutathione and neurotransmitters production, and the general availability of the methyl group for a variety of biochemical reactions. While elevated homocysteine is considered by many to be an independent risk factor for dementia,[10,11] lowering homocysteine with synthetic forms of B vitamins (e.g., folic acid) has not been shown to slow dementia progression.[12] The data linking MTHFR polymorphism to AD risk is conflicting. A few studies have suggested that the MTHFR C677TT mutation is three times more prevalent in AD patients than in controls, while other studies have found no relationship between MTHFR genotype and impaired cognition.[13,13a,13b] This suggests we have a lot more to learn about the methylation cycle and its complexities. The associations between methylation defects and dementia may be illuminated by genome-wide SNP analysis as it becomes more widely available and affordable (see Chapter 38).

Chronic Exposure to Toxins

Environmental exposures that have been proposed—though not proven—to increase AD risk include those to aluminum, lead, mercury, organophosphate pesticides, and extremely-low-frequency electromagnetic fields.[14-17]

CASE STUDY

A 91-year-old man was brought by his wife to the author's clinic with a chief complaint of progressive memory loss during the past several years. Upon initial assessment we learned that the patient was a strong and physically healthy 3-war veteran. He lacked a number of important AD risk factors such as cardiac disease and family history of AD; however, he had been eating swordfish at least twice weekly for many decades. The patient's Mini-Mental State Examination (MMSE) score was 23/30. Mercury Tri-Test (blood, urine, and hair testing) was ordered based on a clinical suspicion of mercury toxicity.[18] The results revealed a total mercury level nearly 10 times higher than the Centers for Disease Control's average level for healthy individuals, with predominance of methylmercury, an organic form found in fish. The patient's wife removed swordfish and other high-mercury fish

TABLE 11.1   **Risk Factors of Alzheimer Disease (AD)**

Risk Factor	Comments
Advanced Age	Advanced age is the most important risk factor in AD; 10% of persons who are 65 years old develop AD. The incidence at 85 years is as high as 50%.[163]
APOE-ε4	Individuals with two APOE-ε4 genes are at least eight times more likely to develop A. The *APOE4* gene exerts its maximal effect on people in their 60s.[164]
Body Weight	U-shaped risk distribution—obesity likely due to inflammatory and insulin resistance factors and underweight due to poor nutritional factors.[165-167]
Cardiovascular Disease (CVD)	Hypoperfusion leads to mitochondrial dysfunction and neuronal death.[168]
Diabetes and Insulin Resistance	In AD, brain glucose utilization and energy production are impaired.[169] Diabetes is a risk factor not only for strokes and vascular dementia but also for AD.[170]
Family History of AD	Three- to four-fold increased AD risk among those with first-degree relatives with the disease.[171]
Education	Higher education is associated with lower risk of AD later in life.[172]
Glutathione (GSH) low	Numerous studies have shown low neuronal GSH level in patients with AD.[99-101]
Hypertension	Numerous studies have linked midlife hypertension to AD risk.[45,173,174]
Hormonal Imbalances	• Low estrogen[175] • Cortisol deregulation[63,64] • Low DHEA and pregnenolone are common in AD patients • Hypothyroid and can cause dementia-like symptoms
Methylation Defects	MTHFR mutations and high homocysteine levels—see text
Minimal Cognitive Impairment (MCI)	10%–15% will progress to dementia. Patients with MCI function normally in daily activities requiring nonmemory cognitive abilities such as thinking, understanding, and decision making.[176]
Sleep Apnea	One of the more recently found factors, likely due to nocturnal hypoxia.[177]
Smoking	Surprisingly mixed findings; nicotine may have protective effects making association less clear.[178]
Chronic Stress	See text
Toxicities	Mercury, lead, organophosphates, and others—see text
Traumatic Brain Injury (TBI)	AD risk is doubled in patients who have experienced TBI early in life.

TABLE 11.2   **Nutritional and Minerals/Vitamins Risk Factors of Alzheimer Disease (AD)**

Consuming High Glycemic Index Diets	High glycemic foods are well known to have proinflammatory effects; this is addressed in detail in a separate chapter.
Low Omega-3 Dietary Content	See text for details.
Low B12 and B6	Well-known risk factors clearly associated with AD risk.[13]
Niacin (B1) Deficiency	Causes Wernicke–Korsakoff: dementia, sight and muscular coordination problems, confabulations, and hallucinations
Thiamine (B3) Deficiency	Causes pellagra: dementia, diarrhea, and dermatitis
Selenium Deficiency	Studies have suggested that low selenium levels increase AD risk.[179,180] One study demonstrated a direct correlation between plasma selenium concentration and cognitive function.[181]
Vitamin E Insufficiency	Numerous studies have associated low Vitamin E levels with AD, but the data is mixed.[182,183]
Copper Excess	Studies have shown free copper, not bound to ceruloplasmin, is increased in patients with AD and correlates negatively with cognition.[184,185] Dietary copper is in organic form and is processed by the liver to bind to ceruloplasmin. In contrast, inorganic copper from supplements and from unfiltered drinking water in areas where copper pipes are used can bypass the liver and enter metabolism as free copper readily delivered to and deposited in the brain.[186]
Zinc Insufficiency	Zinc intake has been thought to decrease available copper and may therefore have a protective role. In a recent systematic review, low zinc intake was attributed to AD risk.[187]
Vitamin D Deficiency	A meta-analysis of 37 studies found that adults with low serum vitamin D concentrations (<50 nmol/L) had poorer cognitive function and greater risk of AD than adults with higher vitamin D concentrations; AD patients have lower vitamin D concentrations than controls.[188] More recently, a large cohort study found an increased risk of all-cause dementia and AD among elderly adults with low serum Vitamin D concentrations.[189]

from his diet, and the author prescribed comprehensive nutritional detoxification support consisting of alpha-lipoic acid, methylated B vitamins, N-acetyl-cysteine, zinc, and other nutrients. Repeat Mercury Tri-Test showed an 80% reduction in the patient's total mercury level six month later and normal mercury levels four months after that. At a follow-up visit one month after the last mercury test, the patient's wife reported substantial memory improvement and his MMSE score was 27/30.

Differentiating Normal Aging From Mild Cognitive Impairment or Alzheimer Disease

As the mature brain ages, its short-term ability to keep and use information normally declines. This results in cognitive changes such as forgetfulness, distractibility, and reduced efficiency in carrying out tasks.[19] Distinguishing cognitive changes of normal aging from mild cognitive impairment (MCI) or AD is best achieved with specialized screening questionnaires. Screening takes time and skill, and is not routinely performed in busy primary care practices. As a result, an AD diagnosis is frequently delayed by several years until symptoms worsen. Early diagnosis is also delayed because the presenting complaint is rarely "I am losing my memory," even though family members may have this observation. Patients who personally complain of memory loss are not likely to have AD, although they may have MCI. MCI is different from AD in two critical aspects: patients with MCI have (1) normal overall cognition and (2) normal functioning per measures of Activities of Daily Living (ADL).

Most of patients are first seen for memory complaints by primary care providers. However, establishing a diagnosis of MCI or AD requires a comprehensive mental assessment and is better done in a memory clinic.

Screening

Due to the high prevalence of AD, regular screening is recommended for all adults aged more than 65 years,[20] although a screening frequency has not been defined. Several screening methods exist and as no data supports the superiority of one method over another, the choice may be determined by the operator's comfort with each tool and the available time. The Mini-Mental State Examination (MMSE) has been the most popular; however, due to copyright issues, it can no longer be used without obtaining rights from the publisher, Psychological Assessment Resources (PAR). PAR claims that the various free, online versions of the MMSE are all derivatives of the original and thus copyrighted. The MMSE cannot be used to screen for MCI as its sensitivity for MCI is only 18%.[21]

The authors recommend having familiarity with two methods: Mini-Cog and Montreal Cognitive Assessment (MoCa). An abnormal score on either test signifies cognitive impairment and suggests a high probability of MCI or AD diagnosis.

Mini-Cog takes less than 5 minutes to implement. The test consists of three items, recall, and a clock draw. Scoring is either pass or fail; patients who miss two or

more recall items or make any mistake on the clock draw are considering to have failed and should be referred for a more detailed cognitive assessment.

MoCa is a 30-point, 10–15-minute test somewhat similar to the MMSE, but it can be used for diagnosing both MCI and early AD. The patient's total score can be tracked longitudinally as a measure of disease progression. MoCa was validated against the MMSE in 2005.[21] A normal score is considered to be 26/30 or above; one point is added for patients with 12 or less years of education. Before initiating use of the MoCa with patients, a practitioner should have a detailed understanding of the test's instructions and, ideally, have observed its administration by an experienced clinician several times.

Diagnosis

As with any other illness, diagnosis begins with the patient's story. If a comprehensive clinical query and the results of memory or neuropsychological testing provide suspicion of AD, they should be followed by physical examination, laboratory studies, and possibly neuroimaging to rule our reversible causes and to prepare an AD treatment plan.

Physical examination may reveal evidence of stroke, making vascular dementia more likely. While a physical exam is often unrevealing, functional assessment of the tongue, skin, and nails may reveal subtle evidence of vitamin and essential fatty acid deficiencies. Routine laboratory studies should include complete blood count, comprehensive metabolic panel, vitamin B12, folate, thyroid panel, and testing for syphilis and human immunodeficiency virus (HIV). Beyond these, the integrative practitioner may consider investigations for fasting glucose; hemoglobin A1c (HbA1c); free zinc and copper; high sensitivity C-reactive proteins; serum levels of pregnenolone, dehydroepiandrosterone (DHEA), and testosterone in both sexes; and a comprehensive nutritional assessment that may include an oxidative panel and fatty acid analysis. Patients with AD often have hormonal and nutritional abnormalities, as well as increased oxidative stress. There are a number of oxidative stress assays available. The authors prefer assessing reduced glutathione (GSH), lipid peroxides, coenzyme Q10, 8-hydroxy-deoxyguanosine (8-OHdG), cysteine/cystine ratio, and superoxide dismutase (SOD). Total body lead or mercury is assessed only upon suspicion of toxicity from history, examination (i.e., multiple amalgams), or elevated oxidative stress. Testing for heavy metals using serum levels alone is likely to miss cases due to rapid sequestration from blood into tissues.[22] Screening patients for the APOE4 gene remains controversial. Knowledge of a positive APOE4 status can provide motivation to make early lifestyle changes, but it may also cause psychological distress due to the high likelihood of developing AD.

Neuroimaging has become an adjunct tool for AD diagnosis despite the lack of clarity as to which tests should be done. Some prefer special positron emission tomography (PET) scans, others believe magnetic resonance imaging (MRI) scans are more useful, and a combination of these has also been proposed (Fig. 11.1). Authors have not yet embraced routine neuroimaging. National Institute on

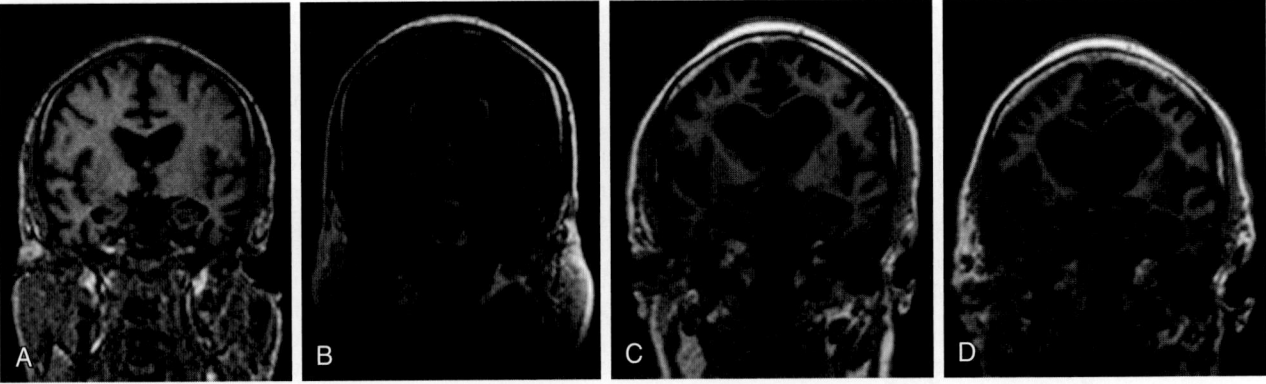

FIG. 11.1 ■ A, Longitudinal serial coronal magnetic resonance imaging (MRI) in patient with bvFTD, demonstrating increasing frontal and temporal atrophy after 1 year of symptoms; B, after three years of symptoms; C, after 7 years of symptoms; D, after 9 years of symptoms. *bvFTD,* Behavioral variant frontotemporal dementia. (From Peterson R, Graff-Radford J. Alzheimer disease and other dementias. In: Daroff RB, Jankovic J, Mazziotta JC, Pomeroy SL, eds. *Bradley's neurology in clinical practice.* 7th ed. Philadelphia, PA: Elsevier; 2016:1380-1421. Courtesy Bradley Boeve.)

Aging provides information on new genetic, laboratory, and imaging strategies for AD diagnosis.[23]

Clinical Course

AD progresses slowly with an average life expectancy of 8–10 years from onset. However, since most patients are diagnosed several years into the disease, the time from diagnosis to death is often much shorter. After confirming the AD diagnosis and ruling out possibly reversible conditions, clinicians should focus on arresting or slowing down the decline, anticipating and palliating dementia-associated symptoms, and providing assistance to family and caregivers to help alleviate caregiver stress.

A number of rating scales have been designed to characterize a patient's level of dementia, predict life expectancy, and improve coordination among providers and caregivers. Clinical Dementia Rating (CDR) is a 5-point scale used to characterize six cognitive and functional areas, including memory, orientation, and personal care. The CDR requires substantial time to administer, yet it is reliable and increasingly used in research and clinical settings.[24]

The Reisberg Functional Assessment Staging Test (FAST) is a validated measure of AD course that is easy to use in clinical settings despite its complex scoring system.[25] The FAST scale is also used to assess eligibility for hospice. Hospice eligibility criteria require patients to have a life expectancy of 6 months or less; however, estimating how long AD patients will survive is challenging. The current AD hospice eligibility criteria (available at http://alzonline.phhp.ufl.edu/en/reading/hospice.php) has been criticized; some clinicians recommend referral for hospice evaluation when the patient's goals are consistent with those of hospice and their symptoms can no longer be adequately managed by caregivers.[26]

INTEGRATIVE THERAPY

Given the numerous pathophysiologic factors of AD, it is not surprising that no monotherapy has been proven

effective in stopping AD progression. A combination of therapies, however, may have important disease-modifying effects, according to anecdotal evidence. In a recently published case series, Bredesen describes a novel "therapeutic system" of diet and lifestyle changes which he prescribed to 10 patients (median age, 68 years) who had been diagnosed with AD, MCI, or subjective cognitive impairment. Nine patients experienced a halting and reversal of memory loss symptoms that had been progressing during the past 1–12 years. Six patients were able to return to work. The program consisted of 25 interventions—not all of which were followed by every patient—addressing key, scientifically based pathogenic mechanisms, for example, personalized stress reduction plans, an inflammation-minimizing diet, and fasting for at least 12 hours at night to enhance autophagy, known to reduce intracellular Aβ secretion. Approximately half of the interventions involved nutritional supplementation. These findings illustrate the potential for comprehensive AD treatment targeting multiple pathophysiological pathways, although they remain to be confirmed via clinical trials.[27]

> While no single treatment has been proven to halt AD progression, multidimensional therapies show promise for disease modifying effects.

Lifestyle Factors

Exercise

Aerobic exercise training has been associated with modest improvements in memory, executive function, attention, and processing speed in nondemented individuals.[28] In AD patients, exercise programs had a positive effect on cognition and ADL.[29]

There are several proposed mechanisms for the effect of exercise on cognition. Exercise increased the gene expression of synaptic plasticity and mitochondria[30-32] and reduced extracellular amyloid proteins in the hippocampus and frontal cortex.[33] AD comorbidities such as hypertension and diabetes are better controlled with exercise. Exercise prescription for early AD should include a combination of aerobic, balance, strength, and stretching exercises practiced for 30–60 minutes per day four to five times per week. As the disease progresses, exercise should focus on balance and strength to prevent falls, sarcopenia, and contractures.

Cognitive Exercise

Cognitive exercises may slow cognitive decline or reduce the risk of dementia. A computerized mental activity training program including games improved cognition in older adults with cognitive complaints.[34-36] Leisure activities including reading and playing board games or musical instruments also decreased dementia risk in the elderly.[37] There is no clear mechanism, but these activities might affect perceptual speed, accuracy, and attention. The amount or frequency of activity may be more strongly associated with cognitive improvement than the type of exercise.[34,37]

Yoga and Tai Chi

Yoga and tai chi are mind-body practices that combine physical and cognitive exercises for stress-reducing effects. Healthy, elderly individuals who practiced yoga daily for 1 month and weekly for 3 months improved their immediate and delayed recall.[38] Among AD patients residing in a long-term care facility, yoga had no impact on cognitive function but improved physical health and reduced the symptoms of depression and agitation.[39]

The series of slowly flowing circular movements, known as *tai chi*, is a martial art form that has been practiced for general health and well-being in China.[40] A few studies have shown a decreased risk of cognitive decline and increased brain volume among tai chi practitioners.[41,42] Tai Chi can be practiced alone or in groups. Like yoga, tai chi is reasonably safe when taught by experienced teachers, requires minimal equipment or space, and is inexpensive when offered in group format.

Optimizing Vascular Disease Risk Factors

A number of longitudinal studies in the elderly support the idea that reducing cardiovascular risk factors may also lower the risk of cognitive decline. In both the Honolulu Asia Aging Study (n = 6000 men) and an osteoporotic fractures study cohort (n = 9704 women), the risk of cognitive decline was relatively lower in individuals without diabetes, hypertension, smoking, excessive alcohol consumption, and poor social networks.[43,44] Poorly managed hypertension in midlife increases the risk of subsequent dementia.[45-47] Results of a large cohort study suggested that use of antihypertensive medications to control hypertension was associated with reduced dementia risk.[48]

Optimizing Gut Health

Increased intestinal permeability is thought to be a common cause of systemic inflammation.[49] In addition, unhealthy changes in intestinal microbial flora, called *dysbiosis*, appear to be an independent factor contributing to inflammation.[50] While research linking these factors to AD has not yet been established, leading clinicians have proposed that optimizing gut health could improve brain function.[51,52] The importance of gut flora in human health will grow quickly, especially with the help of the National Institute of Health (NIH) Human Microbiome Project.

Nutrition

A recent randomized clinical trial (RCT) compared a plant-based, low-fat diet with an antioxidant-rich Mediterranean diet that included mixed nuts (30 g per day) or olive oil (1 L per week) in 447 healthy, elderly volunteers. Over 3 years, those on the poly- and monounsaturated fat-supplemented diet experienced improved memory, frontal functions, and global cognition.[53] Like the antiinflammatory diet (see Chapter 88), a Mediterranean diet is thought to inhibit inflammation. Another recent trial evaluated the MIND diet—a hybrid of the Mediterranean and DASH (see Chapter 89) diets—in 900 elderly participants. Those who followed a MIND diet had a 53% lower risk of developing AD. The Mediterranean diet also had a modest protective effect.[54] The MIND diet is relatively simple, allows a limited intake of animal-based food, and specifies consumption of berries and leafy greens, which have neuroprotective benefits according to animal and human studies (Table 11.3).

Intermittent Fasting

In addition to the aforementioned diets, authors advocate regular intermittent fasting. In recent years, studies have demonstrated that intermittent fasting has a number of beneficial effects of reducing oxidative damage and inflammation, optimizing energy metabolism and bolstering cellular protection. In AD animal models, regular caloric restriction has resulted in an improved clinical and pathological picture.[55] An easy way to practice intermittent fasting is to eat the last meal of the day 3 hours before bedtime, resulting in a 12-hour nighttime fast. If this results in patient waking up at night due to hypoglycemia, then mealtime may be gradually adjusted, allowing the patient to adapt to hypoglycemia and shift to ketogenesis, which is thought to be neuroprotective. Ketogenesis may also be enhanced by medium-chain triglycerides in form of 1 to 2 tablespoons daily of coconut oil or Axona medical food (described in the following section).

Omega-3 Fatty Acids

Omega-3 long-chain polyunsaturated fatty acids, including α-linolenic acid (ALA), eicosapentaenoic acid (EPA), and docosahexaenoic acid (DHA) play essential roles in cell membrane viscosity and in antiinflammatory processes. Humans can synthesize DHA and EPA from ALA. While EPA is antiinflammatory and modulates membrane fluidity and neuronal synaptic plasticity, DHA is the most abundant membrane lipid.[56] Most

---

TABLE 11.3 **Mediterranean-DASH Intervention for Neurodegenerative Delay (MIND) Diet**

Foods to Consume More of	Foods to Avoid or Decrease
Whole grains at least three servings per day	Red meats and red meat products less than four times per week
Green leafy vegetables at least six times per week	Fast/fried food less than once per week
Other vegetable at least one per day (red-orange vegetables preferred)	Butter, margarine less than 1 tablespoon a day
Berries at least twice a week	Cheese once per week or less
Fish at least once a week	Pastries and sweets less than five times per week
Poultry at least two times per week	
Beans at least three times per week	
Nuts at least five times per week	
Olive oil as your primary oil	
Alcohol/wine once per day	

---

epidemiological data clearly demonstrates that increased fish intake lowers the risk for AD development.[57] However, randomized trials of fish oil supplementation have generally failed to produce positive effects on AD prevention or progression.[58,59] Similarly, studies of isolated high-dose DHA (2 g per day) have not shown a benefit.[60] In healthy adults > 65 years, a higher dietary intake of omega-3 polyunsaturated fatty acid was associated with a lower level of plasma amyloid beta (Aβ) 42, which is linked with a reduced AD risk.[61]

Key components of diet for AD prevention and treatment include the following:
1. Low-glycemic index diet.
2. Reduction of proinflammatory foods such as red meat, dairy, and sugar.
3. High amounts of fresh fruits and vegetables including high antioxidant foods such as berries, turmeric, and green tea.
4. High amounts of foods rich in omega-3 fatty acids.
5. Overnight fasting to promote ketogenesis.

Mind-Body Techniques

Chronic Stress

Persistent stress is thought to be a cause of many chronic diseases. Memory function is influenced by stress too. Acute or temporal stress may positively affect stimulus-induced neuroplasticity, while persistent stress impairs synaptic activity.[62] The hypothalamic-pituitary-adrenal (HPA) axis is a central system in stress-mediated processes. Activation of the HPA axis by stress triggers rapid secretion of corticotrophin releasing hormone (CRH) from the paraventricular nucleus (PVN) of the hypothalamus. This influences the release of adrenocorticotrophic hormone (ACTH) from the anterior pituitary, which induces the adrenal gland to release cortisol (see Chapter 94). Cortisol induces stress adaptation in many organs. It also provides negative feedback inhibition to the HPA axis via activation of glucocorticoid receptors in the PVN, amygdala, and hippocampus.[62] HPA axis dysfunction has been shown to contribute to AD risk in many studies;

however, a clinically measurable link, for example with cortisol levels, has failed to produce clear results and is generally not used in practice. A large population-based cohort study showed no relationship between morning serum cortisol levels and cognitive function and annual cognitive decline.[63,64] The dexamethasone suppression test was assessed but not found clinically useful for AD.[65,66] Salivary cortisol level changes from morning to evening were associated with AD and smaller hippocampal volumes.[67,68] It has been proposed that persistently elevated cortisol is directly involved in memory impairment by irreversible hippocampal damage. Decreased hippocampal volume has been observed in patients with Cushing disease, and in one study, hippocampal volume increased after successful treatment of that disease.[69,70] Cortisol blocks glutamate uptake by the glial cell, causing increased accumulation of glutamate in the synapses and activating N-methyl-D-aspartate (NMDA) receptors, resulting in an influx of calcium into the postsynaptic neuron. Excessive cytosolic calcium increases oxidative stress thought to cause neuronal death.[71]

Meditation

Clinical trials have suggested the benefits of meditation as nonmedical intervention for dementia treatment. Transcendental meditation and mindfulness training, practiced twice daily for 20 minutes, improved cognitive flexibility, memory, and verbal fluency in elderly subjects at 12 weeks.[72] In a small, nonrandomized study, 8 weeks of a meditation practice called *kirtan kriya* was shown to improve cognitive function and cerebral blood flow in patients with MCI. Kirtan kriya takes about 12 minutes and consists of breathing, finger movement, and the chanting of primal sounds.[73,74] Tibetan sound meditation daily for 6 weeks improved verbal memory, short-term memory, and processing speed in adults suffering drug-induced cognitive impairment.[75] Mindfulness-based stress reduction programs have not been studied in AD, but may be well-suited for prevention given their success for stress reduction. The choice of mind-body modality will likely be based on local resources and the preferences of the patient and practitioner (see Chapter 100).

Sleep

Seven to eight hours of good quality sleep is recommended for AD patients. Sleep apnea should be excluded or treated. Melatonin use (described in the following section) can be helpful for AD patients with insomnia.

Vitamins and Minerals

B Vitamins

Frank deficiency of vitamin B12 can cause pseudodementia or pseudodepression and is common in the elderly. We recommend a serum level above 500 pg/mL. Alternatively, intracellular B12 levels may be assessed by some functional labs such as Genova and Spectrocell.

While there are no clear guidelines regarding B vitamin and dementia, the authors advocate the use of activated forms of B12 and folate: methylcobalamin and 5-methyltetrahydrofolate (5MTHF) often called *L-methylfolate*. One strategy is to use a therapeutic B complex with high doses of activated B12 and 5MTHF.

DOSAGE

The authors usually use 1000 mcg of methyl B12 and L-methylfolate per day, with doses ranging between 200 mcg and 10,000 mcg of each.

PRECAUTIONS

When supplemented with methylcobalamin, patients with COMT SNPs are at increased risk of side effects of anxiety or agitation due to higher levels of dopamine and norepinephrine. This can often be mitigated with hydroxy or adeno B12 or decreasing dose of methyl B12. B complex is better taken in the morning to avoid sleep disruptions in sensitive patients. In addition to prescribing activated B vitamins, the authors recommend avoiding synthetic folic acid in patients with dementia unless a negative MTHFR status is reported. Data supporting the negative effects of unmetabolized folic acid is slowly growing.[76]

Consider testing all AD or MCI patients for MTHFR SNPs and if positive for either A1289C or C677T use methylfolate (1–10 mg) and avoid synthetic folic acid.

Vitamin E and C

Investigation of vitamin E as a treatment for AD has produced conflicting results. While some trials found cognitive and functional benefits with high dose synthetic α-tocopherol (2000 IU per day), a meta-analysis and Cochrane Review each concluded that there is no clear clinical benefit of high-dose vitamin E and that it should not be used for AD or MCI.[77-81]

Unless nutritional testing indicates vitamin C or E deficiency, we recommend that patients obtain adequate doses from dietary sources including fruits, nuts, and vegetables.

Interactions of different phytochemicals with vitamin C and E and other antioxidants likely provide additional beneficial effects.[82,83] A multivitamin or antioxidant formula should provide mixed tocopherols to contain all eight natural isoforms (instead of synthetic α-tocopherol) with a daily dose of 200–400 IU of vitamin E and 500–1000 mg of vitamin C.

Vitamin D

We recommend assessing vitamin D status in all patients with AD and optimizing and maintaining serum Vitamin D 25 OH levels at 40–60 ng/mL.[84] Vitamin D supplementation (of at least 800 IU) has been shown to reduce the risk of falls.[85]

Selenium

Brazil nuts have a high concentration of selenium (Se), and two Brazil nuts daily are the recommended source.[86,87] Since the levels of selenium in Brazil nuts can vary from 8–83 mcg/g, overdose is possible and patients should be advised accordingly. A typical supplemental dose of selenium is 100–200 mcg.

Zinc and Copper

We recommend free zinc and copper assessment for all patients with AD. In the case of zinc, targeted high normal range is reasonable, which may require supplemental doses of 15–50 mg per day. With copper the reverse is true, and the aim is to keep patients at a low normal or even just under normal levels by removing all supplemental forms of copper, filtering water, or using high-dose zinc and alpha-lipoic acid in an attempt to lower the copper level. There is no need to limit copper rich foods as organic forms of copper contribute little to elevate free copper levels.

Multivitamins in Alzheimer Disease

For supplementation of patients with a poor diet or documented nutritional deficiencies, follow these guidelines:
- No additional copper and iron
- Natural forms of vitamin E 200–400 IU—mixed tocopherols
- Methylated forms of folate—at least 400 mcg
- Activated forms of B12—methyl, hydroxy, or adeno B12—at least 500 mcg
- Zinc at least 15 mg
- Selenium 100–200 mcg

Supplements

Acetyl-L-Carnitine

Acetyl-L-carnitine (ALCAR) is synthesized in the human brain, liver, and kidney; it facilitates fatty acid oxidation, enhances acetylcholine production, and stimulates protein and membrane phospholipid synthesis.[88] In mild cognitive impairment and mild AD patients, the result of a meta-analysis revealed a significant advantage for ALCAR compared to placebo in daily doses of 1.5–3.0 g.[89] However, a Cochrane Review has not found it to be effective.[90] ALCAR appears to increase nerve growth factor (NGF), which is thought to be important for neuronal survival.[91]

DOSAGE

Typical daily dose is 2–3 g.

PRECAUTIONS

Side effects are uncommon, but it can include bloating, abdominal cramps, and particular body odor.

Omega-3 and Fish Oil

Unless a diet is very high in oily fish, the authors recommend supplementation with omega-3 fatty acids. Fish oil appears to be the easiest to obtain, and as long as purification is adequate, it should remove most of contaminants, including mercury. Fatty acid analysis is currently available, and its utilization for patients with AD could be useful; the authors have found that identifying patients with decreased Delta 6 desaturase activity can help balance fatty acids by increasing intake of gamma-linolenic acid through usage of borage, evening primrose, or black current oils. One long-term strategy could be providing a 4:1 Omega-6:3 balanced supplement with at least 1 g of DHA/EPA.

DOSAGE

The typical dose is 1–3 g per day of combined DHA/EPA, and at least 50% should be DHA. We often use a 2:1 DHA:EPA ratio.

PRECAUTIONS

Doses greater than 4 g per day may have a prooxidant effect.

Coenzyme Q10

Coenzyme Q10, a powerful neuroprotective agent, works as a dynamic antioxidant. It is present throughout the brain cell membrane and mitochondria, where it is involved in the production of high-energy phosphate compounds.[92]

DOSAGE

Conversion of ubiquinone to ubiquinol is not universal and thus we prefer use of ubiquinol at 100–200 mg daily.

PRECAUTIONS

Mild gastrointestinal symptoms can occur with 300 mg per day. It can also elevate serum aminotransferase level.

Alpha-Lipoic Acid

Alpha-lipoic acid (ALA) is a natural compound synthesized in the mitochondria.[93] It is believed to induce the oxidative stress response rather than directly act as a free radical scavenger.[94] In addition to inducing the antioxidant system, ALA has been shown to improve glucose handling, increase eNOS activity, and activate Phase II detoxification via the transcription factor Nrf2. ALA also has been proposed to have a chelation effect in the brain on iron and copper.

DOSAGE

Taking 600 mg ALA daily for 2 years or a combination of omega-3 and ALA for 1 year slowed down progression of cognitive decline in AD patients.[95] We routinely use 600 mg 5 days a week, taken with food.

PRECAUTIONS

Because ALA is rather acidic, it can irritate gastric mucosa and should be taken with food.

N-Acetylcysteine and Glutathione

As a glutathione (GSH) precursor, N-acetylcysteine (NAC) has been recently proposed to have an important role in prevention and treatment of AD. Thus it plays an essential role in antioxidant defense and detoxification.[96] NAC does not require an active transporter and can easily cross cell membranes leading to intracellular GSH production.[97] The capacity of NAC to cross the blood-brain barrier has been debated for years, but more recent data seems to suggest that it can indeed cross.[98] A number of studies have shown low neuronal GSH levels in patients with AD.[99-101] In addition to a number of animal model studies, one human RCT showed a possible positive effect on patients with AD.[102] In addition, NAC is a component of several medical foods discussed in the following section, which are trending towards overall benefit. NAC has been used safely in traditional settings, for example, in acute acetaminophen overdose. Intravenous use of NAC or GSH is safe, but expensive and inconvenient. In the past, oral forms of GSH have not been shown to be well absorbed and able to reach the brain. This has been recently changing since introduction of liposomal and other more bioavailable oral and topical forms.

DOSAGE

The authors recommend using NAC at 500–1000 mg per day taken 5 days a week.

PRECAUTIONS

NAC is well tolerated with occasional intestinal side effects.

Botanicals

Huperzine A

Huperzine A is a natural anticholinesterase inhibitor derived from Chinese club moss. A recent meta-analysis, which included 20 RCTs and almost 2000 patients showed positive results on cognitive function and ADLs in patients with AD; however, most of the studies were of poor methodological quality.[103] One recent U.S. based RCT showed slower cognitive decline in patients with AD, but only with the higher dose of 400 mcg twice daily.[46] In addition to anticholinesterase inhibition, huperzine A may have neuroprotective effects that are, as of yet, not well characterized. In 1994, huperzine A was approved by State Food and Drug Administration of China for AD therapy.[104]

Turmeric and Green Tea

Both turmeric and green tea are food-based antioxidants and are consumed in variable amounts in different populations; they have been suggested as possible therapeutic agents for AD. While a number of epidemiological studies show lower risk of dementia in populations consuming high doses of turmeric or green tea, clinical studies are lacking. Given that both foods are recommended as part of an antiinflammatory diet, the authors recommend using them in liberal amounts as foods. Drug interactions at food-based dosages are not common, and both herbs are typically well tolerated; although they can trigger intestinal irritation if taken in larger amounts.[105,106] While epidemiological data for turmeric and green tea being linked to a lower risk of dementia is clear, data on black tea or coffee consumption has provided mixed results.[107,108] Matcha, a powdered form of green tea, is more potent, does not require steeping, and can be mixed with hot or cold water or with other foods. The authors recommend one teaspoon daily in divided doses. Dietary turmeric should be cooked with an oil to enhance absorption. Recipe books on cooking turmeric to maximize its health benefits are available.

Hormones

Dehydroepiandrosterone and Pregnenolone

The adrenal prohormone dehydroepiandrosterone (DHEA) may provide anticortisol effects against the hypercortisolism observed in AD patients.[109] Hippocampal perfusion had a positive correlation with plasma DHEA.[110] However, in a clinical trial of patients with AD using a high DHEA dose, 50 mg twice daily for 6 months, improved cognitive performance was not reported.[111] The same result was observed in healthy elderly women who took 50 mg per day oral DHEA for 1 year.[112]

Melatonin

Low nocturnal melatonin levels and disturbed circadian melatonin rhythms were observed in MCI and AD patients.[113] In healthy elderly, a 1-mg melatonin supplement improved cognitive function and sleep.[114] Cognitive function was improved in AD patients who took melatonin 3 mg per day for 4 weeks.[115] Prolonged-release 2-mg melatonin supplement for 6 months improved cognitive function and insomnia in mild to moderate AD patients.[116] Recently, a meta-analysis of AD patients reported that melatonin (up to 10 mg) nightly over 4 weeks prolonged total sleep time and sleep efficacy, but did not improve cognitive function.[117] Melatonin improved agitation symptoms in dementia patients through the reduction of circadian rhythm disturbance.[118]

Therapies to Consider

Medications (Table 11.4)

Four FDA-approved medications are prescribed to treat the cognitive symptoms of AD. All have neurotransmitter-based effects by either boosting available acetylcholine via acetylcholinesterase inhibition or by antagonizing NMDA-dampening excitatory neurotransmitters.

Data on the effectiveness of these medications is limited. While all agents had a statistically significantly delayed symptom progression in 6-month trials, the effects were small—about 2 or 3 points on the ADAS-Cog Scale (the scale range is 0–70; a higher number indicates a greater cognitive impairment)—and of questionable clinical significance.[125,126] Donepezil is the only FDA-approved medication shown to be effective at 12 months, and patients did not show improvement after 12 months.[127]

The authors prescribe medications only in some cases after detailed discussion with the patient or family. The new high-dose formulation of donepezil (23 mg nightly) has been gaining momentum; however, side effects appear to be more frequent than with the lower dose (10 mg nightly or daily).[128] Fortunately, there appear to be few clinically significant interactions between commonly used AD nutritional supplements and medications. Alkalinizing agents that increase urine pH may decrease clearance of memantine and lead to drug overdose. Ginkgo, commonly used for memory

TABLE 11.4 Medications

Category	Name (Brand)	Approved for (Stage)	Major Side Effects	Comments
Acetylcholinesterase inhibitors	Donepezil (Aricept)	All stages	Bradycardia/heart block, gastrointestinal bleeding, syncope, nausea, diarrhea, headaches	5–10 mg once daily
	Rivastigmine (Exelon)	Mild to moderate		6–12 mg PO or patch
	Galantamine (Razadyne)	Mild to moderate		16–24 mg once daily
N-methyl-D-aspartate (NMDA) antagonist	Memantine (Namenda)	Moderate to severe	Dizziness, headaches, fatigue, diarrhea, constipation, usually well tolerated	5–10 mg twice daily

loss, has a theoretical interaction with liver-metabolized cholinesterase inhibitors, but in a randomized controlled trial of 96 subjects with AD, the combination of donepezil and ginkgo had fewer side effects than donepezil alone.[129]

In addition to Alzheimer-specific medications, most dementia patients with moderate to severe disease are eventually prescribed several medications to manage psychological and behavioral problems including depression, anxiety, agitation, and altered circadian rhythm. Selective serotonin reuptake inhibitors (SSRI) antidepressants are among the most common. The most concerning class of medications used frequently in patients with AD is antipsychotics, both older ones such as haloperidol and newer such as risperidone. While these medications can control agitation, they have severe side effects such as delirium and increased mortality.[130,131] Therefore the authors recommend the following integrative approaches as a first line of treatment for psychological and behavioral problems in patients with AD.

Role of Integrative Therapies for Management of Behavioral Problems

Music. Music is a beneficial intervention in stress-related disorders. Music has been shown to reduce cortisol levels in salivary samples.[132] In dementia patients, music has potential positive effects on agitation and anxiety.[133,134] Music therapy combined with physical exercise or recreational activity also showed a positive synergistic effect in patients with AD.[135,136]

Animal-Assisted Therapy. Animal-assisted therapy (AAT) has been getting attention as a stress-reducing intervention that enhances well-being.[137] In a pilot study, AAT for 3 weeks reduced agitation and increased social interactions in patients with AD.[138] Similarly to music, AAT has been increasingly utilized in nursing homes and assisted living facilities. There is hope that this will translate to lower use of medications.

Reiki. Reiki offers light touch to patients and is believed to reduce stress and stimulate self-healing by optimizing autonomic nervous system and HPA axis. Reiki appears to reduce stress, anxiety, and pain in dementia patients.[139] Caregivers can be easily taught delivering Reiki to patients. One of the authors (MK) assisted in implementing longitudinal Reiki program at a local retirement community, where an integrative team provides Reiki sessions and teaches self-Reiki to staff and residents. A number of treated residents had AD. The program has been well accepted, and our unpublished data showed that some patients and staff members had less anxiety and better life satisfaction. However, we did not assess cognition or observed any functional improvements.

Assisting Caregivers. Dr. Elizabeth Cobbs, one of the most distinguished geriatricians stated, "Supporting and guiding the caregiver may be one of the most powerful 'treatments' we have." If despite the most aggressive care measures, a patient with AD continues to decline, caregiving needs are likely to escalate. Chronic caregiving burden results in poor quality of life, increased risk of acute myocardial infarction, and death.[140-143]

Creating an effective assistance program has proven to be a difficult task, with numerous systematic approaches attempted.[144] While no good answers on the best strategy exist, it is clear that integrative practitioners are well positioned to advocate and teach caregivers self-care. Assuring good sleep, regular exercise, good nutrition, and ongoing social interactions is critical as often all these get disrupted. Logistical support can consist of number of things, including coordinating short-term respite care and covered benefit under hospice so that caregiver can take time off. Educating about AD progression and steps that should be taken at each stage is critical and best started as early as possible. Mind-body approaches such as yoga, meditation, and a Mindfulness-Based StressReduction (MBSR) program recently have been shown to be effective for decreasing caregiver stress and improving mental health.[145,146]

Spirituality

In the prior edition of this chapter, Dr. Dharma Singh Khalsa elegantly summarized the importance of spirituality below.

"Beyond reported improvements in memory, concentration, learning ability, and activities of daily living, patients enrolled in an integrative medical program for cognitive enhancement also note positive changes in what can be described as personal awareness. This awareness sometimes appears as a sense of increased self-knowledge or what many people call spirituality and leads to a feeling of connectedness. Some patients report that this spiritual connection leads to a profound level of wisdom: the combination of age, intelligence, and experience. This wisdom, or maturity, brings greater life satisfaction. These changes are consistent with the work of Benson, Larson, and Matthews, who established that an integrative medical program, including mind-body interactions, enhances spirituality. Spirituality was expressed as experiencing the close presence of a higher power. A preliminary study presented by Dr. Yaku Kaufmann at the 2005 American Academy of Neurology meeting demonstrated that patients with AD who lived a rewarding spiritual lifestyle had slower progression of their illness. This lifestyle was defined as being connected with a spiritual presence in life, whether it took the shape of a family member, close friend, support network, meditation, yoga, or prayer."

Medical Foods
Over the last decade, numerous medical foods claiming efficacy in dementia have appeared. These are Axona, CerefolinNAC, and Souvenaid.[119] Each works differently and all require prescription. Axona and CeferolinNAC are available in United States, but not Souvenaid.

Axona is a form of medium-chain triglycerides (MCT) made of glycerin and caprylic acid. Like all other MCTs, Axona is thought to induce ketogenesis providing ketone bodies to the brain, which is thought to represent a better energy source for the brain as compared to glucose, leading to optimized mitochondrial electron transport. Axona manufacturer, *Accera* has published a single phase II, double-blind, randomized trial of 152 patients showing statistically significant positive result of clinically borderline significance.[120] Axona is taken once daily as a powder mixed with water. Intestinal side effects, mostly gas and diarrhea, are common. The cost of Axona is about $120 per month.

CerefolinNAC is a combination of methylcobalamin 2 mg (B12), L-methylfolate 6 mg and N-acetylcysteine (NAC) 600 mg. It is approved by the U.S. Food and Drug Administration (FDA) for the treatment or prevention of vitamin deficiencies associated with memory loss. The main advantage of CerefolinNAC is once daily dosing in one tablet; however, it does not offer flexibility in dosing of the previously listed nutrients. The cost of CerefolinNAC is about $120 per month. The total cost of each ingredient is a less than that of CerefolinNAC, but the dosages are different.

Souvenaid is designed to promote synaptic formation and function.[121,122] Souvenaid contains uridine monophosphate; choline; phospholipids; EPA; DHA, vitamins E, C, B12, and B6; folic acid; and selenium. It is the most comprehensive formula targeting acetylcholine deficiency, integrity of neuronal membranes, resistance to oxidative stress, and optimal metabolic activity in the brain.[121,122] Several recent clinical trials have shown conflicting results.[121,122] It is not currently available in the United States.

Ginkgo biloba. Although *Ginkgo biloba* has been previously advocated for use in dementia, recent studies reported negative outcomes.[147-149] Despite these negative results, ginkgo clearly has a role in improving microvascular circulation and scavenging free radicals.[150] Authors do not routinely recommend using ginkgo. It may have benefits for patients with a vascular component with history of heart disease, diabetes, transient ischemic attacks, or strokes. Theoretically, ginkgo's risk of increased

bleeding in patients taking Coumadin is probably not clinically significant; however, caution is advised by close monitoring of INR.

Magnesium-L-Threonate. In animal experiments, oral magnesium-L-threonate supplements elevated brain magnesium levels and produced synaptoprotective effects in the hippocampus, including upregulated NMDA receptor signaling and inhibition of TNF-α overexpression. The supplement enhanced short-term synaptic facilitation and long-term potentiation in normal rats and restored deficits in short-term memory and LTP in rats with spared nerve injury.[151,152] In a mouse model of AD, oral magnesium-L-threonate prevented NMDA reception downregulation, synapse loss, and memory decline.[153] Compared to controls, rats treated with the supplement had an improved ability to distinguish between fear contexts and reduced generalization of fear.[154]

L-Alpha-Glycerylphosphorylcholine, Cytidine 5'-Diphosphocholine, and Phosphatidylcholine. Numerous studies have clearly demonstrated the critical importance of adequate dietary choline consumption and that low dietary choline consumption in childhood negatively affects brain development.[155] Phosphatidylcholine (PC), a phospholipid integral to cell membranes, has been more recently tapped as a possible agent for enhancing memory and treating dementia by enhancing a generation of new synapses. Several recent studies have shown that PC improves memory in subjects without memory impairments.[156,157] More recently, novel forms of PC analogues, such as L-Alpha-glycerylphosphorylcholine (alpha GPC) and cytidine 5'-diphosphocholine (CDP-choline), have become available. In contrast to PC, these are water-soluble and have a faster rate of absorption.

Alpha GPC is an actual PC metabolite that in addition to being excellent source of choline, boosts acetylcholine production as well. Daily intake of 1200 mg of semisynthetic derivative of PC alpha GPC has been shown in one RCT to improve all studied measures including MMSE over course of 3 and 6 months. No significant side effects have been reported.[158]

CDP-choline, an endogenous molecule and direct PC precursor, with all benefits on PC and additional protective effect on dopaminergic neurons, is approved for strokes, Parkinson's disease, and other neurological disorders in Japan and Europe, where it is sold under brand name Citicoline. Multiple RCTs using CDP-choline were performed, mostly for vascular dementia. A 2005 Cochrane Review concluded that there is some evidence for positive effect despite mostly short-term and heterogeneous studies.[159]

PC, alpha GPC, and CDP-choline have not been compared side to side or tried in combinations, making it impossible to evaluate which, if any, of these products are preferred. A 2009 Cochrane Systematic Review concluded that there is no obvious benefit of lecithin or PC choline precursors in patients with AD, but due to one study showing strong results, the review concluded that larger studies are needed and moderate benefit can indeed exist.[160]

Intravenous Immunoglobulin Therapy

Intravenous immunoglobulin therapy (IVIG) is a mix of antibodies derived from plasma of healthy donors. IVIG has been used to treat diseases for more than 30 years. It is FDA approved for use in treating several disorders. IVIG is administered intravenously every 2–4 weeks. The initial interest regarding this treatment for use in AD surfaced in 2003 when decreased levels of free antibodies against beta-amyloid in the blood of patients with AD were found.[161] Findings from a recent large phase III trial were disappointing. Primary outcomes were not statistically different from the placebo arm, despite some positive secondary outcomes in some subgroups.[162] Side effects have been described, mostly mild, but have included hypertensive crisis and even stroke, presumably due to increased blood viscosity.

PREVENTION PRESCRIPTION

- Antiinflammatory, Mediterranean, or MIND diets, high in omega-3, with a low glycemic index
- Regular high intake of high antioxidant foods such as green leafy vegetables, turmeric, berries, and green tea
- Patients who prefer a low-fat diet can choose to take oil supplements such as olive, sunflower, safflower, or fish oil.
- Mind-body practices to manage stress, 15–30 min per day
- Regular physical and cognitive exercises
- Advocate building strong social support system to avoid isolation later in life.
- Optimize vascular risk factors: avoid smoking, excessive alcohol use, obesity, prevent or if not possible control hypertension and diabetes.
- Consider high-quality methylated B vitamin complex supplementation for patients aged more than 65 years.

THERAPEUTIC REVIEW

ADDRESS SYSTEMIC ISSUES

- Chronic stress
- Insulin resistance
- Nutritional deficiencies or insufficiencies
- Methylation defects
- Oxidative stress and inflammation
- Increased intestinal permeability and dysbiosis
- Sleep apnea
- Toxic exposures
- Cardiovascular comorbidities such as hypertension

NUTRITION

- Antiinflammatory, Mediterranean, or MIND diets, high in omega-3 with a low glycemic index
- Regular high-intake of high antioxidant foods such as green leafy vegetables, turmeric, blueberries and other berries, and matcha green tea
- One to two tablespoons daily of high-quality coconut oil
- Night time 12-hour fasting

EXERCISE

- Recommend exercise regardless of disease stage
- For early stages—combination of physical and cognitive exercises (e.g., yoga, tai chi)
- Aggressive physical therapy for later stages

MIND-BODY AND BEHAVIORAL

- Meditation: kirtan kriya, Tibetan sound meditation, and other mind-body methods
- Recommend, regardless of disease stage—late stages use music, pet therapy, and Reiki

SUPPLEMENTS

- Acetyl-L-carnitine: 2–3 g per day
- Alpha-lipoic acid: 300–600 mg per day
- N-acetyl cysteine: 500–100 mg per day
- Fish oil: 1–3 g per day of combined DHA/EPA, at least 50% should be DHA
- Huperzine A: 100–400 mcg per day in twice daily dosing. Do not combine with cholinesterase inhibitors.
- Methylated B complex: once per day (unless part of multivitamin)
- Multiantioxidant (could be multivitamin) if poor diet, see Note Box.
- Vitamin D (to maintain serum level of 40–60 ng/mL)
- Ubiquinol (activated coenzyme Q10) 50–100 mg per day

HORMONES

- Assess DHEA and pregnenolone levels and if low use the following:
  - DHEA: 10–100 mg per day
  - Pregnenolone: 10–100 mg per day
- Melatonin: 0.5–10 mg at bedtime. It can help with both sleep and nighttime agitation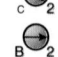

MEDICATIONS

- Discuss risks and benefits—if decision is to proceed, monitor for side effects
- Memantine: start with 5 mg in the morning and slowly increase to 10 mg twice daily
- Donepezil: start with 5 mg every night and increase to 10 mg every night in 4–6 weeks.

TEAM BUILDING

- Hospices and home care agencies
- Therapists providing physical therapy and occupational therapy, yoga instructors, and tai chi teachers
- Geriatric case managers
- Medical house calls programs at http://www.aahcm.org.

Key Web Resources

Alzheimer's Association
The Alzheimer's Association is the world's leading voluntary health organization in Alzheimer's care, support, and research.

http://www.alz.org/index.asp

Alzheimer's Foundation of America
The mission of the Alzheimer's Foundation of America (AFA) is "to provide optimal care and services to individuals confronting dementia, and to their caregivers and families-through member organizations dedicated to improving quality of life."

http://alzfdn.org/

National Institute on Aging, Alzheimer's
Disease Education and Referral Center at NIH
The U.S. Congress created the Alzheimer's Disease Education and Referral (ADEAR) Center in 1990 to "compile, archive, and disseminate information concerning Alzheimer's disease" for health professionals, people with AD and their families, and the public. The ADEAR Center is a service of the National Institute on Aging (NIA), one of the Federal Government's National Institutes of Health and part of the U.S. Department of Health and Human Services. The NIA conducts and supports research about health issues for older people, and is the primary Federal agency for Alzheimer's disease research.

http://www.nia.nih.gov/alzheimers

Dementia.org
Dementia.org is a one-stop resource that provides practical, easy-to-understand information for people with early stages of dementia, people who have not been diagnosed with dementia but want to reduce their risk, friends and family, caregivers, physicians and other health professionals, licensed residential caregiving facilities.

http://www.dementia.org

Mini-Cog
Mini-Cog is validated informant assessment of Alzheimer patients tools.

http://www.alz.org/documents_custom/minicog.pdf.

MoCa
Dr. Ziad Nasreddine created a much quicker comprehensive assessment in order to detect early stage of impairment for the most common neurodegenerative conditions such as Alzheimer disease.

http://www.mocatest.org

CDR
The CDR is a 5-point scale used to characterize six domains of cognitive and functional performance applicable to AD and related dementia.

http://alzheimer.wustl.edu/cdr/Application/Step1.htm

Memory Matrix 1.0
Mem Matrix is a fun game and education for your brain. Memory Matrix helps in improving cognition.

http://tvishitech.com/Memory%20Matrix.html

Matching-3
Swap gems to match jewels in this game.

http://www.popcap.com/games/bejeweled2/online

Brain Fitness
Everyday brain fitness is a complex balance of activities. Visit BrainHQ today to find out what you need to be doing to keep your brain in shape.

http://www.brainhq.com/brain-resources/everyday-brain-fitness

REFERENCES

References are available online at ExpertConsult.com.

CHAPTER 12

HEADACHE

Remy R. Coeytaux, MD, PhD • John Douglas Mann, MD

Headache is one of the most common complaints that brings a patient to the attention of health care providers.[1] Ninety percent of all headaches are either migraine, with or without aura; tension-type headache (TTH); or a mixture of the two. Sixteen percent of adult women and 6% of men suffer from migraine.[2] The remaining 10% of headaches seen by caregivers are secondary to disorders of the tissues of the head and neck, including the cervical spine, sinuses, temporomandibular joints, and dental structures and soft tissue trauma and posttrauma, with primary tumors, infection, and metastatic cancers constituting a small fraction of the possible causes.

"Red flag" symptoms of life-threatening disorders include early morning headaches that awaken the patient; visual dimming or double vision; headaches that are increasing in frequency or severity over weeks to months; headaches made significantly worse by postural changes; explosive onset of new, severe head pain; and headaches associated with mental status changes, focal motor or sensory deficits, syncope, seizures, fever, or stiff neck. Headaches in the setting of systemic illness, weight loss, human immunodeficiency virus (HIV), or known malignancy clearly require thorough investigation. Findings on examination that prompt further diagnostic workup include focal neurological signs, evidence of head or neck trauma, temporal artery tenderness, papilledema, nuchal rigidity, fever, and physical evidence of local or systemic infection or malignancy.

Clinical guidelines are available for pharmacological prevention and treatment of migraine[3-5] and tension-type headache.[6] The emphasis in this chapter is on nonpharmacological, behavioral, nutritional, and complementary therapies that are effective in the treatment or prevention of migraine and tension-type headache.

MIGRAINE PATHOPHYSIOLOGY

Characteristics typical of migraine include subacute onset of throbbing head pain (unilateral or bilateral) associated with nausea and vomiting, photophobia, and sonophobia. Headaches are heralded by visual or other nonpain premonitory symptoms (auras) in about 20% of those with migraine. The duration is usually more than 4 hours and may last up to 72 hours with fluctuating intensity.[7] The precipitating factors can include menses, specific foods, stress or letdown following stress, changes in the weather, infection, fatigue, and bright sunlight.

While the origin of migraine pain is not fully understood, recent evidence points to a role for potent vasodilators, such as substance P and calcitonin gene-related peptide (CGRP), released by peripheral nerve endings of cranial nerve V on blood vessels in the scalp and meninges[8] (Fig. 12.1). This leads to sterile inflammation and edema of blood vessels, with increased sensitivity to mechanical stimulation, resulting in pain. Glutamate, nitric oxide, and vanilloid receptors are also implicated in migraine. Translation of this information to therapy is very active. For instance, CGRP receptor antagonists are currently in phase III clinical trials.[9,10] In the periphery, release of serotonin by platelets in the early stages seems to increase pain and prolong the headache. Centrally, the presence of a "headache generator" in the midbrain and pons is supported by findings from positron emission tomographic studies obtained during migraine attacks. Genetic influences are evident in a majority of patients with one or more family members experiencing migraine. Although the individual attacks of migraine are often stereotypic, variation is not uncommon and comorbid TTH is frequent.

> Patients with migraine often suffer from tension-type headaches (TTH) and other forms of headache. A carefully recorded history of headache symptom characteristics helps establish criteria that lead to diagnoses and helps highlight distinctions that guide specific therapies.

The following sections describe complementary approaches that are potentially useful for integration with conventional therapies in the treatment of migraine (Table 12.1). Conventional approaches rely heavily on pharmaceutical interventions to prevent or abort headaches and are usually prescribed with analgesics and antiemetics. Although these measures are by themselves generally effective in the management of symptoms, they are often expensive; come with significant side effects; and do not address the underlying physical, psychological, and energetic issues that lead to headache. Patients with headache currently use a variety of alternative and complementary therapies,[11] many of which will be reviewed in this chapter.

INTEGRATIVE THERAPY

Lifestyle

Effective management of migraine requires a careful assessment of lifestyle issues related to sleep, nutrition, exercise, stress management, and relationships. Regularizing meal times, developing an exercise routine, and correcting poor sleep can significantly reduce the frequency of migraine.[12,13] Sleep hygiene guidelines are readily

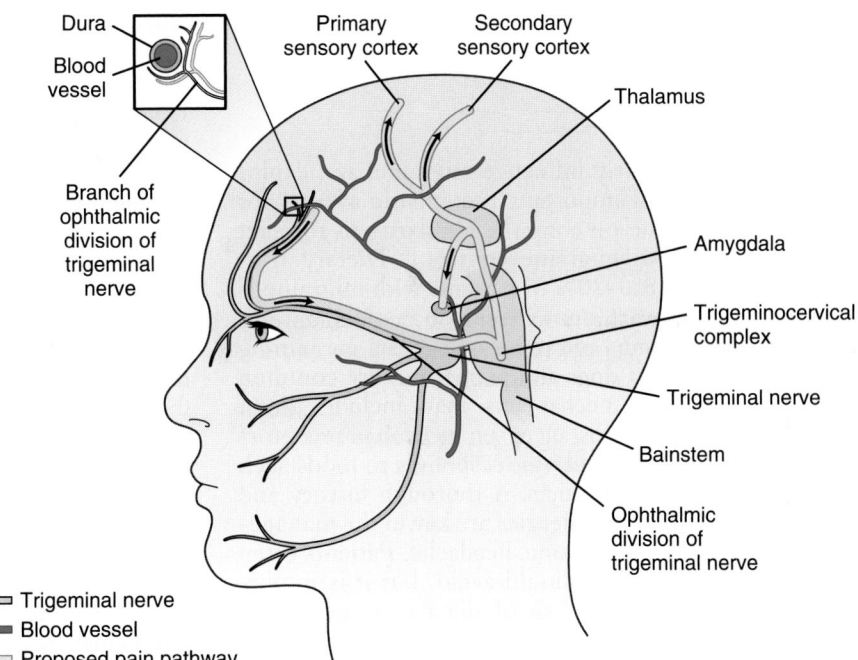

FIG. 12.1 ■ Pathophysiology of headaches. (From Nicolson Stephen E. *Massachusetts General Hospital comprehensive clinical psychiatry.* 4th ed. Philadelphia, Elsevier Inc; 2016:78, 839-851)

Legend:
- Trigeminal nerve
- Blood vessel
- Proposed pain pathway

TABLE 12.1 Summary of Migraine Therapies

Types of Therapy	Specific Examples/Comments
Preventive	
Lifestyle	Sleep hygiene, exercise, stress management
Nutrition supplements—botanicals	Elimination of "food triggers," consideration of food allergy, maintenance of good hydration. Magnesium, riboflavin, coenzyme Q10, omega-3 fatty acids, α-lipoic acid
	Feverfew, petasites, melatonin, and valerian root (sleep); ginger root (nausea)
Pharmaceuticals	Tricyclic antidepressants, β-blockers, calcium channel blockers, anticonvulsants, NSAIDs, botulinum toxin; reduction of the risk of analgesic rebound headache by addressing analgesic polypharmacy
Mind-Body Techniques	
Biofeedback	Motivation required to practice and use as a life skill
Relaxation	Progressive muscle relaxation, focused breathing exercises, guided imagery
Cognitive-behavior therapy	Modification of maladaptive thoughts and reactions to feelings and sensations
Neurolinguistic programming	Alteration of the subjective experience of pain and modification of expectations
Self-hypnosis	Use for both headache prevention and pain control
Mindfulness meditation	Improvements in mood, coping, blood pressure, muscle tone, pain control, and pain perception
Body work	Craniosacral therapy and chiropractic
Bioenergetics	Effectiveness in both preventing and treating migraine
Abortive and Acute	
Pharmaceuticals	NSAIDs, ergot alkaloids, isometheptene, intranasal lidocaine, triptans, valproate, magnesium, narcotics, antiemetics (ginger)
Chiropractic, massage	Use especially for headaches associated with neck discomfort
Acupuncture	Use for severe acute attacks

NSAIDs, nonsteroidal antiinflammatory drugs.

available, easy to implement, and often lead to a decrease in both duration and frequency of migraine.[14]

Nutrition

Dietary choices clearly influence migraine, and exploration of diet is an important therapeutic avenue for improving migraine outcomes[15]; regularity in the diet may be the key to migraine control.[16] Dietary triggers are found in 8%–20% of patients with migraine.[17] Red wines, dark beers, aged cheese, some nuts, onions, chocolate, aspartame, and processed meats containing nitrates (such as hot dogs and pepperoni) are common offenders. Specific mechanisms may include direct effects of ingested substances on neuronal receptors governing headache or allergic responses to foods such as gluten and dairy products. A thorough history and testing for specific food allergies are key in the management of recurrent and chronic headache. Patients often know which foods they should avoid, but it is important to raise the possibility of dietary triggers with patients as these sometimes go unnoticed until they are brought up and discussed. Caffeine is a dietary factor that is particularly important. Caffeine withdrawal can temporarily exacerbate migraine or TTHs, whereas caffeine taken during a migraine can reduce pain in some patients, possibly due to its vasoconstrictive effects on the scalp and meningeal vessels. However, caffeine excess (more than five cups of coffee per day) can contribute to maintaining chronic daily headache, especially when combined with medication excess (see Chapters 31 and 86).

Diets that contain large quantities of omega-6 fatty acids are generally proinflammatory and are likely to aggravate migraine and chronic TTH. In a study of 65 adults with chronic daily headache, of which 85% had chronic migraine, there was significant improvement in headache severity and frequency in those on a high omega-3, low omega-6 fatty acid diet compared to baseline and compared to those on a low omega-6 fatty acid diet alone.[18] The dietary interventions lasted 12 weeks. Food was provided, and all subjects received regular dietary counseling throughout the intervention. Fatty acid supplements were not given. Clinical benefits were most pronounced in the last 4 weeks of the intervention. Most striking were the correlations between clinical improvement and levels of omega-3–derived antiinflammatory lipid mediators. Biochemical endpoints correlated closely with clinical improvement in pain and psychological distress[19] (see Chapter 88).

Obesity and metabolic syndrome have also been found to be associated with migraine and chronic headache, perhaps related to the proinflammatory state associated with these conditions.[20-22] Inflammatory bowel disorders also have a higher incidence of migraine.[23] Treatment implications for migraine in these conditions, while not fully defined, favor integration of dietary choices with other forms of treatment.

Specific nutrients and supplements that have shown promise in headache management are reviewed in the following text.

Supplements

Magnesium

Levels of ionized tissue magnesium are often low in migraine, especially in individuals with menstrual migraine.[24-26] There is limited evidence that suggests that oral supplementation with magnesium may be effective in the prevention of migraine.[27] The mechanisms leading to improvement with magnesium supplementation may include reduction in cerebral cortical neuronal excitability or alteration in magnesium-dependent circadian regulatory mechanisms that are frequently disturbed in migraine.[28-30] One study showed that oral magnesium dicitrate 600 mg given once a day significantly reduced the frequency of migraine compared to placebo.[31] In another study, oral administration of 360 mg of pyrrolidine carboxylic acid magnesium daily for 2 months was associated with greater pain relief than placebo in women with menstrual migraine.[32] Patients with menstrual migraine should continue magnesium for at least 3 months to determine the effectiveness because beneficial effects may be delayed for several cycles.

Preventive benefit can be achieved with oral potassium magnesium aspartate (500–1000 mg/day at bedtime). Magnesium oxide is more readily available and cheaper than other forms, but it is poorly absorbed, especially when combined with calcium, zinc, or iron. Magnesium may cause diarrhea, particularly in those with irritable bowel syndrome, a common comorbid condition. For acute treatment of migraine, 2 g in 100 mL of saline given IV over 30 min appears to be effective and safe in an outpatient setting,[33-35] but the U.S. Food and Drug Administration (FDA) issued a warning in 2013 about potential harm to the fetus associated with prolonged use of IV magnesium sulfate during pregnancy.[36]

DOSAGE

For prevention: potassium magnesium aspartate 500–1000 mg at bedtime

PRECAUTIONS

May cause diarrhea; consider magnesium gluconate as an alternate form

---

Riboflavin (Vitamin B₂)

Patients with migraine have been shown to have reduced phosphorylation potential in brain and muscles, suggesting a mitochondrial defect in electron transport.[37] Riboflavin is a precursor for two coenzymes involved in electron transfer for redox reactions. One hypothesis for the mechanism of action of riboflavin is that it improves mitochondrial energy reserves without changing neuronal excitability.[38] In several clinical studies of riboflavin as a supplement in migraineurs, there were significant preventive effects.[39,40] It may have synergistic preventive effects when used concurrently with a beta-blocker.[38] There are no head-to-head studies comparing riboflavin with other preventive measures. Results in children with migraine are mixed.[41,42]

DOSAGE

The recommended dose of riboflavin is 200 mg twice daily with meals.

PRECAUTIONS

Riboflavin is well tolerated and does not influence metabolism of other agents. Patients may notice that color of their urine turns to intense yellow with daily use. It is safe in pregnancy.

Coenzyme Q₁₀

The rationale for studying coenzyme Q_{10} relates to lower phosphorylation potentials found in patients with a variety of chronic disorders including migraine.[43] The findings of an open-label trial showing reduction in headache frequency at 3 months with daily dosing of 150 mg of coenzyme Q_{10} were confirmed in a double-blind, placebo-controlled, randomized trial in 42 patients with migraine.[44,45] The oral coenzyme Q_{10}, 100 mg three times a day, resulted in a reduction in attack frequency by 47.6% compared to 14.4% in the controls at 3 months. The number of days with headache was also significantly reduced. Like riboflavin, there was no change in headache intensity or duration once a headache occurred. Another clinical trial published in 2011 demonstrated early (but not sustained) benefits associated with coenzyme Q supplementation for the prevention of migraine in children and adolescents.[46] There have been no major recent studies.

DOSAGE

Coenzyme Q_{10}, 150 to 300 mg/day; minimum 3-month trial based on research of Sandor and associates.[24]

PRECAUTIONS

Well tolerated with rare gastrointestinal side effects, is relatively expensive, and safe in pregnancy.

Fish Oil

Rationale for the use of omega-3 fatty acids in migraine prevention includes their antiinflammatory properties, vascular relaxation effects, and inhibition of serotonin release from platelets. Only two studies in the last 15 years specifically address the role of omega-3 supplements in migraine. The American Academy of Neurology (AAN) Guidelines for Headache (2013) ranked the evidence as insufficient to make recommendations.

One study of fish oil capsules for migraine prevention used a randomized crossover design in 27 adolescents with migraine; it compared daily omega-3 fatty acids vs an olive oil control, both given as capsules, with no change in the diet. Each arm was 2 months with a 2-week washout. Both olive oil and omega-3 were associated with a striking reduction in headache frequency compared to baseline and

washout frequencies.[47] There were no measures of compliance or biochemical endpoints and no follow-up.

Another study of fish oil capsules in 96 adults with migraine showed no benefit.[48] The dosing ranged between 2 and 6 g/day, and there was no recommendation to change the usual diet of subjects. Side effects included nausea and symptoms of gastric reflux.

A recent diet-only study of adults with chronic migraine on omega-3-enriched diet for 12 weeks, without supplements, showed significant benefits in headache by week 9 of the intervention, which increased further during the last 3 weeks, compared to a reduced omega-6 diet.[18] It is safe during pregnancy.

DOSAGE

According to the available literature, it is best to increase omega-3 fatty acid levels through nutrition rather than taking it as a supplement.

Daily use of a compound containing 400 mg of riboflavin, 300 mg of magnesium, and 100 mg of feverfew has been shown to be effective in reducing the frequency of migraine in adults.[49]

Botanicals

Feverfew (Tanacetum parthenium Leaf)

Johnson et al. reported a significant increase in migraine severity and frequency when feverfew was stopped in a small group of migraineurs taking it for prevention.[50] In one well-designed study, a 70% reduction in headache frequency and severity was shown in 270 patients with migraine.[51] Variations in the standardization of the dried leaf constituents confound replication studies of this herb. A reproducibly manufactured extract of feverfew has shown preventive efficacy in a double-blind randomized controlled trial (RCT).[52] There are no long-term studies documenting safety and no head-to-head trials with other preventive medications. The mechanism of action in migraine may be related to its inhibiting effects on platelet aggregation and inflammatory promoters, such as serotonin and prostaglandins, or possibly its effect in dampening vascular reactivity to amine regulators of blood flow.

DOSAGE

Oral administration of feverfew up to 125 mg/day of the dried leaf standardized to a minimum of 0.2% parthenolide. Beneficial effects may take weeks to develop.

PRECAUTIONS

Aphthous ulcers and gastrointestinal irritation develop in 5%–15% of users. Abrupt cessation of feverfew occasionally results in agitation and increased headache. It is not recommended during pregnancy due to prolongation of bleeding times.

Butterbur (Petasites hybridus Root)

In a large, three-arm, dose-finding RCT of a standardized extract of the root of this perennial shrub, it was found that migraine attack frequency was reduced by almost 50%. Among those on the highest dose, 68% had a 50% or greater reduction in headache frequency.[53] This effect continued for at least 4 months. One smaller study showed similar results,[54] and another study in 108 children and adolescents with migraine was also positive.[55] One study that compared butterbur root extract to both music therapy and placebo in the prevention of migraine in children had mixed findings, with butterbur demonstrating efficacy compared to placebo in the long-term, but not short-term, follow-up.[56] A systematic review of the published literature on the effectiveness of *P. hybridus* revealed that higher dose extracts (150 mg) were associated with a lower frequency of migraine attacks after 3–4 months compared to a lower dose and placebo.[57] The extract is commonly standardized to 15% of the marker molecule (petasins) and known carcinogens are removed. Drug–herb interactions have not been studied.

> **Dosage**
>
> Butterbur, 50 mg three times a day for 1 month; then 50 mg twice a day
>
> **Precautions**
>
> Unknown effects in pregnancy; excessive belching as a side effect

Supplements for Sleep

Sleep management is a major therapeutic strategy in helping patients gain control over their headaches. Melatonin and valerian root can be used on a temporary basis to improve sleep.

Melatonin

Melatonin is used in the management of migraine to improve sleep and circadian rhythms. Sleep maintenance, as opposed to sleep induction, is improved with melatonin. Melatonin is recommended every night for 4–6 weeks and then tapered off. During that period, a sleep hygiene program can be put into place to reduce the need for the supplement. There are few side effects. Leone and coworkers demonstrated that a daily intake of 10 mg of melatonin for 14 days significantly reduced cluster headache frequency.[58] Others have shown beneficial effects of melatonin in migraine and other types of headache, including migraine prevention in children.[59-61] However, a recently published, double-blind, placebo-controlled, crossover study comparing extended-release melatonin at a dose of 2 mg 1 hour before bedtime did not demonstrate improvement in migraine frequency compared to placebo.[62]

> **Dosage**
>
> Melatonin, 2–12 mg; start at 2 mg and titrate up every 4 days as needed for sleep. Lower doses are needed if taken each evening for several weeks. Higher doses (>15 mg) are needed to acutely induce sleep over several days (jet lag).
>
> **Precautions**
>
> Fatigue, drowsiness, dizziness, abdominal cramps, and irritability

Valerian (Valeriana officinalis Root)

When taken at night for sleep, valerian rarely results in residual drowsiness on awakening. It is nonaddictive and useful as an anxiolytic when given during the daytime (up to 250 mg three times per day). It does not impair psychomotor or cognitive performance.[63] The mechanism of action includes stimulation of the central nervous system gamma-aminobutyric acid (GABA) receptors along with enhanced release and inhibition of reuptake of GABA. In clinical trials, including the use for sleep and anxiety, it has been judged to be safe.[63-66] Gastrointestinal irritation is the most common side effect (15%).

> **Dosage**
>
> Valerian, 100–300 mg of the extract standardized to 0.8% valerenate at bedtime or 250 mg every 6 hours for anxiety
>
> **Precautions**
>
> Very unpleasant smell that may aggravate nausea during migraine. It may cause worsening of tension headache if taken regularly for more than 3 months. It should not be used during pregnancy.

> Magnesium aspartate, in contrast to magnesium oxide, is easily absorbed and rarely causes diarrhea when used for migraine prevention. Avoid giving either preparation at the same time as calcium, zinc, or iron. Dosage: 500–1000 mg each night.

Pharmaceuticals

There is no inherent difficulty in the integration of conventional and complementary approaches in the treatment of headache. Conventional pharmacological therapy includes use of preventive and abortive medications. The pharmaceutical approaches discussed here are the ones for which there is greatest evidence of efficacy and clinical usefulness.[3-5]

Preventive Pharmaceutical Therapies

Application of preventive pharmacological therapies in practice is typically organized around classes of medications, including tricyclic antidepressants, selective serotonin reuptake inhibitors, beta-blockers, calcium channel blockers, anticonvulsants, and other miscellaneous agents. The goals are reduction in headache frequency and severity, improved function, and increased responsiveness to abortive and analgesic agents.

The decision to start preventive therapy is based on the following: (1) headache frequency of more than two per month or more than 3 days per month lost to headache, (2) willingness of the patient to take a medication or supplement daily for at least 3 months, and (3) ability to maintain a headache diary. Medications for prevention are administered according to the half-life and a schedule that minimizes side effects. Effectiveness is best measured by having the patient maintain a headache diary, noting headache frequency and intensity as well as significant life events, such as stressful circumstances, menses, vacations, and major changes. Patients may respond to any of several beta-blockers (e.g., propranolol, atenolol, metoprolol, or timolol), making the choice of an agent highly individualized. It is not possible to predict who will respond to a given agent in advance, although the history of a family member who achieved effective prevention with a given agent may guide initial choices. Comorbid depression, a history of active asthma, and thyroid disease limits the use of beta-blockers, whereas obesity limits the use of tricyclic antidepressants and valproate.

Medications and supplements are prescribed one at a time and tapered up to a maximum dose or until satisfactory benefit is realized at lower doses. Most drugs are started at less than half the predicted maximum dose. Often, patients achieve satisfactory results at doses well below the maximum, particularly with the tricyclic antidepressants. On the other hand, verapamil usually has to be given at doses of at least 320 mg/day for benefit to occur. Magnesium, vitamin B_2, coenzyme Q_{10}, and daily aspirin mix well with conventional preventive agents.

Once improvement is achieved, the medication combination is continued for a period of 3–6 months with periodic gradual reductions in one or more agents to determine the minimum effective dose. Effective preventive agents allow time for patients to work on lifestyle issues, including management of stress, sleep, nutrition, and exercise, as well as to develop life skills, such as relaxation, biofeedback, and self-hypnosis. Preventive agents are also chosen to facilitate the treatment of comorbid depression and sleep dysfunction. As patients improve, diaries that focus on pain are discontinued.

Tricyclic Antidepressants. Amitriptyline, in doses of up to 150 mg at bedtime, starting as low as 10 mg, is effective for prevention. A few patients do well on very low doses such as 10 mg at night. Other useful medications in this group include nortriptyline, up to 100 mg at bedtime. Sleep is often improved, which reduces migraine frequency. Dry mouth, morning drowsiness, and constipation are significant side effects.

Beta-Blockers. Medications in this class that have been shown to be effective for migraine include propranolol, nadolol, timolol, atenolol, and metoprolol. Long-acting formulations have not been formally studied. Side effects include fatigue, depression, insomnia, dizziness, and nausea. Rebound headaches may occur if beta-blockers are suddenly withdrawn. Dosing of propranolol for migraine prevention ranges between 80 and 240 mg/day in two or three divided doses.

Calcium Channel Blockers. Calcium channel blockers shown to be effective include verapamil, nimodipine, flunarizine, and nifedipine. Delayed onset (weeks) of effectiveness is typical, and side effects such as abdominal pain, bloating, weight gain, constipation, and even headache are not uncommon. A typical dose of verapamil is 180 mg twice daily.

Anticonvulsants. The major members of this group prescribed for migraine are sodium valproate, gabapentin (Neurontin), topiramate (Topamax), zonisamide (Zonegran), and levetiracetam (Keppra).[67,68] A typical adult dose of sodium valproate for prevention is 1500 mg/day, with a starting dose of 250 mg twice daily. Side effects include weight gain, alopecia, tremor, and nausea. Sodium valproate is available in 125-, 250-, 500-mg, and sustained-release formulations. Topiramate is the most consistently effective of the four most commonly used drugs in this class, but cognitive side effects and nausea can be limiting. Levetiracetam and zonisamide have the fewest side effects.

Nonsteroidal Antiinflammatory Drugs. Trends toward reduction in migraine frequency have been seen with daily use of aspirin, naproxen, ketoprofen, and tolfenamic acid. Gastric side effects are common, and patient compliance is poor. Dosages include naproxen 500 mg twice daily, aspirin 350–975 mg/day, and ketoprofen 150 mg/day. These drugs are not safe in pregnancy.

Botulinum Toxin. Botulinum toxin has been found to prevent migraine when injected in small quantities at multiple sites into the muscles of the forehead, temples, posterior neck, and the trapezius muscle.[69-73] The early Phase III REsearch Evaluating Migraine Prophylaxis Therapy (PREEMPT) studies showing efficacy have been confirmed.[74-76] The FDA has approved it for treatment of chronic migraine (>15 headache days per month). The positive response rate in those with chronic migraine is more than 60%. The frequency of chronic migraine is reduced significantly, whereas headache intensity remains largely unchanged. Effects last an average of 2–4 months. There is limited evidence on its efficacy in TTH. Side effects are few and can include transient weakness of injected muscles. Dosing is 100–200 units total per injection session. It is injected with a 27-gauge needle over 15–25 sites (~2–10 units per site).

Abortive Pharmaceutical Therapies

The following is a list of medications that, when taken early in the course of migraine, can abort further development of the headache.

Nonsteroidal Antiinflammatory Drugs. Ibuprofen (800 mg) and naproxen sodium (200–400 mg) can block headache progression when given during the first few hours when the headache is building. Ibuprofen in liquid form (200–400 mg) is recommended when nausea occurs early in the headache. Individual variation in responsiveness to nonsteroidal antiinflammatory drugs (NSAIDs) is high; thus, it is worth trying several different agents from this class early in the headache.

Ergot Alkaloids. Now largely supplanted by the triptans, ergot alkaloids can be useful in those who cannot tolerate other abortive methods. A typical dose is ergotamine tartrate, 1 mg orally, 2 mg sublingually, or dihydroergotamine (DHE-45) 2 mg subcutaneously (self-injection) every 4 hours for up to three doses. A nasal inhalational form is also available.

Isometheptene. Isometheptene (Midrin) has a low side-effect profile and modest cost. It is a weak vasoconstrictor of scalp vessels. The dosing is two or three capsules at the start of a headache, then one every 45 minutes for three more doses as needed within 24 hours.

Intranasal Lidocaine. Intranasal lidocaine is effective for most forms of migraine and is particularly useful when given during the aura and when nausea and vomiting are prominent early in the headache.[77] The mechanism may relate to the anesthetizing effects of lidocaine on sphenopalatine ganglia. Lidocaine (4% liquid) is applied with a dropper, 0.25–0.50 mL up each nostril, with the patient supine and the head hyperextended. Side effects include a mild transient burning sensation in the nasal passages and occasional transient numbness in the throat. The nasal spray form of lidocaine is generally ineffective. Repeat dosing can be done hourly for 4–6 hours. Intranasal ketorolac has also shown promise for the acute treatment of migraine.[78]

Triptans (5-Hydroxytryptamine Receptor 1B/1D Agonists). The triptans, on average, are the most effective agents available for aborting migraine.[79-82] They act by blocking the release of inflammatory cytokines from the distal nerve endings of the trigeminal system onto the scalp and meningeal vessels and by their vasoconstrictive effects on scalp vessels. Multiple products are available by prescription, including tablet or melt forms, self-injection kits, and nasal sprays. Efficacy of a single dose is 60%–80% for pain and nausea relief, with a 25%–30% recurrence rate necessitating a second dose. The choice of a triptan depends on patient response, side-effect profile, and preferred route of administration. Long-acting forms, including naratriptan (Amerge) and frovatriptan (Frova), can be effective when recurrence rates are noted with the more rapidly acting triptans. Oral melt formulations and nasal sprays are useful when nausea is prominent early in the headache.

Usual dosing is at 2-hour intervals, if necessary, for a maximum of three doses in 24 hours.

- Sumatriptan (Imitrex): 25-, 50-, and 100-mg tablets; 20-mg nasal spray; and 6- and 4-mg/0.5 mL injection kits

- Naratriptan (Amerge): 1- or 2.5-mg tablets
- Rizatriptan (Maxalt): 5- or 10-mg tablets or melt tablets
- Zolmitriptan (Zomig): 2.5- or 5-mg tablets or melt tablets
- Almotriptan (Axert): 12.5-mg tablets
- Frovatriptan (Frova): 2.5-mg tablets
- Eletriptan (Relpax): 40-mg tablets

Triptans are contraindicated in pregnancy, cardiovascular disease, complex migraine, and poorly controlled hypertension. Cost is a major factor. Rebound headache can occur with daily use. Side effects include transient pressure sensations in the chest, neck, and head. It is ineffective in TTH and occasionally effective in cluster headache. Insurance coverage varies widely.

Mind-Body Techniques

Biofeedback

Biofeedback has demonstrated effectiveness in treating both migraine and TTH without major side effects or adverse interactions with other therapies. Thermal biofeedback, in which patients learn to increase the temperature of their hands through guided imagery and relaxation training, and/or electromyography (EMG) biofeedback, wherein patients learn to relax targeted skeletal muscle groups, have been shown to significantly improve migraine symptoms.[83,84] A meta-analysis of 25 studies showed that biofeedback is comparable to preventive pharmacotherapy,[85] and another meta-analysis of 55 studies revealed that migraine headache frequency and perceived self-efficacy showed strongest improvements in biofeedback patients. Migraine patients experienced significant reductions in headache frequency, intensity, and headache-related disability as well as reductions in interictal symptoms, such as irritation and anxiety, in a study combining thermal and EMG biofeedback and relaxation training.[84] Biofeedback, however, did not appear to provide additional benefit in a study involving 64 patients randomized to relaxation training vs relaxation training plus biofeedback.[86] Multiple studies showed a reduction in medication use and health service utilization for both migraine and TTH patients when using biofeedback techniques.[87,88] Biofeedback may also enhance the effectiveness of preventive, abortive, and rescue migraine medications.[89]

There are no criteria for predicting benefit from biofeedback, and the training requires a significant time commitment (10- to 15-hour-long sessions plus home practice). Pharmacotherapy combined with biofeedback may have variable results. This is an important point because vascular reactivity (a major target in biofeedback training) may be modified by medications used for headache prevention (e.g., beta-blockers), potentially limiting the effects of training. On the other hand, biofeedback could be favorably synergistic with magnesium or topiramate.[90] Biofeedback is indicated in patients intolerant to medications, those oriented toward self-efficacy in pain management, pregnancy, and is especially suited for those willing to regularly practice the techniques.

Relaxation

The category of relaxation includes progressive muscular relaxation, focused breathing exercises, and guided imagery. Holroyd and Penzien reported that these techniques are as effective as biofeedback.[55] Treatment effects were enhanced by beta-blockers and other preventive agents, making integration both feasible and effective. Some patients are able to identify the early stages of a headache in time to deploy focused relaxation or guided imagery to abort the full development of pain. D'Souza et al. demonstrated that relaxation training improved headache frequency and disability associated with migraines among college students compared to written emotional disclosure or a neutral writing group control.[91] These techniques can be taught in groups and then practiced individually using audiotapes. Relaxation appeals to those with an internal locus of control and above-average motivation (see Chapter 94).

Cognitive-Behavioral Therapy

Cognitive-behavioral therapy is a stress-management approach designed to help patients identify maladaptive thought patterns (e.g., self-blame, hopelessness, helplessness, worthlessness, and catastrophizing) as well as emotional states such as anger and anxiety that can precipitate and amplify headaches. Acknowledgment of present-moment and historical emotional states, shifting of habitual thought patterns, and modification of physiological responses are the key steps in this approach. It has been shown to be effective, alone or in combination, with other behavioral therapies for headache.[92] Combining cognitive-behavioral and biofeedback therapies is effective.

Hypnosis

Hypnosis has been shown to reduce the number of headache days and decrease headache intensity among patients with chronic TTH.[93] For abortive therapy, hypnosis is useful in helping patients identify the early stages of migraine so that they can initiate relaxation or self-hypnosis routines. Patient motivation and regular practice is a vital part of this strategy. Self-hypnosis can also be useful in resetting expectations about future successes with treatment, reducing rumination about the past and future, and modifying patterns of negative thought (see Chapter 95).

Mindfulness Meditation

Meditation has been shown to have positive effects on mood, cardiac function, blood pressure, and muscle tone when regularly practiced. Effects are believed to be mediated by the development of nonjudgmental awareness of feelings, thoughts, and sensations combined with a sense of gratitude while optimizing the sympathetic and parasympathetic nervous system balance. Group instruction is based on the work of Jon Kabat-Zinn[94,95] and is taught as an 8-week course, including 2–3 hours of formal training each week, combined with daily practice of at least half

an hour of meditation. Patients report improved sleep and less anticipatory anxiety relating to headache as well as reduction in headache intensity.[96] Home practice is important in maintaining benefits.[97]

Feasibility studies indicate that mindfulness training, specifically Kabat-Zinn's 8-week mindfulness-based stress reduction program, is effective for reducing headache severity in migraine and TTH patients.[98,99] One study of migraine patients also showed reductions in levels of anxiety and migraine-related disability after the 8-week course.[98] Headache-specific mindfulness training may improve outcomes[100,101] (see Chapter 100).

Biomechanical Techniques

Physical Therapy

Physical therapy alone does not appear to be effective in the treatment of migraine, but it can be useful as an adjunct to biofeedback and relaxation training when there is significant reactive muscle tension in the upper body with limitation of head and neck movement.

Spinal Manipulation

Chiropractic and osteopathic manipulation approaches are often used for patients whose migraines have a cervicogenic or musculoskeletal component. One study of 218 patients demonstrated comparable results in reduction of migraine headache frequency and intensity in a prospective, randomized, parallel-group comparison of amitriptyline, spinal manipulation, and their combination.[102,103] A systematic review of manual therapies for the treatment of migraine included four RCTs, each of which suggested that chiropractic spinal manipulation may have prophylactic effectiveness similar to that of propranolol and topiramate.[104] However, many of the studies lacked methodological rigor, necessitating future research. Another review published in the same year found that spinal manipulation, whether performed by a chiropractor, physician, or physical therapist, was not effective as a replacement drug therapy for reducing migraine duration but may be an appropriate adjuvant therapy.[105] A review of 21 articles found evidence in support of effectiveness of spinal manipulation for episodic and chronic migraine but not TTH.[106]

Bioenergetics

Acupuncture

Findings from a systematic review and meta-analysis of acupuncture for migraine prophylaxis involving 22 trials with 4419 participants suggest that acupuncture is more effective than routine care only, but not more effective than sham acupuncture, and that acupuncture is associated with better outcomes and fewer adverse effects than prophylactic drug treatment.[107] A more recent patient-level data meta-analysis of acupuncture for the management of chronic headache (including chronic migraine) concluded that acupuncture is superior to sham acupuncture and medication therapy in decreasing headache intensity and frequency and in improving response rate to treatment.[108] A recently published sham-controlled randomized trial reported similar findings among patients with frequent migraine.[109] The current evidence clearly suggests that acupuncture is effective as an adjunct to usual care in the treatment of migraine, but the degree to which placebo effects contribute to this efficacy is unknown.

Homeopathy for Headache Prevention

There are few prospective studies that have evaluated the effectiveness of homeopathy for migraine treatment or prevention. A systematic review of four RCTs and two observational studies found varying results. The observational studies showed significant improvements in homeopathically treated patients with regard to headache intensity, medication usage, and health service utilization.[75] Three of the four RCTs produced equivocal results, while the remaining RCT showed significant reduction in headache frequency in the homeopathy group.[75] A 2010 study found that patients seeking homeopathic treatment for migraine maintained positive results in terms of headache frequency, quality of life, medication use, and health services utilization for 24 months after study completion.[76] The first prospective pediatric homeopathy study with 159 children in 12 countries showed significant decrease in the frequency, severity, and duration of migraine attacks and reduced absenteeism from school during 6 months of treatment.[110]

Therapies to Consider

Formal evidence of effectiveness of the following treatments in migraine is anecdotal, largely theoretical, empirical, limited, or nonexistent. However, some patients respond favorably to them. Based on their overall safety, they may be considered in an integrated treatment plan. For prevention, consider the following: naturopathy, probiotics, ginkgolide B, tai chi, yoga, craniosacral therapy, and ayurvedic medicine. For acute therapy, consider the following: aromatherapy, Reiki, and therapeutic touch; sleep induction with an oral hypnotic; and lorazepam with haloperidol IV; methylprednisolone IV; and valproic acid.

PREVENTION PRESCRIPTION—MIGRAINE

- Identify and avoid environmental factors that consistently lead to headache, e.g., allergens, fluorescent lights, loud noises, fumes, and dust.
- Implement a sleep hygiene program using a prebedtime routine that signals a time leading to restorative sleep. Avoid excessive as well as inadequate sleep.
- Eliminate foods that lower the threshold for migraine, that is, chocolate, aged and yellow cheese, caffeine, red wine, dark beer, shellfish, and meats processed with nitrates.

- Water/fluid intake should be a minimum of 40–60 oz per day for an adult.
- Maintain an exercise program: aerobic level activity, minimum 30 minutes, three times a week.
- Regularize meals, sleep, exercise, and use of medications for prevention.
- Maintain a diary documenting headache frequency and intensity, response to medications, association with major life changes, stress, and changes in physiological states, such as menses, pregnancy, and illness. Share the diary information with caregivers.

THERAPEUTIC REVIEW

MIGRAINE PREVENTION

Lifestyle

- Regular meals and sleep, sleep hygiene, aerobic exercise three times a week, headache calendar, stress management, and avoiding environmental triggers $A \uparrow_1$

- Consider discontinuation of hormonal birth control method if menstrual migraine is evident or the history is suggestive of cause and effect. Consider nonhormonal birth control such as a copper intrauterine device.

Nutrition

- Elimination of food triggers: wine, aged cheese, cashews, chocolate, processed meats, caffeine $A \uparrow_1$

Biochemical Supplements

- Magnesium aspartate, 500-1000 mg qhs   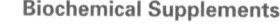 $B \nearrow_1$
- Riboflavin, 200 mg bid $B \nearrow_1$
- Coenzyme Q_{10}, 150 mg daily $B \nearrow_1$

Botanicals

- Feverfew, 125 mg up to tid $B \rightarrow_2$
- Butterbur, 50 mg tid $A \uparrow_1$
- For sleep: valerian root extract, 100-300 mg qhs B_1; melatonin, 6–10 mg qhs $B \nearrow_1$

Pharmaceuticals

- Aspirin, 325 mg daily $C \searrow_2$
- Amitriptyline, 10–150 mg qhs $A \nearrow_2$

- Propranolol, 60–180 mg daily — A 2
- Gabapentin, 300–600 qid — C 2
- Topiramate, 100–200 mg qhs — A 2
- Verapamil, 180–480 mg daily — B 2
- Valproate, 500 mg tid — A 2
- Botulinum toxin, subcutaneous 100 units q3 mo — B 1

Mind-Body
- Biofeedback 10 sessions — A 1
- Cognitive behavioral therapy — A 1
- Hypnosis — B 1
- Mindfulness meditation 8-wk course — B 1

Biomechanical
Consider in cases where muscle tension in the jaw, neck, or shoulder is prominent:
- Chiropractic — C 2
- Massage — C 1

Bioenergetics
- Acupuncture, 6–8 sessions over 8 weeks, repeat as needed — A 1

Acute Migraine Treatment
- Use of specific abortive measures depends on efficacy, cost, side effects, and ease of administration. Use of narcotics and antiemetics is not covered.

Lifestyle
- Darkened, quiet environment, maintain hydration, meals if possible, sleep

Biochemical Supplements and Herbals
- Magnesium sulfate, 2 g IV in 100 mL saline over 30 min — C 1
- Ginger tea for nausea, 8 oz q3 h — C 1
- Aromatherapy (peppermint) — C 1

Pharmaceuticals
- Naproxen sodium, 250–500 mg q4 h — B 2
- Ibuprofen liquid, 200–400 mg q2 h — C 2
- Lidocaine 4% liquid, 0.25 mL in each nostril q1 h — C 1
- Isometheptene (Midrin) 2 tablets at onset, then 1 tablet q45 min × three — B 1
- Triptans. Many available. Dosing routines identical: initial dose at the onset of head pain, followed no sooner than 2 hours by a second dose if necessary. Limit 3 doses in 24 hours — A 2
- Valproate, 1 g IV over 1 h — B 2
- DHE-45, 1.5 mg IV over 30 min preceded by promethazine (Phenergan) 20 mg IV — C 2

Mind-Body
- Self-hypnosis training — C 1
- Practiced biofeedback routine — B 1
- Relaxation — B 1

Biomechanical
- Massage, slow stretch — C 1

Bioenergetic
- Acupuncture — B 1

TENSION-TYPE HEADACHE

TTH may exist in a spectrum with migraine, as shown by positive responses to antimigraine agents in some patients, with or without coexisting migraine. History and physical examination suggest intermittent muscle traction of pain-sensitive tendons and connective tissues of the head and neck. Pain is typically bilateral, nonthrobbing, and band-like, with trigger points at the base of the skull, temples, masseters, and forehead. The pain is typically slow in onset and intermittent with little or no nausea or sensory sensitivity. Positive responses to NSAIDs suggest that inflammatory and myofascial influences dominate, with modest secondary contributions from vascular structures.

Certain pericranial conditions (e.g., brain tumor and central nervous system infection) can present with features of TTH and little else. It is rare for a vascular headache pattern to be the presenting complaint for such conditions. Warning symptoms and signs that suggest the need for head imaging and other studies are reviewed in the first section of this chapter.

INTEGRATIVE THERAPY

There is considerable overlap with migraine in an integrated treatment approach to TTH. Lifestyle issues surrounding stress, sleep, exercise, and diet are central to effective management and all need to be reviewed carefully for both the work and home environments. It is important to remember that individuals with baseline TTH may develop conditions that abruptly amplify the pain. Examples include sinus and dental infections, head trauma, refractive errors, glaucoma, cervical disk disease, depression, and occult hypertension.

A thorough physical examination may lead to discovery of tender areas and trigger points in the head, neck, or shoulders that promote or sustain head pain. Observation of the patient while sitting, walking, and lying down can provide useful clues to musculoskeletal imbalances. Examination of temporomandibular joints is important in all patients because daytime clenching, nocturnal bruxism, and joint disease can all contribute to the pain of TTH.

Patient education in ergonomics, posture, and breathing is often useful in treating TTH. Mind-body approaches can be usefully integrated with conventional therapies. Hypnosis has been shown to reduce the number of headache days and decrease headache intensity among patients with TTH.[111,112] One study of 98 patients with TTH found that when given a choice between medication treatment with amitriptyline or hypnotic relaxation, more participants chose hypnotic relaxation and stayed with their choice when given repeated opportunities to switch to amitriptyline therapy. Seventy-four percent

(74%) of patients in the hypnotic relaxation group and 58% of patients in the medication group had a 50% reduction in the frequency of headaches. TTH patients demonstrated decreased headache frequency after a twice-weekly 6-week mindfulness course.[101]

A combination of sleep hygiene and regularization of daily schedules is effective in reducing pain in motivated and compliant patients. The botanicals for sleep previously described for migraine can be equally effective for those with TTH. Patients should be strongly encouraged to reduce consumption of sugar, caffeine, and red meat along with increasing omega-3 fatty acids to reduce the sympathetic nervous system activity and to enhance the production of antiinflammatory prostaglandins. Detoxification from unneeded drugs is part of effective TTH management. One often overlooked area is dehydration. Poorly hydrated muscles tend to cramp and contract painfully.

Pharmaceuticals have a limited role because of the risk of rebound headache and the tendency to reduce motivation to attend to needed lifestyle adjustments. NSAIDs should be medium- to long-acting and strictly limited to less than 20 doses per week. Muscle relaxants provide limited short-term benefit and tend to lead to psychological dependence and rebound headache. Triptans are rarely effective in TTH.

When TTH occurs daily or almost daily without evidence of an underlying organic condition, analgesic rebound headache is likely, especially when there is use of more than a total of 20 doses of analgesics (NSAIDs and opiates), decongestants, muscle relaxants, and caffeine per week. Caffeine consumption, when greater than three drinks a day, should be tapered slowly over 2–3 weeks along with short-acting analgesics. Pain is managed with patient education, biofeedback, relaxation, slow-stretch exercises, massage, heat, long-acting NSAIDs, and low-dose tricyclic antidepressants given at night (10–50 mg amitriptyline or equivalent).

Chiropractic

There are few older studies of chiropractic or osteopathic manipulation in TTH. Hoyt et al. reported a 50% reduction in headache severity after a single, 10-minute cervical manipulation session.[113] In another study of patients with posttraumatic headache, a 57% reduction in pain intensity and a 64% reduction in analgesic use over a 2-week period was found after two cervical spine manipulation treatments compared with treatment with ice packs.[114] Another group found no difference between chiropractic manipulation vs daily amitriptyline at the end of a 6-week course of treatment in patients with chronic TTH. However, patients who received chiropractic manipulation had fewer headaches on follow-up 6 weeks after the end of treatment.[115] Finally, an RCT comparing soft tissue therapy plus spinal manipulation vs soft tissue therapy plus placebo laser treatment for episodic TTH did not show a statistical difference in outcomes between the two arms.[116] Credible recent studies are lacking.

Acupuncture

A three-arm, randomized controlled trial involving 270 patients with TTH demonstrated that a course of up to 12 acupuncture treatments over 8 weeks was associated with significantly improved clinical outcomes compared to no acupuncture but not when compared to a sham-acupuncture comparison group.[117]

A systematic review that included a meta-analysis of data from five trials that compared acupuncture with a sham acupuncture control demonstrated small but statistically significant benefits for treatment response and other clinical outcomes. The authors of the systematic review concluded that "acupuncture could be a valuable nonpharmacological tool in patients with frequent episodic or chronic tension-type headaches."[118]

Therapies to Consider—TTH

Therapies that promote awareness of mind-body healing connections have the greatest potential for reducing TTH pain. Although evidence supporting the following approaches is sparse, they have proven to be useful in some patients: mindfulness meditation, naturopathy, Reiki, healing touch, magnet therapy, aromatherapy, prolotherapy, tai chi, yoga, traditional Chinese medicine and ayurvedic medicine.

PREVENTION PRESCRIPTION—TTH

- Notice physiological reactions to stressful situations in the home and workplace, especially muscle contraction in the neck and shoulders, breathing patterns, chest sensations, and gastrointestinal responses such as nausea, pain, and diarrhea.
- Develop a daily relaxation routine that focuses attention on posture and muscles of the head and neck.
- Maintain adequate sleep, regular aerobic exercise, and adequate hydration.

- Modify the diet to ensure regular consumption or supplementation of omega-3 fatty acids.
- Be alert to conditions that may contribute to or intensify muscular head pain, such as sinus or dental infection, jaw clenching, tooth grinding, head thrusting, anxiety, and depression.
- Be checked for hypertension at least twice a year.
- Consult a physician if symptoms of weakness, loss of sensation, poor coordination, difficulty with speech, fever, or syncope occur with TTH.

THERAPEUTIC REVIEW—TTH

TENSION-TYPE HEADACHE
- Emphasis is placed on lifestyle and mind-body techniques and reduced reliance on medication.

Lifestyle
- Stress management, sleep hygiene, nutritional choices, ergonomic awareness, regular aerobic exercise

Nutrition
- Increase omega-3 fatty acid per diet or supplements. Reduce sugar, caffeine, red meats, tobacco, alcohol

Sleep and Exercise
- Sleep hygiene
- Aerobic exercise, 30 minutes, three times per week

Supplements and Herbals
- Melatonin, 6–10 mg qhs

- Valerian root, 100–300 mg qhs

Pharmaceuticals
- Time-contingent NSAIDs
- Limit total of NSAIDs, decongestants, and caffeine to less than 20 doses per week

Mind-Body
- Biofeedback and relaxation training
- Stress management, cognitive-behavioral therapy, mindfulness meditation

Biomechanical
- Manipulative therapy, massage, craniosacral therapy

Bioenergetic
- Acupuncture, 6–10 weekly sessions with follow-up as needed

Key Web Resources

NIH National Center for Complementary and Integrative Health (NCCIH). Current practice guidelines, ongoing research and research findings relating to pain, including headache. NCCAM home page links to headache management using complementary approaches.	https://nccih.nih.gov/health/pain/headaches.htm
NIH National Institute of Neurologic Disorders and Stroke (NINDS) website for diagnostic criteria, treatment information, and recently funded research in headache and pain.	http://www.ninds.nih.gov/disorders/migraine/migraine.htm
The American Migraine Foundation website. Academic Headache Centers, guidelines, American Migraine Patient Registry, and Migraine Awareness in Schools.	http://www.americanmigrainefoundation.org/about-us/armr/
Mayo Clinic. Comprehensive information website on migraine.	http://www.mayoclinic.org/diseases-conditions/migraine-headache/basics/definition/con-20026358

REFERENCES

References are available online at ExpertConsult.com.

CHAPTER 13

PERIPHERAL NEUROPATHY

Sunil T. Pai, MD

PATHOPHYSIOLOGY

Peripheral neuropathy or peripheral neuritis is a common neurological disorder that results from damage to the peripheral nerves. It may be caused by diseases of the nerves or may be the result of systemic illnesses. It has various causes, including toxic trauma (Table 13.1), certain prescription medications and chemotherapeutic agents (Table 13.2), and mechanical injury that causes compression or entrapment, for example, carpal tunnel syndrome (see Chapter 70). Even simple pressure on superficial nerves, such as that from the prolonged use of crutches or sitting in the same position for too long, can lead to the disorder. Nutritional deficiencies can cause peripheral neuropathy, as seen in vitamin B deficiency (i.e., from alcoholism, pernicious anemia, isoniazid-induced pyridoxine deficiency, or malabsorption syndromes). Other causes include viral and bacterial infections and other infectious diseases (e.g., human immunodeficiency virus [HIV] infection, Lyme disease), autoimmune reactions (e.g., Guillain-Barre syndrome, chronic inflammatory demyelinating polyneuropathy, multifocal motor neuropathy), cancer (e.g., lymphoma, multiple myeloma), collagen-vascular disorders (e.g., systematic lupus erythematosus, rheumatoid arthritis, polyarteritis nodosa, Sjogren syndrome), endocrinopathies (e.g., hypothyroidism, acromegaly), and rare inherited genetic abnormalities (e.g., hereditary sensory neuropathy types I, II, III, and IV; Krabbe disease; Charcot-Marie-Tooth disease). Despite a thorough history and physical examination, the origin remains a mystery in approximately 50% of cases.[1]

One of the most common causes is diabetes. Peripheral neuropathy is estimated to be present in approximately 40%–60% of individuals with diabetes of 25 years or more in duration.[2] Diabetic neuropathy is now thought to be the most common form of peripheral neuropathy in humans,[3] and the incidence significantly increases with age.[4] Although the exact pathophysiology of diabetic neuropathy has not yet been clearly identified, the origin is multifactorial. Persistent hyperglycemia, oxidative stress, and inflammatory, autoimmune, and microvascular mechanisms are important factors.

Persistent hyperglycemia is the most common primary factor responsible for the development of diabetic neuropathy. It is thought to increase oxidative-nitrosative stress. Oxidative-nitrosative stress activates the polyol pathway, which results in the intraneural accumulation of fructose and sorbitol, and thereby damages the nerves.[5] This polyol pathway hyperactivity is pathogenic because it increases the turnover of cofactors, such as NADPH and NAD^+, leading to a reduction of glutathione. It also increases the production of advanced glycation end products (AGEs), activation of diacylglycerol and protein kinase C (PKC) isoforms, and overactivity of the hexosamine pathway.[6,7,8] Depletion of glutathione may be the fundamental cause of oxidative stress and be related to the accumulation of toxic elements.[9]

Oxidative-nitrosative stress not only activates the above but also instigates and amplifies neuroinflammation. This coupling between oxidative-nitrosative stress and inflammation is because of the activation of TNF-alpha, NF-kappaB along with numerous other interleukins, AP-1 an inhibition of Nrf2, peroxynitrite mediate endothelial dysfunction, altered NO levels, and macrophage migration. These all create proinflammatory cytokines, which are responsible for tissue damage, and debilitating and painful neuropathy.[10-14]

Hyperglycemia alone, however, cannot account for the development of nerve damage because diabetic neuropathy also occurs in patients with well-controlled disease, while other patients with poorly controlled disease have no evidence of neuropathy.[2]

Immunological mechanisms also play a role in the development of diabetic neuropathy. This damage is caused by antineural autoantibodies that circulate in the serum of some diabetic patients. Antiphospholipid antibodies may also be present and may contribute to nerve damage in combination with vascular abnormalities.[15]

Finally, endoneural vascular insufficiency, resulting from decreased nitric oxide or impaired endothelial function, impaired sodium/potassium-adenosine triphosphatase (Na^+/K^+-ATPase) activity, and homocysteinemia, has been found to be a primary cause of diabetic neuropathy.[15-18] Investigators have postulated that ischemia related to endoneural and epineural vascular changes causes nerve damage by thickening the blood vessel wall. Eventually, occlusion of the vessel may occur, leading to vascular permeability, compromise of endoneural blood flow (Fig. 13.1), and microvascular impairment.[19,20] Preclinical and clinical studies have shown a reduction of peripheral perfusion not only in the nervous tissue[21,22] but also in the skin,[23,24] indicating microvascular changes.[24,25]

Other multifactorial mechanisms that are implicated in the development of diabetic neuropathy are body habitus, environmental factors (e.g., alcohol, smoking, exposure to heavy metals), and genetic predisposition.

By these mechanisms, the sensory, autonomic, and motor nerves may all be affected, beginning with the distal lower extremities and spreading to involve the upper extremities as the diabetes progresses.[3] Diabetic neuropathy usually manifests in a "stocking-and-glove" distribution, with sensory loss, dysesthesias, and painful paresthesias, most commonly in the lower extremities. Common symptoms include the following: tingling, prickling, or numbness;

TABLE 13.1 Agents Causing Symptoms Associated With Toxic Neuropathy

Acrylamide (truncal ataxia)	Lead (wrist drop, abdominal colic)
Alcohol	Lucel-7 (cataracts)
Allyl chloride	Mercury
Arsenic	Methylbromide
Buckthorn toxin	Mold (in water-damaged buildings)
Carbon disulfide	Nitrous oxide inhalation
Cyanide	Organophosphorus esters (triorthocresyl phosphate, leptophos, mipafox, trichlorphon) (cholinergic symptoms, neuropathy of delayed onset)
Dichlorophenoxyacetic acid	
Dimethylaminopropionitrile (urinary complaints)	Polychlorinated biphenyls
Biologic toxin in diphtheritic neuropathy (pharyngeal neuropathy)	Tetrachlorbiphenyl
	Thallium (pain, alopecia, Mees lines)
Ethylene oxide	Trichloroethylene (trigeminal neuralgia)
Germanium	Vacor
Hexacarbon (n-hexane) (glue-sniffing; occupational exposure to solvents, glue, or glue thinner)	

Modified from Wyngaarden JB, Smith LH Jr, Bennett JC, eds. *Cecil textbook of medicine.* 19th ed. Philadelphia: Saunders; 1992:2246.

TABLE 13.2 Pharmaceutical Agents Associated With Generalized Neuropathy

5-Azacytidine	Ifosfamide
5-Fluorouracil	Isoniazid[†]
Amiodarone	Metronidazole, misonidazole
Antiretrovirals	Nitrofurantoin*
Aurothioglucose	Penicillamine
Chloramphenicol	Perhexiline
Clioquinol	Phenytoin
Cytarabine	Pyridoxine[†] (in excessive amounts)
Dapsone*	Platinum[†] (cisplatin, oxaliplatin)
Disulfiram	Sodium cyanate
Ethambutol	Statins
Ethionamide	Stilbamidine
Etoposide	Suramin
Gemcitabine	Taxoids (paclitaxel, docetaxel)
Gold	Thalidomide[†]
Glutethimide	Vinblastine
Hexamethylmelamine	Vincristine
Hydralazine	VM-26

*Predominantly motor (neuropathy).
[†]Predominantly sensory (neuropathy).
Modified from Wyngaarden JB, Smith LH Jr, Bennett JC, eds. *Cecil textbook of medicine.* 19th ed. Philadelphia: Saunders; 1992:2247.

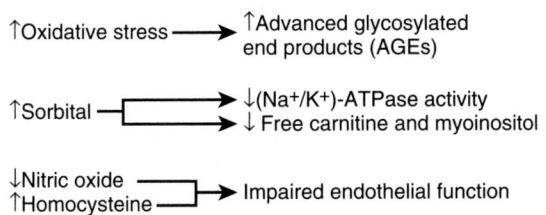

FIG. 13.1 ■ Pathophysiological factors in diabetic neuropathy. ATPase, adenosine triphosphatase; K⁺, potassium; Na⁺, sodium. (From Head K. Peripheral neuropathy: pathological mechanisms and alternative therapies. *Altern Med Rev.* 2006;11:295.)

burning or freezing pain; sharp, stabbing, or electric pain; extreme sensitivity to touch; muscle weakness; and loss of balance and coordination. However, pain intensity is not always associated with the severity of the neuropathy and can occur even without nerve injury.[26,27]

INTEGRATIVE THERAPY

Because diabetic neuropathy is the most common peripheral neuropathy that is encountered in clinical practice, and its symptoms consist primarily of pain, the management of neuropathy involves not only prevention and control of the underlying disease, for example, diabetes, but also alleviation of the resultant painful symptoms. In addition, because the worldwide rise in cancer over the next 20 years has been projected to be 57%,[29] there will be an increase in chemotherapy-induced neuropathy, which is a side effect of such treatments. Although the neuropathological mechanisms are in the end similar, studies are underway on the utilization of natural and adjunctive therapies to lower the incidence and side effects from chemotherapy.

Lifestyle

Nutrition

Good diabetic control can be one of the best preventive measures for peripheral neuropathy. The benefits of near normoglycemia on nerve function in the Diabetes Control and Complications Trial adequately demonstrated that strict glycemic control may reduce the incidence of diabetic neuropathy by up to 64%.[30]

In addition, multiple studies have shown that following a whole-foods, low-fat, high-fiber, plant-based diet combined with exercise can decrease type 1 diabetic medications by up to 40%[31] or eliminate them completely in type 2 diabetes.[32-35] Furthermore, there is growing evidence that oxidative stress due to the previously described mechanisms creates deficits in antioxidant defense, which play a major role in diabetic neuropathy,[6,36] and, therefore, a plant-based diet, which is rich in antioxidants, phytonutrients, and fiber, is vitally important. Plant-based diets are associated with improved glycemic control, lower lipid levels and oxidative stress, and improvement in other physiological and cognitive health factors in type 2 diabetics, and produce better glycemic control compared to a standard ADA diet.[37-41] Maintaining diabetic control and avoiding environmental toxins, such as heavy metals, cigarettes, alcohol, and pollution, are of the utmost importance.

Exercise

Regular exercise, that is, walking for a minimum of 30 minutes three times a week, should be implemented. An optimal regimen consists of daily walks for 30 minutes to 1 hour as tolerated (see Chapter 91).

Although there is inadequate evidence to evaluate the effect of exercise on functional ability in patients with peripheral neuropathy,[42] some evidence indicates that strengthening exercises improve muscle strength in peripheral neuropathy. Most of the studies involved conventional exercises such as cycling, running, and walking. However, patients may be fearful that exercise may exacerbate their symptoms, as well as increase the possibility of injury.[42] Physical limitations of their current state of health can lead to decreased compliance, and, therefore, proper guidance and support must be given.

Movement Therapies: Tai Chi, Yoga

Studies have shown that as little as 6 weeks to 6 months of performing tai chi can improve motor performance (e.g.,

6-minute walk, leg strength, timed up-and-go), enhance balance (the greatest improvements are seen in patients with large sensory losses), improve plantar sensation, decrease glycated hemoglobin (HbA1c), and improve peripheral nerve conduction velocities.[62-66] Tai chi can be used as a safe and effective intervention for patients with peripheral neuropathy.

Movement therapies, such as yoga and tai chi, are usually gentler and less strenuous and, as such, may lead to better compliance. With proper instruction and supervision, these techniques may be valuable lifestyle behaviors to help patients who may not be able to exercise using conventional modalities.

Mind-Body Therapy

Biofeedback

Biofeedback may be used to reduce stress and improve coping skills, which may aid in improving compliance, thereby promoting better glycemic control and reducing the pain associated with diabetic neuropathy.[23,67] Biofeedback has been shown to reduce HbA1c directly and to increase blood flow in the extremities, which, in turn, decreases neuropathic pain, reduces stress levels, improves psychological health, and enhances quality of life.[68-72] The patient should be referred to a behavioral therapist or a psychologist who teaches biofeedback techniques. The recommendation is a minimum of six 1-hour biofeedback sessions at approximately 1-week intervals. Usually, the treatments include sessions of guided imagery or relaxation techniques (see Chapters 94 and 97). During these sessions, the patient wears a biofeedback device that indicates physiological responses, such as electromyographic or electrodermal responses, and a vital sign monitor typically for blood pressure, pulse, or oxygen saturation. The monitoring enables patients to conceptualize how emotion, anxiety, stress, and pain can affect their physiological status.

Once patients gain the ability to alter their physiological state, they are taught to perform the relaxation biofeedback techniques at home, at work, or on the go with the use of biofeedback home-use computer, tablet, or smartphone programs[72] (e.g., emWave Pro, emWave,[2] Innerbalance [HeartMath Institute, Boulder Creek, CA]), audio CDs, DVDs, or guided imagery exercises 10–20 minutes each day, in order to attain the same result without the monitoring equipment (see Chapter 96). Therefore biofeedback is a tool that the patient can use to control certain physiological parameters during times of stress or pain in order to help alleviate symptoms.

Bioelectromagnetics

Physical Vascular Therapy. Pulsed electromagnetic frequency (PEMF) devices have rapidly emerged worldwide as a technology used by both physicians and patients. Physical vascular therapy is the new classification of a patented waveform of the next generation of pulsed electromagnetic therapy (PEMF) devices from a company called BEMER, which holds the patent on this technology and has supported most of the research. With all research, the reader should use caution when the majority of the data come from the makers of a device, drug, or supplement. Although PEMF devices are very popular for commercial use, there are few published studies apart from those on BEMER's patented device, which has been used for over 15 years in Europe. When physical vascular technology is applied via a mat, improvements in microcirculatory characteristics, such as capillary perfusion, venular outflow, or oxygen utilization, can occur.[82]

Increase in microcirculation can improve the transport of cellular and humoral factors of the immune system, leading to decreased pain and increased healing responses. Various case-controlled, pilot, and placebo-controlled studies have shown that the benefits of improving microcirculation include improved blood glucose response and utilization in organ tissue, improved immune response, increased physical rehabilitation response, improved wound healing, decreased pain and neuropathy, and increased pain-free walking due to peripheral arterial disease.

Increasing microcirculation may improve penetration and increase the efficacy of the medications used to treat peripheral neuropathy.[83-90]

In one study of 165 patients with difficult peripheral neuropathic pain that was not controlled adequately with medications, daily use of the device for 2–5 weeks for 25 to 30 minutes was associated with a 61% decrease in pain on a visual analogue scale (VAS). In addition, there was improvement in motor performance (25%), elimination of somatic complaints (5%), elimination of psychological complaints and associated depression (32%), and a significant improvement in the quality of life (75%).[91] Another randomized placebo-controlled study using BEMER vascular technology demonstrated clinically significant improvements in diabetic polyneuropathy and tropic skin lesions of approximately 3 cm^2 in area. Patients were treated with the BEMER vascular therapy mat for 10 minutes twice daily at level 3 (10.5 = microtesla) for 30 days.[92] Furthermore, it has been shown to significantly improve sleep and quality of life and lower pain and fatigue.[93-95] BEMER has been shown to have positive effects on neuropathic pain and diabetic complications and can be used safely as an adjunctive therapy.

Bioenergetics

Acupuncture. Acupuncture and electroacupuncture have been found to be useful for neuropathic pain. Because beta endorphins are involved in the pathogenesis of both painful and painless neuropathy,[98] acupuncture may exert its well-known effect by stimulating the production of endorphins in the central nervous system.[99] Although acupuncture cannot easily be explained by known neurophysiological mechanisms, several studies have examined the effects of acupuncture in the treatment of various types of peripheral neuropathy, including diabetic, HIV-associated, chemotherapy-induced, and neuropathy of mixed origin.[100-106] In randomized controlled studies, case series, and sham studies, acupuncture was shown to improve nerve conduction velocity, decrease numbness and pain (66%–87%), and improve symptoms more effectively than conventional medical treatment in peripheral neuropathy induced by chemotherapeutic drugs (66% vs. 40%), especially in moderate and severe sensory nerve disorders.[107-113] In some cases (67%), patients were able to reduce or stop their pain medications.[114]

Neuroacupuncture has a positive effect on neuropathic pain and often results in the ability to reduce or stop pain medications.

Patients can receive six courses of classical acupuncture analgesia[115,116] to both lower limbs over a 10-week period. In addition to classical acupuncture, a small, clinical, pilot study of biweekly electroacupuncture treatments for 4 weeks demonstrated a reduction in continuous pain from 32.9% to 15.9% and a decrease in the intensity of pain attacks from 59% to 44%.[117] Electroacupuncture may have a positive influence on nerve conduction velocity and may also relieve neuropathic pain.[115] Electroacupuncture is performed in two cycles of five sittings each (10 sessions) at 2-day intervals. Most clinical studies provided one to two treatments per week for 10–20 weeks.

There is clinical evidence that an acupuncture subspecialty called neuroacupuncture (Chinese scalp acupuncture) has remarkable effects on central nervous systems disorders.[118] A more comprehensive mixture of body acupuncture and neuroacupuncture (with or without electrical stimulation) can improve clinical outcomes by using the following protocol. In my clinical experience, this works very well. Neuroacupuncture points are the upper one-fifth sensory area (S 1/5) for the lower limbs, middle two-fifths sensory area (S 2/5) for the upper limbs, and foot motor and sensory areas; ear points: ShenMen, sympathetic, foot; body points: GB-40, GB-34, SP-10, SP-6, ST-44, LR-3, and Bafeng (extra point). Electrical stimulation can be used for the ear and body points at a frequency of 100 Hz at low intensity for 10–15 minutes in order to achieve an enhanced response.[119]

Before such therapies can be recommended, a constitutional evaluation by a practitioner who is trained in acupuncture, or more specifically neuroacupuncture, should be considered because each modality is prescribed on the basis of the unique symptoms and physical characteristics of the patient. A comprehensive review of medical acupuncture and scalp acupuncture for physicians may be found in the various texts by Dr. Joseph Helms[120] and Dr. Jason Hao.[119]

Botanical Medicine

Diabetes, diabetic neuropathy, and its complications all have inflammatory triggers and components, as previously described. Many herbs are used for diabetes (see Chapter 33); however, a few Ayurvedic herbs, such as curcumin,[121-139,141-150] boswellia,[151-169] ginger,[170-189] and black pepper,[190-200] are used to treat the pain of diabetic neuropathy and the other complications and comorbidities associated with diabetes.

Curcumin

Curcumin is the active ingredient found in turmeric at a concentration between 3% and 5%. It is widely used as a spice and food colorant throughout India. For more than 4000 years, curcumin has been used in traditional Ayurvedic medicine to treat a wide variety of ailments. It is one of the most researched natural medicines to date, with more than 7000 published studies.

THE RELEVANT MOLECULAR TARGETS

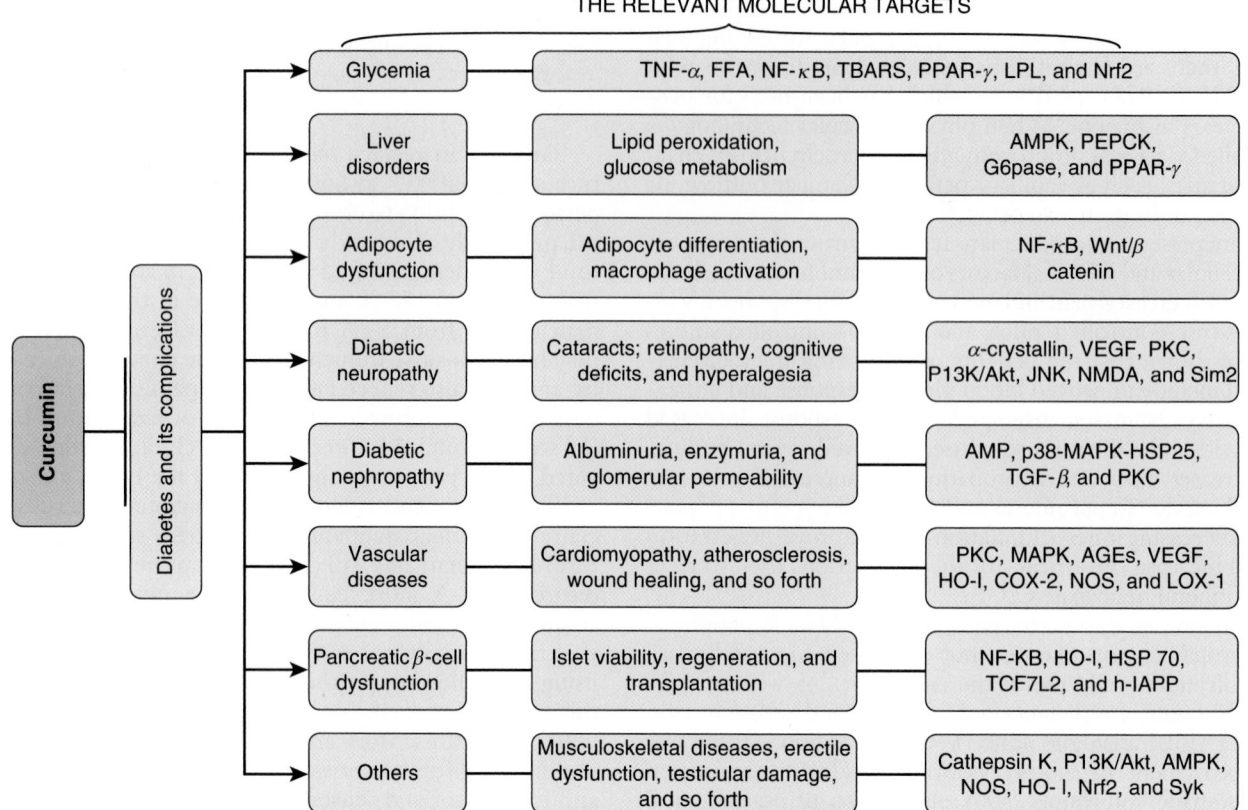

FIG. 13.2 ■ The relevant molecular targets of diabetes and the complications that are modulated by curcumin.

Curcumin has been shown to be beneficial in treating many different inflammatory diseases, including diabetes and its complications, for example, diabetic neuropathy[201] (Fig. 13.2). It reduces inflammation through more than[161] one biological mechanism, including nuclear factor-kappaB (NF-kB), C-reactive protein, cyclooxygenase-2 (COX-2), 5-lipoxygenase (5-LOX), interleukin (IL)-1beta, IL-6, IL-10, IL-12, tumor necrosis factor-alpha (TNF-alpha), interferon-gamma, activator protein-1, macrophage inflammatory protein (MIP), matrix metalloproteinase (MMPs), human leukocyte elastase (HLE), several types of protein kinases, adhesion molecules, and genes involved in inflammation.[137-139,141,142,148] In addition, curcumin has been shown to improve endothelial function,[143,144] reduce vascular inflammation,[145,146] down-regulate adipokines, including resistin, leptin, and monocyte chemotactic protein-1, and minimize osmotic stress by regulating the polyol pathway.[137,202]

Furthermore, it downregulates the p300/CBP HAT activity-mediated gene expression of BDNF and COX-2 in neuropathic pain.[203]

Curcumin also demonstrates antinociceptive activity by attenuating diabetic and chemotherapy-induced neuropathic pain,[147,204-206] and has been shown to provide other benefits for diabetic complications in *in vitro*, animal, and human studies.[139,207] In addition, curcumin not only helps with pain but has also been shown to have neuroprotective benefits through the following actions:

• Suppression of β-amyloid oligomer-induced phosphorylation of tau and degradation of insulin receptor substrate via c-Jun N-terminal kinase (JNK) signaling. This is beneficial in improving cognitive deficits and insulin signaling in Alzheimer's disease.[208,205]

• Effects on malondialdehyde and glutathione, oxidative stress index, total antioxidant state, and nitric oxide levels in the brain and sciatic tissue.[209-211] This is mediated through regulation of TNF-alpha and TNF-alpha receptors.[148,212-214] Curcumin is an effective oral TNF-alpha and NF-kB blocker along with other pro-inflammatory markers in diabetes.[212,213]

• Finally, curcumin may act upon the opioid system for alleviation of diabetic peripheral neuropathic pain.[214]

Therefore, curcumin can be used as a safe analgesic for neuropathic pain while assisting in reversal of insulin resistance, hyperglycemia, hyperlipidemia, obesity, and neurodegenerative disorders, which are common in diabetic patients as well as in the general population.[137,215]

DOSAGE

Curcumin 500 mg four times daily or 1000 mg twice daily is commonly used. Absorption can be enhanced by combining curcumin with black pepper. Many combination products are available, such as Bosmeric-SR [a sustained-release formulation that combines patented Curcumin C3 Complex, Boswellin PS, and gingerols (20%) along with Bioperine (black pepper) to enhance absorption], two caplets orally twice daily.

PRECAUTIONS

Although curcumin is nontoxic to human subjects at high doses,[138] many curcumin supplements may contain contaminants, such as lead, and are not standardized to the curcuminoids that provide health benefits. Curcumin C3 complex is a patented form of curcumin that is standardized to 95% curcuminoids, including curcumin (70%–80%), bidemethoxycurcumin (2.5%–6.5%), and demethoxycurcumin (15%–25%). Curcumin C3 complex has the most research in human studies at major hospitals and universities and thus is a safe and effective form to be recommended.

Cannabinoids

Through the growing changes in the legalization of cannabis and the use of medical cannabis for chronic pain syndromes, one must start to look at the importance of cannabinoid medicine as part of an integrative medicine approach. Two primary types of cannabinoid receptors (CB1 and CB2) exist on cells throughout the body. These receptors are most abundant in the brain (CNS) and peripheral tissues, respectively. Medial cannabis contains both THC (delta-9 tetrahydrocannabinol), the part that is psychogenic, and CBD (cannabidiols), the part that is not. Both have numerous health benefits in diabetes and its complications.[216]

Cannabinoids represent a new class of therapeutic agents for the treatment of chronic pain and other diseases that involve glycine receptor dysfunction.[217] In addition to alleviating pain, studies on the benefits of cannabinoids have included improvement of quality of life and sleep.[218]

Randomized placebo-controlled trials (RCTs) involving cannabis and cannabinoids have been used in different populations of chronic neuropathic pain patients to provide effective analgesia in conditions that are refractory to other treatments.[219]

Although currently not available in the US (due to its THC content), a prescription medication called *Sativex*, which contains THC:CBD in an approximate 1:1 ratio, has been investigated. Multicenter, randomized controlled trials, along with double-blind, randomized, placebo-controlled trials, used the THC:CBD oral spray and demonstrated a significant reduction in pain by 30%.[220-222] Current applications are pending with the FDA for the indication for treatment of peripheral neuropathy with this oral spray. However, with this combination THC:CBD formulation, tolerability of increasing doses of THC in lieu of adequate analgesia was the most common side effect and depression was also a confounding factor.[220-226]

Newer sources of CBD, which are derived from industrial hemp, containing CBD and traces of THC, are currently available. Therefore, without the psychogenic component and without accessibility being an issue, as it is currently legal and available in all 50 states, these are a great alternative option for patients regardless of the federal and state restrictions that may be in place for medical cannabis.[227] With this opportunity available, CBD has now been studied on its own.

Cannabidiol (CBD) decreases inflammation and neuropathic pain in preclinical models of diabetes. CBD exposure enhances the ability of arteries to relax via enhanced production of vasodilatory COX-1/2-derived products acting at EP4 receptors.[228] CBD decreases the autoimmune inflammatory phenotype,[229] is an inhibitor of NF-kappaB and

interferon-beta/STAT pro-inflammatory pathways,[230] and exhibits analgesic [231,232] and antiinflammatory actions[233,234] in chronic diseases and cancer. CBD also has been shown to lower inflammation in oxidative stress,[238] and may be used to modify the development of the neuropathic pain state by restricting the elevation of microglial density and phosphorylated p38 MAPK.[239] Furthermore, CBD has been shown to inhibit paclitaxel-induced neuropathic pain without diminishing nervous system function or chemotherapy efficacy.[240]

A patient's perception of cannabis and CBD extracts depends greatly on their age, their socioeconomic and cultural beliefs, the location and atmosphere of the dispensary, and federal and state restrictions. Many of my patients are simply afraid to try medical cannabis for one or a combination of these reasons, and, therefore, I preferentially use CBD products to provide health benefits without the other issues related to medical cannabis.

CBD is nontoxic in nontransformed cells, does not induce changes in food intake, does not induce catalepsy, does not affect physiological parameters (heart rate, blood pressure, and body temperature), does not affect gastrointestinal transit, and does not alter psychomotor or psychological functions. No toxicity or side effects have been demonstrated in subjects taking up to 600 mg in a single dose for chronic use. Even higher doses of up to 1500 mg/day of CBD have been shown to be well-tolerated in humans.[227,241-243]

DOSAGE

CBD from industrial hemp oil (high CBD, trace THC). Legal in US without need for a medical card; 5–15 mg bid to tid, with coconut oil (to improve absorption) and stevia (optional for improved taste), held sublingually for 2–3 minutes then swallowed. Doses may be increased weekly for improved response.

CBD:THC from medical cannabis. Ratios of CBD:THC vary according to the strains and dispensary. High CBD low THC is preferred (e.g., 20:1), or similar to the prescribed drug worldwide ratio of 1:1. Administration the same as previously but start with lower doses. 1–2 mg bid to tid to start and increase dose as tolerated. Check state regulations on the legality to prescribe for peripheral neuropathy or chronic pain conditions.

PRECAUTIONS

CBD and medical cannabis products should be validated by third party laboratories and checked for microbial content, pesticides, herbicides, solvents, and percentage amounts of CBD and THC per unit batch or amount acquired. Avoid cannabinoid use in pregnancy and breast-feeding.

CBD may also potentiate many prescription pain medications, NSAIDs, anticonvulsants, and antidepressants and, therefore, reduction of those medications should be monitored as necessary. Acute glucocorticoid use may be potentiated by CBD, and chronic CBD use may downregulate the glucocorticoid response.[244]

Geranium Oil (Pelargonium spp.)

A patented formulation of geranium oil, Neuragen PN, has been clinically studied. It contains a proprietary blend of five essential oils and six homeopathic ingredients. A multicenter, double-blind, crossover trial and a randomized, double-blind, placebo-controlled clinical trial showed a significant reduction in neuropathic pain in 93% of patients within 30 minutes of the application of Neuragen PN. In addition to the immediate reduction of neuropathic pain, 70%–80% had lasting relief up to 8 hours.[245,246] Geranium oil provides significant pain relief in as little as 5 minutes and lasts up to 8 hours. Therefore, geranium oil can be used as monotherapy or used in conjunction with other treatments for diabetic neuropathy for breakthrough pain or immediate pain relief.

DOSAGE

Neuragen PN is highly concentrated, and, therefore, one only needs to apply one to two drops to the affected area, rub in, and allow to absorb. It can be applied several times a day but no more than five times daily. For efficient application to wider areas, or for extremely sensitive skin, it is recommended to dilute four or five drops in 1 tablespoon of carrier oil, such as grapeseed oil or jojoba oil, before application. Neuragen PN is now also available in a gel for easy application. Pain relief may be immediate, but it is usually noticed within 30 minutes. If pain relief is not experienced with the first application, repeat the application over a period of 3 days.

PRECAUTIONS

As with any essential oil, only a few drops are needed because it can irritate the skin. For patients with sensitive skin, it is best mixed with carrier oil first before direct application is attempted. Wash hands after use, and avoid contact with eyes and open sores. Discontinue if rash occurs.

Evening Primrose Oil

Evening primrose oil (EPO) is extracted from the seeds of Oenothera biennis. EPO is a rich source of omega-6 essential fatty acids, primarily gamma-linolenic acid (GLA) and linoleic acid, which are both essential components of myelin and the neuronal cell membrane.[247] GLA has demonstrated positive results in the treatment of experimental diabetes and may be more beneficial than docosahexaenoic acid (DHA) in preventing diabetic neuropathy.[248-250] GLA is converted to prostaglandin E1 (PGE1) preferentially over PGE2. PGE1 has antiinflammatory, antiplatelet, and vasodilating properties. In patients with diabetes, however, levels of PGE1 are decreased, and levels of PGE2 and thromboxane are increased,[251] and therefore, inflammation, vasoconstriction, and platelet aggregation tend to be promoted.[253] Supplementing the diet with GLA has been shown to augment the production of PGE1 (by bypassing the blocked enzymatic step delta-6-desaturase) that is seen in patients with hyperglycemia.[254-256]

Two of three randomized controlled trials showed positive effects of GLA in diabetic neuropathy.[247] Two trials with GLA at 360 mg/day for 6 months and 480 mg/day for 1 year demonstrated statistically significant improvements in neuropathy scores, nerve conduction velocities, and action potentials. Therefore, EPO may be helpful for mild to moderate diabetic peripheral neuropathy.

DOSAGE

The dose is 360 mg/day of GLA from EPO (the most researched source of GLA, as opposed to borage oil or black currant oil), and it may be increased up to 480 mg/day. Obtain high-quality oil (preferably certified organic), packaged in light-resistant containers, refrigerated, and marked with a freshness date to avoid rancidity.

PRECAUTION

EPO may increase the effectiveness of ceftazidime, chemotherapy agents, and cyclosporine, and may interact with phenothiazines and cause an increase in seizures. Patients taking antiplatelet agents or anticoagulants should use EPO cautiously or not at all. Theoretically, the use of nonsteroidal antiinflammatory drugs (NSAIDs) may counteract the effect of EPO.

Supplements

Many supplements have been shown to be helpful for the symptoms of diabetes (see Chapter 33) and, in particular, peripheral neuropathy. The supplements with the best results for peripheral neuropathy are discussed here.

Acetyl-L-Carnitine

Acetyl-L-carnitine (ALC) is an acetylated form of L-carnitine, which is an amino acid that is responsible for the transport of fatty acids into a cell's mitochondria. ALC is far superior to normal L-carnitine in terms of bioavailability in that it is absorbed by the gastrointestinal tract, enters cells, and crosses the blood–brain barrier more readily than does unacetylated carnitine.

Peripheral neuropathy is a common side effect of chemotherapeutic drugs, which belong to the platinum, taxane, vinca alkaloid, and proteasome inhibitor families. Animal studies have shown the benefits of ALC as a specific protective agent when it is given concomitantly and after treatment for chemotherapy-induced neuropathy due to cisplatin, oxaliplatin, paclitaxel, and vincristine, without any interference with the antitumor activity of the drugs.[257-259] ALC has been shown to reduce pain significantly in diabetic neuropathy.[260-262] Furthermore, studies in humans showed that ALC, given as a 1-g/day infusion over 1–2 hours for at least 10 days, improved chemotherapy-induced peripheral neuropathy in up to 73% of patients.[263] Patients with chemotherapy-induced peripheral neuropathy who were treated with oral ALC (1 g three times a day) for 8 weeks showed sensory improvement (60%) and motor improvement (79%), and their total neuropathy scores, including neurophysiological measures, improved (92%), with symptomatic improvement persisting for a median of 13 months after ALC treatment.[264] In addition to chemotherapy-induced peripheral neuropathy, multiple long-term (1-year) randomized, double-blind, placebo-controlled studies showed that ALC improves pain, nerve regeneration, and vibratory perception in patients with chronic diabetic neuropathy.[265,266] ALC appeared to work more effectively in patients with type 2 diabetes, with a shorter duration of neuropathy than in patients with type 1 diabetes.[252]

DOSAGE

The recommended dose is 500 mg orally twice a day to 1000 mg orally three times a day. Better pain control is seen at the higher dose regimen.

PRECAUTIONS

ALC may cause nausea, vomiting, diarrhea, headache, bladder irritation or infection, unusual body odor, stuffy nose, and rash. Other side effects associated with ALC include restlessness and difficulty sleeping.

Alpha-Lipoic Acid (ALA)

Alpha-lipoic acid (ALA), also known as thiotic acid, is approved for clinical use in the management of diabetic neuropathy in Germany, and has been extensively used there in medical practice since 1959.[266] ALA is a universal antioxidant, exerting direct (scavenges free radicals) and indirect (participates in the process of recycling other natural antioxidants, thereby increasing glutathione, vitamins C and E, and coenzyme Q10) antioxidant activity.[267-270] ALA chelates transition metal ions (e.g., iron and copper) and effectively mitigates toxicities associated with heavy metal poisoning.[271] Investigators have established that ALA protects against lipid peroxidation and increases the activity of antioxidant enzymes (e.g., catalase and superoxide dismutase) in peripheral nerves. By decreasing oxidative stress through the inhibition of hexosamine and AGE pathways, ALA normalizes impaired endoneural blood flow and impaired nerve conduction velocity.[272,273]

Several studies have established the neurogenerative and neuroprotective effects of ALA. The efficacy and safety of ALA in peripheral and autonomic diabetic neuropathy have been demonstrated in many randomized, double-blind, placebo-controlled trials.[274-288] A meta-analysis provided evidence that treatment with ALA significantly improves both positive neuropathic symptoms and neuropathic deficits to a clinically meaningful degree in diabetic patients with symptomatic polyneuropathy.[289] Further studies have shown that the oral forms of ALA are effective for peripheral neuropathy.[290] ALA has been shown to be effective for diabetic mononeuropathy of the cranial nerves with full recovery of all of the patients in the study.[291] The studies ranged from a minimum treatment of 3 weeks to 2 years, and, therefore, 3 weeks is likely to be the minimum treatment time. Although greater improvements were seen with higher doses, so were adverse effects such as gastrointestinal upset and headaches.[289]

Most studies on ALA used parenteral doses ranging from 600 to 1800 mg, which demonstrated more rapid response than oral doses at the same dose range, and found a continuous daily improvement in symptom scores beginning on the eighth day of treatment.[289] Unfortunately, the parenteral form of ALA is not currently available as a prescribed therapy in the United States, and only the oral form is available in various doses. In most studies, 600 mg seems to be the starting dose. To obtain similar results, patients should use high-quality products from manufacturers that source ALA from Europe (Germany or Italy).

DOSAGE

ALA is given orally at 600–1800 mg daily. Start with 600 mg daily, and increase up to 1800 mg daily in divided doses if needed.

PRECAUTIONS

Although no evidence has indicated that ALA affects glycemic control, case studies have shown improved glucose handling in diabetic patients.[271] As a precaution, patients who are predisposed to hypoglycemia, including those receiving hypoglycemic agents, should have blood glucose levels monitored closely. In addition, because ALA acts as a chelator, monitor for possible mineral deficiencies. Gastrointestinal upset may occur at higher doses. Rarely, this supplement may cause rash.

B Vitamins

Benfotiamine: Vitamin B1. Benfotiamine, also known as S-benzoylthiamine-O-monophosphate, is a lipid-soluble derivative of vitamin B1 (thiamine) and is absorbed up to 3.6 times more than water-soluble forms. Vitamin B1 is associated with a 120-fold greater increase in the levels of metabolically active thiamine diphosphate. Its lipid solubility allows it to penetrate the nerves more readily. It has been found to provide a higher bioavailability of thiamine than its water-soluble counterparts.[292-294] Benfotiamine reduces advanced glycation end-products (AGE) by 40%, which has been shown to prevent macro- and microvascular endothelial dysfunction in individuals with type 2 diabetes.[295-300]

Studies have shown that benfotiamine improves neuropathy scores significantly,[301,302] increases nerve conduction velocity,[303-305] and reduces HbA1c and pain.[306] On the Russian market, it is one of the most studied drugs for neuropathic pain.[306] In addition, it lowers inflammation and may be useful for ameliorating the analgesic effect of mu-opioid agonists on neuropathic pain.[307-309] In a randomized, placebo-controlled, double-blind pilot study and phase III clinical study, investigators demonstrated a pronounced effect on the decrease in pain[310,311] in conjunction with the previously described benefits. Benfotiamine may also be beneficial in preventing diabetic nephropathy[312] and retinopathy.[313] Therapeutic benefits can be seen as early as 3 weeks, with the most significant improvements occurring in patients taking the highest-dose of benfotiamine, that is, 600 mg/day at 6 weeks.[310,311,314]

DOSAGE

The recommended dose of benfotiamine is 150–300 mg twice daily specifically for diabetic peripheral neuropathy.

Methylcobalamin: Vitamin B12. Methylcobalamin is the active form of vitamin B12. In a small double-blind, placebo-controlled trial of type 1 and 2 diabetes with neuropathy, the patients given oral methylcobalamin at a dose of 500 mcg three times daily showed significant improvements in somatic and autonomic symptoms compared to placebo.[316] A review of several clinical trials on the use of methylcobalamin alone or in combination with other B vitamins found overall symptomatic relief of neuropathy symptoms that was more pronounced than electrophysiological findings.[317] In addition, supplementation of 1500 mcg/day methylcobalamin for 2 months resulted in improved vibratory perception thresholds and heart rate variability (a sign of improvement in autonomic neuropathy) in patients with diabetes.[318]

DOSAGE

For the best bioavailability and absorption, the recommended dose is 500 mcg three times daily or 1500 mcg daily of methylcobalamin or 5-adenosylcobalamin. Most generic vitamins contain cyanocobalamin, which may not be as effective or as beneficial.

B-Complex Multivitamin. Vitamins B1 (thiamine), B6 (pyridoxine), and B12 (cobalamin) play an important role in the pathogenesis of peripheral neuropathy in deficiency syndromes, such as those resulting from alcoholism or pernicious anemia, isoniazid-induced pyridoxine deficiency, and malabsorption syndromes. If peripheral neuropathy is caused by deficiency syndromes, use B-100 complex (a multivitamin that usually contains 25–100 mg of thiamine, riboflavin, niacin, pyridoxine, and pantothenic acid and may also include other vitamins such as folate) for ease of administration and intake of all B vitamins.

DOSAGE

B-complex multivitamin (B-100), one tablet once or twice daily, is taken for peripheral neuropathy caused by deficiency syndromes. The B vitamins methylcobalamin and 5-adenosylcobalamin (vitamin B12), and the 5-methyltetrahydrofolate (5-MTF) form of folate should be used in these formulations.

PRECAUTIONS

Avoid excessive doses of vitamin B6 (pyridoxine). Doses higher than 250 mg/day can cause reversible nerve damage.

In prescribing B-complex vitamins, make sure that the patient is not already taking another vitamin supplement that may contain B vitamins. Vitamin B3 (niacin) in doses greater than 300 mg/day may cause headache, nausea, skin tingling, and flushing. Vitamin B6 in doses greater than 250 mg/day may cause reversible nerve damage.

Fish Oil: Omega-3 Fatty Acids

Similar to EPO (GLA), omega-3 fatty acids are also essential for healthy nerve cell membranes and blood flow.[319] Omega-3 fatty acids have been found to have neuroprotective effects against experimental diabetic neuropathy, reduce neuropathic pain, proinflammatory cytokine production, and other metabolites and benefit macrovascular and microvascular functioning in diabetics.[320-325] In a case series, omega-3 fatty acids were shown to decrease pain and improve function, and, in a randomized, double-blind, placebo-controlled trial, were found to be protective against paclitaxel-induced peripheral neuropathy.[326,327] Furthermore, a clinical study of diabetic patients with neuropathy who consumed 1800 mg eicosapentaenoic acid (EPA) daily for 48 weeks reported significantly decreased cold and numb sensations and improved vibrational perception, in addition to improved vibratory threshold. Circulation, measured in the dorsalis pedis artery, and lipid profiles also significantly improved.[328]

DOSAGE

Doses are EPA, 1000–2000 mg/day, and DHA, 500–1000 mg/day. The natural triglyceride form provides superior absorption and bioavailability, up to 70% more than preparations with ethyl ester forms.[329] For patients who are vegan or allergic to fish, a plant-based form of EPA and DHA called NutraVege is available. It contains Echium plantagineum oil (stearidonic acid, a precursor of EPA), and algal DHA and GLA. High-potency fish or plant oils should be used to obtain the clinical dose.

PRECAUTIONS

Possible blood thinning effects may occur with higher doses. Patients taking anticoagulant medications should be closely monitored.

Pharmaceuticals

Capsaicin

Capsaicin, which is an extract of chili peppers, when applied topically, has been demonstrated to relieve neuropathic pain by affecting sensory fibers, especially C fibers,[330] and by depleting endogenous neurotransmitter stores associated with pain transmission, such as substance P, vasoactive intestinal peptide, cholecystokinin, and somatostatin.[331] Capsaicin does not reverse, stabilize, or lessen neuropathy but decreases the pain that occurs from it. It can result in a burning sensation with the first few weeks of use. Successive applications, however, result in a dose-dependent degeneration and desensitization of afferent fibers, blocking further action potential conduction.[330] Patients should be advised to continue use, if the pain is tolerable, for at least 4–6 weeks before the full benefits are appreciated.

A Cochrane Database Systematic Review showed that capsaicin, either as repeated application of a low-dose (0.075%) cream or a single application of a high-dose (8%) patch, may provide a significant degree of pain relief to some patients with painful neuropathic conditions.[332] In addition, patients with postherpetic neuralgia and painful HIV-associated distal sensory polyneuropathy were studied in randomized, double-blind, multicenter trials using a high-concentration capsaicin dermal patch successfully for up to 1 year; this patch is now available by prescription.[333-335]

DOSAGE

Capsaicin cream is available over the counter (Capzacin HP, Zostrix HP). Various strengths range from 0.025% to 0.1%, although clinical studies use the 0.075% strength. The cream is applied to the affected area up to three or four times daily for at least 4–6 weeks. Clinical trials show that application must take place three or four times a day for improvement.[332] Using it daily, twice daily, or on an as-needed basis is likely to be ineffective.

The capsaicin 8% patch (Qutenza) is by prescription only and is applied in a physician's office. The painful area is pretreated with anesthetic, and the patch is applied for 1 hour and then removed. One patch provides relief for up to 3 months. Follow insert directions for specific application procedures.

Antidepressants

The Neuropathic Pain Special Interest Group of the International Association developed evidence-based guidelines for the pharmacological treatment of neuropathic pain using first-line treatment options, including tricyclic antidepressants (TCAs), dual reuptake inhibitors of serotonin and norepinephrine, and calcium channel $\alpha2$-δ ligands.[336] The results of a systematic review defined clinical success as a 50% reduction in pain. Investigators found that TCAs were the most effective analgesics, followed by traditional anticonvulsants and the newer-generation anticonvulsants, respectively.[337] However, the review concluded that the efficacy of most of these pharmacological treatments is limited because, for any particular drug, only 30% of treated patients experience analgesia.[338] With these low analgesic response rates and the risk of side effects, the use of integrative therapies and dietary supplements is therefore recommended in a trial of benefit before treatment with pharmaceuticals.

Tricyclic Antidepressants. TCAs, such as amitriptyline (Elavil, Endep), nortriptyline (Aventyl, Pamelor), and desipramine (Norpramin), have been commonly used as the mainstay for the palliation of pain secondary to diabetic neuropathy.[339] Many placebo-controlled, randomized controlled trials found TCAs to be efficacious for several different types of neuropathy.[340] TCAs work by increasing the postsynaptic concentration of norepinephrine. Because the inhibitory pathways in the spinal cord use norepinephrine as a neurotransmitter, TCAs are believed to increase the inhibitory influence on nociceptive transmitting neurons.[341] Selective serotonin reuptake inhibitors (SSRIs), such as fluoxetine and paroxetine, have also been used; although they are better tolerated than TCAs, they have little or no efficacy in relieving pain.[342-344]

Serotonin Norepinephrine Reuptake Inhibitors.
- Venlafaxine (Effexor)
- Duloxetine (Cymbalta)

Although both drugs have been used traditionally as antidepressants, studies on venlafaxine and duloxetine have demonstrated beneficial treatment for reduction of painful diabetic neuropathy with better tolerability and fewer side effects than TCAs.[346-350] Although these studies are positive and duloxetine has been granted US Food and Drug Administration (FDA) approval for the treatment of neuropathic pain, the effects have been found to be less than 12 weeks in duration, and therefore the long-term efficacy and safety are unknown.

Anticonvulsants

- Gabapentin: First-line choice
- Pregabalin (Lyrica): First-line choice

Gabapentin has been shown to be highly efficacious in the treatment of various painful neuropathic conditions, including postherpetic neuralgia and diabetic neuropathy.[352] Based on the reviewed randomized controlled trials, gabapentin shows good efficacy, a favorable side effect profile (especially when compared with phenytoin and carbamazepine), and fewer drug interactions; therefore, it may be a first-choice treatment in painful diabetic neuropathy, especially in older adults.[353,354] The number needed to treat (NNT) was reported as 5.8.[355] The precise mechanism of action of anticonvulsants to account for their analgesic effects is unknown. Anticonvulsants modulate both peripheral and central mechanisms through sodium channel antagonism, inhibition of excitatory transmission (e.g., N-methyl-d-aspartate receptor), or enhancement of gamma-aminobutyric acid–mediated inhibition.[356]

Pregabalin is a selective high-affinity ligand for the α2-δ subunit of the voltage-gated calcium channel,[357] which plays a role in the pathological changes that are believed to be associated with neuropathic pain in humans.[358,359] Double-blind, placebo-controlled trials have shown that pregabalin is effective in the treatment of diabetic peripheral neuropathy and postherpetic neuralgia, and that it produces significant improvement in various pain scores and reduced sleep interference.[360,361] The FDA has approved pregabalin for the management of neuropathic pain associated with diabetic peripheral neuropathy and postherpetic neuralgia. Pregabalin is structurally and mechanistically related to gabapentin but differs from gabapentin in exhibiting linear pharmacokinetics with increasing doses and low intersubject variability. These properties may make pregabalin easier to prescribe and could impart a more effective dose range with potentially fewer side effects. Although pregabalin has become a first-line agent in the treatment of diabetic peripheral neuropathy and postherpetic neuralgia, all of the studies were less than 13 weeks in duration, and, therefore, the long-term durability of the response and safety are unknown. The NNT was 6.3.[362] Physicians should also consider cost before prescribing this agent.

Gabapentin

> **DOSAGE**
>
> A single bedtime dose of 300 mg of gabapentin for 2 nights can be followed by 300 mg given twice daily for an additional 2 days. If the patient tolerates this twice-daily regimen, the dose can be increased to 300 mg three times a day. Additional titration upward can be carried out in 300-mg increments as side effects allow. Total daily doses greater than 3600 mg are not currently recommended.[345] A possible combination with 10–25 mg of TCAs (see earlier) can be added for patients with sleep disturbance.
>
> **PRECAUTIONS**
>
> The most serious concern with gabapentin is leukopenia. This drug can also cause somnolence, dizziness, ataxia, and fatigue. Taper dose over 7 days or longer to discontinue.

Pregabalin (Lyrica)

> **DOSAGE**
>
> Pregabalin is taken at 50–150 mg daily, divided into two or three doses. After an initial daily dose of 150 mg, it should be titrated with the patient's response and tolerability over 2 weeks to a maximum of 300 mg daily. Pregabalin dosage adjustment should be considered in cases of renal impairment.[363]
>
> **PRECAUTIONS**
>
> The most common side effects are dizziness, somnolence, headache, dry mouth, and peripheral edema.

Analgesics

Simple analgesics, such as acetaminophen, aspirin, naproxen, and ibuprofen, may be used in conjunction with anticonvulsants and antidepressants; however, the response is very poor. Caution must be taken because many NSAIDs received black box warnings and can cause fatal cardiac and gastrointestinal events. Do not exceed the recommended daily dose because of the risk of renal and hepatic toxicity, particularly in diabetic patients.

Narcotic analgesics are also suboptimal agents for pain control. Owing to their significant central nervous system and gastrointestinal side effects, coupled with the problems of tolerance, dependence, and addiction, these agents should rarely be used, if ever. If a narcotic analgesic is considered, the analgesic tramadol (Ultram), which binds weakly to opioid receptors, may provide some symptomatic relief.

> **DOSAGE**
>
> Tramadol, 50–100 mg, is taken every 6 hours as needed for pain; the maximum dose is 400 mg per day. Caution should be used with the combination of tramadol, antidepressants, and anticonvulsants, owing to increased seizure risk.

Biomechanical Modalities

Electrical Stimulation

Electrical stimulation modalities, such as transcutaneous electrical nerve stimulation (TENS)[364] and application of spinal cord stimulators,[365] have been used successfully to alleviate the pain and discomfort associated with peripheral neuropathy. TENS portable units that generate a biphasic, exponentially decaying wave form (pulse width 4 msec, 25–35 V, more than 2 Hz) should be used for 30 minutes daily for 4 weeks. A study showed that percutaneous electrical nerve stimulation (PENS), in addition to decreasing pain, improves the patient capacity for physical activity, sense of well-being, and quality of sleep, while reducing the need for oral nonopioid analgesic medication.[366] PENS is similar to electroacupuncture in that electrical stimulation is delivered via disposable acupuncture-type needles. It differs from electroacupuncture in that it is delivered along the peripheral nerves that innervate the region of neuropathic pain, rather than being delivered at acupuncture points or along meridians. Although the use of alternating low and high frequencies of 15 and 30 Hz at 30-minute intervals three times a week is recommended, the patient should be evaluated by a health care professional who is familiar with electrical stimulation techniques for adjustment of frequencies and time intervals as tolerated.

Neural Blockade

Local anesthetic peripheral and sympathetic blocks provide useful diagnostic information but tend to confer only temporary therapeutic benefits in patients with peripheral neuropathy.[367]

Surgery

Entrapment neuropathies, such as carpal tunnel syndrome, may be relieved by surgical decompression (see Chapter 70). In addition, compression or entrapment from cancers may be addressed by removal of the tumor directly.

Therapies to Consider

Agaricus brasiliensis

Agaricus brasiliensis (AbS) is native to Brazil and is widely grown in Japan because of its medicinal properties. AbS has traditionally been used for the prevention of a range of diseases, including cancer, hepatitis, atherosclerosis, hypercholesterolemia, dermatitis, and diabetes.[368-370] Randomized, double-blind, placebo-controlled trials have shown that AbS improves insulin resistance in type 2 diabetes.[371] Furthermore, in animal studies, it has been shown to reduce inflammatory mechanisms and lower diabetic neuropathic pain.[372]

Tocotrienols

Tocotrienols, more specifically delta and gamma isomers that are derived from annatto and palm, are an important part of Vitamin E, which is now being extensively researched for its antihyperlipidemic, antidiabetic, antiinflammatory, anticancer, and immune-supportive actions.[373-376] In human and animal studies, tocotrienols have been shown to improve diabetes and to reduce neuropathic pain.[377] Current clinical trials are underway to investigate neuroprotection by tocotrienols in type 1 and type 2 diabetes mellitus (VENUS). Note that tocotrienols are very temperature sensitive, therefore, these products should be kept refrigerated,[378] and should not be taken with other forms of Vitamin E (e.g., alpha-tocopherols) for the best absorption.[379-381] Tocotrienols may be started at a dose of 125 mg bid or tid.

PREVENTION PRESCRIPTION

- Eat a whole-foods, low-fat, high-fiber, plant-based diet.
- Avoid environmental toxins such as heavy metals, cigarette smoke, alcohol, pesticides, and herbicides.
- Prevent adult-onset diabetes by maintaining an ideal weight and staying physically fit and active.

- If possible, avoid specific toxins (see Table 13.1) and pharmaceutical agents that are known to cause neuropathy (see Table 13.2).
- Avoid doses of vitamin B6 (pyridoxine) greater than 250 mg/day.
- If taking the chemotherapeutic medications cisplatin, paclitaxel (Taxol), or vincristine, consider acetyl-l-carnitine, 1 g three times daily for 8 weeks.

THERAPEUTIC REVIEW

LIFESTYLE AND NUTRITION

- Daily exercise that consists of walking for at least 30 minutes per day three times per week should be implemented. If walking is not possible because of painful peripheral neuropathy, gentler forms of exercise, such as yoga or tai chi, three times a week for 30–90 minutes are therapeutic. A whole-foods, low-fat, high-fiber, plant-based diet with strict glycemic control should be strongly advised. Environmental and other toxins, such as heavy metals, cigarette smoke, alcohol, and pollution, should be avoided.

MIND-BODY THERAPY

Biofeedback

- Recommendation is for at least six 1-hr biofeedback sessions at approximately 1-week intervals. Thereafter, relaxation biofeedback techniques can be performed at home with the use of biofeedback home-use programs (e.g., emWave Pro, emWave 2, Innerbalance [HeartMath Institute]), audio CDs, or guided imagery exercises (for 10–20 minutes each day).

Bioenergetics

- Pulsed electomagnetic field (PEMF): BEMER vascular therapy mat for 10 minutes twice daily at level 3 (10.5 = microtesla) for 30 days.
- Acupuncture and neuroacupuncture points: upper one fifth sensory area (S 1/5) for the lower limbs, middle two fifths sensory area (S 2/5) for the upper limbs, and foot motor and sensory areas; ear points: ShenMen, sympathetic, foot; body points: GB-40, GB-34, SP-10, SP-6, ST-44, LR-3, and Bafeng (extra point). Electrical stimulation can be used for the ear and body points at a frequency of 100 Hz at a low intensity for 10–15 minutes for an enhanced response. Patients can receive 2 treatments per week for 10 weeks.
- Electroacupuncture: This treatment can be performed in two cycles of five sittings each (10 sessions) at 2-day intervals.

BOTANICALS

- *Curcumin longa, Boswellia serrata*, ginger, and black pepper (e.g., Bosmeric-SR, two caplets twice daily) or Curcumin C3 complex: 1000 mg three times daily.
- Cannabidiols (CBD) from industrial hemp oil: 5–50 mg tid, with coconut oil (to improve absorption) and stevia (optional for improved taste), held sublingually for 2–3 minutes then swallowed. Doses may be increased weekly for improved response.
- CBD:THC from medical cannabis. High CBD low THC is preferred (e.g., 20:1), or for more pain control, a ratio of 1:1, which is similar to the prescribed drug in other countries. Administration is the same as previously, but start with lower doses. 1–2 mg bid to tid and dose up as tolerated.

- Geranium oil (*Pelargonium* spp.): For topical pain relief, apply a few drops (i.e., Neuragen PN) to the affected area several times a day.
- Evening primrose oil (EPO; *Oenothera biennis*): 360 mg orally daily of GLA from EPO. The dose may be increased up to 480 mg orally daily.

SUPPLEMENTS

- Acetyl-L-carnitine (ALC): 500 mg orally twice daily to 1000 mg orally three times daily. ALC is used for both chemotherapy-induced and diabetic peripheral neuropathy.
- Alpha-lipoic acid: 600–1800 mg orally daily; start with 600 mg orally daily and increase up to 1800 mg orally daily in divided doses if needed.
- Benfotiamine: Lipid-soluble vitamin B1, 150–300 mg twice daily specifically for diabetic peripheral neuropathy.
- Methylcobalamin or 5-adenosylcobalamin: Better-absorbed vitamin B12, 500 mcg three times daily or 1500 mcg daily.
- B-complex multivitamin (B-100): One tablet once or twice daily for peripheral neuropathy caused by deficiency syndromes.
- Fish oil (omega-3 fatty acids): Eicosapentaenoic acid (EPA), 1000–2000 mg/day, and docosahexaenoic acid (DHA), 500–1000 mg/day or a vegetarian plant-based option (i.e., NutraVege 2x).

PHARMACEUTICALS

For topical relief:
- Capsaicin cream 0.075%: Apply to the affected area up to three or four times daily for at least 4–6 weeks.
- Capsaicin patch (8%): One patch to area for 1 hour (after preanesthetic application) and then remove.

It is applied in a doctor's office under supervision.

For acute pain management, consider:
- Analgesics: Nonsteroidal antiinflammatory drugs (NSAIDs) as usually prescribed for pain, as well as narcotics.

For chronic pain management:
Antidepressants
- Amitriptyline or nortriptyline: 10 mg orally at night; titrate the dose upward to 25 mg orally at night as side effects allow (usual range: 50–300 mg/day).
Anticonvulsants
- Gabapentin (first-line choice): 300 mg orally at night for 2 days, then 300 mg orally twice daily for 2 days; can be increased to 300 mg orally three times daily as tolerated, with increases in 300-mg increments as side effects allow; maximum daily dose, 3600 mg.
- Pregabalin: 50 mg three times daily. After an initial daily dose of 150 mg, it should be titrated according to the patient's response and tolerability over 2 weeks to a maximum of 300 mg daily.

BIOMECHANICAL THERAPY

- Transcutaneous electrical nerve stimulation (TENS): Use of a TENS portable unit for 30 minutes daily for 4 weeks is recommended.
- Percutaneous electrical nerve stimulation (PENS): This modality can be used three times a week; stimulation is delivered along the peripheral nerves that innervate the region of neuropathic pain.
- Neural blockade: This provides only temporary therapeutic benefit.
- Surgery: Surgical decompression may relieve symptoms in carpal tunnel syndrome; with neuronal entrapment from cancer, removal of the tumor itself may also be helpful.)

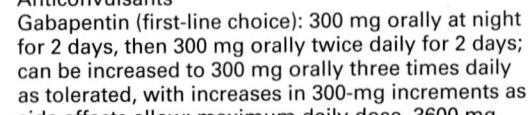
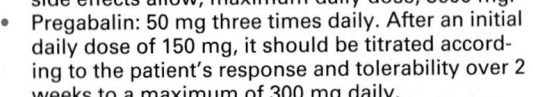
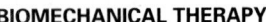

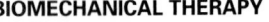

Key Web Resources

National Institute of Neurological Disorders and Stroke. This page has information about organizations that support neuropathic conditions, as well as up-to-date clinical trials.	http://www.ninds.nih.gov/disorders/peripheralneuropathy/peripheralneuropathy.htm
MedlinePlus, National Library of Medicine. Simplified information is provided for patients about neuropathy and its associated conditions with definitions.	http://www.nlm.nih.gov/medlineplus/ency/article/000593.htm
WebMD. This page on understanding peripheral neuropathy contains the basics for patients.	http://www.webmd.com/brain/understanding-peripheral-neuropathy-basics
The Foundation for Peripheral Neuropathy. Public charity providing information on research and treatment options for patients and health care providers.	https://www.foundationforpn.org

Disclosure: Dr. Pai has financial interests in the company that produces Bosmeric-SR.

REFERENCES

References are available online at ExpertConsult.com.

CHAPTER 14

MULTIPLE SCLEROSIS

Bradly Jacobs, MD, MPH, ABOIM • Surya Pierce, MD

PATHOPHYSIOLOGY

Multiple sclerosis (MS) is the most common cause of chronic neurological disability in young adults, with a prevalence that varies geographically from 1 to 2.5 per 1000.[1]

Although its origin and exact mechanisms remain uncertain, MS is a complex disorder that is characterized by axonal injury, inflammation, and demyelination. The triggers for axonal loss are thought to be caused by inflammatory demyelination of the myelin sheath and ATP-related hypoxia of the neurons causing neurodegeneration. Progressive neurological disability is the result of this axonal damage and loss. Demyelination impairs the transmission of nerve impulses and results in fatigue, weakness, numbness, locomotor difficulty, pain, loss of vision, and other health problems. In general, MS is viewed as an autoimmune disorder that transpires when internal antibodies mistakenly direct their "attack" against the body's own nerve cells.

Research suggests that MS is more correctly thought of as one end of a spectrum of central nervous system (CNS) disorders, and is the byproduct of a malfunctioning physiological immune response, the original purpose of which is protective. According to this view, all individuals are endowed with the potential ability to evoke an autoimmune response to CNS injuries (viral, bacterial, toxin, or direct injury). The inherent ability to control this response, so that its effect is beneficial, is limited, and correlates with an individual's inherent ability to resist autoimmune disease induction.[2]

Because of the wide variation in disease presentation and the development of treatment protocols, it is useful to categorize MS patients into the following four groups[3]:
1. Relapsing-remitting (RR) disease occurs at onset in 80% of cases, and is characterized by acute attacks followed by remissions with a steady baseline between attacks. Patients with a definite diagnosis of relapsing-remitting MS should be considered for disease-modifying therapy.
2. In 50% to 80% of patients with RR disease, progressive deterioration with less marked attacks occurs within 10 years of onset. The disease in these patients is called secondary progressive phase MS (SP-MS).
3. Primary progressive MS (PP-MS) occurs in 10% to 15% of patients and is characterized by progressive deterioration from the outset without superimposed relapses.
4. Approximately 6% of patients with PP-MS also experience relapses in parallel with their disease progression and are said to have progressive-relapsing MS (PR-MS).

ETIOLOGY

Research into the causes of MS has been rendered difficult by the marked variation in the disease expression. It is unclear whether MS is one disease with variable symptoms or whether the different subtypes represent unique causes.[4] At present, four major theories for the cause of MS are recognized: immunological, environmental, infectious, and genetic.

Immunological Factors

The theory that MS is an organ-specific autoimmune disease, although unproven, is widely accepted. Antibodies against antigens that are located on the surface of the myelin sheath cause demyelination, either directly or by complement-mediated processes. Investigators have suggested that priming of myelin-reactive T cells occurs as part of the disease process in MS. Primed T cells that are reactive to myelin antigens may develop a phenotype that makes them more resistant to regulatory processes. The concept that autoantigens can drive B-cell clonal expansion and contribute to autoimmunity has been demonstrated in other autoimmune diseases. The role of B cells in the recovery from inflammatory demyelination has also been hypothesized.[5]

The hygiene theory claims that childhood exposure to infectious agents is beneficial to the maturing immune system through modulation of T-helper cells, that is, Th1 and Th2. Indeed, research has found that autoimmune conditions, including MS, are less prevalent in parts of the world where infectious agents, such as helminths and toxoplasmosis, are endemic. Furthermore, case reports have documented a reduction in disease severity following travel to developing countries. Extrapolating from phase 1 trials on patients with inflammatory bowel disease, investigators conducted a phase 1 study enrolling five patients with MS and treating them with nonpathogenic helminths (*Trichuris suis* [pig whipworm]), given twice monthly for 3 months. The intervention was well tolerated with no adverse events, and patients experienced an average reduction of brain lesions from 6.6 to 2.0 on MRI, which then increased to 5.8 lesions 2 months after the intervention was discontinued.[6] Another study using similar helminths showed that the treatment was well tolerated but that no benefit was seen.[7] A 50-patient, phase 2, randomized study in Germany is now ongoing.[8,9]

Environmental Factors

Several decades of research have documented that the incidence of MS increases with increasing distance from the Equator. Possible explanations for this finding include genetic predisposition in population groups, dietary factors, and levels of the active form of vitamin D. Evidence indicates that the timing of the exposure to an environmental agent plays a role, with exposure before puberty predisposing a person to the development of MS later in life.[10] A dietary influence on MS was first reported by Swank et al. in 1952,[11] who noted that people living in colder climates tend to consume diets that are higher in fat compared to those living in more tropical regions, and that this dietary difference was linked to a higher incidence of MS in the colder regions.[11]

The relationship between mercury from dental fillings and MS is very controversial.[12,13] At present, there are insufficient data to render an opinion. However, exposure to cigarette smoke has been demonstrated to be a clear risk factor for developing MS, as well as increasing the severity of the illness.[16,17] These findings suggest the possibility of environmental toxins or pollutants in the pathogenesis of MS.

Infectious Agents

At least 16 different infectious agents have been implicated as causes of MS; however, none has been definitely associated with the disease. At present, three agents are receiving the most attention: human herpesvirus-6, *Chlamydia pneumoniae*, and Epstein-Barr virus.

Genetic Factors

Although most cases of MS are sporadic, susceptibility to MS is substantially affected by genetic factors. For example, clear associations exist between certain subtypes of the major histocompatibility human leukocyte antigen (HLA)-DRB1 gene and susceptibility and the disease course in MS.[18] However, the aggregate contribution of germline genetic variants to the disease expression of a given patient with MS may be modest. This concept is highlighted by the observation that the clinical expression of MS may be quite different between monozygotic twin siblings who both have the disease. It is therefore likely that several postgermline events influence the clinical expression of MS.[19]

DIAGNOSIS

The hallmark for the clinical diagnosis of MS is neurological dysfunction that is disseminated in space and time. Objective evaluation includes magnetic resonance imaging (MRI), evaluation of cerebrospinal fluid, and evoked potential testing (measuring the electrical activity of the brain in response to stimulation of sensory nerve pathways). The pathological hallmark of MS is the presence of demyelinated plaques involving the periventricular white matter, optic nerves, brainstem, and cerebellum or spinal cord white matter (Figs. 14.1 and 14.2).

INTEGRATIVE THERAPY

Lifestyle

Smoking Cessation

As previously mentioned, tobacco smoke exposure is a risk factor for developing MS and is associated with a worse prognosis. Smokers with MS should be offered appropriate counseling and supportive measures to quit smoking.

> In addition to being a major risk for other diseases, tobacco smoking is probably the most important disease-specific, modifiable risk factor for patients with multiple sclerosis who smoke.

Exercise

During the 1990s, people with MS were instructed to avoid strenuous physical activity due to fears that it may worsen their neurological status, such as occurs when MS patients get overheated. However, current research has demonstrated that physical activity is safe and well tolerated and has the same health benefits as in the general population. In addition, physical fitness and exercise have been associated with improved muscle strength, spasticity, cognition, reduced fatigue, and may even have neuroprotective properties.[20–22,25,26]

Sunshine

There is an increased prevalence of MS in extreme latitudes. Furthermore, case-control studies have found that sunlight is associated with a reduced risk of MS diagnosis and mortality.[27,29] Whether this association with sunlight is entirely attributable to vitamin D is unclear.

Mind-Body Therapy

Psychosocial Factors

Depression is common in MS, and death by suicide occurs seven times more frequently than in the general population. Combining counseling with body work therapies can be highly effective in countering depression in MS patients.

Psychological stress has been clearly identified as a trigger for relapses of MS and possibly contributes to disease progression.[30–32] Furthermore, coping styles may affect susceptibility to the harmful effects of stress in MS.[33] Given the relatively modifiable nature of life stress and coping, patients with MS should be encouraged to learn some form of stress reduction, stress management, or coping techniques (see Chapter 94).

> Stress and coping strategies should be addressed in every patient with multiple sclerosis and may affect both the relapse frequency and disease progression.

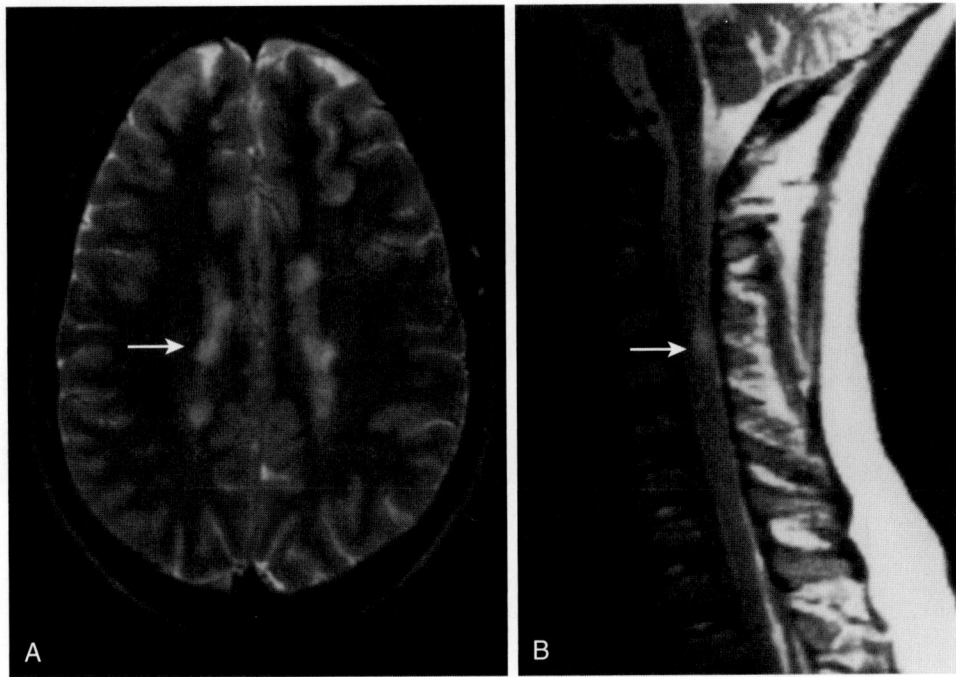

FIG. 14.1 ■ Multiple sclerosis. **A**, T2-weighted magnetic resonance imaging (MRI) of the brain showing multiple lesions located in the white matter characteristic of multiple sclerosis *(arrow)*. **B**, T1-weighted MRI of the spine indicating a demyelinating plaque of multiple sclerosis in the mid-cervical region *(arrow)*. (From Johnson MV. Demyelinating disorders of the CNS. In: Kliegman RM, Behrman RE, Jenson HB, eds. *Nelson Textbook of Pediatrics*. 18th ed. Philadelphia: Elsevier; 2007.)

Yoga

Yoga techniques have been shown to improve circulation, balance, the ability to relax, flexibility, and eyesight, and to reduce muscle tension—all features typically affected by MS.[34] A systematic review identified seven randomized clinical trials that evaluated the effect of yoga on MS and documented a clinical benefit on mood and fatigue.[36] In the absence of a specific yoga class for MS patients, an individualized yoga program that is developed closely with a qualified yoga teacher or therapist is likely to produce similar benefits.

Mindfulness Meditation

Mindfulness meditation involves paying attention in a systematic manner with the intention of being awake and receptive to the present moment rather than focusing on the past or future. The Chinese characters depicting mindfulness meditation use the character for presence over the character for heart, implying that the intention is to bring presence of heart. The goal is to cultivate moment-to-moment awareness of personal thoughts, emotions, body, and surroundings. It has been successfully applied to a range of health issues that directly or indirectly relate to people living with MS (see Chapter 100). An 8-week mindfulness-based intervention demonstrated significant improvement in measures of nonphysical quality of life, depression, fatigue, and anxiety compared with usual care in patients with MS.[37] A 2014 systematic review identified three studies using mindfulness for MS and found benefits for quality of life, pain,

fatigue, single leg standing balance, anxiety, and depression, with benefits persisting for 6 months after the intervention.[38]

Nutrition

While there is a paucity of clinical data regarding the role of specific diets in the treatment of MS, it is likely that dietary factors influence the course of MS via modulation of inflammation.[39] The following are nutritional and dietary recommendations for patients with MS that generally target inflammation:

- In general, eating a diet relatively high in omega-3, polyunsaturated fatty acids is associated with positive health effects and may be recommended to most individuals. Primary sources of foods rich in omega-3 essential fatty acids include cold-water fish, nuts, seeds, and dark green leafy vegetables, which reduce inflammation by their effect on prostaglandins and leukotrienes (see Chapter 88).[40] Evidence is mixed on the benefit of omega-3 fatty acid supplementation for people with MS,[42-44] possibly due to the variability in formulations and dosages (see Supplements section).
- Avoid trans fats. This is done by avoiding processed or packaged foods. The FDA has stated that trans fats are "not generally recognized as being safe." There is clear evidence of excess risk for all-cause death and cardiovascular events with the consumption of trans fats. Beginning in 2018, the FDA will ban food manufacturers from producing foods with trans fats.

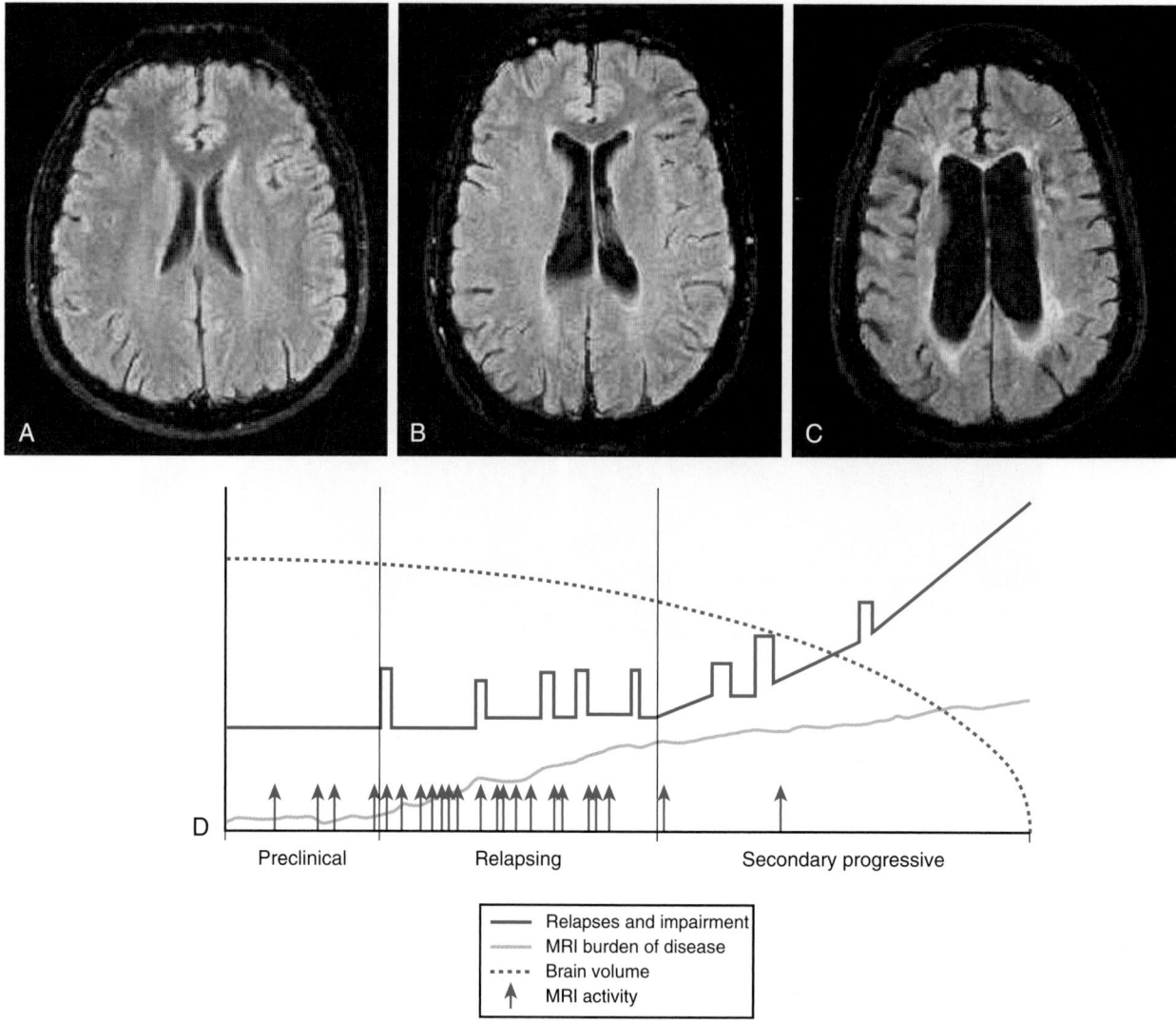

FIG. 14.2 ■ Changes in magnetic resonance imaging (MRI) with disease duration. **A–C,** Comparison of three scans from patients with different disease durations, indicating the appearance of atrophy and ventricular dilation with time. **D,** As brain atrophy appears, a decline in the number of gadolinium-enhancing lesions is commonly seen. (From Lublin FD, Miller AE. Multiple sclerosis and other inflammatory demyelinating diseases of the central nervous system. In: Bradley WG, Daroff RB, Fenichel GM, Jankovic J, eds. *Neurology in Clinical Practice.* 5th ed. Munich: Butterworth-Heinemann; 2008.)

- Many practitioners recommend that patients with active symptoms should observe the effects of a structured *elimination diet*. This involves elimination of common or suspected food allergens or triggers for at least 2 to 4 weeks followed by a systematic rechallenge (see Chapter 86). Case reports have noted gluten sensitivity manifesting as optic neuritis,[45] and an increase frequency of gliadin and gluten IgA antibodies in MS.[46] Patients should keep a daily journal to monitor changes from baseline. Given that instituting an elimination diet can be challenging, some patients and practitioners opt for autoimmune antibody testing while recognizing that these tests have variable sensitivity and specificity.

Energy Medicine

Magnet Therapy

Magnetic therapy is simply the therapeutic application of magnets and can be delivered in many forms. In a 12-week, randomized trial, subjects with MS laid down on a metal mat for 8 minutes twice daily. The device delivered low-frequency, pulsed electromagnetic field therapy. Another study had subjects with MS wear wristwatch-size, magnetic pulsing devices called Enermed for 10 to 24 hours daily for 2 months. Another device also delivered low-frequency magnetic stimulations at 37.5 mT and a sequence of pulses at 4 to 7 Hz three times weekly for 2 months. These studies demonstrated consistent benefits in reducing fatigue but no benefit for depression in subjects with MS.[53]

Supplements

Vitamin D

Observational studies have shown that vitamin D levels positively correlate with a reduced risk of developing MS,[54] and that lower levels of vitamin D are associated with higher MS disease disability and activity[55] as well as relapse rates.[56] A 2015 study demonstrated that Europeans with genetically lowered vitamin D levels were twice as likely to develop MS.[57] A pilot randomized trial documented an inverse relationship between vitamin D levels and MS disease activity on MRI.[58] One study found that serum vitamin D3 levels greater than 100 nmol/L were associated with a 53% risk reduction of developing new lesions on MRI.[59] There are currently two ongoing clinical trials to evaluate the effect of supplemental vitamin D in patients with a clinically isolated episode of MS,[60,61] and there are two clinical trials evaluating the effect of high-dose vitamin D3 (10,000 to 14,000 IU/daily) in patients with RR-MS who are also receiving interferon-beta.[62,63] Among patients living with MS and who have normal renal function, dosages of 10,000 units daily have been used without evidence of toxicity.[64,65]

DOSAGE

Titrate for a serum level greater than 80 ng/mL to achieve immunomodulatory effects. Titrate vitamin D3 up to 4000 to 10,000 IU units daily. Doses in the higher end of this range should be monitored with serum levels for vitamin D and calcium.

PRECAUTIONS

Watch for the theoretical risk of hypercalcemia; however, recent dose-escalation safety studies have not validated this concern.

Thiol-based Antioxidants

Alpha-lipoic acid (ALA), N-acetylcysteine (NAC), and glutathione (GSH) are powerful antioxidants that scavenge free radicals such as reactive oxygen and reactive nitrogen species. Given our understanding of the role of oxidation in MS disease progression and severity, and the association of reduced glutathione levels in patients with MS, these compounds merit further investigation. Studies using the classic animal model for MS (*experimental autoimmune encephalomyelitis* [or *EAE*] mice) report a consistent reduction of disease severity and inflammation with ALA, and inhibition of acute EAE in mice through the scavenging of free radicals.[66] Human studies examining mediators of inflammation using ALA have documented mixed results.[67] There is limited data on humans using these compounds; however, multiple studies are now underway evaluating the effect of thiol-based antioxidants on MS disease progression in humans.

DOSAGE

- ALA: 600 mg twice daily.
- NAC: 600 mg three times daily.
- Glutathione: 600 to 800 mg intravenously diluted in 10 to 20 mL of sterile water and infused over 15 to 20 minutes two to three times weekly. (Glutathione is not absorbed orally.)

PRECAUTIONS

- ALA: In general, quite well tolerated and safe. At higher doses can infrequently cause nausea, vomiting, and skin irritation at the IV site when given intravenously.
- NAC: Infrequently causes nausea, vomiting, and diarrhea.
- GSH: Rapid infusion can provoke respiratory distress, coughing, rhinorrhea, and vertigo.

Magnesium

Magnesium is required for adequate levels of metabolized vitamin D products to be maintained in the circulation. At 800 mg/day, magnesium also has a mild effect on the muscle spasticity that is often associated with MS.

DOSAGE

600 to 1200 mg/day

PRECAUTIONS

Individual tolerance for magnesium is variable. Advise patients to decrease the dose if diarrhea develops.

B-Complex Vitamins

B vitamins have been shown to aid cognitive function, act as antioxidants, and decrease the production of inflammatory cytokines.

DOSAGE

Varies by preparation.

Vitamin B$_{12}$

Deficiency of vitamin B$_{12}$ and errors in vitamin B$_{12}$ metabolism are known to cause demyelination of the CNS.[68] High doses of vitamin B$_{12}$ given intramuscularly have been shown to improve brainstem nerve function in chronic, progressive MS.[69] Teaching patients self-injection of vitamin B may be a cost-effective way of improving overall well-being.

DOSAGE

Oral doses are 1000 to 2000 mcg/day in the form of methylcobalamin. Intramuscular doses of hydroxycobalamin are 1000 mcg/day for 5 days, then twice weekly for 4 weeks, and then twice monthly.

Biotin

High-dose biotin (300 mg daily; 10,000% of the adequate daily intake) is thought to prevent both demyelination by triggering myelin synthesis and neurodegeneration by replenishing ATP in hypoxic neurons.[70]

Biotin has traditionally been marketed for hair and nails. Biotin is a water-soluble B-vitamin called vitamin B7. One of its main functions is to facilitate fatty acid synthesis, and it avidly crosses the blood–brain barrier. Biotin is an essential coenzyme for five essential carboxylases, including acetyl-CoA-carboxylase (ACC). ACC is highly expressed in oligodendrocytes, which play a major role in myelin synthesis, and is the rate-limiting factor in the synthesis of malonyl-CoA, a critical building block for fatty acid synthesis. The current theory is that high dose biotin may markedly increase myelin repair through this mechanism.[70]

A group of French investigators published a proof-of-concept case series of 23 adults with progressive MS receiving 100 to 300 mg of biotin daily for up to 36 months (mean 9.2 months). They reported that more than 90% of the subjects experienced improvements over baseline in disability and the progression of MS. Improvement occurred 2 to 8 months after treatment commenced.[71] Results from a multicenter, randomized, blinded study were presented at the American Academy of Neurology in April 2015.[72] Investigators reported a statistically significant difference between the proportions of subjects who experienced a reduction in disability in the active group (12.5%) compared to the placebo group (0%), as well as a significant difference in disease progression.[72]

DOSAGE

300 mg daily.

PRECAUTIONS

None documented; biotin is generally well tolerated.

Botanicals

Ashwagandha (*Withania somnifera*)

Ashwagandha is an Ayurvedic herb (see the discussion on Ayurveda later), also known as winter cherry, that is sometimes called Indian ginseng in reference to its rejuvenating and tonic effects on the nervous system. Ashwagandha's antiinflammatory, antioxidant, anxiolytic, and antidepressant activities all make this herb an important supplement for patients with MS.[73,74]

DOSAGE

1 to 2 g of the whole herb in powdered form two or three times a day.

PRECAUTIONS

Some Ayurvedic herbs have been found to have high levels of contaminants such as lead. By knowing the supplier's source of the herb, you can be sure your patient is not taking a contaminated product.

Curcumin (Diferuloylmethane)

One of the principal biologically active ingredients in turmeric (Curcuma longa plant; an Indian spice) is curcumin, a lipophilic compound that easily crosses membranes. Curcumin is a turmeric extract from the root of the Curcuma longa plant. Studies with EAE mice have consistently shown inhibition of oxidation and inflammation through upregulation of the nuclear translocation of nuclear factor-E2-related factor (Nrf2), and inhibition of nuclear-factor kappa-beta (NF-kB), respectively. Specific pathways affecting inflammation include decreased T-cell production of IFN-gamma and inhibition of Th1 and Th17 differentiation. A 2-year randomized, blinded, clinical trial examining the effect of curcumin as an adjuvant to IFN-B1a has completed recruitment and is now ongoing.[78] This compound has a proven safety record in humans, with dose escalation studies up to 8 g daily, and is well tolerated.[79] Whether the documented effectiveness in animal models will translate into humans has yet to be determined.

DOSAGE

500 mg to 3 g twice daily. For enhanced bioavailability, curcumin should be bound to a lipophilic compound or formulated with black pepper. Examples of formulations include standardization of 95% curcuminoids bound to black pepper extract (*Piper nigrum*, Bioperine®), or a preparation standardized to 70% to 80% curcumin, 15% to 25% desmethoxycurcumin, and 2.5% to 6.5% bisdemethoxycurcumin in a lipophilic emulsion.

PRECAUTIONS

Higher doses may cause abdominal fullness or discomfort. It may increase blood levels of sulfasalazine by threefold.

Ginkgo biloba

Ginkgo has antioxidant effects and inhibits platelet-activating factor (PAF), which results in antiinflammatory properties and possible inhibition of glutamate excitotoxicity, thereby improving cognition. Three randomized trials found that ginkgo improved cognitive performance[67]; however, the largest randomized study published to date (120 persons) found no benefits in cognitive performance.[80] In evaluating the herb's effect on fatigue, a 4-week, pilot, randomized study found benefits; however, no effect was found on attention/concentration nor visual-spatial memory.[81]

DOSAGE

The EGb-761 formulation should be used when possible, standardized to 24% flavone glycosides, 7% proanthocyanidins, and 6% terpene lactones at 120 mg twice daily.

Cannabinoids

Cannabinoids are psychoactive compounds with medicinal properties. Tetrahydrocannabinol (THC) and cannabidiol (CBD) are the most studied cannabinoids. CBD has substantially less psychoactive properties than THC. Synthetic cannabinoids (e.g., dronabinol) are closely related to THC. Based on systematic reviews, the evidence published to date indicates that oral cannabis extract is clearly effective, and THC is most likely effective in reducing pain (excluding central neuropathic pain) and spasticity symptoms. They are probably not effective in improving tremor or signs of spasticity.[82] There is insufficient evidence for effects on urge incontinence or bladder symptoms.[82] Sativex oromucosal spray (unavailable in the US) is probably effective for spasticity symptoms, pain, and urinary frequency, and probably ineffective for signs of spasticity, incontinence episodes, and tremor.[82] There is insufficient evidence for these outcomes with inhaled cannabis.[82] Prior to recommending this therapy, physicians should counsel patients about the potential legal issues and unwanted side effects.

DOSAGE

The dose varies considerably depending on potency and patient tolerance. The dose of synthetic THC (e.g., dronabinol) varies from 2.5 to 10 mg daily. THC-CBD combination oral extracts, as capsules or mouth spray (e.g., Sativex which contains 2.7 mg THC and 2.5 mg CBD per spray), are used at doses varying from 2.5 to 120 mg daily.[82]

PRECAUTIONS

Generally well tolerated. Significant laboratory findings or serious adverse events have not been reported in clinical research. Mild to moderate side effects are common and include dizziness, drowsiness, and memory or concentration difficulties. Less frequently, research subjects reported nausea, constipation, dry mouth, or increased appetite.[53]

Green Tea Polyphenol Epigallocatechin-Gallate

Epigallocatechin-gallate (EGCG) is an antioxidant that accumulates within the mitochondria of neurons and decreases apoptosis of neurons undergoing oxidative stress.[83] EGCG administered as 95% pure capsules 200 mg three times daily was administered to patients with MS over 12 weeks and was found to improve muscle metabolism during moderate exercise among men, possibly because of sex-specific effects on autonomic and endocrine control.[84] In 2015, investigators conducted both a 10-person phase 1 case series study and a 13-person phase 2 randomized study using a Japanese product (polyphenon E) containing 50% EGCG at 400 mg twice daily. Results from the phase 1 study showed a 10% increase in N-acetyl aspartate levels (a marker of the number of neurons and their mitochondrial energy production), suggesting a neuroprotective benefit. One person experienced hepatotoxicity. The phase 2 study used a different product, and five of seven participants randomized to active treatment experienced hepatotoxicity, requiring discontinuation of the study. The same investigators will be conducting a phase 2 randomized trial with 48 participants using the 95% pure EGCG formulation.[85] There are several other studies listed on the clinicaltrials.gov website, and most of these focus on safety and neuroprotective effects.

DOSAGE

EGCG 95% pure 200-mg capsules three times daily.

PRECAUTIONS

Until safety studies report otherwise, we do not recommend the use of high concentration EGCG compounds due to the documented hepatotoxicity risk.

Hormones

Estrogen and Oral Contraceptives

Estrogen has been found to have neuroprotective and immunomodulatory effects in women with active MS. Most patients with MS who become pregnant experience a significant decrease in symptoms, with mild exacerbation during the postpartum period.[86] Research has shown that estriol causes an immune shift from T-helper 1 to T-helper 2 cells. Studies have documented a reduction in symptoms and a decrease in gadolinium-enhancing lesions on MRI in women with MS who are treated with estriol or high dose ethinylestradiol.[87-91]

DOSAGE

Ethinylestradiol 40 μg and desogestrel 125 μg as oral contraceptive therapy

PRECAUTIONS

The concerns are the same as with all high-dose estrogen therapies.

Testosterone

Testosterone has also been found to have immunomodulatory and neuroprotective effects, as well as ameliorating MS symptoms, in men with active MS.[86,92,94]

DOSAGE

Use micronized testosterone from compounding pharmacies. For men: 10 g of gel containing 100 mg testosterone

PRECAUTIONS

Contraindications include polycythemia, benign prostatic hypertrophy (BPH), and prostate cancer. Serum testosterone levels should be monitored. Some patients experience skin dermatitis with topical application.

In a pilot, crossover study of 10 men with active MS who were receiving 10 g of gel containing 100 mg testosterone daily for 12 months, investigators reported improved cognitive function, slowing of brain atrophy on MRI, and no significant adverse events; however, no changes in new lesions were identified on MRI.[94]

Pharmaceuticals

Corticosteroids

Evidence indicates that the administration of high-dose corticosteroids during MS relapses can improve the associated disabling symptoms, and oral and intravenous therapy have been found to have similar efficacy.[95-97] Corticosteroids do not affect overall long-term functional recovery or outcomes.[95] Plasma exchange is indicated for patients with severe attacks that are refractory to high-dose corticosteroids.

DOSAGE

Methylprednisolone, 1 g/day intravenously (or an equivalent oral regimen). Prednisone, 1250 mg orally daily for 3 to 5 days. Low-dose oral dosage regimens vary. The most common regimen is prednisone 60 mg orally once a day for 5 days, then 40 mg orally for 5 days, followed by 20 mg for 5 days, 10 mg for 5 days, and finally 5 mg for 5 days.

While generally well tolerated within the context of acute treatment, some people experience euphoria, psychosis, irritability, insomnia, depression, gastritis and ulceration, and osteoporosis from repeated use. High-dose corticosteroids may be associated with defects in long-term memory.[98-100] High-dose corticosteroids given outside of a relapse in order to prevent disability progression may actually contribute to worsening of disability progression in some patients upon discontinuation of therapy.[101]

Disease-Modifying Treatments

Patients with a definite diagnosis of relapsing-remitting MS should consider disease-modifying therapies (listed in the following) recognizing that these therapies address the signs and symptoms of MS and are not curative. Their benefits include reduction in relapse rates and frequency of new brain lesions; however, the effect on progression to disability is uncertain. The choice of therapy should be based on patient preferences, values, and disease severity. When considering therapy, treating clinicians often recommend natalizumab for more rapidly progressive disease in patients who prefer a robust effect over safety. Interferon beta injectable formulations and glatiramer acetate are preferred for patients who value safety over effectiveness and ease of administration. Oral therapy with dimethyl fumarate should be considered for patients who value convenience and believe the robust effectiveness and safety findings from two large, multicenter, randomized, blinded trials, and one study (the CONFIRM study) suggesting noninferiority compared with glatiramer. Biotin is the newest compound under evaluation as a potential disease-modifying treatment (see the Dietary Supplements section in this chapter). It is convenient, and initial findings suggest that it is very well tolerated and may be effective.

Fumaric Acid

Fumaric acid appears to have neuroprotective and immunomodulatory (not immunosuppressive) properties through nuclear factor (erythroid derived-2)-like2 (NRF2) activation. NRF2 concentrates in the cell cytoplasm causing immunoregulatory as well as cytoprotective effects via upregulation of antioxidant proteins.

In two large, phase 3, randomized clinical trials (CONFIRM [n = 1430] and DEFINE [n = 1200]), subjects with active MS were allocated dimethyl fumaric acid (BG-12) 240 mg two or three times daily, glatiramer acetate, or placebo for 48 weeks to 2 years, with primary endpoints being assessed at 2 years. Both studies showed reduction in relapse rates and in the development of new brain lesions identified on MRI. In the DEFINE trial, active treatment groups experienced a 50% reduction in the annualized relapse rate compared to placebo (0.17 and 0.19 vs. 0.36, respectively). Furthermore, 27% of the active treatment groups experienced a relapse compared to 46% of the placebo group, 36% had a relative risk reduction in disability progression compared to placebo, and there was a significant reduction in the average number of new or enlarging lesions on MRI in the active groups compared to placebo.

The CONFIRM trial randomized people to BG-12 240 mg twice or three times daily, subcutaneous glatiramer acetate 20 mg daily, or placebo in a 1:1:1:1 ratio. At 2 years, the annualized relapse rate was significantly lower in the active treatment groups (0.22, 0.20, 0.29, respectively, compared to 0.40 in the placebo group), and the number of new or enlarging brain lesions on MRI were also significantly lower in the active treatment groups compared to placebo. No significant differences were identified between the two active classes of treatment. Adverse events were mild to moderate and included flushing and gastrointestinal events (diarrhea, nausea, or abdominal pain), which decreased over time.[104,105]

DOSAGE

Dimethyl fumarate (*BG-12, Tecfidera*) 240 mg twice daily, then increase to 240 mg three times daily.

PRECAUTIONS

Laboratory testing for lymphocytopenia should be done at baseline and every 4 to 6 months thereafter because cases of progressive multifocal leukoencephalopathy have been found to occur in patients with preexisting lymphocytopenia. Patients may experience flushing, diarrhea, nausea, or abdominal pain.

Interferon Beta

Interferon beta-1b was the first disease-modifying agent to be approved in the United States. The 5-year data suggest a 33% reduction in relapse frequency and new or enlarging brain lesions on MRI in patients treated with high-dose IFNB-1b (250 mcg) compared to placebo. Disease progression was slower with high-dose IFNB-1b compared to placebo (35% versus 46%, respectively).[106] In addition, all-cause mortality was lowered by 46% among those receiving 50 mcg or 250 mcg of IFNB-1b every other day compared to placebo (17.9, 18.0, and 30.6%, respectively).[107] Earlier commencement and duration of therapy have been shown to improve survival. While the published 5-year data is promising, the long-term benefit of lifelong IFNB remains unclear because the published studies provided treatment for 2 years, at which time point there was unblinding and therefore substantial loss to follow up at 5 years. Of note, one third of patients developed neutralizing antibodies that reduced drug effectiveness.

DOSAGE

Interferon beta-1b (*Betaseron, Extavia*) 50 mcg or 250 mcg every other day by self-injection subcutaneously.

Interferon beta-1a (*Avonex, Rebif*) 22 mcg or 44 mcg three times weekly by self-injection subcutaneously.

Pegylated interferon beta-1a (*Plegridy*) 125 mcg once every 2 or 4 weeks subcutaneously or 30 mcg weekly by intramuscular injection.

PRECAUTIONS

Injection site reaction, headache, fever, flu-like symptoms, pain, diarrhea, constipation, lymphocytopenia, elevation of liver enzymes, myalgias, depression, and anxiety may occur. Caution when using concurrent potentially hepatotoxic medications.

Glatiramer Acetate

Glatiramer acetate (GA) is a synthetic copolymer of tyrosine, glutamate, alanine, and lysine that resembles the myelin sheath components and therefore induces GA-specific T-helper 2 cells, which secrete antiinflammatory cytokines in the CNS through cross-recognition with myelin autoantigens. Research suggests that GA promotes neurogenesis, is neuroprotective, and has antiinflammatory properties.

> **DOSAGE**
>
> Glatiramer (*Copaxone, Glatopa*) 20 mg subcutaneously daily or 40 mg three times weekly.
>
> **PRECAUTIONS**
>
> Glatiramer is well tolerated by most patients. Local injection site reaction is the most prominent adverse reaction. Cases of hepatotoxicity have been reported.

Natalizumab

Natalizumab is a selective adhesion molecule inhibitor used for the treatment of relapsing forms of MS. It was withdrawn from the market shortly after U.S. Food and Drug Administration approval because of the development of progressive multifocal leukoencephalopathy. Consequently, this drug is available only through a restricted program under a risk evaluation and mitigation strategy (REMS) called the TOUCH prescribing program.

Therapies to Consider

Traditional Healing Systems

Traditional Chinese Medicine. Traditional Chinese medicine (TCM) is a codified ancient healing system with a holistic approach that employs therapies such as acupuncture, herbs, and behavioral recommendations. In general, it views MS as representing a heterogeneous group of causes and disease processes. From a TCM perspective, patients with MS often exhibit the signs of spleen deficiency with dampness blocking the channels, or liver or kidney deficiency. In the hands of an experienced practitioner familiar with MS, TCM can be a safe and effective modality. Additionally, separate aspects of TCM, such as acupuncture, are often used for MS-related symptoms. Use of acupuncture has been reported in up to 35% of MS patients.[108]

Ayurveda. Ayurveda is among the oldest existing healing traditions. In explaining disease and healing processes, it relies on the interplay of the three *doshas*, or cardinal humors: *vata* (formed of ether and air), *pita* (formed of fire and water), and *kapha* (formed of earth and water). The Ayurvedic description of MS is analogous to that of biomedicine: an excess of pita (inflammation) burns up the kapha (myelin) and results in an excess of vata. For MS, the reduction of pita (inflammation) and the replenishing of the kapha (myelin) are often targeted with medicinal oils, diet, herbs, and lifestyle changes.

PREVENTION PRESCRIPTION

- Eliminate tobacco
- Engage in stress reduction practice regularly, such as mindfulness or yoga
- Exercise regularly
- Ensure adequate sleep
- Get adequate sunlight
- Monitor vitamin D3 levels
- Eat an antiinflammatory diet (see Chapter 88)
- Evaluate whether you might have food intolerances (e.g., dairy, wheat, corn, etc.) through conducting a 1-month elimination diet (see Chapter 86)
- Consider high-dose biotin 300 mg daily

THERAPEUTIC REVIEW

LIFESTYLE

- Smoking cessation   A↑₁
- Exercise
  - For muscle strength, spasticity, fatigue   B⊘₁
  - For cognition   C→₁
- Regular childhood sunshine exposure   B⊘₁

MIND-BODY THERAPIES

- Yoga for mood and fatigue   B⊘₁
- Mindfulness meditation for QOL, pain, anxiety, depression, fatigue   A↑₁

MAGNETIC THERAPY

- Fatigue   B⊘₁
- Depression   B⊘₁

NUTRITION

- Antiinflammatory diet   C→₁
- Elimination diet   C→₁

SUPPLEMENTS

- Omega-3 fatty acids (antiinflammatory)   C→₁
- 400 to 600 mg docosahexaenoic acid + 400 mg EPA
- Vitamin D (achieve levels just over 80 nmol/L)   B→₂
- Thiol-based antioxidants (NAC, ALA, GSH)   C⊘₂
  - N-acetylcysteine: 1000 mg twice daily
  - Alpha-lipoic acid: 600 to 1200 mg daily
  - Glutathione 600 to 800 mg IV two to three times weekly
- Biotin 300 mg daily   B⊘₁

BOTANICAL

- Ashwagandha, 1 to 2 g of the whole herb in powdered form two or three times a day   C⊘₂

Cannabinoids

Spasticity Symptoms and Pain

- Oral cannabinoids extract
- Synthetic THC *(dronabinol)* 2.5 to 10 mg daily

Spasticity Symptoms, Urinary Frequency, and Pain

- Oromucosal spray *(Sativex)* 2.7 mg THC/2.5 mg CBD spray at a dose of 2.5 to 120 mg daily
- Curcurmin 500 mg to 3 g twice daily
- Ginkgo biloba, standardized 24% flavone glycosides, 7% proanthocyanidins, and 6% terpene lactones, 120 mg twice daily
- Fatigue
- Cognition (no effect)
- EGCG 95% pure, 200-mg capsules three times daily

HORMONES

- Estriol oral 4 mg twice daily
- Oral contraceptives in women: ethinylestradiol 40 mcg and desogestrel 125 mcg
- Pregnancy

- Testosterone in men: 10 g of gel containing 100 mg of testosterone

PHARMACEUTICALS

Acute Relapse

- Corticosteroids oral or IV

Disease-Modifying Therapy for Relapsing-Remitting MS

- Pig whipworm (*T. suis*) oral
- Dimethyl fumaric acid (BG-12) oral 240 mg twice or three times daily
- Interferon beta-1b and -1a injection
  - 1b 50 mcg or 250 mcg every other day by self-injection subcutaneously
  - 1a 22 mcg or 44 mcg three times weekly by self-injection subcutaneously
- Pegylated 1a 125 mcg once every 2 or 4 weeks subcutaneously or 30 mcg weekly by intramuscular injection
- Glatiramer acetate injection: 20 mcg daily subcutaneously
- Natalizumab: 300 mg intravenously every 4 weeks

Key Web Resources

Multiple Sclerosis Foundation. This not-for-profit organization seeks to provide "a comprehensive approach to helping people with MS maintain their health and well being" through programming and education. The website provides a wide variety of information including disease basics, support group contacts, articles on complementary and alternative medicine therapies, online forums, and links for health professionals. In addition, they engage in regular fundraising events that help fund MS research.

http://www.msfocus.org/default.aspx

National Multiple Sclerosis Society. The Society's mission is to "mobilize people and resources to drive research for a cure and to address the challenges of everyone affected by MS." The website features updates on fundraisers and research, a multimedia library, and advocacy and research-oriented resources.

http://www.nationalmssociety.org

REFERENCES

References are available online at ExpertConsult.com.

CHAPTER 15

PARKINSON'S DISEASE

Adam D. Simmons, MD

CLINICAL SIGNS AND SYMPTOMS OF PARKINSON'S DISEASE

Parkinson's disease is a progressive neurodegenerative disorder. Individuals with Parkinson's disease often exhibit a characteristic tremor, a shuffling gait, and masked facial expression. However, the effects of Parkinson's disease are much more widespread.

Preclinical

Parkinson's disease likely starts many years before it is first recognized by either physicians or patients, with subtle and nonspecific early symptoms. Typically, Parkinson's disease progresses slowly; however, the rate of progression is highly variable. In retrospect, many individuals can recall the development of early signs years before they first suspected they had Parkinson's disease. Commonly, early symptoms include constipation in addition to a decreased sense of both smell and taste. Sleep difficulties, such as REM (rapid eye movement) behavior disorder and restless legs syndrome, may also predate motor symptoms by many years. Family members may have noted a decrease in the range of facial expressions, a softness and flatness in the voice, and a more passive personality. Some individuals diagnosed with Parkinson's disease are found to have suffered from late-onset depression for several years prior to diagnosis.

Early Symptoms

While the cardinal features of Parkinson's disease are described as resting tremor, rigidity, bradykinesia, akinesia, postural instability, flexed posture, and "freezing" episodes, these symptoms do not typically present all at once. The early motor signs of Parkinson's disease may be subtle and nonspecific, and are often recognized only in retrospect. A decrease in arm swing or stride length on one side while walking may lead to shoulder, upper back, low back, or hip pain. Decreased fine motor coordination may cause difficulty with buttons and clasps. Thus, getting dressed in the morning may become slower as Parkinson's disease develops. Additional movements may slow and decrease in amplitude. For example, handwriting often becomes smaller and more difficult to read. When tremors first develop, they are often intermittent and most obvious during stressful situations.

As the disease progresses, physical signs become more obvious, and tremor is often more constant. However, tremor may be absent altogether in a proportion of patients, particularly those with a later age of onset.

Parkinsonian tremor is typically present only at rest. A proportion of individuals learn to control tremors by keeping their hands active. As walking becomes more difficult, individuals with Parkinson's disease tend to become more sedentary. Difficulty with initiating movement, in combination with worsening balance, may make rising from soft chairs and car seats an arduous process. As the disease advances, akinesia (lack of movement) and bradykinesia (slowness of movement) continue to become more prominent, and posture may become more stooped. Individuals with Parkinson's disease may attribute these signs to weakness or stiffness of the limbs or body.

Nonmotor Symptoms

In addition to the more well-known motor symptoms, individuals with Parkinson's disease experience a wide range of nonmotor symptoms. Occasionally, these symptoms may be even more disabling than the motor symptoms. The nonmotor symptoms of Parkinson's disease are categorized broadly as psychiatric, autonomic, sleep-related, and sensory (Table 15.1).

Advanced Disease

Unfortunately, some symptoms of advanced Parkinson's disease are not responsive to any currently available medications or surgery. Motor freezing, or episodes when individuals feel that their feet are "glued to the floor," is typically difficult to treat with medications. However, specially modified canes and walkers, which use a laser to project a red line for patients to step over, have utility in breaking these episodes. Other strategies include walking to a rhythm, that is, a marching song. Safety modifications in the home, such as grab bars in the bathroom and kitchen, can help prevent falls and extend patient independence. As fine motor skills diminish, switching to garments without buttons and shoes with Velcro or elastic laces can help with getting dressed. Individuals with low voice volume may benefit from the Lee Silverman Voice Therapy (LSVT) program.[1]

Risk Factors

Epidemiological studies have identified factors that increase the risk of developing Parkinson's disease. By design, such studies are unable to identify definitive causes. While Parkinson's disease is generally more common in industrialized societies, it is observed at a greater frequency in rural areas.[2] Exposure to pesticides,[3] heavy metals,[4] some dairy products,[5] and drinking well water have been shown to increase the risk of Parkinson's disease.[6]

TABLE 15.1	Nonmotor Symptoms in Parkinson's Disease
Psychiatric	Depression Anxiety Apathy Dementia Hallucinations Impulse control disorders
Autonomic	Constipation Orthostasis (lightheadedness on standing) Excessive sweating Urinary incontinence
Sleep Disorders	Insomnia REM behavior disorder Restless legs syndrome Excessive daytime sleepiness Fatigue
Sensory	Impaired sense of smell and taste Blurred vision Numbness and tingling Pain

Large doses of the pesticide rotenone has been shown to cause Parkinsonian syndrome in laboratory rats used experimentally as a model for studying Parkinson's disease.[7] Ironically, rotenone is currently allowed in organic farming practices, although typical exposure rates have not been shown to cause Parkinson's disease.

Trichloroethylene (TCE) is a degreaser used as a dry cleaning solvent to clean metal in factories and in some household cleaning agents. A recent study of twins reported that occupational exposure to TCE increased the risk of Parkinson's disease by five-fold.[8]

Increasing exposure to cigarettes and coffee are correlated with a lower risk of developing Parkinson's disease.[4] While smoking is not recommended as a preventive measure, both nicotine patches[9] and caffeine[10] are being investigated as possible therapies.

PATHOPHYSIOLOGY

The underlying cause of Parkinson's disease remains elusive. The variety in the constellation of symptoms and rate of progression suggest Parkinson's disease is a collection of similar disorders rather than a single entity. A single etiology, therefore, is unlikely to be identified. The variety of epidemiological risk factors indicates multiple competing factors, including genetics, diet, and toxic exposures, among others that have yet to be identified, may contribute to the pathogenesis of Parkinson's disease. The balance of such factors likely determines individual risk of developing Parkinson's disease.

Lewy Bodies

The hallmark pathology of Parkinson's disease is the death of dopaminergic neurons in the brainstem and the presence of intraneuronal inclusions known as Lewy bodies. Lewy bodies contain multiple constituents. However, research has focused on aggregations of the protein

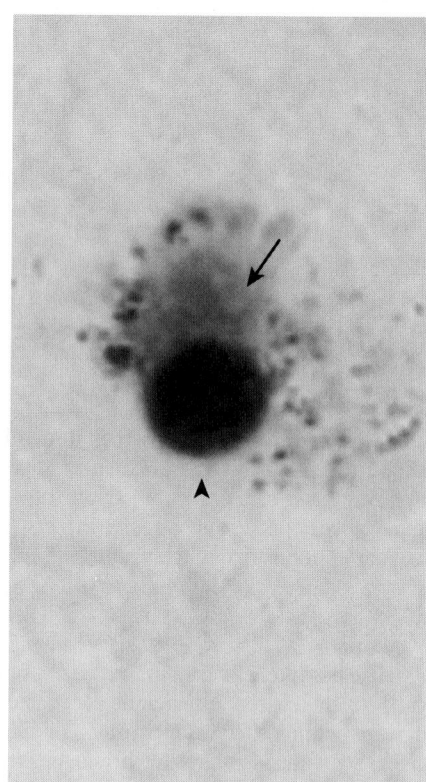

FIG. 15.1 ■ A combination of a pale body (*arrow*) and a small Lewy body (*arrowhead*) in melanized projection cells of the substantia nigra. (Reproduced from Braak H, Del Tredici K, Rüb U, et al. Staging of brain pathology related to sporadic Parkinson's disease. *Neurobiol Aging.* 2003;24:197–211.)

alpha-synuclein bound to the intracellular chaperone protein ubiquitin[11] (Fig. 15.1).

The Braak Hypothesis

A German pathologist, Hideo Braak, conducted an extensive and detailed study of the progression of Lewy body pathology in Parkinson's disease.[12,13] His findings demonstrated the first signs of PD pathology appearing in the CNS are Lewy bodies in the olfactory bulb and the dorsal motor nucleus of the vagus nerve. From there, evidence of Lewy body formation and neuronal cell death spreads rostrally from the medulla. It is not until the substantia nigra is severely affected that patients develop the stereotypical motor symptoms of PD. This evolution and Braak's proposed staging system supports the concept of a preclinical stage of Parkinson's disease. Braak's study also indicates Parkinson's disease is not simply a disease of dopamine deficiency, with other neurotransmitters also affected, including the serotonergic, histaminergic, and noradrenergic systems. These other neurotransmitters are thought to be involved in the etiology of many of the nonmotor symptoms of Parkinson's disease.

The Mitochondrial Hypothesis

A recurring theme in hypotheses of the etiology of Parkinson's disease is dysfunction of the mitochondria. Damage to mitochondrial complex I has been reported in individuals with Parkinson's disease.[14] Impaired energy metabolism in the mitochondria of dopaminergic neurons may lead to production of reactive oxygen species,[15] with the resulting oxidative damage to cell proteins, lipids, and DNA eventually leading to cell death.[16]

Alpha-Synuclein

Recent studies indicate a central role for the protein alpha-synuclein in the pathogenesis of Parkinson's disease. It has long been known that alpha-synuclein can be found bound to ubiquitin within Lewy bodies in areas of the brain affected by Parkinson's disease.[17] However, unbound alpha-synuclein may be more harmful to neurons.[18] In conjunction with dopamine, alpha-synuclein enhances neuronal susceptibility to death from oxidative stress.[19] Evidence is mounting that alpha-synuclein becomes capable of transmitting PD pathology when misfolded, much like the misfolded prion proteins responsible for the transmission of Creutzfeld-Jacob ("mad cow") disease.[20-22]

INTEGRATIVE THERAPY

An integrative and multidisciplinary approach to treating Parkinson's disease should start with optimizing general health through exercise and diet. Some patients will choose to take supplements for their potential neuroprotective benefits, while others will prefer to wait for definitive studies. Pharmaceuticals will eventually be required to help control the motor symptoms of Parkinson's disease. A thorough discussion of the treatment of the nonmotor symptoms of Parkinson's disease can be very lengthy and beyond the scope of this chapter. Modalities from alternative medical systems will also be covered.

Nutrition

A large, prospective population-based study in Rotterdam, the Netherlands, found a higher dietary intake of omega-3 fatty acids was associated with a decreased risk of PD.[23] The effect was entirely due to the intake of plant-based α-linolenic acid rather than fish oils. Even without a preventive effect, fish oil may still have benefit for patients with Parkinson's disease. A separate double-blind, placebo-controlled study of patients with Parkinson's disease and major depression found improved mood symptoms in patients taking fish oil, with or without antidepressants.[24] Additionally, fish oil supplements were shown to reduce the risk of sudden cardiac death in otherwise healthy men in the Physician's Health Study.[25]

Nutrition Suggestions for Patients With Parkinson's Disease

- Eat foods high in fiber to lessen constipation.
- Foods high in omega-3 fatty acids may be beneficial.
- Eat colorful fruits and vegetables for dietary sources of antioxidants.

Exercise

Aerobic Exercise

Aerobic exercise has a multitude of benefits for people with or without Parkinson's disease. A systematic review including multiple exercise modalities found significant benefit for people with Parkinson's disease.[26] Improvements were found in physical functioning, health-related quality of life, strength, balance, and gait speed. Additionally, a large cohort study demonstrated individuals with regular exercise had a better quality of life, better mobility, better physical function, less progression of disease, less caregiver burden, and less cognitive decline.[27] Data from animal studies have indicated aerobic exercise may be neuroprotective and slow the progression of Parkinson's disease.[28,29] Furthermore, exercise has utility in reducing depression and anxiety,[30] both common issues in Parkinson's disease. Forms of exercise that have been studied range widely from aerobic walking,[31] tango dancing,[32] and playing video games on a Nintendo Wii.[33] There is no clear evidence to suggest one form of exercise has greater benefit over another. Therefore, choosing an exercise program that is enjoyable enough to be continued is considered the best strategy.

Tai Chi

Tai chi is a martial art that started in ancient China as a means of self-defense. However, over time it became primarily used for health purposes. Tai chi emphasizes the cultivation of internal energy, qi, through the meditative properties of paying close attention to the details of movements. There are many different styles of tai chi, but all involve slow, relaxed, graceful movements, with each movement flowing into the next. The body is in constant motion and posture is important. Individuals practicing tai chi must concentrate, put aside all distracting thoughts, and breathe in a deep and relaxed but focused manner. In the Chinese community, people commonly practice tai chi in nearby parks, often in early morning before going to work.[34]

The largest published study of tai chi in Parkinson's disease demonstrated a significantly reduced risk of falling.[35] Other studies evaluating objective improvements in laboratory measures of gait or balance have not shown measurable differences.[36] However, one of the same researchers did report improvements in some of the nonmotor symptoms of Parkinson's disease.[37] There is sufficient evidence to suggest tai chi is a safe and effective exercise for reducing falls and improving general well-being in Parkinson's disease.

Benefits of Exercise in Parkinson Disease

Aerobic exercise has multiple benefits including:
- Increasing energy levels
- Decreasing depression and anxiety
- Potentially slowing disease progression
- Tai chi and yoga may help maintain and improve balance.

Supplements

N-Acetyl Cysteine

While there is evidence that glutathione can be transported actively across the blood–brain barrier, it is unable to cross passively or in large volumes.[38] Therefore, endogenous production is likely the primary source of brain glutathione stores. N-acetyl cysteine is a precursor to glutathione that is able to cross the blood–brain barrier.[39] It may, therefore, be a more effective way of increasing intraneuronal glutathione levels than intravenous infusions of glutathione. In animal studies, N-acetyl cysteine has been shown to increase glutathione levels in the brain.[40] N-acetyl cysteine has also been shown to protect against cell death in animal models of Parkinson's disease.[41] Although associated with the smell of rotten eggs, it is typically well-tolerated.[42]

DOSAGE

1200 to 2400 mg per day

PRECAUTIONS

Frequent side effects include nausea, vomiting, and diarrhea.[43]

Glutathione

Glutathione is a potent, naturally occurring intracellular antioxidant. Glutathione levels are significantly reduced in the substantia nigra of patients with early Parkinson's disease.[44] Glutathione has been trialed as a twice daily intravenous infusion in a small open label study.[45] A more recent double-blinded study of intravenous infusions three times a week demonstrated a positive trend early but worsening of symptoms after treatment cessation.[46] A phase II clinical trial of an intranasal delivery system for glutathione, that bypasses the blood–brain barrier, is being conducted at Bastyr University.[47] However, there is currently insufficient enough evidence to support the use of glutathione in the treatment of Parkinson's disease.

N-acetyl cysteine is a precursor of glutathione and can help replenish reduced glutathione levels as a result of reactive oxygen species that play a role in the pathogenesis of PD.

Co-Enzyme Q10

Coenzyme Q10 (CoQ10), or ubiquinone, is the electron receptor of mitochondrial complexes I and II. CoQ10 levels are significantly reduced in the mitochondria of individuals with early Parkinson's disease.[48] A randomized controlled trial in patients with Parkinson's disease reported a statistically significant slowing of the decline in a clinical rating scale (UPDRS) at the highest dose of 1200 mg of CoQ10 with 1200 IU of vitamin E.[49] However, a second and larger trial using 1200 mg and 2400 mg doses of CoQ10, in addition to 1200 IU of vitamin E, was halted due to a lack of beneficial effect. The authors concluded that CoQ10 was safe; however, there was a trend toward worse outcome in the treatment groups.[50]

CDP-Choline

CDP-choline, or citicoline, is an intermediate in the synthesis of phospholipids, which are essential components in the assembly and repair of cell and mitochondrial membranes. Therefore, CDP-choline may have neuroprotective qualities as well as therapeutic effects in Parkinson's disease.[51,52] Several studies have investigated using CDP-choline as a supplement to levodopa. CDP-choline reportedly allows reductions in levodopa doses by up to 50% without any reduction in symptom control.[53,54] CDP-choline may enhance dopaminergic therapy in Parkinson's disease through multiple mechanisms, including decreased reuptake of dopamine leading to increased levels at the synaptic cleft. Additionally, CDP-choline activates tyrosine-hydroxylase and induces increased dopamine production.[55]

DOSAGE

750 to 1500 mg orally per day

PRECAUTIONS

CDP-choline use without lowering levodopa doses can lead to increased dyskinesias and other levodopa-induced side effects.

Vitamin D

Vitamin D is a secosteroid hormone that has modulating effects on immune and neural cells in addition to its classical actions on calcium and bone metabolism.[56] Vitamin D can be obtained from dietary sources as well as manufacture by the skin with exposure to sunlight. Vitamin D deficiency has been shown to be markedly more common in patients with Parkinson's disease.[57,58] Additionally, vitamin D deficiency is associated with an increased risk of developing Parkinson's disease. Individuals with serum 25-hydroxyvitamin D concentrations greater than 20 ng/mL were reported to have a 65% lower risk of developing Parkinson's disease than those with levels below 10 ng/mL.[59] Vitamin D has been demonstrated to be neuroprotective in animal models of Parkinson's disease.[60,61] Administration of 1,25-dihydroxyvitamin D3 reportedly increases glial cell line-derived neurotrophic factor (GDNF) mRNA and protein levels in the striatum of rats.[62] GDNF has shown promise as neuroprotective agent in animal models of Parkinson's disease.[63] A preliminary study demonstrated a trend toward improved balance with vitamin D supplementation;[64] however, further studies are required to determine the efficacy of vitamin D supplementation in treating Parkinson's disease.

Vitamin E

Vitamin E (tocopherol) has been investigated by one of the longest studies of neuroprotection in Parkinson's disease. Ten-year follow-up data from the DATATOP study found no evidence that 2000 IU doses of vitamin E have efficacy in slowing the progression of Parkinson's disease.[65] Additionally, 14-year data from the Nurses Health Study found no association between reduced risk of developing Parkinson's disease and vitamin E supplementation. However, the consumption of nuts, which contain high levels of vitamin E, was found to be associated with a reduced risk of developing Parkinson's disease. Nut consumption may have served as a marker of a healthier diet.[66]

Vitamin B$_6$ (pyridoxine)

Vitamin B$_6$ can increase peripheral conversion of levodopa to dopamine and should therefore be avoided in individuals taking carbidopa/levodopa. The decarboxylase inhibitor carbidopa can be used to prevent this effect, but may not be effective with high doses of vitamin B$_6$.[67]

Creatine

Creatine monohydrate is a supplement often used to improve athletic performance, increase muscle mass, and serve as an intracellular energy source. In a small 12-month trial, creatine was found to marginally slow the progression of Parkinson's disease.[68] However, a much larger follow-up study (NET-PD) was halted at 5 years due to a lack of benefit. These findings do not support the use of creatine monohydrate in patients with Parkinson disease.[69]

Botanicals

Green Tea (EGCG)

Epidemiological studies have indicated drinking three cups of tea per day may decrease the risk of developing Parkinson's disease by 28%. While other caffeinated beverages, such as coffee, also are linked with a reduced risk of Parkinson's disease,[4] there is evidence that other constituents may account for at least some of the observed beneficial effects.[70] In addition to caffeine, green tea contains multiple polyphenols, catechins, and flavonols.[71] The potent antioxidant EGCG is the most studied component to date. Moreover, green tea may be beneficial in Parkinson's disease as an inhibitor of both apoptosis and of toxic alpha-synuclein fibrils in addition to its antioxidant effects.[72-74]

DOSAGE

3 cups per day

PRECAUTIONS

Green tea can be a strong diuretic.

Curcumin

Curcumin is a phenolic compound with antiinflammatory properties that is found in the spice turmeric. Turmeric is commonly used in Indian and Asian foods, particularly curries. Curcumin has been used also for centuries in the Ayurvedic medical tradition in India. Curcumin has been shown to be a potent antioxidant that can attenuate loss of glutathione in cultured dopaminergic cells.[75] It has also been shown to reduce cell loss in an animal model of Parkinson's disease.[76] Additionally, curcumin reportedly protects against apoptosis in a cultured dopaminergic cell line,[77] with the aggregation of alpha-synuclein and level of toxic misfolded variants reduced.[78]

DOSAGE

Studies in people with Parkinson's disease have not yet to be reported. However, typical doses of curcumin for other conditions range from 400 to 600 mg curcumin in capsules three times a day, to 3 g turmeric root daily in divided doses.[79] As an alternative to taking curcumin capsules, patients may incorporate increased amounts of turmeric into their diet.

PRECAUTIONS

Curcumin may cause mild stomach upset at high doses of several grams.

Mucuna Pruriens

Mucuna pruriens (velvet bean or cowhage) is a leguminous plant that has been used for centuries in Ayurvedic medicine for the treatment of Parkinson's disease. Mucuna pruriens contains levodopa as well as two components of the mitochondrial electron transport chain; coenzyme Q10 and nicotine adenine dinucleotide (NADH).[80] In a single-dose, randomized controlled trial, a mucuna seed powder formulation had comparable efficacy to levodopa in reducing Parkinsonian symptoms.[81] This formulation had a quicker onset and caused less dyskinesias than levodopa. The results of an open-label study of another formulation, HP-200, in 60 patients over 12 weeks indicated Mucuna pruriens was well tolerated and helped alleviate Parkinsonian symptoms.[82] Currently, neither formulation is commercially available.

ACUPUNCTURE

There have been few studies of the efficacy of acupuncture in patients with Parkinson's disease. Two meta-analyses of the current literature concluded that there is not sufficient evidence to support or refute the use of acupuncture in Parkinson's disease.[83,84] Both reviews suggested that larger randomized controlled trials were warranted, particularly as some studies with design flaws reported promising results. For Parkinson's disease, acupuncture may be particularly useful in the treatment of some nonmotor symptoms or associated symptoms, such as back and joint pains. An open label study of acupuncture in 20 patients with Parkinson's disease reportedly statistically significant improvements in sleep.[85] Additionally, 85% of patients reported subjective improvements in at least one individual symptom. A separate pilot study of acupuncture in Parkinson's disease demonstrated positive trends toward decreased nausea, improved sleep, greater ease of activities of daily living, and improved quality of life.[86]

PHARMACEUTICALS

Levodopa

Levodopa remains the gold-standard therapeutic agent in Parkinson's disease. Levodopa is an amino acid that easily crosses the blood–brain barrier, where it is converted into dopamine to increase neuronal supply. Levodopa is combined with a decarboxylase inhibitor, carbidopa, in the US to prevent conversion in the peripheral bloodstream.

Levodopa remains the most effective treatment for the majority of the motor symptoms of PD, with the possible exception of tremor. However, the administration of levodopa is often delayed in the mistaken belief that early treatment will shorten the number of years that it will remain effective.[87]

Two new, long-acting, formulations of carbidopa/levodopa are now available. Rytary™ is a capsule containing a combination of immediate-release and extended-release carbidopa/levodopa beads. Duopa™ is a gel formulation of carbidopa/levodopa that is continuously pumped through a PEG tube directly into the small intestine.

DOSAGE

Carbidopa/levodopa 25/100 mg three times a day (early disease). As the disease progresses, patients may take up to 2 g levodopa per day in divided doses as frequently as every 2 hours.

PRECAUTIONS

Levodopa may cause lightheadedness, fatigue, nausea, confusion, hallucinations, dyskinesias, and lower extremity edema. However, levodopa tends to cause fewer side effects for the amount of benefit compared to other dopamine agonists.

Dopamine Agonists

Ropinirole, pramipexole, and the rotigotine patch are the primary dopamine agonists used in the US. All have very similar efficacy and are very effective at primarily treating the motor symptoms of Parkinson's disease. Dopamine agonists act as a replacement for decreased dopamine levels in the brain by directly stimulating dopamine receptors and are often used in early Parkinson's disease to delay the introduction of levodopa and risk of developing dyskinesias.[88] Extended release formulations of both ropinirole and pramipexole are available.

DOSAGE

Ropinirole: start: 0.25 mg three times a day; maximum of 24 mg per day
Pramipexole: start: 0.125 mg three times a day; maximum of 4.5 mg per day
Rotigotine: start: 2 mg/24 hr patch once a day; maximum of 8 mg/24 hr patch once a day

PRECAUTIONS

Both dopamine agonists have a similar range of side effects. The most common are sleepiness, fatigue, nausea, and lower extremity swelling. Patients have fallen asleep while driving without first feeling sleepy.[89] There is also an increase in obsessive and compulsive behaviors that may rarely cause serious problems (i.e., gambling, sexual obsessions). Milder impulse control problems are common.[90]

Rasagiline

Rasagiline is a highly-selective monoamine oxidase type B (MAO-B) inhibitor that slows the endogenous breakdown of dopamine and its precursor, levodopa. Unlike rasagiline's older cousin, selegiline, no amphetamines are produced during the degradation of rasagiline. This difference is significant because amphetamines are considered to be neurotoxic. Rasagiline can be used as a stand-alone treatment in early Parkinson's disease, although its symptomatic effects are typically mild. In later disease, rasagiline can extend the length of action of levodopa and reduce "off" time.

Recent studies have indicated that rasagiline may be neuroprotective via antiapoptotic effects. In a study using a delayed start design, rasagiline was found to slow the progression of the clinical symptoms of Parkinson's disease.[91,92]

DOSAGE

Rasagiline 1 mg orally, once per day

PRECAUTIONS

Rasagiline usually is very well tolerated with few side effects. Despite being an MAO inhibitor, there are no food restrictions and rasagiline can be used with many antidepressant medications. However, rasagiline should not be taken with tramadol or medications containing dextromethorphan. Rarely, rasagiline may cause a dangerous excess of serotonin (serotonin syndrome), with symptoms including flushing, sweating, tremors, diarrhea, and elevated blood pressure.

COMT Inhibitors

Entacapone and tolcapone both inhibit the degradation of dopamine and levodopa by blocking the enzyme, catechol-O-methyl transferase (COMT). Entacapone is used more frequently as there have been rare cases of liver failure with tolcapone. Accordingly, hepatic enzymes must be monitored carefully during tolcapone treatment. Entacapone can increase the length of action of levodopa when taken concurrently. However, because entacapone has no effect on its own, it is also available as a combination pill with carbidopa/levodopa.

DOSAGE

Entacapone 200 mg taken with each dose of carbidopa/levodopa; maximum of 1600 mg per day (8 doses)

PRECAUTIONS

Entacapone can potentiate the side effects of levodopa, including dyskinesia, lightheadedness, confusion, and hallucinations. Although not dangerous, patients will often be concerned if they are unaware that entacapone may turn the urine a dark orange or yellow color.

Amantadine

Amantadine is an antiviral medication used to treat and prevent influenza infections. Amantadine was serendipitously found to reduce Parkinson's disease motor symptoms when it was given prophylactically in a nursing home. Amantadine can be used as a standalone treatment or in combination with rasagiline for the early symptoms of Parkinson's disease, including tremor.[93,94] Amantadine can also be used to reduce dyskinesias, fidgety movements that are a side-effect of levodopa, later in the course of the disease.

DOSAGE
100 mg twice a day to three times a day

PRECAUTIONS
Amantadine may cause confusion and hallucinations, particularly in the elderly. Fatigue, lower extremity edema, lacy rash (levido reticularis), and lightheadedness are other common side effects.

Zonisamide

Zonisamide is an antiepileptic medication that has been found to have efficacy in treating Parkinson's disease. Zonisamide has specific efficacy for reducing tremor and is posited to work by several mechanisms. Zonisamide has been found to stimulate dopamine synthesis and may also directly inhibit the indirect pathway through delta opioid receptors.[95] Zonisamide has also been shown to reduce neuronal and astroglial cell loss in animal models of Parkinson's disease.[96,97]

DOSAGE
25 mg to 100 mg per day as one dose or divided into two doses

PRECAUTIONS
Kidney stones can occur in up to 1% to 2% of patients taking zonisamide,[98] and patients taking zonisamide should be advised to keep well-hydrated. Other side effects include weight loss, dry mouth, fatigue, and nausea.

Anticholinergic Medications

Anticholinergic medications are rarely used as a primary treatment for Parkinson's disease due to the high incidence of side effects, such as hallucinations, confusion, drowsiness, dry mouth, urinary retention, and blurry vision. However, trihexyphenidyl can be very effective in treating tremor refractory to other medications.

DOSAGE
Trihexyphenidyl 6 mg to 15 mg per day in three divided doses

SURGERY

Deep Brain Stimulation Surgery

Deep brain stimulation surgery for Parkinson's disease involves the placement of a permanent electrode into the basal ganglia for continuous, high-frequency electrical stimulation. Deep brain stimulation is considered in patients who remain responsive to levodopa, but its effects are not maintained. Surgical candidates may appear to cycle rapidly from feeling "frozen" to being wildly dyskinetic without spending much time in a comfortable state. Other patients may be considered for surgery if they are unable to tolerate sufficient doses of levodopa due to side effects. In a study of 255 patients that fit these criteria, deep brain stimulation surgery was shown to be more effective than optimal medical management.[99] This study found patients who received deep brain stimulation were more likely to experience a clinically significant improvement in motor function (71% vs. 32%). On average, the deep brain stimulation group gained 4.6 hours of time with good motor function per day. However, serious adverse events were more common with deep brain stimulation. In a similar study, significant improvements in motor function were observed at four years after surgery.[100]

MIND-BODY CONNECTION

Depression and anxiety are extremely common in Parkinson's disease, with approximately 20% to 40% of surveyed patients reporting these conditions.[101,102] Depression in Parkinson's disease is frequently unrecognized, in part due to the significant overlap of outward manifestations.[103] In Parkinson's disease, depression may decrease quality of life more than motor symptoms.[104] Accordingly, it is important to screen for these disorders and initiate counseling if identified.

Increased stress levels have been found to exacerbate the symptoms of Parkinson's disease in a temporary fashion. While there is no significant clinical evidence for or against their use, mindfulness-based stress reduction programs may be considered. A study of an 8-week mindfulness-based intervention reported an increase in grey matter density following the intervention.[105] Other mind-body exercises, such as yoga and Qi Gong, should be also be considered for stress reduction.

PREVENTION PRESCRIPTION

For the treatment of Parkinson's disease, risk reduction rather than prevention is the goal.
- Engage in regular aerobic exercise.
- Drink 3 cups of tea per day, preferably green tea.
- Maintain a diet high in antioxidants and omega-3 fatty acids.
- Eat a handful (not a canful) of nuts daily (rich in vitamin E and in B vitamins).
- Reduce exposure to pesticides. Wash all fruits and vegetables carefully, including those that are grown organically.
- Reduce exposure to heavy metals. Test and filter well water as appropriate.
- Reduce exposure to industrial solvents and dry cleaning.

THERAPEUTIC REVIEW

The following is a summary of the therapeutic options for Parkinson's disease. As Parkinson's disease has a variety of manifestations and symptoms, the ladder approach to treatment may not always work but may be appropriate for mild motor symptoms. Because Parkinson's disease is a chronic and progressive disease, the majority of patients will eventually need to be treated using strategies from multiple rungs of the ladder below.

Category	Items	Rating
Remove Exacerbating Medications	If other medical conditions allow, stop all medications that may induce Parkinsonism such as neuroleptic drugs, metoclopramide, and prochlorperazine. Amlodipine, lithium, valproate, and amiodarone are more rarely implicated and typically more difficult to discontinue.	
	Reduce exposures to pesticides.	
	Have well water tested to reduce exposures to heavy metals.	
Mind-Body Therapy	Facilitate optimism. The placebo effect is very strong in Parkinson's disease.	B↗1
Exercise	Encourage regular aerobic exercise.	A↑1
	Consider Tai Chi for stress management and improving balance.	B↗1
Nutrition	A high fiber diet may help with constipation.	B↗1
	Encourage foods rich in omega-3 fatty acids, such as salmon, walnuts, pumpkin seeds, and flax seeds.	C→1
	Use turmeric in cooking.	C→1
	Drink 3 cups of tea per day, preferably green tea.	B↗1
Neuroprotection	Rasagiline 1 mg daily.	B↘2
	N-acetyl cysteine 600 mg twice daily.	C↘2
	Encourage regular aerobic exercise.	B↗2
Therapeutic Supplements	CDP-Choline 500 to 1250 mg daily. Reduce carbidopa/levodopa dose to 30%–50% if given together.	B↘2
Acupuncture	Acupuncture may help with the nonmotor and pain symptoms of Parkinson disease.	B↗1
Pharmaceuticals	The overall strategy is to initiate treatment with an MAO inhibitor and then trial either amantadine or a dopamine agonist in patients without cognitive impairment. Treatment should be initiated with carbidopa/levodopa in patients with prominent gait impairment, significant rigidity, or cognitive impairment.	
	Rasagiline: 1 mg daily.	A⊘2
	Amantadine: 100 mg twice daily to three times daily.	B→2
	Dopamine agonists	A⊘2
	Ropinirole: start with 0.25 mg TID and titrate up to a maximum of 24 mg per day.	
	Pramipexole: start with 0.125 mg TID and titrate up to a maximum of 4.5 mg per day.	
	Rotigotine patch: start with 2 mg/24 hr and titrate up to a maximum of 8 mg/24 hr.	
	Carbidopa/levodopa IR: titrate up from carbidopa/levodopa 25/100 half tablet three times daily up to carbidopa/levodopa 25/250 QID as necessary.	A⊘2
	For tremor-predominant Parkinson's disease, start with:	
	Zonisamide: 25 mg to 100 mg daily.	B→2
	Trihexyphenidyl–titrate up from 1mg daily to twice daily then three times daily, to a maximum of 15 mg per day.	B→2
	If carbidopa/levodopa wears off early consider:	
	Rasagiline: 1 mg daily (if not already being used).	A⊘2
	Entacapone: 200 mg with each dose of carbidopa/levodopa up to 8 doses per day.	A⊘2
	Rytary™ (carbidopa/levodopa) with dose conversion according to a chart found in the prescription insert.	A⊘2

Category	Items	Rating
	If dyskinesias develop and are causing the patient problems, trial decreasing the dose of carbidopa/levodopa or division into smaller but more frequent doses. If this is not possible, consider adding:	
	Amantadine 100 mg twice daily to three times daily.	B2
Surgery	Consider deep brain stimulation surgery targeting either the subthalamic nucleus or the globus pallidus internus for patients who respond to levodopa yet have severe motor fluctuations with rapid wearing off or dyskinesias.	A3
	Consider the Duopa™ pump for patients who respond to levodopa yet have severe motor fluctuations with rapid wearing off or dyskinesias but are not candidates for neurosurgery.	B3

Key Web Resources

Purpose	URL
American Parkinson Disease Association. Local and national Parkinson's disease events	http://www.apdaparkinson.org
The Michael J. Fox Foundation for Parkinson's Research. News about current Parkinson's disease research	https://www.michaeljfox.org
National Parkinson Foundation. Clinical, research, education and outreach programs	http://www.parkinson.org
EWG Guide. List of the most and least contaminated crops	http://www.ewg.org/foodnews
US Environmental Protection Agency. Information on water testing, filtering, and safety	http://www.epa.gov/safewater
In-Step Mobility Products, Inc. U-Step walkers and canes with laser light	http://www.ustep.com
LSVT Global. Lee Silverman Voice Technique: LOUD & BIG therapy programs	http://www.lsvtglobal.com

REFERENCES

References are available online at ExpertConsult.com.

SECTION III

INFECTIOUS DISEASE

SECTION OUTLINE

16 OTITIS MEDIA

17 CHRONIC SINUSITIS

18 VIRAL UPPER RESPIRATORY INFECTION

19 HIV DISEASE AND AIDS

20 HERPES SIMPLEX VIRUS

21 CHRONIC HEPATITIS

22 URINARY TRACT INFECTION (UTI)

23 LYME DISEASE

CHAPTER 16

OTITIS MEDIA

David K. Becker, MD

PATHOPHYSIOLOGY

Otitis media (OM) is a generic term for inflammation of the middle ear. Middle ear infections occur when fluid accumulates in the middle ear as a result of the body's inflammatory response to viral or bacterial infection. Occasionally, sterile fluid may accumulate due to dysfunction of the eustachian tube (Fig. 16.1), a finding more common in children as the eustachian tube occasionally fails to function sufficiently due to small size or abnormal shape. Otitis media is divided into 3 categories for clinical and research purposes: acute OM (AOM), OM with effusion (OME), and chronic OM with effusion (chronic serous OM or CSOM).[1] AOM is the most commonly diagnosed subtype and commonly occurs as part of, or a complication of, upper respiratory tract infection. The OME designation can be confusing as middle ear effusions occasionally present without signs of inflammation. Effusions may also occur as part of the healing process following AOM (which can last weeks to months) or as a complication of eustachian tube dysfunction. CSOM may be associated with auditory and speech impairments.[2] The tympanic membrane is a thin, sensitive layer of skin that, when inflamed or under pressure, can be a source of significant pain (see Fig. 16.1). Infectious causes of AOM include viral (influenza, adenovirus, others) and bacterial pathogens (nontypeable *Haemophilus influenzae, Streptococcus pneumoniae, Moraxella catarrhalis*),[3,4] with earache and fever common presenting symptoms. Factors that may predispose to an increased frequency of OM include atopy (allergic rhinitis and cow's milk allergy), exposure to prenatal and postnatal tobacco smoke,[5] and exposure to air pollution.[6]

INTEGRATIVE THERAPY

An integrative approach to otitis media begins with primary prevention—reducing the risk factors that contribute to otitis. For management of acute or chronic OM, the goal is selecting a treatment approach that balances the relative risks and benefits of the range of options available that may help relieve symptoms and supporting the body's natural healing response. Finally, secondary prevention options should be considered for the reduction of recurrence and sequelae of repeat infections. Commonly used therapies for otitis include biologically based therapies (including pharmaceuticals), manual and body-based therapies, and homeopathy. It may be helpful to review with families the epidemiology and natural history of upper respiratory infections (URIs). The majority of young children have at least 6 URIs per year.[7] URIs are common, frequently occur back to back, and can be frustrating for patients and families despite being a normal part of childhood experience. Because at least 80% of cases of AOM resolve without antibiotic treatment,[8] the majority of patients can be observed without antibiotics, with treatment focused on symptom relief and supporting the body's healing response. Caution is warranted for careful observation for rare but significant complications of AOM, including mastoiditis, tympanic membrane perforation, and meningitis.

Nutrition

A number of nutritional interventions have been studied for recurrent acute otitis media (ROM). An interesting cross-sectional study found increased odds of pneumococcal carriage among children consuming a diet high in processed sweets, with a diet higher in fruits and berries found to be associated with a decreased risk of AOM (odds ratio, 1.36; 95% CI 1.03–1.9; P = 0.03).[9] A small pilot study of 8 children administered 1 tsp of cod liver oil with vitamin A plus a selenium supplement found that study participants received antibiotics for 12% fewer days than controls.[10]

Biochemical

Pharmacies and natural health stores abound in remedies marketed for the treatment of symptoms associated with OM. Over-the-counter products containing pharmaceutical agents for management of cough and congestion in young children have been strongly discouraged by the U.S. Food and Drug Administration due to concerns regarding potential harm and lack of efficacy.[11] Acetaminophen and ibuprofen can be effective in reducing fever and pain but can also have significant side effects. However, strong epidemiological evidence indicates acetaminophen may be associated with subsequent development of asthma if used with high frequency.[12] Judicious use is warranted.

> Ibuprofen and/or acetaminophen can be used for pain relief in children with acute otitis media. But be careful with over-prescribing acetaminophen as some data suggests excessive use may increase the risk of asthma.

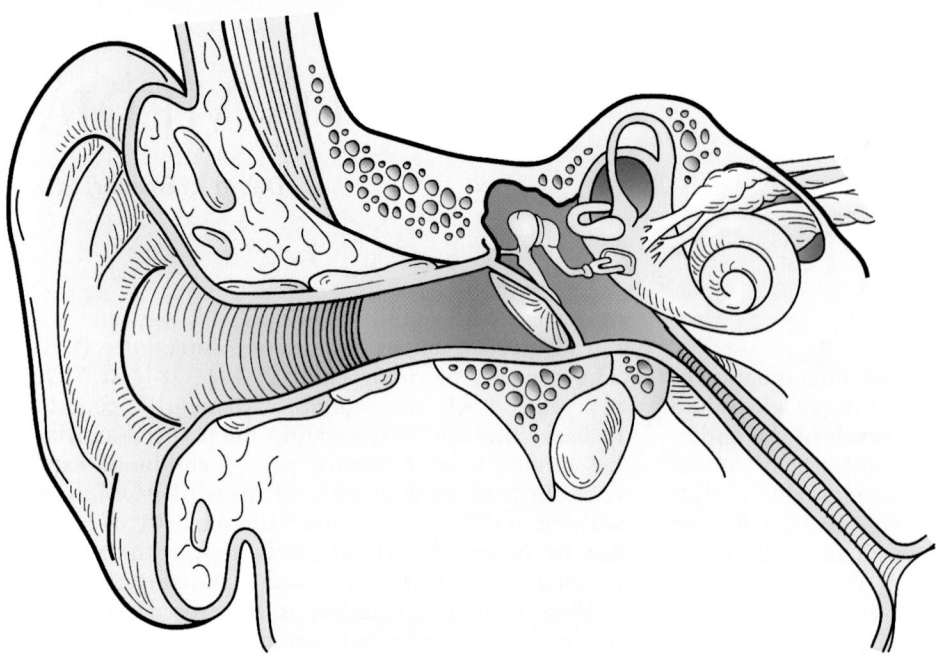

FIG. 16.1 ■ Anatomy of the ear.

Botanicals

Combination Herbal Extract Ear Drops

Botanically based topical ear drops are available from a wide variety of manufacturers. Guidance on specific brands or herbal combinations is limited by a lack data and variability in the contents of products. A specific product combination used in previous studies included the following ingredients: garlic *(Allium sativum)*, mullein flower *(Verbascum thapsus)*, calendula flower, St. John's wort *(Hypericum perfoliatum)*, lavender, and vitamin E in an olive oil base. In two separate trials of children aged 5–18 years, this combination was found to be effective as topical anesthetic drops in relieving pain.

Other botanical remedies for upper respiratory tract infections may have benefit in children with uncomplicated URI's and associated middle ear effusions[7] (see Chapter 18).

Supplements

Xylitol

Several trials have evaluated the efficacy of xylitol in preventing AOM episodes. A Cochrane review found "fair evidence" that xylitol reduces AOM occurrences by up to 25% among children attending day care.[13] However, a negative trial using a dose of 5 g three times a day suggests higher doses and frequency may be necessary.[14]

DOSAGE

The conclusions of a Cochrane review suggest 8–10 mg of xylitol in 5 divided doses daily may be necessary.

PRECAUTIONS

Xylitol has few adverse effects but, when they do occur, they generally present as stomach upset and diarrhea. Xylitol is a polyol sugar that is avoided in the FODMaPs diet that has been reported to be beneficial for irritable bowel syndrome (see Chapter 90).

Vitamin D

Low vitamin D levels have been reported to be associated with poor health outcomes by numerous epidemiological studies. Two prospective controlled trials of vitamin D supplementation in children with a history of ROM both reported a significantly reduced subsequent incidence of AOM among children with low initial levels of vitamin D.[15,16] Of note, neither study attempted to achieve unusually high vitamin D levels. On average, vitamin D levels after the intervention were between 23 and 36.8 ng/mL.

DOSAGE

In those with ROM and low vitamin D levels, supplementation with vitamin D3 should be administered to raise serum levels to a level >25 ng/mL. Generally, 1000 IU of vitamin D are required to raise serum levels by 8–10 ng/mL.

Probiotics

Two comprehensive review studies and a recent randomized trial failed to provide evidence to support probiotics as an effective preventive strategy for AOM.[17–19] The studies included in the reviews used different probiotic strains in varying quantities, which highlights the complexity of this research field. Another review suggests that probiotics may reduce the colonization of *Streptococcus pneumonia*, but no direct reduction in AOM incidence has yet been shown.[20] Research in this area is growing but limited by the immense diversity of the microbiome. While there are not yet data that clearly support the use of probiotics for the treatment or prevention of OM, the safety profile and potential benefit mean a treatment trial in some circumstances is reasonable.

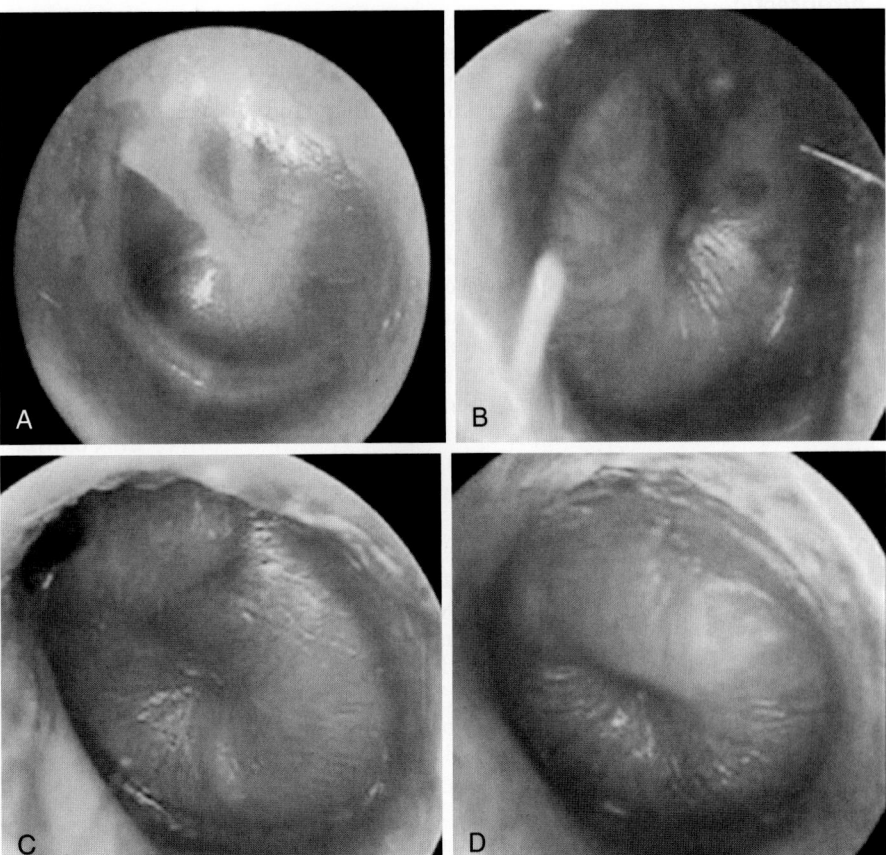

FIG. 16.2 ■ A, Normal TM. B, TM with mild bulging. C, TM with moderate bulging. D, TM with severe bulging. (Courtesy of Alejandro Hoberman)

Pharmaceuticals

The widespread use of antibiotics for AOM has come under much-needed critical review over the past 5–10 years. While concerns regarding antibiotic resistance were of primary interest among conventional critiques, other concerns, including effects on the microbiome, have now gained recognition as well. Current guidelines from the American Academy of Pediatrics (AAP) emphasize the use of otoscopy to confirm the presence of acute erythema *and* purulent effusion causing *significant* bulging of the tympanic membrane as the most specific signs of a bacterial infection warranting antibiotic treatment to prevent significant complications, particularly in younger children[2] (Fig. 16.2). Most cases of AOM do not have this combination of findings and can be observed and followed for resolution without the use of antibiotics as the initial treatment.

The most sensitive sign to support the use of antibiotics in acute otitis media is a bulging tympanic membrane with erythema and purulent effusion on otoscopy (see Fig. 16.2).

Should the use of antibiotics be indicated, first-line treatment should cover the most common bacterial pathogens, including *S. pneumoniae*, *Haemophilus influenzae*, and *Moraxella catarrhalis*.

DOSAGE

Amoxicillin at 80–90 mg/kg/day in divided doses twice daily is the first-line treatment for AOM.[2] Second-line options include amoxicillin-clavulanate and third-generation cephalosporins, including IM ceftriaxone in refractory cases.

PRECAUTIONS

Overprescribing of antibiotics may result in growing resistance of microbial organisms. Diarrhea and GI intolerance are the most common side effects seen.

Biomechanical

Osteopathy

Two small studies have evaluated the efficacy of osteopathic manipulation in the management of ROM and/or CSOM.[21,22] In Degenhardt and Kuchera's uncontrolled pilot study, eight children received weekly manipulative treatment for 3 weeks concurrent with traditional management. During a 1-year follow-up, only one child required surgical tube placement and 5 children had no recurrences.

A second, controlled study of 57 children aged 6 months to 6 years with at least 3 episodes of AOM in the prior 6 months evaluated the efficacy of a series of 9 osteopathic sessions over a 6-month period. Children in the treatment group had significantly fewer surgical procedures and fewer episodes of AOM. No follow up beyond the 6-month trial period was conducted, and there was a dropout rate of 25%. No adverse reactions were reported.

Chiropractic

The literature on chiropractic intervention for OM is comprised primarily of case reports, case series, and commentaries. A comprehensive review by Pohlman and Holton-Brown of both the osteopathic and chiropractic literature was published in 2012.[23] Of the 49 publications reviewed, only 3 were clinical trials and only one of those was a chiropractic intervention. This study randomized 20 patients aged 6 months to 6 years into treatment and sham spinal manipulation arms. However, data from this study could not be analyzed as the validity of the otoscopy and tympanometry was poor. Pohlman and Holton-Brown, citing the limited quality of data in addition to the absence of series adverse reactions, concluded that there was inadequate evidence to support or refute the use of spinal manipulation in children with ROM or CSOM.

Surgery

Updated AAP guidelines for the management of OM note the controversial nature of surgical intervention for ROM or CSOM.[2] There is a lack of consensus among otolaryngologists regarding recommendations for surgery, with roughly a third each saying they would "never," "sometimes," or "often or always" place tympanostomy tubes for a hypothetical case of a 2-year-old with recurrent AOM. Tympanostomy tube insertion has been demonstrated to reduce subsequent bouts of AOM and improve disease-specific quality of life measures (including hearing loss and speech impairment). Careful weighing of the risks and benefits is warranted. The AAP concluded that "clinicians may offer tympanostomy tubes for ROM" (defined as 3 episodes in 6 months or 4 episodes in 1 year).

Therapies to Consider

Homeopathy

A handful of small studies have suggested the benefit of homeopathy in the treatment of AOM (PIR).[8] While quality studies are lacking, the safety profile of homeopathic remedies is excellent provided the products used are truly homeopathic and do not contain physiologically active quantities of natural health products. Hopefully, controlled trials comparing homeopathic remedies with other treatment modalities will help clarify relative benefit (see Chapter 115).

PREVENTION PRESCRIPTION

PRIMARY PREVENTION PRESCRIPTION

- Encourage and facilitate exclusive breast-feeding for at least 4–6 months.
- Educate families about, and advocate for, limiting exposure to air pollution and tobacco smoke.
- Avoid unnecessary antibiotic exposure.
- Guide families on how to make nutritious food choices, including creative ways to get adequate whole grains, fruits, vegetables, healthy proteins, and oily fish.

- Vaccination for *Pneumococcal* and *Haemophilus* influenza infections may be efficacious in the prevention of some AOM episodes.

SECONDARY PREVENTION PRESCRIPTION

- Consider one or more of the following for prevention of recurrent AOM and OME:
  - Primary prevention measures
  - Vitamin C: 100–500 mg daily
  - Vitamin D: 1000 IU daily
  - Probiotics: at least 10 billion organisms daily of Lactobacillus and Bifidobacteria
  - Omega-3 fatty acids: at least 1 g of DHA and EPA combined, daily
  - Xylitol: at least 5 g, five times daily

THERAPEUTIC REVIEW

ENVIRONMENTAL
- Address potential allergens and triggers of upper respiratory inflammation (tobacco smoke, cow's milk protein).

BOTANICALS
- Herbal extract ear drops: use 2–3 drops in infected ear every 4 hours as needed for pain.

MANIPULATIVE AND BODY-BASED METHODS
- Consider osteopathic or chiropractic treatments for patients who are being considered for surgical intervention.

PHARMACEUTICALS
- Use antibiotics judiciously in younger patients and those with marked signs of inflammation and increased middle ear pressure. Amoxicillin at 80–90 mg/kg/day in divided doses twice daily is the first-line choice
- Acetaminophen or ibuprofen for pain relief.

SURGERY
- Myringotomy tubes may be considered in cases with hearing loss and/or speech delay.

Key Web Resources

American Academy of Pediatrics (AAP) section on complementary and integrative medicine. Includes access to newsletter and list serve.	http://www2.aap.org/sections/chim/
National Center for Complementary and Integrative Health. Includes evidence on a variety of topics related to pediatrics and integrative medicine.	https://nccih.nih.gov/
Pediatric Complementary and Alternative Medicine Research and Education (PedCAM) Network from the Department of Pediatrics at the University of Alberta in Canada.	http://www.pedcam.ca/

REFERENCES

References are available online at ExpertConsult.com.

CHAPTER 17

CHRONIC SINUSITIS

Robert S. Ivker, DO

PATHOPHYSIOLOGY

Prevalence

Since 1981, chronic sinusitis has been ranked among the most common chronic diseases in the United States. It is currently the most common respiratory condition in the world. According to the National Center for Health Statistics (a division of the Centers for Disease Control and Prevention [CDC]), approximately 40 million Americans of all age groups suffer from this ailment.[1] Chronic sinusitis affects nearly 15% of the population, corresponding to one out of every seven individuals. Furthermore, 22% of all women between the ages of 45 and 64 years are reported to have chronic sinusitis (compared to 15% of men in this age group), an incidence approximately equal to that of hypertension. Sinusitis is second only to arthritis among the most common chronic diseases affecting women in this age group. In men in this age group, sinusitis ranks fourth behind hypertension, hearing impairment, and arthritis. It was the primary reason for nearly 12 million physician office visits in 1995,[2,3] and over 200,000 sinus surgical procedures were performed in 1994[4] (the current number is more than 300,000). Medical costs for diagnosing and treating this condition are estimated to be greater than $10 billion annually.

When sinusitis is considered together with allergic rhinitis (the fourth most common chronic condition), asthma, and chronic bronchitis (the eighth and ninth most common conditions, respectively), respiratory disease resulting from these ailments affects more than 90 million people—nearly one out of every three Americans—and thus constitutes our first environmental epidemic. In the 1960s, none of these four respiratory conditions were among the top 10 chronic health problems.

Etiology

The modern-day plague of *air pollution* is insidiously destroying the respiratory tract of those breathing polluted air. According to the Environmental Protection Agency (EPA), 60% of Americans currently live in areas where the air quality makes breathing a risk to their health. A 1993 study performed by the EPA and Boston's Harvard School of Public Health reported that 50,000 to 60,000 deaths a year are caused by particulate air pollution.[5] A subsequent study in 1995 bolstered the earlier findings while concluding that people who live in highly polluted cities die earlier (approximately 10 years sooner, a 15% decrease in life expectancy) than if they had been breathing healthier air. In addition to particulates, other components of toxic air include carbon monoxide, ozone, sulfur dioxide, nitrogen dioxide, hydrocarbons, and lead.

The nose and sinuses are lined by the respiratory epithelium. By virtue of the histological and physiological characteristics of its outermost lining, the *ciliated mucous membrane* or *mucosa*—serve as the body's *air filter*, *humidifier*, and *temperature regulator* as well as *protector of the lungs*. This continuous mucous membrane that extends from just inside the nostrils to the alveolar sacs in the lungs is a connected porous protective shield for the body's air portal. The respiratory epithelial mucosa serves as a vital component of the immune system and acts as the first line of defense against bacteria, viruses, pollen, animal dander, cigarette smoke, dust, chemicals, automobile exhaust, and other potentially harmful air pollutants. The majority of its function of filtration, humidification, and temperature regulation occurs in the nose and in the four pairs of paranasal sinuses (maxillary, ethmoid, frontal, and sphenoid) comprising the entrance and vestibule of the respiratory tract.

Although the human body is a self-healing organism, the self-rejuvenating process typically requires a period of rest and recovery. The primary challenge preventing healing of the respiratory mucosa is continuous respiration of approximately 20,000 breaths per day. When the air that we breathe is polluted and dry, as indoor air tends to be, especially during the winter months, the mucous membrane can easily become mildly inflamed from the chronic irritation in addition to one or more of the etiological factors listed later. Without the opportunity for rest and recovery, chronic irritation often leads to *chronic inflammation*, the underlying pathophysiological process of chronic sinusitis. Chronically inflamed mucosa is weak and therefore more vulnerable to cold viruses, the most common trigger for sinus infections. The mucosa may also become hyperreactive and more sensitive to a wide variety of allergens, foods, and chemicals.

Nothing is more important to optimal physical well-being than the quality of the air breathed and the ability to breathe it. Pollutant-laden air often has far less than the optimal 20% oxygen or negative ion content (3000 to 6000 ions/cm³), thus adding to its effect as a chronic irritant in causing inflamed and hypersensitive mucous membranes. Chronically inflamed mucosa often results in increased mucus secretion (rhinorrhea and postnasal), head and nasal congestion with some degree of obstruction of the ostia, headaches, and nasal allergy.

Symptoms and Diagnosis. *Chronic sinusitis* is defined as persistent or recurrent episodes of infection or inflammation of one or more sinus cavities that produce the majority or all of the following symptoms and signs: headache, facial pain, head congestion, purulent postnasal drainage or rhinorrhea, and fatigue.[6] Purulent mucus does not always indicate infection; however, it does always indicate some degree of inflammation. Although most otolaryngologists rely on computed tomography scanning for the definitive diagnosis of sinusitis, a good history and physical examination to detect the presence of most or all of the defining signs and symptoms of chronic sinusitis can provide a reliable diagnosis of acute sinusitis in primary care settings. Patients who are most debilitated by chronic sinusitis typically have some degree of fungal sinusitis. Unfortunately, even in 2015, no consistently reliable laboratory tests are available for the definitive diagnosis of chronic sinusitis. As *Candida* is a normal inhabitant of the body, the identification of *Candida* overgrowth can be challenging with laboratory testing alone. Accordingly, clinicians should consider the use of patient history, Dr. William Crook's *Candida* Questionnaire and Scoresheet (see Fig. 17.1), and the therapeutic response to antifungal treatment to confirm the diagnosis of fungal sinusitis.

Risk Factors for Acute and Chronic Sinusitis

- Infections: the common cold causes inflammation and ciliostasis.[7] Candidiasis, yeast overgrowth, or fungal sinusitis may cause severe respiratory and systemic inflammation.
- Environment (both indoor and outdoor air pollution and pollen)
- Lifestyle (diet, cigarettes, and other sources of smoke)
- Allergies: Half of chronic sinusitis sufferers have allergies to pollen or food.
- Food sensitivities
- Emotional stress, particularly repressed anger and grief (unshed tears)
- Dry air: Air with less than 30% relative humidity occurs in an arid or semiarid climates or as the result of forced-air heating systems, air-conditioning (particularly in cars), oxygen therapy, or wind.
- Cold air: the ideal temperature is greater than 65°F.
- Occupational hazards: those at highest risk include automobile mechanics, construction workers (especially carpenters), painters, beauticians, firemen, airport, and airline personnel.
- Gastroesophageal reflux disease
- Dental infection: infection of the upper teeth may spread to the maxillary sinuses.
- Malformations (polyps, cysts, deviated septum)

Fungal Sinusitis

Since the early 1990s, I have treated the patients who have presented with the most severe and challenging cases of chronic sinusitis using an antifungal regimen. A landmark Mayo Clinic (Rochester, MN) study,[8] published in September 1999, reported an immune system response to fungus, rather than to bacterial infection, as the cause of the majority of cases of chronic sinusitis. The investigators reached this conclusion after studying 210 patients with chronic sinusitis and identifying 40 different species of fungus, including *Candida*, in the mucus of 96% of participants. Similar organisms were identified in a control group of normal healthy volunteers. The investigators concluded that the immune

response to these fungi in patients with chronic sinusitis is markedly different from that of healthy people and that this unusual immune reaction is responsible for the chronic inflammation, pain, and swelling of the mucous membranes associated with sinusitis. These investigators termed the condition "allergic fungal sinusitis." However, the investigators failed to speculate on the possible impact of previous multiple courses of broad-spectrum antibiotics on the immune response to fungal organisms in these patients. The resultant profound disruption of the normal bacterial flora of the mucosa likely contributed to the immune response observed. However, this issue was not addressed, and this study concluded simply by stating, "we must begin looking at chronic sinusitis as more than simply a bacteriological and/or anatomical problem, but as a dysfunction of the immune system mediated by a fungus."

Between October, 1999, and February, 2000, my colleagues and I[9] conducted a study with 10 patients of an allergist-immunologist, who were symptomatic despite aggressive conventional treatment for chronic sinusitis (four of the patients also had asthma). The study consisted of five group sessions with follow-up evaluations at 1-year and again at 7.5 years. Dr. William Crook's *Candida* Questionnaire and Scoresheet (Fig. 17.1) was used as part of baseline measurements, and all 10 patients scored in the "probably yeast-connected" category or higher. All patients were treated with the Sinus Survival Program (currently called the Respiratory Healing Program, shown in the following) in addition to fluconazole. Statistically significant improvement was observed 1 month following the introduction of fluconazole and again at the end of the 5-month study. Although asthma outcomes were not measured, three of the four asthmatic patients reported marked improvements in asthma symptoms, and they were able to reduce treatment dosage or stop inhaler use. At both the 1-year and 7.5-year follow-up assessments, improvements in sinusitis symptoms and quality of life were either maintained or enhanced in all participants. This is the only published *long-term* study of the treatment for fungal sinusitis.

> **Note**
>
> An allergic inflammatory response to fungal organisms is an important etiological factor in chronic sinusitis.

INTEGRATIVE THERAPY

The Respiratory Healing Program

Although antibiotics have been the mainstay of conventional medical treatment for chronic sinusitis, often followed by sinus surgery if the problem has not resolved, these therapeutic modalities increasingly offer only temporary relief and fail to resolve or cure chronic sinusitis. In a study of 161 children with acute sinusitis, researchers concluded that "antimicrobial treatment offered *no benefit* in overall symptom resolution, duration of symptoms, recovery to usual functional status, days missed from school or child care, or relapse and recurrence of sinus

---

Candida Questionnaire and Score Sheet

This questionnaire is designed for adults, and the scoring system isn't appropriate for children. It lists factors in your medical history that promote the growth of *Candida albicans* (Section A), and symptoms commonly found in individuals with yeast-connected illness (sections B and C).

For each "Yes" answer in Section A, circle the point score in the box at the end of the section. Then move on to sections B and C and score as directed. Filling out and scoring the questionnaire should help you and your doctor evaluate the possible role of candida in contributing to your health problems. Yet, it will not provide an automatic "Yes" or "No" answer.

SECTION A: HISTORY POINT SCORE:

(1) Have you taken tetracyclines (Sumycin, Panmycin, Vibramycin, Minocin, etc.) or other antibiotics for acne for one month or longer? 25
(2) Have you, at any time in your life, taken other "broad spectrum" antibiotics* for respiratory, urinary, or other infections for 2 months or longer or in shorter courses 4 or more times in a 1-year period? 20
(3) Have you taken a broad spectrum antibiotic* — even in a single course? 6
(4) Have you, at any time in your life, been bothered by persistent prostatitis, vaginitis, or other problems affecting your reproductive organs? 25
(5) Have you been pregnant:
    2 or more times? 5
    1 time? 3
(6) Have you taken birth control pills:
    For more than 2 years? 15
    For 6 months to 2 years? 8
(7) Have you taken prednisone, Decadron, or other cortisone-type drugs by injection or inhalation:
    For more than 2 weeks? 15
    For 2 weeks or less? 6
(8) Does exposure to perfumes, insecticides, fabric shop odors, and other chemicals provoke:
    Moderate to severe symptoms? 20
    Mild symptoms? 5
(9) Are your symptoms worse on damp, muggy days or in moldy places? 20
(10) Have you had athlete's foot, ringworm, jock itch, or other chronic fungus infections of the skin or nails? Have such infections been:
    Severe or persistent? 20
    Mild to moderate? 10
(11) Do you crave sugar? 10
(12) Do you crave breads? 10
(13) Do you crave alcoholic beverages? 10
(14) Does tobacco smoke really bother you? 10

TOTAL SCORE, SECTION A:

* Including ampicillin, amoxicillin, Augmentin, Keflex, Ceclor, Bactrim, Septra, Levaquin, Zithromax, and many others. Such antibiotics kill off "good germs" while they are killing off those which cause infection.

SECTION B: MAJOR SYMPTOMS

For each of your symptoms, enter the appropriate figure in the point score column:
Not at all 0 points
Occasional or mild 3 points
Frequent and/or moderately severe 6 points
Severe and/or disabling 9 points
Add total score and record it in the box at the end of this section.

POINT SCORE:

(1) Fatigue or lethargy
(2) Feeling of being "drained"
(3) Poor memory or concentration
(4) Feeling "spacey" or "unreal"
(5) Depression
(6) Numbness, burning, or tingling
(7) Muscle aches
(8) Muscle weakness or paralysis
(9) Pain and/or swelling in joints
(10) Abdominal pain
(11) Constipation
(12) Diarrhea
(13) Bloating
(14) Troublesome vaginal discharge
(15) Persistent vaginal burning or itching
(16) Prostatitis
(17) Impotence

FIG. 17.1 ■ *Candida* **Questionnaire and Score Sheet.** (From Crook WG. *The yeast connection: a medical breakthrough.* 3rd ed. Jackson, TN: Professional Books; 1986.)

Continued

(18) Loss of sexual desire
(19) Endometriosis or infertility
(20) Cramps and/or other menstrual irregularities
(21) Premenstrual tension
(22) Spots in front of the eyes
(23) Erratic vision

TOTAL SCORE, SECTION B:

SECTION C: OTHER SYMPTOMS
For each of your symptoms, enter the appropriate figure in the point score column:
Not at all 0 points
Occasional or mild 1 point
Frequent and/or moderately severe 2 points
Severe and/or disabling 3 points
Add total score and record it in the box at the end of this section.

POINT SCORE:

(1) Drowsiness
(2) Irritability or jitteriness
(3) Incoordination
(4) Inability to concentrate
(5) Frequent mood swings
(6) Headache
(7) Dizziness/loss of balance
(8) Pressure above ears, feeling of head swelling, and tingling
(9) Itching
(10) Other rashes
(11) Heartburn
(12) Indigestion
(13) Belching and intestinal gas
(14) Mucus in stools
(15) Hemorrhoids
(16) Dry mouth
(17) Rash or blisters in mouth
(18) Bad breath
(19) Joint swelling or arthritis
(20) Nasal congestion or discharge
(21) Postnasal drip
(22) Nasal itching
(23) Sore or dry throat
(24) Cough
(25) Pain or tightness in chest
(26) Wheezing or shortness of breath
(27) Urinary urgency or frequency
(28) Burning on urination
(29) Failing vision
(30) Burning or tearing of eyes
(31) Recurrent infections or fluid in ears
(32) Ear pain or deafness

TOTAL SCORE, SECTION C:

TOTAL SCORE, SECTION A:

TOTAL SCORE, SECTION B:

GRAND SCORE:
The Grand Total Score will help you and your doctor decide if your health problems are yeast-connected. Scores in women will run higher as 7 items in the questionnaire apply exclusively to women, whereas only 2 apply exclusively to men.

IF YOUR SCORE IS: SYMPTOMS ARE:

180 (women) 140 (men)	almost certainly yeast-connected
120 (women) 80 (men)	probably yeast-connected
60 (women) 40 (men)	possibly yeast-connected
Less than 60 (women) 40 (men)	probably not yeast-connected

FIG. 17.1 ■ cont'd

symptoms."[10] For the growing number of patients who have failed to respond to repeated courses of broad-spectrum antibiotics and surgery, postoperative patients, and the growing numbers of individuals who elect not to have (or are not candidates for) surgery or to take antibiotics, the Respiratory Healing Program has consistently produced successful outcomes.

The *goal* of this integrative holistic treatment program for chronic sinusitis is to address the primary cause (inflammation) by healing the chronically inflamed mucous membrane. Although this is a relatively complex problem with multiple risk factors contributing to chronic inflammation, what makes this approach so effective is that each of these factors is either mitigated or eliminated.

Components of the Respiratory Healing Program for Chronic Sinusitis

- Treating and preventing sinus infections and colds
- Practicing nasal hygiene—spraying, steaming, and irrigating
- Eating a healthy, antiinflammatory, and hypoallergenic diet in combination with antiinflammatory and antioxidant vitamins and supplements
- Improving indoor air quality
- Treating yeast overgrowth or fungal sinusitis
- Detoxification
- Treating allergies
- Strengthening and restoring balance to the immune system
- Healing the issues in your tissues: mental, emotional, spiritual, and social health factors

If the patient closely adheres to the first seven components listed here, he or she will usually experience significant improvement within 1 to 2 months, regardless of the duration of chronic sinusitis. Depending on the patient—the severity of the condition, the level of commitment, and my sense of the patient's capability—I typically introduce the first five components at the first session, followed a month later by detoxification and recommendations for strengthening immunity and mitigating allergies. The third and fourth sessions, 2 and 3 months into the program, are focused on mental and emotional health and on spiritual and social health, respectively.

The keys to curing chronic and fungal sinusitis are becoming a highly skilled practitioner in the *art of preventive medicine* (specifically preventing sinus infections) and making a commitment to *healing one's life*. My more than three decades of experience in treating extremely challenging cases of chronic sinusitis have made it apparent that mental, emotional, social, and spiritual factors have a profound impact on the degree of inflammation and immune dysfunction. Specifically, repressed anger may be the single most significant cause, with unshed tears (grief resulting from the perceived loss of love) (see Chapters 99 and 102). To have the greatest therapeutic benefit, the following recommendations should be practiced on a daily basis and incorporated into one's lifestyle. From the foregoing published study and statistics I have derived from

patient questionnaires since 1990, more than 90% of patients who make at least a 3-month commitment (and three to four office visits) to the Respiratory Healing Program experience significant improvements in their symptoms of chronic sinusitis, with the majority of patients ultimately cured.

INTEGRATIVE THERAPY: TREATING AND PREVENTING SINUS INFECTIONS AND COLDS*

Natural Antibiotics

Garlic

Allimed® or Allimax® (both 100% pure allicin, the active ingredient in garlic) is my first choice treatment for sinus infections because studies have shown it to be highly effective as an *antibacterial*,[11,12] *antiviral* (kills cold viruses),[13] and *antifungal*.[14] In my practice, it has been consistently effective in treating and preventing sinus infections and colds. However, garlic needs to be taken in therapeutic doses. Allimed (450 mg/capsule) and Allimax (180 mg/capsule) are both available in a liquid form for children.

Dosage

For treating a sinus infection: Allimed, two capsules three times daily for 10 days; or Allimax, five capsules three times daily for 10 days.

For treating colds and preventing sinus infections: at the first sign of a cold, Allimed, two capsules (or Allimax, five capsules) three times daily for 2 to 3 days; then one capsule (or Allimax, two capsules) twice daily for 2 to 3 days if symptoms have subsided.

EchinOsha and Elderberry

The commercial formulation EchinOsha with elderberry contains two antiviral herbs, *Echinacea*[15] and elderberry[16] (also effective with the influenza virus), in addition to osha root, which helps to strengthen the immune system. This preparation is contraindicated during pregnancy and in patients with autoimmune disease.

Dosage

EchinOsha, for treating colds and flu: 1 to 2 teaspoons every 2 to 4 hours for as long as symptoms are present; or *Echinacea* extract, 2 drops four to five times a day.

Yin Chiao

This antiviral Chinese herb is available in health food stores.

Dosage

For treating colds: three to five tablets or capsules (300 to 500 mg each) four or five times a day in the first 48 hours.

*(Editor's Note: Dr. Ivker has financial ties to some of these products which are sold through his website.)

TABLE 17.1 **Physical and Environmental Health Components of the Sinus Survival Program**

Measure	Preventive Maintenance	Treatment
Sleep	7–9 hr; no alarm clock	8–10+ hr/day
Negative ions or air cleaner	Continuous operation; use ions, particularly with air conditioning	Continuous operation
Room humidifier, warm mist	Use during dry conditions, particular during winter when central heat is on and in summer if air conditioner is on	Continuous operation
Saline nasal spray	Use daily, particularly if exposed to dirty or dry air	Use daily every 2–3 hr
Steam inhaler	Use as needed if exposed to dirty or dry air	Use two to four times/day; add eucalyptus oil
Nasal irrigation	Use as needed if exposed to dirty or dry air	Use daily, two to four times/day, after steam
Water, filtered	Drink 1/2 oz/lb body weight; with exercise, drink 2/3 oz/lb	1/2–1/3 oz/lb of body weight
Diet	Emphasize fresh fruit and vegetables, whole grains, fiber; limit sugar, dairy, caffeine, and alcohol	No sugar, dairy, alcohol
Exercise, preferably aerobic	Minimum of 20–30 min three to five times/wk; avoid outdoors with high pollution or pollen levels and extremely cold temperatures	No aerobic exercise; moderate walking allowed; avoid outdoors with high pollution or pollen levels and cold temperatures

Modified from Ivker RS. *Sinus survival: the holistic medical treatment for sinusitis, allergies, and cold.* 4th ed. New York: Tarcher/Putnam; 2000.

Grapefruit Seed Extract

In capsule or liquid form, grapefruit seed extract, which is antifungal and antiviral, is available in health food stores.

Dosage

250 mg three times daily or 10 drops in water three times daily (the liquid form has an unpleasant taste).

Nasal Sprays

Sinus Survival Spray

This saline nasal spray that contains purified water with Himalayan salt, aloe vera, berberis aquifolium, and potassium sorbate. The combination of aloe and Himalayan salt has an antiinflammatory effect, and the berberis is antiviral (Table 17.1).

Dosage

Every 1 to 2 hours with infection; apply a dab of peppermint oil to the *outside* of the nostrils following each application. Use for both treatment and prevention on a daily basis.

Nasal Rescue (Ionic Silver Spray)

This is highly effective in killing bacteria, viruses, or fungi. It contains ionic silver.

Dosage

Every 15 to 20 minutes for maximum effectiveness; apply a dab of peppermint oil to the outside of the nostrils following each application. Use only for treating infection.

Nasal Hygiene (see Table 17.1)

Steam Inhaler

This acts as a decongestant[17,18] and mucolytic. Highly medicinal eucalyptus oil, peppermint oil, and tea tree oil should be added to the steam. Use three to four times a day for at least 15 to 20 minutes if treating an infection, and once or twice daily preventively for treating chronic inflammation.

Irrigation

Perform three to four times a day for treating a sinus infection, immediately following the use of the steam inhaler.[19,20] A pulsatile irrigator is the most effective irrigating device and the only device shown to remove the biofilms. Irrigation is one of the best methods for quickly eliminating (and preventing, once or twice daily) sinus infections, in addition to treating chronic and fungal sinusitis (see Chapter 113).

Antiinflammatory and Antioxidant Vitamins and Supplements

Vitamin C

A regimen of 3000 to 5000 mg three times a day with meals is followed, for its antiinflammatory and antioxidant effects. Use this high dosage until symptoms subside, and then reduce to 2000 mg three times a day. Vitamin C is most effective if taken in the form of Ester C or a mineral ascorbate (for better absorption and gastrointestinal tolerance), rather than ascorbic acid. Dosage should be reduced if diarrhea occurs.[21-26]

Vitamin D-3

I recommend 50,000 units daily for 3 days and then reduce to 10,000 daily for the remainder of the treatment.

Vitamin D-3 is a potent immune strengthener. Studies have demonstrated that most illnesses are accompanied by a deficiency in vitamin D.[27-31]

Grape Seed Extract

Patients should take 300 mg in the morning on an empty stomach. Grape seed is a powerful antioxidant, antiinflammatory, and antihistamine.[32-34]

Fish Oil

Eicosapentaenoic acid (EPA) 1000 to 3000 mg/docosahexaenoic acid (DHA) 500 to 900 mg per day. Fish oil contains a combination of omega-3 and omega-6 fatty acids and is an excellent natural antiinflammatory.[35-37]

Sleep

Sleep of 9 to 10 hours or more has been shown to have benefit in treating sinus infections, with 7 to 9 hours beneficial for prevention. Adequate sleep is perhaps the most effective, convenient, and least expensive way to strengthen the immune system.

Diet

Patients should predominantly eat organic vegetables and fruits as well as nongluten grains (brown rice, quinoa, millet, buckwheat, and amaranth), fiber, and protein; they should *avoid* sugar, dairy, wheat, other carbohydrates (especially gluten grains), caffeine, and alcohol. Sugar weakens immunity, and wheat, dairy, and gluten grains are the most common causes of food allergy (often a trigger of sinus infections).

Patients should also drink at least ½ oz of filtered water per lb of body weight (e.g., 160 lbs = 80 oz/day). For colds, patients should drink lots of warm or hot liquids; ginger root or peppermint tea is recommended, possibly including ginger, honey, lemon, cayenne, cinnamon, and a teaspoon of brandy (see Chapter 18).

Emotional Factors

Treat the emotional cause. Sinus infections may be influenced by repressed anger or unshed tears. I recommend the safe release of anger, as well as reflecting on feelings of grief or some sense of loss. The feeling of grief or loss is typically not as obvious as anger, but it's probably there, just a bit deeper. Journaling is another excellent method for releasing either or both of these painful emotions (see Chapter 98).

Improving Indoor Air Quality (see Table 17.1)

Ideal air quality is rated according to clarity (freedom from pollutants), humidity (between 35% and 55%), temperature (between 65° and 85°F), oxygen content (21% of total volume and 100% saturation), and negative ion content (3000 to 6000 .001 micron ions per cm³). Air that is clean, moist, warm, oxygen-rich, and high in negative ions is healing to the mucous membrane (see

Table 17.1). To create optimal indoor air, I recommend the following:
- A negative ion generator[38-40]: used as an air cleaner and placed in rooms in which patients spend the bulk of their time, particularly the bedroom and office
- Furnace filter: an electrostatic or pleated filter (e.g., Filtrete by 3M)
- Air duct and furnace cleaning
- Carpet cleaning
- Use of a humidifier: a warm-mist room unit, particularly during the winter months
- Plants, particularly those able to remove formaldehyde (boston fern, chrysanthemums, striped *Dracaena*, dwarf date palm) or carbon monoxide (spider plant)

Treating Yeast Overgrowth and Fungal Sinusitis

The majority of severe and unresponsive (to conventional treatment) cases of chronic sinusitis require anti-*Candida* antifungal treatment. Although very similar in its holistic scope, the comprehensive treatment program for fungal sinusitis or yeast overgrowth and candidiasis is more challenging than the regimen for simple chronic sinusitis (i.e., without a significant degree of candida overgrowth), chiefly because of the restrictive *Candida*-control diet. The treatment program depends upon how sick the patient is, which can be reliably determined through medical history and Dr. Crook's *Candida* Questionnaire & Scoresheet (see Fig. 17.1). If yeast symptoms are confined to the gastrointestinal tract or vagina, the program is shorter and simpler than if yeast toxins have spread throughout the body and are causing recurrent sinus infections in addition to inflammation in other parts of the body (e.g., myalgia, arthralgia, mental "fog," or severe fatigue). In the case of systemic inflammation, which is most often the situation in patients with severe chronic sinusitis, curing the condition can take from 6 months to 1 year.

The treatment program for fungal sinusitis consists of four components. I recommend integrating all four of the following components simultaneously for the best possible outcomes:
1. Reduce the overgrowth of *Candida*.
2. Eliminate the fuel for the growth of *Candida* organisms through diet. Starve them!
3. Restore normal bacterial flora in the bowel.
4. Strengthen the immune system.

Reducing the Yeast Overgrowth

Until recently, I relied heavily on the prescription antifungal Diflucan (Fluconazole) to kill *Candida*. The dosage I prescribe is 200 mg daily for 6 weeks, followed by 200 mg every other day for 3 weeks. Although Diflucan is effective, it often results in a *die-off*, or Herxheimer's reaction, which usually occurs during the first two weeks of treatment and typically lasts for 2 days to 1 week. Diflucan is so effective in killing yeast that dying organisms release a "flood" of toxins into the bloodstream that can cause fatigue, headaches, congestion, increased mucus drainage, nausea, loose stools, flulike aches and pains, and any other symptom (usually resulting from inflammation) that yeast toxins are known to produce. Distilled water (both drunk and used as an enema), vitamin C, and ibuprofen all have benefit in reducing die-off symptoms.

Although for a short time patients may possibly feel worse after starting treatment with Diflucan, they may also choose to look at the "regression" resulting from die-off as a confirmation of the diagnosis of *Candida* overgrowth, as well as a hopeful sign that they are eliminating yeast and will be feeling much better very soon. Following die-off, the majority of patients experience a level of health significantly greater than they had before the *Candida* overgrowth.

Prescription drugs, however, rarely provide the entire solution. In addition to antifungal supplements and probiotics, patients must also be prepared to adhere strictly to dietary recommendations.

In 2004, I demonstrated antifungal supplements, Allimax and Allimed, to be nearly as effective as fluconazole, although not as fast acting. Antifungal supplements have no harmful side-effects (antifungal drugs have a minimal risk of liver toxicity), and the die-off reaction is usually less severe. Allimed contains the same 100% pure allicin, called allipure, as Allimax; however, each capsule of Allimed is 450 mg rather than the 180 mg capsules of Allimax. Allimed is available only through practitioners and is expensive. Allimed can be used as first-line treatment for mild to moderate candidiasis, or in conjunction with fluconazole in severe cases. Antifungal supplements also work well in treating sinus infections, as noted earlier, because they are highly effective antibacterial agents.

Other antifungal supplements with utility in treating chronic sinusitis include the following:

- Candex or Candisol. This supplement contains an enzyme that destroys the cell wall of candida organisms and reduces die-off symptoms. It is particularly helpful in patients who have both sinusitis and asthma. Not infrequently, die-off symptoms worsen asthma and make breathing more difficult. Candex and Candisol are well tolerated and consistent components of the *Candida* treatment program. Candex is readily available in most health food stores. Candisol, which has a higher strength of the active ingredient, is available only through practitioners.
- Flora Balance or Latero Flora. This unique strain of bacteria, *Bacillus laterosporus B.O.D.*, is available in some health food stores as Flora Balance or through physicians as Latero-Flora. It has been tested extensively and found to be highly effective for gastrointestinal dysfunction, food sensitivities, and candidiasis.
- Grapefruit seed extract. Can be taken in liquid or capsule form, this supplement is also available in most health food stores.

I take an aggressive approach to treating fungal sinusitis and usually use several of the products described previously in combination (but not all of them together), along with either fluconazole or Allimed.

Numerous products available in health food stores can help to eliminate *Candida*. The majority of products contain caprylic acid, garlic, pau d'arco, plant tannins, grapefruit seed extract, oregano oil, and other herbs that act directly on *Candida* or indirectly by strengthening the immune system, although the majority of these products do not work as quickly as the regimen recommended previously. Patients may find it helpful to *rotate* antifungal supplements and not continue the use of the same product for longer than approximately 2 months.

Eliminating the Fuel for Candida *Through Diet*

In addition to strengthening the immune system, diet is the foundation of any antifungal treatment program. As each individual has a unique body chemistry, no two *Candida*-control diets will be exactly the same. Moreover, every physician who treats candidiasis and fungal sinusitis has somewhat different dietary recommendations. However, the majority of individuals with yeast overgrowth are far more susceptible to food allergies, and the following basic principles apply to almost any patient who opts for a *Candida*-control, hypoallergenic, and antiinflammatory diet:

1. A diet consisting primarily of protein and fresh organic vegetables, with a limited amount of complex carbohydrates and fat-containing foods, and a small amount of fresh fruit.
2. Sugar and concentrated sweets are always avoided.
3. The minimum time frame for maintaining the diet is 3 to 6 months, although the diet can be less restrictive the longer it is followed.
4. The best practice is to rotate acceptable foods and not eat a particular food more than once every 3 or 4 days. This is especially true for grains.
5. Changing one's diet can be a challenge. The more involved the patient is in the process, including planning, shopping, and cooking, the easier and more rewarding it will be.

Note: For the first 21 days, avoid starch and high sugar foods, including fruit. Also avoid yeast and mold foods (see later).

Foods to Include at the Onset of the Diet

Vegetables. Vegetables should be eaten freely and comprise 50% to 60% of total diet. Vegetables may be eaten raw or lightly steamed and should be organic and clean (washed well). Vegetables with high water content and low starch are preferable. The following are recommended:

- Green leafy: all lettuce, spinach, parsley, cabbage, kale, collard greens, watercress, beet greens, mustard greens, bok choy, and sprouts
- Other low-starch vegetables: celery, zucchini, summer squash, crookneck squash, green beans, broccoli, cauliflower, brussels sprouts, radish, bell pepper (green, red, yellow), asparagus, cucumber, tomato, onion, leek, garlic, and kohlrabi
- Moderately low starch: carrot, beet, rutabaga, turnip, parsnip, eggplant, artichoke, avocado, water chestnuts, peas (green, snow peas), and okra

Protein. Protein should be eaten predominantly at breakfast and lunch with no less than 60 g per day including antibiotic- and hormone-free meats; fresh or deep-water ocean fish; raw organic seeds and nuts; and acceptable proteins such as fish, canned fish (salmon and tuna—no more than two times per week), turkey, ground turkey, chicken, lamb, wild game, Cornish hens, eggs (limit two to four per week), and seeds and nuts (almonds, cashews, pecans, filberts, pine nuts, Brazil nuts, walnuts, pistachios, sunflower seeds, raw or dry roasted sesame seeds, pumpkin seeds).

Complex Carbohydrates. Complex carbohydrates include starchy vegetables, legumes (introduced after the first 21 days), and whole grains. These should only be consumed in sufficient quantities to maintain energy (ideally, one serving a day or less), with restriction varied according to food allergies, which can be determined with food rotation. Following are the recommended sources:

- Starchy vegetables: new and red potatoes, sweet potatoes, yams, winter squash (acorn, butternut), pumpkin
- Legumes: lentils, split peas, black-eyed peas, beans (kidney, garbanzo, black, navy, pinto, lima, adzuki)
- Nongluten grains: brown rice, millet, quinoa, buckwheat, and amaranth, sprouted or cooked, organic and clean; available in bulk at health food stores; grains rotated every four days; tasty as breakfast cereals, in salads and soups, and in casseroles and stir-fry; stored away from light and heat in airtight containers; other whole grains (with gluten) that should be eaten in only limited amounts: barley, spelt, wild rice, corn, oats, cornmeal, bulgur, couscous

Flaxseed Oil. Flaxseed oil should be taken as 1 to 2 tablespoons daily on grains or vegetables or as a salad dressing, *not* heated or used for cooking. Flaxseed oil should be kept refrigerated and away from light. Other acceptable oils (cold-pressed) include extra virgin olive oil, canola, walnut, and macadamia nut used within 6 weeks of opening.

Foods to Include After 21 Days

Fruits. Fruits are introduced into the diet slowly as one serving per day until patients are sure they do not make symptoms worse. One starts with melons, berries (blueberries, raspberries, huckleberries, blackberries), lemon, and grapefruit (only after first 21 days of the diet) and then chooses from among most other fresh fruits, all of which are generally sweeter than the first group. These include apple, pear, peach, orange, nectarine, apricot, cherry, and pineapple. Fruit juices should be very diluted to at least 1:1 with water. Freshly squeezed fruit juice is considered best. Full-strength juices, canned fruit juices, and all dried fruits are avoided.

Yeast and Mold-Containing Foods. Yeast and mold-containing foods are allowable only if the patient is not allergic. However, these should be introduced very gradually (no more than one particular food every 3 to 4 days) and not until at least 3 weeks into the diet. Yeast and mold-containing foods include the following: fermented dairy products such as yogurt, kefir, buttermilk, low-fat cottage cheese, and sour cream; fermented foods such as tofu, tempeh, miso, and soy sauce; and raw almond butter, and raw sesame tahini.

Foods to Avoid

- Refined sugar and sugar-containing foods: cakes, cookies, candy, doughnuts, pastries, ice cream, pudding, soft drinks, pies, etc.; anything containing sucrose (table sugar), fructose, maltose, lactose, glucose, dextrose, corn sweetener, corn syrup, sorbitol, and mannitol; honey; molasses; maple syrup; date sugar; barley malt; rice syrup; NutraSweet; and saccharine; table salt (often contains sugar; sea salt preferred).
- To diminish sugar cravings: chromium picolinate, 200 mcg twice daily; biotin, 500 to 1000 mcg twice daily; and a yeast-free B-complex, 50 mg twice daily, only if the patient is not already taking a comprehensive multivitamin; craving also eliminated by 4 days without any sugar
- Milk and dairy products: all cheeses (unsweetened soy milk and butter allowed, but not in excess)
- Bread and other yeast-raised baked items, including cakes, cookies, and crackers; whole grain cereals; pastas; tortillas; waffles; and muffins
- Beef and pork
- Mushrooms: all types
- Rye and wheat (avoided for first 3 weeks)
- Grapes, plums, bananas, dried fruit, canned fruit, and canned vegetables
- Alcoholic beverages
- Caffeine: both tea and coffee (herbal tea and green tea allowed)
- White or refined flour products, packaged or processed and refined foods
- Fried foods, fast foods, sausage, and hot dogs
- Vinegar, mustard, ketchup, sauerkraut, olives, and pickles (raw apple cider vinegar allowed)
- Margarine, preservatives (e.g., in frozen vegetables)
- Refined and hydrogenated oils
- Leftovers (can be frozen for later)
- Rice milk (high carbohydrate content)

This diet is meant to be a guide. Responses to this diet will vary greatly depending upon the severity of candidiasis, food allergies, and type of medication (if any) the patient is taking to eliminate *Candida*. The majority of individuals who closely adhere to this diet will experience a significant improvement within 1 month. If the diet is followed for 3 to 4 weeks, in addition to taking medication or antifungal supplements, and the patient reports no improvement, the diet should be changed back to a basic vegetable (low-starch) and protein diet, and food allergy or leaky gut syndrome should be highly suspected. The offending food is often one eaten every day and for which the patient has developed a craving. If new foods are reintroduced very gradually, such as every 3 to 4 days, then the offending food should be easily detected from symptoms that arise after eating it.

Initially many patients complain, "there's nothing to eat on this diet." Losing 8 to 10 pounds of body weight during the first month is not unusual. Many different nutritious and tasty choices are available, however, and weight loss will stabilize unless patients are significantly overweight. A key factor in successfully maintaining the diet lies in finding desirable recipes. *Candida*-control diet cookbooks are relatively easy to locate in most health food stores.

This *Candida*-control, hypoallergenic, and antiinflammatory diet is essentially the same diet I recommend to all my patients with chronic sinusitis, although it need not be quite as restrictive if fungal sinusitis is not a significant factor.

My basic dietary recommendations are to avoid milk and dairy products, sugar, wheat, caffeine, and alcohol,[41-46] as well as to increase intake of fresh organic vegetables and fruits, whole grains, fiber, and protein.

Restoring Normal Bowel Bacterial Flora

The best way to restore normal bacterial flora in the bowel is through the administration of probiotics, specifically those containing *Lactobacillus acidophilus* and *Bifidobacterium bifidum*. The probiotic should contain a minimum of two billion CFUs (colony forming units); however, I've recently been recommending preparations with 20 billion CFUs. Patients should start taking a probiotic supplement at the very beginning of the treatment program for fungal sinusitis. Intestinal bacteria can be restored through a multitude of *Lactobacillus acidophilus* and *Bifidobacterium bifidum* products available in health food stores.

Many yogurt products do not contain a high amount of viable organisms by the time they reach the consumer. This is especially true of highly processed yogurt products and those with many additional ingredients. Individuals who are sensitive to dairy products, as well as those with chronic respiratory disease, should not use yogurt as a consistent source of beneficial bacteria because milk protein may contribute to inflammation of the mucous membrane. Brands of yogurt that have added sweeteners should be avoided.

Strengthening the Immune System

Immune strengthening is a vital aspect of treating *Candida* overgrowth and fungal sinusitis. The three steps described previously can all contribute in varying degrees to a stronger immune system.

Both regular aerobic exercise[47] and, especially, adequate sleep, in addition to the recommendations for strengthening mental, emotional, social, and spiritual health (see later), can have a profound impact on creating a strong immune system. The combined effect of these aspects of the Respiratory Healing Program can potentially have a far greater effect on immune function than can any single supplement or food.

Improvements in chronic sinusitis may become evident within 2 to 3 weeks of beginning the *Candida* treatment program; however, a period of 3 months to 1 year in the most severe cases is usually required to complete the healing process. Practitioners should strongly recommend that patients maintain a healthy diet without reverting back to excess sugar and alcohol or an excess of any food.

Detoxification

In conjunction with treating *Candida* overgrowth (particularly because these organisms release massive amounts of toxins as they die), a detoxification process should be initiated (see Chapter 106). Options for detoxification include the following:

Water

Patients are advised to drink copious amounts of water (filtered or distilled), at least half an ounce per pound of body weight.

UltraInflamX-360

The core medical food drink UltraInflamX-360 (Metagenics, San Clemente, California) reduces inflammation and promotes accelerated detoxification. This highly researched nutraceutical contains patented, proprietary ingredients. Published research is available in the literature,[48-50] in addition to clinical trials from the Functional Medicine Research Center in Gig Harbor, Washington. I recommend a 3-month course of UltraInflamX-360 with the following regimen:
- First week: one scoop twice daily
- Second and third weeks: two scoops twice daily
- Following the third week, for 3 days only: no food eaten, and two scoops taken four to five times per day
- Fourth, fifth, and sixth weeks: two scoops twice daily
- Seventh, eighth, and ninth weeks: two scoops once daily
- Tenth, eleventh, and twelfth weeks: one scoop daily

Natural Cellular Defense

Natural Cellular Defense (NCD, Waiora, Boca Raton, Florida) is a detoxifier, alkalinizer, and immune strengthener composed of a mineral (clinoptilolite zeolite) micronized and purified by a patented process and suspended in sterile water. NCD is approved by the U.S. Food and Drug Administration and generally recognized as safe (GRAS). NCD removes heavy metals, dioxins, and petrochemical and other environmental toxins. As an alkalinizer (raises digestive pH), NCD assists immune function by eliminating many bacteria and viruses in the GI tract, as well as *Candida*, which thrives in a more acidic environment.

Colon Hydrotherapy

I recommend *colonic treatments* as a rapid method of removing excess *Candida* from the bowel and mitigating die-off effects. Much more effective than an enema, colon hydrotherapy is best performed on a weekly basis (twice during the first week) for 6 weeks in conjunction with taking an antifungal drug. Hydrotherapy can help cleanse the bowel of *Candida*, toxins, and dead yeast organisms while assisting the inflamed lining of the bowel to begin the healing process. Colonic treatments can also significantly enhance the detoxification process by stimulating the liver to release toxins (the liver is the primary detoxification organ in the body), while also helping to flush the small bowel with water absorbed by the body through the colon. These treatments need to be performed by trained colon hydrotherapists, who are usually found in most cities by calling the office of a naturopath or chiropractor.

Far-Infrared Sauna

Although I have had no experience either personally or with patients who have used a far infrared (FIR) sauna, numerous reports and references[51-53] regarding the efficacy of far infrared (FIR) sauna for detoxification have been published. Several FIR sauna devices are portable, convenient, and economical and can be used in the privacy of the patient's home.

The primary advantage of the FIR sauna is that a conventional sauna heats the air in the chamber to a very high temperature, which in turn heats the body. The FIR sauna works differently. Neither oxygen nor nitrogen molecules in the air can block the FIR wave, thus allowing the FIR wave to penetrate the body to a depth of approximately 2 inches without injuring the skin with hot air.

Mind-Body Therapy

Mental and Emotional Health Recommendations

Most sufferers of chronic sinusitis have repeatedly heard the message, "You're going to have to live with it" from their physicians, or have come to this conclusion themselves. This belief often adds to already existing feelings of anger, sadness, fear, and possibly hopelessness. Essential mental and emotional components of the Respiratory Healing Program include the following: modifying beliefs and attitudes through *affirmations* and *visualizations*; creating a *goal list* and an *ideal life vision* (developing clarity about personal and professional objectives); learning to express painful emotions, especially through the *safe release of anger*, *journaling*, and finding more *humor*, *optimism*, and *play* in life.

Physical problems with the nose and sinuses bioenergetically correspond to mental and emotional issues associated with self-evaluation, truth, intellectual abilities, openness to the ideas of others, the ability to learn from experience, emotional intelligence (the ability to identify, experience, and express feelings), and feelings of adequacy. These issues are all associated with the sixth ("third eye") chakra in Ayurvedic medicine. I have found most patients with chronic sinusitis to be high achievers, perfectionists who set very high standards of performance for themselves and tend to be unforgiving of themselves and others for making mistakes. The repressed anger felt by most sinus sufferers is often self-directed. Assisting the patient to achieve a heightened sense of awareness of the possible contributing factors can help to begin the process of healing.

Mental and Emotional Health Practices

- Affirmations
- Visualizations[54]
- Goal or ideal vision list

These first three should be practiced daily for 10 to 20 minutes. Affirmations are most effective when written, recited, and visualized.
- Anger release (safely): punching (a punching bag, sofa, or pillow), screaming, stamping; while simultaneously exhaling the "shhhh" sound; highly therapeutic for chronic sinusitis
- Journaling[55]
- Optimism
- Humor
- Biofeedback
- Psychotherapy: cognitive therapy and family therapy
- Play
- Energy medicine modalities: healing touch, Reiki, qi gong, or craniosacral therapy

Spirituality

Spiritual and Social Health Recommendations

Integrative holistic medicine is based on the belief that *unconditional love is life's most powerful healer*. Its corollary, *the perceived loss of love is our greatest health risk*, is also the spiritual cause of chronic sinusitis and all disease. Healing the spirit is by far the most powerfully therapeutic component of the Respiratory Healing Program. Spiritual health is simply learning to love one's self in body, mind, and spirit. The first step in the Respiratory Healing Program is to love and nurture the sinuses (i.e., to heal the chronically inflamed mucous membrane). To heal the self spiritually involves connecting to a higher power (God, Spirit, or whatever term one is comfortable with) in a personal way and becoming attuned to this energy. By engaging in this spiritual healing process, individuals experience a profound reduction in feelings of fear and a greater capacity for unconditional love of self and of others. They are also better able to identify special talents and gifts. This awareness helps them to fulfill their life's purpose while fully experiencing the power of the present moment. The spiritual practices I recommend most are *prayer*, *meditation*,[56] *gratitude*, and *spending time in nature*.

Relationships with others are the crucible that most strongly determines the spiritual health of each person. Optimal *social health* consists of a strong positive connection to others in community and family and intimacy with one or more people. It is often much easier to feel a connection with Spirit during moments of solitude than it is to express that connection through interactions with others. At the same time, relationships offer the greatest opportunities for spiritual growth and for learning how to receive and impart unconditional love. *True spiritual health is a balance between the autonomy of the self and intimacy with others.*

On the basis of a growing number of relationship studies, researchers have concluded that social isolation is statistically just as dangerous as smoking, high blood pressure, high cholesterol, obesity, or lack of exercise. A separate study has shown that marital conflict can weaken immunity.[57]

The primary opportunities available to each person for improving social health include *forgiveness*,

PREVENTIVE PRESCRIPTION

1. Become more *aware* of the quality and quantity of the air you are breathing, water you are drinking, the food you are eating, exercise and sleep you are getting, and, most importantly, the stress you are experiencing. Close below the surface of stress lies *anger*, with yourself or others; and deep within your heart you will find *shame, fear,* and *grief* for your perceived loss of love from early childhood.

2. Pay more *attention* to how each of the foregoing factors affects the condition of your sinuses.

3. Once you have learned what factors contribute most to the way your sinuses feel, then determine which of the recommendations in the earlier integrative therapy section are consistently effective in improving the way you feel. The *daily practices* that are most helpful to nearly every sinus sufferer are adequate sleep and water intake, elimination of dairy products and a significant reduction in sugar intake, use of a saline/aloe nasal spray, inhaling medicinal eucalyptus oil, nasal irrigation (any method), journaling, anger processing, and a spiritual or meditative practice.

4. *Repeat* to yourself several times a day:
   - I'm always doing the best I can. There are no mistakes, only lessons.
   - I am totally accepting of myself exactly as I am.
   - I am here now in this present moment.
   - I am here to love and be loved.

5. Remember that you are a unique individual with a different set of needs, desires, beliefs, and gifts than anyone else. As you heighten your level of *self-awareness,* your intentions will be clear and you will be much better able to care for yourself, heal your life, and potentially cure your chronic sinusitis.

THERAPEUTIC REVIEW

LIFESTYLE

- Sleep: Adequate good quality sleep can help improve immune function.
- Use a negative ion generator as an air cleaner in the bedroom and office.
- Saline nasal spray: Use daily every 2 to 3 hours. Saline sprays containing aloe vera are most helpful.
- Steam inhaler: Use this device for 15 to 20 minutes two or three times daily.
- Medicinal eucalyptus oil: This can be added to the steam for optimal benefit or inhaled from a tissue several times a day.
- Nasal irrigation: Use one of several methods for nasal irrigation, although a pulsatile irrigator is most effective. Perform two to three times daily. This modality is best performed following steam inhalation therapy.
- Exercise: Engage in regular aerobic exercise three to five times per week for at least 30 minutes.

NUTRITION

- Avoid milk and dairy products, sugar, wheat, caffeine, and alcohol.
- Increase intake of fresh organic vegetables and fruits, whole grains, fiber, and protein.
- Increase water intake (filtered or distilled) to at least ½ oz/lb of body weight.
- If candidiasis is suspected (e.g., history of multiple antibiotics), strict adherence to a *Candida*-control diet is recommended. This diet avoids yeast-containing foods, such as breads, and foods that promote yeast growth such as refined sugars, processed foods, cheeses, peanuts, vinegar, and alcoholic beverages.

SUPPLEMENTS

- Vitamin C: 1000 to 2000 mg three times daily
- Vitamin D-3: 5000 to 10,000 I.U. daily
- Grape seed extract: 100 to 300 mg daily in the morning on an empty stomach
- Selenium: 100 to 200 g daily
- Essential fatty acids: 2 tablespoons/day of flaxseed oil and 1 to 4 g docosahexaenoic acid/eicosapentaenoic acid daily.

BOTANICALS

- Garlic as 100% pure allicin (Allimed or Allimax): 450 mg daily preventively or 900 mg three times per day for treating a sinus infection or fungal sinusitis
- Echinacea: 2 dropperfuls four to five times per day for treating a sinus infection
- Grapefruit seed extract: 250 mg twice daily for treating a sinus infection or fungal sinusitis

PHARMACEUTICALS, SURGERY, AND *CANDIDA* OR FUNGAL SINUSITIS TREATMENT

- Fluconazole or other antifungal drugs, if the history and symptoms indicate *candida* or yeast overgrowth and fungal sinusitis
- *Candida*-control diet
- Antifungal supplements
- Probiotics containing *Lactobacillus acidophilus* and *Bifidobacterium bifidus*
- Surgery (polypectomy), usually indicated for nasal polyps (A, 3)

MIND-BODY THERAPY

- Affirmations, visualizations, goals, or ideal life vision list, practiced daily for 10 to 20 minutes
- Anger release (safely)
- Journaling
- Biofeedback
- Psychotherapy
- Energy medicine modalities: healing touch, reiki, Qi gong, or craniosacral therapy

SPIRITUALITY

- Prayer, meditation
- Gratitude, intuition, spiritual practices: observing a weekly Sabbath; fasting; practices around earth, air, fire, water
- Forgiveness, communication exercises: shared vision, attentive listening
- Support groups

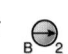

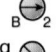
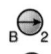
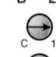
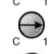

friendships, selfless acts and altruism, support groups,[58] and especially *marriage, committed relationships*, and *parenting*. Practicing forgiveness is particularly challenging for, and most helpful to, the typical patient with chronic sinusitis. Much of patient anger, which often precipitates a sinus infection, is ultimately self-directed for making perceived mistakes. In learning to forgive themselves, such patients are able to expand their capacity to forgive others and thereby heighten intimacy in their relationships (see Chapter 99).

> The three primary components of the Respiratory Healing Program for treating, preventing, and curing chronic sinusitis are as follows: reduce or eliminate inflammation of the mucous membrane, stop infection, and strengthen immunity.

Key Web Resources

Author-sponsored site that offers holistic medical treatment options and educational programs available through the author's practice, *Fully Alive Medicine,* in Boulder, CO.	http://www.fullyalivemedicine.com
Author-sponsored site that provides products and educational resources for patients engaged in the Respiratory Healing program.	http://www.sinussurvival.com

REFERENCES

References are available online at ExpertConsult.com.

CHAPTER 18

VIRAL UPPER RESPIRATORY INFECTION

Bruce Barrett, MD, PhD

Humanity's most frequent illness, the common cold, is caused by acute viral infection of the upper respiratory tract.[1-4] Acute respiratory infections (ARIs) are often classified as being caused either by influenza, the most serious of the common viruses, or other viruses (noninfluenza ARI). In the United States, noninfluenza ARI accounts for more than 20 million clinic visits and 40 million lost days of school and work, with total costs estimated at $40 billion, making noninfluenza ARI the seventh most expensive illness.[5-7] Influenza causes an annual mid-winter epidemic that varies year to year, but can be a major cause of hospitalization and death.[8-10]

Although colds are often considered a nuisance rather than a major public health threat, even rhinovirus, the least pathogenic of the common cold viruses, may cause death among elderly and immunocompromised individuals.[11-13]

On average, children experience four to six symptomatic colds per year, in addition to several asymptomatic infections. For adults, the average is two to three symptomatic colds per year and perhaps one or two asymptomatic infections.[14-16] Some individuals are particularly prone to colds, whereas others get them infrequently.[17] Numerous factors appear to be involved, but overall, susceptibility remains poorly understood.

Although there still is no good proven cure for the common cold, a number of treatments have been reported to have symptom-reducing benefit in one or more randomized controlled trials (RCTs).[18-24] In terms of prevention, behavioral strategies such as hand washing, regular exercise, and smoking avoidance are widely accepted to be at least somewhat effective.[25-31] Immunization is considered impractical, as there are hundreds of strains of viruses. Our own research indicates training in mindfulness-based stress reduction may serve to reduce incidence, duration and impact of viral ARI.[32-36]

Pathophysiology

As an *illness*, the common cold is characterized by nasal congestion and drainage, sneezing, sore or scratchy throat, cough, and general malaise.[37-39] Cough may or may not be present and tends to occur later in the disease, occasionally lasting for weeks after other symptoms have resolved. The severity of symptoms varies markedly, from barely noticeable to truly debilitating.[40] While true fever is atypical for most viruses, feelings of feverishness and chilliness are common.[41]

> There is no proven cure for the common cold. Even the most positive previous trials have reported only modest symptomatic benefit, with little or no duration of benefit.

As an infectious *disease*, viral ARI is characterized by the replication of viruses in the nasopharyngeal epithelium,[42] leading to a cascade of local and systemic immune responses.[43-45] Viral replication triggers cytokine-mediated local inflammatory reactions, in addition to the recruitment of white blood cells. Parasympathetic neural pathways activate and coordinate local responses. Blood vessels dilate and capillaries leak, causing edematous tissue and transudates in the nasal passages.[46] Mucous glands are activated, resulting in mild to copious exudative discharge. Inflammatory changes in the respiratory epithelium may persist for days or weeks after viral shedding dies down. Activation of inflammatory mechanisms leading to bronchial constriction makes viral ARI the most frequent cause of asthma exacerbation.[47]

Rhinovirus is the single most common etiological agent, but accounts for less than half of all ARIs.[48-50] Other causative viruses include adenovirus, coronavirus, enterovirus, influenza virus, parainfluenza, and respiratory syncytial virus (RSV).[4,51] Metapneumovirus[52,53] and bocavirus[54-56] are now known to cause ARI illness in both children and adults. There are likely additional viruses that are as yet undiscovered; even the best research laboratories fail to identify an etiological agent in up to one quarter of individuals with obvious colds. A small number of bacteria, such as streptococcus and *Haemophilus influenza*, may cause common cold syndrome.

Respiratory viruses follow seasonal patterns. Influenza and RSV infections only occur during the winter months, with rhinovirus colds typically observed in the fall and spring. Adenovirus infection appears year-round. Parainfluenza mini-epidemics are episodic, while sporadic outbreaks of atypical agents, such as *Bordetella pertussis*, further complicate the epidemiology of ARI.

The spectrum of illness varies greatly within and among agents. In general, influenza causes the most severe illness and is therefore often classified separately from other viral ARIs. Nevertheless, the majority of illness episodes caused by influenza are indistinguishable from those caused by other viruses, with a significant number of influenza infections reported to be asymptomatic.[57-62] Less than a quarter present with the classic "influenza-like illness" symptoms of rapid onset, fever, cough, headache, and myalgia. Despite a coordinated system to provide influenza vaccine (flu shots) each fall, influenza is implicated in as many as 20,000 deaths each year.[8,9,63]

Psychosocial Influences

Common colds are influenced by a variety of biological, psychological, and social factors. Numerous cross-sectional and prospective epidemiological studies have provided relatively consistent findings.[14-16] Colds occur most frequently among infants and children, and among adults in contact with them. Children who are in preschool daycare have more colds than those who are not, but have fewer colds during subsequent school years.[64,65] While moderate regular exercise protects against infection, excess activity, such as running a marathon, increases risk temporarily.[31,66-68] Poor mental health has been shown to be associated with increased risk.[69,70] Stress, both acute and chronic, is known to increases ARI risk.[71-73] Sheldon Cohen first demonstrated this by showing that perceived stress predicted not only whether volunteers would become sick when exposed to rhinovirus, but whether and to what extent they would shed virus.[74-76] Childhood socioeconomic status,[77] number and quality of social relationships,[78] and negative emotion[79,80] have also been shown to predict viral shedding, as well as severity and duration of cold symptoms. Subsequent studies have corroborated these findings.[62,71,81-84] Building on this background, my research team conducted a randomized trial finding that training people in mindfulness-based stress reduction can lead to substantive reductions in ARI illness episodes.[32-36] An earlier study by Dr. Rakel and I on placebo effects and the influence of doctor–patient interaction indicated that empathetic patient-oriented clinicians may be able to positively influence common cold outcomes.[85]

> The common cold is an excellent example of how the mind and body interact. Stress can increase susceptibility while social support can reduce incidence. Perceived empathy of caregivers may also reduce illness severity and duration.

INTEGRATIVE THERAPIES

There are hundreds of reported treatments for the common cold.[18-23,27,86] Globally, botanical remedies have been the mainstay of treatment. Descriptions of herbal therapies for common cold fill countless pages of notes and treatises by physicians, anthropologists, and ethnobotanists.[87-90] However, relatively few of these traditional remedies have been adequately tested for pharmaceutical properties and clinical effectiveness. The present section will review several botanicals that are widely used or have been evaluated by randomized controlled trials (RCT). The next section will cover the use of nonbotanical complementary treatments, such as vitamin C and zinc. Finally, this chapter will briefly describe conventional therapies, such as antihistamines, decongestants, and cough medications.

Botanicals

Andrographis (*Andrographis paniculata* or *Justicia paniculata*)

Andrographis is indigenous to Asia, with traditional use most prominent in India. Of the 28 *Andrographis* species, *A. paniculata* is most commonly used for the treatment of ARI. According to Ayurvedic tradition, Andrographis is attributed to many important medicinal properties and is used for the treatment of constipation, digestion, fever, pain, sore throat, snake bite, and to clean the blood. In the West, andrographis is most commonly used as a common cold treatment or preventative.

Various laboratories have reported antimicrobial,[91] antihyperglycemic,[92,93] antiinflammatory,[94] immunomodulatory,[95,96] and psychopharmacological[97] effects attributable to andrographolide, flavonoids,[98] and other phytochemical constituents. There have now been at least eight RCTs published including more than 1000 subjects that have evaluated various andrographis derivatives in the treatment of ARI, including pharyngitis.[99-106] Systematic reviews by Coon and Ernst[107] and Poolsup et al.[108] conclude the following:

> *"Collectively, the data suggest that* A. paniculata *is superior to placebo in alleviating the subjective symptoms of uncomplicated upper respiratory tract infection. There is also preliminary evidence of a preventative effect.* A. paniculata *may be a safe and efficacious treatment for the relief of symptoms of uncomplicated upper respiratory tract infection; more research is warranted."[107]*

> *"Current evidence suggests that* A. paniculata *extract alone or in combination with* A. senticosus *extract may be more effective than placebo and may be an appropriate alternative treatment of uncomplicated acute upper respiratory tract infection."[108]*

The most recent trial, not included in the reviews referred to previously, also reported positive results.[109] Based on published evidence, and with no evidence of serious safety concerns, it seems reasonable for adults to seek relief from ARI symptoms with andrographis-based cold remedies. There is insufficient evidence to favor specific products, dosing regimen, or particular standardization procedures for phytochemical content. For pregnant women and children, it seems prudent to recommend against the use of andrographis because there is little data from studies in these populations to exclude risk of harm.

> **DOSAGE AND STANDARDIZATION**
>
> The majority of clinical trials used products standardized to 4 or 5 mg andrographolide per tablet. A reasonable dose regimen would be two to four of these tablets, three times daily, for the first few days of a cold.
>
> **PRECAUTIONS**
>
> There are no known side effects of andrographolide; however, as with all medicinal treatments, caution and careful use are recommended.

Astragalus (*Astragalus membranaceus; Astragalus mongholicus*)

Astragalus is an important medicinal plant in traditional Chinese medicine.[110] While there are dozens, if not hundreds, of reported uses, astragalus extracts are commonly used for both the treatment and prevention of the common cold.[111] While antiviral activity has been reported, immunomodulation is the purported mechanism of action. Indeed, several studies have reported the effects of astragalus on the immune system, from enhanced immunoglobulin production to restoration of lost T-cell activity.[112-116] Astragalus root contains astragaloside, flavonoids, and saponins, which are variously thought to be involved in various hypothesized mechanisms of action. Unfortunately, due to a lack of human ARI trials, no clear recommendations can be made for or against the use of astragalus for the treatment or prevention of common cold, and no specific doses or precautions have been reported.

Carrageenan

Carrageenans are linear sulfated polysaccharides deriving from Irish moss (*Chondrus crispus*) and other seaweed and algae. Carrageenans are widely used in the food and cosmetics industry for the thickening, stabilizing, and gelling of a wide variety of products, including toothpaste. During the past decade, a carrageenan-based nasal spray has been tested as common cold treatment, with positive results reported.[117] Eccles et al. reported reductions in inflammatory cytokines levels and symptoms in a randomized trial among N = 35 young adults.[118] Fazekas et al. reported an RCT among N = 153 children, which found reductions in viral load and time to viral clearance, but no symptomatic benefit.[119] Ludwig et al. reported an RCT among N = 211 adults, where "alleviation of symptoms was 2.1 days faster in the carrageenan group in comparison to placebo (p = 0.037)." It appears that all of these studies were sponsored by the same company, Marino Med, and that their product is available in Europe but not the United States. While these results are certainly intriguing and carrageenan nasal spray is likely safe, further research is required before specific recommendations can be made regarding its use for the treatment of URI.

Dosage

The formulation used in the trial above was Iota-Carrageenan (0.12%) in a saline solution, one spray in each nostril, three times daily for 4 days.

Chamomile (*Matricaria chamomilla; Matricaria recutita*, German chamomile; *Chamaemelum nobile*, Roman chamomile)

Chamomile has been used widely as a botanical remedy for centuries for a variety of purposes, including dysmenorrhea, gingivitis, hemorrhoids, infantile colic, indigestion, insomnia, nausea, vaginitis, and topically,

for a variety of skin conditions.[120] In the United States, chamomile is most often used as a calmative or sedative, and for the treatment of irritable bowel syndrome. However, chamomile is also used for acute respiratory infection and hence merits inclusion in the present review. As a common cold remedy, chamomile can be taken as an infusion (chamomile tea) or as an inhalation by boiling the flowering tops. A study evaluating inhaled vapors from boiling chamomile reported benefit but was of insufficient quality to reach firm conclusions.[121]

Dosage

Although there is limited evidence, a cup or two of chamomile tea as supportive treatment for the common cold is safe and may be beneficial.

Precautions

While there are no known dose-dependent adverse reactions, allergic sensitivity, including several cases of anaphylaxis, has been reported.[122]

Echinacea (*Echinacea angustifolia; Echinacea purpurea; Echinacea pallidae*)

All dozen species from the genus *Echinacea* are indigenous to North America. Native communities discovered many medicinal uses, later transferring their knowledge to European settlers.[123] In the 1920s, Echinacea was introduced into Germany, where it has been popular ever since. Today, echinacea extracts are widely used in America, Europe, and elsewhere, particularly for the prevention and treatment of the common cold.[124] A considerable body of evidence exists regarding the uses of echinacea, including 24 randomized trials including more than 3000 participants,[125] and dozens of in vitro and animal studies.[126-128] While there is consensus that various echinacea extracts display immunologic activities, such as promoting macrophage activation and inducing cytokine expression,[129-137] there is considerable disagreement concerning which of the many echinacea-derived phytochemicals are involved. Various alkylamides, glycoproteins, polysaccharides, and caffeic, cichoric, and caftaric acids have all been implicated. Differing extracts from all three species and from various plant parts have shown immunoactivity in laboratory models. To my knowledge, no credible head-to-head, dose-finding, or viral load outcome studies have been reported, with very little pharmacokinetic information available.[138,139] A comprehensive safety review notes a number of reported allergic reactions but suggests no dose-dependent adverse effects or major drug interaction concerns.[140]

Randomized clinical trials testing echinacea extracts for the prevention and treatment of common cold were first conducted in Europe, with several early trials reporting positive result.[141-148] More recent trials in the US and elsewhere have reported mixed results, with higher quality trials finding no benefit.[149-153] I directed two of those trials. The first was flatly negative[154]; however, the second observed some positive trends.[155] Preventive trials have all trended in beneficial directions, but none have individually demonstrated clearly positive results.[156] Systematic reviews of the two dozen reported trials vary in their interpretation of the evidence.[157-163] Our recent Cochrane review[125] and JAMA publication[156] found no clear benefit among treatment trials but noted that prevention trials consistently favored some benefit. Not included in those reviews, a recent head-to-head trial of an echinacea tea against the antiinfluenza drug oseltamivir in influenza-like illness found the echinacea preparation to be equally effective.[164] A recent review argued that positive trials may be due to inadvertent unblinding, with either placebo effect or participant reporting bias contributing to false positive results.[165] It is also possible that negative studies have gone unreported, thereby yielding publication bias.

Given that echinacea extracts appear safe and that the vast majority of published trials have reported positive trends, it seems reasonable to cautiously support the use of echinacea in adults, particularly those with favorable personal experience and positive expectations.[166]

DOSAGE AND STANDARDIZATION

Positive trials have used differing formulations, with preparations made from the leaf and flower of *Echinacea purpurea* most widely used. However, preliminary evidence suggests that alkylamides from the roots of *E. purpurea* and *E. angustifolia* may have the greatest bioavailability and immunoactivity.[139,167,168] While there is a lack of consensus regarding standardization criteria, the majority of experts agree that echinacea extracts should be used as early as possible in the course of a cold, with multiple doses per day for the first few days of symptoms. Beyond that, no specific doses or precautions have been identified.

PRECAUTIONS

My own opinion is that use in children should be discouraged, as the best pediatric RCT found no positive effects but did report a slight increase in the incidence of skin rash among patients randomized to echinacea.[169] While there is a modest case control study finding no adverse effects in pregnancy,[170] I caution against its use as the risks are theoretically substantive.

There is greater evidence regarding echinacea, zinc, and vitamin C than any single conventional therapy. Unfortunately, there is a negative trial for every positive one.

Elderberry (*Sambucus nigra*)

Preliminary research indicates elderberry extracts may have antiinflammatory and antiviral antiinfluenza properties.[171-173] A Norwegian RCT among N = 60 volunteers reported potential symptom reduction benefit in influenza-like illness.[174] To my knowledge, those findings have not been replicated. With only one small limited trial and no good safety data, the use of elderberry for

the treatment of URI is intriguing but unlikely to become widely adopted.

Garlic (*Allium sativum*)

Garlic is widely used as a food and flavoring. Medicinally, there are hundreds of reported uses of garlic. The most prominent of these is moderation of cholesterol and other lipids, for which modest beneficial activity has been reasonably established.[175-178] While in vitro studies have reported antibacterial and antiviral effects, only one relevant human trial of the efficacy of garlic in treating the common cold has been reported.[179] Josling reported a RCT in which 146 participants were randomized to daily garlic or placebo capsules for 12 weeks.[180] Dramatic between-group differences were observed, with 65 colds in the placebo group and 24 in the garlic group (p < 0.001), with an average cold duration of 5.0 days among those taking placebo versus 1.5 days among those taking garlic (p < 0.05). While the study was reportedly double-blind, proof of blinding was not provided. The active treatment was "an allicin-containing garlic supplement" dosed at "one capsule daily." No further information on extraction methods, phytochemical composition, or amount of garlic was provided. Nevertheless, it may be reasonable to tentatively support the use of garlic as the risk of side effects is low, cardiovascular benefits are likely, and garlic is tasty.

DOSAGE

My personal recommendation is to use fresh garlic in cooking as much and often as palatable while being conscious of the cardiovascular and cold-prevention benefits of garlic.

Ginger (*Zingiber officinale*)

Ginger root is also very widely used as a food flavoring as well as for its medicinal properties. There is reasonable evidence supporting its effectiveness as an antinausea agent[181-183] and in the treatment of vertigo,[184] dysmenorrhea,[185-187] and knee osteoarthritis.[188] In the ARI setting, one small trial of a ginger and goldenrod combination reported small benefits.[189]

To my knowledge, no other trials of ginger root in the treatment of URI have been completed. Nevertheless, as ginger is widely used as a treatment for colds and flu, and as I personally happen to use ginger as a common cold remedy, it is included in this review.

DOSAGE

Buy a nice ginger root at the local grocery store, shave off the peel and slice the root thinly using a sharp knife, being careful not to cut one's fingers. Drop the sliced ginger into boiling water and steep for 5 minutes, then add honey and lemon to taste. Sip slowly, and *feel* the ginger work! (Dr. Barrett's personal recipe)

Ginseng (*Panax ginseng, Panax quinquefolium*)

Asian (*P. ginseng*) and American (*P. quinquefolium*) ginseng are used for a wide variety of purposes. The genus name *Panax*, chosen by Linnaeus, in fact derives from the same root word as Panacea, the Greek goddess of healing. The most widespread medical theory supporting the use of ginseng derives from traditional Chinese medicine.[190] Ginseng is thought to have "adaptogenic" attributes, which bring balance, homeostasis, and healing.[191-193] Some evidence of the effectiveness of a *P. ginseng* extract in preventing common cold comes from an Italian trial among N = 227 individuals followed for 12 weeks.[194] A Korean preventive trial evaluating *P. ginseng* among N = 100 individuals reported 12 cases of ARI (25%) in the ginseng group, compared to 22 (45%) in the placebo group.[195] A series of Canadian studies of a polysaccharide-rich *P. quinquefolium* extract reported immunomodulatory changes.[196-198] An RCT among N = 198 elderly nursing home residents reported reductions in both cold and flu episodes.[199] A second preventive trial using the same formulation among N = 323 subjects reported a statistically significant 13% difference in incidence in cold and flu episodes during 4 months of observation.[200,201] The proprietary formula used in this series of research has been approved for use in Canada. In the U.S., it would seem reasonable for preventive-minded people to use small doses of ginseng extracts (either *P. ginseng* or *P. quinquefolium*) regularly during the cold and flu season; however, as evidence is modest and safety not established, the use of ginseng in pregnancy and among children is not advised. Evidence is insufficient to recommend specific dosing or side effects.

DOSAGE

For prevention during times of high risk, take 100 mg daily. For acute infection, consider 100 mg twice daily for 9 days.

PRECAUTIONS

Ginseng is generally well tolerated but may cause insomnia, tachycardia, and elevated blood pressure.

Goldenseal (Hydrastis canadensis)

Goldenseal is among the top selling botanicals in the United States. In addition to cold remedies, *Hydrastis* extracts are found in treatments for allergy and in digestive aids, feminine cleansing products, mouthwashes, shampoos, skin lotions, and laxatives.[120] Goldenseal is combined with echinacea in many cold therapies. However, there are currently no RCTs evaluating the efficacy of goldenseal, either alone or in combination with echinacea. The phytochemical constituent berberine is pharmacologically active, and in overdose can cause significant toxicity, including cardiac arrhythmia and death.[202] Goldenseal is contraindicated in pregnancy and lactation. Berberine-rich extracts are included in many traditional Chinese medicines. The demand for goldenseal has led to overharvesting and to the substitution of other plants containing berberine or similar compounds. Given these considerations, I do not recommend goldenseal for the prevention or treatment of the common cold.

Lemon (Citrus limon)

Originally from India, the lemon tree is now cultivated throughout the world and used as a food, flavoring, and botanical remedy. Medicinal uses include the prevention and treatment of scurvy. Lemon is also used for malaria, rheumatic arthritis, and fever, in addition to numerous other indications. Lemon juice and lemon-flavored teas are used for the prevention and treatment of colds, coughs, and flu. While rigorous evidence of the effectiveness of lemon is lacking, lemon is generally recognized as safe and to have important nutritional value as a source of vitamin C (ascorbic acid), thereby making lemon a good choice for those who derive symptomatic comfort.

Peppermint (Mentha piperita)

Peppermint and other members of the mint family are widely used for a variety of medicinal purposes, including coughs and colds, as well as for a variety of gastrointestinal purposes. When treating colds, mint teas and infusions are taken internally, while mint oils are applied topically. Peppermint oil is composed primarily of menthol, menthone, and menthyl acetate. Menthol especially has been extracted and included in various topical cold remedies classified as "menthol rubs." While neither mint teas nor menthol rubs have been subjected to rigorous randomized controlled trials evaluating their efficacy in treating the common cold, both applications seem reasonable from a cost, risk, and potential benefit perspective, at least in adults. More concentrated preparations, such as peppermint oil, should not be applied to the mucosa of infants or young children, as direct inflammatory toxicity can result. Bronchospasm, tongue swelling, and even respiratory arrest have been rarely reported.[202,203]

Umckaloabo (Pelargonium sidoides)

Various preparations of this South African plant have been used for centuries following ethnobotanical tradition.[204-207] Antiviral effects, including antiinfluenza activity, have been reported.[208,209] Three RCTs in adults (N = 746) and three RCTs in children (N = 819) have yielded somewhat inconsistent yet generally positive findings.[210-212] A 2013 Cochrane review concluded that "*P. sidoides* may be effective in alleviating symptoms of acute rhinosinusitis and the common cold in adults, but doubt exists. It may be effective in relieving symptoms in acute bronchitis in adults and children, and sinusitis in adults."[213] Scientific interest in Pelargonium is relatively recent, and conclusions to date are tentative. However, umckaloabo seems a reasonable choice for adults looking for a natural treatment for cough, cold, or bronchitis. No specific formulation or dose regimen can be recommended.

DOSAGE

The formulation used in the above research was Eps 7630, which is an 11% aqueous ethanolic extract available in Europe. In America, the most commonly available form is a 1X homeopathic dose through a variety of brand names. The effectiveness of homeopathic doses is unknown.

PRECAUTIONS

While no dose-dependent adverse effects are known, gastrointestinal disturbance and hepatotoxicity have been reported,[214] and the results of a previous study indicated that allergic reactions may be a relatively frequent problem.[215]

There are several trials supporting the use of Andrographis, pelargonium (umckaloabo), and intranasal carrageenan gel. These are ones to watch!

Vitamins, Minerals, and Home Remedies

Chicken Soup

Hot chicken soup is the epitome of traditional cold remedies, and its use is supported by many personal testimonies. Chicken soup as a cold remedy is somewhat supported by at least two human studies, one reporting inhibited neutrophil chemotaxis[216] and the other indicating increased nasal mucus velocity and decreased nasal airflow resistance.[217] No RCTs using patient-oriented outcomes have been reported. Personally, I would be much more enthusiastic if the chicken industry adopted more responsible sanitary, environmental, and animal welfare policies. In the meantime, the use of soup made from free-range chickens and substantial quantities of wholesome organic vegetables can be cautiously supported, although I personally prefer soup with vegetables only.

Honey

Honey is widely used as a food and flavoring, and has been advocated as a treatment for cough and other ARI symptoms, particularly for children. A 2012 Cochrane review found two trials including 265 children.[218-220] While the quality of the trials was considered mediocre, the authors concluded that "honey may be better than 'no treatment' and diphenhydramine in the symptomatic relief of cough but not better than dextromethorphan."[218] These may not be fair comparators, as diphenhydramine is not known to have antitussive properties and dextromethorphan and other OTC drugs are not recommended for children.[23] Nevertheless, honey may be a reasonable choice for cough in children aged 2 to 10 years as it is safe and tastes good. Honey does contain large amount of glucose and fructose, so tooth-brushing afterwards is recommended. Honey is not recommended for infants due to the risk of *Clostridium botulinum* infection.

DOSAGE

Consider adding a teaspoon of honey to ginger, chamomile, or peppermint tea.

Consider adding a teaspoon of honey for cough and a squeeze of lemon to a tea made with one or more of the botanicals discussed as having positive evidence against viral URI.

Dry Saunas and Hot Baths

In 1990, Ernst et al. reported a nonrandomized 6-month prevention trial in which, "25 volunteers were submitted to sauna bathing, with 25 controls abstaining from this or comparable procedures. In both groups the frequency, duration and severity of common colds were recorded for 6 months. There were significantly fewer episodes of common cold in the sauna group. This was found particularly during the last 3 months of the study period when the incidence was roughly halved compared to controls. It is concluded that regular sauna bathing probably reduces the incidence of common colds, but further studies are needed to prove this."[221] The research community apparently did not heed Dr. Ernst's sage advice as, to my knowledge, there have been no subsequent trials testing the therapeutic properties of hot water bathing in the prevention or treatment of common cold. However, in 2010, Pach et al. reported a trial evaluating hot dry sauna as a treatment for the common cold, in which N = 157 individuals were randomized to wearing a winter coat in a hot dry sauna or wearing a coat in the sauna at room temperature.[222] Trends towards symptomatic benefit and reduced medication use were noted at various time points during the 7 days of treatment; however, the overall conclusion was that "inhaling hot air while in a sauna has no significant impact on overall symptom severity of the common cold."[222] Despite the limited research on hot baths and the disappointing results of the previous dry sauna trial, these are modalities that I would personally recommend, should the opportunity exist, as long as one is reasonably healthy and the facilities are clean. However, I do not recommend wearing a winter coat in the sauna as I do not consider this proper attire. An optional bathing suit may perhaps be more appropriate, and certainly easier for laundering. There is no data regarding the optimal frequency, duration, or temperature of saunas and baths for the prevention or treatment of URI.

PRECAUTIONS

Although saunas and hot baths are generally safe and potentially therapeutic, adequate hydration and care when standing up are important because heat-induced peripheral vasodilation can lead to orthostatic hypotension, dizziness, and increased fall risk.

Inhaled Hot Moist Air

One widespread traditional cold remedy involves the inhalation of hot moist air, often with a botanical or other additive. As noted above, benefits of inhalation of vapors from chamomile tea were reported by a previous clinical trial.[121] The most recent Cochrane review evaluated six heterogeneous RCTs with a total of 394 trial participants reporting mixed results.[223] While it seems reasonable to recommend humidification when the air is dry, and perhaps advocate the inhalation of hot moist air for those that find it comforting, it should be noted that water boils at around 100 °C, and inhalation of vapors near this temperature may cause significant thermal damage. Be careful!

Hot Toddy

I have been impressed by the number of people, including several physicians, who have come up after a lecture to tell me that their favorite cold remedy was some form of a hot alcoholic beverage, such as a "hot toddy" or hot buttered rum. While to my knowledge no trials have tested any of these remedies, testimonies of symptomatic benefit should not be totally disregarded. At a societal level, there is a well-known inverse relationship between moderate regular consumption of alcoholic beverages and the number and severity of colds.[28] Those who consume one or two drinks daily have fewer and less severe colds than both those who drink heavily and fewer colds than those who do not drink alcohol at all. One study found this relationship to be most pronounced for red wine.[224] Personally, I like to add a bit of rum to a cup of hot orange juice as a nighttime cold remedy. However, this would be contraindicated among those with alcohol use disorders, in children, pregnant women, and individuals who need to use a motor vehicle or who operate hazardous machinery.

Nasal Saline

What could be more healthful and therapeutic than a mild saltwater rinse of the nasal cavities? While saline nasal lavage is a longstanding tradition in many cultures, it is only recently that Western biomedicine has begun to integrate this practice. Currently, there are a number of positive trials among individuals with allergic rhinitis and chronic sinus symptoms, including one at the University of Wisconsin Department of Family Medicine.[225]

A 2015 Cochrane review evaluated the results of five RCTs, two in adults (N = 205) and three in children (N = 544), all comparing nasal saline to routine care of common cold.[226] These authors concluded, "nasal saline irrigation possibly has benefits for relieving the symptoms of acute URTIs. However, the included trials were generally too small and had a high risk of bias, reducing confidence in the evidence supporting this." In the largest adult trial, Adam et al. randomized 140 individuals to one of three groups: hypertonic saline, normal tonic saline, or no treatment (two squirts per nostril, three times per day.) No significant differences were observed between groups in terms of duration or severity of symptoms.[227] On the other hand, the largest pediatric trial published to date reported significant improvements in breathing and reductions in nasal secretions.[226] In addition to trials designed to test nasal saline, there is some evidence from trials using saline as a placebo. For example, Diamond et al. reported a trial in which 955 participants were randomized to one of three doses of nasal ipratropium, to the "placebo" saline vehicle, or to no treatment at all.[228] The nasal saline vehicle yielded greater benefit compared to no treatment than did any of the ipratropium doses when compared with each other or with saline.

Overall, nasal saline is a remedy with potential benefit and virtually no cost or significant risks. I suggest twice daily treatment for the first few days of a cold (see Chapter 113).

Probiotics

Probiotics are live bacteria that are thought to support healthy gastrointestinal function. Several trials have demonstrated benefit for antibiotic-associated diarrhea[229] and have indicated benefit for irritable bowel syndrome and other conditions.[230-234] Interestingly, there is now reasonably strong preliminary evidence that probiotics may also prevent or ameliorate ARI illness. This evidence includes more than a dozen trials testing the efficacy of probiotics in preventing cold and flu illness episodes.[235-243] One RCT was conducted among elderly individuals,[240] and two involved children.[239,242] One of these was aimed at preventing diarrheal illness but instead provided evidence of cold and flu prevention.[242] Two recent meta-analyses reviewed more than a dozen RCTs including more than 3000 participants and noted "significantly fewer numbers of days of illness per person"[244] among those receiving probiotics versus placebo, concluding that "the results implied that probiotics had a modest effect in common cold reduction."[245] Various formulations are available without prescription and, to my knowledge, there are no significance concerns regarding adverse effects. Until further evidence becomes available, we can be cautiously optimistic and perhaps even advocate probiotics for preventing or treating common cold; however, no specific products or dose regimens can be singled out as particularly effective (see Chapter 105).

Vitamin C (Ascorbic acid)

The use of vitamin C for the prevention and treatment of the common cold became widespread after double Nobel laureate Linus Pauling promoted his belief in this therapy in the 1950s and 1960s.[246] By the early 1970s, three major trials conducted in Toronto by T.W. Anderson indicated preventive effectiveness.[247-249] Over the next few decades, more than 30 trials including more than 12,000 participants have been reported.[250,251] Interestingly, approximately half of these trials reported positive results, far more than would be expected by chance; however, this was not enough to convince more skeptical scientists. While there is no clear consensus regarding the reasons why some trials found benefit and others did not, it seems reasonable to tentatively conclude some preventive effectiveness, as concluded by a recent Cochrane systematic review:

> *"Regular supplementation trials have shown that vitamin C reduces the duration of colds, but this was not replicated in the few therapeutic trials that have been carried out. Nevertheless, given the consistent effect of vitamin C on the duration and severity of colds in the regular supplementation studies, and the low cost and safety, it may be worthwhile for common cold patients to test on an individual basis whether therapeutic vitamin C is beneficial for them."[250]*

The evidence supports modest preventive effectiveness for doses of 200 mg to 500 mg daily. Benefits of larger doses for prevention, or as treatment for new onset colds, is supported by some trials and systematic reviews,[252] while other trials have reported contradictory results.[253] Given the generally accepted safety of ascorbic acid at doses up to a few grams per day over short periods, it seems reasonable to cautiously support its use in treating URI, particularly among individuals those positive experiences and expectations (very high doses, such as the 18 grams per day that Linus Pauling was reportedly taking up to his death at age 93 in 1994, have not been tested in trials and cannot be supported). Regular intake of vitamin C rich foods, however, can be enthusiastically supported because greater intake of fresh fruits and vegetables has been associated with many health benefits in dozens of large observational studies and has no known risks.

Vitamin D

In combination with calcium, vitamin D is widely recommended as a preventive or treatment for osteopenia and osteoporosis. Interest in vitamin D for a wide variety of other health concerns has blossomed over the past decade. Vitamin D for common cold prevention and treatment has been advocated, bolstered by the fact that vitamin D levels are low and ARI incidence is high during winter months.[254] Unfortunately, enthusiasm has not been matched by evidence. To my knowledge, there is only one good quality RCT evaluating vitamin D for preventing colds.[255] Although the results trended towards slight benefit, the general interpretation was negative.[256]

Zinc. In some ways, the story of zinc for the treatment of colds is similar to that of vitamin C. Reportedly, the physician George Eby noticed rapid recovery from an ARI in a child hospitalized and given zinc for unrelated reasons. This observation was followed by an RCT that reported positive results in 1984 (but had methodologic flaws).[257] Since then, a dozen trials with more than 1300 participants have been conducted using various zinc preparations.[258-263] Trials testing zinc acetate in doses of 75 mg or more have tended to report the most positive results.[264] The most recent Cochrane review was generally positive,[259] and many authorities now recommend zinc as a treatment for common cold.[265] However, there are concerns regarding adverse effects, such as unpleasant taste and/or nausea. While zinc is an essential mineral, with many known protective effects when ingested in foods in appropriate doses,[266,267] use of relatively high doses during acute illness may confer minimal risks. Advocates recommend frequent dosing (every 2 to 3 hours) for the first 2 or 3 days of a cold, a dosing regimen that some patients may not find convenient. Nasal irritation is common, and loss of sense of smell has been reported.[268] My personal recommendation is to tentatively support the use of oral or nasal zinc preparations among those who have experienced benefit and/or express positive feelings about the treatment but to not recommend use among children or pregnant women.

DOSAGE

Zinc gluconate, one table or lozenge containing 9–24 mg of elemental zinc, up to every 2 or 3 hours while awake, for the first few days of ARI illness.

PRECAUTIONS

Zinc can inhibit the absorption of other minerals (copper) if used for extended periods of time. Nasal formulations have been associated with the loss of smell.

Among 13 trials of zinc including 1400 participants, approximately half reported positive and half reported negative results.

Mind Body

Placebo, Meaning, and Mind-Body Effects

During the past two decades I have read reports of hundreds of trials and dozens of systematic reviews and become increasingly convinced of the importance of mind-body effects, otherwise described as placebo or meaning effects.[269-273] Positive thinking, suggestion, expectancy, and belief in the therapeutic value of a given remedy can be a powerful healing force. While regular exercise, balanced nutrition, and tobacco cessation are clearly associated with fewer and less severe illness episodes, so too are positive mental health attributes such as favorable psychological profile and healthful social relationships. Psychological predispositions, especially sociability and a positive emotional style, are predictive of both symptomatic and physiological outcomes. For the integrative clinician, this means that understanding an individual's belief system may be a crucial part of the therapeutic encounter. If a patient already believes in a safe therapy, reinforcing that belief may enhance the therapeutic response. If patients are wary of a mentioned remedy, clinicians should not press the issue. Remember that reassurance, empathy, empowerment, and positive prognosis can all be usefully employed in the clinical encounter.

Pharmaceuticals and Conventional Cold Products

Antihistamines

Drugs blocking the effects of histamine have been sold as cold remedies for more than a century but, interestingly, have been subjected to less in terms of rigorous RCT research than alternatives such as vitamin C, zinc, and echinacea. Nevertheless, there is reasonable evidence of the modest benefit of first generation antihistamines, such as diphenhydramine, clemastine fumarate, and chlorpheniramine, in reducing nasal drainage.[274-277] However, effects appear to be more attributable to anticholinergic mechanisms than antihistamine effects, and second generation "nonsedating" antihistamines do not seem to provide benefit.[278] For adults who do not mind the potential sedating or membrane-drying effects, or those with allergic responses, a first generation antihistamine may be a reasonable choice. For children, where there is no positive evidence whatsoever, antihistamines should be reserved for allergic rather than infectious rhinitis.

Decongestants

The oral decongestant, pseudoephedrine, has been tested in several clinical trials and appears to have minor benefit in reducing nasal congestion and drainage.[279-282] Side effects, including anxiety, dizziness, insomnia, and palpitations, are fairly common. More worrisome is the potential risk of elevated blood pressure and cardiac arrhythmia. Phenylpropanolamine, for decades a popular over-the-counter decongestant, was taken off the market after studies indicated an association with increased mortality, particularly among elderly individuals.[283]

The topical intranasal decongestant, oxymetazoline, has been shown to decrease nasal airway resistance as well as mucus production and drainage.[284-287] Intranasal phenylephrine has been less extensively studied but likely has similar effects. Unfortunately, these proven benefits come at the risk of nasal membrane dryness and discomfort. Oxymetazoline should be used for no more than 4 days as rebound nasal congestion can occur.

Cough Suppressants

Dextromethorphan, the active ingredient in cough remedies designated with "DM," is widely used as an over-the-counter cough suppressant. Codeine, and to a lesser extent hydrocodone, are prescribed for cough and are thought to work through similar opioid-mediated mechanisms. As such, these medications have side effects including sedation, constipation, and, potentially, respiratory suppression. While most patients and clinicians agree that these remedies work, there is considerable debate over effect size and mechanism of action due to a lack of appropriate evidence.[288-290] The best systematic review of cough remedies for children and adults concluded: "there is no good evidence for or against the effectiveness of OTC medicines in acute cough."[291] Benzonatate (Tessalon perles) is licensed as a prescription antitussive but appears to have been given this indication despite a lack of good evidence.

Analgesics/Antipyretics

There is no doubt that acetaminophen and nonsteroidal antiinflammatories (NSAIDs), such as aspirin, ibuprofen, and naproxen, are effective in treating pain and fever that may accompany the common cold. However, some reports suggest that viral shedding may be prolonged by analgesics.[292,293] While limited use for pain reduction is eminently reasonable, the widespread use of NSAIDs for general common cold symptoms is not justified, as evidence-of-benefit is marginal, and many thousands of individuals die each year from NSAID-attributable gastrointestinal hemorrhage and congestive heart failure.[294-296]

Anticholinergics

Ipratropium nasal spray has been evaluated by several good quality RCTs regarding its efficacy in the amelioration of the symptoms of infectious and allergic rhinitis.[297,298] These trials, including a dose-response trial among 955 individuals with community-acquired common cold,[228] reported definite benefit in terms of reduced nasal congestion and drainage. Common side effects include headache, uncomfortable nasal dryness, and nosebleed.

Combination Formulas

The multibillion-dollar market in cold remedies is dominated by numerous products containing combination formulas. Loopholes in FDA regulations have allowed pharmaceutical companies to mix various decongestants, antihistamines, analgesics, and antitussives, and then market these products under a variety of brand names and questionable claims. While there is some evidence of the effectiveness of these products from several RCTs,[274,299] very few if any of currently marketed products have been tested in large, well-controlled RCTs. Personally, I recommend against using any combination cold formula, with a possible exception for those who are convinced that a specific formula works for them. Perhaps most importantly, clinicians as well as parents should be made aware that no cold formula has ever been proven to work in children. In my opinion, acetaminophen (paracetamol) is the only currently justifiable treatment of pain in children.

Antivirals

Dozens of phase I and II trials using experimental rhinovirus infection models have reported benefit for several different antiviral drugs.[300-304] None, however, have demonstrated safety or efficacy in the treatment of community-acquired colds and therefore none can currently be recommended. Nevertheless, this remains an active area of research; safe and effective antiviral cold treatments may become available in the future.

> Conventional treatments, such as antihistamines, decongestants, and cough remedies, may help slightly with some symptoms but do tend to have side effects.

PREVENTION PRESCRIPTION

- Do not smoke
- Exercise regularly
- Wash hands frequently
- Eat a balanced nutritious diet, including foods containing vitamin C and zinc

- Maintain supportive social relationships
- Reduce exposure to people with colds
- Reduce stressors and/or negative responses to stress
- Antibiotics should not be used for the treatment of cold symptoms in children or adults.
- There is some evidence for the effectiveness of andrographis (400 mg twice daily), vitamin C (200–500 mg daily), ginseng (100 mg daily), and probiotics in the prevention of colds. As the evidence is weak, consider these treatments only during high-risk times.

There is no good evidence of the effectiveness of any treatment, conventional or integrative, in children. While children can suffer side effects, they are less likely than adults to benefit from the placebo effect. Dr. Barrett says, "Don't drug the kids!"

THERAPEUTIC REVIEW

Below is a summary of therapeutic options for common cold. None are proven beyond reasonable doubt to be safe and effective. Nevertheless, these are all reasonable options given best current evidence of benefit and harm.

TREATMENT OF COMMON COLD

Botanicals

- Andrographis. Consistent preliminary evidence of benefit, no major concerns of harm. No good reason to pick one formulation or dose regimen over another. A common dose is 400 mg of dried herb, or extract containing 5 to 20 mg of andrographolide, up to three times daily for the first few days of illness. B_1
- Echinacea. Contradictory evidence, with several positive trials. Evidence on prevention is more consistent than that for treatment. No serious concerns of harm but should be avoided in pregnancy. Use three or four times daily for the first few days of a cold. No strong reason to pick one formulation over another B_1
- Pelargonium/Umckaloabo. Contradictory evidence, with a few positive trials. No serious concerns of harm. Use three or four times daily for the first few days of a cold. No strong reason to pick one product over another B_1

Supplements

- Vitamin C. Contradictory evidence, with several positive trials. Water-soluble vitamin. Necessary nutrient. Very safe in reasonable doses. B_1

- Zinc. Contradictory RCT evidence, with several positive trials, particularly with higher doses of zinc acetate. Use lozenges frequently for the first couple days of a cold. Side effects may include bad taste or nausea. B_2
- Astragalus, chamomile, garlic, ginger, ginseng, lemon, peppermint, hot baths, hot moist air, nasal saline, and chicken soup are all unproven but safe supportive therapies. C_1

Pharmaceuticals

- First generation (sedating) antihistamines may decrease nasal congestion but may cause drowsiness. B_2
- Intranasal decongestants appear to be effective in decreasing nasal congestion and drainage but quite often cause nasal dryness or irritation, and, rarely, insomnia, palpitations, or elevated blood pressure. B_2
- Oral decongestants may be effective in decreasing nasal congestion but may cause insomnia, palpitations, or elevated blood pressure. B_2
- Intranasal ipratropium appears to be effective in decreasing nasal congestion and drainage but may cause headache, nasal irritation, or nosebleed. B_2
- Antivirals for true influenza of no more than 36 hours duration may reduce symptom severity, duration, and infectivity A_2

Key Web Resources

REFERENCES

References are available online at ExpertConsult.com.

CHAPTER 19

HIV Disease and AIDS

Stephen Dahmer, MD • Benjamin Kligler, MD

PATHOPHYSIOLOGY

The human immunodeficiency virus (HIV) is a highly contagious lentivirus (family Retroviridae) that causes the potentially life-threatening condition acquired immuno-deficiency syndrome (AIDS). Since 1981, when the first case of AIDS was reported in the United States, the disease has become a global pandemic, resulting in an estimated 65 million infections and 25 million deaths worldwide. Currently, approximately 0.8% of the world is considered to have people living with HIV/AIDS (PLWHA).[1]

Many PLHWA are unaware that they are infected with the virus, and an estimated 10%–60% of individuals with early HIV infection will not experience symptoms. In April 2013, the USPSTF recommended that clinicians screen all adolescents and adults aged 15–65 years for HIV infection. Younger adolescents and older adults who are at increased risk should also be screened. They also recommend screening all pregnant women, including those who present in labor with unknown HIV status.[2]

In practice, the possibility of acute HIV infection should be considered in patients who present with any ill-defined febrile illness. Suspicion should be heightened for those presenting with HIV-consistent symptoms, including diarrhea, rash, lymphadenopathy, aseptic meningitis, and mucocutaneous ulcers. In the United States, the rec-ommended algorithm for screening involves an initial fourth generation combined antigen/antibody immuno-assay with confirmatory immunoassay of a second type followed by HIV viral testing if there is a discrepancy.[3] Since 1997, home testing kits have been available for patients to test themselves, and a new smartphone testing device could also soon be available.[4]

Two types of HIV have been characterized: HIV-1 and HIV-2. HIV-1 was discovered first; it is more contagious and virulent and, therefore, the cause of the majority of HIV infections globally. HIV-2 has poor capacity for transmission and is largely confined to West Africa.

Since 1996, AIDS has been transformed into a serious but manageable chronic illness by the widespread use of antiretroviral medications (highly active antiretroviral ther-apy [ART or HAART]). Many of the current challenges in the management of HIV-positive patients pertain to mini-mizing the possibility of developing viral resistance while maximizing quality of life by preventing or controlling the adverse effects associated with the use of antiretrovirals. A newer challenge is the prevention and treatment of chronic disease as life expectancy increases. For all patients with early HIV infection, genotypic drug resistance testing as well as hepatitis B and C serologies should be performed because they can influence treatment choice.[5]

INTEGRATIVE THERAPY

PLWHA have a strong history of being active regarding their health care. Since early in the epidemic, they have advocated for effective, available treatments. AIDS activ-ists have long promoted the idea that individuals living with HIV should not only have access to all potentially effective therapies but also the right to make informed choices about which treatments to use, including comple-mentary therapies (as recently popularized in mainstream culture by the movie *Dallas Buyers Club*).

People with HIV disease typically use integrative approaches for several reasons. First is to promote health-ier functioning of the immune system. Second is for a claimed antiviral effect of the therapy. Third is to treat an HIV-associated symptom or condition. Fourth is to miti-gate one or more side effects of antiretroviral medications, as in the use of glutamine supplements for protease inhibi-tor (PI)–associated diarrhea. Finally, many use integrative therapies simply to improve their quality of life or gain a sense of empowerment by being involved in their own care.

Lifetime use of complementary and alternative medi-cine (CAM) by PLWHA ranges from 30% to 90%, with national studies suggesting CAM use around 55% and practitioner-based CAM about 15%. Vitamins, herbs, and supplements are the most common, followed by prayer, meditation, and spiritual approaches. CAM use is predicted by the length of time since HIV diagnosis as well as a greater number of medications/symptoms. CAM is often used to address limitations or problems with anti-retroviral therapy.[6] Although the advent of effective phar-maceutical treatment for HIV has led to a decrease in the use of CAM, rates of use nevertheless remain high. In a cohort of HIV-positive adults (N = 642) followed semian-nually in the Nutrition for Healthy Living (NFHL) study between 1995 and 1999, HAART use increased from 0% to 70%, but ingested CAM use decreased only from 71% to 52%.[7] The investigators concluded that most people with HIV at this point apparently feel that "CAM thera-pies complement, rather than replace ART [and that] physicians should routinely ask about ingested CAM therapy use in HIV-positive patients."[7]

In a recent survey of 1000 randomly selected infectious disease (ID) practitioners, 75% felt that CAM and integra-tive medicine modalities are useful.[8] Despite acceptance and persistent use of CAM, assessment of these popular

CAM therapies among HIV-positive populations continues to be problematic. Approximately 20% of the existing studies have assessed the reliability and 3% assessed the validity of the CAM instruments employed, making evidence-based recommendations very problematic.[9]

Pharmaceuticals

Antiretroviral Therapy

Over the past two decades, ART has radically altered the natural history of HIV infection, and advances continue to evolve.[10] Opportunistic diseases have become less common, and mortality has declined to the point that HIV-infected individuals now have a near-normal life expectancy (Table 19.1).[11] More than 50% of deaths in PLWHA receiving ART are now related to conditions other than AIDS.[12] It is recommended that all HIV-positive individuals start ART regardless of CD4 count to both reduce the risk of disease progression and prevent transmission.[13] Those starting ART should be willing and able to commit to treatment and understand the benefits and risks of therapy and the importance of adherence. The recommendation for those with CD4 count > 500 cells/mm³ is based on expert opinion with the stated caveat that patients may choose to postpone therapy, and providers, on a case-by-case basis, may elect to defer therapy on the basis of clinical and/or psychosocial factors.

In 1987, a drug called AZT became the first-approved treatment for HIV disease. Since then, approximately 30 drugs have been approved, with more under development. These medications fall into several classes. The first category is the antiretrovirals, used for their specific activity against HIV. These agents are currently divided into six groups: (1) the nucleoside reverse transcriptase inhibitors (NRTIs), which include zidovudine (Retrovir), emtricitabine (Emtriva), abacavir (Ziagen), didanosine (Videx), stavudine (Zerit), and lamivudine (Epivir);

(2) the PIs, which include indinavir (Crixivan), nelfinavir (Viracept), amprenavir (Agenerase), and numerous others; (3) the nonnucleoside reverse transcriptase inhibitors (NNRTIs), which include rilpivirine (Edurant), efavirenz (Sustiva), and nevirapine (Viramune). Newer classes include (4) entry inhibitors (including fusion inhibitors), such as enfuvirtide (Fuzeon) and maraviroc (Selzentry); (5) integrase inhibitors, such as raltegravir (Isentress) and dolutegravir (Tivicay); and (6) multiple-class combination drugs, such as efavirenz + tenofovir + emtricitabine (Atripla), which are technically not a separate class of HIV medications but combinations of the previously mentioned classes into one single pill with specific fixed doses of these medicines. Currently, the most common approach is to use these agents in combinations of at least two drugs (4/5th of the preferred initial regimens for ART-naive patients are integrase based) to reduce the possibility of viral resistance.

Consensus has shifted multiple times in deciding the optimal time to start ART therapy, with the most recent recommendations leaning strongly toward early ART for all PLWHA. Released at the time of publication were results from the Strategic Timing of Antiretroviral Treatment (START) study, the first large-scale randomized clinical trial to establish that earlier antiretroviral treatment benefits all HIV-infected individuals; 4685 patients with HIV from 35 different countries were followed for an average of 3 years, and serious AIDS events as well as serious non-AIDS events and death were recorded. As of March 2015, a total of 41 (0.6 per 100 patient years) of those events were found in the early treatment group and 86 (1.25 per 100 patient years) in the delayed group (Hazard ratio Arm A/B [95% confidence interval; CI]= 0.47 [0.32–0.68]).[14]

The second category of pharmaceuticals, used less widely since the advent of effective antiretroviral medications, comprises the prophylactic agents used for prevention of specific HIV-related opportunistic infections.

TABLE 19.1 When to Start Antiretroviral Therapy

Measure	Recommendation
Specific Conditions	
Symptomatic HIV disease	**Antiretroviral therapy recommended regardless of CD4 cell count**
Pregnancy	
High HIV-1 RNA level (> 100,000 copies/mL)	
Rapid CD4 count decline (> 100 cells/mm³ per year)	
Active hepatitis B or C*virus coinfection	
Active or high risk for cardiovascular disease	
HIV-associated nephropathy	
Symptomatic primary HIV infection	
Age > 60 years	
Risk for secondary HIV transmission is high	
CD4 cell count ≤ 500 cells/mm³	**Antiretroviral therapy recommended**
CD4 cell count > 500 cells/mm³	**Antiretroviral therapy should be considered†**

*Active co-infection with HCV or HBV requires treatment with specific antiretroviral regimens.
†New recommendations for HIV patient care include offering ART to all patients regardless of CD4 cell count, changes in therapeutic options, and modifications in the timing and choice of ART in the setting of opportunistic illnesses such as cryptococcal disease and tuberculosis.
From Thompson MA. Antiretroviral treatment of adult HIV infection: 2010 recommendations of the International AIDS Society-USA panel. *JAMA* 2010;304:321–333.

These drugs include trimethoprim-sulfamethoxazole (Septra, Bactrim) for prophylaxis of *Pneumocystis carinii* pneumonia and toxoplasmosis and azithromycin and rifabutin for prophylaxis of *Mycobacterium avium* infection.

People living with HIV/AIDS must be more than 95% adherent to their treatment plans in order for them to remain effective. This means that missing more than one dose per month may reduce effectiveness of therapy.

Pre- and Postexposure Prophylaxis

Currently, no vaccine or cure for HIV is publicly available. Interesting areas of research include CpG 7909 and stem cell transplant ("Berlin patient"). Unfortunately, all stem cell transplant HIV recipients to-date have relapsed. The universally recommended method for the prevention of HIV is to avoid blood-to-blood contact and to practice safe sex. On July 16, 2012, the U.S. Food and Drug Administration (FDA) approved Truvada (emtricitabine/tenofovir disoproxil fumarate) as the first drug to reduce the risk of HIV infection in uninfected individuals who are at high risk and/or engage in sexual activity with HIV-infected partners. Truvada is taken daily as preexposure prophylaxis (PrEP) in combination with safer sex practices to reduce the risk of sexually-acquired HIV infection. When taken consistently, PrEP has been shown to reduce the risk of HIV infection by up to 92%.[15] Postexposure prophylaxis (PEP) can be prescribed for people who have recently been exposed to HIV; it involves starting ART no more than 72 hours (3 days) after exposure. Two to three drugs are usually prescribed (preferred regimen is Raltegravir [Isentress] 400 mg po twice daily PLUS Tenofovir/Emtricitabine 300/200 mg [Truvada] po once daily), and they must be taken for 28 days. PEP is not always effective; it does not guarantee that someone exposed to HIV will not become infected.[16]

A trial using a three-drug combination pill of the brand name Complera that includes emtricitabine 200 mg, rilpivirine 25 mg, and tenofovir disoproxil fumarate 300 mg once daily with food for 28 days in 100 HIV-infected men resulted in no acquisition of HIV at 12 weeks.[17]

Lipodystrophy

In a separate category, on November 10, 2010, the FDA approved Egrifta (tesamorelin) to treat HIV patients with lipodystrophy (associated with many ART medications), a condition in which excess fat develops in different areas of the body, most notably around the liver, stomach, and other abdominal organs. Although it may decrease visceral abdominal fat in PLWHA, it has not been shown to provide any clinical benefit (e.g., decrease in cardiovascular risk or improved quality of life); it is nonformulary, and the estimated 30-day price is $2042.[18] Long-term safety is yet another concern, and a 10-year observational study is currently underway.[19]

Smoking

According to Centers for Disease Control and Prevention (CDC) estimates in 2009, 42% of HIV-infected Americans in care smoked cigarettes (one of the highest rates of smoking for any subgroup).[20] Smoking poses a special hazard to PLWHA beyond its already well-established negative effects on the health.[21] Evolving science supports the idea that HIV infection is associated with a chronic state of persistent inflammation (regardless of CD4/viral load) and that this inflammation increases the risk for illnesses for which smoking is already a well-established cause. Additionally, smoking inhibits effective CD4+ T lymphocyte function and thereby increases the risk for certain infections (e.g., pulmonary).[22] Quit rates are 37% lower for HIV-infected smokers than for subjects in the general population.[20]

Nutrition

Early research in the 1980s showed that decreases in body weight, body mass index, and body fat percentage may be the first signs of declining nutritional status resulting from HIV disease and may begin even during the early asymptomatic phase of HIV infection. PLWHA experience HIV-associated wasting and lose body mass despite nutritional intake that should be adequate for their height and weight. In a study of nutritional status in 108 HIV-positive patients, both with and without AIDS, body weight, serum cholesterol level, and CD4+ level progressively decreased over a 6-month period and HIV-associated wasting persisted.[23] This study also found a significant relationship between low serum cholesterol—a marker for poor nutrition—and adverse patient outcome.

Nutrition counseling and intervention in the early stages of HIV disease constitute important components of a prevention-oriented treatment plan because these measures may help forestall adverse nutritional changes in HIV-positive patients. Although definitive data supporting specific nutritional recommendations are scarce, reasonable suggestions include the following: a diet high in omega-3 essential fatty acids such as flaxseed and fish oils; small, frequent meals to ensure adequate intake of calories and to reduce the likelihood of malabsorption; avoidance of simple sugars, which may inhibit immune function on a short-term basis as shown by some studies; and avoidance of large amounts of alcohol and caffeine. In 227 HIV-infected patients, adherence to a Mediterranean dietary pattern was favorably related to cardiovascular risk factors in patients with fat redistribution[24] (see Chapter 88).

Another purpose for which nutritional interventions are widely used is to address the problems with malabsorption experienced by many HIV-positive patients. Common recommendations include the use of *Lactobacillus*, *Bifidobacterium*, and other "friendly bacteria" to maintain proper balance of intestinal flora (see Chapter 105) and the use of whole food-based nutrition to prevent the development of subclinical vitamin deficiencies or promote higher intake of the supplements discussed in the following sections. Although these recommendations have not yet been shown to affect the course of HIV disease progression, all are safe and reasonable to include in an integrative treatment plan.

Supplements

Multivitamins

Many clinicians have routinely recommended multivitamin supplementation for HIV-positive patients. A double-blind, placebo-controlled study of multivitamin (vitamins B, C, and E) supplementation in 1078 HIV-positive pregnant women in Tanzania demonstrated that over a 6-year follow-up period, women taking multivitamins had significantly less progression to World Health Organization (WHO) stage 4 disease or died compared with women given placebo (relative risk = 0.71).[25] Subjects in the multivitamin group also had significantly higher CD4+ and CD8+ cell counts and significantly lower viral loads. Adding vitamin A to this multivitamin regimen did not improve the outcome and, in fact, reduced the benefit of multivitamin therapy on some of the outcome measures.

Vitamin A

Vitamin A supplementation has been extensively studied for ameliorating infection with HIV in adults and for possibly reducing the likelihood of vertical HIV transmission. An association between lower vitamin A levels, lower CD4+ counts, and higher risk of progression to AIDS was reported.[26] A study in African women demonstrated a connection between vitamin A deficiency and increased maternal-to-fetal transmission of HIV.[27] However, other prospective trials, including one with 341 HIV-positive patients followed over 9 years, demonstrated no significant difference in the risk of AIDS progression with vitamin A levels.[28] Trials of high-dose vitamin A supplementation also failed to show an effect on CD4+ or CD8+ counts, viral loads, lymphocyte responsiveness to mitogens, or progression of disease.[29] The association between vitamin A deficiency and increased vertical transmission of HIV initially reported in Kenya was not borne out in subsequent U.S. studies. The Women and Infants Transmission Study (WITS), a large prospective ongoing cohort study, found that vitamin A level does not correlate with increased risk of HIV vertical transmission in North America.[30] The investigators suggested that vitamin A supplementation in addition to prenatal vitamins is not necessary.

DOSAGE

15,000 IU of **mixed carotenoids**

PRECAUTIONS

Chronic intake of preformed vitamin A can be toxic, leading to hair loss, confusion, liver damage, and bone loss.

Vitamin B₁₂

Supplementation with a B-complex vitamin may be beneficial in HIV-infected patients. Lack of vitamin B_{12} has been associated with peripheral neuropathy and myelopathy; a 9-year prospective cohort study in 310 patients found vitamin B_{12} levels to be an early and independent marker of HIV disease progression, and time to development of AIDS was found to be 4 years less on an average in subjects observed to have lower vitamin B_{12} levels.[31] Despite equivocal results of intervention trials using B_{12} supplementation, supplementation continues to be widely used in HIV disease.

DOSAGE

100–1000 mcg daily

PRECAUTIONS

No significant adverse effects of B_{12} supplementation have been reported.

Antioxidants: Vitamins C and E, Selenium, and α-Lipoic Acid

Vitamins C and E both have been explored for a role in the treatment of HIV disease owing to their antioxidant properties. Other substances including selenium and α-lipoic acid are commonly used for the same purpose. In addition, vitamin C has been shown in vitro to inhibit viral replication at high doses.[32] On the basis of this finding, intravenous vitamin C has been widely used to achieve the high serum levels necessary for antiviral activity. No evidence supports this aggressive approach, although anecdotally it has not been proved to be as dangerous as was initially feared. α-lipoic acid has theoretical, yet clinically unsubstantiated, use in HIV for HIV-related dementia, hepatoprotection, peripheral neuropathy, and lipodystrophy.

The role of antioxidant supplements in general in HIV disease requires further study. A 2009 review of 19 studies showed that evidence to support standard selenium supplementation in patients with HIV is both limited and insufficient, yet although the available evidence for selenium supplementation is weak, its low toxicity and side-effect profile seem to pose minimal risks, especially at low doses.[33] Vitamins E and C at more standard doses are safe and may decrease lipid peroxidation and enhance the immune system; however, conclusive evidence on the effects of these vitamins in HIV disease is still lacking. Higher doses of vitamin E should be avoided as elevated serum levels could potentially increase the risk of cardiovascular disease in PLWHA.[34]

DOSAGE

Vitamin E 400 units daily; vitamin C 500–2000 mg one to three times daily; selenium 55–70 mcg daily; α-lipoic acid 20–50 mg daily

PRECAUTIONS

Concomitant administration of high doses of vitamin C can reduce steady-state indinavir plasma concentrations.[35]

Vitamin D

While best known for its effects on bone health, vitamin D deficiency has also been associated with muscle weakness, more than a dozen types of internal cancers, multiple sclerosis, and type 1 diabetes mellitus. Most recently, there has been peaked interest in its immunomodulatory actions, especially related to PLWHA.[36,37] Observational studies conducted in PLWHA who are not taking ART have reported associations between vitamin D deficiency and susceptibility to tuberculosis, upper respiratory tract infection, and oral candidiasis, raising the possibility that supplementation might reduce susceptibility.[38] Although its clinical effects are still under investigation, the high potential for benefit of vitamin D coupled with its excellent safety profile and the high prevalence of deficiency in the U.S. population suggest that we should encourage supplementation in PLWHA regardless of ART.

DOSAGE

Because the IOM has doubled the safe upper limit from 2000–4000 IU of vitamin D per day, in our practice we have moved toward recommending 1000–2000 IU of D_3 daily in summer and 2000–4000 IU of D_3 daily in winter.

PRECAUTIONS

Vitamin D toxicity can cause hypercalcemia and anemia. Symptoms include fatigue, gastrointestinal (GI) intolerance, bone pain, and a metallic taste.

N-Acetylcysteine

Because of the strong evidence that depletion of glutathione levels correlates with progression of HIV infection, much interest has been focused on the use of the nutritional supplement N-acetylcysteine (NAC) as a means to replete intracellular glutathione levels.[39] Despite its early promise, however, NAC has not been proven beneficial in the treatment of HIV disease. One randomized controlled trial failed to show any influence of NAC on T-cell counts or disease progression.[40] Despite the lack of evidence supporting its use, this supplement is commonly used.

DOSAGE

The dose of NAC is 600–1200 mg daily.

PRECAUTIONS

Can cause GI adverse effects including nausea, abdominal pain, and irregular bowel movements.

l-Carnitine

l-Carnitine (ALCAR) may be helpful in mitigating some of the adverse effects of antiretroviral medications, including peripheral neuropathy and dyslipidemia. Acetylcarnitine acts to facilitate transport of essential fatty acids across cell membranes and thus may have a role in normalizing intracellular lipid metabolism and regulating peripheral nerve function and regeneration. Decreased levels of carnitine have been found in HIV-positive people; in addition, patients with AIDS experiencing neuropathy with zidovudine or didanosine therapy had significantly lower levels of acetylcarnitine than those with AIDS but without neuropathy.[41] One open trial of oral acetyl-l-carnitine supplementation (1500 mg twice daily) for up to 33 months in 21 HIV-positive patients with established antiretroviral-induced neuropathy found an improvement in neuropathic grade in 76% of patients.[42] HIV RNA load and CD4+ and CD8+ cell counts were not altered. An increased proliferation of peripheral blood mononuclear cells in vitro was noted after oral supplementation with l-carnitine; a significant decrease in triglyceride levels was also noted.[43]

DOSAGE

Give 2000–3000 mg of l-carnitine orally daily for HIV-positive patients with peripheral neuropathy or high triglyceride levels.

PRECAUTIONS

Can cause GI distress and body odor. Urine, breath, and sweat can have a fishy odor; further study of this supplement is needed to substantiate the possible benefits.

l-Glutamine

l-Glutamine supplementation has been shown in animal models to speed proliferation of colonocytes. Glutamine deficiency is also hypothesized to play a role in the process of HIV-associated wasting.[44] Many patients taking PIs experience chronic diarrhea as a medication side effect. A randomized trial involving 35 HIV-positive men with PI-induced diarrhea found that when added to a regimen of fiber and probiotic supplementation, l-glutamine (30 g/day) significantly decreased the frequency of diarrhea and the need for antidiarrheal medications.[45] Anecdotally, many patients find glutamine to be helpful in mitigating this side effect even at lower and more easily administered doses.

DOSAGE

Give 2000 mg daily of l-glutamine in two or three divided doses, with the dose titrated upward as needed to 40 g daily.[46]

PRECAUTIONS

Patients with cirrhosis and seizure disorder should avoid glutamine as it can potentially worsen these conditions.

Calcium Carbonate

Several studies to date have shown that calcium carbonate supplementation can help reduce the frequency of PI-associated diarrhea.[47,48] The dose typically used is

500 mg twice daily, although some clinicians report that a higher dose may be more effective. This treatment has no reported interactions or adverse effects.

DOSAGE

Usual dose of calcium carbonate is 500 mg twice daily.

PRECAUTIONS

As we further elucidate the effect of calcium supplementation on cardiovascular risk, the decision to supplement should be made based on risks and benefits stratified to individual patients.[49]

Omega-3 Polyunsaturated Fatty Acids

Patients under ART have a unique dyslipidemia (elevated triglycerides and nonhigh-density lipoprotein-cholesterol [non-HDL-C] and low HDL-C) with insulin resistance (characterized by hypoadiponectinemia). Dyslipidemia along with other possible factors (inflammation related to the viral infection itself) are reported to increase risk of cardiovascular disease in PLWHA. One study randomized 51 patients in a placebo-controlled, double-blind trial to receive either two capsules of Lovaza fish oil twice daily or two capsules of placebo. After 12 weeks, the omega-3 group noted slightly decreased plasma triglycerides and induced antiinflammatory effects by increasing the formation of antiinflammatory leukotriene B5.[50] Fifty-four subjects with HIV and elevated serum triglycerides (higher than 150 mg/dL) were randomly assigned to a control group or an intervention group and given supplemental omega-3 fatty acids for 13 weeks. The investigators documented dramatically reduced serum triglycerides, decreased arachidonic acid in the phospholipid fraction, and reduced de novo lipogenesis associated with the metabolic syndrome in the intervention group.[51]

DOSAGE

Dose is 4 g/day of docosahexaenoic acid and eicosapentaenoic acid, the main essential fatty acids found in fish oil.

PRECAUTIONS

High doses (more than 6 g) can increase free radical production and can have an antiplatelet effect.

Zinc

Adequate zinc is necessary for immune function, and zinc deficiency is estimated to occur in more than 50% of HIV-infected adults. A prospective, randomized controlled clinical trial involving 231 HIV-infected adults with low plasma zinc levels revealed that zinc supplementation for 18 months reduced the likelihood of immunological failure by four-fold while controlling for age, sex, food insecurity, baseline CD4+ cell count, viral load, and ART (relative rate, 0.24; 95% CI, 0.10–0.56).[52]

DOSAGE

Doses generally suggested are 50–75 mg per day for men and 40–60 mg per day for women on zinc picolinate.

PRECAUTIONS

High doses can inhibit the absorption of other minerals, most significantly copper. Zinc should be taken with meals to avoid nausea and vomiting.

Chromium

Chromium is an essential micronutrient, and its deficiency has been reported to cause insulin resistance, hyperglycemia, and hyperlipidemia. A randomized, double-blind, placebo-controlled trial enrolled 52 HIV-positive subjects with elevated glucose, lipids, or evidence of body fat redistribution who also had insulin resistance. Chromium was tolerated without side effects and resulted in a significant decrease in the following: Homeostatic Model Assessment-Insulin Resistance (HOMA-IR, an insulin resistance indicator) (median [interquartile range; IQR]; pre, 4.09 [3.02–8.79]; post, 3.66 [2.40–5.46]; $p = .004$); insulin (pre, 102 [85–226]; post, 99 [59–131] pmol/L; $p = .003$); triglycerides, total body fat mass (mean ± standard error of mean [SEM]; pre, 17.3 ± 1.7; post, 16.3 ± 1.7 kg; $p = .002$), and trunk fat mass (pre, 23.8 ± 1.9; post, 22.7 ± 2.0%; $p = .008$).[53]

DOSAGE

The dose is 400 mcg/day chromium-nicotinate.

PRECAUTIONS

There are at least three reports of kidney damage in patients who took chromium picolinate.

K-PAX Immune Support Formula

In 2006, a double-blind, placebo-controlled, randomized clinical trial of 40 HIV-infected patients showed that a broad-spectrum micronutrient supplement could produce a statistically significant 24% increase in the mean CD4+ cell count of individuals taking stable HAART ($p = .01$).[54] The micronutrient supplement tested (K-PAX Immune Support Formula, Mill Valley, California) included 33 ingredients and was consumed twice daily with food. The supplement is currently paid for by the New York AIDS Drug Assistance Program. For ingredients of the immune support formula used in the research, see Table 19.2.

DOSAGE

Four capsules twice per day (for less than 120 lbs) or eight capsules twice per day (for more than 120 lbs)

PRECAUTIONS

No significant adverse effects of or interactions with K-Pax have been demonstrated to date.

TABLE 19.2 **Immune Support Formula for HIV Infection Found in K-PAX Formulation**

Micronutrient	Total Daily Dosage	Micronutrient	Total Daily Dosage
N-Acetylcysteine (NAC)	1200 mg	Calcium	800 mg
Acetyl l-carnitine	1000 mg	Magnesium	400 mg
α-Lipoic acid	400 mg	Selenium	200 mcg
β-Carotene	20,000 units	Iodine	150 mcg
Vitamin A	8000 units	Zinc	30 mg
Vitamin C	1800 mg	Copper	2.0 mg
Vitamin B_1	60 mg	Boron	2.0 mg
Vitamin B_2	60 mg	Potassium	99 mg
Pantothenic acid	60 mg	Iron	18 mg
Niacinamide	60 mg	Manganese	10 mg
Inositol	60 mg	Biotin	50 mcg
Vitamin B_6	260 mg	Chromium	100 mcg
Vitamin B_{12}	2.5 mg	Molybdenum	300 mcg
Vitamin D	400 units	Choline	60 mg
Vitamin E	800 units	Bioflavonoid complex	300 mg
Folic acid	800 mcg	l-Glutamine	100 mg
		Betaine HCL	150 mg

From Kaiser J, Campa A, Ondercin JP, et al. Micronutrient supplementation increases CD4 count in HIV-infected individuals on highly active antiretroviral therapy: a prospective, double-blinded, placebo-controlled trial. *J Acquir Immune Defic Syndr.* 2006;42:523–528.

Botanicals

Chinese Herbal Approaches

In the traditional practice of Chinese medicine, herbal formulas are typically individualized to suit a given patient's condition, rather than standardized as a treatment for a given "disease." In the United States, however, the use of standardized formulas for certain conditions has become quite popular. Earlier, small randomized controlled trials of two such Chinese herbal formulae (Enhance and Clear Heat, formulated by Health Concerns in California) showed a trend (statistically nonsignificant) toward fewer symptoms in the treatment group than in the placebo group.[55] However, a more recent, prospective, placebo-controlled, double-blind study of a different Chinese formula in 68 HIV-infected adults with CD4+ cell counts lower than 0.5 × 109/L found no significant differences between the intervention and placebo groups regarding viral loads, CD4+ counts, symptoms, or quality of life scores. No significant therapy-related toxicities were reported, although patients taking Chinese herbs reported significantly higher gastrointestinal disturbances (79% vs 38%; $p = .003$) than those receiving placebo. The investigators concluded that this particular Chinese herbal formula was not effective when administered in a Western medicine setting.[56]

A study of 18 volunteers evaluated the safety and efficacy of CKBM-A01, a Chinese herbal medicine (combination of herbs including wu wei zi [Schisandrachinensis], ginseng *[Panax ginseng]*, hawthorn [*Fructus crataegi*], jujube [*Ziziphus jujube*], soybean [Glycine max], and *Saccharomyces cerevisiae* [baker's yeast]), and patients' quality of life. Although CKBM-A01 appeared to be safe, it provided no significant improvement in quality of life in asymptomatic HIV-infected patients and no significant improvement in the treatment of HIV infection based on CD4+ cell counts and viral loads.[57] Well-controlled, long-term follow-up studies of use of these Chinese herbal preparations are needed before Western practitioners can recommend them with confidence.

PRECAUTIONS

Significant concerns remain regarding possible herb–drug interactions, given the large number of herbs in most Chinese formulae, especially in those patients concurrently taking conventional antiretroviral medications.

Milk Thistle

Elevation of liver function tests (LFTs) in patients taking ART is common, especially in those coinfected with hepatitis C. Numerous in vitro studies have found that silymarin speeds the regeneration of hepatocytes after a chemical injury.[58] A significant improvement in liver function in patients with alcoholic hepatitis was noted after treatment with milk thistle extract.[59] At present, no firm evidence specifically links the hepatoprotective function of silymarin with liver damage from antiretrovirals. However, clinical experience suggests that milk thistle may help normalize LFTs allowing patients to continue on an effective ART regimen. Contrary to a widely held popular belief among patients with HIV disease and many practitioners, milk thistle has no documented antiviral effect either in HIV disease or hepatitis C.

TABLE 19.3   **Red Flags of Integrative Therapies (Think Twice Before Moving Forward)**

- You are discouraged from consulting others or information you bring to the visit is belittled
- Information about the therapy focuses on financial success or popularity rather than how it works
- Claims that a treatment can be used for a long list of illnesses without explanation of how results vary depending on how the conditions are related
- Rationale relies predominantly on testimonials
- Information is focused on comparisons with similar products, which have not been adequately studied
- Qualifications of practitioners/providers/promoters are not readily offered
- Information packets/handouts mix opinions and facts
- The treatment is unjustifiably expensive, and no clear explanations are given
- Available studies of the product have not been published or are published only in the newsletter/publication created by the manufacturer/seller

DOSAGE

The dose is 240 mg twice daily of standardized milk thistle (silymarin) extract.

PRECAUTIONS

Silymarin is well tolerated. It can occasionally have a laxative effect.

Red Rice Yeast Extract

Hyperlipidemia is a common side effect of treatment with PIs. A standardized extract of Chinese red rice yeast can reduce cholesterol levels by up to 20% in certain patients. One randomized controlled trial showed a significant decrease in lipids with the use of this supplement, with no significant toxicity.[60] Red rice yeast has not been tested specifically in PI-related hyperlipidemia. No significant adverse effects have been reported to date in patients using this supplement (see Chapter 27).

DOSAGE

The dose is 1200 mg of red rice yeast orally twice daily.[61]

PRECAUTION

Because this supplement can contain statin-like compounds, it is prudent to monitor liver function similarly for red rice yeast extract over the long term.

Herb–Supplement–Medication Interactions

An extremely active and important area of current research covers the questions of possible interactions among herbal medicines, supplements, and anti-HIV medications. In particular, herbs and supplements that induce elements of the cytochrome P-450 system have been found to potentially lead to lowered serum levels

of PIs. For example, St. John's wort—an herb commonly recommended for depression—induces cytochrome P-450 activity and can lead to a decrease in indinavir levels of up to 57%; nevirapine levels can also be affected.[62] Garlic, commonly used for elevated cholesterol levels, can have similar effects through increased cytochrome P-450 activity.

Databases are slowly becoming available that provide information regarding known herb–drug and supplement–drug interactions, and practitioners caring for patients taking antiretrovirals should regularly consult these sites to provide informed counseling to patients regarding their concomitant use of herbs and supplements. One example of a free online search database is offered by Medscape: http://reference.medscape.com/drug-interactionchecker.

> People living with HIV/AIDS on protease inhibitors should use grapefruit juice with caution, if at all.
> St. John's wort increases cytochrome P-450 activity and can reduce serum levels of medications metabolized by this system. It can decrease indinavir levels up to 57%.[54]

Mind-Body Therapy

Research in psychoneuroimmunology has clearly linked psychological stress to impaired immune function. Although a specific link between T-cell count or function and stress reduction in HIV disease has not been clearly established, one study did find a trend toward increased T-cell count in subjects practicing a mind-body approach, and other studies found improvement in natural killer cell function and other immune parameters. Stress reduction approaches studied to date in HIV-positive patients include biofeedback, meditation, systematic relaxation, hypnosis, and cognitive-behavioral stress management training. A review of several mind-body applications from the literature follows.

Progressive Muscle Relaxation and Biofeedback

Ten HIV-positive men who were asymptomatic but had T-cell counts lower than 400 were enrolled in a randomized, 10-week study in which the experimental group received a 1-hour training session twice weekly in progressive muscle relaxation and biofeedback-assisted relaxation.[61] The subjects were expected to practice the techniques daily. Follow-up at 1 month after the intervention was completed showed decreased anxiety and improved mood and self-esteem and increased T-cell counts, as shown by the State Anxiety Inventory, the Profile of Mood States, the Self-Esteem Inventory, and a basic T-cell count. The extremely small sample size limits the generalizability of these findings.

The differing effects of guided imagery, progressive muscle relaxation, and no intervention were tested on 69 participants in an uncontrolled study over a span of 6 weeks.[63] Subjects were instructed in their particular intervention and then expected to continue daily practice for the duration of the study. The outcome showed improved quality of life scores for the guided imagery group but no change in the group practicing progressive muscle relaxation.

Mindfulness and Stress Reduction

Forty-eight HIV-1–infected adults were randomized to either an 8-week mindfulness-based stress reduction (MBSR) program or a 1-day control stress reduction education seminar. Findings provided an initial indication that mindfulness meditation training can buffer CD4+ T-lymphocyte declines in HIV-1–infected adults independent of antiretroviral medication use.[64]

A small, nonrandomized study examined the effects of a structured, 8-week, MBSR program on perceived stress, mood, endocrine function, immunity, and functional health outcomes in HIV-positive adults. Although functional and quality of life outcomes were not significantly affected, natural killer cell activity and number significantly increased in the MBSR group compared with the comparison group.[65]

Another study of stress management training focused on both CD4+ counts and quality of life measurements in 45 HIV-infected and AIDS patients (30 in the intervention group and 15 in the control group).[66] This study found a lower mean stress level and a trend toward higher CD4+ counts in the intervention group. The intervention led to immediate increases in emotional well-being and perceived quality of life, but these outcomes were not sustained at a 6-month follow-up. The presence of illness-related intrusive thinking was higher in the control group at follow-up, whereas that of the intervention group actually decreased.

Further studies are needed to distinguish whether any one of the mind-body approaches is more effective than others in patients with HIV disease. Generally, these strategies are considered extremely safe. The one exception to this general rule is that patients with a history of psychosis or unstable behavior should avoid hypnosis and undertake other deep relaxation approaches with caution because these practices may increase the risk of relapse in certain patients (see Chapters 94 and 100).

Spirituality

Spirituality is an important resource that individuals use to cope with HIV disease. A growing body of evidence is supporting its effect on disease progression, more positive health behaviors, and quality of life.[67] An integrated perspective utilizing a spiritual assessment is prudent in assisting PLWHA in coping with the challenges of the disease (see Chapter 114).

Therapies to Consider

Acupuncture

Acupuncture has been widely used both to enhance immune function and general well-being in HIV-positive patients and to treat specific HIV- or medication-related symptoms. One randomized controlled trial that examined amitriptyline plus acupuncture found no benefit of standardized acupuncture over sham (placebo) acupuncture in the treatment of HIV disease–related peripheral neuropathy.[68] Methodological challenges in studying acupuncture make it difficult to demonstrate a small positive effect of an acupuncture intervention. Specifically, to construct a valid placebo intervention (i.e., sham acupuncture) that does not in itself carry a therapeutic benefit beyond that of placebo is difficult. In addition, individualized strategies both for specific symptoms and for overall health may have higher efficacy than that of standardized treatment protocols more amenable to study in such trials; however, these individualized strategies are extremely difficult to study in blinded trials. Thus, a trial such as this one examining standardized acupuncture treatment versus individualized choice of points may fail to show efficacy because of the lesser efficacy of the standardized approach.

Massage Therapy

Massage therapy has been shown to reduce anxiety levels. Massage therapy is proposed to have a positive impact on the quality of life and immune function through stress mediation. The ability of massage to produce significant effects in the treatment of PLWHA deserves further study. A randomized trial of massage therapy in HIV-exposed neonates showed a significant benefit; other evidence is all anecdotal.[69] Although massage therapy has not been proved to affect CD4+ levels per se, evidence showed that daily massage in HIV-positive men improved natural killer cell function and increased CD8+ cell counts.[70] A Cochrane Systematic Review examined the safety and effectiveness of massage therapy on quality of life, pain, and immune system parameters. The investigators concluded that some evidence supports the use of massage therapy to improve quality of life among PLWHA, particularly in combination with other stress management modalities, and that massage therapy may have a positive effect on immunological function.[71] The benefits in terms of mood and decreased anxiety and the lack of adverse effects make massage therapy a reasonable choice for the HIV-positive patient.

Hypnosis

Painful HIV distal sensory polyneuropathy (HIV-DSP) is the most common nervous system disorder in HIV patients. The symptoms adversely affect quality of life and often diminish capacity for independent self-care. To date, no interventions have been shown to be consistently effective in treating the disorder.[62] Volunteers receiving three weekly brief hypnosis interventions were followed for a total of 17 weeks. At exit, 26 out of 36 (72%) had improved pain scores with mean pain reduction in those individuals being 44%. Improvement was found irrespective of whether or not participants were taking pain medications. There was also evidence for positive changes in affective state and quality of life.[72]

Therapies to Know About

Medical Cannabis

A DEA Schedule 1 substance, medical cannabis cannot be prescribed in the United States; however, 28 states and the District of Columbia (more than 24.6 million Americans) permit, in varying degrees, use of cannabis with a licensed physician recommendation.[73] Medical cannabis as a treatment option is not widely accepted in the medical community, yet the best current evidence supports HIV neuropathy with three high-quality randomized controlled clinical trials establishing the pain relieving efficacy of cannabis.[74-76] A calculated NNT of 3.6 for herbal cannabis in HIV neuropathy is beaten only by amitriptyline when compared to currently available modalities.[77] A 2007 article in the *New England Journal of Medicine (NEJM)* stated that "clinicians and patients who are comfortable with the concept of therapeutic cannabis use can explore its usefulness in ameliorating painful peripheral neuropathy, especially in situations in which other approaches have failed."[78]

DOSAGE

Start at 1–5 mg mixed major cannabinoids (THC and CBD) depending on patient history of previous cannabinoid use and titrate slowly to alleviate neuropathic pain while avoiding unwanted side effects (see the following).

PRECAUTIONS

The most common side effects are sedation, dizziness, dry mouth, nausea, and disturbances in concentration. Medical cannabis used for chronic pain over one year appears to have a reasonable safety profile.[79] The only absolute contraindications are acute psychosis and other unstable psychiatric conditions. Cannabis use during pregnancy is not recommended. Drug interactions are a concern, with special attention paid to other therapies metabolized by CYP1A2, CYP3A4, and CYP2D6.[80] Smoking should be actively discouraged, and alternative routes of cannabis delivery—tincture, vaporized, sublingual, oral medication—should be used when appropriate on a case-by-case basis.

Dinitrochlorobenzene

Dinitrochlorobenzene (DNCB) is a chemical used to develop color photographs. Some HIV-positive individuals have used a very dilute solution to a small patch of skin to enhance the immune system function. Applying DNCB should produce redness, itching, and even blisters. If symptoms are too intense, the dosage is lowered, and if mild, the dosage is increased. DNCB is absorbed through the skin and has immunomodulatory effects, which may include the stabilization of CD4+ cell levels. A small Brazilian trial of 35 individuals not on ART using DNCB over an 18-month period experienced significant weight gain and increases in CD4+ when compared to control.[81] A DNCB starter kit costs between $25 and $50 and is not regulated.

DOSAGE

DNCB is available as a liquid solution in four strengths: 10%, 2%, 0.2%, and 0.02%. The solution is applied on the skin once a week to a 2-inch square area. Then the area is bandaged and kept dry for 10 hours. After the first skin response (a red, itchy rash), the strength of the DNCB solution is lowered

PRECAUTIONS

There is very little research to support the benefits of DNCB, and there has been no recent research. No study on DNCB has started with more than 35 patients, and many patients dropped out of the studies. The first application of DNCB may produce a chemical "burn" in addition to the normal itchy rash. The rash occurs each time DNCB is applied and lasts for a few days. Some people have persistent scarring or rashes where they apply DNCB. It may also cause sensitivity to other chemicals.

PREVENTION PRESCRIPTION

- Encourage routine HIV testing for all adults. CDC recommends that health care providers test everyone between the ages of 13 and 64 at least once as part of routine health care. Younger adolescents and older adults who are at increased risk should also be screened. They also recommend screening all pregnant women, including those who present in labor with unknown HIV status.

- Be aware and educate on the prompt treatment of HIV exposure with PEP. Make sure that your practice has a PEP protocol in place.

- Discuss PrEP for those at high risk: http://www.cdc.gov/hiv/pdf/prevention_PrEP_factsheet.pdf.

- Behavioral risk reduction counseling is an important part of the management of HIV-infected patients. At each visit, review the patient's understanding of HIV transmission and sexual/drug use activities.

- Inquire about tobacco use and encourage cessation.

THERAPEUTIC REVIEW

It is now recommended that all HIV-positive individuals start ART regardless of CD4 count to reduce the risk of disease progression and prevent transmission of HIV. This approach does not preclude the use of integrative strategies as supportive adjuncts and to alleviate certain disease- or medication-related symptoms.

PHARMACEUTICALS

- Consultation with a physician familiar with the rapidly changing range of medication options is recommended for proper choice of pharmaceutical approaches.

NUTRITION

- Nutritional consultation early in the course of HIV infection should be recommended.
- Adequate calorie consumption and an emphasis on whole foods, Mediterranean diet, and a high intake of omega-3 essential fatty acids are important elements.
- Absorption issues should be considered as well.

SUPPLEMENTS

- Multivitamin daily, emphasizing vitamins B, C, D, and E and avoiding additional vitamin A or any other unnecessary vitamin supplementation.

- ALCAR: 2000–3000 mg daily, especially in peripheral neuropathy or lipid disturbance.
- l-Glutamine: 2000 mg daily, especially in chronic diarrhea or malabsorption syndromes.
- Calcium carbonate supplementation: 500 mg twice daily for PI–induced diarrhea.

BOTANICALS

- Milk thistle extract: 240 mg twice daily in patients with elevated values on LFTs or coinfection with hepatitis C.
- Red rice yeast: 1200 mg twice daily for hyperlipidemia.
- High level of awareness among practitioners regarding possible interactions between herbal medicine, especially cytochrome P-450 inducers, and antiretroviral medications.
- Medical cannabis: 1–5 mg to start; titrate to alleviate neuropathic pain while avoiding side effects.

MIND-BODY APPROACHES

- Biofeedback, deep relaxation therapy, visualization, cognitive-behavioral stress reduction training, or other mind-body strategies.
- Strongly consider exploring a spiritual assessment.

KEY WEB RESOURCES

National HIV/AIDS Clinicians' Consultation Center. UCSF/ San Francisco General Hospital–based AIDS Education & Training Centers clinical resource for health care professionals: toll-free numbers linking physicians to expert clinical advice on HIV/AIDS management and managing health care worker exposures to HIV and hepatitis B and C, as well as consultation on antiretroviral use in pregnancy, labor and delivery, and the postpartum period.

http://www.nccc.ucsf.edu/

The Body, a subsidiary of HealthCentral Network. Community-oriented commercial website in English and Spanish has information on prevention and treatment, coverage of major HIV/AIDS conferences, online community discussion threads, and an extensive ask-the-experts feature.

http://www.thebody.com/index.html

Johns Hopkins Medicine. A comprehensive HIV guide for clinicians is available from Johns Hopkins and requires signing up for an account (free).

https://www.hopkinsguides.com/hopkins/index/Johns_ Hopkins_HIV_Guide/All_Topics/A

This website links people to HIV testing, treatment, mental health, and substance abuse services, housing, and other resources.

http://locator.aids.gov/

National Institutes of Health HIV/AIDS Prevention & Service Provider Locator. This U.S. Department of Health and Human Services project offers the latest federally approved information on HIV/AIDS clinical research, treatment and prevention, and medical practice guidelines for people living with HIV/AIDS, their families and friends, health care providers, scientists, and researchers.

http://www.aidsinfo.nih.gov

The National AIDS hotline is available in English and Spanish, 24 hours a day, 7 days a week. The number is 1-800-CDC-INFO (1-800-232-4346)

REFERENCES

References are available online at ExpertConsult.com.

CHAPTER 20

HERPES SIMPLEX VIRUS

Maret Rossi • Bradly Jacobs, MD, MPH, ABOIM

The herpesvirus family is a group of more than 100 double-stranded DNA viruses,[1] eight of which are known to commonly infect humans: herpes simplex 1 (primarily known as herpes labialis), herpes simplex 2 (primarily known as herpes genitalis), human herpesvirus type 3 (varicella-zoster virus), human herpesvirus type 4 (includes Epstein Barr virus), human herpesvirus type 5 (cytomegalovirus), human herpesvirus type 6 (includes roseolovirus), human herpesvirus type 7 (HHV-7), and human herpesvirus type 8 (includes Kaposi's sarcoma-associated virus).[2] Each form of the virus manifests in different ways, but all have a symptomatic active period followed by a latent or inactive period. The symptom-free latent period can last for months to years to even a lifetime, meaning symptoms may never reappear. In this chapter, we focus on herpes simplex virus as approximately 90% of individuals worldwide are reported to have antibodies against HSV-1, HSV-2, or both.[3]

EPIDEMIOLOGY

HSV-1 and HSV-2 can infect system of the body; however, generally HSV-1 targets the orolabial regions, while HSV-2 predominantly affects the anogenital region. Although the prevalence of HSV-1 has decreased in recent decades, there is an increased frequency of HSV-1 targeting the genital region, with HSV-1 the more prevalent form of the two. There are approximately 500,000 new primary HSV-1 infections annually in the U.S,[4] and by the age of 20, approximately 50% of the American population will be infected.[5]

According to the Sexually Transmitted Diseases Surveillance report of the Centers for Disease Control and Prevention (CDC) for 2013, the prevalence of HSV-2 among the US population decreased from 21% in the years 1988–1994 to 15% in the years 2007–2010.[6,7] Of note, 87% of 14–49 year olds in the US never received a clinical diagnosis.[8] Further, prior HSV-1 infection increases the likelihood of asymptomatic HSV-2 infection by three-fold. HSV-2 is a sexually transmitted disease, and its prevalence is positively correlated with sexual activity and inversely with socioeconomic status.[9] African Americans are at a four-fold higher risk of HSV infection compared with Caucasians, with women at a two-fold higher risk compared with men.[10]

CLINICAL MANIFESTATION

Although generally asymptomatic, HSV-1 infections typically manifest as oral and labial lesions and occasionally as facial lesions.[11] Initial areas frequently become erythematous and then develop into a cluster of fluid-filled blisters (vesicles) that eventually weep then crust over (one of the hallmarks of HSV infection).[12] Primary infections resulting in oral viral shedding can last 23 days (mean, 7–10 days), with neutralizing antibodies appearing on days 4–7. Children with symptomatic first infection may have a high fever (101 to 104°F), sore throat and mouth, malaise, tender cervical lymphadenopathy, and inability to eat.[13] Recurrent oral-labial lesions occur in approximately 30% of individuals with serological evidence of HSV-1 herpes, with 40% of these individuals experiencing more than one recurrence annually. Initial symptoms prior to lesions manifest may include pain, tingling, and itching.[14]

In contrast, HSV-2 infections primarily appear in the anogenital region. HSV-2 infection manifests as macules and papules that form small blisters and may transform into painful ulcers that crust over prior to healing.[15] The initial episode is typically the most severe and may last longer than subsequent outbreaks. Symptoms may include fever, malaise, headaches, dysuria, and tender inguinal lymph glands.[16] Lesions and viral shedding may persist for 3 weeks in the initial episode. Recurrent outbreaks are typically less intense and last approximately 8 to 10 days, similar to that of herpes labialis.[17] Individuals can typically expect to have 4–5 recurrent outbreaks within 1 year of the primary infection.[18]

As viral titers are 100 to 1000 times greater when visible herpes lesions are present, the rates of transmission via viral shedding increase when an individual is symptomatic. To infect an individual, herpes simplex virus travels through microscopic breaks in oral or genital mucosal tissue and replicates within epithelial cells upon entry.[19] After this active period, the virus is transported to sensory neurons in regional ganglia where it remains in a dormant phase until reactivation.[20] It is important to note that even when latent, herpes virus remains transmissible to others. Known triggers of herpes simplex include facial trauma, surgery, fever, and exposure to UV light, as discussed later in this chapter.[21]

There is no known cure for herpes simplex infections.[22] The goal of treatment during acute episodes is to decrease the viral activity, and the goal during recurrent episodes is to prevent the return of an outbreak.

> Herpesvirus shedding can be transmitted after the skin lesions have healed, but viral shedding is greatest when an individual is symptomatic. Condoms reduce transmission only by 30% since other skin areas are likely shedding the virus.

INTEGRATIVE THERAPY

Lifestyle

As herpes is highly contagious and sexually transmitted, patients should avoid sexual contact during an outbreak to prevent transmission of genital herpes and kissing to prevent oral herpes infection. Patients should wash hands frequently to reduce self-inoculation of the eyes and face. Should patients have sexual contact, they should be advised to use condoms. However, condom usage is reportedly associated with only a 30% reduction in transmission, most likely because lesions may be located in areas outside the region covered by the condom.[23]

When considering triggers that increase viral shedding and/or incident outbreaks, patients should consider all factors that increase allostatic load and/or impair innate immune function, such as enhanced perceived stress, acute infections, excessive exercise, poor sleep quality, and poor nutrition. Other triggers include marked emotional stress, HIV infection, and immunosuppressive medications. In addition, triggers of HSV-1 reactivation include environmental trauma, such as wind exposure; ultraviolet light; and physical trauma, such as local injury to the face or lips.[24] Consequently, regular use of sun protection (hats, sunblock) and lip balm are important prevention strategies. See Table 20.1 for a summary of potential triggers of Herpes simplex virus reactivation.

Nutrition

Lysine and Arginine

Lysine is an essential amino acid that is not naturally produced by the body. Many clinical trials have reported that lysine-rich diets and lysine supplements reduce the recurrence, severity, and healing period of herpes simplex virus infections. Conversely, arginine appears to be an antagonist of lysine. Griffith et al. demonstrated in an in vitro study that herpes simplex virus uses arginine for replication.[25] Miller et al. observed that lysine competes with arginine for intestinal absorption, transport to cells, and reabsorption at the renal tubule, and it degrades arginine by activating arginase.[26,27] Therefore, it is recommended to avoid arginine-rich foods, such as nuts, grains, chocolate, and refined sugars, and increased intake of a lysine-rich diet of meat, fish, and dairy.[28] The arginine and lysine ratio of selected foods is presented below[30] (see Table 20.2 for dietary considerations in herpes simplex virus infection).

Supplements

Lysine

One may consider supplementing a low-arginine diet with oral lysine. A double-blind, crossover clinical trial, randomly assigned 41 patients to receive lysine hydrochloride (624 mg or 1248 mg per day) or placebo for 24 weeks, and then the alternate treatment for an additional 24 weeks. All patients received a diet high in lysine and low in arginine. Patients in the high-dose group reported significantly fewer recurrences of herpes simplex virus in the lysine period than the placebo period, with lower dose of lysine showing no benefit.[31] In a separate randomized, double-blind clinical trial, 114 patients with orofacial, genital herpes, or both received 1000 mg lysine hydrochloride or placebo three times a day for 6 months. Of the 52 who completed the trial, 74% in the lysine group reported the treatment to be effective or very effective compared with only 28% in the placebo group. The authors reported that lysine significantly reduced healing time, severity, and incident outbreak frequency.[32] Overall, the effectiveness of maintaining a high lysine diet and taking supplemental lysine by mouth is supported by modest clinical evidence.

DOSAGE

1 g orally, three times daily

PRECAUTIONS

May cause GI distress at high doses (>10 g daily). May modestly raise LDL cholesterol levels.

Vitamin C

Ascorbic acid (Vitamin C) has been studied since 1936 due to its success in boosting immune function and inactivating a wide range of viruses in vitro, including herpes.[26] In a small double-blind clinical trial 42 years later, patients with herpes simplex outbreaks were administered a protocol of 200 mg vitamin C and 200 mg water-soluble flavonoids (apparently from citrus) or a lactose placebo to be taken three times daily for 3 days. Symptom remission was 57% shorter in the active treatment group compared with placebo (4.2 vs. 9.7 days; p < 0.01).[34] Investigators and biological plausibility suggest that treatment is most effective when initiated during the prodromal stage.

DOSAGE

Acute treatment 500 mg two times daily

PRECAUTIONS

GI distress with single doses greater than 1000 mg

TABLE 20.1	Potential Triggers of Incident Herpes Simplex Virus Reactivation
Acute infection	
HIV infection	
Immune suppressing medication	
High perceived stress	
Poor sleep quality	
Poor nutrition	
High emotional stress	
Blunt trauma or burn to face, lip, mouth, or genital area	
Excessive exposure to wind, sun, arid climate	
Fever	

TABLE 20.2 **Dietary Considerations in Herpes Simplex Virus Infection**

Foods	Quantity of food	Ratio of Arginine to Lysine	Quantity of Lysine
Low Arginine to Lysine Ratio (Helpful foods)			
Yoghurt	1 cup	0.35	700 mg
Cheese	3 oz.	0.4	1650 mg
Milk, whole	1 cup	0.45	600 mg
Cheese, cheddar	3 oz.	0.49	1497 mg
Cheese, ricotta	½ cup	0.50	1600 mg
Avocado	1 medium	0.50	100 mg
Tuna (3 oz)	½ can	0.6	2400 mg
Halibut, baked	3 oz.	0.65	2083 mg
Salmon	3 oz.	0.65	2014 mg
Sardines, canned in oil	3 med	0.65	814 mg
Chicken (baked light meat)	3 oz.	0.71	2232 mg
Pork	3 oz.	0.83	1586 mg
High Arginine to Lysine Ration (Foods to avoid)			
Almonds	18 nuts	4.7	145 mg
Peanut	¼ cup	3.0	363 mg
Cashews	10 nuts	2.6	185 mg

Zinc

Zinc is a mineral that is essential in cellular processes such as immunity and protein folding.[35] Topical zinc has been considered as a treatment for reducing symptoms, preventing recurrence, and shortening duration of outbreaks of oral and genital herpes. In a 2013 controlled clinical trial, 100 patients with herpes genitalis were allocated to one of four groups: one group of ten people received placebo and the remainder were allocated to receiving one of three groups, each containing a different concentration of topical $ZnSO_4$ (1%, 2%, or 4%). Treatment was initiated on day 1, then administered every 5 days for 1 month, then every 10 days for 2 months, and finally every 15 days for 3 months for a total of a 6-month protocol. At the end of the study, 80% versus 33%, 20%, and 3% of patients (placebo administration vs. 1%, 2%, and 4% topical $ZnSO_4$ administration, respectively) experienced recurrent outbreaks over the study period. Out of the three concentrations, 4% $ZnSO_4$ proved most effective and was well-tolerated.[36]

A trial of 200 patients with acute herpes simplex lesions applied a 0.25% zinc sulfate in a saturated solution of camphor water eight to ten times per day beginning within 24 hours of an outbreak. Investigators reported that lesions usually disappeared within 3–6 days, and the earlier treatment began the shorter the duration of symptoms.[37] A double-blind randomized trial assigned 46 patients with oral or facial herpes with symptoms of less than 24-hour duration to receive either zinc oxide-glycine cream or placebo. Treatment was applied every 2 hours for the lesser of 21 days or symptom resolution. Treatment was associated with a 23% reduction in symptom duration (5.0 vs. 6.5 days; p

< 0.02) in addition to a statistically significant reduction in symptom severity.[38]

There is moderate evidence to suggest that topical zinc formulations have utility in reducing the severity and duration of symptoms, and potentially the recurrence frequency, of oral/facial herpes infection. The greatest evidence is for formulations containing zinc sulfate, and reasonable evidence exists for zinc oxide-glycine and zinc monoglycerolate. There is only limited evidence evaluating oral zinc supplementation. We therefore favor using topical formulations for oral herpes infection.

DOSAGE

0.25%–4% zinc sulfate topical cream applied at initial onset of symptoms (ideally), then every 5 days for 1 month, then every 10 days for 2 months, and finally every 15 days for 3 months; although this protocol was well tolerated in one study, lower concentrations (0.25% every 30–60 minutes until lesions disappear) have been found to be effective.

PRECAUTIONS

Zinc sulfate solutions at higher concentrations (e.g., 4%) may cause pain, irritation, itching, and dryness.

Botanicals

Propolis

Propolis is a resin-like substance collected by bees from various plants, such as conifer and poplar trees.[39] It has antioxidant effects that boost the immune system, with evidence indicating it may aid in the recovery process of HSV-1 and -2 infection. In a randomized, single-blind, controlled multicenter study, 90 adults diagnosed with recurrent genital herpes (HSV-2) received a specific 3% propolis ointment (Herstat or Cold Sore FX), an acyclovir ointment, or a placebo. Ointments were applied to the affected area four times daily for 10 days. Investigators reported a statistically significant reduction in symptom severity and duration, as well as wound healing as determined by the study dermatologist, with propolis treatment. They further reported reductions in coexisting vaginal superinfections compared with both acyclovir and placebo groups.[40] In another study, the application of the same specific 3% propolis ointment (Herstat) to areas affected by HSV-1 infections five times daily at the start of symptoms reduced the symptom duration by 3–4 days and reduced pain.[41]

DOSAGE

3% propolis ointment applied four to five times daily for 10 days

PRECAUTIONS

Do not use for patients with allergies to bee products.

Lemon Balm

The lemon-scented herb, lemon balm (*Melissa officinalis*), belongs to the mint family and has been used therapeutically for centuries.[42] Due to its antiviral properties, lemon balm has been investigated as a method of treating herpes simplex virus. In a double-blind, randomized clinical trial, 66 patients with herpes labialis (HSV-1) applied a 1% topical ointment of lemon balm oil (70:1 extract) to the affected area four times daily starting with prodromal symptoms and continuing 2–3 days after lesions had healed. The results demonstrated that lemon balm oil ointment not only shortened the healing period (4.94 vs. 4.03 days) but also prevented infection spread and reduced burning, stabbing, and tingling symptoms.[43] An in vitro study investigated the phytochemical mechanism of *Melissa officinalis* and its antiviral effects on HSV-1 and HSV-2, finding that its inhibitory activity was due to lemon balm extracts inhibiting the virus prior to adsorption but not after penetration.[44] Therefore, it is recommended that lemon balm be applied as soon as one experiences prodromal symptoms in order to ensure the most effective and successful results. Finally, an in vitro study conducted in 2014 examined the effects of an aqueous extract of lemon balm and its phenolic compounds caffeic acid, p-coumaric acid, and rosmarinic acid on acyclovir-resistant strains of herpes simplex virus I. The study investigators reported lemon balm extract inhibited cell penetration of drug-sensitive and drug-resistant HSV strains by 80% and 96%, respectively.[45]

DOSAGE

Apply a topical 1% ointment of lemon balm oil to the affected area four to five times daily from the start of prodromal symptoms until 2–3 days after lesions have healed. The majority of previous studies used the product, Lomaherpan, which is a 1% dried lemon balm extract cream.

Sangre de Grado

Croton lecheri is a large tree that grows in the upper Amazon region of Colombia, Ecuador, and Peru; a dark red resin, where the name Sangre de Grado is derived, oozes from its bark.[46] Traditionally, Sangre de Grado has been used orally to treat diarrhea and promote gastrointestinal function. Recently, the powdered dry extract has been found to contain a novel proanthocyanidin called SP-303 that if applied topically may reduce genital and anogenital herpes lesions. A multicenter, double-blind, placebo-controlled clinical trial explored the efficaciousness and safety of Virend, a topical antiviral agent containing 15% SP-303, on recurrent genital herpes of AIDS patients. The trial reported that 41% of patients treated with Virend experienced complete healing of lesions versus 14% of patients in the placebo group (p = 0.05), with 50% of patients receiving active treatment compared with 19% of patients receiving placebo found to be culture negative (p = 0.06).[47]

DOSAGE

15% SP-303 ointment applied three times daily for 21 days

Aloe Vera

Aloe vera (*Aloe barbadensis*) is a cactus-like plant that grows in hot, dry climates and has been used for its medicinal properties by many cultures for millennia. A systematic review by Vogler and Ernst reviewed two randomized, double-blind clinical trials by the same author who studied the efficacy of a topical formulation in treating genital herpes. They concluded that there is limited evidence supporting its use.[48] The first study randomized 120 patients to receive either aloe vera cream (aloe vera extract 0.5% in hydrophilic cream), aloe vera gel, or placebo three times daily for 5 days. The aloe vera cream was associated with a statistically significant reduction in healing time (4.8 days vs. 7.0 days and 14.0 days, respectively) and a higher number of cured patients (70% cured patients vs. 45% and 7.5%, respectively).[49] The second study randomized men to aloe vera extract 0.5% in a hydrophilic cream or placebo. The results of this trial corroborated the results of the first trial in finding that the aloe vera cream group experienced significantly shorter healing times (4.9 days vs. 12 days, p < 0.001) and a higher number of cured patients (66.7% vs. 6.7%, p < 0.001) than those in the placebo group.[50]

DOSAGE

0.5% aloe vera extract in hydrophilic cream applied three times daily for 5 days

Acupuncture

There is robust evidence regarding the benefits of acupuncture in reducing anxiety, perceived stress, insomnia, depression, pain, and improving overall well-being and quality of life. Each of these factors has been associated with triggering incident HSV outbreaks. Consequently, acupuncture should be considered as an adjuvant therapy that may reduce recurrent infection rates through intermediate pathways.

Mind-Body Therapies

In addition to physical discomfort, receiving a diagnosis of oral and particularly genital herpes can cause emotional, psychological, and psychosexual distress including depression, anger, guilt, and/or anxiety.[51] In fact, the psychological component can become more disruptive to the patient's quality of life than the physical component.[52]

Relaxation Training

In 1985, adults living in a senior home were taught progressive muscle relaxation three times weekly for 1 month compared with social support, and a reduction in HSV antibodies that persisted 1 month beyond the intervention was documented.[53]

Hypnosis

In a pilot crossover study, 21 patients with genital HSV received 6 weeks of self-hypnosis using immune function imagery by listening to an audiotape recording of a live session. The study reported a 40% reduction in recurrent episodes (p = 0.05), with patients experiencing improved mood and reduced depression and anxiety.[54]

Other Mind-Body Interventions

In a study, 62 HIV-positive men coinfected with genital herpes were randomly assigned in a ratio of 2:1 to either a 10-week cognitive behavioral stress management class or wait-list control. Investigators reported that HSV-2 IgG antibodies were significantly reduced within the treatment group and remained unchanged in control group.[55]

There is a paucity of published literature on the effect of meditation, psychotherapy, and social support for people with recurrent HSV infection. Nonetheless, these therapies have been shown to improve quality of life and well-being, and as such will undoubtedly help people living with this condition.

Pharmaceuticals

There is no known curative therapy for HSC infection. Therefore, the mainstay of conventional treatment remains antiviral pharmaceutical medical therapy (acyclovir, famciclovir, valacyclovir) designed to inhibit DNA synthesis and viral replication.[56] Of note, many of the treatment guidelines for oral herpes have been extrapolated from genital herpes clinical research and guidelines.[57]

Antiviral medications have been shown to significantly reduce the severity and duration of symptoms during primary infection, reduce recurrent outbreaks frequency when taken prophylactically, and are extremely well tolerated. In comparative studies, these medications have

been shown to be noninferior in effectiveness. While acyclovir is considerably less expensive, valacyclovir is dosed less frequently and thus associated with greater patient adherence to treatment regimens.[58]

Topical anesthetic agents, such as viscous ziladent, benzocaine, and lidocaine, are available for the management of painful oral lesions resulting from HSV-1 infection and have been shown to provide limited short-term relief. Topical antiviral medications (e.g., penciclovir, docosanol) for HSV-1 oral lesions have demonstrated modest benefit in improving symptom severity and duration.[59]

> Herpes simplex is an intracellular virus that responds best to oral antiviral medications. Topical antivirals have only modest benefit.

Primary Uncomplicated HSV Infection

DOSAGE

The typical duration of treatment is 7–10 days. For maximal clinical benefit, treatment should commence within 72 hours of symptom onset. Any of the following medications can be prescribed, with factors for consideration including cost and dosing frequency.

Acyclovir: 200 mg five times daily or 400 mg three times daily
Famciclovir: 250 mg three times daily
Valacyclovir: 1000 mg twice daily

PRECAUTIONS

Dosage adjustments for renal insufficiency.

Recurrent Uncomplicated HSV Infection

Treatment strategies depend on patient's quality of life (i.e., recurrence frequency and severity of symptoms) and risk of exposing an uninfected sexual partner as viral shedding may occur in the absence of symptoms. Treatment options include no treatment, episodic treatment (at onset of recurrence), and chronic suppressive therapy (typically 1-year treatment followed by observational period). No treatment and episodic treatment are typically reserved for individuals with infrequent recurrences of minimal symptom severity, and those with no risk of viral transmission to an unexposed partner. For individuals experiencing frequent outbreaks (arbitrarily defined in research studies as greater than six episodes annually) or at risk of viral transmission, chronic suppressive therapy has been shown to be highly effective in improving overall quality of life and reducing outbreak frequency, symptom duration, and severity when compared with episodic therapy. A study randomized 156 patients with recurrent genital HSV to 12 months of either acyclovir 400 mg twice daily, 200 mg five times daily for 5 days at onset of symptoms, or placebo. Chronic suppressive therapy increased the number of days before recurrent outbreak and reduced symptom duration to 250 days and 0.32 days per month, respectively, compared to 28 days and 4.18 days per month with episodic treatment and 23 days and 4.72 days with placebo, respectively.[60]

Health professionals should discontinue chronic suppressive antiviral therapy once a year to determine whether continuation is necessary. To optimize the effectiveness of episodic therapy, it is important that patients maintain medication supply on-hand so that treatment can commence within 24 hours of the onset of prodromal symptoms (paresthesia, tingling, pain, redness).

DOSAGE

Chronic suppressive therapy. A 12-month treatment course of any of the following:
- Acyclovir (400 mg twice daily)
- Famciclovir (250 mg twice daily)
- Valacyclovir (500 or 1000 mg once daily)

Episodic therapy. To increase effectiveness, commence treatment within 24 hours of prodromal symptoms (pain, tingling, paresthesia). Oral herpes treatments differ from genital herpes and are therefore distinguished below. Treatment options include any of the following:
- Acyclovir:
  - Oral herpes: 200 mg or 400 mg five times daily for 5 days
  - Genital herpes: 800 mg three times daily for 2 days; 800 mg twice daily for 5 days; or 400 mg three times daily for 5 days
- Famciclovir:
  - Oral herpes: 750 mg twice daily for 1 day; or 1500 mg as a single dose
  - Genital herpes: 1000 mg twice daily for 1 day; or 500 mg once, then 250 mg twice daily for 2 days
- Valacyclovir:
  - Oral herpes: 2 g twice daily for 1 day
  - Genital herpes: 500 mg twice daily for 3 days or 1000 mg once daily for 5 days

PRECAUTIONS

Dosage adjustments for renal insufficiency

Therapies to Consider

Black Tea Extract

Black tea, derived from the leaves of the *Camellia sinensis* plant, is rich in theaflavins. Two studies have examined the effect of black tea extract on HSV-1 in vitro. The results of the first found that a concentration of 75 μM was not toxic to cultured cells and yet exhibited potent dose-dependent anti-HSV-1 effects, inhibiting > 99% of viral production.[61] The other observed that black tea extract at concentrations of 0.14 μM reduced HSV-1 virions in human cells by interfering with the attachment, penetration, and DNA replication of HSV-1.[62] This preliminary evidence is intriguing and supports further research in humans. Given the overall health benefits of black tea, people with HSV may consider drinking black tea daily and observe whether they experience any benefits against herpes virus symptoms.

Rhubarb and Sage

In a double-blind, comparative, randomized trial, 145 patients diagnosed with herpes labialis received rhubarb-sage cream, sage cream, or Zovirax cream (topical formulation of acyclovir). Healing period was 6.7 days in the rhubarb-sage cream group, 7.6 days in the sage cream group, and 6.5 days in the Zovirax cream group.[63] Further studies are required to determine the utility of rhubarb and sage together as a topical treatment for herpes simplex virus infection.

PREVENTION PRESCRIPTION

INCIDENT INFECTION PREVENTION

- Engage in honest dialogue with potential sexual partners regarding HSV status
- Avoid sexual contact during times of excess stress or when other triggers exist that increase the quantity of viral shedding
- Use a condom during sexual encounters to reduce risk of viral transmission

REDUCE RECURRENT OUTBREAKS

- Avoid trauma to skin (excessive sunlight and wind, physical trauma)
- Maintain good sleep quality
- Manage perceived and objective stress levels
- Evaluate whether a high lysine and low arginine diet alters outbreak frequency
- Consider daily use of Lysine supplementation, 1000 mg three times daily
- Consider chronic suppressive antiviral pharmaceutical therapy if outbreaks are frequent or quality of life is affected.
  - Acyclovir (400 mg twice daily)
  - Famciclovir (250 mg twice daily)
  - Valacyclovir (500 or 1000 mg once daily)

Elderberry

Hippocrates called the elder tree his "medicine chest" back in 400 CE. In recent years, preliminary evidence indicates favorable antimicrobial and antiviral effects of elderberry. In a 2005 interview Madeleine Mumcuoglu, MD, an Israeli virologist, explained her findings of elderberry neutralizing the activity of hemagglutinin spikes on the surface of the herpesvirus: "When these hemagglutinin spikes are deactivated, the viruses can no longer pierce cell walls or enter the cell and replicate."[64] A 2011 study reported that the flavonoids in a standardized elderberry extract (*Sambucus nigra L.*) bound to several bacteria and viruses in vitro.[65] Elderberry has become a common recommendation for cold and flu relief; however, its effect on herpes simplex virus 1 and 2 has not yet to be elucidated. However, there are anecdotal reports of patients claiming benefit in reducing the duration and severity of herpes genitalis symptoms.

THERAPEUTIC REVIEW

HERPES

Acute Treatment

- Supplements
  - Lysine: 1 g, three times daily — B 2
  - Vitamin C: 500 mg two times daily for 3 days — B 2
  - Zinc sulfate. Topical solution 0.0025%–0.25% applied at initial onset of symptoms (ideally) — B 2
    a. Apply every 30–60 minutes until lesions disappear—OR—
    b. Every 5 days for 1 month, then after every 10 days for 2 months, and finally every 15 days for 3 months
- Botanicals
  - For oral and genital
    - Propolis 3% topical ointment: four times daily for 10 days — B 2
  - For oral
    - Lemon Balm oil 1% topical ointment or cream (70:1 extract) — B 2
    - Apply to affected area four times daily until 3 days after lesions healed.
  - For genital
    - Propolis 3% topical ointment: four times daily for 10 days — B 2
    - Sangre De Grado: 15% SP-303 ointment applied three times daily for 21 days — B 2
    - Aloe vera 0.5% extract in hydrophilic cream: three times daily for 5 days — B 2
- Acupuncture to improve sleep, perceived stress, and anxiety — B 1
  - Once weekly, typically 20–45 minutes per treatment, individualized treatment protocol encouraged.

- Mind-Body Therapies
  - Self-hypnosis once weekly — B 1
  - Progressive muscle relaxation training program — C 1
  - Cognitive behavioral therapy training — C 1
  - Other—meditation, psychotherapy — C 1
- Pharmaceutical
  - Primary infection: Ideally start within 72 hours of symptom onset. Treat for 7–10 days. Choose from following based on dosing and cost: — A 2
    - Acyclovir: 200 mg five times daily or 400 mg three times daily
    - Famciclovir: 250 mg three times daily
    - Valacyclovir: 1000 mg twice daily
  - Episodic therapy for oral: Prescribe medication for on-demand use. Commence treatment within 24 hours of onset prodromal symptoms (pain, tingling, paresthesia). — A 2
    - Acyclovir: 200 mg or 400 mg five times daily for 5 days
    - Famciclovir: 750 mg twice daily for 1 day; or 1500 mg as a single dose
    - Valacyclovir: 2 g twice daily for 1 day
  - Episodic therapy for genital: Treatment options include any of the following: — A 2
    - Acyclovir: 800 mg three times daily for 2 days; 800 mg twice daily for 5 days; or 400 mg three times daily for 5 days
    - Famciclovir: 1000 mg twice daily for 1 day; or 500 mg once, then 250 mg twice daily for 2 days
    - Valacyclovir: 500 mg twice daily for 3 days or 1000 mg once daily for 5 days

Key Web Resources

Purpose:	URL:
CDC 2015 STD Treatment Guidelines for Genital Herpes	http://www.cdc.gov/std/tg2015/herpes.htm
HerpeSite. Noncommercial website focused on nonbiased information, empowerment, and support to people living with herpes.	http://www.herpesite.org/
University of Maryland Medical Center. Provides content licensed from A.D.A.M.—an integrative medicine content provider.	http://umm.edu/health/medical/altmed/condition/herpes-simplex-virus
Longwood Herbal Task Force. Has conducted extensive literature review on range of dietary supplements and botanicals. Limitation is last update was in 2003; however, excellent resource for identifying older studies	http://www.longwoodherbal.org/

REFERENCES

References are available online at ExpertConsult.com.

CHAPTER 21

CHRONIC HEPATITIS

Tina M. St. John, MD

PATHOPHYSIOLOGY

Characterized by hepatonecrosis and inflammatory cell infiltration, hepatitis is most commonly caused by viral and toxic agents. Deemed chronic when persisting for longer than 6 months, hepatitis triggers an ongoing inflammation that often leads to fibrosis and eventually cirrhosis, with a concomitant increased risk of hepatocellular carcinoma.

Chronic hepatitis may develop due to a variety of etiologies, either in isolation or combination (Table 21.1). The majority of individuals develop chronic hepatitis without a recent recognizable acute clinical illness or obvious symptoms. The condition is typically insidious and slowly progressive, declaring itself clinically only after cirrhosis develops with accompanying signs and symptoms.

Hepatitis C is the most common cause of chronic viral hepatitis in the United States, accounting for approximately 75% of all cases.[1,2] Given its high prevalence and clinical implications, chronic hepatitis C (CHC) is the focus of this section. Integrative treatments aimed at controlling chronic hepatic inflammation and its sequelae underlying the pathogenesis of CHC are applicable to other liver conditions that share a similar pathophysiology.

The hepatitis C virus (HCV) is hepatotropic but minimally cytopathic. The detrimental effects of chronic infection arise predominantly from ongoing inflammation, which causes marked oxidative stress. In the presence of ongoing hepatonecrosis, connective tissue is laid down as the body attempts repair. Accumulation of extracellular connective tissue leads to fibrosis, which progresses predictably (Table 21.2). Cirrhosis is the final stage of the fibrotic process, characterized by diffuse hepatocyte damage, nodular regeneration, and aberrant architecture accompanied by impaired hepatocyte function and impeded portal blood flow. The histological hallmarks of chronic hepatitis are hepatic necrosis, mononuclear infiltration, and fibrosis, which serves as the primary indicator of hepatic injury. Fibrosis and cirrhosis are assessed directly with liver biopsy or indirectly with noninvasive testing, including transient elastography and blood markers, such as platelet count, hyaluronic acid, procollagen type 3 N-terminal peptide, and tissue inhibitor of matrix metalloproteinase-1.[3]

Chronic inflammation due to *hepatitis infection* results in free radical production, *fibrosis, cirrhosis*, and hepatocellular carcinoma.

Advanced fibrosis and cirrhosis are associated with increased risk of hepatocellular carcinoma (HCC). CHC is the leading cause of HCC in the United States, with a 2% to 8% incidence per year among individuals with HCV-related cirrhosis.[4] Liver cancer incidence in the United States tripled between 1975 and 2005 before stabilizing from 2007 through 2010.[5,6] Although the 1-year, cause-specific survival for HCC has increased from 25% in 1992 to 47% in 2004,[5] overall 3-year survival remains at approximately 17%.[7]

With the recent introduction of direct-acting antivirals (DAAs), curative-intent treatment is recommended for all adults with CHC.[8] Fibrotic stage, however, is a primary consideration in determining the relative urgency of antiviral treatment. Approximately 5% to 20% of individuals with CHC develop cirrhosis over 20 to 30 years.[9-11] The results of prospective observational studies and outcome modeling projections indicate the risk of CHC disease progression to severe fibrosis or cirrhosis is minimal at 10 to 15 years in individuals with persistently normal alanine aminotransferase (ALT) levels, but greater than 30% to 40% in those with elevated serum ALT levels and portal fibrosis.[9,12] Because clinical findings and liver enzyme levels do not predictably correlate with hepatic histological features, cirrhosis cannot be ruled out based on clinical and laboratory assessments alone.[13,14] Nonhistological factors associated with accelerated CHC progression are shown in Table 21.3. Viral load is notably absent as it has not been found to correlate with disease progression.

Reducing Free Radicals

The primary care provider has an important role in promoting constitutional, hepatic, and immunological health and wellness. Factors that potentially influence CHC disease progression and may be affected by integrative interventions fall into two primary arenas: oxidative stress and immunological function.[21-30] Chronic inflammation leads to an overabundance of oxygen-derived free radicals. The influence of free radicals in a given inflammatory reaction depends on the balance between the production and inactivation of these reactive metabolites. To the extent that one can influence the balance favorably toward decreased oxidative stress, one can potentially limit or reduce damage caused by an overabundance of free radicals.

Enhancing Liver Detoxification

As the interface between the digestive tract and the rest of the body, the liver orchestrates metabolic homeostasis and detoxifies endogenous waste products and pollutant xenobiotics. A two-phase detoxification process

TABLE 21.1 Common Etiologies of Chronic Hepatitis

Etiological Category	Specifics
Hepatitis viruses	Hepatitis C Hepatitis B (+/– hepatitis D)
Toxins and medications	Ethanol Methyldopa Isoniazid Nitrofurantoin Amiodarone
Acquired metabolic disorders	Nonalcoholic steatohepatitis
Autoimmune disease	Autoimmune hepatitis
Inborn metabolic disorders	Wilson's disease Hemochromatosis Alpha$_1$-antitrypsin deficiency
Biliary diseases	Primary and secondary biliary cirrhosis Primary sclerosing cholangitis Biliary tree anomalies
Cryptogenic	—

TABLE 21.2 Stages of Liver Fibrosis

Stage	Characteristics
0	No fibrosis
1	Confined to enlarged portal zones
2	Periportal or portal–portal septa with intact architecture
3	Architectural distortion (septal fibrosis, bridging) without obvious cirrhosis
4	Probable or definite cirrhosis

TABLE 21.3 Nonhistological Factors Associated with Accelerated Fibrosis Progression Among People with Chronic Hepatitis C[8,15-20]

Genotypic male
Age > 40 years at the time of initial infection
Heavy alcohol use
Daily marijuana use
Obesity and/or insulin resistance
Genotype 3 infection
Coinfection with HIV and/or HBV
Organ Transplant

HBV, hepatitis B virus; HIV, human immunodeficiency virus.

TABLE 21.4 Substances That Support Phase II Detoxification[31,32]

Detoxification Pathway	Required Nutrients
Glutathione conjugation	Dietary glutathione Vitamins B$_2$, B$_6$, and C N-acetylcysteine Glycine, cysteine, glutamine, and methionine Zinc, copper, manganese, and selenium
Amino acid conjugation	Glycine, taurine, glutamine, arginine, and ornithine Magnesium
Methylation	S-adenosylmethionine Vitamin B$_{12}$ and folic acid Choline Molybdenum
Sulfation	Sulfur-rich foods B vitamins Taurine, methionine, cysteine, and glutathione Zinc, copper, manganese, selenium, and molybdenum
Acetylation	Vitamins B$_1$, B$_2$, B$_5$, and C Acetyl coenzyme A
Glucuronidation	Glucuronic acid and glutamine Magnesium Vitamins B$_3$ and B$_6$

neutralizes and eliminates these chemicals. For optimal function, the phases of detoxification must be balanced and supported by adequate dietary intake to provide the necessary system elements. Phase I of the detoxification pathway is chemical neutralization, predominantly mediated by the cytochrome P-450 system. This system of heme-derived enzymes catalyzes redox reactions for a wide variety of endogenous and exogenous substrates. Enzymatic P-450 neutralization yields free radicals that can damage hepatocytes. These oxygen-derived chemicals are removed by hepatic antioxidants. One of the most important of these is glutathione, which is also used in phase II of the detoxification process. High levels of toxin exposure can deplete hepatic glutathione and hamper both phases of the detoxification process.

Phase II of the detoxification process is elimination, which typically involves a conjugation reaction that renders the toxin water-soluble, thereby facilitating excretion through bile or urine. The six pathways of phase II detoxification are glutathione conjugation, amino acid conjugation, methylation, sulfation, acetylation, and glucuronidation.[31] Many experts consider glutathione conjugation the most important of these pathways. Table 21.4 provides a list of substances required for phase II detoxification (see Chapter 106).

INTEGRATIVE THERAPY

The choice of therapeutic modalities used in an integrative approach to CHC management depends on numerous factors, including the patient's liver status, goals, and comorbidities. Regardless of the modalities chosen, the fundamental goals of integrative CHC management are as follows: decrease hepatic inflammation to limit disease progression; support and enhance hepatic detoxification capacity; support healthy immune function; decrease the risk of cirrhosis, hepatocellular carcinoma, and extrahepatic complications; and support and enhance quality of life.

Pharmaceuticals

Guidelines from the American Association for the Study of Liver Diseases and the Infectious Diseases Society of

America in collaboration with the International Antiviral Society–USA (AASLD/IDSA/IAS–USA) state that, "[Antiviral] treatment is recommended for all patients with chronic HCV infection, except those with short life expectancies that cannot be remediated by treating HCV, by transplantation, or by other directed therapy."[8] The benefits of virological cure include reduced hepatic inflammation and morbidity; potential improvement in hepatic fibrosis; reduced risk of HCC and liver-related mortality; and partial or complete remission of extrahepatic manifestations of CHC.[33-37]

Pharmacological treatment of CHC has evolved rapidly since 2011. Direct-acting antiviral therapy has replaced the previous standard treatment regime of peginterferon plus ribavirin.[8] Compared to peginterferon plus ribavirin, newer interferon-free DAA regimens are better tolerated with fewer contraindications, require a shorter duration of treatment, and are markedly more effective at inducing sustained viral response (SVR). Clinical trial data indicate that DAA-based CHC treatment leads to an SVR in 80% to 100% of patients.[38-45] The drawbacks of DAA therapy include affordability and drug interactions.[46-48]

> The introduction of direct-acting antiviral therapy has revolutionized the treatment of HCV. Although costly compared to previous regimes, DAA therapy requires a shorter duration, has fewer side effects, and is effective in 80%–100% of patients.

The decision to initiate therapy is based on the following considerations: patient's personal preferences, liver status, and comorbidities; the likelihood of disease progression; and potential risks and benefits. It is recommended that all people with CHC—treatment-naïve or experienced, including those with compensated or decompensated cirrhosis—should be considered for antiviral therapy. There is differential priority and urgency, however, based primarily on the relative risk of complications and likelihood of HCV transmission to others. Individuals at the greatest risk of complications are considered highest priority for treatment as they are likely to derive the greatest benefit from virological cure (Table 21.5).

Risk factors can be used to predict the likely natural history of CHC. The clinical course in a given individual, however, is inherently unpredictable. The decision to initiate antiviral treatment and the timing of such therapy must be individualized. For patients with minimal fibrosis who are asymptomatic, opting to defer curative-intent therapy for a short period is unlikely to represent a major health risk. Supportive management and regular follow-up are the cornerstones of care for all individuals with CHC, regardless of their treatment decisions.

Direct-Acting HCV Antivirals

In the United States, DAAs are the mainstay of recommended first-line CHC treatment. DAAs are used in combination to reduce the likelihood of treatment failure due to preexisting or evolving antiviral resistance.[49] Ribavirin may be added to combination DAA therapy in some situations for the same reason.[50] The specific antiviral

TABLE 21.5 Clinical Factors That Increase Priority for Antiviral Hepatitis C Treatment[8,38,51]

Advanced fibrosis or compensated cirrhosis
Liver transplant candidate or recipient
Coexisting liver disease (e.g., hepatitis B, NASH)
HIV coinfection
Severe or debilitating extrahepatic manifestations
Type 2 diabetes mellitus

HIV, human immunodeficiency virus; NASH, nonalcoholic steatohepatitis.

regimen and duration of treatment for a given patient depends on HCV genotype and subtype, past treatment experience, presence of cirrhosis (with or without decompensation), comorbidities (e.g., HIV, renal disease), and the presence of genetic viral variations that could influence treatment response.[8,38,51]

Since the first HCV DAAs were approved by the U.S. Food and Drug Administration in 2011, additional agents continue to be introduced at a rapid pace. Currently, FDA-approved DAAs for combination treatment of CHC include protease inhibitors (simeprevir, paritaprevir, and grazoprevir); polymerase inhibitors (sofosbuvir and dasabuvir); and NS5A inhibitors (ledipasvir, ombitasvir, daclatasvir, velpatasvir, and elbasvir). Protease inhibitor ritonavir lacks anti-HCV activity but is used to boost levels of some HCV DAAs by inhibition of CYP3A4 enzymes. The swiftly changing pharmacological landscape in CHC is driving a concomitant flux in treatment recommendations. Table 21.6 summarizes current AASLD/IDSA/IAS–USA recommended and alternative therapies for HCV genotype 1, 2, and 3 infections, which account for 98% of cases of CHC in the U.S.[52]

DOSAGE
See Table 21.6.

PRECAUTIONS
The side effect profile of HCV DAAs is markedly better than peginterferon plus ribavirin. A number of clinically relevant drug interactions, however, warrant scrupulous attention. Interference or enhancement of drug absorption, metabolism, or elimination may affect bioavailability, potentially leading to toxicity or subtherapeutic drug levels. Prescription and over-the-counter medications as well as certain herbs are known to interfere with specific DAAs. Medications and drug classes of particular concern include antiretrovirals, immunosuppressants, proton pump inhibitors, anticonvulsants, statins, phosphodiesterase inhibitors, calcium channel blockers, benzodiazepines, ethinyl estradiol, amiodarone, gemfibrozil, rifampin, azole antifungals, St. John's wort, and milk thistle.[38,46,53] As research examining specific DAA and herb or supplement interactions is often lacking, many experts recommend avoiding all such therapeutics during antiviral treatment. As specific interactions vary among the DAAs, it is critical to crosscheck all medications, herbs, and supplements taken against the prescribing information to minimize the risk of drug-related complications during treatment.

TABLE 21.6   AASLD/IDSA/IAS–USA Recommended and Alternative Direct-Acting Antiviral Regimens for Chronic Hepatitis C due to Genotypes 1, 2, and 3[8]

Genotype	Cirrhosis*	RAV Considerations[†]	Antiviral Regimen: Recommended (R) or Alternative (A)[‡]	Duration (weeks)
			Initial Treatment	
1a, 1b	+ or –	Elbasvir RAVs absent (relevant for 1a only)	R: daily fixed-dose elbasvir (50 mg)/grazoprevir (100 mg)	12
1a	+ or –	eblasvir RAV present	A: daily fixed-dose elbasvir (50 mg)/grazoprevir (100 mg) plus weight-based ribavirin[§]	16
1a, 1b	+ or –	–	R: daily fixed-dose ledipasvir (90 mg)/sofosbuvir (400 mg)	12
1a, 1b, 2	+ or –	–	R: daily fixed-dose sofosbuvir (400 mg)/velpatasvir (100 mg)	12
3	–	–	R: daily fixed-dose sofosbuvir (400 mg)/velpatasvir (100 mg)	12
3	+	+/– Y93H RAV	R: daily fixed-dose sofosbuvir (400 mg)/velpatasvir (100 mg); add weight-based ribavirin[§] if Y93H RAV is present	12
1a	–	–	R: daily fixed-dose paritaprevir (150 mg)/ritonavir (100 mg)/ombitasvir (25 mg) plus twice-daily dosed dasabuvir (250 mg) and weight-based ribavirin[†]	12
1a	+	–	A: daily fixed-dose paritaprevir (150 mg)/ritonavir (100 mg)/ombitasvir (25 mg) plus twice-daily dosed dasabuvir (250 mg) and weight-based ribavirin[†]	24
1b	+ or –	–	R: daily fixed-dose paritaprevir (150 mg)/ritonavir (100 mg)/ombitasvir (25 mg) plus twice-daily dosed dasabuvir (250 mg)	12
1a, 1b	–	–	R: daily simeprevir (150 mg) plus sofosbuvir (400 mg)	12
1a, 1b	+	Q80K variant absent (relevant for 1a only)	A: daily simeprevir (150 mg) plus sofosbuvir (400 mg) with or without weight-based ribavirin[§]	24
1a, 1b, 3	–	–	R: daily daclatasvir (60 mg[¶]) plus sofosbuvir (400 mg)	12
3	+	+/– Y93H RAV	R: daily daclatasvir (60 mg[¶]) plus sofosbuvir (400 mg); add weight-based ribavirin[§] if Y93H RAV is present	24
1a, 1b	+	–	A: daily daclatasvir (60 mg[¶]) plus sofosbuvir (400 mg) with or without weight-based ribavirin[§]	24
2	–	–	A: daily daclatasvir (60 mg[¶]) plus sofosbuvir (400 mg)	12
2	+	–	A: daily daclatasvir (60 mg[¶]) plus sofosbuvir (400 mg)	16 to 24
			Retreatment After Prior Treatment Failure with Peginterferon and Ribavirin	
1a, 1b	+ or –	Elbasvir RAVs absent (relevant for 1a only)	R: daily fixed-dose elbasvir (50 mg)/grazoprevir (100 mg)	12
1a	+ or –	Eblasvir RAV present	A: daily fixed-dose elbasvir (50 mg)/grazoprevir (100 mg) plus weight-based ribavirin[§]	16
1a, 1b	–	–	R: daily fixed-dose ledipasvir (90 mg)/sofosbuvir (400 mg)	12
1a, 1b	+	–	R: daily fixed-dose ledipasvir (90 mg)/sofosbuvir (400 mg) plus weight-based ribavirin[§]	12
1a, 1b	+	–	A: daily fixed-dose ledipasvir (90 mg)/sofosbuvir (400 mg)	24
1a	–	–	R: daily fixed-dose paritaprevir (150 mg)/ritonavir (100 mg)/ombitasvir (25 mg) plus twice-daily dosed dasabuvir (250 mg) and weight-based ribavirin[§]	12
1a	+	–	A: daily fixed-dose paritaprevir (150 mg)/ritonavir (100 mg)/ombitasvir (25 mg) plus twice-daily dosed dasabuvir (250 mg) and weight-based ribavirin[§]	24
1b	+ or –	–	R: daily fixed-dose paritaprevir (150 mg)/ritonavir (100 mg)/ombitasvir (25 mg) plus twice-daily dosed dasabuvir (250 mg)	12
1a, 1b	–	–	R: daily simeprevir (150 mg) plus sofosbuvir (400 mg)	12

Continued

TABLE 21.6 **AASLD/IDSA/IAS–USA Recommended and Alternative Direct-Acting Antiviral Regimens for Chronic Hepatitis C due to Genotypes 1, 2, and 3[8]—cont'd**

Genotype	Cirrhosis*	RAV Considerations[†]	Antiviral Regimen: Recommended (R) or Alternative (A)[‡]	Duration (weeks)
Retreatment After Prior Treatment Failure with Peginterferon and Ribavirin				
1a, 1b	+	Q80K variant absent (relevant for 1a only)	A: daily simeprevir (150 mg) plus sofosbuvir (400 mg) with or without weight-based ribavirin[§]	24
1a, 1b, 2	+ or –	–	R: daily fixed-dose sofosbuvir (400 mg)/velpatasvir (100 mg)	12
3	–	+/– Y93H RAV	R: daily fixed-dose sofosbuvir (400 mg)/velpatasvir (100 mg); add weight-based ribavirin[§] if Y93H RAV is present	12
3	+	–	R: daily fixed-dose sofosbuvir (400 mg)/velpatasvir (100 mg) plus weight-based ribavirin[§]	12
1a, 1b	–	–	R: daily daclatasvir (60 mg[‡]) plus sofosbuvir (400 mg)	12
2	–	–	A: daily daclatasvir (60 mg[‡]) plus sofosbuvir (400 mg)	12
2	+	–	A: daily daclatasvir (60 mg[‡]) plus sofosbuvir (400 mg)	16 to 24
1a, 1b	+	–	A: daily daclatasvir (60 mg[¶]) plus sofosbuvir (400 mg) with or without weight-based ribavirin[§]	24
3	–	+/– Y93H RAV	R: daily daclatasvir (60 mg[¶]) plus sofosbuvir (400 mg); add weight-based ribavirin[§] if Y93H RAV is present	12
3	+	–	R: daily daclatasvir (60 mg[¶]) plus sofosbuvir (400 mg) with weight-based ribavirin[§]	24

*Cirrhosis refers to compensated cirrhosis unless otherwise noted.
[†]Resistance-associated variants (RAVs) represent HCV genetic variations that can adversely affect treatment response with certain DAA regiments. Pretreatment testing is recommended before using these regimens.
[‡]Recommended regimens are favored for most patients in a given subgroup, based on optimal efficacy, favorable tolerability and toxicity profiles, and duration. Alternative regimens are those that are effective but have, relative to recommended regimens, potential disadvantages, limitations for use in certain patient populations, or less supporting data than recommended regimens. For some groups, data are insufficient to recommend a specific regimen; alternatives are considered equivalent.
[§]Weight-based ribavirin: 1000 mg daily if <75 kg or 1200 mg daily if >75 kg in two divided doses.
[¶]Daclatasvir dose may need to be adjusted if used with cytochrome P450 3A/4 inducers or inhibitors.

Ribavirin

Ribavirin is a guanosine analog with in vitro and in vivo activity against a variety of viruses. Although it has little in vivo effect against HCV in isolation, adding ribavirin to DAA therapy reduces the risk of developing antiviral resistance during treatment, thereby leading to improved therapeutic response.[54,55]

DOSAGE

See Table 21.6.

PRECAUTIONS

Ribavirin is associated with two serious adverse effects; hemolytic anemia and birth defects. Monitoring hemoglobin and hematocrit throughout therapy is essential, as is scrupulous use of reliable birth control during and for 6 months after the completion of treatment.[54,55]

Treatment Response

HCV viral load determines virological response. Quantitative HCV RNA testing within the 12 weeks before initiating DAA-based therapy, at week 4 of treatment, and 12 weeks after completion of antiviral therapy is recommended. The majority of individuals have undetectable HCV RNA at week 4 of DAA therapy; however, treatment response may be delayed in those with cirrhosis. In such cases, repeat testing at week 6 is recommended. While evidence-based guidelines for the cessation of DAA-based HCV treatment have not been established, AASLD/IDSA/IAS–USA recommends discontinuing treatment if there is a 10-fold or greater increase in HCV RNA levels from baseline at week 6 of treatment.[8]

Hepatitis A and B Vaccination

Patients with documented CHC not previously immunized and without serological evidence of immunity should be vaccinated against hepatitis viruses A and B. Superinfection in a patient with CHC may cause acute fulminant disease. In the absence of an acute fulminant episode, new infection superimposed on preexisting chronic liver disease may accelerate disease progression and negatively affect prognosis.

Supplements

Glutathione

The potent antioxidant glutathione serves numerous crucial functions, including detoxification and cytotoxic

T lymphocyte (CTL) activation.[56] Glutathione is predominantly produced intracellularly in the liver from cysteine, glutamate, and glycine. Glutathione levels are frequently below normal levels in patients with CHC.[57-59] One study found that CHC patients with the lowest glutathione levels had the highest viral loads and greater degrees of liver damage compared to patients with the highest glutathione levels.[59]

Absorption of intact oral glutathione is limited as it is hydrolyzed by intestinal gamma-glutamyl transferase.

Optimal glutathione levels are achieved by consuming a diet rich in foods with high levels of sulfur-containing amino acids (e.g., asparagus, avocados, broccoli, spinach, garlic, and unprocessed meats) and may be enhanced by supplements that promote glutathione production, such as vitamins C and E, N-acetylcysteine (NAC), selenium, and silymarin.

Vitamin C

Vitamin C is a powerful antioxidant and antiinflammatory, functions that may help limit chronic inflammation and oxidative stress associated with CHC. A study published in 2008 noted an inverse relationship between plasma vitamin C and aspartate aminotransferase (AST) levels among patients with CHC.[60] Vitamin C also has immunomodulatory and anticarcinogenic functions, and has been found to preserve intracellular reduced glutathione concentrations and improve overall antioxidant capacity.[61,62]

DOSAGE
The typical vitamin C dosage is 200 mg to 250 mg twice daily, although recommendations vary widely. The tolerable upper intake limit (UL) is 2000 mg/day.[63]

PRECAUTIONS
Vitamin C modulates iron absorption and transport. High doses should be avoided in patients with hemochromatosis or other conditions with the potential for iron overload. High-dose vitamin C is contraindicated in patients with a history of kidney stones or renal insufficiency. Excessive doses may result in bloating and/or diarrhea.

Vitamin E

Vitamin E is a fat-soluble antioxidant that supports optimal glutathione levels. Research data on vitamin E in the setting of chronic hepatitis are mixed. Two small studies of CHC patients found vitamin E supplementation led to reduced ALT levels in roughly one-half of study participants.[64,65] However, another study in which CHC patients took supplemental vitamin E, selenium, and vitamin C daily found no effect on ALT, HCV viral load, or oxidative markers after 6 months of treatment.[66] Some studies have indicated that vitamin E may have a role in interrupting the fibrotic process.[67,68]

DOSAGE
The typical dose is 400 IU/day of d-alpha tocopherol.

PRECAUTIONS
High-dose vitamin E may potentiate the effects of antithrombotic drugs and some herbs (e.g., garlic and ginkgo). Patients with vitamin K deficiency should avoid high-dose vitamin E. The UL for vitamin E is 1500 IU/day.[63]

Selenium

The essential nutrient selenium exerts potent antioxidant activity via its roles in the formation and function of selenium-dependent glutathione peroxidases. Selenoproteins serve as important regulators of tissue redox status, inflammation, and immune responses. Selenium deficiency has been linked to innate, humoral, and cell-mediated immunosuppression.[69] Significantly reduced selenium levels have been found among patients with CHC, with greater deficiencies observed in cirrhotics compared to those with lesser fibrosis.[70-73] Thus there is at least a theoretical role for supplemental selenium in limiting CHC-related disease progression, although efficacy has yet to be proven. Similarly, the potential role of selenium in HCC prevention among patients with chronic viral hepatitis remains uncertain. A large Taiwanese study conducted in the late 1980s and early 1990s examining selenium levels in 7342 men with chronic hepatitis B or C and development of HCC found selenium levels were lowest in men with CHC. Participants with the highest selenium levels were 38% less likely to develop HCC compared to participants with the lowest selenium levels.[74] Another large-scale, contemporaneous Chinese study found a similar protective effect among patients with chronic hepatitis B infection.[75] Subsequent studies, however, have failed to definitively demonstrate a chemoprotective effect associated with selenium supplementation and HCC risk.[76,77]

DOSAGE
The typical selenium dose is 200 mcg/day in the form of high-selenium yeast or L-selenomethionine.

PRECAUTIONS
The UL for selenium is 400 mcg/day,[63] although adverse reactions are uncommon at doses less than 900 mcg/day.[78] Symptoms associated with selenium toxicity include hair and nail brittleness and loss, rash, fatigue, irritability, nausea, vomiting, and diarrhea.[79]

S-Adenosylmethionine

S-adenosylmethionine (SAMe) is synthesized in all body tissues but highly concentrated in the liver. SAMe serves as the primary methyl group in transmethylation reactions, which are integral to phase II hepatic detoxification and biosynthesis of nucleic acids, phospholipids, proteins, and other essential molecules. Available in the U.S. as a nutritional supplement, SAMe is used medicinally in Europe for liver disorders, depression, osteoarthritis, and fibromyalgia.

SAMe has been shown to have hepatoprotective effects in animal models of experimental injury; however, the few results from human studies have been less definitive.[80,81] A placebo-controlled, 2-year study of 123 patients with alcoholic cirrhosis found 200 mg of oral SAMe daily significantly improved survival and delayed the need for liver transplantation.[82] SAMe has been shown in animal models to protect against the development of HCC,[83-85] although efficacy has not yet been established in humans with cirrhosis. Studies of patients with viral hepatitis and other chronic liver conditions have found that SAMe has utility in alleviating associated symptoms, such as itching, jaundice, and fatigue, and reduces liver enzyme and bilirubin levels.[86,87] SAMe has also been used for decades in Europe to treat depression, a common complaint among CHC patients. A 2013 literature review concluded that the proof of concept is solid, but additional study data are required before SAMe can be confidently recommended as first-line or adjuvant therapy for depression.[88]

The high cost of SAMe, its relative instability, and lack of conclusive data to support its use in CHC preclude its recommendation for regular use. Some clinicians recommend a combination of methionine, trimethylglycine, vitamin B_{12}, and folic acid to support endogenous SAMe production.

DOSAGE

The typical dose of SAMe for liver disease is 800 mg twice daily on an empty stomach.

PRECAUTIONS

Mild gastrointestinal upset, anxiety, hyperactive muscle movement, and insomnia have been reported as side effects of SAMe use. Patients with depression and bipolar disorder should be closely monitored while taking SAMe.

Alpha-Lipoic Acid

Alpha-lipoic acid (ALA) is a fatty acid antioxidant. A key metabolite in mitochondrial energy production and a potent free radical scavenger, ALA is used medicinally in many European countries, primarily to treat liver disorders and neuropathy. The effect of ALA in raising cellular glutathione levels is thought to be important in CHC due to relative glutathione deficiency.[89,90] ALA also helps recycle and regenerate other antioxidants, including vitamins E and C.[91] Results from studies of animal models indicate that ALA may impede fibrosis progression associated with chronic hepatitis by reducing production of reactive oxygen species.[92,93]

ALA is costly and has not been well studied in clinical trials among people with chronic viral hepatitis. Therefore its routine use is not recommended. In patients with unexplained spikes in liver enzymes, however, ALA may be advisable to reduce oxidative stress.

DOSAGE

ALA dosage is 500 to 600 mg/day.

PRECAUTIONS

No side effects have been reported with ALA doses up to 1000 mg/day.

Glutamine

Glutamine is a conditionally essential amino acid. Although normally synthesized in adequate amounts, endogenous glutamine production may be inadequate during periods of metabolic stress. Glutamine is crucial for many metabolic functions, including protein and glutathione synthesis, energy production, maintenance of optimal antioxidant status, and immune function. Glutamine regulates the expression of several genes and activates numerous proteins.[94] l-Glutamine is an immunonutrient and the preferred substrate for energy production in enterocytes and lymphocytes. Glutamine influences production of some T-cell-derived cytokines and is important for optimal lymphocyte proliferation.[95-97] Notably, lymphocytes are unable to produce glutamine. If glutamine stores are depleted by ongoing immunological demands, glutathione production will therefore be inadequate. Glutamine is an important nutritional supplement when metabolic stress renders endogenous synthesis inadequate.

DOSAGE

Glutamine doses of 2 to 4 g/day are used during periods of metabolic stress or poor dietary intake. Glutamine supplements should be taken between meals.

PRECAUTIONS

Glutamine supplementation should be approached with caution in patients with hepatic or renal insufficiency.[98]

Zinc

The essential mineral, zinc, serves numerous important biochemical roles, including functioning as an essential cofactor in healthy immunological function and supporting antioxidant systems. As zinc deficiency is uncommon in developed countries, routine zinc supplementation is unnecessary for most CHC patients but may be a consideration for individuals who are nutritionally deprived.

DOSAGE

The typical zinc dosage is 15 mg/day. The UL for zinc is 40 mg/day.[99]

PRECAUTIONS

Long-term ingestion of high-dose zinc may deplete copper stores, interfere with iron function, and lead to microcytic anemia. Ingestion of large amounts of zinc (>30 mg/day) may cause acute toxicity with nausea, vomiting, diarrhea, anorexia, abdominal cramps, a metallic taste, headache, and drowsiness.

Iron

People with CHC should avoid iron overload. Increased hepatic iron stores are associated with higher degrees of inflammation and more severe hepatic fibrosis in patients with CHC compared to patients without iron overload.[100,101] Iron supplements should be avoided among patients with CHC except in cases of documented deficiency. Iron-binding supplements may be beneficial in patients with increased serum iron levels.

Botanicals

Milk Thistle (*Silybum marianum*)

Milk thistle is the most commonly used supplement among CHC patients.[102] The active component of milk thistle, silymarin, has reported antioxidant, antiinflammatory, antifibrogenic, antiproliferative, and immunomodulatory effects in addition to stabilizing hepatocyte cell membranes against free radical attack.[103-105] Silymarin is a potent antioxidant. It has been reported to raise hepatic and intestinal glutathione levels by 50% in animal studies[106] and to increase levels of the antioxidant enzymes superoxide dismutase, glutathione peroxidase, and catalase in other animal models.[107,108] Silymarin also has antifibrotic properties. Among silymarin users in the Hepatitis C Antiviral Long-Term Treatment against Cirrhosis (HALT-C) trial, researchers found reduced fibrosis progression but no significant difference in clinical outcome compared to nonusers.[109] A separate U.S. multicenter, double-blind, placebo-controlled trial among 154 CHC patients previously unsuccessfully treated with interferon-based therapy found no significant differences in serum ALT levels, viral load, or quality of life between participants taking 420 mg or 720 mg of oral silymarin 3 times daily for 24 weeks compared to those taking a placebo.[110] An earlier randomized, double-blind, 12-month trial of 177 Egyptian patients with CHC, however, found patients taking oral silymarin reported improved symptoms and general well-being, although no effect was noted in HCV viremia, ALT, or serum and ultrasound markers of hepatic fibrosis.[111] Combination treatments with milk thistle as a principal component are currently being evaluated. In a small study of CHC patients treated with a 3-month course of a combination of silybin phospholipids and vitamin E, researchers found a significant reduction in serum aminotransferase levels.[112] Other clinical studies of the effects of silymarin on chronic liver disease have yielded mixed results.[113-115] A 2005 Cochrane systematic review of 13 randomized trials and a 2014 meta-analysis of randomized controlled trials of silymarin in CHC patients both concluded there is lack of high-quality evidence of efficacy.[116,117] The difference between laboratory observations and clinical efficacy may be attributable to issues such as limited absorption of oral silymarin, relatively low blood levels, and HCV-specific alterations in hepatic silymarin uptake and enterohepatic cycling.[103,110,118]

In summary, research data indicate that many actions of silymarin may theoretically be beneficial for chronic hepatitis patients. Clinical data to support this supposition, however, remain lacking with regard to CHC.

Given that milk thistle has no known serious adverse effects, many clinicians believe the potential for benefit justifies use of this supplement despite the current lack of robust, supportive clinical evidence.

DOSAGE

The typical milk thistle dosage for chronic hepatitis is 300 mg three times daily, or 210 mg of silymarin three times daily. Silymarin-phosphatidylcholine is absorbed more effectively than regular standardized milk thistle and requires less frequent dosing (240 mg twice daily). Alcohol extracts should be avoided in patients with hepatitis.

PRECAUTIONS

Side effects of milk thistle are reportedly rare. Reported adverse reactions include stomach pain, nausea, vomiting, diarrhea, headache, rash or other skin reactions, and joint pain. Allergic reactions may occur in patients with hypersensitivity to ragweed or plants in the daisy family.

Milk thistle should be discontinued at least 1 week prior to beginning DAA-based antiviral therapy (particularly simeprevir and elbasvir/grazoprevir) and avoided throughout treatment due to the risk of drug–herb interactions.[8]

Licorice Root (*Glycyrrhiza glabra* and *uralensis*)

Licorice root preparations have been an accepted treatment for hepatitis in Japan since the 1960s. Glycyrrhizin (an aqueous extract of licorice root) acts primarily as an antiinflammatory and cytoprotective agent.[119] Although the antiviral properties of glycyrrhizin have been demonstrated in vitro, they do not appear to be clinically relevant.[119-121] Some clinical studies reporting benefit have used a form of intravenous glycyrrhizin called Stronger Neo-Minophagen C (SNMC; 0.2% glycyrrhizin, 0.1% cysteine, and 2% glycine). A nonrandomized, retrospective Japanese study reported that long-term SNMC treatment (3 to 5 times weekly for 13 to 15 years) among patients with viral hepatitis led to significantly reduced incidence of cirrhosis and hepatocellular carcinoma.[122] A review article published in 2005 noted, however, that SNMC "improves liver function in patients with chronic hepatitis" but does not reduce mortality.[119] A Cochrane review of medicinal herbs for HCV infection concluded that glycyrrhizin did not demonstrate significant beneficial effects.[123] A 2014 review similarly concluded that evidence of clinical efficacy remains lacking.[124]

Despite promising animal model data and anecdotal experience supporting the parenteral use of glycyrrhizin, robust clinical data demonstrating efficacy are scant. Moreover, oral licorice root preparations remain virtually unstudied.

DOSAGE

The recommended dosage of oral licorice root depends on the form: 250 to 500 mg three times daily for solid dry powder; 1 to 2 g three times daily for powdered root; or 2 to 4 mL three times a day for fluid extracts.

PRECAUTIONS

High-dose glycyrrhizin may lead to an aldosterone effect with potassium loss, water retention, and hypertension. Use may potentiate the effects of diuretics, certain cardiac medications (e.g., digitalis), and corticosteroids. Glycyrrhizin should be used cautiously in the setting of hypertension, ascites, renal insufficiency, and cardiac failure. A diet high in potassium-rich foods is recommended for patients taking a licorice root preparation. Blood pressure and potassium levels should be monitored regularly.

Schisandra (*Schisandra chinensis*)

Schisandra has long been used in traditional Chinese and Kampo medicine for liver disorders. Medicinal substances derived from the fruit of the plant include schisandrine A, B, and C, and several gomisins. Schisandra is a potent free radical scavenger, a characteristic that may explain the hepatoprotective effects observed with this botanical. Gomisin A has been found to promote hepatocyte growth factor, limit lipid peroxidation, and inhibit apoptosis in acute hepatic injury animal models.[125,126] Gomisin A also acts as an antiinflammatory, preventing the release of arachidonic acid by macrophages.[127] Laboratory evidence suggests that gomisin A may have anticarcinogenic effects[128,129]; however, published clinical trial data examining schisandra use in CHC patients are lacking.[130]

DOSAGE

The typical dosage for Schisandra extract is 100 mg twice daily.

PRECAUTIONS

Schisandra lignans have been reported to induce phase I drug metabolism[131] and competitively inhibit the methylation pathway of phase II detoxification in animal models.[132] Caution should be used if medications metabolized by the cytochrome P-450 system are given with schisandra. Side effects are uncommon and include dyspepsia, anorexia, and urticaria.

Astragalus (*Astragalus membranaceus*)

Astragalus is an important immunomodulatory herb in Chinese medicine.[133] In vitro studies have demonstrated that astragalus promotes B-cell proliferation and antibody production and enhances CTL activity.[134] Astragalus also acts as an antioxidant, increasing superoxide dismutase and decreasing lipid peroxide activity. Astragalus is reported to have protective effects against toxins in animal models.[135] An astragalus injection solution was found to have an inhibitory effect on experimental hepatic fibrogenesis, possibly due to its antioxidant properties.[136] A small trial among patients with chronic hepatitis B found astragalus supplementation was associated with decreased serum fibrosis markers and liver enzymes.[137] A 2009 meta-analysis of clinical trials from English and Chinese literature concluded that astragalus and certain other traditional Chinese botanicals may have activity against HCC, although the authors noted

a potential publication bias due to a lack of randomization in the studies evaluated.[138] Whether these agents have a chemoprotective role in patients with chronic viral hepatitis at increased risk for HCC remains a matter of conjecture.

DOSAGE

The typical dosage of astragalus powder is 4 to 7 g daily and typically provided in herbal concoctions.

PRECAUTIONS

Doses greater than 28 g/day may cause immune suppression. Astragalus should be avoided in patients with autoimmune disease or receiving immunosuppressive therapy due to its immunostimulatory effects. As astragalus may contain selenium, ingestion of large amounts may lead to selenosis. Astragalus may potentiate the effects of antithrombotic and anticoagulant medications. Side effects of astragalus use are uncommon.

Herbal Concoctions and Traditional Chinese Medicine

Traditional Chinese medicine (TCM) has long described healing remedies for chronic liver maladies. Integrative TCM relies on individualized constitutional diagnosis and treatment in parallel with biochemical, histological, and other diagnostic methods. Because constitutional diagnostic methods are used in formulating treatment plans, individualized herbal concoctions containing several botanicals are commonly used. Herbal concoctions for chronic hepatitis are likely to include varying doses and combinations of the botanicals discussed previously in addition to others. Herbal concoction prescriptions are modified according to a patient's changing signs and symptoms. Referral to a qualified TCM practitioner with experience treating chronic hepatitis may be beneficial for patients who opt to forego antiviral therapy.

Mind-Body Therapies

Research is beginning to catch up with clinical experience regarding the negative effects of psychosocial stress on health, particularly with respect to the roles of glucocorticoids and catecholamines. Stress activates the hypothalamic-pituitary-adrenal axis, leading to increased glucocorticoid secretion. The sympathetic nervous system is similarly activated by stress, which increases catecholamine levels.[139] Both groups of substances cause specific cytokine responses that influence the inflammatory response, with human studies demonstrating alterations in a number of immunomodulators related to acute experimental stress.[140,141] A small study in Japan found an association between chronic psychosocial stress related to type 1 personality and increased hepatitis C severity.[142] Stress has been shown to induce interleukin-6 and tumor necrosis factor-alpha within the liver, thus augmenting the hepatic inflammatory response.[143] Evidence suggests that repetitive stress may aggravate chronic inflammatory diseases to a greater extent than acute stressors.[144] Thus mind-body therapies that alleviate psychosocial stress may enhance the liver-specific and overall health of patients living with chronic hepatitis.

Therapeutic modalities that enhance balance and increase a sense of control, meaning, and purpose may decrease the degree to which psychosocial stress contributes to a patient's disease process. Chronic illness is a stressor in and of itself. Whatever we can do to help patients minimize or alleviate this and other stressors in their lives is healing in the broadest and truest sense (see Chapter 94).

Examples of modalities that may help alleviate stress and enhance peacefulness include meditation, prayer, journaling, counseling, support groups, behavioral therapy, hypnosis, and visualization, as well as art, music, and dance therapy. Relaxation techniques, such as deep breathing, biofeedback, and others, may also merit discussion. Clinicians should offer therapeutic approaches that suit a patient's personality, culture, and belief system.

Lifestyle Interventions

Measures to Reduce Toxin Exposure

Exposure to exogenous toxins increases hepatic workload and oxidative stress. When the liver is already in a state of chronic inflammation, this additional burden may exacerbate ongoing injury and accelerate disease progression.

Reduce Dietary Toxins. Oral intake of toxic xenobiotics can be minimized by avoiding prepackaged, ready-to-eat foods, processed meats, and canned foods. Encourage organically grown foods, but keep in mind that such products may not be affordable for some patients.

Avoid Alcohol. Alcohol abstinence is one of the most important recommendations a clinician can make for patients with CHC. Even low levels of alcohol intake in patients with HCV has been associated with accelerated fibrosis and increased risk of cirrhosis and HCC.[145-147] Clinicians must be prepared to offer patients with alcohol addiction or dependence with information about local services that provide psychosocial support in becoming alcohol-free. Alcohol in over-the-counter products (e.g., mouthwash, cold preparations, and tinctures) is also to be avoided (see Chapter 83).

Avoid Tobacco Products. All tobacco products (chewing tobacco, cigars, pipes, and cigarettes) introduce an array of toxins into the body and should be avoided. Smoking reduces glutathione levels due to the additional burden of detoxifying nicotine and neutralizing free radicals produced by tobacco toxins. Smoking increases the risk of hepatocellular carcinoma[148,149] and has been linked to accelerated CHC fibrosis.[150]

Avoid Unnecessary Drugs and Supplements. Pharmaceuticals, botanicals, and supplements that are metabolized by the liver can dramatically increase the xenobiotic burden on the liver. Additionally, some of these products have hepatotoxic potential (Table 21.7). All products with hepatotoxic potential should be avoided or prescribed with caution and closely supervised.

Recreational drug use is an important topic to discuss with all chronic hepatitis patients as these drugs increase the toxic burden on the liver. Many patients with CHC smoke marijuana to alleviate disease-related symptoms. Daily cannabis use, however, has been reported to significantly accelerate hepatic fibrosis progression.[151] Smoking marijuana may also contribute to steatosis, an independent risk factor for CHC progression.[152] A study among HIV–HCV coinfected patients, however, failed to demonstrate a relationship between marijuana use and CHC progression.[153] Asking about marijuana use in the same manner as other lifestyle issues opens the door to a candid discussion.

Avoid Environmental and Occupational Toxin Exposure. Pesticides, herbicides, and other toxic chemicals can damage hepatocytes and elevate liver enzyme levels.[154-157] Home exposure to paint and lacquer, glues, epoxy, and other toxins should be minimized.

Exercise

Exercise enhances portal blood flow, decreases fatigue,[158] improves overall well-being, and may alleviate depression,[159] a common finding in patients with CHC. Moderate exercise has also been shown to improve immune response.[160,161] Encourage a realistic exercise program

TABLE 21.7 Common Pharmaceuticals and Botanicals with Hepatotoxic Potential	
Type	**Specific Agents**
Pharmaceuticals	Acetaminophen
	Alpha-methyldopa (Aldomet)
	Amiodarone (Cordarone)
	Carbamazepine (Tegretol)
	Diclofenac (Voltaren, Cataflam)
	Fluconazole or ketoconazole (Diflucan, Nizoral)
	Hydralazine (Apresoline, Novo-Hylazin)
	Ibuprofen (Advil, Motrin, Nuprin)
	Nitrofurantoin (Macrodantin)
	Phenytoin (Dilantin)
	Sulfa medications (especially Septra or Bactrim)
	Amoxicillin (Amoxil)
	Chlorpromazine (Thorazine)
	Ciprofloxacin (Cipro)
	Duloxetine (Cymbalta)
	Statins/HMG-CoA reductase inhibitors (Caduet, Crestor, Lescol, Lipitor, Mevacor, Pravachol, Simcor, Vytorin, Zocor)
Botanicals	Barberry (*Berberis vulgaris*)
	Comfrey (*Symphytum officinale*)—Should never be taken internally
	Golden ragwort (*Senecio aureus*)
	Groundsel (*Senecio vulgaris*)
	Huang qin (*Scutellaria baicalensis*)
	Kava-kava (*Piper methysticum*)
	Pennyroyal (*Mentha piperita officinalis*)
	Sassafras (*Sassafras albidum*)
	Senna (*Cassia senna*)
	Valerian (*Valeriana officinalis*)
	Wall germander (*Teucrium chamaedrys*)
	Wood sage (*Teucrium scorodonia*)
	Ma-huang (*Ephedra equisetina*)
	Jin bu huan (*Lycopodium serratum*)

that takes into account the patient's current activity level and interests and progresses gradually.

Encourage Healthy Body Weight. Steatosis increases the rate of hepatic fibrosis in CHC patients.[162,163] Although genotype 3 disease is most closely associated with steatosis risk, elevated BMI has been shown to be an independent predictor of nonalcoholic steatosis.[164] Overweight and obese patients should be encouraged to engage in a sensible, sustainable weight-reduction program. Management of metabolic syndrome, high triglycerides, and obesity is a priority as insulin resistance is common among CHC patients.[165]

NUTRITION

The liver is the master processor of nutrient and metabolic homeostasis, and one's diet can make these jobs easier or more difficult. A diet including a variety of fresh fruit and vegetables supplies the necessary nutrients to support hepatic synthetic and detoxification functions. High-quality protein supports hepatic synthetic functions and the immune system. Low dietary fat helps prevent or counter hepatic steatosis, a condition that accelerates CHC progression. Avoiding excessive carbohydrates helps stabilize glucose metabolism, which is often disturbed in CHC patients due to insulin resistance (see Chapters 88 and 87).

Encourage Regular Consumption of Cruciferous Vegetables

Cruciferous vegetables include cabbage, broccoli, cauliflower, Brussels sprouts, kale, mustard greens, collard greens, kohlrabi, rutabaga, turnips, bok choy, arugula, horseradish, radish, wasabi, and watercress. These vegetables are good sources of vitamin C, selenium, folate, carotenoids, lignans, flavonoids, and indole-3-carbinol, which can increase the activity of certain phase I and II detoxification enzymes.[166,167]

Encourage Regular Consumption of Fruit

Fruit is a rich source of vitamins C, E, and K, folate, selenium, magnesium, potassium, carotenoids, flavonoids, lignans, terpenoids, and fiber. Adequate amounts of a variety of fruit help ensure an adequate supply of substrates needed for detoxification and biosynthesis. Berries—especially black raspberries, elderberries, blackberries, and blueberries—contain high concentrations of antioxidants.[168] Peaches, mangoes, and melons are also rich in antioxidants. Citrus fruit contains high concentrations of the phytochemical D-limonene, a strong inducer of phase I and II of the detoxification system.[169]

Avoid Foods That Inhibit the Detoxification System

Certain foodstuffs inhibit the detoxification system. Grapefruit contains naringenin, an inhibitor of cytochrome P-450 3A4 of the phase I detoxification system.[170] Capsaicin from hot peppers, eugenol from clove oil, and quercetin from onions also slow phase I detoxification. Patients with chronic liver disease are best advised to limit intake of these foodstuffs accordingly.

Encourage Adequate Protein Intake

Adequate protein intake is essential for healthy immune function and detoxification. Liver disease and chronic inflammation increase the body's requirements for protein, particularly in the presence of cirrhosis. Furthermore, phase II of the detoxification system is especially vulnerable to inadequate protein intake. Healthful sources of complete proteins include eggs, lentils, nuts, lean meats, fish, poultry, and soy. Encourage lean white meat and fish over red meat.[171] Recommended daily protein intake (in grams) should be calculated by multiplying body weight (in pounds) by a factor 0.5 to 0.7.

Encourage Healthful Dietary Fat Intake

When counseling patients regarding healthful dietary fat intake, focus on two major points: limiting dietary fat to no more than 30% of caloric intake and limiting intake of omega-6 polyunsaturated fats and trans fats. Limiting overall fat intake is important as high-fat diets—particularly in combination with reduced protein and carbohydrates—increase the risk of steatosis and cirrhosis among patients with chronic hepatitis.[172,173]

Most primary care clinicians are accustomed to promoting the consumption of unsaturated fats over saturated fats in order to improve cardiovascular health. Patients with chronic liver disease, however, have additional pathophysiological concerns. Unsaturated fats are more volatile (polyunsaturated fats more so than monounsaturated fats) and prone to oxidation than saturated fats. As hepatic oxidative stress is typically high in patients with CHC, the additional stress of large quantities of unsaturated fats may exacerbate hepatocyte injury. Reduced intake of polyunsaturated omega-6 fatty acids (e.g., safflower oil, sunflower oil, corn oil) is particularly important. Encourage the use of predominantly monounsaturated fats such as olive, canola, and peanut oils for cooking. Also encourage the consumption of omega-3 fatty acids to help reduce inflammation.[174] Finally, all patients should be advised to avoid trans fats (see Chapter 88).

Encourage Dietary Fiber

Dietary fiber helps bind toxins in the gut, resulting in bowel excretion of toxins without hepatic processing. A European cohort study involving more than 477,000 participants found dietary fiber, particularly from grain and vegetable sources, had a protective effect against the development of HCC in patients with chronic hepatitis B and/or C.[175] Encourage whole-grain and vegetable sources of dietary fiber.

Encourage Green Tea

Catechin polyphenols in green tea have antioxidant, antiangiogenic, and antiproliferative properties that may help reduce hepatic inflammation, slow chronic hepatitis disease progression, and attenuate HCC risk.[171,176-178] A 2009 meta-analysis found a significantly decreased risk of primary liver cancer associated with long-term consumption of green tea.[179]

DOSAGE

Two or three cups of green tea daily.

PRECAUTION

Caution patients against the use of highly concentrated green tea extracts as cases of fulminant hepatitis have been reported.[180,181]

Encourage Coffee

Regular coffee contains caffeine, chlorogenic acids, and a broad array of other compounds that collectively have hepatoprotective effects. Drinking coffee is associated with slower CHC disease progression, decreased fibrosis severity,[182-184] and reduced risk of cirrhosis and HCC.[185]

DOSAGE

Two to four cups of filtered, regular coffee daily.

PRECAUTION

Whereas filtered coffee appears to be hepatoprotective, unfiltered coffee (boiled or pressed) may cause elevations of serum liver enzyme levels.[185-187]

PREVENTION PRESCRIPTION

HEPATITIS C PRIMARY PREVENTION

- Do not share needles or other drug paraphernalia.
- Do not share personal care items that may be contaminated with blood, including toothbrushes, razors, and manicure and pedicure equipment.
- Do not get a tattoo with an unsterilized stylus; be certain new ink and new or sterilized ink pots are used.
- Avoid contact with blood during sexual activity.
- If you have multiple sexual partners, use latex condoms correctly and consistently at every sexual encounter.
- Use universal body fluid precautions.

HEPATITIS C SECONDARY PREVENTION

- Abstain from alcohol, tobacco products, street drugs, and unnecessary medications and supplements.
- Avoid environmental toxins, including pesticides, herbicides, and other toxic chemicals.
- Achieve and maintain a healthy body weight.
- Exercise regularly.
- Establish and maintain ongoing health care to include immunizations, CHC disease progression monitoring, and HCC screening, as indicated.

THERAPEUTIC REVIEW

SCREENING

The Centers for Disease Control and Prevention recommends one-time, hepatitis C antibody screening for anyone born during 1945 through 1965 due to the high prevalence of the disease in this age group.[188] The CDC also recommends anti-HCV screening for individuals who have one or more of the following risk factors:

- current or former use (even if only once many years ago) of injected street drugs
- receipt of blood, blood products, or an organ transplant before 1992, or clotting factors prior to 1987
- receipt of blood, blood products, or an organ transplant from a donor who later tested positive for hepatitis C
- long-term renal dialysis
- HIV infection
- persistent ALT elevation
- born to a mother with active HCV infection
- accidental exposure to HCV-positive blood
  The AASLD/IDSA/IAS–USA recommends annual HCV screening for individuals who currently inject illicit drugs and HIV-positive men who have unprotected sex with men.[8] Routine screening is not recommended for pregnant women, healthcare workers, first responders, or nonsexual household contacts. Screening is discretionary for individuals who may be at increased risk of hepatitis C related to tissue transplantation; past incarceration; body piercings and/or tattoos; current or former recreational drug use taken other than orally or parenterally (e.g., intranasally or subcutaneously); and a history

of multiple sex partners, sexually transmitted infection, or a sexual partner of someone with hepatitis C.

Hepatitis screening tests detect HCV antibodies. A reactive result indicates HCV exposure, but further testing is required to differentiate past versus active infection[189] because approximately 15% to 25% of people spontaneously resolve HCV infection.[190] People with a positive antibody screen should be tested for HCV RNA, which is typically detectable within 2 to 3 weeks of the initial infection. A positive result indicates active HCV infection, while a negative result indicates there is no active infection.

INITIAL EVALUATION AND MANAGEMENT

Individuals newly diagnosed with hepatitis C require additional testing to evaluate current disease status and factors that may influence disease progression and/or treatment decisions.[8,38]

Laboratory

- HCV genotype testing is recommended for any patient considering antiviral therapy because HCV genotype affects the regimen choice, duration of treatment, and probability of successful viral clearance.[8,38]
- HIV and hepatitis B testing is recommended as coinfection influences disease progression and treatment.
- Obtain baseline markers of liver status (e.g., AST, ALT, albumin, bilirubin, INR, CBC, and platelet count).
- Order noninvasive blood markers for fibrosis (e.g., Fibrotest, Fibrosure) if there is no clinical evidence of cirrhosis to evaluate hepatic fibrosis.

- Obtain baseline HCV viral load for patients who will begin antiviral treatment within 12 weeks. Defer pretreatment viral load testing if the period between testing and treatment initiation will be > 12 weeks.

Radiology

- Assess hepatic fibrosis with imaging studies (ultrasound, CT, or transient elastography) if there is no clinical evidence of cirrhosis. Consider a liver biopsy if imaging studies are inconclusive and/or inconsistent with noninvasive blood markers of fibrosis.

Lifestyle

- Reduce environmental (e.g., tobacco) and dietary toxin exposure.
- Abstain from alcohol and illicit drug use. Refer for alcohol/drug dependence counseling and treatment as needed.
- Achieve and maintain healthy body weight.
- Exercise regularly.
- Counsel patients about reducing the risk of HCV transmission.

Nutrition

- Include six to seven daily servings of fruits and vegetables (particularly cruciferous vegetables). ⊘ B₁
- Limit grapefruit and other inhibitors of the detoxification system. ⊘ B₁
- Limit fat intake (no more than 30%; aim for 10%–20%). ⊘ B₁
- Eliminate trans fats (hydrogenated and partially hydrogenated oils). ⊘ A₁
- Use olive, canola, or peanut oil in cooking. ⊘ C₁
- Increase intake of omega-3 fatty acids (cold-water fish, nuts, flaxseed). ⊘ B₁
- Decrease intake of omega-6 fatty acids (vegetable oils). ⊘ B₁
- Increase fiber intake. Consider supplementation with methylcellulose or psyllium if dietary fiber intake is inadequate. ⊘ C₁
- Ensure adequate protein intake. ⊘ B₁

Pharmaceuticals

- Vaccinate patients without immunity to hepatitis A or B. ⊘ A₁
- Discuss antiviral treatment options with all patients, including duration of therapy, regimens, and potential risks and benefits.
- Encourage antiviral treatment for patients with clinical factors that increase risk of HCV-related complications as they are most likely to realize short-term, high-impact benefits from viral cure (see Table 21.5). ⊘ A₁

- Patients undergoing antiviral treatment should discontinue all nonessential herbs, supplements, and medications during therapy.

Mind-Body

- Encourage lifestyle choices that reduce psychosocial stress.
- Explore relaxation and meditative techniques tailored to the patient's personality, belief system, and culture to help reduce stress.

Supplements

- Selenium: 200 mcg daily ⊘ C₂
- Iron-free multivitamin with minerals: one daily ⊘ C₁
- B-complex: one daily ⊘ C₁
- Vitamin C: 200–250 mg bid ⊘ C₁
- Vitamin E (D-alpha tocopherol): 400 IU daily ⊘ C₂
- Precautions: Avoid iron supplementation and excess vitamin A.

Botanicals to Consider

- Silymarin-phosphatidylcholine: 240 mg bid ⊘ C₁
- Licorice root: 200–500 mg dry powder tid, 1–2 g powdered root tid, or 2–4 mL fluid extract tid ⊘ C₂
- Schisandra: 100 mg of extract bid ⊘ C₁
- Astragalus: 4–7 g of powder qd ⊘ C₁

Monitoring

- See patients who are not receiving antiviral therapy at least twice yearly to monitor for signs of progression and/or extrahepatic disease manifestations.
- Monitor AST/ALT ratio; a ratio > 1 indicates probable disease progression to advanced fibrosis or cirrhosis.[191] Refer for gastroenterology or hepatology consult.
- Consider repeat liver fibrosis evaluation as clinically indicated.

Consultations

- Infectious disease consultation and comanagement is highly recommended for patients with HCV–HIV coinfection.
- Hepatology consultation is recommended for CHC patients with decompensated cirrhosis, hepatitis B coinfection, or another comorbid hepatic condition.
- Nutrition consultation is recommended for patients with cirrhosis.

Key Web Resources

REFERENCES

References are available online at ExpertConsult.com.

CHAPTER 22

URINARY TRACT INFECTION (UTI)

Amy B. Locke, MD, FAAFP, ABIHM

Pathophysiology and Epidemiology

Urinary tract infections (UTIs) are common, with an estimated life time incidence of approximately 53% in women and 14% in men.[1] The higher prevalence in women is thought to be related to urethral length. For those who have had a prior infection, the risk of another increases dramatically. One study found a recurrence rate of 44% within 1 year among women with a history of UTI.[2] The most common causative pathogens include gram negative organisms, in particular *Escherichia coli* (*E. coli*), which account for 80% of infections.[3] Many recurrent infections may actually represent reinfection with the same organism.[4] Despite clearing the bacteria from the urine, the colon may act as a reservoir for pathogenic bacteria.

A simple UTI, or cystitis, involves bacterial colonization of the bladder. Complicated UTIs usually involve structural or anatomic factors, underlying disease states such as diabetes that hinder treatment, or drug-resistant bacterial strains. Ascending infections into the kidneys are not uncommon, particularly with complicated UTIs; pyelonephritis requires urgent medical attention to avoid damage to renal structures and sepsis. Factors that increase the likelihood of progression include delayed treatment, unrecognized infection, asymptomatic bacteriuria in pregnancy, anatomical factors, and systemic diseases that lower immune function, such as diabetes.

Asymptomatic bacteriuria does not require treatment outside of pregnancy. Although bacteriuria is more common in diabetics,[5] treatment has not been shown to alter outcomes.[6,7] A 2015 Cochrane review found no benefit of treatment across diverse populations and diagnoses.[8] The United States Preventive Services Task Force (USPSTF) recommends screening for bacteriuria in pregnancy (A-grade recommendation) and against screening for others (D-grade recommendation).[9] The rapid treatment of pregnant women with both clinically diagnosed UTI and asymptomatic bacteriuria is essential due to the high risk of pyelonephritis.

Clinical Presentation

The majority of episodes of lower urinary tract infection present with a combination of dysuria, urinary urgency, and frequency. Gross hematuria, suprapubic discomfort, and cloudy urine are not uncommon. Symptoms of fever, myalgia, or low back/flank pain should prompt consideration of pyelonephritis. A history of dysuria, urinary frequency, and absence of vaginal discharge reportedly indicates a 90% probability of UTI.[10] Physical examination findings may consist of suprapubic tenderness; however, a physical examination is not required in the evaluation of UTI.

Laboratory testing frequently comprises urinalysis only. Urinalysis may reveal the presence of nitrites, leukocyte esterase (LE), and/or hematuria. The presence of nitrites with either LE or hematuria has a reported positive predictive value of 92%, but a negative predictive value of 76% when all three are absent.[11] Urine culture is not required for the diagnosis and treatment of simple UTI but may be helpful in patients with recurrent symptoms in order to exclude other etiologies, such as interstitial cystitis or when there is concern regarding the presence of drug resistant organisms. If performed, greater than 100,000 colony forming units of a single organism confirms the diagnosis of UTI.

The differential diagnosis of dysuria includes *Chlamydia trachomatis* cervicitis and interstitial cystitis, among others, in women. Prostatitis and urethritis should be excluded in the treatment of men with UTI. Treatment via phone for those with recurrence is generally considered acceptable. Many practices have a nurse triage protocol that allows recommendations, including prescriptions, to be provided without an office visit. Patients with frequent complicated UTIs, women with pyelonephritis in, and men with UTI may benefit from further evaluation by a urologist or further imaging.

Risk Factors

A number of factors that may predispose an individual to recurrent UTIs that vary across the age spectrum (Table 22.1). Younger women who are sexually active, have a history of UTIs as children, have had a new partner in the last year, use condoms (particularly those with spermicidal lubrication), or use diaphragms are at increased risk.[12,13] The frequency of intercourse has also been demonstrated to be an independent risk factor.[12] An inverse relationship between voiding after intercourse and risk of UTI has been shown by some studies but not others.[14] Tight clothing, tampon use, and soap preference have not consistently been shown to be related to recurrence in case control trials.[12] Delayed urination in college-age women has been reported to be significantly associated with infection risk in some studies but not others.[12,15] Physiological changes during pregnancy are associated with a significant increase in the frequency of UTI.

Postmenopausal women with recurrent UTI are more likely to be affected by diabetes, history of premenopausal UTI, urge incontinence, sexual activity,

TABLE 22.1   Risk Factors for Urinary Tract Infection

Young Women	Older Women	Men	General
Higher frequency of intercourse	Diabetes	Lack of circumcision	Foreign bodies
History of UTI as child	History of premenopausal UTI	Penetrative anal intercourse	Nephrolithiasis
Condom use	Urge incontinence	Female partner with UTI	Catheters
Spermicide use	Sexual activity	Prostatic hypertrophy	Family history of recurrent UTI
Diaphragm use	Incomplete bladder emptying		Decreased fluid intake
Pregnancy	Cystocele		Dysfunctional Elimination
Delayed urination			
Lack of voiding after intercourse			

incomplete emptying of the bladder, and the presence of a cystocele.[16,17] Children may have increased rates with bowel and bladder dysfunction, termed Dysfunctional Elimination Syndrome,[18] as well as vesicoureteral reflux.

Some risk factors cross all age ranges, including family history of recurrent UTI[12] and foreign bodies, such as renal stones and catheters. Family history of recurrent UTI may be associated with increased risk due to the relationship between specific phenotypes and bacterial adherence to the bladder wall.[19] Antibiotic use is a risk factor for UTI, presumably due to its effect on vaginal flora. Altered vaginal flora from *Lactobacillus* to *E. coli* is associated with an increased risk of recurrent infection.[20] This may explain the risk associated with spermicide use, as it increases colonization by *E. coli*.

Risk factors that predispose men to simple UTI include penetrative anal intercourse, a female partner with UTI, and lack of circumcision.[21] The risk of UTI in uncircumcised males has recently been estimated to be much higher than previously thought, with a relative risk increase of approximately 23%.[22] Obstructive symptoms, such as those due to prostatic hypertrophy, predispose to complicated UTI.

INTEGRATIVE THERAPIES

Nutrition

In general, a diet high in fruits and vegetables, whole grains, and healthy fats will promote good health and may strengthen the immune system. In addition, some foods and food components are thought to have a direct impact on the frequency of UTI.

Bladder Irritants

Many believe that certain foods cause irritation of the bladder. Lower urinary tract symptoms may increase with consumption of certain foods;[23] however, the relationship with UTI risk has yet to be clearly established, with case-control studies evaluating dietary factors reporting negative results.[14] Possible irritants include caffeine, simple sugars and starches, tobacco, alcohol, and some food additives. For those with recurrent infections, a trial diet to avoid these substances may result in a reduction in the frequency of urinary infections.

Garlic and Onions

Garlic has been used as an antimicrobial agent throughout history for a wide range of conditions. Previous studies have evaluated its effect on a broad range of organisms, including viral, bacterial, fungal, and parasitic infections. Garlic appears to be active against common urinary pathogens.[24] The most active ingredient of garlic is thought to be the sulfur-containing compound, allicin.[25] There are, however, nearly 100 compounds present that may act synergistically. In animal models of urinary pseudomonas, garlic appears to decrease bacterial counts and prevent renal damage.[26] Human trials of garlic for urinary tract infection are currently lacking. Garlic may be have utility in the treatment of acute or recurrent infections.

Chopping or mashing garlic cloves 10 minutes prior to eating or cooking seems to maximize the release of allicin, thereby increasing effectiveness. Raw consumption is preferred to cooking, as the highest allicin content may be found in raw garlic. Cooked garlic, however, may also have significant health benefits.

Onions also contain allicin and may have utility in the treatment and prevention of urinary pathogens, although no trials have so far been reported. Onions contain a large number of compounds thought to promote health, including flavonoids such as quercetin.

Fluids

Many practitioners recommend significant fluid intake to flush the urinary system with the aim of preventing UTIs. The effectiveness of this approach, however, has not been consistently proven by previous literature. Several studies have reported an association between decreased fluid intake and susceptibility to UTI,[27,28] while others have not supported this finding.[12,14] A review concluded that combination of fluid intake, frequent voiding, and complete bladder emptying may have greater benefit than simply drinking larger volumes.[29] There is no harm in this recommendation, and it may indeed be helpful. Fluid intake may play a role in dealing with constipation, which particularly plays a role in UTIs in children.

Supplements

Probiotics

Due to the colonic bacterial reservoir of pathogenic strains likely involved in recurrent UTIs,[4] it is a logical extension to maximize intestinal health. Probiotic treatments have been evaluated in a number of studies; however, consistent results are lacking. Theoretically, *Lactobacillus* strains provide a barrier in the vagina and on the perineum that prevents bladder colonization. *Lactobacillus* strains outcompete pathogenic strains and affect their adhesion.[30] A 2013 meta-analysis found *Lactobacillus* species to be effective in preventing UTI but noted small study sizes.[31] The most efficacious strains according to previous literature appear to be *L. rhamnosus* GR-1 and *L. reuteri* RC-14 (previously known as *L. fermentum*).[32] A randomized trial comparing these strains (1 billion CFU orally bid) to trimethoprim/sulfamethoxazole (TMP/SMX) found the antibiotic to be superior; however, many regard the results of this study as evidence that these species have benefit in treating UTI.[33] The probiotic arm had no change from baseline in antibiotic resistance, whereas the antibiotic arm developed 100% resistance to TMP/SMX and high resistance rates to a number of other antibiotics.

Several studies have found *L.* GG to be less effective.[32] The optimal dosing of probiotics is unclear, but is likely to be at least in the one billion colony forming unit (CFU) range. Probiotics can be given orally or vaginally.

DOSAGE

Two billion colony forming units daily of *Lactobacillus rhamnosus* and *reuteri*.

PRECAUTIONS

The risks associated with the use of probiotics in immunocompetent individuals is exceedingly small.

The best studied species of probiotic are *Lactobacillus rhamnosus* and *reuteri*. Products containing these strains are increasingly available. Patients should be counseled regarding identifying products containing these specific species.

Vitamin C (Ascorbic acid)

Vitamin C may or may not have a role in the prevention of recurrent UTI. In a single blind randomized trial of pregnant women, 100 mg of ascorbic acid reduced UTI rates by more than half over 3 months (29.1% vs. 12.7%).[34] In a case control study, intake of vitamin C was found to be correlated with protection against UTI in college age women; however, the amounts of vitamin C taken were not noted.[14]

DOSAGE

Optimal dosage is unknown. Consider 100 mg daily.

PRECAUTIONS

Diarrhea and GI upset may occur with high doses.

D-Mannose

D-Mannose is a simple sugar found in fruits. D-Mannose is not broken down in the bloodstream and is concentrated in the bladder where it prevents bacterial adherence to the bladder wall. The cellular receptors of uroepithelial cells, to which bacteria such as *E. coli* bind, are composed of D-mannose.[35] When taken as a supplement, D-mannose binds to bacterial receptors, blocking the ability of bacteria to adhere to the epithelial cell wall.[35] Animal studies have reported the efficacy of D-mannose in decreasing bacteriuria within 1 day.[36]

The safety of D-mannose has been studied in long-term studies in mice without evidence of harm[37] and has been used in humans for the treatment of a rare carbohydrate deficient glycoprotein syndrome.

Recent trials have begun to evaluate the efficacy of D-mannose in humans when taken for UTI prophylaxis. No studies have evaluated its efficacy as an acute treatment. A study of 308 women comparing nitrofurantoin and 2 g daily of d-mannose reported equally efficacy compared to no treatment.[38] A pilot study evaluated 250 mg d-mannose in combination with 500 mg cranberry extract, a gelling compound made of 1 billion *Streptococcus thermophilus* ST10 and 250 mg tara gum, and two species of *Lactobacillus* (2.5 billion *L. plantarum* LP01 and 1 billion *L. paracasei* LPC09).[39] In this small trial of 33 women, there was a statistically significant reduction in symptoms of recurrent UTI with the use of D-mannose. Accordingly, D-mannose is considered to have promise as a potentially safe supplement for the treatment of UTI.

DOSAGE

Optimal dosage is unknown. Consider 2 g daily for prevention.

PRECAUTIONS

Loose stools and abdominal bloating may occur at high doses.

Other Supplements

Other supplements that have been evaluated for the prevention of recurrent UTI include weekly to monthly bladder instillation of high dose hyaluronic acid and chondroitin.[40]

Botanicals

Cranberry (*Vaccinium macrocarpon*)

Cranberry juice and powder have successfully been used to prevent urinary tract infection. The use of cranberry dates back to Native American tribes who used it for the treatment of urinary conditions. Historically, cranberry was thought to work by acidifying urine, yet recent studies have shown effects with minimal change in urine pH.[41] The presumed active compounds, proanthocyanidins (PACs), inhibit bacterial adhesion to the bladder wall and decrease bacterial virulence.[42,43] In a small trial, a dose of 72 mg of PAC was effective against *E. coli* infection, with the effect appearing to be dose dependent.[42] The optimal dose of cranberry for the treatment of UTI is currently unknown.

Heterogeneity among the results of previous studies has made practical advice difficult, with variations in the dose and type of cranberry product making comparisons particularly challenging. A 2012 Cochrane review evaluated 24 randomized trials using cranberry juice or capsules and found some evidence that cranberry juice may decrease the frequency of UTI in susceptible women but found a high dropout rate, likely related to difficulty adhering to daily juice consumption.[44] In several trials, cranberry was found to be similarly effective to antibiotics. Optimal dosing could not be determined by these studies, with the authors concluding that cranberry juice should not be recommended and cranberry extract should be studied more thoroughly. A more recent trial in postsurgical patients found a 50% reduction in UTI compared to placebo among women administered two capsules bid (equivalent to two 8-oz glasses of cranberry juice daily).[45]

Other trials have examined recurrent UTI in a more general population of women. In a randomized control trial, cranberry juice was compared to cranberry powder and a placebo in sexually active women.[46] The incidence of recurrent UTI was found to be reduced by approximately 30% in both cranberry groups. The doses used in this study were 250 mL of cranberry juice three times daily and concentrated cranberry juice tablets twice daily. The size of the tablets used was not disclosed. A separate trial used only 30 mL of cranberry-lingonberry concentrate daily, with a 20% risk reduction in recurrence observed.[47] Small studies that have shown success with cranberry tablets have used 400 to 800 mg doses twice daily.[48,49] The size and design of these studies may limit extrapolation to larger populations. A trial randomizing older women to 500 mg of cranberry extract or 100 mg of trimethoprim found equal efficacy in the prevention of UTI[50]; however, a trial in younger women comparing 500 mg of cranberry extract to TMP/SMX found cranberry to be inferior.[51] Cranberry was also associated with a significantly lower rate of antibiotic resistance. Further studies are required to determine the most effective doses and frequency of cranberry supplementation.

Although cranberry products are frequently used to treat acute infection, the efficacy of this approach has not been studied.[52]

DOSAGE

16 oz (500 mL) of unsweetened cranberry juice daily or cranberry extract 500 mg daily to 400–800 mg bid.

PRECAUTIONS

Moderate interaction with warfarin is possible.

Many cranberry beverage products on the market contain only a small amount of cranberry juice and a significant amount of sweeteners. These may have a minimal impact on the urinary tract and a potentially negative impact on overall health.

Uva Ursi (*Arctostaphylos uva ursi*)

Uva ursi, or bearberry, leaf has long been used for urinary symptoms, although there is little human data regarding its efficacy in treating UTI. The active compound of uva ursi is thought to be arbutin, which is converted into hydroquinone following consumption.[53] Alkaline urine is thought to be necessary for the efficacy of uva ursi, with in vitro studies indicating activity against typical pathogens.[54]

A preliminary trial reported the effectiveness of uva ursi in preventing recurrent UTI when combined with dandelion root and leaf.[55] In this trial, women took an extract for 1 month and were then followed for 1 year. During that time, 18% of women in the placebo group (27 individuals) and 0% in the treatment group (30 individuals) developed a UTI.

DOSAGE

3 g dried herb daily or as one cup of an infusion (3 g dried herb steeped in 150 mL of cold water for 12–24 h) four times daily.

Hydroquinone derivative 400–800 mg up to four times daily.

PRECAUTIONS

Unfortunately, due to potential toxicity when used long term, uva ursi cannot be recommended for the purpose of prophylaxis. The toxicity of uva ursi may be related to the component hydroquinone and the inhibition of melanin,[56] although tannins may also play a role. The most common side effects of uva ursi include nausea and gastrointestinal distress. Rarer and more serious side effects may include hepatotoxicity, retinal disease,[56] seizure, cyanosis, and death. These risks are more pronounced with high doses and prolonged use. Many experts recommend limiting the use of uva ursi to acute infections for no longer than 1 week at a time and no more than five courses per year,[57] although others have argued that longer use may be safe.[58] Uva ursi is not considered safe in pregnancy or children. Uva ursi can turn urine a greenish-brown color and interfere with urinalysis.

Berberine

Berberine is an alkaloid found in a number of plants. Common in the traditions of traditional Chinese medicine, Ayurvedic medicine, and Native American healing, plant species that contain berberine include goldenseal (*Hydrastis canadensis*), oregon grape (*Berberis aquifolium*), bayberry (*Berveris vulgaris*), coptis (*Coptis chinensis*), and tree turmeric (*Berberis aristata*). A small number of studies of this compound have been reported. Some have used specific plants and others have used isolated berberine. In vitro studies have demonstrated berberine sulfate causes inhibition of *E. coli* adhesion to epithelial cells.[59] Studies using berberine for other indications have not reported toxicity or significant side effects.[60]

DOSAGE

Optimal dose unknown.

PRECAUTIONS

Berberine is not considered safe in pregnancy or for infants due to the risk of kernicterus.[61] Berberine may also effect the cytochrome P450 system and, subsequently, the serum levels of other substances.

Goldenseal (*Hydrastis canadensis*)

Goldenseal is a woodland herbaceous plant native to North America. There is little data to support the use of goldenseal in the treatment of UTI. However, goldenseal root has been used for antimicrobial purposes. A study of goldenseal extract demonstrated in vitro activity against a number of common urinary pathogens[62]; however, in vivo studies have not been reported. Flavonoids present in goldenseal have been posited to act synergistically with berberine.[63] There is concern of overharvesting and dwindling populations in the forests of Eastern North America.

Other traditional herbal preparations that have been used for urinary tract infections include stinging nettles, marshmallow root, echinacea, burdock, slippery elm, dandelion, and lovage. Some of these, such as *Echinacea angustifolia*, have been studied in the treatment of other conditions. For example, although Echinacea has been identified as an immune stimulator, it has not been studied in UTI. Others have little research regarding their clinical uses.

Pharmaceuticals

Antibiotics

Simple cystitis in women may be treated with 3 days of any of several antibiotics, including TMP/SMX and ciprofloxacin; however, current guidelines[7] recommend using fluoroquinolones as a second line due to the potential development of resistance and potential harm. Other acceptable antibiotics include nitrofurantoin for 5 days. Amoxicillin is not recommended due to high resistance rates. Optimal therapy often depends on antibiotic resistance rates in the individual's community. Complicated UTIs require a longer course of antibiotics. Pregnant women and those with chronic disease, such as diabetes, should be treated for 7 days. Men with UTI are also typically treated for 7 days.

Recurrent UTI may be treated with prophylactic antibiotics daily or postcoital. Either approach has been shown to decrease the frequency of UTIs. Prophylactic antibiotics are usually continued for 6 to 12 months before a trial period of cessation. In a Cochrane review, 6 and 12 months of prophylactic treatment were found to have equal efficacy.[64] Postcoital antibiotics appear to be as effective against recurrent UTIs as daily therapy among individuals with symptoms related to intercourse.[64]

DOSAGE

Nitrofurantoin ER 100 mg bid for 5 days. Trimethoprim/sulfamethoxazole one tablet DS (160/800 mg) bid for 3 days. Fosfomycin 3 g one dose. Ciprofloxacin 250 mg bid for 3 days.

Prophylactic doses are typically administered once daily at the same dose used for treatment. Common choices include nitrofurantoin, TMP/SMX, and ciprofloxacin daily.[65] Postcoital doses are provided as one tablet at the time of intercourse.

PRECAUTIONS

Frequent or long-term use of antibiotics may be associated with medication side effects, bacterial resistance, and risk of disruption to normal bacterial flora.

Phenazopyridine

Phenazopyridine (Pyridium) can provide pain relief from dysuria and bladder spasms. Phenazopyridine is available over the counter and by prescription.

DOSAGE

100–200 mg bid for 2 days.

PRECAUTIONS

This medication may turn urine a dark orange color, which may interfere with urinalysis.

Estrogen

Systemic estrogen replacement does not appear to have an effect on the frequency of UTIs in postmenopausal women[66,67]; however, topical estrogens may be beneficial for postmenopausal women with recurrent UTI.[67,68] Successful studies have used estriol or estradiol in various forms.[69] Generally, studies have used a daily dose for 2 weeks and then twice weekly.

In a randomized trial, 0.5 mg of vaginal estriol nightly for 2 weeks followed by two times weekly for 8 months compared with placebo resulted in a significant reduction in the frequency of UTI (0.5 vs. 5.9 episodes per patient year). Vaginal estriol was found to be less effective than daily nitrofurantoin in preventing recurrent UTI.[70]

DOSAGE

25 mcg vaginal estradiol every day for 2 weeks followed by two times weekly. Estradiol vaginal ring inserted every 12 weeks. 0.5 mg vaginal estriol every day for 2 weeks followed by two times weekly.

PRECAUTIONS

Vaginal estrogen may be absorbed systemically at high doses, prompting the need for endometrial protection. In general, the safest approach is to use the lowest effective dose for the least amount of time needed.

Other Therapies to Consider

Behavioral Changes

Certain behaviors are thought to be associated with an increased risk of urinary tract infection, many of which are associated with irritation of the urethra or reflux of urine back into the bladder from the urethra. These include intercourse, tight clothing, holding of urine, and irritants such as bubble bath, douche, or other products. Many of these associations have no evidence base, but addressing them is associated with little risk of harm. For those with dysfunctional voiding, pelvic floor training is beneficial for improving muscle relaxation.

Acupuncture

In a randomized trial of acupuncture compared to no treatment, women with a history of recurrent UTI had a 50% reduction in UTI compared to the control group (73% vs. 52% with no UTI over 6 months).[71] The treatment group received biweekly acupuncture sessions over 4 weeks and were followed for 6 months. There was a reduction in bladder residuals in the treatment group of 50% compared to baseline, with no change observed in the control group. An earlier study by the same research team reported similar results with a partial response with sham acupuncture compared to a no-treatment control.[72]

Mind-Body Skills

Although no specific mind-body skills have been evaluated for the prevention or treatment of UTI, mental and spiritual health are important components of overall health, including a healthy immune system. They, along with other foundations of health such as nutritional status, adequate sleep, and physical activity, are essential for optimal health. Attention to techniques to improve these factors, whether through yoga, mindfulness, social connectedness, or other strategies, will likely help limit susceptibility to infectious processes.

Biofeedback

In a subgroup of women who suffer from dysfunctional voiding, pelvic floor therapy was reported to decrease the frequency of recurrent UTIs.[73] Dysfunctional voiding is defined as increased external sphincter activity during voluntary voiding. This occurs in individuals without neurological deficits.

> Pelvic floor relaxation training with biofeedback can be a useful intervention for those who have dysfunctional voiding with incomplete bladder emptying.

Children with overactive bladder and/or dysfunctional voiding also respond to biofeedback techniques aimed at decreasing recurrent UTI.[74] Biofeedback has utility in the treatment of dysfunctional elimination syndrome, which is a frequent cause of childhood UTI.[75] Diaphragmatic breathing combined with pelvic floor muscle retraining has also been shown to have efficacy in the treatment of children with UTI.[76]

PREVENTION PRESCRIPTION

- Encourage a plant-based diet high in garlic and onions.
- Remove possible bladder irritants such as caffeine, alcohol, and simple sugars.
- Encourage adequate fluid intake.
- Monitor stress and focus on foundations of health such as optimal diet, physical activity, sleep, mental, and spiritual health.
- Encourage frequent voiding and avoidance of holding urine.
- Avoid constipation.
- Consider changing method of birth control if frequent UTI is associated with the use of spermicides, condoms, or diaphragm use.
- Urinate after intercourse.

THERAPEUTIC REVIEW

Below is a summary of therapeutic options for acute treatment and prevention of UTI. If a patient presents with severe symptoms or a history suggestive of a complicated UTI, antibiotic therapy should be initiated immediately. For patients with mild to moderate symptoms, a ladder approach may be more appropriate. Patients should be counseled to seek further care if their symptoms worsen or do not resolve.

ACUTE INFECTION

Nutrition
- Encourage garlic consumption

Supplements
- D-mannose: ¾ tsp three times daily

Botanicals
- Cranberry: 16 oz of unsweetened juice daily or extract 400 mg bid
- Usa ursi, hydroquinone derivative: 400–840 mg up to four times daily or 3 g of dried root daily

Pharmaceuticals
- Nitrofurantoin ER: 100 mg bid for 5 days
- Trimethoprim/sulfamethoxazole: one tab DS bid for 3 days
- Fosfomycin: 3 g for 1 day
- Ciprofloxacin: 250 mg bid for 3 days
- Phenazopyridine: 200 mg bid for 2 days (Symptom management only)

RECURRENT INFECTIONS
- Remove exacerbating factors

- Eliminate use of spermicides, trial change of birth control method
- Urinate after intercourse

Nutrition
- Encourage garlic consumption
- Encourage adequate fluid intake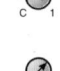

Supplements
- Probiotics: one billion colony forming units daily of *Lactobacillus rhamnosus* and/or *fermentum*
- D-Mannose: 2 g daily
- Vitamin C: 100 mg daily

Botanicals
- Cranberry: 16 oz of unsweetened juice daily or extract 400 mg bid
- Uva ursi
- Other herbal products that have potential benefit include berberine containing plants and echinacea

Pharmaceuticals
- Trimethoprim/sulfamethoxazole: one tablet DS daily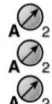
- Nitrofurantoin: 100 mg daily
- Ciprofloxacin: 250 mg daily
- Vaginal estrogen: daily for 2 weeks, followed by twice weekly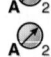

Other Therapies
- Biofeedback for those with dysfunctional voiding
- Acupuncture

Key Web Resources	
National Center for Complementary and Integrative Health. Dietary and herbal supplements page	https://nccih.nih.gov/health/supplements
National Institute of Diabetes and Digestive and Kidney Diseases	Urinary Tract Infections in Adults: http://www.niddk.nih.gov/health-information/health-topics/urologic-disease/urinary-tract-infections-in-adults/Pages/facts.aspx#eating Urinary Tract Infections in Children: http://www.niddk.nih.gov/health-information/health-topics/urologic-disease/urinary-tract-infection-in-children/Pages/facts.aspx

REFERENCES

References are available online at ExpertConsult.com.

CHAPTER 23

LYME DISEASE

Ather Ali, ND, MPH, MHS

EPIDEMIOLOGY

Lyme disease is a multisystem infection caused by the spirochetal bacterium *Borrelia burgdorferi*.[1,2] *B. burgdorferi* sensu lato is the only species known to cause human infection in North America, whereas pathogenic species in Europe and Asia include *B. burgdorferi* sensu stricto, *B. garinii*, and *B. afzelii*, among others.[1-3,3a] A number of other genospecies of *B. burgdorferi* have been identified, although the public health importance of these is not well defined.[3]

In 1977, Lyme disease was characterized by Steere et al. and named for the geographic area (Lyme, Old Lyme, and Haddam, Connecticut) where 39 patients presented with arthritic symptoms of previously unknown cause,[4] although individual cases of Lyme borreliosis were described in Europe as early as 1883.[3]

Lyme disease is the most common vector-transmitted disease in the United States.[3] Approximately 30,000 cases of Lyme disease are reported to the Centers for Disease Control and Prevention (CDC) each year, although the CDC notes that these rates reflect overdiagnosis of cases as well as overall underreporting, noting that approximately 300,000 diagnoses of Lyme disease are made in the United States each year.[3] The vast majority (95%) of reported cases occur in the northeastern and midwestern areas of the United States in 14 states (Connecticut, Delaware, Maine, Maryland, Massachusetts, Minnesota, New Hampshire, New Jersey, New York, Pennsylvania, Rhode Island, Vermont, Virginia, and Wisconsin), with higher rates among children aged 5–15 years and adults older than 50 years.[3] Fig. 23.1 illustrates the distribution of Lyme disease in the United States; Vermont has the highest incidence of Lyme disease (108 cases per 100,000).[6] Lyme borreliosis also occurs in some Asian countries and throughout Europe.[1,3]

The principal vectors for transmission of *B. burgdorferi* in the United States are nymphal deer ticks (*Ixodes scapularis* and *pacificus*) during the late spring or summer months.[8] Infected ticks need to be attached for at least 24–48 hours to be able to transmit the organism.[8] Bites from Ixodes ticks are usually painless and are often unrecognized. Fig. 23.2 illustrates stages in the life cycle of the deer tick.

Ixodes ticks may also transmit *Anaplasma phagocytophila*, *Babesia microti*, *Borrelia miyamotoi*, *Ehrlichia* species, and Deer tick virus (a type of Powassan virus), either separately or in conjunction with *B. burgdorferi*.[9] The impact of coinfections on the clinical course of Lyme disease can range from self-clearing fevers to life-threatening illnesses.[2]

Infected persons do not transmit Lyme disease to others; no epidemiological or clinical data currently confirm sexual or congenital transmission of *B. Burgdorferi* between humans,[10] despite widespread concern.

Uncomplicated Lyme disease is generally treatable, with a favorable prognosis.[3]

Clinical Course

Lyme disease is classified into three stages; early localized Lyme disease, early disseminated Lyme disease, and late Lyme disease.[10] Early localized Lyme disease is characterized by a rash (erythema migrans, see Fig. 23.3) appearing at the site of the tick bite typically between 7 and 14 days following the bite.[10] Erythema migrans is usually asymptomatic but may become pruritic or painful.[2] Systemic symptoms sometimes may accompany the rash and include fever, myalgia, headache, fatigue, and localized lymphadenopathy.[10]

Early disseminated Lyme disease may manifest as multiple erythema migrans, usually appearing 3–5 weeks following the tick bite. Neurological findings, including meningitis and cranial nerve palsies, may present. Other symptoms can include fatigue, flulike symptoms, carditis (manifested as heart block), and syncopal episodes.[2,10]

Late Lyme disease occurs weeks to months after initial infection and is characterized by arthritis, usually affecting the large joints including the knee, and can be mono- or oligoarticular. Neurological complications may develop, including polyneuropathy, encephalitis, and encephalopathy.[10,12]

Chronic Persistent Symptoms, Chronic Lyme Disease, Posttreatment Lyme Disease Syndrome, and Medically Unexplained Symptoms

Fatigue, arthralgia, and myalgia may persist after initial treatment for Lyme disease,[2] with reported frequencies varying between 0%–50% in published studies[11] and reported rates of 10%–20% in recent trials. Steere reports that 10% of patients with Lyme arthritis develop persistent synovitis that can last for months or years after initial antibiotic treatment.[13] The impact of persistent symptoms is great; health-related quality of life is often severely compromised.[14,15]

> Risk factors for posttreatment Lyme disease syndrome include delays in initial diagnosis, higher severity of symptoms at treatment, and the presence of neurological symptoms at the time of initial treatment.[11]

In a cohort in Westchester County, NY, Asch et al. found that 53% of patients reported persistent symptoms

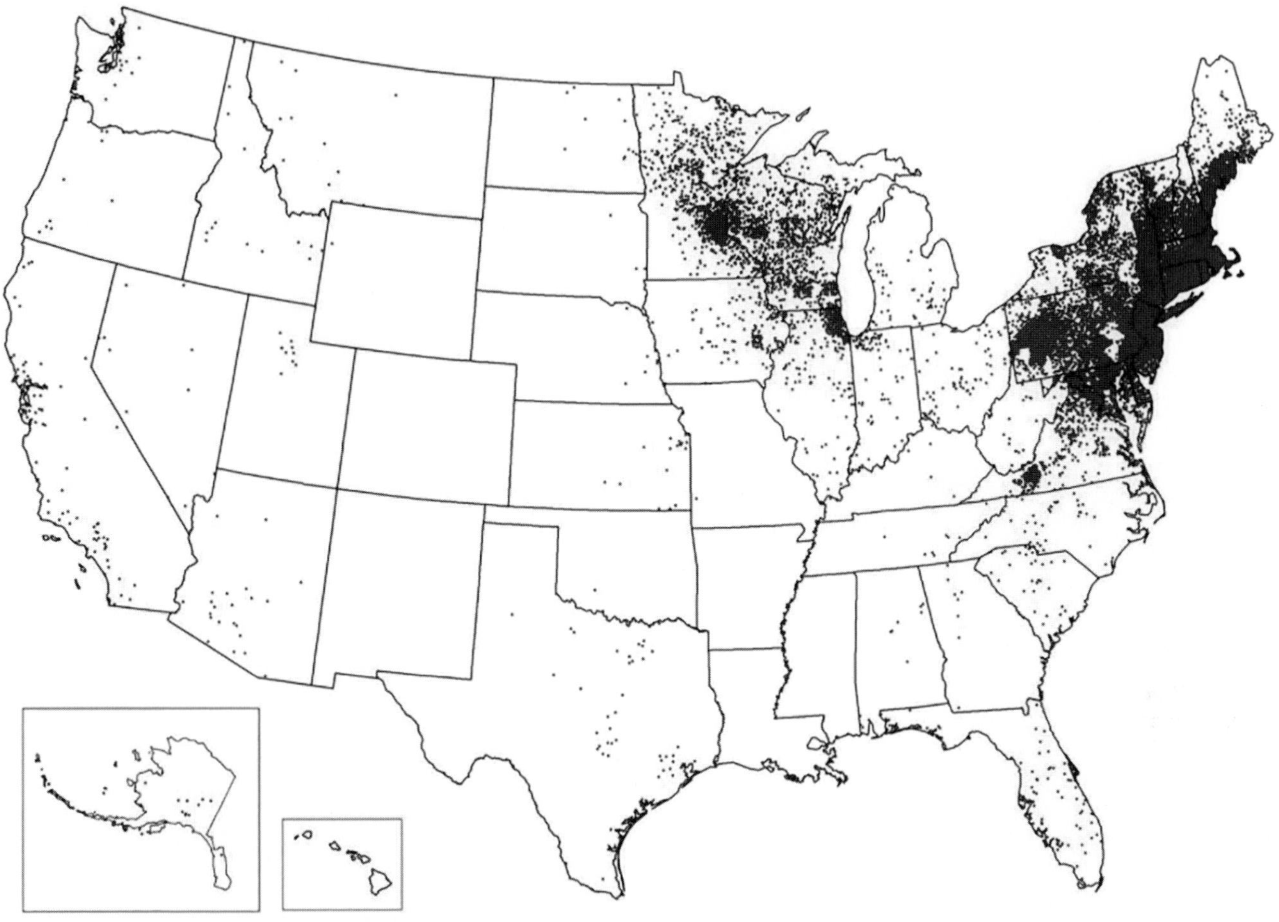

1 dot placed randomly within county of residence for each confirmed case

FIG. 23.1 ■ **Distribution of Lyme Disease.** The distribution of Lyme disease corresponds to the distribution of the Ixodes ticks that transmit *Borrelia burgdorferi*. (From the Centers for Disease Control and Prevention, Division of Vector-Borne Diseases: Lyme disease maps: http://www.cdc.gov/lyme/stats/maps/map2013.html.)

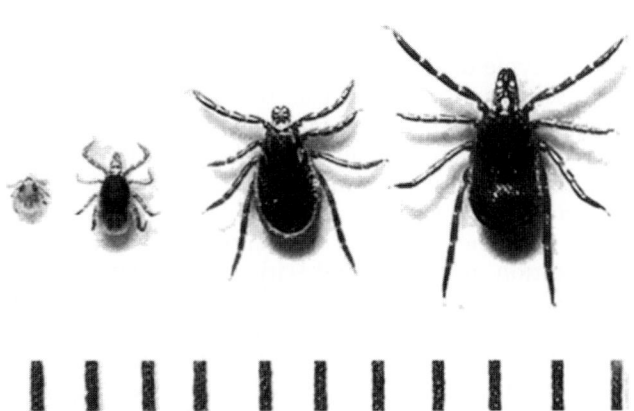

FIG. 23.2 ■ Various stages of the life cycle of the deer tick Ixodes scapularis, the vector for Lyme disease in the northern United States. The larval stage is shown on the left, followed by the nymphal stage, the adult female, and the adult male on the right. Most infections are transmitted from ticks at the nymphal stage. (Originally published in Murray TS, Shapiro ED. Lyme disease. *Clin Lab Med*. 2010;30:311).

following initial treatment for Lyme disease, and noted that antibiotic treatment within 4 weeks of initial infection was associated with a greater likelihood of full symptom resolution.[16] In a pediatric cohort, 23% of children developed refractory arthritis after initial treatment.[17] These children were subsequently treated with nonsteroidal antiinflammatory drugs, intraarticular steroid injections, or disease-modifying antirheumatic drugs. None developed chronic arthritis or recurrent infections.[17] Of note, polymerase chain reaction (PCR) testing of joint fluid can detect *B. burgdorferi* DNA for several weeks after spirochetes are killed[18] and thus may not be a good test for effectiveness of treatment. Chandra et al. found significantly higher levels of antineural antibody reactivity in persons with persistent Lyme symptoms compared with post-Lyme healthy and normal healthy controls, suggesting chronic symptoms may be related to a differential immune response[19]; however, a recent follow-up study did not find similar proportions of antineural antibodies in chronic fatigue patients with similar symptomology.[20] Other potential mechanisms of posttreatment symptoms include autoimmunity, potential genetic predisposition, and inflammatory genotypes of *B. burgdorferi* as well

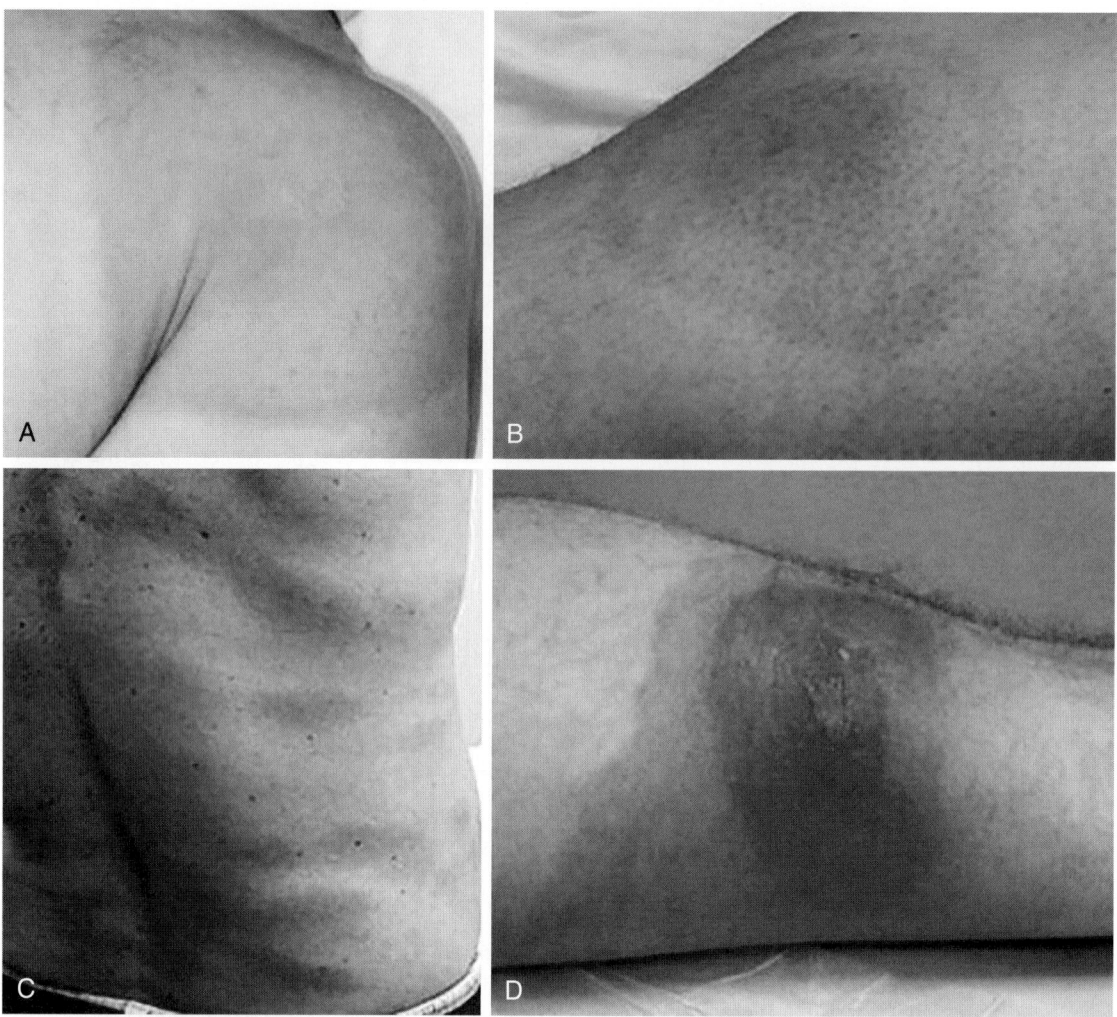

FIG. 23.3 ■ *Erythema migrans* **Rash of Lyme Disease.** A, Typical macular lesion on left shoulder. B, Bull's eye lesion on lateral thigh with central punctum. C, Multiple lesions on back. D, Lesion with vesicular center on posterior thigh. (Courtesy Juan Salazar, MD, University of Connecticut Health Center. In: Ferri FF, editor: *Ferri's Clinical Advisor*. Philadelphia, Elsevier; 2016:755.)

as speculation regarding antibiotic-tolerant persistent organisms.[11]

Chronic Lyme disease is a label used for a constellation of nonspecific symptoms, such as fatigue, night sweats, sore throat, lymphadenopathy, arthralgia, myalgia, palpitations, abdominal pain, nausea, diarrhea, sleep disturbance, poor concentration, irritability, depression, back pain, headache, and dizziness, with or without serological or clinical evidence of previous infection by *B. burgdorferi*.[21-25] The diagnosis of chronic Lyme disease is nebulous; no standard definition exists, though it is understood to be distinct from "post-Lyme disease syndrome" or "late Lyme disease" in which arthralgia and other symptoms persist after documented *B. burgdorferi* infection.[21,26,27]

Patients are frequently diagnosed with chronic Lyme disease based on nonstandard interpretations of serology or other testing that has limited validity and reliability, or more often, based on clinical symptoms alone[26] or occasionally attributing symptoms to chronic coinfections.[28] Chronic Lyme disease is diagnosed throughout the United States, including areas

where Lyme disease is not endemic.[24,29,30] Often, persons self-diagnose using lists of multiple nonspecific symptoms found on the internet. Treatment usually includes regimens of multiple antibiotics, often administered parenterally, frequently continuing for months or years in opposition to standard guidelines for treatment of Lyme disease.[26] This approach is far longer in duration and associated with substantially greater risks than standard treatment for any other spirochetal infection and virtually all infectious agents treated with antibiotics. Chronic Lyme disease regimens often result in considerable out-of-pocket expenses (often amounting to tens of thousands of dollars per year), patient distress, and potential harm,[31] as well as increasing risk of selecting for antibiotic resistant bacteria.[24] Some attribute chronic Lyme disease symptoms to drug-resistant reservoirs of *B. burgdorferi*, including atypical intracellular cystic or spherical forms.[32,33] However, no research has correlated the presence of these organisms with persistent symptoms, nor has the eradication of these been associated with improvement in symptoms.[34]

Despite the challenging political controversy regarding persistent Lyme symptoms, research has been unable to associate chronic symptoms with the presence of spirochete infection. Further, no association between the eradication of Lyme infection and improvement of symptoms has been observed.

One survey found that 2.1% of Connecticut-based primary care physicians diagnose and treat chronic Lyme disease, while the majority were unsure or did not believe in the existence of chronic Lyme disease.[4] A 2014 survey found that less than 5% of Public Health faculty members reported expertise in Lyme disease or posttreatment Lyme disease syndrome.[35] The predominant infectious disease, pediatric, and neurology organizations discount chronic Lyme disease as a distinct clinical entity, while other academic, professional, and advocacy organizations argue the contrary. This issue has become politicized with acrimonious debate among academic organizations and advocacy groups.[36]

Chronic Lyme disease symptoms may resemble other medically unexplained symptoms (also known as functional somatic syndromes), including chronic fatigue syndrome, irritable bowel syndrome, fibromyalgia, sick building syndrome, and chronic unexplained pain,[15,37,38] as well as neurological conditions such as amyotrophic lateral sclerosis[39] or multiple sclerosis.[40] The lack of clear pathophysiology in medically unexplained conditions often results in extensive and expensive diagnostic workups and significant iatrogenic complications.[41,42] Like many chronic conditions in which persons are suffering from pain, psychiatric comorbidities are prevalent and often overlooked.[29,42-44] At least 13% of outpatient visits are attributable to medically unexplained symptoms.[42,45] Suffering is often exacerbated by a self- or provider-validated cycle that attributes common somatic complaints to serious conditions.[44] Significant symptomatic and objective overlap occurs in these conditions in addition to high rates of cooccurrence of different syndromes.[44,46,47]

In one qualitative study, patients identifying with chronic Lyme disease reported significant declines in health status and dissatisfaction with healthcare in mainstream settings.[15] In one sample, nearly half of chronic Lyme disease patients were diagnosed with fibromyalgia.[48] Occasionally, persons with other defined medical conditions (including cancer) are misdiagnosed as having chronic Lyme disease.[49] Many syndromes present with similar constellations of nonspecific symptoms such as muscle weakness, arthralgias, and general fatigue.[50] Patients with these conditions regularly seek out complementary and alternative medicine (CAM) therapies and providers.[15,51-54]

1. Persons suffering from chronic persistent symptoms often present with debilitating and severe symptoms. Patients should not be dismissed or disregarded because the pathophysiology of their symptoms is unknown. Effective symptomatic treatments can significantly improve quality of life.
2. In most conditions, CAM patients and providers are promoting less-invasive therapies than the mainstream standard-of-care. Lyme disease is an unusual case where CAM patients and providers are often seeking more invasive and elaborate interventions than conventionally provided.

Diagnosis

Lyme disease is diagnosed according to historical and physical findings; serology is used to support the diagnosis in persons without erythema migrans. Early Lyme disease is generally diagnosed based on the presence of erythema migrans; persons at this early state will likely be seronegative, as erythema migrans appears before an adaptive immune response develops.[55] In a case series in Maryland, 87% of patients with early Lyme disease presented with erythema migrans[56]; 70% of the Lyme disease cases reported to the CDC between 2003 and 2005 presented with erythema migrans.[57] The FDA does not recommend serological testing in early Lyme disease because of the low sensitivity of tests in early manifestations.[58]

The CDC criteria for diagnosis of Lyme disease are (1) erythema migrans alone or (2) at least one late manifestation plus laboratory confirmation of infection. Laboratory confirmation, by this definition, includes isolation of *B. burgdorferi* from a clinical specimen or the presence of IgM or IgG antibodies to *B. burgdorferi* in serum or cerebrospinal fluid.[59] The CDC recommends a two-tier process when testing blood for evidence of Lyme disease. Initial testing using an enzyme-linked immunosorbent assay (ELISA) or immunofluorescent assay (IFA) is followed by a Western blot for confirmation.[59] It is important to note that the CDC criteria for Lyme disease are not intended for use by clinicians to make a diagnosis of Lyme disease. Rather, they are intended for national surveillance data,[60] although the majority of cases in practice do fulfill this definition.[55]

ELISA testing is associated with many false positives,[61] thus the need for confirmation of a positive or equivocal ELISA by Western Blot. A negative ELISA, on the other hand, does not warrant further serology.[26,59,62] Western blot testing is more specific, that is, it will likely be positive when a person is truly infected. IgM antibodies will appear first, typically within 1–2 weeks of initial infection. IgG antibodies appear later, usually within 2–6 weeks after the onset of erythema migrans. At least 90% of persons with late Lyme disease have positive IgG antibodies.[63] These may remain elevated following successful antibiotic treatment and symptom resolution.[55] Steere et al. reported that 16% of a large cohort had systemic symptoms of Lyme disease without initially presenting with erythema migrans that later demonstrated positive serology.[64] Of note, persons who fit into this rubric should have objective symptoms, such as arthritis or facial palsy, as opposed to arthralgia.

The sensitivity of two-tier testing is greatest in late Lyme disease. In the acute phase of erythema migrans, sensitivities range from 29% to 40% and increase to 97% in those with arthritis (with specificity at 99%).[1] Of note, there is considerable variability between the different commercial assays that are FDA-cleared, especially for the detection of IgM antibodies.[1]

It is not recommended to screen persons without objective evidence of Lyme disease for possible exposure to Lyme disease.[55,62] Seropositivity indicates past exposure and does not prove an active infectious process[65] and should not be used to diagnose active Lyme disease. Serological testing is most useful in persons with a high pretest probability: persons in which Lyme disease is likely based on history and clinical presentation. In this population, positive serology supports the diagnosis of Lyme disease. In late Lyme disease, a positive IgG result is nearly always observed. In persons with low prior probability of Lyme disease, serological testing will result in more false positive results.

Testing of ticks for *B. burgdorferi* is generally advised to determine whether antibiotic therapy should be initiated.[66]

Strict use of the standard diagnostic criteria will minimize false positives but may result in atypical presentations being missed.[67] Less stringent diagnostic criteria incorporating broader clinical symptoms have been proposed and are in use by a minority of clinicians[68]; however, no literature is available assessing the diagnostic accuracy of these alternative criteria.

Recent advances in Lyme disease testing can potentially improve the sensitivity and specificity of current diagnostic methods, although these advances have not translated to better standards of care.[62] A number of unconventional (not FDA-cleared) direct-to-practitioner lab tests exist that claim to improve upon standard Lyme disease assessment and diagnosis; however, it is beyond the scope of this chapter to review them all. These are often propriety tests developed and marketed by a single laboratory. These tests are regularly paid for out-of-pocket by patients, often with extensive markups by practitioners. Besides marketing materials from the laboratories themselves, there is minimal independent data assessing the validity of these tests. Literature from one representative test included an advertisement for the test that superficially resembled a peer-reviewed journal article. The article promoted incorporating the lab's novel testing into existing diagnostic algorithms, and claiming that the novel tests have relevance by "...clarifying clinically ambiguous cases, and confirming therapeutic success." No data justifying these claims are presented, although the choices of immunological markers appeared reasonable.

The alternative tests report positive results at much higher rates than conventional serology. Despite the documented shortcomings of conventional serology (such as low sensitivity during early infection and subjective interpretation of bands)[62] that can result in false negatives and the appeal of tests that claim more sensitivity, the alternatives cannot be endorsed at this time. Tests that provide unique interpretations of Western blot results do not increase sensitivity, but rather decrease specificity.[62] It is unknown whether the higher rates of positive results from alternative tests are due to more true positives or whether the results are (1) impacted by selection effects (where people more likely to be infected are sent to alternative labs), (2) less precise or accurate than conventional testing, (3) false positives,[62] (4) affected by confirmation bias, or (5) a combination thereof. Unfortunately, no independent data is available that assesses these factors.

Due to the high out-of-pocket cost and uncertain benefit of these tests, none of these invalidated tests[69] can be recommended without documenting adequate human testing, at minimum ensuring (1) high sensitivity and specificity in diagnosing Lyme disease according to established criteria, (2) minimal intrasample variability, assessed independently,[63,70,71] and (3) comparative effectiveness in relation to and in addition to standard ELISA and Western blot testing.

> If a tick is engorged or likely attached for >72 hours, consider treating with a single dose of 200 mg of doxycycline. This can reduce the risk of Lyme by 87%. Only 1%–3% of tick bites in endemic areas result in infection. The number of tick bites needed to be treated to prevent one case of erythema migrans is 50 (number needed to treat, NNT = 50). If the tick is not engorged or is known to be attached for less than 72 hours, consider reassurance.[2]

INTEGRATIVE THERAPY

Persons with Lyme disease typically seek CAM for three major reasons. Some seek CAM therapies in addition to conventional therapies—a *complementary* or *integrative* approach. Some believe that conventional therapies are ineffective or dangerous and seek more "natural" *alternatives* to mainstream therapies. Some present after learning about chronic Lyme disease through the internet or advocacy groups promoting treatment protocols employing a myriad of long-term antimicrobials (often parentally),[68,72] nutritional supplements, botanicals, and other unconventional therapies, such as hyperbaric oxygen[73] or antifungals.[15,74]

Since the evidence that differentiates chronic Lyme disease from other medically unexplained conditions is unclear, this section will focus on acute Lyme disease as defined and diagnosed using standard criteria.[26]

Risk Reduction

Reducing the risk of tick bites in endemic areas and proper removal of ticks within 48 hours following a bite are the most effective means to reduce the incidence of Lyme disease (see *Prevention Prescription*).

No major lifestyle interventions such as specific diets or exercise regimens have been shown to reduce risk of contracting Lyme disease.[75] "Immune boosting" formulas or other natural products have not been shown to affect the incidence of Lyme disease.

ACUTE INFECTION

Pharmaceuticals

Lyme disease is best treated with antibiotics. Treatment within 4 weeks of symptom onset is strongly associated with complete recovery.[16] Coinfections should be addressed as warranted. Persons experiencing late Lyme disease symptoms with neurological, rheumatological, or cardiac manifestations should be treated by an appropriate specialist. It is important to note that no credible alternatives exist to prompt antibiotic treatment; the risks of inadequate treatment are progression to more severe symptomology and greater risk of long-term sequelae.

Antibiotics

Doxycycline is the first-line therapy in early Lyme disease; it is effective for the treatment of erythema migrans as well as for human granulocytic anaplasmosis (HGA) that may occur concurrently with early Lyme disease. Patients experiencing carditis or arthritis can use these regimens as well.[2]

In persons with early Lyme disease with cranial nerve palsy (without clinical evidence of meningitis), oral doxycycline, amoxicillin, or cefuroxime axetil can be used.[2,76]

DOSAGE (ADULTS)[2,26]

Doxycycline: 100 mg twice per day for 14 days (range: 10–21 days)

Amoxicillin: 500 mg three times per day for 14 days (range: 14–21 days)

Cefuroxime axetil: 500 mg twice per day for 14 days (range: 14–21 days)

PRECAUTIONS

Doxycycline should not be used in children aged <8 years or in pregnant or lactating women. Amoxicillin and cefuroxime axetil have also demonstrated efficacy in treating early Lyme disease, are effective for the treatment of early Lyme disease, and can be used in children aged <8 years.[2,26]

Late Lyme arthritis can be treated with somewhat longer regimens than those used in early Lyme disease. Some persons may not respond or require intravenous antibiotics. For persons with recurrent or persistent arthritis, the Infectious Disease Society of America recommends additional 4-week courses of oral antibiotics for persons whose symptoms have improved with initial oral treatment and intravenous therapy for persons not experiencing substantial improvement on oral antibiotics.[26]

DOSAGE

Doxycycline: 100 mg twice per day for 14 days (range: 14–21 days)

Amoxicillin: 500 mg three times per day for 14 days (range: 14–21 days)

Cefuroxime axetil: 500 mg twice per day for 14 days (range: 14–21 days)

PRECAUTIONS

Doxycycline can increase photosensitivity; avoid exposure to sunlight, sunlamps, or tanning beds while using doxycycline. A sunscreen (minimum SPF 15) can also be helpful. Do not take iron supplements, multivitamins, calcium supplements, antacids, or laxatives within 2 hours before or after taking doxycycline.

Supplements

Probiotics

Antibiotic-associated diarrhea occurs in approximately 25% of patients[77]; probiotic therapy may mitigate this.[78] As probiotic effects vary by indication and strain, recommendations generally need to be strain specific. The strains most likely to be effective in treating antibiotic-associated diarrhea are *Lactobacillus GG, Bifidobacterium lactis Bb-12, Lactobacillus acidophilus La-5,*[79] *Lactobacillus sporogenes,* and *Saccharomyces boulardii.*[78] Some evidence supports the use of *S. boulardii* in treating *Clostridium difficile* colitis.[80]

DOSAGE

Five to forty billion colony forming units/day[78] throughout the duration of antibiotic treatment[81] or 200 g of a specific yogurt product containing *Lactobacillus rhamnosus GG, Bifidobacterium lactis Bb-12,* and *Lactobacillus acidophilus La-5*[79]

PRECAUTIONS

Probiotics are generally safe; however, case reports of endocarditis and sepsis in immunocompromised patients exist.[82] In addition, caution should be exercised in patients with a central venous catheter or who have compromised intestinal mucosa.[77]

CHRONIC PERSISTENT SYMPTOMS

It is important to assess whether Lyme disease has been adequately treated and that the patient actually had objective evidence of Lyme borreliosis. Persons without an initial diagnosis of Lyme disease using objective criteria should be discouraged from pursuing a diagnosis of chronic Lyme disease. Persistent symptoms may not be due to continued active borreliosis; rather, such patients can be treated with symptomatic and antiinflammatory measures. Antibiotic-refractory arthritic symptoms may also be autoimmune in origin or attributed to persistent infection.[11,18]

For persons with unexplained symptoms with a low prior probability of Lyme disease, the value of alternative testing is minimal as true positives will be rare. If test results are positive, there are psychological benefits from a diagnosis supporting a defined medical process, whether or not the diagnosis is accurate. This potential benefit may be outweighed by the high possibility of negative externalities from identifying with cases of severe, lifelong debilitation (prevalent in the popular media)[83,84] coupled with highly-invasive and potentially harmful treatments of unclear benefit. Clearly, there is benefit in a true positive identification of Lyme disease with subsequent treatment resulting in symptomatic relief, thereby reducing the likelihood of long-term sequelae.

A number of unconventional methods are purported to treat acute, or more often, persistent infection. Some, purporting to detect "vibrations" in the body (such as the Rife machine) or electrodiagnostic devices (such as the Vegatest) have no scientific basis nor any validity in treating Lyme disease (or any other disorder). Some elaborate alternative protocols exist[85,86] but have not been systematically assessed in controlled trials. Other common herbal therapies with some evidence for antimicrobial activity that are safe include *Artemisia annua,* olive leaf, goldenseal (*Hydrastis canadensis*), and grapefruit seed extract, although they have not demonstrated antispirochetal activity. Some other common interventions in Lyme disease protocols include chaparral (*Larrea divaricata*)[87] and colloidal silver[88] that have significant risks of toxicity and harm; these should be actively discouraged.[15]

The following are a sampling of integrative therapies that can be antiinflammatory or analgesic with a high potential benefit-risk ratio. As there are a paucity of clinical trials assessing CAM interventions in persons with persistent symptoms following Lyme borreliosis, therapies that are safe and have demonstrated efficacy in inflammatory conditions or medically unexplained conditions (such as fibromyalgia) that symptomatically resemble chronic Lyme disease were chosen. A more comprehensive list of potential therapies can be found in the fibromyalgia and chronic fatigue syndrome chapters (Chapters 47 and 48).

It is critical to acknowledge and address the real suffering and debilitating symptomology of patients,[83,84] regardless of whether the etiology of their symptoms is clear or ambiguous.[15] The benefits of a salutogenic patient-practitioner relationship are described in Chapter 3.

Pharmacological

Antiinflammatory Treatments

Nonsteroidal antiinflammatory drugs (NSAIDS), intraarticular steroid injections, or disease-modifying antirheumatic drugs (DMARDS) have all been used to treat persistent symptoms associated with Lyme disease.[17]

Antibiotics

Five randomized controlled trials have been conducted in patients with post-Lyme disease syndrome using long-term antibiotic regimens.[14,24,89-91] Krupp et al. demonstrated improvements in fatigue in persons treated with intravenous ceftriaxone after 28 days compared to placebo, without improvement in cognitive function or a laboratory measure of infection.[89] Six of the 52 patients that began the interventions (11.5%) discontinued the study due to adverse events; of these, four patients (three on placebo) required hospitalization due to line sepsis.[89] None of the other studies have demonstrated significant benefit for long-term antibiotic treatment in patients with ongoing subjective symptoms following standard treatment of initial Lyme disease.[14,91a]

Case reports documenting symptomatic relief using long-term antibiotic therapy are common,[92] and Cameron et al. reported significant improvements in quality of life in patients experiencing persistent Lyme disease symptoms when treated with amoxicillin for 3 months,[93] although this study has been criticized for a number of methodological flaws that may render its conclusions moot.[94] Of note, a number of antibiotics used to treat Lyme disease exhibit antiinflammatory effects, including macrolides and tetracyclines,[95] while B-lactams[96] and tetracyclines[97] exhibit neuroprotective effects. Thus symptomatic relief using antibiotics can be achieved through

other pharmacological actions besides antimicrobial effects.

PRECAUTIONS

The risks of long-term antibiotic therapy are well documented including anaphylaxis and biliary complications, resulting in cholecystectomy[98] as well as fatal sepsis[31] and infection of intravenous catheters.[24] Longer courses of antibiotics increase the risk of adverse events.[18] NSAIDS, DMARDS, and intraarticular injections also pose considerable risk and may be undesirable if treatments with a better risk-benefit ratio exist.

If the presence of persistent borreliosis cannot be established using objective criteria, nonpharmacolgical therapies are initially recommended for symptomatic relief. Pharmaceuticals can be considered if nonpharmacological means do not provide adequate relief. Antibiotics should only be used if active borreliosis is confirmed.

Gabapentin

In an open pilot study in 10 patients with neuroborreliosis, 10 patients were treated with gabapentin (starting at 300 mg/day and increasing to a maximum tolerated dose). Weissenbacher et al. reported that pain symptoms improved in 90% of patients and sleep quality and general health improved in 50% of patients.[99]

DOSAGE

300 mg/day titrating up to a maximum tolerated dose within 4–12 weeks. In the study by Weissenbacher et al., the average dose associated with pain reduction was 700 mg.[99]

PRECAUTIONS

Gabapentin is associated with a variety of adverse effects, including depression and increasing the risk of suicide.[100] Abrupt discontinuation of gabapentin can cause withdrawal symptoms.[99]

Herbal

The herb *Uncaria tomentosa* (Cat's claw) is prominent in a number of alternative protocols for Lyme disease.[85] It has antioxidant, antiinflammatory, and immunostimulant activity.[101] No evidence exists for specific antispirochetal activity. In a randomized trial in persons with rheumatoid arthritis, a specific extract of *Uncaria tomentosa* demonstrated efficacy in reducing painful joints.[102]

DOSAGE

60 mg daily in three divided doses of an extract free of tetracyclic oxindole alkaloids.[102]

PRECAUTIONS

Can cause headache, vomiting, and dizziness.

Lifestyle

Antiinflammatory Diet (See Chapter 88)

The antiinflammatory diet is characterized by emphasizing omega-3 fatty acids (found primarily in deepwater fish) and minimizing omega-6 fatty acids, with an emphasis on unprocessed whole grains, beans, and fruits and vegetables. Fish oil, especially EPA, is often added as a supplementary measure. There is significant overlap between the antiinflammatory diet and the Mediterranean diet in reducing risk of cardiovascular disease.[103,104]

Antiinflammatory diets have demonstrated clinical benefits in persons with inflammatory diseases such as rheumatoid arthritis.[103,105] More extensive antiinflammatory dietary measures, such as a gluten-free vegan diet, have been shown to reduce inflammatory markers in patients with rheumatoid arthritis[106] as well as improve symptoms.[107]

Aerobic and Weight-Bearing Exercise

Moderate aerobic exercise has been shown to improve physical function, mood, symptom severity, and self-efficacy in fibromyalgia patients,[108] as well as energy in patients with unexplained fatigue.[109] Other trials have confirmed the benefits of aerobic exercise and muscle strengthening for fibromyalgia,[110-112] as well as hydrotherapy[113] and walking.[114] Pain, the most characteristic symptom of fibromyalgia, was reduced in persons exercising at low-to-moderate intensity two or three times per week with positive effects on depressed mood, quality of life, and physical fitness.[115] Aerobic exercise, performed twice weekly over 8 months, can alleviate symptoms as well as demonstrate antiinflammatory effects.[116]

Multiple systematic reviews indicate that, among myriad treatments proposed for fibromyalgia, mild-to-moderate intensity aerobic and weight-bearing exercise (including aquatic exercise)[117] has consistently shown to be effective in alleviating, pain, fatigue, depression, and improving health-related quality of life in persons with fibromyalgia.[118-122]

> DOSAGE
>
> Mild aerobic exercise with weight training two to three times weekly for at least 4 weeks.[118] Initiate at 15 minutes and increase to 30 minutes as tolerance grows.

Supplements

Probiotics

Preliminary studies suggest the efficacy of probiotic strains in treating chronic fatigue syndrome-associated anxiety[123] using *Lactobacillus casei* strain Shirota (LcS). Some chronic Lyme disease protocols include probiotics.[72] Some probiotics have antiinflammatory properties that are strain- and species-specific and may be used symptomatically.[124,125]

> DOSAGE
>
> 24 billion colony forming units of *Lactobacillus casei* strain Shirota (LcS); available in a fermented milk commercial product (Yakult).

Omega-3 Fatty Acids

Omega-3 fatty acid intake is inversely associated with major depression,[126,127] a strong comorbidity with chronic fatigue syndrome and fibromyalgia.[128] Further, serum levels of EPA are significantly lower in chronic fatigue syndrome patients than in normal controls.[129] Omega-3 fatty acid supplementation has some evidence for efficacy in treating a number of nonspecific symptoms associated with persistent Lyme disease, including fatigue, arthralgias,[130] depression,[131] and anxiety.[69]

> DOSAGE
>
> 2500 mg of omega-3 fatty acids (with 50% or more EPA), consistent with a case series[132] documenting clinically significant pain reduction and improved function associated with a variety of conditions including fibromyalgia.

Intravenous Micronutrient Therapy

A clinical trial of a popular intravenous formula (the Myers' cocktail)[133-135] found both a large treatment effect and a large placebo effect in improving pain, mood, and global function, with effect sizes comparable to FDA-approved drugs for fibromyalgia.[134] Contextual factors and the therapeutic relationship are important factors in the overall effectiveness of a therapy, especially with subjective outcomes such as in chronic pain syndromes,[136,137] and perhaps stronger with alternative therapies associated with elaborate rituals and distinct contexts.[138] There is an ethical imperative to provide therapeutic options that are safe and effective for symptomatic relief, with appropriate informed consent, without endorsing approaches that are unsafe or ineffective.[139] There is emerging literature on the psychobiology of the placebo effect, with clinically significant effects demonstrated in a variety of contexts.[138,140] Intentional use of placebo in clinical practice is routine[141] with complex ethical implications.[138]

> DOSAGE
>
> Weekly slow intravenous infusions (over 10 minutes) of Myers cocktail. Persons responding to the Myers' cocktail should experience significant symptomatic relief within 4 weeks. The Myers' cocktail contains 5 mL magnesium chloride hexahydrate (20%), 3 mL calcium gluconate (10%), 1 mL Hydroxocobalamin (1000 mcg/mL), 1 mL pyridoxine hydrochloride (100 mg/mL), 1 mL dexpanthenol (250 mg/mL), 1 mL B-complex 100 (contains 100 mg thiamine HCl, 2 mg riboflavin, 2 mg pyridoxine HCl, 2 mg panthenol,100 mg niacinamide, 2% benxyl alcohol, 5 mL vitamin C [500 mg/mL], and 20 mL sterile water).

Acupuncture

Acupuncture[142,143] (and sham acupuncture[144]) have been shown to symptomatically improve pain associated with fibromyalgia. Although analgesic effects often do not differ from placebo acupuncture,[145] the therapy has minimal risk,[144] reduces anxiety,[145] and may be effective for fatigue[146] in chronic disease.[147]

> **DOSAGE**
>
> 20-minute individualized session weekly.

Massage Therapy

Various forms of massage have demonstrated short-term beneficial effects in treating fibromyalgia symptoms in randomized trials.[148,149] Despite the lack of a complete understanding of the mechanisms, massage has clearly been shown to improve osteoarthritis pain.[150-155] Massage therapy has been evaluated and found efficacious as an adjunct treatment for pain secondary to cancer,[156-168] low back pain,[169-172] procedural pain,[173,174] rheumatoid arthritis,[175,176] and fibromyalgia.[177,178] It also has been shown to be beneficial for patients with chronic pain following spinal cord injury.[179] In a randomized, open-label clinical trial, a series of classical Swedish massage therapy sessions was found to be as effective as conventional analgesia for chronic rheumatic pain.[175]

> **DOSAGE**
>
> Swedish or other massage approach (30–60 minutes) one to two times weekly.

Mind-Body Therapy

Psychological trauma is associated with persistent Lyme disease symptoms[180] and fibromyalgia,[181] and chronic stress tends to exacerbate symptoms.[182,183] Mind-body therapies are especially attractive in cases where psychological trauma predates the onset of symptoms, as both somatic and psychological benefits are often seen.[184] Cognitive-behavioral therapy has demonstrated good evidence in improving function in adults[185] and adolescents with fibromyalgia.[186]

Tai Chi

Two randomized trials demonstrated significant benefits of tai chi, a Chinese mind-body practice involving meditation, deep breathing, and slow, gentle, graceful movements[187,188] for fibromyalgia. Tai chi has also shows promise in improving symptoms of rheumatoid arthritis.[74,189]

> **DOSAGE**
>
> Group course with experienced teacher twice weekly for at least 12 weeks.

Mindfulness Meditation

A number of trials have assessed the effects of various regimens of mindfulness meditation with promising results in outcomes ranging from pain severity, physical function, and tender point threshold[190-194] in persons with fibromyalgia.

Mindfulness-based stress reduction (MBSR) is a standardized protocol of mind-body therapies that involves mindfulness meditation, patient education, and group support[195-197] developed by Kabat-Zinn et al. at the Stress Reduction Clinic of the University of Massachusetts Medical Center. Several randomized trials have demonstrated the benefit of MBSR for a variety of chronic conditions with improvements in psychological and somatic measures.[198-208]

> **DOSAGE**
>
> The standard 8-week course of MBSR consists of an instructor delivering group instruction for 2.5 h/wk (consisting of meditation practice, group discussions, and mindfulness skill-building activities),[197] a single half-day meditation retreat, and daily practice of 30–45 minutes 6 days per week.[195] Internet-delivered interventions have also demonstrated promise.[209,210]

Therapies to Consider

If chronic persistent symptoms continue without resolution and other conditions are definitively ruled out, other complementary therapies can be considered such as trigger-point injections, chiropractic manipulation, and myofascial release therapy, all of which demonstrate some evidence of efficacy.[185]

PREVENTION PRESCRIPTION FOR LYME DISEASE

REDUCE RISK FOR TICK BITES IN ENDEMIC AREAS

- Clear brush and trees, remove leaf litter and woodpiles, and keep grass mowed.
- Wear light-colored clothing that covers the skin to aid in identifying and protecting from tick bites. Tuck pant legs into socks when outdoors in vegetated areas.
- Apply tick and insect repellents containing 20%–30% DEET [N,N-diethyl-3-methyltoluamide],[3] although excessive doses have been reported to cause neurological complications in children.[211]

- Permethrin, a synthetic pyrethroid applied to clothing, is effective in killing ticks. Toxicities have been reported at high doses.[211,212]
- A plant-based insect repellant containing oil of lemon eucalyptus has been shown to protect from mosquitoes but has not demonstrated efficacy against ticks.[211]
- The most effective methods shown to reduce risk of Lyme disease in endemic areas are the use of protective clothing and using tick repellents on the skin and clothing.[213]
- Check skin for ticks after being outdoors in the late spring and summer months in endemic areas. Fig. 23.4 illustrates the life cycle of ticks that can transmit Lyme disease.
- Bathe within 2 hours after spending time in vegetation.[3,214]
- Pesticides are effective, but recommendations are tempered due to environmental concerns and risk of harm to children and wildlife.

REDUCE RISK FOR LYME DISEASE AFTER A TICK BITE

- Remove ticks using fine-tipped tweezers and a steady motion, grasping the tick as close as possible to the skin. Pull directly away from the skin. Do not use petroleum jelly, nail polish, or heated instruments to remove a tick.
- Monitor for signs and symptoms of Lyme disease after a tick bite.
- Consider antimicrobial prophylaxis (200 mg doxycycline in a single dose for adults or 4 mg/kg up to a maximum dose of 200 mg for children aged >8 years, and 250 mg of amoxicillin in children aged <8 years) if a tick is attached for more than 48 hours in an endemic area, although risk of *B. burgdorferi* infection is low; 1.2% of untreated children in a large cohort developed Lyme disease after a tick bite in a highly endemic area. Treatment subsequent to symptom onset is associated with complete recovery.[215]

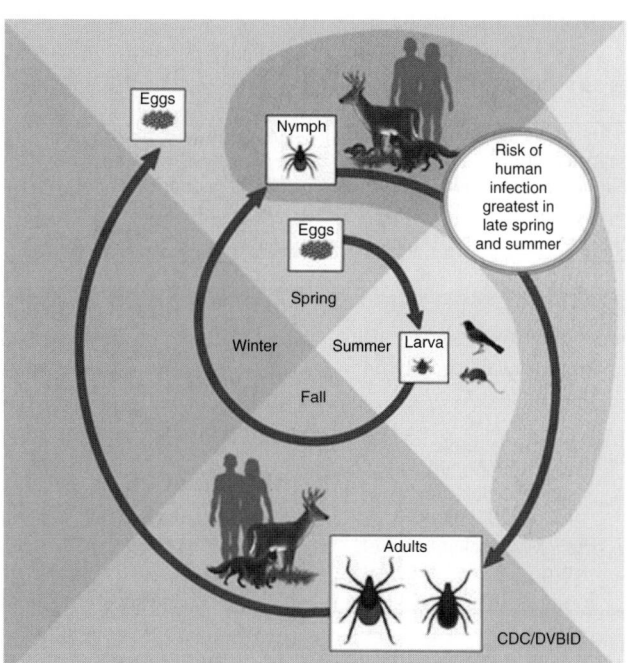

FIG. 23.4 ■ Life cycle of blacklegged ticks that can transmit anaplasmosis, babesiosis, and Lyme disease. (From the Centers for Disease Control and Prevention, Division of Vector-Borne Diseases: Life cycle of hard ticks that spread disease: http://www.cdc.gov/ticks/life_cycle_and_hosts.html.)

THERAPEUTIC REVIEW

EARLY LYME DISEASE	ADULT DOSING	
Doxycycline	100 mg twice per day for 14 days (range, 10–21 days)	A 2
Amoxicillin	500 mg three times per day for 14 days (range, 14–21 days)	A 2
Cefuroxime axetil	500 mg twice per day for 14 days (range, 14–21 days)	A 2

EARLY LYME DISEASE WITH NEUROLOGICAL MANIFESTATIONS	ADULT DOSING	
Doxycycline	100 mg twice per day for 14 days (range, 14–21 days)	A 2
Amoxicillin	500 mg three times per day for 14 days (range, 14–21 days)	A 2
Cefuroxime axetil	500 mg twice per day for 14 days (range, 14–21 days)	A 2
Probiotics: *Lactobacillus GG, Lactobacillus sporogenes, Bifidobacterium lactis Bb-12, Lactobacillus acidophilus La-5,* or *Saccharomyces boulardii*	5–40 billion CFU/day throughout the duration of antibiotic treatment or 200 g of a specific yogurt product containing *Lactobacillus rhamnosus GG, Bifidobacterium lactis Bb-12,* and *Lactobacillus acidophilus La-5*[79]	B 1

CHRONIC PERSISTENT SYMPTOMS	ADULT DOSING	
NSAIDS, intraarticular steroid injections, DMARDS	Varies as needed	B 3
Antibiotics (long term, intravenous)	Varies, only when borreliosis is confirmed	C 3

CHRONIC PERSISTENT SYMPTOMS	ADULT DOSING	
Gabapentin	300 mg/day titrating up to a maximum tolerated dose within 4–12 weeks (average dose, 700 mg)	B 2
Uncaria tomentosa (cat's claw)	60 mg daily in three divided doses of an extract free of tetracyclic oxindole alkaloids	B 2
Antiinflammatory diet		B 1
Aerobic and weight-bearing exercise	15–30 minutes two to three times weekly for at least 4 weeks	A 1
Probiotics: *Lactobacillus casei* strain Shirota	24 billion colony forming units of available in a fermented milk product	C 1
Omega-3 fatty acids	2500 mg of omega-3 fatty acids (with 50% or more EPA) per day	B 1
Intravenous micronutrient therapy	37 CC infused weekly of the Myer's cocktail	C 2
Acupuncture	20-minute individualized session weekly	B 1
Massage therapy	Swedish or other massage approach (30–60 minutes) one to two times weekly	B 1
Tai chi	Group course with experienced teacher twice weekly for at least 12 weeks	A 1
Mindfulness meditation, mindfulness-based stress reduction	Group course with weekly meeting and daily practice	B 1

Key Web Resources

Lyme Disease: Centers for Disease Control and Prevention	http://www.cdc.gov/lyme
Lyme Disease Tick Map (iTunes app)	http://itunes.apple.com/us/app/lyme-disease-tick-map/id369913510?mt=8
University of Rhode Island Tick-Encounter Resource Center	http://www.tickencounter.org/

ACKNOWLEDGMENT

The helpful suggestions from Carlos Oliveira, MD, and technical support from Theresa Weiss, MPH, are appreciated.

REFERENCES

References are available online at ExpertConsult.com.

CARDIOVASCULAR DISEASE

SECTION OUTLINE

24 HYPERTENSION

25 HEART FAILURE

26 CORONARY ARTERY DISEASE

27 DYSLIPIDEMIA

28 ARRHYTHMIAS

CHAPTER 24

HYPERTENSION

Gregory A. Plotnikoff, MD, MTS • Jeffery Dusek, PhD

Hypertension is the most important risk factor for cardiovascular morbidity and mortality in industrialized countries. At least 65 million Americans have blood pressures that place them at significantly higher risk of coronary artery disease, heart failure, renal failure, thoracic and abdominal aneurysms, myocardial infarction, and stroke. Hypertension is also associated with cognitive dysfunction, erectile dysfunction, and loss of vision. The higher the pressure, the greater the risk of complications.[1]

However, hypertension frequently is asymptomatic; in the absence of symptoms, elevated blood pressure may not hold particular significance for patients. In many cultures of the world, if there is no pain, there is no disease. This means that clinicians face three key challenges. First, is there a shared awareness? Is hypertension even an issue for the patient? Second, will the patient accept any intervention to treat an abstract number? Third, will the patient accept a long-term intervention with no immediate benefit? For these reasons, patients benefit when integrative clinicians initially explore the meanings, beliefs, and interpretations the patient brings to their experience of numbers from ambulatory blood pressure measurements. The patient's answers should both guide the clinician's approach and foster a working partnership (see also Chapter 3).

Hypertension prevention and treatment represents an ideal opportunity to codevelop a customized action plan that addresses logical options regarding diet, exercise, supplementation, smoking cessation, and mind-body self-care skills development. Additional insights may also come from both Ayurvedic and traditional East Asian medicine traditions. This chapter will address how each of these individual interventions can contribute to improved health and well-being.

> A reduction in systolic blood pressure of 5 mmHg is reportedly associated with a 7% reduction in all-cause mortality.

There is no question that every clinician must be well versed in the treatment of hypertension. However, at the time of writing this chapter, considerable confusion exists regarding optimal hypertension management. For this reason, a brief review of the controversies is warranted.

In 2014, JAMA published the eighth report of the Joint National Committee on Prevention, Detection, Evaluation, and Treatment of High Blood Pressure (JNC 8).[2] This was greatly anticipated as the previous report, termed JNC 7, was published in 2003. Nine new recommendations were made, the most controversial of which was to redefine the goal blood pressure for those greater than 60 years of age to < 150/90 mmHg. For all others aged over 18 years, the goal blood pressure was recommended as < 140/90. This same goal was recommended for patients with chronic kidney disease or diabetes.

Significant confusion followed the publication of JNC 8. Critics noted the marked lack of consistency with JNC 7; the lack of consensus among the JNC 8 committee members, with 5 of 17 authors quickly publishing a dissent[3]; and the lack of clarity in definable quality measures in hypertension by which to grade physicians. The American Heart Association (AHA) and American College of Cardiology (ACC) continue to recognize JNC 7 and are currently preparing their own guidelines.

The confusion follows from the mixed conclusions of the two JNC reports. The 2003 JNC 7 report defined a normal BP as less than 120 mmHg systolic and less than 80 mmHg diastolic. The report similarly defined stage 1 hypertension as 140–159 mmHg systolic and 90–99 mmHg diastolic. In between normal and stage 1 values is a category the JNC 7 report termed prehypertension. This new term was introduced to heighten awareness of both risk and opportunities for prevention. The JNC 7 report also noted that the BP treatment goal is less than 130/80 mmHg for persons with diabetes or renal disease and hypertension[1] (Table 24.1). In marked contrast, JNC 8 did not define a "normal" blood pressure, eliminated the stages of hypertension, and revised upward the thresholds for treatment, including for those persons with comorbidities.

How could this happen? JNC 7 recommendations were based upon expert consensus derived from a thorough but nonsystematic literature review that included observational studies. In contrast, JNC 8 recommendations followed from a formal systematic review by methodologists who were restricted to consideration of randomized controlled trials (RCTs) with more than 100 hypertensive participants who were followed for at least 1 year. This eliminated approximately 98% of all previously published clinical studies of hypertension treatment, including observational studies, systematic

TABLE 24.1 **JNC 7 and JNC 8: Goal Blood Pressures**

	JNC 8	JNC 7
Ages 18–59 years	< 140/90	< 140/90
Ages ≥60 years	< 150/90	< 140/90
Diabetes mellitus or chronic kidney disease	< 140/90	< 130/80

reviews, and meta-analyses.[4] The JNC 8 committee also restricted their analysis to three questions. First, does initiation of antihypertensive pharmacological treatment at a specific threshold improve health outcomes? Second, do attempts to reach specified blood pressure goals lead to improvements in health outcomes? And, third, do various antihypertensive drugs or drug classes differ in regards to health outcomes? The panel did not address whether therapy-associated adverse effects and harms resulted in significant changes in important health outcomes.

The JNC 8 recommendations were graded based upon the quality of evidence reviewed. Not considered for the first two questions were any RCTs that included participants with a normal blood pressure (such as persons with diabetes). Studies considered for the third question were limited to those that examined one class of medication versus another. This eliminated all single agent placebo-controlled trials from consideration.

Based upon such a rigorous evidence-based review, only two grade A "strong" recommendations could be made. First, for those ≥ 60 years of age, antihypertensive pharmacological therapy should be initiated at a threshold of ≥ 150 mmHg systolic blood pressure or ≥ 90 mmHg diastolic blood pressure with a goal blood pressure of < 150 mmHg systolic and < 90 mmHg diastolic. Second, for those < 60 years of age, pharmacological therapy should be initiated at a diastolic blood pressure ≥ 90 mmHg with a treatment goal of achieving a pressure < 90 mmHg.

Likewise, only three Grade B "moderate" recommendations could be made. For the general nonblack population, including those with diabetes, initial therapy should include a thiazide diuretic, a calcium channel blocker (CCB), an angiotensin converting enzyme inhibitor (ACEi), or an angiotensin receptor blocker (ARB). For the general black population, initial therapy should be a thiazide diuretic or CCB. For those aged ≥ 18 years with chronic kidney disease, the initial or add-on pharmaceutical should be an ACE or ARB to improve kidney outcomes.

Grade C or "weak" recommendations were based upon RCTs with major limitations, such as the presence of post hoc analyses of non-prespecified subgroups. Only one recommendation was possible; for blacks with diabetes, initial therapy should be a thiazide diuretic or a CCB.

Every other recommendation made by the JNC 8 committee was labeled grade E, the category representing consensus expert opinion. This means that the evidence base from the gold standard of randomized-controlled trials was too weak to make a definitive recommendation. Further, any other clinical intervention for the prevention and treatment of hypertension fails the strictest definition of "evidence-based" practice. Given contradictory clinical trial data, these guidelines will likely remain controversial.[5]

> JNC 8 recommends blood pressure treatment for those ≤ 60 years of age at 140/90 mmHg. For those older than 60 years, treatment is recommended at 150/90 mmHg. First line therapy can be with a thiazide diuretic, ACE, ARB, or CCB. In the black population, a thiazide or CCB should be used. In those with kidney disease, an ACE or ARB is recommended.

Although observational studies and association studies have demonstrated a strong relationship between lower blood pressures and reduced risk, all the way down to very low blood pressures, evidence from RCTs does not indicate any patient benefit from treatment *with pharmaceuticals* to achieve lower blood pressures. Two significant implications exist for integrative practitioners and their patients. First, JNC 8 widens the range of acceptable blood pressures for patients. Second, JNC 8 reduces the pressure to prescribe pharmaceuticals for patients who decline or wish to avoid pharmaceuticals. In fact, JNC 8 explicitly supports the role of conventional risk modifications including reducing sodium intake, increasing exercise, moderating alcohol consumption, losing weight, and following the Dietary Approaches to Stop Hypertension (DASH) eating plan. The American Heart Association has gone even farther. In 2013, it affirmed that all individuals with blood pressure levels > 120/80 mmHg should consider trials of alternative approaches as adjuvant methods to help lower blood pressure when clinically appropriate.[6]

Because many persons wish to avoid pharmaceutical therapies, integrative clinicians are often sought who can counsel from an evidence base regarding the most appropriate treatment options available. This chapter's purpose is to expand the range of logical, nonpharmaceutical for both the prevention and treatment of hypertension. The intent is to support integrative clinicians in their capacity to codevelop an evidence-informed, customized action plan with their patient.

Nonpharmaceutical approaches to the treatment of hypertension, which include and go beyond the basic lifestyle modification recommendations found in the JNC 8 report, are provided in the following.

INTEGRATIVE THERAPY

Lifestyle Modification

Smoking Cessation

Smoking cessation should be part of every comprehensive lifestyle modification plan. Cigarette use is reportedly associated with a 4 mmHg increase in systolic blood pressure and a 3 mmHg increase in diastolic blood pressure compared with placebo.[7] Persons with hypertension who smoke, however, are at an additional increased risk of cardiovascular events compared with those with hypertension that do not smoke. This risk includes both ischemic and hemorrhagic stroke, and correlates directly with the number of cigarettes smoked.[8,9] Progressive muscle relaxation training,[10] hypnotherapy,[11] and acupuncture[12] may have utility in assisting smoking cessation. Electronic cigarettes are not considered smoking cessation devices.[13]

Nutrition

Mediterranean Diet

The efficacy of the Mediterranean diet in preventing or treating hypertension was evaluated among 9408 men and women enrolled in a prospective cohort study from 1999–2005. The study documented that, after adjustment for major hypertension risk factors and nutritional covariates, the degree of adherence to the Mediterranean diet over 6 years was associated with modest blood pressure reduction. For those with high adherence, mean systolic pressure declined by 3.1 mmHg (95% confidence interval [CI], −5.4 to 0.8) and mean diastolic blood pressure by 1.9 mmHg (95% CI, −3.6 to −0.1).[14]

Beyond hypertension, a systematic review of 35 different experimental studies demonstrated that the Mediterranean diet has favorable effects on lipoprotein levels, endothelium vasodilatation, insulin resistance, metabolic syndrome, antioxidant capacity, myocardial and cardiovascular mortality, and cancer incidence in obese patients and in those with previous myocardial infarction.[15] Additionally, the NIH-AARP study of 214,284 men and 166,012 women demonstrated that, over 10 years, adherence to the Mediterranean diet was associated with approximately a 20% reduction in all-cause mortality in both men and women. In comparing high to low conformity adherence in men, hazard ratios of cardiovascular and cancer mortality were 0.78 (95% CI, 0.69–0.87) and 0.83 (95% CI, 0.76–0.91), respectively. Similarly, a 12% reduction in cancer mortality was demonstrated in females (P = 0.04).[16] From the HALE (Healthy Aging: Longitudinal Study in Europe) study of persons aged 70–90 years, adherence to the Mediterranean diet and a healthful lifestyle was associated with a more than 50% lower rate of all-cause and cause-specific mortality[17] (see Chapter 88).

The Dietary Approaches to Stop Hypertension (DASH) Diet

The DASH diet (Dietary Approaches to Stop Hypertension) trial enrolled 459 participants and provided each with all food for 11 weeks. For the first 3 weeks, the participants were provided a control diet low in fruits, vegetables, and dairy products, with a fat content typical of the average diet in the United States. Participants were then randomly assigned to receive either 8 weeks of the control diet rich in fruits and vegetables or a "combination" diet rich in fruits, vegetables, and low-fat dairy products with reduced saturated and total fat. Sodium intake and body weight were maintained at constant levels. For the 326 participants with prehypertension, the DASH diet resulted in reduced systolic and diastolic pressures of 3.5 mmHg (P < 0.001) and 2.1 mmHg (P = 0.003), respectively. Among the 133 subjects with level I hypertension, the DASH diet reduced systolic and diastolic blood pressure by 11.4 and 5.5 mmHg more than the control diet (P < 0.001 for each).[18] These results have since been replicated in numerous settings (see Chapter 89).

Olive Oil

One of the main components of the Mediterranean diet is olive oil, which provides both high levels of monounsaturated fatty acids (MUFA), principally oleic acid, and healthy polyphenols. Oleic acid has been shown to have antihypertensive effects in laboratory animals.[19] Phenolic compounds in olive oil prevent lipoperoxidation, induce favorable changes in lipid profile, improve

endothelial function, and have antithrombotic properties.[20] In the Prevención con Dieta Mediterránea (PREDIMED) study of 772 asymptomatic persons 55 to 80 years of age at high cardiovascular risk, participants allocated to Mediterranean diets supplemented with either nuts or virgin olive oil demonstrated mean reductions in systolic pressure of 5.9 mmHg compared to those allocated a control low-fat diet (CI, −8.7 to −3.1 mmHg) and 7.1 mmHg (CI, −10.0 to −4.1 mmHg), respectively.[21]

Olive oil represents a logical substitute for butter and partially hydrogenated vegetable oils. The Food and Drug Administration (FDA) allows manufacturers to state on labels that consuming approximately two tablespoons (23 g) of olive oil a day may reduce the risk of heart disease. As a general recommendation, use organic, cold-pressed, extra-virgin olive oil for cold cooking, such as salad dressings and vegetable dips.

The consumption of a diet rich in polyphenols, including those found in olive oil and cocoa beans, appears to be important for hypertension prevention and control.[22] Polyphenols can induce nitric oxide (NO)-mediated endothelium-dependent relaxation in most arteries, including the coronary arteries. Polyphenols can also induce endothelium-derived hyperpolarizing factor (EDHF)-mediated arterial relaxation.[23,24]

Cocoa (Theobroma cacao)

In observational studies, regular intake of cocoa-containing foods has been shown to be associated with lower cardiovascular mortality. In a cohort of 470 Dutch men followed for 15 years, cocoa intake was inversely associated with blood pressure and positively associated with reduced risk of both cardiovascular and all-cause mortality. The first published meta-analysis of cocoa reviewed five randomized controlled studies of cocoa administration (n = 173) with an average intake of 100 g daily (500 mg of polyphenols) for a median duration of 2 weeks demonstrating reductions in pooled mean systolic and diastolic blood pressure values of 4.7 mmHg (95% CI, −7.6 to −1.8 mmHg; P = 0.002) and 2.8 mmHg (95% CI, −4.8 to −0.8 mmHg; P = 0.006), respectively, compared with controls. Of the five studies cited, only two trials enrolled hypertensive patients.[25]

Following this report, the authors enrolled 44 adults with untreated upper-range prehypertension or stage 1 hypertension in a prospective 18 week randomized-controlled trial of either 6.3 g (30 kcal) per day of dark chocolate containing 30 mg of polyphenols or matching polyphenol-free white chocolate. Low-dose dark chocolate intake reduced the prevalence of hypertension from 86% to 68%, with mean systolic BP decreasing by 2.9 (1.6) mmHg (P < .001) and diastolic BP by 1.9 (1.0) mmHg (P < 0.001). This was accomplished without changes in body weight or plasma levels of lipids, glucose, and 8-isoprostane (a measure of oxidative stress). The decrease in BP was also accompanied by a sustained increase in vasodilatative nitric oxide donor S-nitrosoglutathione levels by 0.23 (0.12) nmol/L (P < 0.001). In comparison, the polyphenol-free white chocolate intake was not associated with any changes in BP or plasma biomarkers.[26]

The benefit of flavonol-containing cocoa appears to also extend to persons with diabetes. A 30-day, thrice-daily consumption of flavanol-containing cocoa (321 mg flavanols per dose) versus a matched product with 25 mg of flavanols per dose in 41 persons treated for diabetes reportedly increased baseline brachial artery flow-mediated dilatation by 30% (P < 0.0001) without evidence of tachyphylaxis or decline in glycemic control.[27]

A 2010 pooled meta-analysis included 13 trials (15 treatment arms) and reported the most significant findings in hypertensive and prehypertensive subgroups (SBP, –5.0 ± 3.0 mmHg; P = 0.0009; DBP, –2.7 ± 2.2 mmHg, P = 0.01) compared to placebo. However, blood pressure was not reduced below 140 mmHg systolic or 80 mmHg diastolic. Daily flavanol dosages ranged from 30 mg to 1000 mg in the active treatment groups (dark chocolate with 50%–70% cocoa).[28]

> Consider recommending ¼ of a standard-sized dark chocolate bar consisting of 70% cocoa daily to help lower blood pressure.

Red Wine

Although alcohol consumption may cause multiorgan damage and raise blood pressure, red wine consumption is inversely associated with mortality due to cardiovascular diseases.[29] Previous studies have shown this effect even intakes as high as 300 mL of wine per day.[30] Risk reduction is greatest for red wine at low to moderate intake.[31] One possible explanation is that red wine is an extremely rich source of bioactive polyphenols. Noteworthy compounds include the flavonoids (quercetin, catechin, and epicatechin), proanthocyanidins, anthocyanins, and phenolic acids including gallic, caftaric, and caffeic acid in addition to the trihydroxystilbene termed resveratrol. These compounds are not found in white wines as the fermentation process for white wines, unlike for red wines, does not include the polyphenol-rich grape skins, seeds, and stems.[32] Each polyphenol may play some role in preventing or treating hypertension. For example, quercetin, catechin, and resveratrol promote nitric oxide production by vascular endothelium. Although animal studies have reported many potentially beneficial effects with oral administration of quercetin or resveratrol, they have not documented a reduction in blood pressure.[33,34]

Omega-3 Fatty Acids

A diet rich in cold-water fatty fish or grass fed animals is also rich in omega-3 polyunsaturated fatty acids (PUFA) that may prevent the development of hypertension. Omega-3 fatty acid deficiency contributes to development of hypertension in animal models.[35] This also appears to be true for humans. A 20-year follow-up study of a cohort of 4508 adults aged 18–30 years without hypertension at baseline documented an inverse association between long-chain omega-3 intake and development of hypertension. For the highest intake quartile compared to the lowest, after adjustment for potential confounders, the hazard ratio was just 0.65 (95% CI, 0.53–0.79; P [trend] < 0.01).[36] A double-blind, placebo-controlled intervention of 4 g of omega-3 fatty acids for 8 weeks in patients with chronic kidney disease with an initial supine blood pressure of 125.0/72.3 mmHg demonstrated significant reductions in 24 hour systolic (–3.3 ± 0.7 mmHg) and diastolic (–2.9 ± 0.5 mmHg) blood pressures in addition to a 24% reduction in serum triglyceride levels.[37] A recent meta-analysis of 70 RCTs confirmed blood pressure reduction in both hypertensive and normotensive subjects, with the strongest effects of eicosapentaenoic acid (EPA) and docosahexaenoic acid (DHA) supplementation observed in untreated hypertensive subjects (systolic blood pressure, –4.51 mmHg, 95% CI, –6.12 to –2.83; diastolic blood pressure, –3.05 mmHg, 95% CI, –4.35 to –1.74). A confounder to randomization for clinical trials is that blood pressure reduction may be most pronounced in persons with the CYP4F2 V33M polymorphism.[38]

> Supplementation of ≥2 grams per day of EPA + DHA (fish oil) appears necessary to reduce diastolic pressure.[39]

Fiber

A meta-analysis of 25 randomized controlled trials published up to the year 2004 documented that supplemental intake of dietary fiber significantly reduced both systolic and diastolic in hypertensive patients. The degree of reduction was significant: systolic –5.95 mmHg, (95% CI, –9.50 to –2.40) and diastolic –4.20 mmHg, (95% CI, –6.55 to –1.85). The authors suggested that at least 8 weeks of supplementation was required to achieve the maximal blood pressure reduction.[40] A 2007 study in hypertensive, overweight patients of psyllium powder dosed at 3.5 grams 20 minutes before each meal documented significant systolic and diastolic pressure reduction compared to controls.[41]

Flax Seed

Flax seed is a common dietary supplement that contains short-chained omega-3 fatty acids, lignans, and fiber. A 2013 prospective, double-blinded, placebo-controlled, randomized trial (n = 110) evaluated daily ingestion of 30 g of milled flaxseed or placebo over 6 months. The mean reduction in systolic blood pressure was approximately 10 mmHg and in diastolic was 7 mmHg. Participants with an initial systolic blood pressure ≥ 140 mmHg had significantly greater reductions.[42] A 2015 meta-analysis of 11 studies (14 trials) did not demonstrate as profound a reduction in blood pressure following flax seed supplementation. The data reviewed indicated that flaxseed supplementation slightly reduced systolic blood pressure (–1.77 mmHg; 95% CI, –3.45 to –0.09 mmHg; P = 0.04) and diastolic blood pressure (–1.58 mmHg; 95% CI, –2.64 to –0.52 mmHg; P = 0.003).[43]

Inorganic Nitrates

Both the Mediterranean and the DASH diets contain foods that are rich in inorganic nitrates, a source of the vasodilator, nitric oxide, via transformation by symbiotic bacteria. Reduced nitric oxide production has been linked to hypertension, endothelial dysfunction, and insulin resistance.[44] Foods that support nitric oxide production via nitrate content include root vegetables, such as beets, carrots, and turnips in addition to dark greens, celery, and leeks (Fig. 24.1). Four weeks of a beetroot juice intervention in a randomized, placebo-controlled study of 68 patients with hypertension aged 18–85 years reduced 24-hour ambulatory systolic and diastolic BP by 7.7 mmHg and 5.2 mmHg, respectively, (95% CI, 4.1–11.2 and 2.7–7.7; P < 0.001 for both) as well as blood pressures measured in clinic and at home.[45] No tachyphylaxis was observed. The authors also noted that the intervention, compared to placebo, improved endothelial function by ≈20% (P < 0.001) and reduced arterial stiffness by 0.59 m/s (95% CI, 0.24–0.93; P < 0.01). Supplementation with 250 mL a day of beetroot juice was well tolerated. The necessary dose and time required for the effect of beetroot on blood pressure is currently unknown. A follow-up 1-week intervention with nitrate-rich beetroot juice reported increases in all measures of serum and urinary nitrates but did not reduce blood pressure.[46]

Exercise

Both JNC 7 and JNC 8, as well as the American Heart Association and the American College of Sports Medicine, recommend aerobic endurance exercise for the primary prevention, treatment, and control of hypertension. Blood pressure reductions of approximately 5–7 mmHg systolic can follow an isolated exercise session (acute) or following exercise training (chronic). Reductions in blood pressure can last up to 22 hours following endurance exercise. The higher the initial blood pressure is, the greater the response.

The American College of Sports Medicine recommends the following exercise prescription for those with high BP:
- Frequency: on most, preferably all, days of the week. Intensity: moderate intensity (40%–60% VO_2R).
- Time: ≥30 min of continuous or accumulated physical activity per day.
- Type: primarily endurance physical activity supplemented by resistance exercise.[47]

Weight Loss

A 2008 meta-analysis of all weight loss studies demonstrated that dietary interventions to reduce body weight resulted in better blood pressure reduction than either of the prescription drugs orlistat and sibutramine. Weight loss of 4 kg (10 pounds) by diet was associated with a mean reduction in systolic blood pressure of approximately 6 mmHg. Similar weight loss with orlistat reduced systolic blood pressure by approximately 2.5 mmHg. Sibutramine treatment reduced body weight but did not lower and may have even elevated, blood pressure. The authors noted that no prospective studies demonstrate mortality or other patient-relevant end points can be lowered by weight reduction.[48]

Dietary Supplements

Dietary supplements represent low-cost, low-toxicity interventions that may be helpful in reducing blood pressure. However, when reviewing the medical literature, one must be aware of several limitations in the quality of research in this area. First, few studies measure and report serum levels at baseline and following the study period. This failure to document the presence or absence of a serum or intracellular deficiency or functional insufficiency means dosing is blind. If one size does not fit all, then studies are at high risk of false negative results due to underdosing. Additionally, treatment of a patient population with preexisting sufficient levels presumably means that additional dosing is unlikely to confer benefit. Further, adherence to the intervention protocol cannot be assessed without measurement of serum levels. Second, few studies intervene

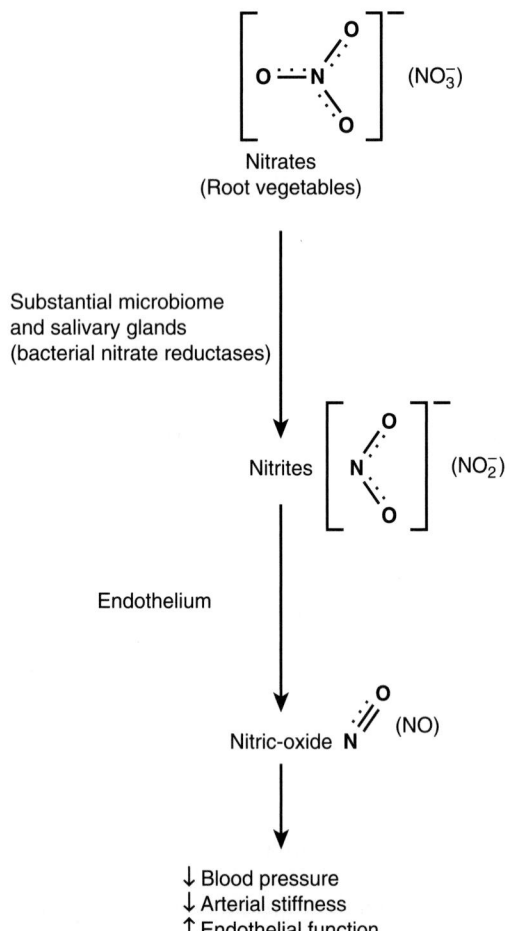

FIG. 24.1 ■ Dietary nitrate–nitrite–NO pathway.

with a dose based on the achievement of a targeted serum level. Most dosing is extrapolated from in vitro or epidemiological studies of intake in large populations. Individual variability in uptake and metabolism are not considered when calculating dosing. Third, differences in the bioavailability and function of different forms of a dietary supplement may exist. Accordingly, the majority of interventional nutrition research does not answer the very important clinical question, "does replenishment of a deficiency to a given serum level result in an improved clinical outcome?" Evidence-based, patient-centered care requires significantly better clinical studies.

CoQ10

Coenzyme Q_{10} (CoQ_{10}, ubiquinone, or ubiquinol) is a crucial cofactor in the electron transport chain and oxidative phosphorylation for production of adenosine triphosphate (ATP). The highest tissue concentration of CoQ10 is found in the heart, with the highest cellular concentration on the inner membrane of the mitochondrion. CoQ10 has been shown to be a potent antioxidant. Reduced levels are associated with aging, hyperthyroidism, cardiovascular disease, total parenteral nutrition, aerobic training, and ultraviolet exposure.[49] Statins and some beta blockers, such as propranolol, can reduce endogenous production of CoQ10 by as much as 40%.[50] A 2015 meta-analysis of eight clinical trials documented significant reduction in serum levels of CoQ10 with the use of all statins.[51] Supplementation can reduce oxidative stress and hyperinsulinemia, two significant drivers of hypertension.[52]

Low serum levels of CoQ10 were first associated with hypertension in 1975.[53] Since then, several studies have reported that supplementation can significantly reduce both systolic and diastolic hypertension without affecting aldosterone, sodium, or potassium levels or plasma renin activity. A trial involving 109 symptomatic hypertensive patients supplementation with CoQ10 (75–360 mg/day) to achieve a serum level of $> 2.0\mu g/mL$ reported a substantial reduction in mean systolic (from 159 to 147 mmHg) and diastolic (94 to 85 mmHg) blood pressures with concomitant improvement in New York Heart Association (NYHA) functional class and medication requirements. After an average of 4.4 months, 37% of patients were able to discontinue one antihypertensive drug, 11% discontinued two drugs, and 4% discontinued three drugs. Only 3% required the addition of one antihypertensive drug, and none required the addition of more than one antihypertensive drug. Importantly, 25% of all patients were able to control their blood pressure with only CoQ10 supplementation.[54]

> Statin drugs and some beta-blockers (propranolol) can reduce the endogenous production of CoQ10 by as much as 40%.

A 2007 meta-analysis of 12 clinical trials (n = 352 patients) concluded that CoQ10 supplementation in hypertensive patients can lower systolic blood pressure by up to 17 mmHg and diastolic blood pressure by up to 10 mmHg without significant side effects. In three randomized, double-blind controlled trials (n = 120), mean systolic pressure in the treatment group decreased by 16.6 mmHg (P < 0.001) from a mean of 167.7 mmHg (95% CI, 163.7–171.1 mmHg). The mean diastolic blood pressure decreased by 8.2 mmHg (P < .001) from 103 mmHg (95% CI, 101–105 mmHg) before treatment. In comparison, the placebo arms demonstrated minimal and statistically insignificant reductions in systolic and diastolic pressures. In the open-label, uncontrolled trials included in the analysis, patients were treated at doses of 60 to 120 mg daily for 6 to 12 weeks. Mean systolic blood pressure declined by 13.5 mmHg (95% CI, 9.8–17.1 mmHg; P < 0.001) and mean diastolic by 10.3 mmHg (95% CI, 8.4–12.3 mmHg; P < 0.001). This meta-analysis noted that in many of the studies included, patients were able to discontinue medication.[55]

DOSAGE

Dose to achieve a serum level of > 2.0μg/mL. This will require 75–350 mg a day taken with meals that contain some fat.

PRECAUTIONS

Side effects are infrequent and include abdominal discomfort, nausea, vomiting, diarrhea, anorexia, rash, and headache. CoQ10 has an antiplatelet effect so can theoretically increase the risk of bleeding with antiplatelet or anticoagulant agents. As excretion is via the bile, accumulation may occur in patients with hepatic impairment or biliary obstruction.

Vitamin D

Calcitriol, also known as 1,25-dihydroxyvitamin D, is the activated secosteroid hormone form of vitamin D that has receptors on nearly every tissue, including vascular smooth muscle cells[56] and renin-producing juxtaglomerular cells.[57] Calcitriol regulates hundreds of genes including the renin gene and thus the renin–angiotensin system (RAS) that controls blood pressure. Observational data from both the Health Professionals Followup Study (613 men) and the Nurses Health Study (1198 women) found low vitamin D status with was significantly associated with increased risk of incident hypertension over 4–8 years. For those with a serum 25 (OH) D level < 15 ng/mL compared to those with a level > 30 ng/mL, the RR for men was 6.13 (95% CI, 1.00–37.8) and for women was 2.67 (95% CI, 1.05–6.79).[58] In 2010, the Intermountain Heart Collaborative Study Group of 41,504 patients reported that vitamin D deficiency (<30 ng/mL) was associated with highly significant (P < 0.0001) increases in the prevalence of hypertension and associated cardiac risk factors of diabetes, hyperlipidemia, and peripheral vascular disease. Vitamin D deficiency was also strongly correlated (P < 0.0001) with coronary artery disease, myocardial infarction, heart failure, stroke, and death.[59]

Despite the potential benefits of vitamin D in improving cardiovascular health, few prospective trials support the hypothesis that vitamin D replenishment to normal levels reduces blood pressure. Among 148 elderly women with a mean 25-(OH) D serum level of 10 ng/mL (severe deficiency), 800 IUs of vitamin D3 supplementation per day for 8 weeks raised serum levels by 12 ng/mL and reduced systolic pressure by 7 mmHg compared to placebo. In contrast, among 189 men and women with a mean baseline level of 13 ng/mL, a single dose of 100,000 IU of vitamin D3 raised serum levels to a mean of 20 ng/mL at 5 weeks compared to placebo but had no effect on blood pressure.

Prior to the 2015 DAYLIGHT study with 534 participants, the largest prospective trial had enrolled 438 participants with a mean BMI of 35, mean 25 (OH) D level of 23.2 ± 8.5 ng/mL, systolic pressure of 124 ± 15 mmHg, and diastolic pressure of 75.4 ± 9.7 mmHg and randomized participants into three treatment groups: placebo, 20,000 IUs, or 40,000 IUs of oral cholecalciferol per week. At the end of 1 year, the low dose group had increased serum 25 (OH) D to a mean of 40 ng/mL, and the high dose group increased levels to a mean of 55 ng/mL with no significant change in blood pressure.[60] Of note, the main objective for this study was to study the effect of vitamin D supplementation on weight change, so the study was not designed and powered to detect effects on blood pressure. In the DAYLIGHT study, participants with prehypertension or stage I hypertension were enrolled and randomized to 400 IU or 4000 IUs per day. The median 25-hydroxyvitamin D level at baseline was 15.3 ng/mL. After 6 months, both the low-dose and high-dose arms demonstrated significantly improved vitamin D status but no significant reductions in either systolic or diastolic blood pressures.[61] Of note, vitamin D supplementation does not appear to reduce adiposity.

Future studies will need to address whether there is a threshold serum level needed to reduce the risk of incident hypertension or reduce already elevated pressures. Additionally, the duration of vitamin D sufficiency required for the prevention or reduction of hypertension needs to be defined.

Magnesium

Magnesium is a well-understood and frequently used intervention for hypertension in preeclampsia. Neither the JNC 7 nor JNC 8 guidelines recommend oral supplementation of magnesium. However, in addition to the potentially high magnesium intake associated with either a Mediterranean or DASH diet, several studies have reported that low dietary intake of magnesium correlates strongly with high blood pressure. The Women's Health Study followed 28,349 female United States health professionals aged ≥45 years without hypertension for almost 10 years. Magnesium intake, after adjustment for age and randomized treatment, was found to be inversely associated with the risk for incident hypertension. The highest quintile of intake (median, 434 mg/day) had a relative risk of 0.87 (95% CI,

0.81–0.93; P for trend < 0.0001) compared with those in the lowest quintile (median, 256 mg/day). Further adjustment for other risk factors slightly attenuated this inverse association.[62] The Honolulu Heart Study reported that of 61 nutritional substances studied, magnesium intake had the strongest inverse association with BP.[63]

Despite the inverse relationship between dietary magnesium and hypertension prevalence observed in epidemiological studies, clinical intervention studies have failed to demonstrate consistent benefit. As noted above, several limitations exist in the literature. For magnesium, few studies have measured baseline serum levels, with even fewer measuring intracellular magnesium levels. Serum magnesium levels do not reflect intracellular magnesium.[64]

Additionally, there are many forms of magnesium that may have different bioavailability and physiological activity. Accordingly, "one-size fits all" magnesium studies of varying dosing and varying type of magnesium prevent any meta-analysis of existing randomized trials. Despite these limitations, magnesium appears to be beneficial in reducing blood pressure and to be nontoxic.

A recent clinical trial enrolled 48 patients with mild uncomplicated hypertension and randomized them to 12 weeks of 600 mg/day of oral magnesium pidolate and lifestyle recommendations or lifestyle recommendations as a control. Mean 24-hour systolic pressures declined by 5.6 ± 2.7 mmHg (P < 0.001) and diastolic pressures declined by 2.8 ± 1.8 mmHg (P = 0.002) compared to controls.[65] In 82 diabetic hypertensive adults with documented hypomagnesemia receiving captopril but not diuretics, supplementation with 2.5 g magnesium chloride over 4 months decreased systolic pressure by 20.4 ± 15.9 mmHg compared to 4.7 ± 12.7 mmHg with placebo (P = 0.03). The magnesium intervention reduced diastolic pressure by 8.7 ± 16.3 mmHg versus 1.2 ± 12.6 mmHg in the placebo group. The adjusted odds ratio between serum magnesium and blood pressure was 2.8 (95% CI, 1.4–6.9). A threshold serum level for effect was not reported.[66]

DOSAGE

Natural sources of magnesium include pumpkin seeds, nuts, coffee, quinoa, spinach, bran cereal, buckwheat, and beans.

Dietary or supplementation intake doses of 400–800 mg of nonoxide forms of magnesium (malate, glycinate, taurate, etc.) are required to achieve normal intracellular and serum potassium levels.

PRECAUTIONS

Magnesium supplementation may cause loose bowel movements. Start at a low dose (120–200 mg) and slowly increase as tolerated.

Botanicals

Garlic (Allium sativum)

Garlic has been widely promoted for antihyperlipidemic effects; however, the results of both animal and human studies have indicated a blood pressure-lowering effect. Two separate meta-analyses published in 2008 demonstrated significant blood pressure lowering effects in persons with hypertension. The first meta-analysis included 11 of 25 studies from the systematic review. These demonstrated a mean decrease in the hypertensive subgroup of 8.4 ± 2.8 mmHg for SBP (P < 0.001) and 7.3 ± 1.5 mmHg for DBP (P < 0.001).[67] The second meta-analysis included 10 trials in the analysis, of which three had patients with elevated blood pressures. For hypertensive participants, the garlic interventions reduced systolic pressure by a mean of 16.3 mmHg (95% CI, 6.2–26.5) and diastolic pressure by a mean of 9.3 mmHg (95% CI, 5.3–13.3) compared with placebo.[68] Since then, the results of a 12-week randomized controlled trial of aged garlic extract in 79 patients with uncontrolled systolic hypertension indicated 480 mg (1.2 mg of S-allylcysteine) is both acceptable and effective at lowering systolic blood pressure (reduced by 11.8 ± 5.4 mmHg compared with placebo; P = 0.006).[69]

DOSAGE

The dose for raw garlic cloves is half to two cloves per day. Supplements may help avoid garlic breath. Consider a standardized dose containing 4000 mcg of allicin or 1.2 mg of S-allylcysteine.

PRECAUTIONS

Adverse effects include the following: diaphoresis; dizziness; mouth, esophagus, and stomach irritation; nausea; and vomiting. Allergic reactions are rare. Dosages greater than for culinary use may increase the risk of bleeding if taken with anticoagulants or antiplatelet agents.

Hawthorn (Crataegus monogyna)

Hawthorn as an herbal extract is a cardiovascular tonic popular in Europe that has been in use since at least the first century AD. Hawthorn is a short deciduous tree whose leaves, berries, and flowers contain high concentrations of flavonoids. Extracts are used for their positive inotropic and vasodilatory properties. Three clinical trials for blood pressure reduction have demonstrated very mild effects.[70-72] Hawthorn is most often used for early-stage congestive heart failure.

DOSAGE

The German Commission E Monographs cites the use of standardized extracts containing 30–169 mg of proanthocyanidins (18.75%) calculated as epicatechin or 3.5–19.8 mg of flavonoids (2.2%) calculated as hyperoside taken in two to three individual doses for a total dose of 750–1500 mg of Hawthorn per day.[73]

PRECAUTIONS

Transient side effects including dizziness, gastrointestinal complaints, headaches, and heart palpitations have been reported.[74] Results from the HERB-CHF trial of Crataegus extract WS1442 documented that participants treated with hawthorn extract were 3.9 times more likely to experience progression of heart failure at the start of hawthorn therapy compared to placebo. The observed increase in risk diminished over time.[75]

Herbs that require close monitoring in the treatment of patients with hypertension include licorice, ephedra, and Panax ginseng, which all have the capacity to significantly raise blood pressure.

Mind-Body Therapy

Despite numerous historical reports of decreases in BP attributed to mind-body practices,[76-81] a Cochrane Review[82] raised concerns regarding the impact of these interventions on blood pressure as many studies were conducted in the 1980s and 1990s, and the methodological quality of these studies was inconsistent. Specifically, not all studies were randomized controlled trials, the enrollment criteria were not specific to age group, cardiovascular risk factors, or type of hypertension, and the degree of blood pressure reduction varied widely. This important meta-analysis of randomized controlled trials concluded, somewhat surprisingly, that mind-body practices produced only modest benefits in reducing SBP, even though the investigators reported a roughly 5.5 mmHg reduction in SBP and a 3.5 mmHg reduction in DBP. Regarding the potential clinical significance of this reduction, SBP reductions between 2 and 5 mmHg have been shown to result in decreased mortality from stroke (14%), coronary heart disease (9%), and total mortality (7%).[83]

Since 1995, additional well-designed randomized controlled trials have demonstrated the efficacy of mind-body interventions, including relaxation response elicitation,[84,85] biofeedback,[86-89] transcendental meditation,[90,91] mindfulness based stress reduction (MBSR)[92,93] yoga,[94,95] qi gong,[96,97] and tai chi,[98] on reducing systolic blood pressure (SBP) or diastolic blood pressure (DBP). Although several of the more recent studies are limited by small sample sizes, many now address the mechanistic and biological mechanisms by which these approaches reduce BP. Additionally, the overall consistency of positive results indicates that, as a whole, mind-body interventions do positively affect both SBP and DBP. Aggregating the findings of these studies shows average reductions of approximately 10 mmHg and 7 mmHg for SBP and DBP, respectively.

Relaxation Response

Relaxation response (RR) is one of the most accessible means of discovering and developing mind-body self-care skills.[83] The efficacy of RR in treating hypertension has been demonstrated by a 8-week intervention trial in older adults (mean age, 66.8 years) with elevated SBP and normal DBP who were taking at least two antihypertensive medications.[84] Participants were blinded to hypothesis and were randomly assigned to one of two interventions to reduce BP: group 1 (relaxation response intervention; n = 61) or group 2 (intensive lifestyle modification; n = 61). Clinic SBP decreased by 9.4 mmHg and 8.8 mmHg in the relaxation response and lifestyle modification groups, respectively (P < 0.0001), without a difference observed between groups. In a second phase of the study, participants who achieved a clinic assessed SBP of less than 140 mmHg and had at least a 5 mmHg reduction from baseline entered an antihypertensive medication elimination protocol, with 44 subjects in the relaxation response group and 36 in the lifestyle modification group qualifying for the protocol. Participants in the relaxation response group were more likely to eliminate an antihypertensive medication successfully than were those in the lifestyle modification group (odds ratio, 4.3; 95% CI, 1.2–15.9; P = 0.03). The relaxation response intervention not only led to an important decrease in BP comparable to that of intensive lifestyle modification, but also resulted in a significantly greater capacity for participants to eliminate an antihypertensive medication without increasing BP (see Chapter 94).

Biofeedback

Reduced blood pressure is presumed to be a treatment effect of biofeedback training due to increased parasympathetic tone and/or reduction in adrenal hormone production. The first clinical trial to suggest that biofeedback was effective in persons with hypertension was published in 1981. In this 8-week study of 38 persons, the intervention group demonstrated significantly lower blood pressure, muscle tension, serum aldosterone, and urinary cortisol levels compared to controls.[78] However, a 2010 systematic review of 36 biofeedback trials found no persistent effectiveness in hypertension management.[99] Since then, the results of one pilot study have indicated that biofeedback training was effective at attenuating blood pressure elevations due to psychosocial stressors and emotional activation.[87] This interpretation was supported by an earlier clinical trial of biofeedback for 4 weeks with 20 participants.[88] A 2015 randomized trial enrolled 59 adults for 16 weeks of biofeedback training with real-time BP feedback signals or, as the control group, training with pseudofeedback signals. A large percentage of both groups demonstrated a greater than 5 mmHg reduction by 9 weeks that persisted for 8 weeks after completing the study.[85] The investigators interpreted this as the result of repeated practice in BP self-regulation (see Chapter 96).

> Reducing the breathing rate to 6 breaths per minute lowers blood pressure and enhances heart rate variability. This is considered the ideal breathing rate for inducing cardiovascular benefits.

Transcendental Meditation

Two studies examined the effect of a 12-week proprietary transcendental meditation (TM) intervention on BP in medicated African Americans. In the first study,[89] 111 individuals (mean age, 67 years) were randomized to TM, progressive muscle relaxation (PMR), or health education. The findings indicated that TM resulted in a clinic-based 10.6 mmHg reduction in SBP and a

6.6 mmHg reduction in DBP, significantly greater than the 4.0 mmHg and 2.1 mmHg reduction for PMR and greater than the 1.5 mmHg reduction in SBP and 0.6 mmHg increase in DBP among the health education group. In a more recent study enrolling younger subjects (mean age, 48.5 years),[90] the TM intervention (n = 54) resulted in a clinic-based 1.6 mmHg reduction in SBP and a 4.2 mmHg reduction in DBP at the end of the 12-week intervention. PMR (n = 52) led to a 1.77 mmHg increase in SBP and a 1.4 mmHg reduction in DBP, whereas health education (n = 44) resulted in a 2.0 mmHg increase and a 0.5 mmHg decrease in DBP. Overall, the results of these well-controlled trials indicate a significant effect of the TM intervention on BP (see Chapter 100).

Mindfulness-Based Stress Reduction

Two recent studies examined the impact of mindfulness-based stress reduction (MBSR) on unmedicated individuals with elevated blood pressure or prehypertension but not reaching the stage 1 hypertension designation (140 mmHg/80 mmHg). In the first study,[91] adults were randomized to either 8 weeks of MBSR or progressive muscle relaxation (PMR). Both MBSR (n = 21) and PMR (n = 17) were conducted in group settings for 2.5 hours per week with 45 minutes of mandatory homework practice. Results indicated a 4.8 mmHg reduction in SBP with MBSR, which was significantly larger than the 0.7 mmHg reduction in the PMR group (P = 0.016). Results indicated a 1.9 mmHg decrease in clinic DBP with MBSR, which was significantly larger than the 1.2 mmHg increase in the PMR group (P = 0.008). No significant differences in daytime ambulatory measures of either SBP (3.1 mmHg decrease vs 1.5 mmHg decrease in MBSR and PMR groups, respectively) or DBP (4.1 mmHg decrease vs 2.2 mmHg decrease in MBSR and PMR groups, respectively) were observed between interventions. In the second study, termed HARMONY,[92] unmedicated, stage 1 hypertensive adults were randomized to MBSR (n = 46) or a wait-list (WL; n = 41), with ambulatory BP at 12 weeks serving as the primary outcome. The 24-hour ambulatory measures of SBP (MBSR, −0.4 ± 6.7 mmHg vs WL, −.04 ± 7.8 mmHg) and DBP (MBSR, 0.04 ± 4.9 mmHg vs WL, −0.4 ± 4.6 mmHg) did not significantly differ between groups. The pattern of these results provides some doubt as to whether MBSR has a measurable impact on clinic blood pressure and any impact on ambulatory blood pressure.

Yoga

The first study to explore whether a yoga intervention could affect BP was conducted in unmedicated persons with hypertension who were 35 to 65 years old.[93] The 33 subjects were equally randomized to yoga intervention, treatment with antihypertensive medications, or a no-treatment control. Yoga resulted in large reductions in clinic-based SBP (33.3 mmHg) and DBP (26.3 mmHg), comparable to the impact of antihypertensive medications on SBP (24.0 mmHg) and DBP (9.9 mmHg). Both active interventions were superior to the smaller reductions exhibited in the no-treatment group (SBP, 4.2 mmHg; DBP, 2.0 mmHg). Since then, several small studies have been conducted, which suggest that yogic practices, as a daily discipline, reduce blood pressure; however, clinical significance has not been demonstrated. A recent study of iyengar yoga versus dietary modification reported significant reductions in blood pressure in both arms at 12 weeks.[94] A recent systematic review noted that 17 trials met the inclusion criteria but only two RCTs were of acceptable methodological quality. Significant reductions in systolic or diastolic blood pressures were reported by 11 and 8 trials, respectively, compared with pharmacotherapy, breath awareness, no treatment, or usual care. The authors noted that the evidence for yoga was supportive but inconclusive and needed more rigorous studies.[100]

Qi Gong

Numerous studies have examined the effect of a qi gong intervention on BP. However, only two have been published in English. In the first study,[95] 58 unmedicated individuals (mean age, 56 years) were randomized to either a 10-week qi gong intervention or a wait list control group. Qi gong led to a significant reduction in clinic-based SBP and DBP (approximately 10 mmHg and approximately 3 mmHg, respectively) compared with increases in SBP and DBP (approximately 3 mmHg and approximately 1 mmHg, respectively) in the wait list control group. In the second study,[96] 36 unmedicated participants were equally divided randomly to a 8-week qi gong intervention or a wait list control. Qi gong was associated with significant reductions in clinic-based SBP and DBP (approximately 12 mmHg and approximately 10 mmHg, respectively) compared with increases in SBP and DBP (approximately 2 mmHg and approximately 2 mmHg, respectively) in the wait list control group. As both studies included a wait list control group, further placebo-controlled studies are now required. Nevertheless, particularly if one considers the numerous studies published in Chinese, some support exists for considering a qi gong intervention for hypertension as recommended in a recent systematic review.[101]

Tai Chi

The impact of a tai chi intervention has been evaluated in a group of 76 people with stage 1 hypertension or high-normal BP and no medications (mean age, 51.6 years).[97] The 12-week intervention had a large impact on SBP (15.6 mmHg reduction) and DBP (8.8 mmHg reduction) relative to the sedentary control condition (n = 37; 6.4 mmHg increase in SBP and 3.4 mmHg increase in DBP). Tai chi resulted in significant reductions in BP relative to a sedentary control.

Despite important methodological concerns raised by meta-analyses of earlier studies, more recent evidence examining the impact of various mind-body approaches on BP supports clinically relevant and persistent reductions.

Although several of the more recent studies were limited by small sample sizes, the overall consistency of the positive reported results indicates that, as a whole, mind-body interventions do positively affect both SBP and DBP. Many mind-body studies now address the mechanistic and biological mechanisms underlying the efficacy of these approaches in reducing BP. Understanding the antihypertensive effects of these therapies may increase the appropriate use of these therapies in clinical contexts.

THERAPIES TO CONSIDER

Earthing

Electrical grounding, also referred to as "earthing," represents an easy and comfortable therapy with potential benefit in enhancing overall health, including blood pressure. Grounding follows from direct physical contact with the earth, such as walking barefoot on grass or a beach, or indirect contact through use of a grounded blanket. Either means results in rapid transfer of electrons from the earth to the body and equalization of the electrical potential of the body with that of the planet. Proponents assert that such equalization may have antiinflammatory activity because reactive oxygen species (ROS), also known as free radicals, have one or more unpaired electrons and damage DNA and/or cellular proteins and lipids by creating chain reactions of electron stealing in order to satisfy their need for a paired electron. The lack of antioxidants (electron donors) is believed to worsen cellular damage. Thus proponents claim that electron replenishment via grounding to the negatively charged earth may minimize the impact of oxidative stress.[102]

Evidence of the association between hypertension/cardiac health and grounding comes from small studies reporting improvements in blood viscosity,[103] parasympathetic tone, diurnal rhythms, inflammation, and heart rate variability.[104,105] No definitive benefits or harms have been documented.

Ayurveda

Practitioners may use diet, lifestyle adjustments, herbs, breathing exercises, massage, and yoga to balance doshas pertinent to the experience of hypertension, such as a state of excess pitta. For many persons with hypertension, a pitta-pacifying diet of cooling foods may be beneficial. Foods that may lead to imbalanced pitta states include coffee, alcohol, hot, spicy, and oily foods, which can include many nuts and fermented or pickled foods. These may be particularly challenging in hot summer months. Yoga may also have beneficial effects on hypertension. A recent systematic review of 17 qualifying RCTs noted that 11 reported significant reductions in systolic blood pressure and 8 reported significant reductions in diastolic blood pressure, with yoga compared to pharmacotherapy, breath awareness or reading, health education, no treatment, or usual care.[106]

Traditional Chinese and East Asian Medicine

Practitioners may identify persons with the Western diagnosis of hypertension as having one or more Eastern diagnoses, such as yin deficiency of liver and kidney, ascendant liver yang, phlegm stagnation, or blood stagnation. Persons with a Western diagnosis of hypertension may be treated for an Asian pattern with acupuncture, moxibustion, or herbs in order to tonify, expel phlegm and wind, clear heat, resolve blood stasis, or clear dampness. Commonly used herbs in multiherb formulas include gou teng (*Uncaria* species), niu xi (*Cyathula* species), tian ma (*Gastrodia* species), chuanxiong (*Ligusticum sinense)*, fu ling (*Poria cocos* wolf), zexie (*Alismatis* species), and ju hua (chrysanthemum). The Chinese herb danshen (*Salvia miltiorrhiza*), commonly used for cardiovascular issues, should not be used concurrently with warfarin.[107] Use of any herbal medicines with Western cardiovascular pharmaceuticals warrants close monitoring. Acupuncture may provide positive effects with enhanced regulation of the autonomic nervous system and achievement of a balanced constitutional state. Currently, insufficient evidence exists to support the use of acupuncture,[108,109] moxibustion,[110] or ancient multiherb formulas[111,112] in the treatment of the Western diagnosis of hypertension.

PREVENTION PRESCRIPTION

Per Michael Pollan: "Eat food. Not too much. Mostly plants." These three guidelines minimize intake of unhealthy fats including hydrogenated vegetable oils, limit intake of unhealthy sugars including high fructose corn syrup, and significantly increase intake of potassium, magnesium, calcium, inorganic nitrate, and soluble fiber.

- Exercise for at least 30 minutes a day at least 4 days per week.
- Limit alcohol consumption.
- Do not smoke.
- Breathe: incorporate mind-body practices into your daily routine.

THERAPEUTIC REVIEW

DIETARY

- Follow the DASH diet eating plan with its emphasis on foods rich in potassium, magnesium, calcium, and nitrates A_1
- Reduce dietary sodium to less than 2.4 grams per day (1 tsp) A_1
- Limit alcohol to two drinks or less per day for men and one drink or less per day for women A_1
- Consider 10 to 30 grams per day of 70% cacao dark chocolate B_1
- Consider 30 grams per day of flax seed B_1
- Consider 30 grams per day of dietary fiber B_1

EXERCISE

- Aim for 30 minutes a day of aerobic exercise A_1

WEIGHT LOSS

- Aim for a weight loss of at least 10 pounds (4.5 kg) if overweight A_1

DIETARY SUPPLEMENTS

- Maintain a serum 25-OH-vitamin D greater than 40 ng/mL C_1
- Ensure 1000 mg a day of EPA and DHA by fish or krill oil A_2
- Consider CoQ10 to achieve a serum level > 2.0 µg/mL B_2
- Consider absorbable magnesium at 6 mg/kg. B_2

BOTANICAL

- Consider a trial of garlic at 4000 mcg allicin or 1.2 mg of S-allylcysteine B_2
- Consider the tonifying effect of hawthorn 750–1500 mg per day B_2

MIND-BODY

- Attempt to practice any of these approaches for approximately 20 minutes daily. Overall evidence for each intervention are as follows:
  - Mind-body
  - BB
  - Biofeedback
  - TM
  - Yoga
  - Qi gong
  - Tai chi

PHARMACEUTICAL

- Follow the JNC 7 guidelines that emphasize thiazide diuretics as first line agents or JNC 8 guidelines that also allow the use of calcium channel blockers, angiotensin converting enzyme inhibitors, or angiotensin receptor blockers A_2

OTHER THERAPIES

- Consider Ayurvedic assessment for dietary and other means of balancing one's dosha (constitutional state) C_1
- Consider traditional East Asian medicine, including acupuncture, for balancing one's constitutional state C_1

NOTE

- With use of all therapies, including pharmaceuticals, an organized system of regular follow-up and review with self-monitoring and appointment reminders appears to be effective adjuncts for blood pressure control[113]

Key Web Resources

American Heart Association Hypertension Risk Calculator. This calculator calculates BMI and provides a visual guide of risk followed by inquiries into the steps patients may wish to take to reduce blood pressure. The calculator will demonstrate the degree of improved risk with every positive step entered.

http://www.heart.org/HEARTORG/Conditions/HighBlood-Pressure/WhyBloodPressureMatters/Assess-Your-High-Blood-Pressure-Related-Risks_UCM_301829_Article.jsp#.V7Xn6_krJpg

Your Guide to Lowering High Blood Pressure with DASH. This National Heart, Lung and Blood Institute website contains DASH diet instructions.

http://www.nhlbi.nih.gov/health/resources/heart/hbp-dash-index

DASH Diet Recipes. These websites provide free access to numerous recipes that are consistent with the DASH diet.

http://www.mayoclinic.org/healthy-lifestyle/recipes/dash-diet-recipes/rcs-20077146

https://www.pinterest.com/karilmullins/dash-diet-recipes/

The Eighth Report of the Joint National Committee on Prevention, Detection, Evaluation, and Treatment of High Blood Pressure (JNC 8). Free downloadable version of the JNC 8 report.

http://jama.jamanetwork.com/article.aspx?articleid=1791497

REFERENCES

References are available online at ExpertConsult.com.

CHAPTER 25

HEART FAILURE

Russell H. Greenfield, MD

Much has changed within a relatively short time span with respect to the management of chronic heart failure (HF). Sadly, much remains largely unchanged. Pharmacological and technological advances for the treatment of HF have helped set the stage for the most recently updated treatment guidelines developed jointly by the American College of Cardiology Foundation (ACCF) and the American Heart Association (AHA) in 2013.[1] Promising research findings have provided much needed hope for a breakthrough; however, the reality remains that the morbidity, mortality, and escalating financial burden to society associated with HF continue to be unacceptably high. The statistics are sobering: at 40 years of age, the lifetime risk of developing HF for both men and women is 20%.[2] Incidence rates worsen with advancing age, increasing from approximately 20 per 1000 persons aged 65–69 years to more than 80 per 1000 persons aged ≥ 85 years.[3] It is estimated that over 5 million individuals in the U.S. currently have clinical HF,[4] with one in five Americans predicted to be aged >65 years by the year 2050.[5] Thus the prevalence of HF in the U.S. is expected to increase dramatically, particularly as more people survive heart attacks. HF is the most frequent Medicare diagnosis-related group.[6] A conservative estimate of the direct and indirect costs associated with HF in the United States in 2010 was $39.2 billion.[7] Experts believe that renewed attention and energy should be applied towards addressing HF, at least equal to that directed towards cancer.

Few, if any, medical problems represent as substantial a burden on our health care system as HF yet offer so true a picture of both the need and potential benefit of an integrative approach to care. The single best way to treat HF is to prevent its development because once established, HF follows an inexorable progression toward greater infirmity and death, typically within a few short years. Prevention, prevention, prevention must be our mantra with respect to HF management. Lifestyle and dietary measures that promote optimal heart health should be encouraged early in life, and improved access to preventive medical care across socioeconomic strata should be mandated. Careful surveillance for early signs of hypertension, diabetes, obesity, mood disorders, and coronary artery disease is essential in addition to aggressive treatment of these comorbidities with the use of safe and effective available interventions.

Integrative treatment of heart failure focuses primarily on prevention.

For people who have already developed symptomatic HF, the emphasis rests squarely on conventional medical therapy with physiological goals of lowering both preload and afterload, maintaining stable left ventricular function, limiting activation of the renin-angiotensin-aldosterone system, and inhibiting release of neurohormonal factors. Therapeutic goals should emphasize optimizing both functional capacity and quality of life. Complementary medical therapies with promise of efficacy and evidence of safety can be employed as adjuncts, to the benefit of some patients.

HF is a complex clinical syndrome that results from structural or functional impairment of ventricular filling or ejection of blood,[1] and exists in various different forms including acute and chronic, congestive, right- and left-sided, in addition to systolic and diastolic. Cardinal manifestations of HF include fatigue, shortness of breath, and fluid retention. As a proportion of patients present without signs or symptoms of fluid overload, the term "heart failure" is generally preferred over "congestive heart failure." While many different disorders may cause or contribute to the development of HF, the majority of cases involve left ventricular dysfunction. This chapter focuses exclusively on chronic systolic HF, a disorder marked by impaired left ventricular ejection fraction (<45%) in which cardiac output is insufficient to meet metabolic demands. This condition is now referred to as HF*r*EF (heart failure with reduced ejection fraction), as opposed to HF*p*EF (heart failure with preserved ejection fraction).[1]

HF*r*EF most commonly develops as a consequence of long-standing cardiovascular disease, particularly hypertension or coronary artery disease, leading to ischemic cardiomyopathy. Once considered to be solely a manifestation of the mechanical inability of the heart to pump blood adequately throughout the body, the pathophysiology of HF*r*EF is now recognized to be multifactorial. Initially positive neurohormonal compensatory mechanisms, believed to involve angiotensin II, norepinephrine, aldosterone, natriuretic peptides, vasopressin, and endothelin[8] among other compounds, ultimately become maladaptive and contribute to clinical deterioration (Table 25.1).[9–12] In the most severe form of HF*r*EF, pulmonary edema develops as backward pressure within congested capillaries becomes high enough to allow fluid leakage into lung tissue thereby compromising gas exchange and creating a life-threatening situation. Death most often results from progressive cardiac decompensation, respiratory failure, or cardiac dysrhythmia (sudden cardiac death).

Several classification systems for HF have been proposed, owing in part to myriad clinical presentations.

TABLE 25.1 Pathophysiological Features

- Increased calcium entry into myocytes
- Myocyte hypertrophy and loss with interstitial fibrosis, with resulting ventricular hypertrophy and dilation (structural remodeling)
- Reduced wall motion
- Increased myocardial energy expenditure
- Systemic vasoconstriction
- Sodium retention and circulatory congestion
- Increased circulating catecholamines
- RAAS activation
- Increased levels of tumor necrosis factor-alpha and atrial and B-type natriuretic peptides

RAAS, renin-angiotensin-aldosterone system.
Data from references [6–9].

TABLE 25.2 New York Heart Association Functional Classification System

NYHA Class	Description
I	Physical activity not limited by symptoms such as shortness of breath, fatigue, or palpitations
II	Physical exertion mildly limited, with symptoms of shortness of breath, fatigue, or palpitations developing with typical daily activities
III	Physical activity severely curtailed; symptoms of shortness of breath, fatigue, or palpitations developing with almost any kind of activity
IV	Symptoms and physical discomfort present even at rest

NYHA, New York Heart Association.
From The Criteria Committee of the New York Heart Association. *Nomenclature and Criteria for Diagnosis of Diseases of the Heart and Great Vessels.* 9th ed. Boston, Mass: Little & Brown; 1994.

The New York Heart Association (NYHA) system (Table 25.2)[13] defines the level of illness according to exercise capacity and symptoms, whereas the ACCF/AHA stages of HF (Table 25.3)[14] emphasize development and progression of the disease, and can be used to describe both individuals and populations.[1] Together, the NYHA functional classification and the ACCF/AHA stages of HF provide complementary diagnostic information regarding the presence and severity of HF, and serve to help guide therapeutic intervention.

INTEGRATIVE THERAPY

The critical message regarding management of HF*r*EF cannot be overemphasized—do everything to prevent the disease from developing in the first place. Integrative means to help prevent or, at least, aggressively treat disorders that contribute to development of HF (including hypertension, coronary artery disease, diabetes, mood disorders, and dyslipidemia) can be found under the appropriate chapter headings in this text. The aims of treatment for established HF*r*EF are straightforward:

TABLE 25.3 2005 ACCF/AHA Stages of Heart Failure

ACCF/AHA Stage	Description
A	At risk for HF but without structural heart disease or HF symptoms
B	Structural heart disease but without signs or symptoms of HF
C	Structural heart disease with prior or current symptoms of HF
D	Refractory heart failure requiring specialized intervention

ACCF, American College of Cardiology Foundation; AHA, American Heart Association; HF, heart failure.
From Hunt SA, Abraham WT, Chin MH, et al. 2009 focused update incorporated into the ACC/AHA 2005 guidelines for the diagnosis and management of heart failure in adults: a report of the American College of Cardiology Foundation/American Heart Association Task Force on Practice Guidelines. *J Am Coll Cardiol* 2009; 53:e1-e90.

prevent progressive cardiovascular deterioration; minimize symptoms; enhance quality of life; and increase survival rates. Fig. 25.1 is a flow chart of approaches to the treatment of HF*r*EF. Fig. 25.2 is a treatment algorithm for HF*r*EF according to disease stage.

Herbs and Supplements

Be sure to advise patients that the agents discussed in the following paragraphs do not act quickly, and that 4 to 6 weeks or more may pass before clinical benefit, if any, is evident. These remedies offer the greatest promise of clinical benefit in patients with less severe disease (ACCF/AHA stages A to C, NYHA classes I to III). Thus the use of these agents is not considered appropriate for acutely worsening HF.

Botanicals

Hawthorn (*Crataegus oxycantha*)

Long a favored herbal remedy in Europe, hawthorn is a slow-acting cardiac tonic whose active constituents are considered to be flavonoids, such as vitexin and rutin, and oligomeric proanthocyanidins. The German Commission E specifically recommends only the leaf and flower of the hawthorn plant be used therapeutically.

Numerous beneficial effects have been ascribed to hawthorn based on both animal and human studies,[15–17] including:

- Increased coronary artery blood flow
- Enhanced pumping efficiency of the heart (improved contractility)
- Antioxidant activity
- Phosphodiesterase inhibition
- Angiotensin-converting enzyme (ACE) inhibition
- Antidysrhythmic effects (lengthens the effective refractory period, unlike many cardiac drugs
- Mild reduction in systemic vascular resistance (lowered blood pressure)

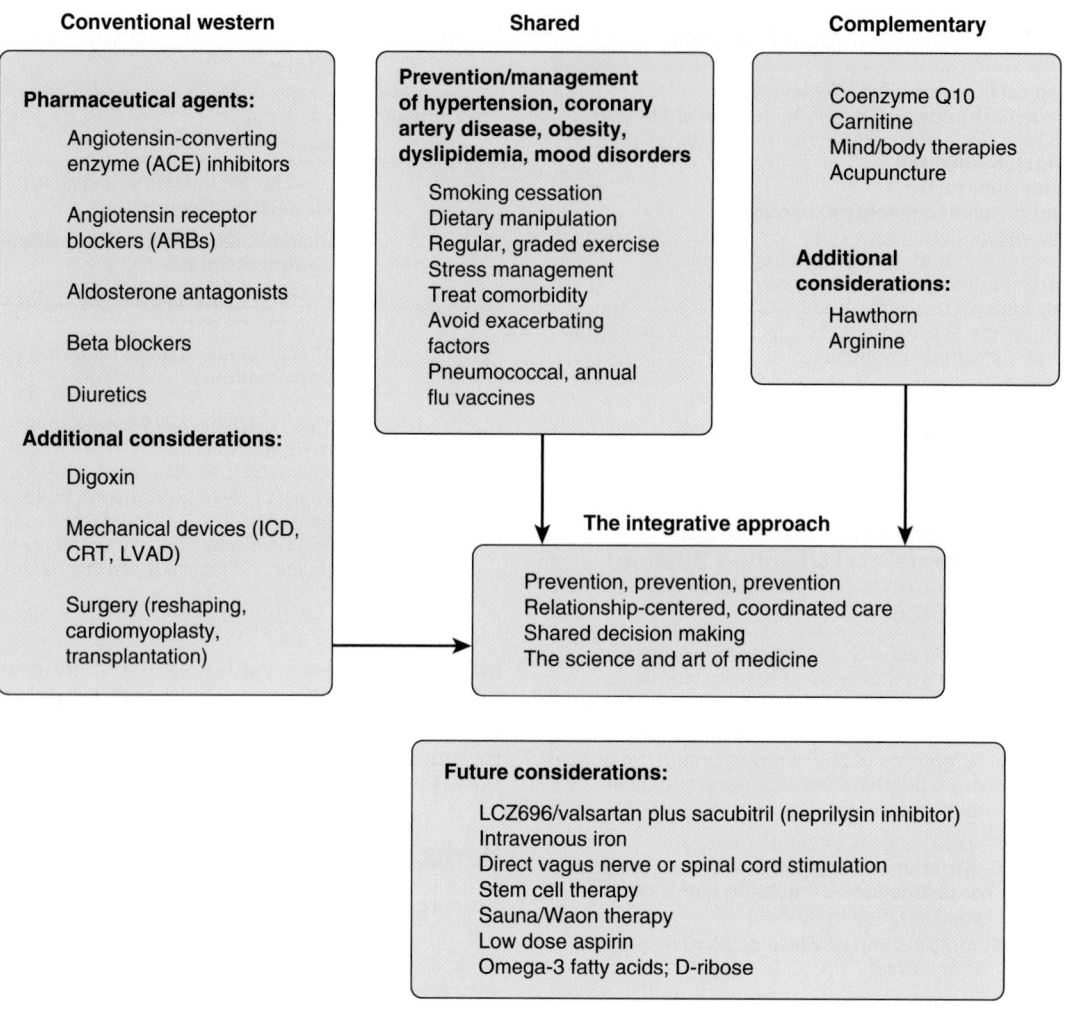

Conventional western

Pharmaceutical agents:

Angiotensin-converting
enzyme (ACE) inhibitors

Angiotensin receptor
blockers (ARBs)

Aldosterone antagonists

Beta blockers

Diuretics

Additional considerations:

Digoxin

Mechanical devices (ICD,
CRT, LVAD)

Surgery (reshaping,
cardiomyoplasty,
transplantation)

Shared

**Prevention/management
of hypertension, coronary
artery disease, obesity,
dyslipidemia, mood disorders**

Smoking cessation
Dietary manipulation
Regular, graded exercise
Stress management
Treat comorbidity
Avoid exacerbating
factors
Pneumococcal, annual
flu vaccines

Complementary

Coenzyme Q10
Carnitine
Mind/body therapies
Acupuncture

**Additional
considerations:**

Hawthorn
Arginine

The integrative approach

Prevention, prevention, prevention
Relationship-centered, coordinated care
Shared decision making
The science and art of medicine

Future considerations:

LCZ696/valsartan plus sacubitril (neprilysin inhibitor)
Intravenous iron
Direct vagus nerve or spinal cord stimulation
Stem cell therapy
Sauna/Waon therapy
Low dose aspirin
Omega-3 fatty acids; D-ribose

FIG. 25.1 ■ **Therapeutic Options for HFrEF.** *CRT,* cardiac resynchronization therapy; *ICD,* implantable cardioverter-defibrillator; *LVAD,* left ventricular assist device. Data for this figure was found from references [202–210].

Reviews of placebo-controlled trials have reported both subjective and objective improvement in patients with mild forms of HF (NYHA classes I and II).[16,18,19] In one study, hawthorn was compared to the ACE inhibitor, captopril, for the treatment of HF. At the end of the trial period, improved exercise capacity compared with baseline measurements was observed in both treatment groups, with no statistically significant difference between the two treatments. However, a relatively low dosage of captopril was administered in this study.[20] Other studies of hawthorn in patients with HF have reported improvements in clinical symptoms, pressure-rate product, left ventricular ejection fraction, and patients' subjective sense of well-being.[21–25] A 2008 systematic review suggested significant improvements in symptoms and physiological outcomes associated with the use of standardized extracts of hawthorn among patients with HF.[26] However, the majority of the studies with positive results did not include treatment with drugs now accepted as standard medical therapy, such as ACE inhibitors and beta blockers. Subsequent studies evaluating hawthorn in the setting of chronic HF in combination with current standard medical therapy

have reported less successful outcomes. In one trial, the standardized hawthorn extract, WS 1442, was added to conventional medical therapy for HF that included ACE inhibition and beta blockade over 6 months. No significant improvement following treatment with hawthorn was observed in a 6-minute walking test, the primary end point, or secondary end points including quality of life and NYHA classification. However, a modest improvement in left ventricular ejection fraction was observed.[27] The results of the SPICE study, a large 24-month, randomized clinical trial of hawthorn in patients with NYHA heart failure classes II and III and left ventricular dysfunction, indicated no statistically significant benefit of hawthorn on the composite end point of cardiac death, nonfatal myocardial infarction, and hospitalization for worsening disease. There was a trend toward reduced cardiac mortality in the treatment group, most notably for those with significantly impaired left ventricular function.[28] Most concerning, however, are the results of a retrospective safety analysis of the use of hawthorn in NYHA class II to III HF over 6 months.[29] The analysis revealed that hawthorn not only failed to impede progression of disease but appeared to increase

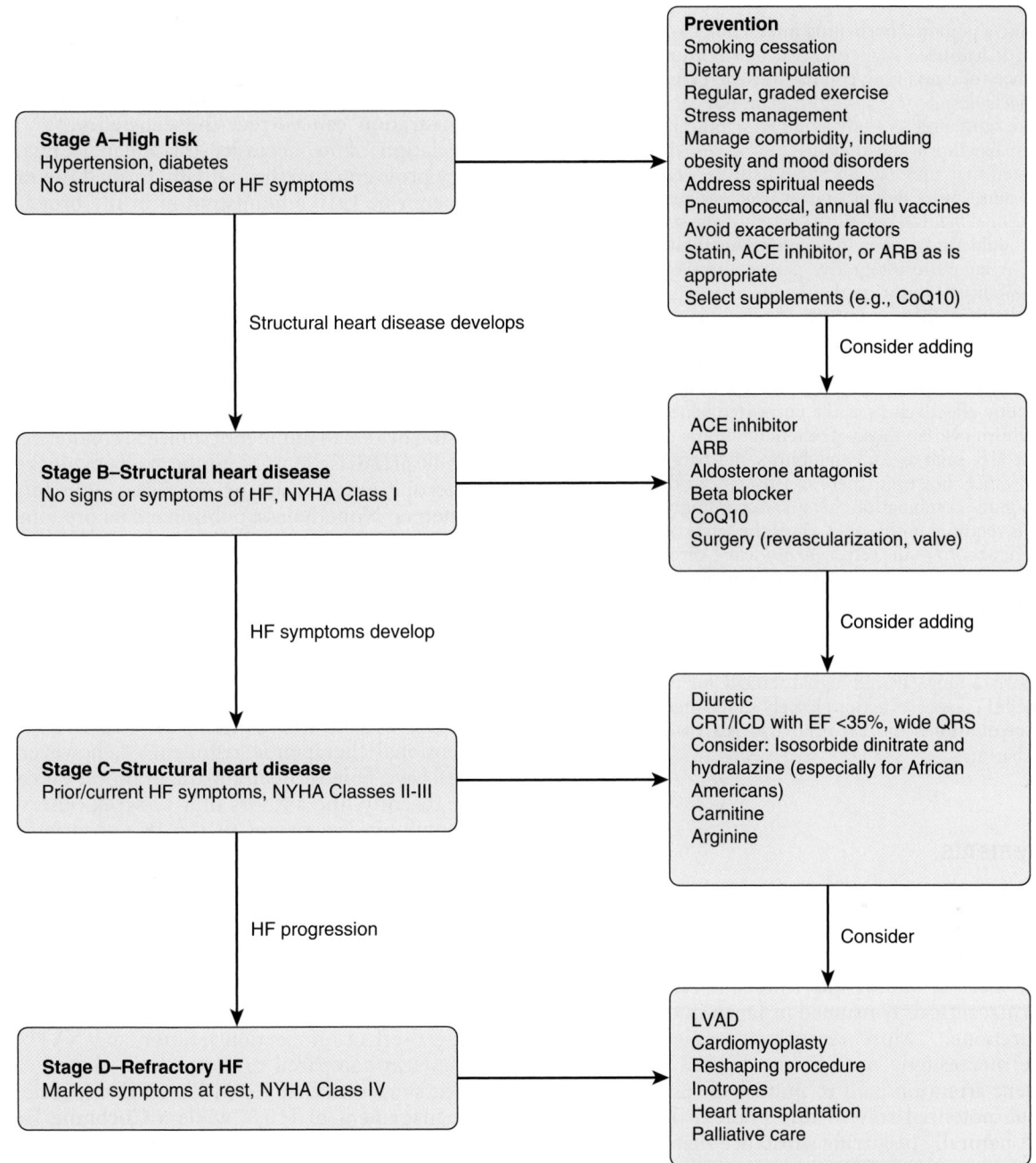

FIG. 25.2 ■ **Clinical Pathway of HF*r*EF Management.** ACE, angiotensin converting enzyme; ARB, angiotensin receptor blocker; CoQ10, coenzyme Q10; CRT, cardiac resynchronization therapy; EF, ejection fraction; HF, heart failure; ICD, implantable cardioverter-defibrillator; NYHA, New York Heart Association. (Adapted from: Yancy CW, Jessup M, Bozkurt B, et al. 2013 ACCF/AHA guideline for the management of heart failure: executive summary. *Circulation.* 2013;128:1810-1852.)

the risk of early HF progression. Hospitalization rates were higher, and death rates were slightly higher, in those receiving hawthorn compared with placebo.[29] In light of the previously good safety record of hawthorn, these findings are puzzling and quite concerning.

DOSAGE

Hawthorn is usually standardized to its content of flavonoids (2.2%) or oligomeric proanthocyanidins (18.75%). The recommended daily dose, according to previously reported studies, ranges from 160 to 1800 mg; however, most practitioners believe therapeutic efficacy is greater with higher doses (600 to 1800 mg/day). Noticeable improvement may not occur for 6 to 12 weeks.

PRECAUTIONS

With the exception of the one study described previously where hawthorn was associated with early HF progression, few side effects have been associated with the use of hawthorn. Practitioners should remember that hawthorn has a mild hypotensive effect. A previous significant concern regarding a potential herb–drug interaction has largely been allayed. It had been suggested that hawthorn may enhance the activity of digitalis glycosides, thus increasing the risk of side effects despite the hawthorn plant not containing digitalis-like substances. A study found no significant interaction between hawthorn and digitalis[30]; however, the investigators noted that these agents should still be combined with caution until more definitive data becomes available. Most conventional medical practitioners reflexively state that hawthorn should not be given to people taking digitalis for heart failure. A far more integrative perspective would consider the possibility of lowering the therapeutically effective dosage of digitalis, thereby minimizing the side effects associated with its use, by combining digitalis with an appropriate dose of hawthorn. Similarly, , combination therapy may permit the use of lower doses of hawthorn with no reduction in therapeutic effectiveness as the purported beneficial actions of hawthorn overlap those of other commonly used medications in HF, such as ACE inhibitors and beta blockers. In each instance, however, there is a paucity of data available to help guide combination therapy. Accordingly, further research is required in this area. Until the safety and effectiveness of hawthorn in the setting of guideline-directed medical management of HFrEF are clearly proven, its clinical indications should be considered rare.

Hawthorn, a long-favored herbal remedy for mild forms of chronic HF, possesses actions largely supplanted by conventional medications, and has been associated with untoward risk of harm.

Supplements

Coenzyme Q10

Coenzyme Q10 (sometimes abbreviated as CoQ10) has long been used as a nutritional supplement for cardiovascular disease, and at one time was one of the top six pharmaceuticals consumed in Japan under the name ubidecarenone.[31] More recently, coenzyme Q10 has become increasingly used in the United States, with significant attention paid to published research examining the potential role of this agent in HF management. A naturally occurring substance that behaves like a vitamin, coenzyme Q10 is present in small amounts in most diets. Coenzyme Q10 is also synthesized within the body from tyrosine, partially through a pathway shared with cholesterol synthesis. Coenzyme Q10 is found in highest concentrations within the mitochondrial membranes of organs with significant energy requirements, particularly the heart, where it acts as a carrier of both electrons and protons, and interacts with enzymes intricately involved with energy production.[32-35] Coenzyme Q10 also possesses antioxidant[36] and membrane-stabilizing[37] effects.

The concentration of coenzyme Q10 within the plasma and myocardium is lower in patients with cardiac failure compared to controls, regardless of etiology.[38-40] The more severe the degree of HFrEF according to the NYHA functional classification system, the greater the deficiency of coenzyme Q10.[41-44] Whether a reduced coenzyme Q10 concentration is causal, as may be the case in idiopathic dilated cardiomyopathy, or secondary, as is likely with ischemic cardiomyopathy, remains unclear. Regardless, demonstrated myocardial deficiency of coenzyme Q10, the knowledge that exogenous administration can correct the deficiency,[40,45] and an appreciation of its necessity for adequate myocardial energy provision together initially formed the rationale for coenzyme Q10 administration in the broad setting of HF.

The first clinical application of coenzyme Q10 in cardiovascular disease was reported in 1967.[46] Since that time, numerous studies evaluating the utility of coenzyme Q10 use in the setting of chronic HF have been published. Unfortunately, the studies are of highly variable quality due to the following limitations: uncontrolled or of short duration (weeks to a few months); inclusion of a small number of subjects; conducted before the widespread use of ACE inhibitors, beta blockers, and aldosterone antagonists; or measured only functional parameters. Nonetheless, published data predominantly indicates a supportive role for coenzyme Q10 in HF, with beneficial effects on ejection fraction,[47-49] end-diastolic volume index,[48,50] development of pulmonary edema and hospitalization rate,[51] and symptoms.[49,52,53] Research suggests that withdrawal of CoQ10 supplementation results in worsening cardiac function and symptoms,[54] and at least two studies have reported a survival benefit when coenzyme Q10 is added to a conventional therapeutic regimen[55,56]; however, some studies have failed to demonstrate clinical efficacy.[57,58] More recently, the authors of a 12-week observational trial combining coenzyme Q10 with a proprietary maritime pine bark extract in a small number of patients with NYHA class II to III HF reported improvements in ejection fraction and treadmill walking distances.[59] The Q-SYMBIO trial reported benefits of 300 mg of CoQ10 daily in the setting of HF at both 16 weeks and 2 years of follow-up.[60] A separate study of coenzyme Q10 combined with 10 mg of atorvastatin reported a mildly beneficial effect on ejection fraction and NYHA functional status compared to atorvastatin alone.[61] A 2013 analysis suggested that CoQ10 has a therapeutic role in the management of HF,[62] while a Cochrane Database review suggested no firm conclusions could yet be made due to the poor quality of existing research.[63] CoQ10 may help reduce the incidence of atrial fibrillation in patients with HF.[64] Clearly, however, large multicenter trials are required to determine the true efficacy of coenzyme Q10 in the treatment of HF.

DOSAGE

Most CoQ10 supplements are provided in the oxidized state (ubiquinone), which is reduced to ubiquinol following ingestion. While no clear advantage of one over the other has been proven, both oxidized and reduced forms of coenzyme Q10 are available in supplement form.[65] The optimum dosage of coenzyme Q10 in the setting of HF has yet to be undetermined. Studies have used doses ranging from 30 to 600 mg/day; however, most practitioners initially prescribe 100 to 200 mg daily. Softgel capsules of coenzyme Q10 may provide superior bioavailability.[66]

PRECAUTIONS

Coenzyme Q10 appears to be remarkably free of significant side effects. The most common adverse reaction is gastrointestinal upset (epigastric discomfort, loss of appetite, nausea, and diarrhea), occurring in less than 1% of all studied subjects.[67] Caution is advised for patients receiving anticoagulation therapy because there are case reports of possible procoagulant activity in patients taking warfarin, perhaps due to the structural similarity of coenzyme Q10 to menaquinone.[68-70] On the other hand, patients taking 3-hydroxy-3-methyl-glutaryl-coenzyme A (HMG-CoA) reductase inhibitors (statins) may benefit from supplementation with coenzyme Q10. As alluded to earlier, cholesterol and coenzyme Q10 partially share the mevalonate pathway, the biosynthetic pathway disrupted by statin drugs. Cholesterol production and the endogenous pathways for coenzyme Q10 production may both be compromised by HMG-CoA reductase inhibition.[71-75] Studies have indicated that supplemental CoQ10 may help reduce the incidence of statin-associated myopathy[76,77]; however, this approach remains controversial.

Carnitine

Carnitine, another vitamin-like substance, acts as a carrier of the fatty acids required for energy production from the cytoplasm to mitochondria. Carnitine is synthesized from the amino acid, lysine, but it is also available in small amounts from foods such as red meat (see brief discussion under Precautions). Organs with the highest concentrations of carnitine (those with high levels of fatty acid metabolism, including the heart and skeletal muscle) are incapable of synthesizing carnitine.[78] Myocardial carnitine is concentrated within the left ventricle.[79,80] Levels of carnitine are reportedly low in patients with HF,[81,82] and depletion of myocardial L-carnitine appears to affect cell membrane function adversely, leading to impaired myocardial contractility.[83-85]

Only the L-form of carnitine should be used therapeutically; the DL-form has yet to be proven safe. Investigators have suggested that propionyl L-carnitine (PLC; created through the esterification of L-carnitine) is most effective in the setting of heart disease due to its highly lipophilic nature.[86] PLC has been shown to improve muscle metabolism,[87] to stimulate the Kreb's cycle,[88] and to improve heart contractility[89,90] in animal models. Studies of L-carnitine in humans with ischemic heart disease or peripheral vascular disease have reported enhanced cardiac performance and increased exercise tolerance.[91-93]

Preliminary human trials using PLC in the setting of HF have provided promising results.[94] Long-term administration of PLC has been shown to improve ventricular function, reduce systemic vascular resistance, and increase exercise tolerance.[95,96] Acute administration of PLC reportedly lowered pulmonary artery and capillary wedge pressure in a study of patients with HF,[97] while a statistically significant reduction in 3-year mortality was reported in a separate study.[98] A well-conducted study reporting no significant benefit of PLC in HF did, however, reveal a trend toward beneficial effects in patients with relatively preserved heart function (ejection fraction between 30% and 40%) and demonstrate the safety of PLC.[99]

DOSAGE

The dosage of PLC used in the majority of previous study was 2 g/day (range, 1 to 3 g/day) in two to three divided doses.

PRECAUTIONS

Current literature strongly suggests that PLC is safe for patients with HF. L-Carnitine has been reported to cause an unpleasant body odor at extremely high doses. However, the majority of studies using PLC have reported no significant side effects or major toxicity,[78] although an effect on peripheral thyroid hormone action has been posited.[100] Concerns over the safety of carnitine have focused on dietary sources, including meat and eggs, and the production of TMAO (trimethylamine-N-oxide) by gut bacteria. TMAO has been linked to increased risk of acute coronary events and the progression of HF.[101,102] The contribution of carnitine supplementation toward the production of TMAO has yet to be elucidated.

L-Arginine

L-Arginine is an essential amino acid with vasodilatory effects that may enhance coronary artery blood flow and lessen cardiac workload. Use of L-arginine has been associated with improved hemodynamics and decreased endothelial dysfunction,[103-107] improved exercise tolerance,[103,108,109] improved kidney function,[110] and enhanced quality of life.[111] L-arginine may protect against the development of cardiorenal syndrome, a condition where kidney or heart dysfunction adversely affects the other organ system in the setting of HF.[112] There is promising evidence supporting a role for arginine in the management of HFrEF[113]; however, there is a lack of data to support its regular use in clinical practice.

DOSAGE

The typical dose recommended in HF is 2 g three times daily.

PRECAUTIONS

L-Arginine increases potassium levels when used in combination with other potassium-sparing drugs[114] and may increase the incidence of recurrent herpetic lesions. The results of a clinical trial cast doubt on the utility of arginine therapy after myocardial infarction, and even indicated such an intervention may increase mortality in older patients.[115]

Pharmaceuticals

Angiotensin-Converting Enzyme Inhibitors

Early institution of maximal therapy with ACE inhibitors saves lives. Numerous studies have shown that treatment with ACE inhibitors slows progression of HF and can improve quality of life and long-term prognosis.[116-118] The biggest limitation of this class of agents is that many patients are not receiving maximal beneficial dosages. Such undertreatment stymies anticipated therapeutic benefits. ACE inhibitors should strongly be considered in all patients with reduced ejection fraction to help prevent symptomatic HF, as well as in those with HFrEF unless contraindicated.

DOSAGE

Initial and maximal dosages for commonly used agents are as follows[1]:

- Captopril: 6.25 to 50 mg three times daily
- Enalapril: 2.5 to 20 mg twice daily
- Fosinopril: 5 to 40 mg daily
- Lisinopril: 2.5 to 40 mg daily
- Perindopril: 2 to 16 mg daily
- Quinapril: 5 to 20 mg twice daily
- Ramipril: 1.25 to 10 mg daily
- Trandolapril: 1 to 4 mg daily

PRECAUTIONS

Many physicians remain wary of the potential side effects of ACE inhibitors, such as hypotension, kidney problems (increased creatinine levels), and electrolyte disorders (hyperkalemia). A safe and effective approach is to start at a low dose before slowly increasing the dosage and periodically checking electrolyte levels. All patients with a verified diagnosis of HF able to tolerate ACE inhibitors should be prescribed these agents, with dosage maximized appropriately. Some patients may develop a chronic, dry cough with ACE inhibitor therapy that may limit utility. In this instance, angiotensin receptor blockade and vasodilator therapy are appropriate considerations. Efforts should first be made to ensure that cough is not secondary to the development of HF with congestion.

Angiotensin Receptor Blockers (ARBs)

Angiotensin II subtype I receptor blockers provide more complete blockade of the renin-angiotensin system than ACE inhibitors and have been shown to decrease morbidity and mortality to a degree similar, but not superior, to that of ACE inhibitors. ARBs have fewer side effects than ACE inhibitors and, in carefully selected cases, may be of benefit when combined with ACE inhibitors as part of standard therapeutic regimens.[119–123] This last point bears a warning; ACE inhibitors should only be combined with ARBs with considerable caution as studies have reported increased morbidity and mortality, and no significant all-cause mortality benefit, particularly among patients also receiving an aldosterone antagonist.[1,122,123] ARBs are a reasonable alternative for patients who are unable to tolerate ACE inhibitor therapy.[122,124]

DOSAGE

Initial and maximal dosages for commonly used agents are as follows[1]:

- Candesartan: 4 to 32 mg daily
- Losartan: 25 to 150 mg daily
- Valsartan: 20 to 160 mg twice daily

PRECAUTIONS

Aside from the cautions noted above, ARBs are typically well tolerated.

Aldosterone Antagonists

Aldosterone mediates sodium retention, cardiac remodeling, myocardial fibrosis, and baroreceptor dysfunction.[125] Studies evaluating spironolactone, a diuretic and nonselective aldosterone antagonist, have reported reductions in both the need for hospitalization and the risk of sudden death when spironolactone is added to standard conventional medical therapy.[126–129] Eplerenone is a more selective aldosterone antagonist that has also been shown to reduce morbidity and mortality in HF. Although the benefits of aldosterone antagonism in HF are well established, this form of therapy remains underused by physicians, perhaps due to concerns regarding hyperkalemia.[130] Data indicate an important role for spironolactone even in patients with NYHA class I to II HF.[131] All patients with advanced HF*r*EF (left ventricular ejection fraction <35%) should be considered for aldosterone antagonist therapy.[132,133]

DOSAGE

Initial and maximal dosages for commonly used agents are as follows[1]:

- Spironolactone: 12.5 to 50 mg daily
- Eplerenone: 25 to 50 mg daily

PRECAUTIONS

Spironolactone and eplerenone are known to promote potassium and magnesium retention. Adequate kidney function should be confirmed prior to the initiation of aldosterone antagonists, with frequent electrolyte level monitoring. Avoid concomitant use of these agents with trimethoprim-sulfamethoxazole or ciprofloxacin in elderly patients due to increased risk of hyperkalemia.[134]

Beta Blockers

Once considered contraindicated in the setting of HF, beta blockade has clearly been shown to have benefit in all but the most severe functional classes of HF when added to a regimen of ACE inhibitors or ARBs. Beta blockers enhance left ventricular systolic function and have been shown to decrease hospitalization rates and reduce the incidence of sudden cardiac death.[135–141] They not only affect the mechanical action of the heart but also provide autonomic balance and counteract specific neurohormonal processes that contribute to progressively worsening heart function through cardiac remodeling.[142–144] Beta blockade combined with ACE inhibition is considered a cornerstone of HF*r*EF management.

Three beta blocking agents have been shown to have benefit in the clinical setting of HF, although the most beneficial agent in specific instances remains unclear. Treatment should be initiated at low doses and gradually titrated upward.[145]

DOSAGE

Initial and maximal dosages for commonly used agents are as follows[1]:

- Bisoprolol: 1.25 to 10 mg daily
- Carvedilol: 3.125 to 50 mg twice daily
- Carvedilol CR: 10 to 80 mg daily
- Metoprolol succinate extended release: 12.5 to 200 mg daily

PRECAUTIONS

Side effects include hypotension and bradycardia.

Angiotensin-converting enzyme (ACE) inhibitors, angiotensin receptor blockers (ARBs), beta blockers, and aldosterone antagonists are each associated with positive impacts on HF-related mortality.

Cardiac Glycosides (Digoxin)

Digoxin has been a mainstay of the conventional Western medical armamentarium since the days of William Withering, who first explored the benefit derived from use of the leaves of the common foxglove plant (Digitalis purpurea) more than 100 years ago. Until relatively recently, digoxin was commonly employed in the treatment of supraventricular dysrhythmias (atrial fibrillation) and HF, particularly when HF was associated with hypertension, valvular disease, or coronary artery disease.

Digoxin is known to be a positive inotrope (increases the pumping efficiency of the heart); however, more recent work has demonstrated beneficial neurohormonal activity. Administration of digoxin does not appear to affect overall mortality when added to current standard medical therapy, although digoxin may improve symptoms, enhance exercise capacity, improve patient quality of life and clinical status, and reduce hospitalization rates in some instances.[146–150]

However, the use of digoxin in the setting of HFrEF is not without risk, with a 2013 study reporting a major increase in all-cause mortality (72%) in a community cohort of patients with new systolic HF who were administered digoxin in combination with beta blockers.[151]

DOSAGE

The initial and maximal dose is as follows[1]:
• Digoxin: 0.125 to 0.25 mg daily in most patients

PRECAUTIONS

Although useful, digoxin has a very narrow therapeutic window and toxicity is common. Few physicians initiate digoxin therapy early in the course of HF, with most prescribing it only in moderate to severe disease, and then only as second- or third-line therapy. Digoxin can be used both in the setting of acute cardiac decompensation and as part of chronic maintenance therapy. Digoxin should not be prescribed as monotherapy—patients with HF should almost always be taking an ACE inhibitor in combination with other medications as previously described. Lower doses of digoxin are often necessary in patients with renal insufficiency.

Isosorbide Dinitrate and Hydralazine

Few therapies underscore the notion that no two people are alike as clearly as the combination of nitrates and hydralazine. Combined use of hydralazine and isosorbide dinitrate was the first treatment shown to improve survival in HF, though it was subsequently found to be less effective than ACE inhibition in direct comparisons.[145] African Americans with HF, however, generally do not respond as favorably to ACE inhibitors or beta blockers as nonAfrican-Americans, and appear to have less nitric oxide activity than nonAfrican-Americans. The Reevaluation of the Veterans Administration Cooperative Study on Vasodilator Therapy of Heart Failure (V-HeFT trial)[152] reported a significant reduction in mortality among African Americans receiving nitrates and hydralazine. Subsequently, the African-American Heart Failure Trial (A-HeFT) evaluated the same fixed combination of isosorbide dinitrate and hydralazine in addition to standard therapy.[153] The study was stopped early due to a reduction in mortality with combination therapy of 43%. The vasodilatory effects of this therapy are mediated by increased nitric oxide levels as a result of the effects of isosorbide dinitrate as a nitric oxide donor and hydralazine as an inhibitor of the breakdown of nitric oxide. In 2005, the U.S. Food and Drug Administration approved the use of BiDil (a fixed-dose combination of isosorbide dinitrate and hydralazine) for the treatment of HF in African Americans. More recent data indicate a possible role for isosorbide dinitrate and hydralazine as an add-on therapy for patients of any race with advanced HF.[154]

DOSAGE

Initial and maximal dosages is as follows[1]:
• Hydralazine/isosorbide dinitrate (BiDil): 37.5 mg hydralazine/20 mg isosorbide dinitrate to 75 mg hydralazine/40 mg isosorbide dinitrate three times daily

PRECAUTIONS

Headaches and dizziness have been reported, as has hypotension.

Diuretics

Diuretics help lessen cardiac workload by decreasing preload yet the efficacy of these agents in prolonging survival was not demonstrated until 2006.[155,156] The most commonly used diuretics in the setting of HF are loop diuretics, such as furosemide, which are especially beneficial once fluid retention has developed.

DOSAGE

Initial and maximal dosages for commonly used agents are as follows[1]:
• Bumetanide: 0.5 to 10 mg daily
• Furosemide: 20 to 600 mg daily
• Torsemide: 10 to 200 mg daily

PRECAUTIONS

Periodic blood tests are required to evaluate electrolyte balance, particularly potassium and sodium levels. Diuretics may increase renin and aldosterone levels, thereby worsening the neurohormonal milieu. Benefits of therapy usually outweigh risks, however, because diuretic therapy may reduce morbidity and mortality in addition to improving the symptoms of HF.[155]

Biomechanical Therapy

The risk of sudden cardiac death in the setting of HF is markedly increased, likely due to an increased incidence of ventricular dysrhythmias. With an eye toward preventing sudden cardiac death, biomechanical approaches are increasingly being used in the treatment of HF.

Evidence supporting the use of cardiac resynchronization therapy (CRT, a form of biventricular pacing) to correct dyssynchronous ventricular contraction and associated incomplete ventricular filling, and implantable cardioverter defibrillators (ICDs) either separately or combined, is compelling with data strongly suggesting improved quality of life and reduced mortality, particularly among patients with stage C disease.[157-167] The use of CRT combined with an ICD in asymptomatic or mildly symptomatic patients with heart disease, reduced ejection fraction, and a wide QRS complex was associated with a 34% reduction in the risk of death or HF events as compared with the use of ICD alone.[167] CRT and ICD are recommended for patients with a left ventricular ejection fraction of less than 35%, NYHA class III to IV symptoms, and a QRS complex duration of more than 0.12 seconds.[1,6,145] The utility of this approach may be expanding in light of evidence indicating potential health benefits across the spectrum of HF presentations, even among patients with mild disease.[168] Drugs remain the mainstay of HFrEF treatment; however, mechanical device therapy is now offering significant benefits to a major subset of patients. The placement of left ventricular assist devices (LVADs), cardiomyoplasty, revascularization for ischemic heart failure, reshaping procedures utilizing titanium anchors, and heart transplantation represent some of the most drastic surgical interventions for the treatment of HF. LVADs may have utility in prolonging life in patients with advanced HFrEF; however, there is concern that LVADs may contribute to declines in cognitive function and impair health.[169]

> The most significant recent change in conventional medical treatment for chronic HF is the increased reliance on device therapy, particularly mechanical circulatory support.

Bioenergetics

Acupuncture

Investigators have posited that acupuncture may ameliorate conditions that worsen the prognosis for patients with HF, particularly among those with high sympathetic activity.[170,171] A pilot study of acupuncture offered to 17 subjects with stable NYHA class II to III HF receiving appropriate medical therapy reported no benefit with respect to ejection fraction but a marked improvement in 6-minute walk test results in the active group.[172] These results are intriguing; however, further studies are required to validate the use of acupuncture in the treatment of HF.

Mind-Body Therapy

Depression is an independent risk factor for HF and is extremely prevalent among patients with established disease.[173,174] Depression-specific activation of inflammatory cytokines occurs in people with HF and may lead to worsening morbidity and mortality rates.[175,176] Norwegian data indicate that moderate to severe depression increases the risk of HF by 40%.[177] Numerous

studies have reported that providing adequate means of stress reduction can help relieve depression and anxiety, reduce the risk of developing cardiovascular disease, and improve the health and well-being of patients with established HF.[178-184] Some of the benefits of mind-body therapies may be related to impacts on the autonomic nervous system.[185] Despite a lack of studies evaluating the treatment of depression among patients with HF, this is becoming an active area of interest.[186] A study evaluating the utility of biofeedback in treating advanced HF reported increased cardiac output and reduced systemic vascular resistance compared with controls.[187] A more recent small trial examining the effects of transcendental meditation compared with health education in African Americans with HF reported improvements in 6-minute walk scores, depression scores, and measures of quality of life after 6 months, in addition to a reduced hospitalization rate.[188]

Health benefits of mind-body therapy were reported by the SEARCH (Study of the Effectiveness of Additional Reductions in Cholesterol and Homocysteine) trial, which examined the effect of training in mindfulness meditation and coping skills in association with support group discussion in more than 200 adults with HFrEF.[189] Although medical management was not maximized in a small percentage of subjects, measures of anxiety and depression were significantly lower in the active group at the end of the study period. The study found no impact on hospitalization or death rates, but symptom improvement persisted to a 12-month follow-up. A small study of older patients with HF receiving maximal medical therapy reported improvements in neurotransmitter levels and quality of life measures after listening to 30-minute meditation tapes twice daily at home for 12 weeks.[185]

Additional studies supporting the benefits of mind-body approaches for patients with HF include those focusing on freeze-frame stress management,[190] behavior modification,[191] relaxation response training,[192,193] and tai chi.[194,195]

Lifestyle

Community education regarding the adverse effects of smoking, excessive alcohol intake, and obesity must continue and expand. Assistance with tobacco and alcohol cessation, as well as weight management planning, should be made readily available across socioeconomic classes. It is worth noting that recent data indicate moderate alcohol intake (defined as up to one glass of wine, one 12-ounce beer, or a single shot of liquor each night) is associated with reduced risk of HF in both women and men. Higher intakes are associated with increased all-cause mortality, although not specifically an increased risk of HF.[196]

A diagnosis of HF is not a contraindication to participating in exercise. Studies have shown that appropriate, graded exercise programs can improve function and quality of life among patients with HF.[197-200] Lack of improvement after fitness training is associated with a poor prognosis.[201] Results of the HF-Action trial[202] were disappointing, reporting at best a modest impact on hospitalization and mortality rate with regular exercise; however, the results reinforced the safety of regular exercise and cardiac rehabilitation for patients with HF. The combination of physical exertion and a healthy diet can help patients maintain optimal body weight and thereby lessen strain on the heart. Sufficient rest is also important, with a target of at least 7 hours of sleep each night considered prudent. The diagnosis and treatment of obstructive sleep apnea can help reduce morbidity and mortality in the setting of HF.[203]

Regular participation in spiritual or religious practices may protect against heart disease.[204–207] Many patients struggle with their spirituality once a diagnosis of HF is made, a struggle that adds to an already stressful situation and perhaps leads to increased morbidity.[208,209] The burden of symptoms, mood disorders, and spiritual challenges associated with HF has been equated to those experienced by people with cancer.[210] Attention to spiritual needs can help patients adjust to their new circumstances, address specific regrets with regard to prior lifestyle choices, and search for present meaning and future hope.[211,212] Religious practice is one of many aspects of spiritual care; in one study it was gratitude, rather than religiosity per se, that was found to account for improved mood, better sleep, reduced fatigue, and lower levels of inflammatory markers related to cardiac health in people with asymptomatic (stage B) HF.[213] Patients who come to accept their diagnosis of HF appear to enjoy better quality of life compared with those who have not.[214]

Nutrition

Adhering to an antiinflammatory diet (see Chapter 88) may help prevent the development of HF and slow progression of established disease. While avoidance of red meat is not necessary, processed meats may be harmful. A recent study demonstrated an increased risk of incident HF and HF-related mortality among patients with a high intake of processed meats, such as cold cuts and sausage.[215] Patients with stage C HF typically require additional measures to maintain health. Fluid and sodium (salt) restriction has long been believed to positively affect cardiac function and symptoms in patients with HF; however, sodium restriction is currently the subject of intense debate. In fact, the most recent HF guidelines consider sodium restriction reasonable but not mandatory for patients with symptomatic HF to help reduce congestive symptoms.[1]

Supplementation with B vitamins, especially thiamine, should be considered,[216–218] as should micronutrient supplementation, including magnesium.[219–222] The safety of high-dose vitamin E in patients with established cardiovascular disease remains unknown.[223]

PREVENTION PRESCRIPTION

- Do not smoke. If you do smoke, get help to quit.
- Follow an antiinflammatory or Mediterranean-style diet.
- Participate in regular physical fitness activities.
- Manage stress in healthy ways.
- Aim for ~7 hours of sleep each night.
- Maintain a healthy weight for height.
- Work with your doctor to manage medical conditions that may lead to heart failure, especially high blood pressure, coronary artery disease, high cholesterol levels, mood disorders, and diabetes.
- Attend to your spiritual side.
- Have the pneumococcal vaccination and annual flu vaccination.
- Avoid overuse of nonsteroidal antiinflammatory medications (NSAIDs).

THERAPEUTIC REVIEW

All patients with heart failure should be started on a combination of an angiotensin-converting enzyme (ACE) inhibitor and beta blocker where appropriate, with consideration given to aldosterone antagonist therapy and ARBs. *Be careful to avoid complications such as hyperkalemia.* Aggressive treatment of comorbidities should be considered.

REMOVAL OF POTENTIAL EXACERBATING FACTORS

- Try to discontinue nonsteroidal antiinflammatory drugs and first-generation (nondihydropyridine) calcium channel blockers.

STRESS MANAGEMENT AND MIND-BODY THERAPY

- Promote proper attention to mood and stress management, and offer instruction in tools such as meditation, relaxation response, and tai chi.

SLEEP

- Consider the possible presence of obstructive sleep apnea and manage appropriately.

GRADED EXERCISE

- Enroll patients in a certified cardiac rehabilitation program.

NUTRITION

- Encourage an antiinflammatory diet or Mediterranean-style diet.
- Urge fluid and salt restriction.

SPIRITUALITY

- Inquire about and address needs in an open fashion, and use pastoral care services as appropriate.

BIOENERGETICS

- Acupuncture

SUPPLEMENTS

- Coenzyme Q10: 100 to 200 mg daily

- Propionyl-L-carnitine: 1 to 3 g daily

- Arginine: 2 g three times daily

BOTANICALS

- Hawthorn: 600 to 1800 mg daily (exercise caution of using with digoxin)

PHARMACEUTICALS

- ACE inhibitors

- ARBs

- Beta blockers

- Aldosterone antagonists

- Isosorbide dinitrate in combination with hydralazine

- Diuretics

- Digitalis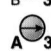

SURGERY

- Cardiac resynchronization therapy or implantable cardioverter defibrillator

- Left ventricular assist device

- Cardiomyoplasty

- Reshaping procedures

- Heart transplantation

Key Web Resources

American Heart Association. HF information primarily for patients	http://www.heart.org/HEARTORG/Conditions/HeartFailure/Heart-Failure_UCM_002019_SubHomePage.jsp
American Heart Association. Succinct review of noteworthy changes found in 2013 HF guidelines	http://newsroom.heart.org/news/acc-aha-update-guideline-for-management-of-heart-failure
Consumerlab.com. Natural product reviews (subscription required)	http://www.consumerlab.com
Natural Medicines Comprehensive Database. Evidence-based assessment of vitamins, supplements, and herbs (subscription required)	http://naturaldatabase.therapeuticresearch.com/home.aspx?cs=&s=ND

REFERENCES

References are available online at ExpertConsult.com.

CHAPTER 26

CORONARY ARTERY DISEASE

Stephen Devries, MD, FACC, FAHA

INTEGRATIVE APPROACHES TO CARDIOVASCULAR DISEASE

Despite the many advances in treatment and prevention, cardiovascular disease remains the leading cause of premature death and disability in the United States.[1] Nevertheless, 70% of cardiovascular disease is preventable through lifestyle changes alone.[2] Clearly, we have work to do.

An integrative approach acknowledges the great value and potentially life-saving benefits of modern pharmacology and procedures while also recognizing the limitations of these approaches when used in isolation. An integrative approach is ideally suited to the prevention and treatment of coronary disease because it addresses many of the root causes, especially those influenced by lifestyle. The goal of this chapter is to provide a perspective on the utility of a broader spectrum of therapies beyond those that constitute conventional cardiovascular care.

PATHOPHYSIOLOGY

What triggers a cardiovascular catastrophe? For many years, it was believed that a cardiovascular event occurred after many years of progressive narrowing of the coronary artery. According to this view, myocardial infarction develops as a result of progressive accumulation of cholesterol deposits on the lining of the coronary arteries, leading to complete cessation of blood flow. This theory held that over time, cholesterol deposits accumulate and ultimately stop blood flow, leading to myocardial infarction. In more recent years, this paradigm has been largely upended and replaced by a more complex, and less intuitive, picture.

Angiographic studies have revealed, quite surprisingly, that acute coronary events often arise from "mild" coronary lesions that are far less than 50% obstructive.[3] The explanation for this paradoxical finding is that vulnerable plaques, those most likely to rupture and evolve into a complete thrombotic occlusion, are those with large lipid cores and thin fibrous caps.[4] Surprisingly, the majority of plaques with the largest lipid cores are not severely stenotic (lipid-laden deposits may enlarge the artery and do not always reduce blood flow). Conversely, some of the most severely stenotic plaques are not necessarily the ones with the largest lipid cores and therefore may not be the most "vulnerable."

A useful way of thinking about this concept and conveying it to patients is that a mild coronary lesion can be considered a "fault line" that appears quite passive and

harmless in a quiescent phase. However, like any fault line, these seemingly harmless plaques may erupt at any moment, causing a potentially lethal cardiac event.

This scenario has implications for both the detection and treatment of coronary disease. With regards to detection, a mildly stenotic coronary lesion is not flow limiting and therefore would not be expected to result in chest pain or provoke abnormal findings on cardiac stress testing. This is the explanation for the anecdote familiar to most clinicians and patients about the individual who sailed through a stress test with "normal" results only to suffer a cardiac catastrophe a short time later.

The fact that a coronary event can rapidly develop from "mild" angiographic lesions emphasizes the need to prevent coronary lesions from developing rather than focus on reducing the severity of stenoses with interventional procedures.

The triggers of coronary artery disease are both genetic and environmental. Genetic factors include inherited metabolic disorders, including dyslipidemia and diabetes. Environmental and lifestyle factors include nutritional imbalance; sedentary lifestyle; stress and depression; smoking; and air pollution. These areas will be explored in detail later in this chapter.

> A mild coronary lesion can be considered a "fault line," which may appear quite passive and harmless in a quiescent phase. However, like any fault line, these seemingly harmless plaques may erupt at any moment causing a potentially lethal cardiac event.

INTEGRATIVE THERAPY

Nutrition

Nutrition is perhaps the most powerful therapy available for the prevention and treatment of coronary disease.

Mediterranean Diet

The power of nutritional therapy is highlighted by the striking results of the Lyon Diet Heart study.[5] In this study of individuals who survived myocardial infarction, patients were divided into two groups distinguished only by dietary intervention. The control group was advised to consume a "prudent" diet consisting of reduced cholesterol and total fat. The intervention group was advised to eat a Mediterranean-style diet. Patients in this group were counseled to eat more vegetables and fruit, to eat more nuts and fish, to use olive oil and the canola-based margarine as their predominant cooking oils, and to reduce intake of red meat and refined carbohydrates.

The study was intended to last 5 years but was stopped short at 27 months due to a strikingly helpful effect in the Mediterranean diet group.

At that point, a 73% reduction in cardiovascular events, including myocardial infarction and cardiac death, was observed in the Mediterranean-style diet group. A longer-term follow-up study was published 5 years later, demonstrating a durable benefit of the Mediterranean-style diet with a 72% reduction in cardiovascular events after 5 years.[6]

A Mediterranean-style diet has also proven beneficial for primary prevention of cardiovascular disease. A study stratified 7447 individuals at increased risk of, but without manifest, heart disease to one of two dietary arms (either added nuts or added olive oil) with comparisons to a control group (planned to be a low fat diet but, ultimately, resembled the baseline diet). No significant difference in fruit and vegetable intake was observed between the Mediterranean diet groups and controls. The study was terminated prematurely due to the finding of a clear benefit in the two Mediterranean diet groups, with a 30% reduction in cardiovascular events observed thought to be predominantly attributable to fewer strokes.[7]

The substantial benefits of the Mediterranean diet are not surprising given the proven benefits of its component parts. High consumption of vegetables and fruit are the cornerstones of the Mediterranean-style diet. Daily consumption of vegetables in the Lyon study averaged 427 g (approximately five servings).[8] Increased intake of vegetables, particularly dark green leafy vegetables, has been shown to be associated with substantially reduced risk of coronary heart disease. Each daily serving of dark green leafy vegetables, for example, has been linked to a 23% reduction in coronary heart risk.[9] Fruit intake in the Lyon study averaged 271 grains (approximately two servings; see Chapter 88).

> The results of the Lyon Mediterranean diet study underlie my personal recommendation of five servings of vegetables per day and two servings of fruit.

Whole Grains

Another key constituent of the Mediterranean diet is the avoidance of refined grains and an emphasis on the consumption of whole grains. Refined grains, typically void of fiber, are deleterious in a number of ways. As compared to whole-grain, refined grains result in greater release of glucose into the circulation, triggering higher insulin levels and a greater tendency toward atherosclerosis. Higher sugar intake is associated with reduced levels of HDL and increased levels of the more atherogenic small dense LDL[10] (see Chapter 87).

The method of grain preparation has important health implications. Boiled whole grains (i.e., oat, quinoa, barley) are typically a healthier choice than bread made from the flour of whole grains. Examples of whole grains include barley, buckwheat, quinoa, polenta, and brown rice. A meta-analysis demonstrated a 21% lower risk of cardiovascular events with 2.5 servings per day of whole grains consumed compared to the absence of whole-grain foods in the diet.[11] Consuming pulverizing grains, even whole grains, results in higher blood glucose levels than intact grains.[12] Therefore, boiled whole grains are typically a healthier choice than bread made from the flour of whole grains.

Fish

Fish is another component of a healthy diet, with benefits for both primary and secondary prevention of heart disease. In the Chicago Western Electric Study, more than 35 grams of fish intake per week (approximately three servings) was associated with a 38% reduced risk of cardiac death.[13] The Diet and Reinfarction Trial (DART) similarly demonstrated a 29% reduction in all-cause mortality among males instructed to eat fish compared to those who did not after only 2 years.[14] Accordingly, substituting chicken or fish for red meat has been shown to reduce the risk of coronary heart disease.[15]

Nuts

Nuts have potent benefits for the reduction of coronary heart disease. Increased nut consumption has been linked to longevity, with a 21% improved survival over 5 years in those with the highest versus lowest levels of nut consumption.[16] Four servings of nuts per week (30 g/serving, or ~1 large handful/serving) have been shown to reduce the risk of coronary heart disease by 37%.[17] Increasing consumption of nuts to two handfuls per day reduces LDL cholesterol by as much as 10% in those with baseline values of greater than 160 mg/dL.[18]

> The success of nutritional interventions is greatly enhanced when patients perceive nutrition as a priority of their health care practitioner. At every clinical encounter with a patient, I recommend inquiring about the number of servings of vegetables and fruit consumed every day and the type of grains, quantity of fish, and number of servings of nuts consumed on a weekly basis. Emphasizing the importance of diet during each clinic visit allows obstacles to be identified and progress to be celebrated.

Exercise

Patients often inquire about "natural" methods for prevention and treatment of heart disease. In concert with dietary changes, there is no therapy more potent than the addition of regular exercise. Surprisingly, exercise intensity appears to be less important than frequency and consistency. In the Health Professionals Follow-Up Study, walking for 30 minutes per day was associated with an 18% reduction in the occurrence of cardiovascular disease.[19] In the Women's Health Initiative observational study, exercise of as little as 4.2 metabolic equivalent (MET) hours per week resulted in a 27% reduction in heart disease risk. The benefits of exercise were even greater for a higher levels of exercise (32.8 MET hours per week).

Although aerobic exercise is generally emphasized for cardiovascular health, resistance training also adds considerable benefit. Resistance training for at least 30 minutes per week resulted in a 23% lower risk of heart disease compared no resistance training in males.[19]

Therefore, a reasonable prescription for exercise could start at 30 minutes of brisk walking every day in addition to two to three sessions per week of light resistance training interspersed with stretching. More vigorous workouts of longer duration are likely to be of even greater benefit. Of course, individual prescriptions need to take into account the patient's general health history and cardiovascular status. Stress testing prior to beginning a program may be appropriate for those with a history of heart disease or those with multiple cardiovascular risk factors, particularly those who have been previously sedentary.

Pharmaceuticals

In addition to nutrition and exercise as "foundations" of heart health, patients with symptomatic coronary artery disease should receive treatment informed by American Heart Association/American College of Cardiology (AHA/ACC) guidelines. Proven medical therapy for symptomatic coronary disease includes aspirin, nitrates, beta-blockers, and calcium channel blockers. Angiotensin-converting enzyme inhibitors are also potent antihypertensives and may provide additional cardiovascular prevention above and beyond their antihypertensive properties. Statin therapy should be considered an essential component of treatment for patients with established vascular disease and those at high risk of vascular disease due to its lipid-lowering effects and a host of "pleiotropic" or nonlipid beneficial metabolic effects. A detailed discussion of these therapies is beyond the scope of this chapter but can be found in the AHA/ACC guideline statements (http://my.americanheart.org/professional/guidelines.jsp).

Tables 26.1 and 26.2 provide information on the interactions of pharmaceuticals and supplements.

Antiplatelet and Anticoagulant Therapies

Aspirin is the most widely prescribed over-the-counter therapy in cardiology. Aspirin is a mainstay of therapy for patients with established cardiovascular disease, and is frequently recommended for individuals at high risk of cardiovascular disease. However, dosing remains a challenge because higher doses have greater antiplatelet activity and are associated with an increased risk of gastrointestinal bleeding. A useful tool to balance the

benefits and risk of aspirin therapy is provided by the Agency for Healthcare Research and Quality (see Key Web Resources).[20]

Patients receiving warfarin may consult integrative practitioners for recommendations regarding alternative options, including those in atrial fibrillation wishing to discontinue warfarin. Patients frequently inquire about the possibility of replacing warfarin with over-the-counter products, including nattokinase, fish oil, and vitamin E, among others. Unfortunately, no studies reported to date have supported the use of botanicals or herbs as replacements for warfarin in patients considered to be at high thrombotic risk.[21]

Angioplasty/Stenting

Angioplasty and stenting are commonly regarded as the most potent interventions available in cardiology. It would be logical to assume that mechanical opening of a severely stenotic coronary artery would reduce the likelihood of myocardial infarction. Surprisingly, however, angioplasties and stents have not been shown to reduce the risk of myocardial infarction or prolong life in the vast majority of patients who receive these therapies (those who are asymptomatic or with stable coronary disease). Survival benefit from angioplasties and stents appears to be confined to patients in the midst of acute myocardial infarction or unstable angina. In the more chronic setting, the benefit of angioplasty and stenting is restricted to the amelioration of chest pain.

This counterintuitive finding was demonstrated by the COURAGE trial, where treatment of stable coronary patients with a catheter-based intervention did not prevent myocardial infarction or improve survival compared to initial treatment with medical therapy alone.[22] The absence of a survival benefit for catheter-based interventions in stable coronary patients was confirmed in a subsequent meta-analysis of eight trials including a total of 7229 patients.[23]

The explanation for the lack of expected outcomes following angioplasty and stenting in patients with stable disease has yet to be elucidated; however, this lack of efficacy is likely due to mechanical interventions generally being directed at one or two of possibly hundreds of "vulnerable" plaques that exist in an individual's coronary tree.

Research shows that when conversations regarding the risks and benefits of catheter-based interventions are more fully explained by cardiologists, patients are less likely to choose an invasive approach.[24]

Lipid Management

Lifestyle changes are the foundation of a solid prevention program, and it should be recognized that the role of lipid management is subordinate to optimizing lifestyle measures.

Nevertheless, lipid management is an extremely important consideration for both primary and secondary prevention. Of the lipid parameters, the priorities for

TABLE 26.1	Important Herbal and Supplement Interactions with Antiplatelet Drugs and Warfarin	
Agents	**Herb or Supplement**	**Effects of Interaction**
Antiplatelet drugs (aspirin, ticlopidine, NSAIDs, clopidogrel)	Caffeine	Antiplatelet effect
	Cordyceps fungus	Platelet antagonism
	Curcumin	Antiplatelet effects
	Dong quai	Platelet antagonism
	Feverfew	Inhibition of platelet aggregation
	Fish oil	Platelet antagonism
	Garlic	Inhibition of platelet aggregation
	Ginger	Prolongation of bleeding time
	Ginkgo	Antiplatelet activity, hemorrhage
	Green tea	Antiplatelet effects
	Guggul	Antiplatelet activity
	Horse chestnut	Antiplatelet activity
	Policosanol	Antiplatelet activity
	Resveratrol	Inhibition of platelet aggregation
	Vitamin E	Antiplatelet activity
Warfarin	Coenzyme Q10	Decrease in INR
	Dong quai	Elevation of PT and INR
	Fenugreek	Possible increase in INR
	Fish oil	Elevation of INR
	Garlic	Elevation of INR
	Ginkgo	CNS hemorrhage
	Ginseng	Decrease in INR
	Green tea	Decrease in INR
	L-Carnitine	Potential increase in INR
	St. John's wort	Decrease in INR

CNS, central nervous system; INR, international normalized ratio; NSAIDs, nonsteroidal antiinflammatory drugs; PT, prothrombin time.
From Burleson K. Coronary artery disease. In: Rakel D, ed. *Integrative Medicine*, 2nd ed. Philadelphia: Saunders; 2007:302.

TABLE 26.2	Important Herbal and Supplement Interactions with Other Cardiovascular Drugs	
Cardiovascular Drug	**Herb or Supplement**	**Effects**
Digitalis	Hawthorn	Potentially increased serum levels
	Herbal laxatives	Decreased absorption
	Psyllium	Hypokalemia
	St. John's wort	Decreased serum levels
Amiodarone	—	See precautions for digoxin, warfarin, statins, or herbs with hepatic effects
Propranolol	Guggul	Decreased bioavailability
Clonidine	Yohimbine	Both alpha$_2$-antagonists
Calcium channel blockers	Guggul	Decreased bioavailability
Cyclosporine	St. John's wort	Decreased serum levels
Statins	Red rice yeast	Magnified side effects

From Burleson K. Coronary artery disease. In: Rakel D, ed. *Integrative Medicine*, 2nd ed. Philadelphia: Saunders; 2007:303.

prevention in order of importance are LDL, HDL, and triglycerides. Total cholesterol is not considered the most useful endpoint as it is a summated term that may either underestimate or overestimate risk. Note that a third of heart attacks occur in individuals with a total cholesterol under 200 mg/dL[25] (see Chapter 27).

Low Density Lipoprotein

Among all lipid parameters, control of LDL is of primary importance because it is most closely associated with cardiovascular risk. Nevertheless, the optimal method of measuring LDL for determining cardiovascular risk remains controversial. Low-density lipoprotein is an apolipoprotein that carries the bulk of circulating cholesterol. Traditional measurement of LDL-C, the basis for most treatment decisions, assesses only the cholesterol content of this complex molecule.

However, mounting evidence suggests that the cholesterol content of LDL may not be the best indicator of cardiovascular risk. Instead, quantification of the number of LDL particles appears to more closely correlate with cardiovascular risk than conventional measurement of LDL cholesterol.

In order to better understand how cholesterol concentration relates to LDL particle number, consider the following example: imagine filling two bathtubs with cholesterol to the same level designated by the LDL-C value. For the purpose of this example, we will designate an LDL-C of 125 mg/dL as corresponding to filling the bathtub halfway with cholesterol balls. In one tub, 100 large balls are used to fill the tub halfway. In the second tub, 2000 small marbles are used to fill the tub to the exact same halfway mark. At first glance, both tubs, filled halfway to the same level of 125 mg/dL, might appear to represent equal cardiovascular risk. However, the person with 2000 smaller particles has a much higher risk of cardiovascular disease than the other individual with an identical LDL-cholesterol but with many fewer particles. In other words, risk is much more closely associated with the number of LDL particles than the concentration of cholesterol.[26]

Several tests are available for the quantification of atherogenic particles (the vast majority of which are LDL particles). The most readily available method for estimating the number of atherogenic particles is non-HDL cholesterol, a simple term that is calculated by subtracting HDL-C from total cholesterol. Calculation of non-HDL cholesterol is particularly helpful when triglycerides exceed 200 mg/dL, an environment where the formation of small, dense LDL is more likely. A more accurate reflection of the number of atherogenic particles, however, is ApoB. ApoB takes advantage of the fact that each atherogenic particle contains exactly one molecule of ApoB.[27] Therefore ApoB has been shown be closely associated with cardiovascular risk than LDL-C. Another option for quantification of atherogenic particles is LDL particle number, a proprietary test that has been shown in the Framingham Offspring Study to more closely predict cardiovascular risk than LDL-C.[26] Treatment goals for ApoB and LDL particle numbers are not currently well established but are commonly set as percentile rankings for the given population (i.e., <5th percentile for a very high-risk patient).[28]

The most potent treatment available for reducing LDL cholesterol, ApoB, and LDL particle number are prescription HMG-CoA reductase inhibitors, or statins. These medications are capable of lowering LDL cholesterol by more than 50% and have been proven to reduce the likelihood of a cardiovascular event by approximately a third in both primary and secondary prevention studies. Studies of statins have reported an overall but inconsistent mortality benefit.[29]

Statin-Related Myalgias

Despite the proven benefits of statins in high-risk individuals, statin therapy is not without risk. Myalgias are a particularly frequent adverse reaction that may be more common than described in the package inserts of these medications. An observational study of statins in clinical practice revealed that muscle-related adverse reactions occur in as many as 11% of patients receiving statins.[30] The potential for adverse muscle-related symptoms increases with increased doses.

A survey of patients who reported muscle-related symptoms to their physician while taking statins revealed a sobering finding: in only 29% of cases did physicians consider the possibility of a link between the patient complaining of muscle pain and the use of statins.[31] In 47% of cases, the clinician dismissed the possibility of such a link. Patients feeling that their symptoms are not being acknowledged by their physician may explain why more than 50% of patients stop taking statins after only 1 year.[32]

> Alternatives to the use of prescription statins can play an important role when:
> • Patients are unable to tolerate prescription statins due to adverse reactions
> • Patients are philosophically opposed to the use of prescription statins

Options for the treatment of patients with intolerance to prescription statins include (1) reducing the dose of the prescription statin; (2) changing to a different prescription statin; or (3) using nonprescription lipid therapy.

Surprisingly, cutting the dose of a statin in half generally reduces the efficacy of the statin to lower LDL-C by only 7%.[33] Nevertheless, adverse reactions, particularly myalgias, are often improved or eliminated by lowering statin dose.[30] Therefore, for mild myalgias related to statin use, dosage modification may eliminate adverse reactions without sacrificing appreciable lipid control.

Prolongation of the dosing frequency of prescription statins may also have benefit. Rosuvastatin, which has the longest half-life of any available statin, has been shown to retain potent effectiveness in lowering LDL-C levels when dosed as infrequently as one or two dosages per week.[34,35] In one study, a mean rosuvastatin dose of 10 mg given once a week resulted in a mean reduction in LDL-C of 23%.[35]

Another option for patients unable to tolerate prescription statins is to switch to a different statin. Reactions can be idiosyncratic, and one brand may be well tolerated when others are not. Rosuvastatin and pravastatin may be better tolerated in some individuals, possibly due to their hydrophilic nature. Fluvastatin may also be considered as it has a unique metabolic pathway among statins (mostly by 2C9), which may explain the findings of a large survey reporting fluvastatin to have the lowest risk of myalgias of all statins.[30]

> Water soluble statins, such as rosuvastatin and pravastatin, may cause a lower frequency of statin-related myalgia in some patient population. Fluvastatin may also cause fewer muscle symptoms due to its unique metabolism.

High Density Lipoprotein

HDL is protective against atherosclerotic disease due to its role in removing LDL from plaque (reverse cholesterol transport) in addition to its antioxidant function. The average serum HDL-C levels in men and women are 40–45 mg/dL and 50–55 mg/dL, respectively. Low HDL is associated with significantly increased cardiovascular risk, even in individuals with low LDL.[36] However, studies evaluating the efficacy of pharmacological therapies in raising HDL, including niacin and cholesteryl ester transfer protein (CETP) inhibitors, have been disappointing.[37]

Lifestyle measures are the primary strategies to raise HDL and include weight loss, exercise, and smoking cessation.[38] Reducing intake of added sugar and food with high glycemic load also has utility in raising HDL.[10]

Alcohol is effective at raising HDL levels, and this effect may explain the lower risk of cardiovascular events associated with moderate alcohol intake (one serving/day).[39] All forms of alcohol, including white and red wine, beer, and hard liquor, have been shown to raise HDL. The cardiovascular benefits of alcohol need to be balanced against the potential for accidents and abuse, as well as the increased risk of breast cancer associated with alcohol intake in women.

The most potent pharmacological agent available for boosting HDL-C is niacin. The HDL-raising effect of niacin is dose-related, with an increase of 20%–30% observed at the highest doses of around 2000 mg/day.[40,41] The ability of niacin to further reduce vascular risk in patients already receiving a statin, however, has yet to be demonstrated. Despite an increase in HDL levels when niacin was added to background statin therapy, no improvement in cardiovascular outcomes was observed in two large studies.[42,43]

TABLE 26.3	Nonprescription Therapies for Reducing LDL-C
Product	**LDL-C Reduction**
Psyllium (10 g/day)	7%[48]
Sterol/stanol (2.0 g/day)	12%[53]
Niacin (up to 2 g/day)	15%–20%
Red yeast rice (2400 mg/day)	20%–30%

SUPPLEMENTS

When none of the dosing options for prescription statins are tolerated (or the patient refuses to consider a prescription statin), nonprescription therapies may be particularly useful. In order of increasing efficacy, the following nonprescription therapies are useful for control of LDL cholesterol: fiber, stanols/sterols, niacin, and red yeast rice (Table 26.3).

In contrast, herbal or botanical preparations often used for cholesterol management that have been shown to have modest or no benefit include policosanol,[44] garlic,[45] and guggulipids.[46]

Fiber

The water-soluble fraction of fiber, soluble fiber, reduces the absorption of cholesterol in the intestinal tract. Therefore additional fiber, either in food or in supplements, can aid in cholesterol management. Each gram of dietary fiber reportedly decreases LDL-C by approximately 2 mg/dL.[47]

DOSAGE

Supplementation with psyllium, totaling 10 g per day, can reduce LDL-C by 7%.[48]

Stanols/Sterols

Plants do not contain cholesterol but are rich in phytosterols and stanols. Sterols and stanols reduce cholesterol by competing with dietary and biliary cholesterol for intestinal absorption. These agents are capable of reducing LDL-C by up to 12%, when used either as monotherapy or as an adjunct to statin therapy.[49] There is no significant difference in the LDL-lowering effect of stanols/sterols when administered in supplement form or as enriched foods.[50]

DOSAGE

Stanols/sterols 2.0 g/day as a single dose.

PRECAUTIONS

Generally well-tolerated but may cause GI distress.

Niacin

Niacin, a B vitamin, has favorable effects on serum lipids. At higher doses, niacin can reduce LDL cholesterol by 15%–20%, increases LDL particle size to more favorable forms, increases serum HDL, and lowers serum levels of Lp(a). "No flush" or "flush-free" niacin (inositol hexaniacinate) should be avoided because these products do not contain the active form of niacin and, consequently, have no significant lipid-altering properties for most individuals.[51] Care should be taken to avoid niacinamide and nicotinamide, products whose name resembles niacin but have no lipid-altering properties. As previously noted, evidence to date does not support the addition of niacin to statin therapy. The use of niacin as monotherapy in patients unable to tolerate statin therapy remains a therapeutic option.

DOSAGE

The typical starting dose is 500 mg per day, titrated upward in 500-mg increments every 6–8 weeks as required to a maximal daily dose of 2000 mg per day. Liver function should be checked after each dose adjustment.

PRECAUTIONS

Although niacin has ideal lipid-altering properties, its use is limited by frequent adverse reactions, which are typically annoying but harmless. The most common adverse reaction to niacin is flushing, which can occur in up to 50% of individuals and is particularly common when initiating therapy or increasing dosage. The best strategy to reduce the risk of flushing involves taking niacin with food, typically dinner, and to use aspirin or nonsteroidal antiinflammatory agents immediately prior to its use. Additional relief from flushing may be possible by taking niacin with applesauce as an after dinner snack. The reason why applesauce may be beneficial in reducing flushing is unknown, but may be attributable to a high concentration of pectin, a soluble fiber known to delay gastric emptying.[52]

Strategies to Reduce Niacin Flush

- Take niacin with dinner, or after dinner with apple sauce
- Take aspirin or a nonsteroidal antiinflammatory with niacin
- Avoid "no flush" niacin as it is ineffective

Red Yeast Rice

Red yeast rice is the most effective over-the-counter therapy for the treatment of elevated LDL cholesterol and reduces LDL-C levels by 20%–30%.[53,54] The combination of red yeast rice, fish oil, and therapeutic lifestyle changes has been proven to lower LDL-C by 42%, a reduction comparable to simvastatin 40 mg. This supplement, taken in pill form, is a fermentation product resulting from growing the yeast, *Monascus purpureus*, on rice. Red yeast rice contains a family of cholesterol-lowering molecules known as monacolins, the most prevalent of which is monacolin K (better known by the chemical name lovastatin).

The concentration of monacolins varies widely between different preparations of red yeast rice.[55] Further, some brands have been shown to contain citrinin, a potentially nephrotoxic fermentation by-product.[55] Therefore it is recommended that practitioners become familiar with a particular brand of red yeast rice and advise patients to continue taking the same brand to increase the likelihood of a consistent result.

Red yeast rice may be a useful option for patients who are not able to tolerate prescription statins, typically due to myalgias. In a study of patients unable to take prescription statins due to the development of myalgias, 93% of those taking red yeast rice were free of significant muscle symptoms with an average LDL-C reduction of 21%.[56] A multicenter trial of 116 patients demonstrated a 27% overall reduction in LDL-C (combined results from doses of 1200 and 2400 mg/day). Doubling the dose of red yeast rice from 1200 to 2400 mg/day has been shown to confer an additional 4.6% reduction in LDL-C.[54]

Long-term studies of red yeast rice have also been reported. A Chinese study of 4870 patients who suffered myocardial infarction were followed for nearly 5 years, with a significant reduction in cardiovascular events and a 33% reduction in total mortality compared to placebo observed at the end of the study period.[57]

DOSAGE

1200 mg twice daily is the typical (and maximal) dose. A lower starting dose of 600 mg twice daily can be used in patients with a history of statin intolerance.

PRECAUTIONS

The amount of active ingredient varies between brands. In addition, a few brands have been shown to contain citrinin, a potential nephrotoxin. Obtain baseline liver and renal function tests and repeat labs 2 months after initiating therapy and twice a year thereafter. Consumerlabs.com has evaluated red yeast rice brands for potency and the presence of citrinin.

Fish Oil

High triglycerides are associated with an increased risk of cardiovascular disease in both men and women but, interestingly, the risk is higher in women.[59] The mechanisms underlying this increased risk is not well understood, but likely related to an association between high triglycerides and a predominance of small, dense LDL particles.

Beyond lifestyle changes, the most effective pharmacological treatments for elevated triglycerides include fibrates (gemfibrozil and fenofibrates) and fish oil. Fish oil has been shown to reduce triglyceride levels by 50% in patients with baseline levels exceeding 500 mg/dL.

Results from studies evaluating omega-3 for the prevention of cardiovascular disease have been mixed.[60,61] The lack of an observed benefit of omega-3 in recent meta-analyses may be confounded by the inclusion of studies using low dose therapy, as well as an overall increase in background dietary omega-3 intake.

Currently, the effectiveness of fish oil in preventing cardiovascular disease remains uncertain. A strong recommendation should be made for intake of at least two fish meals per week. Fish oil supplementation is considered a stronger recommendation for patients who do not regularly eat

DOSAGE

If fish oil is used for the prevention of cardiovascular disease, approximately 1000 mg of combined eicosapentaenoic acid (EPA) and docosahexaenoic acid (DHA) is recommended.

For treatment of elevated triglycerides, doses of 1000 mg to 4000 mg of combined EPA and DHA are required. This can be achieved with either over-the-counter fish oil or prescription omega-3 products. Particularly with over-the-counter preparations, care should be taken to dose fish oil according to combined EPA and DHA content rather than the amount of "total" fish oil listed on the front of over-the-counter products. For example, if the label lists EPA 300 mg and DHA 200 mg and the serving size is two capsules, then the dose would be four capsules daily to obtain 1000 mg of EPA/DHA.

Vegan preparations of long chain omega-3 fatty acids are available, typically consisting of DHA alone. Vegan omega-3 preparations are usually not highly concentrated and may require multiple pills to achieve the desired total DHA dose.

PRECAUTIONS

Fish oil may have a mild anticoagulant effect and should be used with caution in patients taking warfarin. Fish oil may cause mild GI upset, which may be relieved by storing fish oil in the freezer prior to use.

FISH OIL DOSING

- Dosage should specify EPA and DHA content (rather than total fish oil).
- Advise patients to check the nutrition label of products to confirm EPA and DHA content.
- The typical dosage for prevention is approximately 1000 mg of combined EPA and DHA.
- The typical dosage for treatment of hypertriglyceridemia is 1000–4000 mg of combined EPA and DHA.

Coenzyme Q10 (CoQ10)

- **Not controversial**: CoQ10 is a mitochondrial membrane bound compound involved in electron transport and energy production. Therapy with statins lowers the level of circulating CoQ10.
- **Controversial**: Supplementing patients who take statins with CoQ10 reduces the risk of statin-related adverse side effects.

Despite the logic inherent in correcting deficient levels of CoQ10, most reported studies to date have not supported treatment with CoQ10 for the prevention of statin-related adverse reactions.[62,63] Nevertheless, study findings remain inconclusive due to small sample sizes that may be inadequate to demonstrate benefit. The few studies reported benefit have used CoQ10 at doses of 100–200 mg/day.[62]

Further confounding the potential role of CoQ10 is uncertainty regarding the diagnosis of statin intolerance, with only 36% of patients with a diagnosis of statin intolerance found to have reproducible statin-related side-effects with repeat challenges.[63]

Evaluation of the effect of CoQ10 deficiency on statin-related myalgias is difficult because blood levels of CoQ10 typically decrease with statin therapy, while tissue levels are not consistently affected.[64] The majority of circulating CoQ10 is found in LDL, and therefore any intervention that lowers LDL will obligatorily also lower CoQ10.[64]

Therefore, the role of CoQ10 in patients treated with statins remains questionable. What does appear clear is that no significant adverse reactions have been reported with CoQ10 at dosages that far exceed the most common dose range of 100 to 200 mg/day.[65]

DOSAGE

100–200 mg/day can be considered for treatment of mild myalgias in patients taking statins (although lowering the dose of statin or changing to a different type of statin is likely to be more effective). CoQ10 has no intrinsic lipid-altering properties and has not been reported to reduce the likelihood of developing coronary artery disease.

There is, however, stronger evidence that CoQ10 may be useful as an adjunct in the treatment of systolic heart failure. A prospective, randomized trial of 420 patients conducted over 2 years reported that CoQ10 100 mg three times daily resulted in a significant improvement in total mortality, cardiovascular mortality, and New York Heart Association functional class[66] (see Chapter 25).

Vitamin D

Receptors for vitamin D have been identified in heart muscle cells and within arterial walls. Activation of these receptors has many beneficial functions related to blood pressure regulation and normal arterial function.[68]

Accordingly, vitamin D deficiency has been associated with increased cardiovascular risk. The Framingham Offspring Study evaluated individuals without known cardiovascular disease and found that a vitamin D level less than 15 ng/mL was associated with a 62% increase in cardiovascular risk. The link between vitamin D deficiency and cardiovascular risk was especially prominent in those with hypertension.[69]

Vitamin D deficiency also appears to play a role in statin intolerance. The development of myalgias appears to be more prevalent among vitamin D deficient patients. In one study, the average vitamin D level in those with statin-related myalgias was 21 ng/mL, as compared to those without myalgias with an average level of 30 ng/mL.[70] This finding was supported by the observation that patients with statin-related myalgias may experience resolution of their symptoms with vitamin D replacement.[71,72]

DOSAGE

Although the relationship between vitamin D and cardiovascular disease remains incompletely understood, available data indicate levels above 30 ng/mL are desirable. For patients who are vitamin D deficient, replacement can be achieved with daily dosing of over-the-counter vitamin D_3 (doses of 1000 to 5000 IU per day, depending on severity of baseline deficiency).

PRECAUTIONS

Excess vitamin D may cause hypercalcemia, and levels should be rechecked to assess adequacy of treatment and reduce toxicity.

Folic Acid

Folic acid, vitamin B6, and vitamin B12 have been studied in patients with coronary disease because they reduce the circulating level of homocysteine. Elevated homocysteine levels have previously been linked to increased risk of both coronary heart disease and stroke.[73]

Unexpectedly, randomized trials of folic acid, B6, and B12 have failed to demonstrate a benefit for secondary prevention despite the achievement of reduced homocysteine levels (the NORVIT trial, 3749 individuals following myocardial infarction given regimens containing folic acid 800 mcg; and HOPE-2 trial, 5522 patients with vascular disease or diabetes taking folic acid 2500 mcg).[74,75] Of note, a trend toward harm in the group administered a combination of folic acid, B6, and B12 was observed in the NORVIT trial.

It is unclear why folic acid has failed to reduce the occurrence of cardiovascular events. One explanation is that folic acid is simply a marker, as opposed to a target, of increased risk. An alternative explanation is that folic acid causes harm by unknown mechanisms that offset the benefits of homocysteine reduction.

Although folic acid supplementation has not proven useful, foods rich in folate, particularly dark green leafy vegetables, are strongly associated with cardiovascular benefit. One study reported a 23% reduction in the development of coronary heart disease with each daily serving of green leafy vegetables.[9] Therefore foods rich in folate should be encouraged.

Folic acid supplementation has not proven useful for the prevention of cardiovascular events. However, foods rich in folate, particularly dark green leafy vegetables, are associated with significant benefit.

Vitamin E

Vitamin E has been postulated to reduce the risk of coronary disease due to its potent antioxidant properties. An early study, the Cambridge Heart Antioxidant Study (CHAOS), showed benefit in reducing nonfatal myocardial infarction with a median follow-up of approximately 1.5 years.[76] Subsequent studies of longer duration (3.5–8 years) and larger sample sizes (9541–14,641 patients), have failed to confirm a beneficial effect, with no reduction in cardiovascular events with vitamin E.[77-79] These trials have used 400–800 IU of alpha tocopherol per day, predominantly from synthetic sources.

Vitamin E exists in eight isomers: four tocopherols and four tocotrienols. One concern in vitamin E studies is that they generally evaluated only the isolated alpha tocopherol fraction of vitamin E. Some experimental data suggest that gamma and delta tocopherol may be more beneficial than the alpha isomer used in clinical trials.[80,81]

Evidence to date does not support the use of the synthetic alpha tocopherol isomer of vitamin E for the prevention of cardiac disease. Additional research is required to evaluate the effect of mixed tocopherols and tocotrienols on the incidence of cardiovascular events.

Mind/Body

One of the areas where an integrative approach stands to contribute most to the field of cardiology is in appreciation of the role of the mind/body connection in heart health. Although many people are intuitively aware that thoughts and emotions can influence the body, most conventional medical encounters do not include assessment of the patient's emotional state, let alone offer therapies directed at mind-body interventions.

The emotional states most commonly linked to heart disease are stress, anxiety, and depression. Of equal importance is the known association between happiness and heart health.

The link between stress and anxiety with heart disease is strong and far reaching. So much so that anxiety disorders diagnosed early in life, by age 20, independently predict a doubling of heart risk more than 30 years later.[82]

The mechanism by which stress affects cardiac function is unclear but knowledge is increasing rapidly in this area. Stress clearly leads to an increase in catecholamine levels, which are known to increase blood pressure and heart rate, and therefore increase cardiac work.[83] Psychological stress provoked by mental arithmetic produced severely reduced coronary blood flow, identical to that typically observed with strenuous exercise.[83] The cortisol response to mental stress has also been linked to plasma levels of cardiac troponin T, a marker of cardiac injury.[84]

A particularly extreme manifestation of stress on heart health is the recently described Takotusbo cardiomyopathy. In this fascinating but potentially lethal condition, psychological stress has been shown to lead to marked increases in circulating catecholamine levels.[85] The increase in circulating catecholamine triggers acute heart failure typically requiring maximal cardiac support. Antecedent psychological stressors documented to trigger "stress cardiomyopathy" include death of a parent, surprise birthday party, fear of a medical procedure, and public speaking.[86] Interestingly, cardiac function often completely recovers, following the acute phase of Takotsubo cardiomyopathy.

Perhaps less well recognized is the influence of stress on circulating serum lipid levels. Both acute and chronic stress have been linked to unfavorable lipid responses. Within hours of acute psychological stress, total cholesterol levels have been shown to increase by 7 mg/dL and LDL cholesterol by 5 mg/dL.[87] Furthermore, the acute lipid response to stress was observed in individuals diagnosed with hypercholesterolemia 3 years later, suggesting stress may be a contributing cause to chronic dyslipidemia.[87]

Just as emotional factors may contribute to the development of heart disease, they can also be harnessed to promote heart health. Meditation practiced by individuals with coronary disease over 5 years has been demonstrated to reduce the combined risk of a cardiovascular event or death by 48%.[88] The mechanism of risk reduction by meditation likely includes a decrease in cardiovascular workload, as demonstrated by the ability of meditation to ameliorate the expected increase in heart rate associated with infusion of isoproterenol[83] (see Chapter 100).

A separate study reported that patients assessed as "optimists" had a 55% reduced risk of cardiovascular death, adjusted for traditional risk factors, compared to their less upbeat peers.[89]

A wide range of therapies are available to assist patients with cardiac disease to better manage their stress and anxiety. In addition to more conventional treatments with psychoactive medication or referral for cognitive behavioral therapy, the palette available to the integrative practitioner includes meditation, yoga, biofeedback, healing touch, Reiki, massage, and acupuncture. There is no one resource that is generically superior to another. Instead, referral should be made based on individualized assessments including the patient's prior knowledge or history with a particular approach, the patient's philosophical inclination, local expertise, and cost. This "matching" process is truly one of the arts of integrative medicine.

OTHER THERAPIES

Enhanced External Counterpulsation (EECP)

Enhanced external counterpulsation is a noninvasive method of improving blood flow to the heart and reducing anginal symptoms. This treatment involves repetitive leg compressions with a pneumatic device that drives blood backward into the aorta and increases coronary blood flow. A study of 1097 patients with coronary disease reported 73% of patients had improvement in the severity of angina at the completion of treatment, with sustained benefit observed after 2 years.[90] A separate study examined 363 patients with severe angina and depressed left ventricular function. After treatment, 72% of patients had a reduction in the severity of angina from severe to mild or none with benefit maintained after 2 years.[91]

Protocols generally involve 35 one-hour sessions of treatment over 5 weeks. Patients referred for this treatment historically have been those with refractory angina who have exhausted medical therapy and mechanical revascularization options.

Chelation Therapy

Chelation therapy has been proposed as a treatment for atherosclerotic vascular disease. The hypothesized mechanisms of benefit include the binding of calcium to atherosclerotic plaques and reduced oxidative stress leading to improved vascular function. A double-blind, placebo-controlled chelation trial jointly sponsored by the National Institute of Health and National Center for Complementary and Alternative Medicine studied 1708 patients with past history of myocardial infarction. Chelation therapy was found to significantly decrease the primary endpoint by 18% (combined total mortality, cardiovascular events, revascularization, and hospitalization for myocardial infarction).[92] Diabetics, a prespecified subgroup, had particular benefit with a 39% reduction in the primary end-point. These provocative study results are clearly hypothesis-generating. Additional studies are required to determine the reproducibility of these results and elucidate the underlying mechanisms (see Chapter 107).

PREVENTION PRESCRIPTION

- Nutrition (Mediterranean diet)
- Weight management
- Smoking cessation if needed
- Social connection
- Exercise (aerobics and resistance training)
- Tools for management of stress/anxiety
- Lipid management

THERAPEUTIC REVIEW

NUTRITION

Mediterranean-Style Style Diet A_1

- 5 servings of vegetables/day
- 2 servings of fruit/day
- Whole grains, eliminate refined carbohydrates
- 2 servings of fish/week
- Reduce red meat
- Nuts frequently

EXERCISE

- 30 min/day walking or a minimum of 30 min 3x/week of more intensive aerobics A_1
- Resistance training at least 30 min/week

SMOKING CESSATION A_1

LIPID MANAGEMENT

For LDL-C

- Fiber supplements: (e.g., Psyllium, 10 g/day) B_1
- Stanols/sterols: 2.0 g/day B_1
- Niacin: 500–2000 mg/day A_2
- Prescription statins: dose varies A_2
- Red yeast rice: 1200–2400 mg/day divided BID B_2

For HDL-C

- Exercise A_1
- Weight loss A_1
- Reduced intake of carbohydrates A_1
- Niacin 500–2000 mg/day A_2

For Triglycerides

- Exercise A_1

- Weight loss A_1
- Reduced intake of carbohydrates A_1
- Fish oil: 1000–4000 mg EPA/DHA per day A_2
- Fibrates: fenofibrate 45–150 mg/day A_2

To Reduce Statin Related Myalgias

- Consider CoQ10 100–200 mg/day B_1
- Replete vitamin D deficiency B_1
    - Goal is level > 30 ng/mL

STRESS/ANXIETY REDUCTION

- Breathing exercises C_1
- Biofeedback C_1
- Meditation B_1
- Yoga C_1
- Acupuncture C_1
- Cognitive behavioral therapy B_1
- Anxiolytics B_2

ANTIANGINAL THERAPY

- ASA 81–325 mg daily A_2
- β-Blockers (e.g., metoprolol succinate, usual dose 50–200 mg daily) A_2
- Nitrates (e.g., isosorbide mononitrate, usual dose 30–120 mg daily) A_2
- Calcium channel blockers (e.g., amlodipine 2.5–10 mg daily) A_2
- Angioplasty/stent (for angina) A_3
- EECP B_2

Key Web Resources

American Heart Association Practice Guidelines	http://professional.heart.org/professional/Guidelines Statements/searchresults.jsp
Natural Medicines Database. This site is an excellent resource for detailed information regarding supplements including scientific basis (or lack thereof), adverse reactions, and interactions with drugs/supplements	http://www.naturaldatabase.com
ConsumerLab. This site summarizes testing information regarding the content and purity of commonly recommended supplements	http://www.consumerlab.com
Aspirin Guidelines from the Agency for Healthcare Research and Quality. Guidelines for aspirin use for the primary prevention of cardiovascular disease	http://www.ahrq.gov/professionals/clinicians-providers/resources/aspprovider.html
10-year CV Risk Calculator from the National Heart, Lung and Blood Institute. Risk assessment tool for estimating the 10-year risk of having a heart attack	http://cvdrisk.nhlbi.nih.gov/calculator.asp

REFERENCES

References are available online at ExpertConsult.com.

CHAPTER 27

DYSLIPIDEMIA

Mark Houston, MD, MS, MSc

INTRODUCTION

The combination of a lipid-lowering diet and scientifically proven nutraceutical supplements significantly reduces total low-density lipoprotein (LDL) cholesterol, triglycerides (TG), and very low density lipoprotein (VLDL); decreases LDL particle number (LDL-P); increases LDL particle size and total and type 2 b high-density lipoprotein (HDL); and improves HDL functionality. In addition, inflammation, oxidative stress, and vascular immune dysfunction are decreased. Prospective clinical trials demonstrated reductions in coronary heart disease (CHD) and cardiovascular disease (CVD) with optimal nutrition and/or administration of nutraceutical supplements, such as omega-3 fatty acids (FAs), red yeast rice (RYR), alpha-linolenic acid (ALA), and niacin. A combined program of nutrition and nutraceutical supplements represents a scientifically valid alternative for patients who prefer nondrug therapies or who are intolerant to statins or other drugs for the treatment of dyslipidemia. This will be the primary focus of this chapter.

This approach to decrease dyslipidemia-induced vascular disease recognizes and treats the various steps that are involved in the development of atherosclerosis and CHD.

PATHOPHYSIOLOGY

Dyslipidemia is one of the top five risk factors for CVD, along with hypertension, diabetes mellitus (DM), smoking, and obesity.[1]

There are an infinite number of vascular insults, but only three finite responses of the vascular endothelium, vascular smooth muscle (VSM), and cardiac smooth muscle to these insults. These three responses include inflammation, oxidative stress, and vascular immune dysfunction.[2-4] These pathophysiological processes lead to endothelial dysfunction (ED) and VSM and cardiac dysfunction.

The vascular consequences include CVD, CHD, myocardial infarction (MI), and cerebrovascular accidents (CVAs).[4]

Genetics, epigenetics, chronic inflammatory micro- and macronutrient intake, obesity (visceral obesity), chronic infections, toxins, tobacco products, DM, lack of exercise, and some specific pharmacological agents, including many of the older beta-blockers and thiazide or thiazide-like diuretics, contribute to dyslipidemia.[5,6]

Several genetic phenotypes, such as apolipoprotein E (APOE), result in variable serum lipid responses to diet, as well as contribute to CHD and MI risk.[7,8] In addition, HDL proteomics that affect paraoxonase-1 (PON-1) and scavenger receptor B-1 (SR-B1) increase CVD.[9] The sortilin I allele variants on chromosome 1p13 increase LDL and CHD risk by 29%.[10]

Recent studies suggest that increasing dietary cholesterol intake will not significantly alter serum total or LDL cholesterol levels or CHD risk.[5,6]

Some saturated fats, depending on their carbon chain length, may have minimal influences on serum lipids and CHD risk, whereas mono- and polyunsaturated fats have a favorable influence on serum lipids and CHD risk. Reducing refined carbohydrate intake, such as sugars, bread, white potatoes, white rice, starches, and low-fiber carbohydrates, may be more important in improving serum lipids and lipid subfractions than saturated fats and cholesterol. Refined carbohydrates have more adverse effects on insulin resistance, atherogenic LDL, small LDL, LDL-P, VLDL, TG, total HDL, HDL subfractions, and HDL particle number (HDL-P), thus contributing to CHD risk more than saturated fats.[5,11-17]

Postprandial hyperglycemia, hypertriglyceridemia, and endotoxemia coupled with inflammation, oxidative stress, and immune vascular dysfunction are highly associated with atherosclerosis.[18-21] This is metabolic endotoxemia.

The validity of the "Diet–Heart Hypothesis," implicating dietary saturated fats, cholesterol, and eggs as causative of CHD and MI, has been questioned.[12-14] Trans-FAs have definite adverse effects on serum lipids and increase CVD, CHD, and MI risk, but omega-3 FAs and monounsaturated fats improve serum lipids and reduce CVD risk.[5,11-17] Trans fats suppress transforming growth factor beta (TGF-B) responsiveness, which increases the deposition of cholesterol into cellular plasma membranes in vascular tissue.[16]

TESTING

Expanded lipid testing is the best method to determine risk for CHD and the optimal treatments.

Expanded lipid profiles that measure lipids, lipid subfractions, particle size and number, and APOB and APOA are preferred over standard lipid profiles that measure only the total lipid levels.

These expanded lipid profiles, such as lipoprotein particles (LPP, Spectracell Laboratories, Houston, Texas), nuclear magnetic resonance (NMR, Liposcience, Burlington, North Carolina), Berkeley Heart Labs, Boston Heart Labs, and vertical auto profile (VAP, Atherotech, Birmingham, Alabama), improve serum lipid analysis and CHD risk profiling.[24,25]

LDL-P is the primary lipid parameter that drives the risk for CHD and MI as well as coronary artery calcification as measured by computed tomography (CT) angiography.[26,27] Dense LDL type B or LDL type 3 and type 4 have secondary roles in CHD only if the LDL-P is elevated.

Dysfunctional HDL[28-31] may be inflammatory and atherogenic and lose its atheroprotective effects especially in patients with DM, metabolic syndrome, and obesity.[31]

> LDL-P drives the risk for CHD and MI. Once the LDL-P is normal, the LDL size is not important as a risk factor (Fig. 27.1).

Oxidation and inflammation of APOA-1 often result in higher levels of HDL that are dysfunctional and not protective.[31] The ability to evaluate HDL functionality, either directly or indirectly, measuring reverse cholesterol transport, cholesterol efflux capacity,[29] or myeloperoxidase (MPO)[30-31] will improve the assessment and treatment of dyslipidemia-induced vascular disease, CHD, and MI. At this time, only serum MPO is available clinically to measure HDL function.

An understanding of the pathophysiological steps in dyslipidemia-induced vascular damage is mandatory for optimal and logical treatment (Fig. 27.2). The ability to interrupt all of the various steps in this pathway will allow more specific treatments to reduce vascular injury,

improve vascular repair systems, and maintain and restore vascular health.

Native LDL, especially large type A LDL, is not usually atherogenic until modified. However, there exists an alternate pinocytosis mechanism that allows macrophage ingestion of native LDL, which accounts for up to 30% of foam cell formation in the subendothelium during chronic inflammation or infections.[32-33] LDL must be modified from its native form in most clinical circumstances for it to be atherogenic. This modification makes the LDL a foreign substance that is recognized by macrophages, which then mount an immunological and inflammatory response that damages the vascular system.

Decreasing LDL modification, the atherogenic form of LDL cholesterol, by lowering the various forms of LDL modification such as oxidized LDL (oxLDL), glycated LDL (glyLDL), glycooxidized LDL (gly-oxLDL), and acetylated LDL (acLDL), modifying the uptake of modified LDL into macrophages by the scavenger receptors (CD36 SR), and decreasing the inflammatory, oxidative stress, and autoimmune responses will reduce vascular damage beyond treating the LDL cholesterol level.[34-40] There are numerous mechanistic pathways that can be treated to interrupt dyslipidemia-induced vascular damage and disease (Table 27.1). Reduction in high-sensitivity C-reactive protein (hs-CRP), an inflammatory marker, reduces vascular events independent of reductions in LDL cholesterol through numerous mechanisms.[39]

> Modified LDLs, such as oxidized and glycated LDL, are atherogenic, whereas native LDL is not in most clinical situations. The one exception is that even native LDL may be atherogenic due to pinocytosis by macrophages in the setting of chronic infections or inflammation.

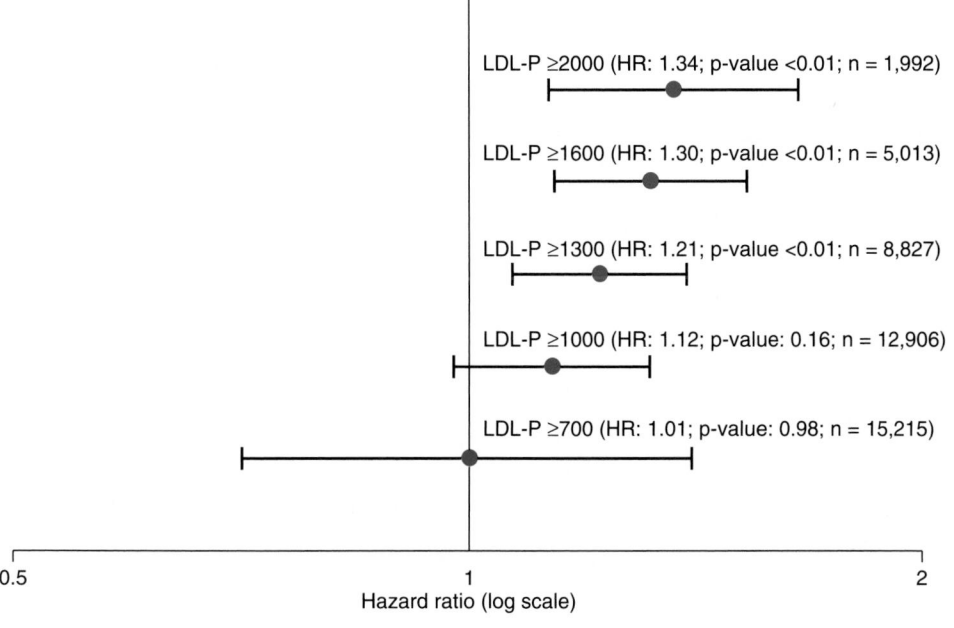

FIG. 27.1 ■ **Risk for future CHD events by LDL-P.** Hazard ratios (HRs) for future CHD events across LDL-P thresholds are adjusted for baseline demographics, comorbidities, and LDL-C. Median follow-up was 10.1 months. Sample sizes indicate the number of patients with LDL-P levels at or above the designated thresholds. (Part 1: assessment of CHD incidence by LDL-P). (From Toth PP, Grabner M, Punekar RS, et al. Cardiovascular risk in patients achieving low-density lipoprotein cholesterol and particle targets. *Atherosclerosis.* 2014;235:585-591.)

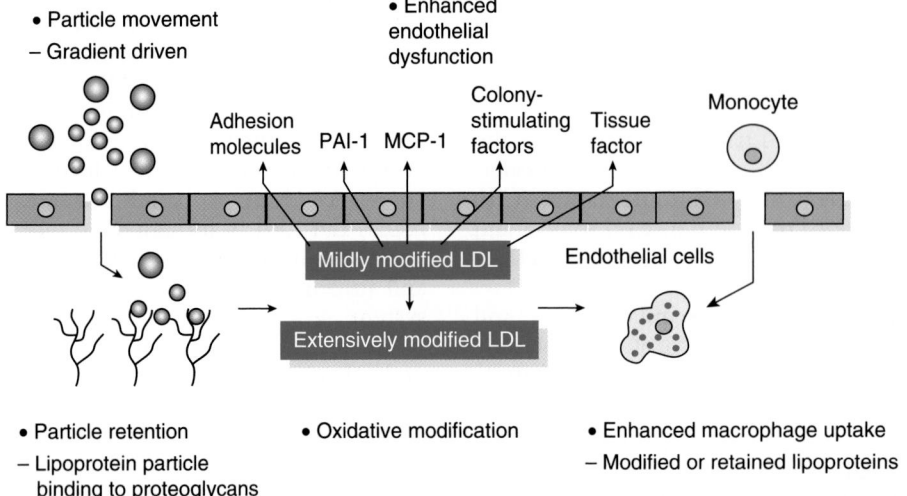

FIG. 27.2 ■ The various steps in the uptake of LDL cholesterol, modification, macrophage ingestion with scavenger receptors, foam cell formation, oxidative stress, inflammation, and autoimmune cytokines and chemokine production.

TABLE 27.1   Mechanisms for Treatment of Dyslipidemia-Induced Vascular Disease

Mechanism	Treatment/Nutrients
Improve endothelial function and repair	Aged garlic
Modify caveolae, caveolin-1, lipid rafts, membrane microdomains, unesterified cholesterol, and cholesterol crystals	Lycopene, omega-3 fatty acids, and statins
Increase eNOS and nitric oxide	Resveratrol, flaxseed, omega-3 fatty acids, NAC, taurine, pycnogenol, grape seed extract, pomegranate, aged garlic
Modify pattern recognition receptor (PRR) activation and toll-like receptors	Niacin, EGCG, pantethine, resveratrol, MUFA, curcumin, pomegranate, aged garlic, sesame, gamma/delta tocotrienols, lycopene
Decrease cholesterol crystals, LDL phospholipids, oxLDL, APO-B, and 7-ketosteroids that activate the PRR	Omega-3 fatty acids and statins
Decrease LDL burden	Niacin, RYR, plant sterols, sesame, tocotrienols (gamma/delta), pantethine, GLA, citrus bergamot, EGCG, omega-3 fatty acids, flaxseed, MUFA, aged garlic, resveratrol, curcumin, orange juice, soluble fiber, soy, lycopene, astaxanthin, fiber
Reduce cholesterol absorption	Plant sterols, soy, EGCG, flax seeds, sesame, garlic, fiber
Increase cholesterol bile excretion and upregulate LDL receptors	EGCG, sesame, tocotrienols, curcumin, policosanol, plant sterols
Decrease LDL particle number	Niacin, omega-3 fatty acids, statins
Decrease APO-B	Niacin, omega-3 fatty acids, plant sterols, EGCG, astaxanthin
Decrease LDL modification/oxidation	Niacin, EGCG, quercetin, pantethine, resveratrol, red wine, grape seed extract, MUFA, curcumin, pomegranate, garlic, sesame, gamma/delta tocotrienols, lycopene, polyphenols, flavonoids, oleic acid, glutathione, citrus bergamot, tangerine extract, policosanol, RBO (ferulic acid gamma-oryzanol), coenzyme Q10, vitamin E, polyphenols, and flavonoids
Inhibit LDL glycation	Carnosine, histidine, rutin, pomegranate, organosulfur compounds
Increase LDL size (type B to type A)	Niacin, omega-3 fatty acids, plant sterols
Reduce inflammation	Niacin, omega-3 fatty acids, flaxseed, MUFA, plant sterols, guggulipids, resveratrol, glutathione, quercetin, curcumin, aged garlic

TABLE 27.1 Mechanisms for Treatment of Dyslipidemia-Induced Vascular Disease—cont'd

Mechanism	Treatment/Nutrients
Decrease LDL signaling	Plant sterols
Decrease modified LDL macrophage uptake by scavenger receptors	Resveratrol, N-acetyl cysteine (NAC), aged garlic
Decrease CAMs, macrophage recruitment, and migration	NAC, resveratrol, luteolin, glutathione, and curcumin
Alter macrophage phenotype	Omega-3 fatty acid, plant sterols, sterolins, and glycosides
Modify signaling pathways	Plant sterols and phytosterolins
Increase reverse cholesterol transport	Lycopene, niacin, plant sterols, glutathione, wogonin, resveratrol, various flavonoids and anthocyanins, alpha-linolenic acid
Increase total HDL and HDL 2 b levels and convert HDL 3 to HDL 2 and 2 b (increase size)	Niacin, omega-3 fatty acids, pantethine, red yeast rice, MUFA, resveratrol, curcumin, pomegranate, astaxanthin, citrus bergamot
Improve HDL function. Reduce inflammation, oxidative stress, and immune dysfunction	Quercetin, pomegranate, EGCG, resveratrol, glutathione, lycopene
Increase APO A-1 lipoprotein	Niacin
Increase PON-1 and PON-2	EGCG, quercetin, pomegranate, resveratrol, glutathione
Decrease VLDL and TG	Niacin, RYR, omega-3 fatty acids, pantethine, citrus bergamot, flaxseed, MUFA, resveratrol, astaxanthin
Lower Lp(a)	Niacin, NAC, gamma/delta tocotrienols, omega-3 fatty acids, flax seed, CoQ10, vitamin C, L-carnitine, L-lysine, L-arginine, almonds
Reduce foam cell and fatty streak formation	Resveratrol, NAC, phytosterolins
HMG-CoA reductase inhibition	RYR, pantethine, gamma/delta tocotrienols, sesame, EGCG, omega-3 fatty acids, citrus bergamot, garlic, curcumin, GLA, plant sterols, lycopene, soy, statins

INTEGRATIVE THERAPY

Many patients cannot or will not use pharmacological treatments, such as statins, fibrates, bile acid resin binders, or ezetimibe, to treat dyslipidemia.[5] Statin-induced or fibrate-induced muscle disease with myalgias or muscle weakness, abnormal liver function tests, neuropathy, memory loss, mental status changes, gastrointestinal (GI) disturbances, glucose intolerance, and DM are some of the reasons that patients may require the use of nutritional supplements.[41-45] Many patients who are on prolonged, high-dose statins have other clinical symptoms and/or lab abnormalities such as chronic fatigue, exercise-induced fatigue, decrease in lean muscle mass, reduced exercise tolerance, and reductions in coenzyme Q10, carnitine, vitamin E, vitamin D, omega-3 FAs, selenium, free T3 levels (hypothyroidism), and steroid or sex hormones.[5,41-53]

Treatment approaches that combine weight loss, reductions in visceral and total body fat, increases in lean muscle mass, optimal aerobic and resistance exercise, use of scientifically proven nutrition, and nutraceutical supplements alone or integrated with drug therapies offer not only improvement in serum lipids but also reductions in inflammation, oxidative stress, immune dysfunction, and ED and VSM dysfunction. In addition, surrogate markers for vascular disease or clinical vascular target organ damage, such as CHD and carotid intimal medial thickness (IMT), were reduced in many clinical trials using a nonpharmacological approach.[5]

Nutrition

Nutrition is an important treatment for dyslipidemia, CHD risk factors, and the prevention and treatment of CVD. Numerous epidemiological studies and prospective clinical trials,[54-81] including the Framingham Heart Study,[54,55] Seven Countries Study,[56,57] Pritikin diet studies,[58-60] Ornish Lifestyle Heart Trial,[61-64] Omni Heart Trial,[55] Portfolio diet,[65-68] Mediterranean diet,[69-73] Lyon Diet Heart Study,[72] Indian Heart Study,[74] PREDIMED study,[73-76] and Paleolithic diet, have clearly established the relationship between diet, serum lipids, inflammation, and CVD, including CHD and stroke. The reader is referred to these excellent studies for review as this information will not be included in this chapter.

Although many questions still exist regarding optimal intakes of fats, which types of fats, types and quality of protein, as well as the dietary intakes of complex and refined carbohydrates, most studies clearly indicate that trans-FAs and refined carbohydrates have an adverse effect on serum lipids and cardiovascular outcomes.[81] Some saturated fats may be adverse, others neutral, and some potentially beneficial. The monounsaturated FA (MUFA) and omega-3 FA are consistently beneficial for dyslipidemia and CVD. A vegetarian diet with increased complex carbohydrates and fiber and lower dietary cholesterol is also beneficial. Intake of lean, wild, and organic types of protein and cold-water fish improves lipids and CHD risk factors (see Chapter 88).

THE MAMMALIAN CELL MEVALONATE CHOLESTEROL PATHWAY AND PP (PYROPHOSPHATE)

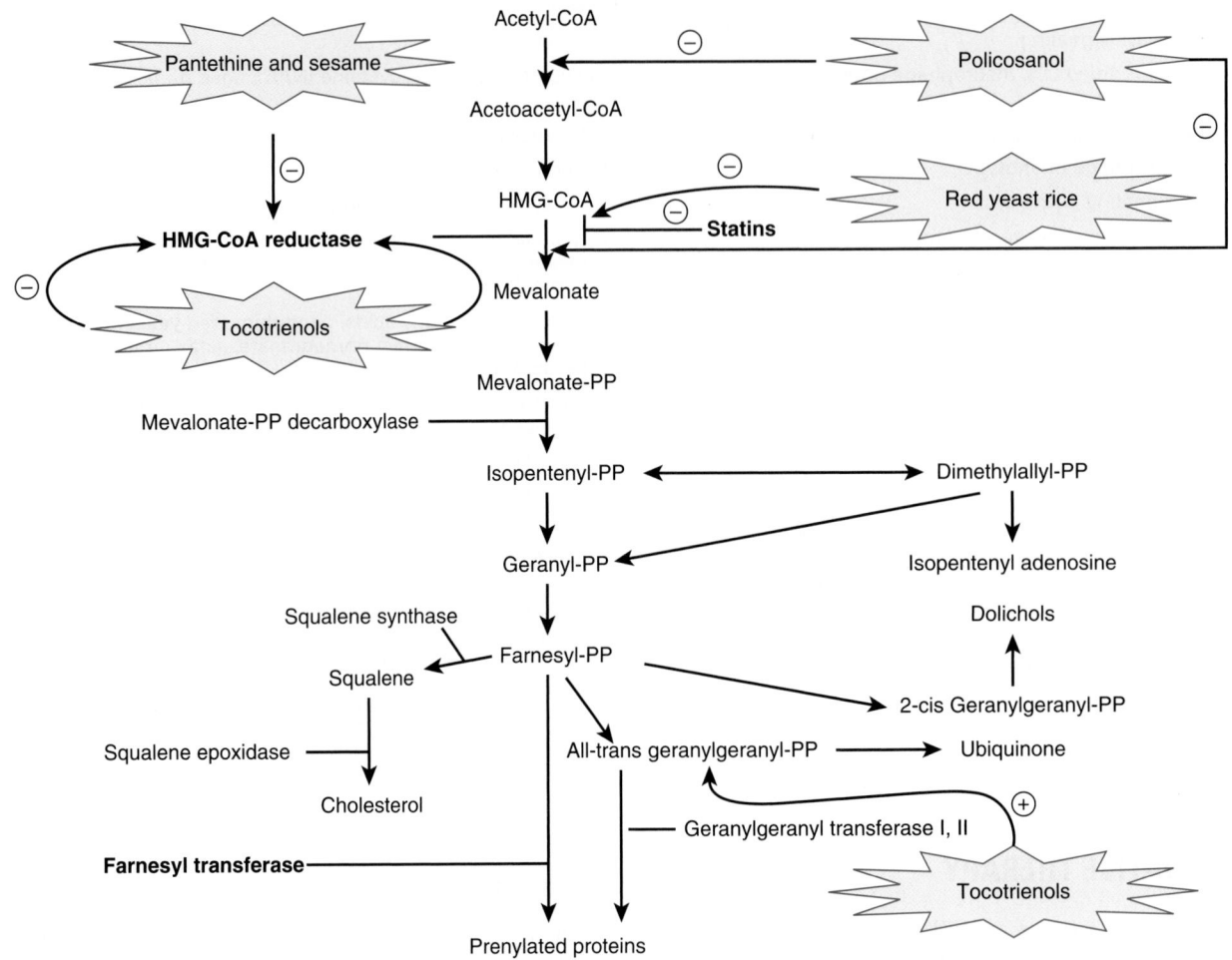

FIG. 27.3 ■ Proposed mechanisms of action of nutraceuticals and statins in the cholesterol pathway.

Nutraceutical Supplements

Nutraceutical supplement management of dyslipidemia has not been frequently reviewed.[5,6,82] New important scientific information and clinical studies are required to understand the present role of these natural agents in the management of dyslipidemia.[5,6,82]

Clinical trials showed excellent reductions in serum lipids and CHD with niacin, omega-3 FAs, RYR, fiber, and ALA.

Smaller studies that have used surrogate vascular markers showed improvements in carotid IMT and obstruction, coronary artery plaque progression, coronary artery calcium score by electron beam tomography (EBT) and CT angiography, as well as a decrease in generalized atherosclerosis and improvement in endothelial function.[5,82-84] The proposed mechanisms of action of some of the nutraceutical supplements on the mammalian cholesterol pathway are shown in Fig. 27.3.

Niacin (Vitamin B3)

Niacin has a dose-related effect (1–4 g/day) in reducing total cholesterol (TC), LDL, APOB, LDL-P, TG, and

VLDL and increasing HDL and LDL size from small type B to large type A, especially the protective and larger HDL 2 b particle and APOA-1.[5] Niacin also increases the HDL-P (the predominant protective lipid parameter) and HDL function with improvements in reverse cholesterol transport.[57-59] Niacin has a logarithmic dose-response on HDL, with smaller doses having a large effect. The effect on LDL reduction is a linear dose-response that requires higher doses.[85]

The changes are dose related, varying from 10% to 30% for each lipid level.[5,86,87] Niacin inhibits LDL oxidation, increases TG lipolysis in adipose tissue, increases APO-B degradation, and reduces the fractional catabolic rate of HDL APO A-1. Niacin inhibits platelet function, induces fibrinolysis, decreases cytokines and cell adhesion molecules (CAMs), lowers Lp(a), increases adiponectin, inhibits cholesterylester transfer protein (CETP), and increases reverse cholesterol transport.[5,85-87] However, despite an improved lipid profile, there is variable improvement in endothelial and microvascular function.[90]

Randomized clinical trials such as the Coronary Drug Project, HATS trial, ARBITER 2, Oxford Niaspan Study, FATS, CLAS I and CLAS II, and AFRS have shown reductions in coronary events, decreases in coronary atheroma (plaque), and decreases in carotid IMT.[5,86,87,90-94] The recent negative findings in the AIM-HIGH study[95,96] do not detract from these positive clinical trials, as this study has numerous methodological design flaws and was not powered to statistically determine CVD endpoints. The recent HPS-THRIVE trial of 26,000 patients using 2 grams of extended-release niacin plus the antiflushing agent laropiprant daily or placebo on top of a background therapy of simvastatin with or without ezetimibe did not reduce cardiovascular events despite a 17% increased HDL and 20% decreased LDL.[97,98] Whether the inhibition of flushing by laropiprant or some other unknown effect of this agent interfered with the HDL function and the cardiovascular (CV) outcomes is not clear. However, the recommendation not to use niacin in the face of the other many positive studies is clearly premature.

DOSAGE

The effective dosing range is from 500–4000 mg/day. It should be titrated slowly starting at 100 mg/day and increased each week by 100–200 mg/day. Sustained-release niacin is preferred. Only vitamin B3 niacin is effective in dyslipidemia.

The nonflushing niacin (inositol hexanicotinate; IHN) does not improve lipid profiles and is not recommended.[5,99]

PRECAUTIONS

The side effects of niacin include hyperglycemia, hyperuricemia, gout, hepatitis, flushing, rash, pruritus, hyperpigmentation, hyperhomocysteinemia, gastritis, ulcers, bruising, tachycardia, and palpitations.[5,86,87] Elevations in homocysteine should be treated with vitamin B6, B12, and folate. Niacin-induced flushing is minimized by increasing the dose gradually, taking it on a regular basis without interruption, consumption with meals, avoiding alcohol within 4 hours of ingestion of niacin, consumption of 81-mg baby aspirin, and supplemental quercetin (500 mg), and apples, apple pectin, or applesauce.

Red Yeast Rice

RYR (*Monascus purpureus*) is a fermented product of rice that contains monacolins, which inhibit cholesterol synthesis via 5-hydroxy-3-methylglutaryl-coenzyme A (HMG-CoA) reductase and thus has "statin-like" properties (13 natural statins).[5,82,102-124] RYR also contains ergosterol, amino acids, flavonoids, trace elements, alkaloids, sterols, isoflavones, and monounsaturated FAs that improve the lipid profile.

RYR administered orally to adult subjects with dyslipidemia at 2400 mg/day reduced LDL-C by 22% (p < 0.001) and TG by 12% with little change in HDL.[5,82,102] RYR reduces the risk of abdominal aortic aneurysms (AAA) by suppressing angiotensin II levels.[103] RYR also is effective in mouse models against obesity-related inflammation, insulin resistance, and nonalcoholic fatty liver disease (NAFLD).[104] RYR in conjunction with berberine improves insulin resistance, glucose, and lipids in subjects with or without metabolic syndrome.[114,117,123] RYR,

policosanol, and artichoke leaf extract decrease and RYR with plant stanols reduce LDL-C significantly.[105,111,112] RYR with berberine, policosanol, astaxanthin, coenzyme Q10, and folic acid reduced LDL cholesterol (LDL-C) by 21.1%, similar to pravastatin 10 mg/day, with a simultaneous 4.8% increase in HDL cholesterol (HDL-C) over 8 weeks.[120]

RYR inhibits tumor necrosis factor (TNF)-alpha and metalloproteinase (MMP)-2 and MMP-9,[107] suppresses caveolin-1, increases endothelial nitric oxide synthase (eNOS) expression, improves abnormal hemorheology,[106] increases adiponectin,[113] improves the leptin-to-adiponectin ratio,[120] lowers hs-CRP, improves vascular remodeling parameters such as MMP-2 and MMP-9,[115] reduces expression of tissue factor oxLDL, and reduces thrombosis in animal models by suppressing nicotinamide adenine dinucleotide phosphate oxidase and extracellular signal-regulated kinase activation.[118] In a recent placebo-controlled Chinese study of 5000 subjects over 4.5 years, an extract of RYR reduced LDL by 17.6% (p < 0.001) and increased HDL by 4.2% (p < 0.001).[124] CV mortality fell 30% (p < 0.005) and total mortality fell 33% (p < 0.0003) in the treated subjects. The overall primary endpoint of MI and death was reduced by 45% (p < 0.001). A recent meta-analysis and clinical trials of RYR for dyslipidemia and CVD endpoints confirmed these positive findings.[109,110,121,122]

DOSAGE

The recommended dose is 800–4800 mg/day of a standardized RYR.

PRECAUTIONS

A highly purified and certified RYR must be used to avoid potential renal damage induced by a mycotoxin, citrinin.[5,82,102] No adverse effects have been reported such as myalgias or liver dysfunction with long-term use nor is there any interference with the cytochrome (CY)P450 enzymes.[118] Although reductions in coenzyme Q10 may occur in predisposed patients and those on prolonged high-dose RYR, because of its weaker "statin-like" effect, this is not as likely as with statins. RYR is an excellent alternative for patients with statin-induced myopathy[5,82,102,116,124] and for statin-intolerant patients with or without type 2 DM in conjunction with the Mediterranean diet to effectively manage their dyslipidemia.[119]

Plant Sterols (Phytosterols)

The plant sterols are naturally occurring sterols of plant origin that include B-sitosterol (the most abundant), campesterol and stigmasterol (4-desmethyl sterols of the cholestane series), and the saturated stanols.[5,82,125-129] The plant sterols are much better absorbed than the plant stanols. The daily intake of plant sterols in the United States is about 150–400 mg/day mostly from soybean oil, various nuts, and tall pine tree oil.[82] These have a dose-dependent reduction on serum lipids.[126] TC is decreased 8%, and LDL is decreased 10% (range, 6%–15%) with no change in TG or HDL on doses of 2–3 g/day in divided doses with meals.[5,82,125-129] A recent meta-analysis of 84 trials showed that an average intake of 2.15 g/day reduced LDL by 8.8% with no improvement in serum lipids at higher doses.[126]

The mechanism of action is primarily to decrease the incorporation of dietary and biliary cholesterol into micelles due to the lower micellar solubility of cholesterol, which reduces cholesterol absorption and increases bile acid secretion. In addition, there is an interaction with enterocyte adenosine triphosphate (ATP)–binding cassette transport proteins (ABCG8 and ABCG5) that directs cholesterol back into the intestinal lumen.[5,82,125] The only difference between cholesterol and sitosterol consists of an additional ethyl group at position C-24 in sitosterol, which is responsible for its poor absorption. The plant sterols have a higher affinity than cholesterol for the micelles. The plant sterols are also antiinflammatory and decrease the levels of proinflammatory cytokines such as hs-CRP, interleukin (IL)-6, IL-1b, TNF-alpha, phospholipase (PLA) 2, and fibrinogen, but these effects vary among the various phytosterols.[129,130]

Some studies have shown a reduction in atherosclerosis progression and reductions in the progression of carotid IMT and carotid plaque, but the results have been conflicting.[5,82] Patients that have the rare homozygous mutations of the ATP-binding cassette are hyperabsorbers of sitosterol (absorb 15%–60% instead of the normal 5%) and will develop premature atherosclerosis.[82] This is a rare autosomal recessive disorder termed *sitosterolemia*. There are no studies on CHD or other CVD outcomes to date with phytosterols.

DOSAGE

The recommended dose is 2–2.5 g/day (average, 2.15 g/day).

PRECAUTIONS

The plant sterols can interfere with absorption of lipid-soluble compounds such as fat-soluble vitamins and carotenoids like vitamins D, E, and K and alpha-carotene.[5,82]

Soy

Numerous studies have shown mild improvements in serum lipids with soy at doses of 30–50 g/day.[5,82,131,132] TC falls 2%–9.3%, LDL decreases 4%–12.9%, TG decreases 10.5%, and HDL increases up to 2.4%. However, the studies are conflicting due to differences in the type and dose of soy used in the studies, as well as nonstandardized methodology.[5,82,131,132] Soy decreases the micellar content and absorption of lipids through a combination of fiber, isoflavones (genistin, glycitin, diadzin), and phytoestrogens.[5,82,131,132] Soy also reduces sterol regulatory element-binding protein (SREBP) and HMG-CoA reductase, increases LDL receptor density, and increases the antioxidant activity of superoxide dismutase (SOD) and catalase.[133] The greatest reduction is seen with soy-enriched isoflavones with soy protein.

DOSAGE

The dose is 30–50 g/day.

PRECAUTIONS

None.

Green Tea Extract and Green Tea (EGCG)

Catechins, especially EGCG, may improve the lipid profile by interfering with micellar solubilization of cholesterol in the GI tract and reducing absorption.[5] In addition, EGCG reduces FA gene expression, inhibits HMG-CoA reductase, increases mitochondrial energy expenditure, reduces oxLDL, increases PON-1, upregulates the LDL receptor, decreases APO-B lipoprotein secretion from cells, mimics the action of insulin, improves ED, activates nuclear erythroid 2-related factor 2 (Nrf2), increases heme oxygenase-1 (HO-1) expression, decreases inflammation, displaces caveolin-1 from cell membranes, increases nitric oxide, reduces endothelial inflammation, and decreases body fat.[5,134-137]

A meta-analysis of 14 trials shows that EGCG at 224–674 mg/day or 60 oz of green tea a day reduced TC by 7.2 mg/dL and LDL by 2.19 mg/dL (p < 0.001). There was no significant change in HDL or TG level.[138]

DOSAGE

The recommended dose is a standardized EGCG extract at 1000 mg/day or 60 oz brewed green tea a day.

PRECAUTIONS

Caution regarding the stimulatory effects of caffeine if tea is consumed.

Omega-3 Fatty Acids

Observational, epidemiological, and controlled clinical trials have shown significant reductions in serum TG, VLDL, decreased LDL-P, increased LDL and HDL particle size, as well as major reductions in all CVD events.[5,139-146] The DART trial demonstrated a decrease in mortality of 29% in men post-MI, and the GISSI prevention trial found a decrease in total mortality of 20%, in CV deaths of 30%, and in sudden death of 45%. The Kuopio Heart Study demonstrated a 44% reduction in fatal and nonfatal CHD in subjects in the highest quintile of omega-3 intake compared to the lowest quintile.[5,139,140] Omega-3 FA reduced CHD progression, stabilized plaque, and reduced coronary artery stent restenosis and coronary artery bypass grafting (CABG) occlusion.[5,141] In the JELIS study, the addition of 1.8 grams of omega eicosapentaenoic acid (EPA) to a statin resulted in an additional 19% relative risk reduction (RRR) in major coronary events and nonfatal MI and a 20% decrease in CVA.[5,142]

There is a dose-related reduction in VLDL of up to 50% and in TG of up to 50% with little to no change or decrease in TC, LDL, or APO-B and no change to a slight increase in HDL.[5,143-146] However, the number of LDL particles decreases and LDL particle size increases from small type B to large type A (increase of 0.25 nm). The antiatherogenic HDL 2 b also increases by up to 29%. The rate of entry of VLDL particles into the circulation is decreased and APOCIII is reduced, which allows lipoprotein lipase to be more active.[27] There is a decrease in remnant chylomicrons and remnant lipoproteins.[5,144] Patients with LDL more than 100 mg/dL have reductions in total LDL, and those that are below 80 mg/dL have mild increases.[145] However, in both cases, the LDL-P decreases, the dense LDL-B increases in size to the less atherogenic LDL-A particle, and APO-B levels decrease. There is a net decrease in the concentration of cholesterol carried by all atherogenic particles and decreases in nonHDL cholesterol. Omega-3 FA are antiinflammatory, antithrombotic, lower blood pressure (BP) and heart rate, improve heart rate variability,[5,139] decrease FA synthesis, increase FA oxidation, and reduce body fat and weight.[5] Omega-3 FAs are one of the only substances that lower lipoprotein-associated phospholipase A2 (Lp-LPA2).[27] Insulin resistance is improved without any significant changes in fasting glucose or hemoglobin A1c with long-term treatment.[147] Doses of 3 g/day of combined EPA and docosahexaenoic acid (DHA) at a 3:2 ratio with gamma linoleic acid (GLA) at 50% of the total EPA and DHA content and 700 mg of gamma/delta tocopherol at 80% and 20% alpha tocopherol per 3 grams of DHA and EPA are recommended.[5] DHA and EPA may have variable but favorable effects on the various lipid levels.[5,143,144,147] EPA does not usually increase LDL, is less effective in lowering TG than DHA, and does not alter the LDL or HDL particle size.

Although DHA may increase total LDL, it increases LDL and HDL size and lowers TG more.[146] New free FA forms of omega-3 FAs have a fourfold greater area under the plasma n-3 polyunsaturated FA (PUFA) curve than prescription Lovaza and thus a more potent reduction in TG levels.[147] The data on krill oil and dyslipidemia are limited to only two studies in humans.[148,149] The first study[148] showed a dose-related response of LDL-C reduction of up to 39%, TG reduction of 27%, and HDL elevation of 60%.[148] Another study[149] showed minimal reductions in TG of 10%, but the decrease was not sustained during long-term treatment. These findings with krill oil are very disparate, and the studies are not confirmatory. Krill oil is not recommended at this time for the treatment of dyslipidemia.

DOSAGE

The dose is 1000–4000 mg/day with a 3:2 ratio of EPA to DHA.

PRECAUTIONS

High doses for prolonged periods can have a prooxidant effect.

The combination of plant sterols and omega-3 FAs is synergistic in improving lipids and inflammation.[98]

Flax

Flax seeds and flax lignan complex with secoisolariciresinol diglucoside (SDG) and increased intake of ALA from other sources such as walnuts have been shown in several meta-analyses to reduce TC and LDL by 5%–15%, Lp(a) by 14%, and TG by up to 36% with either no change or a slight reduction in HDL.[5,150-152] These properties do not apply to flaxseed oil. In the Seven Countries Study, CHD was reduced with increased consumption of ALA. In the Lyon diet trial at the end of 4 years, intake of flax reduced CHD and total deaths by 50%–70%.[5] Flax seeds contain fiber, lignins, and phytoestrogens, which decrease the levels of 7 alpha-hydroxylase and acyl-CoA cholesterol transferase.[5,150-152] Flax seeds and ALA are antiinflammatory, reduce hs-CRP, decrease TG, increase HDL, decrease insulin resistance and the risk of type 2 DM, reduce visceral obesity and systolic BP, increase eNOS, and improve ED. Flax decreases VSM hypertrophy, reduces oxidative stress, and increases cholesterol efflux in macrophage-derived foam cells by decreasing stearoyl-CoA desaturase-1 expressions and farnesoid X receptor's mechanisms of action, which retard the development of atherosclerosis.[5,150-154]

DOSAGE

The dose of flaxseed is 14–40 g/day.[5,150-154] Chia seeds (*Salvia hispanica*) are the richest botanical source of ALA at 60% weight/volume.[153] The dose of chia seeds is 25 g/day.

PRECAUTIONS

None.

Monounsaturated Fatty Acid

MUFAs, such as olives, olive oil, and nuts, reduce LDL by 5%–10%, lower TG by 10%–15%, increase HDL by 5%, decrease oxLDL, reduce oxidation and inflammation, improve ED, lower BP, decrease thrombosis, and reduce the incidence of CHD (Mediterranean diet).[5,155-159] MUFA reduce CD40L gene expression and its downstream products (IL23A, adrenergic B-2 receptor, oxLDL receptor 1, IL-8 receptor) and related genes involved in atherogenic and inflammatory processes in vivo in humans.[159] MUFA are one of the most potent agents to reduce oxLDL in humans.

DOSAGE

The equivalent of 3–4 tablespoons (50 grams) a day of extra-virgin olive oil (EVOO) in MUFA content is recommended for the maximum effect in conjunction with omega-3 FAs.

PRECAUTIONS

None. The caloric intake of this amount of MUFA did not result in any weight gain in the PREDIMED study and resulted in a significant reduction in CVD.[73]

Sesame

Sesame at 40 g/day reduces LDL by 9% through inhibiting intestinal absorption, increasing biliary secretion, decreasing HMG-CoA reductase activity, and upregulating LDL receptor gene expression, 7 alpha-hydroxylase gene expression, and SREBP 2 gene expression.[161,162]

DOSAGE

A randomized placebo-controlled crossover study of 26 postmenopausal women who consumed 50 grams of sesame powder daily for 5 weeks had a 5% decrease in TC and a 10% decrease in LDL-C.[161]

PRECAUTIONS

None.

Tocotrienols

Tocotrienols are a family of unsaturated forms of vitamin E termed *alpha, beta, gamma,* and *delta.*[5] The gamma and delta tocotrienols lower TC by up to 17%, LDL by 24%, APO-B by 15%, and Lp(a) by 17% with minimal changes in HDL and APO A-1 in 50% of subjects at doses of 200 mg/day given at night with food.[5,163-165] The gamma/delta form of tocotrienols are antioxidants and also inhibit cholesterol synthesis by suppression of HMG-CoA reductase activity by two posttranscriptional actions.[5,163-165] These include increased controlled degradation of the reductase protein and decreased efficiency of translation of HMG-CoA reductase mRNA. These effects are mediated by sterol binding of the reductase enzyme to the endoplasmic reticulum membrane proteins called INSIGs.[164] The tocotrienols have natural farnesylated analogs of tocopherols, which give them their effects on HMG-CoA reductase.[164] In addition, the LDL receptor is augmented. Increased intake of alpha-tocopherol (>20% of total tocopherols) may interfere with the lipid-lowering effect.[5,163] Tocotrienols are metabolized by successive beta oxidation then catalyzed by the CYP450 enzymes 3A4 and CYP4F2.

The combination of a statin with gamma/delta tocotrienols further reduces LDL cholesterol by 10%.[163] The tocotrienols block the upregulation of HMG-CoA reductase secondary to competitive inhibition by the statins.[5,163] Carotid artery stenosis regression has been reported in about 30% of subjects given tocotrienols over 18 months. They also slow progression of generalized atherosclerosis.[5,165]

DOSAGE

The recommended dose is 200 mg of gamma and delta tocotrienol at night with food.

PRECAUTIONS

The tocotrienol dose is very important, as increased dosing will induce its own metabolism and reduce effectiveness, whereas lower doses are not as effective.[5] Also, concomitant intake (less than 12 hours) of alpha-tocopherol reduces tocotrienol absorption.

Pantethine

Pantethine is the disulfide derivative of pantothenic acid and is metabolized to cystamine-SH, which is the active form in treating dyslipidemia.[5,166-170] More than 28 clinical trials have shown consistent and significant improvement in serum lipids. TC was decreased by 15%, LDL by 20%, APO-B by 27.6%, and TG by 36.5% over 4–9 months. HDL and APO A-1 was increased by 8%.[5,166-171]

The effects on lipids are slow, with peak effects at 4 months, but may take up to 6–9 months.[5,166-171] In addition, pantethine reduces lipid peroxidation of LDL and decreases lipid deposition, intimal thickening, and fatty streak formation in the aorta and coronary arteries.[5,166-171]

Pantethine inhibits cholesterol synthesis and accelerates FA metabolism in the mitochondria by inhibiting hepatic acetyl-CoA carboxylase, increases CoA in the cytoplasm, which stimulates the oxidation of acetate at the expense of FA and cholesterol synthesis, and increases Krebs cycle activity.[5,166-171] In addition, cholesterol esterase activity increases and HMG-CoA reductase activity decreases.[5,166-171] There is 50% inhibition of FA synthesis and 80% inhibition of cholesterol synthesis.[5] The lipid effects are additive to statins, niacin, and fibrates.

DOSAGE

The recommended effective dose is 300 mg thrice a day or 450 mg twice a day with or without food.[5,166-171]

PRECAUTIONS

None.

Garlic

Numerous placebo-controlled clinical trials and a meta-analysis in humans show reductions in TC of 17 mg/dL and reductions in LDL of about 9 mg/dL at doses of 600–900 mg/day over 2 months with a standardized extract of allicin and ajoene.[5,175-182] Many studies have been poorly controlled and used variable types and doses of garlic, which have given inconsistent results.[5,175,176] Aged garlic (AGE) has shown the best results related to improvement in serum lipids as well as lowering BP, improving endothelial function and arterial elasticity, decreasing coronary artery calcium and plaque progression, and lowering hs-CRP.[5,84,175-182] Eating whole crushed garlic may also be effective, but the most recent studies have used an AGE, which maintains potency and reduces odor. Garlic reduces intestinal cholesterol absorption, inhibits enzymes involved in cholesterol synthesis, and deactivates HMG-CoA reductase.[5,175] In addition, AGE reduces VSM proliferation and transformation, decreases oxidative stress and inflammation, decreases oxLDL, prevents entry of lipids into the arterial wall and macrophages, increases eNOS and NO, increases glutathione, glutathione reductase, and superoxide dismutase, has fibrinolytic activity, and has antiplatelet activity.[5,84,175] AGE has been used in these studies alone or in conjunction with B vitamins, folate, arginine, and statins.[176-179]

DOSAGE

The preferred dose of aged garlic (AGE; Kyloic acid) is 600 mg twice a day.

PRECAUTIONS

Common side effects include bad breath, body odor, and GI distress. Garlic can inhibit platelet function and should be used with caution in those on anticoagulant medications.

Resveratrol

Resveratrol reduces oxLDL; inhibits acyl-coA cholesterol acyltransferase (ACAT) activity and cholesterol ester formation; increases bile acid excretion; reduces TC, TG, and LDL; increases PON-1 activity and HDL; inhibits NADPH oxidase in macrophages; and blocks the uptake of modified LDL by CD36, a scavenger receptor (SR).[183,184] N-acetyl cysteine (NAC) has this same effect on CD36 DR and should be used in conjunction with resveratrol.[183]

DOSAGE

The dose of trans-resveratrol is 250 mg/day and that of NAC is 1000 mg twice a day.

PRECAUTIONS

None.

Curcumin

Curcumin, a phenolic compound in turmeric and curry,[5,185] induces changes in the expression of genes involved in cholesterol synthesis such as the LDL receptor mRNA, HMG-CoA reductase, SREBP, cholesterol 7 alpha-hydroxylase, peroxisome proliferator–activated receptor (PPAR), liver X receptor (LXR), and affects the expression of genes involved in leukocyte adhesion and transendothelial migration to inhibit atherosclerosis.[5,185-188] In one human study of 10 patients consuming 500 mg/day of curcumin, HDL increased by 29% and TC fell by 12%.[5,185] A recent meta-analysis of five studies of 133 subjects did not indicate a significant effect of curcumin on any of the lipid parameters.[188] Larger randomized clinical trials are needed to determine the lipid-lowering effects and potential reduction in CV effects with curcumin.

DOSAGE

The dose is 500–1000 mg twice a day.

PRECAUTIONS

High doses can cause GI upset.

Berberine HCl

Berberine HCl is an alkaloid present in roots, rhizomes, and stem barks of selected plants.[189-191] In a study of 32 dyslipidemic patients, 500 mg/day of berberine HCl decreased TC by 29%, LDL-C by 25%, and TG by 35% in 3 months.[190] Berberine increases hepatic LDL-R and suppresses PCSK9 expression that increases hepatic LDL excretion and is additive to statins in its lipid-lowering effect.[189,190] Berberine has additive LDL-lowering effects with statins[189] and ezetimibe.[191] A meta-analysis of berberine that included 11 randomized trials of 874 subjects showed significant reductions in TC, LDL, and TG and an increase in HDL without any serious adverse effects.[192]

DOSAGE

The recommended dose is 500 mg qd to bid.

PRECAUTIONS

Can cause kernicterus in newborns. Nursing mothers should avoid it. Berberine is more effective and has fewer adverse effects compared with ezetimibe monotherapy.[191]

Pomegranate

Pomegranate increases PON-1 binding to HDL and levels of PON-2 in macrophages. It is a potent antioxidant that increases total antioxidant status (TAS), lowers oxLDL, decreases antibodies to oxLDL, inhibits platelet function, reduces glycosylated LDL, decreases macrophage LDL uptake, and reduces lipid deposition on the arterial wall.[193-198]

These changes impede the progression of carotid artery IMT and lower BP especially in subjects with the highest oxidative stress, known carotid artery plaque, and the greatest abnormalities in TG and HDL levels.[193-198]

DOSAGE

The recommended dose is 8 oz of pomegranate juice or 1–2 cups of pomegranate seeds a day.

Citrus Bergamot

Citrus bergamot has been evaluated in several clinical prospective trials in humans. At doses of 1000 mg/day, this compound lowers LDL by up to 36%, TG by 39%, and increases HDL by 40%.[199-203] Citrus bergamot inhibits HMG-CoA reductase, increases cholesterol and bile acid excretion, binds to the ACAT receptor, and lowers oxLDL.[199-203] Favorable effects on glycemic parameters include reductions in glucose via AMPK and the GLUT4 receptor, reduction in reactive oxygen species (ROS), and weight loss. The active ingredients include naringin, neroeriocitrin, neohesperidin, poncerin, rutin, neodesmin, rhoifolin, melitidine, brutelidine, and vitamin C.[199-205]

DOSAGE

The dose is 1000 mg daily.

Lycopene

Lycopene is an acyclic carotenoid with a high concentration in tomatoes and other rose-colored vegetables and fruit. It has been shown in tissue culture to inhibit HMG-CoA reductase; induce Rho inactivation; increase PPAR gamma, LXR receptor, and RXR activities; increase reverse cholesterol transport and efflux with ABCA1, APO A-1 expression, and caveolin-1 expression; increase HDL 2 and 3; improve HDL functionality; reduce serum amyloid A; decrease CETP; increase PON-1; and reduce inflammation in humans.[206-208] This reduces intracellular cholesterol and lowers cholesterol in lipid domains, which alter membrane-induced cellular signal transduction. The two unconjugated double bonds in the lycopene molecule have high activity against ROS. Higher serum lycopene levels are associated with reductions in carotid IMT and carotid atherosclerosis.[209]

DOSAGE

The doses are lycopene 20 mg/day and astaxanthin 15 mg/day.

Probiotics

Mixed high-dose probiotics at 60–100 billion organisms a day reduce TC by 9%, LDL-C by 8%, and TG by 10%.[211-214] Probiotics precipitate bile salts and deconjugate bile salts with bile salt hydrolase (BHL). They are also incorporated into cell membranes as well as being assimilated into cholesterol itself.

Combinations

A prospective open-label human clinical trial of 30 patients for 2 months showed significant improvement in serum lipids using a proprietary product with a combination of pantethine, plant sterols, EGCG, gamma/delta tocotrienols, and phytolens.[215] TC fell 14%, LDL decreased 14%, VLDL dropped 20%, and small dense LDL particles fell 25% (types III and IV).[215] In another study using the same proprietary product with RYR 2400 mg/day and niacin 500 mg/day, TC fell 34%, LDL decreased by 34%, LDL-P fell 35%, VLDL dropped 27%, and HDL increased 10% (verbal communication, unpublished data).[216]

Studies indicate an RRR of CVD mortality with omega-3 FAs of 0.68, with resins of 0.70, and with statins of 0.78.[217] Combining statins with omega-3 FAs (EFA) decreases CHD 19% more.[142] The combination of gamma/delta tocotrienols and a statin reduces LDL cholesterol an additional 10%.[163] Plant sterols with omega-3 FAs have synergistic lipid-lowering and antiinflammatory effects.[146] A combination of RYR, bitter gourd, chlorella, soy protein, and licorice resulted in significant reductions in TC, TG, and LDL as well as BP in 228 subjects in a controlled clinical trial.[218] AGE alone or in combination with B vitamins, folate, arginine, coenzyme Q10, or statins improves lipids and other markers of endothelial function, vascular elasticity, NO, inflammation, hs-CRP, coronary artery calcium, and plaque regression.[5,84,175-179] Future studies are needed to evaluate various other combinations on serum lipids, surrogate vascular endpoints, and CHD and CVD morbidity and mortality.

PREVENTION PRESCRIPTION

- Nutrition: encourage a traditional Mediterranean diet
- Exercise: 60 min/day for at least 4 days/week with 40 minutes of resistance training and 20 minutes of interval aerobic training

- Maintain an ideal weight

THERAPEUTIC REVIEW

This approach to lipid management to decrease vascular disease utilizes a more functional and metabolic medicine approach with a broader treatment program that addresses the multitude of steps involved in dyslipidemia-induced vascular damage (see Table 27.1). This is a valid alternative for patients who are statin-intolerant, cannot take other drugs for the treatment of dyslipidemia, or in those who prefer alternative treatments.

TESTING

- Evaluate global CV risk with a risk scoring system (see Key Web Resources for a risk calculator)
- Use advanced lipid testing that evaluates LDL-P, LDL particle size, HDL-P, MPO, SAA, and hs-CRP (Table 27.2).
  - LDL-P drives CHD risk

- Reverse cholesterol transport (RCT) and cholesterol efflux capacity (CEC) and HDL-P drive reductions in CHD risk
- HDL is often dysfunctional with inflammation and oxidative stress
- HDL levels more than 85 mg/dL are often dysfunctional
- Measuring MPO and hs-CRP help define dysfunctional HDL

LIFESTYLE

- Identify underlying causes of dyslipidemia; remove and treat them

NUTRITION

- Encourage a Mediterranean-style diet

EXERCISE

- 60 min/day for at least 4 days/week with 40 minutes of resistance training and 20 minutes of interval aerobic training

NUTRITIONAL SUPPLEMENTS

Start with RYR, plant sterols, berberine, and omega-3 FAs. Others are added as needed based on specific needs for lipids as discussed.

- RYR 2400–4800 mg at night with food
- Plant sterols 2.5 g/day
- Berberine 500 mg/day to twice a day
- Omega-3 FAs with EPA/DHA at a 3:2 ratio 4 grams/day with GLA at 50% of the total EPA and GLA and gamma/delta tocopherol
- Niacin (nicotinic acid B3) 500–3000 mg/day as tolerated pretreated with quercetin, apples, and aspirin 81 mg. Take with food and avoid alcohol. Never interrupt therapy.
- AGE Kyolic standardized 600 mg twice a day
- MUFA 20–40 g/day (EVOO 4 tablespoons a day)

- Gamma/delta tocotrienols 200 mg hs
- Sesame 40 g/day
- Pantethine 450 mg bid
- Lycopene 20 mg/day and astaxanthin 15 mg/day
- Trans-resveratrol 250 mg/day with NAC 500 mg twice a day
- Citrus bergamot 1000 mg/day
- Probiotics standardized 15–50 billion organisms bid
- Curcumin 500–1000 mg twice a day
- EGCG 500–1000 mg bid or 60–100 ounces of green tea a day
- Pomegranate 1 cup of seeds/day or 6 ounces of juice a day

PHARMACEUTICALS

- Integrative treatment with statins such as rosuvastatin or a bile acid sequestrant such as colesevelam hydrochloride may be added to the previous nondrug therapies and lifestyle suggestions.

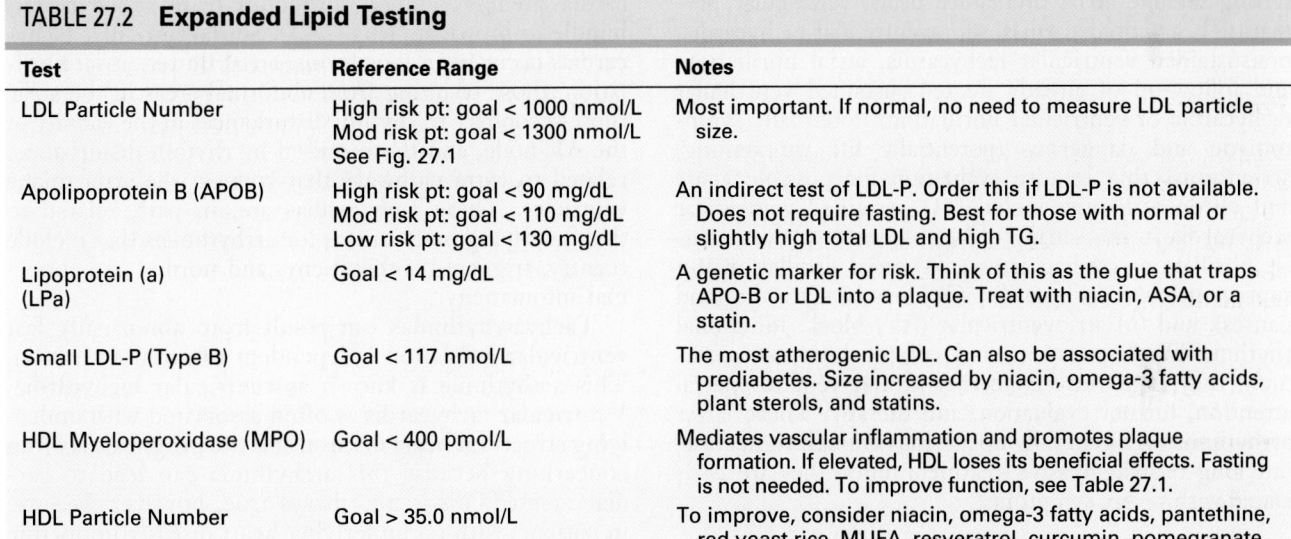

TABLE 27.2 **Expanded Lipid Testing**

Test	Reference Range	Notes
LDL Particle Number	High risk pt: goal < 1000 nmol/L Mod risk pt: goal < 1300 nmol/L See Fig. 27.1	Most important. If normal, no need to measure LDL particle size.
Apolipoprotein B (APOB)	High risk pt: goal < 90 mg/dL Mod risk pt: goal < 110 mg/dL Low risk pt: goal < 130 mg/dL	An indirect test of LDL-P. Order this if LDL-P is not available. Does not require fasting. Best for those with normal or slightly high total LDL and high TG.
Lipoprotein (a) (LPa)	Goal < 14 mg/dL	A genetic marker for risk. Think of this as the glue that traps APO-B or LDL into a plaque. Treat with niacin, ASA, or a statin.
Small LDL-P (Type B)	Goal < 117 nmol/L	The most atherogenic LDL. Can also be associated with prediabetes. Size increased by niacin, omega-3 fatty acids, plant sterols, and statins.
HDL Myeloperoxidase (MPO)	Goal < 400 pmol/L	Mediates vascular inflammation and promotes plaque formation. If elevated, HDL loses its beneficial effects. Fasting is not needed. To improve function, see Table 27.1.
HDL Particle Number	Goal > 35.0 nmol/L	To improve, consider niacin, omega-3 fatty acids, pantethine, red yeast rice, MUFA, resveratrol, curcumin, pomegranate, astaxanthin, and citrus bergamot.

Key Web Resources

National Heart, Lung, and Blood Institute 10-year cardiac risk assessment tool — http://cvdrisk.nhlbi.nih.gov/calculator.asp

HealthPartners shared decision-making tool: "Statins: Should I Take Them?" — https://www.healthwise.net/healthpartners/Content/StdDocument.aspx?DOCHWID=aa44406#av2388

REFERENCES

References are available online at ExpertConsult.com.

CHAPTER 28

ARRHYTHMIAS

Brian Olshansky, MD

Cardiac arrhythmias are slow (brady), fast (tachy), or irregular heart rhythm disturbances (ectopy, atrial fibrillation, and others). Arrhythmias may be a normal phenomenon related to change in autonomic tone; examples include sinus arrhythmia, sinus bradycardia, and sinus tachycardia. Arrhythmias should be evaluated and treated for the following interrelated reasons: (1) to eliminate symptoms, (2) to prevent imminent death and hemodynamic collapse, and (3) to offset long-term risk of serious symptoms and death. This chapter focuses on an approach to evaluate and treat arrhythmias by using an integrative approach.

Common arrhythmias encountered in an office-based setting include atrial premature beats, ventricular premature beats, bradycardias, supraventricular tachycardia, nonsustained ventricular tachycardia, atrial fibrillation, and follow-up of already treated sustained ventricular tachycardia or ventricular fibrillation. Potentially symptomatic and dangerous (potentially life threatening) arrhythmias that require evaluation for possible acute and chronic therapy include (1) sustained ventricular tachycardia in the setting of heart disease, (2) ventricular fibrillation (cardiac arrest), (3) atrial fibrillation, (4) supraventricular tachycardia, (5) sinus bradycardia (and pauses), and (6) atrioventricular (AV) block. Junctional rhythm, AV dissociation, and ectopic beats are common; they may cause concern and may require special attention, further evaluation, and therapy. These latter arrhythmias are generally not serious enough to necessitate long-term aggressive treatment unless they are associated with severe symptoms.

PATHOPHYSIOLOGY

Types and Mechanisms

Heart rhythm disturbances have multiple potential mechanisms and causes. The heart rhythm is a mechanical response to electrical activation of specialized fibers and the atrial and ventricular myocardia. Electrical activation is generally initiated in the sinus node and then leads to activation through various atrial conductive pathways to the AV node, the His–Purkinje system, and the ventricles. The sinus node may be activated slowly as a result of damage to this structure or because of autonomic effects. Increased vagal tone, for example, slows the sinus node rate. Abnormalities in conduction disturbances throughout the normal pathways can also lead to heart block and bradyarrhythmia.

The autonomic nervous system can influence the sinus node either to slow it or to speed it. The autonomic nervous system can also influence other tissue in the heart to make it more automatic, accelerate faster, and overtake normal sinus node activation. This influence can lead to activation resulting from an ectopic focus.

Tachyarrhythmia

Common rhythm disturbances causing an increase in heart rate are known as tachycardias. Tachycardias include sinus tachycardia, which can be a normal response to stress and exercise or an inappropriate acceleration for no apparent reason. Supraventricular tachycardias are less common but require tissue above the His bundle to propagate (Fig. 28.1). Supraventricular tachycardias occur in various forms: atrial flutter, atrial fibrillation, those resulting from abnormal areas in the atria, those secondary to rhythm disturbances in the vicinity of the AV node, and those caused by rhythm disturbances related to extra pathways that connect the atria to the ventricles. These tachycardias are, in part, related to the underlying mechanisms for arrhythmias that include reentry, triggered automaticity, and normal and abnormal automaticity.

Tachyarrhythmias can result from abnormally fast ventricular activation independent of atrial activation. This arrhythmia is known as ventricular tachycardia. Ventricular tachycardia is often associated with underlying structural heart disease, and the prognosis is often concerning because this arrhythmia can lead to cardiac arrest. This is not always true, however, because in patients with no underlying heart disease (idiopathic cause), ventricular tachycardia can have a benign prognosis. Another serious ventricular arrhythmia is ventricular fibrillation. This rhythm disturbance causes cardiac arrest and, without electrical countershock, is fatal.

Other arrhythmias include ventricular ectopic beats, which can manifest as single ectopic beats; bigeminy (every other beat); trigeminy; quadrigeminy; in a fixed coupled fashion; or unrelated to other beats, couplets, triplets, and other forms of nonsustained ventricular tachycardia.

Many potential problems are related to heart rhythm disturbances. Abrupt change in the heart rate, especially with marked slowing or acceleration, can lead to hemodynamic compromise, syncope, and other related symptoms. Rhythm disturbances that are extraordinarily fast or that originate in the ventricles and are associated with structural heart disease can be premonitory signs of cardiac arrest. However, most rhythm disturbances that are seen in clinical practice are benign.

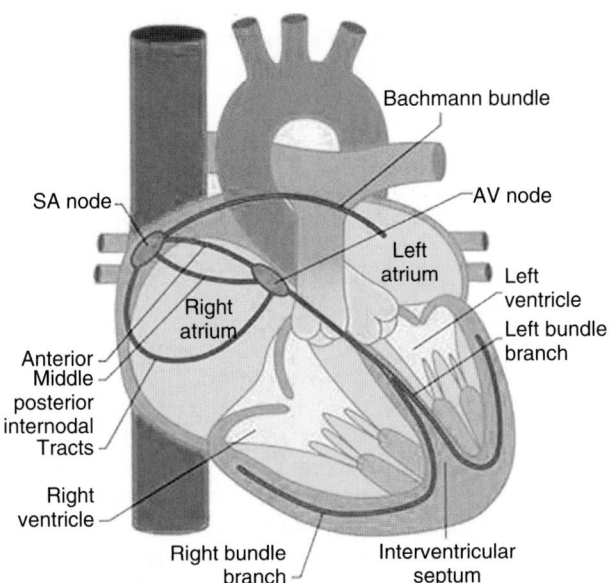

FIG. 28.1 ■ Cardiac anatomy. Cardiac anatomy comprises electrical and structural components. The electrical impulse that directs cardiac contraction originates in the sinoatrial *(SA)* node and is rapidly conducted through the atria by specialized conduction tracts. The impulses merge at the atrioventricular *(AV)* node, where, after a brief pause, they are rapidly conducted into the ventricles through the bundle of His, which is composed of specialized Purkinje cells. Blood moves from the atria into the ventricles through the tricuspid and mitral valves, respectively, during diastole. During systole, blood from the ventricles is pumped into the pulmonary artery and aorta through the pulmonic and aortic valves, respectively. (From Marks AR. Cardiac function and circulatory control. In: *Goldman-Cecil medicine*. Philadelphia, Elsevier; 2016:53, 262-267.e3)

Ectopic Beats

Ectopic beats that trigger palpitations frequently are the result of ventricular ectopic activity (premature ventricular contractions [PVCs]), atrial ectopic activity (premature atrial contractions [PACs]), and atrial arrhythmias such as atrial fibrillation. Ventricular ectopy and atrial ectopy, when not associated with serious underlying structural heart disease, are relatively benign. Although the risk of death may be slightly increased in any patient with PVCs (up to doubling of mortality), the risk remains low in persons with a normal heart. The reason to treat ectopic beats is not to prevent death, but rather to prevent symptoms. Asymptomatic atrial and ventricular ectopy in a patient with no underlying heart disease does not require treatment.

In a study of 1139 patients with normal ventricular ejection fraction and no history of heart failure, participants with the most PVCs compared to those with the least had a 31% increased risk of death.[1]

Symptomatic atrial and ventricular ectopy, however, becomes a major problem to treat in clinical practice for several reasons. First, no good, safe, medical therapies are available.[2-14] Drugs used to suppress ectopy frequently can be proarrhythmic and increase the risk of sudden

death or increase the severity of the arrhythmias, and these agents can have numerous other serious complications. Second, the problem can be highly symptomatic and concerning to the patient, with potentially a tremendous impact on quality of life. Third, the degree of symptoms from benign arrhythmias varies tremendously, and patients who are highly symptomatic may require several types of therapeutic interventions, which can extend as far as drug therapy and even radiofrequency catheter ablation approaches. In some patients, caffeinated beverages, chocolate, and even high sugar levels can trigger ectopic activity.[15,16]

Atrial Fibrillation

Atrial fibrillation is a complex arrhythmia with myriad presentations and therapeutic intervention possibilities. The general approach to atrial fibrillation is threefold: (1) cardiac ventricular rate control, (2) rhythm control, and (3) prevention of thromboembolic events. Although atrial fibrillation is associated with a doubling in mortality, this is not generally the reason for treatment. However, treatment is directed at prevention of symptoms, with treatment of the arrhythmia alone yet to be shown to decrease mortality (it may even increase mortality). Atrial fibrillation occurs in more than 2.2 million U.S. residents.

The most important aspect of the history is to inquire about the ingestion of stimulants such as caffeine, simple sugars, chocolate, pseudoephedrine, ephedra, guarana, ginseng, gotu cola, yohimbe, and others.

People with paroxysms of atrial fibrillation, or at least those patients who present to physicians, are highly symptomatic. Perhaps these patients do not represent the great majority of patients with atrial fibrillation; however, the number of patients with paroxysmal fibrillation who never frequent a health care provider is unknown. In addition, patients with symptomatic atrial fibrillation are not always symptomatic during atrial fibrillation. They often have symptoms when they are in normal sinus rhythm and can be asymptomatic during atrial fibrillation. The presence of persistent paroxysmal or permanent atrial fibrillation frequently inspires long-term treatment and consideration of the threefold treatment approach.

Palpitations

Palpitations are among the most common complaints associated with arrhythmias; the differential diagnosis is extensive. Palpitations can be intermittent or sustained, regular or irregular, and even unrelated to an arrhythmia. Catecholamine excess alone can cause a sensation of palpitations without an arrhythmia even being present.[17]

Some causes of palpitations include the following: anxiety; severe viral syndrome; alcohol; stimulants (cocaine, methamphetamine); stimulant medications including pseudoephedrine; drinks containing caffeine, theobromine, or theophylline; poor sleep (or an irregular sleep cycle); and several supplements (including *Ginkgo biloba*, ephedra, ginseng, guarana, horny goat weed, yohimbe, and others). Hormonal changes and excess thyroid hormone can also lead to palpitations.

Palpitations can represent somatization of a psychiatric disorder. Of 125 outpatients referred for ambulatory electrocardiographic monitoring to evaluate palpitations, 34% had an arrhythmia, whereas 19% had a psychiatric disorder, particularly major depression or a panic disorder.[18] Those with psychiatric disorders were younger, more disabled, and more hypochondriacal about their health. Their palpitations were more likely to last longer than 15 minutes, were accompanied by other symptoms, were more intense, and were associated with more emergency room visits. Several reports have confirmed the high incidence of psychiatric conditions in association with palpitations.[19,20] Nevertheless, careful evaluation of palpitations must rule out organic disease.

Palpitations are only rarely the result of a life-threatening process, although they can be associated with or represent manifestations of underlying ventricular dysfunction or other structural heart disease. Palpitations in a patient with heart disease, especially coronary artery disease, should raise suspicion that the palpitations are the result of an arrhythmia.[21,22]

Approach to the Patient

Perspective

Arrhythmias may have little meaning if they have no prognostic significance, do not alter hemodynamics or cardiac function, and are not symptomatic. Routine screening of an asymptomatic patient is not recommended. Patients typically seek medical care for palpitations, an arrhythmia associated with symptoms, a symptom thought to be caused by an arrhythmia, or nonspecific symptoms that may result from an arrhythmia.

Initial Evaluation and Diagnosis of the Arrhythmia

The initial evaluation includes a careful, circumspect, and complete history (directed toward the symptoms and any potential relationship with an arrhythmia, as well as an assessment of potential responsible conditions), a physical examination, and a 12-lead electrocardiogram at baseline and, if possible, during the arrhythmia. An unhurried, careful, and complete history is the key to appropriate further evaluation, and the clinician should resist the urge to perform expensive, unnecessary, or potentially risky tests. Several issues should be addressed in the history (Table 28.1).

The electrocardiogram recorded during the arrhythmia or while the patient is symptomatic determines the need for further evaluation and treatment. An ambulatory monitor or an event monitor may be needed, in selected patients, to secure a diagnosis. If the symptoms are sporadic, but occur daily, use of an ambulatory (Holter) monitor is the best approach.[23-26] An event recorder or transtelephonic monitor can help make the diagnosis in a patient with less frequent palpitations. Transtelephonic devices are small, lightweight, and inexpensive.

TABLE 28.1   Historical Features of Importance in the Evaluation of the Patient

- Which arrhythmia is present?
- Does the arrhythmia cause symptoms?
- Does the arrhythmia have prognostic significance?
- Is the problem life threatening?
- Does the patient require hospital admission or extensive testing?
- Is specialist consultation required and, if so, how urgently?
- Is treatment required?

The memory feature allows recording of data without the need for immediate access to telephone transmission. One such device is a small patch *(Zio Patch)* that is worn for 2 weeks with a summary of the results sent to the clinician.[27] An implantable monitor (Reveal, Medtronic, Minneapolis, MN) is also available.[28] The device can record events triggered by the patient or by preselected criteria automatically. The device can record up to 42 minutes of data. If episodes are associated with exercise or physical or mental stress, or when an arrhythmia cannot be documented with ambulatory or transtelephonic monitoring, exercise testing may secure a diagnosis.

Risk Assessment

The clinician should determine whether an arrhythmia has prognostic importance: Is it a premonitory sign of death? Several conditions, including ventricular tachycardia and the Wolff-Parkinson-White syndrome (Fig. 28.2), are potentially life threatening. Not all ventricular tachycardias are life threatening; a patient without heart disease, for example, who has idiopathic sustained ventricular tachycardia (*not* idiopathic ventricular fibrillation) has little chance of dying. In contrast, even a single episode of nonsustained ventricular tachycardia in a patient with coronary artery disease and poor left ventricular function, as a result of prior myocardial infarction, may be associated with a poor prognosis.[29]

Rarely, an asymptomatic arrhythmia must be urgently treated. Symptoms and their relationship with the arrhythmia require careful assessment. A correlation of the arrhythmia and symptoms is preferred, although not always possible.

Indications for Inpatient Management

Hospital admission is required if the patient has significant underlying heart disease (e.g., cardiomyopathy with congestive heart failure or coronary heart disease with active ischemia), if the arrhythmia is life threatening and requires rapid reversion (e.g., rapid tachyarrhythmias, polymorphic ventricular tachycardia, prolonged QT interval in a patient with syncope), or if the arrhythmia is uncontrolled or highly symptomatic. Hospital admission is preferred for older patients, who may have not only underlying heart disease, but also other chronic illnesses, such as kidney or liver disease that may affect antiarrhythmic therapy.

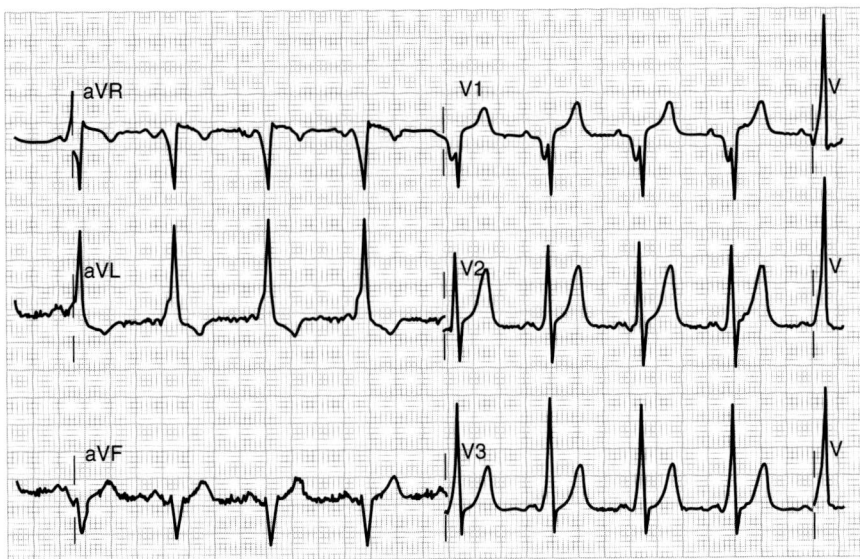

FIG. 28.2 ■ Six leads of an echocardiograph of a patient with Wolff-Parkinson-White syndrome showing delta waves.

Referral to a Specialist

A cardiologist is frequently needed to help manage the complex patient with an arrhythmia; for example, a temporary pacemaker may be needed for a patient with symptomatic bradycardia. Referral to an electrophysiologist may be necessary to institute aggressive acute therapy, such as intravenous amiodarone for life-threatening ventricular tachycardia, antitachycardia pacing for acute reversion of an arrhythmia, for placement of an implantable cardioverter defibrillator (ICD), or to reprogram a pacemaker or an ICD (Table 28.2).

INTEGRATIVE THERAPY

The need for long-term therapy must be carefully individualized to each patient because the severity and importance of symptoms are highly variable. The symptoms associated with any arrhythmia can have an impact on lifestyle, occupation, driving, and other important daily activities. These issues must be considered for every patient and are evaluated as part of a diagnostic and therapeutic approach.

Diet

Gastric Distention

Dietary interventions in some cases can influence some arrhythmias. A large meal can distend the stomach and stimulate vagal afferents thus leading to vagal efferent activation, causing atrial fibrillation in patients who have vagally mediated atrial fibrillation, hypotension, and bradycardia.

Food as a Trigger

Some foods may even act as triggers, and patients will often report some evidence for this. Alcohol is one of the major triggers for atrial fibrillation and ventricular ectopy.[30,31] Caffeine is frequently another trigger for

TABLE 28.2	**Reasons for Referral to a Specialist**

- Resuscitated ventricular fibrillation
- Sustained ventricular tachycardia
- Atrial fibrillation that is difficult to control or refractory to standard therapies
- Nonsustained ventricular tachycardia
- Symptomatic supraventricular tachycardia that is difficult to control
- Sinus bradycardia (sick sinus syndrome, tachy-brady syndrome)
- Second-degree atrioventricular block
- Unexplained ventricular ectopy in the athlete or in a symptomatic patient
- Syncope with a suspected arrhythmic mechanism
- Patients with devices (pacemakers, implantable defibrillators) who are unstable
- Uncontrolled rhythm problems

ectopic beats but not necessarily atrial fibrillation.[15,16] Restriction of alcohol and caffeine may have no effect on arrhythmias. If this is the case, restriction will be of no benefit and may adversely influence the patient's lifestyle. Specific food allergies can trigger a reaction and cause palpitations. Trans fats, particularly of the 18-2 type (found in doughnuts, fried foods, and artificial cheese such as in processed pizza), have been associated with cardiac arrest.[32,33] In contradistinction,[34] omega-3 fatty acids may improve outcomes[34,35]; however, current data do not indicate an antiarrhythmic effect.[36] Fat balance appears to have an effect on cardiovascular health.[37] Alcohol consumption may enhance the effects of omega-3 fatty acids while also potentially triggering atrial fibrillation.[38,39]

The effects of diet on the autonomic nervous system are complex. Several foods increase sympathetic nervous system tone. High levels of sodium also increase the effects of catecholamines and influence ventricular ectopy.[40-45] Caffeine, theophylline, and theobromine present in coffee, tea, and chocolate may be inciting factors, or they may possibly have positive benefits.[46-49] Data indicating that coffee causes atrial fibrillation are questionable.[50,51] Trial and error with these food substances is worthwhile; however, there's no particular reason to eliminate all these foods if they do not have an effect on the arrhythmia. Patients may complain that a specific food triggers a rhythm disturbance by an unknown mechanism. This is not uncommon and is possibly related to some type of allergic reaction or other related issue.

> Gastric distention from large meals, excessive caffeine, alcohol, high levels of sodium, trans fats, severe fluctuations in blood sugar levels, and, possibly, food allergies are potential dietary triggers of cardiac arrhythmias.

Botanical Stimulants of Arrhythmia

Specific supplements can trigger arrhythmias. Ma huang, from the Chinese ephedra plant, contains catecholamines including ephedrine that can initiate ectopic rhythm disturbances and cause life-threatening problems.[52,53] Investigators have even suggested that ambrotose, ginkgo, and other commonly used substances may exacerbate or even cause arrhythmias.

Diet and Anticoagulation

Diet is very important in arrhythmia management, especially in patients who require anticoagulation for atrial fibrillation or other arrhythmias. If the diet changes markedly with significant alterations in vitamin K levels, the prothrombin time will fluctuate tremendously (Table 28.3).

> A balanced diet, low in fat and high in roughage that will lead to a moderate level of blood sugar and as little stress as possible on the gastrointestinal tract, may improve the arrhythmias.

Exercise

Exercise and physical exertion can trigger various arrhythmias. Maintaining excellent physical health through exercise, however, decreases the effects of the sympathetic nervous system on the heart and heart rhythm and improves outcomes in almost all circumstances. The sympathetic nervous system often has a major contributory role in the genesis of serious and benign atrial and ventricular arrhythmias. Exercise performed regularly, with enhancement of aerobic capacity, decreases sensitivity to catecholamines, reduces circulating catecholamine levels, decreases sympathetic nervous system tone, and enhances vagal tone. All these effects increase heart rate variability, which decreases the risk of sudden death and the potential for catecholamine-initiated or sympathetically initiated atrial and ventricular arrhythmias (see Chapter 96). Exercise can also modulate other potential rhythm disturbances, such as sinus

TABLE 28.3	**Therapeutic Review for Nonvalvular Atrial Fibrillation**

1. Address underlying triggers
The most important triggers are hyperthyroidism, hypertension, obesity, alcohol toxicity, obstructive sleep apnea, and a recent pulmonary infection. Also perform an echocardiogram for structural heart disease or congestive heart failure (CHF).

2. Everyone needs rate control
Have a goal of <80 beats/min at rest and <110 beats/min with activity. A 24-hour ambulatory monitor is the most accurate tool to assess this. Rate control will improve symptoms and prevent tachycardia-associated cardiomyopathy.
- Use a beta-blocker if your patient has CHF or coronary artery disease (CAD)
- Use a nondihydropyridine calcium channel blocker (verapamil, diltiazem) in those with lung disease (chronic obstructive pulmonary disease [COPD] and asthma)
- If more rate control is needed, consider adding digoxin, which can work synergistically with beta-blockers and calcium channel blockers.

3. Should I refer to cardiology for rhythm control?
Two large studies on rate vs. rhythm control (the AFFIRM and RACE trials) reported mortality was slightly better with rate control; however, there are some exceptions.
Rhythm control should be considered for the following:
- Younger individuals (<65 years)
- CHF
- Persistent symptoms despite rate control

4. If rhythm control is required, should drugs or ablation be used?
Ablation is more successful but is associated with greater risk. If drugs are not successful, follow with ablation. Amiodarone has the benefit of providing both rate and rhythm control but has liver, lung, and thyroid toxicity.

5. When should I anticoagulate and which anticoagulation drug should I use?
Use the CHA2DS2-VASc and HAS-BLED scores found in "Key Web Resources" to determine the need and risk of anticoagulation. A CHA2DS2-VASc score of 2 or more and a HAS-BLED score of ≤3 warrants anticoagulation with warfarin or a novel oral anticoagulant (NOAC).
- Use warfarin in those with end-stage kidney disease or on dialysis.
- If a NOAC is used in those with chronic kidney disease, the dose needs to be reduced.
- Dual antiplatelet therapy (e.g., aspirin [ASA] and clopidogrel) is no longer recommended due to the risk of bleeding.

tachycardia. Especially in young women, inappropriate sinus tachycardia and postural orthostatic tachycardia syndrome are potential problems.[54] Inappropriate sinus tachycardia is a condition in which the sinus node appears to be hyperactive; the cause is not completely known. It may be, in part, related to abnormal sympathetic nervous system stimulation but may also be an intrinsic problem with the sinus node. Increasing exercise decreases the potential for this problem. Exercise appears to be beneficial in treating many arrhythmias, but it must be used with caution. For patients with malignant arrhythmias, exercise therapy must be prescribed and supervised by a qualified physician who is knowledgeable about the risks, benefits, and methods of monitoring the patient.

Lifestyle

Lifestyle has a major impact on arrhythmias.[55-57] Cigarette smoking and other forms of nicotine have no potential benefit and may be harmful for any individual.[56,58] Nicotine use can exacerbate the risk of sudden death and malignant and benign arrhythmias of all types. Although alcohol may have a beneficial effect on cardiovascular mortality, myocardial infarction, and cholesterol, it has no benefit on any form of arrhythmia. The combination of alcohol and nicotine is even more likely to trigger an arrhythmia.

Mind-Body Therapy

Autonomic variations can occur with numerous lifestyle interventions, including meditation and other mind-body therapies.[59,60] The influence can be profound and may occur by several potential mechanisms: (1) change in autonomic function, (2) placebo effect, (3) direct effect on the rhythm, (4) change in perception of the importance of the arrhythmias to the patient, and (5) shifting of the attention from the arrhythmia to some other issue.

Biofeedback can decrease the number, frequency, and severity of palpitations related to arrhythmias. The effects of biofeedback have been known for some time.[61-65] Another issue is the simple process of developing awareness that a patient can learn to identify a rhythm disturbance as not a potentially noxious experience. The interpretation of the severity of the rhythm disturbance amplifies the severity of the effects on symptoms. Having a patient face the problem can actually empower the patient to improve his or her perception of the arrhythmia and its implications. Ultimately, properly used psychosocial therapy can reduce the risk of death.[66] Biofeedback devices can also be used to enhance heart rate variability (see Chapter 96).

Meditation

Meditation has been shown to be associated with a decreased risk of sudden death in high-risk patients because of a reduction in ventricular fibrillation.[59,60] Meditation may affect the autonomic nervous system in a beneficial way.[67] It may also change the perception of the arrhythmia for patients who have a benign problem.

Meditation and relaxation techniques may also be useful for individuals who have an ICD for life-threatening rhythm disturbances. If the device is activated frequently, it can cause tremendous grief. Meditation and relaxation techniques can improve outcomes in such patients. These techniques may also allow for better patient acceptance of the shocks (see Chapter 100).

Relaxation appears to have a positive benefit. For years, physicians have used benzodiazepines to treat rhythm disturbances, such as atrial fibrillation and supraventricular tachycardia, by inducing relaxation. If a patient comes into an emergency room with such an arrhythmia and is allowed to relax, the rhythm will often stop spontaneously (see Chapter 94).

Acupuncture

Data suggest that acupuncture may be antiarrhythmic for atrial fibrillation.[68] Although acupuncture may affect other arrhythmias beneficially, current data are far from definitive.[69] Acupuncture can also trigger inappropriate shocks in patients with ICDs, and this therapy should be avoided in these patients.[70]

Supplements

Coenzyme Q10

Coenzyme Q10, at a dose of 100–300 mg a day, may decrease episodes of atrial fibrillation by an unknown mechanism. Coenzyme Q10 can also have an effect on ventricular and atrial ectopy.[71]

L-Carnitine

l-Carnitine, at a dose of 3 g a day or more, can improve mitochondrial function and left ventricular function and may prevent some atrial and ventricular arrhythmias. Several small randomized controlled trials of carnitine have reported a reduction in risk of sudden cardiac death and total death in patients with cardiomyopathy. The mechanism is not clear, but it may be attributable to carnitine improving the mitochondrial and myocardial function.[72-74] Carnitine has no known adverse effects. It may reduce ischemia and reperfusion-induced arrhythmias and raise the ventricular fibrillation threshold (of unclear significance).[75]

Magnesium

Magnesium, approximately 1 g a day as a salt (e.g., magnesium sulfate), has been associated with a decrease in arrhythmias. Magnesium can decrease triggered activity and can slow conduction in the AV node.

Magnesium supplementation administered to patients in congestive heart failure in a double-blind, placebo-controlled trial showed improvements in arrhythmias. Individuals taking 3.2 g per day of magnesium chloride equivalent to 384 mg per day of elemental magnesium had between 23% and 52% fewer occurrences of specific arrhythmias over a 6-week follow-up period.[45] Although some data suggested that magnesium had a beneficial effect on atrial fibrillation,[76] other data did not support its use.[77] Magnesium may also be associated with reduced risk of sudden death in women.[78]

Copper and Zinc

Three cases were reported in which ventricular premature beats disappeared, and PVCs decreased, after copper supplementation at a dose of 4 mg per day.[43] Investigators discovered that zinc made the arrhythmias worse and that extra zinc can lead to copper deficiency. The use of copper has a potential problem, however, in that high copper levels can lead to atherosclerosis.

Selenium

A deficiency in selenium can cause heart problems including arrhythmias. No good data, however, are available to suggest that selenium supplementation in patients with low selenium levels will improve arrhythmia status.[40,79]

Potassium

Potassium supplementation is extraordinarily important, especially if a patient is taking drugs that lower potassium levels. Potassium has been implicated in all types of rhythm disturbances, and potassium deficiencies can lead to torsades de pointes. Anyone with long QT interval syndrome, and specifically those patients who take drugs that lower potassium levels, clearly should take potassium supplements. This can also be done through potassium in the diet, including fruits and vegetables that contain high potassium concentrations (see Chapter 89).

Omega-3 Fatty Acids

Omega-3 fatty acids appear to influence several myocardial channels that can affect arrhythmias.[80-84] Specifically, omega-3 fatty acids appear to have an effect on calcium and potassium channels.[85] In men with symptomatic PVCs, omega-3 fatty acids were shown to decrease the risk of PVCs by approximately 70% when supplementation was in the form of fish oil,[86,87] but data are conflicting.[88]

Fish oil was also shown in the second Gruppo Italiano per lo Studio della Sopravvivenza nell'Infarto Miocardico (GISSI2) prevention trial to be associated with a decreased risk of total death and sudden death. This study included 11,324 Italians who had had a myocardial infarction within the preceding 3 months. These patients were randomized to approximately 850 mg of omega-3 polyunsaturated fatty acids (n = 2836), vitamin E (n = 2830), or neither (n = 2828). Patients who were given fish oil had a 45% reduction in sudden death and a 20% decrease in mortality.[85]

The Lyon Diet Heart Study and the Physicians' Health Study both showed a benefit to the use of fish oil. The Diet and Reinfarction Trial (DART) included 2033 men with acute myocardial infarction who were randomized to receive or not to receive advice on diets: decreased fat intake to 30% of total energy, at least two weekly portions (200–400 g) of fatty fish (or 1.5 g fish oil capsules if unable to take fish), and cereal fiber to 18 g daily. Patients who were given "fish advice" survived substantially longer and significantly better.[89]

These data inspired the Fatty Acid Antiarrhythmia Trial, a randomized, placebo-controlled trial of 3 g of fish oil compared with cod-scented olive oil, to look at the incidence of recurrent ventricular arrhythmias in patients who had ICDs and were at risk for sudden death. Many of these patients had malignant ventricular arrhythmias leading to shocks from their device. The aim of this study was to decrease the number of shocks. Fish oil was found to be effective in this study, but data were conflicting.[90]

The data on fish oil in arrhythmias and improving outcomes in patients with heart disease are extensive.[91-93] Although the data in some cases conflict, fish oil is associated with improved autonomic influences,[94-96] reduction in atrial fibrillation[97] (especially after cardiovascular surgery,[98] but not in all studies[99]), reduction in risk of all-cause mortality, reduction in symptomatic ventricular ectopy, and reduction in depression (depression is associated with increased mortality after myocardial infarction).[100] Although some data show benefits for atrial fibrillation,[101] a placebo-controlled study found no value of fish oil.[102]

In addition, data on patients after myocardial infarction have not shown benefit, likely because present therapy is already so good.[103] The higher-risk patients may be the ones who benefit the most.[104] Concerns also exist about the toxins in some of the supplements, including dioxins, polychlorinated biphenyls, polybrominated diphenyl ethers, and chlorinated pesticides.[105]

Omega-3 fatty acids are available in various forms, not only fish oil.[106] Certain plant oils can be metabolized into omega-3 fatty acids, including flaxseed oil, which also has other potential benefits,[107] including those on mood. Because omega-3 fatty acids can improve mood, they may also have an autonomic affect that can decrease the sensation of arrhythmias or decrease arrhythmias altogether.

> For dosing omega-3 fatty acids, educate the patient to read labels. If you are recommending 1000 mg of omega-3 fatty acids, the user needs to look at the amount of eicosapentaenoic acid (EPA) and docosahexaenoic acid (DHA) per serving size. If the label notes 300 mg of EPA and 200 mg of DHA per two capsules (serving size), the patient would need to take four capsules daily to obtain 1000 mg of omega-3 fatty acids.

Vitamins

A long-standing case of sick sinus syndrome was reported to resolve with supplementation of 800 units per day of vitamin D.[108] However, it was not clear that vitamin D was the cause of this change.

Data indicate that vitamin C given postoperatively to patients at risk for atrial fibrillation and to patients who undergo coronary artery bypass graft surgery may lead to a marked reduction in atrial fibrillation[109-113]; however, these data have not been confirmed. Although the underlying mechanism is unknown, vitamin C appears to have antiarrhythmic properties and can prevent atrial fibrillation, at least in some patients. The mechanism may be by clearance of free radicals or by an antiinflammatory effect.

Botanicals

Many of the original antiarrhythmic drugs were derived from herbal therapy: quinidine (a stereoisomer of quinine from cinchona bark), lidocaine, amiodarone (from khellin, derived from the herb *Ammi visnaga*), and digoxin (from foxglove) are a few.[114,114a-c] Data suggest that several other herbal preparations may have antiarrhythmic effects.

Ciwujia or Siberian ginseng (*Acanthopanax senticosus* harms), which is used for athletic performance and weight loss, may have antiarrhythmic effects. Ciwujia was studied in isolated rat hearts with transient coronary occlusion.[115] Ciwujia extract reduced reperfusion-induced ventricular fibrillation and ventricular tachycardia. It also reduced the number of cells with abnormal action potential configurations. Ciwujia may reduce the incidence of malignant arrhythmias.[115] Siberian ginseng can cause an apparent increase in digoxin levels.[116] Whether this finding represents a false serum elevation, whether ginseng converts to digoxin in vivo, or whether ginseng alters the metabolism of digoxin is unclear.

Angelica and *Ginkgo biloba* may have a protective influence during myocardial ischemia and reperfusion.[117] In a rat model, the incidence of ventricular premature beats and the total incidence of arrhythmia were greatly reduced.[118]

Licorice root has been shown to have an antiarrhythmic property.[119] Zhi gan cao (prepared licorice) injection can antagonize arrhythmias induced by chloroform, catecholamines, aconitine, strophanthin-K, and barium chloride. Licorice root may slow the heart rate, prolong PR and QT intervals, and antagonize the positive chronotropic response induced by catecholamines. Another component of licorice, sodium 18 beta-glycyrrhetinate, strongly counteracts arrhythmia induced by chloroform, lengthens the appearance time of arrhythmia induced by $CaCl_2$, slightly retards the heart rate of rats and rabbits, and partly antagonizes the acceleration effect of isoproterenol on rabbit hearts. The clinical significance of these experimental findings is unclear.[120]

Various herbs are now considered potentially useful by some practitioners to treat ventricular and supraventricular arrhythmias. Motherwort contains butenolide, glycosides (stachydrine), and alkaloids. A dose between 4 and 5 g of motherwort can decrease palpitations, presumably by a mild beta-blocking affect, although the exact mechanism that motherwort exerts on the heart to decrease ectopic beats is unclear. No randomized controlled trial has been performed using motherwort.

> Think of motherwort as the "beta blocker" of the botanicals.

Khella (*Ammi visnaga*) has significant antiarrhythmic effects. In the 1950s, a compound known as khella was derived from the *Ammi visnaga* plant and used to treat angina resulting from coronary heart disease, with significant improvement in those patients. Khella has also been used over the years by naturopaths to decrease palpitations. Khella is the original substance from which a very potent antiarrhythmic drug, amiodarone, was derived.[121-123]

Hawthorn berry has been used to treat atrial fibrillation and may also have an effect on other rhythm disturbances.[116] Hawthorn contains hyperoside (vitexin, rhamnose), rutin, and oligomeric procyanidins. A dose of 160–900 mg of the water ethanol extract is recommended. Exactly how this herb works is unknown, but it may act on the sodium-potassium adenosine triphosphatase pump similar to digoxin. More likely, hawthorn acts as a phosphodiesterase inhibitor. Hawthorn may reduce the risk of sudden death and help treat patients in heart failure, and may have other benefits.[124,125]

Rhodiola may have had some antiarrhythmic effects in a rat model in which arrhythmias were induced by epinephrine and calcium chloride.[126] Rhodiola can increase the ventricular fibrillation threshold,[127] and although this effect may be beneficial, the meaning is uncertain. The antiarrhythmic effect of rhodiola may result from activation of the opioid system and stimulation of kappa-opioid receptors.[128]

Data suggest that garlic, agrimony, celery, ginger, berberine, corkwort, *Stephania tetandra* root, astragalus, *Fissistigma glaucescens*, xin bao, bu xin, yu zhu, and mai dong, among others, are antiarrhythmic under various experimental conditions and for various arrhythmias. At the present time, however, the data are not definitive enough to recommend treatment with any of these herbal therapies for a specific arrhythmia.

Pharmaceuticals

The standard first-line drug therapy approach for benign PVCs, PACs, and episodes of atrial fibrillation is often a beta-adrenergic blocking drug. This class of drug alters the autonomic nervous system tone on the heart, although the effectiveness of this approach is unclear. Good data suggest that it is not effective whatsoever. Further, side effects are common when using these therapies for ectopic beats.

For atrial fibrillation, various antiarrhythmic drugs are available.[129] Their use depends on the underlying heart disease, link to the episodes, age of the patient, severity of symptoms, and the difficulty in maintaining sinus rhythm (see Table 28.3)

For ventricular ectopy and PVCs, if beta-blockers do not work, various antiarrhythmic drugs can be used including, for normal hearts without any evidence of ischemic heart disease, class IC antiarrhythmic drugs such as propafenone and flecainide.[6,7] One concern about these antiarrhythmic drugs, like any antiarrhythmic drug, is they can triple the mortality rate if underlying heart disease is present. The use of these drugs is never completely safe, and they can have other so-called proarrhythmic effects.[2-9]

Numerous other antiarrhythmic drugs can be used, but each one of them has significant side effects. The use of these drugs is discouraged for benign ventricular ectopy unless the patient is severely symptomatic.

Although antiarrhythmic drugs can suppress arrhythmias, the important issues of proarrhythmia and side effects must be considered. All antiarrhythmic drugs have the potential to increase ectopy or induce, or aggravate, monomorphic ventricular tachycardia, torsades de pointes, ventricular fibrillation, conduction disturbances, or bradycardia. This is known as proarrhythmia.[2-9] The use of antiarrhythmic drugs should be reserved for clinicians who are expert in their use.

The risk of proarrhythmias from medication is greatest in those who need the most protection, specifically those patients with depressed left ventricular function with an ejection fraction less than 30%.

Risk-to-Benefit Ratio

The goal of therapy for any arrhythmia is to eliminate symptoms or prevent a potentially serious outcome, primarily a life-threatening arrhythmia and sudden death. These goals must be balanced against the risks associated with antiarrhythmic therapy, including proarrhythmia and the side effects of individual drugs.

No study has shown that ventricular ectopy suppression in any group of patients with asymptomatic arrhythmia improves survival. The only reason to treat is to suppress symptoms from arrhythmias as long as treatment does not worsen arrhythmias and the prognosis.

Ablation Therapy

Another potential treatment that is nonpharmacological is ablation therapy. Occasionally, ablation therapy can be used to remove focal triggers for rhythm disturbances in the atrium or ventricles for eliminating PACs and PVCs.

Occasionally, a patient with ventricular bigeminy does not perfuse with the PVC and therefore has an underlying rapid ventricular rate without adequate perfusion, especially during the PVC. Such a patient can develop tachycardia-mediated cardiomyopathy, and heart failure will ensue. This problem can be eliminated by treating the PVC. Ablation therapy is also used to treat various supraventricular tachyarrhythmias. In fact, atrial fibrillation, especially when paroxysmal, can be treated by ablating focal ectopic beats that often originate from the pulmonary veins.

CONCLUSION

Arrhythmia management is complex and multifaceted. Treatment depends on the arrhythmia, its implications, the symptoms, and the effect on the patient. Patients with serious rhythm disturbances must be referred to a specialist, especially if the arrhythmias are potentially life threatening. If not, an approach to improve outcomes should involve change in lifestyle and exercise. Following these dietary recommendations may be useful. If this is not enough, mind-body effects can be substantial. Consider meditation. Acupuncture can have beneficial effects as well. Several herbal preparations may influence the presence of an arrhythmia; however, care must be taken because some supplements, such as ma huang, can worsen an arrhythmia or even create a new, life-threatening one.

PREVENTION PRESCRIPTION

- Avoid arrhythmia triggers if identified and definable (e.g., excess caffeine intake).
- Encourage regular aerobic exercise as long as it does not trigger arrhythmias.
- Urge risk factor reduction to prevent the development of structural heart disease (treatment of hypercholesterolemia, hypertension, smoking, or excess ethanol intake).
- Moderate balanced caloric intake and maintenance of appropriate weight.
- Prevent stress. Incorporate meditation, yoga, and bioenergy techniques.
- Maintain a regular sleep-wake cycle with at least 7–8 hours of sleep nightly.
- Encourage two to three servings of fish a week and, if unable, consider supplementing with 1–2 g of fish oil.
- Avoid the use of drugs or supplements that stimulate or mimic the effect of catecholamines (e.g., over-the-counter decongestants, ephedra [ma huang], and caffeine).

THERAPEUTIC REVIEW

The treatment of arrhythmias cannot be easily standardized and does not fit into any clearly defined algorithmic pathway. The reason for this is the diverse presentations of arrhythmias, the complexity of management, the great span of problems ranging from completely benign to clearly life threatening, the lack of randomized controlled clinical data in some instances, the difficulty in diagnosing problems, and the overlap with many other syndromes. Despite these caveats, some rational common sense recommendations can be set forth to manage patients who have suspected cardiac arrhythmias.

FOR PATIENTS WITH PALPITATIONS

- Diagnosis is crucial, and arrhythmias can range from sinus rhythm through various types of ectopy to supraventricular or ventricular tachycardia.
- If no arrhythmia is documented, consider anxiety or panic attacks and treat accordingly.

- Encourage stress reduction techniques such as meditation and yoga. B 1

FOR PATIENTS WITH SYMPTOMATIC ECTOPY OR PREMATURE VENTRICULAR CONTRACTIONS

Lifestyle

- Determine the severity of the symptoms and their relation to the arrhythmia. Assess underlying conditions.
- Determine the risk to the patient.
- For proven benign ectopy, discuss the risks of drug therapy and suggest alternatives first.

Nutrition

- Eliminate dietary or other apparent triggers (caffeine, alcohol, trans-fatty foods, blood glucose fluctuations). B 1

Mind-Body Therapy

- Promote mind-body interventions such as meditation, yoga, Reiki, or qi gong.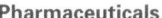
- Counsel the patient about the benign nature of the condition. Patients who understand will be able to tolerate the arrhythmia better.

Exercise

- Determine the relation to exercise, and consider a tailored exercise program.

Supplements and Botanicals

- Suggest omega-3 fatty acids: 2–3 g/day of eicosapentaenoic acid plus docosahexaenoic acid essential fatty acids
- Magnesium supplementation: 300–1000 mg daily
- Consider herbal approaches: motherwort, 4–5 g of dried above-ground parts daily
- Consider carnitine: 3 g daily and then coenzyme Q10: 100–300 mg daily with a meal

Pharmaceuticals

- Drug therapy: only if resistant to foregoing measures
- Beta blockade (titrated upward): consider extended-release metoprolol (Toprol XL), 50, 100, or 200 mg daily; or atenolol, 50–100 mg daily
- Calcium channel blockers (diltiazem or verapamil): 120–360 mg daily
- Antiarrhythmic drugs: used as last resort (if no structural heart disease, flecainide, propafenone, sotalol are the first choices; then amiodarone, but only in resistant, highly symptomatic cases; risks may outweigh benefits)

Ablation Therapy

- Suggest ablative therapy for motivated patients willing to take the excess risk (counsel patients that symptoms are benign)

FOR PATIENTS WITH PAROXYSMAL ATRIAL FIBRILLATION

Lifestyle and Risk Factors

- Correlate symptoms with the arrhythmia. Determine the presence of underlying conditions, including hyperthyroidism.
- Assess the risk to the patient and the need for rate control, anticoagulation, and maintenance of sinus rhythm (see Table 28.3).

Nutrition

- Determine triggers, if possible. If a relationship is determined, eliminate caffeine, alcohol, and any potentially offending drug.

- If arrhythmia occurs at night, consider changes in diet (no large meals causing gastric distention).

Exercise

- If arrhythmia is exercise related, consider an exercise program.

Mind-Body Therapy

- Promote mind-body interventions such as relaxation techniques.
- Counsel patients and educate them about the disease process.

Acupuncture

- Suggest acupuncture (not well tested but perhaps effective).

Supplements and Botanicals

- Omega-3 fatty acids: 2–3 g of fish oil daily.
- Magnesium supplementation: 300–1000 mg daily.
- Coenzyme Q10: 100–300 mg daily with a meal.
- Hawthorn berry: 160–900 mg daily.
- Motherwort: 4–5 g daily.

Pharmaceuticals

- Beta blockade (to control rhythm and rate): see earlier for dosage.
- Calcium channel blockade (to control rate, diltiazem or verapamil): 120–360 mg daily.
- Digoxin (little effect, but may help in combination with a beta blocker and is safe if used carefully at appropriate doses).
- Antiarrhythmic drugs depend on the patient and the conditions. The risk-to-benefit ratio is complex and depends on other diagnosed conditions, symptoms, and antiarrhythmic drugs. Amiodarone is the most effective drug but has the greatest risk of side effects. Propafenone and flecainide can triple the risk of death in patients with underlying heart disease and are contraindicated in patients with coronary disease or impaired ventricular function.

Ablation Therapy

- Ablation of the pulmonary veins or parts of the left atrium.
- Ablation of the atrioventricular node with a pacemaker (patient remains in atrial fibrillation) not completely effective.
- Ablation of other inciting arrhythmias.

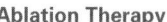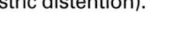

Key Web Resources

CHA2DS2-VASc Score for Atrial Fibrillation Stroke Risk. This tool calculates the need for anticoagulation to reduce the risk of stroke in patients with atrial fibrillation.

http://www.mdcalc.com/cha2ds2-vasc-score-for-atrial-fibrillation-stroke-risk/

HAS-BLED Score. Determines the risk of bleeding for those patients who may benefit from anticoagulation.

http://www.mdcalc.com/has-bled-score-for-major-bleeding-risk/

Surgical Risk Prediction. This tool assesses surgical risk of patients seen for preoperative physical examinations.

http://riskcalculator.facs.org/RiskCalculator

Risk Assessment Tool for Estimating 10-Year Risk of Developing Hard Coronary Heart Disease. This tool from the National Cholesterol Education Program assesses 10-year cardiovascular risk.

http://www.nhlbi.hin.gov/health-pro/guidelines/current/cholesterol-guidelines/quick-desk-reference-html/10-year-risk-framingham-table

emWave by HeartMath. This biofeedback tool helps enhance heart rate variability.

http://www.heartmath.com

Integrative Medicine Program, University of Wisconsin School of Medicine and Public Health. This is a patient handout on omega-3 fatty acids.

http://www.fammed.wisc.edu/sites/default//webfm-uploads/documents/outreach/im/handout_omega3_fats_patient.pdf

NOACs for Nonvalvular Atrial Fibrillation

NOAC	Dosage	Benefits/Risks Compared to Warfarin
Dabigatran (Pradaxa)	Creatinine clearance (CrCl) ≥ 30 = 150 mg bid CrCl 15–30 = 75 mg bid	Less intracranial and fatal bleeds Higher rate of GI bleeds
Rivaroxaban (Xeralto)	20 mg/day with evening meal CrCl 30–50 requires close monitoring CrCl ≤ 30: Avoid the use of NOACs	Less intracranial and fatal bleeds
Apixaban (Eliquis)	5 mg bid ↓dose to 2.5 mg bid if any two of the following: Age ≥ 80 Weight ≤ 60 kg Serum Cr ≥ 1.5 mg/dL	Less intracranial bleeds same GI bleeds. One study showed bleeding risk to be similar to ASA in those who were unsuitable for warfarin.

Adapted from Prystowsky EN, Padanilam BJ, Fogel RI. Treatment of atrial fibrillation. *JAMA.* 2015;314:278-288 and Moss JD, Cifu AS. Management of anticoagulation in patients with atrial fibrillation. *JAMA.* 2015;314:291-292.

REFERENCES

References are available online at ExpertConsult.com.

SECTION V

ALLERGY/INTOLERANCE

SECTION OUTLINE

29 ASTHMA

30 THE ALLERGIC PATIENT

31 FOOD ALLERGY AND INTOLERANCE

287

CHAPTER 29

ASTHMA

John D. Mark, MD

PATHOPHYSIOLOGY

Asthma is a common chronic respiratory disorder characterized by episodes of airway obstruction and reversibility. Asthma affects more than 25 million persons in the United States, of which approximately 18 million are adults.[1] Asthma is known to be a complex inflammatory process caused by many factors including genetic predisposition, environmental exposures, viral infections, and other host factors such as lack of breastfeeding, second-hand smoke exposure, and prenatal stress.[2] The symptoms of asthma are usually recurrent episodes of wheezing, dry cough, chest tightness, and breathlessness. This chronic inflammation leads to bronchial hyperresponsiveness to various stimuli and results in the clinical manifestations and severity of asthma as well as subsequent responses to treatment.

Research into the immunological basis of asthma has shown that in susceptible individuals, chronic inflammation of the airways occurs and is characterized by infiltration of mast cells, eosinophils, and T-helper cell type 2 (Th2) CD4+ T-lymphocytes. Eosinophils are recruited via a chemical gradient due to the release of chemotactic agents, such as interleukin (IL)-5, and induce epithelial damage. This Th2 response within the lung then triggers an aberrant injury-repair mechanism that may lead to airway remodeling.[3] Finally, Th2 cells induce the production of allergic antibody immunoglobulin E (IgE), ultimately resulting in the clinical manifestation of allergy and asthma.

Risk Factors and Triggers

Investigators believe that asthma often begins in childhood and may result from an interaction of several factors (Fig. 29.1). Studies of case-controls and genomic linkages have identified 10 genomic regions and more than 100 genes associated with allergy and asthma. There are consistently replicated regions on the long arms of chromosomes 2, 5, 6, 12, and 13. This wide heterogeneity illustrates that the basis of asthma is both genetic predisposition and gene-by-environmental interactions.[4] Thus the natural course of asthma varies considerably according to asthma phenotype and various environmental influences.

Asthma symptoms can be triggered by a variety of exposures (Table 29.1). Infections with viruses, such as respiratory syncytial virus and rhinovirus, have been thought to be triggers not only because they cause airway swelling and obstruction, but also because they influence cellular responses of the immune system increasing, thereby increasing susceptibility to asthma. The lung microbiome may also play a significant role in both the etiology of asthma and in asthma control. Certain viral and bacterial infections may alter the asthma phenotype. Recent studies have shown that bacterial colonization of the airways in neonates with *S. pneumonia*, *H. influenza*, and *M. catarrhalis* are associated with an increased risk of pneumonia and bronchiolitis in early childhood independent of current asthma.[5] Once microbes become established in the lungs, a balance to maintain homeostasis may occur. Any imbalance in the microbial community may cause airway disease, such as asthma. Establishment of the lung microbiome is not static but dynamic and may affect the relationship between the microbiota and lung-specific immunity.[6]

Other key factors associated with poor asthma control include overestimation of asthma control by patients and physicians, improper technique in using inhaled medications, and nonadherence to therapies (particularly controller medications). These factors may lead to increased exacerbations, more hospitalizations, and higher mortality rates.[7] Understanding current asthma guidelines, measuring lung function, and monitoring medication use, in addition to improving adherence and education, may improve asthma control (Fig. 29.2).

INTEGRATIVE THERAPY

Lifestyle

Environment

Reducing exposure to environmental triggers, such as dust mites and cockroaches, to which many patients with asthma are sensitive is important. House dust mites, which are microscopic insects that live off dead skin cell flakes, are all around us despite being too small to see. The mites and their waste products can be allergenic. To limit exposure to dust mites, particularly in the bedroom where they are most common, one should (1) enclose pillows and mattresses in airtight polyurethane covers or use fiberfill products instead of down or foam pillows, (2) remove carpeting (hardwood or linoleum floor is better) and curtains, (3) wash sheets and stuffed toys (for pediatric patients) in hot water every week, and (4) clean bedrooms frequently with a vacuum that has a high-efficiency particulate air (HEPA) filter. Cockroaches and their feces are also a recognized trigger for asthma, so cleanliness is important to decrease their presence. In addition, it helps to wash floors and counters frequently to eliminate cockroach debris. Other important control measures include eliminating exposure to tobacco smoke and removing pets from the home.

Asthma is a chronic airway inflammation

Environmental risk factors/Genetic predisposition

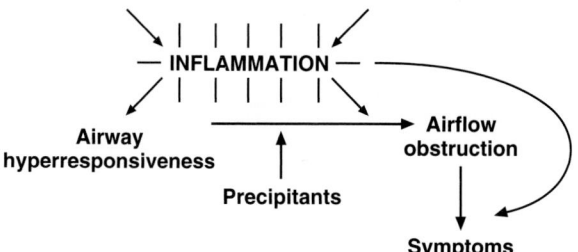

FIG. 29.1 ■ Asthma severity may change with environment, activities, and other factors. When the patient is well, monitoring and treatment are still needed to maintain control.

TABLE 29.1	**Triggers of Asthma Symptoms**

- Allergens, such as house dust mites, pets, and pollens
- Colds and viral infections
- Exercise
- Gastroesophageal reflux disease (stomach acid flowing back up the esophagus)
- Medications and foods
- Emotional anxiety
- Air pollutants, such as tobacco smoke, wood smoke, chemicals, and ozone
- Occupational exposure to allergens, vapors, dust, gases, and fumes
- Strong odors and sprays, such as perfumes, household cleaners, cooking fumes, paints, and varnishes

---

Nutrition

Diet therapy or nutritional advice is the most common "alternative" therapy prescribed by nonallopathic physicians for patients with asthma. In theory, diet can modulate intestinal flora (gut microbiome), affect immune maturation, and interact with underlying genetic dispositions in the development and even the origin of asthma. Nutrition, including the type of foods (saturated fats, amount of fiber), may influence the gut microbiome; studies have shown that having fewer bacterial species, such as *Lactobacilli*, *Bacteroidetes*, and *Bifidobacteria*, in addition to having more coliform bacteria, such as a *Clostridia* and *Enterococci*, may lead to allergic sensitization.[8] Clinicians have long thought that eliminating certain "allergenic" foods and decreasing exposure to foods, such as dairy products (believed to be associated with increased mucus production), will help improve chronic asthma symptoms and their severity; however, studies have not supported this theory.[9] Avoidance of certain foods or food types is a common practice. Food-induced asthma is rare; however, many patients feel that certain foods can trigger asthma exacerbations, so an elimination diet may be used.[10] The easiest way to conduct an elimination diet is to pick a food to which the patient appears to be sensitive, such as nuts or eggs, and then eliminate it from the diet for 2 weeks. At the end of 2 weeks, gently reintroduce the food into the diet. If a significant change occurs, such as bloating or headaches, the

patient may indeed be sensitive to that particular food (see Chapter 86). Epidemiological studies have indicated that dietary habits influence lung function, with populations with a higher intake of polyunsaturated fatty acids (omega-6 fatty acids) shown to have a higher prevalence of asthma, eczema, and allergic rhinitis, and those with increased intake of omega-3 fatty acids to have a lower prevalence of atopy and asthma.[11] The use of the Mediterranean diet, which includes high consumption of fruits, vegetables, olive oil, whole grains, regular fish intake (with decrease in meat), has been posited to have utility in both preventing and treating asthma.[12,13]

The following are the nutritional recommendations for patients with asthma:
1. Eliminate potential allergens:
   a. Any food associated with a history of intolerance (gastrointestinal disturbance or eczema)
   b. Sulfites (especially in dried fruits)
   c. Food additives (aspartame, benzoates, and yellow dye no. 5)
   d. Dairy products (for a trial period, as mentioned previously)
2. Increase intake of fruits and vegetables because they are rich in antioxidants, levels of which have been shown to be low in patients with chronic lung problems such as asthma.
3. Increase intake of omega-3 fatty acids by eating cold-water fish (e.g., sardines, herring, and salmon) and reduce intake of omega-6 fatty acids by eliminating vegetable oils and instead using olive oil (see Chapter 88).

If intake of dairy products is decreased or eliminated (especially in children), a calcium supplement should be considered.

Exercise

Although exercise can induce symptoms in patients with asthma, numerous studies have shown that asthma can be better controlled in patients who exercise regularly. No study has yet reported the superiority of one type of exercise over another. Investigators have long assumed that swimming may be beneficial as the environment is moister and cold, dry air may exacerbate asthma symptoms. However, studies have not supported this concept. Instead, any type of exercise performed on a regular basis that does not increase symptoms should be encouraged. In addition, studies have reported that swimming in highly chlorinated pools or indoor pools with possible mold exposure may exacerbate asthma symptoms.[14] A recent Cochrane review concluded that the overall quality of studies regarding water-based exercise and asthma was low but did observe clear differences between water-based exercise and comparator treatments.[15] The older the patient, the greater the efficacy of exercise regimens in managing asthma. This effect may, in part, be attributable to improved self-image and overall health associated with regular exercise in adults.

STEPWISE APPROACH FOR MANAGING ASTHMA LONG TERM

The stepwise approach tailors the selection of medication to the level of asthma severity or asthma control.
The stepwise approach is meant to help, not replace, the clinical decisionmaking needed to meet individual patient needs.

Assess control:

Step up if needed (first, check medication adherence, inhaler technique, environmental control, and comorbidities)

Step down if possible (and asthma is well controlled for at least 3 months)

		STEP 1	STEP 2	STEP 3	STEP 4	STEP 5	STEP 6
	At each step: Patient education, environmental control, and management of comorbidities						
0–4 years of age		**Intermittent asthma**	**Persistent asthma: daily medication** Consult with asthma specialist it step 3 care or higher is required. Consider consultation at step 2.				
	Preferred treatment[†]	SABA* as needed	Low-dose ICS*	Medium-dose ICS*	Medium-dose ICS* + Either LABA* or montelukast	High-dose ICS* + Either LABA* or montelukast	High-dose ICS* + Either LABA* or montelukast + Oral corticosteroids
	Alternative treatment[††‡]		Cromolyn or montelukast				
		If clear benefit is not observed in 4–6 weeks, and medication technique and adherence are satisfactory, consider adjusting therapy or alternate diagnoses.					
	Quick-relief medication	• SABA* as needed for symptoms: intensity of treatment depends on severity of symptoms. • With viral respiratory symptoms: SABA every 4–6 hours up to 24 hours (longer with physician consult). Consider short course of oral systemic corticosteroids if asthma exacerbation is severe or patient has history of severe exacerbations. • Caution: frequent use of SABA may indicate the need to step up treatment.					
5–11 years of age		**Intermittent asthma**	**Persistent asthma: daily medication** Consult with asthma specialist it step 4 care or higher is required. Consider consultation at step 3.				
	Preferred treatment[†]	SABA* as needed	Low-dose ICS*	Low-dose ICS* + Either LABA*, LTRA* or theophylline(b) OR medium-dose ICS	Medium-dose ICS* + LABA*	High-dose ICS* + LABA*	High-dose ICS* + LABA* + Oral corticosteroids
	Alternative treatment[††‡]		Cromolyn, LTRA* or theophylline[§]		Medium-dose ICS* + Either LTRA* or theophylline[§]	High-dose ICS* + Either LTRA* or theophylline[§]	High-dose ICS* + Either LTRA* or theophylline[§] + Oral corticosteroids
			Consider subcutaneous allergen immunotherapy for patients who have persistent, allergic asthma.**				
	Quick-relief medication	• SABA* as needed for symptoms. The intensity of treatment depends on severity of symptoms: up to 3 treatments every 20 minutes as needed. Short course of oral systemic corticosteroids may be needed. • Caution: Increasing use of SABA or use >2 days/week for symptom relief (not to prevent EIB*) generally indicates inadequate control and the need to sleep to step up treatment.					
≥12 years of age		**Intermittent asthma**	**Persistent asthma: daily medication** Consult with asthma specialist it step 4 care or higher is required. Consider consultation at step 3.				
	Preferred treatment[†]	SABA* as needed	Low-dose ICS*	Low-dose ICS* + LABA* OR medium-dose ICS*	Medium-dose ICS* + LABA*	High-dose ICS* + LABA* AND consider omalizumab for patients who have allergies[††]	High-dose ICS* + LABA* + oral corticosteroids[§§] AND consider omalizumab for patients who have allergies[††]
	Alternative treatment[††‡]		Cromolyn, LTRA* or theophylline[§]	Low-dose ICS* + Either LTRA* theophylline,[§] or zileuton[‡‡]	Medium-dose ICS* + Either LTRA* theophylline,[§] or zileuton[‡‡]		
			Consider subcutaneous allergen immunotherapy for patients who have persistent, allergic asthma.**				
	Quick-relief medication	• SABA* as needed for symptoms. The intensity of treatment depends on severity of symptoms: up to 3 treatments every 20 minutes as needed. Short course of oral systemic corticosteroids may be needed. • Caution: Use of >2 days/week for symptom relief (not to prevent EIB*) generally indicates inadequate control and the need to sleep to step up treatment.					

* **Abbreviations:** EIB, exercise-induced bronchospasm; ICS, inhaled corticosteroid; LABA, inhaled long-acting beta$_2$-agonist; LTRA, leukotriene receptor antagonist, inhaled short-acting beta$_2$-agonist.

† Treatment options are listed in alphabetical order, if more than one.

‡ If alternative treatment is used and response is inadequate, discontinue and use preferred treatment before stepping up.

§ Theophylline is a less desirable alternative because of the need to monitor serum concentration levels.

** Based on evidence for dust mites, animal dander, and pollen; evidence is weak or lacking for molds and cockroaches. Evidence is strongest for immunotherapy with single allergens. The role of allergy in asthma is greater in children than in adults.

†† Clinicians who administer immunotherapy or omalizumab should be prepared to treat anaphylaxis that may occur.

‡‡ Zileuton is less desirable because of limited studies as adjunctive therapy and the need to monitor liver function.

§§ Before oral corticosteroids are introduced, a trial of high-dose ICS + LABA + either LTRA, theophylline, or zileuton, may be considered, although this approach has not been studied in clinical trials.

FIG. 29.2 ■ **Stepwise Approach for the Long-Term Management of Asthma.** (From the Department of Health and Human Services: Guidelines (from the National Asthma Education and Prevention Program, Expert Panel Report 3, updated Sept 2012. National Heart, Lung, and Blood Institute; National Institutes of Health; U.S. Department of Health and Human Services.)

Mind-Body Therapy

Breathing Exercises

Breathing exercises and breathing retraining have been used in the management of asthma (Buteyko, yoga, physical therapy). One specific form of breathing therapy, known as the Buteyko breathing technique, has been posited to have benefit in treating asthma by decreasing respiratory rate and allowing the carbon dioxide concentration in the lungs and blood to rise, thus resulting in bronchodilation. This technique dates back to 1952, when Dr. Buteyko theorized that "hidden" hyperventilation caused asthma symptoms. In vitro studies have indicated low alveolar carbon dioxide pressures may result in bronchoconstriction and greater airway resistance. Results of other studies suggest that the Buteyko breathing technique may be beneficial in treating asthma but were limited by small samples sizes. A study measuring end-tidal carbon dioxide (ETCO$_2$) found no correlation between ETCO$_2$ and breath-holding time, with the investigators postulating that the Buteyko breathing technique may help by improving the biomechanics of breathing.[16] A systematic review concluded that "no reliable conclusions can currently be drawn concerning the use of breathing exercises for asthma in clinical practice."[17] A larger randomized controlled trial reported that the use of the Buteyko technique for 6 months was associated with improved asthma control, and those using Buteyko had an additional benefit of reduced inhaled corticosteroid use[18] (see Chapter 92).

Yoga

Yoga embodies many of the previously discussed therapies for improving the health of patients with asthma. Yoga has a cardiovascular component because it is a form of exercise. This mind-body method involves using regulated breathing exercises (pranayama), with relaxation and meditation also included in many yoga practices. One study reported that yoga reduced airway hyperresponsiveness and improved some aspects of quality of life.[19] In a separate study of 132 adults with mild asthma who were randomized into a yoga group and a control group, the yoga group had significantly improved lung function after 8 weeks. Both groups continued their regular pharmacological treatments.[20] Although promising, a recent review of yoga and asthma studies including 14 randomized controlled trials with 824 patients reported that yoga was associated with improvements in asthma control, quality of life, peak expiratory flow rates, and the ratio of forced expiratory volume in 1 second compared to psychological interventions. However, the authors concluded that no effect was robust enough against all potential sources of bias and could not be used as a routine intervention but may be considered as an ancillary or alternative therapy for asthma.[21]

Biochemical

Botanicals

The use of botanicals is one of the oldest and most widely used therapeutic approaches in asthma care worldwide. Although the amount of knowledge and information regarding herbal or botanical treatment of asthma is large, a significant portion is not based on well-designed or well-performed clinical studies.[22] There have been several systematic reviews that continue to show the lack of high quality randomized controlled studies using botanicals in the treatment of asthma.[23,24] The use of herbal remedies is reportedly associated with lower adherence to conventional medications, particularly inhaled corticosteroids.[25] Many of the botanicals used for the treatment of asthma are similar to pharmaceuticals in terms of chemical properties. Further, many are used traditionally, and tradition varies by culture.

Boswellia (*Boswellia serrata*). *Boswellia* (also known as salai guggal or Indian frankincense) is a botanical used frequently in Ayurvedic medicine and traditionally used for inflammatory disorders, such as asthma and arthritis. Boswellic acid, the major constituent of *Boswellia*, is thought to inhibit 5-lipoxygenase and leukotriene synthesis, and this may be the mechanism for its antiinflammatory properties. *Boswellia* may enhance the effectiveness of conventional leukotriene modifier medications (see later). A small placebo-controlled study in adults reported that subjects taking *Boswellia* had fewer asthma exacerbations and improved lung function.[26]

DOSAGE

A common dosage recommendation is 300 mg three times/day.

PRECAUTIONS

Few precautions have been reported other than occasional gastrointestinal effects, such as epigastric pain, heartburn, nausea, and diarrhea.

Coleus (*Coleus forskohlii*). Coleus is a fairly uncommon botanical in the United States but has a long history of use for respiratory and asthma problems in India in the Ayurvedic medicine tradition. A member of the mint family, *Coleus forskohlii* grows wild on the mountain slopes of Nepal, India, and Thailand. Traditionally, coleus was used for numerous purposes including treatment of rashes, asthma, bronchitis, insomnia, epilepsy, and angina. Coleus is thought to act much like theophylline and has been studied as an effective bronchodilator. Coleus has been shown to increase intracellular cyclic adenosine monophosphate levels and stabilize cells that release histamine, although its clinical value is still to be determined. One study showed that an inhaled dose of forskolin powder from an inhaler device increased lung function by improving forced expiratory volume in 1 second (FEV$_1$) in patients with asthma.[27] However, another study compared the efficacy of oral forskolin versus inhaled beclomethasone for mild or moderate persistent adult asthma and found no statistically significant difference between the forskolin and beclomethasone treatment groups in any lung function parameter at baseline or after treatment.[28]

Dosage

A common dosage recommendation for coleus is 50 mg two or three times/day of an extract standardized to contain 18% forskolin or a 10-mg dose using an inhaler device.

Precautions

No precautions have been reported; however, coleus should be used with caution in patients receiving antihypertensive (beta blocker) or anticoagulant therapy. Pregnant women should not take coleus or any derivative.

Ma Huang (*Ephedra sinica*). Ma huang, also known as Chinese ephedra and Chinese joint fir, has been commonly used as an asthma remedy in China for thousands of years. The pharmaceutical ephedrine (derived from *Ephedra sinica*) was used in asthma therapy until the advent of more specific beta-agonist medications. Ma huang may be part of many combinations of other botanicals, including licorice and other antiinflammatory agents. Botanicals and supplements containing ephedra alkaloids have now appeared in many preparations for losing weight and increasing energy.

Precautions. Ephedra is not recommended for use in the treatment of asthma due to warnings from the U.S. Food and Drug Administration (FDA) and reports of serious side effects, particularly when used in combination with caffeine and other stimulants, such as bitter orange.

Ma huang botanicals and combination products have serious potential for side effects. Deaths associated with the use of ma huang have been reported. Central nervous system problems, such as nausea, vomiting, sweating, and nervousness, in addition to palpitations, tachycardia, hypertension, anxiety, and myocardial infarction, have been reported.[29]

Complications, including death, have been reported when ma huang is taken at high doses or with caffeine-containing products. Deaths have been reported with just one use of ma huang.

Licorice (*Glycyrrhiza glabra*). Licorice, also known as liquorice, sweet wood, and sweet root, has been used as a cough remedy and asthma treatment. The active ingredient is glycyrrhizin, also known as glycyrrhizic acid. The effect of licorice in treating asthma derives antiinflammatory effects and the enhancement of endogenous steroids. Licorice is also thought to be an expectorant, aiding in the expulsion of mucus from the bronchial passages, and a demulcent, which can be soothing to irritated airways and bronchioles.

Dosage

Licorice is available in several forms such as dried root, which can be used as an infusion or decoction. The dried root dose is usually 1.0 to 5.0 g three times per day. If a licorice tincture is used (1:5 strength is common), the dose is 2 to 5 mL three times a day. Finally, the standardized extract (containing 20% glycyrrhizic acid) dose is 250 to 300 mg three times a day.

Precautions

The side effects of licorice are minimal if less than 10 mg of glycyrrhizic acid is taken daily and prolonged use is avoided. Long-term use, however, can cause headache, hypertension, dizziness, edema, and other signs of aldosteronism (through the binding of mineralocorticoids). Licorice may also cause low serum potassium and should be avoided in patients taking cardiac glycosides, blood pressure medications, corticosteroids, diuretics, or monoamine oxidase inhibitors. A deglycyrrhized licorice (DGL) is available, but its effectiveness has not been well studied and may not be as effective as other products containing glycyrrhizin.

Pycnogenol. Pycnogenol (a proprietary mixture of water-soluble bioflavonoids extracted from French maritime pine) has been used for its antiinflammatory properties in conditions such as asthma. Pycnogenol is a blend of several bioflavonoids, including catechin, epicatechin, taxifolin, oligomeric procyanidins, and phenolic fruit acids such as ferulic acid and caffeic acid. This preparation is thought to exert its effect by blocking leukotrienes and other cytokines that increase inflammation and cause asthma symptoms. A study in children with asthma reported that Pycnogenol improved pulmonary function and reduced the need for rescue medications.[30] In a more recent study of 76 adults using Pycnogenol in addition to inhaled corticosteroids (ICS) or ICS alone, the Pycnogenol group had better control of signs and symptoms of allergic asthma and a reduced need for medications, predominantly a reduction in the strength of ICS required.[31]

Dosage

Pycnogenol is supplied in 30-, 50-, and 100-mg tablets. The usual dosage is 30 to 100 mg/day for maintenance therapy. The manufacturer recommends 1 mg/kg/day.

Precautions

No serious side effects have been reported; however, Pycnogenol is recommended to be taken with or after meals because it has an astringent taste. Minor side effects, including gastrointestinal discomfort, headache, nausea, and dizziness, have been reported, which resolve when the botanical is discontinued.

Herbal Mixtures. Japanese combination herbs and remedies (Kampo), such as Saiboku-to, blend black cumin, chamomile, cinnamon, cloves, rosemary, sage, spearmint, and thyme into a botanical combination that reduces asthma symptoms. This combination is thought to be effective due to antiinflammatory properties of blocking 5-lipoxygenase and inhibiting platelet-activating factor (PAF).[32] PAF is produced by several inflammatory cells, including eosinophils, and is thought to cause airway hyperreactivity, microvascular leaks, increased airway secretions, and epithelial permeability. Other trials using traditional Chinese medicine herb mixtures have reported potential utility in improving asthma control. These mixtures include ASHMI (a traditional herbal mixture) and Ding Chuan Tang, with both shown to improve asthma control and airway reactivity.[33,34] However, a Cochrane review of 27 studies using various herbal treatments (1925 subjects) found that the studies varied considerably and noted small sample sizes along with poor reporting quality and a wide variety of treatment regimens. Although the studies did provide some insight into the long-term efficacy and harm profiles of these various treatments, no recommendation for their standard use in the treatment of asthma could be made.[35]

DOSAGE

Combination herbal preparations are usually prepared as a tea and taken two to four times/day, depending on the particular mixture and brand used.

PRECAUTIONS

No side effects have been reported with these combination therapies.

Supplements

Vitamin and Mineral Overview

In addition to botanical and herbal preparations, vitamins and minerals are frequently used for the long-term treatment of asthma. As with most of the treatments mentioned thus far, few studies support the use of supplements despite their use historically for the treatment of asthma and chronic respiratory symptoms.

Vitamin C

Vitamin C has been extensively studied in asthma; however, results have been mixed. It has been proposed that vitamin C may be protective because it is involved in the metabolism of histamine, prostaglandins, and cysteinyl leukotrienes, which all have been associated with exercise-induced bronchoconstriction (EIB). A recent meta-analysis concluded that vitamin C slowed decreases in lung function compared to control treatment in a subset of patients.[36] Another review of studies for using vitamin C for both asthma and exercise-induced bronchoconstriction analyzed 11 trials with over 400 subjects (only one study involved children). The authors concluded, by rating the quality of the studies, that there was no significant difference between vitamin C and placebo.[37]

DOSAGE

The recommended dose of vitamin C is 250 to 500 mg once or twice a day.

Vitamin D

As with vitamin C, numerous studies have examined vitamin D levels and their correlation with asthma. Recent studies have demonstrated important roles of vitamin D outside of bone health, particularly in asthma and immune function. Because all cells in the body have vitamin D receptors, vitamin D may play an integral part in immune function and affect Th1 and Th2 cytokines, which play a role in the development of atopy and asthma.[38] Vitamin D deficiency has been linked to asthma in children and shown to be correlated with

severity of symptoms, increased exacerbations, and need for asthma medications.[39] In a survey of 616 children, serum vitamin D levels were associated with airway reactivity, hospitalizations, and the use of antiinflammatory drugs.[40] However, a study in adults (n = 207) with persistent asthma and vitamin D deficiency did not show a benefit in the prevention of asthma exacerbation when vitamin D was added to inhaled steroids.[41] Lower vitamin D levels have also been shown to be inversely associated with recent upper respiratory tract infections, which are a common trigger of acute asthma.[42] Taking supplemental vitamin D for the prevention of upper respiratory tract infections may help decrease asthma exacerbations.

DOSAGE

The recommended dose for vitamin D depends on patient age and the presence of vitamin D deficiency. For bone health, the recommended dose of vitamin D is 400 IU per day for children under the age of 1 year and 600 IU per day for those above the age of 1 year. However, many practitioners use doses up to 4000 IU per day with monitoring of serum levels of 25-hydroxyvitamin D (25[OH]D).

PRECAUTIONS

The safe vitamin D dosing range is unknown; however, an excess of vitamin D may cause abnormally high serum levels of calcium that may damage bones, soft tissues, and kidneys.

Vitamin E

Vitamin E refers to eight tocopherols with variable antioxidant properties that are present in foods in differing amounts. Of these, α-tocopherol has been reported to have beneficial effects on lung function and wheezing in asthma. However, dietary supplementation with α-tocopherol reportedly has no effect on FEV1, asthma symptoms, or bronchodilator use in adults with mild-to-moderate asthma.[44] In epidemiological studies, intake of vitamin E by diet or supplementation has been associated with fewer pulmonary problems, with poorly controlled asthma shown to be associated with low vitamin E levels.[45]

DOSAGE

The recommended dose of vitamin E is 400 units/day of mixed tocopherols.

PRECAUTIONS

The risk of all-cause mortality may be increased with prolonged use of doses greater than 400 units daily.

Magnesium

The role of magnesium in decreasing bronchospasm has been evaluated by both the conventional medical and the complementary and alternative medicine communities. Intravenous magnesium is now commonly used for serious asthma symptoms (status asthmaticus). The use of oral magnesium has also been studied. In adults, magnesium was shown to decrease symptoms but not to improve pulmonary function in one study and to have no benefit in another.[46] In a more recent study of 55 adults taking 340 mg of magnesium a day for 6 months, objective measurements of lung function, including bronchial reactivity to methacholine and peak flow measurements, improved in addition to subjective measures of asthma control and quality of life.[47]

DOSAGE

The recommended dose of magnesium is 200 to 400 mg/day. Magnesium gluconate and magnesium glycinate are the forms least likely to cause diarrhea.

PRECAUTIONS

Oral preparations of magnesium may cause diarrhea.

Selenium

Selenium is a potent antioxidant used in the treatment of many inflammatory conditions, including asthma. Selenium is incorporated into glutathione peroxidase, which may protect cells against oxidative stress. Studies have reported that increased selenium levels are associated with a reduction in the prevalence of asthma.[48] The results of studies using selenium supplementation have been inconsistent regarding the control or treatment of chronic asthma. This inconsistency may result from the complex relationship between selenium and asthma, as selenium can augment the oxidative stress that accompanies asthma but also exert significant effects on various immune responses.[49]

DOSAGE

The recommended dose of selenium is 100 to 200 mcg/day.

PRECAUTIONS

When selenium is consumed in amounts exceeding 400 mcg/day, symptoms of toxicity may appear including nausea, vomiting, abdominal pain, fatigue, irritability, and weight loss.

Fish Oil

The use of antiinflammatory medications is now standard in the asthma treatment. If patient diets could be altered to decrease the propensity for the development of inflammatory precursors, conditions such as asthma would be less problematic. The inclusion of adequate amounts of dietary omega-3 essential fatty may limit leukotriene synthesis by blocking arachidonic acid metabolism. Because omega-3 fatty acids have the potential to resolve inflammation, omega-3 fatty acid intake is hypothesized to improve asthma by reducing.[50] A rich source of omega-3 fatty acid is fish oils. As eating cold-water oily fish (mackerel, sardines, herring, salmon, and cod) is not common in most Western diets, the use of fish oil capsules has become increasingly standard. Epidemiological studies have shown diets high in cold-water oily fish to significantly reduce the risk of asthma and improve pulmonary function. The vegetarian sources of omega-3 fatty acids (flaxseed oil, canola oil, and soy oil) are used even less

in most diets, so the study of fish oil in asthma has been primarily investigated.

In one prospective study, dietary supplementation of omega-3 fatty acids in infants at high risk of developing asthma was associated with a small reduction in wheezing episodes in the first 18 months; however, this association was no longer present by age 5.[51,52]

DOSAGE

One 500-mg capsule of fish oil is taken two to three times/day. Benefit may not be evident for several months.

Pharmaceuticals

Bronchodilators

Bronchodilators have long been used to help alleviate bronchospasm and difficulty with breathing associated with asthma "attacks." Bronchodilators belong to several different classes. Commonly used beta agonists include albuterol, salmeterol, and formoterol. Levalbuterol is similar to albuterol and has been purported to have fewer cardiovascular side effects. The methylxanthines (theophylline and aminophylline) are used as second- or third-line drugs because they have more significant side effects, and their use requires serum level monitoring.

DOSAGE

- Albuterol: two to four puffs of a metered-dose inhaler (MDI) one to three times/day, as needed, or via nebulizer (unit dose) every 4–6 hours as needed
- Levalbuterol: one inhalation vial (three strengths) per nebulizer three times/day or two puffs one to three times/day by MDI as needed
- Salmeterol or formoterol (long-acting beta-agonist): one actuation of a dry powder inhaler (DPI) twice a day
- Methylxanthines (theophylline): dosage dependent on age and weight

PRECAUTIONS

Beta agonists may cause rapid or irregular heartbeat, insomnia, and nervousness. Anticholinergic medications have few side effects, except for occasional dry mouth or headache. The theophylline-type medications may cause tremor, shakiness, nausea, and vomiting. Overdose of methylxanthines can cause serious problems, such as seizures and cardiac arrhythmias.

Antiinflammatory Medications

Antiinflammatory medications are considered the most important components of the pharmacological approach to asthma care. Several categories of these medications are available, usually listed as steroidal and nonsteroidal. The steroidal MDIs and DPIs include fluticasone, beclomethasone, mometasone, ciclesonide, and budesonide. Newer proprietary preparations that have been shown to reduce the need for higher doses of the steroidal preparations include combinations of an inhaled steroid (fluticasone, budesonide, or mometasone) with a long-acting bronchodilator (salmeterol or formoterol). Oral preparations, such as prednisone, prednisolone, and methylprednisolone, are also available. Nonsteroidal medications include the leukotriene inhibitors montelukast and zafirlukast. These medications act by blocking certain pathways involved in airway inflammation once exposure (allergic, irritant, infectious, emotional, or exercise) has occurred. The oral steroids are considered the most potent agents and have the greatest potential for significant side effects.

DOSAGE

The dosage of leukotriene inhibitors differs according to the specific type used. The dosage of montelukast, for example, is 10 mg/day for adults and 5 mg/day for children (chewable tablets). For a child younger than 5 years, 4 mg/day is recommended (not to be used in children younger than 12 months).

Dosages for steroidal inhalers are usually two puffs (or one actuation of the DPI) twice/day. Oral steroids are usually taken at 1 to 2 mg/kg or 20 to 40 mg/day (adults) for varying amounts of time. A short "burst" of treatment may be prescribed for 3 to 5 days in total.

PRECAUTIONS

Nonsteroidal medications have few side effects. Leukotriene inhibitors may cause headache or mood changes. Liver function should be monitored as some nonsteroidal medications may cause hepatic dysfunction. The steroidal medications, particularly oral preparations, may cause decreased height velocity (in children), immune suppression, hypertension, cataracts, and hirsutism (if taken long-term or at high dose). The inhaled forms have less common side effects and have been studied long-term in children[53]; however, they may cause hoarseness, cough, and oral candidiasis unless a spacer is used or thorough mouth rinsing is practiced. Combination medications (corticosteroids plus a long-acting beta agonist such as fluticasone and salmeterol) have a black box warning given by the FDA due to the possibility that some patients may have worsening of symptoms when using these types of medications, including increased asthma exacerbations and even death.

The newer antiinflammatory steroidal inhalers, used alone or in combination with a long-acting bronchodilator, constitute the most innovative and effective pharmacological approach to chronic asthma care.

Biomechanical Approaches

Massage

Massage therapy is an ancient treatment, dating back to the second century in China. It was referred to as the *art of rubbing* and was common until pharmaceuticals began to be heavily used instead, starting in the 1950s. Massage now commonly consists of using variable pressure, tension, and vibration on various parts of the body. Few studies have investigated the efficacy of massage, with studies performed before the 1990s limited by sampling issues, lack of controls, sample size, and inappropriate use of statistical analysis.[54,55] However, improvements in pulmonary function have been reported after massage in children with asthma.[56] A more recent open parallel-group, randomized controlled trial study of 60 children with asthma (30 in each group) was conducted using 20 minutes of massage by parents at bedtime for 5 weeks. The massage group was found to have significant improvements in lung function (FEV1 and FEV1/FVC). The study also demonstrated good compliance by the parents in performing massage, with many continuing to use massage after the study was completed.[57]

DOSAGE

The time and duration of massage therapy for the average patient with asthma are not known. The study that reported improvement in asthma symptoms used once-a-day massage for 30 days. Massage can be performed by a family member or friend who has been taught massage techniques or by a massage therapist.

Osteopathy

Osteopathy is another system of medical care that embraces the body as a whole and in which structure and function are closely interrelated. One main premise is that because osteopathy emphasizes that all body systems, including the musculoskeletal system, operate in unison, a disturbance in one system can alter functions of other systems. The main categories of osteopathic manipulative treatment (OMT; e.g., craniosacral, strain-counterstrain, and myofascial) involve more than 100 different individual treatments. OMT has been used for the treatment of both chronic and acute symptoms of asthma. OMT has demonstrated utility in increasing vital capacity and rib cage mobility, improving diaphragmatic function, clearing airway secretions, and improving autoimmune function. Studies of the efficacy of OMT in treating asthma have been small with poor methodology.[58] A study of 140 pediatric asthma subjects, where 90 subjects received OMT (specifics not provided) and 50 subjects received a sham (light tough) therapy reported a significant improvement in peak flow in the OMT group.[59] A study of the effectiveness of osteopathic manipulative treatment in pediatric asthma has been posted through the European Institute for Evidence Based Osteopathic Medicine on ClinicalTrials.gov (NIH).[60]

DOSAGE

The findings of an osteopathic practitioner determine the most appropriate form of OMT. Again, the form chosen may affect any part of the body depending on physical examination. Often, helping the patient use various parts of the chest in breathing may help.

Chiropractic

Chiropractic, the third largest regulated health care profession in North America, has been involved in health care for conditions such as asthma since the late 1800s. The theory of chiropractic care is based on the idea that the properly adjusted body, particularly the spine, is essential for health, with influence on life force and good health attained through the use of spinal manipulation therapy for the removal of subluxations.[61]

Although studies on chiropractic treatments in asthma have reported overall improvements in lung capacity, quality of life, and respiratory symptoms, a meta-analysis of these studies, including three randomized controlled trials, concluded that there was insufficient evidence to support the routine use of chiropractic adjustments in the treatment of asthma.[62]

DOSAGE

The dosage of chiropractic care depends on the practitioner.

PRECAUTIONS

Reported complications of chiropractic manual treatments have been documented, but none were found in relation to the treatment of asthma. Chiropractic care often involves repeated use of radiographs, thus making frequent radiation exposure an issue for some patients.

Mind-Body Therapy

Mind-body therapies have been used in the treatment of asthma in various ways. They are at times referred to as *cognitive-behavioral therapies* and encompass several approaches. No single therapy has been shown to be superior over another; however, some therapies appear to be more acceptable to individual patients. Discussing several types of therapy with patients and their families will enhance the success of mind-body interventions. Research in this area started in the early 1960s, and approaches have included relaxation therapy, breathing exercises, biofeedback, and hypnosis, and guided imagery.

The theory behind the use of these therapies is the inflammatory process can be modulated by the autonomic nervous system through emotions. Numerous studies in both children and adults have shown higher levels of anxiety and, at times, panic when asthma symptoms are perceived. In addition to anxiety, stress has been shown to influence the immune response and may promote a higher sympathetic activity, augment IgE production, cause a shift from a Th1 to a Th2 allergic-type response, and promote airway inflammation without overt symptoms.[64] Stress has also been shown to enhance airway inflammation in asthma by modulating immune cell function through neural and hormonal pathways.[65,66,67]

Hypnosis and Guided Imagery

Hypnosis has been used for achieving relaxation, relieving pain, helping with physical discomfort (even chronic pain), and altering moods. Hypnosis is multidimensional and helps patients develop a heightened focus on an idea or image. The process may be brief or may involve complex instructions depending on the subject, the goal, and the therapist. Hypnosis has been shown to be effective in patients whose asthma is mild and those whose symptoms have an emotional component. Studies on hypnosis have reported decreases in symptoms and medication use, as well as improvements in pulmonary function, in "motivated" patients.[68]

Guided imagery involves a form of self-hypnosis in which the patient uses an image of her or his own creation after an initial relaxation period to help reduce asthma symptoms. This method is particularly effective in children with an active and vibrant imagination. Children can often be taught this technique in less than half an hour, with improvements in asthma symptoms observed after a few practice sessions. Guided imagery starts with initial relaxation (using diaphragmatic breathing, known as "belly breathing") and then progresses to an imagery session. The subject develops an image and then focuses on taking control or command of the perceived airway or lung problem by using this image. An example is moving from a closet to the outdoors, where the child is able to breathe again. This emotion-mediated format enables disclosure and subsequent reframing for the child and allows independence from the chronic illness (see Chapters 95 and 97).

DOSAGE

As with relaxation, these therapies have the greatest effect if used often, and particularly if used when asthma symptoms are initially mild. This approach prepares the patient for dealing with worse symptoms during an attack.

Disclosure and Journaling

Much like the findings in rheumatoid arthritis, there is evidence to suggest that just having the patient with asthma discuss their symptoms may decrease the severity and frequency of the asthma. Journaling, in which one writes about asthma in a journal three to five times a week for 20 to 30 minutes, has been shown to reduce both symptoms and medication use. In one study, patients wrote in their journals about a stressful event that they had not discussed with others or that had been unresolved, while the control group just about daily events only.[69] The investigators reported a 13% improvement in lung function, as measured by the FEV_1, in patients who wrote about a stressful experience compared with the control group. In a more recent study, adults aged 18 to 80 years with asthma (n = 154) were instructed to use several integrative medicine interventions consisting of nutritional manipulation, yoga techniques, and journaling. The treatment group showed significant improvement in several areas of the Asthma Quality of Life Questionnaire[70] (see Chapter 98).

Other Therapies to Consider

The most appropriate placement of bioenergetic modalities, including traditional Chinese medicine (TCM), healing touch and prayer, and homeopathy, in the stepwise approach to asthma care is challenging. These modalities are suitable for all treatment plans, from the most mild to the most severe cases of asthma. These methods should be used in conjunction with the previously discussed therapies if patients have moderate or severe symptoms and are considered the appropriate first-line treatments in interested patients with mild or intermittent asthma.

Traditional Chinese Medicine

TCM has been practiced for several thousands of years and takes many forms. The basis of TCM is the understanding of the connections between the body, mind, and spirit in health and disease. The belief in an unseen vital energy that affects patient health and the flow of energy or qi (chi) through the appropriate channels is the basis of this practice. Practitioners can affect energy flow or intensity by manipulating balance through the use of acupuncture, Chinese herbs, diet, and physical therapy. TCM can successfully treat many medical conditions.

Acupuncture and other forms of TCM are thought to be beneficial in the treatment of asthma. Clinical observations indicate acupuncture and individually mixed Chinese herbs are effective, although clinical trials have not supported these observations. The National Institutes of Health 1997 Consensus Development Conference on Acupuncture recommended acupuncture for many conditions, including asthma.[71] A study of children with asthma (n = 26 in both the acupuncture and control groups) using asthma diaries as the primary outcome reported a significant reduction in asthma symptoms, in addition to a reduced need for beta-agonist and inhaled steroid use, after 10 weeks of acupuncture treatments. However, no differences were observed between the groups at 8 months after the completion of acupuncture.[72] In another small study, 52 asthmatic children were randomly selected to receive 10 laser sessions (3 sessions/week) on traditional Chinese acupoints. A significant reduction in asthma symptoms, improvement in lung function (FEV1), and subsequent reduction in the use of inhaled steroids was observed with the use of acupuncture, indicating improved asthma control.[73] In a recent review of acupuncture in children, a total of 32 articles were assessed for eligibility, resulting in seven studies (n = 410) being included. The authors concluded that the efficacy of acupuncture was unclear and larger randomized controlled studies are required.[74]

DOSAGE

The dosage of acupuncture is practitioner-dependent, and the effects of TCM usually take several treatments to appear.

PRECAUTIONS

Adverse side effects of acupuncture are rare but have been reported, including pneumothoraces.

Homeopathy

Homeopathy is considered an energy medicine because it is not based on the usual physical laws found in science, but rather on the premise that the use of "remedies" that would cause the same symptoms (principle of like cure) and are very dilute (the more dilute, the more potent; law of dilution) represents the most powerful treatments. Practitioners believe that dilution in water actually imparts healing energy, and this energy, combined with the patient's vital force or energy, is used in healing.

A recent prospective, observational, longitudinal study of individualized homeopathic medicines used adjunctively in 30 children with asthma reported statistically significant improvements in the severity and frequency of nocturnal asthma attacks or awakenings, the use of inhalers and oral corticosteroids, and PFT parameters at 3 and 6 months.[76] A review of homeopathy in the treatment of respiratory allergies and asthma evaluated evidence from controlled trials considered to be of high quality. The authors concluded that homeopathy may be helpful in combination with conventional therapies in the treatment of respiratory allergies and asthma.[77] A review of studies of homeopathy in treating asthma (6 trials with a total of 556 subjects were included) concluded there is currently insufficient evidence to reliably assess the potential utility of homeopathy in treating asthma.[78]

Homeopathic remedies depend on the particular patient's symptom pattern and should be individually assessed by an experienced homeopath to select the correct constitutional remedy. Some of the most commonly used homeopathic remedies are as follows:

- *Arsenicum album*: used for asthma with restlessness and anxiety
- Ipecac: used for chest constriction and cough
- *Pulsatilla*: used for chest pressure and air hunger
- *Sambucus*: used for asthma symptoms that awaken one during the night

DOSAGE

Dosage depends on the individual and on the guidance of the practitioner (see Chapter 115).

PRECAUTIONS

Homeopathy is thought to be safe, owing to the extreme dilution, and the treatments are inexpensive.

PREVENTION PRESCRIPTION

- Eliminate potential allergens and triggers in the environment.
- Increase fruit and vegetable intake, along with that of omega-3–rich fats, which are found in cold-water fish, nuts, greens, and ground flaxseed.
- Follow an exercise regimen, and consider other types of activities that incorporate both exercise and meditation, such as yoga and martial arts.
- Take controller medications, such as inhaled steroids and leukotriene-modifier medication, routinely until asthma is no longer persistent and medications can be safely decreased or discontinued.
- Consider adding a multivitamin with antioxidants (vitamins C, D and E, B-complex, selenium) to the diet.

- Botanicals may be helpful in controlling and decreasing asthma symptoms but are best taken under the guidance of a health care provider with experience in using them.
- Mind-body therapies, such as relaxation, visualization, and self-hypnosis, may decrease

asthma exacerbations and reduce the need for asthma medications.
- Stress reduction in the home, work place, and school may prevent or decrease asthma symptoms and airway inflammation.

THERAPEUTIC REVIEW

The following is a summary of therapeutic options for treating asthma. If a patient is having persistent symptoms (daily wheezing, shortness of breath, difficulty sleeping, or difficulty exercising) or severe symptoms (even if intermittent), it is best to prescribe more aggressive therapy, such as beta-agonists or antiinflammatory medications, as controller medications. For patients with mild to moderate or intermittent symptoms, this stepwise approach may be considered.

LIFESTYLE

- As with many chronic illnesses, asthma prevention is considered the best approach. Unfortunately, changing a patient's lifestyle, including their environment, is challenging. Due to cultural and regional differences in the United States, patient populations differ in how they approach chronic illness and the way they use medical care.

ENVIRONMENTAL

- Reducing exposure to asthma triggers can be therapeutic in itself. House dust mite reduction, frequent cleaning, use of HEPA filters, avoidance of second-hand smoke, and removal of all pets from the home will help decrease airway "irritability." A₁

NUTRITION

- Asthma symptoms often diminish following elimination of allergenic-type foods, such as dairy products (at least for a trial period); shellfish; and foods with nitrites, sulfites, added food coloring, and artificial sweeteners. Patients should consider increasing intake of organic fruits and vegetables for their antioxidant contribution, as well as foods rich in omega-3 fatty acids while decreasing those containing omega-6 fatty acids (vegetable oils). B₁

SUPPLEMENTS

- Magnesium: 200 to 400 mg/day B₂
- Fish oil: 1 g (eicosapentaenoic acid plus docosahexaenoic acid) twice daily B₂
- Vitamin D: 400 units for children younger than 4 years of age and 600 units daily for adults B₂
- Vitamin C: 250 mg twice daily B₂
- Vitamin E: 400 units a day or less of mixed tocopherols B₂

MIND-BODY THERAPY

- These techniques can be beneficial in the treatment of asthma, and breathing and relaxation are excellent places to start. B₁
- Guided imagery and hypnosis therapies are readily available in most communities and also help decrease symptoms, medication use, and physician or urgent care visits. Usually, these methods should

be used regularly (once or twice daily) until familiar to the patient. They can then be used as needed for asthma symptoms. B₁
- Journaling is also recommended, and patients should spend at least 20 minutes writing about their asthma or other stressors in their lives three times per week. B₁
- Cognitive therapies should not be used in place of medications, particularly if symptoms are moderate or severe. If the patient is using a peak flow meter, these therapies can be used while peak flow values are in a safe range.

EXERCISE

- Exercise not only has benefits in managing asthma (three to five periods of exercise lasting a minimum of 20 minutes per week), but also improves self-esteem, weight loss, and cardiovascular health. Exercise should be used with caution in patients with exercise-induced asthma. B₁

BOTANICALS

- Coleus: 50 mg three times/day  C₂
- Kampo (also known as Kanpo) is a mixture of Japanese herbs found in powder form, such as Easy-Breather Tea (Yama's Herbs, New York): 3 rounded teaspoons in warm water two to three times/day B₂
- Pycnogenol: 30 to 100 mg/day or 10 mg/kg/day, taken two to three times/day  B₂

PHARMACEUTICALS

- For patients with mild to moderate symptoms that are persistent, starting with pharmaceutical agents with antiinflammatory properties, such as fluticasone two puffs of a 110 metered-dose inhaler (110 mcg/inhalation) twice daily, or budesonide one actuation twice daily, will improve symptoms in the majority of patients while the other interventions mentioned previously can be started. For acute symptoms, albuterol two puffs twice daily or levalbuterol two puffs twice daily should be considered. These medications should be considered first-line therapy for patients with persistent or severe symptoms. A₂
- Other medications, such as leukotriene modifiers (montelukast 10 mg daily), may also be considered.  A₂

BIOMECHANICAL APPROACHES

- As adjuncts to other modalities and depending on patient preference, massage, osteopathic manipulative treatment, and chiropractic therapies may be very beneficial. All three have different approaches and regimens. Finding a practitioner familiar with treating patients with asthma is the key. B₂

Key Web Resources

Prevent Asthma Attacks. This website has links to many asthma education and asthma resources, including the American Lung Association	http://www.noattacks.org/asthma-resources
Allergy and Asthma Network. This nonprofit patient education and advocacy organization provides consumer-friendly information about asthma and allergies.	http://www.aanma.org/
Guidelines for the Diagnosis and Management of Asthma. The National Institutes of Health, through the National Heart, Lung and Blood Institute, has published evidence-based guidelines for the treatment of asthma, including several extensive sections on patient and family education and environmental control.	http://www.nhlbi.nih.gov/health-pro/guidelines/current/asthma-guidelines
Allergy Solutions, Inc. This company sells products for patients with allergies and asthma, including HEPA filters, and pillow and mattress covers.	http://www.allergysolution.com/default.asp

REFERENCES

References are available online at ExpertConsult.com.

CHAPTER 30

THE ALLERGIC PATIENT

Randy J. Horwitz, MD, PhD

Allergic diseases are a ubiquitous part of modern life. Nearly 18 million people suffer from allergic rhinitis. If we add in drug allergies, food allergies, and allergic asthma, over 20% of U.S. citizens—approximately 50 million people—are estimated to suffer from an allergic condition, and they annually spend $8 billion on prescription drugs for treatment of allergic symptoms.[1] A nationwide survey found that more than half (54%) of all U.S. citizens test positive to one or more allergens.[2] Although acute and chronic allergic diseases may not rank as a leading cause of mortality in the general population, they do constitute a leading cause of work and school absenteeism, generating a significant social and economic burden.

The incidence of allergies (and asthma) is increasing at a dramatic rate.[3] Although both genetic and environmental factors are implicated in this rise, the rapidity of the increase favors environmental contributors—either directly or via epigenetic mechanisms. This hypothesis warrants a more careful consideration of modifiable factors that may alter allergic reactivity—factors which are ideally suited to an integrative approach.

This chapter considers general integrative approaches to the patient with atopy or environmental allergies, whether seasonal or perennial. Separate chapters in this volume deal with some of the more prominent allergic and allergy-related conditions, including asthma (see Chapter 29), atopic dermatitis (see Chapter 72), and food allergies (see Chapter 31). Some commonalities link these seemingly disparate disorders, however, and knowledge of these common principles may be helpful in devising treatment recommendations for patients with allergies.

PATHOPHYSIOLOGY

The wide range of allergic conditions observed in the clinical setting and described in the literature may lead one to believe that a seemingly infinite number of discrete mechanisms are responsible for allergic symptoms. Despite the diversity in end-organ effects, however, much of the underlying pathophysiology in allergic diseases is remarkably similar. In addition, such knowledge enables the physician to recognize, and even anticipate, adverse reactions. For example, knowing that some patients with an anaphylactic reaction or an asthma exacerbation may experience a late-phase allergic response compels the physician to continue intensive therapy until the reaction has completely subsided.

The term allergy, in common usage, connotes a variety of reactions that range from mildly debilitating to life threatening. Patients are notorious for classifying *any* untoward adverse reaction as an "allergy," a practice that is often promulgated by the harried health care staff and unwieldy electronic health records. In conventional medicine, however, we recognize that the term "allergy" specifically describes a precise cascade of biochemical reactions that, in genetically predisposed (or atopic) individuals, may result in certain physical symptoms, such as rhinorrhea, sneezing, wheezing, bronchoconstriction, and even life-threatening vasodilation and hypotension (anaphylaxis).

Underlying this reactivity is a phenotypic predilection toward activation of type 2 helper T cell (Th2) reactivity (and suppression of Th1 reactivity) in atopic individuals. The classification of helper T cells into these two categories is based upon the types of cytokines they produce following stimulation (Table 30.1). Th1-type cytokines tend to produce inflammatory responses that are responsible for killing intracellular parasites and for perpetuating autoimmune responses. Interferon gamma (IFN-g) is a key Th1 cytokine. The Th2-type cytokines are implicated in allergic diseases and include interleukins 4, 5, and 13, which are associated with the promotion of IgE and eosinophilic responses in atopy, and interleukin-10, which exerts more of an antiinflammatory activity. In a healthy individual, we expect a balance of Th1 and Th2 responses, depending upon the provocative pathogen. In those with atopy or asthma, we typically see an overexuberant Th2 profile.

Much research has been focused upon modification of this Th2 phenotype, either in the prenatal period or in early childhood. If successful, such an intervention would likely reduce the prevalence of allergic diseases, or at least mitigate some of the more harmful sequelae of allergic reactions. Researchers have examined prenatal and postnatal infection exposure, early and late food introduction, and even household pet exposures as predictors of atopy in later life. Unfortunately, despite several provocative studies, there is no recognized intervention that will accomplish this goal. In many cases, studies have actually prompted a complete reversal of conventional and accepted recommendations, as was the case with peanut avoidance in the prevention of peanut allergies.[4] Lacking clear-cut allergy prevention guidelines, we are forced, at present, to temper and modify the allergic response in atopic individuals.

The pathophysiology of the allergic reaction has been well described. There are at least four classically defined mechanisms of pathophysiology as defined by Gell and Coombs; however, most allergic reactions involve more than one type of mechanism. For the purposes of this chapter, we will focus upon the IgE-mediated type 1 reaction, which is responsible for the more common clinical allergic conditions, including allergic rhinitis and allergic asthma.

The type I reaction, or the classic IgE allergic hypersensitivity reaction, is a two-step process by which a

TABLE 30.1   Type 1 Helper T cell (Th1) versus Type 2 Helper T cell (Th2) Phenotypes

	Th1 cells	Th2 cells
Proposed function	Cell-mediated immunity & inflammation; intracellular pathogens; autoimmunity	Allergy/asthma; extracellular parasites; antibody-mediated immunity
Cytokines elaborated	IL-2: development of regulatory T cells and expansion of T cell repertoire IFN-g: activates macrophages, enhances IgG production and Th1 cell production	IL-4: enhances IgE production; inhibits Th1 responses IL-5: promotes eosinophil survival IL-10: inhibits antigen presenting cell function IL-13: enhances IgE and mucus production
Association with medical conditions	Autoimmune diseases Some viral infections Some bacterial infections	Allergic diseases Asthma Some parasitic infections
Differentiation from Th0 cells triggered by	IL-12	IL-4

IFN-g, interferon gamma; *Ig*, immunoglobulin; *IL*, interleukin.

genetically susceptible (i.e., atopic) individual initially becomes allergic to a substance via a process known as *sensitization* (Fig. 30.1).

During the initial stage of sensitization, the individual develops significant amounts of immunoglobulin E (IgE) antibodies against an inhaled, ingested, or injected substance, such as pollen. Long-lived memory B cells, which are capable of producing more of this specific IgE antibody immediately when stimulated, appear in the circulation, largely through the action of Th2 cytokines. The newly formed IgE antibody binds either to circulating blood basophils or to mast cells located in the mucosal layers of the skin, the gastrointestinal tract, and the respiratory system. Millions of IgE molecules of different specificities (directed against different allergens) are present on the surface of each mast cell and basophil, with their concentration often determined by the degree of exposure. This explains why many people suffer seasonal allergy symptoms. An individual is considered sensitized only after sufficient levels of IgE antibodies directed against a specific substance have been produced and are bound to the surfaces of these cells. The process of sensitization does not produce any of the symptoms that we equate with allergic disease—in fact, a person is usually unaware of these initial molecular and cellular changes; not until reexposure to the allergen do allergic symptoms manifest.

> Immunoglobulin E (IgE) acts as a bridge that cross-links a specific antigen on the surface of mast cells and basophils to release mediators that foster inflammatory activity.

The second step in the allergic process is the *reactivity* phase. This occurs when a sensitized person is reexposed to the allergen, which now acts as a bridge, cross-linking specific IgE molecules on the surface of each basophil or mast cell. This bridging phenomenon induces changes within the cell, typically through the action of complex protein kinase cascades. Ultimately, this cross-linking process leads to degranulation of the mast cell or basophil, a process that releases both preformed mediators (e.g., histamine, serine proteases, and proteoglycans) and newly synthesized compounds (e.g., eicosanoids and cytokines). The activities of these mediators of allergic inflammation

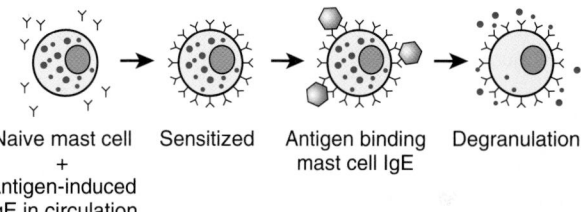

Naive mast cell   Sensitized   Antigen binding   Degranulation
+   mast cell IgE
Antigen-induced
IgE in circulation

FIG. 30.1 ■ Allergic Sensitization and Reactivity (Degranulation). The process of sensitization and degranulation in mast cells begins with production of antigen-specific immunoglobulin E *(IgE)* in genetically predisposed individuals. Initial binding of specific IgE to the naive mast cell surface "primes" the cell for activity. Subsequent binding of a specific allergen to the mast cell triggers complex intracellular biochemical events, leading to degranulation and subsequent mediator release.

are readily observable in a patient experiencing an allergic reaction. Histamine dilates blood vessels and thus causes localized edema in tissues such as the skin and mucosal membranes, as well generalized urticaria. Cytokines can chemotactically attract diverse cells to the "site of attack," as is the case in an asthma exacerbation, when Th2 cells and eosinophils infiltrate and populate the lungs. In an allergic exacerbation, clinical symptoms vary from negligible rhinorrhea to sudden death (severe anaphylaxis) depending on the degree of exposure and the sensitivity of the person exposed to the allergen. Most cases lie somewhere between these extremes. Although the cellular and molecular events for all immediate hypersensitivity reactions are similar, differences in target organ responses ultimately dictate the clinical patterns of disease activity once a reaction has been induced.

Allergic reactions also produce an inflammatory reaction; indeed, one of the most important research findings from the past few decades is the recognition that most of the pathophysiological processes of diverse allergic reactions have a common inflammatory pathway. Elucidation of this pathway has resulted in more precise, targeted therapies with which to control allergic inflammation. In the past, treatment with systemic corticosteroids was the only antiinflammatory intervention available. Although remarkably effective, these steroids provide relief at the expense of severe, long-term adverse effects, including osteoporosis, myopathy, and even psychiatric disturbances. The development of inhaled corticosteroids has

TABLE 30.2   **Antiallergy Activities of Select Compounds**

Class	Examples	Activity	Notes
Antihistamine	Loratidine Cetirizine Diphenhydramine	Block H1 receptors on target tissues	Works best prophylactically; may be sedating
Bioflavonoid	Quercetin Fisetin Cromolyn	Basophil/mast cell degranulation inhibition	Works best prophylactically; poor absorption
Supplements	Magnesium Vitamin C	Unclear; may relax bronchial smooth muscle (mag) or reduce oxidative stress (vit C)	Vitamin C is good preexercise; magnesium primarily used acutely
Botanicals	Stinging nettle Butterbur	Autocoid downregulation of histamine activity; inhibition of NF-kB	Antihistamine activity; blocks NF-kB
Nutritionals	Fish oil	Reduces leukotriene production in arachidonic acid cascade	Use correlates with increases in omega-3 content of cell membranes
TCM	ASHMI (Antiasthma Herbal Medicine Formula)	Reduces numbers and severity of asthma flares in people and animal models	Novel antiinflammatory mechanism as yet undefined

NF-κB, nuclear factor-κB.

mitigated some of these effects; however, these therapies still have adverse consequences. Fortunately, the identification of biochemical intermediates and enzymes in the inflammatory cascade has reduced the need for such powerful and nonspecific drugs and led to targeted therapies for interrupting the allergic inflammatory cascade, or at least controlling the allergic symptoms, until the triggered reaction eventually attenuates on its own.

Although analogues for specific pharmacological activities exist in the conventional and integrative therapeutic realms, it is the overall approach to treatment that more clearly differentiates the two approaches to care. Whereas a conventional physician tends to treat each disease state (and symptom) separately and specifically, an integrative practitioner may additionally consider measures to diminish an atopic predisposition. These additional therapies are described in this chapter and in the chapters on specific allergic diseases (Table 30.2).

INTEGRATIVE THERAPY

Nutrition

Specialized Allergen Avoidance Diets

The avoidance of specific foods or food additives that are found to be responsible for gastrointestinal or anaphylactic allergic reactions, such as peanuts in sensitive individuals, is an obvious and effective intervention. Such elimination diets are useful for both true food allergies and even for food sensitivities (see Chapter 86). However, food avoidance is also useful when one is attempting to control less severe, nongastrointestinal allergies. For example, patients who are troubled by recurrent sinus infections or mild to moderate refractory asthma symptoms often benefit from certain dietary modifications. Usually, these avoidance diets are specific to an individual, but some common classes of foods have been popularly linked to allergic exacerbations, such as dairy products, wheat, and even animal proteins. These foods seem to be associated with a worsening of allergic symptoms in many patients, although published clinical data in this area are scant. It

is important to remember that despite a shared diagnosis, allergic diseases are remarkably heterogeneous between individuals, so typically, one size does not "fit all."

A handful of small studies refute the association between milk and mucus production or allergic symptoms,[5] but biologically plausible hypotheses support such an association.[6] For example, certain types of milk (from specific breeds of cow) contain a protein called β-CM-7, which has been shown to stimulate mucus glands in the human digestive tract.[7] As these same glands are found in the upper and lower respiratory tract, milk proteins may increase phlegm production. In any case, a brief trial (4–6 weeks) of dairy avoidance is helpful to discern such an association in selected individuals and is widely used.

Omega-3 Fatty Acids

Alterations in the dietary intake of fats are known to affect the fatty acid composition of cell membranes.[8,9] This fact is especially pertinent to inflammatory conditions because catabolism of cell membrane–derived fats is an initial step in inflammatory mediator production through the arachidonic acid cascade. Omega-3 supplementation decreases the ratio of omega-6 to omega-3 fatty acids in the inflammatory cell lipid membrane, thus creating less substrate for mediator production.[8,9] This process, in turn, decreases the production of many potent bioactive compounds (e.g., leukotrienes) that are intimately involved in allergic inflammation. The level of inhibition of leukotriene production by dietary modification rivals that of pharmacological agents, such as zileuton[10] (see Chapter 88). Clinical trials of fish and plant omega-3 acid supplementation in the treatment of asthma and allergic diseases have been inconsistent, likely owing to the heterogeneity of the disease and huge variation in the form and dosage of fats. Despite this, a significant proportion of subjects respond favorably, making increased dietary omega-3 intake (or a trial of omega-3 supplementation) a useful clinical intervention.[11]

Several published studies have used doses of 3.2 g eicosapentaenoic acid (EPA) and 2.2 g docosahexaenoic acid (DHA) daily as a supplement to a standard diet.[8]

In one clinical trial, 26 patients with asthma were placed on defined diets of varying omega-3 to omega-6 content.[12] More than 40% of subjects showed marked improvement in airway hyperresponsiveness when they consumed a diet with an elevated omega-3 content. These responders to dietary interventions could be readily identified through analysis of the leukotriene composition of their urine, a measure that predicted which patients were likely to improve with dietary intervention.[12] Interestingly, a similar evaluation of urinary leukotrienes was used in the development of leukotriene inhibitors (e.g., montelukast), and a differential responsiveness was observed among subjects.[13] In practice, a trial of fish oil at this dose is useful in assessing responsiveness. Decreases to 1500–2000 mg EPA daily are then possible, with monitoring of clinical parameters.

Dietary Antioxidants. The association between dietary antioxidant intake and the allergic response has been the subject of much study over many years. Because oxidation reactions are commonplace among inflammatory processes (allergies included), the hope was that antioxidants would either prevent the development of allergic disease or mitigate the severity of the reactions. Many positive and negative reports exist in the literature, fairly equally divided, thus precluding definitive and global conclusions. Some findings are worthy of mention, however, particularly a few examining vitamin C and selenium intake.

A food frequency questionnaire was used to examine 4500 school-aged children in Korea and found that children with elevated vitamin C consumption had fewer allergic rhinitis symptoms.[14] A case-control study, also using a food frequency questionnaire, found that apple consumption and dietary selenium intake were negatively associated with asthma prevalence in a 1500-person cohort.[15] Interestingly, selenium functions as a cofactor for glutathione peroxidase, which helps prevent peroxidation of cell membranes by consuming free peroxide in the cell. In one report, children with asthma had significantly lower red blood cell glutathione peroxidase activity than that of a healthy control group.[16] Finally, patients with asthma have higher amounts of oxidized glutathione in their airways, a finding perhaps indicating that patients with asthma are subject to greater oxidative stress.[17]

Studies examining whole food consumption, as opposed to individual antioxidant supplements, found that higher intakes of cooked vegetables, tomatoes, and fruits in children were protective factors for symptoms of shortness of breath and wheeze during a 12-month observation period.[18] Consumption of citrus fruits, in particular, had a protective role for these symptoms, which may be related to vitamin C intake. In the same study, consumption of bread, butter, and margarine were all associated with an increased risk of shortness of breath and wheezing.[18] These findings are not universally accepted, however, because data in the literature are conflicting.

Finally, no conclusive consensus evidence indicates that antenatal supplementation of any vitamin or mineral during pregnancy will reduce the probability of atopy or asthma later in life for children.[19,20] By definition, these studies are difficult to perform, and the number of confounding variables is extremely high.

Supplements

Many supplements are commonly used for the treatment of allergic rhinitis and asthma. The most promising of these are the flavonoids, which are plant pigments that give fruits and vegetables their brilliant colors. The benefits of these compounds have been demonstrated in both *in vitro* and animal studies, with human studies just beginning. Unfortunately, it is very difficult to absorb orally administered flavonoids owing to their unique chemistry. The addition of several compounds to flavonoid formulations (e.g., bromelain, vitamin C) are aimed at increasing systemic absorption. Some flavonoids have already been adopted by the pharmaceutical industry and are available as prescription medications. An example of this is cromolyn, which is commercially sold under the trademark of Intal. There are other over-the-counter products that are also promising, including quercetin, fisetin, and Pycnogenol. As this group has shown remarkable in vitro activity against allergic inflammation, it is worth considering each in some detail.

Quercetin

Quercetin is a bioflavonoid obtained from diverse sources, including apples, buckwheat, onions, and citrus fruits. Most data supporting the role of quercetin in attenuating allergic reactivity have been obtained from in vitro studies, as well as from animal models of allergic disease. In vitro studies have shown that quercetin stabilizes the membranes of mast cells and reduces the release of preformed histamine.[21,22] In animal models, quercetin is able to suppress anaphylactic responses in sensitized rats,[23] and it inhibits asthmatic inflammation in guinea pigs and rats.[24]

Quercetin must be used as a preventative—taken before allergen exposure. Thus the activity of quercetin is similar to that of cromolyn, a drug that is often prescribed for allergy and asthma prophylaxis (see later). Quercetin also inhibits the production of enzymes responsible for manufacturing the potent leukotrienes.[25] Practitioners usually recommend that quercetin be used regularly during an individual's entire allergy season, or year-round for those with perennial allergies.

Quercetin is similar to cromolyn in its mechanism of action. Both are basophil and mast cell stabilizers.

Dosage

The dose of quercetin is usually 400–600 mg of a coated tablet one to three times daily between meals (adjust dose for clinical response). Quercetin is not soluble in water, however, so it is a poorly absorbed nutrient. Bromelain, a protein-digesting enzyme extracted from pineapples, increases the absorption of quercetin, as does vitamin C. Therefore quercetin is typically sold blended with one or both additives.

Precautions

None are reported.

Pycnogenol

Pycnogenol is a proprietary antioxidant–bioflavonoid mixed extract isolated from the bark of the maritime pine (*Pinus pinaster*). Pycnogenol has a variety of biological activities, ranging from blood pressure reduction to mitigation of elevated blood glucose. In terms of allergic diseases, it has been shown to be efficacious in a murine model of airway inflammation,[26] as well as in a clinical trial of children with asthma.[27] In this study, Pycnogenol improved asthma symptoms and pulmonary function and decreased rescue inhaler use. In addition, there was a significant reduction of urinary leukotriene production in the treated group.[27] More recent studies have explored the use of Pycnogenol in people with allergic rhinitis.[28] When taken well in advance of the "allergy season," Pycnogenol improved both nasal and ocular symptoms with no significant adverse events.

DOSAGE

Pycnogenol is available from many sources; however, as a proprietary preparation, all products bearing the name "Pycnogenol" come from one common source (Fig. 30.2). The recommended dose used in asthma studies is 1 mg/lb body weight in two divided doses. For allergic rhinitis, the recommended dose is 100 mg given once per day, which may be at the low end. As with many of these interventions, I tend to use the higher dose, gauge response, then try a dose reduction while observing clinical response.

PRECAUTIONS

None are reported. Pycnogenol can be added to existing allergy/asthma regimens.

Fisetin

Fisetin is another bioflavonoid compound that is very active against allergic inflammation, at least in in vitro and in animal models. It is found primarily in strawberries, but also in apples, persimmons, and onions. Fisetin has gained some attention in the scientific community due to its memory-enhancing capabilities in rodents.[29] However, bioavailability is the biggest issue with fisetin, as with other flavonoids. Most studies of fisetin involving memory enhancement or asthma were performing using intravenous or intraperitoneal formulations. However, several studies used oral preparations.[29] A biological mechanism for the action of fisetin in attenuating allergic inflammation has been proposed, and it is more complex

than that of other bioflavonoids. This compound appears to potently inhibit nuclear factor-kappaB (NF-κB)—a transcription factor, or on-off switch, responsible for the expression of many inflammatory genes (e.g., IL-1, IL-2, IL-6, IL-8, tumor necrosis factor, adhesins, major histocompatibility class I, inducible nitric oxide synthase, and COX-2).[30] Accordingly, fisetin may produce antiinflammatory effects in many reactions that transcend allergic disease. In animal models, fisetin potently inhibited asthma flares in sensitized animals following exposure to allergens. The antiinflammatory effect of fisetin rivaled corticosteroids.[30]

DOSAGE

Typical oral doses for animals ranged from 5–25 mg/kg, and intraperitoneal doses were 0.3–3 mg/kg, in the presence of a chemical carrier (DMSO). Commercial doses for humans are at the lower end of this range and typically are 100–200 mg daily for the oral compound.

PRECAUTIONS

None are reported. Fisetin can be added to existing allergy/asthma regimens.

Magnesium

Magnesium is a standard of care in the emergency treatment of acute asthma exacerbations, and it is usually administered as an intravenous solution, but occasionally in a nebulized form (the jury is still out as to the comparative efficacies of the two routes).[31] Magnesium has been shown to improve forced expiratory volume in 1 second (FEV_1) and reduce ICU admissions in that setting.[32] Inverse associations have also been reported between intracellular (RBC) magnesium levels and asthma severity.[33] Despite this association, little convincing literature supports a role for long-term magnesium replenishment in the care of mild to moderate asthma. Some published reports note an improvement in asthma symptoms in subjects with higher magnesium intake,[34] while others link dietary magnesium intake with an increased risk of asthma and wheezing in children.[35] A recent 6-month study of magnesium supplementation (340 mg daily) in adults with mild-to-moderate asthma produced improvements in bronchial hyperreactivity, peak flow measures, and quality of life indices, without significant effects on other markers of asthma control nor inflammatory markers.[36]

DOSAGE

Magnesium glycinate seems to be less irritating to the gastrointestinal system. The typical dose is 400–500 mg daily.

PRECAUTIONS

Side effects are primarily gastrointestinal. At standard doses, magnesium can produce laxative effects, which are readily reversible with dose reduction.

Some forms of magnesium supplementation have prominent laxative effects. The clinician should be wary of prescribing magnesium citrate, oxide, or hydroxide in a patient for whom diarrhea is a problem. Start with 250 mg daily and build up to 400–500 mg daily.

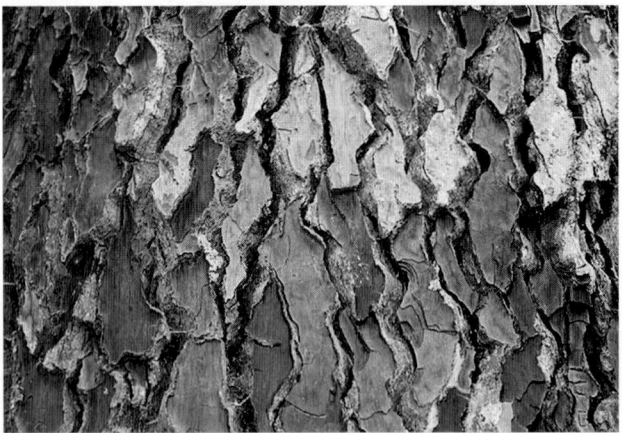

FIG. 30.2 ■ Pycnogenol is a proprietary antioxidant-bioflavonoid mixed extract isolated from the bark of the maritime pine (*Pinus pinaster*).

Other Botanicals

Butterbur (Petasites Hybridus)

Butterbur has traditionally been used to treat migraine headaches but also asthma and bronchitis because it is thought to reduce mucus production. A study of 132 people with seasonal rhinitis (hay fever) found that an extract of butterbur was as effective as cetirizine (Zyrtec), a commonly prescribed, mildly sedating antihistamine, and had fewer side effects (especially less sedating). The study lasted only 2 weeks and required four to five doses of the herb daily.[37] More recently, the mechanisms of butterbur action were more carefully delineated in a mouse model of asthma.[38] In this study, butterbur was shown to inhibit leukotriene activity and reduce allergic airway inflammation and bronchial hyperreactivity by specifically inhibiting allergic cytokine formation (including interleukins 4 and 5). An open trial of butterbur in the treatment of asthma in adults reported decreased beta agonist use, but it was a poorly designed study.[39]

> **DOSAGE**
>
> Petasites extracts are typically standardized to contain a minimum of 7.5 mg of petasin and isopetasin. The adult dosage ranges from 50 to 100 mg twice daily for the treatment of migraine headaches. A high-quality, standardized product prepared in Germany is Petadolex. It is prepared using a carbon dioxide extraction, and its content of pyrrolizidine alkaloids is lower than the limits of detection (the German government requires content to be less than 1 mg daily by dosage). In the previously cited rhinitis study, participants took one butterbur extract tablet (standardized to 8.0 mg of total petasin per tablet) four times daily. The 50-mg Petadolex tablet is standardized to contain 7.5 mg petasins and may also be used up to four times daily in adults.
>
> **PRECAUTIONS**
>
> The main concern in using butterbur is finding a preparation that is free of harmful pyrrolizidine alkaloids. These compounds are capable of causing toxic reactions in humans—primarily venoocclusive liver disease.

Stinging Nettle (Urtica Dioica)

Stinging nettle has a long history of use as an antiallergy preparation, and it is also used in the treatment of prostatic hypertrophy. The "stinging" hairs and leaves of this plant contain histamine, serotonin, acetylcholine, and 5-hydroxytryptamine, compounds that typically are the *cause* of allergic symptoms. Some investigators attribute the antihistaminic properties of ingested nettles to an autocoid or feedback inhibition of histamine and histamine-related compounds. Studies have revealed that nettle extract also inhibits the release of tryptase, a mast cell mediator of allergic inflammation, as well as other proinflammatory mediators, such as cyclooxygenase-1 (COX-1), COX-2, and prostaglandin D_2 synthase (PGDS).[40] A more important activity, however, may be the inhibitory effect of nettle on the transcription of inflammatory genes. Nettle extracts have been shown to inhibit the activity of NF-κB—the transcriptional activator (described previously), which functions as an on-off switch for inflammatory genes.[41]

Clinically, few trials have been conducted. In one randomized double-blind study, 57% of patients rated nettles to be effective in relieving allergic rhinitis symptoms and 48% reported that nettles equaled or surpassed previously used allergy medications in effectiveness.[42]

> **DOSAGE**
>
> The typical dosage is 300 to 350 mg of a freeze-dried extract used one to three times daily, as needed.
>
> **PRECAUTIONS**
>
> Rare allergic reactions and possible gastrointestinal upset have been reported.

Pharmaceuticals

Cromolyn

Cromolyn is a prime example of a drug whose active ingredient was isolated from a botanical source with a historical record of effectiveness. Isolated from an extract of the khella plant (*Ammi visnaga*), cromolyn has demonstrated potent mast cell–stabilizing activity in vitro. When used prophylactically in advance of allergenic exposure, cromolyn can markedly reduce the rate and degree of mast cell degranulation and thus allergic symptoms. Cromolyn is available by prescription in a nebulized form for inhalation (Intal), as a liquid for oral use in gastrointestinal allergic conditions (Gastrocrom), and without a prescription as a nasal preparation for allergic rhinitis (NasalCrom). Unfortunately, it is no longer available as a metered-dose inhaler in the United States. Nebulized cromolyn is useful in treating children with asthma and was a mainstay of asthma antiinflammatory medications prior to the development of inhaled corticosteroids.

> **DOSAGE**
>
> For the treatment of allergic rhinitis, the dosage is one spray of nasal spray (NasalCrom) into each nostril three to four times/day until the condition improves and then one spray in each nostril every 8 to 12 hours. This preparation can also be used prophylactically approximately 20–30 minutes before allergen exposure (e.g., exposure to a cat). For asthma, one ampule (20 mg) is used by nebulizer three to four times daily.
>
> **PRECAUTIONS**
>
> Cromolyn is quite safe, and adverse reactions are extremely rare.

Antihistamines

Antihistamines bind to the H_1 histamine receptor and inhibit allergic reactions at the level of the target organs; that is, they do not prevent the initiation of the classic allergic response but can inhibit (or at least reduce) the effects of histamine, a key biochemical mediator of allergy. Many different chemical classes of antihistamines are available, but most clinicians prefer the first- and second-generation pharmaceutical agents.

First-generation antihistamines are safe, over-the-counter preparations that are effective in reducing allergic symptoms, but at the expense of significant central nervous system effects. First-generation compounds tend to be highly lipophilic and readily cross the blood–brain barrier thus causing mild-to-marked sedation. In addition, anticholinergic effects, such as urinary retention, may prevent the use of these drugs in patients with prostatic hypertrophy or urinary hesitancy from other causes. Because of the longer history of use of first-generation antihistamine products, many practitioners recommend them in certain higher-risk circumstances, such as in pregnancy. Examples of first-generation compounds are diphenhydramine (Benadryl), clemastine (Tavist), and chlorpheniramine (Chlor-Trimeton).

Second-generation antihistamines typically have fewer anticholinergic and antimuscarinic side effects than first-generation agents and appear to be equally effective. The mechanism of action is similar for first- and second-generation drugs, although more research has focused on the presumptive antiinflammatory activity of the second-generation compounds. For example, desloratadine downregulates various inflammatory mediators, including the generation and release of IL-4 and IL-13 by human basophils.[43] Examples of second-generation antihistamines include cetirizine (Zyrtec), loratadine (Claritin), and fexofenadine (Allegra).

Although many advertisements have been devoted to identifying specific and superior uses for differing brands of antihistamines (e.g., better efficacy in treating urticaria or rhinitis), much of this information represents marketing efforts because large head-to-head published comparisons of drugs for specific allergic conditions are lacking.

Finally, topical antihistamines are available as nasal sprays. Although systemic absorption is less than with oral preparations, similar adverse effects can occur. Bitter taste limits use in many patients. Examples of topical antihistamines include azelastine (Astepro) and olopatadine (Patanase).

Dosage

The standard dose of antihistamine varies with the particular compound. Follow the label directions.

Precautions

Patients should not operate heavy machinery or automobiles while they are taking even mildly sedating antihistamines, including cetirizine (a second-generation compound). A study conducted in 2000 compared driving coordination in subjects administered standard doses of a first-generation antihistamine (diphenhydramine) with subjects given alcohol, fexofenadine, or a placebo. Remarkably, diphenhydramine had a greater impact on driving performance than alcohol.[44] In addition, urinary retention, confusion, dizziness, drowsiness, dryness of mouth, or convulsions (seizures) may be more likely to occur in older adults who take the older antihistamines.

Prolonged used of medicines with anticholinergic side effects has been associated with a higher risk for memory loss due to the inhibitory effect of acetylcholine.[45]

Nasal Corticosteroids

Topical (nasal) corticosteroids are relative newcomers to the allergic rhinitis pharmacopeia. They are regarded as first-line therapy for moderate to severe rhinitis symptoms, especially nasal congestion, for which they seem to outperform antihistamines.[46] A brief period (perhaps weeks) often elapses before maximal effects are appreciated. These drugs function as topical antiinflammatory agents and reduce allergic inflammation locally in the nasal mucosa and sinus passages. Many of the newer preparations are regarded as safe because they exhibit first-pass metabolism and thereby lessen the possibility of systemic absorption and long-term adverse effects. As of 2013, two formulations are available as over-the-counter products: Flonase (fluticasone) and Nasacort (triamcinolone). More are expected to follow.

Dosage

The dosage varies with each preparation. Typically, one spray in each nostril daily is sufficient for maintenance. Occasionally, this dose is doubled for short periods (i.e., during peak allergy weeks).

Precautions

Common side effects include epistaxis (up to 10%). Concern also exists about growth rate declines in prepubescent children; however, this observation has been noted in very few reports. Higher rates of posterior subcapsular cataracts have also been reported. Concerns about systemic absorption of these steroid compounds and the long-term effects remain, although several studies have demonstrated only mild adrenal inhibition.

I have observed cases of septal perforation as a result of improper spraying of corticosteroids in the nares. Advise patients to aim the "nozzle" of the canister or bottle away from the nasal septum (i.e., toward the outside of the nostril). Use of the opposite hand for each nostril will naturally aim the mist away from the septum.

Immunotherapy

Allergic desensitization is an effective adjunct to drug therapy in selected patients. It is generally reserved for those individuals who show no response to other therapies or for whom life-threatening reactions can occur with unpredictable frequency (e.g., insect sting anaphylaxis). Immunotherapy in the United States historically consisted of the subcutaneous administration of gradually increasing amounts of allergic material given at regular intervals ("allergy shots"). The mechanism by which the injections diminish allergenic sensitivity is not completely clear; however, their effectiveness has been demonstrated in cases of allergic rhinitis and for some types of asthma as well. This therapy is believed by some to be a last resort because the potential for an adverse reaction is always present and the reaction itself can be life threatening. From 1985 to 1993 in the United States, 52.3 million administrations of immunotherapy resulted in 35 deaths. These numbers equate to a mortality incidence of less than 1 per million, which is quite low but still unacceptable for patients treated for a nonlife-threatening condition such as allergic rhinitis.[47] Moderate to severe systemic reactions are fairly common and warrant close patient supervision immediately after the administration of a desensitization injection.

Sublingual Immunotherapy

A newer immunotherapy modality that is rapidly gaining acceptance in the United States is sublingual immunotherapy (SLIT). Popularized in Europe years ago, when subcutaneous immunotherapy was deemed too dangerous for regular use, sublingual immunotherapy is similar to the subcutaneous route except that the allergen extract is provided as drops that the patient self-administers under the tongue (sublingually) on a daily basis. Many subspecialists decried this newer therapy as it opened the treatment of allergic diseases to nonallergists. However, it is gaining acceptance among younger practitioners and medical consumers alike. The sublingual route has been shown to be efficacious in numerous studies, and it is considered very safe, with few mild reactions reported and no deaths.[48] SLIT therapy is usually initiated with a full dose (or a very short dose escalation schedule), with the first dose given under medical supervision. Dosing continues once daily and is self-administered by the patient at home.

Over the past several years in the United States, there has been "off-label" use of regular injectable liquid allergen extracts for sublingual immunotherapy, but this is somewhat controversial.

SLIT therapy can be used for foods as well as for aeroallergens. The efficacy of this method depends upon appropriate allergen testing and careful extract dosing. Although considered very safe, as with any active immunotherapy, there is still a risk of anaphylaxis.

DOSAGE

In 2014, the FDA approved three commercially available SLIT products: Oralair, a once-daily sublingual tablet that contains a mixture of freeze-dried extracts from the pollens of five grasses; Grastek, a single-species Timothy grass pollen sublingual tablet; and Ragwitek, a short ragweed pollen sublingual tablet. These products are designed to be initiated a few months before the start of the grass (or ragweed) pollen season and are continued throughout the season.

Mind-Body Therapy

Numerous studies have documented the value of mind-body approaches to many allergic conditions. Classic studies from the late 1960s demonstrated that many patients with moderate to severe asthma exhibit severe symptoms when they are exposed to saline mists that they believed were potent allergens. Even more remarkable was their prompt recovery with use of a saline inhaler that they believed to be a beta agonist.[49,50] Even standard skin test reactions that produce classic wheal-and-flare reactions to subcutaneously introduced allergens can be modulated by mind-body techniques. In one study, patients with dust mite sensitivity who were skin tested after viewing a humorous video demonstrated lower wheal-and-flare reactivity to dust mite allergen than did patients viewing a control video (weather documentary).[51] Finally, a randomized controlled trial examined the effectiveness of the addition of self-hypnosis to a pharmacological regimen for allergic rhinitis. Allergic symptoms in 79 patients with "hay fever" showed significant improvement over the course of two pollen seasons compared with those in control groups[52] (see Chapter 95).

Traditional Chinese Medicine

Until recently, relatively few controlled studies have examined the role of acupuncture or Chinese herbs as part of a traditional Chinese medicine (TCM) approach to allergies. Now, however, owing to several ground-breaking studies from the Mount Sinai Hospital in New York, this is perhaps the most exciting area for future innovation. Researchers there purified and dissected several ancient Chinese herbal formulations for both asthma and food allergies and uncovered some remarkable results.

An herbal preparation, tested in an animal model of asthma, was shown to be as effective an antiinflammatory agent as corticosteroids, but through a novel mechanism and with potentially fewer adverse effects.[53] Through a series of carefully designed experiments, the group was able to test the compound, which they call ASHMI (Anti-asthma Herbal Medicine Intervention), on 90 adults with mild–moderate asthma.[54] They compared their formulation to daily prednisone over a 4-week period and determined that the TCM herbal compound was safe, well tolerated, and as effective as the corticosteroid at improving peak flow, FEV1, symptoms, and reducing the need for bronchodilators. However, ASHMI did not affect serum cortisol levels or cause weight gain, relative to the corticosteroid. This herbal blend is expected to enter the marketplace soon.

A similar research initiative by the same workers led to the discovery of a Chinese formula that was completely protective in an animal model of peanut allergy.[55] The therapy also proved to be long lasting. This finding is remarkable because few, if any, therapies exist for this potentially fatal condition.

A human study demonstrated the superiority of a regimen of acupuncture plus Chinese herbs (versus placebo) in the treatment of seasonal allergic rhinitis.[56] The study assessed rhinitis symptoms with several validated scales, which showed significant improvements in quality of life and symptom control in patients who received a standard regimen of acupuncture along with a standardized herbal decoction. The therapy was found to be well tolerated and safe in this study population. Finally, a recent meta-analysis evaluated the efficacy of traditional Chinese herbal medicine for the treatment of persistent allergic rhinitis. The list of acceptable studies was pared down to seven, involving a total of 533 patients. Although nasal symptom scores were significantly reduced with herbal medicine, no other outcomes (i.e., objective measures) were affected.[57]

PREVENTION PRESCRIPTION

- Use environmental modification, including reduction of dust mite allergen: encase mattress and pillows, remove carpeting if possible, and replace curtains with shades or blinds
- Remove allergenic pets from the home, or at least from the bedroom
- Consider buying a high-efficiency particulate air (HEPA) filter
- Plan activities to avoid exposure to early morning peak pollen counts

- Resist the temptation to open the windows; use the air conditioner and change furnace filters often
- Follow an antiinflammatory diet. Avoid processed foods, partially hydrogenated oils, white sugar, and flour. Replace vegetable oils with olive or canola oil for cooking. Avoid excessive amounts of saturated fat
- Consider a 4-week elimination diet to see if it impacts symptoms. Start by eliminating dairy or wheat

THERAPEUTIC REVIEW

The following is a summary of general therapeutic options for allergies (e.g., allergic rhinitis). If a patient presents with severe respiratory or anaphylactic symptoms, stabilizing pulmonary function or allergen exposure risk with potent conventional therapies is prudent before introducing supplements or botanical preparations. For the patient with mild to moderate allergy symptoms, however, this stepladder approach is appropriate.

REMOVE ENVIRONMENTAL TRIGGERS FROM THE HOME

- With perennial allergens (e.g., dust mites), tell the patient to wash bedclothes weekly in hot water, encase mattresses and pillows in mite-impermeable covers, and remove carpeting from rooms (especially bedrooms). Regular vacuuming of carpeted areas (by someone without allergies) is also suggested.
- Pet-sensitive individuals are a special case. The ideal solution, removal of the pet from the household, is typically not an option with pet lovers. In this case, removing pet access to the bedroom is helpful. Regular washing of the pet may or may not be of benefit
- A high-efficiency particulate air (HEPA) filter is useful for light, floating allergens, such as cat allergens; it is less effective with dog allergens.

AVOID PEAK POLLEN EXPOSURE OUTDOORS

- Outdoor pollens are ubiquitous; avoidance is nearly impossible. Pollen-sensitive patients can avoid significant exposure by limiting outdoor activities between 5 and 10 a.m. and on dry, windy days when airborne pollen levels are highest.

NUTRITION

- Decrease dairy (milk protein) and total protein intake. Plant proteins may be preferable.
- Consume fats rich in omega-3 found in cold-water fish, nuts, greens, and ground flaxseed. Consider the addition of pharmaceutical-grade (distilled) fish oil capsule or liquid supplements.
- Increase water intake dramatically to maintain adequate hydration.
- Increase intake of natural bioflavonoids and antioxidants by eating more organic fruits (especially brightly-colored berries) and vegetables.

MIND-BODY THERAPY

- Clinical hypnosis may markedly attenuate allergic reactivity.
- Consider a trial of homeopathy, which is particularly helpful in individuals with multiple chemical or drug sensitivities. This form of therapy is safe for adults and children.

TRADITIONAL CHINESE MEDICINE

- Acupuncture therapy with or without Chinese herbal therapy can be used for allergic rhinitis. Most studies used artificially standardized regimens; individualized therapy may be more efficacious.
- Chinese herbal therapy and acupuncture can be helpful for asthma control, especially the latest compounds from Mt Sinai School of Medicine (ASHMI; Antiasthma Herbal Medicine Intervention).

SUPPLEMENTS

- Pycnogenol: 100 mg twice daily
- Fisetin: 100 mg once or twice per day
- Quercetin: 400–600 mg one to three times daily
- Magnesium glycinate: 400 mg daily
- Vitamin C: 250 mg twice daily

BOTANICALS

- Freeze-dried stinging nettles: 300–500 mg one to three times/day
- Butterbur (Petadolex): 50–100 mg twice daily

PHARMACEUTICALS

- Cromolyn sodium: nasal spray, one spray/nostril three to four times daily; nebulizer, 20 mg (one ampule) two to four times daily
- Second-generation antihistamines (oral)
    - Loratadine: 10 mg daily
    - Fexofenadine (Allegra): 180 mg daily or 60 mg twice daily
    - Cetirizine (Zyrtec): 5–10 mg daily
- Nasal antihistamines
    - Azelastine (Astepro), olopatadine (Patanase): one to two sprays/nostril twice daily
- Nasal corticosteroids (may be added if other natural and pharmacological interventions fail or if nasal congestion or recurrent sinusitis is a prominent problem)
    - Fluticasone nasal (Flonase): 1–2 sprays/nostril daily
    - Triamcinolone (Nasacort): 1–2 sprays/nostril daily
    - Budesonide nasal (Rhinocort): 1–2 sprays/nostril daily

IMMUNOTHERAPY

- This is typically reserved for those patients with more severe or refractory symptoms, life-threatening allergic reactivity, or coexisting conditions (e.g., asthma, sinusitis)
- Consider sublingual immunotherapy (SLIT) before subcutaneous immunotherapy.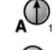

Key Web Resources

Purpose	URL
American Academy of Allergy Asthma and Immunology: professional allergy organization providing general info, updated research news, patient handouts.	http://www.aaaai.org/
This is the blog of Ves Dimov, an allergist at Cleveland Clinic. He has been posting since he was a Fellow and regularly reports on the latest clinical and research findings. Of general interest—not just for allergists.	http://allergynotes.blogspot.com
One of the best sources for analyses of the latest health-related articles. Well-written and researched; your patients are reading this!	http://www.nytimes.com/pages/health/index.html
NeilMed is a great source of nasal irrigation supplies and information for patients and also sends samples to healthcare practitioners.	http://www.neilmed.com

REFERENCES

References are available online at ExpertConsult.com.

CHAPTER 31

FOOD ALLERGY AND INTOLERANCE

Alan R. Gaby, MD

Food allergy is well recognized in clinical medicine as a cause of acute attacks of asthma, urticaria, and angioedema and as a contributing factor in some cases of eczema and rhinitis. These types of allergic reactions are called immediate or type 1 hypersensitivity reactions and are mediated by immunoglobulin E (IgE). The diagnosis and treatment of type 1 hypersensitivity reactions is well covered in standard medical texts, and a detailed discussion of this type of allergy is beyond the scope of this chapter.

Another type of food reaction, often referred to as "hidden" or "masked" food allergy, was described as early as the 1930s[1,2] and 1940s,[3,4] and has been described in the medical literature hundreds of times since then.[5] Hereinafter, unless otherwise specified, the term "food allergy" in this chapter will refer to hidden food allergy. Many integrative-medicine practitioners, including the author of this chapter, have observed that food allergies are a common cause of, or triggering factor for, a wide range of physical and mental disorders and that working with food allergies is an essential component of the practice of medicine. According to one estimate, as much as 60% of the population suffers from undetected food allergies.[6] Symptoms and disorders that have been reported to have a significant food allergy component are listed in Table 31.1.

> Hidden food allergies appear to be a common cause of, or triggering factor for, a wide range of physical and mental disorders.

Many doctors are not convinced that food allergy is a common problem, and some doubt that it even exists. Skeptics emphasize that many of the conditions said to be related to food allergy fluctuate in severity and have a significant psychological component. Consequently, it may be difficult to distinguish a true food reaction from a conditioned (psychogenic) response or a spontaneous exacerbation of symptoms. Moreover, there is no generally accepted mechanism to explain how foods could cause such a wide range of seemingly unrelated symptoms and conditions.

Proponents of the food allergy-disease connection point out that hidden food allergies are often overlooked because they are difficult to identify. Unlike type 1 hypersensitivity reactions, which usually trigger immediate symptoms and are therefore relatively easy to identify, hidden food reactions are often delayed for hours or even days. Moreover, hidden food reactions do not necessarily occur every time the offending food is consumed, but may depend on factors such as coingestion of other allergens, the method of cooking or processing of food, coexisting

stressors, and hormonal cycles. Identifying a cause–effect relationship between ingestion of specific foods and the development of symptoms is further complicated by the tendency of people to become addicted to the foods to which they are allergic and to experience transient relief after ingesting foods that are later demonstrated to be the cause of their chronic symptoms. Thus patients are often unaware that they have food allergies, and medical histories and diet diaries are frequently of little or no value for identifying specific allergens.

NOMENCLATURE

It has been argued that food-induced symptoms should not be called allergic reactions unless an immune-mediated mechanism can be demonstrated and that in the absence of such demonstration, terms such as intolerance or sensitivity would be more appropriate. However, the more we learn about physiology, the more apparent it becomes how blurred the lines are between the immune system and various other bodily systems (such as the endocrine, nervous, and cardiovascular systems). Some mediators of food-induced symptoms (e.g., platelet activation) could reasonably be considered to be within the domain of any of these systems, including the immune system.[7,8]

In the primary care setting, it is often difficult or impossible to identify the mechanisms underlying food-induced symptoms. Moreover, it is not clinically useful to attempt to delineate these mechanisms in many cases (although there are some important exceptions, as discussed in the section on differentiating food allergy from other food reactions). Notwithstanding concerns about its scientific accuracy, use of the term "allergy" has some advantages. In particular, it helps patients understand that food reactions can involve a wide array of different tissues and organs, and that in many instances even very small doses of an offending agent can evoke symptoms. For these reasons, the author tends to refer to food reactions as allergies unless a nonimmune-mediated mechanism is suspected (as in, for example, gastrointestinal reactions to fermentable carbohydrates or pseudoallergic reactions to food-derived salicylates or histamine).

PATHOPHYSIOLOGY

Why an Epidemic of Food Allergies?

When the author was in elementary school in the 1950s, virtually none of the children had attention deficit-hyperactivity disorder (ADHD). Today, ADHD is very

TABLE 31.1 Symptoms and Conditions That May Be Caused or Exacerbated by Food Allergy

Cardiovascular

Angina

Arrhythmias

Hypertension

Thrombophlebitis

Dermatological

Acne vulgaris

Dermatitis herpetiformis

Eczema

Pruritus

Purpura

Status ulcers

Urticaria

Ear, Nose, and Throat

Hearing loss

Hoarseness

Meniere's disease

Nasal polyps

Nosebleeds (epistaxis)

Olfactory dysfunction

Otitis externa

Otitis media

Sinusitis

Sore throat

Taste disorders

Vasomotor rhinitis

Vertigo

Gastrointestinal

Abdominal pain

Constipation

Crohn's disease

Diarrhea

Eosinophilic esophagitis

Gallbladder disease

Gastritis

Gastroesophageal reflux disease

Irritable bowel syndrome

Nonulcer dyspepsia

Pancreatitis

Peptic ulcer

Proctitis

Pruritus ani

Rectal bleeding

Ulcerative colitis

Vomiting

Neurological

Ataxia

Epilepsy

Migraine

Multiple sclerosis

Restless legs syndrome

Neurological

Tension-type headache

Ophthalmological

Conjunctivitis

Uveitis

Pediatric

Colic

Enuresis

Growing pains

Psychiatric

Anxiety

Attention deficit-hyperactivity disorder

Autism

Bipolar disorder

Depression

Dysthymia

Panic attacks

Schizophrenia

Pulmonary

Asthma

Chronic obstructive pulmonary disease

Cough

Renal

Glomerulonephritis

Nephrotic syndrome

Rheumatological

Juvenile rheumatoid arthritis

Psoriatic arthritis

Rheumatoid arthritis

Systemic lupus erythematosus

Vasculitis

Urological

Dysuria

Urethritis

Urinary frequency

Urinary tract infections

Miscellaneous

Aphthous ulcers

Candidiasis (*Candida*-related complex)

Edema

Fatigue

Food cravings

Halitosis

Insomnia

Obesity

Recurrent infections

Teeth grinding (bruxism)

Thrombocytopenia

Vaginitis

common and appears to be related in many cases to food allergy. In addition, the frequency of anaphylactic reactions to peanuts and other foods has been increasing in recent years.[9]

While one can only speculate on the reasons for the increased prevalence of allergies, possible culprits include alterations in immune function induced by environmental pollutants[10] and vaccinations, multiple antigenic exposures from the 2700 additives in our food supply, and genetic engineering of foods.[11,12] In particular, hybridization techniques have been used since the 1950s to produce new strains of wheat to increase crop yield.[13] Genetic modification has introduced new immunogenic proteins into modern wheat, which may explain, in part, the apparent increases in the prevalence of celiac disease and nonceliac gluten sensitivity in recent decades.

It has been suggested that immunoglobulin G (IgG) is involved in at least some food reactions[14,15]; however, that possibility has not been well studied. The results of one study suggested that the innate immune system (for example, Toll-like receptor 2) plays a role in the pathogenesis of nonceliac gluten sensitivity, whereas the adaptive immune system does not seem to be involved.[16] In contrast, both the innate and adaptive immune systems appear to contribute to type 1 hypersensitivity reactions. Whether the innate immune system plays a role in hidden allergy to food proteins other than gluten has not been investigated. Aside from these preliminary clues, the molecular mechanisms underlying hidden food allergy are poorly understood.

Specific Adaption

Another way of looking at the pathophysiology of food allergy is through the conceptual framework elucidated by Theron Randolph regarding the adaptation of patients to foods to which they are sensitive.[17] Randolph, a pioneer in the field of hidden food allergy, referred to this process as specific adaptation (SA), which he considered to be analogous to, though distinct from, the general adaptation syndrome (GAS) response to stress, as described by Hans Selye. A schematic representation of these types of adaptation is presented in Fig. 31.1.

Stage 1 of SA (which corresponds to the alarm stage of the GAS) is the preadaptive/nonadapted stage. In this stage, repeated exposure of a susceptible individual to an allergenic food results in progressively increasing sensitivity to the food, although symptoms are typically absent or mild at this point. Stage 2 of SA corresponds to the adaptation/resistance stage of the GAS. Initially, the patient is relatively symptom free (stage 2a, addicted/adapted), but may have adapted to the allergenic food by becoming addicted to it. He/she may have learned subconsciously to consume the food at regular intervals to avoid withdrawal symptoms. With continued exposure, the patient progresses to stage 2b (addicted/maladapted), in which ingestion of the food causes various physical and mental symptoms. However, the patient remains addicted and is usually unaware that the food is causing problems. It is at this stage that patients typically consult a health care practitioner. Stage 3 of SA (postadaptive/nonadapted) corresponds to the exhaustion stage of the GAS. In this stage, exposure to the food, even in low doses, produces acute symptoms. Some patients approach stage 3, but few actually reach it.

Patients who are in stage 2b can be reverted to a nonadapted stage 1 by means of an elimination diet, after which exposure to the allergenic food results in a rapid and exaggerated reaction. Thus an elimination diet followed by individual food challenges can be used diagnostically to demonstrate the etiology of patient symptoms.

RESEARCH VALIDATION

This section reviews several clinical trials that demonstrate the role of food allergy in the etiology of common

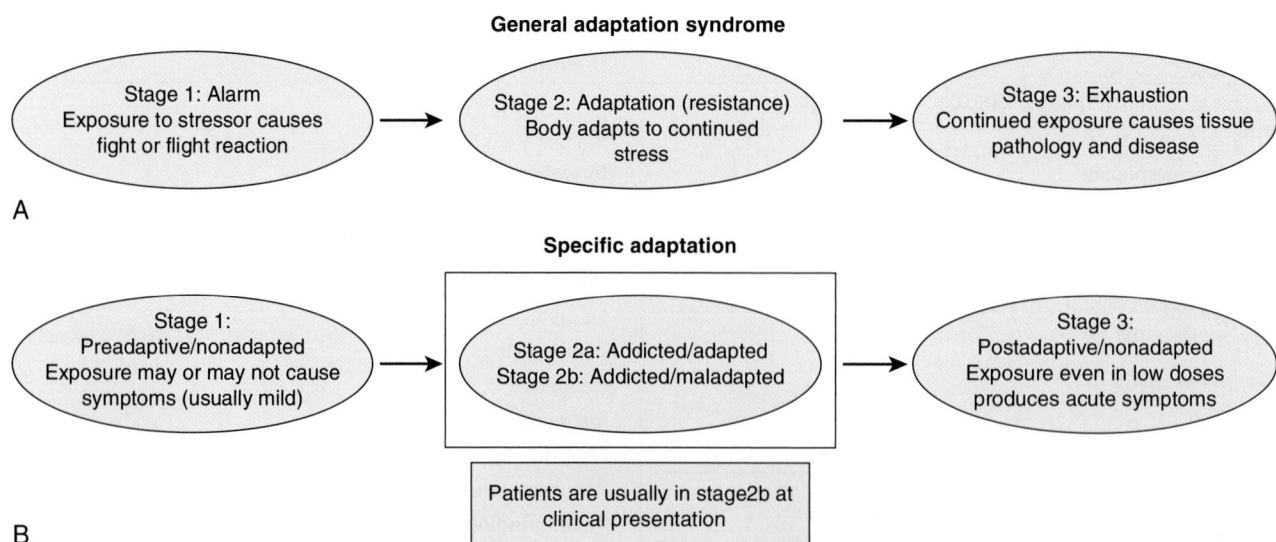

FIG. 31.1 ■ Stages in the development of hidden food allergy (specific adaptation) as contrasted with the general adaptation syndrome.

clinical conditions. These studies were chosen for review either because the findings were confirmed by double-blind, placebo-controlled food challenges or because the observed improvements were substantially greater than those obtainable with conventional medical approaches.

Migraine

Sixty patients with chronic, frequent migraines (mean duration of illness, 18.5 years) consumed an elimination diet for 5 days consisting only of two low-risk foods (usually lamb and pears) and bottled spring water. Migraines disappeared within 5 days in most cases. Each patient then tested one to three common foods per day, with evaluation of symptoms and acute pulse changes (which are thought by some investigators to indicate allergic reactions). Foods that most frequently caused reactions were wheat (78%); orange (65%); egg (45%); tea and coffee (40% each); chocolate and milk (37% each); beef (35%); corn, cane sugar, and yeast (33% each); mushrooms (30%); and peas (28%). When an average of 10 (range, 1–30) foods were avoided, all patients improved. The number of headaches in the treated group fell from 402 per month to 6 per month, with 85% of patients becoming headache free.[18]

Rheumatoid Arthritis

Fifty-three patients with rheumatoid arthritis were randomly assigned to a diet that excluded common allergens or to their usual diet (control group). After 1 week, the patients on the exclusion diet began reintroducing one food at a time, and any foods that produced symptoms were removed from the diet. After a total of 6 weeks, the diet group had significant improvements in subjective and objective measures of disease activity compared with the control group.[19] Long-term follow-up of 100 rheumatoid arthritis patients who underwent diet therapy at the same clinic revealed that one-third remained well on diet alone (without any medication) for up to 7.5 years after starting treatment.[20]

Irritable Bowel Syndrome

Twenty-one patients with irritable bowel syndrome followed a strict elimination diet consisting of a single meat, a single fruit, and distilled or spring water for 1 week. Symptoms disappeared in 14 patients (67%). Subsequently, individual food challenges identified the following symptom-evoking foods: wheat (64% of patients), corn (36%), dairy products and coffee (29% each), tea (21%), and citrus fruits (14%). Jejunal biopsies were normal in all patients who reacted to wheat, indicating the absence of celiac disease. Six patients underwent double-blind food challenges; in each case, the food reaction was confirmed.[21]

Nonceliac Gluten Sensitivity

Sixty-one adults without celiac disease or type 1 hypersensitivity to wheat (i.e., negative wheat-specific IgE test) who believed that gluten was the cause of their intestinal and extraintestinal symptoms were randomly assigned to receive, in double-blind fashion, 4.4 g per day of gluten or placebo (rice starch) in capsules for 1 week. After a 1-week washout period on a gluten-free diet, each participant was crossed over to the other treatment for an additional week. Compared with placebo, gluten significantly increased overall symptoms ($p < .04$). Abdominal bloating ($p = .04$), abdominal pain ($p < .05$), foggy mind ($p < .02$), depression ($p = .02$), and aphthous stomatitis ($p < .03$) were significantly more severe with gluten than with placebo. These results confirm that gluten can trigger both intestinal and extraintestinal symptoms in nonceliac patients with self-reported gluten sensitivity.[22]

DIAGNOSIS
Medical History

Food allergy should be considered in the differential diagnosis of all of the symptoms and conditions listed in Table 31.1. The likelihood that a patient has food allergies appears to increase in proportion to the number of symptoms and conditions the patient has that could be due to food allergy. In addition, the index of suspicion should be increased in patients who have a childhood history of colic, recurrent ear infections, sore throats, runny nose, "growing pains," asthma, eczema, or "getting sick all the time," and in those with a family history of allergy. On questioning, patients may report that they feel worse after eating and better when they fast. However, many patients with food allergies also have reactive hypoglycemia, which generally has the opposite pattern with respect to meals (i.e., better after eating, worse when fasting). When patients have both reactive hypoglycemia and food allergies, it may be difficult to draw diagnostic conclusions from the symptom pattern in relation to meals. As previously noted, patients may be unaware that they have food allergies, and dietary histories and diet/symptom diaries are frequently of little or no diagnostic value.

> Many patients with chronic illnesses are unaware that they have food allergies, and diet histories are often of little or no value for identifying symptom-evoking foods.

Physical Examination

Physical signs of allergy (food or inhalant) may include pallor of the nasal mucosa, general pallor, "allergic shiners" (edematous dark circles under the eyes), generalized edema, Dennie's lines (horizontal creases across the lower eyelids), and ecchymoses. Signs seen primarily in allergic children include the "allergic salute" (wiping or rubbing the nose with an upward movement of the hand) and an "allergic crease" (a single horizontal crease across the lower portion of the nose from repeated allergic saluting).

Other Diagnostic Tests

Conventional skin-prick tests, scratch tests, and blood tests for food-specific IgE antibodies are of value for identifying IgE-mediated type 1 hypersensitivity reactions, but these tests have repeatedly been found to be unreliable for diagnosing hidden food allergies.

IgG4 Antibody Testing

Blood tests that measure food-specific IgG4 antibodies are also commercially available; however, the reliability of these tests is in doubt for a number of reasons. First, some commercial laboratories have reported widely divergent results when sent split samples of the same blood. Second, various microorganisms and other contaminants may be present in the food samples from which the test antigens are prepared. Therefore, the presence of antibodies to a food extract may, in some cases, indicate nothing more than previous exposure to common bacteria and fungi. Third, some allergic reactions are not due to native food proteins but to polypeptides produced during the process of digestion or to glycosylation products produced during cooking. Those antigens would not be among the ones measured by blood tests. Fourth, while there is evidence that antibodies within the IgG4 fraction act as symptom-evoking antibodies, the IgG4 fraction also appears to contain blocking antibodies, which may prevent allergic reactions.[23] Consequently, the theoretical basis for measuring IgG4 antibodies as a diagnostic test for food allergies is open to question. Fifth, as previously noted, some food reactions are not mediated by antibodies and would therefore not be identifiable by antibody testing. The author is not aware of any published research that addresses the incidence of false-positive and false-negative results from IgG antibody tests. However, clinical experience suggests that the frequency of incorrect test results (i.e., those that conflict with the results of elimination and rechallenge) is unacceptably high, with one study reporting that IgG blood testing was of no value for identifying specific food sensitivities in children with attention deficit-hyperactivity disorder.[24]

ALCAT Testing

Another blood test, known as antigen leukocyte antibody test (ALCAT), measures platelet aggregation and morphological changes in white blood cells after whole blood is mixed with various food extracts. In one study, the incidence of false-positive results using this test was 24.3% and the incidence of false-negatives was 30.9%,[25] suggesting that this test is unreliable for diagnosing food allergies. In addition, when split samples of the same blood were sent under different names to a laboratory that performs the ALCAT test, only 34% of the tests performed showed the same results.[26]

Food Extract Testing

Provocative testing is used by some practitioners to diagnose food allergies. This procedure involves intradermal or sublingual administration of various dilutions of food extracts. A similar procedure is used to "neutralize" or desensitize allergies. Although the efficacy of food extract injection therapy has been

demonstrated in a double-blind study,[27] others have failed to find a beneficial effect.[28] Accordingly, provocative testing and neutralization remain controversial techniques.

INTEGRATIVE THERAPY

Elimination Diet

Hidden food allergies can usually be "unmasked" by means of an elimination diet, followed by individual food challenges.[29] After a patient has been on a hypoallergenic diet for a period of time (usually 2–3 weeks), chronic symptoms often disappear or improve and the body reverts from a state of "waterlogged" allergy-addiction to one of increased alertness and sensitivity. In this hypersensitive state, ingestion of an offending food results in a rapid and exaggerated reaction, allowing the patient to identify previously unsuspected allergens.

> In most cases, hidden food allergies can be identified by means of an elimination diet, followed by individual food challenges.

The author has prescribed elimination diets for more than 2000 patients. The diet used in the vast majority of cases is described in detail in Appendix A, Allergy Elimination Diet (available online at ExpertConsult.com) and is a modification of an elimination diet developed by William Crook.[18] It excludes all foods that contain refined sugar, wheat, dairy products, corn, eggs, citrus fruits, coffee, tea, alcohol, and food additives other than vitamins. Patients also exclude any foods to which they know or strongly suspect they are allergic (even foods that are normally allowed on the diet) and any foods they eat three or more times a week. The reason that frequently eaten foods are eliminated is that individuals with an allergic constitution may develop hidden allergies to foods they eat frequently (even foods that are not common allergens). Patients who find it too difficult to eliminate otherwise permitted foods that they have been eating frequently may consume those foods on a rotating basis (i.e., no more than every 4 days) during the elimination phase.

Alternatives to refined sugar (such as honey, maple syrup, and barley syrup) are permitted or prohibited on an individual basis depending on whether the patient is suspected to be sensitive to simple sugars. Tap water is excluded if the patient is thought to be highly sensitive. When tap water is excluded, the patient is advised to use spring or distilled water bottled in glass or hard (non-leaching) plastic containers.

This method of selecting which foods to avoid seems to be reasonably effective at excluding the most common allergens, as well as most other foods to which a particular patient is likely to be sensitive. Allergenic foods that are not initially excluded can frequently be detected by the patient during the elimination phase (after the body has become hyperalert from excluding the major allergens), particularly if those foods are being consumed on a rotating basis. Foods that clearly evoke symptoms during the elimination phase are removed from the diet.

A marked diuresis is common during the early part of the elimination diet, as chronic allergic edema begins to resolve. Approximately 25% of patients experience "withdrawal" symptoms within a few days of starting the diet. Withdrawal symptoms may include fatigue, irritability, headaches, malaise, and increased hunger. These symptoms typically resolve after 1–3 days, and the patient begins to feel better than before starting the diet. In most cases, withdrawal symptoms are not severe and do not require treatment. If symptoms are too uncomfortable, patients may obtain relief by taking buffered vitamin C (sodium ascorbate or calcium ascorbate) at a dose of 1000 mg up to four times per day. Withdrawal symptoms may also be ameliorated by taking alkali salts (such as sodium bicarbonate and potassium bicarbonate in a 2:1, 1:1, or 1:2 ratio) at a dose of 1/4 to 1/2 teaspoon dissolved in 6–8 ounces of water three to four times per day, as needed.

Clear symptomatic improvement is usually evident after 10–21 days on the elimination diet, although some patients improve more quickly. In a small proportion of patients, improvement is not seen until the fourth week on the diet.

Editor's Note

The author offers his recommendations on how to do an elimination diet in Appendix A (available online at ExpertConsult.com). Also see Chapter 86 for further discussion and recommendations.

Individual Food Challenges

Patients are typically advised to continue the elimination diet for 3 weeks, after which they undergo individual food challenges. Food challenges may be started sooner if the patient has experienced marked improvement for at least 5 days and has been on the diet for at least 10 days. Patients who have not improved after 3 weeks are encouraged to continue the elimination diet for an additional week. If no improvement is seen after 4 weeks, patients are given the option of returning to a healthful diet or undergoing individual food challenges. Occasionally, patients who have not shown clear improvement on the elimination diet discover from individual challenges that specific foods exacerbate their symptoms.

Methods of testing individual foods are described in Appendix A. Allergic reactions to foods typically occur within 10 minutes to 12 hours of ingestion, although the onset of joint pain may be delayed by as much as 48 hours. Typically, one new food is tested per day. However, if the patient's chief complaint is arthritis, new foods are tested every second day. Challenge foods

that evoke symptoms are removed from the diet, and the patient waits until the symptoms have largely disappeared before testing the next food. Foods that do not trigger symptoms are also removed from the diet for the remainder of the testing period, but they may be consumed again after the individual food challenges have been completed. If the patient is uncertain whether or not a food has triggered symptoms, that food should be retested 4–5 days later. Occasionally, it is not clear whether a reaction is due to the most recently tested food or to a delayed reaction to a previously tested food. In that case, both foods should be retested at a later time.

Some patients feel so much better on the elimination diet that they choose not to undergo the individual food challenges. This can lead to confusion regarding which foods truly need to be avoided because waiting too long (such as more than 6 weeks) before undergoing food challenges may decrease a person's reactivity to allergenic foods and therefore decrease the probability that challenges with these foods would provoke symptoms. However, as long as the patient is consuming a balanced diet that contains adequate amounts of all macronutrients and micronutrients, there does not appear to be any harm in continuing the elimination diet indefinitely.

Alternative Elimination Diet

In cases where multiple food allergies are suspected, patients can be placed on a highly restrictive diet (usually lamb, pears, and spring water) for 5 days, followed by individual food challenges (up to three different foods per day). The advantage of this approach is that it may result in rapid clearing of symptoms and it allows for rapid retesting of foods. However, such an approach requires a highly motivated patient.

Elimination-and-Rechallenge Diets in Clinical Practice

Some patients are able to undertake the elimination-and-rechallenge program successfully by simply reading the information provided in Appendix A (available online at ExpertConsult.com).

More often, patients find the prospect of markedly changing their diet to be overwhelming. This reaction to being shown the elimination diet is due, in part, to a lack of familiarity with alternative foods and, in part, to their knowledge (conscious or unconscious) that they are addicted to substances such as sugar, wheat, dairy products, coffee, or alcohol.

To enhance compliance, I informed patients that the elimination diet is a diagnostic test of finite duration; that withdrawal symptoms are transient; and that identifying hidden allergens may allow the patient to regain control of his or her health. The staff nutritionist spent as much time as necessary to teach patients the specifics of the program (usually 30–60 minutes), and patients were encouraged to phone the office if they had questions or problems. About 80%–90% of patients who were taught the elimination diet completed it successfully; of those, more than two-thirds experienced significant clinical improvement. In many cases, identification and avoidance of allergenic foods resolved chronic issues that had failed to respond to any other treatment.

Differentiating Food Allergy From Other Food Reactions

Some food reactions are mediated by the immune system, others are nonimmune mediated, and in others the mechanism is uncertain. The various mechanisms underlying food reactions are summarized in Chapter 86. As previously mentioned, in many cases it is both difficult and not clinically useful to determine whether a food reaction is a true allergy or whether it occurs through a nonimmune-mediated mechanism. However, there are some important exceptions.

Pseudoallergy

Pseudoallergic reactions are hypersensitivity reactions to food additives or to compounds that occur naturally in foods.[30] Examples of pseudoallergens include salicylates, histamine, sulfites, benzoates, and tartrazine (FD&C Yellow #5). Pseudoallergic reactions appear to involve direct (as opposed to antibody-mediated) activation of mast cells or a pharmacological effect (as in the case of histamine intolerance). Distinguishing pseudoallergy from allergy has two advantages. First, identifying a pseudoallergen as an etiological factor may help the patient devise a more focused and effective diet. For example, if the pattern of food reactions suggests sensitivity to salicylates or histamine, the patient can be directed to information on how to follow a low-salicylate or low-histamine diet. Second, pseudoallergic reactions are often dose dependent in contrast to allergic reactions, which may occur even with low-level exposures. Awareness of this dose–response relationship may allow for a less restrictive diet.

Reactions to Fermentable Carbohydrates

Some patients with irritable bowel syndrome (IBS) are intolerant to one or more types of fermentable, poorly absorbed carbohydrates, which can cause symptoms by exerting an osmotic effect in the gastrointestinal tract.[31] These carbohydrates are collectively called FODMaPs, which is an acronym for fermentable oligosaccharides, disaccharides, monosaccharides, and polyols (see Chapter 90). FODMaPs include fructose, lactose, sorbitol, fructans (fructooligosaccharides, inulin), and galactooligosaccharides. Several studies have demonstrated that consumption of a low-FODMaPs diet improves symptoms in patients with IBS.[32-35] Fructans are present in relatively high concentrations in gluten grains, and some IBS patients who are intolerant to fructans erroneously attribute their gastrointestinal symptoms to gluten sensitivity.[36]

FODMaPs intolerance should be considered in patients whose food-induced symptoms are limited to the gastrointestinal tract. As with pseudoallergy, identifying FODMaPs as etiological agents may lead to a more effective diet plan, and awareness that the reactions are dose dependent may allow for a less restrictive diet.

Celiac Disease versus Nonceliac Gluten Sensitivity

As previously mentioned, many patients who experience gluten-induced intestinal or systemic symptoms do not have celiac disease. To provide appropriate dietary recommendations and follow-up, it is important to distinguish celiac disease from nonceliac gluten sensitivity. In people with celiac disease, strict avoidance of gluten is essential because ingestion of even small amounts may increase the risk of developing intestinal lymphoma, nutrient deficiencies, and other complications. In contrast, patients with nonceliac gluten sensitivity may experience symptoms if they eat gluten, but they do not appear to be at increased risk for serious complications.

> In patients who react to gluten, it is important to distinguish between celiac disease and nonceliac gluten sensitivity.

Some of the differences in clinical presentation and laboratory findings between celiac disease and nonceliac gluten sensitivity are listed in Table 31.2. Awareness of these differences may help the clinician determine whether a small-bowel biopsy or genetic and serological testing for celiac disease is necessary.

Precautions With Elimination Diets

As previously noted, exaggerated reactions may occur when individual foods are reintroduced after the patient has been on an elimination diet for a few weeks. While life-threatening or severe anaphylactic reactions to food challenges are uncommon, they have been known to occur, particularly in patients with a history of severe asthma or severe atopic dermatitis.[17,37,38] In addition, some patients with atopic dermatitis who had not previously experienced acute problems from ingesting cow's milk became sensitized to cow's milk after its removal from the diet. Symptoms such as urticaria, dyspnea, vomiting, cough, or rhinoconjunctivitis have occurred in such patients after a cow's milk challenge, even if they had been avoiding cow's milk for years.[39]

Patients considered at risk for severe reactions should either not undergo diet therapy or should have food challenges performed under the guidance of an experienced practitioner in a hospital or other properly equipped setting. Patients considered at risk for moderately severe reactions who are conducting individual food challenges at home should have epinephrine and other rescue medication close at hand.

Individuals who abuse alcohol are at risk of developing delirium tremens when they withdraw from alcohol.

TABLE 31.2 **Prevalence of Various Clinical and Laboratory Findings in Patients With Celiac Disease (CD) and Nonceliac Gluten Sensitivity (NCGS)**

Clinical or Laboratory Finding	CD	NCGS
Constipation	7%	51%
Diarrhea with weight loss or steatorrhea	67%	25%
Severe vitamin D deficiency (serum 25[OH]D < 10 ng/ml)	30%	0.8%
Iron-deficiency anemia	20%	2.4%
Presence of two or more nutritional deficiencies (vitamin D, iron, vitamin B$_{12}$, zinc)	20%	0.8%
Serology (tTG [IgA/IgG], DGP, EMA)[26,48-51]	Usually positive, relatively high sensitivity and specificity	Usually negative
HLA type DQ2 and/or DQ8	Nearly 100% (negative test makes it very unlikely that a person has celiac disease)	Approximately 30%–40% of the general population
Intestinal permeability[16]	Tends to be increased	Tends to be normal or decreased

DGP, deaminated gliadin peptide antibodies; *EMA*, antiendomysium IgA antibodies; *HLA*, human leukocyte antigen; *tTG IgA/IgG*, tissue transglutaminase IgA/IgG antibodies.
Modified from Kabbani TA, Vanga RR, Leffler DA, et al. Celiac disease or non-celiac gluten sensitivity? An approach to clinical differential diagnosis. *Am J Gastroenterol.* 2014;109:741-746.

These individuals should not attempt an elimination diet until they have completed an alcohol detoxification program. It would be prudent to observe similar precautions with people who abuse cocaine, narcotics, or other drugs.

Some patients with food allergies, particularly those with multiple allergies, may develop a fear of eating, which can lead to malnutrition. The practitioner should assess the nutritional adequacy of these patients' diets and should provide dietary and psychological counseling when necessary.

> Patients with food allergies should receive appropriate counseling to ensure that their diet is nutritionally adequate.

After Testing

The information provided in this paragraph relates to hidden food allergies and does not apply to type 1 (immediate) hypersensitivity reactions. Most foods become progressively less reactive the longer they are avoided, although a small percentage of food allergies are permanent (i.e., the food provokes symptoms even after many years of avoidance). Adults should avoid allergenic foods for at least 6–12 months before attempting to reintroduce them into their diet. Some children are able to resume eating allergenic foods after as little as 3 months. Previous allergens that are successfully reintroduced should, in most cases, be consumed no more than once every 3–4 days. More frequent consumption of these foods may eventually cause the allergy to return.

Highly allergic patients may fare best if they follow a rotary diversified diet in which no food is eaten more often than every 4 days. Some practitioners recommend rotating food groups (e.g., legumes every other day) in addition to rotating specific foods (e.g., soy on day 2,

lentils on day 4). While most of the patients the author has worked with did not need to follow a strict rotation diet, it would be prudent for all individuals with allergies not to eat the same foods every day.

Patients who need to avoid common foods should receive appropriate counseling to ensure that their diet is balanced and not nutritionally deficient.

"Allergic to Everything"

Some patients react to so many foods that they find it difficult to consume a nutritionally adequate diet. In these patients, symptom-evoking foods may be tolerated to some extent if they are consumed as part of a 4- or 5-day rotation diet. However, patients with multiple allergies represent a major challenge, and their clinical outcomes are often less than satisfactory. Many such patients also have multiple chemical sensitivities and inhalant allergies. Avoiding such exposures as much as possible and administering desensitization therapy for foods, inhalants, and other substances may be worthwhile. Comprehensive treatment of patients with multiple sensitivities is beyond the scope of this chapter and may require referral to a physician trained in environmental medicine. Many such physicians are members of the American Academy of Environmental Medicine. Information about this organization is available below under Key Web Resources.[40]

Other Treatments

Total Allergic Load

Patients with food allergies often improve when their total allergic load is decreased by identifying and avoiding inhalant and chemical allergens and by undergoing desensitization therapy when appropriate. Similarly, sensitivity to inhalants and chemicals may decrease when patients begin avoiding allergenic foods.

Nutritional Supplements

Specific nutritional supplements may be of benefit for the prevention and treatment of certain conditions that are often caused or triggered by food allergy. For example, magnesium[41] and riboflavin[42] often reduce the frequency of migraine episodes, and omega-6 fatty acids have been found to be of benefit for patients with eczema.[43] However, there is no clear evidence that nutritional supplements reduce allergic reactivity per se.

Anti-Candida Program

In the author's experience, an anti-*Candida* program, consisting of dietary modifications and prescription or herbal antifungal agents, sometimes decreases allergic reactivity in patients who have clinical evidence of a syndrome that has been called chronic candidiasis, *Candida*-related complex, or *Candida* hypersensitivity syndrome. Although other practitioners have reported similar observations, the existence of this syndrome remains controversial. An anti-*Candida* program may work by decreasing intestinal inflammation and permeability, thereby decreasing the absorption of allergenic macromolecules. The evaluation and management of chronic candidiasis is described elsewhere.[44,45]

PREVENTION PRESCRIPTION

- Encourage breastfeeding: In observational studies, atopic dermatitis developed less frequently in children who had been breastfed than in those who had been formula fed.[46,47] Whether breastfeeding would prevent other conditions associated with food allergy is not known.

- Consider introducing eggs and peanuts between 4 and 11 months of age. Early introduction of peanuts and eggs has been associated with less IgE allergy to these foods later in life.[47a]

- Avoid unnecessary chemical exposures: In some patients, food allergies develop or become worse after exposure to toxic or allergenic chemicals, presumably as a result of stress on, or injury to, the immune system.

- Follow a rotary diversified diet: People with an allergic constitution tend to become allergic to foods they consume frequently. Including a wide range of foods in the diet and not eating the same foods every day may reduce the risk of developing hidden food allergies.

THERAPEUTIC REVIEW

TESTING

- Conduct a thorough medical history and physical examination to assess the likelihood that the patient has food allergies.
- When appropriate, prescribe and supervise an elimination diet followed by individual food challenges.

NUTRITION

- Work with the patient to devise a nutritionally adequate, diverse diet that avoids the symptom-evoking foods identified during the testing period.

NUTRITIONAL SUPPLEMENTS

- Various nutritional supplements may be useful for specific conditions that have a food allergy component (e.g., magnesium for the prevention of migraines or asthma attacks, probiotics for the treatment of irritable bowel syndrome, and fatty acids for the treatment of eczema). While there is no clear evidence that nutritional supplements can prevent food-allergic reactions per se, an individualized program of hypoallergenic nutritional supplements may improve clinical outcomes in allergic patients.

LIFESTYLE

- Integrative approaches such as avoiding stress and engaging in regular physical exercise may improve the overall health of allergic patients, although there is no clear evidence that these lifestyle factors decrease allergic reactivity per se.

Key Web References

International Chronic Urticaria Society. Information on a low-salicylate diet.	http://chronichives.com/useful-information/low-salicylate-diet
International Chronic Urticaria Society. Information on a histamine-restricted diet.	http://chronichives.com/useful-information/histamine-restricted-diet
My Food My Health. The FODMAPS recipes, diet, and meal plan.	https://myfoodmyhealth.com/meal-plans-diets/fodmaps-14-day-diet-plan
American Academy of Environmental Medicine. Provides information for those with multiple environmental sensitivities that extend beyond food.	http://www.aaemonline.org/

REFERENCES

References are available online at ExpertConsult.com.

METABOLIC/ENDOCRINE DISORDERS

SECTION OUTLINE

32 INSULIN RESISTANCE AND THE METABOLIC SYNDROME

33 DIABETES MELLITUS

34 HYPOTHYROIDISM

35 POLYCYSTIC OVARIAN SYNDROME

36 OSTEOPOROSIS

37 AN INTEGRATIVE APPROACH TO OBESITY

38 MTHFR, HOMOCYSTEINE, AND NUTRIENT NEEDS

39 ADRENAL FATIGUE

INSULIN RESISTANCE AND THE METABOLIC SYNDROME

Edward (Lev) Linkner, MD • Corene Humphreys, ND

DEFINING METABOLIC SYNDROME

The terms "syndrome of insulin resistance (IR)" and "the metabolic syndrome" were coined in the 1980s by Gerald Reaven, MD, an endocrinologist at Stanford Medical School in California. Other names used to describe the condition include syndrome X, prediabetes, dysmetabolic syndrome, and cardiometabolic syndrome.[1]

Metabolic syndrome is associated with a constellation of risk factors for atherosclerosis and type 2 diabetes mellitus (DM) including[2]:

- Elevated fasting glucose
- Elevated triglycerides
- Reduced high-density lipoprotein (HDL) cholesterol
- Hypertension
- Central obesity

The presence of three or more of these risk factors defines the metabolic syndrome. Following a joint scientific statement by several major organizations, a set of defined cut off values were determined for all components, with the exception of waist circumference (Table 32.1).[3] According to the National Cholesterol Education Program Adult Treatment Panel III, a waist circumference of more than 40 inches (101 cm) in men and more than 35 inches (89 cm) in women is a defining criteria for metabolic syndrome.[4] These values apply to Western cultures only. For information regarding other ethnic groups, readers should refer to the 2010 article by Lear et al.[5] that outlines existing and proposed waist circumference and waist-to-hip ratios.

Additional abnormalities posited to define the metabolic syndrome include endothelial dysfunction, and procoagulant and proinflammatory states.[6]

IR is the most common clinical finding associated with metabolic syndrome and is thought by many investigators to represent the predominant mechanism underlying the pathogenesis of this condition. IR is defined as decreased cellular sensitivity to insulin and varies according to cell type, organ, and particular metabolic pathway.[1] Research suggests that IR is associated with an inflammatory state and the activation of inflammatory pathways sustains IR and ultimately leads to the development of metabolic syndrome.[7]

PREVALENCE

The incidence of metabolic syndrome has reached epidemic proportions, with nearly 35% of all U.S. adults and 50% of those aged 60 years and older estimated to have metabolic syndrome in a 2015 report. Data from the National Health and Nutrition Examination Survey (NHANES) 2003 to 2012 reported a prevalence of metabolic syndrome of 33% (95% confidence interval [CI], 32.5% to 33.5%), with a significantly higher prevalence in women compared with men (35.6% vs 30.3% respectively; $P < 0.001$). When stratified according to ethnicity, the highest prevalence of metabolic syndrome is observed among Hispanics (35.4%; CI, 34.2% to 36.6%), followed by nonHispanic whites (33.4%; 95% CI, 32.6% to 34.2%) and blacks (32.7%; 95% CI, 31.5% to 33.9%). Overall, an increasing prevalence with advancing age has been reported for all ethnic groups. The prevalence of metabolic syndrome was reported as 18.3% among individuals aged 20 to 39 years and to be significantly higher at 46.7% among individuals aged 60 years or older.[8]

The increased prevalence of IR, metabolic syndrome, and type 2 DM is thought to be attributable to the global rise in the prevalence of obesity. Visceral fat is now considered to be involved in a number of metabolic, endocrine, and immune functions, all of which have been shown to increase risk of cardiovascular disorders.[11] Metabolic syndrome is reportedly associated with a twofold increased risk of cardiovascular disease (CVD) and a four-fold increased risk of type 2 DM compared to individuals without the condition[4] (Table 32.2).

PATHOPHYSIOLOGY

The etiology of IR and the metabolic syndrome is multifactorial and encompasses genetics, nutrient deficiencies, and metabolic defects in addition to lifestyle and environmental factors. The pathophysiology of the metabolic syndrome involves a complex cascade of events that occur intracellularly. Insulin is a major hormone whose action is required for proper tissue development, growth, and maintenance of glucose homeostasis.[12] Insulin also affects lipid metabolism by increasing hepatic and adipose lipid synthesis. IR is characterized by decreased responsiveness in the tissues to appropriate circulating levels of insulin and is considered the major contributor to the pathogenesis of metabolic syndrome (Fig. 32.1). Accordingly, IR in muscle tissues causes reduced glucose disposal from the bloodstream, and hepatic IR causes increased glucose production. Impairment of insulin secretion by pancreatic beta cells is a critical feature of the metabolic syndrome that leads to hyperglycemia due to defective insulin secretion and timing of the insulin response to glucose.[13]

TABLE 32.1 Criteria for the Clinical Diagnosis of the Metabolic Syndrome[3,6]

Measure	Categorical Cut Points
Elevated waist circumference	Greater than 40 inches (102 cm) in men or greater than 35 inches (88 cm) in women
Elevated triglycerides (drug treatment for elevated triglycerides is an alternate indicator)	150 mg/dL or greater
Reduced HDL cholesterol (drug treatment for reduced HDL cholesterol is an alternate indicator)	Less than 40 mg/dL for males and less than 50 mg/dL for females
Elevated blood pressure (drug treatment for hypertension is an alternate indicator)	Systolic 130 mm Hg or greater and/or diastolic 85 mm Hg
Elevated fasting glucose (drug treatment for diabetes mellitus is an alternate indicator)	100 mg/dL or greater

Modified from Alberti KG, Eckel RH, Grundy SM, et al. Harmonizing the metabolic syndrome: a joint interim statement of the International Diabetes Federation Task Force on Epidemiology and Prevention; National Heart, Lung, and Blood Institute; American Heart Association; World Heart Federation; International Atherosclerosis Society; and International Association for the Study of Obesity. *Circulation.* 120(16):1640-1645, 2009 and Aguilar M, Bhuket T, Torres S, Liu B, Wong RJ. Prevalence of the metabolic syndrome in the United States, 2003-2012. *JAMA.* 313(19):1973-1974, 2015.
HDL, high density lipoprotein.

TABLE 32.2 Abnormalities Associated With Insulin Resistance[9,10]

Some Degree of Glucose Intolerance
- Impaired fasting glucose
- Impaired glucose tolerance

Abnormal Uric Acid Metabolism
- ↑ Plasma uric acid concentration
- ↓ Renal uric acid clearance

Dyslipidemia
- ↑ Triglycerides
- ↓ High-density lipoprotein cholesterol
- ↓ Low-density lipoprotein particle diameter
- ↑ Postprandial lipemia

Hemodynamic Changes
- ↑ Sympathetic nervous system activity
- ↑ Renal sodium retention
- ↑ Blood pressure (50% of patients with hypertension have insulin resistance)

Hemostatic Changes
- ↑ Plasminogen activator inhibitor-1
- ↑ Fibrinogen

Endothelial Dysfunction
- ↑ Mononuclear cell adhesion
- ↑ Plasma concentration of cellular adhesion molecules
- ↑ Plasma concentration of asymmetric dimethyl arginine
- ↓ Endothelial-dependent vasodilatation

Reproductive
- Polycystic ovarian syndrome
- Low testosterone in men

Data from Corona G, Monami M, Rastrelli G, et al. Testosterone and metabolic syndrome: a meta-analysis study. *J Sex Med.* 2011;8:272-283 and Reaven G. Metabolic syndrome: pathophysiology and implications for management of cardiovascular disease. *Circulation.* 2002;106:286-288.

The key targets of insulin action are predominantly skeletal muscle (75%), followed by cardiac muscle, adipose tissue, and the liver. In the liver, insulin inhibits the production and release of glucose in healthy subjects by inhibiting gluconeogenesis and glycogenolysis. Defects in glucose transport or in the hexokinase II pathway may represent the principle mechanism underlying the inhibition of muscle glycogen synthesis. *In vivo* studies using nuclear magnetic resonance spectroscopy have demonstrated defects in muscle glycogen synthesis are caused by a defect in muscle glucose itself.[14] The glucose transporter 4 (GLUT4) is the major carrier of glucose into the cell. Stimuli, such as insulin and exercise, promote GLUT4 activity by embedding it into the cell membrane. Peroxisome proliferator–activator receptors (PPARs) are nuclear hormone receptor transcription factors that cause target genes to be expressed and play essential roles as regulators of insulin action[13] (Fig. 32.2).

Previous definitions of IR generally considered the condition exclusively in terms of the negative effects on glucose metabolism. Such effects include hyperglycemia following a high carbohydrate meal and over-stimulation of pancreatic beta cells to produce more insulin. Eventually, pancreatic beta cells become unable to produce sufficient insulin to maintain normal blood glucose levels. This inability of beta cells to produce sufficient insulin underlies the transition from IR to type 2 DM.[15] It is important to emphasize that IR

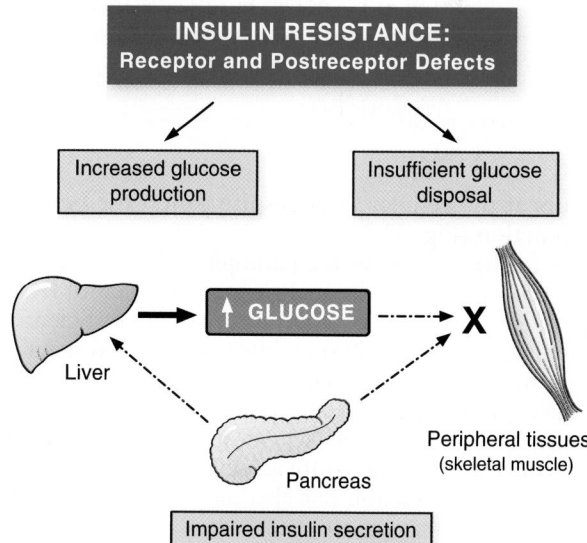

FIG. 32.1 ■ **Sites of the Three Major Pathogenic Defects That Lead to Type 2 Diabetes Mellitus.** Insulin resistance in muscle causes reduced glucose disposal from the bloodstream, and hepatic insulin resistance causes increased glucose production. Impairment of insulin secretion by pancreatic beta cells is a critical feature that leads to hyperglycemia when insulin secretion and the timing of the insulin response to glucose are defective.

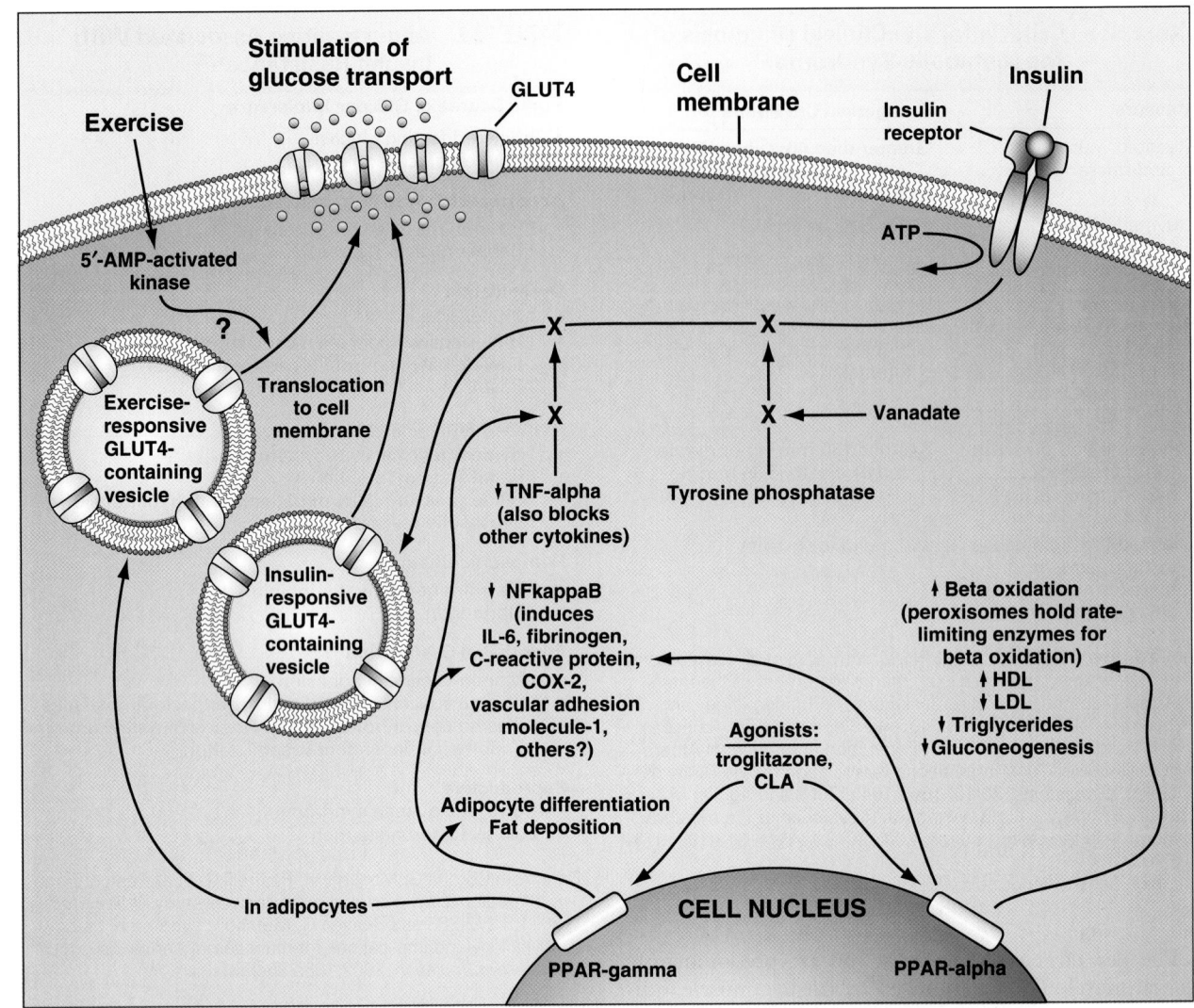

FIG. 32.2 ■ Insulin Signaling Pathways. AMP, adenosine monophosphate; ATP, adenosine tri-phosphate; CLA, conjugated linoleic acid; cox, cyclooxygenase; glut, glutamine transporter; HDL, high-density lipoprotein cholesterol; LDL, low-density lipoprotein cholesterol; NF-κβ, a B cell–specific transcription factor; PPAR, peroxisome proliferator-activator receptor; TNF, tumor necrosis factor.

occurs at the cellular level despite pancreatic beta cell dysfunction (Fig. 32.3).

As further studies of the pathophysiology of IR have been reported, the traditional glucocentric view of IR has evolved to include the "lipocentric" concept. Scientists have discovered that abnormalities in fatty acid metabolism cause inappropriate build-up of fat in muscle tissue, the liver, and other organs. Lipotoxicity, associated with increased plasma free fatty acid levels, is a hallmark of IR. Subsequently, these lipids are associated with not only an abnormal accumulation but also increased fat oxidation with further damage to the cell.[16,17]

IR may involve the insulin receptor itself. The insulin receptor belongs to the receptor tyrosine kinase family which also includes insulin-like growth factor-1 receptor (IGF-1R) and the insulin receptor-related receptor (IRR). Therefore impairment of insulin-stimulated glucose uptake may also result from the upregulation of inhibitors of these signaling pathways. Furthermore, protein-tyrosine phosphatases (PTPases) may also have a role as negative regulators of the insulin-signaling cascade. A combination of the downregulation and upregulation of certain receptors may be a key element of IR pathophysiology.[13]

Chronic, low-grade inflammation has also been posited to have a central pathogenic role in IR. Research has shown that proinflammatory cytokines and acute-phase reactants are associated with many features of the metabolic syndrome. These inflammatory cytokines promote IR through site-specific serine phosphorylation of insulin substrates.[16]

Therefore, IR, predominantly in skeletal muscle, manifests as a reduction in insulin-stimulated glycogen synthesis resulting from decreased glucose transport. Once this occurs, lipid accumulates in many cells, most importantly in the liver and pancreas, causing oxidative stress and deleterious changes to cellular metabolism. These multiple defects in insulin signaling have been posited to underlie downstream impaired glucose metabolism in

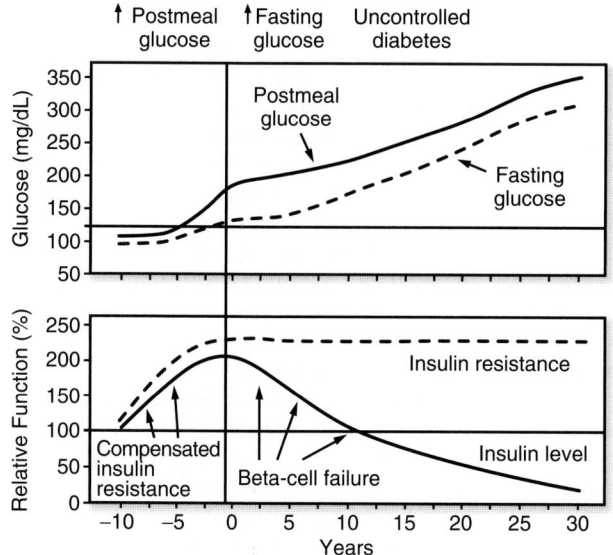

FIG. 32.3 ▦ Natural history of diabetes, depicting rising blood glucose levels with progressive beta cell dysfunction.

TABLE 32.3 Comorbidities of the Metabolic Syndrome

Alzheimer's disease[22]
Atrial fibrillation[23]
Baldness[24]
Breast cancer[25]
Cardiovascular risk[30]
Chronic fatigue syndrome[31]
Chronic kidney disease[32]
Cognitive impairment[33]
Colorectal cancer (men)[26]
Coronary artery disease[34]
Depression[35]
Endometrial cancer[27]
Erectile dysfunction[36]
Gestational diabetes[37]
Gout[38]
Hypothyroid and subclinical hypothyroidism[39]
Kidney stones[40]
Nonalcoholic fatty liver disease[41]
Pancreatic cancer[28]
Peripheral artery disease[42]
Psoriasis[43]
Sleep apnea[44]
Thyroid cancer[29]

most tissues[13,18] (Table 32.3). These pathways are summarized in Fig. 32.4.

Impact of Environmental Toxins on Metabolic Syndrome and Type 2 Diabetes MellitusNew research points to the role of environmental toxins as etiological factors in the pathogenesis of IR and type 2 DM. The organic compound bisphenol A (BPA) has been found to have an association with IR and type 2 DM. BPA is used to make polycarbonate and epoxy resins and is primarily found in food and beverage containers. BPA has been used commercially since 1957, with more than 90% of U.S. residents estimated to have detectable levels in urine. Findings from the 2003–2008 NHANES report revealed an association between BPA and prediabetes, independent of traditional risk factors.[19] Based on experimental studies, BPA appears to affect glucose metabolism through a number of pathways including insulin resistance, pancreatic beta cell dysfunction, adipogenesis, inflammation, and oxidative stress.[19] Other pollutants, such as air pollution[20] and traffic-related pollution,[21] have also been implicated in IR and increased risk of mortality attributable to type 2 DM.

Persistent organic pollutants (POPSs) may also play a role in the pathogenesis of the metabolic syndrome and type 2 DM. POPs are a class of compounds characterized by low water and high lipid solubility, an ability to persist in the environment, and a cause of biomagnification in the food chain. Pesticides, solvents, and foods from animals, such as seafood, are the main sources of POPs. Because POPs are lipophilic, these substances are highly resistant to degradation and have an estimated half-life of 7 to 10 years.[45] Some of the most common POPs found in humans include dioxins, polychlorinated biphenyls, dichlorodiphenyldichloroethylene, transnonachlor, hexachlorobenzene, and hexachlorocyclohexanes.[46] In the 1999–2002 NHANES report, higher concentrations of POPs (mainly pesticides and herbicides) were associated with an increased prevalence of type 2 DM. Subjects in the highest category (more than the 90th percentile) of exposure, as compared with the lowest category (less than

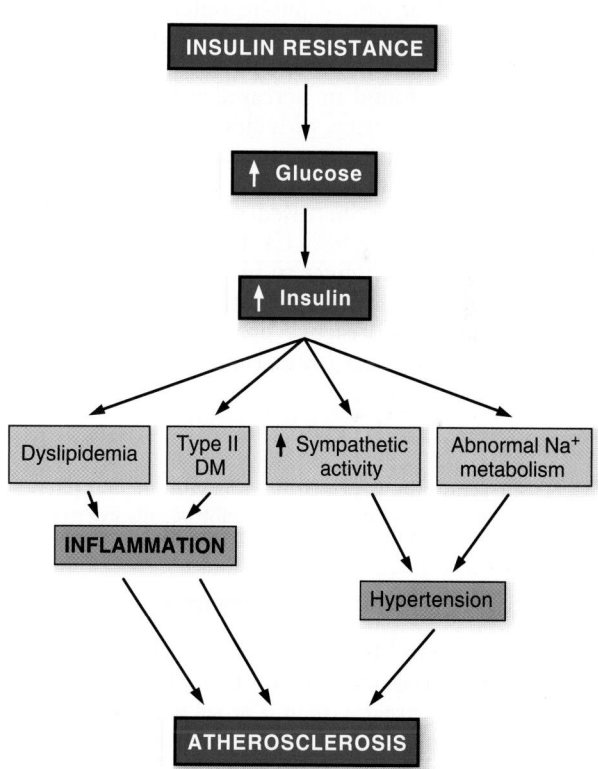

FIG. 32.4 ▦ **Summary of Insulin Resistance and Its Effects.** DM, diabetes mellitus; Na+, sodium.

the 25th percentile), had a 38-fold (P < 0.001) increased prevalence of type 2 DM. Obesity was not found to be a risk factor for type 2 DM in individuals with undetectable levels of persistent organic pollutants.[47] A year later, the same research group reported a positive correlation between POPs (in particular organochlorine pesticides) and the metabolic syndrome.[48] According to a *Lancet* editorial, the findings from the study by Lee et al. might imply that "virtually all of the risk of diabetes conferred by obesity is attributable to persistent organic pollutants, and that obesity is only a vehicle for such chemicals."[46] In a 2013 review of the epidemiological evidence of an association between POPs and diabetes, Magliano et al.[45] concluded that there is an independent relationship between POPs exposure and diabetes in the general population as well as occupationally exposed and high-risk populations.

Inorganic arsenic is another environmental toxin that appears to be associated with the metabolic syndrome and type 2 DM. The primary sources of inorganic arsenic are contaminated drinking water due to naturally occurring arsenic in rocks and soils, and food.[49] Organic arsenic is predominately derived from the ingestion of fish and shellfish, and is considered nontoxic as it is excreted unchanged in the urine. Results from the 2003–2004 NHANES cross-sectional study revealed a positive association between increasing levels of total urinary arsenic and type 2 DM. Subjects with type 2 DM had 26% higher total arsenic levels than subjects without DM. In the fully adjusted model comparing the 80th and 20th percentiles of total urine arsenic (16.5 vs 3.0 g/L), the odds ratio for type 2 DM was 3.58.[50] No association was observed between organic arsenic and type 2 DM. The investigators suggested that 8% of public water systems in the United States exceed the U.S. Environmental Protection Agency's standard of 10 mcg/L for drinking water.[50] Wang et al.[51] also found an increased prevalence of metabolic syndrome in subjects with elevated hair arsenic levels. After adjustment for confounding variables, subjects with hair arsenic in the 2nd tertile (0.034 mcg/g) had a statistically significant increased risk of metabolic syndrome (odds ratio, 2.54; 95% CI, 1.20 to 5.39; P < 0.015). Inorganic arsenic is thought to increase the risk of type 2 DM by stimulating increased expression and secretion of high sensitivity C-reactive protein (hs-CRP), which in turn activates nuclear factor kappa-beta via the Rho-kinase pathway.[52]

Metabolic syndrome is primarily an environmental phenotypic disorder (92%) rather than a genotypic disorder (8%).

Nonalcoholic Fatty Liver Disease

Nonalcoholic fatty liver disease (NAFLD) has been defined as the accumulation of fat in the liver (hepatic accumulation of greater than 5% of liver weight confirmed by magnetic resonance spectroscopy or liver biopsy) in the absence of other specific causes of liver infiltration, such as recent or significant alcohol ingestion, hepatic viral infections, or other causes of liver disease.[53,54] NAFLD is now the most common chronic liver disease worldwide, affecting both adults and children with an estimated prevalence of 20% to 35% in the general population.[55]

Traditionally NAFLD has been viewed as a histological continuum from pure fatty liver (steatosis) through nonalcoholic steatohepatitis (NASH) to liver fibrosis, potentially leading to liver cirrhosis associated with increased risk of hepatocellular carcinoma.[53] The histological progression of NAFLD begins with micro–macro vesicular steatosis, which primarily affects the perivenular regions, and may extend to panacinar distribution. The diagnosis of NASH is informed by the presence of fatty infiltration accompanied by inflammation associated with one of three additional features on liver histology: hepatocyte ballooning; Mallory hyaline; or fibrosis.[54,56] IR is considered the initial injury to the liver, which leads to increased uptake and synthesis of free fatty acids and impaired inhibition of adipose tissue lipolysis with resultant steatosis. Following initial fatty infiltration, the liver becomes increasingly vulnerable to multiple hits including gut-derived bacterial endotoxins, cytokine and adipokine imbalance, mitochondrial dysfunction, oxidative stress, lipid peroxidation, Kupffer cell activation, and hepatic stellate cell activation.[58] These multiple hits are proposed to stimulate hepatocyte injury and the progression from steatosis to NASH and ultimately fibrosis and cirrhosis (Fig. 32.5).[59]

Single nucleotide polymorphisms (SNPs) appear to be associated with NASH but not simple steatosis. NASH confers an increased risk of cirrhosis and secondary malignancy, partly attributable to genetic predisposition.

Immunological events are believed to play a role in the development and progression of NASH, and to be associated with hepatic apoptosis and fibrogenic responses. Additionally, impaired regeneration of hepatic progenitor cells appears to be a unifying pathophysiological pathway for NASH, with resultant dysregulated adipokine production and fibrosis.[53] In recognizing simple steatosis and NASH as two discrete entities with different etiologies, clinicians can identify and more closely monitor patients at greatest risk of liver fibrosis and cirrhosis, and individualize therapeutic interventions.

The Interrelationship Between Nonalcoholic Fatty Liver Disease and IR

NAFLD is considered the hepatic manifestation of metabolic syndrome, as IR is currently considered the fundamental underlying pathogenetic mechanism underlying the development of hepatic steatosis. Additionally, all key components of metabolic syndrome (abdominal obesity, impaired fasting glucose, dyslipidemia, and elevated blood pressure) have been identified as major risk factors for the development and progression of NAFLD.[55] Based on epidemiological studies, cardiovascular disease is the leading cause of death in NAFLD patients, followed by malignancy and liver disease, respectively. These findings imply NAFLD is a strong risk factor for cardiovascular disease and cardiovascular-related mortality.[61,62]

The prevalence of NAFLD is estimated to be 50% to 100% in obese and overweight patients, and 30% to 50% in patients with metabolic syndrome.[55] NAFLD combined with metabolic syndrome is reportedly correlated with greater severity of liver disease and increased likelihood of NASH, independent of age, sex, and body weight. Given the high prevalence of NAFLD, it has

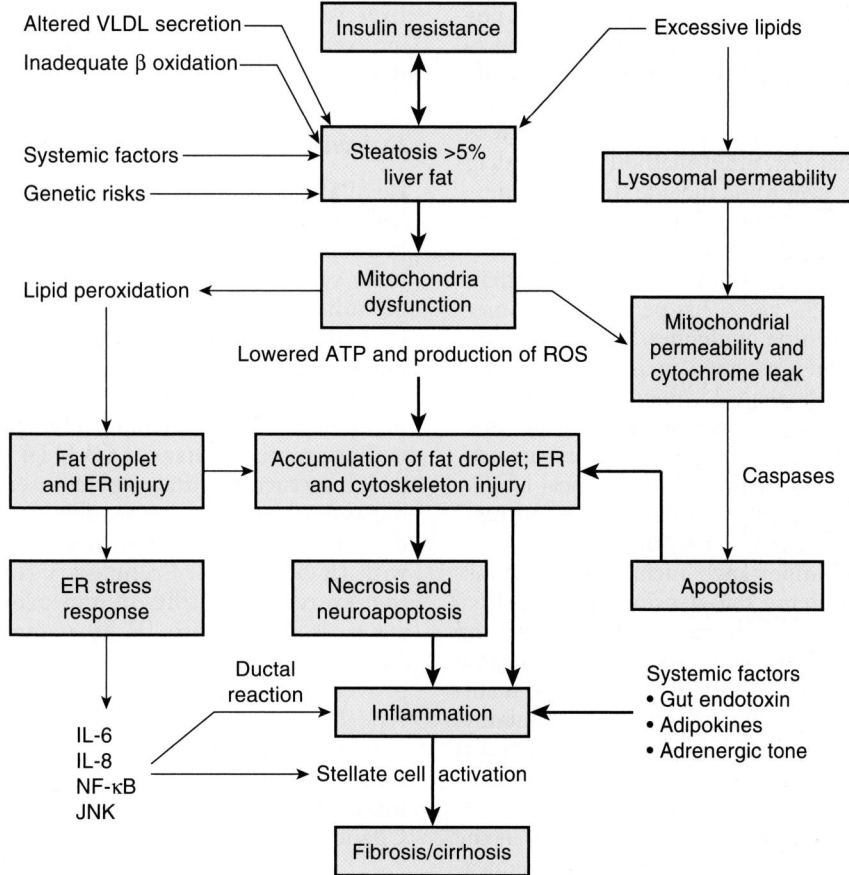

FIG. 32.5 ■ Illustration of Molecular Events Involved in the Pathogenesis of Nonalcoholic Fatty Liver Disease. ATP, adenosine triphosphate; ER, endoplasmic reticulum; IL, interleukin; JNK, c-Jun-N-terminal kinase; NF-κβ, nuclear factor kappa beta, a B cell–specific transcription factor; ROS, reactive oxygen species. (Reprinted with permission from Xiao J, Fai So K, Liong EC, Tipoe GL. Recent advances in the herbal treatment of non-alcoholic fatty liver disease. *J Tradit Complement Med.* 2013;3(2):88-94.)

been proposed that NAFLD be incorporated into diagnostic criteria for the metabolic syndrome.[55]

In the hepatic IR state, fatty infiltration is characterized by an increase in free fatty acids (FFAs) from sources including diet, adipose tissue, and de novo lipogenesis. Persistently increased glucose and hyperinsulinemia stimulate de novo lipogenesis by upregulating a number of transcription factors, which increase the activity of lipogenic enzymes. Fructose and high-fructose corn syrup have been identified as sugars that stimulate lipogenesis more profoundly that glucose. Ordinarily, FFAs are transported to the mitochondria for beta-oxidation or undergo esterification for excretion in VLDL or storage as fat droplets. IR-induced upregulation of FFAs causes direct hepatotoxicity via a number of intracellular responses. Excess FFAs activate the endoplasmic reticulum stress response, cause leakage during mitochondrial beta-oxidation, and lipid peroxidation in mitochondria (primarily), microsomes, and peroxisomes leading to reduced intracellular antioxidant capacity and increased oxidative stress. These mechanisms promote cellular apoptosis, a self-protective cellular response and key pathogenic event in NAFLD. Prolonged and increased levels of reactive oxygen species generated from mitochondrial dysfunction ultimately lead to steatosis and hepatic fibrosis.[58]

DIAGNOSIS

Metabolic syndrome can be diagnosed using the criteria described in Table 32.1. Outside a research laboratory, standard of practice for the diagnosis of the metabolic syndrome is to conduct a 2-hour glucose and insulin tolerance test (GITT), which can easily be ordered through any outpatient laboratory. The protocol is as follows: (1) 2 days of carbohydrate loading, (2) blood sampling for fasting glucose and insulin measurements, and (3) consumption of a 75-g glucose drink. Thereafter, blood specimens for glucose and insulin measurements are obtained (but not always necessarily) at half-hour intervals for the first hour, followed by a final specimen 2 hours later. In the majority of patients, fasting and 2-hour measurements are sufficient. Essentially, this protocol is the standard glucose tolerance test (GTT) with concomitant insulin testing. A caveat of this approach is that clinicians should ensure the laboratory used is familiar with diagnostic procedures involving insulin, which is a very unstable hormone in vitro. False-negative diagnoses are possible if only a fasting insulin specimen is obtained. Regular drawing of blood specimens for the measurement of insulin is required to maintain test functionality. Clinician are required to understand the effect of insulin on managing blood glucose levels following glucose consumption. Baseline fasting insulin levels should normally be less than 15 microunits/mL and less than 30 microunits/mL at 2 hours following consumption of a 75-g glucose load.

Although the 2-hour GITT is considered the most accurate and functional test, other methods for the diagnosis of the metabolic syndrome include the following:

- Triglyceride-to-HDL cholesterol ratio (TG:HDL-C)—a healthy ratio is less than 2.
- Glycosylated hemoglobin (HbA1c): values for patients with IR are between 5.7 and 6.4 as per the 2010 American Diabetes Association guidelines.[63]
- Fasting insulin: When assessed in isolation, normal values should be less than 15 microunits/mL (140 pmol/L); however, a normal fasting insulin result does not rule out IR. Reference ranges are laboratory specific, so clinicians must check with the clinical laboratories for specific values. In addition, what is "normal" and what is "healthy" can be vastly different.

Other markers of importance include elevated hs-CRP, uric acid, small dense low-density cholesterol (sd LDL-C), and inflammatory markers such as IL-6 and IL-8, TNF-alpha, PAF-1, and adiponectin. Because NAFLD is hypothesized to represent the hepatic manifestation of IR, the measurement of gamma-glutamyl transpeptidase (GGT) levels should also be considered as this transaminase enzyme is the most sensitive in detecting liver toxicity.

For the majority of clinicians, the 2-hour GITT is the most valuable in terms of diagnosis and patient education, particularly for normal-weight individuals suspected to have metabolic syndrome and women with polycystic ovarian syndrome.

INTEGRATIVE THERAPY

Lifestyle intervention offers the greatest promise for the prevention and management of the metabolic syndrome.

Lifestyle Factors

Although the pathogenesis of IR is multifactorial, lifestyle factors are known to have a profound effect on blood glucose homeostasis. According to statistics reported in 2009, at least 92% of type 2 DM cases are related to lifestyle choices.[64] Lack of exercise, central adiposity, and a diet high in refined carbohydrates and saturated fats and low in fiber represent key lifestyle characteristics associated with IR and type 2 DM. Knowler et al.,[65] researchers in the Diabetes Prevention Program, compared lifestyle modification with diet and medication in more than 3000 patients with prediabetes. The investigators assigned patients to three groups who received one of the following: (1) metformin 850 mg twice daily, (2) a lifestyle modification program with goals of at least 7% weight loss, or (3) placebo. After 3 years of follow-up, the metformin group contained 31% fewer diabetics, and the lifestyle modification group contained 58% fewer subjects with diabetes compared with the placebo group.

Exercise, weight loss, and a healthy diet are key lifestyle interventions for reducing IR and the risk of developing type 2 DM.[7]

Exercise

Regular exercise is a vital component of a holistic medical treatment plan and has been shown to reduce the incidence of IR by half.[66] Patients with IR and metabolic syndrome are recommended to partake in 30 to 60 minutes of moderate-intensity aerobic workouts (e.g., brisk walking) at least five times per week. Resistance training should also be encouraged up to twice weekly.[7] Exercise offers a number of physiological and mental/emotional benefits. One physiological benefit is that exercise enhances GLUT4 transporter activity, which in turn facilitates glucose entry into cells while bypassing the need for insulin.[67] This effect has been demonstrated both in healthy individuals and those with IR or T2DM. Preliminary research also suggests that exercise has utility in improving the inflammatory state associated with IR by reducing levels of proinflammatory chemokines.[68] Yoga is another modality proven to help reduce oxidative stress in patients with type 2 DM. Yoga combined with standard care reportedly improves glycemic control and reduces body mass index.[69] Other benefits of regular workouts include increased lean muscle mass and reduced body fat (see Chapter 91).

Weight Management

Excessive food consumption, particularly dietary fat and foods with a high glycemic index, is a key contributor to the pathogenesis of IR and metabolic syndrome.[2] Although the majority of patients with IR are overweight, a small subgroup of patients has a normal body mass index. These patients are termed *metabolically obese*, normal-weight individuals and share the same risks of developing type 2 DM and cardiovascular disease due to increased visceral fat.[70] Increased visceral fat is associated with increased release of free fatty acids and initiates a self-perpetuating cycle leading to the development of increased IR. Affected patients are said to be "bathed in cortisol" and have the appearance of Cushing syndrome. As previously mentioned, this type of fat affects other organs by causing dysfunction and increasing inflammation. Adipose cells are not, as previously believed, passive depots for energy but are rather hormonally active by secreting adipokines. Adipose cells have also been shown to secrete TNF-alpha, adiponectin, resistin, leptin, and other inflammatory mediators, all of which are involved in the promotion and exacerbation of IR. Hu et al.[71] reported sedentary behaviors (particularly watching television) are associated with significantly elevated risks of visceral adiposity, irrespective of exercise levels. Studies have reported that even small percentages of weight loss (6 to 10%) can significantly improve IR and reduce the risk of developing type 2 DM by 58%.[65,72] Weight reduction (coupled with exercise) has also been shown to improve histological disease activity in patients with NAFLD.[58]

As little as 10% weight loss can reverse fatty infiltration of the liver.

The speed of chewing has also been shown to have an impact on diabetes risk. Fast eating is reported associated with a more than two-fold increased risk of type 2 DM compared with slower eating.[73] Eating quickly has also been positively associated with body mass index, increased body weight, and weight gain based in a nationwide survey of middle-aged women.[74]

Nutrition

For patients with insulin resistance, the focus should be on diets rich in whole grains rather than refined grains, fish and white meat instead of red meat, and plenty of fruits and vegetables along with nuts, legumes, and soy. In 2002, researchers from the Harvard School of Public Health published a set of nutritional guidelines known as the Alternative Healthy Eating Index (AHEI) with an emphasis on the foods listed previously. Results from the Whitehall II Prospective Cohort Study showed that adherence to the AHEI in a middle-aged population was associated with a reversal of the metabolic syndrome after 5 years (odds ratio 1.88; 95% CI, 1.04 to 3.41). This effect was more pronounced in subjects with central obesity and elevated serum triglycerides.[75]

The Mediterranean and low glycemic index/load diets are considered the most effective nutritional regimens for the treatment of metabolic syndrome, insulin resistance, and NAFLD.

Mediterranean Diet

Much has been written about the Mediterranean diet, which is rich in vegetables, legumes, soy products, fish, and essential fatty acids. This type of diet is also low in refined carbohydrates and "junk foods," as well as in red meat, which is rich in saturated fats.[55] The beneficial effects associated with adherence to the Mediterranean diet relate to the nutrient-dense properties of the foods (i.e., vitamins, minerals, phytochemicals, and fiber).[55] In a randomized trial, Esposito et al.[76] compared a Mediterranean diet with a standard diet in 180 patients with metabolic syndrome. After 2 years, only 40 out of 90 subjects on the Mediterranean diet still had features of metabolic syndrome compared with 78 out of 90 participants in the standard diet group. A recent paper by Salas-Salvadó et al.[77] also demonstrated a significant reduction in the incidence of type 2 DM with adherence to a Mediterranean diet. In this trial, nondiabetic subjects aged 55 to 80 years old were randomly assigned to either a low fat diet (control group), a Mediterranean diet supplemented with 1 L/week of free virgin olive oil, or a Mediterranean diet supplemented with 30 g/day of nuts. All diets were ad libitum. After 4 years, the incidence of type 2 DM was 18% in the control group, 10% in the Mediterranean plus olive oil group, and 11%

in the Mediterranean plus nuts group. When pooling the Mediterranean diet groups, there was a 52% reduction in the incidence of type 2 DM when compared with the control group. Of particular interest was the fact that the reduced incidence of type 2 DM occurred in the absence of any significant alterations in body weight or physical activity. Adherence to the Mediterranean diet has also been associated with reduced risk of metabolic syndrome in NAFLD patients[55] (see Chapter 88).

Low-Glycemic Index Foods

The glycemic-index is a system for classifying carbohydrate-containing foods based on glycemic response. Carbohydrates range from simple sugars to starches and can all be converted to glucose. The rate at which conversion occurs is determined by saccharide chain length, with longer chains constituting complex carbohydrates. The glycemic index value for carbohydrates can vary by more than fivefold, with starchy foods having a higher glycemic index than nonstarchy foods such as fruits, vegetables, and legumes. Diets that favor high-glycemic index foods are associated with increased 24-hour glucose and insulin levels in addition to higher levels of C-peptide and glycosylated hemoglobin. These effects have been demonstrated in both nondiabetic and diabetic individuals.[78]

Research has shown that a combination of exercise and a low-glycemic index diet in obese subjects with prediabetes not only improves postprandial hyperinsulinemia but also reduces pancreatic beta cell stress. Conversely, exercise in combination with a high-glycemic index diet impairs beta and intestinal K cell function despite a similar reduction in weight loss. These findings emphasize the importance of diets rich in low-glycemic index foods that support beta cell preservation, a key factor in the prevention of type 2 DM[79] (see Chapter 87).

Fiber

Dietary fiber, either from whole foods or dietary supplements, is a vital component of the treatment plan for IR and metabolic syndrome. Fiber helps reduce blood pressure as well as total and LDL cholesterol levels, and it modifies inflammatory markers. When taken with meals, soluble fibers, such as psyllium, have been shown to improve postprandial glycemic index and increase insulin sensitivity. Psyllium appears to work by reducing glucose absorption from the intestine and increasing GLUT-4 protein expression in muscles. Regular consumption of dietary fiber also promotes weight reduction by enhancing satiety. Oats and barley are other examples of soluble fiber that have U.S. Food and Drug Administration (FDA)-approved health claims for reducing the risk of heart disease.[4]

Cooking Techniques

Cooking methods can also have an impact on biochemical markers associated with IR and metabolic syndrome. High-heat-treated foods typically found in the Western diet generate harmful compounds known as Maillard reaction products. These compounds have been found to reduce insulin sensitivity and increase plasma cholesterol and triglycerides.[80] Mild cooking techniques such as steaming, poaching, and stewing are recommended instead of roasting, barbecuing, broiling, or frying.

Therapeutic Foods

Blueberries are rich in phenolic compounds and anthocyanins and have been demonstrated to have certain health benefits, including improved cognition and reduced cardiovascular and cancer risk. Preliminary research suggests blueberries may also exhibit antidiabetic effects. In a double-blind, placebo-controlled randomized trial, consuming the equivalent of two cups of fresh blueberries a day improved IR in nondiabetic and obese insulin-resistant individuals.[81] Consuming this quantity of blueberries has also been shown to reduce blood pressure, oxidized LDL cholesterol, and lipid peroxidation in patients with metabolic syndrome.[82]

Apple cider vinegar (20 g diluted in 40 g of water) has been shown to reduce postprandial fluxes in glucose and insulin following a carbohydrate-rich meal. Acetic acid in vinegar acts similarly to medications such as acarbose and metformin by suppressing disaccharidase activity and increasing glucose-6-phosphate concentrations in skeletal muscle.[83] Other forms of vinegar, such as white vinegar in a vinaigrette sauce, can also be used to lower postprandial glucose (20 to 28 g white vinegar mixed with 8 g olive oil).[84,85] Another first step would be to promote the patient's own acid production by stopping unnecessary chronic usage of antacid medications if possible.

Foods and Substances to Avoid or Consume in Moderation

Table 32.4 provides a list of foods and substances that should be avoided, given their direct or indirect role in affecting glucose and insulin metabolism.

Research has shown that low to moderate alcohol consumption (one to two standard drinks per day) increases insulin sensitivity and reduces insulin concentrations in nondiabetic postmenopausal women. However, regular consumption in this cohort also increased levels of the steroidogenic hormones DHEA-S and estrone sulfate, which are possible risk factors for breast cancer.[86] Alcohol appears to have a U-shaped relationship with metabolic syndrome, with nondrinkers and heavy drinkers having a similar risk profile. This curious finding may be attributable to increased levels of HDL cholesterol observed in heavy drinkers.[87] As the potential risks may outweigh the benefits, teetotalers should not be encouraged to start drinking to reduce their risk of developing type 2 DM. Smoking should be avoided as it is a known health hazard and shown to be associated with an increased risk for type 2 DM.[88]

Mind Body

Stress Management

Relaxation techniques are valuable in the treatment of IR because they promote stabilization of adrenal gland

TABLE 32.4 Foods to Avoid in Patients With Insulin Resistance and the Metabolic Syndrome

Food/Substance	Metabolic Effect
Refined Starchy Foods	Instant rice, potatoes, white breads, pasta, cereals such as Rice Krispies and corn flakes, corn chips, and canned foods have a high glycemic index and are known to impair glucose metabolism and increase insulin secretion.[78]
Fast Foods	These foods are calorie rich, given their high sugar and fat content, and contribute to weight gain, insulin resistance, and hyperlipidemia.[2]
Sugar Sweetened Beverages	Soft drinks, fruit drinks, iced tea, and energy and vitamin water drinks are often rich in fructose corn syrup and are associated with weight gain and an increased risk of IR and type 2 DM.[89] Consuming one to two drinks/day is associated with a 26% increased risk of developing type 2 DM.[90]
Artificial Sweeteners	Artificial sweeteners, such as aspartame, saccharin, and sucralose, are associated with obesity and a twofold increased risk of type 2 DM.[91]

DM, diabetes mellitus.

function. Stress management lowers both cortisol levels and blood pressure, increases DHEA, improves immunity, and reduces anxiety and depression. Patients are therefore less likely to abuse their bodies and tend to feel better about themselves following the use of relaxation techniques. A prescription with an individualized approach involving meditation, relaxation techniques, prayer, visualization, and other stress-reducing modalities is indicated in patients with IR or type 2 DM.[92]

> Stress management and exercise are key components of therapies for IR and type 2 DM.

Depression

The results of a 2009 study by Takeuchi et al.[93] indicate the metabolic syndrome may be a predictive factor for the development of depression but not anxiety. Multivariate analysis indicated that an increase in waist circumference was the main factor influencing the relationship between metabolic syndrome and new-onset depression. Skilton et al.[35] also found a positive association between depression (versus anxiety) and metabolic syndrome. In light of their research, the investigators posited screening for depression in patients with the metabolic syndrome.

Supplements

Numerous nutritional supplements have demonstrated a beneficial effect on glucose and insulin metabolism. Patients with IR and metabolic syndrome should include a multivitamin as a core component of their health regime. Certain nutrients, including antioxidants, may be required in therapeutic doses to ensure a physiological effect in the management of IR and metabolic syndrome.[94-96] Supplementation with the following nutraceuticals should be guided by overall health and dietary habits along with laboratory parameters and current IR status.

Vitamin B6

A deficiency in vitamin B6 is associated with a decrease in several important enzymes that contribute to gluconeogenesis (the generation of glucose from nonsugar substrates).[97] In patients taking metformin for polycystic ovarian syndrome, vitamin B6 and folate have been shown to counteract increases in homocysteine levels.[98]

DOSAGE

The recommended dose of vitamin B6 is 50 mg to 100 mg/day.[99]

PRECAUTIONS

None have been reported at the recommended dose. Higher doses (>150 mg) may cause reversible neuropathy.

Folic Acid

The combination of IR and elevated plasma homocysteine levels is associated with cardiovascular risk. Research has shown that patients with this combination of risk factors also have altered or reduced folate levels, which are thought to lead to the progression of hypertension.[100] High dose supplementation with folic acid has been shown to protect against microvascular complications associated with metabolic syndrome[101] and improve metabolic profiles in women with polycystic ovarian syndrome.[102] Patients heterozygous or homozygous for the methylenetetrahydrofolate reductase single nucleotide polymorphism (MTHFR C677T) may benefit from supplementation with L-5-Methyltetrahydrofolate rather than folic acid.

DOSAGE

The recommended dose of folate is 500 mcg to 5 mg/day.[99-102]

PRECAUTIONS

None have been reported. The administration of high doses of folic acid to patients with a concomitant vitamin B12 deficiency may correct megaloblastic anemia but increase the risk of irreversible neurological damage.[103]

Vitamin B12

Research has demonstrated a negative correlation between B12 status and body mass index.[104] In patients with metabolic syndrome, the administration of folate and vitamin B12 reportedly decreases IR and improves endothelial function. Homocysteine levels have also been shown to improve with folate and vitamin B12, affirming the beneficial effect of these treatments on cardiovascular disease risk factors.[105] Because metformin has been shown to impair vitamin B12 status, practitioners should assess and monitor B12 levels in patients receiving metformin.[106]

DOSAGE

The recommended dose of vitamin B12 is 500 mcg/day.[107]

PRECAUTIONS

None have been reported at the recommended dose.

Vitamin C

Individuals with metabolic syndrome have been found to have significantly lower levels of vitamin C compared to healthy individuals.[108,109] A deficiency of vitamin C is thought to be associated with a greater resistance to fat mass loss.[110] High doses of vitamin C have also been found to reverse the adverse effects of free fatty acids on vascular function.[111,112]

DOSAGE

The recommended dose of vitamin C is 1000 to 2000 mg/day.[113]

PRECAUTIONS

Take with food to reduce the risk of diarrhea.

Vitamin D

Supplemental (and dietary) vitamin D has been shown to reduce the development of metabolic syndrome.[114] In a study of young adults, an inverse relationship between blood glucose, IR, and serum 25-hydroxy (OH) vitamin D was demonstrated.[115] Other research has confirmed that serum 25(OH) D levels positively correlate with insulin sensitivity.[116,117] Ford et al.[118] also reported significant inverse relationships between serum vitamin D levels and abdominal obesity, elevated triglycerides, and hyperglycemia. Visceral fat reduces the absorption of vitamin D from the skin.

DOSAGE

The recommended dose of vitamin D is 300 to 2000 IU/day.[119,120] Dosing may also be guided by the season of the year and serum 25(OH) D levels (the preferred range is 30 to 60 ng/mL or 75 to 150 nmol/L).[121]

PRECAUTIONS

Monitor serum calcium levels in patients taking thiazide diuretics and vitamin D supplements, as this combination may cause hypercalcemia.[122]

Vitamin E

Vitamin E supplementation has demonstrated hepatoprotective effects in patients diagnosed with NAFLD (including those with NASH when accompanied with pharmacological medications).[58,123]

DOSAGE

The recommended dose is 400 IU per day (or 200 IU twice daily) of alpha tocopherol or 400 mg of mixed tocotrienols.[123-125]

PRECAUTIONS

Exercise caution in patients taking anticoagulants, as chronic high dosing may affect blood clotting and induce symptoms of muscular weakness and fatigue (reported at doses of 720 mg alpha tocopherol per day).[126]

Biotin

High-dose biotin is considered an important vitamin for preventing and treating IR and obesity.[127] When given in quantities 10 times greater than the physiological range, biotin directly activates an enzyme that mimics the action of nitric oxide. Biotin has also been shown to improve glycemic control by reducing excessive hepatic glucose output.[128]

DOSAGE

The recommended dose of biotin is 3 mg three times a day.[127]

PRECAUTIONS

None have been reported.

Chromium

The trace element chromium is an important nutrient that helps prevent IR and dyslipidemia associated with obesity.[129] Chromium also appears to have important effects on skeletal muscle IR.[128] Chromium has been found to improve insulin sensitivity and increase glucose disposal in women with polycystic ovarian syndrome.[130]

DOSAGE

The recommended dose of chromium is 200 to 1000 mcg/day.[130-132]

PRECAUTIONS

Take chromium supplements half an hour before or 3 to 4 hours after thyroid or levothyroxine medications, as chromium may bind to these medications and reduce absorption.[133]

Magnesium

Intracellular magnesium plays a vital role in regulating insulin action, insulin-mediated glucose uptake and vascular tone.[134] Higher intakes of magnesium are associated with increased insulin sensitivity and a reduced risk of developing metabolic syndrome.[135-137] Conversely, low dietary intake of magnesium is associated with an increased risk of developing IR and type 2 DM.[138,139]

DOSAGE

A dose of 100 mg/day is recommended to reduce the risk of developing type 2 DM.[140] A dose of 382 mg/day is required to improve metabolic profiles and blood pressure.[134,141] Dosing can also be guided by assessing red blood cell magnesium levels.

PRECAUTIONS

High-dose magnesium may cause gastric irritation and diarrhea.[142]

Zinc

Recent research has reported an inverse relationship between serum zinc concentrations and insulin resistance.[143] The antioxidant capacity of zinc is thought to underlie its valuable effects on IR.[144] Two randomized controlled trials reported a reduction in fasting glucose and insulin in addition to other markers of IR in obese prepubescent children following zinc supplementation.[145,146]

DOSAGE

The recommended dose of zinc is 20 mg/day.[146]

PRECAUTIONS

None reported at the recommended dose.

Alpha lipoic acid

Alpha lipoic acid (ALA) is a potent antioxidant that is considered important for the treatment of metabolic syndrome. The mechanisms by which ALA exerts its effects include protection against oxidative stress-induced IR, inhibition of hepatic gluconeogenesis, and increased peripheral glucose use.[147] ALA may also exert modest reductions in plasma nonesterified fatty acid concentrations.[148] When administered solely or in combination with the angiotensin receptor blocker irbesartan, ALA has been shown to improve endothelial function and reduce IL-6 and PAF-1 levels in subjects with metabolic syndrome.[149]

DOSAGE

The recommended dose of ALA is 100 mg three times daily before each meal.[149]

PRECAUTIONS

None reported.

Coenzyme Q10

Coenzyme Q10 (CoQ10) is required for adenosine triphosphate (ATP) synthesis and is therefore important for the conversion of carbohydrates to energy.[150] By enhancing the functioning of the mitochondrial enzyme glycerol-3-phosphate dehydrogenase, CoQ10 helps with glycemic control.[128] A study by Singh et al.[151] reported reductions in systolic and diastolic blood pressure, fasting and 2-hour plasma insulin, and triglycerides with the use of CoQ10 supplementation. Markers of oxidation, such as lipid peroxides, malondialdehyde, and diene conjugates, were also lowered by CoQ10, indicating a decrease in oxidative stress. Many patients with IR and metabolic syndrome are treated with statin drugs, and these medications have been found to lower plasma and tissue levels of CoQ10.[152]

DOSAGE

The recommended dose of CoQ10 is 120 mg/day (or 60 mg twice daily).[151]

PRECAUTIONS

CoQ10 may decrease the anticoagulant effect of warfarin. Monitor clotting time regularly, particularly within the first 2 weeks of taking CoQ10.[153]

Acetyl-L-Carnitine

The amino acid, carnitine, plays an important role in energy metabolism, largely through its effects on fatty acid oxidation. Carnitine deficiency has been associated with various conditions, including obesity and type 2 DM.[154] When fatty acids are unable to enter the cell, triglycerides accumulate in the cytosol; an important contributor to the pathogenesis of IR. The administration of acetyl-L-carnitine to patients with type 2 DM and to healthy persons have been shown to improve insulin-mediated glucose disposal.[155]

DOSAGE

The recommended dose of carnitine is 1 to 2 g/day between meals.[156]

PRECAUTIONS

None have been documented at the dose recommended.[156]

Omega-3 Fatty Acids

Long term supplementation with omega-3 fatty acids has been shown to improve postprandial lipoprotein metabolism by decreasing triglycerides and increasing HDL-cholesterol.[2] Omega-3 fatty acids have also demonstrated improvements in endothelial function and arterial stiffness, with an accompanying reduction of the proinflammatory cytokine, IL-6.[157]

DOSAGE

The recommended dose is 1 g/day of eicosapentaenoic acid and docosahexaenoic acid (EPA and DHA). For patients with elevated triglycerides, the dose is 2 to 4 g/day of EPA and DHA.[157-159]

PRECAUTIONS

None have been reported at the recommended dose.

Botanicals

Ginseng (Panax ginseng)

The herb *Panax ginseng* has numerous medicinal effects, including antiinflammatory and antioxidant properties, and has also been used in the treatment of type 2 DM. Ginseng is thought to control and prevent type 2 DM by increasing insulin sensitivity and enhancing insulin secretion.[160] Another proposed mechanism of action lies in the herb's ability to modulate glucose activity by increasing GLUT-4 transporter activity.[161]

DOSAGE

The recommended dose is 100 to 200 mg/day (standardized to contain 4% ginsenosides).[162,163]

PRECAUTIONS

Ginseng may decrease the effectiveness of warfarin.[164]

Green Tea (Camellia sinensis)

Green tea supplementation has been shown to improve whole blood glutathione and plasma antioxidant capacity and reduce plasma iron in adults with metabolic syndrome.[165] Based on the research by Basu et al.,[166] supplemental green tea in patients with metabolic syndrome is thought to reduce serum amyloid alpha, an independent cardiovascular disease risk factor. Green tea may also maintain normal body composition by stimulating thermogenesis and enhancing fat oxidation.[167]

DOSAGE

Green tea extract (270 mg to 460 mg/day of epigallocatechin gallate).[165-167]

PRECAUTIONS

Green tea may decrease the effectiveness of warfarin.[168] Do not combine with ephedrine or other stimulants.[169]

Milk Thistle (Silybum marianum)

Milk thistle is considered an important herb in the treatment of hepatic disorders and also appears to play a beneficial role in maintaining normal glucose and lipid metabolism. Liver dysfunction impairs the efficiency of postprandial hepatic glucose storage and is thought to trigger hyperinsulinemia due to reduced liver clearance of insulin.[170] Phase III clinical trials have determined silymarin (the active component of milk thistle) to be the best medication for NAFLD due to its effects in lowering aminotransferase levels and reducing steatosis severity, liver ballooning, and fibrosis. Milk thistle has also been shown to act as an insulin sensitizer in studies of patients with NAFLD.[171]

DOSAGE

Give 420 to 600 mg/day (standardized to contain 70%–80% silymarin).[172,173]

PRECAUTIONS

Exercise caution in patients taking drugs metabolized by cytochrome, the P-450 isoenzymes CYP3A4 and CYP2C9, because the silibinin content of milk thistle may inhibit these hepatic isoenzymes.[174]

Pharmaceuticals

While lifestyle modification is the preferred approach to managing IR and metabolic syndrome, at times prescription drugs are necessary. The problem with such medications is that they do not correct underlying nutrient deficiencies. Medications often merely "treat" the results of the disease; that is, they reduce high serum lipid or glucose levels or high blood pressure but do not treat the overall patient. Although no FDA-approved prescription drugs exist for IR, many of the medications used for type 2 DM have studied as treatment of metabolic syndrome. Some of these medications may not specifically address IR or may have unhealthy side effects. For example, 3-hydroxy-3-methyl-glutaryl-coenzyme A (HMG-CoA) reductase inhibitors (statins) lower serum CoQ10, and metformin reduces folic acid and vitamin B_{12} levels but may increase homocysteine levels. Statin administration is also associated with a dose-dependent increase in insulin resistance.[175] Of importance is the fact that pharmaceutical drugs do not correct diet and lifestyle issues. Pharmaceuticals can be an appropriate complementary option when required. Following is a list of medications grouped according to their physiological action. There are a number of brands in each category, and many can be used in combination with each other. Even though these medications are usually used for type 2 DM, they are often prescribed for IR (although they may need to be prescribed "off-label"). It should be noted that medications approved for type 2 DM are the main medications being investigated for the treatment of NAFLD.[58]

Oral Medications

Insulin Sensitizers. Biguanides (e.g., metformin) are the most commonly used front-line medications.

These drugs work by reducing glucose output from the liver (most likely by decreasing gluconeogenesis).[176]

Thiazolidinediones help improve body cell sensitivity to insulin by stimulating the nuclear receptor, peroxisome proliferator activated receptor (PPAR-gamma). These receptors are primarily found in fat cells and, to a lesser extent, in liver and skeletal muscle.[176]

Agents That Slow the Digestive/Absorptive Process. Alpha-glucosidase inhibitors help slow down the absorption of carbohydrate into the bloodstream following a meal, thereby reducing postprandial glucose peaks.[177]

Medications That Increase Insulin Production and Decrease Glucose Production. Dipeptidyl pepdiase-4 (DPP-4) inhibitors are a newer class of drugs that work by inhibiting the breakdown of incretin hormones glucagon-like peptide-1 and glucose dependent insulinotropic peptide. Increased levels of these hormones result in improved glucose-dependent insulin secretion, suppressed glucagon secretion, and reduced gastric emptying.[178]

Sodium-Glucose Transporter-2 (SGLT-2) Inhibitors. These medications work by a novel insulin-independent mechanism by blocking the reabsorption of glucose in the proximal convoluted tubules of the kidneys, thereby resulting in increased glucosuria and weight loss (due to loss of 300 to 400 kcal/day).[179]

Bile Acid Sequestrants. Colesevelam is a second-generation bile acid sequestrant and the only drug in this class that is approved for the treatment of hyperlipidemia and type 2 DM.[180] Bile acid sequestrants work by binding bile acid in the intestinal lumen, thus impeding bile acid reabsorption in the terminal ileum and increasing fecal bile-acid output.[181] A small study reported the efficacy of colesevelam in improving impaired fasting glucose levels.[182]

Surgery

The most dramatic, but at times successful, option for the treatment of type 2 DM is bariatric surgery. While the majority of studies have focused on bariatric surgery for type 2 DM,[183-189] there is research to support the use of this procedure in obese patients. In a nonrandomized, prospective, controlled study, bariatric surgery proved to be more efficient than usual care in the prevention of type 2 DM in obese persons. Subjects were divided into patients who underwent bariatric surgery (1658) and obese matched controls (1771). No participants had type 2 DM at baseline. After 15 years, type 2 DM developed in 392 participants in the control group compared with 110 in the bariatric surgery group, corresponding to incident rates of 28.4 cases per 1000 person-years and 6.8 cases per 1000 person-years, respectively (adjusted hazard ratio with bariatric surgery, 0.17; 95% CI, 0.13 to 0.21; P < 0.001).

PREVENTION PRESCRIPTION

- Maintain a healthy body weight. People with an increase in visceral (truncal) fat are at higher risk.
- Exercise of 30 minutes/day is recommended on most days of the week for patients with appropriate weight and 60 minutes/day on most days of the week for those needing to lose weight.

- Manage stress and increase the relaxation (parasympathetic) response.
- Follow a low-glycemic load, Mediterranean-type diet.
- Take a high quality multivitamin that includes minerals and B-group vitamins.

THERAPEUTIC REVIEW

LABORATORY EVALUATION

- 2-hour glucose and insulin tolerance test to measure glucose and insulin levels after a glucose load.
- Serum lipid measurements (looking for increased triglyceride level, decrease in high-density lipoprotein cholesterol level, and normal or slightly increased low-density lipoprotein cholesterol level).
- Fasting glucose higher than 100 mg/dL.
- High-sensitivity C-reactive protein, a marker of inflammation, and gamma-glutamyltranspeptidase, a marker of liver toxicity.

LIFESTYLE

- Encourage an exercise routine that consists of moderate intensity workouts and resistance training.   A①₁
- Encourage goals to achieve appropriate weight.   A①₁
- Encourage the patient to stop using nicotine-containing products.   B⊘₁

NUTRITION

- Low-carbohydrate, Mediterranean-type diet with a focus on low-glycemic index foods.   A①₁
- High-fiber diet including soluble fibers, such as psyllium, oats, and barley.   B⊘₁
- Decreased consumption of red meat and fried foods.   B⊘₁

MIND-BODY THERAPIES

- Encourage lifestyle choices to reduce stress and anxiety. Recommend a relaxation technique tailored to the individual.   B⊘₁

- Note: The preceding recommendations highly outweigh those that follow for the treatment of IR and metabolic syndrome.

SUPPLEMENTS

- High-quality multivitamin with minerals and B-group vitamins.   B⊘₁
- Omega-3 fatty acids (eicosapentaenoic acid/docosahexaenoic acid) 1 to 4 g/day to reduce inflammation, blood pressure, and triglyceride levels.   B⊘₁
- Chromium picolinate: 200 to 1000 mcg/day.   B→₂
- Vitamin C: 1000 to 2000 mg/day.   B→₂
- Vitamin D: 300 to 2000 IU/day.   B⊘₁
- Alpha-lipoic acid: 100 to 300 mg/day.   B⊘₁
- Coenzyme Q10: 60 to 120 mg/day.   B→₂
- High risk individuals may need to consider additional supplementation as outlined in the body of the text.

BOTANICALS

- American ginseng: 100 to 200 mg/day.   B→₂
- Milk thistle: 420 to 600 mg/day.   B→₂

PHARMACEUTICALS

- Metformin: 500 to 2500 mg each morning or twice daily.   A⊘₂
- Pioglitazone: 15 to 45 mg/day.   A⊘₂

Key Web Resources

The National Diabetes Information Clearinghouse (NDIC) provides information on insulin resistance and prediabetes	https://www.niddk.nih.gov/health-information/diabetes/types/prediabetes-insulin-resistance
Myhealthywaist.org offers education and tools regarding the importance of reducing large waistlines	http://www.myhealthywaist.org
Educational resources on lipids and health	https://www.lipid.org/lipidacademy
Calorie needs calculator from the Mayo Clinic	http://www.mayoclinic.com/health/calorie-calculator/NU00598
Fitday is a website that provides online education, tools, and record-keeping to help meet weight loss and exercise goals	http://www.fitday.com

---

REFERENCES

References are available online at ExpertConsult.com.

CHAPTER 33

DIABETES MELLITUS

Matthew Moher, MD

Type 2 diabetes mellitus represents a global epidemic that is predicted to intensify. The number of individuals with type 2 diabetes mellitus (DM) worldwide was 30 million in 1985, 171 million in 2000, and 220 million in 2009.[1] As of 2014, type 2 DM is estimated to affect 387 million individuals worldwide,[2] representing a worldwide prevalence of 8.3%. From 1990 to 2008, the prevalence of DM doubled, and had not declined by 2012.[3] From 1998 to 2009, the prevalence of DM rose a staggering 230% in Canada alone and is predicted to continue rising. The CDC estimates 40% of Americans will develop DM in their lifetime.[4]

Type 2 DM is common in both the developed and developing worlds.[5,6] The increasing prevalence of DM is attributed to rising obesity rates, sedentary lifestyles, aging populations, and improved survival of individuals with the disease.[7]

Type 2 DM is also associated with huge health care costs. In a special report from 2009 entitled, *An Economic Tsunami: the Cost of Diabetes in Canada*, the estimated cost of type 2 DM in 2010 was $12.2 billion and projected to increase by a further $4.7 billion by 2020.[8]

The silver lining is that type 2 DM is largely preventable, with epidemiological studies predicting primary prevention of diabetes in America could reduce the risk of all-cause and cardiovascular mortality by up to 9.0%.[9]

PATHOPHYSIOLOGY

The pathophysiology of type 2 DM is complex and fundamentally consists of hyperglycemia, insulin resistance, and impaired insulin secretion[4] (see Fig. 33.1 for a general overview).

Carbohydrate intake and subsequent absorption of glucose into the blood triggers insulin release from the beta cells of the pancreas. Insulin stimulates the uptake of glucose into cells via the GLUT-4 glucose transporter. Insulin resistance (IR) may ensue after chronic exposure to high serum glucose levels. Steroid administration and physical inactivity may also contribute.[10] The development of type 2 DM is thought to be characterized by peripheral cells becoming unable to efficiently uptake glucose in response to insulin in combination with beta islet cell dysfunction and decreased insulin production.

Insulin functions in stimulating cellular glucose uptake, decreasing hepatic gluconeogenesis, and increasing adipose tissue triglyceride synthesis, glucagon regulation, and vascular tone. These important functions of insulin are all impaired in type 2 DM.

Diabetes is referred to as "starving amidst the feast." IR refers to impaired glucose transport into muscle cells that accounts for the "starving" amidst the hyperglycemia

"feast." Additionally, cellular starvation feedback mechanisms exacerbate hyperglycemia by stimulating hepatic gluconeogenesis and fat breakdown.

IR also contributes to the production of free fatty acids and inflammatory cytokines. Inflammatory markers shown to be elevated in DM include C-reactive protein, IL-6, plasminogen activator inhibitor-1 (PAI-1), and tumor necrosis factor (TNF)-alpha, in addition to white cell count.[11-13]

Adiponectin is an antiinflammatory cytokine that has been shown to reduce plasma levels of free fatty acids. High adiponectin is associated with improved lipid profiles, glycemic control, and reduced inflammation.[14] DM has shown to be correlated with a reduction in adiponectin.[15]

> Adiponectin is a hormonal protein produced by adipose tissue. Contrary to common sense, low levels (not high) of adiponectin are bad and result from a proinflammatory state. Adiponectin levels can be increased with exercise and weight loss.

While studies on type 2 DM pathophysiology have previously focused on IR, the role of the pancreas has become increasingly recognized. Beta islet cells are well known to produce insulin; however, these are not the only pancreatic islet cells. Alpha islet cells produce glucagon, considered a counterpart of insulin. The interaction between insulin and glucagon is usually very tightly regulated; however, increased glucagon further exacerbates the hyperglycemic state in type 2 DM as a result of IR and impaired insulin secretion.[16]

Genetics also contribute to the pathogenesis of type 2 DM. Medical genomics is considered to be a field of active research with great potential. Genomic single-nucleotide polymorphisms (SNPs) have been shown to be associated with DM risk.[17-20] Genetic risk may also interact with environmental factors.

Inorganic arsenic exposure in drinking water increases risk of type 2 DM.[21] Bisphenol A, used in hard plastics and resins, has also been linked to DM.[22] Pesticide exposure, specifically organophosphates and chlorinated pesticides, may also be associated with increased risk.[23]

INTEGRATIVE THERAPY

Lifestyle

Diabetes is largely preventable. The principles of preventative management apply a holistic therapeutic approach to patients with established DM.

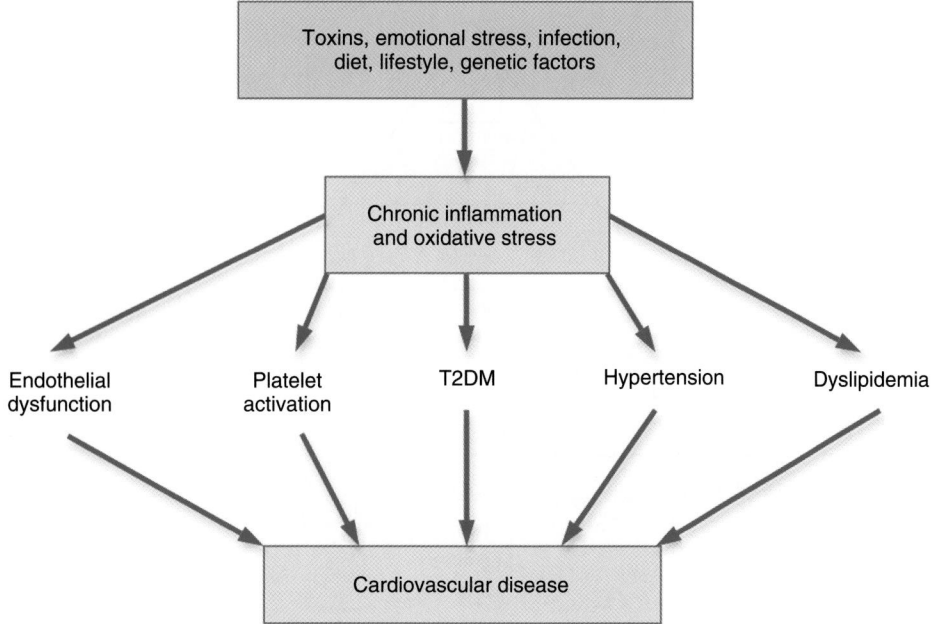

FIG. 33.1 ■ Pathophysiology of type 2 diabetes mellitus and inflammatory disorders. T2DM, type 2 diabetes mellitus.

Four large epidemiological, long-term studies are widely cited in support of lifestyle intervention as the cornerstone of type 2 DM prevention.

In 2001, the Finnish Diabetes Prevention Study (DPS) investigated 522 middle-aged, overweight subjects with impaired glucose tolerance over 4–10 years. The lifestyle intervention consisted of counseling aimed at reducing weight, total intake of fat, and intake of saturated fat, and increasing intake of fiber and physical activity. Annual oral glucose tolerance testing indicated DM to be largely preventable in this cohort of high-risk individuals.[24]

In 2002, the Diabetes Prevention Program (DPP) investigated 3234 overweight high-risk individuals with impaired glucose intolerance (mean age, 51 years) over a 3-year period. Similar lifestyle interventions to the Finnish study were found to be superior to metformin in terms of diabetic prevention.[25]

The China Da Qing Diabetes Prevention Study, involving 577 high-risk individuals identified by a region-wide clinic screening process of >110,000 individuals, reported similar results over 6 years of lifestyle intervention.[26]

More recently, the 2011 nationwide Zensharen Study for Prevention of Lifestyle Diseases involving 641 overweight Japanese middle-aged persons with impaired glucose tolerance reported lifestyle modifications regarding weight loss, diet scrutiny, and exercise were associated with a decreased risk of type 2 DM.[27]

Smoking

Several studies, including meta-analyses, have shown smoking is a preventable risk factor for type 2 DM.[28,29] Mechanisms underlying the association between smoking and type 2 DM include impaired insulin sensitivity, glucose tolerance, and the metabolic syndrome.

Exercise

Exercise is tantamount in both the prevention and management of type 2 DM. Large cohort studies over 15–20 years have reported decreased cardiovascular risk and all-cause mortality in diabetics who undertake regular physical activity.[30-32] Both aerobic exercise and resistance training reduce HbA1c in patients with type 2 DM.[33]

Studies indicate regular yoga can reduce HbA1c and fasting blood glucose levels. Hatha yoga is reported to have most evidence in reviews. In fact, Hatha yoga has shown to reduce HbA1c to the same effect as regular aerobic exercise.[34,35]

Health care providers can support patients by encouraging 30 to 60 minutes of moderate-intensity aerobic activity on most days of the week. The American Heart Association, the American Diabetes Association, and the American College of Sports Medicine recommend at least 150 minutes of moderate-intensity aerobic activity per week for patients with diabetes[36] (see Chapter 91, Writing an Exercise Prescription).

Nutrition

Nutrition, exercise, and lifestyle are the tripartite cornerstones of integrative diabetic management. Evidence supports the use of all three of these important modalities.

Nutrition therapy alone has been shown to improve glycemic control and lower HbA1c levels by 1%–2%.[37,38] This powerful evidence comes from multidisciplinary efforts between general practitioners, registered dietitians, and educators to individualize diet plans with regular follow-up. Dietitians and diabetic nurse educators are valuable resources with clear benefit in DM management.[39-41]

In general, diets incorporating the principles of food guides, such as the Healing Foods Pyramid (Fig. 33.2), are a good starting point for clinicians and patients.

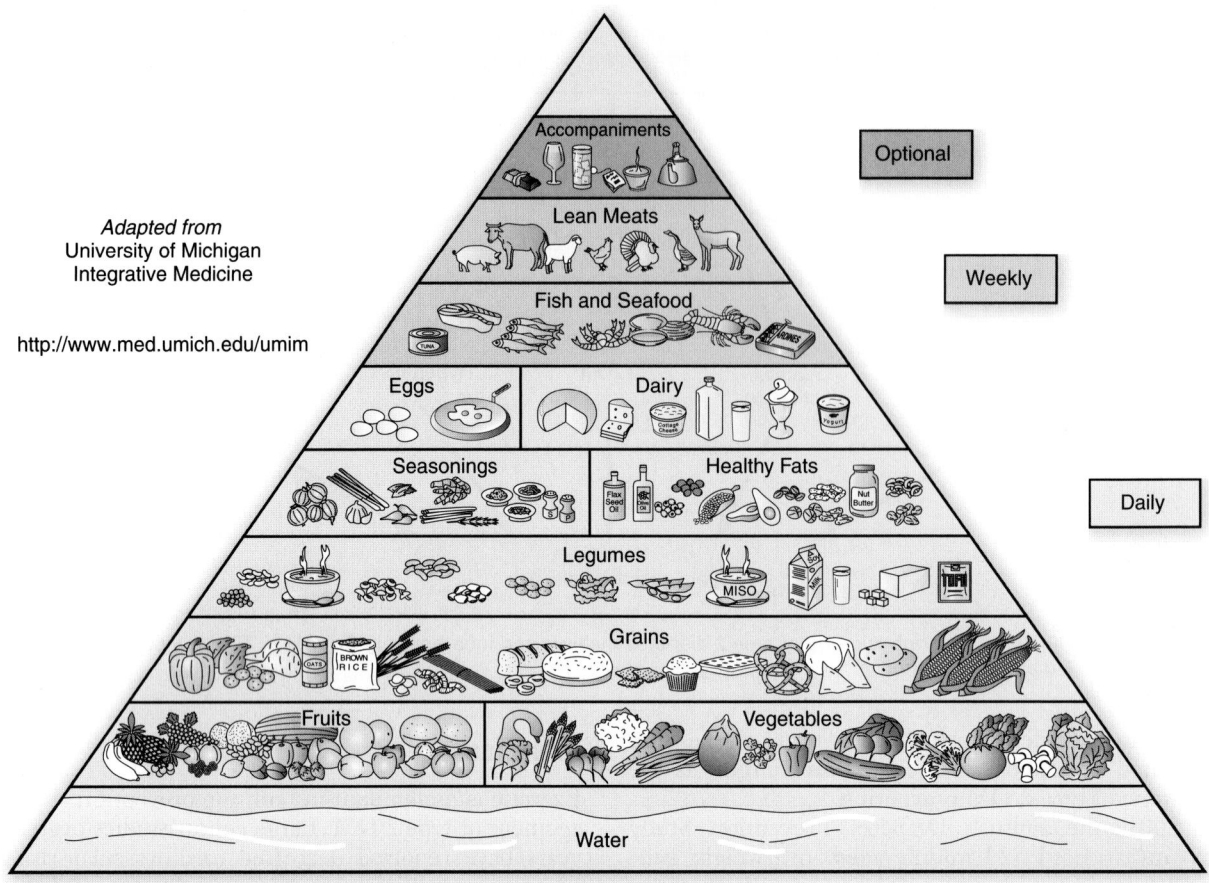

Adapted from
University of Michigan
Integrative Medicine

http://www.med.umich.edu/umim

FIG. 33.2 ■ University of Michigan integrative medicine health foods pyramid. (Reproduced from Regents of the University of Michigan. Developed by Monica Myklebust, MD, and Jenna Wunder, MPH, DR, 2008.)

Education regarding glycemic index (GI) takes this approach a step further. Glycemic index refers to blood glucose spikes following the intake of certain foods. High GI foods, such as table sugar, have greater effects on blood glucose levels and generate wide swings in insulin levels, eventually contributing to IR. A large multicenter meta-analysis demonstrated that diets containing low GI foods can reduce HbA1c by 0.43%.[42] GI tables are widely available online (http://www.diabetes.ca/diabetes-and-you/healthy-living-resources/diet-nutrition/the-glycemic-index).

Another important concept is glycemic load (GL). GL is based on GI but also incorporates the quantity of carbohydrate in a typical serving size. For example, bananas have a low GI (52) but a high GL (10.5) due to high carbohydrate content by weight). Conversely, watermelon has a high GI (72) but low GL (3.6) (see Chapter 87).

Specific Foods

Fiber

Soluble dietary fibers, such as psyllium, oats, beans, and eggplant, have been shown to lower postprandial blood glucose.[43] Pulses, such as lentils, chickpeas, and beans, also lower blood glucose.[44] Soy, walnuts, and other nuts have

demonstrated similar benefits.[45-47] Almonds in particular have been shown to reduce both HbA1c and postprandial blood glucose levels in small trials.[48,49] A growing body of research supports the beneficial effects of vegetarian and vegan diets for patients with type 2 DM.[50-52] In addition to vegetable protein, whole grains are also rich in minerals and antioxidants. In a large prospective cohort study, fiber from whole grains improved glycemic control in patients with type 2 DM.[53]

Alcohol

Light to moderate alcohol consumption may be beneficial in DM. Studies have shown decreased risk of type 2 DM and death due to CAD in established diabetics.[54] The majority of studies included in this review favored red wine, indicating the antioxidant effects of resveratrol to be a potential mechanism. Further, moderate alcohol consumption has been linked with higher adiponectin levels. Adiponectin, described previously, supports glucose homeostasis and improves insulin sensitivity.

The resveratrol and alcohol in red wine may raise adiponectin levels and maintain insulin sensitivity.

Dietary Fat

Diets higher in saturated versus polyunsaturated fats have been shown to be associated with increased HbA1c and IR in patients with type 2 DM.[55] The quality of fat is important. Research supports selective fat intake, favoring mono-unsaturated and polyunsaturated fats such as omega-3, which have been shown to prevent cardiovascular disease.

The Mediterranean diet captures the beneficial effects of macronutrient selectivity. A rigorous 4-year trial and subsequent 8-year follow-up comparing a low carbohydrate Mediterranean diet versus a low fat diet reported a reduction in HbA1c, decreased requirement for the initiation of diabetes medications, and an increase in cases of diabetes remission.[56,57]

Other foods that may be of benefit include chia (*Salvia hispanica*), which is rich in alpha-linoleic acid, and onions (*Allium cepa*). Magnesium deficiency has been shown to be a risk factor for type 2 DM.[58] Magnesium is found in dark green leafy vegetables, nuts, whole grains, and coffee. Moderate caffeine intake in the form of coffee or green tea may decrease risk of type DM according to a systematic literature review and meta-analysis.[59]

Mind-Body Therapy

Mindfulness

A plethora of literature is amassing in support of the health benefits of mindfulness, with 52 papers published in 2003, rising to 477 by 2012. Nearly 100 randomized controlled trials (RCTs) of mindfulness were published in 2014. Mindfulness has been shown to reduce stress, blood pressure, and even mitigate cardiovascular risk. A particularly interesting study involving PET scans of Buddhist monk brains during meditation provided concrete evidence that meditation can induce neurophysiological changes[60] (see Chapter 100).

Cognitive-Behavioral Therapy

Cognitive-behavioral therapy helps patients gain insight into the habits and patterns that affect their thoughts and actions and the ways in which these thoughts and actions affect their health and lives. A sizeable body of research has established the benefits of cognitive-behavioral therapy on glycemic control and self-care. In a systematic review of 25 trials in type 2 DM, 12 trials involving 522 patients used glycemic control as an outcome measure. In those trials, participants who received 6 to 16 group or individual counseling sessions had s 0.76% reduction in HbA1c levels compared to placebo.[61,62]

Biofeedback

Biofeedback training can strengthen the mind-body connection by helping patients learn to control specific bodily functions, including muscle tension, skin temperature, sweating, breathing, heart rate, and even regional brain waves. In a published study, researchers randomized 39 patients with well-controlled type 2 DM to receive 10 weekly individual sessions of skin temperature and electromyograph biofeedback or 3 group education sessions. Biofeedback was associated with improved glycemic control and a decrease in HbA1c levels by 0.8%.[63] This finding may seem surprising; however, biofeedback trials have reported changes in plasma cortisol, peripheral vasoconstriction, and other markers of sympathetic nervous system activity.

Sleep Hygiene

Several studies have linked poor sleep hygiene with DM risk. Systematic and meta-analyses of these studies have confirmed that too short, too long, or interrupted sleep compared to 8 hours of uninterrupted sleep significantly increases DM risk.[64]

Herbalism

Herbalism is the most ancient practice of medicine, indeed as old as human beings. Even chimpanzees have been shown to use plant medicines for the treatment of certain gastrointestinal ailments.

As an example, metformin, a derivative of the French lilac, has been used to treat DM since the middle ages.

Personally, I advise consultation with professional herbalists, preferably registered under their respective regional guild, to ensure prescription quality. In general, I value tincture extracts more than capsules of ground material due to greater potency and bioavailability. For patients who prefer over-the-counter medications or are unable to afford a herbalist consultation, I would recommend the use of products that are standardized extracts.

Table 33.1 includes a review of literature regarding commonly used plants and supplements. Below are plant medicines that have been trialed for at least 3 months (the lifespan of a RBC is 120 days) and demonstrated reductions in HbA1c levels of at least 0.5% in patients with type 2 DM.

Botanicals

Coccinia cordifolia

Coccinia cordifolia, or ivy gourd, is a perennial herb of the cucumber family. It is native to India but spreads easily and is now distributed worldwide. It is an important Ayurvedic diabetes medicine with additional choleretic, laxative, antiinflammatory, and demulcent properties. The leaves appear to have insulinomimetic effects on lipoprotein lipase, glucose-6-phosphatase, and other glycolytic enzymes. A double-blind, placebo-controlled RCT of 60 diabetics aged 35–60 years was performed, with the treatment arm consisting of 1 g ivy gourd extract for 90 days. The results demonstrated significant decreases in fasting, postprandial blood glucose, and HbA1c levels compared to placebo.[65]

DOSAGE

Dried leaves or extracts at doses equivalent to 15 g can be taken with meals.

PRECAUTIONS

Ivy gourd is well-tolerated but may cause nausea, drowsiness, and headaches.

TABLE 33.1 **Glycemic Effects and Cardiovascular Benefits of Different Treatments for Type 2 Diabetes Mellitus**

Therapy	Effects	Cardiovascular Benefits
Arsenic exposure avoidance	Arsenic exposure increased risk by 358% in population studies	—
Emotional stress avoidance	Emotional stress increased risk by 60% to 236% in population studies	CV and all-cause mortality
Egg avoidance	Egg consumption increased risk by 50% in two population studies	CV disease
Coffee	Reduced risk by 40% in meta-analysis	Lipids, CV mortality
Leafy green vegetables	Reduced risk by 14% in meta-analysis	BP, lipids, all-cause mortality
Moderate alcohol consumption	Reduced risk by 50% in meta-analysis	Lipids, CV and all-cause mortality
Avoidance of sugar-sweetened beverages	Sugar-sweetened beverages increased risk by 26% in meta-analysis	—
Treatment of periodontal disease	Periodontal disease increased risk by 150% to 225% in population studies	MI and stroke risk
Lifestyle intervention	HbA1c decreased 0.3% in meta-analysis	BP, lipids
Regular exercise	HbA1c decreased 0.6% in meta-analysis	BP, lipids, CV and all-cause mortality
Low-glycemic diet	HbA1c decreased 0.5% in meta-analysis	Lipids, CV disease
Beans and pulses	HbA1c decreased 0.5% in meta-analysis	BP, lipids
Chia	—	BP, C-reactive protein
Cognitive-behavioral therapy	HbA1c decreased 0.78% in meta-analysis	—
Biofeedback	HbA1c decreased 0.8% in one trial	—
Treatment of vitamin D deficiency	May decrease type 2 DM risk	Endothelial function
Chromium	HbA1c decreased 0.6% in meta-analysis	—
Alpha-lipoic acid	Decreased diabetic neuropathy	? Liver, CV disease
Omega-3 fatty acids	—	Lipids, platelets, CV disease
Magnesium	HbA1c decreased 0.3% in meta-analysis Reduces type 2 DM risk 16%	Lipids, endothelial function
L-Carnitine	? Insulin sensitivity	Lipids, lipoprotein(a)
Benfotiamine		Endothelial function
Vitamin K$_2$	? Stimulates beta cells	CV disease
Avoidance of selenium	Selenium may increase risk 55%	—
Avoidance of high-dose vitamin B$_6$, vitamin B$_{12}$, folate	These vitamins may increase nephropathy	Increased CV disease
Berberine	HbA1c decreased 0.9% in one trial	—
Cinnamon	HbA1c decreased 0.5% in one trial	—
Ginseng	Improved glucose parameters	—
Fenugreek	HbA1c decreased 1.4% in one trial	—
Ivy gourd	HbA1c decreased 0.6% in one trial	—
Momordica charantia	Improved glucose parameters in four trials	—
Prickly pear cactus stem	Improved glucose parameters in one trial	—
Pycnogenol	HbA1c decreased 0.8% in one trial	—
Metformin	HbA1c decreased 1.0%	CV and all-cause mortality
Sitagliptin	HbA1c decreased 1.25%	—
Sulfonylurea	HbA1c decreased 1.0%	May increase risk
Pioglitazone	HbA1c decreased 1.25%	—
Bariatric surgery	Curative in 78% of patients	? CV and all-cause mortality
Insulin	Dose-dependent	—

BP, blood pressure; CV, cardiovascular; DM, diabetes mellitus; HbA1c, glycosylated hemoglobin; MI, myocardial infarction.

Salacia Reticulate

Salacia reticulate, or kothala himbutu, was investigated in a double-blind, crossover RCT of an herbal tea containing kothala himbutu extract in 51 patients with controlled DM over 3 months. This study reported significantly lower HbA1c levels in the treatment arm.[66]

DOSAGE

Three times daily before meals. In the previous trial, the tea was manufactured by Siddhalepa Ayurveda Hospitals, Ratmalana, Sri Lanka and prepared in accordance with a patented formula (international patent application no. PCT/IB00/00405).

PRECAUTIONS

Side effects are dose-dependent and predominantly include gastrointestinal disturbances, such as gas, bloating, abdominal pain, and diarrhea.

Touchi (Soy)

Water-extracted touchi, a traditional Chinese food (soybean extract), has been shown to exert a strong inhibitory effect on rat intestinal alpha-glucosidase. Touchi was also investigated in a 3-month, double-blind, randomized trial of 36 diabetics. Treatment consisted of 0.3 g of touchi in the form of tea preprandially for 3 months and resulted in a reduction in HbA1c levels by 0.5% vs placebo.[67]

DOSAGE

0.3 g in tea before meals.

PRECAUTIONS

Well tolerated orally but may cause mild gastrointestinal upset.

Gynostemma Pentaphyllum

Gynostemma pentaphyllum is a Vietnamese herb used as a tea to treat DM. A double-blinded RCT of 24 drug-naïve patients with diabetes treated with 6 g tea daily for 12 weeks vs placebo reported a reduction in plasma glucose and a decrease in HbA1c levels of 2%.[68]

DOSAGE

6 g in tea daily.

PRECAUTIONS

Generally well tolerated but may cause nausea and diarrhea.

Marine Collagen Peptides (Gelatin)

Marine collagen peptides from fish hydrolysate, a traditional Chinese medicine, were investigated in an RCT of 100 patients with diabetes compared to a control group. This trail reported that administration of 13 g of marine collagen peptides for 3 months significantly lowered LDL, free fatty acids, and markers of inflammation, such as C-reactive protein and nitric oxide, in addition to reducing HbA1c levels and increasing adiponectin levels.[69]

DOSAGE

13 g as a capsule daily.

PRECAUTIONS

May cause an unpleasant taste, bloating, gas, or heaviness in the stomach.

Silymarin (Milk Thistle)

The antioxidant flavonoid silymarin, an extract of milk thistle (*Silybum marianum*), has demonstrated good results in several rigorous trials. As an adjunct to glibenclamide, silymarin was investigated at a dose of 200 g/day in 52 patients with diabetes for 120 days. This randomized, placebo-controlled, double-blinded trial reported reductions in HbA1c levels and body-mass index.[70,71]

DOSAGE

200 g/day extract.

PRECAUTIONS

Well tolerated but may have a laxative effect or cause gastrointestinal symptoms.

Citrullus Colocynthis

Citrullus colocynthis, also known as the schrad fruit, is a traditional medicine of Iran. A clinical trial investigating 25 patients with diabetes treated with 100 mg fruit capsules versus control reported significant reductions in plasma glucose and HbA1c levels.[72]

DOSAGE

100 mg fruit capsules.

PRECAUTIONS

High doses may cause irritation of the gastric mucosa resulting in bloody diarrhea and colitis. Nephrotoxicity has also been documented.

Cinnamon

Cinnamon is a culinary spice made from the bark of *Cinnamomum* sp. trees. The aqueous extract appears to improve insulin receptor function by multiple mechanisms in addition to increasing glycogen synthase activity. However, the results of clinical trials have been inconsistent, with the majority of trials being small and insufficiently powered. A proportion of trials have reported the benefit of cinnamon in reducing HbA1c levels.[73] A trial compared *Cinnamomum aromaticum* (cassia cinnamon) 500 mg twice daily with usual care in 109 patients with type 2 DM for 90 days. This trial reported mean reductions in HbA1c levels of 0.83% in the cinnamon group and 0.37% in those receiving usual care, a difference that reached statistical significance.[74] A Cochrane meta-analysis of 10 RCTs did not demonstrate the efficacy of 2-g *Cinnamomum cassia* in reducing HbA1c levels.[75] However, a separate meta-analysis concluded that cinnamon can reduce plasma blood glucose levels.[76] More investigation is required regarding this.

DOSAGE

The optimal dose of cinnamon for the treatment of type 2 DM is unclear; however, 1- to 2-g doses are commonly prescribed (1 teaspoon of cinnamon is equivalent to 4.75 g). The majority of over-the-counter cinnamon preparation are a combination of cassia and Ceylon cinnamon.

PRECAUTIONS

Stomatitis and perioral dermatitis have been reported with the use of cinnamon.

Fenugreek

Trigonellafoenum graecum, or fenugreek, is a legume used extensively in India, North Africa, and the Mediterranean. The defatted seeds of fenugreek have been used to treat diabetes for centuries in Ayurvedic and other healing systems. A component of fenugreek, 4-hydroxyisoleucine, has been shown to increase pancreatic insulin secretion and inhibit glucosidase activity, with studies reporting effects on satiety, gastric emptying, and insulin receptor function. Fenugreek may also have lipid-lowering effects and several studies have posited hypoglycemic effects. In 42 patients with diabetes poorly controlled with sulfonylureas, 2.1 g fenugreek extract tid for 12 weeks reduced HbA1c and fasting blood glucose levels compared to placebo.[77]

DOSAGE

Until further evidence provides clear guidance, practitioners may use crude powder or extracts at doses equivalent to 20 to 30 g of crude seeds. This dose can be titrated according to meal size and individual results.

PRECAUTIONS

Fenugreek may cause gastrointestinal intolerance, with diarrhea, dyspepsia, abdominal distention, and flatulence.

Supplements

Table 33.1 describes the glycemic effects and cardiovascular benefits of different treatments for type 2 DM.

Vitamin D

25(OH)D levels have been shown to be lower in type 2 DM and obesity. Studies have reported that vitamin D levels are associated with increased risk of type 2 DM, by virtue of insulin sensitivity and beta cell activity. However, while studies are supportive of the use of vitamin D supplementation in the management of type 2 diabetes, others remain inconclusive. A review of eight trials reported no glycemic benefit of vitamin D supplementation.[78]

Chromium

This trace element has several effects on carbohydrate and lipid metabolism. A complex containing trivalent chromium has been shown to influence glucose tolerance. Evidence suggests that chromium acts to reduce tissue lipid content and that chromium responders are more likely to be more obese, more insulin resistant, and have poorer glycemic control regardless of baseline chromium status.[74] A meta-analysis of 41 trials evaluating the glycemic effects of various formulations identified 14 trials of chromium including patients with type 2 DM.[75] However, the evidence was determined to be difficult to interpret because of low study quality and differences in formulation and dose, with the best results reported by trials evaluating chromium picolinate or brewer's yeast at doses of at least 200 mcg daily. In these trials, a mean reduction in HbA1c of 0.6% compared with placebo was reported.

DOSAGE

A dose of 200 to 1000 mcg daily is recommended.

PRECAUTIONS

Chromium has no known side effects.

Alpha-Lipoic Acid

Also known as *thioctic acid*, alpha-lipoic acid (ALA) is a potent lipophilic antioxidant that is found in most eukaryotic cells. ALA also acts as a cofactor for several mitochondrial and cytosolic enzymes, with the right-sided enantiomer being the active form. In addition to its antioxidant activity, ALA can also regenerate other antioxidants via reduction reactions, including vitamins C and E, coenzyme Q10, and glutathione. ALA also chelates mercury, arsenic, iron, and other metals that act as free radicals. ALA is present in trace amounts in organ meats and some vegetables, but these amounts are negligible compared with usual therapeutic doses.

ALA has been used to treat several diseases in Europe and Japan since the 1950s. A large body of preclinical research supports the potential benefit of ALA in liver disorders, cardiovascular disease, cancer prevention, and neuropsychiatric disorders, and for heavy metal and general detoxification.

Good evidence indicates that ALA reduces painful diabetic neuropathy. First used parenterally, ALA in oral form has been shown to be effective in a multicenter trial involving 181 patients with type 2 DM who received varying doses for 5 weeks. All doses provided an overall reduction in symptoms of 50%, with the lowest dose (600 mg daily) causing the fewest side effects.[76] This finding may be related to reduced lipid peroxidation in neuronal cell membranes or improved endothelial function and microvascular blood flow.[77] ALA may also improve insulin sensitivity through enhanced GLUT4 translocation and glucose uptake in muscle and fat cells.[78] This last effect was observed by trials of intravenous ALA and has yet to be firmly established with the oral form; however, this study provides further support for the use of ALA in patients with type 2 DM.

The majority of published trials have used regular ALA (an R-S racemic mixture). R-Lipoic acid is marketed as a superior product because it is the endogenously produced form; however, there is a lack of evidence from clinical trials to support this claim. A sustained-release form of ALA is marketed as superior based on the short half-life of regular ALA; however, data to indicate whether peak or total levels are most important, and evidence of the safety and efficacy of this product are similarly lacking. At this time, regular ALA is the only recommended form.

DOSAGE

The most appropriate dose for neuropathy is 600 mg daily; however, a dose of 50 to 100 mg is sufficient for antioxidant purposes. Absorption is greatest on an empty stomach.

PRECAUTIONS

The most common side effect of ALA is nausea; however, insomnia, fatigue, diarrhea, and rashes have also been reported.

Omega-3 Fatty Acids

Fish and other marine species are the main sources of eicosapentaenoic acid (EPA) and docosahexaenoic acid (DHA) in the human diet. Alpha-linoleic acid is an omega-3 precursor found in walnuts, flax, and other grains. Although omega-3 fatty acids have no effect on glycemic control, these fats have antiinflammatory, antithrombotic, and antiarrhythmic effects that appear to prevent and treat cardiovascular disease. For this reason, omega-3 fatty acids offer important benefits to patients with type 2 DM.

A Cochrane systematic review of 23 trials involving 1075 patients who used omega-3 fatty acids at an average dose of 3.5 g daily reported improved lipid parameters and platelet function.[79] Small trials have reported improvements in endothelial function, with one study reporting significant improvements in impaired flow-mediated dilatation with the consumption of 2 g of omega-3 fatty acids.[80]

DOSAGE

The majority of cardiovascular benefits of omega-3 fats occur at doses of 1000 mg (EPA and DHA) daily; however, higher doses are often used.

PRECAUTIONS

Fishy repeats and mild gastrointestinal upset are the only side effects of omega-3 fatty acid supplementation. Although bleeding in aspirin or warfarin users is often cited as a reason for caution, the literature contains no specific reports of this effect.

Magnesium

Magnesium affects insulin secretion and action in addition to influencing lipid parameters and endothelial function. A systematic review identified nine trials that evaluated magnesium supplementation for 4 to 16 weeks in 370 patients with type 2 DM and noted improvements in fasting glucose and high-density lipoprotein cholesterol. In the five trials of sufficient duration to evaluate HbA1c, a nonsignificant reduction of 0.31% (95% CI, –0.81 to 0.19) was reported.[81] A separate review of magnesium for the prevention of type 2 DM found seven cohort studies and reported an overall benefit, with an average daily dose of 100 mg decreasing the risk of type 2 DM by approximately 16%.[82] The accuracy of routine tests in reflecting total magnesium body stores remains unclear.

DOSAGE

Usual starting doses are approximately 100 mg daily and can be increased as desired or to bowel tolerance. Magnesium is available as oral liquid or tablets, transdermal lotion, or Epsom salts, as well as in parenteral formulations.

PRECAUTIONS

Gastrointestinal intolerance, mainly diarrhea, is the most common side effect. Chelated magnesium (magnesium glycinate) causes less diarrhea than do other forms of magnesium.

Antioxidants

Individuals who consume diets rich in antioxidants are at greatly reduced risk of type 2 DM; however, commonly-used antioxidant supplements do not appear to have the same preventive effect. In 8171 women who were followed for 9.2 years in the Women's Antioxidant Cardiovascular Study, only a mild benefit of vitamin C in the prevention of type 2 DM was indicated by a nonsignificant trend, whereas vitamin E increased the risk of type 2 DM and beta-carotene offered no benefit.[83] The Prevention of Progression of Arterial Disease and Diabetes (POPADAD) trial reported no significant benefit in 1276 Scottish adults administered a low-dose mixed antioxidant supplement or placebo for 8 years.[84]

The benefits of antioxidant-rich foods are likely attributable to the dozens of phytomedicines they contain, components that are currently poorly understood. Although antioxidants and multivitamins are commonly prescribed by integrative practitioners as "insurance against deficiency," this practice may not be safe. High doses of vitamins have been shown to interfere with absorption and use of lesser-known but potentially more powerful antioxidants in food. High profile examples include tocopherols and carotenoids. Whole food supplements may be a reasonable alternative approach. In one study, an antioxidant supplement derived from pomegranate, green tea, and ascorbic acid improved lipid parameters and markers of oxidative stress in a placebo-controlled trial involving 114 patients with type 2 DM conducted in Turkey.[85]

Vitamin E

Vitamin E is one of the most commonly used specific antioxidants; however, there is a lack of evidence to support its use in patients with type 2 DM. Negative results reported by large cardiovascular and cancer trials have been the subject of media reports, controversy, and debate among integrative medicine practitioners. Alpha-tocopherol supplementation did not decrease the risk of type 2 DM in the large Alpha-Tocopherol Beta-Carotene (ATBC) cancer trial,[86] and a separate small trial reported prooxidant effects shortly after ingestion of a single 1200-unit dose.[87]

Although several tocopherols and tocotrienols have vitamin E–like activity, the majority of vitamin E supplements contain alpha-tocopherol only. Some investigators have posited that the negative results of vitamin E trials are attributable to decreased absorption of other, more potent molecules of this family whose absorption is inhibited by alpha-tocopherol supplementation.[88] In fact, one study found no difference between the effects of alpha- and gamma-tocopherol on markers of oxidative stress and inflammation in patients with type 2 DM.[89] Other trials have reported that gamma-tocopherol increases blood pressure[90] and has no effect on platelet function.[91]

Greater benefit from alpha-tocopherol has been demonstrated among individuals who are homozygous for a haptoglobin gene variant that has been shown to increase oxidative stress and is present in 3% to 4% of the population. In an Israeli double-blind study involving 1434 people with type 2 DM who were homozygous for haptoglobin-2, alpha-tocopherol reduced the risk of a combined cardiovascular end point by more than 50%.[92] This is an example of how genetics may improve future treatment outcomes in personalized medicine.

Vitamin E supplements containing mixed tocopherols and trienols are increasingly available; however, clear dosing guidelines for their use for type 2 DM have yet to be published. Vitamin E has no known side effects.

L-Carnitine

L-Carnitine shuttles fatty acids into mitochondria and has been proposed as a potential therapy for type 2 DM based on its potential effects on intracellular lipid accumulation. A pilot study found no improvements in glycemic control after 4 weeks of L-carnitine use in 12 patients with type 2 DM;[93] however, several trials have reported that L-carnitine improves lipid parameters and significantly reduces lipoprotein (a), an important independent inherited cardiac risk factor for which few effective therapies exist.[94]

DOSAGE

The usual dose is 500 to 1000 mg three times daily.

Benfotiamine

Postprandial endothelial dysfunction has been proposed as a link between metabolic syndrome and atherosclerosis. This state is associated with oxidative stress, hyperglycemia, hypertriglyceridemia, and altered nitric oxide function, and been attributed to glucose-protein complexes in food, named advanced glycation end products (AGEs). These complexes are formed at high temperatures and activate AGE-specific receptors, which stimulate monocytes and endothelial cells and ultimately promote inflammation.

Benfotiamine is a synthetic analogue of thiamine with significantly greater bioavailability. Benfotiamine activates transketolase, an enzyme that helps clear AGEs, thus improving postprandial endothelial function. In a pilot study, 350 mg of benfotiamine after meals completely eliminated vascular measures of postprandial endothelial dysfunction in 13 patients with type 2 DM.[95]

This important finding has not been replicated since it was reported in 2006; however, there is a substantial clinical need for corroborating evidence. Several trials have indicated that benfotiamine improves diabetic neuropathy,[96,97] an unsurprising finding considering the neurological symptoms observed in cases of thiamine deficiency. While one trial reported no improvement in markers of diabetic nephropathy,[98] a separate trial reported improvements in microalbuminuria.[99]

DOSAGE

The 350-mg dose used in the pilot study is higher than found in most formulations.

PRECAUTIONS

While early evidence is very promising, it is probably premature to recommend the widespread use of synthetic thiamine analogues because long-term safety data are not available.

Vitamin K

This fat-soluble vitamin exists as phylloquinone (K1) in plants, menaquinone (K2) in animals, and a fermented soybean product known as *natto*. Vitamin K2 is considered more biologically active and is a cofactor for the carboxylation of proteins. Vitamin K2 is involved in the production of osteocalcin, which strengthens bones by forming a protein scaffold. Vitamin K2 is also involved in the production of matrix Gla protein, which prevents vascular calcification by repairing smooth muscle and endothelium. Vitamin K2 is receiving growing attention as a target for the treatment of diverse disorders in addition to its established role in coagulation factors biosynthesis.

Early studies indicate that vitamin K2 stimulates beta cell proliferation and enhances insulin sensitivity. Vitamin K deficiency, as suggested by low levels of carboxylated osteocalcin, is also associated with an increased risk of type 2 DM.[100] Recommending vitamin K2 for glycemic control is premature; however, its endothelial and cardiovascular benefits make it an appealing addition to an integrative type 2 treatment plan.

DOSAGE

The starting dose of vitamin K2 is typically 100 mcg daily; however, higher doses have been commonly used.

PRECAUTIONS

Patients taking warfarin require close monitoring and dose adjustment after starting vitamin K2; however, vitamin K2 ultimately reduces the fluctuations in international normalized ratio observed in vitamin K2-deficient patients.[101] Vitamin K has no other known side effects.

Risks of Specific Supplements

Although evidence indicates selenium has insulin-like actions and may delay microvascular complications, integrative practitioners should be aware of the association between selenium and the risk of type 2 DM. In the Nutritional Prevention of Cancer trial, 1202 individuals with localized melanoma were randomized to receive selenium or placebo for cancer prevention. After a mean follow-up duration of 7.7 years, selenium users developed type 2 DM more often (hazard risk, 1.55; 95% CI, 1.03 to 2.33), with the greatest risk observed in individuals with the highest baseline selenium levels (hazard risk, 2.70; 95% CI, 1.30 to 5.61).[102] Selenium supplementation should only be considered in patients with low baseline selenium levels. The maximum daily dose is 200 mcg. The mechanisms underlying the difference in effects of inorganic and organic forms of selenium on the risk of type 2 DM risk have yet to be elucidated.

Practitioners should exercise caution when using B vitamins in patients with nephropathy. In the Canadian Diabetic Intervention with Vitamins to Improve Nephropathy (DIVINe) trial, 238 patients with type 1 DM or type 2 DM were administered a tablet containing folic acid 2.5 mg, vitamin B_6 25 mg, and vitamin B_{12} 1 mg daily or placebo for approximately 3 years for the treatment of elevated homocysteine levels. Although the treatment group had lower plasma homocysteine levels, worse kidney function and a higher incidence of cardiovascular events were observed in this group.[103] The investigators postulated that this finding may be attributable to increased cell proliferation induced by folic acid, increased methylation from folic acid and vitamin B_{12}, or nitric oxide-related mechanisms. Earlier reports noted poorer cardiovascular outcomes associated with B vitamins, indicating further studies are required to clarify this issue.

Pharmaceuticals

The standard approach to treating type 2 DM is focused on improving glycemic control, as reflected by serum levels of HbA1c. This approach is based on the assumption that all reductions in HbA1c are of equal benefit, regardless of how they are achieved. However, more recent evidence contradicts this assumption.

Recent systematic reviews clearly indicate that different drugs have different effects on real-world clinical measures of morbidity and mortality, independent of their ability to lower blood glucose. Growing recognition of this important gap in our understanding of type 2 DM treatment has created confusion for patients and caregivers. Bridging this gap will be crucial for providing more effective integrative treatment in the future.

Metformin

Metformin is a biguanide that is structurally similar to guanidines that were originally discovered in extracts of *Galega officinalis* (French lilac). Metformin has been in use since the 1950s, thus making it one of the oldest, and perhaps most effective, oral hypoglycemic drugs. Although its exact mechanism of action is unclear, metformin improves insulin sensitivity and reduces hepatic gluconeogenesis.

Metformin is the only diabetes medication shown to reduce cardiovascular mortality (OR, 0.74; 95% CI, 0.62 to 0.89) in systematic reviews,[104] and as such should be considered first-line treatment for diabetes.

DOSAGE

The typical dose range is 500 to 1000 mg twice daily.

PRECAUTIONS

Other than mild occasional nausea and diarrhea, the only drawback of metformin use is impaired vitamin B_{12} absorption in the terminal ileum, which may lead to vitamin B_{12} deficiency.[105] Metformin may also cause lactic acidosis in patients with renal insufficiency or alcoholism.

Sulfonylureas

Sulfonylureas increase insulin secretion by pancreatic beta cells by binding to membrane channels. Sulfonylureas drugs have also been used for several decades but do not appear to improve cardiovascular outcomes. The use of sulfonylureas is limited by their potential to cause weight gain and association with more frequent hypoglycemic episodes, which can lead to arrhythmias and cardiac ischemia.[106] A systematic review found that glyburide was almost twice as likely as other sulfonylureas to cause hypoglycemia; however, cardiovascular outcomes were identical for all drugs in this class.[107] Patients using sulfonylureas and metformin in combination are reportedly at greater risk of cardiovascular mortality than patients using metformin alone.[108]

DOSAGE

The usual dose of glyburide is 2.5 to 10 mg twice daily.

PRECAUTIONS

Glyburide may cause hypoglycemia and weight gain.

Thiazolidinedione

Thiazolidinediones increase insulin sensitivity by activating peroxisome proliferator-activated receptor gamma, a nuclear receptor with salutary effects on fatty acid balance, adipocyte differentiation, adiponectin, and other factors involved in glucose and lipid metabolism. The use of rosiglitazone has decreased dramatically since it was found to increase the risk of heart attacks by more than 40% in patients with type 2 DM, possibly because of drug-related increases in LDL or congestive heart failure. Pioglitazone (Actos) is the only drug in this class currently licensed for the treatment of type 2 DM. The impact of pioglitazone on cardiovascular outcomes remains unclear; however, a systematic review did find that it improves glycemic control with a mean reduction in HbA1c levels of 0.58%.

DOSAGE

The dose of pioglitazone is 15 to 30 mg once daily.

PRECAUTIONS

The average weight gain associated with the use of pioglitazone is 7 lb, and mild edema is commonly noted. A further issue with long-term pioglitazone use is osteoporosis, with a meta-analysis of 10 trials involving 13,715 participants demonstrating fracture risk is more than doubled with the use of pioglitazone (OR, 2.23; 95% CI, 1.65 to 3.01).[109] Pioglitazone may increase cardiovascular risk.

Incretins

Incretins are hormones produced in the small intestine during a meal that enter the vasculature and trigger insulin release by pancreatic beta cells. The two incretins are glucagon-like peptide (GLP-1) and gastric inhibitory peptide (GIP). A newer class of drugs that inhibit dipeptidyl peptidase-4 (DPP-4), an enzyme that degrades GLP-1 and GIP, have demonstrated efficacy in increasing insulin and decreasing glucagon levels.

Sitagliptin. Sitagliptin (*Januvia*) is a dipeptidyl peptidase-4 inhibitor.

DOSAGE

The recommended dose of sitagliptin is 100 mg once daily.

PRECAUTIONS

The only side effects noted in trials are nasopharyngitis and headache; however, the long-term safety of sitagliptin remains unclear because DPP-4 degrades dozens of other enzymes and sitagliptin has not been evaluated in long-term trials. The impact of sitagliptin on cardiovascular events and mortality remains unclear; however, meta-analyses indicate that the use of sitagliptin is associated with HbA1c reductions by 0.7%.[110]

Exenatide and Liraglutide. Exenatide (Byetta) and Liraglutide (Victoza) are GLP-1 analogues. In comparison trials with insulin and other oral hypoglycemic, exenatide and liraglutide have been shown to reduce HbA1c by approximately 1.0% without causing hypoglycemia or weight gain.[111] Liraglutide has also been approved for weight loss.

DOSAGE

The dose of exenatide is 5 mcg twice daily for 1 month and increased to 10 mcg twice daily as required. A once-weekly injection is available as a 2 mg weekly subcutaneous dose. The dose of liraglutide is 0.6 mg subcutaneous injection daily for 1 week and then increased to 1.2 mg daily.

PRECAUTIONS

Reported side effects include diarrhea, nausea, and vomiting. Cases of pancreatitis have been reported. Data regarding cardiovascular outcomes are not currently available.

Insulin, sulfonylureas, and thiazolidinedione all cause weight gain. Metformin, incretins, and sodium-glucose cotransporter 2 inhibitors are weight neutral or can help with weight loss.

Sodium-Glucose Cotransporter 2 Inhibitors

This new class of medicines inhibits the reabsorption of glucose in the kidney, thereby encouraging the excretion of glucose via the urine. Sodium-glucose cotransporter 2 inhibitors have been found to reduce HbA1c levels by 0.5 to 0.8% and result in mild weight loss.[79]

DOSAGE

- Dapagliflozin (*Farxiga*); 5–10 mg by mouth every morning.
- Canagliflozin (*Invokana*); 100–300 mg before breakfast.
- Empagliflozin (*Jardiance*); 10–25 mg by mouth every morning.

PRECAUTIONS

Sodium-glucose cotransporter 2 inhibitors may increase the risk of lower urinary tract infections and should be avoided in patients with a GFR < 45.

Insulin

Although insulin administration can be lifesaving, insulin is a proinflammatory hormone. Every effort should be made to optimize glycemic control; however, it is probably best to use the lowest possible doses of exogenous insulin to achieve this goal. Insulin-dependent patients with type 2 DM can often greatly reduce their dose requirements by following an integrative treatment protocol, as described in this chapter.

One important mechanism underlying the risk of type 2 DM is stimulation of insulin-like growth factor-1 (IGF-1) and other growth hormones. IGF-1 levels predict cancer risk, with the first indication that insulin users may be at increased risk of cancer published in 1967.[112] For reasons that are unclear, patients with type 2 DM are at a 20% increased risk of breast cancer[113] and a 30% increased risk of colon cancer.[114] Research indicates glargine, a long-acting insulin analogue, may be more carcinogenic due to greater stimulation of IGF-1 compared to other types of insulin. The hope is that the International Study of Insulin and Cancer, funded by Sanofi-Aventis (the makers of glargine), will clarify this issue. Many insulin protocols, regimens, and analogues are available; however, their use is beyond the scope of this chapter. Practitioners should be aware that, although these regimens may allow patients to take their insulin in a more convenient or practical manner, there is a lack of evidence demonstrating any approach is superior to another. Short-acting insulin analogues are commonly used; however, meta-analyses indicate these therapies do not provide any advantage over regular human insulin.[115] Similarly, there is no evidence to suggest the long-acting insulin analogues, glargine and detemir, are superior to regular insulin.[116] Continuous infusion pumps represent a newer technology that may be superior; however, their benefit has been demonstrated only among patients with type 1 DM.[117]

Other Drugs That Improve Outcomes

Angiotensin-Converting Enzyme Inhibitors. ACE inhibitors have been shown to have efficacy in preventing and treating type 2 diabetes. Accordingly, the integration between seemingly disparate physiological systems may have a powerful impact on health and disease. The precise mechanisms underlying the effect of the renin-angiotensin system on glucose metabolism remain unclear; however, multiple lines of evidence exist. Angiotensin II is known to mediate vasoconstriction and hypoperfusion of skeletal muscle and pancreatic islets. Angiotensin II also appears to affect insulin signaling and glucose transport by mechanisms that have yet to be elucidated. In a systematic review of 13 trials involving 93,451 patients with hypertension, the use ACE inhibitors reduced the risk of incident type 2 DM by an impressive 26%.[118] A number of ACE inhibitors are available, with ramipril being the most widely studied at a recommended dose of 2.5 to 10 mg once daily.

Statins. Statins are universally recommended for patients with type 2 DM; however, their effectiveness in treating type 2 DM is increasingly complicated. As a drug class, 3-hydroxy-3-methyl-glutaryl-coenzyme A (HMG-CoA) reductase inhibitors are known to improve lipid parameters. However, the clear cardiovascular benefits of statins are more strongly associated with antiinflammatory effects. The absolute risk reduction observed with statins is compelling in people who have already had a cardiovascular event; however, the effectiveness of statins is limited in patients who have not. Patients with type 2 DM fall somewhere in between these two patient populations, with the higher baseline vascular risk among patients with diabetes making statin therapy more appropriate.[119]

Red yeast rice is a natural source of several statin compounds and may represent a reasonable alternative for patients who are unable to tolerate or do not wish to use a statin drug.

Unfortunately, recent evidence indicates some statins increase the risk of type 2 DM. In a meta-analysis of 13 trials involving 91,140 adults, the overall increase in type 2 DM risk was 9% (95% CI, 1.02 to 1.17).[120] Subgroup analysis revealed that different statins have very different effects. Simvastatin, atorvastatin, and rosuvastatin increased the risk of type 2 DM, whereas pravastatin reduced the risk.[121] This finding indicates pravastatin may be a more appropriate choice in patients with type 2 DM until this issue has been resolved. The recommended dose of pravastatin for the treatment of type 2 diabetes is 20 to 80 mg once daily.

Bariatric Surgery

Various surgical procedures can induce weight loss by resecting, tightening, shrinking, or bypassing the stomach and upper digestive tract. These forms of so-called bariatric surgery lead to profound weight loss and may be the most important advance in the treatment of type 2 DM in decades. Although surgery is not the most philosophically appealing solution to the worldwide epidemic of type 2 DM and other metabolic diseases related to obesity, it is increasingly recognized by governments and insurers worldwide.

In a review of 103 clinical trial treatment arms involving 3188 patients with type 2 DM, 78% had complete resolution of clinical and laboratory manifestations of diabetes postoperatively, with significant improvements observed in 87% of patients with a reported average weight loss of 38.5 kg.[122] Long-term reductions in all-cause morbidity and mortality are increasingly reported.

Short-term complications include gastric dumping syndrome, hernias, wound infections, and pneumonia. The most important long-term consideration following bariatric surgery is nutrient malabsorption.

Deficiencies of vitamins A, C, D, K, and B_{12}, and folate, iron, selenium, calcium, zinc, and copper should be expected following bariatric surgery.[123] All patients who have undergone bariatric surgery should take a daily multivitamin and multimineral supplement. Anemia, hyperparathyroidism, and peripheral neuropathy are common postoperatively. Patients who report vague symptoms following bariatric surgery should be evaluated for nutrient deficiency and reminded of the importance of supplementation.

PREVENTION PRESCRIPTION

- Reduce stress.
- Obtain 6 to 8 hours of restful sleep per night.
- Eat a low-glycemic Mediterranean diet that includes whole grains, vegetable protein, vegetables, and some fruit, coffee, and moderate alcohol.
- Practice daily exercise, aerobic or resistance.

- Manage weight and treat obesity.
- Avoid air pollution by maintaining a safe distance from high-traffic roads at work and home.
- Practice a form of mindfulness or meditation.
- Treat prediabetes with aggressive lifestyle intervention and consider metformin 500 to 1000 mg twice daily.

THERAPEUTIC REVIEW

LIFESTYLE

- Consider referral to a comprehensive lifestyle program if available.   A↑₁

EXERCISE

- Encourage daily aerobic or resistance exercise.   A↑₁

DIET

- Low-glycemic diet and moderate carbohydrate reduction.   A↑₁
- Avoidance of sugar-sweetened beverages and juices.   A↑₁
- Consumption of more lentils, beans, pulses and soy, chia and other whole grains, onions and green leafy vegetables, almonds, walnuts, and other nuts.   A↑₁
- Moderate coffee and wine consumption.   A↑₁

MIND-BODY THERAPY

- Ask about and treat disordered sleep, stress, anxiety, and depression.
- Discuss stress reduction options and facilitate the chosen modality.

SUPPLEMENTS

- Alpha-lipoic acid: 50 to 100 mg daily.   B↗₁
- Chromium: 200 to 1000 mcg daily.   A↑₁
- Benfotiamine: 350 mg with meals.   B→₂
- Omega-3 fatty acids: 1 to 4 g daily.   B↗₁
- L-Carnitine: 500 to 1000 mg three times daily.   C→₁
- Magnesium: 200 to 500 mg daily.   A↗₂
- Vitamin K: 100 mcg daily (caution with warfarin).   B↘₂

BOTANICALS

- Cinnamon: 1 to 5 g ground bark with meals or equivalent extract.   A↑₁
- Fenugreek (*Trigonella foenum-graecum*): 30 g seed powder or equivalent extract with meals.   B↗₁
- Touchi, water extract (soy) 0.3 g in tea daily.   B↗₁
- Marine collagen peptides: 13 g daily.   B↗₁
- Silymarin: 200 g daily.   B↗₁
- Ivy gourd (*Coccinia indica*): 15 g powdered dried leaves or equivalent extract.   B→₂
- *Salacia reticulate* (kothala himbutu): premanufactured tea daily.   C↘₂
- Gynostemma pentaphylum: 6 g in tea daily.   C↘₂

PHARMACEUTICALS

- Metformin: 500 to 1000 mg twice daily.   A↗₂
- Add other drug classes as required to achieve optimal glycosylated hemoglobin levels.

SURGERY

- Bariatric surgery for morbidly obese patients.   A→₃

Key Web Resources

Fooducate helps track food with the goal of weight loss.	http://www.fooducate.com/
Glooko. This app allows patients to download blood sugar readings and keep a log based on nutrition and medications used.	https://www.glooko.com/
Myfitnesspal. Monitors activity and allows user to set weight loss goals.	https://www.myfitnesspal.com/
Glycemic Index Foundation: Provides eating plans that help control diabetes and lower serum triglyceride levels.	http://www.gisymbol.com/
Diabetes Connect: A community website for the education and discussion of diabetes care.	http://www.diabeticconnect.com/
National Center for Complementary and Integrative Health: Information about an integrative approach to diabetes.	https://nccih.nih.gov/health/diabetes

ACKNOWLEDGMENT

The author would like to acknowledge Richard Nahas, MD, the author of this chapter in the previous edition, because some of the material from the previous edition has been used in this chapter.

REFERENCES

References are available online at ExpertConsult.com.

CHAPTER 34

HYPOTHYROIDISM

Leslie Mendoza Temple, MD, ABOIM • Pooja Saigal, MD

PATHOPHYSIOLOGY

Normal Thyroid Physiology

Thyrotropin-releasing hormone (TRH) from the hypothalamus increases release of thyroid-stimulating hormone (TSH) from the anterior pituitary gland. TSH stimulates the thyroid gland to release the prohormone thyroxine (T4) alongside the active metabolite triiodothyronine (T3); this yields 20% of the body's available T3. Thyroid hormone transporters transport circulating T4 into cells of various peripheral organs, where type 1 deiodinase (D1) and type 2 deiodinase (D2) catalyze intracellular conversion of T4 to T3; this yields the remaining 80% of the body's available T3. T4 and T3 suppress both TRH and TSH secretion via negative feedback. Type 3 deiodinase (D3) clears T4 and T3 by catalyzing the conversion of T4 to reverse T3 (rT3) and T3 to T2. In a single day, the human body generally produces T4:T3 in a ratio of 5:2; however, the half-life of T4 is much longer than that of T3, so the physiological serum ratio of T4:T3 in the human body is 14:1.[1,2] In a healthy individual, thyroid hormones, enzymes, and nutritional cofactors (to be described in this chapter) will influence and are influenced by other members of the endocrine system, notably the hypothalamus, pituitary, adrenal glands, ovaries, and testes.

Pathophysiology of Hypothyroidism

Hypothyroidism is the insufficient synthesis of thyroid hormone necessary for metabolic processes throughout the body. Worldwide, iodine deficiency is the most common cause of **primary hypothyroidism**. In iodine-sufficient countries, autoimmune destruction of the gland (Hashimoto disease) is the leading cause of primary hypothyroidism. The second leading cause is iatrogenic, including surgery, radioactive iodine, medications (e.g., lithium, amiodarone), overconsumption of goitrogens, and external beam radiation. Primary hypothyroidism accounts for approximately 95% of cases compared with less than 5% from secondary and tertiary types. One must evaluate and treat for other causes of hypothyroid-like symptoms that can trigger body stress, including adrenal insufficiency, hypogonadism, anemia, anxiety, depression, toxic exposures, and food sensitivities or allergies.

Secondary hypothyroidism results from decreased TSH secretion from pituitary tumors (adenomas most common), pituitary surgery, or other pituitary diseases, such as Sheehan syndrome. **Tertiary hypothyroidism** results in decreased TRH secretion because of infiltrative processes in the brain such as sarcoidosis, infection, or congenital

defect. TSH levels may vary from low, normal, or even slightly elevated values, whereas the free T4 (FT4) level remains low. Generally, serum TSH concentrations are low in patients with pituitary disease and normal or high in those with hypothalamic disease. Clinical correlation and magnetic resonance imaging (MRI) of the hypothalamus and pituitary are necessary for proper diagnosis. **Transient hypothyroidism** may occur after abrupt withdrawal of long-term thyroid hormone therapy or from silent or subacute thyroiditis. **Resistance to thyroid hormone (RTH)** is a rare autosomal dominant inherited syndrome of decreased end-organ sensitivity to thyroid hormone.

Subclinical Hypothyroidism

In subclinical hypothyroidism (SCH), TSH is elevated but FT4 is in the normal range. The thyroid gland is stimulated to work harder but is still keeping up with the body's metabolic needs. The prevalence of SCH is variable, with 8% of women and 3% of men affected, increasing to 15%–18% in women aged more than 60 years.[3] In addition, 2%–5% of patients with SCH progress to overt hypothyroidism per year.[4]

In SCH, the clinical decision to prescribe thyroid hormone is based mainly on the presence of symptoms and lab results. If a patient is symptomatic, checking thyroid peroxidase antibodies (TPO Ab) and thyroglobulin antibodies (Tg Ab) may help identify an autoimmune cause (Hashimoto disease) and the risk for progression to overt hypothyroidism. If antibodies are positive and the patient is symptomatic, then treatment with low-dose thyroid hormone may be indicated. If the patient has symptoms, yet has negative antibodies and no other possible causes, a low dose of thyroid hormone may still be warranted for several months' trial.

> Subclinical hypothyroidism is when the TSH is elevated but FT4 is normal. Do not consider treating unless the patient is symptomatic, has underlying heart disease, or the TSH is >10 mIU/L.

Possible consequences of untreated SCH are coronary atherosclerosis, elevated low-density lipoproteins (LDLs), and progression to overt hypothyroidism.[5] Statin-induced myopathy may be associated with mild thyroid insufficiency, so thyroid hormone may be useful for high-risk cardiovascular patients starting statin medication, particularly if the TSH is elevated.[6,7]

The risks for cardiac arrhythmias (atrial fibrillation) and osteoporosis must be weighed against the benefits of receiving thyroid hormone therapy,[4] but clinical monitoring of pulse rate and symptoms of hyperthyroidism (e.g., anxiety, insomnia, palpitations, diarrhea, weight loss, irritability), as well as periodic bone density testing in appropriate patients, would likely reduce these risks.

Other abnormal laboratory findings in hypothyroidism may include increased creatine phosphokinase, elevated cholesterol and triglycerides, and normocytic or macrocytic anemia.

Clinical Presentation

Common symptoms of hypothyroidism can include fatigue, dry skin, cold intolerance, hair loss, concentration problems, constipation, weight gain, carpal tunnel symptoms, dyspnea, hoarseness, and menorrhagia. Physical signs are manifested by obesity, dry, coarse skin; brittle nails; cool extremities; thinning of the lateral eyebrows and hair; myxedema; delayed tendon reflexes; and diminished hearing.[8] In addition to the physical findings described, basal metabolic rate may be estimated using axillary temperature measurements and assessment of Achilles tendon reflexes (ATRs). A series of morning basal body temperatures less than 97.4°F and delayed ATRs may enhance the clinical diagnosis.[9]

Laboratory Studies

The laboratory evaluation of hypothyroidism remains a controversial topic in the medical community. Minimal evaluation should include TSH, FT4, and TPO Ab. Some clinicians monitor free T3 (FT3) and rT3 levels, which will be discussed later in the chapter. Additional testing may include measuring nutritional cofactors and related hormone pathways, e.g., urinary iodine levels and adrenal gland function, although these tests are not commonly performed in conventional endocrinology with respect to hypothyroidism.

Timing of Blood Collection

In individuals with intact endogenous thyroid function, circadian fluctuation yields the highest TSH secretion between 10 p.m. and 4 a.m. and lowest secretion between 10 a.m. and 6 p.m.; T3 levels peak at 3 a.m.[1,10] However, in patients receiving oral thyroid hormone replacement therapy, serum TSH is lowest about 14 hours after ingestion, FT4 peaks 4–6 hours after ingestion, and FT3 serum peaks 2–4 hours after ingestion. Though these fluctuations may be blunted by endogenous hormone production, it is prudent to check thyroid function tests several hours after thyroid hormone replacement therapy is dosed to capture peak FT4 and FT3 levels and to rule out supratherapeutic dosing regimens.[1] Thus if thyroid hormone replacement therapy is taken at night, then thyroid function tests should be drawn in the morning, preferably prior to caffeine consumption. Alternatively, if thyroid hormone replacement therapy is taken in the morning, then thyroid function tests should be drawn in the afternoon. In general, testing at a consistent time of day is best for serial comparisons.

Optimal Lab Values and Treatment Targets

Every individual has an endogenously set TSH concentration that corresponds to their optimal thyroid function. The normal TSH reference range proposed by the American Association of Clinical Endocrinologists (AACE) and the American Thyroid Association (ATA) is wide, ranging from 0.4 to 4.0 mIU/L. Some investigators suggest lowering the upper limit of serum TSH reference range to 2.5 mIU/L. This narrower TSH reference range may be appropriate when TSH is utilized as a target for therapeutic purposes in overt hypothyroidism, though it may lead to overdiagnosis when TSH is utilized for initial diagnostic purposes.[1,4,11,12]

> The ideal TSH range is controversial. Consider using the broader range of 0.4–4.0 mIU/L for diagnosis and an upper limit of 2.5 mIU/L to guide replacement therapy.

In patients with subclinical hypothyroidism, AACE and ATA guidelines suggest levothyroxine (LT4) supplementation when TSH is greater than 10 because of an increased risk for heart failure (HF) and cardiovascular mortality. They also state that LT4 supplementation may be considered when TSH is greater than the laboratory upper limit but less than 10 if patients have symptoms suggestive of hypothyroidism, positive TPO Abs, evidence of atherosclerotic cardiovascular disease (ASCVD), HF, or associated risk factors for these diseases[1,2,13]

AACE and ATA guidelines recommend treatment for SCH or hypothyroidism if TSH is greater than 2.5 in all females during the preconceptual period or if TSH is greater than trimester-specific reference ranges during pregnancy (0.1–2.5 mIU/L in the first trimester, 0.2–3.0 mIU/L in the second trimester, and 0.3–3.0 mIU/L in the third trimester).[1,2,13]

TSH normalization is usually the goal of thyroid hormone replacement therapy, with improvement of the patient's symptoms being paramount. However, it should be noted that overtreatment with thyroid hormone to achieve subnormal TSH levels is not advised because TSH levels of less than 0.1 are associated with increased risk for osteoporosis and atrial fibrillation. FT4 and FT3 may also be tested and should achieve levels within normal laboratory reference ranges during therapy. Unfortunately, FT3 levels are difficult to interpret because the target reference range, yielding normal physiological function, is uncertain and performance of T3 assays is limited.[1]

An algorithm summarizing diagnosis of hypothyroidism and indications for therapy is shown in Figs. 34.1 and 34.2.

Environmental Toxins and Endocrine Disruptors

Multiple factors such as a low-salt/low seafood diet; high goitrogen consumption; exposure to chlorine, bromine, fluoride, mercury, perchlorate, and certain medications; and heavy metal toxicity can negatively influence the

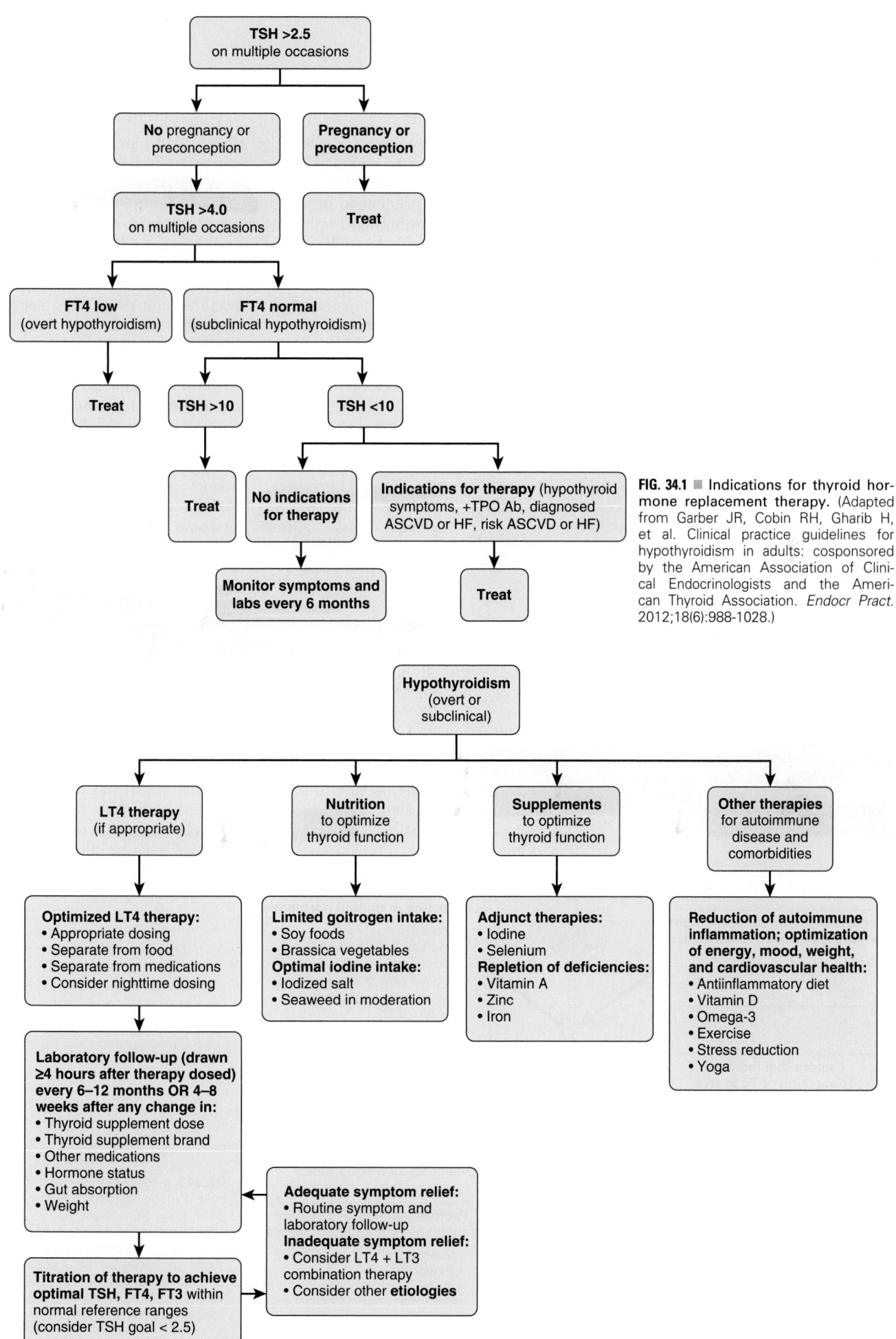

FIG. 34.1 ■ Indications for thyroid hormone replacement therapy. (Adapted from Garber JR, Cobin RH, Gharib H, et al. Clinical practice guidelines for hypothyroidism in adults: cosponsored by the American Association of Clinical Endocrinologists and the American Thyroid Association. *Endocr Pract.* 2012;18(6):988-1028.)

FIG. 34.2 ■ Hypothyroidism Treatment Algorithm.

iodination steps necessary for thyroid hormone production.[14] Functional laboratory testing can further elucidate toxic environmental exposures, including heavy metal testing, food sensitivities, and chemical residues that may interfere with thyroid hormone production. Testing and treatment for these conditions vary and may require further training for the clinician or referral to an experienced clinician.

INTEGRATIVE THERAPY (FIG. 34.3)

Tenets of an integrative, functional medicine approach for improving thyroid health:[14]

- Reduce chronic stress from physical, emotional, nutritional, and environmental sources that can promote a dysfunctional immune system, particularly in patients with positive antithyroid antibodies.
- Provide nutrients that are needed for adequate T4 manufacture, proper T4 to T3 conversion, and optimal T3-binding activity to intracellular receptors.
- Exercise and follow a heart-healthy nutrition program to increase energy and maintain weight (or at least stop gaining weight).
- Use appropriate testing, monitoring, and medications to treat hypothyroidism.

Exercise

Along with a heart-healthy, antiinflammatory nutrition plan, exercise is absolutely critical for hypothyroid patients to maintain healthy weight (or stop gaining weight), elevate mood, modify cardiac risk, and increase bone density, especially in the face of a decreased metabolic rate (see Chapter 91).

Nutrition

Diet

Optimization of endogenous thyroid function is important to compensate for inadequacies of exogenous LT4 therapy. In the setting of autoimmune hypothyroidism, it is prudent to pursue an antiinflammatory diet to reduce autoimmune inflammation and optimize cardiovascular health (see Chapter 88). At present, studies are lacking to determine the efficacy of an antiinflammatory dietary pattern on the course of hypothyroidism. Studies thus far have demonstrated that specific elimination diets, such as a gluten-free diet or lactose-free diet, do not change the natural history of autoimmune hypothyroidism, even in individuals with known sensitivities to specific dietary components. However, a 1-month elimination–rechallenge trial of these diets may be safe and helpful in ameliorating gastrointestinal symptoms and possibly others in the hypothyroid individual.[1,15,16]

Brassica Vegetables. Patients should avoid eating abnormally high levels of Brassica vegetables (e.g., cabbage, turnips, Brussels sprouts, rutabagas, broccoli, cauliflower, bok choy). Millet, peaches, peanuts, pine nuts, strawberries, spinach, and cassava root have small levels of goitrogens as well. These foods are rich in dietary sulfhydryl and thiocyanate compounds that can adversely impact the iodination of thyroglobulin if consumed in high amounts, thus inhibiting the uptake of iodine by the thyroid gland.[17] An observational study of 37 healthy subjects looked at a high daily soybean intake of 30 grams or more over 1–3 months. The subjects had within normal range increases in TSH levels and more hypothyroid-like symptoms that normalized 1 month after soybean cessation.[18] There has been a case report of an 88-year-old woman who was in a coma because of severe myxedema, which was a result of consuming 2–3 pounds of raw bok choy daily for several months.[19] When eaten raw, Brassica vegetables release the

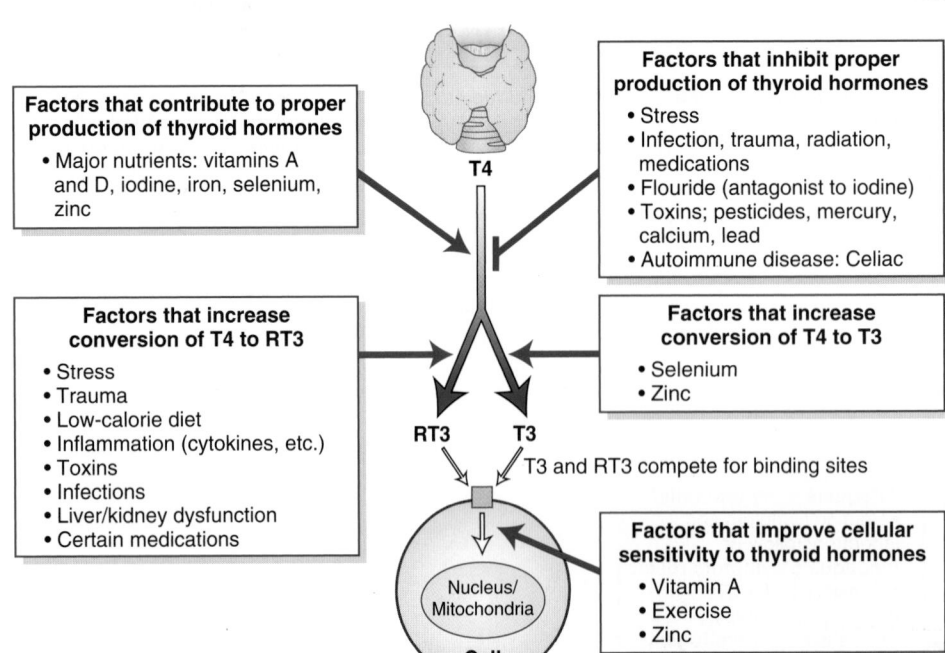

FIG. 34.3 ■ Factors that affect thyroid functions. (Reprinted with permission from Brand JS, Jones DS. Clinical approaches to hormonal and neuroendocrine imbalances. In: Jones DS, ed. *Textbook of functional medicine.* Gig Harbor WA: The Institute for Functional Medicine; 2006:593-604.)

enzyme myrosinase, which accelerates the hydrolysis of glucosinolates. Cooking mostly deactivates the myrosinase in these vegetables.[20] When eating a reasonable amount of soy and Brassica vegetables, steaming or cooking these foods briefly may help reduce their goitrogenic effect while preserving their nutrient content.[21,22]

> Steaming or cooking Brassica vegetables and soy briefly may help reduce the goitrogenic effect of myrosinase while preserving their nutrient content.

Soy. The overall evidence suggests that soy, particularly the isoflavone genistein, does not significantly alter thyroid function in iodine-replete, euthyroid patients. In vitro and in vivo studies account for a majority of the evidence for soy's goitrogenic effects.[23,24] In infants fed noniodine-fortified, soy-based formula, goitrogenic effects were seen, but the problem was easily solved with iodine repletion.[25] Soy isoflavones can aggravate hypothyroidism in iodine-deficient adults as well. Isoflavones are iodinated by thyroid peroxidase, which may be the mechanism for their competitive interference with thyroid hormone production.[26,27] Adequate supplementation of at least 150 mcg of iodine and 200 mcg of selenium may counteract this risk.

TABLE 34.1 Iodine Content of Selected Foods

Food	Content (mcg)
Salt, iodized, 1 teaspoon	400
Bread made with iodate dough conditioner and continuous mix process, 1 slice	142
Bread, made with regular process, 1 slice (most widely available)	35
Haddock, 3 oz	104–145
Shrimp, 3 oz	21–37
Egg, 1	18–26
Cottage cheese 2%, ½ cup	26–71
Cheddar cheese, 1 oz	5–23
Ground beef, 3 oz	8

Adapted from U.S. Department of Agriculture. *Composition of foods, USDA Handbook No. 8 Series.* Agricultural Research Service. Washington, DC; 1976-1986.

For adults on thyroid hormone replacement therapy who enjoy eating soy often or take daily soy supplements, the dosage of thyroid hormone may require more frequent surveillance and higher dosing. Ideally, soy foods and thyroid medication should be taken several hours apart.[28]

Supplements

Several minerals and trace elements are essential for proper thyroid function and metabolism. The clinician and patient should be wary of supplements marketed as thyroid supports given the risk for adulteration with T4 and T3 products.[29] The clinician should monitor hormone levels closely for patients on nutritional supplementation (whether adulterated or clean) because this can potentially reduce pharmaceutical thyroid hormone needs. Should the clinician recommend nutritional supplements, only manufacturers with regularly maintained certifications for Food and Drug Administration (FDA)–required current good manufacturing practices (cGMPs) should be recommended.

> **Iodine:** Too much or too little can cause hypothyroidism; too much iodine given too quickly in a hypothyroid patient can also cause hyperthyroidism. Iodine supplementation with kelp or iodine tablets may be recommended but only for short term after urine testing for iodine deficiency.

Iodine Deficiency

Underconsumption of iodine deprives the thyroid gland of manufacturing active thyroid hormones through the organification of iodine. Repleting with iodine is the treatment of choice for iodine deficiency, achieved with varying success in areas of the world by the iodination of refined salt. Iodine lost from salt is estimated to be 20% from production site to table, with another 20% lost during cooking.[30] Thus iodine should also come from sources such as fresh ocean fish, seaweed, and unrefined sea salt (Tables 34.1 and 34.2). Short-term iodine repletion with supplements is discussed in the following section for appropriate patients. A minimum of 150 mcg of iodine should be consumed on a daily basis (200 mcg for pregnant women and 290 mcg for lactating women).[31]

TABLE 34.2 Commonly Used Seaweed Preparations

Type of Seaweed	Common Use	Amount to Meet Minimum Iodine Dose of 150 mcg/day	Amount to Meet Maximum Iodine Dose of 1100 mcg/day
Nori	Sushi wrapper, rice balls	9 g/day	69 g/day
Wakame	Miso soup	2 g/day	17 g/day
Dulse	Seaweed chips, soups, sauces	2 g/day	15 g/day
Kelp/Kombu	Hot pot dishes, soups	9 mg/day	710 mg/day

Minimum and maximum daily iodine amounts are based on U.S./Japanese source values.
Adapted with permission: Teas J, Pine S, Critchley A, et al. Variability of iodine content in common commercially available seaweeds. *Thyroid.* 2004;14(10):839.

Iodine Testing

If a patient is suspected to have iodine deficiency because of dietary restrictions (e.g., seafood avoidance, low salt consumption), iron deficiency, medication use, or heavy metal toxicity, iodine testing may be useful. Since public health programs to iodize salt have occurred worldwide, it may be assumed that most individuals are iodine replete in targeted countries. However, cases of iodine deficiency have been identified in the United States, a country that has largely eradicated iodine deficiency. The **24-hour urine iodine test** (unprovoked) is the standard test for checking iodine status, although it is a cumbersome test for the patient.[32]

Some clinicians use the **iodine loading test**, a provoked measure of body iodine stores. The test consists of consuming 50 mg of an iodine/iodide combination followed by a 24-hour urine collection. A normal iodine loading test results if 90% or more iodine was excreted in the urine. If the test resulted in a 75% excretion rate, this would imply that the body needs more iodine.[33,34] If an iodine deficiency is noted from this test, some clinicians have used kelp tablets or iodine/iodide replacement (Lugol solution or Iodoral). Iodine supplementation should be recommended for short term only with iodine sources coming from food thereafter.

The **iodine skin patch test** is unreliable and should not be used in isolation for determining iodine status. The test consists of painting a 3 × 3 inch square of iodine tincture on the inner forearm or abdomen at bedtime. A normal body iodine level is supposedly diagnosed if the orange color of the patch takes longer than 24 hours to disappear. If the patch disappears in 10 hours or less, it implies a significant iodine deficiency. However, the iodine skin patch test fails to consider the differences in an individual's skin moisture, ambient temperature, and atmospheric pressure, all of which may affect iodine evaporation rate and patch color intensity in the skin.

> The 24-hour unprovoked urine iodine test is the standard test for checking iodine status, although a spot urine iodine test may still be useful and easier for the patient to perform.

Iodine Excess

The tolerable upper intake level (UL) for adults is 1100 mcg/day (1.1 mg/day).[35] The UL is the highest level of daily intake that is likely to pose no risk for adverse health effects to almost all individuals in the general population. Chronic overexposure to iodine reduces organic binding of iodine by the thyroid gland. A daily iodine intake of 10 times (>1500 mcg/day) the minimum daily adult requirement may cause iodine goiter in some people, especially in individuals with underlying thyroid abnormalities such as Hashimoto disease.[36-39]

Difficulty arises in determining the cumulative daily dose of iodine one is exposed to in food (i.e., kelp, seafood, food preservatives) and iodine-containing substances (i.e., medications, contaminated drinking water, topical antiseptics) over time.

Some practitioners believe in using iodine doses well above the tolerable UL to overcome measured deficiencies for hypothyroidism and even other conditions such as breast cancer.[40,41] The evidence based on this practice needs larger studies to address concerns with potential iodine excess from supplementation or overzealous consumption of iodine-rich foods such as seaweed.

Hence, iodine supplementation should be maintained at a safe level. Levels that are more than adequate (median urinary iodine excretion, 200–299 mcg/L) or excessive (median urinary iodine excretion, >300 mcg/L) may be unsafe, especially for susceptible persons with autoimmune thyroid diseases or iodine deficiency, where iodine repletion should be cautious and for short term with follow-up testing.[42]

Patients who are closely monitored with documented iodine deficiency should receive dietary or medical iodine replacement even if the dose exceeds the UL. The UL is not meant to be applied to individuals who are treated with the nutrient under medical supervision or to individuals with predisposing conditions that modify their sensitivity to the nutrient.[35] The best dosage and duration of oral iodine replacement varies with the individual patient. A dosing regimen is suggested in the following section.

The clinician must use caution in recommending high doses of iodine in a person with a low iodine state as this can temporarily trigger an iodine-induced hyperthyroidism (Jod-Basedow phenomenon) or an iodine-induced hypothyroidism state (Wolff-Chaikoff effect). Patients should be counseled to report side effects that are consistent with either a worsened hypothyroid state or conversely, a hyperthyroid state when taking iodine supplements or kelp tablets.

DAILY DOSAGE: DIETARY IODINE FOR THE GENERAL POPULATION

- Adult men: 150–1100 mcg
- Adult women: 150–1100 mcg
- Pregnant women: 220–1100 mcg
- Lactating women: 290–1100 mcg[31,35]
- Iodized salt equivalent: up to 2.75 teaspoons per day (based on 400 mcg of iodine per 1 teaspoon). Caution: not for individuals on low-sodium diets.

DAILY DOSAGE: IODINE TABLETS OR DROPS FOR DOCUMENTED IODINE DEFICIENCY:

- For documented iodine–deficient adults through a 24-hour urinary iodine test, monitor closely for iodine toxicity if prescribing oral iodine/iodide and use it for short term only. Iodine should then be replaced by food sources, and substances that deplete iodine stores should be avoided when possible. See Table 34.1 for selected foods high in iodine.
- **Lugol solution:** Two drops contain 5 mg iodine and 7.5 mg iodide as potassium iodide. Sig: Two drops po daily for 1–3 months, then retest.
- **Iodoral tablet:** Each 12.5 mg tablet contains a combination of 5 mg iodine and 7.5 mg iodide as potassium iodide.[43]
- **Sig:** ½–1 tablet po daily for 1–3 months, then retest.

PRECAUTIONS

Monitor for signs of iodine toxicity: brassy taste in the mouth, increased salivation, gastrointestinal upset, and acne. Chlorophyll tablets may ease the metallic taste side effect.[34]

TABLE 34.3   Selenium Content of Selected Foods

Food	Content (mcg)
Brazil nuts, unblanched, dried, 1 oz (6–8 nuts)	543
Halibut, Atlantic, or Pacific, ½ filet (159 g weight)	88
Pearled barley, raw, 1 cup	75
Wheat flour, whole grain, 1 cup	74
Lobster, 3 oz	62
Sardines, Atlantic 3 oz	45
Couscous, 1 cup	43

Adapted from U.S. Department of Agriculture, Agricultural Research Service. *USDA National Nutrient Database for Standard Reference, Release 23. Nutrient Data Laboratory.* Available at: http://www.ars.usda.gov/ba/bhnrc/ndl. Accessed 2010.

Selenium

Selenium is an essential trace element required for the deiodination of T4 to active T3 hormone.[40,41] At least 55 mcg per day of selenium is recommended for adults. Eating 4 raw brazil nuts per day provides approximately 300 mcg of selenium, which is within the tolerable UL. Table 34.3 shows high selenium containing foods.[44] Selenium supplementation may help normalize suboptimal T4 and T3 levels.[45]

A meta-analysis of 9 trials found evidence that selenium supplementation was associated with a significant decrease in TPO-antibody titers at 6 and 12 months. Thyroglobulin antibody titers decreased at 12 months. Selenium supplementation was also associated with improvement in mood or well-being compared with placebo. In other meta-analyses, however, the evidence has been mixed on whether selenium has positive or null effects on thyroid function or quality of life.[46-49]

DAILY DOSAGE: SELENIUM

- Adult men: 55–400 mcg
- Adult women: 55–400 mcg
- Pregnant women: 60–400 mcg
- Lactating women: 70–400 mcg[28,35]

PRECAUTIONS

The UL for adults is 400 mcg per day based on the risk for selenosis.[50,51] Excessive intake of selenium (selenosis) can cause discoloration of the skin, deformation and loss of nails, reversible baldness, excessive tooth decay and discoloration, garlic breath odor, weakness, lack of mental alertness, and listlessness.[52]

Vitamin A

Vitamin A is a fat-soluble vitamin obtained directly from animal sources (preformed vitamin A known as retinol) or synthesized from beta-carotene from plant sources. Beta-carotene is a provitamin A precursor that is converted to retinol in the gut. In persons with vitamin A and iodine deficiency from malnutrition, hypothyroidism risk can be reduced with vitamin A supplementation.[53] Vitamin A is involved in T4 manufacture and for intracellular receptor formation for T3.[54] In the United States, vitamin A deficiency is most often associated with excess alcohol intake and strict dietary restrictions. Vegetarians who avoid dairy and eggs should be able to meet their vitamin A requirements through beta-carotene by eating at least 5 servings of fruits and vegetables daily. At least 3–6 mg of beta-carotene daily (equivalent to 833–1667 IU of vitamin A) may maintain blood levels in the range associated with a lower risk for chronic diseases. The highest yielding sources of carotenoids are carrots, cantaloupes, sweet potatoes, and spinach. Most Americans consume enough retinol in milk, margarine, eggs, meat, liver, and fortified ready-to-eat cereals.[55]

DAILY DOSAGE: VITAMIN A (PREFORMED, RETINOL)

- 1 mcg retinol = 3.33 IU vitamin A (on a label) = 12 mg beta-carotene (from food)
- Adult men: 900–3000 mcg (≈ 3000–10,000 IU) preformed vitamin A
- Adult women: 700–3000 mcg (≈ 2300–10,000 IU) preformed vitamin A
- Pregnant women: 770–3000 mcg (≈ 2500–10,000 IU) preformed vitamin A
- Lactating women: 1300–3000 mcg (≈ 4300–10,000 IU) preformed vitamin A.[28,35]

PRECAUTIONS

Too much preformed vitamin A can lead to toxic symptoms, namely birth defects, liver abnormalities, reduced bone mineral density, and central nervous system disorders. There is no published UL for carotenoids.[35]

Zinc

Abnormal zinc metabolism has been linked to hypothyroidism.[56,57] Zinc participates in more than 300 enzymatic reactions, along with multiple functions in transport, immunity, metabolism, and cell structure. Zinc is involved in the conversion of T4 to T3 through the deiodinase enzyme and helps synthesize retinol-binding protein, which transports vitamin A to body tissues. Zinc is an important factor in T3 binding to intracellular receptors in the body. Severe zinc deficiency often accompanies vitamin A deficiency in malnutrition or severe dietary restriction. For most Americans, a majority of zinc in the diet comes from meat, fish, poultry, fortified breakfast cereals, dairy, oysters, liver, dry beans, ginger, soy, and nuts. Good protein intake correlates with zinc intake.[58] The UL for zinc is 40 mg/day for adults.[35]

In a randomized, double-blind, controlled trial, 68 female hypothyroid patients were randomized to one of four treatment groups receiving 30 mg zinc gluconate and 200 mcg selenium as high-selenium yeast, zinc-placebo, selenium-placebo, or placebo-placebo for 12 weeks. Mean serum FT3 levels rose significantly in the zinc-selenium and zinc-placebo groups ($p < .05$). Mean serum FT4 increased and TSH dropped significantly ($p < .05$) in the zinc-selenium group. Total T3 (TT3) and total T4 (TT4) decreased significantly in the selenium-placebo group ($p < .05$). Mean FT3:FT4 ratio increased significantly in the zinc-placebo group ($p <$

.05). Hence, the clinician should choose to optimize these and other micronutrients before adjusting thyroid medication doses if a deficiency is suspected.[59]

DAILY DOSAGE: ZINC

- Adult men: 11–40 mg
- Adult women: 8–40 mg
- Pregnant women: 11–40 mg
- Lactating women: 12–40 mg[31,35]

PRECAUTIONS

Doses greater than 40 mg/day can lead to copper deficiency and gastrointestinal irritation.

Iron

Iron deficiency impairs thyroid hormone synthesis by reducing the activity of thyroid peroxidase. In a deficient state, iron supplementation may improve the efficacy of iodine supplementation.[60] A trial conducted in an iodine-sufficient area in China demonstrated that nonpregnant and pregnant women in their first trimester who had iron deficiency experienced a dramatically increased risk for mild or severe hypothyroidism.[61] Animal sources provide the most potent iron content, with liver, seafood, organ meats, and poultry in descending order of potency. Vegetarian sources of iron are most potent in dried beans, iron-fortified cereal/bread, blackstrap molasses, spinach, peas, and dried apricots. Concomitant intake of vitamin C-rich food or as a supplement enhances the gastrointestinal absorption of iron. Lab evaluation should include serum ferritin which reflects the body's iron storage pool and is the carrier protein for iron.[58] The UL for iron is 45 mg/day for adults.[35]

DAILY DOSAGE: IRON

- Adult men and postmenopausal women: 8–45 mg/day
- Adult premenopausal women: 18–45 mg/day
- Pregnant women: 27–45 mg/day
- Lactating women: 9–45 mg/day[31,35]

PRECAUTIONS

Long-term overdose of iron can create an abnormal accumulation in the liver. Hemochromatosis may occur, causing tissue damage. Iron overload can also favor oxidation of LDL cholesterol and the generation of free radicals, which may also damage body tissues.[58]

Omega-3

Omega-3 fatty acids alter signal transduction via changes in cell membrane lipid composition; furthermore, they modulate gene transcription. Through these mechanisms, omega-3 fatty acids may alter TSH receptor activity, signal transduction, and thyroid hormone synthesis and release; omega-3 fatty acids may also affect thyroid follicular cell proliferation and differentiation. Studies are lacking to determine effects of omega-3 supplementation, plasma concentration, or erythrocyte cell membrane concentration on onset and progression of autoimmune hypothyroidism. One study did show less severe symptoms of hypothyroidism, more rapid response to LT4 therapy, significantly lower TSH, and significantly higher FT4 and FT3 in individuals with higher plasma free fatty acid concentrations compared with those with lower concentrations. A follow-up study demonstrated that administration of omega-3 fatty acids in the form of purified eicosapentaenoic acid (EPA) prevented hypothyroidism based on laboratory and histopathological parameters in rats that were given 1-methyl-2-imidazolethiol to induce hypothyroidism.[62] Further research in human subjects is necessary, but data are promising and warrant consideration of dietary or supplemental omega-3 fatty acids in individuals with autoimmune hypothyroidism. Furthermore, omega-3 fatty acids may also be considered for cardiovascular benefits given the correlation between hypothyroidism and cardiovascular morbidity.

DAILY DOSAGE: OMEGA-3

Adults: 1000 mg/day

Vitamin D

The vitamin D receptor and vitamin D activating enzyme are expressed by immune cells; vitamin D is thus able to regulate inflammatory cytokine production and inflammatory cell proliferation in a pattern that enhances innate immunity and inhibits autoimmune inflammation. Vitamin D deficiency plays a known role in the onset and progression of several autoimmune diseases. Some studies have shown higher incidence of vitamin D deficiency in individuals with autoimmune hypothyroidism and those with TPO antibodies; however, data are mixed, and several studies do not control for confounders. Furthermore, effects of vitamin D deficiency may be more pronounced in certain subgroups of individuals with specific vitamin D receptor polymorphisms. Efficacy of vitamin D supplementation in preventing onset or progression of autoimmune hypothyroidism has not yet been studied in humans, though rat models are promising. Given the potential role of vitamin D in autoimmune hypothyroidism and the many other known benefits of vitamin D optimization, it is prudent to ensure that vitamin D levels are at goal in individuals with autoimmune hypothyroidism and in those with TPO antibodies.[63,64]

DAILY DOSAGE: VITAMIN D

Adults: 400–4000 IU/day titrated to achieve serum 25(OH)D level of 30–50 ng/mL[65]

Probiotics

Hypothyroidism slows gut motility and therefore leads to symptoms of constipation, bloating, and flatulence. Furthermore, small intestinal bacterial overgrowth is also more prevalent in individuals with hypothyroidism.

Probiotic therapy and antibiotic decontamination may be considered to treat alterations in gut flora, as this has been found to reduce the aforementioned gastrointestinal symptoms. Such therapies have not been found to change thyroid function based on measurement of TSH and thyroid hormone levels, though this has not been adequately studied[66,67] (see Chapter 105).

Botanicals

Seaweed

Seaweed is a rich source of naturally occurring iodine and is a good source for meeting daily iodine requirements. It may aggravate thyroid conditions if too much is ingested, which is seen in Asian populations that regularly consume seaweed.

Seaweed iodine content varies by many factors, posing a challenge in terms of determining safe consumption levels. The part of seaweed used, cooking method, genus, geographic location, climate, and stage of growth, all play a role in seaweed's iodine content. Iodine content is lowest in certain genus of seaweed such as nori and dulse. Iodine is also lowest in seaweed harvested and dried on the beach or free-floating in bunches. Iodine level can be reduced by boiling seaweed for 15 minutes and discarding the water. Iodine content is highest if the seaweed is harvested from young plants, stored in water- and air-tight containers, and eaten roasted rather than boiled.[68] Exercise caution in patients on blood thinners taking bladderwrack, an edible brown kelp, which may have some anticoagulant activity.[69] Depending on local pollution levels, edible seaweeds may contain heavy metals such as arsenic and cadmium. Hence, selection of high-quality kelp and seaweed from reputable harvesters is ideal to reduce the risk for toxic ingestion.[70] Table 34.2 outlines commonly used seaweed preparations and iodine content based on US and Japanese source values.[68] There has been recent concern about nuclear fallout affecting seaweed harvested in Japan after the Fukushima Daiichi nuclear disaster in March 2011. Measurements of radioactive isotopes in water, bottom sediment, and marine organisms returned to pre-Fukushima background levels by 2–2.5 years after the disaster. Thus it appears safe to purchase seaweed harvested during or after 2014.[71-74]

Guggulu (Commiphora mukul)

Some animal studies have shown that the Ayurvedic herb guggulu, a gum resin of the *Commiphora mukul* tree, may stimulate thyroid function. It seems to increase T3 synthesis by increasing conversion of T4 to T3.[75-77] Asian studies have shown that guggulu may also improve the hyperlipidemia that often accompanies hypothyroidism.[78]

However, a double-blind, randomized control trial in the United States showed that hyperlipidemic patients on a standard Western diet who took a standardized dose of guggulu experienced a rise in LDL cholesterol levels compared with placebo. TSH levels were not significantly different after treatment with guggulu.[79]

It is important to consider the differences in medical traditions of Ayurvedic, Western medicine, and diet with respect to these differing results. More research is necessary to study the effects of guggulu in the context of a holistic Ayurvedic treatment plan versus its incorporation as a single ingredient in a conventional Western medicine regimen. Take great care in recommending Asian-source Ayurvedic herbs because some brands commonly found in the United States were found to have significant levels of lead, mercury, and arsenic.[80]

Pharmaceuticals

Approach to Thyroid Hormone Replacement Therapy (E-Table 34.4)

The goals of thyroid hormone replacement therapy include resolution of clinical signs and symptoms of hypothyroidism, normalization of labs, and avoidance of iatrogenic hyperthyroidism. Treatment based on symptoms alone is not accurate; symptoms lack sensitivity and specificity given the indolent nature of hypothyroidism and many other conditions that may cause similar symptoms. Monitoring of laboratory tests is therefore necessary with titration of therapy to achieve therapeutic ranges as discussed previously.[1]

The conventional therapy for thyroid hormone replacement in hypothyroidism remains LT4 alone.[81] The initial LT4 dose should be weight-based (1.6 mcg/kg/day); alternatively, the initial dose should be 50 mcg/day in patients older than 50 years or those with known cardiovascular disease. The half-life of LT4 is 7 days; thus, thyroid function testing should be pursued when steady-state concentrations are achieved about 4–8 weeks after initiation of therapy. Thyroid function testing should also be reassessed 4–8 weeks after adjustment in therapy as well as after treatment of malabsorptive disorders, significant changes in weight, or change in hormonal status (e.g., pregnancy, menopause, exogenous hormone therapy).[1]

The brand of LT4 therapy prescribed is an important consideration. As of 2007, the FDA requires all LT4 preparations to maintain doses within 95%–105% of stated potency. Given this permissible degree of variation, studies have shown lack of bioequivalence between similar doses of different LT4 formulations.[82,83] Patients should therefore be advised to maintain therapy on one specific brand name or one specific generic formulation. For patients who are given generic therapy, patients and providers must both be aware of the potential for pharmacies to switch from one generic formulation to another, which requires repeat dose titration.[1]

Preparation of levothyroxine sodium is now also a consideration. LT4 is conventionally available as a solid tablet. However, gelatin capsules for LT4 supplementation have recently become available under the brand name Tirosint; these capsules contain levothyroxine sodium as a liquid dissolved in glycerin and water. The gelatin capsule formulation excludes dyes and excipients (fillers), therefore conferring a lower risk for allergic reactions compared with standard LT4 tablets. If allergic reaction is a concern and cost prohibits switching to the gelatin capsule formulation, the practitioner may alternatively consider achieving the therapeutic dose by utilizing whole and half tabs of the 50 mcg solid tablet formulation, which does not contain dyes (though it still contains excipients). The gelatin capsule formulation may also have better absorption than standard solid tabs in individuals with reduced stomach acid or when taken alongside espresso coffee, though definitive studies are lacking. If malabsorption is a concern and cost prohibits switching to the gelatin capsule formulation, the practitioner may alternatively consider increasing the dose of the solid tablet formulation. Both approaches require follow-up thyroid function tests in 4–8 weeks.[1]

Optimal time for LT4 ingestion is controversial. Temporal relation to food and medication should be considered. LT4 absorption in the gut is inhibited by food, fiber, soy, espresso coffee, and several medications (e.g., ferrous sulfate, calcium carbonate, bile acid sequestrants, sucralfate, phosphate binders, aluminum-containing antacids). Thus, LT4 should be ingested on an empty stomach and separated from medications.[1] Time of day is also a consideration. Two small studies revealed statistically significant improvements in hourly measurements of thyroid function tests when LT4 was dosed in the evening instead of the morning. Circadian variation in all thyroid hormones was preserved; however, there was no significant difference in subjective symptoms between the two groups.[84,85] Thus evening administration of LT4 may be considered, but advantages are unclear. All in all, timing of LT4 dosage should be tailored around individual patient preferences with ingestion in the morning at least 1 hour before food or ingestion at night at least 3 hours after food; LT4 should be separated from other medications and supplements by at least 4 hours.[1]

Patients should be reminded to store LT4 per the instructions on the product insert at 68°F–77°F, protected from light and moisture.[13]

> Timing of LT4 dosage should be tailored around individual patient preferences. To optimize absorption, LT4 may be ingested in the morning at least 1 hour before food or at night at least 3 hours after food; LT4 should be separated from other medications and supplements by at least 4 hours.[1]

Excessive Thyroid Hormone Dose Requirements

Oral LT4 therapy is largely absorbed in the ileum. Celiac disease, *Helicobacter pylori* gastritis, atrophic gastritis, inflammatory bowel disease, lactose intolerance, intestinal giardiasis, and other malabsorptive disorders should be considered in patients who require unexpectedly high doses of LT4 (i.e., doses greater than 2 mcg/kg per day). These conditions are associated with poor LT4 absorption, and celiac disease and autoimmune atrophic gastritis are more prevalent in individuals with autoimmune thyroid disease. Appropriate treatment of the diagnosed malabsorptive disorder

tends to cause a reduction in LT4 dose requirements because of improved absorption in the gut, although such treatment (including gluten- or lactose-free diet) may not change the natural history of the hypothyroidism itself. Therefore when appropriate therapy is initiated for a malabsorptive disorder, thyroid function tests should be monitored and the LT4 dose should be adjusted accordingly. Of note, in patients with lactose intolerance, a lactose-free LT4 preparation should be considered.[1,5,16]

Inadequate Response to Thyroid Hormone Replacement Therapy

Several studies have shown that LT4 supplementation may achieve normal TSH levels without achieving normal FT3 levels or resolution of hypothyroid symptoms. As previously mentioned, it must be kept in mind that the physiologically optimal FT3 range is uncertain and that the differential diagnosis for hypothyroid symptoms is broad. That being said, several etiologies have been proposed for low FT3 levels and persistent hypothyroid symptoms despite normal TSH.

Adequate thyroid hormone production and symptom resolution requires an intact hypothalamic pituitary thyroid axis. This includes intact hypothalamic production of TRH and pituitary production of TSH. This also includes intact thyroid gland production of T4 and 20% of the body's T3; this endogenous thyroid function is particularly important to compensate for inadequacies of exogenous LT4 therapy, which may not yield adequate FT3 levels or replicate circadian thyroid hormone patterns. Finally, this axis also includes intact peripheral conversion of T4 to produce the remaining 80% of the body's T3.

Perturbations at any level of the hypothalamic pituitary thyroid axis may lead to inadequate FT3 levels and persistent hypothyroid symptoms. At the level of the central nervous system, it has been proposed that LT4 therapy inhibits the hypothalamic release of TRH and pituitary release of TSH via negative feedback, therefore suppressing any remaining endogenous thyroid function. At the level of the thyroid gland, it is known that athyreotic individuals do not have any endogenous production of T4 or T3 to compensate for inadequacies of LT4 therapy. At the level of peripheral organs, T4 transporter mutations may compromise T4 movement into cells, thus preventing peripheral conversion of T4 into T3. Finally, at the level of thyroid hormone clearance, it has been proposed that LT4 therapy upregulates D3, which clears T4 and T3 by catalyzing conversion of T4 to rT3 and T3 to T2. Unfortunately, assays to measure transporter function, intracellular T4, and deiodinase function are not yet available.[1]

Some clinicians check the rT3 level, which is believed to be metabolically inactive. Elevated rT3 levels may improve with resolution of the underlying trauma, stress, infection, or malnutritive factors that promoted its formation. In addition to elevated rT3 levels, sick individuals may also have a low-normal TSH, low T4, and low T3. This euthyroid-sick syndrome is thought to be a compensatory mechanism to prevent excessive tissue catabolism during severe illness, unlike the above-mentioned pathological perturbations. Many mechanisms contribute, including ectopic T3 production with negative feedback, central hypothyroidism with low TSH production, reduced thyroid hormone–binding proteins, and increased D3 activity. Adding zinc and selenium to nutritional supplementation or in the diet may help improve a high rT3 level.[48,86] In a study of athyreotic patients versus euthyroid controls, the average FT3 to FT4 ratio was 0.32 in those with normal thyroid function.[87] Setting a treatment target for thyroid hormone replacement based on FT3 to FT4 ratio is not well-established but may provide partial guidance in dosing and overall treatment.

In complex cases, the clinician should consider RTH syndrome, which is characterized by low FT4 to FT3 ratios, low rT3, constipation, growth retardation, and skeletal dysplasia, with referral to an endocrinologist.[88]

In general, thyroid function should not be assessed, and thyroid replacement therapy should not be initiated during severe illness unless thyroid dysfunction is highly suspected.[1]

LT4 + LT3 Combination Thyroid Hormone Replacement Therapy

The use of combination LT4 plus liothyronine (LT3) therapy instead of LT4 alone has been controversial.[89-93] Thus far, data are limited and inconclusive on efficacy and safety of combination therapy. Existing studies have utilized a variety of dosing regimens that do not closely replicate physiological T4:T3 ratios. Furthermore, they have not sufficiently studied specific population subgroups, such as athyreotic individuals. Finally, symptomatic relief has been noted in only a few studies and might be attributed, at least in part, to placebo effect in patients who seek combination therapy.[2]

In patients who achieve normal TSH levels without achieving resolution of hypothyroid symptoms, combination therapy may be considered. The ATA and European Thyroid Association (ETA) guidelines recommend that "LT4 and LT3 combination therapy might be considered as an experimental approach in compliant LT4–treated hypothyroid patients who have persistent complaints despite serum TSH values in the reference range, provided they have previously been given support to deal with the chronic nature of their disease and associated autoimmune diseases have been ruled out." It should be noted that combination therapy is not appropriate in pregnancy, during which exclusive T4 supplementation is crucial for fetal brain development.[2]

Combination therapy regimens should attempt to replicate human physiology, including a T4:T3 ratio of 14:1 and a circadian peak T3 level at 3 a.m. Combination therapy should also account for pharmacokinetics of LT4 and LT3; the half-life of LT4 is 7 days, whereas that of LT3 is much shorter at 1 day; FT4 peaks 4–6 hours after LT4 ingestion and FT3 peaks 2–4 hours after LT3 ingestion. Thus, in accordance with ETA

guidelines, if combination LT4 and LT3 therapy is initiated, the total LT4 plus LT3 dose should be equal to the weight-based starting dose that one would use for isolated LT4 therapy, as described previously (1.6 mcg/kg per day or 50 mcg/day if age is more than 50 years or known cardiovascular disease). The T4:T3 dose ratio should be between 13:1 and 20:1. The LT4 dose should be given once daily; the LT3 dose should be divided into two doses daily (bedtime and morning). If available formulations result in unequal doses when the total LT3 dose is divided, the larger of the two doses should be given at bedtime.[1,2]

To achieve the abovementioned therapeutic regimen, combination therapy is best given as isolated LT4 alongside isolated LT3, each of which can be titrated separately to achieve laboratory endpoints. Isolated LT3 is commercially available as a generic formulation and as a brand name formulation (Cytomel). Combination therapy can also be achieved with use of reliable compounding pharmacies. Proponents of combination therapy have also promoted use of sustained release combination products or desiccated porcine thyroid (e.g., Armour [Forest Pharmaceuticals], Nature-Thyroid [RLC Labs], WP Thyroid [RLC Labs]) containing natural T3 and T4 plus other iodinated compounds.[9,92,93] It should be noted that available synthetic and natural preformulated combination preparations do not provide the aforementioned physiological ratios of T4 and T3. For example, the concentration of T4:T3 in desiccated porcine thyroid is 4.2:1, which yields supraphysiological levels of T3 when ingested by humans.[1,2]

During combination therapy, there is a concern for transient thyrotoxicosis 2–4 hours after the LT3-containing supplement is ingested. Therefore it is prudent to check thyroid function first thing in the morning (after ingestion of the nighttime LT3 dose and prior to ingestion of the morning LT3 dose) to ensure that FT4 and FT3 levels are never outside of laboratory reference ranges, even at their peak. TSH should always be maintained within normal range.

Patients should be counseled about the paucity of conclusive data regarding safety, symptomatic relief, and physiological benefit from combination therapy. They should be counseled about short-term and long-term risks for supratherapeutic thyroid supplementation; they should also be instructed to monitor for symptoms of hyperthyroidism during combination therapy. Finally, patients should be informed that if they do not experience relief of hypothyroid symptoms, or if they do experience hyperthyroid symptoms during the trial of combination therapy, then LT4 monotherapy should be resumed.[2]

> A trial of combination LT4 plus LT3 therapy may be considered in LT4-compliant patients who achieve normal TSH levels without resolution of hypothyroid symptoms. TSH, FT4, and FT3 should always be maintained within normal reference ranges. Other conditions that may contribute to hypothyroid symptoms should be ruled out.

THYROID (T4) HORMONE DOSAGE

Most patients should be treated with LT4 alone. The dose should be weight based (1.6 mcg/kg per day); alternatively, the initial dose should be 50 mcg/day in patients older than 50 years or those with known cardiovascular disease.

Gel formulations *(Tirosint)* may be better absorbed and tolerated in sensitive patients as it is void of dyes and fillers.

COMBINATION THERAPY (T4 + T3) DOSAGE:

Porcine thyroid hormone (e.g., Armour, Nature-Throid, Westhroid) is an older medication used in hypothyroidism.

Desiccated porcine thyroid contains approximately 80% T4 and 20% T3 (4:1 ratio), as well as other iodinated compounds, diiodotyrosine (T2) and monoiodotyrosine (T1), which may play a role in providing additional relief of symptoms.[94,95] Given the short half-life of T3, the total daily dose may be divided into two doses daily (bedtime and morning).

Ideally, the clinician would use T4 (levothyroxine) daily with the addition of T3 *(Cytomel)* dosed twice daily at a ratio of 10–14:1 (T4:T3). So if the patient is on 110 mcg total thyroid, they would be dosed 100 mcg of T4 at night and 5 mg of T3 in morning and 5 mg T3 at night.

PRECAUTIONS

Vegetarians, vegans, and patients who avoid pork because of allergies, religious, or other reasons should be informed of the source of this hormone. Close monitoring of symptoms and thyroid function tests are very important when caring for patients who are taking porcine thyroid replacement; tests should ideally be drawn several hours after ingestion of therapy with the goal of keeping TSH, FT4, and FT3 within normal reference ranges. The T4:T3 ratio in these preparations is 4.2:1 compared with the physiological serum ratio of 14:1; patients should be counseled about the potential risks associated with supraphysiological levels of T3. Recommended thyroid hormone dosages are shown in E-Table 34.4.

---

1 grain (60 mg) desiccated porcine thyroid = 100 mcg T4 and 25 mcg T3.

Therapies to Consider

Traditional Chinese Medicine

In the traditional Chinese medicine (TCM) system, the diagnosis and treatment of individuals with a conventional medicine diagnosis of hypothyroidism depends on the history, tongue, and pulse diagnosis. Hypothyroidism is generally considered to be a deficiency of spleen and/or kidney "yang" energy, especially if characterized by cold sensation, lack of appetite, fatigue, and weight gain. Weight gain is the evidence of "dampness," which is a complication of spleen or kidney yang deficiency. The spleen and kidney are considered too weak to transform excess dampness, causing accumulation of fat and swelling. It is important to appreciate that these findings are classic and may not adequately describe an individual's complete Chinese medicine diagnosis.[96]

Herbal treatment in hypothyroidism aims to strengthen qi and yang deficiency. Qi and yang tonics may include codonopsis, astragalus, epimedium, curculigo, cinnamon bark, and cuscuta, to name a few.[97]

TCM therapies include acupuncture, herbs, moxibustion, nutrition, massage, and movement. The therapeutic

effect of these therapies on hypothyroidism may result from promotion of T4 deiodination with production of more active T3.[98-101] Research in this area is necessary to more fully understand TCM's mechanisms of action in the treatment of thyroid disease.

Stress Reduction

Stress is known to contribute to centrally driven hypoactivation of peripheral glands; furthermore, it is known to contribute to primary gland dysfunction in the setting of autoimmune disease.[102] However, several studies have failed to find an association between psychosocial stress and onset of autoimmune hypothyroidism or emergence of TPO antibodies. Although stress was not found to cause hypothyroidism, hypothyroidism was found to cause stress. This is because of the secondary depressive symptoms, fatigue, and the diagnosis of a chronic disease. Practitioners should screen patients with hypothyroidism for psychological symptoms; moreover, they should provide education about expected symptoms and the natural history of hypothyroidism. Despite current lack of evidence, stress reduction may be advised to optimize hypothalamic–pituitary–thyroid axis function and to help address comorbid psychological symptoms[103-105] (see Chapter 94).

Yoga

One study has demonstrated increased thyroid gland release of thyroid hormones after Yoga therapy in euthyroid men.[106] Another study demonstrated improvement in quality of life scores across physical, psychological, and social parameters after Yoga therapy in hypothyroid women.[107] Both studies involved 1-hour daily Yoga sessions for one month, including specific asanas (stretches and poses) and pranayama (breath practice). Each study included a pose that imparted pressure onto the thyroid gland, including sarvāngāsana (shoulder stand, as demonstrated in Fig. 34.4) and jalandhara bandha (sitting position with chin tucked into throat, as demonstrated in Fig. 34.5), respectively. Of note, contraindications to such poses include spinal osteoarthritis, cervical disk disease, neck injury, hypertension, glaucoma, stroke, and vertebrobasilar syndrome. Inversion poses like the shoulder stand should be avoided in women while menstruating and after the first trimester of pregnancy in accordance with yogic texts.[108-109]

The aforementioned poses may stimulate thyroid gland function via increased perfusion because of the locked position of the chin. Other potential mechanisms for the benefits of yoga may include rebalancing of neurotransmitters, shifting towards parasympathetic state, and promotion of mastery over the mind, body, and emotional self. Further research is needed to identify which specific yogic practices are most efficacious for hypothyroid symptoms and which subpopulations may benefit most. Autonomic balance promoted by yoga may also address the increased sympathetic tone and cardiovascular risk associated with hypothyroidism, though this area also requires future research.[110-111] It is reasonable for practitioners to recommend a trial of yoga therapy to those patients who are interested in this.

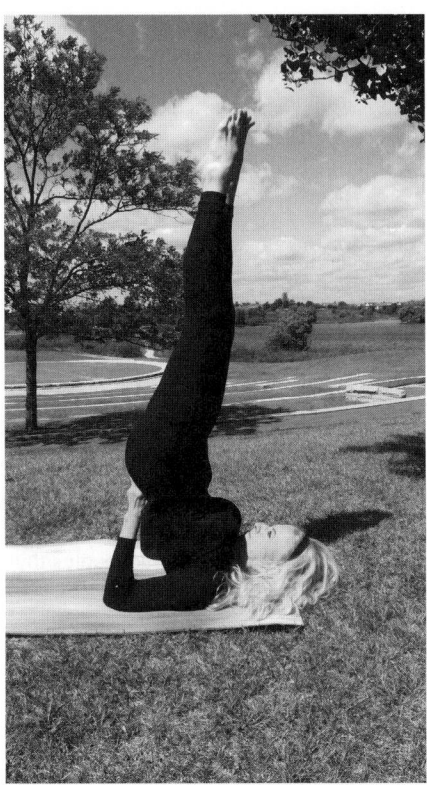

FIG. 34.4 ■ Sarvāngāsana (shoulder stand).

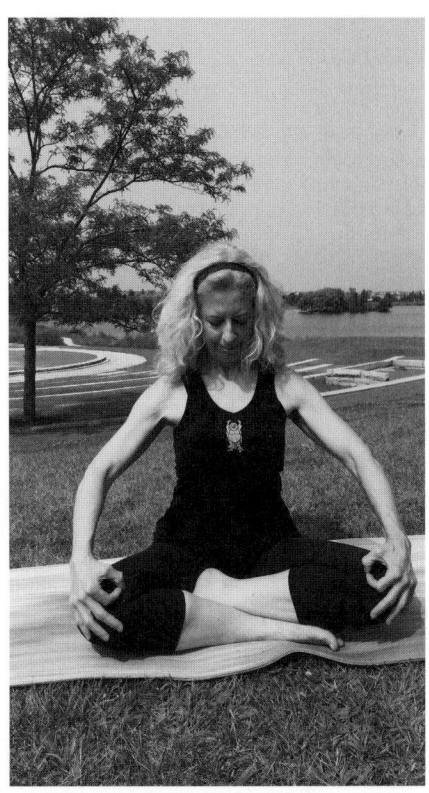

FIG. 34.5 ■ Jalandhara bandha (sitting position with chin tucked into throat).

PREVENTION PRESCRIPTION

- Consume a diet with adequate amounts of iodine, selenium, iron, vitamin A, vitamin D, and zinc.
- Do not consume excessive amounts of iodine for long periods of time.

- Avoid substances that block thyroid hormone synthesis, such as chlorine, bromine, perchlorate, mercury, certain medications, and radiation to the head and neck area when possible

THERAPEUTIC REVIEW

Following is a summary of therapeutic options for hypothyroidism.

EXERCISE

- Maintain a regular aerobic and weight-bearing exercise routine.

NUTRITION

- Separate and avoid excessive amounts of goitrogenic foods and substances which may interfere with thyroid activity.

  Vegetables from the *Brassica* family (cabbage, turnips, Brussels sprouts, rutabagas, broccoli, cauliflower, bok choy); millet, peaches, peanuts, pine nuts, strawberries, spinach, and cassava root. Cook vegetables briefly to reduce goitrogenic substances.

  Medications/Toxins: lithium, thionamides, amiodarone, interferon-α, interleukin (IL)-2, cholestyramine, perchlorate, expectorants, aluminum hydroxide, raloxifene; heavy metals, fluoride, bromine

  Topical antiseptics (betadine), radiocontrast dyes

- Eat a heart-healthy, antiinflammatory diet to maintain proper body weight and reduce cardiovascular risk.

VITAMINS AND MINERALS (PREFERABLY CONSUMED IN FOOD)

- Iodine*: 150–1100 mcg/day
- Iron: 8–45 mg/day
- Selenium: 55–400 mcg/day
- Vitamin A**: 2300–10,000 IU/day
- Zinc: 8–40 mg/day
- Vitamin D: 1000–2000 IU/day

BOTANICALS

- Seaweed: total iodine content should not exceed 1100 mcg/day for the general population unless on targeted megadose therapy. See Table 34.2 for assistance in determining allowable grams/day depending on the variety of seaweed.
- Guggulu: consider using in the context of an Ayurvedic treatment regimen and not as an isolated treatment for hypothyroidism or hyperlipidemia. Take care to avoid heavy metal toxicity in certain Asian-sourced formulations.

PHARMACEUTICALS

- Levothyroxine alone (T4): gold standard of therapy
- Synthetic combination T3 + T4: consider if T4 alone fails to control symptoms adequately; may use compounded formulations
- Desiccated porcine thyroid: consider if synthetic or compounded T3 + T4 fails to control symptoms adequately or based on patient preference/physician experience

TRADITIONAL CHINESE MEDICINE (TCM)

- Qi and yang tonics: includes codonopsis, astragalus, epimedium, curculigo, cinnamon bark, and cuscuta.

A TCM practitioner with a strong background and certification in Chinese herbal medicine should prescribe these combinations.

YOGA

- Advise yoga therapy with emphasis on thyroid-enhancing poses like the shoulder stand (Sarvāngāsana) or jalandhara bandha poses if the patient has no contraindications.

  Yoga practice may still be helpful even without challenging poses like the shoulder stand for the purposes of stress reduction, meditation, enhanced flexibility, and strength.

Key Web Resources

The U.S. National Library of Medicine and the National Institutes of Health provides patient information for the conventional diagnosis and treatment of thyroid disease.	http://www.nlm.nih.gov/medlineplus/thyroiddiseases.html
The American Thyroid Association provides patients and physicians with guidelines for the conventional diagnosis and treatment of thyroid disease.	http://www.thyroid.org
This patient advocate website provides a forum for patients to discuss integrative therapies for managing thyroid disease through novel testing, nutrition, supplements, and alternative thyroid medication use.	http://www.thyroid.about.com

REFERENCES

References are available online at ExpertConsult.com.

CHAPTER 35

POLYCYSTIC OVARIAN SYNDROME

Melinda Ring, MD

Polycystic ovarian syndrome (PCOS) is the most common female endocrine disorder, affecting 10% of women of reproductive age, yet it is frequently overlooked.[1,2] PCOS affects young women and is associated with oligo-ovulation (which leads to oligomenorrhea in more than 75% of affected patients), infertility, acne, and hirsutism. It also has notable metabolic sequelae, including an elevated risk of diabetes and cardiovascular disease, and attention to these factors is important.[3] The heterogeneous nature of PCOS and the diversity of presentations requires a symptom-based approach to treatment because PCOS manifests differently depending on many interacting factors, including environmental exposures, genetics, and lifestyle (Fig. 35.1). This chapter discusses the pathophysiology and integrative approaches to treatment of women with PCOS.

PATHOPHYSIOLOGY

When PCOS was first described (as Stein-Leventhal syndrome) in the 1930s, the presence of cysts in the ovaries was believed to be a defining factor in the origin of the syndrome.[4] Since then, research has shown that, in fact, cysts are only one potential expression of what begins as a disorder of the endocrine system. On pelvic ultrasound, 90% of women with biochemical features of PCOS will have characteristic changes; however, 20% to 30% of women without hormonal disturbance due to PCOS will have similar ultrasound features.[5] Our current understanding, albeit incomplete, is the phenotypic expression of PCOS results from primary hormone imbalances. The three prevalent theories for the pathogenesis of PCOS are as follows:

1. Hypothalamic–pituitary dysfunction results in gonadotropin-releasing hormone and luteinizing hormone dysfunction, which then has downstream effects on ovarian hormone production.
2. A primary ovarian defect (with or without an adrenal defect) in steroidogenesis results in hyperandrogenism.
3. A metabolic disorder characterized by peripheral insulin resistance exerts adverse effects on the hypothalamus, pituitary, ovaries, and, possibly, the adrenal gland.

A number of variables, including genetic factors and lifestyle choices, contribute to the wide range of manifested symptoms of PCOS and make the diagnosis challenging unless clinicians are aware of PCOS as a potential cause. A typically chronic time course assists in diagnosis, with symptoms often developing in adolescence and advancing over time. However, this pattern may be disrupted by lifestyle factors, including weight loss impacting on frequency of ovulation, and contraceptive hormones masking symptoms, thereby complicating the diagnosis.[6]

Criteria for PCOS have been debated among leading organizations since 1990. The differences in criteria reflect the controversy over the origin of the syndrome, as well as its heterogeneous manifestations (Table 35.1).[7,8,8a] However, current diagnostic criteria have unifying trends. All require the presence of at least one of the stigmata of ovarian disease; a history of anovulation or the finding of classic polycystic ovaries on ultrasound. All three criteria are consistent in terms of the inclusion of hyperandrogenism, determined by either clinical (hirsutism or acne) or laboratory findings. Finally, all guidelines require exclusion of hormonal disorders that may mimic PCOS. Although insulin resistance has been noted consistently among women with PCOS, it is not included in any of the current diagnostic criteria.

Based on current data, evaluation for PCOS should include a search for both primary markers and secondary dysfunction. History and physical examination should focus on symptoms and signs, such as oligomenorrhea, acne, hirsutism, and central obesity, as well as searching for manifestations of other confounding diseases. Laboratory tests should include androgen levels (dehydroepiandrosterone [DHEA] sulfate and total and free testosterone measured by equilibrium dialysis) and tests to rule out alternative diagnoses as warranted (e.g., congenital adrenal hyperplasia, androgen-secreting tumors, Cushing syndrome, 21-hydroxylase–deficient nonclassic adrenal hyperplasia, androgenic or anabolic drug use or abuse, syndromes of severe insulin resistance, thyroid dysfunction, or hyperprolactinemia). Laboratory testing for antimüllerian hormone is a newer diagnostic tool that, in combination with measurement of luteinizing hormone levels, has been shown to have high sensitivity and specificity for the diagnosis of PCOS. Polycystic ovaries contain an increased amount of antral follicles, which produce antimüllerian hormone.[8b]

The ratio of total testosterone to dihydrotestosterone (TT/DHT) has demonstrated potential as a new biomarker for an adverse metabolic phenotype in PCOS patients. A study of 275 premenopausal PCOS patients and 35 BMI-matched, healthy controls found a correlation between a high TT/DHT ratio and various adverse hormonal, lipid, and glucose metabolism parameters in patients with PCOS.[8c]

The presence of metabolic syndrome and cardiovascular risk should also be evaluated in patients suspected to have PCOS (e.g., insulin resistance measurement by oral glucose tolerance tests, including glucose and

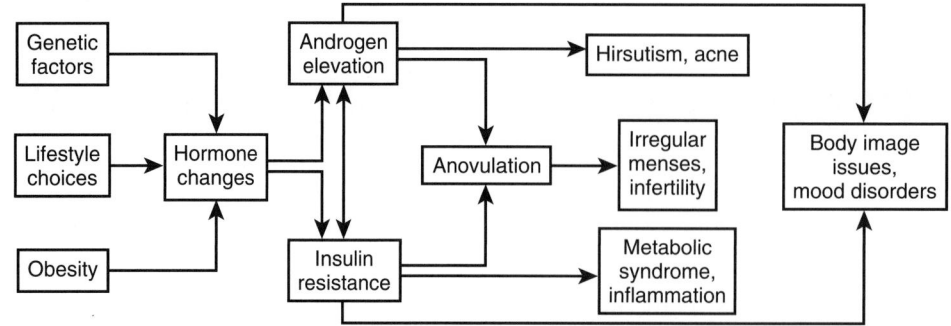

FIG. 35.1 ■ Proposed relationships leading to phenotypic expression of polycystic ovarian syndrome.

TABLE 35.1	Differing Criteria for Polycystic Ovarian Syndrome Among Organizations			
Organization	Criteria	Ovarian Dysfunction	Ovarian Morphology	Hyperandrogenism
National Institutes of Health (1990)[6]	Both of the following and exclusion of related disorders	Oligo-ovulation (less than six menses per year)		Clinical or biochemical (not specified)
Rotterdam Group (2003)[7]	Any two of three of the following and exclusion of related disorders	Oligo-anovulation (nonspecified)	Polycystic ovaries (>12 follicles 2 to 9 mm, or ovarian volume >10 mL)	Clinical or biochemical (free testosterone or free testosterone index)
Androgen Excess Society (2006)[8]	Hyperandrogenism as critical, with addition of at least one ovarian marker and exclusion of related disorders	Oligo-anovulation and/ or polycystic ovaries	Oligo-anovulation and/ or polycystic ovaries	Clinical or biochemical (free testosterone)

insulin levels, and measurement of lipids and inflammatory markers such as C-reactive protein and fibrinogen). Pelvic ultrasound also has utility in supporting the diagnosis of PCOS.

A thorough clinical assessment is critical both to confirm the diagnosis and to identify risk factors for long-term health maintenance. This information helps clinicians prioritize integrative approaches when creating a management plan by elucidating the primary metabolic targets. Treatment plans should take into equal consideration each woman's unique concerns, such as weight management, acne, hair loss, or infertility.

INTEGRATIVE THERAPY

A holistic approach to PCOS addresses the impact of the syndrome on patient mental state and sense of self in addition to immediate symptoms and risk management.

Lifestyle

Weight Management

Weight management plays a central role in the expression of symptoms and long-term consequences of PCOS. A reported 50% to 70% of women with PCOS are obese and should be informed that even 5% to 10% loss of body mass is associated with significant improvements

in clinical metabolic and hormonal markers.[9-11] Guiding women in this arena can be challenging because insulin resistance may inherently make weight loss more difficult, and women are often frustrated by repeated failed attempts to lose weight. Current evidence suggests that the approaches described in the next sections may be most successful.

Physical Activity

Exercise is an important lifestyle approach in PCOS, with diverse benefits including improved insulin sensitivity and preservation of lean body mass. A significant relationship exists between PCOS and inappropriate diet and low physical activity.[11] A 2010 systematic review of exercise therapy in PCOS identified eight studies (five randomized controlled and three cohort) involving moderate intensity physical activity (aerobic and/or resistance) for 12 to 24 weeks.[12] The most consistent reported improvements included improved ovulation, reduced insulin resistance (9% to 30%), and weight loss (4.5% to 10%). Because the optimal exercise regimen for PCOS has yet to be defined, current recommendations for interval training and full-body exercise should be used (see Chapter 91).

A study published in *Human Reproduction* compared the effects of exercise versus a low-calorie diet in 40 women with PCOS.[13] The exercise group had higher ovulation rates, better insulin sensitivity, and greater reduction in waist measurements despite less absolute weight loss.

Nutrition

Macronutrients

Although caloric restriction is clearly required for weight loss, to date only a few, small studies have examined the impact of macronutrient composition in PCOS. Several studies ranging from 1 to 6 months that compared a high-protein and low-carbohydrate diet with a high-carbohydrate and low-protein diet have reported no significant differences in weight loss, circulating androgens, glucose metabolism, or leptin levels.[14,15] Conversely, two pilot studies reported that low-carbohydrate diets were associated with improved depression scores and self-esteem ratings, in addition to lower fasting insulin levels and lower rates of acute insulin response to glucose.[16,17] None of these studies took into account the glycemic index of carbohydrates or the source of protein (animal versus plant based), which may be important factors in insulin resistance and hormone regulation. In 2010, the first study examining the impact of glycemic index in overweight and obese premenopausal women with PCOS (n = 96) randomized women to either an ad libitum low-glycemic index diet or a macronutrient-matched healthy diet and followed the women for 12 months or until they achieved a 7% weight loss. The attrition rate was high in both groups (49%). Of the women who completed the study, those on the low–glycemic index diet demonstrated greater improvements in insulin resistance (p = 0.03), menstrual cyclicity (95% compared with 63%; p = 0.03), and serum fibrinogen concentrations (p < 0.05).

A randomized controlled clinical trial of 48 women diagnosed with PCOS found that following the DASH (Dietary Approaches to Stop Hypertension) diet for 8 weeks led to a significant reduction in serum insulin, triglycerides, and very-low-density lipoprotein cholesterol levels, and significant increases in plasma total antioxidant capacity (TAC) and total glutathione (GSH). The diet in this study consisted of 52% carbohydrates, 18% proteins, and 30% total fats.[17a] At this point, no firm recommendations can be given regarding macronutrient content, although trends indicate women may do best on a low-carbohydrate diet with inclusion of low–glycemic index, high-fiber carbohydrates (see Chapter 87).

Soy

Soy intake in PCOS is a controversial topic. Soy is a plant food and complete protein, meaning that it has all the required amino acids. Soy is also low in fat and contains essential fatty acids, numerous vitamins, minerals, and fiber. Foods containing soy include soy milk and cheese, tofu, tempeh, miso, soy sauce, and edamame. Soy contains phytoestrogens, which has led to debate regarding the benefits versus risks of soy consumption in PCOS.

Currently, very few studies have evaluated soy intake in patients with PCOS. One study reported favorable results regarding the utility of soy in improving cholesterol among patients with PCOS.[18] In this study, 12 obese women with PCOS and high insulin and high cholesterol levels consumed 36 g of soy each day for 6 months. The results demonstrated reduced low-density lipoprotein cholesterol levels following the consumption

of soy. However, the investigators noted no effect on weight loss, hormones, or menstrual cycle. Conversely, many animal studies have demonstrated that soy intake can negatively affect fertility. A review of seven soy intervention studies performed in women using 32 to 200 mg/day of isoflavones demonstrated increased menstrual cycle length.[19] Current evidence does not imply that soy prevents ovulation; however, soy may delay ovulation.

> Further studies of soy consumption in polycystic ovarian syndrome (PCOS) are required. Women with PCOS who struggle with infertility, consume few calories, or eat a poor diet may wish to consider avoiding or limiting the consumption of soy products. Otherwise, moderate to low intake of soy (once a day or several times a week) can be part of a healthy diet for women with PCOS.

Omega-3 Fatty Acids

Inflammation has been identified in patients with PCOS, whether as a consequence or a contributing factor remains unclear.[20,21] In comparison with control subjects, patients with PCOS have decreased fibrinolytic activity, higher levels of plasminogen activator inhibitor-1, and increased C-reactive protein levels (in both obese and nonobese women), all of which are markers of inflammation.[25,26] These findings indicate interventions to reduce cardiovascular risk should be more aggressive in women with PCOS who have increased C-reactive protein levels. Including omega-3 fatty acids may have utility in managing the inflammatory component of PCOS in addition to supporting cardiovascular health (see Chapter 88). The lignans in flaxseeds may provide additional benefit through promoting estrogen elimination.

Supplements

Inositol Family

Investigations into the cause of insulin resistance in PCOS led some researchers to investigate whether derangements in insulin signal transduction could be overcome by oral administration of D-chiro-inositol (DCI), a mediator of insulin action that is naturally formed in the human body from the metabolism of pinitol and myoinositol (commonly known as inositol) in the diet. In several early studies, evidence favored a benefit of DCI in improved insulin sensitivity, triglyceride, and testosterone levels, in addition to improving blood pressure, ovulation, and weight loss.[22,23] In a separate study, 44 obese women with PCOS were randomly assigned to receive placebo or DCI (1200 mg once a day) for 8 weeks. Supplementation with DCI resulted in an improvement in insulin resistance (p = 0.07), a 55% reduction in the mean serum free testosterone concentration (p = 0.006), and an increase in ovulation from 27% to 86% compared with placebo (p < 0.001). The more readily commercially available D-pinitol (D-chiro (+)-O-methyl inositol) has been shown to raise DCI serum levels; however, results of clinical end points, such as impact on insulin sensitivity, have been mixed.[24,25] In an important study of this nutrient in diabetic patients, 600 mg of pinitol twice per day for 3 months lowered blood glucose levels by 19.3%, lowered average glucose levels by 12.4%, and significantly improved insulin resistance.[29] In another study, 25 women received inositol for 6 months. Twenty-two of the 25 (88%) had a single spontaneous menstrual cycle during treatment, of whom 18 (72%) maintained a normal ovulatory activity. Ten pregnancies (40% of patients) occurred during this study.

DOSAGE

DCI: 600 mg daily in patients weighing less than 60 kg (130 lb) or 1200 mg daily in patients weighing more than 60 kg. Pinitol: 600 mg twice daily.

PRECAUTIONS

No interactions with herbs and supplements are known. There is concern that high consumption of inositol may exacerbate bipolar disorder.

Chromium

Chromium is an essential trace mineral that enhances the action of insulin. Although supplementation with chromium has been shown in studies to improve blood glucose control in type 2 diabetes mellitus, little research has focused specifically on patients with PCOS.[26] A pilot study of six women with PCOS concluded that 1000 mcg per day of chromium for as little as 2 months improved insulin sensitivity by an average of 38% (statistically significant) and decreased baseline insulin by 22% (not statistically significant).[27]

DOSAGE

Chromium picolinate: 600 to 1000 mcg in divided doses daily. Picolinate, a byproduct of the amino acid tryptophan, is combined to support absorption of chromium. Dietary sources include Brewer's yeast, liver, mushrooms, wheat germ, oysters, and some fresh fruits.

PRECAUTIONS

The adequate daily intake of chromium for women ranges from 20 to 45 mcg depending on age. Laboratory animals have tolerated 350 times this dose without adverse effects, although there is concern regarding mutagenicity with prolonged use. In humans, short-term use of chromium at 1000 mcg daily is safe; however, these doses are not recommended in pregnancy or renal insufficiency. Prolonged use should be avoided due to concerns regarding adverse effects.

Vitamin D

Vitamin D plays a role in insulin resistance and egg follicle maturation and development. In a small trial of 13 women with PCOS and vitamin D deficiency, normal menstrual cycles resumed within 2 months of vitamin D repletion with calcium therapy in seven of the nine women who had irregular menstrual cycles.[28] Two women subsequently had established pregnancies. The authors of the study posited that abnormalities in calcium balance may be responsible, in part, for arrested follicular development in women with PCOS and may contribute to the pathogenesis of PCOS. Vitamin D also plays a key role in glucose regulation, notably in decreasing insulin resistance,[29,30] and low levels of vitamin D have been negatively correlated with the incidence of type 1 and type 2 diabetes.

DOSAGE

Vitamin D_3: 2000 units daily. Higher doses may be prescribed based on serum 25-OH vitamin D levels. Overweight individuals have a greater risk of vitamin D deficiency because the bioavailability of vitamin D, a fat-soluble vitamin, may be reduced in fat tissue.

PRECAUTIONS

Vitamin D is well tolerated. Gastrointestinal side effects are most commonly reported.

N-Acetylcysteine

Many studies of N-acetylcysteine (NAC) have reported benefit in diabetes, with several demonstrating benefit in PCOS. NAC has multiple actions, including increasing levels of glutathione (an antioxidant), lowering inflammatory markers such as tumor necrosis factor-alpha, and improving insulin sensitivity.[31,32] A study in clomiphene-resistant patients demonstrated improved ovulatory rates (49.3% vs. 1.3%) and pregnancy rates (21% vs. 0%).[33] A prospective randomized placebo-controlled study of 60 women with PCOS aged 25–35 years undergoing intracytoplasmic sperm injection (ICSI) found that NAC improved oocyte and embryo quality. This study also compared the effects of NAC and metformin on oocyte quality, with the results indicating NAC represents an alternative to metformin for women with PCOS undergoing ICSI.[33]

DOSAGE

Give 1200 to 1800 mg/day in divided doses.

PRECAUTIONS

NAC is well tolerated, with occasional reports of nausea.

Selenium

Selenium is an essential micronutrient involved in antioxidant reactions, such as catalyzed by glutathione peroxidase. Studies have suggested selenium also possesses insulin-like actions, and has a potential role in fat and carbohydrate metabolism. A recent randomized, double-blind, placebo-controlled study of 70 women aged 18–40 years with PCOS found that selenium supplementation led to significantly decreased levels of serum insulin (–29 vs. 9 pmol/L), serum triglycerides (–0.14 vs. 0.11 mmol/L) and VLDL-C concentrations (–0.03 vs. 0.02 mmol/L) compared with placebo.[33a] Researchers from this study hypothesized these effects were attributable to inhibition of COX2 expression and inflammatory cytokines, including TNF-alpha and IL-1. Further studies are required to assess the potential benefits and toxicities associated with long-term selenium intake.

DOSAGE

Give 200 microgram per day for 8 weeks.

PRECAUTIONS

No side effects were reported by any PCOS study participants who were taking selenium supplementation. While one study demonstrated selenium intake up to 200 mcg/d for up to 16 weeks is safe for patients over 18 years of age, other studies have reported adverse side effects of hair loss and dermatitis.

Botanicals

Cinnamomum cassia

Cinnamomum cassia (not *Cinnamomum zeyanicum* or *Cinnamomum verum*) has been studied in vitro and in humans for its effects in lowering glucose levels in patients with diabetes.[34-36] A pilot study published in the July 2007 issue of *Fertility and Sterility* reported that 1/4 to 1/2 teaspoon of cinnamon powder reduced insulin resistance in 15 women with PCOS.

DOSAGE

The dose is 1 to 6 g powdered cinnamon (1/4 to 1 teaspoon) or 200 to 300 mg cassia extract.

PRECAUTIONS

Cinnamon is well tolerated. Gastrointestinal side effects are most common.

Licorice

Licorice root and glycyrrhetinic acid have antiandrogen effects that may support treatment goals in PCOS. Licorice root as part of a traditional Chinese medicine formula has also been associated with reduced serum testosterone and ovulation induction in women with PCOS.[37,38] Additionally, licorice is synergistic with spironolactone, with its effects on potassium loss, hypertension, and fluid retention counteracting the opposing actions of spironolactone. A study of 32 hirsute women with PCOS administered 100 mg of spironolactone per day, with half also receiving 3.5 g/day of a licorice root extract standardized to 7.6% glycyrrhetinic acid for 2 months.[39] Licorice use was associated with amelioration of orthostatic symptoms, polyuria, and systolic blood pressure drops, particularly during the first 2 weeks of treatment.

DOSAGE

Glycyrrhiza glabra: 500 mg standardized to 6% to 15% glycyrrhizin (approximately 3.0 to 8.0 g of crude plant material).

PRECAUTIONS

Few adverse events have been reported at lower doses or normal consumption levels. A no-observed effects level has been proposed as purified glycyrrhizin, 2 mg/kg/day. The acceptable daily intake for glycyrrhizin is recommended as 0.2 mg/kg/day. Toxicity from excessive licorice ingestion is well established, including hypokalemia, hypertension, and fluid retention. Licorice is contraindicated in pregnancy.

Chaste Tree Berry (*Vitex Agnus-castus*)

Vitex is one of the most popular botanicals for PCOS, although data from well-conducted studies are not available. *Vitex* is believed to shift the estrogen–progesterone balance in favor of progesterone through increased luteinizing hormone levels and mild inhibition of follicle-stimulating hormone secretion. *Vitex* also reduces prolactin secretion, which may inhibit fertility when elevated. A small study involving women with fertility disorders examined pregnancy rates following the administration of a chaste berry–containing herbal blend versus placebo twice daily for 3 months.[40] Women with secondary amenorrhea or luteal insufficiency in the active treatment group achieved pregnancy twice as often as in the group receiving placebo. However, the total number of patients conceiving was small (15 women).

Two other publications explored the benefits of a *Vitex*-containing blend on progesterone levels, basal body temperature, menstrual cycle length, pregnancy rate, and side effect profile.[41,42] Both were double-blind, placebo-controlled trials of a proprietary nutritional supplement containing chaste berry, green tea, L-arginine, and vitamins and minerals. The treatment group (n = 53) demonstrated increased mean midluteal progesterone levels, particularly among women with very low pretreatment levels. Cycle length and luteal basal body temperatures improved significantly. After 3 months, 14 women in the treatment group were pregnant (26%) compared with 4 of the 40 women in the placebo group (10%; p = 0.01). The results of these studies are difficult to extrapolate given the proprietary nature of the supplements, although the trends toward improvement with no side effects warrant further consideration. Several small studies in the German literature have also reported a benefit of *Vitex* for acne, with self-reports of improvements of up to 70%.[43]

DOSAGE

Vitex products are available in many different forms, including fresh and dried berries, capsules containing powdered chaste berries, and liquid preparations, such as extracts and tinctures. The German Commission E recommends 30-40 mg of dried fruit extract daily, 2.6-4.2 mg of dry native extract (standardized to 0.6% casticin or agnuside), or 40 drops of tincture. Fluid extract ([1:1] g/mL) dosage ranges from 0.5-1.0 mL daily.

PRECAUTIONS

Animal and human studies indicate *Vitex* may interfere with oral contraceptives and hormone therapy. Based on in vitro data, *Vitex* may also interact with dopamine agonists (e.g., bromocriptine, levodopa). Use during pregnancy is not recommended.

Complementary Healing Approaches

Acupuncture

Acupuncture has the potential to influence PCOS through its effects on the sympathetic nervous system, the endocrine system, and the neuroendocrine system.[46,47] In a 2009 study, one group of women with PCOS was treated for 4 months with electroacupuncture, another group of women was given heart rate monitors and told to exercise three times a week, and a third control group was educated about the importance of exercise and a healthy diet but received no instructions. The investigators found that women who received acupuncture or who exercised had decreased sympathetic activity. The women who received electroacupuncture treatments also had more regular menstrual cycles, reduced testosterone levels, and reduced waist circumference. Experimental observations from animal and clinical studies indicate acupuncture exerts beneficial effects on insulin resistance and ovulation. Although research studies are limited, acupuncture may be considered as an adjunctive therapy in many women for its direct impacts on PCOS parameters in addition to associated mood disorders and stress.

Mind-Body Therapy

Women with PCOS have a significantly increased prevalence of depression and anxiety.[48-50] Mood disorders may be directly related to biochemical imbalances (altered androgen levels or insulin resistance), and may be exacerbated by stress related to body image issues and infertility. Addressing these concerns through mind-body approaches, self-care, and cognitive-behavioral therapy should be encouraged for all women. A randomized, controlled trial has shown that women with PCOS who participated in an 8-week mindfulness and stress management program experienced significant reductions in stress, depressive, and anxiety symptoms, along with an increase in life satisfaction and quality of life. The results of this study indicate mindfulness techniques can be used to supplement PCOS care to the benefit of patient mental health[58] (see Chapter 100).

Pharmaceuticals

Medication decisions should be based on the predominant symptoms and goals of individual patients. Major classes of pharmaceutical treatments for PCOS include insulin sensitizers, weight loss medications, and hormone modulators.

Insulin Sensitizers

Metformin improves insulin resistance and hyperandrogenism.[51] Metformin is also associated with regulation of menstruation and ovulation, and may benefit up to 79% of women attempting to conceive. Metformin is considered weight neutral, as opposed to many other medications used for glucose regulation.

DOSAGE

Start with 500 mg daily for 1 week, titrate to 500 mg twice daily in week 2, and as required thereafter. The maximum daily dose is 2.5 g in two or three divided doses.

PRECAUTIONS

Side effects are predominantly gastrointestinal and include nausea and diarrhea. Metformin should be avoided if creatinine clearance is less than 30 mL/minute.

Thiazolidinediones are less thoroughly studied in PCOS compared with metformin. This class of medications is associated with weight gain, thus making it an unattractive choice for many women struggling with PCOS. Studies of troglitazone (now off the market due to hepatotoxicity), pioglitazone, and rosiglitazone have demonstrated improvements in insulin sensitivity, hyperandrogenemia, and ovulatory rates. Given the potential for adverse effects, this class of medications is best reserved for patients with established diabetes mellitus.

Weight Loss Medications

Orlistat, given with an energy-restricted diet, has been shown to improve insulin resistance in addition to lowering free testosterone in obese women in some, but not all, studies.[52-54] As the trials were short term (3 to 6 months), further studies are required to determine the utility of orlistat for the treatment of patients with PCOS.

DOSAGE

A dose of 120 mg three times daily containing fat (during or up to 1 hour after the meal) was used for 3-6 months in previous studies. Omit dose if meal is occasionally missed or contains no fat.

PRECAUTIONS

Orlistat may cause fat-soluble vitamin deficiency and greasy stools.

Hormone Modulators

Oral Contraceptives. Oral contraceptive pills (OCPs) are first-line options for symptoms of androgen excess, such as hirsutism and acne, in accord with the 2008 Endocrine Society Clinical Practice Guidelines. OCPs reduce luteinizing hormone secretion and thus ovarian androgen secretion; additional reductions in free androgen concentration occur through increased levels of sex hormone–binding globulin.[55] OCPs provide additional benefit by protecting against endometrial hyperplasia in amenorrheic women with excess estrogen exposure.

DOSAGE

Appropriate choices include OCP preparations containing 30 to 35 mcg of ethinyl estradiol combined with a progestin with minimal androgenicity, such as norethindrone, norgestimate, desogestrel, or drospirenone.

PRECAUTIONS

Risks and side effects of OCPs are similar to those for women without PCOS. OCPs may increase cardiovascular risk factors, such as inflammatory markers and insulin resistance. Absence of pregnancy should be documented before OCPs are initiated. In patients with no menstrual period for 6 or more weeks, withdrawal bleeding should be induced by administration of 5 to 10 mg of medroxyprogesterone acetate daily for 10 days before initiation of OCP treatment (to minimize breakthrough bleeding when starting the pill).

Although the oral contraceptive pill (OCP) helps many women overcome the troublesome symptoms of polycystic ovarian syndrome (PCOS), these drugs have been associated with an increased risk of cardiovascular disease in the general population.[56,57] The risk of cardiovascular disease is associated with increased age, smoking, and hypertension. Additional concerns include a negative impact on inflammatory markers and diabetes risk. Further studies are required in the PCOS population to assess the long-term benefit-to-risk ratio of using OCPs. For now, increased awareness and regular follow-up of metabolic and cardiovascular markers are critical for all patients taking the OCP.

Progestins. Progestins are appropriate for women who require endometrial protection but are not interested in, or appropriate for, the OCP. Cyclic progestins promote withdrawal bleeding and prevent endometrial hyperplasia.

DOSAGE

Synthetic progestin: medroxyprogesterone acetate 5–10 mg orally daily for 7 to 10 days every 1 to 2 months. Bio-identical progestin: micronized progesterone 200–400 mg orally daily for 10 days every 1 to 2 months. Bio-identical progesterone cream has not been evaluated in research studies, and whether such creams can provide consistent levels sufficient for uterine protection is unclear.

PRECAUTIONS

Sedation or confusion may occur.

Antiandrogens. Antiandrogens, which block androgen binding to its receptor, are often used off label for hirsutism.[58] The most commonly prescribed antiandrogen is spironolactone. Flutamide is another option despite an association with greater side effects.

DOSAGE

Spironolactone, 50 to 200 mg/day; flutamide, 250 mg two to three times a day.

PRECAUTIONS

Contraception is essential as an antiandrogens, such as spironolactone, may be teratogenic if pregnancy occurs. Discontinuation 3 months before conception is therefore recommended. If spironolactone is used alone, endometrial protection may be required.

Clomiphene Citrate. Clomiphene citrate is an antiestrogen and an effective option for ovulation induction for women with PCOS. Approximately 80% of women with PCOS ovulate in response to clomiphene citrate, and approximately 50% conceive.

DOSAGE

The strategy is to use the lowest dose of clomiphene possible to initiate ovulation, starting with 50 mg/day for 5 days (usually days 5 to 9). If no follicle development occurs with this dose, the dose or duration of treatment can be increased.

Statins. There is debate in the literature regarding the cardiovascular and endocrine benefit of statins in women with PCOS. The results of an initial study of 40 patients with PCOS randomly assigned to atorvastatin at 20 mg daily or placebo were promising.[59] After 12 weeks, the researchers reported an absolute reduction in free androgen index (–32.7%) and total testosterone (–24.6%), and increased sex hormone–binding globulin (+13.7%) in the atorvastatin group compared to the placebo group. Patients in the atorvastatin group had lower serum insulin levels and homeostasis model of insulin resistance (HOMA-IR) values compared to the placebo group. Conversely, a study published in 2010, in which 20 patients with PCOS who had low-density lipoprotein levels higher than 100 mg/dL took atorvastatin at 40 mg/day or placebo for 6 weeks of treatment, reported reductions in androgen levels, biomarkers of inflammation, and blood pressure.[60] However, atorvastatin worsened hyperinsulinemia and failed to improve endothelial function in women with PCOS. Until the potential benefit of statins in PCOS has been fully evaluated, reserving statin use for the treatment of hyperlipidemia rather than the treatment of hyperandrogenemia or insulin resistance seems prudent.

DOSAGE

Doses are as per usual recommendations for hyperlipidemia.

PRECAUTIONS

Statins are considered to have teratogenic potential in pregnancy. The usual concerns regarding liver and muscle issues apply.

Surgery

When severe symptoms are not controlled with the therapies described above and a patient has morbid obesity, bariatric surgery may be considered. Results of two small studies on the effects of bariatric surgery have been published.[61] A retrospective study evaluated 30 women with PCOS who underwent laparoscopic Roux-en-Y gastric bypass. Postoperative benefits included resolution of menstrual irregularity (100%), improvement in hirsutism (75%), resolution of type 2 diabetes, and ability to cease medications for hypertension (78%) and hyperlipidemia (92%). These results were confirmed in a prospective study evaluating 17 women with PCOS.

Surgery may also be performed for ovulation induction in the management of clomiphene citrate–resistant anovulatory women with PCOS. Various types of ovarian surgery can be employed (e.g., wedge resection, electrocautery, laser vaporization, multiple ovarian biopsies), and all procedures result in an altered endocrine profile postoperatively. A plausible mechanism for the benefit of surgery for patients with PCOS is the restoration of appropriate gonadotrophin release due to rapid reductions in the secretion of all ovarian hormones restoring feedback to the hypothalamus and pituitary. These surgical procedures provide an option, albeit one used less often now, when natural and pharmaceutical approaches are unsuccessful in anovulatory patients with PCOS.

PREVENTION PRESCRIPTION

- Maintain appropriate weight and a regular aerobic exercise routine.
- Avoid excessive amounts of saturated fat such as those found in red meat, fried foods, and dairy.
- Replace vegetable oils with olive or canola oil for cooking.
- Consume omega-3–rich fats found in cold-water fish, nuts, greens, and ground flaxseed.
- Encourage soy-based foods, such as soy milk, edamame, tempeh, miso, soy nuts, and nonge-netically modified tofu. Try to eat 1 to 2 oz of soy-based foods per day.
- Avoid dietary supplements or environmental exposures that may increase circulating hormone levels, such as pesticides, herbicides, and bovine growth hormone–rich dairy products.
- Avoid supplements or drugs that include dehydroepiandrosterone, androstenedione, testosterone, or human growth hormone.

THERAPEUTIC REVIEW

Lifestyle approaches are first-line recommendations for PCOS, both in conventional and integrative medicine approaches. Many women with PCOS do well with attention to diet, exercise, supplements, and acupuncture. A proportion of women require medications to achieve improvements when metabolic derangements are greater.

LIFESTYLE

- Remove exacerbating factors. Minimize exposure to hormone-disrupting chemicals.

NUTRITION

- Promote weight loss to achieve an ideal body weight. Start with achievable goals and provide adequate support.
- Eat 1 to 2 servings of soy-rich foods daily. Each 1 oz serving (approximately the size of the palm of the hand) provides approximately 25 mg.
- Encourage a low-carbohydrate diet that takes into account the glycemic index of foods.
- Encourage foods rich in omega-3 fatty acids (e.g., salmon, nuts, or ground flaxseeds).

PHYSICAL ACTIVITY

- Recommend moderate exertion for 30 to 60 minutes daily.

SUPPLEMENTS

- Vitamin D3: 2000 units daily (dose based on serum 25-OH vitamin D level)
- Chromium picolinate: 1000 mcg daily
- d-*chiro*-inositol/pinitol: 600 mg once or twice per day
- Selenium: 200 mcg per day for 8 weeks

BOTANICALS

- *Cinnamomum cassia:* 1/4 to 1 teaspoon
- Licorice root in conjunction with spironolactone for the amelioration of side effects and complementary action
- Chaste tree berry (*Vitex*): 60 drops of tincture or 175 mg of extract, standardized to 0.6% agnusides

COMPLEMENTARY THERAPIES

- Acupuncture may reduce sympathetic nervous system tone and improve menstruation. It has additional benefits for stress reduction and mood.
- Mind-body therapies can help women cope with stress, depression, and anxiety related to PCOS.

PHARMACEUTICALS

- Insulin sensitizers include metformin at 500 to 1000 mg twice daily.
- If patients are unable to achieve satisfactory weight loss, consider support with orlistat.
- Medications such as clomiphene may be prescribed in consultation with a reproductive endocrinologist for ovulation induction.
- Antiestrogens for hirsutism include spironolactone at 50 to 200 mg/day, or flutamide, at 250 mg two to three times a day.
- Oral contraceptive pills are prescribed for amenorrhea, hyperandrogenism, and uterine protection.

SURGICAL THERAPY

- Consider referral for bariatric surgery for patients with morbid obesity and significant comorbidities despite the measures listed above.
- Ovarian surgery may be indicated for infertility.

Key Web Resources

American Association of Clinical Endocrinologists: This website contains a position statement on metabolic and cardiovascular consequences of PCOS, as well as practice management forms for new and follow-up visits for patients with PCOS.

http://www.aace.com

Womenshealth.gov: This website, from the U.S. Department of Health and Human Services Office on Women's Health, provides patient education materials on PCOS.

https://www.womenshealth.gov/publications/our-publications/fact-sheet/polycystic-ovary-syndrome.html

American Society for Reproductive Medicine: This website describes medical and surgical options for PCOS.

http://www.asrm.org

REFERENCES

References are available online at ExpertConsult.com.

CHAPTER 36

OSTEOPOROSIS

Louise Gagné, MD • Victoria Maizes, MD

Osteoporosis is defined as a generalized skeletal disorder characterized by compromised bone strength, which predisposes individuals to an increased risk of fracture. Osteoporosis is a significant cause of pain, disability, and death throughout the world. Integrative medicine makes use of a range of strategies to reduce the risk of osteoporosis, including an antiinflammatory diet, supplements, stress reduction, and lifelong exercise habits.

EPIDEMIOLOGY AND PATHOPHYSIOLOGY

The incidence of osteoporotic fractures varies by more than 10-fold in different regions of the world. Rates are highest in Europe, Iran, and Argentina and much lower in China, India, and South Africa.[1] More than 10 million people in the United States have osteoporosis and more than 2 million osteoporotic fractures occur each year.[2] Women are at higher risk of osteoporosis than men and account for approximately 75% of all cases; however, men are at greater risk of dying of a hip fracture should they sustain one (20.7% vs. 7.5%).[3] The costs to the U.S. health care system attributable to osteoporosis are significant, totaling more than $16 billion annually. As the population ages, the costs related to osteoporosis prevention and treatment are expected to continue to climb.[4]

Osteoporosis is a multifactorial disease arising from genetic, hormonal, metabolic, mechanical, and immunological factors. Bones provide the support structure for our bodies, protect vital organs, and play a central role in mineral and acid–base balance. The two main types of bone cells are osteoblasts (which synthesize the organic bone matrix and mediate calcification) and osteoclasts (which resorb bone to allow for metabolic requirements and for repair and remodeling).

Bone mass reaches its peak by around 30 years of age, but repair and renewal of bone continue throughout adult life, with approximately 15% of bone mass turning over each year. Bone is dynamic and constantly responding to a range of hormonal, metabolic, neurological, and mechanical signals. Bone loss usually begins in the fourth decade in both men and women. Women typically lose 0.5% to 0.9% of bone density per year during the perimenopause, 1% to 3% during menopausal years, and 1% per year into old age. On average, women lose 35% of their cortical bone and 50% of their trabecular bone over their lifetimes. Men are half as likely as women to experience a fracture as they reach higher peak bone mass, have a larger cortical thickness, and have better preservation of bone microstructure.[3]

Assessing Bone Strength and Fracture Risk

Bone strength is determined by bone quality in addition to bone mass. Bone quality is influenced by bone geometry, microarchitecture, and the properties of constituent tissues. Although a number of techniques, such a quantitative CT and high-resolution MRI, are being studied; no method is readily available to assess bone quality in a clinical practice setting.[5] Bone mass is most commonly assessed using a dual energy x-ray absorptiometry (DEXA) scan.

Osteoporosis is defined as a bone mineral density (BMD) more than 2.5 standard deviations (SD) below the mean for young adults. Osteopenia is defined as a BMD 1 to 2.5 SD below the young adult mean. However, BMD has limitations as the sole predictor of fracture risk. Most fractures occur in individuals with a BMD above the cutoff of 2.5 SD from the mean.[6] Further, BMD is unable to differentiate between cortical and trabecular bone or characterize the three-dimensional structure of bone. Although some studies have shown a strong correlation between low femoral neck BMD and risk of hip fracture,[7] a wide overlap exists between the bone densities of women who will eventually suffer a fracture and those who will not.[8] Overall, less than 60% of the variation in femoral bone strength is related to BMD.[9]

The Fracture Risk Algorithm (FRAX) developed by the World Health Organization (WHO) uses a number of additional risk factors to more accurately predict fracture risk. These risk factors are: history of prior fracture, thinness, smoking, rheumatoid arthritis, excessive alcohol intake, and history of a hip fracture in a parent. FRAX in combination with BMD has been shown to be superior to either FRAX or BMD alone.[6] The North American Menopause Society (NAMS) recommends that BMD be measured in all women 65 years old or older, and in women age 50 and older with one or more FRAX risk factors.[10]

Other risk factors for osteoporotic fracture should also be assessed. These include nutritional deficiencies, high alcohol intake, excessive caffeine consumption, premature menopause, malabsorption disorders, autoimmune disease, small body frame, white/Caucasian or Asian descent, impaired vision, dizziness or balance problems, fainting or loss of consciousness, physical frailty, and use of medications such as corticosteroids, aromatase inhibitors, proton pump inhibitors, anticonvulsants, sedatives, anticholinergics, antihypertensives, heparin, cyclosporine, and medroxyprogesterone acetate.

Role of Inflammation

Chronic inflammation is implicated in the process of aging,[11,12] and posited to play a role in the development of a wide range of diseases, including cardiovascular disease, Alzheimer's disease, diabetes, and cancer.[13,14] Growing evidence indicates that osteoporosis is also, in part, a result of chronic low-grade inflammation.[15-17] Proinflammatory cytokines, such as interleukin-6 (IL-6), interleukin-1 (IL-1), and tumor necrosis factor-alpha (TNF-alpha), promote accelerated bone loss by the activation of osteoclasts, inhibition of collagen production in osteoblasts, and enhanced breakdown of the extracellular matrix.[17] Furthermore, suppression of proinflammatory cytokines appears to support the growth of new bone. For instance, TNF-alpha inhibitors, such as etanercept, have been found to improve BMD in patients with spondyloarthropathy.[18] It is widely recognized that patients with systemic inflammatory conditions, such as rheumatoid arthritis, inflammatory bowel disease, multiple sclerosis, and systemic lupus erythematosus, are at increased risk of bone loss.[19]

Reducing systemic inflammation can help promote bone density and strength.

Fruits and vegetables are rich sources of antiinflammatory and antioxidant compounds, and diets rich in fruits and vegetables are associated with both increased peak bone mass and improved bone health in older populations.[20-23] The bone-building effects of fruits and vegetables may result from several factors including: antiinflammatory and antioxidant phytonutrients; alkalinizing effects; the provision of nutrients such as potassium, vitamin K, and vitamin C; and the presence of other unknown compounds and synergistic effects. Thus an antiinflammatory diet that includes abundant fruits and vegetables, whole grains, legumes, and healthy fats is recommended as the foundation of an integrative bone health plan (see Chapter 88).

Acid–Base Issues

The skeleton plays a key role in acid–base homeostasis.[24] In bone, minute reductions in the local pH can stimulate osteoclast activity while also impairing the activity of osteoblasts.[25] A diet high in animal protein and low in fruits and vegetables tends to produce a chronic low-grade metabolic acidosis that may be harmful to the skeleton.[26-30] Fruits and vegetables generate bicarbonate that can buffer the acidifying effects of animal protein, alkalinize the urine, and significantly lower urinary calcium excretion.[31] In a study by Buclin et al., acid-forming diets increased calcium excretion by 74% as compared to base-forming diets.[32] Balanced diets with adequate protein along with abundant fruits and vegetables are therefore recommended.[33,34]

In addition to effects on acid–base balance, the benefits of plant foods also appear to be related to pharmacologically active components, including specific monoterpenes,[35] flavonoids, and phenols,[36] that may be responsible for the observed beneficial effects on bone.

Muhlbauer described 25 plant foods as "bone resorption inhibitory food items" (BRIFI). These include garlic, rosemary, Italian parsley, sage, thyme, parsley, dill, onion, arugula, prune, fennel, orange, leek, yellow boletus, wild garlic, field agaric, red cabbage, celeriac, red wine, and lettuce.[37]

Microbiome and Bone Health

There is emerging evidence that the human microbiome plays a significant role in many dimensions of health, including brain function, immune response, levels of inflammation, body weight, and cancer risk.[38,39] The gut microbiome has also been shown to influence bone health. In animal studies, prebiotic feeding aimed at enhancing production of short chain fatty acids by intestinal bacteria resulted in increased fractional calcium absorption and increased bone density and strength.[40] A study by Ohlsson et al. found that treatment with probiotics can diminish bone loss related to sex-steroid deficiency in mice.[41] Several human trials in adolescent girls and boys have found that prebiotic supplementation can increase the numbers of bifidobacteria, enhance calcium absorption, and increase bone mineralization.[42,43] In general, a healthy, diverse microbiome can be supported by including cultured and fermented foods in the diet, eating a diet rich in "microbiota-accessible carbohydrates" (MACs),[44] and avoiding unnecessary antibiotics. Ongoing research may clarify how the health of the microbiome can be supported and enhanced in order to sustain bone health.

Vegetarian and Vegan Diets

Plant-based diets are associated with a lower risk of chronic disease and reduced overall mortality.[45] In 2009, the American Dietetic Association issued a position statement stating: "…appropriately planned vegetarian diets, including total vegetarian or vegan diets, are healthful, nutritionally adequate, and may provide health benefits in the prevention and treatment of certain diseases."[46] In practice, vegetarians and vegans are more likely to have low intakes of vitamin D,[47] calcium, vitamin B12, and omega-3 fatty acids. Vegetarian sources of zinc are also less bioavailable. On the other hand, healthy vegetarian diets contain plentiful amounts of magnesium, potassium, vitamin K, and antioxidant and antiinflammatory phytonutrients. A number of studies have shown that vegetarian, and particularly vegan, diets may increase the risk of osteoporosis and bone fractures.[48] In a meta-analysis by Ho-Pham et al., BMD was, on average, 4% lower in vegetarians (all types) and 6% lower in vegans.[49] The EPIC-Oxford study examined fracture risk in more than 34,000 meat eaters, fish eaters, vegetarians and vegans, and reported fracture risk was highest in vegans. However, when only subjects with adequate calcium intakes were included, no differences in fracture risk were observed between any of the groups.[50] A longitudinal study of Asian vegans and omnivores reported a higher rate of bone loss in the omnivore group, with fracture risk found to be the same in both groups. Lower body weight, higher intakes of animal protein and fats, and corticosteroid use were all associated with a greater rate of bone loss.[51] If vegetarians and vegans follow the principles of an antiinflammatory diet and ensure adequate intake of calcium and vitamin D, they should be able to reap the benefits of a plant-based diet without increasing their risk of osteoporosis.

INTEGRATIVE THERAPY

Nutrition and Nutritional Supplements

Calcium

Calcium is an essential nutrient for building and maintaining healthy bones, and 99% of total body calcium is found in bones. However, high calcium intakes do not guarantee strong bones, and lower calcium intakes do not necessarily lead to weaker bones.[56-58] Calcium requirement is determined by the amount of calcium absorbed versus the rate that calcium is lost via the bowels, kidneys, skin, hair, and nails.[59] To improve calcium absorption and/or decrease calcium losses: ensure an optimum intake of vitamin D[60] and vitamin K,[61] increase fruits and vegetables,[31] aim for a balance of essential fatty acids,[62] consider cutting back on animal protein (although protein intake also increases calcium absorption),[31] keep dietary sodium to <2400 mg/day,[63,64] avoid excess caffeine,[65] and eat fewer highly refined carbohydrates.[66]

It is estimated that adequate calcium intake may range from ~450 mg to ~1150 mg depending on the influence of a variety of factors, such as those listed previously. For instance, it is estimated that a low animal protein intake of 20 g/day, coupled with a low sodium intake of 1.15 g/day may lower the amount of calcium required by 390 mg/day. Maximal calcium absorption from optimal vitamin D intake may lower calcium requirements further.[59]

> The collective effects of various dietary and lifestyle factors may help to explain the "calcium paradox," whereby hip fracture rates are less common in developing countries where calcium intakes are lower.[59]

In 2010 the Institute of Medicine (IOM) issued an update of the dietary reference intakes (DRIs) for calcium and vitamin D (Table 36.1). Before recommending supplemental calcium, the sum of all existing dietary sources of calcium, including baseline intake (~250 mg/day), dairy products, fortified beverages, and calcium that may be present in multivitamins or other supplements, should be calculated. The difference between this total and the DRI can then be used to determine if a supplement is required. A meta-analysis by Tang et al. found that men and women over the age of 50 had significantly lower fracture risk and reduced rate of bone loss with 1200 mg of calcium alone or in combination with vitamin D.[67] Some studies have linked the use of calcium

TABLE 36.1   Dietary Reference Intakes for Calcium and Vitamin D

Life Stage Group	Calcium Estimated Average Requirement (mg/day)	Recommended Dietary Allowance (mg/day)	Upper Level Intake (mg/day)	Vitamin D Estimated Average Requirement (mg/day)	Recommended Dietary Allowance (units/day)	Upper Level Intake (units/day)
Infants 0–6 mo	*	*	1000	†	†	1000
Infants 6–12 mo	*	*	1500	†	†	1500
1–3 yr	500	700	2500	400	600	2500
4–8 yr	800	1000	25,000	400	600	3000
9–13 yr	1100	1300	3000	400	600	4000
14–18 yr	1100	1300	3000	400	600	4000
19–30 yr	800	1000	2500	400	600	4000
31–50 yr	800	1000	2500	400	600	4000
51–70 yr (M)	800	1000	2000	400	600	4000
51–70 yr (F)	1000	1200	2000	400	600	4000
Older than 70 yr	1000	1200	2000	400	800	4000
14–18 yr, pregnant or lactating	1100	1300	3000	400	600	4000
19–50 yr, pregnant or lactating	800	1000	2500	400	600	4000

*For infants, adequate intake is 200 mg/day for 0 to 6 months of age and 260 mg/day for 6 to 12 months of age.
†For infants, adequate intake is 400 IU/day for 0 to 6 months of age and 400 IU/day for 6 to 12 months of age.
From Committee to Review Dietary Reference Intakes for Vitamin D and Calcium. In: Ross AC, Taylor CL, Yaktine AL, Del Valle HB, eds. *Dietary reference intakes for calcium and vitamin D*. Washington, DC: National Academies Press; 2011.

supplements with an increased risk of cardiovascular disease.[68] However, several studies have questioned the validity of these findings.[69-71] A study by Langsetmo et al. found that increased calcium intake from diet and supplements may lower mortality in women.[72] When dietary intake is inadequate, calcium supplementation is recommended but should always be part of a broader strategy that includes adequate vitamin D, vitamin K2, and other bone-building foods and nutrients. Even without dairy products, it is possible to meet daily requirements for calcium from vegetarian sources (Tables 36.2 and 36.3).

Vitamin D

One key role of vitamin D, in relation to bone health, is that is necessary for calcium absorption. The hormonally active form of vitamin D (1,25[OH]D) induces active transport of calcium across the intestinal epithelium. Vitamin D also stimulates the absorption of phosphate and magnesium ions, and acts synergistically with vitamin K to directly stimulate bone mineralization. In addition, vitamin D has beneficial effects on skeletal muscle and can reduce the risk of falls and increase muscle strength, function, and balance.[73]

Serum levels of 25-hydroxyvitamin D (25[OH]D) are required to be at least 34 ng/mL for maximal calcium absorption.[60]

Hypovitaminosis D is common in the United States and rates of vitamin D deficiency are rising.[74,75] Breast-fed infants, women, older adults, obese persons, and people with darker skin tones are at higher risk of vitamin D deficiency. An international epidemiological study found that 64% of postmenopausal women seeking medical care for osteoporosis had inadequate vitamin D concentrations (less than 30 ng/mL).[76] Supplementation with 800 IU vitamin D per day is associated with reduced fracture risk and a number of other positive health outcomes.[77] Population-wide screening for vitamin D deficiency in adults age 65 and older has been shown to be a cost-effective public health strategy.[78,79] It may be reasonable to screen patients of all ages for vitamin D deficiency, since inadequacy is also common in younger age groups.[80,81] Supplementation should be given to achieve a serum 25(OH)D of at least 34 ng/mL.[77] The ideal level for bone health may be considerably higher, with a meta-analysis concluding that optimum fracture prevention is not achieved until a level of 40 ng/mL is reached.[82]

Vitamin D can be obtained through sunlight exposure, from a limited number of foods, or from supplements. Sunlight exposure of 10 to 15 minutes without sunblock at the appropriate latitude and season is a good source of endogenously produced vitamin D. Only a few foods are naturally rich in vitamin D. Food sources include fatty ocean fish, such as salmon, sardines, and black cod; sun-exposed mushrooms; and fortified foods including some brands of orange juice, fortified milk substitutes, cow's milk, and some yogurts. Vitamin D supplementation is an inexpensive and reliable way to ensure an optimum serum level.

DOSAGE

In adults, doses of 1500–2000 IU/day may be needed to maintain a serum 25(OH)D level above 30 ng/mL.[83] Vitamin D_3 (cholecalciferol) is the preferred form[84] and should be taken with meals.

PRECAUTIONS

Minimal if kept within therapeutic limits.

TABLE 36.2 Dairy Calcium Sources

Food	Amount (oz)	Calcium (mg)
Milk	8	300
Yogurt	8	275–325
Hard cheeses high in calcium (cheddar, Swiss, Edam, Monterey Jack, Provolone, Parmesan, Romano, part-skim mozzarella)	1	200–300
Soft cheeses low in calcium (Brie, Neufchatel)	1	20–50

TABLE 36.3 Nondairy Calcium Sources

Food	Amount	Calcium (mg)
White beans	1 oz cooked	161
Spinach	½ cup	122
Turnip greens	½ cup	99
Soybeans	½ cup cooked	90
Broccoli	1 cup cooked or fresh	90
Bok choy	½ cup cooked or fresh	80
Almonds	1 oz dry roasted	80
Salmon	3 oz, canned with bones	180
Dried figs	10	269

Essential Fatty Acids

Both omega-6 (n-6) and omega-3 (n-3) fatty acids are essential nutrients that are incorporated into cell membrane phospholipids, where they influence membrane characteristics and become precursors for eicosanoids, such as prostaglandins, leukotrienes, and thromboxanes. Western diets tend to be relatively high in n-6 fats and low in n-3 fats, with typical ratios in the United States being ~16:1 (n-6 to n-3).[85] The ideal ratio is thought to be between 1:1 and 2:1 (n-6 to n-3).[86] The balance between these fats plays an important role in regulating the inflammatory response.

Omega-3 fatty acids are known to have antiinflammatory effects and suppress production of interleukin 1-beta (IL-beta), TNF-alpha, and IL-6.[87] Certain n-6 fatty acids, such as gamma-linolenic acid (GLA), also have antiinflammatory effects. On the other hand, the n-6 fatty acid, linoleic acid (LA), tends to have proinflammatory effects and promotes increased production of IL-beta, TNF-alpha, and IL-6.

Omega-3 fats appear to play an important role in bone health via a number of mechanisms including: increased calcium absorption, antiinflammatory effects, and promotion of osteoblastogenesis in the bone marrow.[88] In animal studies, fish oils rich in omega-3 fatty acids have been found to attenuate bone loss associated with estrogen withdrawal.[89] Animal studies have also shown that the omega-3 fatty acid, eicosapentaenoic acid (EPA), enhances calcium absorption, reduces calcium excretion, and increases calcium deposition in bone.[90] In a study of postmenopausal Korean women, higher red blood cell (RBC) levels of the omega-3 fatty acids, eicosapentaenoic acid (EPA) and docosahexaenoic acid (DHA), were associated with a lower risk of osteoporosis.[91] In elderly women, supplementation with calcium, EPA, and GLA resulted in a decrease in bone turnover and an increase in lumbar and femoral bone density.[90] In the Rancho Bernardo study, higher ratios of n-6 to n-3 fatty acids were associated with lower BMD in the hip for all women studied and lower BMD in the spine for women not on hormone therapy (HT).[92] A study of postmenopausal Chinese women found that higher intake of sea fish, rich in omega-3 fats, as opposed to freshwater fish, was associated with greater bone mass and a lower risk of osteoporosis.[93]

Despite substantial supporting evidence, a systematic review by Orchard et al. found inconclusive confirmation of a positive effect of omega-3 fatty acids on bone health. However, beneficial effects were found in studies conducted over longer periods of time (≥18 months); with the use of a mixture of fatty acids along with calcium; and, in particular, with increased intake of alpha-linolenic acid (ALA) as opposed to eicosapentaenoic acid (EPA) and docosahexaenoic acid (DHA).[94] Although further studies are required, n-3 fatty acids appear to enhance calcium absorption, reduce calcium excretion, and improve mineralization of bone matrix and bone strength.[62] There are also known health benefits to having an optimal proportion of omega-6 and omega-3 fatty acids in the diet.[85] The majority of individuals will need to increase their intake of omega-3 fats and decrease their intake of omega-6 fats to achieve this balance.

Protein

Protein is essential for the growth and maintenance of healthy bones.[95] Protein has anabolic effects on bone by providing the structural matrix of bone, increasing insulin-like growth factor (IGF-1) levels, and increasing intestinal absorption of calcium.[96] Protein also increases urinary calcium losses; however, other components in foods, such as phosphorus in meat and potassium in legumes, can at least partially offset this effect.[97]

Studies of the effect on bone of animal versus plant proteins and high versus low protein intakes have reported conflicting results. Several studies have found that high levels of animal protein in the diet are associated with increased fracture rates and accelerated bone mineral loss.[98-100] In the Nurses' Health Study, protein intakes higher than 95 g/day were associated with significantly higher forearm fracture rates than protein intakes

lower than 68 g/day.[99] A separate study found that lowering protein intakes to current RDA guidelines (0.8 g/kg) resulted in significant reductions in urinary calcium excretion and in markers of bone resorption.[101] A number of studies have also shown that an increased ratio of vegetable to animal protein is protective against fractures.[102,103] On the other hand, the Framingham Osteoporosis Study found that higher protein intakes (60–83 g/d in quartiles 2–4 vs. 46 g/d in the lowest quartile) in elderly men and women were associated with a 37% decreased risk of hip fracture.[104] The Women's Health Initiative data reported that a 20% increase in protein intake (from 15% to 18% of energy intake) improved BMD maintenance and marginally lowered forearm fracture risk.[105] A systematic review by Calvez et al. concluded that, "…no clinical data support the hypothesis of a detrimental effect of HP (high protein) diet on bone health, except in the context of inadequate calcium supply."[106] Other studies have found that, in the presence of adequate dietary calcium and vitamin D, increasing protein intake may have a favorable effect on bone health.[96,107] It is important to note that the majority of studies evaluating "higher" protein diets have examined modest increases in protein intake rather than the effects on bone of protein intakes in the range of 30% of energy intake.

> An adequate but not excessive intake of protein is recommended as part of a balanced diet that includes abundant fruits and vegetables and adequate calcium. Choosing vegetarian sources of protein, such as quinoa and soy foods, is also highly recommended for bone and overall health.

Vitamin K

There are two naturally occurring forms of vitamin K in foods: phylloquinone (K1), synthesized by plants; and menaquinones (K2), synthesized by bacteria. Vitamin K works synergistically with vitamin D to stimulate bone mineralization.[108,109] Menaquinones play a particularly important role in the prevention and therapy of osteoporosis.[108-110] Vitamin K2 is required for gamma carboxylation of osteocalcin, which stimulates the synthesis of osteoblastic markers and inhibits bone resorption by inhibiting the formation and activity of osteoclasts.[111,112]

A number of studies have reported a link between higher vitamin K status and reduction of fracture risk. Booth et al. found that elderly men and women in the highest quartile of dietary vitamin K had a relative risk for hip fracture of 0.35.[113] Women who consume one or more servings of lettuce per day (a source of K1) reportedly have a relative risk of 0.55 for hip fracture.[114] Patients with osteoporotic fractures of the spine and femoral neck have been found to be markedly deficient in K1 and the MK-7 and MK-8 forms of K2.[115,116] A review by Cockayne et al. suggested that the majority of vitamin K intervention studies have demonstrated a reduction in BMD loss and improved bone biomarkers.[117] A 3-year trial of vitamin K2 (mk-7, 180 mcg/day) in postmenopausal women reported preservation of BMD in the lumbar spine and slowing of the rate of bone loss in the femoral neck.[118] On the other hand, the ECKO trial in postmenopausal women with osteopenia used 5-mg vitamin K1 daily did not show any significant change in BMD.[119]

Vitamin K1 comes from plants and vitamin K2 is produced by gut bacteria. Vitamin K works with vitamin D to mineralize the bone.

Subclinical vitamin K deficiency is common, with typical dietary intakes below the levels associated with decreased fracture risk.[120] The DRI for vitamin K is 90 mcg for adult women and 120 mcg for adult men; however, amounts of 254 mcg/day or higher may be required for optimum bone health.[121] A number of researchers have called for unique DRI's for each form of vitamin K because K2 appears to have an important role in the prevention of vascular calcification and cancer.[61] The best sources of K1 are green leafy vegetables, such as lettuce, collards, spinach and kale, and other vegetables rich in chlorophyll, such as broccoli. Sources of vitamin K2 include animal foods, such as cheese, egg yolks, butter, goose liver, chicken liver, chicken and beef. Natto, a fermented soybean food, is a particularly rich source of K2.[122]

DOSAGE

Adequate vitamin K1 can be readily obtained from green vegetables. If supplementation is needed, the mk-7 form of vitamin K2 is recommended because it results in significantly higher and more stable vitamin K serum levels when compared to K1 or the mk-4 form of K2.[123,124] The recommended dose of mk-7 is 45–90 mcg daily. Vitamin K is a fat-soluble vitamin and thus is best absorbed when taken with a fat-containing meal.

PRECAUTIONS

Vitamin K supplements should not be used by patients taking anticoagulants.[125] For others, vitamin K supplementation does not affect coagulation and has an excellent safety profile. The Institute of Medicine does not list a safe upper limit for vitamin K[126] and, in Japan, studies are commonly conducted using doses of vitamin K2 that are 500 times or more higher than the daily recommended intake in the United States, with no significant side effects reported.[127]

Magnesium

In comparison to calcium, the relationship between magnesium and bone health has been much less well studied. Epidemiological studies have linked higher magnesium intakes with increased BMD.[10,128] Low magnesium intakes can decrease the number and function of osteoblasts, increase the number and activity of osteoclasts, and promote inflammation and oxidative stress.[129] Magnesium is also required for the conversion of vitamin D to 1,25-dihydroxycholecalciferol (calcitriol).[129] Some intervention trials of magnesium supplementation have shown an increase in BMD, as well as reduced fracture rates.[130,131] Almost half of the U.S. population does not obtain the daily recommended intake for magnesium.[132] Low magnesium intakes are also associated with a number of other chronic health conditions, such as type 2 diabetes and hypertension.[132] Good sources of magnesium include dark green leafy vegetables; nuts and seeds; legumes; and whole grains. Supplemental magnesium is readily-available singly or in combination with calcium. Magnesium citrate has superior bioavailability and has been recommended as the best form to use.[133]

Trace Minerals

Several trace minerals, including zinc, copper, boron, and manganese, act as cofactors for specific enzymes important for bone metabolism. Serum concentrations of zinc and copper have been found to be lower in osteoporotic women than in controls.[134] A varied, whole foods diet in addition to a good-quality multivitamin/mineral supplement should ensure an adequate supply of these nutrients.

Vitamin C

Vitamin C (ascorbic acid) is a required cofactor for the formation of collagen, a key component of the bone matrix. Vitamin C is also a major water-soluble antioxidant in the body. Plasma levels of vitamin C and other antioxidants have been found to be substantially lower in postmenopausal women with osteoporosis compared with age-matched controls.[135] The Framingham Osteoporosis Study found that elderly men and women in the highest tertile of total and supplemental vitamin C intake had significantly fewer hip and nonvertebral fractures, with a total intake of ~200 mg/day associated with the lowest prevalence of fracture.[136] A case-control study of elderly Chinese individuals found that higher dietary intakes of vitamin C, vitamin E, beta-carotene, and selenium were associated with a lower risk of hip fracture.[137] The best dietary sources of vitamin C are fruits and vegetables, such as papaya, pineapple, oranges, broccoli, and bell peppers. An antiinflammatory diet should easily supply adequate amounts of vitamin C.

Green leafy vegetables are super foods in relation to bone health as they contain vitamin K, magnesium, vitamin C, and calcium.

Soy

Soybeans are good sources of high quality plant protein, phytoestrogens, minerals, vitamins, essential fatty acids, and fiber. However, results from studies of soy foods and soy isoflavones (SI) in relation to bone health have been mixed. A 3-year trial of SI in postmenopausal women demonstrated nil effects other than a modest bone-sparing effect at the femoral neck.[138] On the other hand, a systematic review of SI supplements by Wei et al. found that isoflavones increased BMD by 54% and decreased deoxypyridinoline (DPD), a bone resorption marker, by 23%. The effects were greatest for postmenopausal women receiving an SI dose > 75mg/d.[139] Several large population-based studies of soy food intake have also reported beneficial effects. The Shanghai Women's Health Study found a relative risk of fracture of 0.63 in the highest quintile of soy protein intake (≥13 g/day).[140] This study, which examined food frequency questionnaires of 75,000 Chinese women aged 40 to 70 years old, also found a significant reduction in fracture risk, even in women in the second quintile, at soy protein intakes of 5 g/day (21 mg/day of isoflavones). This study examined the intake of traditionally-eaten whole soy foods, such as tofu and fresh soybeans, rather than isolated isoflavones. The Singapore Chinese Health Study also studied intake of traditional soy foods and found a significant reduction in hip fracture risk for women but not for men with higher soy intakes.[141] However, data from this study also demonstrated that both men and women had significantly lower hip-fracture risk following an overall dietary pattern labeled "vegetable-fruit-soy."[142]

There is reason to believe that a dietary pattern that includes whole soy foods as they have been traditionally eaten is more beneficial to bone health than isolated constituents of soy.[143,144]

DOSAGE

Based on available evidence, 1–2 servings/day of whole soy foods, such as tofu, tempeh, and edamame, are recommended.

Considerations in Childhood, Adolescence, and Young Adulthood

Up to 90% of peak bone mass is attained by age 18 in girls and by age 20 in boys.[145,146] Thus, osteoporosis prevention programs should begin early in life. Peak bone mass is influenced by genetic factors as well as by diet and physical activity during childhood, adolescence, and young adulthood. Regular physical activity and adequate calcium intake are key factors for achieving peak bone mass.[147] Sufficient vitamin D throughout bone-building years is also important.[148]

Botanicals

Numerous in vitro and animal studies, and a smaller number of human trials, have investigated the potential of herbal medicines to enhance bone health.[37] A study of Shen Gu (mixture for nourishing kidney and strengthening bone: *Fructus psoraleae* 16 g, *Radix codonopsis* 16 g, *Rhizoma drynariae* 16 g, *Cortex eucommiae* 16 g, *Radix Rehmanniae preparata* 20 g, *Radix astragali* 20 g, *Radix glycyrrhizae* 6 g; the treatment group was given 25 mL of the formula twice a day for 6 months) in 96 osteoporotic patients found significant favorable effects on bone.[149] The Ayurvedic preparation Reosto (ingredients per tablet: *Terminalia arjuna* 45 mg, *Withania somnifera* 45 mg, *Commiphora wightii* 235 mg, *Sida cordifolia* 45 mg,

Vanda roxburghi 50 mg, *Godanti bhasma* 120 mg, *Kukkutandatvak bhasma* 35 mg; the treatment group received two tablets twice a day for 12 months) has been found to significantly increase BMD.[150] Deng et al. published the first study of Fufang (herbal formula: *Herba epimedii*, *Rehmannia glutinosa*, *Dioscorea batatas*, *Cornus officinalis*, *Cinnamomum cassia*, *Drynaria fortunei*, *Morinda officinalis*; the treatment group received a dose of 10 g/day of dried granules; the doses of each herb are not available) using fracture as one of the primary endpoints. Postmenopausal women were found to have improvements in BMD and an impressive 43% reduction in fragility fractures over a 5-year period.[151] *Dioscorea spongiosa*,[152,153] *Astragalus membranaceus*,[154] walnut extract (*Juglans regia* L.),[155] and curcumin, a compound found in turmeric root (Curcuma longa),[156] have also demonstrated osteoprotective effects in laboratory and animal studies. Further research is required to elucidate the role of botanical medicines in the prevention and treatment of osteoporosis.

Tea (Camellia sinensis)

Tea has antiinflammatory effects, cardiovascular benefits, and cancer protective properties.[157,158] Tea drinking appears to have beneficial effects on bone, with several studies linking tea consumption to modest increases in BMD.[158,159]

Mind-Body Connection

Chronic stress, through activation of the sympathetic nervous system, tends to exert catabolic effects on the body that result in the breakdown of energy stores and body tissues. In animal studies, both chronic stressors and the administration of glucocorticoids have been shown to stimulate bone resorption.[160,161] Major depression[162] and anorexia nervosa[163] are both associated with elevated serum cortisol levels and increased bone loss. Increased sympathetic nervous system activity stimulates resorption of bone by osteoclasts and inhibits bone formation by osteoblasts.[164]

Stress reduction, using mind-body practices, such as meditation, self-hypnosis, guided imagery, breath work, or biofeedback, is highly recommended as part of an integrative plan to support bone health and overall well-being.

Exercise

In addition to high-quality nutrition, exercise is the other major factor required to build and maintain strong bones. Bone is a dynamic tissue that responds to physiological and biomechanical signals. Both general physical activity and mechanical loading contribute to building peak bone mass, beginning in the prepubertal years.[165,166]

Bone density at all skeletal sites is strongly correlated with muscle mass, and muscle mass is strongly linked to physical activity.[167] Muscle mass generally increases until approximately the age of 30 years and begins to decline after 50 years of age. Muscle strength losses tend to be most striking after the age of 70 years. However, regular exercise at any age, even in very old persons, can result in increased muscle strength, balance, and functional capacity.[168,169]

Exercise training programs in premenopausal and postmenopausal women have been consistently shown to prevent or reverse bone loss in both the lumbar spine and the femoral neck.[170] The Bone Estrogen Strength Training (BEST) Study found that postmenopausal women who received 800 mg/day of calcium citrate, along with a structured exercise program, increased their muscle mass by 11% to 21% and BMD by approximately 2%.[171] Even women with established osteoporosis can improve their bone mass with a low-impact exercise program.[172] Fracture risk can also be decreased with exercise programs. Walking for at least 4 hours per week has been found to decrease hip fracture risk by 41%.[173] A separate study of postmenopausal women found a reduced risk of vertebral fractures after a 2-year program of back-strengthening exercises.[174]

In the Senior Fitness and Prevention (SEFIP) study, 246 women older than 65 years were randomized to an 18-month exercise program or a wellness program. Participants in the exercise program demonstrated an increase in BMD at the spine of 1.77% (compared to an increase of 0.033% in controls) and at the femoral neck of 1.01% (compared to a decrease of 1.05% in controls). Further, fewer falls occurred in the exercise group (1.0 per person compared with 1.66 in the control group) and health care costs were lower in the exercise group.[175] A meta-analysis of the effects of exercise on BMD concluded that "mixed loading impact" exercise is associated with significant increases in BMD at the lumbar spine and femoral neck.[176]

DOSAGE

Recommended physical activities include walking, gentle and vigorous aerobic exercise, jumping, running, weight training, and racquet sports. Ideally, individuals should aim for 30 to 45 minutes of exercise, five or more times per week. Weight training is best performed on alternate days. Tai chi may have a number of beneficial effects, including reducing fall frequency, improving balance and strength, and maintaining BMD.[177,178]

Substances That May Be Harmful to Bone Health

Sodium

The mean sodium intake in the US (3500 mg/day) exceeds the recommended intake of <2400 mg/day, and high salt diets are known to increase urinary calcium excretion.[63] The DASH II diet (Dietary Approaches to Stop Hypertension and Sodium Reduction), which included 9.5 servings of fruits and vegetables per day, low fat dairy products, whole grains, and reduced meat and sodium intake, resulted in decreased calcium losses and reduced bone turnover.[179] The bone benefits of the DASH II diet appear to be related to its overall dietary composition rather than to a reduction in sodium intake per se. Increasing calcium and potassium intakes can substantially offset the urinary losses of calcium caused by high sodium intakes.[64] However, a high sodium intake along with a low calcium intake may lead to detrimental effects on bone health.[180] Because many individuals do not obtain adequate calcium in their diets, patients should be advised to stay within the recommended sodium intake of <2400 mg/day.

Caffeine

Some studies have found that excessive caffeine intake is associated with a modest increase in the risk of osteoporotic fracture.[65] The increased risk appears to occur in women who consume >300 mg of caffeine/day or approximately 4 cups of coffee and who also have a low calcium intake. Individuals with optimal calcium intakes should not experience any negative effects of moderate intake of caffeinated beverages on bone health.[181] Furthermore, a study that followed over 60,000 women for 20 years found that those drinking 4 or more cups of coffee per day had slight decreases in BMD but no increased fracture risk.[182] Accordingly, although it is prudent to avoid excessive intake, caffeine does not appear to be a major risk factor for bone disease.

Vitamin A

Vitamin A (retinol) intakes of >5000 mcg/day have been associated with an increased risk of hip fracture[183]; however, more recent data has failed to confirm this effect. An intervention study found no increase in fracture risk among more than 2000 adults who took a controlled, high-dose retinol supplement (25,000 IU retinyl palmitate/day) for up to 16 years.[184]

Smoking

Cigarette smoking is an independent risk factor for low BMD and the negative effect increases with amount and duration of smoking.[185] Smoking also has negative effects on bone health unrelated to BMD.[186] The effect of smoking on fracture risk may be related to lower body mass, earlier age of menopause, estrogen-lowering effects, impaired calcium absorption, or increased production of free radicals.[187] In the Nurses' Health Study, smokers had a relative risk of 1.2 for hip fracture, and this figure rose to 1.4 for those who smoked ≥ 25 cigarettes/day.[188] A meta-analysis involving >59,000 men and women found that smokers have a relative risk of 1.13 for any fracture and a relative risk of 1.6 for hip fractures.[189] Clearly, for many reasons, men and women should be encouraged not to begin smoking. Current smokers who quit will obtain benefits related to bone health after a period of 10 years.[188]

Alcohol

Animal studies showed that chronic heavy alcohol consumption, particularly during adolescence and young adulthood, can significantly damage bone health.[190] On the other hand, low or moderate consumption of alcohol in adulthood appears to have protective effects on bone health.[191,192] Moderate alcohol consumption has recognized cardiovascular benefits[193] but can also increase the risk of breast cancer in women[194] and has other potentially detrimental effects on health.[195] Men may benefit from a daily alcoholic beverage, whereas women should be advised to have fewer than seven alcoholic drinks per week.

Pharmaceuticals

Osteoporosis is best approached with a lifelong, comprehensive prevention program. Women of all ages should be informed of the diet and lifestyle choices listed previously to support bone health, with secondary causes of osteoporosis corrected whenever possible. In addition, pharmacological therapy may be recommended for the prevention or treatment of osteoporosis. Guidelines for initiating therapy currently vary between organizations. The 2010 North American Menopause Society (NAMS) guidelines recommend treatment in postmenopausal women:

* with prior vertebral or hip fracture
* with hip or spine T-scores lower than –2.5
* and with T-scores between –1.0 and –2.5 and a FRAX score that indicate a 10-year hip-fracture risk of ≥3% or an overall osteoporotic risk of ≥20%[196]

The number needed to treat (NNT) is a useful communication tool for discussing the benefit and potential risks of medications. The NNT for osteopenia or osteoporosis depends on the degree of risk for a fracture. This number is especially instructive in osteoporosis because the NNT to prevent one fracture in low risk women tends to be quite high. A useful clinical tool comes from the physicians who created thennt.com. Their review of the literature led to a recommendation against bisphosphonate preventive therapy for women without a history of fracture or very low BMD because no fractures were prevented over a 3-year period and side effects occurred.[197] The same authors recommended the use of bisphosphonate therapy for women with a prior history of fracture or very low bone density. The NNT was 20 to prevent a vertebral fracture and 100 to prevent a hip fracture in the latter group.[198] NNT allows a frank and specific discussion of the potential usefulness of pharmaceuticals for preventing osteoporosis. When the NNT is high or when the number needed to harm (NNH) is low, women with a preference for taking fewer medications or addressing health challenges with a more natural approach may decide to use lifestyle measures and reassess prior to, or instead of, taking a medication.

Role of Estrogen

Bone loss accelerates as estrogen levels fall in the years following menopause. The primary action of estrogen on bone is to inhibit osteoclast activity by increasing the amount of osteoprotegerin produced by osteoblasts.[199] Estrogen also has antiinflammatory effects and suppresses the production of bone-resorbing cytokines. Consequently, at the time of menopause, the concentration of inflammatory cytokines involved in the induction of osteoclastogenesis rises.[200]

Postmenopausal hormone therapy (HT) has beneficial effects on bone, reduces the risk of colon cancer, and can alleviate hot flashes and vaginal dryness. Conversely, women who use HT have an increased risk of cardiovascular disease, stroke, thromboembolic events, and breast cancer.[201] In the WHI trial, women receiving HT with conjugated equine estrogen, either alone or with medroxyprogesterone acetate, had increased BMD and lower fracture rates.[201]

The dose of HT required to enhance bone health without increasing the risks of other diseases remains unknown. For example, a 2-year randomized controlled trial (RCT) of 417 postmenopausal women who received transdermal estradiol at a dose of 0.014 mg per week compared to placebo reported that the active group had increased lumbar and hip bone density as compared to the placebo group. Bone turnover markers were reduced and endometrial hyperplasia was not increased by HT in this study.[202] Because long-term studies of ultra-low dose transdermal estradiol have not been performed, the associations with breast cancer and heart disease are unknown. The NAMS acknowledges the aforementioned limitations of long-term HT and recommends the use of the lowest effective dose possible.[203] The United States Preventive Services Task Force recommends against using HT to prevent chronic disease.[204] Clearly, the use of HT should be individualized based on a careful exploration of the risks and benefits for individual patients.

Bisphosphonates

Bisphosphonates are indicated for both the prevention and treatment of postmenopausal osteoporosis. As an antiresorptive therapy, bisphosphonates reduce fracture risk by inhibiting the activity of osteoclasts and reducing bone turnover, thus increasing bone mass. The most common side effects of bisphosphonates are dyspepsia, nausea, esophagitis, and abdominal pain. Rare but serious adverse effects include atypical femur fractures, esophageal cancer, and osteonecrosis of the jaw. Vitamin D and calcium status should be assessed and addressed prior to initiating the administration of bisphosphonates.

FDA-approved bisphosphonates for the prevention and/or treatment of osteoporosis in the United States include alendronate (Fosamax, Fosamax Plus D), risedronate (Actonel, Actonel with Calcium, Atelvia), etidronate (Didronel), ibandronate (Boniva), and zoledronic acid (Zometa, and Reclast). They are variably dosed daily, weekly, monthly, or yearly, and either orally or intravenously.

Alendronate was the first bisphosphonate studied for osteoporosis, and it has been shown to increase BMD and reduce the incidence of fractures of the spine and hip in women with osteoporosis.[205-207] The usual dose range of alendronate is 35 mg (for prevention) to 70 mg (for treatment) once weekly. Risedronate was studied in two large trials and was shown to increase BMD and reduce vertebral and some nonvertebral fracture rates.[208,209] The usual dose of risedronate is 35 mg once weekly. Ibandronate is convenient in that it may be given as a once-per-month dose of 150 mg, with two studies supporting its use.[210,211] Ibandronate has not been demonstrated to reduce nonvertebral fractures. Of the three oral forms, alendronate has the lowest 3-year NNT for the prevention of vertebral fractures (NNT = 15; Tables 36.4 and 36.5).

Zoledronic acid is an intravenous form of bisphosphonate approved for postmenopausal osteoporosis. The usual dose is 5 mg once a year. Patients find the annual dosing to be more convenient, and it minimizes the gastrointestinal side effects common with oral bisphosphonates. However, intravenous administration is associated with acute phase reaction symptoms, such as myalgia, arthralgia, fever, mild headache, and flu-like symptoms. Zoledronic acid has been found to increase BMD and reduce hip and vertebral fractures.[212]

The choice of bisphosphonate depends on multiple clinical factors as well as patient preferences.[213] If hip fracture prevention is of primary concern, current evidence is strongest for alendronate and zoledronic acid. Annual intravenous administration is associated with better compliance and is preferred by many women over weekly oral administration.[214] Atelvia need not be taken on an empty stomach, easing its administration. In women with high risk of breast cancer, raloxifene (discussed in the following) may represent the most appropriate choice.

The optimal length of bisphosphonate treatment has become clearer since the Fosamax Fracture Intervention Trial Long-Term Extension (FLEX) trial which reported no difference in vertebral fractures between women who continued alendronate for 10 years and those who stopped treatment after 5.[215] The FDA recommends that some patients may be able to stop bisphosphonates after 3–5 years and maintain the benefits of treatment.[216]

Selective Estrogen Receptor Modulators

Selective estrogen receptor modulators (SERMs) act as estrogen agonists or antagonists depending on the tissue. Raloxifene, a second-generation SERM, has been shown to be an estrogen agonist in bone and liver, maintain bone density, and lower LDL cholesterol. It does not stimulate the endometrium and is a potent estrogen antagonist in breast tissue. It has been studied for the prevention and treatment of osteoporosis.[217-220] The 3-year NNT to prevent vertebral fractures is 16 for women with a history of prior fracture and 46 for women at increased risk.[221] Raloxifene also significantly reduces the risk of breast cancer and improves lipid profiles. The usual dose of raloxifene is 60 mg/day. Side effects include hot flashes, deep vein thrombosis, and pulmonary embolism.

Bazedoxifene is a third generation SERM that has been studied and approved for osteoporosis. Bazedoxifene is an agonist in bone and lipid metabolism and an antagonist in breast and endometrium. It has been shown to prevent both vertebral and nonvertebral fractures.[222]

TABLE 36.4 Vertebral Fracture Prevention Studies

Medication	Dose	3-year NNT to Prevent Vertebral Fracture	Trial
Alendronate (Fosamax)	5 mg/day for 2 yr then 10 mg/day	15/34	FIT
Ibandronate (Boniva)	2.5 mg/day or 20 mg eod for 12 doses every 3 months	21	BONE
Risedronate (Actonel)	2.5 or 5 mg/day	20	VERTA-NA
Zoledronic acid (Reclast)	5 mg IV every yr	14	HORIZON
Raloxifene (Evista)	60 mg/day	46/59 (no prior fracture) 16/10 (with prior vertebral fracture)	MORE
Denosumab	60 mg sq every 6 months	21	FREEDOM
Teriparatide (Forteo)	20 mcg sq/day	12	—

BONE, oral iBandronate Osteoporosis vertebral fracture trial in North America and Europe; eod, every other day; FIT, Fracture Intervention Trial; HORIZON, Health Outcomes and Reduced Incidence with Zoledronic Acid Once Yearly; IV, intravenously; MORE, Multiple Outcomes of Raloxifene Evaluation; NNT, number needed to treat; VERTA-NA, Vertebral Efficacy with Risedronate Therapy-North America.
From Ringe JD, Doherty JG. Absolute risk reduction in osteoporosis: assessing treatment efficacy by number needed to treat. *Rheumatol Int.* 2010;30(7):863-869.

TABLE 36.5 Hip Fracture Prevention Studies

Medication	Dose	NNT to Prevent a Hip Fracture	Trial
Alendronate	5 mg/day for 2 yr then 10 mg/day	91	FIT
Risedronate	2.5 or 5 mg/day	91	HIP
Zoledronic acid	5 mg IV/yr	91	HORIZON

FIT, Fracture Intervention Trial; HIP, Hip Intervention Program; HORIZON, Health Outcomes and Reduced Incidence with Zoledronic Acid Once Yearly; IV, intravenously; NNT, number needed to treat.
From Ringe JD, Doherty JG. Absolute risk reduction in osteoporosis: assessing treatment efficacy by number needed to treat. *Rheumatol Int.* 2010;30(7):863-869.

Side effects include hot flashes and leg cramps in addition to venous thromboembolism, a more serious complication. In the United States, bazedoxifene is currently only available in combination with conjugated estrogen for use in preventing postmenopausal osteoporosis.

Calcitonin

Calcitonin is produced by thyroid C cells and acts to inhibit bone resorption by inhibiting osteoclast activity. Calcitonin from salmon was initially approved by the FDA in 1984 to treat osteoporosis in women and is effective in reducing the pain associated with acute compression fractures of the vertebrae. It may reduce the incidence of vertebral fractures. Side effects are usually minor and include flushing, nausea, and diarrhea. Recent data has revealed an increased risk of malignancy which will likely limit the applicability of calcitonin in the treatment of acute fracture pain.[200] Calcitonin is usually dosed as a daily intranasal spray of 200 IU.

Teriparatide

Teriparatide (PTH 1-34) is a medication that includes a sequence of the final 34 amino acids contained in parathyroid hormone. Teriparatide has anabolic effects on bone and stimulates bone formation in addition to bone remodeling. Two large trials, the Fracture Prevention Trial (n = 1637) and the Treatment of Osteoporosis with Parathyroid Hormone (n = 2532) reported a reduced incidence of vertebral and nonvertebral fractures in postmenopausal women following the use of teriparatide.[223,224] The European Study of Forsteo followed three groups of women for a second year of treatment. The women who received a second year of Teriparatide had further increases in bone density, those switched to raloxifene maintained bone density, and those switched to placebo had a reduction in bone density.[225] The 3-year NNT to prevent vertebral fractures was reported to be

12. Teriparatide is administered as a once-daily subcutaneous injection (20 mcg) for a period of up to 2 years, which may then be followed by an antiresorptive agent (in rats, osteosarcoma has occurred with longer treatment duration and higher doses). Side effects include nausea and headaches.

Denosumab

Denosumab is a human monoclonal antibody that binds to RANKL (receptor activator for nuclear factor kappa-B ligand), thereby blocking binding to RANK and inhibiting osteoclast activity, decreasing bone resorption, and increasing bone density. Prescribed at a dose of 60 mg subcutaneously every 6 months, denosumab has been FDA-approved for the treatment (but not prevention) of osteoporosis. The NNT from the Fracture Reduction Evaluation of Denosumab in Osteoporosis Every 6 Months (FREEDOM) trial, which randomized 7868 women, was 21.[226] Side effects include urinary and respiratory infections, cataracts, constipation, rashes, and joint pain. Rare but serious infections observed in the FREEDOM extension trial include osteonecrosis of the jaw and atypical fractures.[227] Because RANK and RANKL are members of the tumor necrosis factor superfamily, concern remains that inhibiting RANKL may increase the risk of cancer.

Pharmaceuticals to Avoid

Many pharmaceuticals can negatively impact bone density. Commonly prescribed medications with this effect include: antidepressants from the selective serotonin inhibitor class, antiseizure medications, breast cancer treatment (aromatase inhibitors and Tamoxifen), chemotherapeutic agents, gonadotropin releasing hormones used for fertility treatment or medroxyprogesterone acetate used for contraception, proton pump inhibitors, steroids, and any excess use of thyroid hormone.

PREVENTION PRESCRIPTION

Recommendations to build and maintain healthy bones:

- An antiinflammatory diet that includes an abundance of fruits and vegetables, healthy fats, whole grains, legumes, and antiinflammatory herbs, teas, and spices
- Adequate calcium intake from diet +/− supplements
- A serum 25-OH vitamin D concentration in the range of 40 ng/mL
- An intake of vitamin K1 and K2 equaling at least 90 mcg for women and 120 mcg for men
- A balanced ratio of omega-6 to omega-3 fatty acids
- Adequate but not excessive protein (0.8 g/kg), including some vegetarian protein sources

- One to two servings per day of whole soy foods
- A good-quality multivitamin and mineral supplement
- Physical activity for 30 to 45 minutes most days of the week that includes weight-bearing, aerobic, and weight-lifting exercise
- A daily mind-body practice
- Avoidance of smoking and avoidance of excess alcohol intake
- Reduction of the risk of falls and, if possible, avoidance of medications that harm bone or increase the risk of falls
- Pharmaceutical therapies that are individualized, with risk and benefits explored with each patient

THERAPEUTIC REVIEW

An integrative approach encompassing diet, exercise, supplements, and mind-body therapies, as well as pharmaceutical medications when indicated, is recommended to prevent and treat osteoporosis. The same strategies that help people build healthy bones will also protect them against heart disease, diabetes, depression, and a host of other chronic conditions.

LAB EVALUATION

- 25-hydroxy vitamin D level
- Dual x-ray absorptiometry bone scan
- Consider high sensitivity C-reactive protein, thyroid-stimulating hormone, calcium, and alkaline phosphatase.

LIFESTYLE

- Avoid first-hand and second-hand smoke exposure.

EXERCISE

- 30 to 45 minutes/day of aerobic, weight-bearing, and weight-lifting exercise (patients with osteoporosis should consult with a health professional to plan an appropriate, safe exercise program)

NUTRITION

- Limit sodium
- Antiinflammatory diet
- Calcium-rich diet (see Table 36.2)
- Adequate protein intake from plant sources more than from animal sources; one to two servings a day of whole soy foods
- Vitamin K–rich foods
- Tea *(Camellia sinensis):* 2 cups a day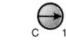

SUPPLEMENTS

- Vitamin D: 1000 to 2000 units/day

- Calcium citrate or carbonate as required such that total daily intake from diet, in addition to supplements, is at least 800 mg/day.
- Multivitamin and multimineral: minerals should include zinc, copper, magnesium, boron, and manganese.

MIND-BODY THERAPY

- Meditation, self-hypnosis, guided imagery, biofeedback, and breath work

PHARMACEUTICALS

Prevention

- For women with osteopenia alone, pharmaceutical treatment is no longer recommended due to NNH exceeding NNT.

Treatment

- Consider a bisphosphonate in women with a previous osteoporotic fracture, or a T-score between 1.0 and −2.5 and FRAX score with 10-year hip fracture risk of ≥3% or overall osteoporotic risk of ≥20%.
- Consider raloxifene in women who fail bisphosphonate therapy due to GI side effects and/or are also at increased risk of breast cancer (for nonvertebral fractures).
- Note: For hip fracture prevention, etidronate and ibandronate (bisphosphonates), and raloxifene (SERM) lack evidence of superiority compared to placebo.
- Consider teriparatide in patients who fail bisphosphonate therapy.
- Consider denosumab in patients who fail bisphosphonate therapy.
- Limit use of calcitonin to treat pain associated with vertebral compression fracture.

Key Web Resources

Bayer HealthCare BEST Strength Training. This is the website of the University of Arizona Center for Physical Activity and Nutrition. Detailed information is available on the Bone Estrogen Strength Training study. A training guide book and continuing education course is available.   http://cals.arizona.edu/cpan/

WHO Fracture Risk Assessment Tool. This tool can be used, with or without BMD, to predict fracture risk in various ethnic/racial groups in the USA (and many other countries).   https://www.shef.ac.uk/FRAX/tool.aspx

National Osteoporosis Foundation: This website provides detailed information for health care professionals and patients about osteoporosis prevention and treatment.   http://www.nof.org

Number Needed to Treat. This website provides evidence-based recommendations for and against medication using NNT and NNH.   http://www.thennt.com/

REFERENCES

References are available online at ExpertConsult.com.

CHAPTER 37

AN INTEGRATIVE APPROACH TO OBESITY

James P. Nicolai, MD • Junelle H. Lupiani, RD • Andrew J. Wolf, MEd

INTRODUCTION

More information on this topic can be found online at ExpertConsult.com.

PATHOPHYSIOLOGY

Definition of Overweight and Obesity

In 2004, obesity was reclassified by Medicare as a chronic disease. Obesity is characterized by an excess of body fat and is most often defined by the body mass index (BMI), a mathematical formula that correlates well with excess weight at the population level. The BMI is measured by taking weight in kilograms divided by height in meters squared (kg/m^2). Worldwide, adults with a BMI of 25 to 30 are categorized as overweight, whereas obesity is classified according to stages or grades (Table 37.1). Grade III obesity was formerly known as morbid obesity; however, the term was appropriately changed for several reasons: morbidity may not occur at a BMI higher than 40 but certainly can be found at BMIs lower than that. BMI can sometimes be inaccurate because it does not distinguish between fat and muscle, nor does it predict body fat distribution. On a population level, however, BMI does seem to track trends in adiposity as opposed to muscularity, and individuals with large muscle mass and resulting high BMIs are easily distinguishable from those with large amounts of adipose tissue.

In a clinical setting, the most valuable measurement strategy for classifying weight other than the BMI is waist circumference. The presence of extreme abdominal fat has been shown to be an independent risk factor for diabetes, high blood pressure, and cardiovascular disease.[6] Waist circumference is obtained by placing a measuring tape in a horizontal plane around the waist at the level of the umbilicus and the superior iliac crests.

Risk of obesity and associated diseases is increased if waist circumference is greater than 40 inches in male patients and greater than 35 inches in female patients.

In children, the term obesity is generally not used because of the potential prejudicial issues that may ensue when a child is labeled with such a title. As a result, being overweight in children is defined conservatively as being at or higher than the 95th percentile of age- and sex-adjusted weight. Children who are at the 85th to 94.9th percentile for weight are considered overweight. Increasing concern about the potentially high numbers of overweight children not classified correctly has prompted an ongoing initiative to revise the definition.

Obesity-Related Health Risk and Morbidity

The disease risk profile based on BMI and waist circumference is described in Table 37.2. Evidence shows that obesity is a proinflammatory state that increases the risk of several chronic diseases, including hypertension, dyslipidemia, diabetes, cardiovascular disease, asthma, sleep apnea, osteoarthritis, and several cancers.[7] Excess weight may also promote gallstone formation, fatty liver, gastroesophageal reflux, menstrual abnormalities, infertility, stress incontinence, gout, carpal tunnel syndrome, and low back pain.[8–12] Obese adults have more annual admissions to hospitals, more outpatient visits, higher prescription drug costs, and worse health-related quality of life than do adults of normal weight.[13]

More information on this topic can be found online at ExpertConsult.com.

Pathogenesis

The challenge with understanding the etiology and pathogenesis of obesity is that this condition is, ultimately, the result of a relatively straightforward series of outcomes (uncontrolled weight gain) achieved by a set of complex and dynamic interactions. The notion that obesity is a direct result of long-term mismatches in energy balance, with daily intake of energy greater than daily output, may not be true. The state of positive energy balance may not be due to too many calories in and not enough calories out, but may be a direct result of a complex set of interactions producing a multitude of genetic, hormonal, and metabolic signals that produce a state of fat storage versus fat burning.[23]

Calories encompass the value that determines this state of energy balance. We eat food, and various metabolic processes in our bodies break it down into energy. The relationship between energy and matter is under the control of the laws of physics, specifically the first law of thermodynamics, proved by Sir Isaac Newton, which states that all energy in the universe is conserved. In relation to food, when more energy is taken in by the body relative to the energy consumed, the surplus is ultimately converted into matter. This works well in a vacuum, but it may not be easily translated into the real world. Although energy intake is relatively determined by food and drink, with each having a particular caloric value, the nature of that matter can vary. Thus calories may not be equal and can translate into differing amounts of energy burned by the body over a fixed period of time. Although a pound of lead and a pound of feathers may drop in a vacuum at the same speed, when a similar experiment is conducted outside, air resistance causes the lead to drop like a stone and the feathers to float to the earth at a leisurely pace. Calories operate in a similar fashion. The calories you eat are absorbed at different rates and have different amounts of fiber, carbohydrates, protein, and fat, along with other chemicals and nutrients that may translate into different metabolic signals that affect the energy equation.[24] Consequently, if it is true that calories are not equal, calorie type may influence energy balance as much as amount. A study from the Harvard School of Public Health confirmed this to be true; overweight patients fed 300 more calories per day actually lost more weight than did their counterparts who were eating food of different composition.[25]

Whereas we are beginning to discover the inherent complexity on the left side of the energy equation (calories in), measuring energy output has always been a much more intricate calculation because of the complex interaction and number of variables that determine how calories are consumed. Energy output is expressed as the sum of various processes, including resting energy expenditure, basal metabolic rate, physical activity, rates of growth, and thermogenesis. Studies have confirmed that macronutrient distribution, endocrine factors, and diverse genetic predispositions may contribute important mitigating influences at any given level of calorie consumption.[2] We are also discovering that the vast microbiome of the gut may play a critical role in how these complex interactions are affected.[27]

Although the pathogenesis of obesity involves a set of complex multifactorial details to explain a relatively simple condition, what should not be forgotten is that human physiology is much the same as it has always been. The increase in obesity prevalence in the past few decades cannot be explained by changes in the human gene pool, but rather by environmental changes and their interactions with us that have not been seen previously in our collective history. An environment that promotes excess food intake of poor quality and discourages physical activity will most surely produce obesity in a species that has adapted itself to survive by responding to caloric scarcity within the confines of a world that demands a significant level of energy expenditure.[13]

TABLE 37.1 Adult Classification of Being Overweight

Classification	Body Mass Index (kg/m²)
Underweight	18.5
Normal weight	18.5–24.9
Overweight/preobese	25.0–29.9
Obese	
Class I	30.0–34.9
Class II	35.0–39.9
Class III	40.0 or higher

Adapted from the National Heart, Lung and Blood Institute, National Institutes of Health. *The Practical Guide: Identification, Evaluation, and Treatment of Overweight and Obesity in Adults.* NIH publication no. 00–4084. Bethesda, MD: U.S. Department of Health and Human Services, 2000.

TABLE 37.2 Classification of Overweight and Obesity and Associated Disease Risk

Classification[a]	BMI (kg/m²)	Obesity Stage	Disease Risk (Relative to Normal Weight and Waist Circumference)[b]	
			Waist Circumference — Men: up to 40 in. (up to 102 cm); women: up to 35 in. (up to 88 cm)	Waist Circumference — Men: more than 40 in.; women: more than 35 in.
Underweight	Lower than 18.5	—	—	—
Normal	18.5–24.9	—	—	—
Overweight	25.0–29.9	—	Increased	High
Obese	30.0–34.9	I	High	Very high
	35.0–39.9	II	Very high	Very high
Extremely obese	40.0 or higher	III	Extremely high	Extremely high

[a]For persons 20 years old and older.
[b]Disease risk for type 2 diabetes mellitus, hypertension, and cardiovascular disease. Increased waist circumference can be a marker for increased disease risk, even in persons of normal weight.
BMI, body mass index.
Adapted from World Health Organization. *Preventing and Managing the Global Epidemic of Obesity.* Report of the World Health Organization Consultation of Obesity. Geneva: World Health Organization; 1997.

Integrative Assessment

Ideally, assessment and treatment of obesity should be done within the setting of a multidisciplinary team designed to manage medical, nutritional, emotional, and exertional components of the desired lifestyle intervention—in this case, weight loss. This ideal setting is often unavailable or unrealistic, however, and in a primary care setting, an obesity management strategy can still be implemented successfully with simple interventions by a single practitioner. Initial goals should focus on modest weight loss of 5%–10% of total body weight over a 12- to 16-week period of time. Such weight loss has been shown in studies to improve blood glucose control in obese patients with type 2 diabetes.[28] Modest weight loss has also been found to prevent the progression of diabetes and cardiovascular disease in those obese individuals with impaired glucose tolerance and insulin resistance[29] (Table 37.3). Improvements can be seen in most obesity-related conditions,

from lipid disorders and hypertension to joint pain, muscle weakness, and lung function, after such a modest 5%–10% reduction in total weight.

An integrative assessment of obesity should include a thorough medical history and physical examination with anthropomorphic measurements, weight history, nutritional and dietary history, assessment of current and past physical activity, diagnostic laboratory evaluation, electrocardiogram (if considering weight loss medications), and screening for current levels of motivation, emotional status, availability of support systems, and potential barriers to treatment.

Current medications should be assessed for their potential promotion of weight gain. Psychiatric medications are notorious for contributing to weight gain and include antipsychotics, some antidepressants, and antiseizure medications. Other commonly used drugs that promote weight include long-acting steroid medications, some oral contraceptives, certain diabetic medications, and drugs for the treatment of blood pressure. A recent study reviewed several trials and summarized drugs associated with weight gain versus weight loss.[31] Weight-neutral alternatives are available and should be considered if weight loss is a priority (Table 37.4).

Weight history should assess the progression of weight gain over time to illustrate the use of any previous weight loss strategies, such as special diets, exercise programs, meal replacements, nutritional supplements, medications, or surgical procedures. The practitioner should understand how much weight was lost and over what period of time, what was the period of weight maintenance, and what promoting factors caused weight regain, if any. "Yo-yo" dieting, consisting of repetitive patterns of weight loss followed by weight regain, may provide information about previous successful strategies, as well as recurrent negative behavioral patterns.

Laboratory testing is an important adjunct to information obtained from a patient's history, and patients should be screened for obesity-related conditions, such as hypothyroidism, liver disease, metabolic syndrome, dyslipidemia, glucose intolerance, insulin resistance, diabetes, and, if

TABLE 37.3 Clinical Identification of Metabolic Syndrome

Risk Factor	Defining Level
Abdominal adiposity	Waist circumference
Men	102 cm (40 inches)
Women	88 cm (35 inches)
Triglycerides	150 mg/dL
HDL cholesterol	
Men	40 mg/dL
Women	50 mg/dL
Blood pressure	130/85 mm Hg or higher
Fasting blood glucose level	110 mg/dL or higher

HDL, high-density lipoprotein.
Third Report of the Expert Panel on Detection, Evaluation, and Treatment of High Blood Cholesterol in Adults (Adult Treatment Panel III): *National Cholesterol Education Program.* Bethesda, MD: National Institutes of Health; 2004. Adapted from National Heart, Lung and Blood Institute, National Institutes of Health.

TABLE 37.4 Medications Associated With Weight Gain

Drug Class	Medications That May Promote Weight Gain	Alternative Drugs That May Be Weight Neutral or Promote Weight Loss
Psychiatric/Neurological		
Antipsychotics	Olanzapine, clozapine, risperidone	Ziprasidone, quetiapine
Antidepressants	SSRIs, tricyclics, lithium	Bupropion, nefazodone
Antiepileptics	Valproate, gabapentin, carbamazepine	Topiramate, lamotrigine, zonisamide
Diabetes Agents	Insulin	Metformin, exenatide,[a] acarbose, miglitol, GLP-1 agonists
	Sulfonylureas	
	Thiazolidinediones	
Steroid Hormones	Hormonal contraceptives	Barrier methods
	Corticosteroids	NSAIDs
	Progestational steroids	
Miscellaneous Agents	Antihistamines	Decongestants, inhalers
	Alpha-antagonists, beta-blockers	ACE inhibitors, calcium channel blockers

[a]Incretin mimetic.
ACE, angiotensin-converting enzyme; NSAIDs, nonsteroidal antiinflammatory drugs; SSRIs, selective serotonin reuptake inhibitors.
Adapted from the North American Association for the Study of Obesity, Obesity Research, Stanford University Libraries, Stanford, CA.

suspected, polycystic ovarian syndrome (PCOS) and Cushing syndrome. Because obesity is a proinflammatory condition, the prudent approach may be to assess inflammatory markers, such as high-sensitive C-reactive protein. Serum 25-(OH) vitamin D levels should be obtained in light of research demonstrating the trend toward significant vitamin D deficiency and decreased bioavailability of vitamin D in the obese population.[32] Vitamin D deficiency is associated with muscle weakness, fatigue, and pain in bones, joints, and muscles, among other things. Normalizing vitamin D status in the obese population should be a priority.

Laboratory tests to consider in the evaluation of obesity include fasting blood sugar (100–125 mg/dL indicates prediabetes); triglycerides (high in metabolic syndrome); high-density lipoprotein (low in vitamin D deficiency); 25-hydroxyvitamin D; thyroid-stimulating hormone (hypothyroidism); cortisol, 8 a.m. spot, or 24-hour urine (Cushing disease); high-sensitive C-reactive protein (inflammation); and serum aspartate aminotransferase, alanine aminotransferase, and gamma-glutamyltransferase (steatohepatitis).

Dietary recall over the course of 1–2 days can provide an idea of food intake, eating patterns, and quality of choices. This approach is limited by the tendency of most people to underreport intake of food, as well as uncertainty about identifying a representative day of eating in an individual's typical routine. Various software programs and online tools are available for performing nutrient analyses of dietary records and for calculating calories, macronutrient and micronutrient profiles, fiber, essential fats, and sources of each. This information can be useful to provide to clients who are undergoing nutritional counseling.

Even when reports of food intake are underreported or somewhat inaccurate, however, viewing the amount of calories one consumes over a 24-hour period can often be surprising and revelatory to the individual who is unaware of portion sizes and the nutritional content of food. Providing patients with a visual illustration of this can be valuable.

Ultimately, for an intervention to be successful, it must closely match the individual's readiness to change. Commitment to such behavioral change is maximized when goals are self-selected and fit with personal lifestyle and values. Gaining clarity on these values is obtained through interactions that allow the practitioner to understand and appreciate the world of the client. Techniques such as motivational interviewing can provide primary care providers with the kinds of counseling tools they need to improve the likelihood that their patients will implement the suggested strategies[33] (see Chapter 101).

Interventions must match readiness to change. Commitment to behavioral change is maximized when goals are self-selected and fit with personal lifestyle and values. Patient ambivalence is universal and should be recognized and acknowledged. Doing so will encourage the patient to argue for, instead of against, change.

INTEGRATIVE THERAPY

In general, the primary clinical intervention for weight management involves lifestyle modification. This includes attention to levels of activity, nutrition, stress management, sleep, sexual activity, relationships, and motivation. Lifestyle modification should be part of any program addressing excess weight, regardless of BMI. More aggressive approaches that include weight loss medications, low-calorie diets with or without liquid meal replacements, and various methods of fasting require a BMI of 30 or higher without comorbidities or BMI of 27 or higher with the presence of one or more comorbid conditions. These strategies require frequent monitoring and, if implemented for longer than 3 months, should be administered by a medical professional trained in supervised weight loss strategies (i.e., a physician certified by the American Board of Bariatric Medicine). For patients who have given serious attempts to their weight loss without appropriate long-term results, surgical interventions should be evaluated as a viable option.

Therapeutic Counseling

Once the assessment has been made and initial treatment goals have been established, a regular visit schedule should be proposed and agreed on by the management team and patient. The more contact patients have with practitioners, the longer they will remain in a program and the greater potential they have to achieve and maintain their weight loss goals. Frequent visits with physicians and ancillary staff (dietitians, exercise physiologists or trainers, and counselors) are recommended and promote greater compliance, as do group support programs.[34-37] Behavioral and nutritional counseling can be conducted by physicians or dietitians and coded for using Current Procedural Terminology (CPT) codes for individuals (97802) or groups (97804). A minimum of one visit per month is encouraged, and weekly or twice-monthly visits are recommended. Programs offering combination visits with a physician followed by ancillary practitioners can allow for efficient delivery of information in a multidisciplinary fashion without having to extend doctor visits. Obese individuals with eating disorders or who have comorbid psychological conditions such as depression or anxiety should be provided with the opportunity for psychotherapy and other counseling by licensed mental health professionals.

Exercise

When consulting with someone who is interested in using exercise as a weight management tool, assessment is essential to setting attainable goals and creating an action plan. For sedentary individuals who are starting an exercise program, the initial goal is simply to start moving. Creating a habit of exercise or movement that emphasizes enjoyment and adherence is an important first step. During this phase, the intensity of exercise is not of paramount importance, but adherence to a modest volume of movement is. Even with modest amounts of movement, one can experience favorable functional changes in strength and endurance that can be a positive and encouraging first step. After a pattern of regular movement has been established and exercise tolerance has improved, the notion of increasing the frequency, duration, and intensity of activity becomes more realistic. Improvements to the thermoregulatory, muscular, and cardiovascular systems of the body operate synergistically to make higher intensities and longer durations more easily tolerated. Ratings of perceived exertion, pedometers, and heart rate monitors are all tools that can be used when making the transition to this next phase of exercise. Although this more detailed phase of exercise prescription is not absolutely needed for managing obesity, it can be very helpful. Exercise has only mild effects on resting metabolic rate, but exercise of sufficient intensity can alter aerobic capacity and improve an individual's capacity to burn calories. Given that most exercise bouts are limited to the 20- to 60-minute window, the productivity of an exercise session can be the key to success.

Aerobic capacity or Vo2max refers to the number of liters of oxygen that can be consumed per minute at maximal aerobic workloads. This workload has been traditionally expressed in terms of metabolic equivalents (METs) or in terms of milliliters of oxygen consumed per minute per kilogram (mL O2/min/kg). The more oxygen someone can consume per minute or the more METs they can produce per minute, the more calories they can burn. For example, two people seem identical on the surface. Both women are 55 years old, are 5 foot 4 inches tall (165 cm), and weigh 165 pounds (75 kg). Subject number 1 can produce 12.8 METs (45 mL O2/min/kg) during a treadmill test, whereas subject number 2 can produce 8 METs (28 mL O2/min/kg) during her treadmill test. Both women achieve maximal heart rates of 165 beats per minute at the end of the tests. Translated into exercise (30 minutes on a treadmill) at a comfortable heart rate for both women (127 beats per minute), the differences are substantial. Subject 1 will burn approximately 13.0 calories per minute for 30 minutes and 390 calories during the 30-minute exercise bout. Subject 2 will burn approximately 8 calories per minute and 240 calories for the 30 minutes. Having a very clear picture of what your clients' abilities are—even determining their aerobic capacity—before creating an exercise prescription is a powerful tool for anyone facilitating weight loss.

During a period of weight loss, clients will inevitably have some losses in lean mass, as well as losses in fat mass. Given the protein-sparing effects induced by resistance training, the addition of resistive muscular work makes sense. Full body exercise routines that engage as many muscles as possible not only save time but also can have beneficial effects on the hormonal response to resistance training.[38] A twice-weekly regimen is sufficient to produce these results.

Nutrition

Diet and its role in weight loss have been studied abundantly over the decades, with evidence to support restriction of calorie-containing macronutrients (carbohydrates, fats, and proteins) as an effective means of achieving weight loss.[39] However, further research suggests that macronutrient-restricted diets may be no better than overall calorie-restricted diets for achieving long-term results.[40-42] Moreover, dietary adherence, rather than type of diet, predicts the greatest success regarding weight lost over time.[43] These three points suggest that personal preference is an important consideration when tailoring individualized dietary interventions for successful weight loss. Assessment tools, such as 24-hour dietary recall and food frequency questionnaires, are important methods for identifying personal preference as a means of recommending dietary approaches to reduce calorie intake.

Popular Diets and Common Weight Loss Programs

Many people seek out recommendations from popular diets and common weight loss programs, most of which have minimal evidence or formal studies to show their effectiveness. However, evidence studying the efficacy of four popular diets (Atkins, Zone, Weight Watchers, and Ornish) for weight loss showed modest reduction in body weight. The study showed that increased adherence was associated with greater weight loss and cardiac risk factor reduction for each diet group.[44] This finding further supports individualized dietary interventions based on personal preference as an important factor in recommending therapy.

Although questions remain about long-term effects and mechanisms, data suggest that a low-carbohydrate, high-protein, high-fat diet may be considered a feasible alternative recommendation for weight loss.[45] Three popular examples are the Atkins diet, the South Beach diet, and the Zone diet. The Atkins diet focuses on eliminating the majority of carbohydrate sources with no modification of fat or protein calories. The South Beach diet offers a 2-week elimination of all carbohydrates followed by the addition of low-glycemic sources in moderate amounts. The Zone diet encourages physical activity, exercise, and hydration and limits carbohydrates. Another popular diet that achieves weight loss, by what is most likely calorie restriction, is the Ornish diet, predominantly a very low-fat vegetarian plan that combines dietary approaches with group support, stress reduction, and moderate exercise. Research from Stanford University in California studied the Atkins, Zone, LEARN (Lifestyle, Exercise, Attitudes, Relationships, Nutrition), and Ornish diets by specifically looking at macronutrient quality and concluded that weight loss diets focusing on macronutrient composition should attend to the overall quality of the diet, including the adequacy of micronutrient intakes. Concerning calorie-restricted diets, those providing moderately low carbohydrate amounts and containing nutrient-dense foods may have a micronutrient advantage.[45]

Each year, millions of U.S. residents enroll in commercial and self-help weight loss programs. Health care providers and their patients know little about the clinical utility of these programs because of the absence of systematic reviews. The University of Pennsylvania in Philadelphia performed an evaluation of major commercial weight loss programs in the United States (eDiets.com, Health Management Resources, Take Off Pounds Sensibly, Optifast, and Weight Watchers).

The outcome of the systematic review showed that use of the major commercial and self-help weight loss programs involved in the trial, with the exception of Weight Watchers, is suboptimal.[46] The study noted limitations related to lack of control for high attrition rates. The investigators also reported that many of the programs were associated with high costs and a high probability that participants will regain 50% or more of lost weight in 1–2 years. This study further supports the need for controlled trials to assess the efficacy and cost effectiveness of commercial weight loss interventions. Additional commercial programs that lack research but continue to gain popularity are Jenny Craig and LA Weight Loss. These programs, like Weight Watchers, provide weight loss services including prepackaged food, planned menus, and psychological support. The limitations are overall cost, sales promotions that encourage on-the-spot commitment to prepaid contracts, and the cost of food and additional vitamins.

In February 2011, the Department of Geriatrics and Metabolic Diseases in Naples, Italy, evaluated the effect of Mediterranean diets on body weight in randomized controlled trials using a meta-analysis. This research found that the Mediterranean diet could be a useful tool to reduce body weight, especially when it is calorie restricted, associated with physical activity, and followed for more than 6 months. The Mediterranean diet was not found to promote weight gain, a finding that removes the objection to its relatively high fat content.[47] This research further supports evidence suggesting that macronutrient-restricted diets may be no better than overall calorie-restricted diets in achieving long-term weight loss. Key components of the Mediterranean diet emphasize exercise, primarily plant-based foods (fruits, vegetables, whole grains, legumes, and nuts), olive oil and canola oil, two or more servings of fish and seafood weekly, and limitations on red meat (Fig. 37.1). The diet also recognizes the importance of enjoying meals with family and friends (see Chapter 88).

The antiinflammatory diet designed by Andrew Weil, MD, based on principles found in the Mediterranean diet, is not intended as a weight loss program, although people have found they have lost weight while adhering to it. General dietary recommendations include eating as much whole, fresh, and unprocessed food as possible (fruits, vegetables, whole and cracked grains, beans and legumes, nuts, avocados, and seeds), with an emphasis on variety of these foods. The diet also limits consumption of processed foods, "fast foods," and foods high in saturated fat sources. The elimination or significant limitation of these foods is most likely an important factor contributing to weight reduction. The diet is based on a 2000 calorie per day plan that provides adequate vitamins, minerals, essential fatty acids, dietary fiber, and protective phytonutrients. At this point, no research has been conducted to study the effects on weight loss associated with the Weil antiinflammatory diet.

Ultimately, dietary restriction as a management strategy for weight reduction can often be used as a sole

MEDITERRANEAN DIET PYRAMID

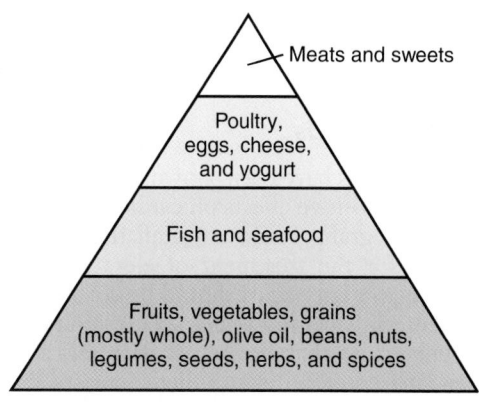

Food groups	Guidance
Meats and sweets	Less often
Poultry, eggs, cheese, and yogurt	Moderate portions, daily to weekly
Fish and seafood	Often, at least two times a week
Fruits, vegetables, grains (mostly whole), olive oil, beans, nuts, legumes, seeds, herbs, and spices	Base every meal on these foods

FIG. 37.1 ▪ **Mediterranean Diet Pyramid.** (From Oldways Preservation and Exchange Trust. www.oldwayspt.org; 2009. Accessed 04.08.11.)

intervention. Evidence suggests, however, that its use in combination with other strategies such as exercise, behavioral therapy, surgery, and pharmacological treatments may increase overall success.

> The best nutritional plan for weight loss is the one to which the patient will adhere.

Pre-Meal Water Loading

Preloading with 500 mL of water 30 minutes before a meal was reported to be associated with a mean weight loss of 2.4 kg after 12 weeks compared to the control group that imagined their stomach's being full 30 minutes before a meal, which lost 1.2 kg, a difference of 1.3 kg.

Those who used the water preload three times a day lost even more, 4.5 kg (~10 lbs) compared to those who only used it zero to one time a day (0.8 kg or 1.7 lbs).[48]

One could also add soluble fiber to the 500 mL of water. The fiber has the added benefit of soaking up water and expanding in the stomach, enhancing the effects of satiety. Fiber also binds to the carbohydrate of the meal, lowering the glycemic index of the foods eaten and also inhibiting the absorption of cholesterol. This is a low-cost, low-harm treatment for overweight patients with diabetes and elevated cholesterol. Examples of soluble fiber to add to the 500 mL of water would include 1–2 teaspoons of psyllium, oat bran, guar gum, ground flax seed, or methylcellulose.

Supplements

Omega-3 Fatty Acids

Omega-3 fatty acids have been shown in various studies to have significant positive effects on cardiovascular health.[49] They are an integral part of an antiinflammatory diet and are indicated for the treatment of elevated triglyceride levels.[50] Omega-3 fatty acids should be considered in the obese patient with cardiovascular comorbidities because clinical studies show that disease risk decreases as the ratio of omega-3 to omega-6 in the diet increases.[51] Supplements are available in prescription form as omega-3-acid ethyl esters under the trade name Lovaza. Omega-3 fatty acids have not been found to help with weight loss but may reduce risk associated with obesity.

DOSAGE

For improvement of cardiac disease risk, the recommended dose is 1–3 g daily, and the ratio of eicosapentaenoic acid (EPA) to docosahexaenoic acid (DHA) should be greater than 1. For the treatment of high triglyceride levels, the recommended dose is higher, at 2–4 g of combined EPA and DHA.

PRECAUTIONS

Individuals with allergies to fish or shellfish should use caution when taking fish oil. Omega-3 fatty acids have antiplatelet and antithrombin effects, which may cause bruising or may interact with additional blood thinning agents. However, the bleeding effects of fish oils taken alone have not been shown to be clinically significant even in large doses.[50] Side effects include a fishy aftertaste and mild gastrointestinal upset.

Vitamin D

Overweight individuals tend to have lower blood levels of vitamin D because excess adipose tissue absorbs and stores this fat-soluble vitamin. In addition, unlike normal-weight individuals who turn over fat tissue, those with relatively immovable fat stores cannot liberate the vitamin D they have. As a general rule, obese individuals are less active outdoors and are exposed to less ultraviolet radiation, a situation that compounds their vitamin D deficiency. Studies have validated that obese individuals tend to have significantly low levels of vitamin D, with symptoms of muscle weakness, muscle aches, bone pains, and fatigue, all of which are potential manifestations of vitamin D deficiency.[52] Additional research has validated the lower comparative bioavailability of vitamin D in obese individuals; they need more of it compared with nonobese subjects.[32] Higher levels of calcium in the presence of adequate serum vitamin D levels has been shown to inhibit fatty acid synthase, an enzyme that converts calories into fat, whereas diets low in calcium increase the enzyme activity by as much as five-fold.[53]

DOSAGE

First, the clinician should determine the patient's serum 25-hydroxyvitamin D levels. Recommended adequate blood levels of vitamin D are between 30 and 60 ng/mL.[54] Supplementation should be adequate to correct deficiencies if present. Obese individuals may need two to three times more vitamin D daily than those needed for normal weight, somewhere between 3000 and 6000 units daily, without posing any risk of toxicity.[53]

PRECAUTIONS

Gastrointestinal effects of larger doses of vitamin D have been reported. This effect may result from the gelatin capsule of prescription formulations and not the preparation itself. These symptoms may be remedied by opening the capsule and ingesting the liquid form. Vitamin D toxicity is often difficult to diagnose. This condition depends on blood levels of calcium (usually above 10.4 mg/dL) and occurs when 25-hydroxyvitamin D levels are usually higher than 200 ng/mL. Hyperphosphatemia and hypercalcemia that occur in vitamin D toxicity can cause constipation, confusion, depression, increased thirst, urination, and electrocardiographic changes, ultimately causing calcification of organs and tissues leading to damage and organ failure.[53]

Green Tea and Green Tea Extract

Animal studies suggested a fat-burning, weight loss, and cholesterol-lowering effect of green tea extracts. This effect seems to be synergistically improved with the addition of exercise. A small Asian study validated significant reductions in body weight, BMI, waist circumference, body fat mass, and subcutaneous fat area after 12 weeks of consuming one bottle of tea with 690 mg catechin antioxidants per day.[56] Another Japanese study found that green tea contains ingredients besides caffeine that stimulate thermogenesis and burn fat.[57]

DOSAGE

Studies found that fat-burning results occurred with tea containing 690 mg of catechins daily. Depending on the brand, the recommended dose consists of two to three cups of green tea per day (for a total of 240–320 mg polyphenols) or 100–750 mg per day of standardized green tea extract. Caffeine-free products are available.

PRECAUTIONS

One cup of green tea typically contains approximately 50 mg of caffeine as compared with 90–150 mg of caffeine for a percolated cup of coffee. Individuals with heart problems, kidney disorders, stomach ulcers, anxiety, and sleep disorders should not take green tea. When considering green tea, pregnant and breast-feeding women should consult their obstetricians.

Individuals who drink excessive amounts of caffeine for prolonged periods may experience irritability, insomnia, heart palpitations, and dizziness. Caffeine overdose can cause nausea, vomiting, diarrhea, headaches, and loss of appetite.

Probiotics

Although there is insufficient evidence available to confidently use probiotics to help with weight loss, there are interesting findings associated with nutrition, types of bacteria, and efficiency of energy storage that may guide future therapy.

A novel study of overweight and normal weight human twins showed that transplanting the stool of each resulted in remarkable changes when it was placed in sterile mice. Bacteria from the overweight twin caused mice to gain more weight. However, when that same strain of mice was fed a high fiber, low fat diet, the obesogenic effect of the stool transplant was negated. [58] This finding indicates nutrition consumed can influence the type of bacteria that grow in the gut, potentially reducing those that are associated with the most weight gain. Obesity is generally associated with more *Firmicutes* and less *Bacteroidetes*. *Firmicutes* are "hard to kill" bacteria with firm outer coats such as *H. pylori*.

The importance of establishing a healthy microbiome from a young age may also influence obesity rates later in life. Cattle are often given antibiotics to increase weight. A Finnish study found this also causes weight gain in humans. This study of 12,062 healthy children evaluated the frequency, age of administration, and type of antibiotics provided. There was a linear trend in weight with the number of antibiotic exposures and a younger age at which antibiotics were given.[27] As with cows, increased weight gain and height were observed, particularly in boys. Administering broad-spectrum antibiotics early and often to children may increase the risk of pediatric obesity (Fig. 37.2).

Caution for Supplements Used for Weight Loss

A study of emergency department visits for adverse events related to dietary supplements found that the most common visits were related to sympathomimetic side effects from weight loss supplements. The main side effects were palpitations, tachycardia, and chest pain. Most supplements used for these purposes contain ingredients that have stimulant properties.[59] Because many patients take these products as a "quick fix" with the impression of safety since a prescription is not needed to obtain them, they will often take excessive doses. Table 37.5 lists the most common ingredients of these products that the clinician should be aware of for patients who present with sympathomimetic side effects.

Common ingredients found in weight loss supplements can cause sympathomimetic side effects, including tachycardia, palpitations, and elevated blood pressure.

Mind-Body Therapy

Mind-body therapies, such as mindfulness and mindful eating programs, meditation, hypnosis, and biofeedback, are popular strategies used to facilitate weight loss plans with a specific target on emotional eating patterns. Stress reduction and improved emotional regulation can potentially allow individuals to make better food choices, feel fuller faster, and recognize abnormal eating habits.

TABLE 37.5	Supplements With Sympathomimetic Effects
Ma huang	This is the plant source of ephedra, which is banned in the US due to its numerous adverse effects.
Guarana	A plant source of caffeine. The seeds contain about 5% caffeine compared to a coffee bean, which contains about 1%.
Caffeine	Coffee bean, tea leaves *(Cemellia sinensis)*, yerba mate, kola nut.
Bitter orange	The peel and fruit contain adrenergic agonists, synephrine, and octopamine, which are similar to norepinephrine.
Hoodia	From a cactus that grows in the South African desert. Traditionally used to suppress appetite. Documented side effects include hypertension and tachycardia.
Ginseng	The three most common ginsengs are American, Panax, and Siberian. American is the most stimulating.

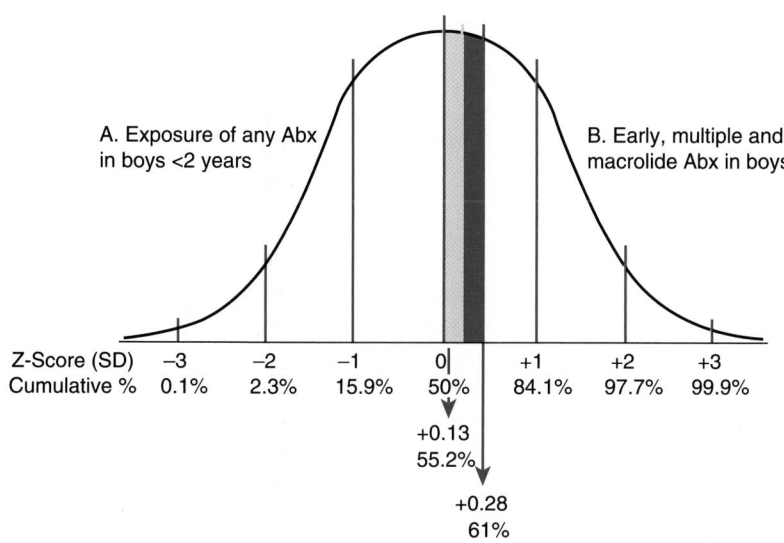

A. Exposure of any Abx in boys <2 years

B. Early, multiple and macrolide Abx in boys

Z-Score (SD)	−3	−2	−1	0	+1	+2	+3
Cumulative %	0.1%	2.3%	15.9%	50%	84.1%	97.7%	99.9%

+0.13
55.2%

+0.28
61%

FIG. 37.2 ■ A, Amount of weight gain associated with any antibiotic in boys aged <2 yrs (increase of 5.2%). B, Amount of weight gain associated with early and multiple antibiotics that included broad-spectrum macrolides (increase of 11%).

By accessing the parasympathetic nervous system more often, the balance of stress hormones, including epinephrine and cortisol, can be shifted in a positive direction. Studies have confirmed that stress-induced cortisol secretion is linked to abdominal obesity, endocrine abnormalities such as increased insulin, metabolic derangements in blood lipids, and hemodynamic changes in blood vessels.[60] Decreasing cortisol levels can aid in a positive strategy to address weight gain proactively.

Unfortunately, the available literature on these therapies in the obese population is relatively scarce. Preliminary studies have reported that mindfulness meditation can reduce episodes of binge eating and nighttime eating disorder.[61] Some studies investigating the role of biofeedback techniques and hypnosis in weight loss showed a mildly positive effect.[62] At present, recommending these strategies to the right individuals who are open to them seems prudent as an adjunct to an ongoing lifestyle management program.

Pharmaceuticals

Pharmacological treatment may be considered an adjunct to lifestyle modification in patients who have not lost at least 1.1 lb (0.5 kg) per week after 3–6 months of implementing their lifestyle program.[63] These medications are appropriate for patients with a BMI 30 or higher or 27 or higher in the presence of comorbid conditions. At present, two classes of drugs are used for weight control: (1) drugs that suppress appetite and augment thermogenesis (phentermine, topiramate, lorcarserin) and (2) drugs that prevent the absorption of fat through the gastrointestinal tract (orlistat). Recent combination medications have been FDA-approved for the treatment of obesity and have begun to be used in this patient population. However, the withdrawal of sibutramine by Abbott Laboratories from both the U.S. and European markets because of an increased risk of stroke and heart attacks has raised concern about the long-term effects of stimulant medications and prompted petitioning for higher standards of review and implementation for weight loss medications.[64]

Phentermine

Phentermine (Adipex-P) is a norepinephrine reuptake inhibitor with schedule IV identification (debated in some medical circles) that has been approved by the U.S. Food and Drug Administration (FDA) for short-term use (12 weeks) since 1959. Phentermine is the most commonly prescribed weight loss medication to date, probably because of its low cost, long history of use, and, contrary to popular belief, low addictive potential. To illustrate this point, the *Drug Abuse Warning Network (DAWN)* report, published in 2006 by the Substance Abuse and Mental Health Services Administration of the U.S. Department of Health and Human Services, showed that anorectics such as phentermine had among the lowest drug misuse or abuse rates per 100,000 emergency room visits, even lower than ibuprofen.[65] Unfortunately, many of the current guidelines for prescribing phentermine reflect recommendations that are more than 50 years old, rather than current evidence of efficacy and safety.[66] Because it

has a molecular structure similar to that of amphetamine, phentermine was originally labeled a schedule IV drug; however, over many decades of clinical use, phentermine has proved to have little to no addictive value, and no abuse or withdrawal syndromes are associated with its use.[65] Continuous use beyond 12 weeks is a common off-label use pattern in bariatric medicine and has validation in the international literature.[67] Putting time limits on medication use for the treatment of a chronic illness such as obesity seems inappropriate when (and only when) the risk of taking the medication is less than the risk of leaving the illness untreated. Weight loss during drug therapy should perhaps not be considered an indication to stop treatment any more than a positive outcome would be for the treatment of other chronic diseases. For this to happen, however, the long-term safety of agents must be assessed and documented in the literature.[68] The literature suggests the effectiveness of phentermine in helping patients lose weight and maintain weight loss for at least a year, if not longer.[69]

DOSAGE

Phentermine is often prescribed in doses of 15–37.5 mg once daily, typically in midmorning. It is occasionally prescribed in half doses given early in the morning then at midmorning, to extend its effects toward evening, when individuals tend to have higher calorie intake. Phentermine has been combined with topiramate (Qsymia) and offered in 3.75/23 mg (phentermine/topiramate), 7.5/46 mg, and 11.25/92 mg to be prescribed once daily and slowly titrated.

PRECAUTIONS

Side effects include insomnia, dry mouth, palpitations, hypertension, and constipation. When considering drug therapy with phentermine (or other stimulant medication), the clinician should conduct a careful review of medical history, drug interactions, and potential side effects. Evaluation of a recent electrocardiogram is recommended to assess cardiac health before administering medications with known stimulant effects, and aggressive regular monitoring (1- to 2-week visits) should be performed during initial treatment to assess vital signs and tolerance to therapy. Longer-term therapy should also prompt regular medical supervision with at least monthly visits.

Contrary to popular belief, phentermine has a low addiction potential.

Lorcarserin

Lorcaserin (Belviq) works as a serotonin 3C receptor agonist (whereas fenfluramine primarily acted as a 2B agonist) to increase food-specific receptors affecting satiety and satisfaction. A year-long study reported a weight loss of 7.3 kg with lorcaserin compared to the control group who lost 3.7 kg. Over 2 years, however, patients gained 25% of their weight back.[70] It is recommended to stop the drug if people fail to lose 5% of their weight after 12 weeks.

DOSAGE

Larcarsarin is prescribed in doses of 10 mg taken twice daily as part of a complete weight loss program including dietary and exercise modification. If using this drug with another serotonin agent, use extreme caution and careful observation.

PRECAUTIONS

Common adverse effects in nondiabetics include headaches, dizziness, fatigue, nausea, dry-mouth, and constipations. In patients with diabetes, side effects include low blood sugar, back pain, cough, and fatigue. There was concern that Belviq may cause heart-valve defects; however, according to research, there was no statistical difference in valvular disease between drug and placebo group at this dose. It is important to take precaution in patients with preexisting heart-valve abnormalities or CHF.

Orlistat

Orlistat (Xenical) works by inhibiting lipases in the gastrointestinal tract such that fat absorption is partially blocked. Orlistat is FDA approved for up to 2 years of continuous use, and it has been shown to be effective for significant and sustainable weight loss, as well as for improving lipid levels, enhancing glucose metabolism, and lowering blood pressure.[71] The discontinuation rate of orlistat is relatively high because of gastrointestinal side effects related to fat malabsorption and roughly equates to 33% in various studies.[72] In one study, lifestyle intervention and orlistat treatment for 4 years delayed the development of type 2 diabetes in obese subjects by 37%, a finding perhaps attributable, in part, to the weight loss achieved.[73] Orlistat is now available in half-strength (60 mg per dose) over-the-counter under the brand name Alli.

DOSAGE

Orlistat is prescribed in doses of 120 mg taken three times daily with meals, and the dose can be omitted when patients ingest a low-fat meal. Starting orlistat once daily with the fattiest meal (usually dinner) and then advancing the dose to three times daily as needed can help lessen the intensity and frequency of side effects.

PRECAUTIONS

Common adverse effects include bloating, flatulence, and fatty or oily stools. Oily spotting, increased fecal urgency or incontinence, and abdominal pain can also be experienced, especially when patients are noncompliant with a low-fat diet. Use of fiber supplements, especially psyllium, can be helpful in reducing side effects. Patients should also take a daily multivitamin, independently of orlistat, to compensate for the potential decreased absorption of fat-soluble vitamins (A, D, E, and K).

Pharmaceuticals for Combined Weight Loss and Type II Diabetes Mellitus

Metformin

Metformin (Glucophage) is indicated for the treatment of type 2 diabetes, but it has also been used off label for the treatment of insulin resistance syndromes, especially in PCOS. Studies have suggested a mild weight loss effect in abdominally obese women with PCOS.[75] Metformin has also been shown to promote weight loss in morbidly obese children and in men with normoglycemic hyperinsulinemia.[76]

DOSAGE

500 mg twice daily. Increase to 1000 mg bid.

PRECAUTIONS

Avoid in those with renal failure as metformin can increase the risk of metabolic acidosis. GI intolerance, including cramping and diarrhea, is the most common side effect.

Liraglutide

Liraglutide is a glucagon-like peptide-1 (GLP-1) hormone that is secreted after a meal. Because it is released by eating food, GLP-1 increases insulin to store energy, reduces glucagon to shut down glucose production by the liver, and slows gastric emptying. Mimicking the effects of this hormone with GLP-1 agonists lowers glucose and can result in weight loss by making people feel full and less hungry. Liraglutide does not affect metabolic energy expenditures. Liraglutide is one of the few diabetes medicines that have also been approved for treating obesity.

DOSAGE

The amount of weight loss and severity of side effects was reportedly dose dependent, with greater amounts of both with the 3.0 mg dosing. However, there was no significant difference in HbA_1C changes between the 3.0 mg and 1.8 mg dosing (0.19% difference). Accordingly, if liraglutide is being used mainly for diabetes control, the dosing of 1.8 mg will likely achieve the sweet spot of least side effects with the most reduction in HbA_1C. However, if it is being used to achieve the most weight loss, titrating up to 3.0 mg would be more likely to achieve this goal. Start at 0.6 mg subcutaneously daily and increase by 0.6 mg every week until you achieve the desired dose, which would be 3 weeks to achieve 1.8 mg and 5 weeks to achieve 3.0 mg.

PRECAUTIONS

As one might expect through its mechanism of action, gastrointestinal intolerance is the main concern with liraglutide. The most common symptom, nausea, is dose dependent, which may explain how it influences weight loss. The other most common side effects are vomiting, dyspepsia, diarrhea, constipation, and abdominal pain. In a study of 846 subjects following for 56 weeks, there were no cases of pancreatitis; however, elevations of serum amylase and lipase levels were common and resolved with discontinuation of the drug.[77] There was a rebound weight gain when the medicine was stopped in the above study and long-term side effects of treatment were not evaluated. In animal studies, liraglutide has been found to increase the risk of thyroid cancer, and there is a concern regarding an increased risk of colorectal cancer. Longer studies are needed to establish the safety of liraglutide with chronic use.

Combination Pharmaceuticals for Weight Loss

Combinations of phentermine with topiramate (Qsymia) and bupropion with naltrexone (Contrave) have been recently approved for weight loss treatment, with studies validating their effectiveness in reducing HbA₁C levels modestly (Table 37.6). Bupropion (Wellbutrin) is a norepinephrine and dopamine reuptake inhibitor that is approved for the treatment of depression and has been shown to have a dose-dependent weight-loss effect in a double-blind, placebo-controlled study. In this study, 83% of patients achieved weight loss of more than 5% of initial body weight when they took 400 mg/day of sustained-release bupropion as compared with 59% of subjects taking 300 mg/day and 46% treated with placebo.[78] Topiramate (Topamax) is an antiepileptic drug that has shown positive weight loss effects during clinical trials in smaller doses than achieved for seizure control.[79]

Surgery

Bariatric surgery is well established as the most effective treatment for obesity; however, it is indicated only for the management of severe obesity, with or without comorbidities, when other therapies have been tried without long-term success.[80] Surgical interventions are currently indicated for patients with a BMI of 40 or higher or 35 or higher with comorbid conditions and reduced quality of life (i.e., hypertension, sleep apnea, or diabetes). Typically, reimbursement for surgical procedures will be granted only after at least a 6-month trial of medically supervised weight loss.

Bariatric surgery rapidly evolved with the advent of laparoscopic approaches in the mid-1990s. Currently, most bariatric surgery is initially attempted in laparoscopic fashion. Surgical weight loss falls into the category of restrictive procedures, malabsorptive procedures, or a combination of the two. Strictly malabsorptive procedures such as jejunoileal bypass and duodenal switch are seldom performed. Purely restrictive procedures include the vertical banded gastroplasty (rarely performed these days), adjustable gastric banding, and vertical sleeve gastrectomy (an emerging procedure). The Roux-en-Y gastric bypass, involving restriction of stomach size along with bypassing a large part of the stomach and duodenum, is an example of a combined restrictive and malabsorptive procedure. Roux-en-Y gastric bypass is still the most popular procedure; however, restrictive techniques are beginning to emerge as competitive procedures that are less invasive and have fewer side effects.

A Cochrane Review compared different surgical procedures, all of which were found to be more effective in promoting weight loss than were nonsurgical methods.[81] Roux-en-Y gastric bypass was more effective than laparoscopic adjustable gastric banding and just as effective as vertical sleeve gastrectomy. Weight loss of up to 33% has been maintained after gastric bypass surgery for up to 10 years, with loss of 50% or more of excess weight achieved with either of the procedures, again an outcome superior to that of nonsurgical approaches.[81] In addition, resolution of comorbidities is often common. Meta-analyses have demonstrated complete resolution of type 2 diabetes in 31%–77% of patients who underwent laparoscopic banding and in 72%–100% of patients who underwent Roux-en-Y bypass.[82] Similar resolution of blood pressure abnormalities has been verified. A Swedish study demonstrated a substantially reduced 10-year mortality rate with bariatric surgery as compared with nonsurgical treatment of obesity.[83]

Bariatric surgery is typically safe, with surgical mortality approaching as low as 0.1%–0.3%, whereas postoperative complications occur in 4%–10% of patients.[84,85] Emerging evidence indicates that bariatric surgery may

---

TABLE 37.6 New Weight Loss Medications and Diabetes

Drug	MOA	↓HbA1C vs. Control	Dose	SE
Phentermine/ Topiramate (Qsymia)	↓Appetite, ↑leptin	0.4%[a]	3.75/23 mg daily × 14 days then 7.5/46 mg daily	Paraesthesia, constipation, dry mouth, insomnia
Lorcaserin (Belviq)	↑Satiety through serotonin activation	0.5%[b]	10 mg bid	Headache, URI, nasopharyngitis, dizziness
Orlistat (Xenical)	↓Fat absorption	0.3%[c]	120 mg with each meal, tid	Oily diarrhea, flatulence, vitamin malabsorption
Bupropion/Naltrexone (Contrave)	↓Appetite, ↑energy expenditure, ↓cravings	0.5%[d]	90/8 mg/d × 1 week, ↑ by one tablet each week until two tablets bid by week 4	Nausea, constipation, headache, dizziness

URI, upper respiratory tract infection.

These medicines are indicated for obesity with a BMI ≥30 or a BMI ≥27 in those with a comorbidity of type II diabetes mellitus, hypertension, or dyslipidemia.

[a]Garvey WT, Ryan DH, Bohannon NJ, et al. Weight-loss therapy in type 2 diabetes: effects of phentermine and topiramate extended-release. *Diabetes Care.* 2014;37(12):3309-3316.

[b]O'Neil PM, Smith SR, Weissman NJ, et al. Randomized placebo-controlled clinical trial of lorcaserin for weight loss in type 2 diabetes mellitus: the BLOOM-DM study. *Obesity.* 2012;20(7):1426-1436.

[c]Miles JM, Leiter L, Hollander P, et al. Effect of orlistat in overweight and obese patients with type 2 diabetes treated with metformin. *Diabetes Care.* 2002;25(7):1123-1128.

[d]Hollander P, Gupta AK, Plodkowski R, et al. Effects of naltrexone sustained-release/bupropion sustained-release combination therapy on body weight and glycemic parameters in overweight and obese patients with type 2 diabetes. *Diabetes Care.* 2013;36(12):4022-4029.

be beneficial for patients with BMIs lower than 35 and comorbidities; however, it is still too early to recommend surgery to such individuals.[86]

Individuals considering bariatric surgery require thorough preparation for the effects of such a procedure on their long-term lifestyle. This preparation should be facilitated by a multidisciplinary team of surgical and nonsurgical practitioners. Coordination of treatment has been cited as one of the most important advances in the care of patients undergoing these surgical procedures.[87] Postoperative challenges include malabsorptive nutritional deficiencies, dumping syndrome that involves profuse diarrhea and stomach pain after overeating refined carbohydrates in patients who underwent bypass procedures, changing dietary patterns to accommodate effects of the procedure, and the physical and emotional changes that occur when experiencing large amounts of weight loss.

Regular access to behavioral experts is essential for patients as they lose weight. Often, maladaptive patterns of eating are a defense mechanism used by patients to deal with elevated levels of emotional stress. When those options are eliminated by a surgical process, the potential for other patterns of behavior to emerge is evident. Having a management strategy to support patients through these psychological adaptations and providing them with proactive alternatives to stress response other than with food can create life-changing opportunities.

PREVENTION PRESCRIPTION

- The basis for prevention of weight gain is learning how to follow an antiinflammatory diet that emphasizes vegetables and fruits from all parts of the color spectrum, whole grains, fish and other sources of omega-3 fatty acids, vegetable protein more than animal sources, monounsaturated fats, and low-fat dairy. To make this a long-term lifestyle change, fruits, vegetables, and high-fiber grains must be used to displace high-calorie processed foods of poor nutritional content (see Chapter 88).
- Fostering a healthy relationship with food and becoming aware of reactive, habitual patterns of eating are vital to preventing weight gain. Learning techniques of mindful eating can facilitate this process.
- Physical activity may play a role in the prevention of weight gain[93]; 30 minutes/day, 5–7 days/ week of any physical activity should be encouraged (see Chapter 91).

THERAPEUTIC REVIEW

All patients should undergo the following assessments. Appropriate therapy can then be determined.

MEDICAL HISTORY

- Assess for comorbid diseases and concomitant medications that induce weight gain.

NUTRITION HISTORY

- Determine previous weight loss attempts and use 24-hour recall and food frequency questionnaires.
- Rule out clinically significant eating disorders (anorexia and bulimia nervosa, binge-eating disorder, nighttime eating syndrome).

ANTHROPOMETRIC MEASUREMENTS

- Weight, height, BMI, waist circumference, body composition, blood pressure, and heart rate

LABORATORY TESTS

- Complete blood count, metabolic profile, fasting lipids, thyroid-stimulating hormone, liver function tests, fasting serum glucose and insulin, hemoglobin A_1c (if diabetic), high-sensitive C-reactive protein, 25-(OH) vitamin D
- Electrocardiogram of starting medications with cardiac effects, unless a recent one (within 12 months) is available for review

GENERAL EVALUATION

- Assess for motivation, importance, and confidence for weight loss, barriers to change, and realistic weight loss goals.
- Assess exercise history, sleep patterns, relevant stressors, and social support.

THERAPEUTIC OPTIONS

BMI 25 or Higher

- Promote a balanced hypocaloric diet and physical activity, and provide behavioral modification counseling.
- Reduce caloric intake from baseline by 500–1000 cal/day to yield a 1- to 2-lb weight loss per week.
- Consider pre-meal water load of 500 mL with one teaspoon of a soluble fiber, such as psyllium, guar gum, ground flax seed, or methylcellulose.
- Encourage purposeful activity for at least 60 minutes daily 6–7 days of the week. Total time may be broken into short bouts of 10–15 minutes each during the initial adoption of an exercise program only.
- Stress management techniques including mind-body therapies, such as meditation, mindful eating, biofeedback, or hypnosis.
- Ensure adequate sleep and treatment of any concomitant sleep disorders.
- Suggest interactive individual or group support sessions for nutrition education and behavioral modification.
- Refer to a dietitian, mental health professional, or exercise specialist as needed.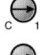

BMI 30 or Higher or 27 or Higher With Comorbid Conditions

- Full liquid fast, protein-sparing modified fast, and pharmacotherapy with dietary intervention are suitable for this BMI level.
- Orlistat, 120 mg orally three times daily, is the first option. This medication is localized to the gut and can be used in combination with phentermine.

- Phentermine can be taken alone (15–37.5 mg daily) or in combination with orlistat (approved for 3-month use by the Food and Drug Administration). **A**₂
- Suggest omega-3 fatty acids at 2–4 g/daily to manage risks associated with obesity. **A**₂
- Treat vitamin D deficiency appropriately to achieve serum 25-(OH) vitamin D levels between 40 and 60 ng/mL. **A**₂

- Other dietary supplements should be used, if at all, on an individualized basis determined by risk-to-benefit ratio and by evaluating the efficacy and safety of each product or combination. **B**₂

BMI 40 or Higher or 35 of Higher With Comorbid Conditions

- Weight loss surgery, if other treatment modalities are ineffective, is suitable for this BMI level. **A**₃

Key Web Resources

NutritionQuest assessment and analysis services: This company is a leader in the field of diet and physical activity assessment, and their Web site is the official source of the Block Food Frequency Questionnaire and other dietary and physical activity questionnaires developed under the guidance of Dr. Gladys Block. Block Assessment Tools are designed and tested for usability and have a long history of validation in various demographic subpopulations. These tools are available in both paper and electronic format.

http://www.nutritionquest.com/assessment

Basal metabolic rate calculator: This tool calculates how many calories your body requires each day.

http://www.calculator.org/calculate-online/health-fitness/basal-metabolic-rate.aspx

Mayo Clinic calorie calculator: This calculator includes individual activity in the calculation.

http://www.mayoclinic.com/health/calorie-calculator/NU00598

FitDay.com: This website allows you to track your nutrition and fitness goals online.

http://www.fitday.com/

The Center for Mindful Eating: This organization helps people learn how to use eating as a mindful process that brings awareness to what we are eating, thus leading to healthier food choices and reduced calorie consumption.

http://www.tcme.org/

REFERENCES

References are available online at ExpertConsult.com.

CHAPTER 38

MTHFR, HOMOCYSTEINE AND NUTRIENT NEEDS

Thomas G. Guilliams, PhD

The science of nutrigenetics defines the interrelationship between a person's genetics and their need for, or utilization of, a particular nutrient. As DNA sequencing and nutritional research have become more sophisticated in the past few decades, numerous clinically-relevant nutrigenetic relationships have come to light. Among the most well known are the various polymorphisms in the gene *MTHFR* that encodes the enzyme methylenetetrahydrofolate reductase (MTHFR) needed to synthesize the active form of folate.* In fact, it is likely that *MTHFR* polymorphisms are the most widely-studied of all nutrigenetic-related polymorphisms, the testing for which is now a common clinical practice. This chapter will not attempt to review the vast amount of published data related to the health risks associated with common MTHFR polymorphism (and other mutations).[1] Instead, after describing the biochemistry related to one-carbon metabolism and the role of MTHFR, we will discuss the utility of testing for common polymorphisms to quantify risk in subjects and discuss the available evidence for the use of nutrient supplements to modify a patient's risk based on their *MTHFR* genetics. We will especially focus on the data involving the supplementation of various folates (food folates, folic acid, folinic acid, and 5-MTHF) to reduce risk in patients related to *MTHFR* genetic status, especially as it relates to elevated homocysteine levels (Hcy).

PATHOPHYSIOLOGY

Methylenetetrahydrofolate Reductase— The Folate Activator

MTHFR is a key enzyme in the one-carbon metabolic pathway that regulates methylation via folate and homocysteine metabolism (Fig. 38.1).[2] Specifically, MTHFR catalyzes the reduction of 5,10-methylenetetrahydrofolate to 5-methyltetrahydrofolate (5-MTHF). MTHFR is a flavoprotein, which uses flavin adenine dinucleotide (FAD, a riboflavin derivative) as a cofactor and nicotinamide adenine dinucleotide phosphate (NAD[P]H, a niacin derivative) as an electron donor. This reaction is irreversible and provides the only endogenous source of 5-MTHF to the cell. The only known function of 5-MTHF is as a methyl donor in the conversion of homocysteine to methionine, a reaction catalyzed by the

enzyme methionine synthase using cobalamin (B12) as a cofactor.[3] Deficiencies in the MTHFR activity lead to reduced cellular availability of 5-MTHF, resulting in elevated serum or urine homocysteine levels.[4] The mechanisms by which MTHFR deficiency influences metabolic dysfunction and disease include the following:

- **Elevated homocysteine.** Elevated plasma total homocysteine (tHcy) is an independent risk factor (or marker) for a wide range of diseases.[5] There are many proposed mechanisms that implicate homocysteine in direct actions on a variety of tissues, although many researchers believe that homocysteine is simply a surrogate biomarker of folate status and/or kidney function and not directly involved in the progression of disease.[6] However, many of the clinical trials in which homocysteine-lowering therapies failed to improve event outcomes were in secondary-prevention populations prescribed a polypharmacy of CVD drugs prior to vitamin consumption (statins, 80%; aspirin, 88%; beta-blockers, 90%; and ACEI, 30%), had baseline tHcy levels below 13 μmol/L, or were unable to achieve posttreatment tHcy levels below 9 μmol/L.[7-9] A wide range of intervention trials have shown that homocysteine-lowering therapies in subjects with mild-to-moderate hyperhomocysteinemia can achieve statistically significant and clinically meaningful benefits.[10-13]

> In 358 older adults studied in a community cohort, those with a homocysteine levels ≥13 μmol/L were almost twice more likely to show decline in memory and global cognitive testing.[10]

- **Increase in the amount or ratio of other folate metabolites.** MTHFR deficiency leads to the likelihood of lower 5-MTHF levels and increasing levels of 5,10-methylenetetrahydrofolate or other nonmethylated forms of folate. While some of these forms are substrates for other metabolic pathways (e.g., for dTMP synthesis; see Fig. 38.1), others may have negative consequences. Some have suggested that elevated 5,10-methylenetetrahydrofolate levels and the subsequent increase in the conversion of dUMP to dTMP may have biological advantages (DNA replication and protection), explaining the high penetration of *MTHFR* polymorphisms in some populations. While no reproductive advantage has yet been attributed to humans with such mutations, recent animal studies have

---

*The gene and the expressed enzyme are both designated with the same letters. The enzyme is designated in capital letters (MTHFR), while the gene is shown in capital italics (*MTHFR*).

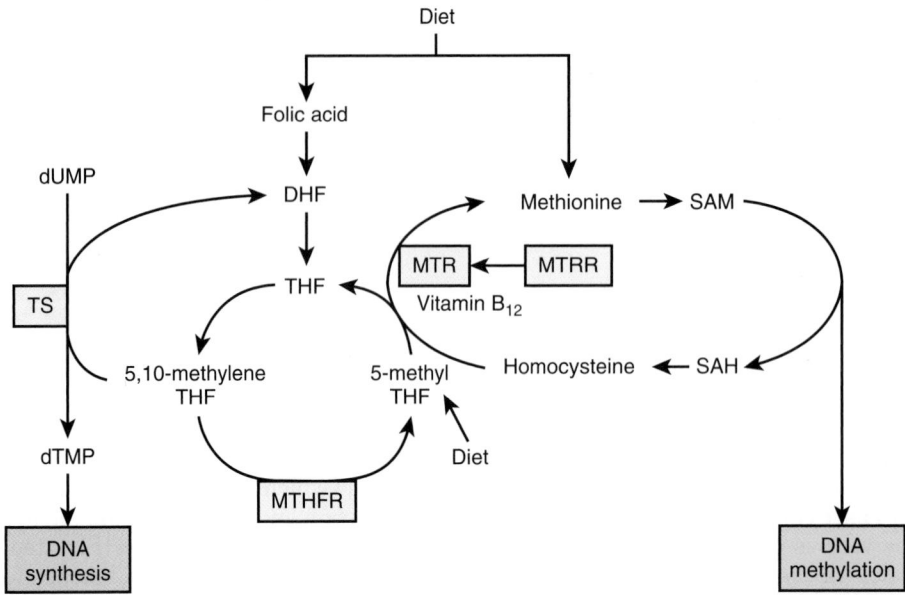

FIG. 38.1 ■ Overview of folate metabolism. Enzymes are provided in boxes. *DHF*, dihydrofolate; *dTMP*, deoxythymidine monophosphate; *dUMP*, deoxyuridine monophosphate; *MTR*, methionine synthase (gene); *MTRR*, methionine synthase reductase (gene); *SAM*, S-adenosylmethionine; *SAH*, S-adenosylhomocysteine; *TS*, thymidylate synthetase; *THF*, tetrahydrofolate.

suggested that protection against malaria may account for the high 677T variant in humans.[14]

- **Lower methionine, S-adenosylmethionine, and overall methylation.** Reduced availability of 5-MTHF results in lower amounts of intracellular methionine available as a precursor for the synthesis of S-adenosylmethionine (SAM), the major methyl-donor for methyltransferase enzymes. Lower levels of methylated metabolites (e.g., methylated proteins or neurotransmitters) may be an immediate consequence of decreased SAM levels, although alterations in DNA and histone methylation can have a long-term effect on gene regulation (epigenetic effects).[15]

Methylenetetrahydrofolate Reductase Mutations and Polymorphisms (Table 38.1)

Over 40 different genetic variants (i.e., mutations) in the *MTHFR* gene have been identified in patients with homocystinuria.[16] Two of these variants, usually called *polymorphisms* due to their relative frequency in the population, have gained particular attention in the research community; both of these are single nucleotide polymorphisms (SNPs). Of these two *MTHFR* polymorphisms, 677C→T and 1298A→C, we will focus mostly on the former where the majority of the risk (and research) exists.

MTHFR 677C→T Polymorphism (a.k.a. C677T)

Kang et al. first described a thermolabile form of the MTHFR enzyme in CHD patients with mild hyperhomocysteinemia in 1991.[17] Several other researchers confirmed the connections between this thermolabile MTHFR enzyme with both elevated homocysteine levels and CVD risk.[18-20] It was later discovered that a common

TABLE 38.1 **Nutrient-Gene Nomenclature**

Nutrigenetics: How a person's genes (i.e., DNA sequence or genotype) impacts their need for, or utilization of, a specific nutrient. Often the particular gene expresses an enzyme that metabolizes the nutrient, uses the nutrient as a cofactor, or is involved in the transport/signaling of the nutrient. The relationship between *MTHFR* genetics and folate is a classic example of nutrigenetics.

Nutrigenomics: How nutrients or their metabolites function to turn on (or off) genes. One of the best examples of this is vitamin D, which activates the vitamin D nuclear receptor (VDR) in the regulation of numerous different genes. Nutri*genetics* and nutri*genomics* are closely related concepts and can influence one another. For instance, genetic differences in the *VDR* gene can impact the need for vitamin D (nutrigenetics) while also influencing the relative genomic impact of vitamin D (nutrigenomics).

Nutrient Epigenetics: Epigenetics describes noncoding alterations in the genome that influence gene expression or cell function. These alterations are semipermanent over many cell divisions and even heritable if they are found in germ-line cells. The two most common types of epigenetic alterations are DNA methylation and histone modification. A person's epigenome is influenced by both nutrigenetic and nutrigenomic mechanisms. For example, cellular 5-MTHF levels can alter the expression of DNA methyltransferase genes (a nutrigenomic effect with epigenetic implications); at the same time, these same folate levels are directly influenced by *MTHFR* genetics (nutrigenetics).[68]

MTHFR single nucleotide difference at base pair 677 (C→T substitution) expressed a protein with a valine (instead of alanine) at amino acid 222, a substitution that alters the active site of the enzyme rendering it thermolabile and less biologically active.[21] The past two decades since this discovery have seen thousands of publications reporting on the population frequencies and differential

TABLE 38.2   **Frequency of the 677C→T Allele in Different Populations Based on Country and Ethnicity**

Area	Sample Number	CC	CT	TT
Europe				
Italy, Sicily	468	29%	51%	20%
Italy, Campania	500	34%	39%	27%
Italy, Veneto				
Italian whites	385	33%	52%	15%
Spain, multicenter				
Spanish whites	601	44%	44%	12%
France, Strasbourg	178	40%	48%	12%
The Netherlands	188	52%	42%	6%
Finland, Helsinki	545	54%	42%	4%
Hungary	378	44%	45%	11%
Russia	587	53%	40%	7%
Middle East				
Israel	210	57%	34%	9%
China				
North, Han	643	31%	49%	20%
South, Han	430	39%	53%	8%
Oceania				
Australia				
Whites	288	51%	41%	8%
Americas				
Mexico	500	18%	50%	32%
USA, Atlanta				
Whites	300	47%	42%	11%
Blacks	298	78%	20%	2%
Hispanics	62	35%	47%	18%
Asian	26	62%	35%	3%
Other, unknown	100	63%	32%	5%
Canada, Alberta				
Whites	240	57%	37%	6%

TABLE 38.3   **Ethnicities and Frequencies of 1298A→C Alleles**

Study Area and Ethnic Group	Sample Number	AA	AC	CC
Africa				
South Africa, Black indigenous	114	62%	34%	4%
Asia				
China	360	67%	31%	2%
China	166	67%	30%	3%
Japan	243	65%	31%	4%
Europe				
Austria	389	47%	43%	10%
Crete	125	46%	44%	10%
Germany	280	46%	44%	10%
Germany	174	51%	39%	10%
Germany, Caucasians	981	44%	45%	11%
Netherlands	403	44%	46%	10%
Netherlands	120	38%	53%	9%
Netherlands	565	44%	46%	10%
Poland	521	61%	34%	5%
Poland	100	55%	41%	4%
United Kingdom	114	43%	47%	10%
United Kingdom	200	47%	42%	11%
United Kingdom	394	54%	38%	8%
Middle East				
Israel, Jewish	397	45%	42%	13%
North America				
United States				
Ashkenazi Jewish	149	54%	38%	8%
Caucasians	159	44%	47%	9%
Hawaii, Caucasians	171	50%	38%	12%
Hawaii, Japanese decent	395	62%	34%	4%
Midwest, unspecified ethnicities	329	50%	42%	8%
Texas, Caucasians	554	48%	45%	7%
Male physicians	344	44%	46%	10%
Canada	129	53%	38%	9%
Canada	119	36%	56%	8%

health risks between subjects expressing both wild-type alleles (homozygous 677CC), those expressing both mutant alleles (homozygous- 677TT), and those that are heterozygous (677CT). Table 38.2 shows the frequency of the 677C→T allele in different populations based on country and ethnicity.

MTHFR 1298 A→C Polymorphism (a.k.a. A1298C)

A few years after the discovery of the thermolabile 677C→T polymorphism, a second common polymorphism was identified in humans. This was also a single nucleotide polymorphism of the *MTHFR* gene at base pair 1298 (A→C), which expressed a protein with an alanine (instead of glutamate) at amino acid 429, a substitution

in the regulatory domain of the enzyme.[22] This enzyme variant is not thermolabile and does not appear to be associated with elevated homocysteine levels, even in homozygous individuals (1298CC).[23] However, individuals who are compound heterozygous for both SNPs (i.e., 1298AC and 677CT) have elevated homocysteine levels similar to homozygous 677TT individuals. The frequency of the 1298A→C polymorphism is highest in populations of European descent; homozygous frequency for the 1298CC ranges from 4% to 12% (Table 38.3).[24]

Health Risks Associated With Methylenetetrahydrofolate Reductase Polymorphisms

The relative chronic disease risk associated with the expression of one or two *MTHFR* 677C→T alleles, or combined with the 1298A→C polymorphism, is not straightforward. While many early case-control studies showed a strong risk for cardiovascular disease, stroke, neural tube defects, Alzheimer's disease, osteoporosis, depression, thrombotic conditions, and a variety of cancers in those expressing the mutant alleles (highest risk usually in homozygous 677TT), many later studies suggested that some or all of the measured risk was dependent on a person's folate status, homocysteine levels, and ethnicity. It is now well understood that the *MTHFR* genotype-to-phenotype expression can be greatly influenced by environmental and dietary factors, as well as other (non-*MTHFR*) genes related to methylation.[4] In other words, clinicians should assess and treat the phenotype of the patient, rather than assume their risk based solely on genotype. Recent meta-analyses and systematic reviews* are available for *MTHFR* genotype-related risk for cardiovascular disease,[25] hypertension,[26] thrombotic conditions,[27] stroke,[28,29] neural tube defects,[30] osteoporosis,[31] Alzheimer's disease,[32] depression and related disorders,[33] and various cancers.[34]

Testing for Methylenetetrahydrofolate Reductase Polymorphisms

There is wide disagreement within the health care community on the utility of testing patients for *MTHFR* polymorphisms. Whereas nearly all published guidelines recommend against the use of *MTHFR* genetic testing, even when homocysteine is elevated (the exception is the American Heart Association, which does recommend *MTHFR* genetic testing when total homocysteine (tHcy) is >13 μmol/L), it is still one of the most common genetic tests ordered by both integrative and conventional medicine physicians. According to a recent analysis of *MTHFR* polymorphism tests performed by 77 different institutions in the United States between 2010 and 2012, only 14.5% were ordered for individuals with previously diagnosed hyperhomocysteinemia (tHcy >13 μmol/L), suggesting that the majority of clinicians that order such tests are unaware of or are disregarding published guideline recommendations for *MTHFR* genetic testing.[35]

> Determining MTHFR genetic status in subjects with a homocysteine level <13 μmol/L is unlikely to alter the clinical recommendation of diet and lifestyle changes; genetic testing in such cases is rarely indicated.

---

*Meta-analysis and systematic reviews have limitations and are often not reflective of the nuances seen in the clinic due to their strict inclusion/exclusion criteria, data adjustments or statistical variances. We suggest that readers consult the references listed if they want to understand these details and judge the merits of their conclusion.

The reason for the discrepancy in the use of MTHFR genetic testing may be rooted in a philosophical difference about how risk should be measured and prevented. Should risk be measured by statistically significant relative risk calculations derived through meta-analysis of the primary end-points of large clinical trials (using hard clinical outcomes like MI or death) or should risk be based on the biochemical vulnerability of reduced methylation that is likely to exist in these patients, especially when correlated to epidemiological data? The community writing the guidelines exclusively considers the former, while it appears integrative clinicians, as well as many conventional clinicians, favor the latter and believe that testing individuals is of some clinical value. Integrative clinicians are also more likely to consider homocysteine levels between 9 and 13 μmol/L as a biomarker of poor methylation, a condition that increases long-term metabolic risk through genomic/epigenetic influences.

As previously mentioned, genotype does not always predict phenotype. Chronic health risk related to an individual's *MTHFR* polymorphism status is highly dependent upon folate intake, actual enzyme activity (best indicated by folate status and homocysteine levels), ethnicity, and other factors that influence methylation outcomes. Nonetheless, knowing a person's *MTHFR* genetics may have potential benefits. In the absence of an individual's historical homocysteine or folate status, clinicians may be able to gauge the potential influence of hypomethylation on a patient's chronic disease risk based on *MTHFR* genetics as well as their diet and supplementation history. While this information alone may not dictate a specific therapeutic strategy, it may help predict future vulnerabilities and explain why certain therapeutic strategies may be more successful than others. Nonetheless, we recommend that analysis for the *MTHFR* polymorphisms be reserved for patients with coronary artery disease, acute myocardial infarction, peripheral vascular artery disease, stroke, depression or venous thromboembolism who have elevated homocysteine levels (>13 μmol/L), or an abnormal methionine-load test.

INTEGRATIVE THERAPY

The therapeutic strategies for lowering risk in individuals with *MTHFR* polymorphisms, particularly in homozygous 677TT individuals, is influenced greatly by a clinician's perspective of the risk related to *MTHFR* genetics, homocysteine levels, and methylation potential. On the basis of folate status–adjusted relative risk data and the failure of homocysteine-lowering therapies to alter primary end-points in large controlled clinical trials, the majority of guidelines recommend against testing *MTHFR* genetics as their authors do not believe there is adequate evidence to recommend any remedial therapies.[36] Our focus in this section is to review the available evidence of measurable differences in therapies based on a patient's *MTHFR* genetics, mostly as it relates to dietary and supplemental changes in folate status. However, in the absence of elevated homocysteine levels or reduced folate status, therapies based solely on *MTHFR* genotype alone may not be warranted.

Dietary and Supplemental Folates

There is a close association between folate status and MTHFR polymorphism/activity status. RBC and plasma folate levels are generally lower in individuals carrying one or two 677C→T alleles, or in compound heterozygous individuals (677CT/1298AC), and conversely, chronic disease risk measurements related to these polymorphisms are higher when folate status is low.[37] Therefore the majority of interventions associated with risk modification in individuals with differing *MTHFR* genotypes have focused on improving folate status through dietary intervention or supplementation, or by homocysteine-lowering therapies through dietary changes and/or supplementation (mostly using folates in combination with other vitamins).

Folate is the generic term for naturally-occurring food folates, folic acid (the fully oxidized monoglutamate form of the vitamin used in dietary supplements and fortified foods), folinic acid, and 5-MTHF. The current recommended daily allowance (RDA) in the United States is measured in Dietary Folate Equivalents (DFE, see the following), although label-claim daily value levels of folate/folic acid are measured by weight in micrograms.* The most recent RDA (1998) is based primarily on the adequacy of red blood cell-folate concentrations at different levels of folate intake, as judged by the absence of abnormal hematological indicators. Use of the DFE reflects a higher bioavailability of synthetic folic acid found in supplements and fortified foods compared to that of naturally occurring food folates.

- 1 mcg of food-derived folate provides 1 mcg of DFE.
- 1 mcg of folic acid taken with meals or within a fortified food provides 1.7 mcg of DFE.
- 1 mcg of folic acid (supplement) taken on an empty stomach provides 2 mcg of DFE.

Without food fortification and supplementation of folic acid, deficiency of folate intake is prevalent in the U.S. NHANES data gathered from 2003 to 2006 show that nearly 90% of Americans consume below the estimated average requirement (EAR) for folate; though after fortification this drops to only 10%.[38] Due to the relationship of widespread folate insufficiency with neural tube defects in early pregnancy, the U.S. instituted

*The FDA has changed to the DV for folates and folic acid in foods and dietary supplements to fix this discrepancy. As of mid-2018, labels must distinguish food-derived folates from folic acid, though it does not specify how to include supplemental 5-MTHF on a food or supplement label as it is neither.

mandatory folic acid fortification of all enriched grain products in 1998.

Plant-derived dietary folates exist mostly in polyglutamate forms, while commercially available folates, such as folic acid, folinic acid, and 5-MTHF, are monoglutamates (Fig. 38.2 and Table 38.4).

Polyglutamate folates from the diet must first be hydrolyzed to their monoglutamate forms by the action of folate hydrolase before being absorbed. Thus when establishing food recommendations, the bioavailability of food-derived folate is commonly estimated at 50% of folic acid (already a monoglutamate).[39] Monoglutamate forms that are not fully reduced (e.g., folic acid) or methylated (e.g., both folic acid and folinic acid) prior to absorption will be reduced and methylated to form 5-MTHF within the mucosa or liver prior to circulation. Once in the target cell, additional glutamate molecules are added to 5-MTHF, to again form a polyglutamate.

Adequate synthesis of 5-MTHF requires sufficient amounts of reduced folates and adequate function of the MTHFR enzyme. Impairment of the MTHFR enzyme can result in elevated conversion of 5,10-methylenetetrahydrofolate to formylated (rather than methylated) folate forms in the cell. Researchers have reported that RBC folate levels in homozygous 677TT individuals contain elevated levels of formylated THF forms and RBC folate in 677CC individuals is exclusively 5-MTHF.[40] Although various studies have suggested that the MTHFR activity in 677TT individuals is reduced by nearly 70% compared to wild-type individuals (677CC), one study showed that only 30% of the RBC folate in 677TT individuals is in the formylated form, a figure which is similar to the approximate 20% increase in homocysteine levels seen in these individuals based on genotype.[25,41]

Three forms of folate are currently used in dietary supplements: folic acid, folinic acid, and 5-methyltetrahydrofolate (5-MTHF). Folinic acid (e.g., calcium folinate) is a 5-formyl derivative of tetrahydrofolic acid (THF). Synthetic 5-MTHF used in medical foods and in dietary supplements (both calcium and glucosamine salt forms are available) is not derived from "natural sources" and is not, as some describe it, a dietary folate. These compounds would be considered bioequivalent (or bioidentical) synthetic analogs (5-MTHF, when naturally found in foods, is mostly in a polyglutamyl, not monoglutamyl form). Commercially available 5-MTHF is organically synthesized using folic acid as a starting material. After reduction to tetrahydrofolate and methylation, a racemic mixture (R,S) of a monoglutamyl 5-MTHF is formed. Crystallization and separation of the two stereoisomers allows for a purified S-form, which is then stabilized using calcium or glucosamine ions (the "S" describes the specific stereochemistry at the #6 carbon; this is often also called the "L" form due to the way this isomer reflects light). Therefore 5-MTHF is sometimes labeled as (6S)-5-methyltetrahydrofolate. Other names include levomefolic acid or L-methylfolate. Unfortunately, this process results in a raw material that is about 200 times more expensive than an equimolar amount of folic acid.

Supplemental folic acid, which must be fully reduced and methylated, is often less capable of increasing serum 5-MTHF levels in 677TT individuals compared

FIG. 38.2 ■ Structure of folic acid (*top*) and reduced folate polyglutamates from foods (*middle*). Table shows the positions and oxidation states of folate one-carbon substitutions. (From Shane B. Folate, vitamin b12 and vitamin B6. In: Stipanuk MH, ed. *Biochemical, physiological, and molecular aspects of human nutrition.* Philadelphia: WB Saunders; 2000.)

One carbon substituent		Position	Oxidation state
Methyl	—CH₃	N-5	Methanol
Methylene	—CH₂—	N-5, N-10	Formaldehyde
Methenyl	—CH=	N-5, N-10	Formate
Formyl	—CHO	N-5 or N-10	Formate
Formimino	HO=CH—	N-5	Formate

TABLE 38.4   Foods Highest in Dietary Folates

- Green leafy vegetables (cooked/boiled)
- Lentils (cooked/boiled)
- Garbanzo beans/chickpeas (cooked/boiled)
- Asparagus (cooked, boiled)
- Spinach (cooked, boiled)
- Lima beans (large, mature seeds, cooked, boiled)
- Orange juice (raw)
- Most commercial products made with flour (fortified with folic acid)

---

to 677CC individuals.[42] Clinical studies comparing the ability of folic acid with 5-MTHF supplementation to change serum folate levels or effect changes in homocysteine in both 677TT and 677CC subjects are limited, as most studies did not recruit sufficient 677TT individuals to reach a statistically significant conclusion.[43] Some studies show no statistical difference, or only slight benefit for 5-MTHF, while others show a statistical benefit for 5-MTHF supplementation, particularly in bioavailability studies. In a recent study comparing a single dose of either 400 mcg of folic acid or equimolar levels of 5-MTHF (416 mcg) in women homozygous for either the CC or TT polymorphism, 5-MTHF supplementation was able to increase plasma folate levels (AUC) by nearly twice that of folic acid in 677TT individuals and by 60% in 677CC subjects.[44] On the other hand, after 13 weeks of folate treatments (using either a folate-rich diet, folic acid, or 5-MTHF) equivalent to 200 mcg of folic acid, each folate form was equally capable of RBC folate benefits and homocysteine lowering in subjects (Italian) with moderate hyperhomocysteinemia (mean baseline level, tHcy 14.1 μmol/L).[45]

Beyond bioavailability and homocysteine-lowering effects, other issues may be important when comparing folic acid versus 5-MTHF supplementation. The first is that high-dose folic acid supplementation (>5 mg/day) results in an increase in serum levels of unmetabolized folic acid.[46] However, this is likely due to overwhelming the capacity of the dihydrofolate reductase (DHFR) enzymes in both the intestine and liver, rather than specific deficiencies in the MTHFR enzyme.[47,48] Nonetheless, while there is no clear evidence of a demonstrable negative consequence for these elevated levels of unmetabolized folic acid, supplementation above 5 mg/day of folic acid, when warranted, should be performed with caution or substituted with 5-MTHF supplementation.[49] The second issue often cited is that high doses of folic acid can mask (not cause) an underlying vitamin B12 deficiency; supplementation with 5-MTHF appears to be less likely to have this consequence, although this has not been confirmed by rigorous clinical trials. Because it is routinely recommend that vitamin B12 be used with any high-dose folate/folic acid supplementation therapy, this issue is of little clinical concern.

In general, pregnant women with a *MTHFR* 677TT genotype are at higher risk for fetal neural tube defects (NTDs); MTHFR A1298A→C polymorphisms play only a minor role in NTD risk.[50] For decades, folic acid was the primary folate used in dietary supplements and in nearly every clinical trial to improve folate status in pregnant women. While no intervention studies using 5-MTHF during pregnancy have been published to date, there are many researchers and clinicians recommending the use of 5-MTHF, rather than folic acid, for preconception and prenatal supplementation.[51] With the exception of additional cost, this recommendation should result in no harm to the mother or child and is likely to increase folate status in these women to a greater extent than a similar level of folic acid.

According to the IOM, the daily recommended intake for folate during pregnancy (defined as a dietary folate equivalent-DFE) is 600 mcg.[52] Technically, this is equal to 300 mcg of a folic acid supplement because the IOM deems 1 mcg of folic acid equal to 2 DFEs. As of December 2014, the daily value (DV) used for folic acid by the FDA to label prenatal supplement (i.e., the 100% DV in the supplement facts box) is 800 mcg, differing both from the 600 mcg DFE recommendation and its 300 mcg folic acid equivalent.[53] Regardless of these discrepancies, NHANES data show that folate/folic acid intake in women of child-bearing age is well below the recommended amount. Therefore we recommend 800–1000 mcg/day of folic acid or 5-MTHF should be added through supplementation starting 8 weeks before conception through the end of breastfeeding. While we do not believe folic acid is either unsafe or ineffective in

such patients, those with MTHFR 677CT or 677TT polymorphisms may realize additional benefits using 5-MTHF rather than folic acid.

DOSAGE

Folic acid: 200 mcg to 5 mg based on starting and target homocysteine levels. Avoid using more than 1 mg of folic acid in 677TT (choose the 5-MTHF form).

5-MTHF: 200 mcg and above based on starting and target homocysteine levels. Consider using in place of folic acid in subjects that are 677TT, 677CT, or compound heterozygous (677CT/1298AC) or when using greater than 5 mg/day of supplemental folate in any subject.

Related Homocysteine Lowering Therapies

Nearly all other diet and nutrient interventions that have been investigated in subjects with *MTHFR* polymorphisms (mostly 677C→T) are related primarily to their ability to lower homocysteine; many of which were investigated in combination with supplemental folate compounds. To the extent that homocysteine lowering is the intended therapeutic goal and 677TT individuals are known to have elevated homocysteine levels, these therapies may be considered helpful in these subjects, although none, except riboflavin, have specifically been shown to directly improve the function of the MTHFR enzyme.

Cobalamin (Vitamin B12)

Cobalamin (B12) is a necessary cofactor for methionine synthase, the enzyme that transfers the methyl group from 5-MTHF to homocysteine using methyl-cobalamin as an intermediate. Vitamin B12 should be used when supplementing folates, especially folic acid. While there are clinicians that prefer one form of B12 over another (cyanocobalamin, methylcobalamin, hydroxocobalamin, or adenosylcobalamin), or claim that one is more effective in subjects with MTHFR polymorphisms, to date, there is no published data to suggest a difference between these forms in such subjects. The biochemistry of cobalamin forms would suggest little in the way of functional differences, although hydroxocobalamin may be favorable in some rare genetic defects in cobalamin metabolism.[54] Oral doses of 1 mg or more are considered equivalent to intramuscular doses for increasing markers of B12 repletion.[55]

DOSAGE

For homocysteine lowering, an oral dose of 1 mg is safe, tolerable, and adequate for most subjects regardless of intrinsic factor or vitamin B12 status. Multivitamin doses starting at 200 mcg are likely adequate for subjects without vitamin B12 insufficiency and normal homocysteine levels.

PRECAUTIONS

There are no safety concerns related to vitamin B12 supplementation and no known toxicity reported for long-term vitamin B12 use; the IOM has set no tolerable upper safety level.

Riboflavin (Vitamin B2)

Riboflavin is the precursor for the MTHFR's stabilizing cofactor, FAD. Low riboflavin levels have been associated with elevated homocysteine, especially in subjects with the *MTHFR* 677TT genotype.[56] Riboflavin supplementation, even as low as 1.6 mg/day, has been shown to reduce homocysteine levels in homozygous 677TT subjects.[57] Riboflavin-5-phosphate is often marketed as an "activated" or natural form of riboflavin to integrative medicine clinicians. As it turns out, this synthetic "bioidentical" form must be dephosphorylated prior to transport into the body and offers no advantages when taken orally.[58,59]

DOSAGE

Oral dose of 2.0–50 mg of riboflavin USP.

PRECAUTIONS

None. Higher doses of riboflavin can result in a harmless intense yellowing of urine (flavinuria).

Pyridoxine (Vitamin B6)

Vitamin B6 is not directly involved in the MTHFR reaction. However, it is a cofactor in the reaction that converts homocysteine to cysteine (transsulfuration pathway) catalyzed by cystathionine β-synthase. Therefore, low vitamin B6 levels can exacerbate the health risk in subjects with low folate and/or MTHFR polymorphisms. Vitamin B6 supplementation has been shown to effectively lower homocysteine levels, especially when added to folate supplementation.[60]

It is common for some manufacturers to include pyridoxal-5-phosphate (P5P) in their formulas, marketing this ingredient as an "active" or "natural" form of supplemental B6. While also being "bioidentical," this ingredient is synthesized from pyridoxine HCl, which increases its cost by approximately seven-fold. When taken orally, P5P must be dephosphorylated prior to absorption and has no clinical advantages over pyridoxine HCl.[61,62]

DOSAGE

Oral dose of 2–50 mg pyridoxine HCl USP. Higher doses are unnecessary for homocysteine-lowering.

PRECAUTIONS

None at the recommended dose. Avoid exceeding the tolerable upper limit (100 mg/day) unless following a therapy known to be safe and effective. Toxic levels (1000 mg a day) can cause sensory neuropathy.

High doses of vitamins B6 (80 mg/day) and B12 (20 mcg a day) can trigger a flare of rosacea with red papules, pustules, and nodules, which can take months to resolve.

Betaine and Choline

Human liver and kidney cells can remethylate homocysteine to methionine using betaine (trimethylglycine) as a methyl donor using the enzyme betaine homocysteine methylstransferase (BHMT). Supplemental betaine (or its precursor choline) have been shown to effectively reduce hyperhomocysteinemia, although studies in patients stratified by MTHFR polymorphisms have not been reported.[63] Higher doses of betaine (~6 grams/day) may be needed to see changes in fasting tHcy,[64] while smaller doses (500–1000 mg) are effective in reducing postmethionine load elevations in homocysteine.[65]

N-Acetylcysteine

Kidney clearance of homocysteine requires that it is unbound, although the majority of homocysteine (75%) in the serum is bound to protein via a disulfide bond. The common dietary supplement ingredient, N-acetylcysteine (NAC), can reduce the disulfide homocysteine-protein bond providing more free homocysteine to the kidney for clearance. The effect is dose-dependent at oral doses between 600 and 1800 mg/day in patients with normal kidney clearance.[66] ESRD patients may require higher doses (5 mg) and several studies have provided NAC intravenously to these subjects.[67]

Side Effects With Methyl Donors

Unpublished clinical reports and online discussions of side effects related to consuming methyl donors have been increasing in subjects of all genotypes. This has often been dubbed as "overmethylation." Symptoms are usually described as headaches, anxiety, palpitations, or unexplained pains after high doses of methyl donors, especially 5-MTHF. While the etiology of this phenomenon has not been investigated, we suggest precaution and gradual dose-escalation, especially in subjects with historically low folate and presumed low methylation. Monitoring changes in tHcy levels or choosing modest targets for tHcy (9–13 μmol/L) may represent a way of mitigating the side effects associated with methyl-donor therapies.

PREVENTION PRESCRIPTION

- Consume a diet high in folate (fruits and vegetables, traditional Mediterranean, or DASH diet).
- If necessary, consider reducing methionine in the diet (methionine increases homocysteine). Foods containing high levels of methionine include eggs, cheese, meats, and soy protein concentrates.
- Monitor homocysteine levels, maintain below 9 μmol/L through diet, and, if warranted, provide daily B-multivitamins.
- Avoid smoking and high consumption of coffee (>6 cups/day).
- Avoid excess alcohol consumption.

THERAPEUTIC REVIEW

Risks associated with MTHFR polymorphisms are greatest in homozygous 677TT and compound heterozygous (677CT/1298AC), and least in 677CT heterozygous individuals. However, in all cases, an individual's phenotype, measured according to homocysteine and folate status, is more predictive of risk compared with the genotype. These recommendations are related both to improving risk related to MTHFR genetics and reducing homocysteine levels.

MTHFR GENETIC TESTING

Should be reserved for patients with coronary artery disease, acute myocardial infarction, peripheral vascular artery disease, stroke, depression, or venous thromboembolism who have elevated homocysteine levels (>13 µmol/L). Patients need only to be tested once, as genotype does not change. In the absence of elevated homocysteine levels or reduced folate status, therapies based solely on *MTHFR* genotype alone may not be warranted.

- MTHFR genetic testing when tHcy >13 µmol/L
- MTHFR genetic testing when tHcy <13 µmol/L

DIET

- Folate-rich diet (Mediterranean/DASH-based, increase vegetables and fruits)
- Low-methionine diet (dietary methionine can elevate homocysteine levels)

SUPPLEMENTS

- Folates: 200 mcg–5 mg/day to normalize homocysteine levels

    - Folic acid: Avoid using more than 1 mg in subjects with *MTHFR* 677TT
    - 5-MTHF: Preferable in subjects with MTHFR 677TT or 677CT/1298AC genotypes, or when using folate therapies above 5 mg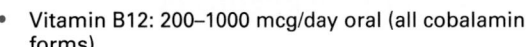

- Vitamin B12: 200–1000 mcg/day oral (all cobalamin forms)

- Riboflavin USP: 2.0–50 mg/day

- Vitamin B6 (Pyridoxine HCl): 2–50 mg/day

- Betaine (trimethylglycine): not to be confused with Betaine HCl (used to deliver HCl for lowering stomach pH): 500 mg–6 g (higher is better)

- Choline: as a precursor to betaine, 3–6 g

- N-acetylcysteine (NAC) to increase free homocysteine for kidney clearance

    - 600–1800 mg/day oral in subjects with normal kidney clearance
    - Up to 5 g/day intravenously in ESRD/dialysis

Key Web Resources

Linus Pauling Institute: Micronutrient Information Center—Folate page	http://lpi.oregonstate.edu/mic/vitamins/folate#genetic-variation-requirements
Genetics Home Reference: MTHFR page	http://ghr.nlm.nih.gov/gene/MTHFR

REFERENCES

References are available online at ExpertConsult.com.

CHAPTER 39

ADRENAL FATIGUE

Jacqueline Redmer, MD, MPH

THE NATURAL STRESS RESPONSE

The human body is well equipped to handle stress. A wide array of hormones and neurotransmitters exist to maintain homeostasis in response to physical and psychogenic stressors. The adrenal glands, which are located at the top of the kidney, are at the center of the body's stress response system. The cortex forms approximately 90% of the adrenal mass, the remaining core being the adrenal medulla. In the adult, the cortex can be morphologically and functionally divided into three layers (the glomerulosa, fasciculata, and reticularis). Each layer has a distinct histological appearance and secretes different steroid hormones (aldosterone, cortisol, and androgens, respectively). The inner 10%–20% of the gland is the adrenal medulla, secreting the catecholamines epinephrine and norepinephrine[1] (Fig. 39.1).

The body responds to physical, emotional, psychological, and biochemical stresses by releasing cortisol. Stress is sensed by the hypothalamus, which then releases corticotropin hormone (CRH). This stimulates the anterior pituitary to produce adrenocorticotropic hormone (ACTH), which triggers receptors in the adrenal cortex to release the appropriate amount of cortisol. When the sympathetic (fight or flight) nervous system is activated, the adrenals respond by releasing epinephrine, norepinephrine, and cortisol, all of which increase heart rate and blood pressure diverting blood to the brain, heart, and skeletal muscle[2] (Fig. 39.2).

Adrenal insufficiency is a well-documented condition in which the adrenals cannot keep up with the stress response of the body. This can happen if there is destruction of the adrenal cortex (primary) or if factors outside of the adrenal glands stimulate them to produce less cortisol (secondary). In primary adrenal insufficiency, the symptoms reflect a loss of glucocorticoid and mineralocorticoid hormones, whereas secondary deficiency usually results only in a loss of cortisol.[3]

Although not widely accepted by allopathic medicine, many alternative medicine practitioners believe that a subclinical adrenal fatigue or burnout can develop when the adrenals have been working hard to keep up with high physical, psychological, or emotional stress demands over time[2,4] (Table 39.1). It is hypothesized that sustained levels of high cortisol may lead to decreased responsiveness in the pituitary and adrenal glands. Changes in hypothalamic-pituitary-adrenal (HPA) axis may be due to the following mechanisms: (1) reduced biosynthesis or release of the respective hormone on different levels of the HPA axis (CRH from the hypothalamus, ACTH from the pituitary, or cortisol from the adrenal glands); (2) hypersecretion of one hormone with a subsequent downregulation of the respective target receptors; (3) enhanced sensitivity to the

negative feedback of cortisol; (4) a decreased availability of free cortisol; and/or (5) reduced effects of cortisol on the target tissue, resulting in a relative cortisol resistance.[5,6]

Adrenal fatigue and chronic fatigue syndrome (now recognized as Systemic Exertion Intolerance Disease) overlap a good deal clinically, and some people view adrenal fatigue as a subset of CFS. A meta-analysis of 19 studies from 2013 on this subject evaluated this relationship. It was found that 24-hour measures of absolute cortisol output did not clearly correlate with fatigue symptoms. However, attenuation of the cortisol diurnal variability, particularly with disruption of waking and circadian rhythms, seems to have more impact on the development of CFS.[9] Other reviews have suggested that HPA axis activity (or dysfunction) may not be at the core of CFS, but instead occur as a result of certain behavioral changes associated with the illness.[10]

DIAGNOSING ADRENAL FATIGUE

In most cases, a diagnosis of adrenal fatigue is based on clinical history and the exclusion of other conditions based on basic lab work. In patients suspected of having adrenal fatigue, however, it may be reasonable to screen for frank adrenal insufficiency. With normal diurnal variations in cortisol, glucocorticoids are lowest at 12 a.m.–1 a.m. and highest at 6 a.m.–8 a.m. In conventional medicine, cortisol adequacy is usually tested for with an 8 a.m. fasting serum cortisol test. In healthy patients, the cortisol level is usually 10–20 mcg/dL. An early morning low serum cortisol concentration less than 3 mcg/dL has a high specificity (100%) and low sensitivity for adrenal insufficiency (36%). Using a higher serum cortisol of 10 mcg/dL as the criterion for adrenal insufficiency increases the sensitivity to 62% and reduces the specificity to 77%. Thus a low morning serum cortisol concentration alone is not a reliable predictor of deficient adrenal function.[11]

Among practitioners, there is controversy regarding the best measurement of cortisol, with many people feeling strongly that salivary, not serum, levels more accurately reflect adrenal function.[12–15] Controversy exists concerning the validity of such testing materials and potential confounding variables, such as dietary interference, salivary viscosity, oral contaminants, and oral diseases such as gingivitis. However, some data suggest that salivary collection is preferable because it adjusts for bioavailable cortisol and is unaffected by cortisol binding globulin level, which rises with oral contraception pills, hypoalbuminemia, cirrhosis, nephrotic syndrome, and pregnancy. Salivary cortisol testing is easy to collect, although testing may not be widely available and testing criteria have not been uniformly accepted.[16]

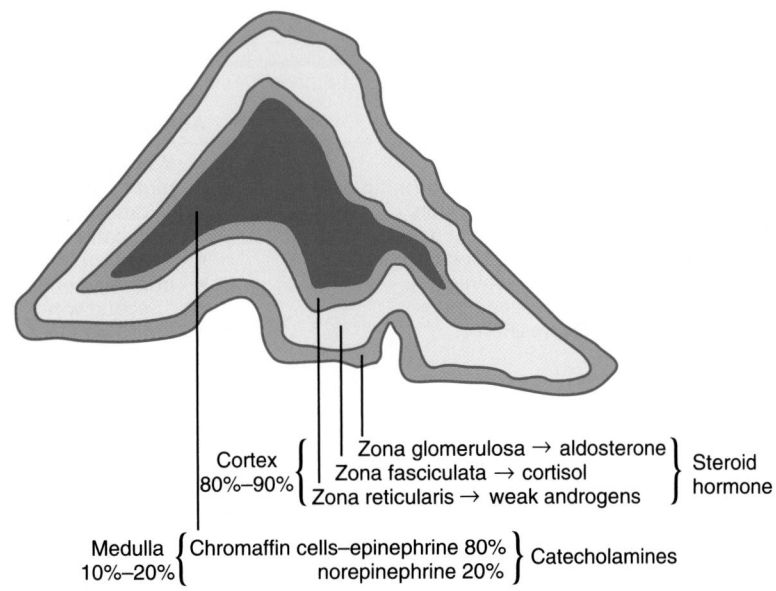

FIG. 39.1 ■ Histology of the adrenal gland. (From White B, Porterfield S. The Adrenal Gland, In: *Endocrine and reproductive physiology*, St. Louis, Elsevier, 2013:147-176.)

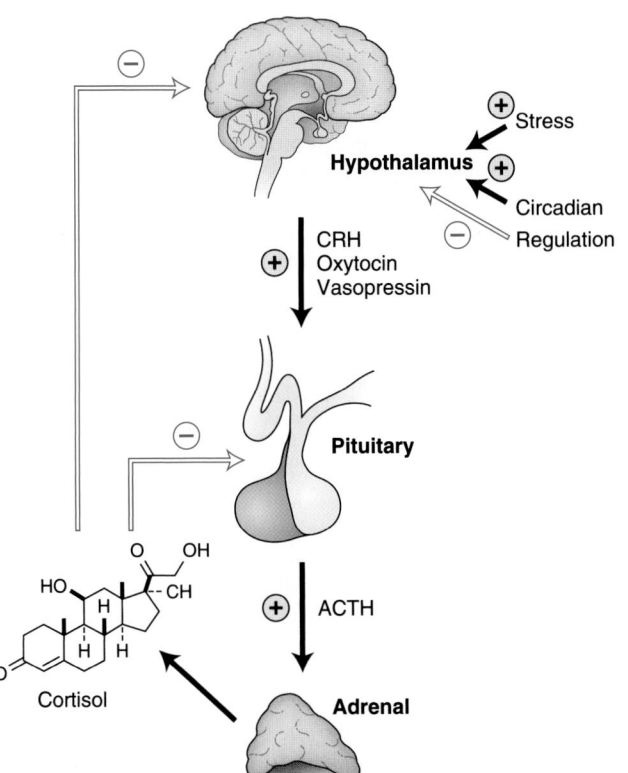

FIG. 39.2 ■ The hypothalamic-pituitary axis. (From Kutikov A. Pathophysiology, evaluation, and medical management of adrenal disorders. In: Wein AJ, Kavoussi LR, Partin AW, Peters CA, editors: *Campbell-Walsh urology*, ed. 11. Philadelphia, Elsevier, 2012:1685-1736.e8.)

When evaluating a patient for adrenal fatigue, consider the following tests to rule out other causes for their symptoms: polysomnography; PHQ-9 testing for depression; and labs including TSH, T3, T4, CBC, ferritin, CMP, magnesium, zinc, and vitamin B12.

Due to the pulsatile nature and diurnal variation of cortisol secretion, many integrative medicine practitioners use a four-point salivary testing technique to assess for patterns suggestive of adrenal fatigue and derangements of the HPA axis. With most protocols, salivary cortisol is checked from 7 a.m.–9 a.m., 11 a.m.–1 p.m., 3 p.m.–5 p.m., and 10 p.m.–12 a.m. These methods assume the assessment of cortisol and DHEA trends is more helpful than a random or 24-hour assessment because of the dramatic variation throughout the day. There is a growing body of evidence supporting the validity of salivary testing for adrenal disorders; however, in general, evidence to support the use and interpretation of four-point testing as a measure of adrenal function remain limited.[17-19] That said, the trends revealed by four-point testing may be informative when assessing a patient for clinical symptoms of adrenal fatigue.

If true adrenal insufficiency is suspected based on an unusually low early morning cortisol level, further testing may include:

ACTH/cosyntropin stimulation test. The ACTH stimulation test is the most commonly used test for diagnosing adrenal insufficiency. In this test, the patient is given an intravenous (IV) injection of synthetic ACTH, and cortisol levels are measured before and after the injection. The normal response after an ACTH injection is a rise in blood and urine cortisol levels. People with Addison's disease or secondary adrenal insufficiency have little or no increase in cortisol levels.[7]

CRH stimulation test. When the response to the ACTH test is abnormal, a CRH stimulation test can help determine the cause of adrenal insufficiency. In this test, the patient is given an IV injection of synthetic CRH, and cortisol levels are taken before and after the injection. People with Addison's disease respond by producing high levels of ACTH, yet no cortisol. People with secondary adrenal insufficiency do not produce ACTH or have a delayed response.[7]

TABLE 39.1 **The Effects of Stress on the Body**

Adrenal Insufficiency Symptoms[7]	Adrenal Fatigue Symptoms[8]	Adrenal Fatigue—Activity Patterns[8]
• Fatigue • Body aches • Weight/muscle loss • Low blood pressure • Lightheadedness • Loss of hair • Nausea/vomiting and diarrhea • Hyperpigmentation	• Fatigue • Difficulty with morning waking • Prone to infection • Craving sweet or salty food • Difficulty concentrating • Hypoglycemia • Decreased libido • Depression	• Waking fatigue, even after an adequate night's sleep • Midmorning low energy—often treated with caffeine or sugar • Afternoon low between 2 p.m. and 5 p.m. • Improved energy after 6 p.m. • "Second wind" around 11 p.m., lasts until 1 a.m.–2 a.m.

INTEGRATIVE THERAPY

Fortunately, many of the harmful effects of chronic stress and adrenal fatigue are reversible, at least to some extent. There are various interventions that can decrease the effects of adrenal fatigue, including nutritional therapies, exercising regularly, supplements, and the incorporation of stress management strategies.

Although lifestyle management alone might not reverse all symptoms of adrenal fatigue, this must be an important component of any treatment plan since unhealthy lifestyle and poor adaptive stress management techniques usually contribute to this condition.

Lifestyle Interventions[8]

Advise patients to:
1. Minimize the sources of psychological, physical, and emotional stress in their lives.
2. Reduce commitments and emphasize unstructured free time in which patients can participate in activities they enjoy.
3. Set a goal to obtain adequate sleep (7–9 hours for adults).
4. Laugh as much as possible. Prescribe laughter therapy. This might include the use of humorous books, movies, stories, YouTube clips, jokes, memories, or anything that makes them laugh.
5. Limit alcohol; in the moment, having a drink feels relaxing but alcohol interferes with sleep and depresses mood.
6. Make good dietary choices; sugar and refined carbs worsen the body's response to stress, even though they may feel satisfying in the short term.
7. Engage in activities that give their lives meaning and purpose.

Nutrition

Patients with adrenal fatigue are encouraged to avoid hypoglycemia because this can raise cortisol levels. Patients should minimize consumption of simple carbohydrates and focus on consuming small, frequent meals. Salt restriction is not necessary[20] (see Chapter 87).

Botanicals

Adaptogens are phytochemicals, which are believed to stabilize physiological processes and encourage homeostasis in the body. Adaptogens helpful in the treatment adrenal fatigue include:

Licorice

Glycyrrhiza licorice appears to have modest glucocorticoid activity and may act synergistically with cortisol. Components of licorice (primarily glycyrrhizin, which is structurally similar to corticoids) can bind to glucocorticoid and mineralocorticoid receptors, weakly mimicking the role of endogenous steroid hormones. There is some evidence that licorice may also reduce the breakdown of hydrocortisone to inactive cortisol products.

DOSAGE

Licorice powdered root 1–4 g daily three times daily.[2,21]

PRECAUTIONS

Licorice, like steroids, can cause salt retention, elevated blood pressure, and hypokalemia. Potassium and blood pressure should be monitored in those taking licorice root. This effect is removed in deglycyrrizinated forms (DGL), but these also lack the active ingredient used for treating fatigue.

Ashwaganda

Ashwaganda is considered to be the preeminent adaptogen in the Ayruvedic medical system. When administered to animals, ashwaganda has been shown to counteract many of the biological changes that accompany severe stress, including changes in blood sugar and cortisol levels.

DOSAGE

Powdered herb 2–3 g twice daily.[2,21]

PRECAUTIONS

Well tolerated at recommended doses. High doses can cause GI intolerance.

Siberian Ginseng

Also known as *Eleutherococcus sentidosus*. Most data on Siberian ginseng has been completed by Russian scientists to improve athletic performance in Olympic athletes and is not available in English. However, one review indicates Siberian ginseng increases the ability to accommodate adverse physical conditions and improves mental performance.

DOSAGE
Variable based on preparation.[21,22]

PRECAUTIONS
Siberian ginseng should be used cautiously in those with heart disease as it can precipitate palpitations, tachycardia, and hypertension. High doses can also cause anxiety and irritability.

Panax Ginseng

While the antistress mechanisms of Panax ginseng are not completely understood, research suggests a variety of actions on both the adrenal glands and the HPA axis. At the level of the brain or HPA axis, ginseng appears to stimulate ACTH and subsequent cortisol production and may also increase binding of corticosteroids to certain regions of the brain.

DOSAGE
Dried root powder 200–600 mg daily.[21]

PRECAUTIONS
The most common side effect is insomnia. Be careful not to give close to bedtime. As with other ginseng's common side effects are related to overstimulation. Ginseng is difficult to grow and harvest. Adulterated products are common so recommend a dependable source.

Rhodiola Rosea

The adaptogenic properites and CNS activities of *Rhodiola* have been attributed primarily to its abilities to influence the levels of the neurotransmitters, serotonin, dopamine, and norepinephrine, by inhibiting the enzyme responsible for their degradation.

DOSAGE
100–300 mg three times daily.[21,22]

PRECAUTIONS
Can cause dry mouth and dizziness.

Supplements

Vitamin B Complex

Studies have shown the B vitamins are protective nutrients for the adrenals, decreasing the stress-induced cortisol response. The B vitamins support sleep quality and are also important cofactors in the production of neurotransmitters.[2,21]

DOSAGE
Consider a B-complex vitamin daily.

PRECAUTIONS
Safe at regular doses.

Vitamin C

Vitamin C is important for numerous physiological functions, including the metabolism of the neurotransmitters dopamine and norepinephrine.[2] The adrenals need more vitamin C than any other organ or tissue in the body, especially during times of stress.[23] For most healthy individuals, the body can only hold and use approximately 250 mg of vitamin C a day, and any excess is lost through urine.

DOSAGE
250 mg twice daily.

PRECAUTIONS
High doses can cause diarrhea.

L-Carnitine

This supplement may be useful for boosting metabolism and increasing energy levels. L-Carnitine helps to move fatty acids into the mitochondria where they are used to produce energy. Several studies have shown that L-carnitine supplementation in healthy, elderly subjects results in a reduction of total fat mass, an increase in total muscle mass, a decrease in fatigue, and improvement in cognitive function. [24,25]

DOSAGE
2 g twice daily.

PRECAUTIONS
May decrease effectiveness of thyroid hormone supplementation.

Dehydroepiandrosterone

Although commonly used for adrenal fatigue, there is minimal evidence to support the use of dehydroepiandrosterone (DHEA). In a study of patient with Sjogren syndrome with fatigue and documented low DHEA levels, replacement with 50 mg of DHEA had no benefit in fatigue scores over placebo.[26]

Adrenal Glandulars

The safety and effectiveness of adrenal glandulars are unknown. Glandular products include ground-up animal adrenal glands (often from pigs), which contain adrenal hormones including cortisol and catecholamines. The dose is not standardized and there is potential for harm (osteoporsosis and hypertension) with long-term use. In general, adrenal glandular supplements are not recommended as they may further suppress the hypothalamic-pituitary-adrenal axis.

Mind-Body Interventions

Very little evidence exists for the use of mind-body techniques in the treatment of adrenal fatigue. However, research shows there are many modalities that can lower cortisol and mediate the effects of stress.

Breathing Practices

Diaphragmatic breathing is relaxing and therapeutic, reduces stress, and is a fundamental procedure of Pranayama yoga, Zen, transcendental meditation, and other meditation practices. Analysis of oxidative stress levels in people who meditate has indicated that meditation correlates with lower oxidative stress levels and lower cortisol levels. One study reported that diaphragmatic breathing after exercise increased antioxidant defense and lowered cortisol levels.[27] Studies have shown that mindfulness based stress reduction programs can also lower cortisol levels in the blood[28] (see Chapters 94 and 100).

Yoga

Yoga has been used in many clinical settings to decrease stress-related illness and concerns. Although the psychological and physiological benefits likely occur in multiple ways, a recent systematic review showed that yoga increases positive affect and self-compassion and leads to lower salivary cortisol levels.[29]

Progressive Muscle Relaxation

Several studies have found lower levels of postintervention heart rate, anxiety, perceived stress, and salivary cortisol, as well as increased levels of self-report levels of relaxation in subjects instructed on progressive muscle relaxation (PMR) versus controls.[30] In a PMR session, patients are instructed to create tension in a specific muscle group, noticing what tension feels like in that area, and then to release this muscle tension and begin to notice what a relaxed muscle feels like as the tension drains away (see Chapter 94).

Biofeedback

Participants in one study were asked to complete a biofeedback training program for 5 minutes a day to decrease heart rate and increase cerebral blood flow. After 28 days, those in the intervention group had significantly lower salivary cortisol than those in the control group.[31]

Bioenergentic Interventions

Reiki

In another study, participants received ten 20-minute reiki sessions over the course of 2.5–12 weeks while being guided through relaxation exercises. Salivary cortisol levels were measured and found to be significantly lower in participants who received reiki and not just instruction in relaxation techniques.[32]

Therapies to Consider

It stands to reason, then, that other modalities which mediate the physiological effects of stress on the body such as hypnosis, imagery, TCM, ayurveda, homeopathy, journaling, and massage would all have the beneficial effect of lowering sympathetic tone, thereby providing supportive treatment for adrenal fatigue.

PREVENTION PRESCRIPTION

Prevent the onset of adrenal fatigue, by encouraging patients to:

• Minimize psychological, physical, and emotional stress
• Reduce commitments and emphasize unstructured free time
• Adopt good self-care patterns and learn stress management techniques

• Set a goal to obtain an adequate sleep (7–9 hours for adults)
• Follow an antiinflammatory, low-glycemic index diet, specifically encouraging sugar and alcohol use in moderation
• Engage in regular physical activity

THERAPEUTIC REVIEW

LIFESTYLE

- Minimize psychological, physical, and emotional stress
- Reduce commitments and emphasize unstructured free time
- Adopt good self-care patterns and learn stress management techniques
- Set a goal to obtain an adequate sleep (7–9 hours for adults)
- Follow an antiinflammatory diet, specifically encouraging sugar and alcohol use in moderation
- Engage in regular physical activity

NUTRITION

- Eat small, frequent meals and minimize simple carbohydrates to avoid hypoglycemia
- No salt restriction

SUPPLEMENTS

- *Glycyrrhiza licorice* powdered root 1–4 g daily three times daily
- Ashwaganda powdered herb 3 g twice daily
- *Panax ginseng* dried root powder 200–600 mg daily
- *Rhodiola rosea* 100–300 mg three times daily
- Vitamin B complex
- Vitamin C 250 mg daily

MIND-BODY

The following mind-body techniques have been shown to reduce cortisol levels
- Breathing practices, including meditation and yoga
- Biofeedback
- Progressive muscle relaxation

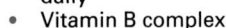
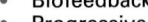

Key Web Resources

Reputable web resources on this topic are limited, which may be due to the variable acceptance of adrenal fatigue within the allopathic community. General information on adrenal insufficiency can be found at:

National Institute of Health Endocrine and Metabolic Diseases: Adrenal Insufficiency and Addison's Disease	http://www.niddk.nih.gov/health-information/health-topics/endocrine/adrenal-insufficiency-addisons-disease/Pages/fact-sheet.aspx

---

REFERENCES

References are available online at **ExpertConsult.com**.

SECTION VII

NEPHROLOGY

SECTION OUTLINE

40 CHRONIC KIDNEY DISEASE

CHAPTER 40

CHRONIC KIDNEY DISEASE

Natalia O. Litbarg, MD

INTRODUCTION

Chronic kidney disease (CKD) is associated with multiple comorbidities, loss of quality of life (QOL), and significant health care costs, and has a high prevalence in most high-income countries (e.g., 5.3% in the UK and 13.7% in the USA) (United States Renal Data System, 2014, http://www.usrds.org/adr.aspx).[1,1a] Early recognition of CKD is important for timely therapeutic interventions and prevention of progression to end-stage renal disease (ESRD).

Definitions

CKD is defined as persistent abnormalities in the kidney structure or function, which are manifested by a decline in glomerular filtration rate (GFR) below 60 mL/min/1.73 m^2 and/or the presence of persistent albuminuria, proteinuria, hematuria, and/or electrolyte imbalances (http://www.kdigo.org/clinical_practice_guidelines/pdf/CKD/KDIGO_2012_CKD_GL.pdf). The prognosis of CKD depends on GFR and the degree of proteinuria (Fig. 40.1). The estimated GFR (eGFR) can be obtained from several formulas using serum creatinine and/or cystatin C levels[2,3](http://nkdep.nih.gov/lab-evaluation/gfr-calculators.shtml). eGFR is very important for the early recognition of CKD because serum creatinine may be "normal" in a patient with diminished muscle mass. In addition, a significant nephron reserve can be lost before either serum creatinine or GFR changes are detectable; this is due to renal compensatory mechanisms such as hypertrophy and hyperfiltration.[4]

Risk Factors

Advancing age, proteinuria, smoking, cardiovascular disease (CVD), certain ethnicities (e.g., African-American, Native-American, and Asian-American), abnormal cholesterol, previous episode(s) of acute kidney injury, exposure to nephrotoxins, and a family history of kidney disease are well-recognized risk factors for developing CKD. In addition, diabetes, hypertension, obesity, and high triglyceride levels have now been identified as early risk factors, which can be present for 30 years or more before a diagnosis of CKD.[5] Many of these risk factors are modifiable and preventable. For example, diabetes and hypertension account for about 44% and 28%, respectively, of all ESRD cases in the US (http://www.cdc.gov/diabetes/pubs/pdf/kidney_factsheet.pdf).

It is likely that many additional risk factors for kidney disease are still not well defined. For example, a lower GFR might be associated with factors in prenatal development (e.g., low birth weight),[6-8] conditions in early life (e.g., formula vs. breastfeeding),[9] or lifetime exposures to environmental toxins (e.g., living near major roads).[10] Atopic diseases have been linked to some idiopathic glomerular diseases.[11]

Pathophysiology

The triggering factors for CKD are diverse; however, endothelial dysfunction, chronic inflammation, and oxidative stress are the main contributors to the progression of CKD from any etiology,[12,13] and are common in the pathophysiology of cardiovascular disease (CVD). Independent of the cause of the initial insult, progression of renal parenchymal injury follows a characteristically uniform pattern,[14] that is, initial loss of nephrons induces adaptive mechanisms, including hypertrophy and hyperfiltration of the remaining functional nephrons. At a certain threshold of renal parenchymal loss, these compensatory mechanisms trigger maladaptive changes and lead to an increase in oxidative stress, production of proinflammatory cytokines, activation of the renin-angiotensin-aldosterone system, and cellular apoptosis (Fig. 40.2), which ultimately promote further nephron damage and loss by glomerulosclerosis, tubular atrophy, and interstitial fibrosis.[15]

Conventional Approach to CKD Management

Any patient with a persistent and unexplained decline in GFR, albuminuria, proteinuria, or hematuria should be referred to a nephrologist, as well as patients with persistent serum electrolytes abnormalities, recurrent nephrolithiasis, hereditary kidney disease, and hypertension that is refractory to treatment with four or more antihypertensive agents (http://www.kdigo.org/clinical_practice_guidelines/pdf/CKD/KDIGO_2012_CKD_GL.pdf).[16] The specific treatment of CKD depends on the underlying causative entity. Glomerular diseases are usually treated based on the renal biopsy diagnosis, and, for the most part, require immunosuppressive and/or cytotoxic medications, while the management of other renal diseases is mostly conservative. The established CKD management of complications is usually according to the Kidney Disease Improving Global Outcomes (KDIGO) guidelines (http://www.kdigo.org/clinical_practice_guidelines/pdf/CKD/KDIGO_2012_CKD_GL.pdf).

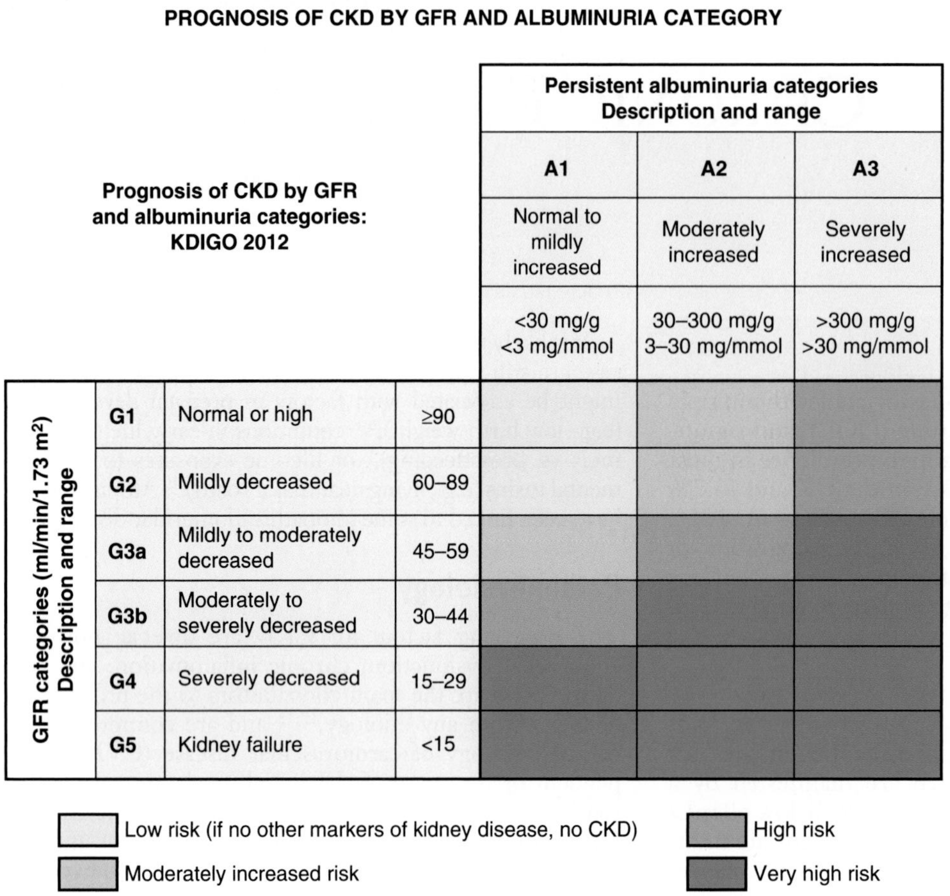

PROGNOSIS OF CKD BY GFR AND ALBUMINURIA CATEGORY

Prognosis of CKD by GFR and albuminuria categories: KDIGO 2012			Persistent albuminuria categories Description and range		
			A1 Normal to mildly increased <30 mg/g <3 mg/mmol	**A2** Moderately increased 30–300 mg/g 3–30 mg/mmol	**A3** Severely increased >300 mg/g >30 mg/mmol
GFR categories (ml/min/1.73 m²) Description and range	G1	Normal or high ≥90			
	G2	Mildly decreased 60–89			
	G3a	Mildly to moderately decreased 45–59			
	G3b	Moderately to severely decreased 30–44			
	G4	Severely decreased 15–29			
	G5	Kidney failure <15			

Low risk (if no other markers of kidney disease, no CKD)   High risk
Moderately increased risk   Very high risk

FIG. 40.1 ■ Prognosis of CKD according to GFR and albuminuria. (From Levey AS, de Jong PE, Coresh J, et al. The definition, classification, and prognosis of chronic kidney disease: a KDIGO controversies conference report. *Kidney Int* 2011;80:17-28.)

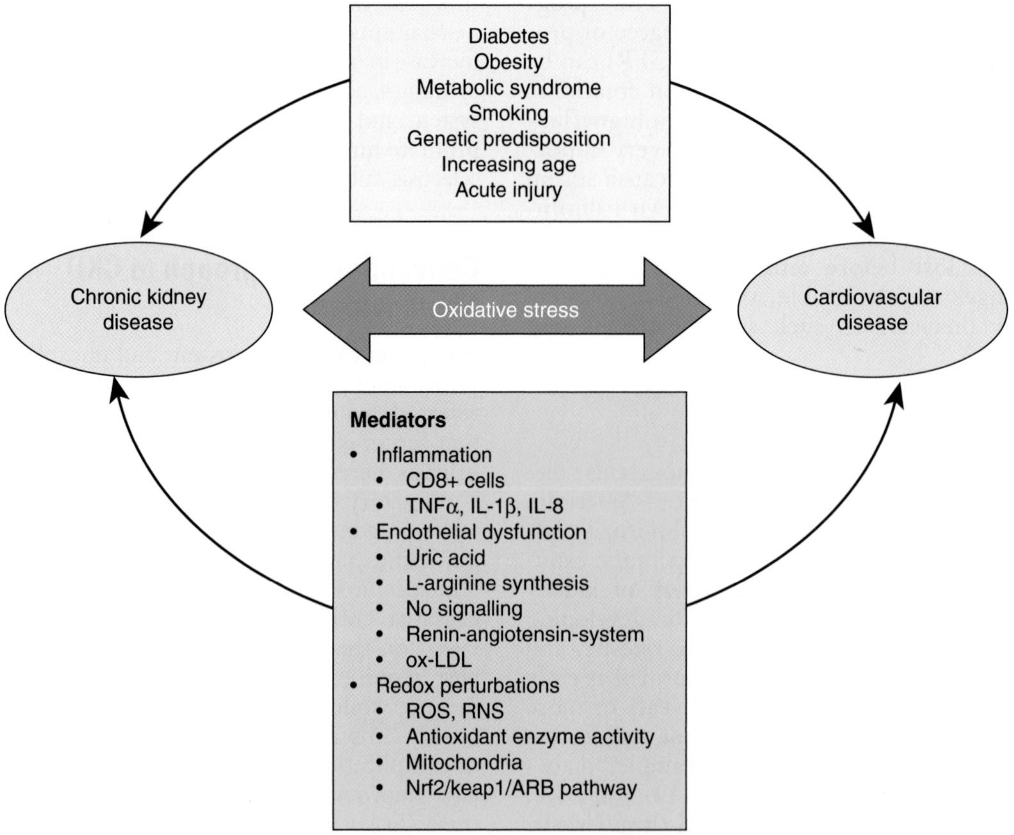

Diabetes
Obesity
Metabolic syndrome
Smoking
Genetic predisposition
Increasing age
Acute injury

Chronic kidney disease ← Oxidative stress → Cardiovascular disease

Mediators
- Inflammation
  - CD8+ cells
  - TNFα, IL-1β, IL-8
- Endothelial dysfunction
  - Uric acid
  - L-arginine synthesis
  - No signalling
  - Renin-angiotensin-system
  - ox-LDL
- Redox perturbations
  - ROS, RNS
  - Antioxidant enzyme activity
  - Mitochondria
  - Nrf2/keap1/ARB pathway

FIG. 40.2 ■ Factors contributing to the progression of CKD and CVD. (From Small DM, Gobe GC. Oxidative stress and antioxidant therapy in chronic kidney and cardiovascular disease. In Morales-Gonzales, JA (ed.): *Oxidative stress and chronic degenerative diseases—a role for antioxidants.* InTech. © 2013 Small DM, Gobe GC. Published in [short citation] under CC BY 3.0 license. Available from: http://dx.doi.org/10.5772/51923.)

Following, the current evidence for integrative strategies in patients with mild to moderate CKD (stage 1–3) is summarized.

INTEGRATIVE THERAPY

Pharmaceuticals

Antihypertensive Agents

According to the 2012 KDIGO guidelines (http://www.kdigo.org) and the Eighth Joint National Committee (JNC 8),[17] angiotensin converting enzyme (ACE) inhibitors and angiotensin receptor blockers (ARBs) are suggested in adult patients with CKD (recommendation grade B). The majority of CKD patients develop volume expansion that requires the use of diuretics. Thiazide diuretics frequently have low efficacy in patients with an eGFR of <45 mL/min/1.73 m^2; therefore, loop diuretics are most frequently used in patients with CKD stage 3 and higher. The addition of aldosterone antagonists or other potassium-sparing diuretics is considered, especially in patients with hypokalemic tendency.[18] However, similar to ACE inhibitors and ARBs, they can increase the risk of hyperkalemia.

Uric Acid-Lowering Agents

Multiple prospective studies, as reviewed by Jalal et al.,[19] involving from 56 to 177,570 subjects who were followed for several years, have demonstrated an association between elevated levels of serum uric acid and the progression of CKD; this was also shown in more recent studies.[20-22] In addition, hyperuricemia was found to be a risk factor for all-cause and CVD mortality,[23] and contrast-induced nephropathy.[24] Treatment of hyperuricemia appeared to lower blood pressure in adolescent patients,[25] patients with immunoglobulin A (IgA) nephropathy,[26] and diabetics with CKD.[27] In four studies involving 50 to 113 patients with CKD and hyperuricemia who were followed from 3 months to 6 years, treatment with allopurinol was associated with decreased progression of CKD.[28,28a-28c]

In five studies involving 60 to 1086 subjects with CKD and hyperuricemia, febuxostat, which is a uric acid-lowering agent with a safer toxicity profile than allopurinol,[29] was associated with better lowering of uric acid levels and a slower decline in renal function.[30-33,33a] In two of these studies, febuxostat had a stronger renoprotective effect than allopurinol.[33,33a] Losartan[34] and irbesartan[35] were also shown to lower uric acid.

There are no recommendations for the treatment of hyperuricemia in CKD in the KDIGO guidelines (http://www.kdigo.org, guideline 3.1.20). The toxicity profile of allopurinol includes severe hypersensitivity reactions, which are rare but potentially lethal. Allopurinol should be started at low dosages (50 mg daily) in patients with CKD and slowly titrated up to achieve the desired lowering of uric acid.[36] A febuxostat dosage of 10–40 mg/day was safe in patients with ESRD who were on dialysis,[37] while the usual doses of 40–120 mg/day have not been studied in patients with an eGFR of <30 mL/min/1.73 m^2. The main associated adverse drug reactions were gout flare-ups[29] (see Chapter 69).

Alkalinizing Therapy

The KDIGO guidelines suggest a correction of serum bicarbonate levels to >22 mmol/L in patients with CKD (grade 2B evidence) (http://www.kdigo.org) in order to improve bone disease and the progression of CKD. Newer data continue to emerge in support of the use of this therapy,[38] and as reviewed by Dobre et al.[39] and Chen et al.[40] The optimal bicarbonate range has yet to be established. Sodium bicarbonate or Shohl's solution can be used, and the base deficit can be calculated (http://www.globalrph.com/bicarb.htm) or replaced empirically and gradually to achieve a bicarbonate level of 22–24 mmol/L. **Caution:** avoid base and sodium overload with bicarbonate supplements,[41] especially in cirrhotic and pregnant patients. Alkalosis has been linked to an increased risk of heart failure in a cohort study[42] and the promotion of vascular calcification in vitro.[43]

Adverse Drug Reactions in CKD

Multiple medications can cause a variety of renal complications.[44-48] The most well recognized are nonsteroidal antiinflammatory drugs (NSAIDs), antibiotics, and chemotherapeutic agents. More recently, acute phosphate nephropathy following exposure to phosphate-containing bowel preparations,[49-52] acute interstitial nephritis associated with proton pump inhibitors,[53,54] and focal segmental glomerulosclerosis (FSGS) and ESRD due to excessive doses of anabolic steroids[55] have been described.

Adverse renal reactions to excipients are less well recognized. A case of silicate nephrolithiasis was reported with nutritional supplements containing silica dioxide.[55a] Sucrose-stabilized intravenous immunoglobulins were associated with acute kidney injury.[56] Aluminum found in commercial drugs, calcium, and iron supplements[57,57a] can cause neurological and bone toxicity in patients with impaired renal function.[58]

Case reports and cohort studies of up to 106 patients highlighted a possible link between various vaccinations and their components (e.g., influenza, hepatitis B, meningoencephalitis, meningococcal C conjugate, tetanus, diphtheria, and poliomyelitis) and glomerular diseases.[59,59a-i]

Nutriceuticals and Supplements

Magnesium

The association between low serum levels of magnesium and increased cardiovascular and all-cause mortality in the general population,[60-62] and in patients with CKD[63-65] is well documented. Hypomagnesemia has also been linked to incident CKD and ESRD,[66] and has been found to contribute to CKD progression in diabetic,[64,67-69] nondiabetic,[70] and post-transplant patients.[71]

The serum concentration of magnesium might be normal in the presence of intracellular magnesium deficiency, especially in patients with CKD.[72] Oral magnesium supplementation can be considered for patients with CKD, especially patients with diabetes, patients with a poor diet, and patients taking diuretics, proton pump inhibitors, and calcineurin inhibitors. Foods rich in magnesium include dark leafy greens, coffee, nuts and seeds, fish, legumes, and whole grains.

Monitoring is required to avoid magnesium overload, especially with magnesium-containing laxatives in patients with CKD.

Vitamin D 25-OH

Expert opinions suggest supplementation with vitamin D 25-OH in CKD stage 3–5 for levels <30 ng/mL (http://www2.kidney.org/professionals/KDOQI/guidelines_bone/Guide7.htm). Multiple observational studies have suggested that vitamin D deficiency is associated with overall and cardiovascular mortality, increased levels of albuminuria, proteinuria, and decreased GFR. However, there is no consensus on the benefits of supplementation, goals for levels, or choice of vitamin D supplements in CKD.[73-83] Although some studies have suggested that there are no adverse effects,[84] caution with vitamin D replacement in CKD is advisable because it can cause increased calcium and phosphate absorption.

Omega-3 Fatty Acids

Several animal[84a,84b] and small clinical studies[85,86,86a-d] and meta-analyses[86e,86f] have suggested beneficial effects of omega-3 fatty acid supplementation on renal function at doses between 0.4–7.7 g/day; however, the evidence is weak and largely based on patients with IgA nephropathy and lupus nephritis.[86c]

Coenzyme Q10 (CoQ10)

Antioxidant CoQ10 has demonstrated renoprotective effects in ischemic, diabetic, and hypertensive animal models of kidney injury.[87-91] In 100 patients who underwent extracorporeal shock-wave lithotripsy, CoQ10 200 mg/day, given for one week before and after the procedure, was associated with a significant increase in GFR and decrease in the urine albumin/creatinine ratio.[92] In a randomized controlled trial of 97 patients with advanced CKD, treatment with hydrosoluble CoQ10 at 180 mg/day appeared to reduce serum creatinine levels and the need for dialysis.[93] Conversely, in a study of 85 patients with CKD stage 3–4, CoQ10 supplementation of 200 mg/day for 8 weeks had no effect on renal function, blood pressure, albuminuria, or proteinuria.[94]

DOSAGE

CoQ10 at doses of 100–200 mg/day appears to be safe in CKD.

N-Acetylcysteine

N-acetylcysteine (NAC) is a precursor of endogenous antioxidants.[15] Furthermore, it might have heavy metal detoxification effects[95-97] and homocysteine-lowering properties. NAC is currently recommended as part of the prevention against acute kidney injury in at-risk patients undergoing intravenous contrast administration (http://www.kdigo.org). The benefits of NAC for renal function preservation have been demonstrated in an animal model[98] and in two small studies performed in patients already on dialysis with residual renal function,[99,100] but not in a placebo-controlled, randomized, open, crossover trial of 20 patients with nondiabetic CKD.[101]

DOSAGE

The commonly prescribed dose of 600 mg twice daily was not associated with side effects in any of the previous studies. Wheat grass is a good nutritional source of NAC.

PRECAUTIONS

NAC should not be prescribed to patients with cystinuria (Cysteine, University of Maryland Medical Center, http://umm.edu/health/medical/altmed/supplement/cysteine#ixzz3YveeNWpy).

PROTOCOL FOR PREVENTING CONTRAST-INDUCED NEPHROPATHY (CONSIDER IN PATIENTS WITH CR > 2.5 MG/DL)

- NAC 1200 mg IV bolus prior to procedure.
- 600 mg orally twice daily for 48 hr after procedure.
- Hydrate with 1 cc/kg (or 0.5 cc/kg in patients with congestive heart failure) normal saline per hour for 12 hours after procedure.

Prebiotics, Probiotics, and Synbiotics

The restoration of intestinal integrity and the microbiome is beneficial in any inflammatory condition.[102,103] In recent years, there has been a greater appreciation of the role of the intestinal microbiome in renal disease.[102,104] Dysbiosis can be caused by CKD due to increased intestinal urea secretion, resulting in excess ammonia, metabolic acidosis, intestinal wall edema, and slow colonic transit, which is frequently complicated by fiber-deficient diets and an increased use of iron and antibiotics.[105] In turn, dysbiosis can contribute to CKD by causing systemic inflammation, endothelial dysfunction, and atherosclerosis, which are related to increased intestinal permeability, bacterial translocation with subclinical endotoxemia, and abnormal colonic bacteria overproduction of uremic toxins.[106-108] Several small studies on probiotic supplementation in patients with CKD stage 3–5 demonstrated variable beneficial results with no adverse effects. The spectrum of benefits included decrease in blood urea nitrogen, creatinine, uric acid, serum uremic toxins levels, improved quality of life, nutritional status, bowel movements, and bacterial dysbiosis.[109-113] In a systematic review and meta-analysis of randomized, controlled trials, patients on probiotics had mildly improved blood pressures.[114,114a] In general, probiotics are considered to be safe; however, they have been linked to cases of sepsis.[115-117] Prebiotics, including inulin, lactulose, and oligofructose, can act synergistically with probiotics to optimize uremic gut dysbiosis. Several studies of prebiotic and synbiotic supplements proved beneficial in patients with ESRD[118,119,119a]; however, no studies are available for the earlier stages of CKD.

Other Supplements and Vitamins With Potential Benefits in CKD

Niacin was found to be beneficial in rats with CKD[120,121] and lowered phosphate levels in patients with CKD.[121a-c] However, when added to statins, niacin did not improve cardiovascular outcome or kidney function, and was associated with higher all-cause mortality in patients with CKD.[122]

High-resistant starch *fiber* supplementation was demonstrated to attenuate oxidative stress, inflammation, and severity of renal dysfunction in a rat model of CKD.[123] High-amylose corn starch (Hi-maize 260) reduced serum levels of uremic toxins in patients with ESRD on hemodialysis, with minimal gastrointestinal side effects.[124]

Vitamin K deficiency is prevalent,[125-127] and a higher than recommended daily intake of vitamin K was associated with a lower risk of all-cause and CVD mortality in advanced CKD;[127] however, the dose and benefit/risk profiles are currently unknown.[128]

Lowering homocysteine levels with *folic acid, vitamin B6,* and *vitamin B12* supplements in patients with CKD (GFR < 60 mL/min) for 5 years was not found to influence cardiovascular outcomes.[128a] A Cochrane systematic review concluded that there was no evidence to recommend the use of *vitamin B* therapy for delaying the progression of diabetic kidney disease. In a single study, *thiamine* was found to be beneficial for reducing albuminuria.[129]

Palmitoylethanolamide (PEA), a derivative of palmitic acid and the commonest fatty acid present in palm tree oil, meats, and dairy products, was shown to be a safe antiinflammatory agent in several animal studies and one observational study in humans,[130] and improved kidney disease in an animal model, as reviewed by Impelizzeri et al.[131]

Short-chain fatty acids (acetate, propionate, and butyrate) are present in high-quality dairy products (e.g., butter and ghee) and are produced by intestinal bacteria.[132,133] Short-chain fatty acid supplementation was found to improve renal function in animals with various models of acute kidney injury.[134-136]

Herbals

Turmeric and Curcumin

The common Asian spice turmeric (*Curcuma longa*) with its most active ingredient curcumin has been used in Oriental medicine for centuries as an antiinflammatory, antioxidant, anticarcinogenic, and antimicrobial agent. Many of these properties have been scientifically confirmed in the last few decades.[137] Numerous studies have demonstrated the benefits of curcumin in various animal models of kidney injury.[137-139] In small randomized trials, turmeric has been shown to reduce proteinuria and serum levels of proinflammatory cytokines in patients with diabetic nephropathy,[140] as well as proteinuria, hematuria, and systolic blood pressure in patients with relapsing or refractory biopsy-proven lupus nephritis[141] without adverse events.

DOSAGE

Generally accepted doses are between 500–2000 mg/day. The bioavailability of curcumin is increased by 2000% by the addition of black pepper[142] (Ayurvedic formulation: 1 part black pepper to 16 parts turmeric).

PRECAUTIONS

Use with caution in doses >600 mg/day in patients at risk of bleeding and hypoglycemia, and in pregnancy, gallbladder disease, and in combination with certain medications. (National Institute of Health MedlinePlus: Turmeric http://www.nlm.nih.gov/medlineplus/druginfo/natural/662.html)

Astragalus

Astragalus membranaceus (huang qi) was found to have renal protective effects in 1804 diabetic patients with nephropathy based on a meta-analysis of studies from China,[143] in a Cochrane review of 22 studies of 1323 participants with CKD,[144] and in a Cochrane systematic review of nine studies in patients with nephrotic syndrome.[145] Small participant numbers and suboptimal methodological and reporting quality prevented definitive conclusions on the basis of these studies. In Chinese medicine, astragalus is used either alone or in combination with other herbs in various doses and forms. Allergic reactions were the most commonly reported adverse events; however, not all studies reported adverse events. Caution is advised in pregnancy.[146]

Cordyceps

Cordyceps sinensis mushroom has been prescribed for centuries in Chinese, Indian, and Tibetan medicine as a tonic.[147] Some animal and human studies have suggested benefits of cordyceps in renal disease.[148] A recent Cochrane review of cordyceps for the treatment of CKD, which included 22 studies with 1746 participants (all published in Chinese), suggested that cordyceps preparations, when used as an adjuvant therapy to conventional medicine, decreased serum creatinine and proteinuria, and increased creatinine clearance, hemoglobin, and serum albumin. The treatment duration ranged from 1 to 6 months, and the doses and preparations varied. The quality of evidence was considered to be low.[149]

DOSAGE

In general, at doses of 1–3 g/day, cordyceps appears to be safe.

PRECAUTIONS

Use with caution in pregnancy/lactation and in patients with autoimmune disease or on immunosuppressive agents.

Rheum officinale

Rhubarb (*Rheum officinale*, or yào yòng dà huáng) root is a common ingredient in virtually all herbal therapies used in Chinese medicine to treat renal failure. In several clinical studies from China, the use of herbal formulations containing *Rheum officinale* was reported to slow the progression of CKD. The study sizes varied from 30–100 subjects, and the etiologies and degrees of renal failure varied. Oral decoction at doses ranging from 1–15 g/day was used for 3 weeks to 40 months.[146,150-153] A Cochrane review of nine studies (682 participants) concluded that the evidence for the efficacy of *Rheum officinale* in improving CKD was scant and of low quality.[154]

PRECAUTIONS

Rheum officinale preparations have high potassium and oxalate content, are reported to cause gastrointestinal problems, electrolyte disorders, and liver toxicity with long-term use,[155] and are even reported to cause AKI.[156]

Tripterygium wilfordii *Hook F*

A Cochrane systematic review found that *Tripterygium wilfordii* Hook F (a traditional Chinese herb léi gōng téng) may have a favorable effect on remission in patients with primary nephrotic syndrome when added to conventional treatment with prednisone or cyclosporine.[157]

DOSAGE

A meta-analysis of four randomized controlled trials with 188 participants found that when used in conjunction with ACE inhibitors, ARBs, or prednisone, it improved remission rates and urinary protein in patients with IgA nephropathy at doses of 60 mg/day or 1–1.5 mg/kg/day.[158]

PRECAUTIONS

Drugs containing *Tripterygium wilfordii* have a narrow therapeutic window, the dose depends on the extraction method, and adequate safety studies are limited. More serious complications include leukopenia, intestinal bleeding, respiratory and liver failure, and even death.[159] Cautious use in geriatric and pediatric populations, and avoidance in pregnancy is recommended.[146]

Ligustrazine

Ligustrazine is a bioactive component contained in Chuan Xiong, a dry rhizome of *Ligusticum chuanxiong*, which is traditionally used in Chinese medicine for the treatment of cardiovascular diseases, headache, and vertigo. It has been used in China for more than 30 years in its purified synthetic form for renal failure, lung fibrosis, and stroke. In a meta-analysis of 25 randomized controlled trials that included a total of 1645 patients with stage 3–4 diabetic nephropathy, treatment with ligustrazine was shown to result in significant therapeutic improvement in blood urea nitrogen, serum creatinine, and urinary protein.[160] Some data from the Chinese literature suggest that ligustrazine might be helpful in nondiabetic CKD, nephritic syndrome (in combination with prednisone), and in the prevention of gentamicin nephrotoxicity (http://www.itmonline.org/arts/ligustrazine.htm).

DOSAGE

Ligustrazine is given as an injection with doses ranging from 40 to 400 mg daily and treatment duration ranging from 10 days to 12 weeks.

PRECAUTIONS

No adverse events have been reported.

Herbal Toxicities

Many herbal remedies can cause significant renal complications (Table 40.1) as described in several reviews.[161-164] Herbal supplements can be contaminated with or contain heavy metals as part of the therapeutic prescription.[165-167] Many herbal supplements have the potential for interaction with prescription medications.[168,169] The KDIGO guidelines recommend that herbal remedies should not be used in patients with CKD (evidence strength 1B) (http://www.kdigo.org/clinical_practice_guidelines/pdf/CKD/KDIGO_2012_CKD_GL.pdf, recommendation 4.4.5). On the other hand, there are very little data comparing the complications caused by herbal medicines and pharmaceuticals.

Nutrition

In multiple studies, healthier diets *rich in plants, whole grains, fiber, calcium, magnesium, and potassium,* such as the Mediterranean diet, have been associated with lower incidence, progression, and mortality in CKD when compared to Western-style diets that are high in fried foods, nondairy animal products, organ meats, cholesterol, and sweetened beverages.[170-176]

Heavy consumption of oxalate-rich juices has been reported to precipitate renal oxalosis and acute kidney injury.[177] Be careful when recommending juicing diets for patients with CKD.

Current guidelines (evidence strength 2C) suggest avoiding high protein intake (>1.3 g/kg/day) in adults

TABLE 40.1 **Herbal Remedies With Nephrotoxic Potential**

Plant Species	Common Name	Toxic Compound	Adverse Renal Effects
Ajuga nipponensis Makino[313]			Acute kidney injury, death
Amanita smithiana, Amanitha proxima, Amanita pseudoporphyria Hongo mushrooms[314-321]			Acute kidney injury, acute tubular necrosis
Aristolochia species[322-327]	Birthwort, pipevine	Aristolochic acid	Aristolochic acid nephropathy with progressive and extensive interstitial fibrosis and proximal tubular atrophy; Fanconi syndrome; urological malignancies
Artemisia absinthium[328]	Wormwood		Rhabdomyolysis and acute kidney injury after ingestion of wormwood oil
Averrhoa carambola[329,330]	Star fruit	Oxalic acid	Acute kidney injury, oxalate nephropathy
Cape Aloes[331]			Acute kidney injury
Cerbera thevetia[332]	Yellow oleander		Acute kidney injury
Cortinarius speciosissimus, Cortinarius orellanus mushrooms[333-337]		Orellanine	Acute kidney injury requiring dialysis; severe tubulo-interstitial lesions with polymorphous cell infiltration, edema, loose fibrosis, and epithelial necrosis
Cupressus funebris Endl.[338]	Morning Cypress	Flavonoids	Acute kidney injury with acute tubular necrosis, acute interstitial nephritis, hemoglobin casts
Ephedra sinica[339-341]	Ma huang, ephedra	Ephedrine	Nephrolithiasis
Glycyrrhiza glabra[342,343]	Licorice	Glycyrrhizin	Hypokalemic nephropathy, hypokalemic rhabdomyolysis with secondary acute kidney injury
Larrea Tridentata[344]	Chapparal or creosote bush		Renal cysts, renal cell carcinoma
Pausinystalia yohimbe[345]	Yohimbe	Yohimbine	Lupus-like syndrome with progressive renal failure
Pithecellobium lobatum, Pithecellobium jeringa, Archidendron pauciflorum[346-350]	Djengkol beans	Djenkolic acid	Acute tubular necrosis, nephrolithiasis, obstructive nephropathy, hematuria
Rumex acetosa[351]	Sorrel	Oxalic acid	Acute kidney injury
Russula subnigricans mushroom[352,353]		cycloprop-2-ene carboxylic acid	Rhabdomyolysis and acute kidney injury
Uncaria guianensis or *Uncaria tomentosa*[354]	Cat's claw Uno de gata		Acute kidney injury attributed to acute allergic interstitial nephritis (renal biopsy not done)

with CKD at risk of progression (http://www.kdigo.org). However, the accumulation of data on the risks of high animal protein intake and the benefits of *animal protein restriction* in patients with CKD is ongoing.[178,179]

Existing guidelines recommend *sodium restriction* to <2 g (or <5 g of sodium chloride)/day in patients with CKD (evidence grade 1C) (http://www.kdigo.org). Recent studies introduced further controversy to these recommendations.[180,181,181a-c] A Cochrane review on dietary salt intake in CKD patients analyzed eight studies (24 reports, 258 participants) and found a gap in critical evidence for the long-term effects of salt restriction on mortality and progression to ESRD, despite the fact that salt restriction considerably reduced blood pressure and proteinuria.[182] Low sodium diets are contraindicated in patients with renal sodium wasting.

Several studies have demonstrated an association of *higher potassium* intake (>2.7–3.3 g/day vs. <1.7 g/day) with lower blood pressures (Mente et al. 2014)[183] and improved renal outcomes in various populations

(Smyth et al. 2014);[180] however, there are no established recommendations for patients with CKD[184] (see Chapter 89).

Hyperphosphatemia in patients with CKD can cause metabolic bone disease, and is associated with an increased prevalence of CVD and mortality. The KDIGO guidelines recommend dietary phosphorus restriction and phosphate binders for hyperphosphatemia (evidence strength 2D) (http://www.kdigo.com). It has been suggested that *inorganic phosphate additives* from processed foods contribute to the progression of CKD in healthy and at-risk individuals,[185] while a vegetarian diet appeared to be beneficial for phosphate balancing in patients with CKD.[186] This can be explained by the significantly lower content and availability of organic phosphates naturally present in plant-based foods (20%–50% absorption) as compared to inorganic phosphate additives in processed foods (90%–100% absorption)[187,188] with a 60% higher content.[189] Inorganic phosphate additives are not indicated on food labels in the US.

Processed foods contain phosphate that is 90%–100% absorbed compared to phosphates naturally found in whole foods, which are 20%–50% absorbed. Therefore, whole foods are safer in patients with CKD.

In two cohort studies, *high dietary fiber* has been associated with better kidney function, and lower inflammation and mortality risk.[190,191] Consumption of *whole grains* that are rich in fiber has been associated with improved glycemic control, circulation, dyslipidemia, and inflammation.[192-195]

In two small studies, *alkalinizing diets*, which are rich in plant-based foods and low in meat and processed foods,[196] have been shown to result in an equal reduction of urine albumin and GFR loss as administration of sodium bicarbonate in patients with CKD.[197,197a] Higher dietary acid load has been associated with lower serum bicarbonate[198] and increased risk of ESRD [199] in the general US population.

Raw nuts are an important source of healthy fats, magnesium, and protein, and their intake in any amount has been found to decrease the risk of mortality related to CKD.[200] **Caution:** excessive intake of nuts should be avoided in CKD due to the potential risk of hyperphosphatemia and oxalate nephropathy.[201] Recommend a handful, not a canful.

High sugar diets contribute to obesity, diabetes, hyperuricemia, and hypertension,[202] and can potentially be damaging to the kidneys.[203] *Artificial sweeteners* have been associated with a decline in renal function in women.[204]

Dietary sources of *probiotics* include fermented dairy products (e.g., yoghurt, lassi, and kefir), vegetables (e.g., kimchi, sauerkraut, olives, and pickles), and soybeans (e.g., miso and natto). Dietary sources of *prebiotics* include chicory root, okra, taro root, dandelion greens, asparagus, bananas, and the garlic and onion family. Caution regarding the amount of salt in fermented products and phosphorus in dairy products should be advised in patients with CKD.

A cohort study of 5746 participants found an inverse relationship between *alcohol* consumption and the risk of developing CKD;[205] however, based on a systematic review, the beneficial role of alcohol consumption on renal function has not been consistently demonstrated.[206]

Multiple case reports have suggested a link between *food sensitivity* and idiopathic glomerular lesions (minimal change disease, membranous glomerulonephritis, type I diabetic nephropathy, IgA nephropathy, and membranoproliferative glomerulonephritis), and some have reported successful outcomes with *avoidance of gluten and/or dairy*[59,207-222,222a] (see Chapter 86).

Environmental Toxins

Large-volume filtration of the blood enhances renal exposure to circulating toxins and renders the kidneys highly susceptible to injury.[223] It is well known that significant exposure to heavy metals, organic solvents, and certain food additives causes nephrotoxicity.[224-235] Recent findings have indicated that even low-dose exposure to toxins

might be associated with kidney disease,[233,236,237] with potential synergy in toxic effects.[238] In Sri Lanka and Central America, the combination of water and dietary pollutants, heavy metals, herbicides, and increased ambient temperatures has been implicated in newly described clusters of CKD of unknown etiology (CKDu).[239-243] Excessive risks of kidney disease have been documented in minority and disadvantaged populations, suggesting disparities in the environmental exposures.[244]

Information on this topic, including information about heavy metals, organic solvents, plastics, pesticides and herbicides, flame retardants, food and cosmetic additives, and air and water pollution, can be found online at ExpertConsult.com.

Diagnosis and Treatment of Environmental Toxicities

Diagnosis of toxicities by environmental pollutants is challenging because the safety margin for exposures is unknown, measurements of levels are not routine, clinical symptoms can be vague, progression of renal disease is multifactorial, and physicians' awareness is low due to the scarcity and controversies in evidence. A thorough history of environmental exposures should be obtained.

Recent studies from China suggest some benefits of lead-chelating therapies with calcium disodium EDTA (ethylenediaminetetraacetic acid) on reducing progression of CKD in patients with high-normal body lead burden[245,246] (see Chapter 107). However, these treatments are cumbersome and serious complications, including renal toxicity[247] and death (due to hypocalcemia), have been reported (http://www.cdc.gov/mmwr/preview/mmwrhtml/mm5508a3.htm). Other chelating therapies that have been studied in heavy metal poisoning include British antilewisite (BAL) or dimercaprol, meso-2,3-dimercaptosuccinic acid (DMSA), 2,3-dimercaaptopropanesulfonic acid (DMPS), and thiamine tetrahydrofurfuryl disulfide (TTFD). Only EDTA and DMSA are FDA approved; however, all have the potential for complications, including chelation of vitamins, renal complications, and neuro- and hepatotoxicity (Food and Drug Administration 14 October 2010). Chelating agents that have been proposed but not studied in CKD include modified citrus pectin (Pectasol), seaweed extract sodium alginate, oral adsorbent activated charcoal, vitamins E and C, selenocysteine, NAC, N-acetylcysteine amide (NACA), and alpha-lipoic acid. However, the only recommendations at this time are avoidance and discontinuation of toxic exposure along with a general healthy lifestyle (see Chapter 108).

Lifestyle Modifications

Weight Loss

Achieving a healthy weight with a body mass index (BMI) of 20–25 is recommended by renal guidelines (www.kdigo.org), and is supported by multiple studies linking obesity with negative outcomes in patients with CKD.[248-251]

Smoking Cessation

Smoking, including secondhand smoking, is a well-recognized risk factor for CKD onset and progression,[252-259] and, in combination with hypertension, is associated with the newly described pathological lesion of nodular glomerulosclerosis.[260-262]

Exercise

For patients with CKD, KDIGO guidelines recommend physical activity that is compatible with cardiovascular health and tolerance, aiming for at least 30 minutes 5 times/week (www.kdigo.org). Exercise in patients with CKD has been shown to improve physical capacity and quality of life,[262a] and, in several studies, has been shown to correlate with slower progression of CKD.[262b-f]

Sleep

Low quality of sleep is common in CKD patients, even in the early stages.[263] An animal model of circadian rhythm disruption was associated with severe renal disease.[264] In human subjects, obstructive sleep apnea (OSA) was associated with increased serum creatinine,[265] cystatin C,[266] urinary albumin,[267,268] accelerated renal function loss,[269] and diabetic nephropathy.[270] Inversely, CKD was also associated with OSA,[271] and CKD progression was accompanied by a worsening of sleep quality.[272]

Stress

Stress can have a negative impact on kidney disease through alterations in the hypothalamic-pituitary-adrenal axis, sympathetic nervous system, and inflammatory cytokines, leading to the development of insulin resistance, metabolic syndrome, obesity, hypertension, type 2 diabetes, and vascular disease.[273]

Mind-Body Therapies

Meditation has been shown to decrease blood pressure, sympathetic activity, and improve quality of life in normal subjects and patients with CKD.[274-279]

Yoga might be beneficial in CKD based on its effects on reducing oxidative stress, psychological stress, and inflammatory conditions.[280] **Caution:** complete inverted poses and fast breathing practices can increase sympathetic activity and raise blood pressure. Yogic cleansing procedures may precipitate electrolyte imbalances and increase the toxic workload on the kidneys.

Tai chi has been found to be beneficial in a small randomized trial of patients with CKD and CVD by improving renal and cardiovascular parameters.[281]

Therapies to Consider

Traditional Chinese Medicine

CKD can be caused by variable element imbalances and deficiencies in traditional Chinese medicine (TCM).[151,282,283,283a] The current evidence of the benefits of TCM in CKD is mostly from small nonrandomized trials.[284] Moreover, the reporting of adverse reactions has been suboptimal.[283a] TCM therapies have been associated with significant adverse reactions, including nephrotoxicity, possibly due to adulteration of herbal remedies with heavy metals, pesticides, and undeclared drugs.[285-287]

Acupuncture

In animal models, *acupuncture* modalities were found to improve hypertension,[288] decrease kidney damage,[289-292] and ameliorate skeletal muscle atrophy in CKD.[293] A small clinical trial found acupuncture to be effective in improving renal function in patients with acute gout attacks and renal damage.[294] Many studies on acupuncture are available exclusively in Chinese.

Ayurveda

Ayurvedic protocols are individualized for each patient with CKD based on variable Dosha imbalances. Multiple Ayurvedic herbs have demonstrated benefits in various animal models of kidney injury.[295-300] There is limited evidence on the efficacy of Ayurvedic detoxification (panchakarma) in humans.[301] Most human studies that have demonstrated benefits of Ayurvedic treatments in CKD are case reports from India,[302-304] with a few multi-patient (67 to 150 subjects) cohort studies.[305-307] Treatment protocols vary; however, the most frequently used herbs are Purnava (*Boerhaavia diffusa*) and Gokshur (*Tribulus terrestris*). Nonherbal Ayurvedic interventions, such as diet, mind-body, and aromatherapy, are likely to be safe; however, the evidence is limited.

Up to 20% of Ayuervedic formulas (up to 40% if Rasa Shastra) were reported to contain unsafe levels of heavy metals,[308,309] and treatments have been reported to cause nephrotoxicity.[310-312]

PREVENTION PRESCRIPTION

- Avoid nephrotoxic medications
- Avoid fluid depletion
- Optimize weight
- Control hypertension, diabetes, and dyslipidemia
- Maintain a balanced, antiinflammatory, low pollutant, alkalinizing diet
- Eat more vegetables, greens, legumes, whole grains, raw nuts, healthy oils, and magnesium-, potassium-, and fiber-rich foods
- Eat less salt, animal protein, simple sugars
- Give preference to organic foods, fish with high omega-3 fatty acids and low levels of mercury
- Avoid processed food, added sugars in all forms, artificial sweeteners, food additives, high-mercury fish, and high-oxalate diet

- Include probiotics and prebiotics in the daily diet
- Avoid exposure to environmental pollutants:
  - Drink pure water
  - Avoid smoking, including secondhand smoking
  - Avoid herbal medicines with heavy metal contaminants
  - Avoid mercury in dental amalgam, herbals, and fish
  - Avoid air pollution by keeping a distance from major roads and industrial sites
- Exercise regularly
- Avoid stress and sleep deprivation, aim for high quality sleep, practice meditation and other mind-body techniques, such as yoga or tai chi
- Maintain proper oral hygiene and treat periodontitis

THERAPEUTIC REVIEW

GENERAL
- Optimize weight, control hypertension, diabetes mellitus, and dyslipidemia
- Avoid potential nephrotoxic medications and volume depletion

DIET
- Maintain a balanced antiinflammatory, low pollutant, alkalinizing diet
- Lower animal protein and sodium
- Avoid sugar, processed food, inorganic phosphate additives, and artificial sweeteners
- Add raw nuts, prebiotics, probiotics, and fiber-containing foods
- Elimination diet (gluten-, dairy-, casein-free) in cases of glomerulonephritis
- Avoid high-oxalate and high-purine diets

LIFESTYLE
- Exercise regularly
- Smoking avoidance/cessation
- Practice mind-body modalities, such as gentle yoga, tai chi, and meditation
- High quality sleep, address obstructive sleep apnea, minimize stress

DETOXIFICATION
- Discontinue exposure to environmental toxins
- Chelation for heavy metal toxicity
- Chelation to decrease heavy metal total body burden
- Dental amalgam removal
- Avoid herbal medicines and fish contaminated with heavy metals

- Avoid plastic food and beverage containers
- Drink pure water

PHARMACEUTICALS
For the management of hypertension, anemia, bone disease, lipids in CKD follow the KDIGO and/or Kidney Disease Outcome Quality Initiative (KDOQI) guidelines (variable levels of evidence)
- Magnesium (not to exceed upper limits of normal)
- Sodium bicarbonate or Shohl's solution (to keep serum bicarbonate levels between 22–24 mmol/L)
- Febuxostat 10–40 mg/day for hyperuricemia
- Losartan 50 mg/day or irbesartan 50–150 mg/day for hyperuricemia with hypertension and type 2 diabetes mellitus
- Allopurinol 50–300 mg/day for hyperuricemia

SUPPLEMENTS
- Omega 3 fatty acids 2–6 g/day
- Vitamin D 25-OH
- Probiotic supplements

HERBALS
- Turmeric (Curcumin) 500–2000 mg/day
- *Astragalus membranaceus* (huang qi)* 15–40 g/day
- *Cordyceps sinensis** 1–5 g/day
- *Ligusticum wallichii* (*Ligusticum chuanxiong*, ligustrazine)* 40–400 mg/day
- *Tripterygium wilfordii* Hook F (lei gong teng)* 12–15 g/day
- Rhubarb root 6–15 g/day

ALTERNATIVE THERAPIES
- Ayurveda
- Traditional Chinese medicine
- Acupuncture

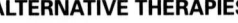
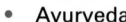

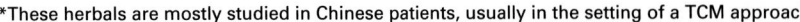
*These herbals are mostly studied in Chinese patients, usually in the setting of a TCM approach.

Key Web Resources

National Kidney Foundation guidelines for CKD management, patient CKD education materials, physician tools including GFR calculators and CME	https://www.kidney.org
Kidney Disease Improving Global Outcomes, international guidelines for CKD management	http://www.kdigo.org
National Kidney Disease Education Program, GFR calculators and formulas	http://nkdep.nih.gov/lab-evaluation/gfr-calculators.shtml
United States Department of Agriculture (USDA) National Nutrient Database for Standard Reference	http://fnic.nal.usda.gov/food-composition
The Environmental Working Group, information on environmental toxins	http://www.ewg.org

ACKNOWLEDGMENTS

I would like to thank Drs. Viorica Khalili and David Rakel for their contributions to this chapter.

REFERENCES

References are available online at ExpertConsult.com.

SECTION VIII

GASTROINTESTINAL DISORDERS

SECTION OUTLINE

41 IRRITABLE BOWEL SYNDROME

42 GASTROESOPHAGEAL REFLUX DISEASE

43 PEPTIC ULCER DISEASE

44 CHOLELITHIASIS

45 RECURRING ABDOMINAL PAIN IN PEDIATRICS

46 CONSTIPATION

CHAPTER 41

IRRITABLE BOWEL SYNDROME

Patrick J. Hanaway, MD

Functional changes in bowel patterns are the hallmark of irritable bowel syndrome (IBS) and were described by Hippocrates as the triad of abdominal discomfort, irregular bowel movements, and various degrees of bloating and rectal urgency. IBS is a chronic relapsing disease in which symptoms vary significantly over time. The undulating course of this symptom complex has limited the ability of studies of the natural history of IBS to distinguish between treatment effects and normal variation. In fact, this is why IBS has been considered to have a more psychosocial overlay. IBS has been considered a "diagnosis of exclusion," defined by the presence of symptoms (abdominal pain/discomfort, bloating, and diarrhea or constipation) and a lack of clearly defined pathology. However, this understanding has evolved significantly over the past 10 years, with the emergence of a view (long-held by integrative and naturopathic physicians) that IBS is multifactorial in nature, involving a dynamic interplay between host factors (genetics and family history), intestinal function (digestion, intestinal permeability, gut microflora, inflammation/immune activation, motility, and visceral sensitivity) in addition to environmental factors, particularly stress and diet.[1,2] This systems-based, integrative approach is, in part, supported by current clinical practices and the consensus of most physicians, though randomized controlled trials (RCTs) are necessary to validate this approach.[3]

PATHOPHYSIOLOGY

The pathogenesis of IBS is multifactorial, with contributions from diet,[4] digestive function,[5] modified permeability,[6] enteric infection,[7] altered GI flora,[8,9] food sensitivities/allergies,[10] visceral hypersensitivity,[11] altered motility,[12] neuroendocrine dysfunction,[13] psychosocial factors,[14] stress,[15] and other factors.[16] Different subsets of patients will present with different functional imbalances, as well as different patterns of interactions between the components of the overall system. This variable presentation may explain why responses to single therapies are so common with IBS. Recent studies of IBS treatments have focused on diet and nutrition, psychoneuroendocrinology, gut microflora, and the immune system, whereas as earlier research predominantly focused on the gut–brain interactions that involve visceral perception and autonomic response.[17] However, more recent studies of postinfectious IBS (PI-IBS), low grade inflammation, small intestinal bowel overgrowth, and altered gut microflora have yielded more effective clinical improvements.[18]

Digestive Function

Digestion of food, through mastication, activation of proenzymes by highly acidic gastric environment, stimulation of the pancreas and gall bladder, and absorption of macro/micronutrients with the support of intact microvilli provide the necessary conditions for digestive function to occur.

Intestinal Permeability

Increased small bowel and colonic permeability has been observed in up to 40% of patients with IBS-D[19] and is associated with visceral hypersensitivity, as well as increased risk of comorbid autoimmune diseases.[20] Alterations in microflora, infections, food allergies, and stressors will all serve to increase permeability promoting symptom exacerbation and acting as trigger for other disease. Permeability issues can be assessed using a "double-sugar" lactulose-mannitol urine test or through the presence of diffusely positive IgG food antibody testing.

Gut Microflora

Studies have increasingly linked the gut microflora to the symptoms and pathophysiology of IBS.[21,22] Findings of these studies include a 3.5-fold increase in patients developing IBS after an enteric infection[23]; increased risk of IBS after antibiotic usage[24]; and multiple molecular studies have demonstrated a decreased diversity of the gut microflora, particularly in aerobic species.[25] Additionally, concerns regarding gut microflora overgrowth in IBS have been raised by the work of Pimentel and colleagues[26] who reported that the eradication of small intestinal bacterial overgrowth (SIBO) using the nonabsorbable drug rifaximin eliminated IBS symptoms in 41% of patients over placebo. This type of overgrowth may provide a better understanding of the bloating and distention common in IBS.[27] Note that while multiple courses of rifaximin can be used safely, it is necessary to understand and treat the underlying cause of SIBO in each patient. For example, proton pump inhibitors may create the conditions required for SIBO.

Immune Dysfunction and Inflammation

Abnormal activation and dysregulated immune function with chronic, low-grade inflammation appears to be an important feature of IBS. Often mediated via mast cells, the role of gastrointestinal flora in immune activation is currently being explored across the continuum of functional bowel disease.[28] The presence of inflammation within the GI tract potentiates activation of visceral perception, motility, and hypersensitivity, even after the original infection has cleared.[29]

Probiotic and dietary prebiotic therapies have been used to correct these deficiencies with good results. Each species and strain of probiotic is unique, with different biochemical effects and specific interactions with the mucosal immune system (see Chapter 105). Additionally, stress has been shown to promote an inflammatory phenotype in patients with IBS. Chronic stress in IBS patients suppresses TH_1 and TH_2 responses and increases IL-6 expression. As stress and inflammation increase, so do symptoms. Accordingly, future treatment strategies should consider each of these phenotypic subsets.[30]

Enteric Nervous System

It is well understood clinically that there is a bidirectional influence of the gut's enteric nervous system (ENS) on the brain's central nervous system (CNS) and vice-versa. We commonly discuss "gut feelings" and recognize stress and emotions affect GI function, modify the gut microbiome, and change symptoms in IBS patients.[31] In addition to elevations in cortisol, patients with IBS have significantly higher postprandial serotonin levels, which are associated with altered gastric emptying, increased small bowel contractions, faster small transit time, and altered pain perception.[32]

Dr. Michael Gershon first described the enteric nervous system (ENS) as the "second brain"[33] that detects nutrients, monitors the progress of digestion, and modulates the pressure/motility of the GI tract. Alterations in the gut–brain axis observed with functional magnetic resonance imaging (MRI)[34] and brain network function testing[35] highlight the role of emotions and mood in the perception of pain in patients with IBS. Recent studies recognize the importance of gut microflora, as well as diet, in bidirectional communication with the brain. That is, brain signaling changes the gut environment while changes in gut microflora can affect both emotions and pain perception through CNS signaling via vagal afferent nerves.[36] Specific mechanisms through which this may occur include short-chain fatty acids (SCFA), bile salts, modified microbiome composition, metabolite production, and protease activity. Imbalances in microbiota composition and metabolism may modify signaling, as well as mucosal permeability (creating potential "downstream" consequences). There is a synergistic effect on signaling when inflammatory mediators are also present, leading to a further increase in visceral hypersensitivity.[37]

Microflora, metabolism, serotonin-producing enterochromaffin cells, and localized inflammation also contribute to gut signaling. Pharmacological approaches have focused on the use of agents to bind enteric serotonin receptors; however, the untoward side effects of these agents have resulted in a high risk/benefit ratio. Integrative medicine takes the root cause of individual imbalances into account, leading to therapies that focus on the

TABLE 41.1	Rome III Criteria for the Diagnosis of Irritable Bowel Syndrome (IBS)

Symptoms present for at least 3 days per month in the last 3 months (with symptom onset at least 6 months previously) and at least two of the following features:
- Pain improved with defecation.
- Onset of pain associated with change in stool frequency.
- Onset of pain associated with change in stool form.

From Longstreth GF, Thompson WG, Chey WD, et al. Functional bowel disorders. Gastroenterology. 2006;130:1480-1491.

TABLE 41.2	"Alarm Signs" in the History of a Patient With Irritable Bowel Syndrome

Weight loss
Fever
Overt or occult blood in stool
Frequent nocturnal bowel movements
Abnormal laboratory tests
Family history of inflammatory bowel disease
Family history or early colon cancer
Onset of symptoms after the age of 50

From Thompson WG, Longstreth GF, Drossman DA, et al. Functional bowel disorders and functional abdominal pain. Gut. 2000;45:S243-S247.

aforementioned areas of diet, digestion, intestinal permeability, gut microflora, inflammation/infection, stress, and mood.

Ninety-five percent of the body's serotonin is in the gut rather than the brain.

Diagnosis

Diagnosis (derived from the Greek words *Dia*, way; and *gnosis*, knowing) is predicated simply upon delineation upon a set of agreed upon criteria, as noted by the symptom-based Rome III determination of IBS (Table 41.1), with diagnostic testing not necessarily required to confirm the diagnosis. However, the multifactorial nature of IBS complicates treatment recommendations. The emphasis on "alarm signs" (Table 41.2) within the Rome classification has not effectively stratified patients at risk because the majority of patients are unlikely to have these signs at the time of evaluation.[38] The Rome III criteria place emphasis on IBS subtypes (IBS-C [constipation], IBS-D [diarrhea], and IBS-M [mixed]) and symptom-based treatment. Recent studies, however, indicate that IBS subtypes do not remain stable over time.[39] Similar to the limitations of the Rome III criteria, subtype stratification does not facilitate integrative treatment based on the underlying physiological changes. IBS is diagnosed according to the exclusion of other disease, so it remains necessary to rule out specific illnesses that may mimic IBS.[40] GI imbalances to consider[41] include celiac disease,

TABLE 41.3 Differential Diagnosis of IBS

Differential Diagnosis	Testing
Infection/parasite	Stool testing for fecal leukocytes, culture, ova, and parasites
Celiac disease	Transglutaminase IgA (tTG IgA) + antideaminated gliadin (DGP IgA) and endomysial (EMA IgA) antibodies Total IgA antibodies
Pancreatic insufficiency	Pancreatic elastase
C. difficile colitis	C. difficile toxin
Food sensitivity	Skin prick testing, elimination diet
Lactose and fructose intolerance	Elimination diet
Small intestinal bacterial overgrowth	Hydrogen breath testing (for lactose or glucose)
Inflammatory bowel disease	Fecal calprotectin, endoscopy
Colorectal cancer	Endoscopy, fecal immunochemical testing for hemoglobin (FIT), and fecal DNA testing (Cologuard)
Dysbiosis	Comprehensive diagnostic stool analysis with microbiology

lactose intolerance, fructose intolerance, food sensitivities, food allergies, small intestinal bacterial overgrowth, dysbiosis, pancreatic insufficiency, acute infection (bacterial, viral), parasitic infection (acute or chronic),[42] *Clostridium difficile* infection, inflammatory bowel disease, and colorectal cancer.

Diagnostic considerations include, first and foremost, an extensive medical history with an understanding of dietary inputs and the utilization of antibiotics, laxatives, fiber, and herbs. In addition, one must elicit the current pattern of bowel movements including frequency, history, abdominal pain, gas, bloating, relationship to meals, and duration. It is surprising how many patients consider their altered bowel movements to be normal. Western medicine does not have a defined norm regarding bowel movement consistency and frequency, while other forms of healing, such as Ayurveda and traditional Chinese medicine, view the regular functioning of the gastrointestinal tract to be a critical barometer of health and well-being, with one to two well-formed bowel movements per day to be the norm.[43]

Etiological factors—infection, parasites, pancreatic insufficiency, celiac disease, food sensitivities, and *C. difficile* infection—should be considered in the differential diagnosis of IBS before the initiation of treatment (Table 41.3).

INTEGRATIVE THERAPY

We must look beyond symptom-based diagnosis and suppression-based treatment to understand the underlying causes of imbalance and illness. Irritable bowel syndrome represents an imbalance within the digestive system. The essential components of that system—nutrition, gut flora, immune system, constitution, thoughts, and environment—work optimally when they are in balance and harmony. This integrative approach highlights the unique needs of the individual patient.

Nutrition

Numerous studies and surveys have reported that the vast majority of individuals with IBS (65%–90%) indicate that their symptoms are triggered by specific foods.[44] A detailed dietary history can often provide insight into common food triggers for IBS, including gluten, lactose, fructose, fatty foods, and fiber[45]; as well as the role of fermentable oligosaccharides, disaccharides, monosaccharides, and polyols (FODMaPs)[46] described in Chapter 90.

Dietary factors can cause all of the symptoms of IBS—pain, bloating, discomfort, and alterations in bowel pattern. Up to 50% of patients with IBS describe a worsening of symptoms after meals,[47] and 84% report symptoms related to one food item eaten.[48] Cordain et al. described the dietary patterns most common today and compared them with the characteristics of ancestral diets,[49] observing significant differences in glycemic load, fiber content, essential fatty acid composition, pH balance, and macronutrient/micronutrient composition. All of these factors have substantial effects on the balance of the commensal flora and nutrient delivery within the gastrointestinal tract. This observation is an important reference point, as are the unique and simple food rules that author Michael Pollan offers—"Eat food. Mostly plants. Not too much."[50] Many IBS patients will experiment with their diet before seeking medical attention, particularly by removing wheat, corn, dairy, eggs, coffee, tea, and citrus.[51]

Dietary approaches provide the most effective means of correcting dysfunction within the gastrointestinal system, and there are many opportunities for the delivery of these tools to patients. However, the profound dietary changes that man has adopted over the past 10,000 years, and accelerated over the past 100 years, have created discord with the nutritional input that our genetic structure has evolved to maximize.[52] This discordance requires a much more complex set of clinical approaches to regain balance and optimal function.

Food Allergies and Sensitivities

Research has noted that food allergies and food sensitivities account for approximately 8%–14% of patients with GI symptoms, though the prevalence of food sensitivity appears to be increasing while the rate of food allergy appears stable.[53] Accordingly, differentiation between food allergy, food sensitivity, and food intolerance is necessary. Food intolerance is poorly defined and will not be considered in this chapter, although intolerance to lactose, fructose, MSG, tyramine, histamine, and other agents may induce IBS symptoms. Food allergy is IgE-mediated and is more prevalent in young children and decreases throughout childhood. Recent reviews have highlighted the increasing prevalence of food allergy; however, there is controversy regarding the diagnostic methodology. IgE-mediated food allergies can be measured but are present only 2% to 4% of the time using the gold standard of Double-Blind Food Challenge.[54] Other studies have reported the prevalence of physician-diagnosed food allergy to range between 6.5%–7.6% among IBS patients.[55] Interestingly, IgE-mediated hypersensitivity responses to food increase in the setting of altered gastric pH.[56] Additionally, changes in IgE-mediated food allergy can have an effect on increasing intestinal permeability, inflammation, and immune response.[57]

Food allergy is distinct from the more controversial term, "food sensitivity"; an IgG-mediated phenomenon that is difficult to assess with current laboratory measures. Typically, the diagnosis of food sensitivity is made with the use of an elimination diet, during which the symptoms resolve when the patient has removed the offending food and symptoms recur when the offending food is returned to the diet (see Chapters 31 and 86). Atkinson et al.[58] used an enzyme-linked immunosorbent assay to evaluate food sensitivity in patients with IBS. A therapeutic diet was administered in one cohort (based on IgG assay results identifying foods to which subjects had raised IgG levels) and a sham diet (i.e., the foods eliminated were not those identified as those to which subjects had sensitivities, according to the IgG assay results) was provided to the control population. A 26% decrease in IBS symptoms was observed when test subjects consumed the therapeutic diet, and symptoms returned when they returned to an unrestricted diet. The diagnostic approach of measuring serum IgG and IgG4 levels is controversial, with conflicting results reported.[59,60] Newer technologies using confocal endomicroscopy have demonstrated that anatomic changes begin within 5 minutes of food challenge in patients with IBS who are positive for clinical food sensitivity.[61] Future studies comparing this technology with IgG testing will help to elucidate the clinical utility of this assessment method. In fact, IgG food antibody testing may be more representative of intestinal permeability (a.k.a. "leaky gut") than specific food sensitivity.

Gluten Sensitivity and Celiac Disease

Approximately 4%–5% of patients with IBS have celiac disease, more than four-fold higher than people without IBS.[62] Antibody testing for celiac disease is quickly becoming a standard of care in patients with IBS. Nonceliac gluten sensitivity (NCGS) is a term used to describe the condition in which gluten leads to a clinical and/or serological reaction that improves with gluten elimination. Biesiekierski et al. demonstrated clinical improvements in IBS following the removal of gluten in patients who were negative for celiac disease. In fact, there was only a small clinical improvement in the subset of patients who were genetically predisposed to celiac disease by HLA DQ2/DQ8.[63] It has also been demonstrated that individuals without celiac disease who have IgG antigliadin antibodies (AGA) feel significantly better when gluten is removed from their diet.[64] However, AGA testing is not definitive for the diagnosis of NCGS due to a high false negativity, thus further clinical trials are necessary. Celiac testing should occur before (or within 4–6 weeks

of) removing gluten from the diet in order to prevent false-negative celiac testing. Increased awareness and understanding of gluten sensitivity has led to an emergence of many "gluten-free" options in the marketplace, but many of them use processed grain flours that may create other problems. Gluten is a fermentable carbohydrate (see FODMaPs in the following) and has been posited to act via prebiotic carbohydrate expression in addition to its roles in mucosal permeability and immunological antigenicity.[65]

Lactose and Fructose Intolerance

The most common form of food intolerance is that to lactose, which affects approximately 25% of adults in the United States and 35%–40% of patients with IBS. Of the IBS patients who restrict lactose in their diets, more than half will have symptom improvement.[66] Sorbitol and fructose intolerances are also quite common. Polyols are sugar alcohols, such as sorbitol, lactitol, and xylitol, which are found in sugar-free products. At least 70% of polyols are not absorbed in healthy individuals.[67] One study found that nearly a third of patients with IBS had significantly more symptoms due to fructose malabsorption and dietary fructose intolerance.[68] A 14-day trial of a fructose-free, lactose-free, sorbitol-free diet should be performed to determine whether symptoms resolve. Foods with these constituents should be added back to a dietary challenge one at a time every 3 days.

> As sorbitol-containing chewing gum can be a common trigger of IBS, clinicians should screen for its use when taking a medical history.

Fermentable Carbohydrates (FODMaPs)

An extension of the idea to avoid simple sugars is the concept of a diet restricting fermentable oligo-, di-, monosaccharides and polyols (FODMaPs). These fermentable substrates (apples, pears, dried fruit, sugar alcohols, mushrooms, avocado, milk, cheese, wheat, rye, onions, artichokes, and inulin) act as prebiotics, and stimulate bacterial growth and gas production. There are several dietary interventions that seek to change prebiotic foods, thus changing gut microbiome expression. As there is no singular gut microbiota across populations, individuals with different microbiota may respond differentially to varied prebiotic foods, as represented by FODMsPs (see Chapter 90), as well as the Specific Carbohydrate Diet (SCD), which has been anecdotally been posited as effective for IBS and IBD.[69]

Fiber

Dietary fiber intake in the United States averages less than 15 g/day, well short of the recommended intake of 25 to 35 g/day, or the 115 g/day found in the paleolithic diet. Although fiber appears to ease constipation symptoms in a proportion of patients, the ability of dietary fiber to improve abdominal pain and diarrhea has been limited. Multiple randomized, controlled trials have failed to demonstrate a benefit of combined soluble and insoluble fiber supplementation for the multiple symptoms of IBS.[70] Soluble fiber and insoluble fiber have been found to have different effects on IBS symptoms. Many studies have been complicated by the use of wheat bran as a source of fiber as wheat bran is a common source of food sensitivity and contains fructans, thus potentially altering symptoms in these studies. Soluble fiber (e.g., psyllium, ispaghula, inulin, and modified citrus pectin) reportedly led to significant improvement, whereas insoluble fiber (corn, wheat bran) worsened clinical outcomes.[71] Soluble fiber is recommended for patients with constipation, with dosages titrated to 20–30 g/day in food or as a supplement. Additionally, soluble fiber increases the production of short-chain fatty acids (SCFA), including n-butyrate, which is a substrate for energy production in the colonic mucosal cells and acts as an antiinflammatory. n-Butyrate and SCFAs can be measured by stool analyses and are essential metabolic products of gut microbiota.

> Soluble fiber (psyllium, ispaghula, inulin, and modified citrus pectin) improves symptoms, whereas insoluble fiber (corn, wheat bran) may worsen symptoms in some cases.

Exercise

Regular physical exercise has been demonstrated to improve stress-coping, enhance well-being, and decrease feelings of depression and anxiety. Physical activity decreases bowel transit time and increases frequency of bowel movements,[72] and structured exercise programs have been shown to improve overall IBS symptoms.[73] Moderate exercise is recommended and encouraged for all patients with IBS.

Sleep

Poor sleep quality is observed in patients with IBS, further compromising their quality of life.[74] Poor sleep predicts symptoms of IBS, rather than vice versa.[75] Good sleep hygiene is an important consideration and often requires supporting the entire family unit to adopt this approach (see Chapter 9).

Supplements

Probiotics

The gastrointestinal (gut) microbiome plays a critical role in the normal development and functioning of the gastrointestinal tract and is broadly influenced by genetics and environment. The fecal microbiota of IBS patients differs significantly from controls due to diet, antibiotics, infection, and stress. Evidence indicates alterations in the gut microbiota in not only the expression of the intestinal manifestations of IBS, but also the psychiatric morbidity that coexists in up to 80% of patients with IBS.[76]

Recent trials have focused on altering gut microflora with the therapeutic use of probiotics; live microbial organisms that are administered in foods or supplements. Probiotics are nonpathogenic, of human origin, resistant to gastric acid and bile, adhere to intestinal epithelium,

and are able to colonize the GI tract.[77] Probiotics appear to decrease fermentation, improve competition against imbalanced and potentially pathogenic flora, and stimulate proper immune functioning. Probiotics have been shown to balance inflammatory cytokines in IBS patients.[78] The human gut microflora plays a critical role in maintaining host health both within the GI tract and systemically through the absorption of metabolites. An "optimal" gut microflora establishes an efficient barrier against the invasion and colonization of the gut by pathogenic bacteria, produces a range of metabolic substrates that in turn are utilized by the host (e.g., vitamins and short-chain fatty acids), promotes development, and provides balance for the immune system.

Earlier studies and clinical experience pointed to the beneficial role of broad-based probiotic therapy, and recent systematic reviews have clearly confirmed that probiotics are effective therapies for IBS, including in the management of global symptoms, abdominal pain, bloating, and flatus.[79] The fecal microflora has been shown to be abnormal in IBS-D,[80] with a loss of bacterial diversity in combination with significantly higher levels of detrimental enterobacteriaceae and lower levels of beneficial fecalibacterium.[81] Changes in the colonic flora may lead to altered fermentation and immune dysregulation of the intestinal mucosa. In patients with IBS-C, altered bacterial fermentation patterns are seen, with lower levels of lactate-utilizing, hydrogen-consuming, methane-generating, and acetate-generating organisms. Sulfate-reducing organisms are increased in IBS-C and produce toxic sulfide compounds and concomitant symptoms.[82]

Information from studies of clinical utility cannot be "transferred" across different strains and different bacteria. The specific species and strain of probiotic is of great importance in the effectiveness of treatment, with strain heterogeneity in clinical studies resulting in heterogeneity among the results. Initial studies have focused on several strains of probiotic, with positive effects reported for the *Bifidobacterium* genus, *Bifidobacterium infantis 35624*, *Lactobacillus plantarum*, *E. coli Nissl 1917*, *Streptococcus faecium*, and (the high potency, 8–strain combination) VSL#3.[83]

> **DOSAGE**
>
> Recommend a mixture of 50/50 *L. plantarum/B. breve* at 25 billion colony-forming units (cfu) twice daily for 6 to 8 weeks; then decrease to 10 billion cfu/day. Other probiotic combinations may be considered on the basis of fecal flora (see Chapter 105).
>
> **PRECAUTIONS**
>
> Avoid in severely immunocompromised patients, including those with severe pancreatic disease.
>
> Altered gastrointestinal flora (i.e., dysbiosis) is considered a critical factor in immune dysregulation and altered function. Correction of dysbiosis is required for successful treatment of IBS.

Prebiotics

Prebiotics are simple carbohydrate molecules that selectively stimulate normal GI flora to proliferate, thus competing with abnormal flora and pathogens for space, food, and adherence. The term, prebiotic, is becoming increasingly problematic as nearly all foods are now recognized to affect the gastrointestinal microbiota. Synbiotics are the combination products of prebiotics and probiotics. Fructooligosaccharides (FOSs) and inulin are the most commonly used supplemental prebiotics at this time, and have been shown to increase bifidobacteria in the stool. Animal studies have reported beneficial effects on microflora balance,[84] and human studies have demonstrated in vivo activation of bifidobacteria[85] but no improvement in IBS.[86] Overall, clinical experience emphasizes the use of foods as prebiotics, with different FODMaP and SCD carbohydrates stimulating differential growth of intestinal microbiota. Thus, it is usually beneficial to balance the gut microbiome with food, probiotics, and antimicrobial agents before promoting the use of supplemental prebiotics.

DOSAGE

See FODMaP diet. Do not recommend prebiotics unless or until there is a rebalancing of the gut flora. Common food sources include apples, pears, dried fruit, mushrooms, avocado, milk, cheese, wheat, rye, onions, artichokes, and inulin.

Pancreatic Enzymes

One of the conditions to be considered diagnostically with IBS is that of pancreatic insufficiency. Pancreatic insufficiency can be a primary process, with depletion of exocrine pancreatic function, or can be secondary to villous atrophy, insufficient cholecystokinin production, or deceased vagal nerve stimulation of the exocrine pancreas. These conditions lead to a decrease in the production of pancreatic elastase in the stool, identification of which can determine the need for supplemental pancreatic enzymes. Laboratory data reveals that 7% of patients with IBS have moderate to severe pancreatic insufficiency.[87] Studies of pancreatic enzyme supplementation in patients with IBS symptoms are now underway.

DOSAGE

Dosing of pancreatic enzymes is standardized according to lipase activity (e.g., Creon 12 = 12,000 IU Lipase activity). Animal glandulars of pancreatin 10× USP have relatively fixed ratios of lipases, proteases, and amylases. Pancreatic elastase can be used to monitor exocrine pancreatic function without being affected by pancreatic enzyme supplementation.

Stool for pancreatic elastase is a relatively inexpensive test to check for pancreatic insufficiency.

Botanical Medicines
Peppermint Oil

Peppermint (*Mentha piperita*) has been used for GI disturbances for millennia. Menthol and methyl salicylate, the main active ingredients, have antispasmodic actions and calming effects on the stomach and GI tract. The physiological effect in reducing smooth muscle contraction and providing relaxation appears to be due to the effect of menthol as a calcium channel blocker on smooth muscle cells.[88] Peppermint also has analgesic properties, mediated through activation of κ-opioid receptors to help block transmission of pain signals. Peppermint oil has been evaluated in a number of randomized trials. A 2006 Cochrane Review confirmed these initial reports, with 79% of IBS patients having alleviation of abdominal pain,[89] and a meta-analysis[90] concluding a beneficial effect after 2 weeks of therapy.

DOSAGE

The recommended dosage of peppermint oil is one to two 0.2 mL (200–400 mg) enteric-coated capsules three times/day between meals. Smaller doses are effective in children (100–200 mg).[91]

PRECAUTIONS

Nonenteric-coated capsules, as well as free peppermint oil, can decrease lower esophageal sphincter tone, resulting in heartburn, although this effect is typically transient. Skin rash has been reported at a rate of approximately 2%.

Ginger

Ginger (*Zingiber officinale*) can be used nutritionally in cooking or as an herbal remedy and has been evaluated in the treatment of postoperative nausea and vomiting. The active gingerols act as an antispasmodic and improve the tone of intestinal muscles. A recent small study demonstrated benefit in both the ginger and placebo groups, with fewer side effects in the ginger group.[92] Ginger is available in many forms, and ginger root tea is particularly helpful after overeating.

DOSAGE

Powdered root, 250–500 mg 3–4 times/day. Prepare ginger tea by chopping a piece of ginger the size of the patient's fifth digit; place in 150 mL of boiling water for 5–10 minutes and strain. Drink one cup before meals.

Aloe

Aloe (*Aloe spicata* and *Aloe vera*) is commonly considered safe for internal ingestion and is used commonly with IBS. Aloe vera is classified by the U.S. Food and Drug Administration (FDA) as a class 1 harsh stimulant laxative because anthraquinones in aloe significantly increase colonic peristalsis. Aloe should be regarded as being in the same class as other anthranoid laxatives, such as cascara (*Cascara sagrada*) and senna (*Cassia senna*). Although these agents may be used for short-term relief of constipation, they are not suitable for use in IBS due to their powerful action and tendency for dependency.[93]

Combination Herbal Therapies

Traditional Chinese Medicine

One of the most often cited studies of integrative medicine in IBS was published by Bensousson et al. in *JAMA*.[94] These researchers demonstrated a beneficial effect of a combination Chinese patent medicine (tong xie yao fang [TXYF]—a generic prescription for presumed spleen qi deficiency and liver–spleen disharmony) used over 16 weeks. Symptoms improved significantly during treatment but returned after the medicine was stopped. However, individualized herbal therapies demonstrated sustained improvement, even at 14 weeks after the individualized herbal medicines were stopped. Thus individualized traditional Chinese medicine (TCM) treatment is recommended. An additional study of TXYF was recently conducted with 120 IBS patients and reported decreased mast cell activation; however, this study did not include a placebo control.[95]

Padma Lax

Padma lax is a complex Tibetan herbal formula for constipation and contains aloe extract, calumba root, cascara bark, frangula bark, rhubarb root (all known laxatives), and other herbs/minerals with antispasmodic and antidiarrheal effects. Several studies have demonstrated the effectiveness of padma lax in constipation-predominant IBS, including a 63% reduction in symptom severity and 90% reduction in the number of patients with severe symptoms.[96,97]

> **DOSAGE**
>
> For IBS with constipation, padma lax two capsules/day for 3 months; decrease dosage to one capsule daily if loose stool is noted.

STW-5

STW-5 is a mixture of aqueous ethanolic plant extracts from *Iberis amara* (clown's mustard), chamomile flower, caraway fruit, peppermint leaves, greater celandine, licorice root, lemon balm leaves, angelica root, and milk thistle fruit. In a 2001 randomized, multicenter study of 208 patients with IBS, STW-5 reduced total abdominal symptoms by approximately 54%, compared with 27% for the placebo, at 4 weeks.[98]

> **DOSAGE**
>
> A common brand name of this product is *Iberogast*. *Iberogast* can be mixed with water in the following dosages:
> Adults and children over 12 years: 20 drops, 3 × day
> Children 6–12 years: 15 drops, 3 × day
> Children 3–6 years: 10 drops, 3 × day
> Children 3 months to 3 years: 8 drops, 3 × day

Mind-Body Therapies

Throughout the past two centuries, IBS was believed to be a nervous disorder that developed in response to external stress and internal neuroses, such as depression and anxiety.[99] Early epidemiological studies demonstrated a 2:1 female-to-male predominance, as well as a higher prevalence of emotional, physical, or sexual abuse in patients with IBS.[100] These vulnerability factors are part of the "enhanced stress responsiveness" that is observed in IBS, manifesting as an inability to turn off the stress response.[101] Higher cortisol levels in morning urine and saliva have been reported in subjects with IBS than in controls, indicating a state of chronic stress.[102] Stress increases intestinal permeability as well as susceptibility to colonic inflammation.[103]

The evolution of mind-body-medicine, research in psychoneuroimmunoendocrinology, and practical tools in heart rate variability biofeedback have increased understanding of the intrinsic relationship between external stressors, emotions, and physiological changes. Integrative treatment of IBS requires an array of therapeutic approaches that treat the patient on mental, emotional, and physical levels.

Mind-body therapy, in the form of relaxation therapy, biofeedback, hypnosis, counseling, or stress management training, has been shown to reduce symptom frequency and severity and to enhance the results of standard medical treatment of IBS. The majority of these therapies focus on correcting maladaptive coping skills that engender emotional stress, which then manifests as GI symptoms.

Stress Management

Lifestyle changes that incorporate stress reduction and stress management strategies, along with progressive muscle relaxation, have proved to be more effective than medical therapy[104] (see Chapter 94).

Hypnosis

Trials conducted in the United Kingdom have reported that weekly hypnosis sessions, in combination with self-hypnosis techniques for 12 weeks, improved the symptoms of abdominal pain, bloating, and disturbed defecation, as well as anxiety scores, but did not alter rectal tone or pain threshold.[105] Specific "gut-directed" hypnotherapy programs are now available (see Chapter 95).

Psychotherapy and Cognitive Behavioral Therapy

Cognitive behavioral therapy (CBT) combines cognitive therapy and behavioral therapy. Behavioral therapy helps patients weaken the connections between troublesome situations and habitual reactions to them. Cognitive therapy teaches how certain thinking patterns cause symptoms. When combined into CBT, these therapies provide powerful tools for eliminating symptoms. CBT, behavioral therapy, hypnosis, and psychotherapy have all been shown to significantly improve symptoms (30%–40%) in patients with moderate to severe IBS in comparison with education or self-administered therapies.[106]

Patients with IBS symptoms often have a combination of mental/emotional stressors and alterations in the psychoneuroimmunological axis. Ensuring a proper gut milieu along with stress management strategies is necessary for optimal gut function.

Acupuncture

In 2006, a Cochrane Review analyzed six RCTs using acupuncture in IBS and concluded there was no evidence to support the use of acupuncture in treating IBS.[107] A more recent study by Lembo et al. demonstrated a benefit of both real and sham acupuncture. It is interesting that the nonspecific placebo effects of acupuncture appear to be therapeutically effective.[108]

Placebo Effects

It has been well documented that RCT research in the treatment of IBS has observed very high placebo response rates. Kaptchuk et al. developed a unique study to evaluate the benefit of openly offering a placebo treatment, which was found to be efficacious![109]

Pharmaceuticals

Oral Cromolyn

Several studies have compared oral cromolyn with a placebo in randomized, double-blind crossover trials. In one study, an 8-week treatment resulted in significant symptom reduction and a long carryover effect in the group initially treated with cromolyn.[110] Two large unblinded studies have compared oral cromolyn with an elimination diet. The largest trial involved 409 patients with well-defined IBS who were monitored for 4 months.[111] Symptom improvement was noted in 60% of patients treated with elimination diet and in 67% of those receiving cromolyn.

DOSAGE

The recommended dose of cromolyn is 200 to 400 mg (1–2 gel caps) four times/day, before meals and 30 minutes before bedtime.

PRECAUTIONS

Cromolyn is well tolerated but may cause diarrhea and headaches.

Antibiotics

The "shotgun" use of antibiotic treatments may lead to significant alterations in the GI microflora, which can be deleterious in the long-term.[112] Most recently, rifaximin (a nonabsorbable antibiotic) has been demonstrated to significantly improve IBS symptoms and is now FDA-approved for the treatment of IBS-D.[113] Rifaximin has also been shown to be useful in the treatment of small intestinal bacterial overgrowth (SIBO), a source of bacterial fermentation, gas, and bloating. SIBO can be diagnosed with a lactulose or glucose breath test. Rifaximin treatment was not found to affect the overall composition of the gut microbiota but diminished potentially detrimental bacteria, such as *Clostridium*, and increased the presence of some species, such as *Faecalibacterium prausnitzii*.[114]

DOSAGE

Rifaximin 550 mg three times/day for 10–14 days in patients with SIBO.

PRECAUTIONS

Rifaximin is not systemically absorbed so most side effects are related to GI function including flatulence, abdominal pain, and stool urgency. Any antibiotic or antimicrobial herb may affect the diversity and quantity of the microbiome and care should be taken to optimize the GI ecosystem in order to replenish a healthy and diverse microbiome.

Antidepressants

A recent meta-analysis reported that tricyclic antidepressants (TCAs) and selective serotonin reuptake inhibitors (SSRIs) significantly lessened abdominal pain and diarrhea in patients with diarrhea-predominant IBS.[115] SNRIs were not effective. Patients able to tolerate TCAs are likely to have symptomatic benefit; however, many patients experience unacceptable side effects.

Therapies to Consider

Betaine Hydrochloride

A basic evaluation of digestion and absorption is often not part of the initial evaluation of GI function in patients with IBS. Factors that affect digestion of food include mastication, hypochlorhydria, and pancreatic insufficiency. Mastication is a simple clinical point to make with patients and is often overlooked. Pancreatic insufficiency and benefit of digestive enzyme supplementation have been discussed previously. Research indicates stomach acid declines with age. Decreased pH limits the activation of peptidases and other critical enzymes necessary for digestion and absorption. Betaine hydrochloride, Swedish bitters, and Gentian violet can be used as supplements to support the reactivation of proper digestion by stimulating gastric acid production.

DOSAGE

325 to 650 mg before a protein-containing meal.

PRECAUTION

Reduce the dose if a warm or burning sensation develops after ingestion.

Osteopathic Medicine

It is often thought that osteopathy and other related manual therapies are used only for musculoskeletal problems. However, recognition of a somatovisceral pathway amenable to manipulation has led to use of these approaches for relief of symptoms in patients with IBS. The somatic areas that are commonly affected include the external oblique muscles (particularly the lower portion), internal oblique muscles, and rectus abdominis muscle; the lower segments of the thoracic spine (T10–T12); the iliocostalis thoracis/lumborum and longissimus thoracis/lumborum muscles; and the quadratus lumborum muscles. Individuals with this somatovisceral connection are often unaware of these tender points until they are discovered by careful palpation. This indirect technique seeks to release the strained somatic segments through initiation of a reciprocal counterstrain of the antagonist muscles (see Chapter 109).

PREVENTION PRESCRIPTION

PRIMARY PREVENTION IN THE FIRST 2 YEARS OF LIFE

- Limit/avoid antibiotics and antimicrobial herbs to maximize opportunity for bowel microflora to develop.
- Practice breastfeeding on demand for the first 12 months of life; avoid formula feeding, if possible.
- Introduction of solid foods—delay introduction of grains until after age 6 months, preferably at 8–10 months of age or when the child's pincer grasp allows them to self-feed.

PRIMARY PREVENTION AT ALL AGES

- Carbohydrates—avoid or minimize simple sugars because they provide the substrate for abnormal bacteria to perpetuate in the GI tract.
- Importance of taking time to eat, preparing food, and eating it with others. Increase vagal tone.
- Learn to reduce stress or the internalization of emotion.
- Paleolithic diet—fewer processed foods, fewer grains, more vegetables.

THERAPEUTIC REVIEW

This is a summary of the therapeutic options for IBS. An initial diagnostic evaluation is necessary to target effective therapies. A celiac panel should be performed in all patients and include tTG IgA and DGP IgA (reflex to EMA IgA) and total IgA. For patients with mild to moderate symptoms of IBS without any clear source of etiology, this ladder approach is appropriate.

MIND-BODY THERAPIES

- Cognitive behavioral therapy
- Hypnotherapy

NUTRITION

- Elimination/challenge diet (see Chapter 86)
- FODMaPs diet (see Chapter 90)
- Some patients may need additional motivation through diagnostic testing (IgG food allergy testing).

SUPPLEMENTS

- Probiotics: 50 billion cfu/day as 25 billion cfu/day of *Bifidobacterium* and 25 billion cfu/day of *Lactobacillus* or *B. infantis* 36524 at 5 billion cfu/day

- Soluble fiber (psyllium, guar gum) 15 g/day with meals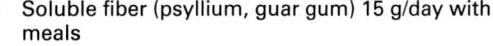

BOTANICALS

- Peppermint oil: one to two enteric-coated capsules three times/day between meals
- TCM herbs: tongxie yaofang
- Tibetan herbs/padma lax for IBS with constipation, two capsules/day for 3 months
- STW-5, 20 drops three times/day for 4 weeks

PHARMACEUTICALS

- Oral cromolyn 200 mg (2 capsules) four times/day before meals and before bedtime
- Antibiotics: rifaximin 400 mg tid for 10 days in patients with evidence of small intestine bowel overgrowth
- Tricyclic antidepressants: such as amitriptyline, 10–25 mg/day with lower doses to start

Key Web Resources

The International Foundation for Functional Gastrointestinal Disorders. A nonprofit education and research organization whose aim is to inform, assist, and support people with functional GI disorders. The website offers patient information as well as recent publications and current research on IBS.	http://www.iffgd.org
The Institute for Functional Medicine. Offers educational opportunities to help health care practitioners develop personalized approaches to understand and find the root cause (i.e., the core clinical imbalances) for a variety of chronic diseases, including IBS.	http://www.fxmed.com
Genova Diagnostics and Doctor's Data Laboratories that perform comprehensive stool and micro-biology testing	https://www.gdx.net/product/gi-effects-comprehensive-stool-test and https://www.doctorsdata.com/comprehensive-stool-analysis-w-parasitology-x3/

REFERENCES

References are available online at ExpertConsult.com.

CHAPTER 42

GASTROESOPHAGEAL REFLUX DISEASE

David Kiefer, MD

Gastroesophageal reflux disease (GERD) occurs when there is abnormal passage of acidic stomach contents, or refluxate, into the esophagus, causing symptoms or complications. GERD is one of the primary causes of the informal name and symptom *heartburn*, and is a common phenomenon. Estimates are that 15% to 20% of people in the United States have heartburn or regurgitation at least once a week.[1-5]

Symptoms of GERD may include any or all of the following: retrosternal burning, acid regurgitation, nausea, vomiting, chest pain, laryngitis, cough, and dysphagia.[3] Injury to the esophagus can include esophagitis, stricture, the development of columnar metaplasia (Barrett esophagus), and adenocarcinoma.[2] A poor correlation exists between the severity of symptoms and the pathophysiological findings in the esophagus.[2] For example, GERD is not the only phenomenon in the differential diagnosis of heartburn. Many individuals with GERD have no endoscopic evidence of esophagitis, and up to 40% of patients with Barrett esophagus did not report heartburn in a clinical study.[2,4] The confusing nature of GERD has limited the development of concrete screening recommendations for advanced disease.

People may turn to complementary and alternative medicine to help with their gastrointestinal symptoms. The 2002 National Health Interview Survey, based on 31,044 interviews in the United States, documented that 3.7% of people used complementary and alternative medicine for stomach or intestinal illnesses,[6] though this percentage had dropped to 1.2% by 2007.[7]

PATHOPHYSIOLOGY

Symptoms of GERD result from the interplay of many factors, including the amount of time the esophagus is exposed to refluxate, the degree of refluxate causticity, and the susceptibility of the esophagus to damage.[4,8,9] Three main mechanisms or factors prevent refluxate from entering the esophagus: the lower esophageal sphincter (LES), the crural diaphragm (which acts as an external esophageal sphincter), and the location of the gastroesophageal junction below the diaphragmatic hiatus.[1,4] Dysfunction or malalignment in any or all of these structures may lead to symptoms of GERD, although the major pathological mechanism is abnormal LES tone.

The LES normally exists in a contracted state and relaxes during the swallow mechanism to allow material into the stomach (Fig. 42.1). The LES also relaxes to vent swallowed air and allow retrograde expulsion of material from the stomach.[4,8] For approximately an hour after meals, people may normally have up to five transient episodes of reflux; however, the symptoms of GERD may develop if these episodes continue.[4,8]

Decreased tone of the LES occurs with many substances, medications, and other factors (Table 42.1).[1,4] Certain beverages may exacerbate symptoms of GERD, with some affecting LES tone. For example, coffee, including instant, decaffeinated, and ground coffee, decreases LES tone initially and, in some people with sustained decreased tone, for up to 90 minutes after ingestion. Caffeinated coffee seems to cause more gastric acid production[10] and greater decreases in LES tone at low pH values.[11] A separate study found an association between pH and titratable acidity and the frequency with which some beverages, such as juices, sodas, coffee, and tea, caused heartburn symptoms in 394 individuals with GERD.[12] Caffeine itself has been shown to have the ability to decrease LES tone.[13]

Symptoms of GERD may result from other factors. For example, increased intraabdominal and gastric pressure, such as from obesity, ascites, pregnancy, or even tight clothes, may lead to GERD.[1,4,14] In addition, GERD may occur when gastric contents are located near the gastroesophageal junction, such as in the recumbent position, while bending over, or in patients with a hiatal hernia.[1] Furthermore, any conditions that decrease the production of saliva may predispose to GERD due to the neutralizing effect of saliva on acid.[1]

Patients report that stress exacerbates GERD, a finding that has been borne out in clinical trials. For example, stress has been shown to increase GERD symptom reports without necessarily being correlated with objective physiological changes, such as increased esophageal acid exposure or duration of acid exposure.[15-17] This phenomenon particularly occurs in people with high levels of anxiety.[16] Other well-known examples are documented worsening of GERD symptoms with job stress[18] and after devastating events, such as the World Trade Center attack in 2001.[19] The enteric nervous system, with innervations throughout the gastrointestinal tract, is now referred to as the *brain–gut axis* and[17] is involved in the contribution of stress to worsening of GERD; however, this system is complex.[8]

Diagnostic testing can be used to determine the cause of patient symptoms and any pathophysiological correlates. For example, barium swallow, upper endoscopy, ambulatory pH, and a trial of proton pump inhibitor

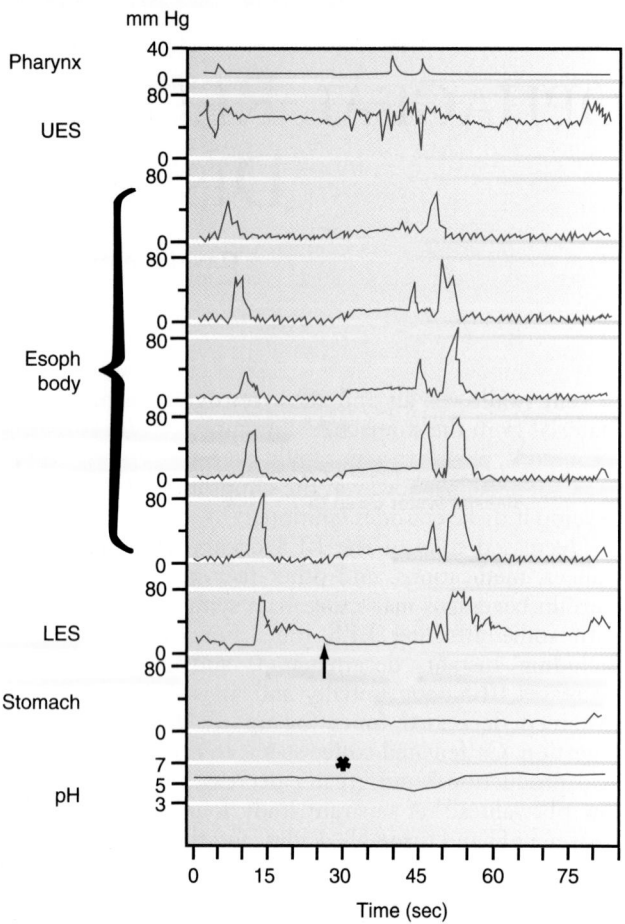

FIG. 42.1 ■ **Normal Swallow Mechanism.** A continuous tracing of esophageal motility showing two swallows, as indicated by the pharyngeal contraction associated with relaxation of the upper esophageal sphincter *(UES)* and followed by peristalsis in the body of the esophagus. The lower esophageal sphincter *(LES)* also displays transient relaxation *(arrow)* unassociated with a swallow. An episode of gastroesophageal reflux *(asterisk)* is recorded by a pH probe at the time of the transient LES relaxation. (From Behrman RE, Kliegman RM, Jenson HB, eds. *Nelson Textbook of pediatrics.* 17th ed. Philadelphia: Saunders; 2004.)

TABLE 42.1	**Factors Associated With Decreased Tone of the Lower Esophageal Sphincter**
Factor	**Examples**
Dietary supplements	Arginine may cause lower esophageal sphincter relaxations through the nitric oxide system Carminative herbs such as peppermint (*Mentha piperita*), spearmint (*Mentha spicata*), and other mint family (Lamiaceae) plants Essential oils (high doses)
Foods and beverages	Alcohol Chocolate (probably through the methylxanthines) Coffee (caffeinated more than decaffeinated) Cow's milk Fat Orange juice Spicy foods Tea Tomato juice
Lifestyle	Smoking
Medications	Aminophylline Anticholinergics Beta-adrenergic agents Bisphosphonates Calcium channel blockers Nitrates Phosphodiesterase inhibitors, including sildenafil
Physiological, by stomach dilation	Acid hypersecretion After meals Gastric stasis Pyloric obstruction
Trauma, irritation, and miscellaneous factors	Esophagitis Scleroderma-like diseases Surgical damage

Data from references 1, 16, 17, and 27.

(PPI) medications are the most commonly used diagnostic tests.[20] Ambulatory pH testing, estimated to have a sensitivity of 79% to 96% and a specificity of 85% to 100% for GERD, may also be used with impedance testing to explore the correlation of symptoms with refluxate volume regardless of acidity (weakly acidic or nonacid reflux).[2,20] One approach is to consider diagnostic testing (upper endoscopy, ambulatory pH, or impedance testing) if a patient is unresponsive to PPI therapy.[20]

Special Considerations for Pediatric Patients

In children, GERD is the most common esophageal disease.[9] In infants, symptoms often peak at 4 months of age and resolve by 12 to 24 months, whereas the clinical course may wax and wane in children, resolving in approximately half of cases.[9] Infants may present with postprandial regurgitation, irritability, arching, choking, gagging, feeding aversion, failure to thrive, obstructive apnea, or stridor. Signs and symptoms in older children include abdominal pain, chest pain, asthma, laryngitis, and sinusitis.[9] Studies in infants with suspected GERD have found both a high incidence of allergy to cow's milk protein[21] and symptomatic improvement when infants with intractable symptoms were changed to a diet free of cow's milk protein.[22]

> Cow's milk protein is a common cause of gastroesophageal reflux disease in infants, and a trial of elimination should be considered.

INTEGRATIVE THERAPY

Lifestyle

In mild cases of GERD, lifestyle modifications are the first line of therapy and can lead to improvement or elimination of symptoms. For example, GERD

TABLE 42.2 Botanical Medicines Useful in Gastroesophageal Reflux Disease

Common Name	Scientific Name (Family)	Mechanism of Action	Dose	Adverse Effects
Chamomile	*Matricaria recutita* (Asteraceae)	Antiinflammatory, antispasmodic	1–3 g (2 g equals 1 tablespoon) of an infusion of the flowers three to four times daily	Occasional allergic reactions in people allergic to plants in the daisy family (Asteraceae)
Licorice	*Glycyrrhiza glabra* (Fabaceae)	Antiinflammatory	Two 380-mg DGL tablets before meals	Mineralocorticoid side effects avoided when DGL form is used
Marshmallow	*Althea officinalis* (Malvaceae)	Mucoprotective	5–6 g of tea daily, in divided doses	Decreased drug absorption
Skullcap	*Scutellaria lateriflora* (Lamiaceae)	Antianxiety	1–2 g of the herb as infusion three times daily, 1–2 mL tincture three times daily	Confusion, stupor, and twitching with high doses
Slippery elm	*Ulmus fulva, Ulmus rubra* (Ulmaceae)	Mucoprotective	1–2 tablespoons per glass of water three to four times daily	Decreased drug absorption
Valerian	*Valeriana officinalis* (Valerianaceae)	Antianxiety	1–2 g root infusion two to three times daily, or a 150-mg capsule two to three times daily	Possibly increased effects of alcohol, barbiturates, and benzodiazepines

DGL, deglycyrrhizinated licorice.

symptoms may improve if smokers quit and if obese patients lose weight.[1,5,23-26] Patients should avoid the foods, supplements, and, if possible, the medications listed in Table 42.1 because of their relaxing effect on the LES. In addition, patients should avoid eating large meals or consuming large quantities of fluids with meals.[1]

If nighttime symptoms are present, patients should elevate the head of the bed by 4 to 6 inches using blocks under the bed posts rather than extra pillows. Use of extra pillows could compress the abdomen and increase intraabdominal pressure, thereby exacerbating symptoms.[1,2,23]

Exercise may benefit GERD indirectly by promoting weight loss; however, it may also have direct effects, with studies independently demonstrating that individuals who are more active have better digestion and less GERD.[25,26]

Demulcent Botanicals

Several types of botanical treatments are useful for GERD (Table 42.2). Demulcent, or mucilaginous, botanical medicines can be used as mucoprotection of the esophageal mucosa, both to soothe irritated tissues and promote healing.[23,27]

Slippery Elm (Ulmus fulva) Root Bark Powder

Slippery elm root bark powder is a demulcent botanical that can be used for symptomatic relief and promotion of healing of the irritated esophageal or gastric mucosa. Most health food stores, integrative pharmacies, and herbal dispensaries with botanical products for sale in bulk supply slippery elm.

DOSAGE

One to two tablespoons of root bark powder should be mixed with a glass of water and taken after meals and before bed. The proportions should be carefully titrated because the preparation can be very thick and difficult for some people to tolerate. To increase palatability, this supplement can be sweetened slightly with honey, stevia, or sugar.

PRECAUTIONS

Slippery elm root bark powder is described by most sources as very safe, although the hydrocolloid fibers may bind simultaneously administered medications and decrease their absorption.[28]

Marshmallow (Althea officinalis)

Marshmallow is another mucilaginous herb for GERD symptomatic relief. Its demulcent properties also make it useful for pharyngitis, wound healing, cough, and bronchitis.

DOSAGE

Marshmallow is usually taken at 5 to 6 g daily, in divided doses, as an infusion of the leaves or root.[29]

PRECAUTIONS

As with slippery elm, a decrease in absorption of orally administered drugs taken simultaneously with marshmallow may occur.[28]

Antiinflammatory Botanicals

Antiinflammatory herbs are often used for GERD symptom relief and to improve healing of the irritated esophageal mucosa.[27] Examples include licorice (*Glycyrrhiza glabra*); meadowsweet (*Filipendula ulmaria*), which also reduces acidity; chickweed (*Stellaria media*); and chamomile (*Matricaria recutita*).

Licorice (Glycyrrhiza glabra)

Licorice is a well-known mucosa antiinflammatory botanical used for GERD, gastritis, and duodenal and peptic ulcers. For long-term use, it should be prescribed as deglycyrrhizinated licorice to prevent the side effects of one of its phytochemicals, glycyrrhizin (see box).

> **DOSAGE**
>
> Two 380-mg tablets of deglycyrrhizinated licorice (DGL) should be taken before meals.[29]
>
> **PRECAUTIONS**
>
> The prolonged use of decoctions or infusions of dried, unprocessed licorice root may cause hypertension, hypokalemia, and edema due to the mineralocorticoid action of the saponin, glycyrrhizin, also called *glycyrrhizic acid*.[28]

Chamomile (Matricaria recutita)

Chamomile is well known for its mild sedative actions and for its antispasmodic effects on the gastrointestinal tract. In GERD, it is used as a nondemulcent antiinflammatory agent.[23,27]

> **DOSAGE**
>
> Chamomile is most commonly prepared as a hot water infusion (tea) of 1 to 3 g (2 g equals 1 tablespoon) of the flowers, steeped in a cup covered with a saucer, taken three to four times daily.[29]
>
> **PRECAUTIONS**
>
> Chamomile is generally well tolerated, although individuals allergic to other plants in the daisy family (*Asteraceae*) may experience an exacerbation of their allergic symptoms with consumption of chamomile.

Antianxiety Botanicals

Many herbal experts recommend botanicals as part of an overall approach to anxiety management, given the connection between anxiety and GERD (see previous). Examples are valerian (*Valeriana officinalis*) and skullcap (*Scutellaria lateriflora*)[27] (see Chapter 6).

Botanical Combinations

Mixtures of botanicals have also been studied either alone or in combination with pharmaceuticals. For example, two reviews have detailed the use of an 8-plant kampo (traditional Japanese medicine) mixture, called *rikkunshito*, for GERD, including PPI-refractory GERD.[30,31]

Pharmaceuticals

Both histamine-2 (H$_2$) receptor antagonists or blockers (H2Bs) and PPIs are commonly used for the symptoms of GERD. A meta-analysis concluded that both H2Bs and PPIs are effective in GERD symptomatic improvement; however, PPIs are significantly more effective than H2Bs.[32] PPIs have also been used in a 1-week therapeutic trial to test and diagnose GERD empirically.[1] The optimal dosing time for PPIs is 30 minutes before a meal, although adherence to the ideal dosing regimen may or may not lead to better symptom control.[33] Some clinicians use H2Bs or PPIs indefinitely to control symptoms.[2] The use of PPIs is particularly important in cases of Barrett esophagus; premalignant changes in the cells of the distal esophagus. The evidence is compelling for a protective effect of PPIs on dysplastic esophageal cells.[34]

Aggressive, long-term acid suppression can decrease the absorption of vitamin B$_{12}$.[1] Consider regular intramuscular injections or sublingual administration of vitamin B$_{12}$ for those individuals requiring long-term treatment with histamine-2 receptor blockers or proton pump inhibitors. Use of these drugs can also lead to iron malabsorption, increased risk of hip and spine fracture, *Clostridium difficile* diarrhea, cardiovascular mortality, and community-acquired pneumonia.[4,5,35]

In one study, between 10% and 40% of people who took PPIs for GERD failed to respond symptomatically, partially or completely, whereas a separate study reported that 85% of patients taking PPIs had persistent GERD symptoms even though 73% of those patients were satisfied with the treatment.[33] Some debate exists regarding the reasons for certain patients not responding to PPIs. Investigators have hypothesized that these patients have functional or nonerosive reflux disease, or weakly acidic or alkaline refluxate.[33]

Some nuances with the prescribing of the two primary classes of pharmaceuticals for GERD, PPIs and H2Bs, are noted in Table 42.3. Box 42.1 describes the protocol for tapering PPIs.

TABLE 42.3 **Comparison of Proton Pump Inhibitors Versus Histamine-2 Receptor Blockers for Gastroesophageal Reflux Disease**

PPIs	H2Bs
Greater rate of healing from esophagitis than H2Bs	Greater rate of healing from esophagitis than placebo
Slight benefit in healing esophagitis with twice the standard dose	
Unclear whether PPIs heal heartburn, as a symptom, more than H2Bs	Both PPIs and H2Bs heal heartburn more than placebo
Complete resolution of heartburn in approximately 40% of patients (compared with 15% for placebo)	

H2Bs, histamine-2 receptor blockers; PPIs, proton pump inhibitors. Data from Kahrilas PJ. Gastroesophageal reflux disease. *N Engl J Med.* 2008;359:1700-1707.

Biomechanical Therapy

Some naturopathic physicians recommend hernial reduction adjustments, an abdominal manipulation technique, when GERD symptoms are complicated by the presence of a hiatal hernia.[23] Although no clinical trials have examined the efficacy of hernial reduction adjustments, referral to an experienced practitioner should be considered for patients with a documented hiatal hernia and symptoms of GERD. Aside from surgery, no documented allopathic interventions exist for the treatment of hiatal hernia.

Mind-Body Therapy

Relaxation training can improve symptoms of GERD by addressing the exacerbation of GERD symptoms due to stress, particularly in patients suffering from chronic anxiety.[33]

BOX 42.1 Helping Taper off a Proton Pump Inhibitor

For those patients who have made positive lifestyle changes and may not need continued chronic acid suppression, it can often be difficult to discontinue proton pump inhibitors (PPIs) because they often cause rebound hyperacidity even if the underlying condition has resolved.[1]

Plan:

1. Slowly taper off the PPI over 2 to 4 weeks (the higher the dose, the longer the taper).
2. While the taper is being completed, use the following for bridge therapy to reduce the symptoms of rebound hyperacidity:
   a. Encourage regular aerobic exercise.
   b. Encourage a relaxation technique, such as self-hypnosis, for gastrointestinal disorders (see Chapter 95) or meditation (see Chapter 100).
   c. Suggest acupuncture one to two times per week.[2]
   d. Add one or more of the following:
      i. Deglycyrrhizinated licorice, two 380-mg tablets, before meals or Sucralfate (Carafate) 1 g before meals
      ii. Slippery elm, 1 to 2 tablespoons of powdered root in water three to four times per day
      iii. A combination botanical product, Iberogast (clown's mustard, German chamomile, angelica root, caraway, milk thistle, lemon balm, celandine, licorice root, and peppermint leaf), 1 mL three times per day[3]
3. If the taper is successful, slowly taper the foregoing supplements (except for positive nutritional changes, exercise, and stress management). If symptoms return, start with one of the foregoing or a histamine-2 receptor blocker. If symptoms are still difficult to control, consider adding back the PPI.
4. Ideally, it is beneficial to avoid long-term acid suppression if possible because this can be associated with malabsorption of vitamin B_{12} and iron,[4] increased risk of community-acquired pneumonia,[5] hip[8,9] and spine[10,11] fracture, *Clostridium difficile* diarrhea,[12] and cardiovascular mortality.[35]

Other Therapies to Consider

Homeopathy

Homeopathy can be a therapeutic consideration. Many of the symptoms associated with GERD, such as indigestion and heartburn, or associated disorders such as hiatal hernia, are mentioned in homeopathy sources and treated with a wide variety of short-term remedies, such as phosphorus, nux vomica, pulsatilla, carbo vegetabilis, arsenicum, bryonia, china, anacardium, argentum, sepia, lycopodium, graphites, and kali bichromium[36] (see Chapter 115).

Traditional Chinese Medicine

Traditional Chinese medicine, which provides a complete assessment based on a unique cultural, diagnostic, and therapeutic approach, may offer relief for patients suffering from GERD. In a study comparing acupuncture with doubling the dose of a PPI for GERD, acupuncture was found to be more effective in reducing symptoms.[37] With treatment suggestions incorporating diet, lifestyle, botanical medicines, and acupuncture or acupressure,[38] traditional Chinese medicine should be considered a therapeutic option based either solely on patient personal preference or on the requirement for adjuncts to incomplete or ineffective allopathic therapies.

Surgery

Surgical treatment is considered by many experts to be an option for people in whom lifestyle modification or adequate medical therapy fails or who are unwilling to take long-term medication.[1,3,39,40] The most common surgical procedure is Nissen fundoplication, either open or laparoscopic, whereby the fundus of the stomach is wrapped wholly (total fundoplication) or partially (partial fundoplication) around the lower esophagus to create an area of high pressure to prevent refluxate from entering the esophagus and causing symptoms. Laparoscopic fundoplication provides long-term disease control similar to that seen with the open approach but with fewer incisional hernias.[40] One review examined health-related quality of life and GERD symptoms after 1 year in four studies involving 1232 people who underwent medical management versus laparoscopic surgical management.[3] Overall, the surgical approach appeared to improve symptoms of GERD more effectively than medical management, although dysphagia (8% to 12% postoperatively),[40] costs after 1 year, and other adverse effects were more pronounced in the surgical group of some studies. One review and meta-analysis concluded that partial laparoscopic fundoplication was associated with less postoperative dysphagia than total fundoplication.[40]

Special Considerations in Pediatrics

The treatment of GERD in infants usually involves dietary interventions such as the normalization of feeding techniques, volumes, and frequency, if these are abnormal.[9] Formula can be thickened with one tablespoon of rice cereal per ounce to decrease the number of regurgitation events, increase calorie density, and reduce the number of crying episodes.[9] One meta-analysis supported the concept that thickened feedings improve GERD symptoms in infants.[41] A short trial of a hypoallergenic diet, in particular to exclude milk and soy, can be helpful in children suspected of having allergies to those foods. Older children with GERD are advised to avoid tomatoes, chocolate, mint, and classically offending beverages (juices, sodas, and caffeinated beverages) and to lose weight, if applicable.

With respect to positioning during meals, infant GERD is worse when infants are seated, supine, or on their side and better when they are prone or carried upright. Due to the risk of sudden infant death syndrome, a prone position cannot be recommended for sleep.[9] Older children may have some relief from GERD when they lie on their left side or with the head of the bed elevated. As with adults, children experience some symptomatic improvement with H2Bs and PPIs; the dose of PPIs is higher per kilogram than for adults (0.7 to 1.5 mg/kg/day).[9]

PREVENTION PRESCRIPTION

- Avoid foods and supplements, and, when possible, medications known to decrease lower esophageal sphincter tone (see Table 42.1).
- Maintain ideal body weight.

- Reduce stress as much as possible through lifestyle change and stress management and mind-body techniques.
- Avoid large meals and consuming large quantities of liquids with meals.

THERAPEUTIC REVIEW

This summary of therapies is for patients with mild to moderate, short-term GERD. Patients with long-standing, more severe GERD should undergo an appropriate diagnostic workup, which may include a referral to a gastroenterologic specialist and for upper endoscopy to exclude esophagitis, ulcers, Barrett esophagus, and adenocarcinoma.

REMOVAL OF EXACERBATING FACTORS

- Avoid foods, supplements, and, when possible, medications known to decrease lower esophageal sphincter tone (see Table 42.1).
- If applicable, quit smoking.
- If applicable, lose weight.

LIFESTYLE

- For nocturnal symptoms, elevate the head of the bed 4 to 6 inches. C 1
- Avoid large meals and consuming large quantities of liquids with meals. C 1

MIND-BODY MEDICINE

- Practice stress management and relaxation techniques. B 1

BOTANICAL MEDICINES

- Deglycyrrhizinated licorice: two 380-mg tablets before meals C 1
- Slippery elm: 1 to 2 tablespoons of powdered root in a glass of water, three to four times daily C 1
- Other botanical medicines that have potential benefit include chamomile, marshmallow, skullcap, and valerian (see Table 42.2).

PHARMACEUTICALS

- Start with a proton pump inhibitor A 2, both for symptomatic relief and for diagnostic purposes.
- Histamine-2 receptor antagonists   A 2
- Over-the-counter antacids, such as calcium carbonate, aluminum hydroxide, and magnesium hydroxide, can be helpful. C 1

SURGERY

- For patients with intractable symptoms, fundoplication should be considered. B 3

Key Web Resources

American College of Gastroenterology clinical updates. This collection of allopathic, evidence-based reviews covers numerous topics relevant to GERD, including diagnosis, management, reflux testing, and surveillance of Barrett esophagus.

http://www.acg.gi.org/physicians/clinicalupdates.asp

University of Wisconsin Integrative Medicine. Patient handouts and video reviews for an integrative approach to GERD management.

https://www.fammed.wisc.edu/integrative/modules/gerd

REFERENCES

References are available online at ExpertConsult.com.

CHAPTER 43

PEPTIC ULCER DISEASE

Joseph Eichenseher, MD, MAT

PATHOPHYSIOLOGY

Each year approximately half a million people in the United States are newly diagnosed with peptic ulcer disease (PUD), with many more millions of undiagnosed cases likely.[1] PUD is caused by disturbances of the gastrointestinal (GI) mucosa. These disruptions are due to the loss of protective elements and/or damaging insults that result in mucosal erosions, most commonly located in the duodenum or stomach. People with PUD commonly complain of epigastric pain (particularly a few hours after meals), bloating, nausea, early satiety, altered bowel habits, and heartburn. Pain is usually improved with food or antacids. PUD may also occur without symptoms, particularly in older adults. Peptic ulcers may cause GI bleeding, which is a potentially life-threatening emergency necessitating urgent endoscopy and intensive care unit consideration. Ulcers may rarely perforate leading to intense pain and acute peritonitis, which is a surgical emergency. Patients with significant weight loss and PUD symptoms should undergo endoscopy to investigate for potential malignant diseases.

The loss of gastrointestinal mucosal integrity is typically multifactorial, with diminished protective elements (predominantly decreased acid buffering, reduced immune system functioning, and slowed wound healing) and increased insults (primarily *Helicobacter pylori* infection, the use of nonsteroidal antiinflammatory drugs [NSAIDs], increased acidity, and inflammation). Treatment efforts are focused on restoring protective factors and reducing harmful affronts.

> Nonsteroidal antiinflammatory drugs, such as ibuprofen or naproxen, should be avoided in patients with a history of peptic ulcer disease (PUD) and minimized in individuals with PUD symptoms who lack a formal diagnosis of PUD.

Peptic ulcers may occur at any time in life, although the incidence gradually increases with age.[2] In the early twentieth century, PUD was diagnosed in men at twice the rate as in women. However, PUD is now nearly equally distributed between genders, although gastric ulcers tend to be more common in women and duodenal ulcers more common in men.[3]

Historically, investigators were aware that smoking, stress, NSAIDs, and family history (risk increases three times with an afflicted first-degree relative)[4] contributed to peptic ulcer formation. However, prior to the late 1970s, allopathic medicine had limited success in treating PUD until the arrival of two revolutionary developments: the invention of pharmaceuticals that reduced the amount of acid the stomach produced; and the discovery of the *Helicobacter pylori* bacterium (Fig. 43.1).

The development of gastric acid-suppressing medications, with the advent of histamine-2 receptor antagonists (H_2 blockers) in the late 1970s and proton pump inhibitors (PPIs) in the 1980s, heralded a new chapter in Western medicine's management of PUD. Previous efforts had focused on reducing risk factors, administering acid buffers (e.g., calcium carbonate) for symptom relief, and surgery (associated with significant morbidity and mortality). With the invention and administration of acid-reducing medications, the majority of cases of PUD are quickly attenuated. This approach has drastically reduced the need for surgery and increased the role of pharmaceuticals in PUD therapy.

H. pylori was identified in 1982, a discovery for which Drs. J. Robin Warren and Barry J. Marshall won the Nobel Prize for medicine in 2005. The more the medical world learns about this unique bacterium, the more our thinking about PUD treatment evolves. *H. pylori* infection has been shown to increase the incidence of PUD by at least four-fold.[5] Rates of *H. pylori* infection vary worldwide according to age and economic status. Younger, more affluent individuals have rates as low as 20%, whereas up to 60% of all individuals in the developing world, and 50% of individuals older than 60 years in the United States, are colonized by the bacterium.[6] Living in the harsh acidic environment of the human stomach, *H. pylori* appears to increase the risk of PUD by directly damaging the protective mucus lining of the GI tract and allowing for increased acidic damage. *H. pylori* also triggers an immune response that causes damaging inflammation. Besides PUD disease, *H. pylori* has been also been linked to increased rates of gastric cancer, dyspepsia, vitamin B_{12} deficiency, iron deficiency, and idiopathic thrombocytopenia (ITP).[7] *H. pylori* may not be without benefits, with some studies indicating a correlation between *H. pylori* colonization and decreased rates of asthma, allergies, GERD, obesity, and esophageal cancer.[7,8] Whether *H. pylori* is predominantly a symbiotic bacteria that has been with humanity for millions of years, occasionally running amok and causing PUD and stomach cancer, or strictly a pathogen that has an increasing niche in the modern world warranting global eradication efforts remains the focus of research efforts. The pending answer to this question will likely guide approaches to PUD treatment in the decades ahead.

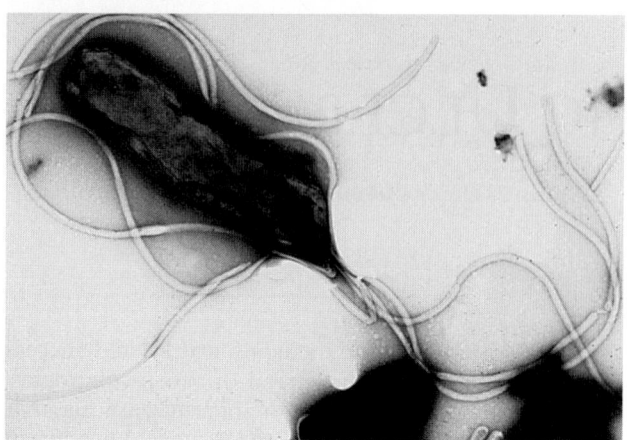

FIG. 43.1 ■ *Helicobacter pylori,* the discovery of which revolutionized medical understanding and management of peptic ulcer disease. (Courtesy Yutaka Tsutsumi, MD.)

Although there have been promising *H. pylori* vaccine studies in animal models, indicating vaccines may eventually become the most powerful tool for treating PUD, successful clinical vaccine trials have yet to be reported. Even with a potential vaccine, complete global eradication of *H. pylori* is logistically challenging, despite *H. pylori* exclusively residing in humans, because there are currently an estimated 4 billion people infected worldwide. Further, only 10% to 20% of *H. pylori*-infected individuals develop PUD.[5] Thus, current treatment efforts should focus on symptomatic carriers. Universal screening of asymptomatic individuals for *H. pylori* is not advised.

H. pylori and NSAIDs, in combination with other risk factors, account for the majority of cases of PUD.[1] The remaining cases are attributable to other independent risk factors and a few clinical "zebras," such as Zollinger-Ellison tumors, carcinoid syndrome, other drugs, radiation, cytomegalovirus, and systemic mastocytosis.

Pharmaceutical acid suppression, and the discovery and subsequent antibiotic treatment of *H. pylori*, resulted in optimism that PUD was on the verge of elimination at the end of the twentieth century. However, due to increasing antibiotic resistance, increased knowledge of the harms of long-term pharmaceutical acid suppression, in addition to evidence of the potential benefits of *H. pylori* infection, there is now a requirement for more judicious use of antibiotics and the incorporation of more integrative PUD approaches in the years and decades ahead.

Diagnosis

The overlapping constellation of PUD symptoms with other diseases, such as gastritis, irritable bowel syndrome, gastroesophageal reflux disease, Crohn's disease, pancreatitis, gallstones, and malignancy, makes the initial diagnosis of PUD challenging, particularly because endoscopy (an invasive, costly procedure) is the current standard for diagnostic testing and the next best tool is a barium GI series (with resulting radiation, cost, and potential inaccuracy). A study reported

that the physical examination finding of epigastric tenderness decreases the likelihood of PUD.[9] Thus, it is not surprising that many practitioners, in addition to patients without signs of serious disease (bleeding or weight loss), hesitate in electing to pursue these invasive diagnostic measures. Accordingly, the majority of cases of PUD may never be diagnosed with certainty. *H. pylori* testing in symptomatic patients increases the number of people diagnosed with *H. pylori* infection, but a positive test result indicates only a bacterial infection, and cannot differentiate between conditions such as gastritis and more serious PUD, although initial management is largely the same. There are various tests for *H. pylori*, but the stool antigen and urea breath tests are consistently the best for determining active infection.

Once a diagnosis of PUD is established, recurrence is reported in up to 74% of patients.[10] PUD management therefore focuses on the prevention and symptomatic treatment, a good fit for an integrative approach (Fig. 43.2).

INTEGRATIVE THERAPY

Nutrition

Dietary constituents were linked to PUD long before the discovery of *H. pylori*, with subsequent research demonstrating certain foods to be protective against *H. pylori* infection. Accordingly, nutrition is considered a key component of ulcer prevention and symptom management.

Meal timing influences PUD, with skipping breakfast[11] and consuming large meals shortly before bedtime shown to increase the risk of PUD.[12]

Fruit and vegetable intake reduces the risk of developing ulcers, with epidemiological studies demonstrating that a diet high in plant-based fiber and vitamin A (e.g., carrots, spinach, mango, sweet potatoes, and apricots) helps protect against PUD.[13] Flavonoids, compounds found throughout the plant world, have been found to be protective against *H. pylori* infection and are present in concentrated amounts in citrus, berries, onions, parsley, green tea, red wine, and dark chocolate.[14] Sulforaphanes, which are phytochemicals found in vegetables such as Brussels sprouts, broccoli, cabbage, cauliflower, bok choy, turnips, and radishes, are also protective against *H. pylori* infection.[15]

Studies have specifically shown that virgin olive oil (30 g daily for 2 weeks) or broccoli sprouts (70 g a day for 8 weeks) have the ability to decrease and potentially eliminate *H. pylori*.[15,16] Foods containing capsaicin (chili) have been shown to be protective against ulcers.[17] Capsules of chilies (fruit of the plant genus *capsicum*) are reviewed in the botanical section of this chapter for acute symptom relief. Other common foods demonstrating protective effects against *H. pylori* include banana, honey, garlic, ginger, okra, pomegranate, and apple.[18-24] There is likely synergy in ingesting combinations of these beneficial foods, a good example of "nutrition is medicine."

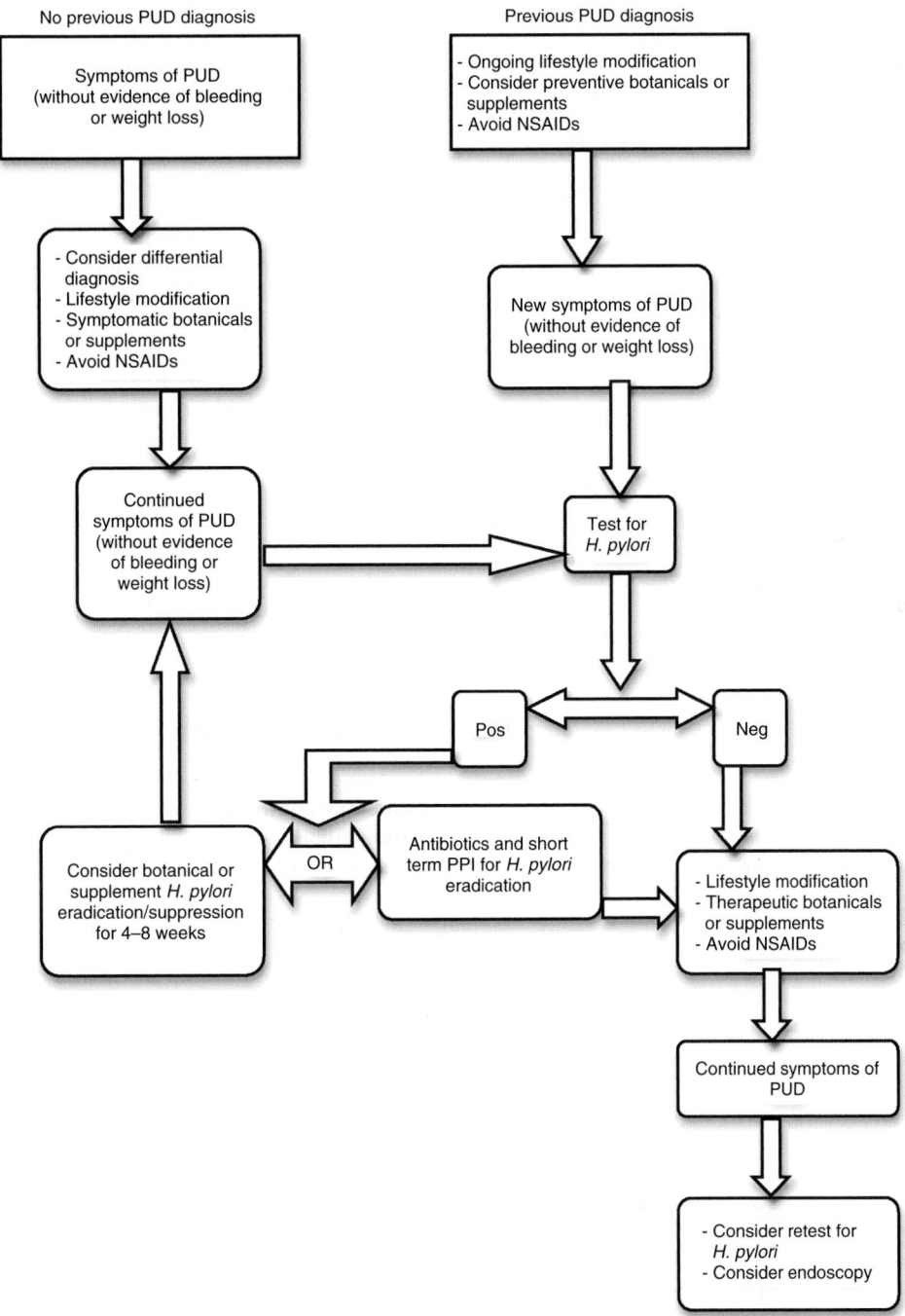

FIG. 43.2 ■ Integrative management flow chart for peptic ulcer disease (PUD). Neg, negative; NSAIDs, nonsteroidal antiinflammatory drugs; Pos, positive; PPI, proton pump inhibitor.

Foods found to be associated with a reduced risk of *Helicobacter pylori* infection include fruits and vegetables rich in carotenoids (yellow, orange), flavonoids (purple and blue vegetables, red wine, and green tea), sulforaphanes (cruciferous vegetables, including cabbage and broccoli), olive oil, garlic, honey, apple, capsaicin (chili), and fermented foods rich in probiotics (yogurt, miso, aged cheese, and sauerkraut).

Milk increases PUD risk, likely due to increased stimulation of acid production.[25] Nonetheless, fermented dairy products and other food with probiotics, such as yogurt, aged cheeses, and sauerkraut, have been shown to be protective against *H. pylori*.[26,27]

Evidence regarding coffee and caffeine, long thought to be risk factors for PUD, is lacking; however, they are known risk factors for reflux disease.

Physical Activity

Multiple studies have demonstrated that regular physical activity, when compared with a more sedentary lifestyle, is protective against PUD.[28,29] One study specifically demonstrated that the risk for duodenal ulcers was 62% less in men who cumulatively walked or ran more than 10 miles per week.[29] Routine exercise should be recommended for almost all patients, particularly those with a previous history of PUD.

Stress Reduction

The relationship between stress and PUD is a classic example of the need for clinicians to keep in mind the social determinants of health (Fig. 43.3), over which our patients have varying degrees of control. Stress is largely a product of the social and environmental milieu, and convincing evidence indicates that stress plays a role in PUD. This connection is established early in life. Childhood stress, in the form of traumatic events, such as an illness of a family member, financial strain, or family conflict, is associated with a nearly 50% higher rate of PUD in adulthood.[30] Studies have also shown that GI ulceration increases with both chronic stress and in times of acute stress, such as during an earthquake or war (e.g., during the bombing of London in World War II).[31,32] A multipronged approach to stress reduction, in comparison with any single method, appears to provide more protection against PUD.[33] As a clinician, recommending individually tailored stress reduction programs, including yoga, tai chi, and other coordinated movements in addition to meditation, focused breathing, and any other culturally applicable relaxation methods, will likely be beneficial (see Chapters 94 and 100).

Sleep

Inadequate sleep is a risk factor for PUD,[11] likely the result of increased stress levels causing immune dysfunction and impaired lifestyle decisions. Maintaining good sleep hygiene is an important component of ulcer avoidance (see Chapter 9).

Tobacco Cessation

Smoking increases rates of PUD up to four times when compared with nonsmokers, likely due to decreased wound healing.[28] Accordingly, smoking cessation is essential in addressing PUD.

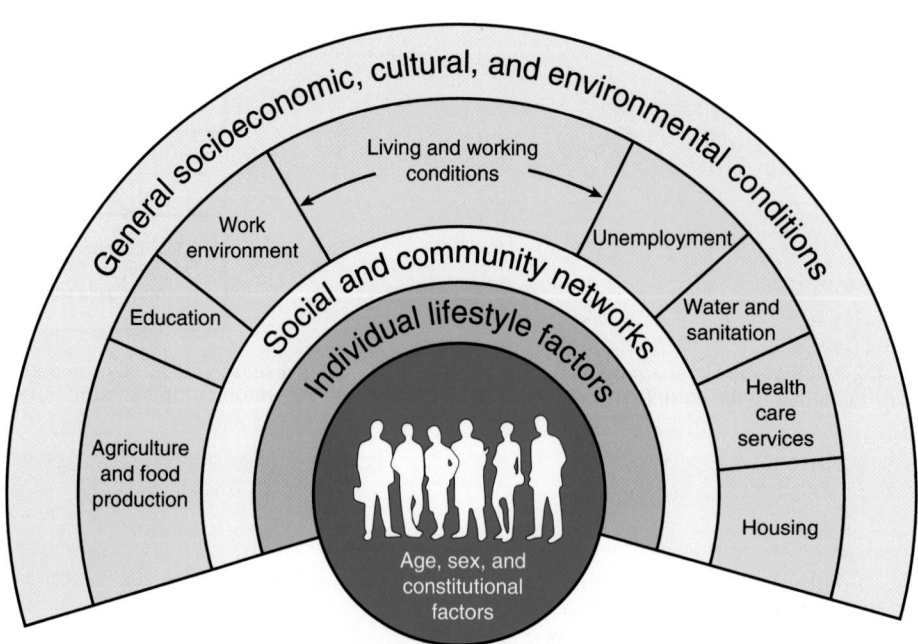

FIG. 43.3 ■ Social determinants of health diagram. (From Dahlgren G, Whitehead M. *Policies and strategies to promote social equity in health.* Stockholm: Institute for Futures Studies; 1991.)

Alcohol Avoidance or Moderation

Alcohol, in large amounts, has been shown to be a risk factor for ulcers, likely as a result of mucosal damage. One epidemiological study reported that individuals who consumed more than 42 drinks per week had a greater than four-fold increase in the incidence of bleeding ulcers compared with individuals who consumed 1 drink per week or less.[34] However, red wine is reported to be protective against *H. pylori* infection, possibly attributable to the activity of bioactive compounds such as flavonoids.[35] Avoiding large quantities of ethanol, particularly higher-percentage drinks, is prudent in patients with a history or symptoms of PUD, whereas moderate red wine consumption should not necessarily be discouraged.

Nonsteroidal Antiinflammatory Drugs

Evidence indicates that NSAID use increases the baseline risk of PUD by up to five times and the risk of bleeding ulcers in patients with established PUD by five times.[36] NSAIDs inhibit prostaglandin production and thus decrease mucoprotective elements in the GI tract. Although evidence indicates that the administration of medications such as sucralfate or misoprostol with NSAIDs can help ease ulcer symptoms and prevent ulcer recurrence,[37,38] NSAIDs should be avoided as much as possible in patients with PUD symptoms or an existing history of PUD disease. As more than 80% of patients taking NSAIDs never develop PUD,[39] these drugs should not necessarily be avoided in asymptomatic patients without a history of ulcers.

Supplements

Probiotics

Certain helpful microorganisms have proven versatile in the treatment of PUD. Probiotics have been shown to reduce ulcer recurrence,[40] and individuals with higher intakes of probiotics have correspondingly lower rates of *H. pylori* infection.[26] Probiotics are likely effective in combating *H. pylori* as a result of increased GI mucus production, competition for mucosal binding sites, and production of compounds with activity against *H. pylori*. Further, results from animal models have indicated probiotics decrease the inflammatory response to *H. pylori*.[41] The majority of reported studies were conducted with *Lactobacillus* strains commonly found in yogurt, yet evidence indicates that other strains of probiotics are also helpful.[42] Thus, incorporating yogurt and other probiotic-containing foods, such as aged cheeses and sauerkraut, into a diet on a regular basis can be beneficial for PUD prevention and avoidance of ulcer recurrence. Many clinical studies have confirmed that probiotics, including both *Lactobacillus* and *Saccharomyces boulardii*, have synergy with antibiotics for *H. pylori* eradication and can decrease antibiotic-related side effects, such as diarrhea, bloating, nausea, and abdominal pain[38,43-45] Although the evidence is weaker, there are numerous studies indicating probiotics alone, without antibiotics, can improve PUD symptoms and suppress (and sometimes eradicate) *H. pylori* infection[46] (see Chapter 105).

DOSAGE

For *H. pylori* antibiotic eradication therapy, available regimens include *Lactobacillus (acidophilus* or GG) capsules, containing at least 1 billion organisms, twice daily, or *Saccharomyces boulardii*, 500 mg twice daily.

A regime of *Bifidobacterium bifidum*, 1×10^{10} CFU, daily for 12 weeks can be used for the suppression of *H. pylori* and PUD symptom relief.

PREVENTION

Probiotic-containing foods or supplements are recommended on a regular basis for patients with a previous history of PUD, a family history of ulcer disease, or other risk factors for PUD.

PRECAUTIONS

Patients sensitive or intolerant to lactose may have GI discomfort with dairy products containing probiotics.

Vitamin C

Ascorbic acid (vitamin C) has been shown to have potential for *H. pylori* eradication; one study demonstrated a 10% eradication rate with 2 weeks of 1000 mg daily.[47] Vitamin C also has additive effects on antibiotic regimens for *H. pylori* eradication.[48] This anti–*H. pylori* capability has been supported by in vitro studies.[49] A 5-year Japanese study demonstrated lower PUD rates in persons taking vitamin C supplementation.[50] A steady dietary intake of vitamin C is recommended for anyone with current symptoms, a previous history or a family history of PUD, or other risk factors for ulcer disease.

DOSAGE

The recommended dose of vitamin C is 500 mg twice daily for *H. pylori* eradication or suppression (in addition to daily dietary intake).

PREVENTION

Eat foods containing vitamin C on a regular basis, including citrus, kiwi, broccoli, strawberry, and cauliflower.

PRECAUTIONS

Dose-related potential adverse effects include kidney stones, diarrhea, nausea, and gastritis. Use with caution in patients with kidney disease.

Zinc

A clinical trial has reported zinc accelerates the healing of gastric ulcers up to three times faster than observed with placebo.[51] This finding has been corroborated by more extensive animal studies.[52] Enhanced healing is likely the result of the fundamental role of zinc in repair of damaged tissue. A compound not available in the United States, zinc acexamate, has been used in East Asia and Europe for PUD and has been found effective in numerous studies.[53]

DOSAGE

The recommended dose of zinc is 40 mg daily for 4 weeks for gastric ulcer treatment.

PRECAUTIONS

Potential side effects include nausea, vomiting, diarrhea, and altered taste. Zinc inhibits the absorption of other minerals, particularly copper.

Polyunsaturated Fatty Acids

Multiple polyunsaturated fatty acids (PUFAs) have been shown to have activity against *H. pylori* in vitro (including alpha-linolenic acid, eicosapentaenoic acid [EPA], gamma-linolenic acid [GLA], and linoleic acid).[54] A clinical study of the administration of 2 g a day of a 1:1 mixture of fish oil (EPA and docosahexaenoic acid) and black currant seed oil (GLA) for 8 weeks cleared *H. pylori* infection in more than 50% of participants.[55] Although elimination rates are significantly lower for PUFAs compared with antibiotics, PUFAs are reasonable to recommend for patients desiring *H. pylori* eradication without antibiotics.

DOSAGE

For *H. pylori* suppression or elimination, 1 g of fish oil and 1 g of GLA-containing oil (evening primrose, black currant seed, borage, or hemp seed oils) daily for 8 weeks.

PRECAUTIONS

PUFAs may cause GI upset. Higher doses of omega-3 fatty acids (more than 3 g/day) may increase the risk of bleeding from anticoagulant effects.

Glutamine

In clinical trials, glutamine has been shown to prevent and cure PUD. A study of patients with burn injury demonstrated that glutamine can help prevent stress ulcers.[56] A separate trial reported more rapid healing of peptic ulcers in patients administered 400 mg of glutamine four times a day.[57] This limited clinical research has also been supported by results from animal studies.[58,59] Glutamine supplementation is likely successful because it is a necessary amino acid for the repair and new growth of cells lining the GI tract. Dietary sources of glutamine include beef, chicken, fish, eggs, wheat, cabbage, beets, beans, spinach, and parsley.

DOSAGE

For PUD treatment, the recommended dose is 400 mg of glutamine powder in water four times daily.

PRECAUTIONS

No significant adverse effects have been reported.

Botanicals

Turmeric (Curcuma longa)

Turmeric has been used for centuries in Chinese and Ayurvedic medicine for the treatment of dyspepsia and epigastric pain. A clinical trial, in which 600-mg turmeric root was administered five times daily to patients with PUD, reported ulcer resolution at 4 weeks and 12 weeks in 48% and 76% of patients, respectively.[60] The same study also demonstrated that turmeric markedly improves symptoms of dyspepsia in 1 to 2 weeks.[60] Turmeric and curcumin, a commercially available turmeric derivative, are known to have activity against *H. pylori* in vitro.[61,62] A clinical trial failed to demonstrate turmeric's ability to eradicate *H. pylori* completely but did observe relief of dyspeptic symptoms.[63] Turmeric has been found to have H_2-blocking properties, which likely also explains much of its healing potential.[64]

DOSAGE

For the treatment of PUD and associated symptoms, the recommended dose of whole turmeric root or powder (capsules) is 600 mg five times daily for 12 weeks.

PRECAUTIONS

Turmeric may cause nausea, diarrhea, heartburn, or kidney stones. Some evidence exists that it may increase the risk of bleeding secondary to antiplatelet activity.

Deglycyrrhizinated Licorice (Glycyrrhiza glabra)

Licorice has been used for medicinal purposes, including the treatment of epigastric pain and dyspepsia, since ancient Egyptian times and for at least 4000 years in China.[65] Deglycyrrhizinated licorice (DGL) does not have the adrenocorticoid effect of glycyrrhiza (sodium retention leading to hypertension) and is less hepatotoxic than the native plant. A small clinical trial demonstrated DGL to be as effective as H_2 blockers for duodenal ulcer resolution at 12 weeks, with fewer episodes of relapse.[66] A robust randomized, double-blinded, placebo-controlled study also reported that 2 months of DGL eliminated *H. pylori* infection in 56% of participants versus 4% for placebo.[67] These effects may be attributable to the bioactive flavonoids found in licorice.

DOSAGE

For PUD, the recommended dose of DGL is 380 mg three times per day for 12 weeks. For *H. pylori* eradication, 150 mg (root extract) daily for 60 days.

PRECAUTIONS

Use with caution in patients with liver disease, renal insufficiency, or hypokalemia. Avoid in pregnancy due to a theoretical risk of preterm labor.

Deglycyrrhizinated licorice (DGL) does not contain the steroid-like component of natural licorice, glycyrrhizic acid, which can induce sodium retention, hypokalemia, and elevated blood pressure.

Mastic (Pistacia lentiscus)

Mastic is a member of the pistachio tree family found throughout the Mediterranean, and its resin has been harvested for more than 2000 years as a spice, for chewing gum, and for medicinal purposes. A double-blind, placebo-controlled trial of 350-mg capsules, taken three times a day for 3 weeks, demonstrated clinically significant improvement of dyspepsia.[68] Mastic has been shown to have activity against *H. pylori* both in vivo and in vitro.[69] A double-blind trial reported that mastic significantly improved duodenal ulcer healing when compared with placebo.[70]

DOSAGE

For dyspepsia, the dose is 350-mg capsules three times a day for 3 weeks. For duodenal ulcer healing, the dose is 500-mg capsules twice daily for 2 weeks.

PRECAUTIONS

Avoid in people with pistachio allergies. Use with caution in patients taking angiotensin-converting enzyme inhibitors because it may cause hypotension.

Cabbage (Brassica oleracea)

Clinical studies in the 1950s demonstrated the effectiveness of cabbage juice for gastric and duodenal ulcer healing when participants drank 1 L of fresh cabbage juice over the course of a day for 10 days.[71,72] Because this research was conducted more than 50 years ago, and in light of subsequently improved diagnostic studies and greater understanding of PUD, further studies of cabbage juice are warranted. However, cabbage should be recommended for the treatment of PUD despite its safety profile and accessibility. Cabbage has been shown to be a rich source of glutamine and sulforaphanes, likely accounting for much of its healing effect.

DOSAGE

For PUD, the recommended dose of cabbage is 1 L of fresh juice (pasteurized juice was found to be ineffective) divided over the course of a day for 10 days.

PRECAUTIONS

Due to its vitamin K content, cabbage may decrease the anticoagulant efficacy of warfarin.

Chili (Capsaicin)

Capsaicin is the active component of chili peppers (the fruits of plants of the genus *Capsicum*). Historically, chilies were thought to exacerbate PUD; however, more recent research has proved the opposite. Epidemiological studies have demonstrated that individuals with higher dietary intakes of capsaicin have correspondingly lower rates of PUD.[17,73] A double-blind trial, in which patients took 2.5 mg of chili pepper in capsules daily for 5 weeks, demonstrated that chili was effective for epigastric pain and other symptoms of functional dyspepsia.[74] Animal models also demonstrated capsaicin, by decreasing gastric acidity, to be protective against ulcer formation.[75]

DOSAGE

For epigastric pain and functional dyspepsia, the recommended dose of chili is 2.5 mg daily of chili pepper capsules (can divide doses) for 5 weeks. For PUD prevention, patients should follow a diet rich in capsaicin, as tolerated.

PRECAUTIONS

Avoid in patients with pepper allergies. Use with caution in patients with diabetes (may cause hypoglycemia) and heart disease (may increase blood pressure). Chilies may cause GI upset. Skin contact may cause irritation.

Cranberry (Vaccinium oxycoccos)

A double-blinded clinical trial in *H. pylori*–positive patients demonstrated the ability of cranberry to suppress and eradicate *H. pylori* in patients who drank 500 mL of cranberry juice for 90 days. Although the study demonstrated only a 14% eradication rate, this rate was many times higher than observed with placebo.[76] In vitro studies of human gastric cells have demonstrated cranberry's ability to impair *H. pylori* adhesion to gastric cell walls, similar to its ability to prevent *Escherichia coli* from binding to the bladder wall in the prevention of urinary tract infections.[77]

DOSAGE

For *H. pylori* suppression or eradication, the recommended dose is 500 mL of cranberry juice daily for 90 days.

PRECAUTIONS

Patients with diabetes should consider sugar-free juice. High doses may cause stomach distress. Cranberry may affect warfarin efficacy.

Neem (Azadirachta indica)

In Ayurvedic medicine, the neem tree has been used for thousands of years for multiple purposes, including for epistaxis, parasites, asthma, diabetes, fever, and epigastric pain. This versatility has earned neem the nickname "the village pharmacy."[78] Clinical studies have reported that 30 mg of neem bark extract, taken for 10 days, reduced gastric acid secretion by 77% while promoting significant duodenal ulcer healing when taken for 10 weeks.[79] Animal studies have demonstrated the antiulcer properties of neem,[80] and elucidated that neem inhibits the proton pump, similar to pharmacological PPIs.[81]

DOSAGE

For duodenal ulcers, the recommended dose is 30 mg bark extract twice daily for 10 weeks.

PRECAUTIONS

Use cautiously in patients with liver disease. Avoid in pregnant women (due to abortifacient properties). Avoid in infants and children due to potential toxicities.

Additional Botanicals

Hundreds of other botanicals have demonstrated activity against *H. pylori* both in vitro and in vivo (animal studies). This list continues to grow, and more clinical trials are needed. Thus, we have limited our scope in this book to agents with convincing results in clinical studies. Over the millennia, most global cultures have developed natural remedies for PUD symptoms, many of which have since been proven to have efficacy in the treatment of *H. pylori* infection, including peppermint (*Mentha piperita*),[82] silver wormwood (*Artemisia ludoviciana*),[82] cinnamon (*Cinnamomum cassia*),[83] yarrow (*Achillea millefolium*),[84] chamomile (*Matricaria recutita*),[84] ginkgo (*Ginkgo biloba*),[21] nutmeg (*Myristica fragrans*),[21] hops (*Humulus lupulus*),[84] goldenseal (*Hydrastis canadensis*),[85] sage (*Salvia officinalis*),[85] green tea (*Camellia sinensis*),[86] red ginseng (*Panax ginseng*),[86] aloe (*Aloe vera*),[14] fenugreek (*Trigonella foenum-graecum*),[87] and mugwort (*Artemisia douglasiana*).[88]

For patients wishing to avoid antibiotics for *H. pylori* eradication, it is reasonable to try a regime of deglycyrrhizinated Licorice (DGL) root extract at a dose of 150 mg daily for 60 days. Cranberry, probiotics, PUFAs, vitamin C, olive oil, and broccoli sprouts all have some evidence for *H. pylori* eradication. There is likely synergy between each of these botanicals, although substantial research has only been conducted on individual agents. Treatment courses should be followed up with *H. pylori* breath testing to determine efficacy.

Pharmaceuticals

Antibiotics

Overwhelming evidence indicates that *H. pylori* eradication with antibiotics, in patients with PUD, dramatically improves symptom resolution and reduces ulcer recurrence.[89] Recommended eradication regimens typically include two to three antibiotics and a PPI, and historically have demonstrated up to 90% eradication rates.[90] However, years after antibiotic treatment of *H. pylori* began, the bacterium has now proven tenacious and to have developed more and more resistance to standard regimens. The majority of studies of traditional three-drug therapies have reported eradication rates lower than 80%, with some less than 50%.[90] Specifically, *H. pylori* has demonstrated marked resistance to metronidazole and clarithromycin, thus necessitating the use of newer

and potentially more toxic antibiotics.[91] Because of the significant geographic differences in resistance patterns, prescribers should ideally be aware of local susceptibilities before patients are administered one of the numerous antibiotic regimens for the treatment of *H. pylori* infection.[92] Widespread destruction of the GI microflora with antibiotics also creates the potential for *Clostridium difficile* infections and other flora imbalances, thus necessitating the administration of antibiotics with probiotics.[93] In light of this trend of increasing resistance and potential harms, it is becoming increasingly practical to consider other methods of *H. pylori* eradication or suppression, such as the integrative therapies discussed in this chapter.

DOSAGE

A typical *H. pylori* eradication regimen is as follows: amoxicillin, 1 g; clarithromycin, 500 mg; and omeprazole, 20 mg; this combination is taken twice per day for 14 days. (Probiotics are also recommended as adjuvant therapy.) If possible, check regional susceptibilities when choosing antibiotics.

PRECAUTIONS

Common side effects of antibiotics used include diarrhea, altered taste, headache, and allergic reactions.

Acid-Suppressing Drugs

Since their introduction in the late 1970s, gastric acid suppression medications (H_2 blockers and later PPIs) have dramatically assisted in the relief of PUD symptoms and ulcer healing. PPIs have been shown to be more effective than H_2 blockers and are more frequently used today.[94] However, accumulating evidence indicates chronic acid suppression (longer than 2 to 3 months) has potential adverse effects, including increased rates of pneumonia, *Clostridium difficile* infection, and bone fracture. These drugs also decrease absorption of certain minerals and nutrients, specifically calcium, vitamin B_{12}, iron, and magnesium.[95-97] Animal models have also demonstrated an increased risk of gastric cancer with extended periods of acid suppression.[96]

There is also concern that long-term use of acid-suppressing therapies is associated with increased rates of myocardial infarction and cardiac mortality.[98,99]

DOSAGE

For PUD and PUD symptoms: PPI (e.g., omeprazole, 20 mg) or H_2 blocker (e.g., ranitidine, 150 mg) once or twice daily, per individual drug, for up to 8 weeks.

PRECAUTIONS

Potential adverse effects of H_2-blockers include nausea, headache, dry mouth, rash, and confusion. PPIs can cause headache and nausea. Extended use may cause the adverse effects discussed earlier.

Long-term pharmaceutical acid suppression (particularly with proton pump inhibitors) is increasingly associated with adverse effects, such as infections, cardiac mortality, and decreased nutrient absorption, and should be limited to 8 weeks or less.

Antacids

Millions of years ago, our ancestors likely figured out that eating chalk or other natural acid buffers relieved epigastric pain and symptoms of PUD. Antacids are still potentially useful today in helping with symptom relief and are found in various nonprescription forms including calcium carbonate, aluminum hydroxide, magnesium hydroxide, and sodium bicarbonate. Theoretically, antacids cause increased gastric acid production due to rebound and, although some studies support this hypothesis, previous studies have demonstrated antacids to be safe at recommended doses.[100]

DOSAGE
For PUD symptoms, patients may take over-the-counter antacids according to individual product instructions.

PRECAUTIONS
High doses of calcium-containing antacids may cause kidney stones, constipation, renal failure, alkalosis, or hypercalcemia. Carbonate-containing antacids may cause alkalosis. Aluminum antacids, in high doses, may cause hypophosphatemia, osteomalacia, constipation, or renal insufficiency. Magnesium antacids should be used in caution in patients with renal disease and may cause hypermagnesemia.

Sucralfate

An older synthetic compound, sucralfate, has been shown to be effective in promoting ulcer healing and has been used since the late 1960s as a PUD treatment. Sucralfate has an impressively complex chemical formula of $C_{12}H_{54}Al_{16}O_{75}S_8$, yet the majority of its beneficial effects are attributed to two properties: its ability to act as an acid buffer and its ability to bind to ulcer sites, thus protecting against further insult. In clinical trials, sucralfate has been shown to be as effective as H_2 blockers for treatment of duodenal ulcers.[101]

DOSAGE
For duodenal ulcers, the recommended dose of sucralfate is 1 g four times daily, 1 hour before meals and bedtime, for up to 8 weeks.

PRECAUTIONS
Sucralfate may cause bezoar formation and constipation.

Acupuncture

Controlled trials have shown that acupuncture is an effective treatment for epigastric pain.[102] Case studies and animal models have also shown acupuncture to have efficacy in the treatment of PUD and for the prevention of ulcer recurrence.[103]

Therapies to Consider

Traditional Chinese Medicine

Massage. In a limited study, 74.5% of patients with PUD who received 20 sessions (every other day) of traditional Chinese medical massage demonstrated complete ulcer resolution.[104] This trial was not randomized, however, and more rigorous investigations are warranted.

Herbs. Yangweishu is a traditional Chinese herbal medicine that is a combination of dang shen (codonopsis root), chen pi (tangerine peel), huang jing (Siberian solomon seal rhizome), shan yao (Chinese yam), xuan shen (ningpo figwort root), and wu mei (mume fruit). Yangweishu was shown in a randomized clinical trial with more than 400 participants to significantly improve ulcer healing and symptom relief when taken with antibiotics compared to antibiotics alone.[105] As formulations vary between manufacturers, clinicians should refer to package labels or TCM consultants for instructions regarding their use. These formulations should not be used by lactating women, during pregnancy, or by children.

Osteopathy

Although adequate clinical trials are lacking, osteopathy may provide symptom relief and prevent PUD. Manual medicine, in theory, can help the GI system to maintain sympathetic and parasympathetic balance, thus reducing excess acid production and restoring homeostasis. Osteopathy may also lead to relief of symptoms by manipulating somatovisceral pathways and is worth considering in patients with access to clinicians experienced in these techniques.

PREVENTION PRESCRIPTION

- Eat a diet rich in fruits and vegetables (particularly those containing vitamins A and C).
- Eat foods containing capsaicin (chili), as well as those with flavonoids and sulforaphanes.
- Eat probiotics: yogurt, sauerkraut, active yeasts, and aged cheeses.
- Avoid nonprobiotic dairy products such as milk.
- Eat breakfast every day, and avoid eating large meals shortly before sleeping.
- Minimize use of nonsteroidal antiinflammatory drugs.
- Avoid smoking cigarettes.
- Avoid excessive alcohol consumption.
- Maintain a moderate exercise routine.
- Obtain adequate sleep.
- Develop and incorporate stress reduction activities.

THERAPEUTIC REVIEW

The following integrative therapeutic options are useful for different niches on the peptic ulcer disease (PUD) spectrum, from prevention, symptom relief, and *H. pylori* elimination to active ulcer healing. Being mindful of the individual end goals of therapy will guide clinical choices. Evidence of a bleeding ulcer or significant weight loss is a reason to refer patients for endoscopy and may constitute a medical emergency.

LIFESTYLE

- Tobacco cessation
- Adequate sleep
- Routine exercise
- Stress reduction interventions
- Abstention from heavy ethanol intake

NUTRITION

- Eat breakfast daily.
- Avoid eating shortly before sleeping.
- Avoid milk.
- Eat probiotic-containing fermented foods, such as yogurt, aged cheeses, miso, and sauerkraut.
- Eat foods containing chili (capsaicin).
- Eat fruits and vegetables, particularly those containing vitamins A and C.

SUPPLEMENTS

- Probiotics during *H. pylori* antibiotic therapy: either *Lactobacillus* (*acidophilus* or GG) capsules, containing at least 1 billion organisms, twice daily; or *Saccharomyces boulardii*, 500 mg, twice daily
- Probiotics for PUD symptom relief and *H. pylori* suppression: *Bifidobacterium bifidum*, 1 × 10^10 CFU, daily for 12 weeks
- Vitamin C for *H. pylori* suppression: 500 mg twice daily
- Zinc for gastric ulcers: 40 mg daily for 4 weeks
- Polyunsaturated fatty acids for *H. pylori* eradication: 1 g of fish oil and 1 g of gamma-linolenic acid–containing oil (evening primrose, black currant seed, borage, or hemp seed oils) taken daily for 8 weeks
- Glutamine for peptic ulcers: 400 mg four times daily

BOTANICALS

- Turmeric for peptic ulcers and PUD symptoms: whole root or root powder (capsules), 600 mg five times daily for 12 weeks

- Deglycyrrhizinated licorice for duodenal ulcers: 380 mg three times per day for 12 weeks
- Deglycyrrhizinated licorice for *H. pylori* eradication: 150 mg (root extract) daily for 60 days
- Mastic for dyspepsia: 350 mg capsules three times a day for 3 weeks
- Mastic for duodenal ulcers: 500 mg capsules twice daily for 2 weeks
- Cabbage for duodenal or gastric ulcers: 1 L of fresh juice divided over the course of a day for 10 days
- Chili (*Capsicum* fruit) for epigastric pain and dyspepsia: 2.5 mg daily of chili pepper capsules for 5 weeks
- Cranberry for *H. pylori* eradication: 500 mL of cranberry juice daily for 90 days
- Neem for duodenal ulcers: 30 mg bark extract twice daily for 10 weeks

PHARMACEUTICALS

- Eliminate nonsteroidal antiinflammatory drugs for patients with PUD
- Antibiotics and proton pump inhibitors (PPIs) for *H. pylori* eradication: amoxicillin, 1 g; clarithromycin, 500 mg; and omeprazole, 20 mg in combination to be taken twice daily for 14 days (check regional bacterial susceptibilities)
- Acid suppression therapy for PUD and PUD symptoms: a PPI (e.g., omeprazole) or histamine-2 (H$_2$) receptor blocker (e.g., ranitidine) once or twice daily per individual drug for up to 8 weeks
- Antacids for PUD symptoms: over-the-counter antacids according to individual product instructions
- Sucralfate for duodenal ulcers: 1 g four times daily for up to 8 weeks

ACUPUNCTURE

- Acupuncture for PUD and/or epigastric pain

THERAPIES TO CONSIDER

- Traditional Chinese medical massage for peptic ulcers
- Traditional Chinese herbs, yangweishu, as an adjuvant for *H. pylori* eradication with antibiotics
- Osteopathy for PUD

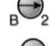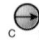

Key Web Resources	
National Digestive Diseases Information Clearinghouse: updated allopathic information on PUD and updates on clinical trials, including ongoing *H. pylori* vaccine trials	http://digestive.niddk.nih.gov/ddiseases/pubs/hpylori/index.aspx
University of Maryland Medical Center: integrative info on PUD for patients	http://ww.umm.edu/altmed/articles/peptic-ulcer-000125.htm
National Center for Complementary and Integrative Health: *H. pylori*-specific information	https://nccih.nih.gov/taxonomy/term/435
Slideshow by 2005 Nobel Prize for Medicine winner, Dr. J. Robin Warren, on the discovery of *H. pylori*	http://www.nobelprize.org/nobel_prizes/medicine/laureates/2005/warren-slides.pdf

REFERENCES

References are available online at ExpertConsult.com.

CHAPTER 44

CHOLELITHIASIS

Ann C. Figurski, DO

Gallstone disease is a common digestive disorder that affects 10%–15% of individuals in developed societies.[1] In the United States, the combination of a diet rich in processed foods and sedentary lifestyle create an environment prone to gallstone formation. Due to the influence of both environment and genetics on gallstone diseases, the occurrence of gallstones varies greatly, ranging from 2%–70% among different populations, with the highest incidence among Pima Indian women older than 30 years of age.[2]

Epidemiological studies have revealed many risk factors for gallstones. Some of these conditions are not modifiable, such as genetics, sex, age, ethnicity, and family history, whereas many conditions can be changed, such as diet, obesity, physical inactivity, medications, and stress.[2,3] Table 44.1 provides a list of conditions that increase the risk of gallstone disease.

PATHOPHYSIOLOGY

Bile aids in the digestion and absorption of lipids from the intestines. Made by the liver, bile is composed of bile acids, cholesterol, and phospholipids. Bile is stored in the gallbladder until the stimulation of its release by cholecystokinin (a hormone released during eating). Conditions that lead to gallstone formation include supersaturation of bile with cholesterol, decreased bile acids that dissolve cholesterol, excess mucus production, and gallbladder dysmotility and stasis (Fig. 44.1). Gallstones are classified as either cholesterol or pigment. In industrialized countries, cholesterol stones account for up to 85%. Most people with gallstones remain asymptomatic. Approximately 20% will develop true biliary symptoms, such as severe pain in the right upper quadrant that can radiate to the back or shoulder.

INTEGRATIVE THERAPY

Lifestyle

Gallstones are part a long list of diseases heavily influenced by lifestyle. A profound rise in the prevalence of chronic conditions, such as diabetes, hypertension, and heart disease, has caused Western medicine to reevaluate its treatments and enhance prevention methods. The causes of these conditions are multifactorial; however, a lifestyle of inadequate physical activity and the standard U.S. diet (highly processed foods) are major contributors. These chronic conditions are not isolated and are all thought to arise from a chronic proinflammatory state caused by these lifestyle factors. Gallstones can be grouped with these other chronic conditions because evidence indicates lifestyle factors, such as diet (macronutrient and micronutrient intake) and exercise, are linked to gallbladder disease.

Maintenance of a Healthy Weight

Obesity, particularly abdominal, is a well-known risk factor for gallstones and associated with increased cholesterol secretion into bile.[2a] The recent trend of rising obesity in children correlates with increasing rates of hospitalizations for pediatric cholelithiasis.[4] Gradual weight loss is important for obese individuals because rapid weight loss may also promote gallstone formation secondary to increased biliary cholesterol and bile stasis. Accordingly, weight loss should not exceed 1.5 kg (3.3 lb) per week in order to avoid this risk.[5]

Exercise

Physical activity is a necessary component of a healthy lifestyle and has a significant impact on many diseases. Studies have also shown that exercise can increase gallbladder motility.[6] In postmenopausal women, physical activity is inversely related to the development of gallstone disease.[7] In one report, women who sat for more than 60 hours a week were 2.32 times more likely to subsequently undergo cholecystectomy.[8] Fortunately, even modest amounts of physical activity have a positive effect, with an observational study of more than 2000 people reporting just 2 hours of activity a week reduced the risk of gallstone disease by 40%.[9]

Stress Reduction

Despite a lack of randomized, placebo-controlled trials, stress is likely to contribute to the development of many diseases. Evidence from animal studies indicates that stress causes gallbladder dysfunction and bile stasis.[3] The general benefits of stress reduction on both mind and body may also extend to the gallbladder. Consider recommending counseling, meditation, or other stress reduction techniques, as appropriate.

Nutrition

Several areas of nutrition overlap in gallbladder disease. For example, vegetarians have a lower rate of cholelithiasis.[10] These findings may be attributable to higher consumption of fruits and vegetables, which are good

TABLE 44.1	Conditions That May Increase the Risk of Gallbladder Disease
Increased cholesterol saturation	Estrogen* (endogenous: pregnancy; or supplemented: hormone replacement therapy, oral contraceptives) Obesity High-cholesterol diet
Decreased bile salts (or increased ratio of secondary bile acids)	Low-fiber diet Ileal inflammation (Crohn disease) Cirrhosis Cystic fibrosis Fibrates Age
Stasis of bile flow	Parenteral nutrition Low-fat, weight loss diets Hypertriglyceridemia (impaired motility) Physical inactivity Ceftriaxone (biliary sludge)[2] Octreotide[2] Stress[3] Iron deficiency anemia[52]

*Estrogen Supplementation

A systematic review of multiple studies found that estrogen supplementation in postmenopausal women increased the likelihood of gallstones.[53] In addition, two randomized, placebo-controlled studies reported an increased risk of biliary disease with supplementation.[54] Both oral and transdermal estrogen supplements can increase biliary cholesterol saturation and decrease cholesterol nucleation time, which may increase risk of gallstones.[55] The Heart and Estrogen/Progestin Replacement Study revealed that supplementation in postmenopausal women with known coronary artery disease resulted in a significant increased risk for biliary surgery.[56] This additional risk should be considered when women elect hormone replacement therapy.

sources of vitamins, minerals, fiber, and antioxidants, all of which have been linked to the inhibition of gallstone formation. In a study of diet differences, patients with gallstones consumed less fish, fruit, fiber, folate, magnesium, calcium, and vitamin C and also ate more cereal, sugar, calories, and saturated fat.[11] Specific dietary components are assessed individually in studies; however, the sum of their effects is likely greater than the individual contributions. Encouraging healthy, well-balanced nutrition (e.g., the Mediterranean diet) full of colorful vegetables and including healthy fats is a good place to start.

Fats

The type of fat consumed is very important in gallbladder disease. The diet should be low in saturated fats but contain sufficient sources of polyunsaturated fats and omega-3 fatty acids. A diet low in total fat may increase the risk of gallstones due to decreased stimulation of bile flow and stasis. Results from animal studies demonstrate that monounsaturated and polyunsaturated fats act as inhibitors of cholesterol cholelithiasis.[12] Fish oil may decrease biliary cholesterol saturation and enhance bile flow.[13] A study comparing fish oil with fibrate therapy in men with hypertriglyceridemia reported that both approaches lowered triglyceride levels, whereas only fish oil increased bile

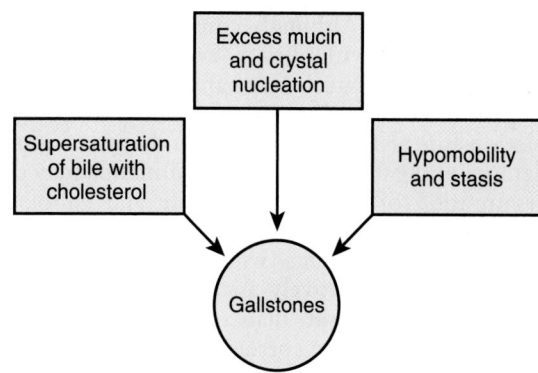

FIG. 44.1 ■ Pathophysiology of gallstones.

acid synthesis. The same study also demonstrated that fish oil increased the ratio of cholic acid to chenodeoxycholic acid, which improves cholesterol solubility.[14] Proinflammatory, arachidonic acid-rich saturated fats increase cholesterol saturation and disrupt the gallbladder epithelium.[15] A separate study revealed that men with the highest consumption of long-chain saturated fatty acids (which includes arachidonic acid) had a 40% increased risk of cholecystectomy.[16] The goal of treatment is to replace saturated fats with the antiinflammatory effects of healthy fats, such as omega-3 fatty acids (see Chapter 88).

Fiber

A higher intake of fiber is associated with a lower prevalence of gallstones. Fiber reduces the absorption of deoxycholic acid by decreasing its formation by intestinal bacteria. Deoxycholic acid is a secondary bile acid that increases the lithogenicity of bile.[17] Water-soluble fiber found in fruits, vegetables, pectin, oat bran, and guar gum can bind this acid and may be helpful in preventing and treating gallstones.[15] A prospective study of 77,000 women demonstrated that individuals consuming the most fruits and vegetables had a 21% reduced risk of gallstones.[18]

A good source of fiber is to mix one teaspoon of ground flaxseed (lignan) into 8 oz of apple juice or applesauce (pectin) and consume daily. This recipe has the added benefit of being a good source of omega-3 fatty acids.[15]

Nuts

In the Nurses' Health Study, a large prospective study, women who consumed nuts frequently had a more than 20% reduced risk of cholecystectomy. This relationship persisted after controlling for multiple confounding variables, including fat intake.[20] Other research showed similar results in men. Men who frequently ate nuts had a reduced risk of gallstone disease. This inverse relationship existed independently of consumption of peanuts, other nuts, or a combination of both.[21]

Simple Sugars

Refined sugars increase the cholesterol saturation of bile and reduce the ratio of beneficial cholic acid to deoxycholic acid.[22] Although consumption of refined sugars is associated with obesity, evidence indicates that simple sugars (monosaccharides and disaccharides) promote gallstone formation independently of obesity.[16] A relationship also appears to exist between glucose intolerance and gallstones. Hyperinsulinemia may cause supersaturation of cholesterol in bile and gallbladder dysmotility. The prevalence of cholesterol gallstones is higher in diabetic patients, with fasting serum insulin levels reported to positively associated with gallstones among women without diabetes.[23] Sugar intake is reported to be positively correlated with serum triglyceride levels and inversely correlated with high-density lipoproteins, and this effect on lipoprotein metabolism may contribute to gallstone formation.[24] Additionally, diets with high glycemic load have been linked to increased rates of cholecystectomy in women[25] (see Chapters 32 and 87).

> Foods associated with a reduced risk of gallstones include fiber-rich fruits and vegetables, whole grains, nuts, coffee, and alcohol in moderation.

Coffee

Individuals with gastrointestinal symptoms are often advised to avoid coffee. Interesting research has demonstrated that coffee can play a role in preventing gallstones, with numerous epidemiological studies corroborating this finding.[2] Coffee and its components have been shown to stimulate cholecystokinin release, enhance gallbladder contractility, and decrease cholesterol crystallization in bile.[26] A large prospective study demonstrated a 40% lower risk of cholecystectomy in men who drank two to three cups of coffee a day over a 10-year period.[27] Other prospective studies have reported intake of caffeinated coffee to be associated with significantly reduced risk of cholecystectomy in women. This is not the case for other caffeinated beverages, with a positive association noted with caffeinated soft drinks.[23] Although some studies have failed to observe this link,[28,29] it is reasonable to continue coffee consumption according to patient preference.

Food Allergy

Interest is growing in food allergies and their effects on health and wellness. A small amount of research, from as early as the 1940s, has described food allergy as a cause of gallbladder disease.[17] In an uncontrolled study of 69 patients with gallstones or postcholecystectomy syndrome, 100% of patients reported symptom resolution after 1 week of initiating an elimination diet. The foods that most commonly evoked symptoms were eggs, pork, onions, fowl, milk, coffee, citrus, corn, beans, and nuts.[30] Thus, clinicians should keep in mind when giving dietary advice to patients with gallstones that simply advising patients to "avoid fatty foods" may be insufficient. An elimination diet may be a good option for those patients with biliary colic who wish to avoid surgery (see Chapter 86).

Water

Drinking six to eight cups of clean water a day will help maintain the water content of bile and prevent crystal agglomeration.[15]

Alcohol

Epidemiological evidence indicates gallstones are among a handful of diseases that are less common among individuals who consume a moderate amount of alcohol (no more than one drink/day for women and two drinks/day for men).[31,32] A large prospective study found that moderate alcohol intake was associated with a decreased risk of cholecystectomy in women.[33] Health benefits are associated with regular consumption of small amounts of alcohol, rather than heavy sporadic drinking. The many hazards and potential health consequences of alcohol consumption must also be considered. Any recommendation for moderate alcohol intake must be evaluated carefully for each person.

Supplements

Vitamin C

Vitamin C (ascorbic acid) is involved in the conversion of cholesterol to bile acids, and vitamin C deficiency has been associated with gallstones in numerous studies.[34,35] Vitamin C supplementation, at a dose of 500 mg four times a day for 2 weeks, has been shown to significantly prolong the time required for cholesterol crystal formation.[36] In an observational study of more than 2000 individuals, the prevalence of gallstones was half that of study participants who did not receive vitamin C supplements.[9] Good sources of vitamin C include red pepper, kiwi, broccoli, strawberries, and citrus.

> **DOSAGE**
>
> The recommended dose of vitamin C is 200 mg twice daily.
>
> **PRECAUTIONS**
>
> Gastrointestinal disturbance may occur, including diarrhea, nausea, vomiting, heartburn, and abdominal cramps. Other side effects include fatigue, flushing, headache, hyperoxaluria, and predisposition to urinary tract stones.[14]

Magnesium

Individuals who consume sufficient magnesium have lower rates of gallstone disease.[11] Additionally, magnesium deficiency is a common mineral deficiency among individuals consuming the standard American diet, also a risk factor for gallstones. A diet rich in magnesium may be a factor in preventing gallstones. Magnesium is found in green leafy vegetables, nuts, coffee, and whole grains. A study reported that men consuming high amounts of magnesium through diet and supplements (average, 454 mg/day) were 28% less likely to have gallstone disease compared with men consuming low amounts (average, 262 mg/day).[37]

DOSAGE

The recommended dose of magnesium is 300 mg daily.

PRECAUTIONS

Gastrointestinal symptoms, such as diarrhea, nausea, and abdominal cramping, may occur with the use of magnesium supplements. Magnesium should be used with caution in patients with renal failure. Toxic levels cause muscle relaxation and loss of deep tendon reflexes.

Vitamin E

Results from animal studies indicate a cholesterol-free diet deficient in vitamin E can lead to cholesterol gallstones.[38] Moreover, when animals were provided a high-fat diet in addition to vitamin E, they did not develop gallstones.[39] Therefore, supplementation with vitamin E may help to prevent gallstones.

DOSAGE

The recommended dose of vitamin E (mixed tocopherols) is 400 units/day.

PRECAUTIONS

Side effects are rare but include nausea, diarrhea, intestinal cramps, fatigue, weakness, headache, blurred vision, rash, and creatinuria. Long-term use may increase cardiovascular risk in persons younger than 65 years old.

Calcium

Calcium preferentially binds secondary bile acids, such as deoxycholic and chenodeoxycholic acid, in the small intestine. These bile acids reduce the solubility of cholesterol, thereby reducing the risk of gallstones once cholesterol is bound and excreted. In a study that monitored the dietary intake of 860 men, calcium intake was inversely associated with gallstone disease.[24]

DOSAGE

Calcium gluconate or citrate: 1000 to 1500 mg/day with meals. Calcium citrate is better absorbed in older adults but costs more.

PRECAUTIONS

Calcium may cause constipation and gastrointestinal irritation. Calcium should not be taken with iron supplements because it decreases iron absorption.

Olive Oil or Gallbladder "Flush"

The gallbladder flush (or liver flush) is a common remedy that is said to cause gallstone passage. Several versions of the treatment exist, including combinations of olive oil, lemon juice, and apple juice. Proponents of this treatment claim that it causes the passage of gallstones. However, chemical analysis of subsequently passed "gallstones" has demonstrated them to be saponified complexes of olive oil, minerals, and lemon juice.[40] Monounsaturated fat in olive oil may stimulate the gallbladder to expel stones; however, these stones may then become lodged in the common bile duct. Ideally, this approach should be avoided until ultrasound evaluation has determined the size and number of stones.

Botanicals: Choleretic Herbs

Herbal medicine has been used to treat gallbladder disease and is a good option for patients with small stones and mild symptoms. Choleretic herbs can stimulate bile production, flow, and solubility.[15,40] These effects can be enhanced by combination with peppermint oil to aid gallstone dissolution. The following list of choleretic herbs may be used individually or mixed in combination as a tea by an herbologist.

Globe Artichoke (Cynara scolymus)

DOSAGE

The recommended dose of globe artichoke is 1 to 4 g of the leaf, stem, or root three times/day. This plant should not be confused with Jerusalem artichoke.

PRECAUTIONS

If used topically, globe artichoke may cause contact dermatitis. Again, caution in those allergic to the *Asteraceae/Compositae* family (ragweed, daisies, marigold).

Milk Thistle (Silybum marianum)

DOSAGE

Standardized 70% silymarin extract, starting at 150 mg twice daily and increasing to three times daily if needed

PRECAUTIONS

Milk thistle may have a laxative effect and should be used with caution in patients allergic to plants in the *Asteraceae/Compositae* family (ragweed, daisies, marigolds).

Dandelion (Taraxacum officinalis)

DOSAGE

Give 4 to 10 g of dried leaf or 2 to 8 g of dried root three times/day. Dandelion tea is made by steeping the same amount in 150 mL of boiling water for 10 to 15 minutes and then straining. One cup of tea should be consumed three times/day. The most convenient dosing is a 1:5 tincture, 5 to 10 mL three times/day.

PRECAUTIONS

Dandelion may cause gastric hyperacidity. If used topically, it may cause contact dermatitis and should be used with caution in patients allergic to plants in the *Asteraceae/Compositae* family (ragweed, daisies, marigolds). Dandelion may also have hypoglycemic effects.

Turmeric (Curcuma longa)

An animal study demonstrated that mice fed a lithogenic diet had a decreased incidence of gallstones of 73% when supplemented with curcumin. Curcumin also reduces biliary cholesterol concentration.[41]

DOSAGE

The recommended dose of turmeric is 450 mg of a curcumin capsule standardized extract or 1.5–3 g turmeric root daily in divided doses.

PRECAUTIONS

Turmeric has blood thinning effects, so patients should be careful if taking other blood-thinning medications. Turmeric should be used with caution in patients allergic to yellow food colorings or plants belonging to the Zingiberaceae (ginger) family.

Botanicals: Gallstone-Dissolving Herbs

Monoterpenes are a class of hydrocarbon molecules found in the essential oils of many plants. These compounds have choleretic properties and inhibit formation of cholesterol crystals.[17] A combination of monoterpenes, predominantly consisting of menthol and pinene, has been shown to be effective for stone dissolution.[42] A double-blind study concluded that the addition of menthol to ursodeoxycholic acid (UDCA) improved outcomes compared with UDCA alone and that menthol was equally effective as the monoterpene combination.[43] The addition of peppermint oil to choleretic herbs should be considered in the treatment of minimal disease with small stones.

Peppermint Oil (Mentha piperita)

DOSAGE

One or two enteric-coated capsules (0.2 mL/capsule) three times/day between meals

PRECAUTIONS

Peppermint oil relaxes the lower esophageal sphincter, and this may lead to reflux or heartburn (enteric-coated capsules may be used to avoid this effect.) Peppermint oil may also cause allergic reactions, flushing, and headache.

Pharmaceuticals

Treatment with bile acids can be used for gallstone dissolution. Bile acids work by inhibiting biliary secretion of cholesterol and increasing bile secretion from the liver. Bile acids may also improve gallbladder motility and are most effective when used in patients with small stones, mild symptoms, and good gallbladder function. Patients with calcified or pigment stones are usually poor candidates for bile acid therapy. Incomplete dissolution and stone recurrence are both significant limitations of bile acid therapy.

Ursodeoxycholic Acid (Ursodiol)

UDCA is a bile acid that lowers bile cholesterol saturation. Numerous studies have demonstrated the utility of UDCA in preventing the formation of gallstones in obese patients undergoing rapid weight loss, either through calorie-restricted diets or bariatric surgery.[44] Maintenance therapy may also be effective in reducing gallstone recurrence.[45]

DOSAGE

The recommended dose of UDCA is 300 mg twice daily.

PRECAUTIONS

Possible adverse effects include hepatic impairment, elevation of liver enzymes, and gastrointestinal upset.

Lifestyle is the key to treatment. Other than surgery, all treatments are associated with a high 5-year risk of recurrence if lifestyle modifications are not employed.

Surgery

Laparoscopic Cholecystectomy

Laparoscopic cholecystectomy is the recommended treatment for patients with symptomatic stones and gallbladder wall inflammation. However, laparoscopic cholecystectomy is not recommended for the majority of patients with asymptomatic gallstones unless they are at risk of gallbladder carcinoma. A major advantage of surgical treatment is the avoidance of recurrence; however, the potential benefits of surgery should be weighed against the potential harms of surgery and anesthesia.

Therapies to Consider

Cholesterol-Lowering Medications

As supersaturation of bile with cholesterol is a key factor in gallstone formation, it has been hypothesized that gallbladder disease can be treated by lowering total cholesterol. Recent studies have indicated cholesterol-lowering medications may help reduce the incidence of cholesterol gallstones. Animal studies have shown that both statins and ezetimibe can prevent cholesterol gallstone formation in mice or prairie dogs[46,47]; however, the limited number of clinical studies have reported conflicting results.[48] At this time, further research is warranted to determine appropriate role of these medications in the treatment of gallstone disease.

Fenugreek

Fenugreek has been shown to lower cholesterol, with animal studies demonstrating a marked reduction in gallstone formation with fenugreek supplementation.[49] Mice fed a lithogenic diet to induce cholesterol gallstones, and those that received fenugreek supplementation along with the lithogenic diet, had a 75% reduction in gallstones.[50] Unfortunately, specific recommendations for the use of fenugreek have yet to be determined due to a lack of clinical studies to support this data.

Piperine

Black pepper (*Piper nigrum L.*) is a very widely used spice, known for its pungent constituent, piperine. Based on the results of recent cellular, animal, and clinical studies, piperine has been found to have immunomodulatory, antioxidant, and antiinflammatory effects, among many others. Results from studies of mice fed a lithogenic diet indicate that piperine can reduce the incidence of cholesterol gallstone formation and reduce biliary cholesterol secretion, as well as have a positive influence on liver function.[51]

Homeopathy

Homeopathy has been used as a safe treatment for more than two centuries despite a lack of scientific evidence. Homeopathy may provide benefit when other treatment options have failed. After consultation, a professional homeopath may recommend various remedies, including Chelidonium, Colocynthis, or Lycopodium.

Acupuncture

Acupuncture, as part of traditional Chinese medicine, can address energy flow through the liver and gallbladder. This technique may be helpful for gallbladder function, as well as for alleviating discomfort caused by gallbladder disease.

Osteopathy

Although manual therapy is effective for treating musculoskeletal complaints, it is also used to treat other body systems. Osteopathy can help to regulate physiology and aid the body in establishing homeostasis. Viscerosomatic reflexes are changes in the musculoskeletal system that reflect visceral disorders. These reflexes are mediated by afferent neurons of the sympathetic nervous system. The use of these reflexes can aid in diagnosis and provide treatment benefit by balancing the nervous system and influencing the viscera. Manual therapy will not cure or prevent gallstones but represent a useful adjunct to other therapies.

PREVENTION PRESCRIPTION

Preventing gallstones is much easier than treating them. The same principles of prevention apply to many common chronic diseases (diabetes, heart disease).

- Maintain a healthy weight, with slow gradual weight loss if body mass index is elevated.
- Exercise. Get moving in a way that is enjoyable and sustainable for you, at least 30 minutes five times weekly.
- Find a stress-reducing practice.
- Encourage a diet high in fiber, vegetables, fruit, nuts, and omega-3 fatty acids.
- Maintain a low intake of saturated fats, refined sugars, and high-glycemic load foods.

- Remember hydration. Drink at least six to eight cups of clean water daily. Consider coffee if you enjoy it, two to three cups daily. A moderate intake of alcohol may be suitable for some patients.
- Consider an elimination diet (see Chapter 86).
- Consider supplementation: vitamin C, 200 mg twice daily; magnesium, 300 mg/day; vitamin E, 400 units/day with meals; calcium, 1000 to 1500 mg/day; and curcumin 450 mg/day.
- Avoid medications associated with gallstone risk including estrogen, ceftriaxone, octreotide, and fibrates. Take precautionary measures if taking these medications, have excessive weight loss, or are receiving total parental nutrition (TPN).

THERAPEUTIC REVIEW

Immediate surgical referral is warranted in the setting of severe recurring symptoms or elevated liver enzymes, amylase, or white blood cell count. In asymptomatic patients or mild cases with normal liver function, the following therapies are recommended.

LIFESTYLE
- Maintain a healthy weight.
- Exercise at least 30 minutes a day, five times a week.
- Participate in stress-reducing activity.

NUTRITION
- Diet should be high in fiber, fruits, and vegetables.
- Consider supplementing with fiber and flaxseed.

- Recommend a diet low in saturated fat, rich in omega-3 fatty acids.
- Drink six to eight cups of water daily.
- Avoid refined sugars.
- Avoid excess intake of legumes.
- Consider an elimination diet.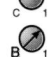

SUPPLEMENTS
- Vitamin C: 200 mg twice daily.
- Calcium: 1000 to 1500 mg/day
- Magnesium: 300 mg/day
- Vitamin E: 400 units/day

BOTANICALS

- Milk thistle (*Silybum marianum*) standardized to 70% silymarin extract: starting at 150 mg twice a day and increasing to three times/day if needed
- Artichoke (*Cynara scolymus*): 1 to 4 g of leaf, stem, or root three times/day
- Turmeric (*Curcuma longa*): 450 mg curcumin capsule, or 3 g root daily
- Peppermint oil (*Mentha piperita*): one to two enteric-coated capsules three times/day between meals

- Dandelion (*Taraxacum officinalis*): 1:5 tincture, 5 to 10 mL three times/day

PHARMACEUTICALS

- Ursodiol (ursodeoxycholic acid): 300 mg twice daily with meals

SURGERY

- Laparoscopic cholecystectomy
- Patients with common bile duct obstruction (elevation of liver enzymes, lipase, and bilirubin, right upper quadrant pain, jaundice, and common bile duct dilation on ultrasound) may require either endoscopic retrograde cholangiopancreatography for stone removal or surgical exploration.

Key Web Resources

National Center for Complementary and Alternative Medicine, National Institutes of Health — http://nccam.nih.gov

National Digestive Diseases Information Clearinghouse, National Institutes of Health — http://digestive.niddk.nih.gov

American Gastroenterological Association — http://www.gastro.org

REFERENCES

References are available online at ExpertConsult.com.

CHAPTER 45

RECURRING ABDOMINAL PAIN IN PEDIATRICS

Joy A. Weydert, MD

PATHOPHYSIOLOGY

Recurrent abdominal pain (RAP) in children was first defined by Apley and Naish in 1958 as consisting of at least three episodes of pain over a 3-month period that are severe enough to interfere with normal activities. RAP is one of the most common reasons to seek medical attention.[1] RAP affects approximately 10% to 15% of all school-aged children and is responsible for 2% to 4% of all pediatric outpatient visits.[2] Fewer than 10% of children with RAP are ever found to have an organic cause for pain; however, substantial morbidity, such as depression, anxiety, lifetime psychiatric disorders, and social phobia, still occurs.[3] Chronic abdominal pain rarely occurs in isolation and is often associated with other chronic pain syndromes, such as chronic headache, fibromyalgia, joint pain/hypermobility, and postural orthostatic tachycardia syndrome (POTS).[4] In addition, RAP is associated with significant health care costs, not only from medical evaluations and medications, but also from missed work and productivity.[5] On average, children with RAP miss 26 days per year of school compared with only 5 days in children who do not have abdominal pain,[6] which has its own long-term consequences. Absenteeism has been identified as a precursor to undesirable outcomes, including poor academic performance, increased rates of school dropout, substance abuse, and violence in adolescents.[7] Parents, teachers, and physicians frequently reinforce pain behavior by excusing children with RAP from chores and other responsibilities, allowing absences from school or providing medications.

The etiology and pathogenesis of RAP has traditionally been considered multidimensional, with biological, psychological, and social factors all playing significant roles in the development of RAP in children. With advances in our understanding of pain physiology, further elucidation of the mechanism's underlying processes will help guide our approach to the treatment of this condition.

A phenomenon known as *central sensitization* is considered the core biological link and final common pathway that leads to chronic pain. Neuroanatomical, neurophysiological, and neurochemical changes occur within nerves of the peripheral (PNS) and central nervous systems (CNS), thereby altering the processing of sensory information. These changes trigger hyperarousal of CNS neurons to otherwise ordinary pain stimuli and leads to heightened experience of pain. Repetitive stimulation of neurons throughout the CNS (spinal column to the cerebral cortex) can lead to upregulation of excitatory receptors and death of the inhibitory interneurons that produce serotonin and endogenous opioids.[8]

The effects of the immune and endocrine systems on the nervous system have been demonstrated and are now widely accepted as part of normal physiology.[9] In addition to the altered physiology of the PNS and CNS caused by trauma or disease, an imbalance in the immune or endocrine systems can promote dysregulation of the nervous system and increased pain through direct effects on neurotransmission (Fig. 45.1).

Immune system dysfunction in children with RAP may be a result of recent viral or bacterial intestinal infection,[10] or from exposure to antibiotics, nonsteroidal antiinflammatory drugs (NSAIDs), steroids, chlorinated water, or a poor diet. These factors disrupt the natural balance of the intestinal microbiota necessary for optimal functioning of the gut. Bacteria interact with intestinal epithelial cells and generate inflammatory mediators that stimulate the sensory nerve endings lying in the gut mucosa. Bacteria also affect intestinal permeability, allowing chemicals and antigens access from the gut lumen into and between the cell walls.[11] Food sensitivity mediated by immunoglobulin G (IgG) antibodies has been identified as a further trigger for RAP. Rather than the classic IgE food allergy response, which is more immediate, IgG-mediated responses are delayed following exposure to a particular antigen,[12] the most common being wheat, dairy, eggs, corn, and soy. This type of food sensitivity creates a low-level, chronic inflammatory response that triggers gut neuronal sensitivity and pain. This response does not, however, trigger excessive levels of calprotectin, a cytosolic protein produced in high levels by granulocytes in inflammatory bowel disease.[13]

Neurotransmitter imbalances, as a result of immune dysregulation, hormone imbalance, or nutritional deficiencies (such as magnesium, iron, zinc, or vitamin B, which are all cofactors in neurotransmitter production), may also contribute to RAP. In the brain–gut axis, which links the neuroendocrine, immune, and enteric nervous systems, the brain and the gut neurons share identical neurotransmitters as they originate from the same cells embryologically. Low levels of serotonin have been associated, not only with depression and headaches, but also with abdominal pain.[14]

Dysregulation of the autonomic nervous system, characterized by increased auditory startle reflex and low vagal tone, has been demonstrated in children with RAP.[15,16]

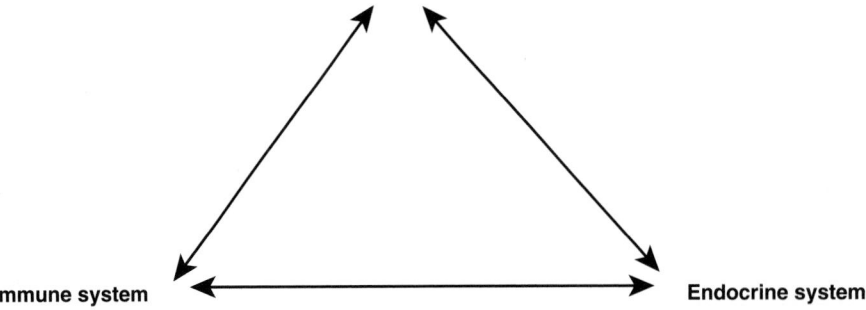

Neurotransmitters/nervous system

(behavior, pain, attention, mood, etc.)

(substance P, glutamate, aspartate, serotonin, etc.)

> [The body needs cofactors—
> **magnesium, zinc, iron, B vitamins,**
> etc.— to work optimally]

Immune system

(neutrophils, autoantibodies, TNF-α, GALT, etc.)

> Approximately 70 % of immune system resides
> in the gut. The gut also synthesizes most of the
> body's neurotransmitters.

Endocrine system

(ACTH/cortisol, estrogen, CRH, vitamin D, etc.)

> Vitamin D is the body's most important hormone.

FIG. 45.1 ■ **Interactions Between Neuroendoimmune Systems.**

Fructose malabsorption, a condition that causes gas, bloating, and cramping, has been found to cause RAP in children found to have fructose intolerance on breath hydrogen testing.[17] The same symptoms have been found in those with yeast overgrowth in the intestinal tract—intestinal candidiasis—typically as a result of oral antibiotic use. Yeast requires a source of carbohydrates to survive and releases carbon dioxide gas during carbohydrate metabolism. Clinically, this process causes abdominal bloating, gas, pain, and intermittent diarrhea that may alternate with constipation.[18,19]

Even obesity has been linked to a greater incidence of constipation, gastroesophageal reflux disease, irritable bowel syndrome (IBS), encopresis, and functional abdominal pain. This association may be related to food choices (processed foods versus whole fruits and vegetables and higher intake of soda with high-fructose corn syrup), physical activity levels, hormonal status, or emotional state.[20] A thorough diet history is important in identifying possible triggers for RAP.

In addition to the previous, other factors known to be associated with a greater incidence of RAP in children include the behavior profile of the patient and genetic vulnerability. A proportion of children may exhibit anxiety, mild depression, withdrawal, or low self-esteem. Investigators have postulated that this behavior profile is frequently fostered within a family structure characterized by parental depression, enmeshment, overprotectiveness, rigidity, and lack of conflict resolution. These factors may influence the way in which RAP is experienced and addressed.[21] Fig. 45.2 displays how each of these factors contribute to the clinical expression of chronic pain.[22]

An understanding of the various pathways that may lead to or perpetuate abdominal pain in children

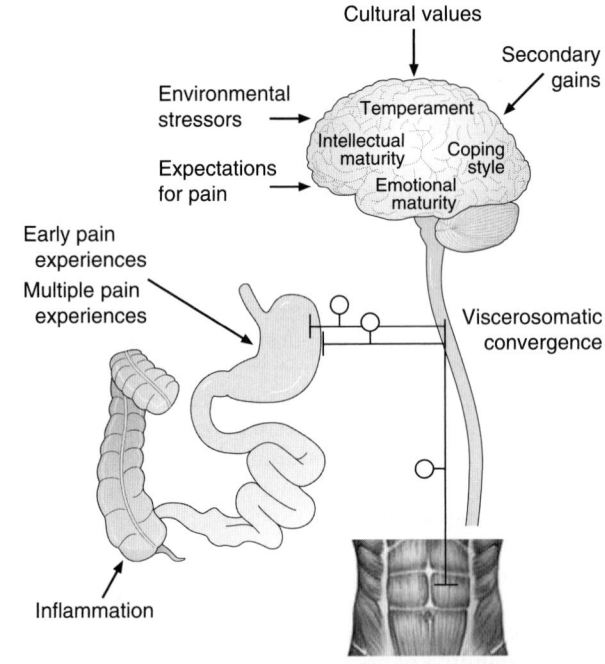

FIG. 45.2 ■ Pathogenesis of visceral hyperalgesia and clinical expression of chronic pain. Primary hyperalgesia develops when sensory neurons with cell bodies in the dorsal root ganglia are recruited and sensitized after early or multiple pain experiences. Secondary hyperalgesia occurs when biochemical changes in pathways from the spinal cord to cerebral cortex result in increased pain perception. *Viscerosomatic convergence* refers to somatic and visceral afferent nerves terminating on the same spinal interneurons, such that the affected individual is unable to define a discrete pain location on the body. Psychological and developmental factors (within the brain) and psychosocial factors (*arrows* pointing to the brain) alter clinical expression of pain. (From Hyams JS, Hyman PE. Recurrent abdominal pain and the biopsychosocial model of medical practice. *J Pediatr.* 1998; 133:473-478.)

will help approach treatment options in an integrative fashion to address any immune imbalances, food sensitivities, nutritional deficiencies, or nervous system dysregulation.

Children with RAP may demonstrate one of the classic presentations, as defined by the Rome Foundation's pediatric Rome III criteria, which may help guide clinical decision making and therapy.[23] To fulfill any of the criteria, the patient typically must experience pain at least once a week for over 2 months and have no evidence of inflammatory, anatomic, metabolic, or neoplastic processes as an underlying cause. Many of these patients may demonstrate evidence of autonomic nervous system imbalance, such as nausea, headaches, lightheadedness, dizziness, or pallor.

1. Functional abdominal pain or syndrome; must include all the following:
   * Episodic or continuous abdominal pain—usually periumbilical
   * Some loss of daily functioning
   * Additional somatic symptoms such as headache, limb pain, or difficulty sleeping
2. IBS; must include all the following:
   * Abdominal discomfort or pain associated with two or more of the following:
     ◦ Improvement with defecation
     ◦ Onset associated with a change in frequency or form of stool
3. Functional dyspepsia; must include all the following:
   * Persistent or recurrent pain or discomfort centered in the upper abdomen
   * Pain not relieved by defecation or associated with change or form of stool
4. Functional constipation; must include two or more of the following:
   * Two or fewer defecations per week
   * At least one episode of fecal incontinence per week
   * History of retentive posturing or excessive volitional stool retention
   * History of painful or hard bowel movements
   * Presence of a large fecal mass in the rectum
   * History of large-diameter stools that may obstruct the toilet
5. Abdominal migraine; must include all four of the following:
   * Paroxysmal episodes of intense, acute periumbilical pain that lasts more than 1 hour
   * Intervening periods of usual health lasting weeks to months
   * Pain interfering with normal activities
   * Pain associated with two or more of the following:
     ◦ Anorexia
     ◦ Vomiting
     ◦ Photophobia
     ◦ Nausea
     ◦ Headache
     ◦ Pallor
6. Cyclic vomiting
   * Two or more periods of intense nausea and unremitting vomiting or retching lasting hours to days
   * Return to usual state of health lasting weeks to months

7. Aerophagia; must include two of the following:
   * Air swallowing
   * Abdominal distention because of intraluminal air
   * Repetitive belching or increased flatus

Serious organic disease can be ruled out by a thorough history, physical examination, and basic laboratory investigations. Pertinent positive results in this evaluation considered "red flags" include the following:

1. A family history of inflammatory bowel disease, ulcer disease, or significant psychosocial disorder
2. Pain that wakes the child from sleep
3. History of weight loss or growth delay
4. Blood in stool or bile-stained emesis
5. A history and physical examination revealing fevers, rashes, joint involvement, or perianal disease
6. Abnormal complete blood count, urinalysis, sedimentation rate, C-reactive protein, or stool for occult blood

If indicated by a positive history, the clinician may consider further testing (i.e., serologic testing for *Helicobacter pylori*, serum transaminases, amylase, lipase, stool for pathogens, and endoscopy).

Use of a comprehensive stool analysis, which assesses intestinal candidiasis, parasites, and the balance of microbiota, may also help direct therapy options. Results of this type of testing will identify the need for pharmaceuticals (i.e., nystatin, fluconazole, or metronidazole) or natural antimicrobial botanicals, such as grapefruit seed extract, olive leaf extract, or oregano oil. These tests may also help guide the choice of probiotics to rebalance the intestinal microbiota.[24]

An evaluation for micronutrient deficiencies (zinc, iron, magnesium, B vitamins, etc.) may also be indicated because these factors play a role in neurotransmitter production and nervous system function.[25]

> Rather than a diagnosis of exclusion, recurrent abdominal pain should be presented as a positive diagnosis, identified as the most common cause of chronic abdominal pain in children. Parents can be reassured that serious disease is unlikely if the history and physical examination are normal.

INTEGRATIVE THERAPY

Nutrition

Diet manipulation has been trialed for years as a treatment for RAP, either through the elimination of certain foods (e.g., lactose-containing foods) or the addition of others (e.g., high-fiber foods). However, studies of dietary interventions have reported varying results.[26,27]

Fiber

Although studies of fiber in the treatment of RAP have been small and the evidence is weak, some investigators have reported that additional fiber may be beneficial in a proportion of children, particularly those with constipation. Increased consumption of fiber goal can

TABLE 45.1 Fiber Content of Various Foods

Foods	Portion Size	Fiber (g)
High Fiber		
All-bran cereal	½ cup	10
Figs, dried	3	10
Kidney beans	½ cup cooked	9
Baked beans	½ cup cooked	8
Broccoli	¾ cup cooked	7
Spinach	½ cup cooked	7
Yam baked in skin	1 medium	7
Whole wheat bread	2 slices	6
Baked potato with skin	1 medium	5
Blackberries	½ cup	5
Apple with skin	1 medium	3.5
Raspberries	½ cup	3.5
Lentils	½ cup cooked	3.5
Whole wheat spaghetti	1 cup	3.5
Wheaties cereal	1 oz	2.5
Low Fiber		
Bagel	1	Less than 1
Cornflakes	1 oz	Less than 1
Grapes	20	Less than 1
Watermelon	1 cup	Less than 1
Lettuce	1 cup	Less than 1

be accomplished by increasing the amounts of fruit, vegetables, legumes, and whole grains in the diet. Breakfast cereals can also be a good source of fiber, particularly cereals made with bran (Table 45.1). If a child has difficulty obtaining adequate fiber through the diet, one teaspoon (2 g) of psyllium powder in 8 oz of cool water or juice may be given up to three times a day. Increased water intake is strongly recommended with increased fiber consumption in order to prevent constipation.

The recommended minimum daily weight of dietary fiber in grams = age of the child + 5. Additional fiber can be added as required.

Food Elimination

Patients should avoid foods that appear to exacerbate pain. If symptoms are suggestive or if the patient has a family history of lactose intolerance, initiate a 2- to 4-week trial of cessation of all dairy products (milk, cheese, yogurt, ice cream, etc.). If no changes are noted after 2 weeks, then consumption of dairy products can be resumed. If improvement is noted, then the patient should slowly reintroduce dairy in small quantities as tolerated. The intake of highly processed foods should be reduced, particularly those with refined carbohydrates (e.g., snacks, candy, and cookies) because the

fermentation of these sugars increases gas production. Studies have demonstrated that the ingestion of various sugars, such as lactose, fructose, sorbitol, and fructose plus sorbitol, increases breath hydrogen measurements and clinical symptoms in patients with RAP.[28,29] Reduced consumption of these sugars caused a reduction in symptoms in 40% to 60% of the subjects studied. Fructose is readily available in sweetened soft drinks and juices, while sorbitol is the leading sweetener used in "sugar-free" foods.

Food allergy has been implicated in abdominal pain; however, testing for the presence of IgE-mediated antibody responses has not demonstrated benefit. However, one study evaluated the efficacy of food elimination based on the presence of IgG antibodies detected by enzyme-linked immunosorbent assay. IgG antibodies cause delayed sensitivity and irritation of the gastrointestinal tract. In a randomized controlled trial (RCT), compliant patients placed on a food elimination diet based on high levels of IgG antibodies had a 26% greater reduction of symptoms compared with patients receiving a sham elimination diet.[30] In a separate RCT, both migraine pain and symptoms of IBS were reduced with food elimination based on IgG food antibodies[31] (see Chapters 31 and 86).

Behavior Modification

Pain behavior is frequently reinforced unknowingly but with good intentions toward the child. Help families recognize that special attention or treatment during pain episodes (i.e., staying home from school, being dismissed from chores or responsibilities, having one-on-one attention from a parent) may foster ongoing pain behavior and diminish self-reliance. Encourage school attendance and completion of personal responsibilities. Physicians can also facilitate a return to a normal lifestyle by offering a thorough explanation of the diagnosis and pathophysiology, reassurance, and options for management and adaptation to the disorder.

Poor sleep can heighten the perception of pain; therefore, working on strategies to promote restorative sleep is important. Eliminate all stimulants in the evening before bedtime, including caffeine, decongestants, television, computer or video games, and arguments. Practice dusk simulation by dimming lights around the house 1 hour before bedtime and shifting to quieter activities. The child should take a warm bath with Epsom salt to relax tense muscles before bedtime. Make sure the bedroom environment is conducive to sleep, that is, dark, quiet, and cool. If the child has difficulty falling asleep, have them practice self-regulation techniques such as controlled breathing or self-hypnosis, discussed later. Also consider using calming herbs such as chamomile.

Botanicals

Chamomile (Matricaria recutita)

The active ingredients in chamomile include the volatile oils alpha-bisabolol and bisabolol oxide and the flavonoids apigenin, luteolin, and quercetin. These constituents have antiinflammatory effects that inhibit phospholipase A, cyclooxygenase, and lipoxygenase pathways.[32] Bisabolol stimulates gastrointestinal tract receptors, thus causing smooth muscle relaxation. Apigenin acts on benzodiazepine receptors in the central nervous system, with anxiolytic effects similar to those of diazepam (Valium) and alprazolam (Xanax) but without the sedative effects.[33,34] Chamomile can be administered as a tea, as an extract, or by capsule in standardized preparations. Glyceride extracts of chamomile can be found for use in children to offset concerns regarding preparations extracted with alcohol. A study in infants with colic used found an herbal tea preparation that included chamomile to be effective in reducing colic episodes.[35]

DOSAGE
- Adults weighing approximately 150 lb: 3 g three to five times per day
- Children weighing approximately 75 lb: 1.5 g three to five times per day
- Children weighing approximately 35 lb: 0.75 g three to five times per day
  One heaped teaspoon of chamomile flowers steeped in hot water yields approximately 3 g. Extracts are supplied as a 1 g/1 mL (1:1) dilution and a 1 g/4 mL (1:4) dilution. Use the following doses as a guide:

150 lb
- 1:1—3 mL three to five times per day
- 1:4—12 mL three to five times per day

75 lb
- 1:1—1.5 mL three to five times per day
- 1:4—6 mL three to five times per day

35 lb
- 1:1—0.75 mL three to five times per day
- 1:4—3 mL three to five times per day

PRECAUTIONS
Chamomile is generally safe, although patients allergic to ragweed, asters, or chrysanthemums should take chamomile with caution. Chamomile is a member of the daisy family and has contributed to allergic reactions in rare cases.

Peppermint (Mentha piperita)

Analysis of peppermint oil typically shows more than 40 different compounds; however, the principal components are menthol, methone, and methyl acetate. Pharmacological studies on peppermint have focused almost entirely on menthol, which has carminative effects (elimination of intestinal gas), antispasmodic effects, and choleretic effects (bile flow stimulant). The mechanism of action of peppermint is thought to be inhibition of smooth muscle contraction by blocking calcium channels.[36] Many studies have been conducted using peppermint oil as a treatment for IBS, including one study in children.[37] Although peppermint did not alter symptoms

associated with IBS, such as urgency of stool, stool patterns, or belching, peppermint was found to reduce associated pain. Peppermint is most widely used as a tea. Due to its calcium channel blockage effects, peppermint may cause relaxation of the lower esophageal sphincter and lead to an increase in heartburn symptoms in some patients. An enteric-coated capsule is available for use in the treatment of IBS. With its delayed release in the small intestine, peppermint has little effect on the lower esophageal sphincter; therefore, it is less likely to cause heartburn.

DOSAGE
- Tea: one to two teaspoons of dried leaves steeped in 8 oz of hot water as needed
- Enteric-coated capsules (200 mg or 0.2 mL):
  - Two capsules three times a day for children weighing more than 100 lb
  - One capsule three times a day for children weighing 60 to 100 lb

PRECAUTIONS
Peppermint is generally regarded as safe; however, hypersensitivity reactions have been reported.

Due to its smooth muscle-relaxing properties, peppermint has the greatest effect on pain related to abdominal spasm.

Ginger (Zingiber officinale)

Ginger contains many volatile oils (sesquiterpenes) and aromatic ketones (gingerols). Gingerols are believed to be the more pharmacologically active constituents of ginger. Historically, ginger has been used as far back as the fourth century BC for stomach aches, nausea, and diarrhea. Ginger has also been used as a carminative, appetite stimulant, and choleretic. Ginger can simultaneously improve gastric motility and exert antispasmodic effects.[38] Studies have shown that ginger's antispasmodic effects on visceral smooth muscle are likely attributable to antagonism of serotonin receptor sites. A double-blind, randomized crossover study reported a significant reduction in nausea and vomiting with the use of ginger in women with hyperemesis gravidarum.[39] Due to its safety profile, ginger is regularly used in pregnancy with no untoward fetal effects.

DOSAGE
- Adults weighing approximately 150 lb: 1 to 2 g dry powdered ginger root per day (10 g fresh)
- Children weighing approximately 75 lb: 0.5 to 1 g dry powdered ginger root per day (5 g fresh)
- Children weighing approximately 35 lb: 0.25 to 0.5 g dry powdered ginger root per day (2.5 g fresh)
  Ginger can improve gastric motility while also exerting an antispasmodic effect. The pharmacist can dissolve ginger capsules in an 8.4% bicarbonate suspension with good stability and bioavailability for use in children unable to swallow pills.

A one-fourth inch slice of fresh ginger root is approximately 10 g. This is equivalent to 1 to 2 g of a dry powder form of ginger that is a more concentrated form found in capsules. Fresh ginger can be brewed as a tea sweetened with honey or can be chopped and added to foods, soups, or salads.

A general rule of thumb for estimating the amount of fresh ginger to use in children is to use the child's "pinky" finger (fifth finger) as the guide to the size of ginger to chop up and steep for tea.

PRECAUTIONS

Ginger is well tolerated when used in typical doses. At higher doses, side effects may include heartburn, abdominal discomfort, or diarrhea. Ginger may have antiplatelet effects and therefore may increase the risk of bleeding in some people.

Slippery Elm (Ulmus fulva)

Slippery elm has demulcent properties that can be used to protect the gastrointestinal tract from irritation. When used internally, slippery elm causes reflex stimulation of the nerve endings in the gastrointestinal tract that produces mucus secretion.[40] This effect may be particularly helpful in children with functional dyspepsia.

DOSAGE

A tea can be made with one cup of boiling water and one tablespoon of powdered bark. Use 2 to 5 mL three times a day.

PRECAUTIONS

No contraindications are associated with slippery elm. Spontaneous abortions have been reported with the use of slippery elm; therefore, it should not be used during pregnancy.

Lemon Balm (Melissa officinalis)

Lemon balm contains volatile oils and constituents that relax muscles, particularly in the bladder, stomach, and uterus, thereby relieving cramps, gas, and nausea. Lemon balm is generally regarded as safe and is one of the components of the product Iberogast, used widely for gastrointestinal problems. A meta-analysis of double-blind, randomized controlled trials conducted on Iberogast found significant improvements compared with placebo in patients with functional dyspepsia.[41]

DOSAGE

- Capsules: 100 to 200 mg dried lemon balm three times daily or as needed.
- Tea: 0.5 to 1.5 g (one-fourth to one teaspoon) of dried lemon balm herb in hot water. Steep and drink up to four times daily.
- Tincture: 0.5 to 1 mL (15 to 30 drops) three times daily.

PRECAUTIONS

Despite a lack of scientific evidence, lemon balm may interact with sedatives and thyroid medications.

Supplements

Probiotics

The human intestinal tract is populated with various microbial species that are nonpathogenic and necessary for normal digestive functioning. Microorganisms, or probiotics, are now recognized as a way to fight disease and improve health. Studies in children have reported a significant reduction in diarrhea symptoms, both from rotavirus infection and antibiotic use, in children following the administration of probiotics.[42,43] Probiotics increase the number of rotavirus-specific IgA-secreting cells and serum IgA levels. Probiotics are thought to help treat RAP by degrading dietary antigens, restoring normal intestinal permeability, and alleviating intestinal inflammation that can trigger pain.[44] Two double-blind, randomized, placebo-controlled trials found that *Lactobacillus* GG reduced the frequency and intensity of pain in children with RAP/IBS when this probiotic was administered over the course of 4 to 8 weeks.[45,46] One of these studies also demonstrated a decrease in the number of patients with abnormal intestinal permeability test results after treatment with *Lactobacillus* GG but not with placebo.

DOSAGE

Use 10 to 100 billion colony-forming units (CFUs) per serving once or twice a day. These preparations can be of a single strain, such as *Lactobacillus* GG, or made of multiple strains, such as *Bifidobacterium bifidus*, *Lactobacillus acidophilus*, or *Lactobacillus reuteri*, to treat both the small and the large intestine.

PRECAUTIONS

Probiotics are considered safe for use. *Lactobacillus* sepsis associated with probiotic therapy has been reported; however, this adverse effect occurred in children considered immunocompromised and at increased risk due to central line placement.

Pharmaceuticals

Despite a lack of controlled studies with established efficacy for many drugs used in functional bowel disorders,[47,48] these agents continue to be prescribed. For this reason, as well as worrisome side effects (for metoclopramide, irritability, and dystonic reactions; for cisapride, arrhythmia, and adverse outcomes in prolonged QT syndrome; for anticholinergics, constipation, blurred vision, tachycardia, and sedation; for tricyclic antidepressants, sedation, agitation, acute mental disturbance, and reduction in seizure threshold), these particular drugs cannot be safely recommended for use in children.

Histamine-2 (H₂) Receptor Antagonists and Proton Pump Inhibitors

For patients with dyspepsia as a primary symptom, histamine-2 (H_2) receptor antagonists and proton pump inhibitors can be used if other strategies are unsuccessful. Studies in children supporting such therapy are few;

however, these drugs may be beneficial and are relatively safe in the short term (6 to 8 weeks).[49]

DOSAGE

- Cimetidine (Tagamet): 10 mg/kg/dose given four times daily. Available as 100 mg over-the-counter (OTC), 200-, 300-, 400-, and 800-mg tablets and a 300-mg/5-mL suspension by prescription
- Ranitidine (Zantac): 2 to 4 mg/kg/dose given twice daily. Available as 75-mg OTC, 150-, and 300-mg tablets; 150-mg granules; and a 75-mg/5-mL suspension
- Famotidine (Pepcid): 0.5 to 3.5 mg/kg/day divided two times a day. Available as 10-mg OTC, 20-, and 40-mg tablets and a 40-mg/5-mL suspension
- Omeprazole (Prilosec): 0.2 to 3.5 mg/kg/day daily or divided twice a day. Available as 10-, 20-, and 40-mg capsules
- Lansoprazole (Prevacid): 1 to 2 mg/kg/day given daily. Available as 15- and 30-mg capsules

PRECAUTIONS

Headaches, diarrhea, abdominal pain, and elevated liver function tests have been reported with the use of histamine-2 (H_2) receptor antagonists and proton pump inhibitors. Prolonged acid suppression can lead to malabsorption of key nutrients, including vitamin B_{12}, iron, magnesium, and calcium.

Cyproheptadine

Cyproheptadine (also known by the brand name Periactin) has antihistamine effects and has been studied through a double-blind, randomized controlled trial conducted over 2 weeks in 29 children. The intensity and frequency of abdominal pain reported by children were significantly improved in the treatment group compared with the control group.[50] Cyproheptadine has historically been used as prophylactic treatment for migraine due to its effects on serotonin and histamine. These effects may have some benefit in children with abdominal migraines over a short period, although further studies are required.

DOSAGE

- Children 7 to 14 years of age: 4 mg two or three times daily (maximum, 16 mg/day)
- Children 2 to 6 years of age: 2 mg two or three times daily (maximum, 12 mg/day)

PRECAUTIONS

The major reported side effects of cyproheptadine are increased appetite and weight gain. Sedation and sleepiness have also been reported.

Biomechanical Therapy

Massage

Massage can ease pain by calming sympathetic arousal, often observed in children with RAP. Decreased sympathetic drive improves gastrointestinal motility. Massage, either of the abdomen directly or indirectly by reflexology, is helpful in alleviating ileus and constipation and can be very comforting overall.[51,52]

Osteopathic Manipulative Therapy

Understanding somatovisceral pathways has led to the treatment of RAP with osteopathic manipulative therapy. Trigger points along the spine and in the large muscles of the back and trunk (e.g., external and internal oblique, rectus abdominis, iliocostalis thoracis, and lumborum muscles) can cause referred pain to the abdominal region that mimics visceral disease. Release of these trigger points through manipulation decreases this reflex effect and therefore lessens pain.[53]

Surgery

Exploratory surgery is not warranted unless strong indications are revealed through history, physical examination, or laboratory investigations.

Bioenergetic Therapy

Traditional Chinese Medicine and Acupuncture

The philosophy of traditional Chinese medicine is that of restoring balance to the body through its flow of energy. Although large clinical trials of traditional Chinese medicine and acupuncture in children with RAP have yet to be reported, one study measured the effects of hand acupuncture in reducing intermittent abdominal pain in 40 children. Pain intensity and medication use were considerably lower in the treatment group.[54] In a randomized, double-blind, placebo-controlled study of Chinese herbs, patients receiving herbs noted significant improvement in bowel symptoms, global well-being, and return to normal life activities compared with the group receiving placebo.[55] Although children may be fearful of needles, many children have reported that acupuncture does not hurt when performed by an experienced professional. Acupressure or electroacupuncture may also be used as alternatives to needles.

Reiki and Healing Touch

As with traditional Chinese medicine, reiki and healing touch are based on the concept of restoring normal energy flow through the body. In patients with disease or pain, this energy may be blocked or stagnant, thus disrupting its normal flow. Through energy work, this energy flow can be restored. Many randomized controlled studies have indicated that energy healing can be effective for pain, anxiety, depression, wound healing, and other problems.[56] Although no specific studies have been conducted in children with RAP, this therapy has no serious side effects and is considered safe (see Chapter 116).

Mind-Body Therapy

It is clear that abdominal pain syndromes are disorders of bidirectional mind-brain-gut interactions and neurobiological processes in the mind-brain-gut inter-actions lead to alterations in motility, sensation, and immune functions.[57]

Because of our current knowledge of the brain–gut axis and associated interactions, it is logical that mind-body therapy be used for the treatment of RAP. Studies published primarily in psychiatric journals have supported the efficacy of interventions that teach stress management, progressive muscle relaxation, coping behaviors, or the use of cognitive-behavioral therapy.[58,59] One study reported significant pain reduction with the addition of biofeedback, cognitive-behavioral therapy, or parental support to fiber therapy in the multimodal treatment of RAP.[60]

Progressive Muscle Relaxation and Breathing Exercises

Both progressive muscle relaxation and breathing exercises, used alone or in combination, are forms of self-regulation that help decrease sympathetic arousal to promote comfort. Progressive muscle relaxation is a way for children to learn to feel the difference between tense and relaxed muscles, and to use this knowledge to cope with abdominal pain. Progressive relaxation reduces anxiety associated with pain by demonstrating the mind-body phenomenon and patient capacity for self-regulation. The benefits of these approaches are that they are easily taught, particularly to school-age children, and can be used anywhere. Scripts can be given to parents to use, or a tape can be made or purchased for home use (see Chapters 94 and 95).

Biofeedback

Biofeedback is a form of relaxation using physiological feedback instruments to reinforce behavior. As relaxation occurs, warmth can be brought to the fingertips, thus increasing distal temperature. Distal temperature can be monitored by sensors placed on the fingers and can reinforce the positive

behavior of relaxation as the temperature rises. Biofeedback may be beneficial in patients who are skeptical regarding the ability of the mind to control body functions. Professionals trained in biofeedback with equipment readily available are best placed to teach this modality.

In a study of heart rate variability biofeedback, children with functional abdominal pain were able to significantly reduce their symptoms by significantly increasing their autonomic balance. The investigators posited change in vagal tone was the potential mediator of this improvement.[61]

Hypnosis and Guided Imagery

Hypnosis and guided imagery allow a state of focused attention in which the mind is more receptive to suggestion. These techniques have been used successfully for all types of pain syndromes, including RAP, and are easily used in children older than 4 years of age (see Chapters 95 and 97).[62,63]

A randomized controlled trial of the use of therapist-directed guided imagery with progressive muscle relaxation reported a significant decrease in the number of days with pain and missed activities compared with controls.[64] A similar study using audio-recorded guided imagery treatment also reported benefit, with treatment effects maintained for more than 6 months.[65] Gut-directed hypnosis therapy has been found to be superior to standard medical therapy in reducing pain scores in children with longstanding abdominal pain in other randomized controlled trials.[66,67]

Psychotherapy

In children or families with significant psychosocial dysfunction, counseling by a child psychiatrist or clinical psychologist may be the best therapy. Cognitive-behavioral family intervention therapy, which often includes teaching specific coping skills, social skills, and relaxation, has been shown to be efficacious in studies of children with RAP.[68,69]

PREVENTION PRESCRIPTION

- Encourage liberal amounts of water and fiber in the form of natural fruits and vegetables to promote daily bowel movements.
- Promote probiotics if the patient has a history of antibiotic, steroid, or nonsteroidal antiinflammatory drug use.
- Ask the patient to practice breathing and relaxation exercises or other self-regulation techniques to reduce stress.

- Encourage healthy sleep habits to promote restorative sleep.
- Consider avoiding high amounts of processed foods and simple sugars, including sorbitol.
- Encourage regular movement and exercise.

THERAPEUTIC REVIEW

Once a child has been thoroughly evaluated and organic disease has been ruled out, any of these therapies can be used in an age-appropriate manner.

NUTRITION
- Avoid foods that have sorbitol and high-fructose corn syrup or are a source of refined carbohydrate because these are poorly digested.

- Prescribe a 2- to 4-wk trial of cessation of all dairy products if the history suggests lactose intolerance (see Chapters 31 and 86).
- Increase fiber by at least 10 g/day through the addition of fruits, vegetables, legumes, and whole grains or with psyllium, one teaspoon/8-oz cool water one to three times daily.
- Increase water intake along with the increase of fiber.

BEHAVIOR MODIFICATION

- Encourage attendance at school and other usual activities.
- Offer strategies to overcome the reinforcement of illness behavior at school and at home.
- Improve restorative sleep.

BOTANICALS

Chamomile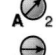

- 3 g three to five times/day (150 lb patient)
- 1.5 g three to five times/day (75 lb patient)
- 0.75 g three to five times/day (35 lb patient)

Peppermint Tea

- One to two teaspoons dried leaves/8-oz hot water as needed
- Enteric-coated capsules (200 mg)
  - Two capsules three times/day (approximately 100-lb patient)
  - One capsule three times/day (60- to 99-lb patient)

Ginger

- 10 g fresh (or 1 to 2 g dry powdered)/day (150-lb patient)
- 5 g fresh (or 0.5 to 1 g dry powdered)/day (75-lb patient)
- 2.5 g fresh (or 0.25 to 0.5 g dry powdered)/day (35-lb patient)

Slippery Elm

- Make tea with one cup boiling water and one tablespoon powdered bark. Give 2 to 5 mL three times a day

Lemon Balm

- 100 to 200 mg capsules three times/day
- 0.5 to 1.5 g tea three times/day
- 0.5 to 1 mL (15 to 30 drops) tincture three times/day

SUPPLEMENTS

- Probiotics: 10 to 100 billion CFUs once or twice/day

PHARMACEUTICALS

- Histamine-2 (H_2) receptor antagonists or proton pump inhibitors for maximum of 6 to 8 weeks if dyspepsia is the primary complaint (see text for dosing)
- Cyproheptadine 2 to 4 mg two to three times/day for abdominal migraine

BIOMECHANICAL THERAPY

- Massage
- Osteopathic manipulative therapy

BIOENERGETIC THERAPY

- Traditional Chinese medicine and acupuncture
- Reiki and healing touch

MIND-BODY THERAPIES

- Progressive muscle relaxation and breathing exercises (see Chapter 92)
- Biofeedback
- Hypnosis and guided imagery (see Chapters 95 and 97)
- Psychotherapy

Key Web Resources

YourChild. This University of Michigan website provides information for parents on abdominal pain in children.

http://www.med.umich.edu/yourchild/topics/abpain.htm

HeartMath and Wild Divine. These websites offer biofeedback devices that can help stimulate parasympathetic activity toward a reduction in abdominal pain.

http://www.heartmath.com
http://www.wilddivine.com

Health Journeys, Kaiser Permanente Healthy Living to Go audio library, and Guided Imagery. These websites are resources for guided-imagery recordings.

http://www.healthjourneys.com
https://healthy.kaiserpermanente.org/health/care/!ut/p/a0/FchBDoMgEADAt_iAzYZEYfFmhH6hhdsGiZlIGELt99seZ9DjC33hO-3cUy18_uxCLD22md9bqnCnLVZ8okd_Nd4zoysVAocj_o9bT-GM6lzVap2M-BamIBCGsgEWPBohoUkKp8UErXjnTZxmGL2lKPpI!/
http://www.guidedimageryinc.com/

"Take a Chill," iZen Garden, Arabian Nights by Relax Kids, and Enchanted Meditation. Relaxation apps for kids

http://itunes.apple.com/us/app/take-a-chill-stressed-teens/id496802813?mt=8
http://itunes.apple.com/us/app/izen-garden-2-portable-zen/id347232643?mt=8
http://itunes.apple.com/app/arabian-nights/id500474568?ign-mpt=uo%3D5
http://itunes.apple.com/us/app/enchanted-meditations-for/id490096965?mt=8

REFERENCES

References are available online at ExpertConsult.com.

CHAPTER 46

CONSTIPATION

Tanmeet Sethi, MD

PATHOPHYSIOLOGY

Constipation is estimated to affect up to 28% of the population of the United States, most commonly older adults, women, and children, and results in more than $6.9 billion in medical costs.[1] Constipation is usually intermittent and self-limiting, although some patients require intervention to achieve resolution. Table 46.1 presents the defining criteria for constipation,[2] but in practical clinical terms, the complaint of constipation and even the diagnosis are often made more subjectively. Asking what patients mean by the statement, "I am constipated," may be the most important first step to management.[3] The majority of patients complaining of constipation describe a perception of difficulty with bowel movements or a discomfort related to bowel movements. The most common terms used by young, healthy adults to define constipation are straining (52%), hard stools (44%), and the inability to have a bowel movement (34%).

Routine diagnostic testing is not recommended for patients with no alarm symptoms and no signs of organic disorder.[4]

Functional constipation is often classified into three distinct categories:

1. Normal-transit constipation: Also known as *functional constipation*, this is the most common type. In functional constipation, stool passes through the colon at a normal rate and bowel movement frequency is normal.[5] In this group of patients, constipation is likely the result of a perceived difficulty with evacuation or the presence of hard stools.[2]
2. Slow-transit constipation: This type of constipation is characterized by prolonged delay of transit of stool through the colon. Patients may complain of abdominal bloating and infrequent bowel movements.[6] The causes are unclear.
3. Pelvic floor dysfunction: These patients have uncoordinated evacuation of stool through the rectum. They are more likely to complain of a feeling of incomplete evacuation, a sense of obstruction, or a need for digital manipulation.[6]

Physicians should keep secondary causes of constipation (the most common being hypothyroidism) in mind, as well as medications that can cause constipation. In one study of more than 20,000 patients, the use of certain drugs was found to be associated with a two- to three-fold increased risk of constipation.[7] Although the list of drugs that can cause constipation is quite lengthy, Table 46.2[7,8] provides some of the most common offenders.

INTEGRATIVE THERAPY

Physical Activity

The generally accepted view is that increasing the amount of physical activity can be a preventive measure for constipation. In fact, a subset of the Nurses' Health Study demonstrated that in more than 62,000 women, physical activity two to six times a week was associated with a 35% decrease in risk of constipation.[9] A previous National Health and Nutrition Examination Survey reported a two-fold increased risk of constipation in persons with a low physical activity level. Despite these findings, data in support of exercise as a treatment for constipation have not been consistent. Nevertheless, many patients who comply with dietary and exercise recommendations have an improvement in symptoms.[10]

Nutrition

Fiber

Although dietary modification may not always succeed, all constipated patients should be initially advised to increase their dietary fiber intake as the simplest, most physiologic, and cheapest form of treatment.[1] Patients should be encouraged to ingest 20 to 25 g of fiber daily by eating whole grain breads, unrefined cereals, plenty of fruit and vegetables, or flax meal or bran. A careful meta-analysis demonstrated that, in 18 of 20 studies, stool weight was increased by adequate fiber supplementation, with fecal transit found to be accelerated.[11,12] Dietary fiber appears to be less effective in severe constipation, particularly the slow-transit variant, in evacuation disorders (fiber may actually worsen these two types), or in constipation secondary to medications.[13-15] In one study, women who engaged in regular physical exercise and had a higher fiber intake (approximately 20 g/day) had a three-fold lower prevalence of constipation compared with women who rarely exercised and consumed approximately 7 g of fiber a day.[9] If ensuring proper intake of fiber is difficult, a commercially packaged fiber supplement may also be used (discussed later under Supplements).

Increasing fiber intake too quickly can cause abdominal bloating or flatulence. To optimize compliance, increase fiber gradually over at least 2 to 3 weeks to 20 to 25 g/day and ensure increased fluid intake to avoid these symptoms.

An example of a 20 g fiber breakfast: half cup bran (10 g) and three dried figs (10 g). Make palatable with one

TABLE 46.1 Rome II Criteria for Functional Constipation

Adults*

Two or more of the following six must be present:

- Straining during at least 25% of defecations
- Lumpy or hard stools in at least 25% of defecations
- Sensation of incomplete evacuation for at least 25% of defecations
- Sensation of anorectal obstruction/blockage for at least 25% of defecations
- Manual maneuvers to facilitate at least 25% of defecations (e.g., digital evacuation, support of the pelvic floor)
- Fewer than three defecations/wk

Infants and Children

- Pebble-like, hard stools for a majority of stools for at least 2 consecutive wk
- Firm stools up to twice/wk for at least 2 wk
- No evidence of structural, endocrine, or metabolic disease

*Loose stools are rarely present without the use of laxatives; criteria for irritable bowel syndrome are not fulfilled.
From Lembo A, Camilleri M. Chronic constipation. *N Engl J Med.* 2003;349:1360-1368.

TABLE 46.2 Medications Associated With Constipation

- Aluminum-containing antacids
- Diuretics
- Antidepressants
- Antihistamines
- Anticholinergics
- Nonsteroidal antiinflammatory agents
- Iron supplements
- Opioids
- Anticonvulsants
- Calcium channel blockers
- Beta-blockers

cup soy or almond milk (1 g fiber), one tablespoon brown sugar for taste, and one tablespoon of cinnamon (slows absorption of sugar).

Examples of other high-fiber foods include 1 large apple or pear (5 g), ½ cup raspberries (9 g), 1 cup Raisin Bran (5 g), 2 Brazil nuts (2.5 g), 23 almonds (3.5 g), 1 cup peas (16 g), 1 cup black beans (15 g), 1 artichoke (10 g), and 1 cup cooked broccoli (5 g).

In pediatric populations, decreased fiber intake has been found to be a risk factor for chronic constipation.[16] One safe and effective dietary fiber recommendation for many children is the *age + 5 = daily grams of fiber* guideline.[17] According to this guideline, the amount of dietary fiber recommended daily is the sum of the child's age in years plus five.

In pregnant women, fiber supplements in the form of bran and wheat fiber have been shown to increase bowel frequency, soften stool, and be better tolerated than stimulant laxatives.[18]

Food Triggers

A large body of evidence indicates that cow's milk and dairy products may be risk factors for chronic constipation in some children.[19-21]

Evidence supports a 4- to 6-week trial of elimination of dairy products as a component of the integrative treatment of childhood constipation.

Fluids

Although the generally accepted approach is to increase fluids both as a preventive measure and as treatment for constipation, supporting data are conflicting.[22] One study reported that increasing fluids with an increased fiber intake (25 g/day) led to greater stool frequency and decreased laxative use compared with increased fiber alone.[23] To date, no studies in children have demonstrated the benefits of increasing fluid intake in states other than severe dehydration.[24] However, carbohydrates and particularly sorbitol, found in some juices such as prune, pear, and apple, can cause increased frequency and water content of stools.[25]

Supplements

Commercially Packaged Fiber Supplements

Commercially packaged fiber supplements include psyllium, methylcellulose, and polycarbophil as bulking laxatives. More information, including dosing, is available in Table 46.3 and is provided later under Pharmaceuticals. Psyllium has demonstrated efficacy in increasing stool frequency and weight and improving stool consistency in idiopathic constipation.[26]

The American College of Gastroenterology Chronic Constipation Task Force systematically reviewed available clinical evidence regarding the use of fiber supplements in chronic constipation and concluded that psyllium was the only fiber supplement with sufficient clinical evidence to support a recommendation for the treatment of chronic constipation.[27]

One double-blind, multicenter study reported psyllium (5.1 g twice daily) as superior to docusate sodium (100 mg twice daily) for softening stools by increasing stool water content with greater overall laxative efficacy in subjects with chronic idiopathic constipation.[27a]

Probiotics

Lactobacillus reuteri, administered at a dose of 108 colony-forming units to infants older than 6 months, has been shown to increase bowel frequency.[28] A high-grade systematic review concluded that the use of probiotics in adults and children augments the number of stools and reduces the number of hard stools.[29] These results were

TABLE 46.3   Agents for Treatment of Constipation in Adults

Type	Generic Name	Dosage	ACG Grade	Comments
Bulking Laxatives	Psyllium (Metamucil)	Titrate up to 30 g/day in divided doses	B	Taken from the ground seed husk of the ispaghula plant; needs to be taken with plenty of water to avoid intestinal obstruction; undergoes bacterial degradation that may contribute to side effects of bloating and flatus; allergic reactions, such as anaphylaxis and asthma, are rare but have been reported
	Methylcellulose (Citrucel)	Titrate up to 6 g/day in divided doses	B	Semisynthetic cellulose fiber relatively resistant to colonic bacterial degradation; tends to cause less bloating and flatus than psyllium
	Polycarbophil (FiberCon)	Titrate up to 4 g/day in divided doses	B	Synthetic polymer of acrylic acid that is resistant to bacterial degradation
Osmotic Laxatives	Magnesium hydroxide (milk of magnesia)	30–60 mL/day	B	Small percentage actively absorbed in the small intestine; remainder draws water into the intestines along an osmotic gradient
	Polyethylene glycol (MiraLax)	17–34 g once to twice/day	A	Organic polymer that is poorly absorbed and not metabolized by colonic bacteria
	Lactulose	15–30 mL once to twice/day	A	Synthetic disaccharide consisting of galactose and fructose linked by a bond resistant to lactase and, therefore, not absorbed by the small intestine; undergoes bacterial fermentation in the colon resulting in formation of short-chain fatty acids; bacteria in the colon can metabolize up to 80 g of lactulose each day; gas and bloating common side effects
Stimulant Laxatives	Sennosides (senna)	8.6–30 mg once to twice/day	B	Anthraquinones are converted by colonic bacteria to their active form, which increases electrolyte transport into the bowel and stimulates intestinal motility; may cause melanosis coli, a benign condition usually reversible within 12 months; no definitive association established between anthraquinones and colon cancer or myenteric nerve damage
	Bisacodyl (Dulcolax)	10–15 mg/day orally 10 mg rectal suppository/day	B	Hydrolyzed by endogenous esterases; stimulates secretion and motility of the small intestine and colon
Stool Softeners	Docusate sodium	50–100 mg once to twice/day	B	Ionic detergents that soften the stool by allowing water to interact more effectively with solid stool; may have modest effects on fluid absorption and secretion; efficacy in constipation not well established
	Docusate calcium	5–45 mL orally nightly	B	Alters stool by being emulsified into the stool mass and providing lubrication for passage of the stool; long-term use may cause malabsorption of fat-soluble vitamins, anal seepage, and lipoid pneumonia in patients predisposed to aspiration of liquids
Emollients	Mineral oil	5–45 mL orally nightly	B	Alters stool by being emulsified into the stool mass and providing lubrication for passage of the stool; long-term use may cause malabsorption of fat-soluble vitamins, anal seepage, and lipoid pneumonia in patients predisposed to aspiration of liquids
Chloride Channel Activator	Lubiprostone	8 mcg twice/day for IBS-C; 24 mcg twice/day for chronic constipation	Not graded	Activates ClC-2 s in the intestine and causes fluid secretion and possible secondary effects on motility; nausea common; administer with food and water; approved for use in adults with chronic constipation and in women older than 18 yr with IBS-C

ACG, American College of Gastroenterology; *bid*, twice daily; *ClC-2*, type-2 chloride channel; *IBS-C*, irritable bowel syndrome with constipation; *PEG*, polyethylene glycol; *po*, by mouth; *qd*, every day; *qhs*, every night.
From Eoff JC III, Lembo A. Optimal treatment of chronic constipation in managed care: review and roundtable discussion. *J Manag Care Pharm.* 2008;14(suppl A):1-15.

statistically significant but clinically only modest. The most thoroughly studied strains for the treatment of constipation are *Bifidobacterium* and *Lactobacillus* (most specifically *Lactobacillus casei Shirota*). A separate prospective trial reported the efficacy of *Lactobacillus* in improving chronic constipation in nursing home residents.[30] Probiotics may be useful in relieving constipation; however, the effect may depend on the probiotic dose, the bacterial strain used, and the population studied.[12] Further studies are required to determine specific recommendations regarding dosing and strain type (see Chapter 105).

Mind-Body Therapy

Behavioral Training in Childhood Constipation

Education for parents and children is an important component of treatment for functional constipation.[30a] The child's fear of a painful bowel movement is the most common motivating factor for fecal retention.

> In childhood constipation, clinicians should explain the physiologic changes that occur as a consequence of chronic constipation, including a diminished ability to recognize the need to stool or that soiling has occurred.[31] Explain that this condition is common and is multifactorial in origin for most children and stress the need to avoid demeaning or embarrassing the child.

Biofeedback

In an instrument-based training program, patients receive auditory or visual feedback, or both, to help train the pelvic floor and relax the anal sphincter while simulating defecation. Biofeedback also improves rectal sensation to assist in proper evacuation.[10] Biofeedback is the preferred treatment for pelvic floor dysfunction, with a reported success rate of 70% to 81% and to be superior to standard treatment (laxatives, fiber, and education).[32-34] Randomized controlled trials (RCTs) have demonstrated that five biofeedback sessions are more effective than continuous polyethylene glycol (PEG) administration for treating pelvic floor dysfunction, with the benefits lasting at least 2 years.[35]

Although biofeedback is not an effective treatment for slow-transit constipation, it should be considered as the first-line treatment for pelvic floor dysfunction. To evaluate for this, do a rectal exam with one hand while placing the other hand on the patient's lower abdomen and have them bear down. The perineum should relax and descend downward. If it does not, suspect pelvic floor dysfunction and remember to screen for a history of sexual abuse.

Hypnotherapy

Substantial evidence supports the use of hypnotherapy in constipation-dependent irritable bowel syndrome, which has considerable overlap with functional constipation.[36] However, there is a lack of specific data on hypnotherapy as a treatment for functional constipation. Until more evidence is available, it may, at times, be reasonable to try hypnotherapy, particularly in patients who have difficulty relaxing the pelvic musculature.

Botanicals

Aloe

Dried latex (aloe latex) from the lining of the inner leaf has historically been used as a laxative. One double-blind RCT of an herbal preparation of aloe, psyllium, and celandin reported a statistically significant advantage of the herbal preparation over placebo.[37] Which part of the preparation was most responsible for the effect was unclear, however, and this preparation is not available in the United States.[37] The anthraquinones in aloe act as a stimulant laxative.

> **DOSAGE**
> A typical dose of aloe is 50 mg aloe extract taken at bedtime.
>
> **PRECAUTIONS**
> It is aloe latex, but not aloe gel, that has a laxative effect.

Traditional Chinese Medicine

Although numerous RCTs have evaluated the efficacy of various components of traditional Chinese medicine in the treatment of constipation, high-level systematic reviews have concluded that methodologic flaws limit their interpretation.[38-40] At least two RCTs have reported the efficacy of a particular formula (yun-chang capsules; also known as the *hemp seed pill*) in treating the functional type of chronic constipation.[41,42] Further studies are required before the use of these components, including Chinese herbs, moxibustion, and auriculotherapy, can be recommended for the treatment of constipation

Abdominal Massage

There is some evidence to suggest that abdominal massage may be a helpful technique in the treatment of constipation. One small 8-week RCT demonstrated an increase in bowel movement frequency, but no decrease in laxative use, with the use of abdominal massage.[42a] The study investigators concluded that this approach may have utility as an adjunctive therapy to the treatment of constipation. However, abdominal massage is considered a long-term treatment due to its delayed effect, which may first be noted after several weeks.

Acupuncture

A large randomized controlled trial of 1075 patients with severe constipation from 15 Chinese hospitals showed that 28 sessions of acupuncture over 8 weeks improved bowel frequency. Surprisingly, the acupuncture had a larger effect after treatment was completed. At 8 weeks, there was an increase in bowel movements by 31.3% compared to sham acupuncture control. And this increased to 37.7% during the 12 weeks of follow up. This improvement following treatment is rarely seen with medications. Often symptoms return after the medication is stopped unless underlying mechanisms have been addressed.[42b]

Perineal Self-Acupressure

Investigators recruited 100 patients with functional constipation according to the Rome III criteria from the community. All patients received educational materials outlining standard treatment approaches, including increased dietary fiber intake, the use of stool softeners, and increased exercise. The patients were randomly assigned (allocation concealment unknown) to no further instruction or to receive a 3- to 5-minute instruction on how to perform perineal massage along with a sex-specific handout. Upon feeling the urge to defecate, patients were instructed to press the perineum, pulsing for 3 to 5 seconds with the goal of breaking up the stool before defecation begins. Clinically relevant improvements in quality of life (p < 0.001) and a bowel function index (p < 0.01) were noted with perineal massage.[42c] Although this is the only RCT of perineal massage reported to date, it provides encouraging support for an intervention that has no toxicity and possible benefit.

Pharmaceuticals

A wide array of laxatives is available to patients. Clinicians must understand how to counsel patients regarding the appropriate use, risks, and optimal dosing of these agents. Dosing and further information on all agents for adults are provided in Table 46.3,[42d] and similar information for children is provided in Table 46.4.[43]

TABLE 46.4   Agents for Treatment of Constipation in Children

Type of Medication	Selected Medications	Recommended Dosage for Maintenance Therapy
Bulk-forming laxatives (OTC)	Methylcellulose (Citrucel) powder	Older than 6 yr: 1–1.5 g/dose Older than 12 yr: 4–6 g/dose
Dietary fiber (OTC) supplement (no systemic absorption)	Psyllium (Metamucil, Perdiem, Serutan, Fiberall, Konsyl)	6–11 yr: ½–1 rounded teaspoon in 8-oz liquid one to three times/day Older than 12 yr: 1–2 rounded teaspoons or one to two packets or one to two wafers one to four times/day or five capsules up to three times/day taken with 8-oz liquid
Osmotic laxative (OTC)	Magnesium hydroxide (Milk of Magnesia [MOM]); liquid, tablets	Younger than 2 yr: 0.5 mL/kg/day 2–5 yr: 5–15 mL/day or in divided doses one to two tablets before bedtime 6–12 yr: 15–30 mL/day in divided doses or three to four tablets before bedtime Older than 12 yr: 30–60 mL/day or in divided doses six to eight tablets before bedtime
	Magnesium citrate	Younger than 6 yr: 2–4 mL/kg/day 6–12 yr: 100–150 mL/day Older than 12 yr: 150–300 mL/day, in single or divided doses
	Magnesium citrate	Used only for bowel cleanout
Lubricants	Mineral oil (OTC)	5–11 yr: 5–20 mL every day or in divided doses Older than 12 yr: 15–45 mL/day every day or in divided doses or 1–4 mL/kg/day
Fiber supplement (OTC); powder, chewable tablets, caplets	Benefiber (partially hydrolyzed guar gum): two teaspoons = 3 g soluble fiber	7–11 yr: ½–1 tablespoon one to three times/day 12 yr–adult: 1–2 tablespoon one to three times/day
Stool softeners (emollients)	Docusate (Colace); liquid, capsule, gel cap (OTC)	Infants and children younger than 3 yr: 10–40 mg/day in one to four divided doses 3–6 yr: 20–60 mg/day in one to four divided doses 6–12 yr: 40–150 mg/day in one to four divided doses Older than 12 yr: 50–400 mg/day in one to four divided doses
Stimulants	Senna (Senokot, Senna-Gen, Senolax, Ex-Lax); granules, syrup, tablets (OTC)	1–5 yr: 5–10 mL/day 5–15 yr: 10–20 mL/day One tablet = 3 mL/granules = 5 mL/syrup
Osmotic enema	Phosphate enema (OTC)	Younger than 2 yr: not recommended 2–11 yr: 2.25-oz pediatric enema Older than 11 yr: 4.5-oz adult enema
Osmotic laxative	MiraLax (polyethylene glycol); GlycoLax	12 yr or older: 17 g (up to measuring line on cap) in 8 oz of water Older than 2–11 yr: 8.5 g (halfway to measuring line on cap) in 4 oz of water

TABLE 46.4 Agents for Treatment of Constipation in Children—cont'd

Type of Medication	Selected Medications	Recommended Dosage for Maintenance Therapy
Stimulant laxative	Bisacodyl (Dulcolax): 5-mg tablet, 10-mg suppository	Older than 2 yr: one half to one suppository or one to three tablets per dose; no liquid form Adolescents: four tablets maximum
Miscellaneous	Glycerin suppository	Children: one infant suppository one to two times/day Children >6 yr: one adult suppository
	Glycerin enema; Enemeez Mini Enema (ingredients: docusate, polyethylene glycol, glycerin)	5–10 mL glycerin in 500 mL normal saline solution 5-mL tubes: one enema/day
Osmotic laxative	Lactulose (Cephulac, Cholac, Chronulac, Constilac, Duphalac, Enulose, Lactulox); crystals, syrup	Infants: 2.5–10 mL/day individual doses Children: 0.6–0.6 mL/kg/dose three to four times/day or 40–90 mL/day in divided doses or 1–3 mL/kg/day in divided doses (maximum, 3 oz/day) Adults: 15–30 mL/day (maximum, 60 mL/day)
	Sorbitol	1–3 mL/kg/day in divided doses, 70% solution

OTC, over the counter.
From Tobias N, Mason D, Lutkenhoff M, et al. Management principles of organic causes of childhood constipation. *J Pediatr Health Care.* 2008;22:12-23; with data from Guandalini S, 2005; *Mosby's pediatric drug consult.* St. Louis: Mosby; 2006; and Pediatric Lexi-Drugs Online. http://lexi.com; 2006 available to subscribers.)

Bulk-Forming Laxatives

Bulk-forming laxatives work naturally to add bulk and water to stools to allow stools to pass more easily through the intestines. These laxatives are safe to take every day and include oat bran, psyllium (e.g., Metamucil), polycarbophil (e.g., FiberCon), and methylcellulose (e.g., Citrucel). Bulk-forming laxatives are most useful in patients with normal-transit constipation, with one study reporting that 80% of this subgroup had resolution of symptoms compared with 35% of patients in the other subgroups.[13]

Stimulant Laxatives

Stimulant laxatives work by stimulating intestinal motility and secretion of water into the bowel. Stimulant laxatives generally take 6 to 12 hours to take effect and may cause abdominal cramping and diarrhea.[5] Products in this class include senna and bisacodyl. Given the poor quality of study design, a lack of placebo-controlled trials, and inconclusive results, the American College of Gastroenterology Chronic Constipation Task Force stated that data were insufficient to make a recommendation regarding the efficacy of stimulant laxatives for the management of chronic constipation, with available data indicated a minimal benefit with these products.[44] Stimulant laxatives may also cause melanosis coli, be habit forming, and have unknown long-term effects on the colon.

Osmotic Laxatives

Saline or osmotic laxatives are hyperosmolar agents that cause secretion of water into the intestinal lumen by osmotic activity. Some of the most commonly used osmotic laxatives are oral magnesium hydroxide (milk of magnesia), oral magnesium citrate, sodium biphosphate (Phospho-Soda), PEG, and lactulose.[5]

Data on the commonly used osmotic laxative, magnesium, are sparse.[45] Despite a lack of evidence, patients and physicians find magnesium helpful and use it routinely.[46]

Use magnesium citrate, 150-mg capsules, to help with constipation. Start with two capsules at bedtime and two in the morning. If no stool occurs the next morning after 4 days, add one capsule (total of three daily) at bedtime. Add one capsule to the evening dose every 4 days until a soft stool is produced each morning. One of the first side effects of magnesium is diarrhea. This helps prevent toxicity from taking too much magnesium. Stop at eight capsules (total of six at bedtime and two in the morning). Use magnesium-containing laxatives cautiously in patients with congestive heart failure and chronic renal insufficiency because of the potential for electrolyte imbalances.

PEG is superior to lactulose in terms of stool frequency per week, form of stool, relief of abdominal pain, and the need for additional products, both in children and adults.[47] Evidence is sufficient to support PEG as a first-line laxative treatment in children, both in terms of efficacy and palatability.[48]

Stool Softeners

These agents, which include docusate sodium, act by lowering surface tension, thus allowing water to enter the bowel more readily. Although stool softeners are generally well tolerated, their efficacy remains in question.[49]

Emollient Laxatives

Mineral oil, the most common example in this category, works by coating and softening the stool. Scant evidence supports the use of mineral oil, which also may lead to depletion of fat-soluble vitamins and increased the risk of aspiration in older adults and children.[50]

Chloride Channel Activators

Lubiprostone and linaclotide are the first agents in this class to be approved by the Food and Drug Administration for the treatment of chronic constipation and constipation-dominant irritable bowel syndrome. These agents work through chloride channels to increase intestinal fluid secretion. Because nausea is the most common complaint, lubiprostone should be taken orally with food and should be avoided in pregnant women and children. Linaclotide is contraindicated in those <6 years old. The safety of lubiprostone has been demonstrated for up to 48 weeks of use.

PREVENTION PRESCRIPTION

- Eat high amounts of fiber-rich foods, including beans, vegetables, fruits, whole grain cereals, and bran.
- Minimize high-fat, low-fiber foods, such as processed foods, dairy products, and meat products.
- Drink an adequate amount of fluid each day to stay hydrated, and increase the amount of water if using higher doses of fiber.
- Engage in regular physical activity to avoid constipation.

- Adopt a good self-care and stress management program to avoid the impact of stress on gut function.
- Stay tuned to the body's natural signals to pass stool.
- Take advantage of the gastrocolic reflex and allow elimination to occur after meals.
- In young children, ensure adequate fiber as they transition to solid foods.

THERAPEUTIC REVIEW

In this summary of therapeutic options for the treatment of constipation, the interventions are presented in a ladder approach from the least to the most invasive options. Although patients with more moderate to severe constipation may travel up the ladder more quickly, the initial approaches are critical for all patients.

ADULTS

Removal of Exacerbating Factors
- Review the patient's medication list and eliminate any medications that may be causing or exacerbating the condition.

Behavioral Training
- If patients experience difficulty in expulsion of stool, they should be advised to place a support approximately 6 inches in height under their feet when they are sitting on a toilet seat, to flex the hips toward a squatting posture.

Nutrition
- Include a gradually increasing amount of fiber in the diet up to 20 to 25 g a day through fruits, vegetables, whole grain breads and unrefined cereals, flax, or bran.   A↑₁
- Encourage increased fluid intake, particularly with the introduction of increased fiber in the diet.   C→₁

Movement
- Encourage regular physical activity.   B↗₁

Perineal Self-Massage
- Dr. Abbott (UCLA) explains the technique in a short video. See below under "Key Web Resources".   B↗₁

Supplements
- Consider adding a commercially packaged fiber supplement, such as psyllium (Metamucil) or methylcellulose (Citrucel). Be sure to take supplements with at least 8 to 12 oz of liquid. Using less fluid can worsen constipation (see Table 46.3).   B↗₁
- Consider a probiotic strain of *Bifidobacterium* or *Lactobacillus* of at least 10⁸ colony-forming units.   B↗₁

Mind-Body Therapy
- Address stress management skills.   C→₁

Biofeedback
- In cases of pelvic floor dysfunction, this is a critical component of therapy.   B↗₁

Pharmaceuticals
- If the foregoing interventions do not resolve symptoms, consider osmotic laxatives with polyethylene glycol (17 to 34 g once or twice daily) as first-line therapy. A↗₂
- For severe cases, a prescription chloride channel activator (lubiprostone, 8 to 24 mcg twice daily for adults; linaclotide, 145 mcg daily 30 minutes before breakfast for adults) may be necessary.   B→₂

CHILDREN

Behavioral Training
- Encourage daily sitting on the toilet, preferably after meals, and avoid embarrassing or punishing the child. Using a stool under the feet can also be used for children during toilet training.

Removal of Exacerbating Factors
- Consider a 4- to 6-week trial of a diet eliminating dairy products. B↗₁

Nutrition
- Ensure an adequate amount of fiber in the diet. Use the age + 5 = daily grams of fiber rule as a general guideline for dosing.   B↗₁
- Increase fluid intake and, in particular, the amount of sorbitol-containing fruit juices (e.g., apple, pear) for osmotic effect. B↗₁

Movement
- Encourage regular physical activity. B↗₁

Supplements
- Consider adding a commercially-packaged fiber supplement if necessary.   B↗₁
- Consider a probiotic strain of *Bifidobacterium* or *Lactobacillus* of at least 10⁸ colony-forming units.   B↗₁

Pharmaceuticals
- If these interventions do not resolve symptoms, consider osmotic laxatives with polyethylene glycol (half to four teaspoons a day, depending on age) as first-line medical treatment (see Table 46.4). A↗₂

Therapies to Consider (or Emerging Therapies)

Fecal transplant therapy: Interest is growing rapidly worldwide regarding the use of fecal microbiota transplantation (FMT) as a "natural" therapy from both patients' and physicians' perspectives. FMT is popular among some patients because it is not associated with the adverse effects of regular medicinal therapy. Although evidence related to chronic constipation is limited to just one trial (n = 3) where chronic constipation was reversed in all patients, [51] it is a therapy to consider in the most refractory patients potentially before extensive surgery.

Key Web Resources

The American College of Gastroenterology	http://www.acg.gi.org/
Patient handout on constipation	http://www.acg.gi.org/patients/pdfs/CommonGIProblems2.pdf
Mayo Clinic patient information on constipation in children	http://www.mayoclinic.com/health/constipation-in-children/DS01138
American Dietetic Association handout for nutrition therapy for constipation	http://nutritioncaremanual.org/vault/editor/Docs/ConstipationNutritionTherapy_FINAL.pdf
Perineal self-acupressure instructional video	http://exploreim.ucla.edu/video/dr-ryan-abbott-on-perineal-self-acupressure-technique-for-chronic-constipation/

REFERENCES

References are available online at ExpertConsult.com.

Adults
- for self message add link to video
- no pharmaceut.

Kids
all except pharmaceuticals

Constipation
2-separate handouts
- 1 for adults
- 1 for child

SECTION IX

AUTOIMMUNE DISORDERS

SECTION OUTLINE

47 FIBROMYALGIA

48 CHRONIC FATIGUE SYNDROME

49 RHEUMATOID ARTHRITIS

50 INFLAMMATORY BOWEL DISEASE

CHAPTER 47

FIBROMYALGIA

Nancy J. Selfridge, MD

PATHOPHYSIOLOGY

Fibromyalgia (FM) is a common cause of widespread pain, occurring in 2%–8% of the general population worldwide. Diagnostic criteria have been through modifications since the American College of Rheumatology (ACR) 1990 criteria were published. Wolfe (2010 and 2011) and Bennett (2013) have devised modified and alternative criteria, respectively, primarily for clinical and epidemiological research.[1,2] Widespread pain of at least a 3-month duration remains a hallmark of the syndrome; however, both sets of criteria can be assessed by patient survey, and both eliminate the tender point count of the 1990 ACR criteria, which was challenging for clinicians to assess reliably. Both tools have high sensitivity and specificity, using the 1990 ACR criteria as the "gold standard." More men meet diagnostic criteria with these newer tools compared to the 1990 ACR criteria.[3] Bennett stresses that diagnostic criteria alone are insufficient for making an accurate diagnosis of FM.[2] Patients benefit from careful evaluation with a thorough medical history and physical examination, which also help establish the foundations of relationship-centered care. FM can coexist with and imitate various autoimmune diseases, hypothyroidism, and some chronic infections such as Lyme disease and hepatitis C. The identification of such disorders as the cause of pain is important to avoid treating these conditions as FM. For coexisting conditions, it is challenging but necessary to determine the contribution of FM to symptoms in order to avoid treating FM with escalating doses of immunosuppressive or disease modifying medications. Laboratory evaluation is guided by the history and physical examination and the evolving differential diagnosis. An exhaustive laboratory and imaging workup is seldom indicated.

Widespread pain for at least 3 months without an identifiable cause is the main diagnostic finding in fibromyalgia.

Central pain sensitization is now considered the primary pathology in FM and is supported by extensive translational neuroimaging research. Functional connectivity on MRI between areas of the brain involved in pain processing and interpretation (dorsolateral prefrontal cortex, anterior cingulate, amygdala, hippocampus, insula, and others) differs in FM patients compared to healthy controls, possibly mediated by altered glutamate and gamma-amino butyric acid (GABA) levels, which will, in turn, affect other neurotransmitter levels.[4-7] When an intervention appears to help reduce pain parameters, functional connectivity appears to normalize.[4,6] Some evidence indicates that familial predisposition and gene polymorphisms may play a role in FM.[8-10] Careful history taking often reveals a significant stressful trigger event or period, such as an accident, a flulike illness, emotional stress, or overwork, preceding the onset of symptoms.[3] The discovery of observable central nervous system (CNS) abnormalities in FM patients stimulates curiosity about the varied ways that the physiology of the stress response might change a brain to manifest as chronic pain and physical symptoms, given certain predisposing variables.

Autonomic dysfunction is present in patients with FM, a likely cause of a variety of symptoms that are occasionally reported as more problematic than pain.[8] Increased sympathetic activity is correlated with increased pain intensity, explaining worsening of symptoms with stress.[11] Several neuroendocrine and immune function alterations have been well documented in FM.[12-18] Although these immunological changes in FM do not meet criteria for immunodeficiency or autoimmune disease, they likely contribute to symptoms.

Research has shown that a subset of patients (approximately 20%) may have biopsy evidence of small fiber peripheral neuropathy.[19,20] It is not yet currently recommended that patients undergo biopsy to detect this problem; however, clinicians should be on the alert for evolving clinical recommendations and guidelines.

Although the precise etiological and pathophysiological roles of the foregoing alterations in neurophysiological, immune, and neuroendocrine functions are unknown, their existence helps dispel any notion that FM is a purely psychosocial disorder. A list of pathological findings in FM patients from recent research is shown in Fig. 47.1.

A sensitive temperament, characterized by high levels of empathy, and a higher than normal sensitivity to environmental factors and emotional cues from others, appears to be a premorbid condition for many patients.[21,22] In addition, FM patients have been shown to demonstrate alexithymia more than healthy controls, with difficulties both in identifying and describing feelings. Further, the degree of alexithymia is correlated with increased pain experience.[23,24] The tension of experiencing stressful triggers and the consequence of living in a society that expects high productivity at the expense of self-care, superimposed on a natural sensitivity and inability to express feelings, may predispose the CNS of FM patients to abnormal sensory

- **Neurophysiological**
  - Reduced levels of hippocampal n-acetyl aspartate
  - Elevated levels of glutamate:
    - o posterior insula
    - o amygdala
    - o posterior cingulate
    - o ventral lateral prefrontal cortex
  - Reduced levels of GABA
    - o Anterior insula
  - Altered functional connectivity between
    - o Insula
    - o DMN€
    - o EAN§
  - Reduced resting connectivity within somatosensory cortex
  - Increased functional connectivity between
    - o Somatosensory cortex
    - o DMN€
  - Small fiber neuropathy (20%)
- **Neuroendocrine**
  - Elevated CSF substance P
  - Impaired growth hormone secretion in response to exercise
  - Excessive sympathetic autonomic tone
  - Reduced IGF-1 levels
- **Immunologic**
  - Elevated CFS Interleukin-8
  - Altered lymphocyte corticosteroid receptors
  - Decreased T cell activation marker expression

FIG. 47.1 ■ Examples of pathological findings of recent translational research on fibromyalgia.[3-8,12-20] €DMN (Default Mode Network) consists of the posterior cingulate, precuneus, medial prefrontal cortex, hippocampal formation, and lateral temporal cortex; it is believed to be engaged in self-referential cognition.[3] §EAN (Executive Attention Network) consists of the dorsolateral prefrontal and posterior parietal cortices and is engaged in executive control over behavior.[3]

processing. High body mass index and reduced physical activity have also been found to be independent risk factors for FM.[25,26]

Despite the fact that the precise mechanism of the disorder remains obscure and is likely quite complex, great hope is contained in the fact that patients with FM can and do respond to a variety of nonpharmacological interventions. This fact may be a testament to the plasticity of the nervous system and its ability to change even in

adults, although we cannot yet evoke reliable changes at will with any given intervention.

INTEGRATIVE THERAPY

General Considerations

Patients with FM are often viewed as difficult or burdensome in busy practices. Patients with other "algo-dysfunctional" syndromes (e.g., chronic chest wall pain, chronic abdominal pain of undetermined origin, irritable bowel syndrome, interstitial cystitis, chronic pelvic pain, dyspareunia, and vulvodynia) present similar challenges: symptoms that are not correlated with physical findings, poorly understood pathophysiology, significant impact on quality of life, and limited response to simple pharmaceutical interventions. Keeping abreast of translational research in FM is onerous in a busy, diverse medical practice. Consequently, well-meaning physicians often communicate invalidating messages to patients both verbally and nonverbally. This is a cognitive and clinical error on the part of the physician. First, evidence of altered neurophysiology and immune function in FM is strong. Second, research indicates that patients experience such invalidation as harmful; invalidation by and mistrust in the physician are correlated with lower quality of life among FM patients.[27] Providing generous listening and affirming the patient's experiences of what often appear to be bizarre or exaggerated symptoms are important because most treatment interventions for FM have demonstrated limited efficacy. Patients experience affirmation as therapeutic, and it is something that all clinicians can provide (see Chapter 3).

> Citing current research that points to a change in the way that the brain processes sensory information, and explaining that FM is a disorder of central nervous system pain sensitization and augmentation associated with neuroendocrine and immune system abnormalities, can help patients move past unreasonable worry and concerns about misdiagnosis.

Promoting the concept that patients can leverage neuroplasticity by trying various integrative interventions and changes in behavior and thinking fosters self-efficacy and seems to support the fact that nonpharmacological therapies have better evidence of efficacy compared with that of medications.[28] Active listening to a patient, demonstrating empathy, and eliciting his/her perspectives may help favorably alter the physiology of the stress response and thus help reduce autonomic dysfunction, pain sensitivity, and other symptoms.[29]

Nutrition

No specific diet has been shown to be effective for FM. However, obesity and being overweight contribute to lower quality of life scores.[30] Motivational interviewing techniques (see Chapter 101) are recommended to move overweight patients toward weight reduction. An increase in dietary antioxidant intake may be beneficial based on evidence of increased oxidative stress and reduced antioxidant enzyme activities in FM patients, although no specific supplements are currently supported by research.[30] An antiinflammatory diet, with increased consumption of whole plant based foods and avoidance of processed foods, may be helpful (see Chapter 88) and likely benefits patients' health in a more general way. Removal of excitotoxins such as MSG and aspartame from the diet may be rational in light of the CNS abnormalities in glutamate and GABA distribution and function observed in FM patients, though research support is mixed.[30] Strict avoidance of trans fats (partially hydrogenated oils, margarine, and shortening) and increased consumption of foods rich in omega-3 fatty acids, calcium, and antioxidants are strongly encouraged and address some of the common deficiencies in the standard U.S. diet.

Exercise

Poor physical fitness is associated with increased symptom severity in FM patients.[26] A 2014 systematic review concluded that diverse forms of exercise have a beneficial effect on physical function and help decrease some of the symptoms of FM.[31] Adherence and attrition have been problematic in many research studies on exercise in FM. Postexercise fatigue and pain and tenderness are frequently severe and can lead to a cycle of muscle disuse.[31,32] Thus, although exercise prescriptions are prudent for all patients with FM, clinicians must think flexibly about exercise and be willing to revise recommendations based on individual patient preferences and experiences. Aquatic exercise appears to provide as much symptom benefit and only slightly less improvement in muscle strength than land-based exercise.[33] Eastern movement practices (tai chi, yoga, qigong) have demonstrated some promise in improving FM symptoms in research; some patients find these forms of body movement easier and more acceptable than conventional exercise.[34-36] Walking exercise can similarly be endorsed as helpful.[37]

Even though activation of the patient through exercise is a most desirable treatment goal, many patients demonstrate resistance. Efforts should be aimed at helping patients both initiate and adhere to an exercise routine. Again, motivational interviewing techniques can be particularly effective in moving resistant patients toward a regular exercise habit. It can be useful to explore our patient's frame by asking, sometimes repeatedly over a long relationship, "What are you finding hard about starting or sticking with an exercise program?" Severe postexercise pain is often cited, but many patients are similar to our usual primary care patients in that they have never embraced an active, exercise-oriented lifestyle. Exploring the patient's present position in the stage of change continuum (precontemplation, contemplation, preparation, action, and maintenance) and focusing on moving to the next stage can help mitigate clinician frustration when patients find it hard to adhere to treatment plans. Current data supports such a broad range of exercise modalities that finding any kind of movement that patients can enjoy regularly and perceive as pleasurable is

intuitively the key to success. Even a cumulative daily 30 minutes of self-selected lifestyle physical activity can provide improvement in FM symptoms[38] (see Chapter 91).

> Evidence suggests that Eastern movement practices, such as tai chi, yoga, and qigong, which include meditative components, may reduce pain and improve function in patients with fibromyalgia.

Bodywork

A variety of bodywork interventions and massage seem to positively affect health-related quality of life for fibromyalgia patients, although pain and other symptoms are not a reliably improved.[39] Though the quality and quantity of evidence is still low, massage and body work interventions are low risk and accessible. Patients can be encouraged to try various modalities if they are so inclined.

Mind-Body Therapy

Meditation

Meditation has been reported to be helpful for a variety of FM symptoms.[40] Results from a recent experimental trial with a wait list control group and a randomized prospective trial supported the practice of mediation.[41,42] Unfortunately, studies are plagued by poor design and methodological flaws. Some of the studies documenting FM symptom improvement with Eastern movement therapies include a strong meditation component, which may substantially contribute to the efficacy of this type of exercise.[34-36] Meditation training increases body awareness and the ability to be comfortable in the present moment and thus can lessen fear of future pain and, with practice, help transform the sensation of pain. Meditation may have additional, as yet undetermined benefits by favorably altering neurophysiology in patients with FM. Meditation is also useful for personal growth, is quite safe, and is accessible in many communities and through online support (see Chapter 100).

Psychotherapeutic and Mind-Body Interventions

Cognitive behavioral therapy (CBT) appears to be somewhat better than pharmacotherapy at improving quality of life and other symptoms in FM patients and is more cost effective.[43,44] Internet-based CBT is reportedly effective for several symptoms, a great advantage in increasing accessibility to this type of intervention.[45] Electromyographic biofeedback, electroencephalographic biofeedback, and hypnotherapy have demonstrated benefit in controlled studies.[46-48] Guided imagery may also be helpful[49] (see Chapter 97).

A randomized controlled study of an Affective Self-Awareness program involving a group intervention of emotional exploration through journaling and meditation demonstrated significant benefit for symptoms and perceived function in patients with FM[50] (see Chapter 102). Anecdotal evidence also supports increasing emotional awareness as a way to mitigate chronic pain.[51,52] Known neurobiological associations between pain and emotion illuminate potential targets for mind-body interventions.[53] Although more research is needed on mind-body interventions, these generally low-risk and low-harm interventions should be part of every treatment plan for patients with FM because of their potential to alter the neurobiological associations between pain and emotion in ways that improve symptoms. When patients are either not receptive to these interventions, or when patients experience increasing disability, it may be helpful for the clinician to explore the following "four Rs" with the patient and encourage self-reflection in journaling if possible[54]:

- Roles: The patient's ability to maintain self-esteem through normal roles as spouse, parent, provider, and so on may be impaired. The work role requires careful evaluation and is often problematic for people who are becoming progressively more symptomatic and disabled. Focus on a simple question as a way of exploring where problems may exist: "In all your roles, are you living for your heart's desires?"
- Reactions: Emotional reactions to events, such as the diagnosis of FM or events that trigger FM, often follow a grieving process.[55] Patients are often stuck in anger and depression and yet may not recognize or be able to easily express their distress.
- Relationships: The patient may often face seemingly insurmountable problems at home or in relationships at work that create repeated stress triggers for symptoms.
- Resources: Psychotherapy, ministers, community programs, self-help groups, and other sources of support and connection may help alter progressive decrease in ability to function. Isolation and alienation clearly make patients symptomatically worse.

Acupuncture

There is low to moderate level evidence that acupuncture and acupoint stimulation temporarily help with some FM symptoms compared to standard treatment or no treatment.[56,57] Electroacupuncture appears to be better than manual acupuncture for most FM symptoms. Studies have been handicapped by small sample sizes and methodological flaws; however, acupuncture has been shown to be safe and well tolerated, and it can be endorsed for patients who wish to try it.

Homeopathy

A 2015 review of complementary and alternative medicine (CAM) therapies for FM summarized three small randomized controlled studies on homeopathic treatments for FM.[58] In these studies, *Rhus toxicodendron*, *Arnica montana*, *Bryonia alba*, and individualized homeopathic remedies were all superior to placebo in treating several symptoms. Though evidence is limited and mechanisms of action remain obscure, homeopathy is considered safe. Patients should be referred to a homeopathic physician for optimum evaluation and treatment

with the understanding that homeopathic remedies may not work well in the presence of certain pharmaceuticals (see Chapter 115).

Supplements

Low evidence of efficacy exists for supplements and natural medicines in the treatment of FM. Further, the use of some common supplements, such as calcium, selenium, and vitamin E, has come under scrutiny as possibly unsafe. Herbal and natural medicines potentially interact with one another and with prescription medications. Thus, a good peer-reviewed and frequently updated database (e.g., Natural Medicines Comprehensive Database; see Key Web Resources) should be used by integrative clinicians to assess available evidence regarding efficacy and harm before recommending supplements and natural medicine therapy. Currently, no natural medicines or supplements have sufficient evidence of efficacy specifically for FM symptoms to strongly recommend them for patients. However, some supplements may be beneficial in select patients for select symptoms based on known or proposed mechanisms of action and evidence of efficacy for other conditions.

Omega-3 Fatty Acids

Use of omega-3 fatty acid supplementation in the form of pharmaceutical grade fish oil, 2–4 g daily in a single dose, may have a modest pain-modulating effect for some patients and may help treat depression in some patients. In general, supplementation with omega-3 fatty acids may also lower cardiovascular risk and help to balance the predominance of proinflammatory omega-6 fatty acids in the typical U.S. diet.

DOSAGE

The recommended dose is 2000 to 4000 mg once daily.

PRECAUTIONS

Omega-3 fatty acids inhibit platelet function and should be discontinued 2 weeks before elective surgical procedures. Use with caution in patients receiving anticoagulant therapy. Choose a pharmaceutical grade product to avoid heavy metal contamination.

Vitamin D

Low vitamin D levels appear to be epidemic at northern latitudes. Although the link between low vitamin D and the pain of FM remains unclear, evidence indicates that low vitamin D levels can be associated with widespread pain.[59] Because of this association, it is not unreasonable to check 25-(OH) vitamin D levels in FM patients at risk for vitamin D insufficiency and supplement with vitamin D to maintain optimal blood levels (40–100 ng/mL) year round. As a general rule, 1000 units of vitamin D_3 (cholecalciferol) will raise serum 25-(OH) vitamin D levels in adults approximately 10 ng/mL. Although overdosing is unlikely, clinicians recommending vitamin D should be aware that vitamin D levels may be higher in patients in the summer if they have sufficient skin exposure to sunlight.

DOSAGE

Cholecalciferol (vitamin D₃) oral supplements in capsule or liquid form can be taken to attain a year round 25-(OH) vitamin D level of 40–100 ng/mL. Seasonal dosage adjustments may be necessary.

PRECAUTIONS

Vitamin D is not to be used in patients who have primary hyperparathyroidism or granulomatous disease, such as sarcoidosis, because of the increased risk of hypercalcemia.

Magnesium

Magnesium may be helpful for some patients with FM, possibly through its muscle-relaxing properties, and it is quite safe.

DOSAGE

The recommended dose is 400–750 mg once daily.

PRECAUTIONS

At higher doses, magnesium may cause abdominal cramping and increased frequency of stools, helping patients recognize when they are taking too much.

S-Adenosylmethionine

S-adenosylmethionine (SAMe) was demonstrated to be safe and effective in alleviating depression when administered to patients who failed to respond adequately to monotherapy with a selective serotonin reuptake inhibitor (SSRI).[60] Although SAMe may have only a modest effect on other FM symptoms, this supplement can be helpful in patients to treat coexisting depressive symptoms.[61]

DOSAGE

The recommended dose is 400–800 mg twice daily.

PRECAUTIONS

SAMe can act as a stimulant and should not be taken close to bedtime because it can cause insomnia. It is expensive.

Botanicals

No adequate controlled trials of botanical treatments have been conducted. In anecdotal reports, many treatments lead to a benefit that wanes with time, a finding that may indicate a short-term placebo effect. Individual patients may benefit from trials of botanicals purported to be helpful for common symptoms of FM, such as low energy, insomnia, and depressed mood.

Turmeric and Ginger

The use of turmeric and ginger in cooking at culinary doses may provide benefit for some patients due to pain-modulating and antiinflammatory properties. At these doses, these spices are likely safe and can be encouraged. When these agents are used at supplement doses, potential side effects and interactions must be considered.

DOSAGE

Ginger may be taken as dried root, starting at 1 g total per day, divided into two or three doses, increasing to up to 4 g daily; or as tea, 1 g of dried root steeped in 150 mL of boiling water for 5 to 10 minutes and strained, one cup up to four times daily.

Turmeric may be taken as powdered root, 0.5–1 g two or three times daily.

PRECAUTIONS

Because turmeric and ginger have platelet-inhibiting activities, they must be used with caution in patients taking anticoagulant therapy and should be discontinued 2 weeks before elective surgical procedures. Both cause gallbladder contraction and may be problematic in patients with gallstones. Ginger may lower blood glucose levels.

Boswellia

Boswellia is an ayurvedic herb that has some documented antiinflammatory and analgesic effects.

DOSAGE

The recommended dose is 500 mg of standardized product three times daily.

PRECAUTIONS

Platelet inhibition and increased bleeding risk are possible with this plant substance. Discontinue 2 weeks before elective surgical procedures.

St. John's Wort

For patients who need treatment for depression and do not wish to use prescription pharmaceuticals, St. John's wort may be helpful.

DOSAGE

The recommended dose is 300 mg up to three times daily of a 0.3% hypericin standardized extract or as tea, steep 2–4 g of the dried herb in 150 mL of boiling water for 5 to 10 minutes and strain, one cup up to three times daily.

PRECAUTIONS

Multiple potential interactions with other drugs occur through stimulation of the cytochrome P-450 enzymes of the liver. The result is lower serum levels of drugs that are cleared by this mechanism.

Pharmaceuticals

Medications can be helpful for FM, although improvement in symptoms is seldom dramatic. In recent reviews, 50% of patients will experience a 30% improvement in symptoms and 30% of patients will experience a 50% improvement, only slightly better than placebo.[62] Side effects are common and interfere with adherence.

Antidepressants

Treating comorbid depression in patients with FM is in their best interest as depression worsens FM symptom severity and prognosis.[63,64] Further, antidepressants can help improve sleep and have modulating effects on pain through norepinephrine and serotonin pathways. Tricyclic antidepressants (TCAs) have been the gold standard of treatment and remain inexpensive and widely available; although they are not FDA approved for FM, amitriptyline is approved for chronic neuropathic pain and has been widely used for FM. Side effects are often prohibitive at higher antidepressant doses. Research on selective serotonin reuptake inhibitors (SSRIs) for the pain of FM has yielded mixed results.[65] The newer dual serotonin and norepinephrine reuptake inhibitors (SNRIs), duloxetine and milnacipran, have compared quite favorably with amitriptyline for the treatment of depression and are FDA approved for FM treatment. These two drugs have been better than placebo for mitigating FM pain and improving function; however, the effect size for these improvements is small, and the clinical significance remains questionable when weighed against common side effects.[62] Clinicians must monitor patients closely and balance improvements in FM symptoms against adverse effects that often interfere with quality of life and functioning. Trazodone may help with sleep and measures of quality of life with a tolerable side effect profile. When combined with pregabalin, trazodone may be helpful in reducing pain as well.[66,67] Although cyclobenzaprine is not an antidepressant, it is closely related to the TCAs, and reviews have supported its use in FM.[62,68]

The clinician should develop a familiarity with several different antidepressants to feel comfortable managing the myriad of possible side effects and potential drug–drug and drug–botanical interactions. For example, patients sometimes add St. John's wort to their prescribed regimens. Serotonin syndrome is a distinct risk when this natural medicine is taken with SSRIs or with SNRIs. Be sure to ask specifically about the use of St. John's wort in patients who are taking these prescription antidepressants.

Tricyclics

DOSAGE

The recommended dose of amitriptyline is 5–10 mg at bedtime initially, titrating upward as needed.

PRECAUTIONS

Excessive sedation, anticholinergic effects, and hypotension may occur.

Selective Serotonin Reuptake Inhibitors

DOSAGE

Fluoxetine is started at 5–20 mg daily and titrated upward as needed. Citalopram is started at 20 mg daily and may be titrated up to 40 mg daily. Escitalopram is started at 10 mg per day and may be titrated up to 20 mg daily.

SSRI PRECAUTIONS

Activation or sedation, induction of mania, hot flushes and sweating, weight gain, sexual dysfunction, and multiple potential drug interactions are possible.

Serotonin and Norepinephrine Reuptake Inhibitors

DOSAGE

Duloxetine is started at 30 mg once daily for 1 week then increased to 60 mg daily. Milnacipran is started at 12.5 mg once daily on the first day, and increased by 12.5 to 25 mg daily for the first week until 50 mg twice daily dosing attained. A dose of 100 mg twice daily may ultimately be necessary for symptom relief.

PRECAUTIONS

Precautions are potentially the same as for TCAs and SSRIs.

Trazodone

DOSAGE

Initiate therapy with 25–50 mg nightly, titrating upward to 300 mg or until the patient reports good sleep and no excess morning grogginess.

PRECAUTIONS

Oversedation, orthostatic hypotension, morning grogginess, and vivid dreams may occur.

Cyclobenzaprine

DOSAGE

Start with 2.5–10 mg at bedtime and titrate up to 40 daily, in divided doses.

PRECAUTIONS

Excessive sedation and an increase in "mental fogging" may occur.

Nonsteroidal Antiinflammatory Drugs

Nonsteroidal antiinflammatory drugs (NSAIDs) continue to be widely used despite evidence that chronic use is associated with health risks. Because of the limited evidence of efficacy and the potential for adverse effects, particularly with long-term use, it is wise to discourage NSAID use for FM and encourage other pain management strategies.

Anticonvulsants

Gabapentin has been used off-label for FM because of its indication for use in chronic neuropathic pain. This agent appears to be safe and efficacious for FM.[69] A similar pharmaceutical, pregabalin, appears to be effective compared with other newer FM drugs and is FDA approved.[62] Both drugs often cause somnolence and dizziness. Significant weight gain with pregabalin is not uncommon and can interfere with adherence. Because significant weight gain can also increase the risk of other chronic diseases, such as hypertension, insulin resistance, and type 2 diabetes, this side effect cannot be considered trivial.

DOSAGE

Gabapentin is started at 300 mg once daily and increased by one tablet to twice per day, then three times per day as tolerated. The maximum dose is 3600 mg daily, although no therapeutic advantage has been shown for neuropathic pain in clinical trials for doses greater than 1800 mg daily. Pregabalin is started at 75 mg twice daily and may be titrated up to a maintenance dose of 450 mg daily, in two divided doses.

PRECAUTIONS

Gabapentin may cause sedation, dizziness, cognitive impairment, and leukopenia, whereas pregabalin may cause sedation, dizziness, weight gain, and thrombocytopenia.

Analgesics

Tramadol

Tramadol is the only opioid that has been shown to have evidence of efficacy in FM.[70] It is a weak μ opioid receptor agonist and also inhibits reuptake of serotonin and norepinephrine. Although studies are limited, tramadol appears to improve pain and quality of life.[62] Because of its mechanism of action, the use of tramadol with antidepressants or St. John's wort potentially causes serotonin syndrome. Tramadol can also cause excessive sedation, and abuse and addiction potential are real. Thus tramadol may be most useful as intermittent therapy for pain exacerbations, avoiding chronic use and dose escalation.

DOSAGE

The recommended dose is 50–400 mg daily in divided doses.

PRECAUTIONS

Sedation, habituation, and serotonin syndrome may occur when prescribed in combination with antidepressants or St. John's wort.

Opioids can induce hyperalgesia, a side effect that FM patients may be more susceptible to because of their baseline centralized pain sensitization. Opioids are not recommended for the treatment of FM.

Cannabinoids

A 2011 systematic review of research on cannabinoids for chronic noncancer pain reported that these drugs may be helpful both for pain and for improving sleep.[71] Two small studies of nabilone have yielded positive outcomes for FM; however, side effects were common. These drugs are not presently approved by the FDA for FM and carry some toxicity potential when they are abused. A cross-sectional survey of FM patients using cannabis compared to nonuser control patients reported some improvement in pain and psychological state, though not in quality of life measures.[72] Patients may ask about the efficacy of cannabis and cannabinoids given the increasing number of states legalizing cannabis for medical and recreational use.

Other Therapies to Consider

Recent reviews of spa therapy and balneotherapy (bathing in hot mineral springs) suggest that these treatments are helpful for multiple symptoms and can have long-lasting effects.[73,74] Patients with access to hot mineral springs and spas can be encouraged to try this modality. Repetitive transcranial magnetic stimulation (rTMS) appears to be promising for improving pain and quality of life for many types of chronic pain, though more research is needed to determine precise protocols for maximum efficacy in treating FM.[75,76] It is expensive ($6,000 to $10,000 for a 4-week course of treatment). Traditional Chinese medicine (TCM) may be helpful for FM, though studies are limited by sample size and methodological flaws.[77] We can encourage and educate patients drawn to explore alternative healing traditions (e.g., TCM, Ayurveda, or shamanism) in a shared decision-making process. Patients may then choose to visit practitioners of the selected therapies to explore the approaches further. If the economic burden is not too great, the addition of this therapeutic modality may be in order.

Another area of potential benefit for patients with FM is emerging from the growing field of energy psychology and energy medicine (see Chapters 103 and 116). Though more research is needed to assess efficacy and to determine mechanism of action, these interventions are safe, and some of them can be learned by the patient and practiced at home.

Summary

Mainstays of a treatment plan for fibromyalgia include an exercise prescription, weight reduction when needed, mind-body types of interventions, treatment of comorbid depression and sleep problems, and judicious trials of other complementary and alternative medicine modalities and conventional pharmaceuticals. However, *every* treatment plan should be individualized and flexible. Fig. 47.2 illustrates a rational approach to an individualized integrative treatment plan for patients newly diagnosed with fibromyalgia.

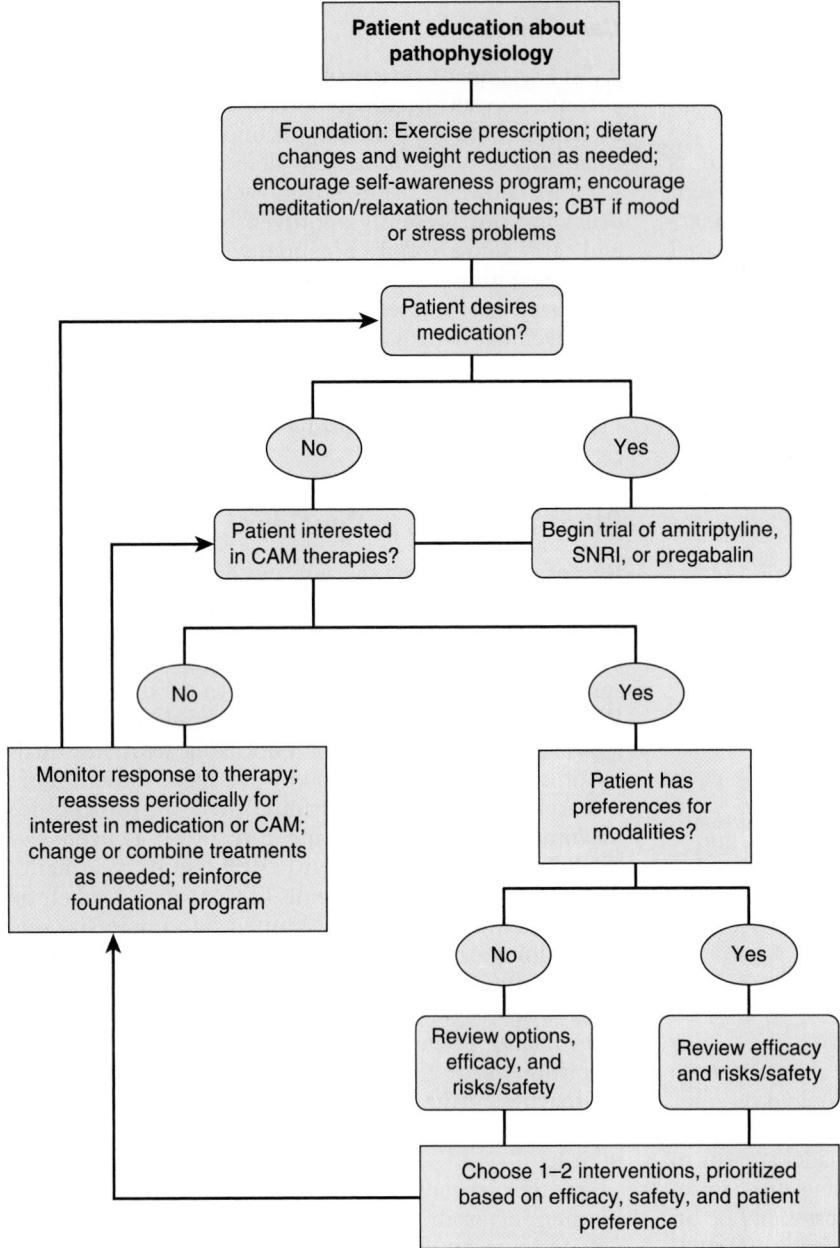

FIG. 47.2 ■ A rational approach to an individualized integrative treatment plan for fibromyalgia.

PREVENTION PRESCRIPTION

No proven preventive strategy exists for FM, but the following may help fortify a susceptible individual against the "slings and arrows of outrageous fortune":

- Exercise and maintain a normal body weight. Combine aerobics, strength training, and stretching. Consider tai chi and yoga. Make exercise a time to play.
- Eat a healthy whole foods diet rich in plant sources of antioxidants. Avoid trans fats and excess caffeine, alcohol, sugars, MSG, and aspartame.
- Honor your temperament and sensitivity. Learn more about yourself and your unique needs and values in work and relationships.

- Journal to stay in touch with your inner feelings and to give voice to negative feelings and stressful events when they arise.
- Put yourself high on the list of things to take care of each day. Consider regular massage therapy or other bodywork to this end.
- Learn to meditate and practice daily. A mindfulness-based stress reduction course is recommended for the structure and support it offers.
- Allow yourself creative outlets such as art, music, dancing, or creative writing.
- Live for your own heart's desires; give yourself permission to figure out what these are.
- If you get stuck in life, find a good psychotherapist.

THERAPEUTIC REVIEW

This summary provides the most helpful options for treating FM symptoms. FM has no documented "cure," and few patients experience complete resolution of symptoms. Despite this dismal fact, the therapeutic benefit of generous listening and affirming the patient's felt experience help. In clinical practice, most patients will report some relief of symptoms with attention and individualized treatment.

NUTRITION

- Weight reduction toward a normal BMI
- A whole foods antiinflammatory diet with ample plant antioxidants, omega-3 fatty acids, and minerals
- Avoidance of trans fats and simple sugars
- Avoidance of MSG and aspartame

EXERCISE

- Exercise prescription tailored to patient preferences and fitness level
- Land- or water-based aerobic exercise, strength training, and stretching
- Encourage patients to try tai chi, yoga, and qi-gong
- 30 minutes of daily cumulative lifestyle activity

MIND-BODY THERAPY

- Mindfulness meditation training and daily practice
- Mind-body self-awareness books and program
- Journaling about emotions and stressors to help increase affective self-awareness
- Cognitive-behavioral therapy for any identified psychological or life struggles

ACUPUNCTURE

- A five-session trial of electro-acupuncture

BODYWORK

- Regular massage therapy or other bodywork

SUPPLEMENTS

- Omega-3 fatty acids (fish oil): 2000–4000 mg daily
- Magnesium: 400–750 mg daily
- Vitamin D₃ (cholecalciferol) to maintain 25-(OH) vitamin D levels between 40–100 ng/mL year round
- S-adenosylmethionine: 800 mg twice daily

BOTANICALS

- Turmeric, ground root: 500–1000 mg two to three times daily
- Ginger, ground root: 1–4 g total daily divided into two to three doses
- Boswellia: 250–500 mg three times daily
- St. John's wort: 300 mg three times daily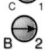

PHARMACEUTICALS

Tricyclic Antidepressants and Similar

- Amitriptyline: 5–50 mg nightly as tolerated
- Cyclobenzaprine: 2.5 mg daily, titrating to 40 mg daily in divided doses as needed
- Trazodone: 25–300 mg nightly as needed

SSRI

- Fluoxetine: 10–20 mg daily
- Citalopram: 20–40 mg daily
- Escitalopram: 10–20 mg daily

SNRI

- Duloxetine: 30 mg for 1 week, increasing to 60 mg thereafter
- Milnacipran: 12.5 mg daily, increasing to 50 mg twice daily by the end of the first week; 100 mg twice daily may be needed

Anticonvulsants

- Gabapentin: 300 mg initially, increasing to a maximum of 1800 mg daily as tolerated
- Pregabalin: 50 mg three times daily, increasing to 450 mg per day over 7 days

Analgesics

- Tramadol: 50–400 mg daily in divided doses

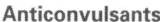

Key Web Resources

Natural medicines database	http://naturaldatabase.therapeuticresearch.com
Emotional awareness program for FM	http://www.unlearnyourpain.com
Exercise videos safe for pain patients	http://www.arthritis.org
Free mindfulness meditation resources	http://www.freemindfulness.org/

REFERENCES

References are available online at ExpertConsult.com.

CHAPTER 48

CHRONIC FATIGUE SYNDROME

Sanford H. Levy, MD, FACP, ABIHM

PATHOPHYSIOLOGY

The pathophysiology of chronic fatigue syndrome (CFS) is not well understood. Some experts believe that CFS and fibromyalgia are part of a single spectrum of disease; in this textbook, fibromyalgia is the subject of a separate chapter. Although this chapter is in the Autoimmune section of this textbook, it is uncertain as to whether CFS is an autoimmune disorder.

Infection is a common precipitant to CFS, based upon patient histories. A hypothesized mechanism is immune system dysfunction, such that interferon continues to be secreted in high amounts even after the resolution of acute infection. Excessive interferon can cause achiness, brain fog, and fatigue. In one 12-month prospective cohort study of 253 patients infected with Epstein-Barr Virus (EBV), Ross River virus, or *Coxiella burnetii*, 28 patients met criteria for CFS at 6 months after onset of infection, with the severity of initial infection found to be a predictor of progression to CFS.[1]

Oxidative stress is a factor, but may well be a consequence rather than an underlying cause. Preliminary research in those with obstructive sleep apnea shows that sleep deprivation increases inflammatory cytokines by 40%.[2] Hypercoagulability is also a factor; researchers performing a variety of assays on 54 patients with CFS/fibromyalgia concluded that 50 of the 54 (92%) had evidence of a hypercoagulable state.[3]

Richard A. Van Konynenburg, PhD, has hypothesized that a methylation cycle block causes depletion of glutathione in some who suffer from CFS. This hypothesis predicts that the key to treatment is to interrupt this vicious cycle by stimulating the enzyme, methionine synthase. This theory was presented in a poster presentation[4] and also in an article published in the *Townsend Letter*,[5] a nonpeer-reviewed medical journal. A search of Medline citations for this author fails to reveal any publications in the peer-reviewed medical literature.

Etiology

The etiology of many cases of CFS is believed to be hypothalamic dysfunction.[6,7] A hypothesis, advocated by Jacob Teitelbaum, MD, is that the energy demands of the body are more than it can meet, so it "blows a fuse" in the hypothalamus and the ensuing fatigue protects the body from harm.[8] Mitochondrial dysfunction is hypothesized to contribute to this imbalance between energy supply and energy demand. Nutritional deficiencies or insufficiencies may contribute to this imbalance. In addition, personality type may also contribute to this imbalance.

The hypothalamic dysfunction is hypothesized to cause disturbances of sleep, hormonal balance, and autonomic control. A vicious cycle is established whereby the sleep disturbance can cause immune dysfunction and further hormonal imbalances.

Stress and exposure to environmental toxins, including pesticides, herbicides, persistent organic pollutants (POPs), and toxic metals (such as mercury, lead, cadmium, and arsenic), are hypothesized to contribute to the development of CFS; 53%–67% of patients with CFS have reported at least one episode of symptom flare after specific chemical exposure.[9] A survey completed 10 years after the Gulf War comparing the health of 1061 deployed veterans to 1128 nondeployed veterans found that their physical health was similar, but deployed veterans had an adjusted odds ratio of chronic fatigue syndrome of 40.6.[10] Hypothesized explanations for this very high odds ratio include stress and exposure to toxins.

Historically, some have proposed that a viral infection is the cause of CFS. In the 1980s, chronic EBV was hypothesized to be the cause of CFS. In the 1990s, HSV 6 was hypothesized as the cause of CFS. However, ongoing research suggests that high viral titers for viruses such as EBV and HSV 6 are a consequence of immune system dysfunction in those with CFS. More recently, researchers have hypothesized xenotropic murine leukemia virus (XMRV) was a cause of CFS. However, methodological issues were identified with the initial positive study, and additional studies seem to rule out a causal link between XMRV and CFS.[11]

Diagnosis

Historically, CFS was defined as more than 6 months of fatigue not relieved by rest and severe enough to interfere with daily activities, not due to another diagnosable cause, and often associated with fever, sore throat, lymphadenopathy, achiness, trouble concentrating, and/or sleep disturbance.[12]

The Institute of Medicine (IOM), in a February 2015 expert committee report, proposed the following diagnostic criteria[13]:

- A substantial reduction or impairment in the ability to engage in preillness levels of occupational, educational, social, or personal activities, that persists for more than 6 months and is accompanied by fatigue, which is often profound, is of new or definite onset (not lifelong), is not the result of ongoing excessive exertion, and is not substantially alleviated by rest, and
- Postexertional malaise, after physical, cognitive, or emotional activity, at least half the time of moderate, substantial or severe intensity, and

- Unrefreshing sleep, at least half the time of moderate, substantial or severe intensity, and
- At least one of the following:
  - Cognitive impairment, at least half the time of moderate, substantial or severe intensity, and
  - Orthostatic intolerance

In this same February 2015 report, the IOM proposed renaming CFS as "systemic exertion intolerance disease," stating that this name provides a more accurate description of the condition.

> The Institute of Medicine, in a February 2015 report, proposed new diagnostic criteria for CFS and renaming of CFS as "systemic exertional intolerance disease (SEID)."

Impact

Chronic fatigue syndrome affects between 836,000 and 2.5 million individuals in the United States,[14] with an estimated total economic cost of $17 to $24 billion.[15] As many as 25% of those with CFS are homebound or bedridden, sometimes for extended periods.[16]

INTEGRATIVE THERAPY

Conventional Treatment

For decades, the standard of care for CFS has been cognitive behavioral therapy (CBT) and graded exercise therapy (GET). Historically, this standard of care was based on small studies. More recently, the large, multiarm PACE trial, described in the following text, has been completed.

A 2008 Cochrane review of 15 studies (n = 1043) of CBT concluded, "CBT is effective in reducing the symptoms of fatigue at posttreatment compared with usual care and may be more effective in reducing fatigue symptoms compared with other psychological therapies. The evidence base at follow-up is limited to a small group of studies with inconsistent findings."[17] While there is strong evidence for the efficacy of CBT, with improvement often sustained for months, various studies have shown that only approximately 30% of people with chronic fatigue syndrome (CFS) recover after cognitive behavior therapy. There is abundant published literature on CBT for treating CFS, with published studies including topics of internet-based CBT; telephone-based CBT; and predictors of a positive response to CBT as a function of practitioner characteristics, patient characteristics, and/or the therapeutic relationship. One study examined outcomes as a function neuropsychological test performance and found that neuropsychological test performance was not related to the change in fatigue, functional impairments, and physical limitations following CBT for CFS, but that underperforming patients did drop out more often.[18] Level of depression may be the most important factor of the cognitive-behavioral model predicting posttreatment

fatigue in CFS.[19] Of note, low cortisol levels, as assessed by measurement of 24-hour urinary free cortisol (UFC), are associated with a poorer response to CBT, based on a study of 84 patients.[20]

The PACE trial is a large, multicenter, four-arm randomized trial of adaptive pacing therapy (APT), cognitive behavior therapy (CBT), graded exercise therapy (GET), and specialist medical care (SMC) for chronic fatigue syndrome, with the first participant randomized on March 18, 2005, and a total of 641 participants. Adaptive pacing therapy involves planning daily activity so as not to overwhelm capacity and worsen fatigue. Preliminary results were published in 2011.[21] A statistical analysis plan for analyzing the results of this trial was published in 2013.[22] A publication reporting on rates of clinical recovery 52 weeks after randomization found that the percentages of participants meeting trial criteria for recovery were 22% (32/143) after CBT, 22% (32/143) after GET, 8% (12/149) after APT, and 7% (11/150) after SMC. This study confirms that recovery from CFS is possible, and that CBT and GET are the therapies most frequently associated with recovery.[23] A publication examining adverse events in the trial, as recorded on three occasions over 1 year in the 641 participants, found that the numbers of adverse events did not differ significantly between trial treatments, but physical deterioration occurred most often after adaptive pacing therapy (APT).[24] Thus, based on a lack of efficacy combined with associated adverse effects, APT is not indicated as a treatment for CFS.

In a 12-week open label trial of 26 patients with CFS, graded exercise therapy had a positive effect on both physical and psychological state.[25] In regard to exercise, a challenge is that overly vigorous exercise is associated with a transient worsening of symptomatology. Thus, the challenge for the practitioner is to incorporate strategies to assist patients to self-monitor and self-regulate energy expenditures, thus maintaining appropriate energy expenditures in coordination with available energy reserves can help improve functioning over time.[26]

> Cognitive behavioral therapy (CBT) and graded exercise therapy (GET) are the conventional standard of care for treatment of CFS.

General Considerations

SHINE Protocol

SHINE is an acronym that can be used as a mnemonic for guiding treatment of CFS—treat the *s*leep disturbance, *h*ormonal imbalances, *i*nfections/immune system dysfunction, *n*utritional deficiencies and insufficiencies, and *e*xercise to tolerance. This acronym was created by Dr. Jacob Teitelbaum to summarize his treatment approach. The details of treatment guided by this approach are outlined in Dr. Teitelbaum's book, *From Fatigued to Fantastic!*[27]

There is published evidence of the efficacy of treatment guided by the SHINE approach. The first publication was a report of a case series.[28] The second, an RCT,[29] showed that at a median follow-up of 101 days, 16 patients in the active treatment group were "much better," 14 "better," 2 "same," 0 "worse," and 1 "much worse." In comparison, at a median follow-up of 98 days, 3 patients in the placebo group were "much better," 9 "better," 11 "same," 6 "worse," and 4 "much worse" (p < 0.0001 Cochran-Mantel-Haenszel trend test).

Many patients with CFS also have symptoms consistent with fibromyalgia. Indeed, some experts consider these two conditions part of the same spectrum of disease. The number of published trials examining interventions for CFS is far fewer than the number of published trials examining interventions for fibromyalgia. Some of the interventions with published evidence of benefit in fibromyalgia may also be of benefit to some who suffer with CFS; I am not citing these published studies in this chapter, as a separate chapter in this textbook devoted to fibromyalgia (see Chapter 47).

There is a growing body of published studies of a variety of unconventional approaches to the treatment of CFS. A systematic review identified a total of 26 RCTs, including 3273 participants, which met the following inclusion criteria: RCTs of any type of CAM therapy used for treating CFS were included, with the exception of acupuncture and complex herbal medicines; studies were included regardless of blinding. Controlled clinical trials, uncontrolled observational studies, and case studies were excluded. The 26 RCTs included study of the following modalities: mind-body medicine, distant healing, massage, tuina and tai chi, homeopathy, ginseng, and dietary supplementation. The authors of this review concluded that studies of qigong, massage, and tuina demonstrated positive effects, whereas distant healing failed to do so. Compared with placebo, homeopathy also had insufficient evidence of symptom improvement in CFS. Seventeen studies tested supplements for CFS. Most of the supplements failed to show beneficial effects for CFS, with the exception of NADH and magnesium.[30] Of the 26 RCTs in this citation, the findings of several are included in this overview chapter; a comprehensive discussion of each of these studies is outside of the scope of this chapter.

While published data is sparse, some patients subjectively feel better after completing a metabolic detoxification regimen. Those with a body burden of toxic metals (lead, mercury, etc.), as measured with a 6-hour urine collection post-provocation with a chelating agent such as DMSA, sometimes subjectively feel better after treatment for the systemic burden of these toxic metals (see Chapter 106).

> SHINE is an acronym that is useful as a general guide to treatment. In addition, some individuals feel better after a course of metabolic detoxification.

Nutrition

Anecdotally, and based upon general principles, an anti-inflammatory, low glycemic load, alkaline diet accompanied by plentiful water intake is optimal for those with CFS.

Exercise

Graded exercise therapy (GET) is considered a conventional treatment for CFS—see the section on conventional treatment previously.

Supplements

Supplements to Treat the Presumed Mitochondrial Dysfunction

Acetyl-L-Carnitine. Carnitine: L-carnitine, acetyl-L-carnitine, or propionyl-L-carnitine may be beneficial and, anecdotally, may also facilitate weight loss in patients who are overweight. The rationale for treatment is that carnitine is essential for mitochondrial energy production; patients with CFS have significantly lower levels of acetyl-L-carnitine, total carnitine, and free carnitine; and those with the lowest levels have the worst functional capacity.[31] In an 8-week crossover trial of 30 CFS patients comparing amantadine with L-carnitine, amantadine was ineffective, but L-carnitine 3 grams per day was beneficial and well tolerated, with the authors reporting a statistically significant clinical improvement in 12 of the 18 studied parameters.[32] In a small, open-label, 24-week study, the clinical global impression of change scale improved significantly in 59% of patients taking acetyl-L-carnitine 2 grams per day and 63% of patients taking propionyl-L-carnitine 2 grams per day.[33]

> **DOSAGE**
>
> 500–1000 mg two to three times per day, typically for an 8-week trial, with gradual tapering of the dose if subjectively effective; discontinue if ineffective.
>
> **PRECAUTIONS**
>
> Carnitine supplements are generally very well tolerated and safe. If one experiences diarrhea, anxiety, agitation, or insomnia, the dose should be decreased.

Coenzyme Q10. There are several published studies showing that Co Q10 supplementation is beneficial in fibromyalgia, but no published trials of Co Q10 supplementation specifically for CFS. In a survey of patients with unexplained chronic fatigue, 69% of 13 subjects reported that Co Q10 was beneficial.[34] Co Q10 is available in supplement form as either ubiquinol, the reduced form, or ubiquinone, the oxidized form. There are divergent opinions amongst experts as to whether one form versus the other is superior.

DOSAGE

100–300 mg daily. Outcomes of supplementation with Co Q10 may be best if dosing is guided by results of serum measurements. Based on the anecdotal experience of Dr. Steven Sinatra, with a focus on treatment of congestive heart failure, an optimal serum level of Co Q10 is considered to be 2.5–3.5 mcg/mL.[35] This blood test is available through commercial labs, such as Quest, but it is expensive and may not be covered by insurance. Note that absorption varies as a function of formulation of Co Q10, and thus the optimal dosage may also vary as a function of the formulation. Data shows that softgels that contain solubilized formulations of soy bean oil or emulsifying agents are more absorbable than powder-based capsules or tablets.[37] Furthermore, Q-Gel, a patented soft gel in which the particle size is reduced from 25–50 microns to 0.4 microns, is more highly absorbable than softgels, as demonstrated by a pharmacokinetic study which showed that the area under the curve was more than twice as high for Q-Gel as compared with softgel capsules with an oil suspension, powder filled hard-shell capsules, or regular tablets.[37] All-Q is a solubilized tablet form of Co Q10 with better bioavailability than Q-SorB (Nature's Bounty) and bioequivalence with Q gel.[38] VESIsorb uses a colloidal delivery system. A study in 20 healthy men and women reported that the area under the curve with this preparation was greater than that for three other oil-based preparations (brand names not specified).[39]

PRECAUTIONS

Generally very well tolerated and safe; however, there are case reports of hypoglycemia and hypotension and of a decrease in the INR in patients on warfarin.

Creatine. Creatine monohydrate is a source of ATP and thus theoretically beneficial in treating the presumed mitochondrial dysfunction in CFS.

DOSAGE

5 g four times a day for 5 days, then 2 g daily for 8 weeks on an empty stomach with a bit of honey. Gradually taper the dose if subjectively effective; discontinue if ineffective.

PRECAUTIONS

Avoid in those with renal failure.

NADH. NADH (also known as *Coenzyme I*) 10 mg daily was reported to be beneficial in a 4-week crossover RCT of 26 patients with CFS.[40]

DOSAGE

10 mg/day for at least 2 months, first thing in the morning, on an empty stomach, half an hour before any food. If no benefit, consider a trial of 20 mg/day. If dose is subjectively effective, gradually taper; if ineffective, discontinue.

PRECAUTIONS

Due to its activating mechanism, it can cause agitation with a caffeine-like effect.

NT Factor Energy Lipids. NT Factor Energy Lipids is a proprietary lipid blend (soy lecithin extract), which contains phosphatidic acid, phosphatidyl-choline (PC), phosphatidyl-ethanolamine (PE), phosphatidyl-glycerol (PG), phosphatidyl-inositol (PI), phosphatidyl-serine (PS), digalactosyldiacylglyceride (DGDG), and monoglactosyldiacylglyceride (MGDG). Benefit was reported in a 12-week clinical trial of elderly patients with severe fatigue.[41]

DOSAGE

¼ teaspoon twice a day for 8 weeks. Treatment can be repeated every 6–12 months.

PRECAUTIONS

None.

Potassium/Magnesium Aspartate. Aspartate is a non-essential amino acid that is converted to oxaloacetate, which is a Krebs cycle substrate. There is published evidence that this compound is effective in fatigue states, with 70%–85% responding to this compound compared, often within 10 days, as compared with a 25% response to placebo.[42,43] The quality of product is important—as presentations by Jacob Teitelbaum, MD, indicate, it must be fully reacted. Dr. Teitelbaum also suggests taking aspartate with malic acid.

DOSAGE

500 mg qid or 1 g bid for 12 weeks, with gradual tapering of the dose if subjectively effective; discontinue if ineffective.

PRECAUTIONS

Caution should be used in those with renal failure.

Ribose (D-ribose). Significant improvement was reported in an uncontrolled study in 41 patients with CFS or fibromyalgia.[44] Significant (statistical and clinical) improvement was also reported in a 3-week open-label, multicenter trial in 203 patients, examining endpoints of energy, well-being, sleep, mental clarity, and pain.[45]

DOSAGE

One scoop (5 g) tid for 4 weeks, with gradual tapering of the dose if subjectively effective; discontinue if ineffective.

PRECAUTIONS

Very safe. If patients feel overenergized or hyperactive when they take ribose, take it with a meal or lower the dose. Anecdotally, this response also suggests the need for adrenal support.

Antioxidants. Because mitochondrial dysfunction increases oxidative stress, this provides a theoretical rationale for supplementation with broad spectrum antioxidants. Anecdotally, some patients report subjective improvement in association with antioxidant supplementation. Consider a whole food antioxidant supplement, such as Fruit 4 Life and Veggies 4 Life, available online or via mail order from Swanson Health Products. Be wary of recommending high-dose individual antioxidants, such as vitamin E in the form of alpha tocopherol or beta-carotene, as high supplemental doses of a single antioxidant may be associated with depletion of other antioxidants, such as gamma tocopherol or alpha carotene.

> Supplements to boost mitochondrial function include carnitine, Co Q10, NADH, potassium/magnesium aspartate, and ribose.

Supplements to Treat the Sleep Disturbance

Anecdotally, the multiingredient product from Integrative Therapeutics, End Fatigue Revitalizing Sleep Formula, may be of benefit. This product is a blend of valerian root extract, passionflower leaf and flower extract, hops flower extract, wild lettuce leaf and leaf extract, Jamaica dogwood root extract, and L-theanine. The recommended dosage is one to four capsules 30 minutes before bedtime.

Additional supplements that may be of benefit in the treatment of insomnia include adenosine, casein tryptic hydroxylate, GABA, glycine, kava kava, L-tryptophan, lavender oil, lemon balm, melatonin, and 5-HTP. For more information on supplements for the sleep disturbance of CFS, see Chapter 9.

Supplements to Treat Hormonal Imbalances

Thyroid. If hypothyroid, consider iodine supplementation and selenium 200 mcg to support conversion of T4 to T3. Note that some multivitamins contain as much as 200 mcg of selenium in the suggested daily dose. Brazil nuts, with approximately 100-mcg selenium per nut, are an alternative to a selenium supplement.

Adrenal. Supplements for adrenal gland support include the amino acid, L-tyrosine 500–1500 mg bid, betaine (TMG) 500–1000 mg/day, pantothenic acid (vitamin B5) 500–1000 mg/day, vitamin B6 100–200 mg/day, and vitamin C 1–2 g tid. In addition to the above supplements, the hormones DHEA and pregnenolone are available over-the-counter in the United States and thus categorized as supplements. Anecdotally, some individuals with CFS report symptom improvement in conjunction with supplementation with these hormones.

Dehydroepiandrosterone (DHEA). In a survey of those with unexplained chronic fatigue, 65% of 17 subjects reported that DHEA was beneficial.[46] It is advisable to measure serum levels of DHEA-sulfate and to supplement only if these levels are suboptimal.

DOSAGE

Jacob Teitelbaum suggests treating if DHEA-S < 150–180 mcg/dL in females and < 350–480 mcg/dL in males, using the following dosing guidelines (doses are once daily):
- Men: 50 mg if level is 0–100 mcg/dL, 40 mg if level is 101–200, 25 mg if level is 201–280, and 10 mg if level is 281–320. The usual supplemental dose in men is 25–50 mg/day.
- Women: 25 mg if level is 0–30 mcg/dL, 15 mg if level is 31–80, 10 mg if level is 81–110, and 5 mg if level is 111–114. The usual supplemental dose in women is 5–25 mg/day.

PRECAUTIONS

Too high a dose in women can cause elevated testosterone levels and can result in acne, darkening of facial hair, and insulin resistance. DHEA supplementation theoretically may increase the risk of breast cancer in women and prostate cancer in men.

Pregnenolone. It is advisable to measure serum levels of pregnenolone and to supplement only if these levels are suboptimal. Sometimes levels are very low, presumably due to high interferon levels (endogenous antiviral) suppressing cholesterol and thus pregnenolone synthesis.

DOSAGE

Dr. Teitelbaum suggests 100–200 mg/day to achieve levels in the upper third of normal; Dr. David Brownstein anecdotally reports success with a lower dose of 10–25 mg daily.

PRECAUTIONS

Supplementation theoretically may increase the risk of breast cancer in women and prostate cancer in men.

Many CFS patients subjectively derive benefit from adrenal and thyroid support, even if measurements of glandular function are within the normal range.

Supplements to Treat the Immune System Imbalance and Infections

Probiotics modulate immune system function, along with many additional mechanisms of action. In a small, open-label study involving 15 patients diagnosed with chronic fatigue syndrome, supplementation with *Lactobacillus paracasei* ssp. *paracasei F19*, *Lactobacillus acidophilus NCFB 1748*, and *Bifidobacterium lactis Bb12* for a period of 4 weeks was found to improve neurocognitive functions, with a trend toward improvement in general symptoms and quality of life.[47]

Chronic candidiasis (yeast overgrowth) is a condition recognized by many integrative practitioners; however, conventional medicine practitioners do not consider this as a true entity. For integrative practitioners, diagnosis is based either on symptom questionnaire scores or on biomarkers in the stool, as measured by specialized laboratories, such as Genova, Metametrix, or Doctors Data. Natural remedies for yeast overgrowth include caprylic acid, garlic, grapefruit seed extract, olive leaf extract, oregano oil, probiotics, and undecylenic acid. Yeast overgrowth that is refractory to treatment may be due to the yeast existing in a biofilm; Interfase has been demonstrated to have efficacy in treating the biofilm.

Supplements to Treat Nutritional Imbalances

Multivitamins. A multivitamin is recommended, at the least for a 2-month trial, with indefinite continuation if effective. The multi, End Fatigue Energy Revitalization System, formulated by Dr. Jacob Teitelbaum and marketed by Integrative Therapeutics, is one option. Dr. Teitelbaum selected the ingredients and the milligram or microgram doses of each ingredient based on his extensive clinical and research experience treating those with CFS.

Amino Acids (Free-Form). Amino acids may be of benefit based on anecdotes. Amino acids may be administered as a customized blend based on the results of laboratory testing to measure amino acid levels, or alternatively administered empirically as a full spectrum free-form amino acid formulation. There are several full spectrum formulations available, including AMINOpowerplus and Total Amino Acid solution.

Iron. Consider supplementing with iron if ferritin levels are < 60 ng/mL. Anecdotally, many individuals with low normal iron stores, as well as those with frankly low iron stores, experience improved energy and improved cognition in association with a ferritin level > 60. In a 12-week RCT of 198 women, aged 18–53, with fatigue, a serum ferritin level < 50 mcg/L (low normal), and a hemoglobin level > 12.0 g/dL (not anemic), those randomized to prolonged release ferrous sulfate 80 mg/day showed a 48% improvement in scores on the Current and Past Psychological Scale for Fatigue, as compared with a 28.8% improvement in the placebo group (p = 0.02). Compared with placebo, iron increased hemoglobin by 0.32 g/dL (p = 0.002) and ferritin by 11.4 mcg/L (p < 0.001).[48] For those who cannot tolerate ferrous sulfate due to gastrointestinal side effects, other OTC forms, such as ferrous bisglycinate or ferrous fumarate, may be better tolerated. For those who cannot tolerate various forms of oral iron, intravenous iron (administered at an infusion center) is safe and effective, and generally covered by insurance.

Methylation Protocol. This is the treatment protocol to address a methylation cycle block if homocysteine levels are elevated. The positive results with this protocol have been presented in a poster,[49] an article in a nonpeer-reviewed medical journal,[50] and in a book.[51]

The protocol includes the following brand name supplements:
1. Activated B12 Guard (hydroxocobalamin) one sublingual lozenge (2 mg) daily.
2. FolaPro (5-methyltetrahydrofolate) ¼ tablet (2 mg) daily.
3. Intrinsi B12/folate (combination of folic acid, 5-methyltetrahydrofolate, folinic acid, cyanocobalamin, calcium, phosphorous, and intrinsic factor) ¼ tablet daily.

4. General Vitamin Neurological Health Formula (a multi with a high ratio of magnesium to calcium, ingredients to support sulfur metabolism, and no iron or copper), ¼ tablet daily, with dose gradually increased to two tablets daily.
5. Phosphatidyl Serine Complex (phospholipids and fatty acids) one soft gel capsule daily.

PUFA (Long Chain Polyunsaturated Fatty Acids). The published data is mixed. In one 3-month RCT, 63 adults with a diagnosis of postviral fatigue, each ill for 1–3 years, were treated with 4 g per day of a blend of linoleic acid, gamma-linolenic acid (GLA), eicosapentaenoic acid (EPA), and docosahexaenoic acid (DHA). At 3 months, 85% of those in the active treatment group assessed themselves as improved over the baseline as compared with 17% in the placebo group (p < 0.0001). Essential fatty acid (EFA) levels were abnormal at the baseline and corrected by active treatment. There were no adverse events.[52] However, a second 3-month trial of 50 patients, using entry criteria of a diagnosis of CFS, and using the same dose and same product (Efamol Marine) as in the previously described trial in patients with postviral fatigue failed to show benefit of treatment. Furthermore, in contrast to the findings in the study of patients with postviral fatigue in which EFA levels were abnormal at baseline, in this study pretreatment red-cell membrane (RBC) EFA of patients showed no significant differences, as compared with those of age-and sex-matched normal controls.[53] Essential fatty acid administration was reported beneficial in a case series of four patients with CFS. These patients consumed a range of 10–18 capsules daily of a supplement (eye q™), for which two capsules provide 186 mg EPA, 58 mg DHA, 20 mg GLA, and 3.2-mg natural vitamin E (in the form of D alpha tocopheryl acetate).[54]

Vitamin B12. Dr. Teitelbaum recommends supplementing with vitamin B12 if the vitamin B12 level is < 540 pg/mL. Hydroxocobalamin and methylcobalamin are activated forms of vitamin B12, and some individuals derive greater subjective benefit from one of these forms as compared with cyanocobalamin. Furthermore, some individuals derive greater subjective benefit from intramuscular or subcutaneous vitamin B12 (cyanocobalamin, hydroxocobalamin, or methylcobalamin) as often as three times a week for 15 weeks, as compared with oral vitamin B12. Dr. Alan Gaby suggests a trial of hydroxocobalamin 1 mg intramuscularly every 4 days for all individuals who suffer from fatigue, independent of baseline vitamin B12 levels, as some individuals may have a defect in transport of B12 across the blood–brain barrier.

Vitamin D. Supplementation with vitamin D3 is recommended at a dose of 1000–2000 IU per day if the 25 hydroxy vitamin D level is < 30 ng/mL. Vitamin D is a fat soluble vitamin, and while the therapeutic window for dosing is wide, high doses of > 10,000 IU daily are potentially toxic. Furthermore, the long-term safety of doses > 2000 IU daily is unknown.

Zinc. There is a theoretical rationale for the use of zinc for treating CFS as some of the symptoms of CFS/FM are similar to symptoms associated with low zinc levels. The typical dose is zinc citrate 30 mg daily or zinc sulfate 220 mg daily. High doses long term can suppress HDL cholesterol and lead to copper deficiency, as zinc and copper compete for absorption in the small bowel.

Botanicals

Myelophil, an extract of a mix of *Astragalus membranaceus* and *Salvia miltiorrhiza*, appears to have a pharmacological effect against fatigue based on results of a pilot 4-week RCT of 36 adults who complained of chronic fatigue. Note the entry criteria for this particular study was chronic fatigue rather than a diagnosis of CFS.[55]

Adaptogens are herbs that support and balance adrenal gland function. Common adaptogens include *Eleutherococcus senticosus*, *Ginkgo biloba*, *Ocimum sanctum* (Holy basil), Maca, *Panax ginseng*, *Rhodiola rosea*, and *Withania somnifera* (Ashwagandha). The medicinal mushroom, *Cordyceps sinensis*, also has adaptogenic properties. Adaptogens may be of benefit in the treatment of CFS; however, there are no published trials.

Medicinal mushrooms that modulate immune system function include *Agaricus blazei*, *Coriolus versicolor*, *Grifola frondosa*, Lion's mane (*Hericium erinaceus*), maitake, reishi (*Ganoderma lucidum*), and shiitake (*Lentinula edodes*). Medicinal mushrooms may be of benefit in the treatment of CFS; however, there are no published trials.

Physical Modalities

Hyperbaric Oxygen

Hyperbaric oxygen therapy may be beneficial in the treatment of CFS based on preliminary data from 16 patients.[56]

Massage Therapy

Intelligent-turtle massage, a traditional Chinese medicine modality, is an effective therapy for relieving the physical symptoms of CFS, based on a RCT of 182 patients.[57]

Mind-Body Therapy

Cognitive Behavioral Therapy

As mentioned in the "conventional treatments" section of this chapter, cognitive behavior therapy (CBT), a form of mind-body therapy, is a conventional treatment for CFS. Mindfulness-based cognitive therapy (MBCT) may offer additional benefits based on the results of a pilot study of a mindfulness-based cognitive therapy (MBCT) intervention adapted for people with CFS who were still experiencing excessive fatigue after CBT. This pilot study included 16 MBCT participants and 19 waiting-list participants; there were significant group differences in fatigue at the 2-month follow-up, and these improvement were maintained up to 6 months posttreatment. The authors of this pilot study concluded that MBCT is a promising and acceptable additional intervention for individuals still experiencing excessive fatigue after CBT for CFS.[58]

Breathing Training

Breathing retraining may offer symptomatic benefit for a subset of patients with CFS who are identified with an asynchronous breathing pattern. In a preclinical study, 5 of 20 patients with CFS were identified with an asynchronous breathing pattern; the session of breathing retraining resulted in an acute decrease in respiratory rate (p < 0.001) and an increase in tidal volume (p < 0.001).[59] It is unknown from this study whether these physiological changes will translate into clinical improvement in symptoms (see Chapter 96).

Guided Imagery

A literature review of 24 articles, of which 8 met criteria, concluded that while guided imagery is a simple, economic intervention with the potential to effectively treat fatigue, findings from the studies to date were inconsistent regarding the effectiveness of guided imagery in treating fatigue.[60]

Self-Management

Brief fatigue self-management training may be beneficial based on the results of a RCT of 111 patients with unexplained chronic fatigue or chronic fatigue syndrome. In the group assigned to two sessions of brief self-management, at 12-month postintervention follow-up, scores on the Fatigue Severity Scale were statistically better than the scores in the attention control group and the usual care group. The limitation of this trial was the high dropout rate (42%–53%).[61]

Counseling

Dr. Jacob Teitelbaum, MD, who has treated hundreds of patients with CFS, has observed that a common psychological profile is one of low self-esteem in childhood, and subsequently a perfectionist and overachiever as an adult. Counseling may be beneficial in this regard, both in terms of assisting the individual in recognizing these traits and guiding the individual as to how to say "no" and achieve adequate rest.[62]

Energy Medicine

Acupuncture

A systematic review of acupuncture and moxibustion treatment for chronic fatigue syndrome in China found that all studies concluded the treatments were effective, with response rates ranging from 78.95% to 100%; however, the qualities of the studies were generally poor, and none of them used a RCT design.[63] In a small, open-label trial of Bo's abdominal acupuncture once a day for 2 weeks in 40 patients with CFS, the authors reported statistically significant improvement in a variety of clinical symptoms.[64] More recently, a two-arm, randomized, controlled, single-blinded trial of acupuncture in 127 individuals with CFS was conducted in China. Sham acupuncture was used in the control group. The treatment regime was two sessions/week for 4 consecutive weeks. Despite considerable positive effects in the control group (sham acupuncture), the experimental group demonstrated significant net-effect sizes at a moderate magnitude in physical and mental fatigue and in the physical component of health-related quality of life.[65]

Qigong

An RCT in which 64 participants were randomly assigned to either an intervention group or a wait-list control group reported that fatigue symptoms and mental functioning were significantly improved in the qigong group compared to controls. Furthermore, telomerase activity increased in the qigong group from 0.102 to 0.178 arbitrary units ($p < 0.05$), and this change was statistically significant when compared to the control group ($p < 0.05$). Thus qigong offers a promising intervention for CFS.[66]

Systems Approaches

Traditional Chinese Medicine

Traditional Chinese medicine (TCM) is widely used in the treatment of CFS in China. The authors of a systematic review of randomized clinical trials identified 23 RCTs involving 1776 participants. The risk of bias of the included studies was high. The types of TCM interventions varied, including Chinese herbal medicine, acupuncture, qigong, moxibustion, and acupoint application. The authors concluded that TCM appears to be effective in alleviating fatigue symptoms in patients with CFS; however, these results are preliminary due to the high risk of bias in the included studies and small study size.[67]

NOTE: See the previous section on energy medicine for citations of studies of acupuncture and qigong.

Pharmaceuticals

There are no FDA-approved pharmaceutical treatments for CFS. Nonetheless, practitioners may prescribe off-label. In a study, which included a survey, 94 CFS patients recruited into an Australian study investigating immunological biomarkers filled out a questionnaire assessing the medicines they were taking. The 94 CFS patients used 474 different medicines and supplements. The most commonly used medicines were antidepressants, analgesics, sedatives, and B vitamins.[68] While RCT evidence of efficacy is lacking for these categories of medications and supplements used to treat CFS, some individuals may nonetheless derive significant symptomatic benefit from an off-label prescription.

Many patients with CFS have generalized achiness (overlap of CFS and FM) and may be treated with one of the FDA-approved pharmaceuticals for fibromyalgia: pregabalin (Lyrica), duloxetine (Cymbalta), or milnacipran (Savella) (see Chapter 47).

Pharmaceutical formulations may be used to treat hormonal imbalances.

Thyroid

Dr. Jacob Teitelbaum recommends a trial of treatment for all individuals with a free T4 < 1.3 ng/dL (below the 50th percentile of the range of normal). Options include the prescription porcine glandular, Armour Thyroid, levothyroxine (synthetic T4), and compounded T4/T3. If CFS is due to hypothalamic dysfunction, as outlined in the etiology section of this chapter, thyroid-stimulating hormone (TSH) is not a valid measure of thyroid function, as in secondary hypothyroidism due to hypothalamic dysfunction, TSH will be low in the hypothyroid individual.

Adrenal

Dr. Jacob Teitelbaum recommends consideration of a trial of low-dose prescription hydrocortisone if the 8 a.m. serum cortisol level is < 16 mcg/dL (below the 50th percentile of the range of normal). Anecdotally, Dr. Teitelbaum reports dramatic responses to hydrocortisone in some patients, and this author too has observed a few dramatic responses. Low-dose hydrocortisone at < 20 mg/day (in two to three divided doses) represents a physiological dose (similar to treating an individual with low normal thyroid function with physiological doses of thyroid medication), and this unconventional approach to treatment is safe.[69]

Gonads

Some practitioners treat with bioidentical testosterone, estrogen, and progesterone when serum levels are below the 50th percentile for a young adult, with anecdotes of positive responses.

Pharmaceuticals may be used to treat coexisting viral infections and parasites; further discussion is outside of the scope of this chapter.

Low-Dose Naltrexone

Giving 1.5–4.5 mg at bedtime, prepared by a compounding pharmacist, may be used to treat immune system dysfunction. The proposed mechanism of action is prolonged upregulation of immune system function, triggered by brief blockade of opioid receptors between 2 a.m. and 4 a.m., and mediated by an increase in endorphin and enkephalin production (www.lowdosenaltrexone.org). There are anecdotes of benefit in those with CFS, and two published trials of benefit in those with fibromyalgia. Low-dose naltrexone is occasionally associated with insomnia during the first week of treatment and may affect thyroid function in those with Hashimoto's thyroiditis.

PREVENTION PRESCRIPTION

- Nutrition: Avoid excess sugar and artificial sweeteners. Consume a low glycemic load diet.
- Sleep: Get 7–8 h of sleep a night.
- Exercise: Choose a physical activity that is fun and feels good.
- Pursue those things that give live meaning and purpose. Follow your bliss![70]

THERAPEUTIC REVIEW

NUTRITION
- Antiinflammatory, low glycemic load, alkaline diet, accompanied by plentiful water intake

EXERCISE
- Graded exercise therapy (GET). Go slow and gradually increase. Consider referral to exercise physiologist or trainer who has experience in working with those with fatigue (see Chapter 91)

MIND-BODY
- Cognitive behavioral therapy
- Mindfulness-based cognitive therapy (MBCT)

SUPPLEMENTS
- Carnitine 500–1000 mg 2–3 times per day
- Coenzyme Q 10 100–300 mg daily
- NADH 10–20 mg daily
- Potassium/magnesium aspartate 1 g bid
- Ribose 5 g tid for 1 month, then bid

- End Fatigue Energy Revitalization System multivitamin one scoop daily
- DHEA 5–10 mg daily in females, 25–50 mg daily in males, if serum DHEA-S levels are suboptimal, with continuation only if subjective benefit and if repeat measurement shows normal level on supplementation
- Iron: If ferritin levels are < 60 ng/mL, with monitoring of level to avoid a level > 150 ng/mL
- Vitamin B12 1 mg as a therapeutic trial, either orally daily or intramuscular twice a week
- Vitamin D: 1000–2000 IU per day of vitamin D3; discontinue in summer months if moderate sun exposure without sunscreen

PHARMACEUTICALS
- Thyroid medication (Armour, levothyroxine, or compounded T4/T3) to achieve a free T4 > 50th percentile; continue only if subjective benefit
- Hydrocortisone, maximum dose of 20 mg daily in divided doses, to achieve serum cortisol > 50th percentile; continue only if subjective benefit
- Naltrexone 1.5–4.5 mg at bedtime, as a therapeutic trial; continue only if subjective benefit

Key Web Resources

Dr. Teitelbaum's website that summarizes the SHINE protocol	http://www.endfatigue.com
The National Academy of Medicine's summary and report the reviews new diagnostic criteria and support of the name change to Systemic Exertional Intolerance Disease (SEID)	http://nationalacademies.org/hmd/reports/2015/me-cfs.aspx
Information on using low-dose naltrexone	http://www.lowdosenaltrexone.org

REFERENCES

References are available online at ExpertConsult.com.

CHAPTER 49

RHEUMATOID ARTHRITIS

Daniel Muller, MD, PhD

PATHOPHYSIOLOGY

Rheumatoid arthritis (RA) is likely caused by a pathological immune response in genetically predisposed individuals to an environmental challenge, probably a viral or bacterial infection.[1] Epidemiological studies have shown that genes encoding the class II major histocompatibility antigens are linked to clinical features of RA. The HLA-DR4 and DR1 proteins present foreign and self-antigens to T cells. These molecules are presumed to play a direct role in the etiology of this autoimmune disease by presenting an "arthritogenic" viral or bacterial antigen to T cells. However, no organism has been definitively linked to the etiology of RA. Recent evidence points to the gut microbiome as playing important roles in health and susceptibility to autoimmune disease.[1] Antibiotic therapy with minocycline is helpful in mild cases of rheumatoid arthritis, although minocycline may act through direct immunomodulatory or antiinflammatory effects rather than through antibacterial activity. Other genes of the immune, endocrine, and neural systems may contribute to the pathogenesis of RA; however, the precise pathophysiological cascade has yet to be defined. RA is an autoimmune inflammatory disease in which immunosuppressive drugs constitute the mainstay of therapy. Certain cytokines, such as tumor necrosis factor (TNF), interleukin (IL)-1, and IL-6, appear to play important roles because inhibitors of these molecules have been shown to decrease disease activity.[2-4] Tofacitinib is a new oral Janus kinase (JAK) inhibitor that acts upstream on intracellular signals to inhibit cytokine production.[5] Similarly, the importance of the roles of cell surface molecules on B and T cells can be shown when these molecules are used as targets for immunomodulatory therapy.[6,7]

Nonsteroidal antiinflammatory drugs (NSAIDs) act to inhibit the enzymes that produce inflammatory prostaglandins, particularly thromboxanes and leukotrienes. The newer NSAIDs preferentially inhibit the cyclooxygenase (COX)-2 enzyme that produces certain of these inflammatory molecules. Unfortunately, these COX-2 inhibitors have increased thrombotic and hence cardiovascular risks, and they may not offer any increased gastroprotection.[8,9] Celecoxib (Celebrex) is still on the market, albeit with increased warnings, while other COX-2 inhibitors have been withdrawn from the market. Omega-3 fatty acids and certain botanicals, such as ginger and turmeric, may also act through decreasing the production or activity of inflammatory prostaglandins.[10-14]

The neural, endocrine, and immune systems all share communication molecules that interact extensively. Molecules from the hypothalamic-pituitary-adrenal axis, particularly cortisol and corticotropin-releasing factor, and from the sympathetic-adrenal-medullary system are linked to disease activity in RA.[15] Corticosteroid drugs have powerful disease-suppressing activity, with equally powerful adverse side effects, such as osteoporosis.[16,17] Prolactin and the estrogenic and androgenic sex hormones have been postulated to play roles as well. Other environmental factors, such as nutrition, coffee, and tobacco, may also contribute to increased risk of RA.[18,19]

Stress and psychological factors have been linked to the etiology of RA and to disease exacerbations.[20] In one study, psychological factors and depression accounted for at least 20% of disability in patients with RA, greater than the 14% attributable to articular signs and symptoms.[21] In another study, helplessness had a direct effect on disease activity.[22]

Study data indicate an increased risk of cardiovascular diseases in patients with inflammatory and autoimmune diseases. Current recommendations include controlling underlying disease, monitoring the ratio of total cholesterol to high-density lipoprotein, the use of statins and angiotensin-converting enzyme inhibitors for antiinflammatory activity, and caution with the use of COX-2 inhibitors and steroids.[23]

Diagnosis

In 2010, new criteria for diagnosing RA were approved by the American College of Rheumatology and the European League against Rheumatism (ACR/EULAR) (Fig. 49.1).[24] Definite RA is confirmed by the presence of synovitis in at least one joint, the absence of a better alternative diagnosis, and a score of 6 or greater (out of a possible 10) from four domains: number and site of involved joints (0–5); rheumatoid factor or anticyclic citrullinated peptide (0–3); elevated sedimentation rate or C-reactive protein (0–1); and duration greater than 6 weeks (0–1). Prior criteria had been criticized for insensitivity to early RA disease. The newer criteria are directed toward instituting more aggressive therapy sooner. Official diagnostic criteria are used for inclusion into studies and do not always reflect diagnoses made in the clinic. In practice, a diagnosis of RA may include earlier diagnostic criteria, such as duration of morning stiffness greater than 1 hour, subcutaneous nodules, x-ray changes, and histological changes in biopsies of synovial tissue. Further, these ACR/EULAR diagnostic criteria do not include newer methods of diagnosis, such as ultrasound and magnetic resonance imaging. Earlier treatment of RA results in better long-term outcomes. These criteria will be used to test whether more aggressive treatment will be helpful in disease in which joint damage has not yet taken place.

Joint involvement (0–5)	
1 med/large joint	0
2–10 med/large joints	1
1–3 small joints	2
4–10 small joints	3
>10 joints (at least 1 small)	5
Serology (0–3)	
Neither Rf nor ACPA positive	0
At least one test low positive	2
At least one test high positive	3
Duration of synovitis (0–1)	
<6 weeks	0
>6 weeks	1
Acute phase reactants (0–1)	
Neither CRP nor ESR abnormal	0
Abnormal CRP or abnormal ESR	1

FIG. 49.1 ■ American College of Rheumatology and European League against Rheumatism (ACR/EULAR) diagnostic criteria for rheumatoid arthritis (RA): 6 out of 10 points or more suggest the diagnosis of RA. *ACPA*, anticyclic citrullinated peptide; *CRP*, C-reactive protein; *ESR*, erythrocyte sedimentation rate; *Rf*, rheumatoid factor. (From Aletaha D, Neogi T, Silman AJ, et al. 2010 Rheumatoid arthritis classification criteria: an American College of Rheumatology/European League against Rheumatism collaborative initiative. *Arthritis Rheum.* 2010;62:2569-2581.)

INTEGRATIVE THERAPY

Exercise

Joint pain can inhibit activity and lead to muscle disuse and atrophy. In turn, muscle atrophy can lead to decreased stability of joints. Light weight training can maintain or even increase muscle strength around joints and can lead to increased joint stability. Stretching muscles can help decrease flexion contractures. Aerobic exercise improves mood, decreases fatigue, and helps control weight gain. Water exercise can be helpful because it is less stressful on joints; however, weight training and walking work better to decrease bone loss (osteoporosis). The Arthritis Foundation provides information on exercise programs (see Key Web Resources). Asian exercise disciplines such as tai chi and yoga can also be beneficial. A form of tai chi called the *range-of-motion (ROM) dance* is particularly suited to persons with disabilities (see Key Web Resources).

Physical and Occupational Therapy

Physical therapy and occupational therapy programs can be invaluable in the treatment of RA. Goals are to improve range of motion and strengthen muscles. Joint protection from deformities can be aided by education and the use of splints, orthotics, ambulatory aids, and other devices. Massage and local heat and cold applications can decrease inflammation, increase circulation, and relax muscles.

Mind-Body Therapy

Self-help courses given through the Arthritis Foundation provide information about diseases and medication and can help in developing coping skills. Simply writing in a journal about positive and negative emotions for 15 minutes a day can be a powerful therapy that relieves symptoms by 25% or more (see Chapter 98).[25]

The benefit of psychological interventions for RA was reviewed in a meta-analysis of 27 studies. Comparisons showed benefit in increasing physical activity and in decreasing pain, disability, depression, and anxiety. Self-regulation techniques, such as goal setting, planning, self-monitoring, feedback, and relapse prevention, were particularly helpful in reducing depression and anxiety.[26]

Meditation and breath awareness are central to yoga practice, and a recent review has documented benefits in RA.[27] A study of meditation in psoriasis, an autoimmune inflammatory skin disease, showed decreased time to clearing the skin disease.[28] Two studies investigated the role of meditation in RA. Pradhan et al.[29] found reductions in psychological stress and increases in measures of well-being at 6 months, but no effects on the progression or activity of RA disease. Zatura et al.[30] reported that both cognitive therapy and meditation were helpful in RA, with better responses in subjects with depression. I continue to recommend this modality for RA (see Chapter 100). The effects of mind-body therapies on depression are important because depression is correlated with pain levels and measures of inflammatory markers.[31]

Nutrition

Food Triggers

Fasting clearly decreases symptoms in RA; however, symptoms rapidly recur with the resumption of food intake.[32] A few people with RA appear to have a food intolerance that exacerbates their disease. Many more people believe that certain foods exacerbate symptoms, but this effect has not been observed in blind trials of food exposure. The offending foods are usually dairy products, wheat, citrus, or nuts. An elimination diet for 2 weeks with the reintroduction of the suspected food can be done with or without the supervision of a physician or a nutritionist (see Chapter 86).

Omega-3 and Omega-9 Fatty Acids

Increased intake of omega-3 fatty acids from cold-water fish, such as salmon, and from nuts, such as walnuts, as well as from flaxseed or hempseed, can provide modest improvement in the control of RA.[10-12,32] The role of saturated fatty acids and trans fats in increasing symptoms is currently unproven. In view of the association of these saturated and trans fats with cardiovascular disease, however, reduction in intake is worthwhile (see Chapter 88).

Cooked vegetables and olive oil have been found to be independently protective against the development of RA. Omega-9 fatty acids in olive oil may confer anti-RA activity.[33]

Coffee

A high intake of coffee (four or more cups a day) has been linked to an increased risk of RA.[18,19] Intake should be decreased to less than this level, or the patient can switch to green tea, for the possible benefit from its antioxidant polyphenols.

Elimination of Tobacco Use

Smoking causes oxidant stress in connective tissues, as evident from the increased wrinkles seen in long-term smokers. One study demonstrated a clear association between smoking and increased risk of RA. In this Swedish population, more than 50% of RA cases could be attributable to smoking in association with certain HLA-DR genes.[34] Patients with RA should be counseled to avoid tobacco.

Supplements

Essential Fatty Acids

Omega-3 fatty acids can be increased by dietary means or through supplementation. Approximate doses for supplementation are eicosapentaenoic acid, 30 mg/kg/day, and docosahexaenoic acid, 50 mg/kg/day.[10-12,32]

Gamma-linolenic acid, 1.4–2.8 g/day, the equivalent of 6–11 g of borage oil daily, has also been shown to be helpful.[11] Effects may not be felt for 6 weeks or more, and continued improvement may occur after many months.

Conjugated Linoleic Acids

One study reported that 3-month supplementation with conjugated linoleic acids (CLAs) led to reductions in standard measures of RA activity (DAS28), morning stiffness, and erythrocyte sedimentation rate. This study provided 2.5 g CLA daily in two capsules containing equal amounts of cis-9, trans-11 CLA, cis-12, and trans-10 CLA.[35]

Antioxidants

Antioxidant vitamins may be helpful in RA, as they seem to be in osteoarthritis. Vitamin E should be taken at 800 units daily as mixed tocopherols, and vitamin C at 250 mg twice per day. Selenium can be found in many foods, including nuts; intake should be at least 100 mcg daily, not to exceed 400 mcg daily.

The recommended intake of calcium to prevent osteoporosis is 1000–1200 mg daily. Adding magnesium, at 400–750 mg daily, and a vitamin D supplement, at 2000 units per day, is probably a prudent approach.[36]

Echinacea should be avoided by patients with rheumatoid arthritis because of anecdotal reports of increased symptoms in persons with autoimmune disease.

Botanicals

Ginger

Ginger (*Zingiber officinale*) may have efficacy in treating RA by inhibiting inflammatory prostaglandins.[13]

DOSAGE

As the dried root, 1 g of ginger two or three times per day to start, increase up to 4 g daily. As tea, 1 g of dried root steeped in 150 mL of boiling water for 5–10 minutes and strained, one cup up to four times daily. Ginger can also be taken in 500-mg capsules at a dose of 1 g two or three times a day.

PRECAUTIONS

Stimulation of increased bile flow can cause pain in the presence of cholelithiasis. Other risks include bleeding, hypertension or hypotension, and hypoglycemia.

Turmeric

Turmeric (curcumin) was shown to have an efficacy similar to that of NSAIDs in an open trial.[13]

DOSAGE

As powdered root, turmeric 0.5–1 g two or three times daily.

PRECAUTIONS

Risks include bleeding, gastrointestinal intolerance, and impaired fertility.

Pharmaceuticals

Nonsteroidal Antiinflammatory Drugs

NSAIDs can be used on a short-term basis with minor risk of gastrointestinal toxicity. The long-term use of NSAIDs, particularly in older adults, poses significant risks for gastrointestinal bleeding. Many NSAIDs are available, with many of the newer ones restricted on some formularies. The classic NSAIDs are ibuprofen (Motrin), at a dose of 800 mg three times daily, and naproxen (Naprosyn), at a dose of 500 mg twice daily. Both have antiplatelet activity. The advantage of using the COX-2 inhibitor, celecoxib, for possible decreased gastrointestinal toxicity has been called into question.[9] Celecoxib shares a lack of antiplatelet effects with other newer NSAIDs. These drugs also have the potential for renal toxicity and are no more effective than older NSAIDs. Data point to the risk of increased thrombosis in patients taking COX-2 inhibitors who have a preexisting increased risk of thrombosis or cardiovascular disease.[8] Two other COX-2 inhibitors have been withdrawn from the market. Celecoxib is used at a dose of 200 mg twice daily.

Corticosteroids

Corticosteroids can rapidly decrease RA symptoms, often within a few hours at high doses. However, both short-term and long-term toxic effects are well known. High and even moderate doses can lead to avascular necrosis of joints, such as the hip, knee, or shoulder; fortunately, this is a rare occurrence. With proper care and early diagnosis of avascular necrosis, disability and joint replacement may be avoided. With long-term corticosteroid use, osteoporosis is a significant risk when doses of prednisone or equivalent are higher than 7.5 mg daily. Other risks include atherosclerosis, diabetes mellitus, cushingoid features, acne, and infection. A minor disease flare can often be treated with a moderately high dose, such as 30–40 mg of prednisone orally and a rapid taper over the course of 1–2 weeks. In some patients, a low dose of corticosteroids appears necessary for optional function; prednisone, 5–7.5 mg daily, is often used for this purpose.[16,17] A common method of treating a flare is to give a long-acting depot preparation such as triamcinolone acetonide (Kenalog), 80 mg intramuscularly. This approach can often control disease for 1–2 months, long enough for the slower-acting disease-modifying antirheumatic drugs (DMARDs) to start working. For disease flares in isolated joints, once infection is ruled out, an intraarticular injection of triamcinolone, 2.5–40 mg, can be given to control local disease.

> A single joint with severely decreased range of motion and increased pain is presumed to be infected until proven otherwise. The patient should be hospitalized overnight for joint aspiration to obtain culture specimens. Blood should also be drawn for cultures, followed by administration of intravenous antibiotics until results of culture are known.

Antibiotics

Antibiotics, particularly minocycline (Minocin) at a twice-daily dose of 100 mg, may be useful in patients with less severe disease.[37] Side effects include gastrointestinal intolerance; dizziness; photosensitivity rash; vaginitis; skin and gingival discoloration; and, rarely, hepatic, lung, and kidney injury. The salutary effects of these agents may not be caused by their antibacterial activity because the tetracyclines also show immunomodulatory and antiinflammatory activities.

Disease-Modifying Antirheumatic Drugs: Overview

DMARDs are also referred to as slow-acting antirheumatic drugs (SAARDs) because they usually take 6 weeks–3 months to show activity. The use of most U.S. Food and Drug Administration (FDA)–approved DMARDs is supported by Cochrane Reviews, including low-dose steroids, hydroxychloroquine, sulfasalazine, methotrexate (with folic acid), azathioprine, leflunomide, cyclophosphamide, etanercept, adalimumab, and infliximab (Fig. 49.2).

Hydroxychloroquine and Sulfasalazine

Hydroxychloroquine (Plaquenil) and sulfasalazine (Azulfidine-EN) are used early in disease when a diagnosis may not be clear or in patients with no characteristic erosive disease. Both drugs have little short-term and long-term toxicity.

DOSAGE

The current accepted dose of hydroxychloroquine is 200 mg twice daily, which carries little risk of toxicity; nevertheless, an ophthalmological examination to test for retinal toxicity is recommended every 6–12 months. To reduce gastrointestinal intolerance, sulfasalazine is usually used in an enteric-coated form; dosing is started at 500 mg a day and raised by one tablet every few days until a dose of 1 g twice daily is reached.

PRECAUTIONS

When used in high doses, hydroxychloroquine carries a risk of retinal toxicity resulting from deposition of the drug into the retina. Sulfasalazine can uncommonly cause rash, hepatotoxicity, and leukopenia.

Methotrexate

Of all of the DMARDs, methotrexate (Rheumatrex) has been shown to be tolerated for longer periods of treatment than any other drug.[3,38] Methotrexate is a folate antagonist and has a multitude of immunomodulatory activities, but its exact mechanism of action in RA is unknown. Doses of methotrexate for RA are usually between 5 and 25 mg given once a week. The dose is usually given orally in tablet form; however, the liquid form can be used orally and is sometimes less expensive. A common practice is to start with 7.5 mg orally once per week, although many practitioners, including myself, recommend starting at higher doses such as 15 mg/week. With the use of higher doses of 20 mg and more, patients are often taught to self-administer the dose subcutaneously once per week to avoid possible problems with gastrointestinal absorption. To decrease side effects, I always prescribe folic acid, 1–2 mg, to be taken each day. A decision to start methotrexate therapy or to raise or decrease the dose should be taken by a practitioner with extensive experience. Methotrexate is the standard by which all other drugs are judged, yet few patients achieve remission and less than a majority will achieve a 50% improvement on composite scores.

Contraindications to use of methotrexate include the following: preexisting hepatic, renal, or pulmonary disease; unwillingness to discontinue alcoholic beverages; and recent malignant disease. Methotrexate has many side effects, the most prominent being hepatitis, bone marrow suppression, pneumonitis, mouth sores, nausea, and headache. A complete blood count, platelet count, and determination of aspartate transaminase, albumin, and creatinine levels are performed initially and then every 2 weeks for 6 weeks after methotrexate therapy is begun. Thereafter, monitoring can be performed every 8–12 weeks. A baseline hepatitis screen and chest radiography are recommended. Tuberculosis skin testing is reserved for patients with strong risk factors or an abnormal appearance on chest radiograph.

Other Immunosuppressive Drugs

Many other immunosuppressive drugs are used in RA. Leflunomide (Arava) is a newer drug that is similar in efficacy to methotrexate.[39] Leflunomide interferes with pyrimidine synthesis, whereas methotrexate interferes

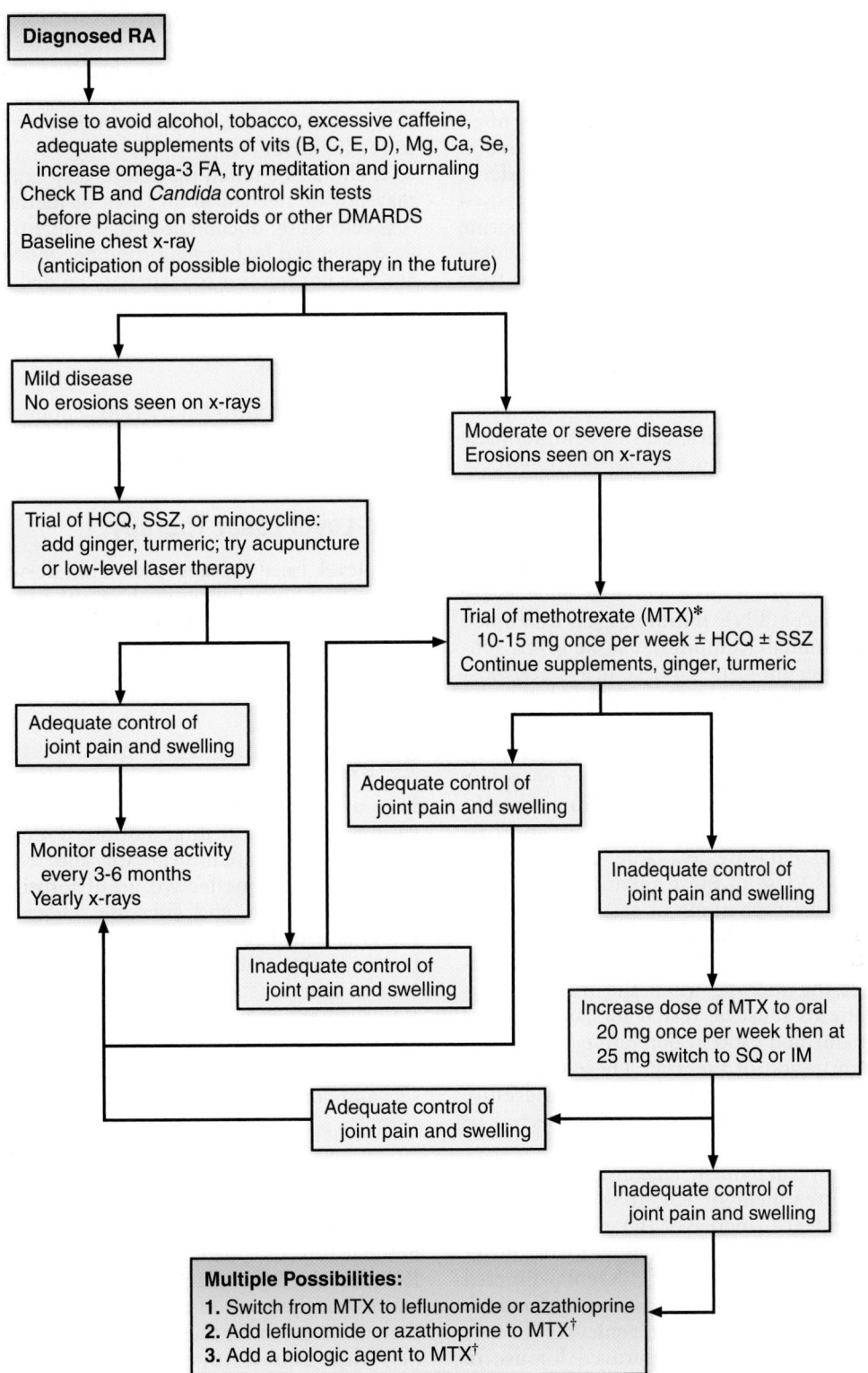

FIG. 49.2 ■ Treatment algorithm for rheumatoid arthritis (RA) in adults. *When starting methotrexate (MTX), add 1 mg of folic acid by mouth daily to decrease side effects, warn patients to avoid alcohol, and schedule laboratory studies (complete blood count, differential, platelets, aspartate aminotransaminase, albumin, creatinine) before starting, then every 2 weeks for 6 weeks, then every 2 months if results are normal. †When adding another disease-modifying antirheumatic drug (DMARD) to MTX, decrease the dose of MTX to 10–15 mg once per week. *Ca,* calcium; *FA,* fatty acid; *HCQ,* hydroxychloroquine; *IM,* intramuscular; *Mg,* magnesium; *Se,* selenium; *SQ,* subcutaneous; *SSZ,* sulfasalazine; *TB,* tuberculosis; *vits,* vitamins.

with purine synthesis. Leflunomide has fewer hepatotoxic effects and possibly little bone marrow toxicity, but is much more likely to cause diarrhea. Azathioprine (Imuran) is metabolized to 6-mercaptopurine and interferes with inosinic acid synthesis. Azathioprine is often substituted for methotrexate; however, its use is associated with gastrointestinal and bone marrow toxicity. Other immunosuppressive drugs less commonly used are mycophenolate mofetil (CellCept), cyclosporine (Neoral), tacrolimus (Prograf), and chlorambucil (Leukeran). Cyclophosphamide (Cytoxan) is often used to treat rheumatoid vasculitis.

Recombinant Biologics

Advances in the therapy of RA have targeted cytokines and cell surface molecules used to communicate between cells of the immune system.[3-7] Etanercept (Enbrel), adalimumab (Humira), and infliximab (Remicade) are TNF inhibitors.[40-42] Etanercept is given subcutaneously once or twice per week, adalimumab is given subcutaneously once every 2 weeks, whereas infliximab is usually given intravenously once every 2 months. Two newer TNF inhibitors, certolizumab (Cimzia) and golimumab (Simponi), can be given subcutaneously once per month.[3,4] These drugs are most often used with another DMARD, usually methotrexate, to reduce the development of autoantibodies. Short-term safety is very high, with little toxicity. As many as 30% of patients may show almost complete remission of symptoms with the combination of methotrexate and an anti-TNF agent. Currently, approximately 15 years of data are available on long-term safety and efficacy.[3,4] Use of these agents carries a risk of life-threatening exacerbations of severe infections, especially sepsis. Patients should temporarily discontinue the anti-TNF therapy during presumed infections and restart the therapy when the infection has resolved. All patients must be tested for latent tuberculosis with the purified protein derivative (PPD) skin test before the initiation of therapy. These drugs also may exacerbate demyelinating disorders; therefore they should be avoided in patients with suspected or proven multiple sclerosis or optic neuritis.

An IL-1 receptor antagonist, anakinra (Kineret), is approved for the treatment of RA. It is given subcutaneously daily and also increases the risk of serious infection. Anakinra is generally thought to have lower efficacy in RA than other biologics. Agents directed toward a cell surface molecule on B cells (rituximab [Rituxan])[6] and a costimulatory molecule on T cells (abatacept [Orencia])[7] have been approved for use in RA. Tocilizumab (Actemra) is directed toward another cytokine, IL-6, and has been approved for use in RA, but is associated with increased risk of neutropenia and increased cholesterol and liver function values. Tofacitinib (Xeljanz) is a new oral Janus kinase (JAK) inhibitor that acts to inhibit cytokine production. Tofacitinib is not a true biologic, but rather a new class of oral medication that acts similarly to a biologic with similar risks to tocilizumab.[5]

It should be noted that these very expensive biologics may not be needed in all cases of methotrexate failure. A recent study documented that triple therapy with sulfasalazine and hydroxychloroquine, added to methotrexate, was not inferior to etanercept added to methotrexate in active RA disease.[43]

Acupuncture

Several small controlled trials of acupuncture in RA have demonstrated decreased knee pain for an average of 1–3 months.[44]

Low-Level Laser Therapy

Low-level laser therapy uses a single-wavelength laser source that likely has photochemical, not thermal, effects on cells. A Cochrane Review suggests that this therapy may be considered for short-term relief of pain and morning stiffness for patients with RA, particularly because it has few side effects.[45]

Surgery

Loss of joint function and intractable pain may be indications for surgical intervention. Synovectomy can be helpful when systemic therapy and intraarticular corticosteroids are ineffective. Joint replacement can help restore function and increase independent activity. Patients with RA have an increased risk of surgical and postoperative complications. Cervical spine disease can lead to spinal instability and risk of neurological injury. Replacement of one joint can result in increased stress on other joints during recovery and rehabilitation. Long-term corticosteroid use can cause fragility of vessels and connective tissue and thus increase the risks of surgery.

Therapies to Consider

The roles of traditional Chinese medicine or Ayurvedic, homeopathy, or spiritual therapies in the management of RA have not been adequately studied.[46] Patients should learn about several different modalities and then record their feelings about these approaches in a journal. They may then choose to visit a practitioner of a selected modality for a trial of the techniques. If the economic burden is not too great, further exploration of therapeutic techniques may be appropriate.

PREVENTION PRESCRIPTION

No proven methods of preventing rheumatoid arthritis exist. However, the following can be recommended:

- Laugh as much as possible. Watch funny movies, read funny books, get up every morning and force yourself to laugh. You'll find it is awkward at first, but it works anyway!
- Journal about stressful events. Make a list of 25 things for which you are grateful.
- Be creative. Do art, dance, play an instrument, beat a drum, write poetry or prose.
- Meditate; I recommend mindfulness meditation.
- Find meaning in life. Ask what gives you the energy to get up in the morning.

- Investigate your personality.[47] Try new things that you are afraid to do.
- If you feel stuck, find a good psychotherapist.
- Exercise. Combine aerobics, strength training, and stretching. Make it a time to play!
- Love people. Hang out with "positive people"; make sure they outweigh the "negative" people in your life. Find "positive" support groups.
- Eat well. Try a vegetarian diet. Make sure to balance your protein intake, and make sure you have adequate vitamin intake.
- Eliminate coffee, smoking, and alcohol. Make high-sugar desserts a small, rare treat.

THERAPEUTIC REVIEW

Evidence is accumulating that current allopathic treatments are successful in slowing joint destruction and in decreasing the mortality associated with rheumatoid arthritis (RA).[3,4,38,43,48] In addition, the rates of extraarticular manifestations of RA, such as Felty syndrome and rheumatoid vasculitis, seem to be decreasing. Therefore, in any but the mildest cases of RA, an integrated approach should include the disease-modifying antirheumatic drugs (DMARDs), usually starting with methotrexate.

EXERCISE

- Muscle strengthening and stretching can be invaluable for maintaining function. Physical therapy can be used initially for instruction; modified yoga or tai chi in the form of the range-of-motion dance can be helpful.

MIND-BODY TECHNIQUES

- Meditation is highly recommended for patients with RA who are willing to devote the daily time to looking more closely at the connections among body, mind, and spirit. Also recommended are relaxation exercises and the development of methods to cope with stress. Tai chi and yoga also may include a meditative component to the training.
- Journaling should be encouraged (see Chapter 98).

REMOVAL OF EXACERBATING FACTORS

- Use of coffee, tobacco, and alcohol should be eliminated.
- If intolerance to dairy products, wheat, citrus, or nuts is suspected, a trial of an elimination diet for 2 weeks with the reintroduction of the suspected food can be undertaken (see Chapter 86).

NUTRITION

- A diet rich in omega-3 fatty acids is achieved by increasing intake of cold-water fish or adding flaxseed meal or flaxseed oil. Olive oil should also be increased in the diet. An antiinflammatory diet is also recommended (see Chapter 88).

SUPPLEMENTS

- Omega-3 fatty acids are recommended; doses for supplementation are eicosapentaenoic acid, 30 mg/ kg/day and docosahexaenoic acid, 50 mg/kg/day, along with gamma-linolenic acid, 1.4–2.8 g/day, the equivalent of 6–11 g of borage oil daily.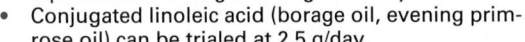
- Conjugated linoleic acid (borage oil, evening primrose oil) can be trialed at 2.5 g/day.
- Vitamin E should be taken at a dose of 800 units daily as mixed tocopherols, and vitamin C can be taken at a dose of 250 mg twice daily. Selenium intake, as nuts or supplements, should be at least 100 mcg daily, not to exceed 400 mcg daily. Recommended intake of calcium is 1.5 g daily; magnesium, 400–750 mg daily, and a vitamin D supplement of 2000 units/ day are also recommended.

BOTANICALS

- Start with ginger, at 1 g twice daily to a maximum of 4 g daily.
- If no effect is seen after 6–8 weeks, the addition of turmeric 0.5–1 g two to three times daily can be trialed.

PHARMACEUTICALS

- NSAIDs are used as little as possible owing to gastrointestinal toxicity. The classic NSAIDs are ibuprofen, 800 mg three times daily, and naproxen, 500 mg twice daily.
- The COX-2 inhibitors decrease but do not eliminate the risk of gastrointestinal bleeding. The dose of celecoxib is 200 mg twice daily.
- Most patients with RA are receiving combinations of drugs. Most patients are given methotrexate therapy unless they have contraindications or side effects.
- A common combination is methotrexate and hydroxychloroquine; sulfasalazine can be added for triple therapy. Corticosteroids in moderately high doses with a rapid taper are often used for exacerbations.
- Commonly, a TNF inhibitor such as etanercept, adalimumab, infliximab, certolizumab, or golimumab is added if methotrexate is only partially effective. If one to two TNF inhibitors are unsuccessful, try rituximab, abatacept, or tocilizumab.
- Leflunomide or azathioprine is often substituted for methotrexate if side effects of methotrexate are intolerable.

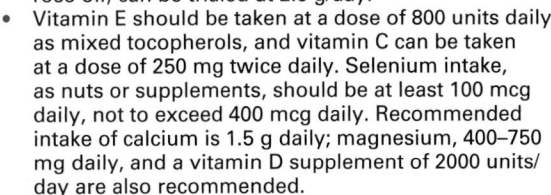

- Methotrexate and leflunomide can be used together with only a modest increase in risk of side effects. The DMARDs and the recombinant biologics have many varied side effects, some of which are only now being defined. New biologics are being developed, including oral formulations. Immunosuppressive pharmaceuticals should be used only with input from a subspecialist rheumatologist.

ACUPUNCTURE

- Acupuncture can be tried for any patient with RA. This modality may be less effective in patients taking corticosteroids.

LOW-LEVEL LASER THERAPY

- Low-level laser therapy can be trialed with little risk of side effects.

SURGERY

- Loss of joint function and intractable pain may be indications for surgical intervention. Synovec-tomy can be helpful when systemic therapy and intraarticular corticosteroids are ineffective. Joint replacement can help restore function and increase independent activity.

CAUTION

Studies have not been conducted on the possible additive effects of ginger, turmeric, vitamin E, and an NSAID for increased risk of hemorrhage. Other commonly used supplements or botanicals such as ginkgo may add further risk. Particular care must be used in patients taking other antiplatelet agents or warfarin sodium (Coumadin). In addition, the interactions of supplements and botanicals with allopathic pharmaceuticals are not fully understood. All health care professionals involved in patient care must be aware of all therapies being used. The addition of any new treatment should prompt increased laboratory monitoring for patients receiving immunosuppressive pharmaceuticals.

Key Web Resources

The Arthritis Foundation, for information on all aspects of RA, treatment, self-help, and other resources	http://www.arthritis.org/about-arthritis/types/rheumatoid-arthritis/
National Center for Complementary and Integrative Health, for further information on integrative therapies	https://nccih.nih.gov/health/RA/getthefacts.htm
The range of motion (ROM) dance from Tai Chi Health is particularly suited to persons with disabilities	http://www.taichihealth.com/indexrom.html

REFERENCES

References are available online at ExpertConsult.com.

CHAPTER 50

INFLAMMATORY BOWEL DISEASE

Alyssa M. Parian, MD • Gerard E. Mullin, MD • Jost Langhorst, MD • Amy C. Brown, PhD

INTRODUCTION AND PATHOPHYSIOLOGY

Inflammatory bowel diseases (IBD), including Crohn's disease (CD) and ulcerative colitis (UC), are autoimmune-based chronic inflammatory diseases that follow a relapsing and remitting course. The pathogenesis of IBD has yet to be fully elucidated; however, studies suggest a multifactorial process involving genetics, environmental exposures, the gut microbiome, and immune dysregulation among others. One accepted theory is that IBD develops due to an exaggerated, uncontrolled immune response to an environmental trigger in the gut microbiota. There has been a rising incidence of IBD worldwide, and experts believe a "westernized diet" is at least partially to blame. A diet high in refined sugars, animal fat, and complex carbohydrates is associated with higher rates of IBD, whereas diets rich in omega-3 fatty acids and fiber protect against development of IBD.[1-5] Alterations in the gut microbiome such as decreased bacterial diversity and an overgrowth of *Bacteroides* species are commonly found in patients with IBD compared to the general population. Aside from diet, gastrointestinal infections[6,7] and antibiotics[8] are known to disrupt the microbiome and have both been recognized as triggers for IBD flares. Aberrations in the mucosal immune system have been implicated in the pathogenesis of IBD. Patients with IBD commonly have increased intestinal permeability, which increases exposure of the intestinal immune system to luminal antigens, triggering further inflammation (Fig. 50.1).[9]

INTEGRATIVE THERAPIES FOR INFLAMMATORY BOWEL DISEASE

IBD is a highly complex chronic inflammatory disease that is amenable to successful modulation by the combination of conventional allopathic medicine and complementary and alternative modalities (CAM). There are many facets of CAM that are highlighted in this text that can mitigate the chronic inflammation of IBD and address the root causation by modifying the triggers for this autoimmune condition. We will utilize a functional medicine approach towards achieving this goal for patients and practitioners. The first goal is to identify preventative risks and to eliminate harmful triggers and mediators of disease. Once the body is in a reboot mode, proper nutrition and lifestyle interventions can help to rebalance the gut ecosystem and mucosal immunity as well as restore vitality and quality of life (QOL).

Nutrition

The gut serves as the body's principle interface between the outside world and immune system. Disruptions in gut integrity and overall function are distorted in autoimmune diseases such as IBD. Orally ingested medications and or nutrients may play a number of roles in propelling or improving symptoms and the course of disease by influencing gut health and mucosal immunity. A number of studies have disclosed the following identifiable and modifiable risks: genetic susceptibility, antibiotic use,[10] hygiene status, diet, infective agent(s) transferred through foods or beverages, recall of bacterial intestinal infections,[10] appendectomy, pollution, smoking, stress,[11] food additives, oral contraceptive use, NSAIDS, and or other environmental factors.[12] However, the relative contributions of individuals factors have yet to be defined. Tetracycline class antibiotics, particularly doxycycline, which is used for acne or other conditions, may be associated with the development of IBD, particularly CD.[13] Overall, disruptions in the delicate balance of gut mucosal and microbial health portend to autoimmunity, but also provide targets to mitigate the onset and course of disease.

Diet is the primary modality that patients use to help modify symptoms. Surveys reveal that a large percentage of IBD patients not only alter their diets but also ask clinicians for dietary advice.[14] Researchers reported that 90% of CD and 71% of UC patients changed their diets following diagnosis.[15] Among patients altering their diets, 73% reportedly experienced improved symptoms of abdominal pain, flatulence, and diarrhea. Despite patient demand for dietary guidance, no diet is currently recommended for IBD in clinical practice guidelines and the online Nutrition Care Manual, which is used by many hospitals, as their diet manual (www.eatright.org) requires extensive updating for IBD.[16]

Enteral nutrition may influence the course of IBD via a number of mechanisms, as illustrated in Fig. 50.2.[15] A systematic review concluded that IBD rates have increased with the spread of the Western diet, specifically a higher intake of total fats, total PUFAs, omega-6 fatty acids, and meat. High-fiber and fruit intakes were shown to be associated with a decreased risk of CD, while high-vegetable intakes were found to be protective against UC.[17] A high fiber diet was revealed in the NHANES study to be associated with a lower risk of CD, but not UC.[5] Only fruit and vegetable fiber (soluble) was associated with this decreased risk, not fiber from insoluble fiber from cereals, whole grains, or legumes. Dixon et al. discuss the possible mechanisms behind the hypothesized link between IBD and carbohydrate, protein, and fat.[18] Alcohol consumption increases IBD risk, perhaps through disruption of the intestinal epithelial barrier resulting in an increased

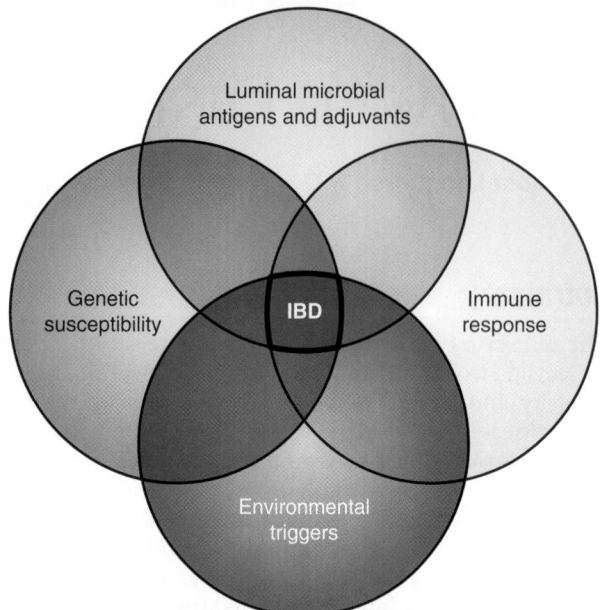

FIG. 50.1 ■ **Pathophysiology of Inflammatory Bowel Disease.** The exact pathophysiology of inflammatory bowel disease remains unknown; however, an interplay of diet, genetics, environmental exposures, the immune system, and the microbiome is believed to contribute. These factors are believed to interact collectively in the pathogenesis of this chronic disease.

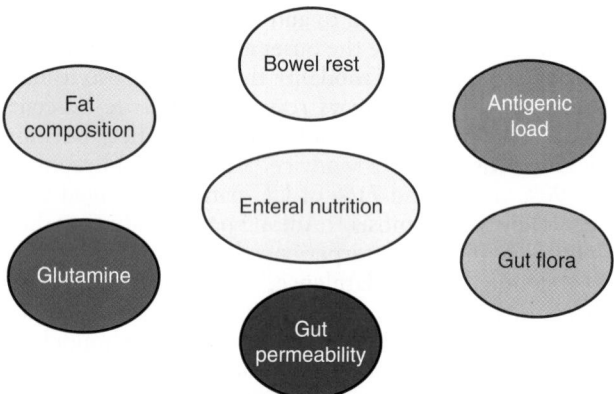

FIG. 50.2 ■ **Mechanisms of Enteral Nutrition for the Induction of Remission of Crohn's Disease (CD).** Enteral nutrition has been shown to induce remission in children and adults with Crohn's disease. The possible mechanisms for the benefit of enteral nutrition for CD include its glutamine content, which has trophic effects upon the small intestine, promotes healing, and improves gut permeability, which decreases the translocation of enteric toxins and food-derived antigens, resulting in the attenuation of inflammation. The presence of prebiotic nutrients in enteric formulations enhances the biodiversity of the gut microbiome and decreases the growth of enteric pathogens, thereby promoting immune regulation. Bowel rest for severe disease, elimination diets, and elemental and polymeric formulations all decrease the antigenic load present in the small intestine, thereby diminishing the translocation of immune-enhancing antigens. Finally, diets that are high in saturated fat content, such as the Western diet, drive inflammation and promote IBD in animal models. In contrast, oral nutritional supplements containing omega-3 fatty acids have been shown to induce clinical remission. In Japan, oral nutrition continues to serve as first-line therapy for CD in children and adults.

intestinal permeability and associated endotoxemia perpetuating inflammation.[19] Researchers suggest that a semi-vegetarian diet may also help because CD patients maintained clinical remission 94% of the time compared to 33% of the time with an omnivorous diet.[20] Coconut-derived medium-chain triglycerides (MCT) oil has been shown to improve bowel damage in animal models and modulate immunity.[21]

Enteral nutrition involves a liquid diet containing nutrients broken down into their small or smallest absorbable units. These liquid formulas are provided to the patient via enteral (gut) or parenteral (vein) routes to provide a partial or exclusive source of nutrients. Three types of enteral formulas are available that vary in their degree of hydrolyzation, palatability, and cost:

1. Polymeric—intact nutrients (carbohydrates, proteins, and lipids) are the most palatable and affordable
2. Semi-elemental—partially hydrolyzed nutrients (peptides, starch polymers, simple sugars, glucose, and fats [primarily MCT; medium-chain triglycerides])
3. Elemental—completely hydrolyzed nutrients (amino acids, monosaccharides, fatty acids, vitamins and minerals), not palatable, and costly.[22,23]

Enteral formulas have a high success rate of inducing remission and ameliorating symptoms without the toxicity seen with pharmaceutical medications. Enteral nutrition is effective for inducing clinical remission in both small and large bowel CD inflammation[23] but not for UC patients.[24] A Cochrane meta-analysis of ten trials involving CD patients found no difference in efficacy between polymeric, semi-elemental diets (n = 146) and elemental diets (n = 188) in obtaining clinical remission.[25] Unlike corticosteroids, enteral therapy may enhance mucosal healing.[26] Researchers have reported improved lactulose/L-rhamnose permeability ratios and cytokine levels[27] with enteral therapy. Additionally, 74% (14/19) of pediatric CD patients on oral polymeric formula experienced endoscopic improvement compared to 33% (6/18) treated with corticosteroid.[28,29] Mucosal healing may be influenced by enteral formulas through lower fecal bacterial concentrations or a lower antigen load crossing the intestinal barrier and triggering inflammation.[30] In a study of 61 CD patients who were induced into remission with drugs, 94% in the home elemental enteral hyperalimentation (HEEH) group (n = 22) maintained remission for 1 year, 63% for 2 years, and 63% at 4 years. Enteral nutrition is the recommended treatment in the United States for children with active CD and for adults suffering from corticosteroid complications or malnutrition.[31]

There is a discrepancy between clinical practice guidelines and practice because a survey of 326 of the 1162 North American Society for Pediatric Gastroenterology, Hepatology and Nutrition members found that 55% used exclusive enteral therapy sparingly, 31% never used it, and 12% used it regularly.[32] Practice guidelines published in the *American Journal of Gastroenterology* for CD state that "corticosteroids are more effective than enteral nutrition to induce remission in active CD patients"[33] based on a Cochrane meta-analysis of only six trials despite identifying 15 eligible trials.[25] However, a PubMed review found that 86% (30/35) of studies supported beneficial results of enteral therapy in CD patients.[34]

In Japan, enteral nutrition is the first line of therapy for both adults and children, and it is also covered by health insurance.[35] After clinical remission with enteral therapy, nightly nasogastric tube feeding followed by a low-fat diet in the day (20–30 g) reportedly resulted in fewer hospitalizations, surgeries, and complications; longer remissions; and lower mortality rates compared to those not receiving enteral therapy.[36,35] The benefits of enteral therapy include improved nutritional status and mucosal healing, higher remission rates, and decreased rates of relapse, hospitalizations, and mortality. CD patients need to be informed of enteral therapy as an available treatment choice because it may be necessary in CD patients with strictures or obstructions and may be particularly useful in managing flares that may precede a recommendation for surgery. Enteral nutrition, as with many other dietary changes, may favorably alter gut microbial balance.[37]

The suggested diet for IBD has a bimodal approach: (1) an elimination diet for symptom control and (2) an antiinflammatory diet for long-term disease control and optimum health. Both of these dietary approaches are covered in depth in Chapters 86 and 88. Popular diets that patients have anecdotally reported to be useful for symptom control and improved quality of life (QOL) in IBD include, but are not limited to, the specific carbohydrate diet (SCD), low-carbohydrate diets, the gluten-free diet, and the yeast-free diet, among others. Essentially, these are all different forms of an elimination diet designed to remove potentially sensitizing foods that trigger symptoms. The SCD and low carbohydrate diets have received the most attention and acclaim from patients and have some research to support their use. The SCD eliminates certain carbohydrates, lactose, and some gluten. It was developed in the 1920s by a pediatrician, Dr. Haas, for celiac disease and published in his 1951 book, *Management of Celiac Disease*.[38] The diet was so successful in reducing Elaine Gottschall's daughter's UC symptoms that she later popularized the SCD in her book, *Breaking the Vicious Cycle: Intestinal Health Through Diet*, and accompanying websites. The current SCD is low gluten because breads are not allowed, and it eliminates disaccharides (lactose, sucrose, maltose, and isomaltose) and digestible saccharides (starches); however, monosaccharides such as glucose, fructose, and galactose are allowed. Foods to avoid include cereal grains, legumes (beans, peas, and lentils), potatoes, and sweeteners. Allowed foods include meat, poultry, fish, eggs, nut flour, peeled vegetables and low-carbohydrate fruits, aged cheese, homemade yogurt, and honey.[34] Essentially, the SCD is an elimination diet that restricts gluten and dairy (lactose-containing foods), two of the highest food offenders in CD. Only two clinical and two case studies have specifically evaluated the SCD in patients. A retrospective study of seven children using the SCD reported that Pediatric Crohn's Disease Activity Index (PCDAI) levels decreased to zero at 3 and 6 months. Each patient's laboratory values, including C-reactive protein, hematocrit, and stool calprotectin, either normalized or significantly improved when measured.[39] Cohen et al.[40] reported the first prospective study evaluating the SCD in nine CD pediatric patients. Six (60%) patients achieved clinical remission by 12 weeks (PCDAI < 10), with improved symptom indices and

capsule endoscopy revealing mucosal healing of intestinal lesions in four (44%) of the subjects at 12 weeks. Two case reports documented improved clinical and endoscopic remission in two adults after 1–2 years on the SCD.[41] In addition to SCD studies, four clinical trials, with weak methodology, have evaluated low-carbohydrate diets in CD. They all support that lower carbohydrate diets (not a SCD) reduce gastrointestinal symptoms in CD.[42-45]

Dietary suggestions based on clinical practice guidelines include, but are not limited to, eating smaller meals, decreasing fiber during active disease and slowly reintroducing it, avoiding dairy products if not tolerate, and avoiding fatty foods (especially fatty meats), beans, peas, nuts, and "scrappy" foods such as raw fruits, vegetables, seeds, and popcorn.[16] During bouts of diarrhea and abdominal pain, a softer diet and sufficient fluids are recommended, whereas high sugar drinks, juices, caffeine, alcohol, and sugar alcohols should be avoided. Obstruction may require a liquid diet or nothing by mouth. Retrospective studies have reported that the top two dietary offenders in a subgroup of CD patients are gluten and casein/lactose[46]; however, wheat (34%; 34/199), milk (31%; 35/144), and yeast (19%; 22/119) were reported to be the foods most likely to cause problems for CD subjects.[47] A cohort survey of 1647 Crohn's and Colitis Foundation Association (CCFA) members (Herfarth, Martin, Sandler, Kappelman, & Long, 2014) revealed that 19% (314) had tried a gluten-free diet, with 66% of them reporting improved symptoms of bloating, diarrhea, abdominal pain, and/or nausea.[48] Such varied responses to diet among IBD patients made it difficult to suggest one type of diet, so IBD patients would appear to benefit from an individualized diet eliminating their particular aggravating foods. Accordingly, the best diet to achieve this aim would be a comprehensive elimination diet as discussed in Chapter 86.

> There is no one particular recommended diet to help alleviate the symptoms and inflammation caused by IBD. Each patient's nutrition plan should be individualized based on disease activity, extent, and phenotype. However, celiac disease and lactose intolerance commonly co-occur with IBD and should be ruled out.

Vitamin-Mineral Supplements in IBD

Patients suffering with IBD frequently have vitamin and mineral deficiencies due to decreased intake or poor absorption secondary to inflamed mucosa. Some vitamins and minerals are believed to have antiinflammatory, immunogenic, and antineoplastic properties. However, serious toxicities are possible with excessive intake of certain nutrients, and caution should be taken regarding interactions between medications and supplements.

Vitamin A

Vitamin A (retinol) is a fat-soluble vitamin important for wound healing[49] and is found to be deficient in up to

44% of IBD patients.[50-52] Vitamin A requires an intact enterohepatic biliary circulation to be adequately absorbed, which is altered in patients with large ileal resections or extensive ileal disease as is commonly seen in Crohn's Disease (CD), which involves the ileum in 80% of cases. Two studies failed to demonstrate a benefit of high-dose vitamin A for maintaining remission in CD, although both studies comprised patients without acute inflammation.[53,54] Supplementation is only recommended to sufficiency in patients with vitamin A deficiency.

Vitamin B12

Vitamin B12 (cobalamin) deficiency is common in IBD patients and has been reported in up to 50% of Crohn's patients.[55-58] Vitamin B12 deficiency can manifest clinically with a variety of signs and symptoms, including nervous system dysfunction or megaloblastic anemia.[57,59,60] The absorption of B12 requires the secretion of intrinsic factor by the stomach, which is essential for the absorption of vitamin B12 in the ileum. Because the ileum is the most frequent location affected in Crohn's disease, there is a significantly increased risk of B12 deficiency and insufficiency among this patient population.[60]

True cobalamin deficiency leads to elevated serum levels of methylmalonic acid (MMA) and homocysteine, which have both been linked to higher risks of cardiovascular disease and stroke. The sensitivity and specificity of serum B12 levels in the diagnosis of B12 deficiency is poor[61-64] and some experts, including NHANES, have recommended that an elevated MMA or homocysteine level be required for an accurate diagnosis of cobalamin deficiency.[61,65] The daily requirement of B12 is 2.4 mcg in the general population.[66] Higher doses are needed if a patient is deficient according to the severity of symptoms. Supplementation via the subcutaneous route is best in patients with ileal inflammation or resection due to poor absorption. However, the malabsorption can be overcome with high doses of oral cobalamin (1000–2000 mcg daily), which are absorbed through passive diffusion or the sublingual route.[66,67]

Vitamin D

Vitamin D has been shown to regulate cell growth and is a key cofactor in the immune system.[68-70] Vitamin D may act as an antiinflammatory and immune regulatory agent. Between 22% and 70% of Crohn's patients and up to 45% of UC patients have been reported to have vitamin D deficiency.[71-74] The Nurses' Health Study has demonstrated two important findings: a lower risk of UC in those with the highest intake of vitamin D supplementation and a lower risk of CD in those with higher vitamin D levels.[75] Patients with CD appear to have less frequent flares and improved disease activity scores with vitamin D supplementation.[76,77] A prospective study showed that CD patients supplemented with vitamin D to sufficiency (30–50 ng/mL) had a decreased risk of hospitalization and surgery.[78] A subsequent prospective, randomized, placebo-controlled study found that daily supplementation with 1200 IU of vitamin D3 decreased the rate of relapse (P = 0.06) in 108 CD patients in remission.[76]

Vitamin D levels (25 hydroxy-D) should be assessed on at least an annual basis in IBD patients and repleted to maintain levels > 30 ng/mL.

Vitamin K

Vitamin K has been shown to play a role in bone health along with magnesium, calcium, and vitamin D. IBD patients with ileitis or those treated with sulfasalazine or antibiotics are at risk of vitamin K deficiency.[78a] Dietary intake of vitamin K has been shown to be lower in IBD patients in several studies. Currently, there is insufficient evidence to support daily vitamin K supplementation. Patients should instead be encouraged to consume green leafy vegetables to obtain vitamin K naturally through the diet.[79]

Vitamin E

Vitamin E has been shown to significantly reduce oxidative stress by preventing the production of reactive oxygen species and terminating chain reactions in cell membranes.[52,80,81] IBD patients have been found to have decreased levels of vitamin E (tocopherol).[82] Several rodent studies and a small human study have shown promise in the treatment of colitis with vitamin E enemas.[83-85] Vitamin E is another fat-soluble vitamin; therefore, large doses can lead to toxicity, and caution needs to be taken with this therapy. Large population-based studies have actually found increased rates of all-cause mortality with high doses of vitamin E supplementation.[86,87]

Vitamin C

Vitamin C or ascorbic acid is an essential water-soluble vitamin that has been found to be low in IBD patients, at least partially due to inadequate intake.[50,52,56] More than 50% of Crohn's patients have been reported to be vitamin C deficient.[56] The wound-healing effects of vitamin C are particularly important.[88] Although excess vitamin C is not life threatening because it is water soluble, high levels may cause diarrhea, nausea, vomiting, abdominal pain, and oxalate kidney stones. Excessive repletion of vitamin C (i.e., intravenous infusions) has not been shown to have any proven health benefits and is not recommended.

Folate

Folate deficiency is observed in up to 26% of CD patients.[50,58] Mesalamines, particularly sulfasalazine and methotrexate, inhibit folate absorption. Folate supplement of 1 mg daily is therefore advised.[89] Folic acid deficiency is associated with elevated homocysteine levels[90] and thromboembolism.[91] Additionally, low folic acid levels are associated with an increased risk of colorectal dysplasia or cancer in IBD patients[92-94] as well as the general population.[95-98] Folate supplementation beyond sufficiency has not been shown to prevent colorectal neoplasia or dysplasia.[99-102] Red cell folate levels are more accurate than serum levels and should be monitored at least annually in patients on the aforementioned medications that predispose to folate deficiency. Low folate levels may also reflect an inherited posttranslational modification of the enzyme methylene tetrahydrofolate reductase (MTHFR), requiring supplementation with folinic acid to sufficiency to bypass the defective metabolic process. Genetic testing for MTHFR mutation is therefore recommended and offered by most commercial laboratories and covered by insurance carriers.

Calcium

Calcium is an essential macronutrient and requires vitamin D for adequate absorption from the intestines. It has been reported that 80% of IBD patients have inadequate calcium intake[50,56] and up to 50% have osteopenia.[103,104] Low magnesium levels, commonly caused by diarrhea, also cause calcium malabsorption. Corticosteroids used to treat IBD are known to inhibit calcium absorption. Calcium deficiency leads to an inability to maintain bone health that eventually causes osteoporosis. Glucocorticoids are also known to accelerate the development of osteoporosis.[79]

The majority of IBD patients likely should be on standard daily calcium supplementation (1000–1500 mg). Because calcium requires vitamin D to be absorbed, IBD patients should be on both calcium and vitamin D supplementation to maintain bone health and prevent osteoporosis, particularly those currently on steroids.[79]

Monitoring of bone health is essential in all patients with IBD because they are at high risk for osteoporosis and bone fractures. To maintain adequate bone health, IBD patients should not smoke cigarettes and should limit or avoid corticosteroid use. Bone homeostasis requires adequate calcium, vitamin D, magnesium, and vitamin K.

Chromium

Chromium deficiency can occur in patients on long-term central parenteral nutrition (CPN),[105] and 10–15 mcg should be added to the daily mix to prevent it. Glucocorticoids have been shown to increase urinary excretion of chromium. Signs of chromium deficiency include a hypochromic microcytic anemia and poor glucose control. Supplementation with chromium up to 600 mcg daily may reverse steroid-induced diabetes.[106]

Iron

Iron is the most commonly deficient nutrient in IBD patients, with a prevalence of approximately 30%.[107] Repletion of iron is clinically challenging in IBD patients. Cholestyramine and antacids impair absorption of iron, whereas ascorbic acid facilitates absorption. Oral iron can be harsh on the GI tract, causing nausea, gastritis, and constipation. There is some evidence that oral iron may increase oxidative stress in the intestines by increasing superoxide anion generation according to Fenton chemistry analysis in animal models.[108] Intravenous iron repletion may be the most effective approach despite a risk of anaphylaxis, particularly in patients with severe deficiency.[109]

Ferric carboxymaltose is a new formulation of iron that can be safely administered at higher doses (1000 mg) to achieve normal levels more rapidly while decreasing the required number of infusions. Due to the decreased number of infusions, patients are more compliant with this therapy. Additionally, ferric carboxymaltose (1000 mg) has been shown to be more effective than standard iron sucrose (200 mg) in improving hemoglobin levels.[110]

Magnesium

Magnesium plays a role in maintaining adequate bone health, parathyroid function, and calcium absorption. Magnesium deficiencies have been reported in patients with diarrhea, high fistula output, malabsorption, or inadequate oral intake. To most accurately measure the body stores of magnesium, a 24-hour urine is required.[111,112] Red blood cell (RBC) magnesium levels also provide an additional measure of intracellular magnesium status. Decreased levels of magnesium in the urine increase the risk of urolithiasis, for which CD patients are already at risk.[113] Magnesium formulations, such as heptogluconate and magnesium pyroglutamate, may have less association with diarrhea than citrate.

Selenium

Selenium is a mineral that plays a vital role in antioxidant functioning by acting as a cofactor for glutathione peroxidase and reducing vitamin E regeneration. Selenium deficiency is associated with cardiomyopathy, hypothyroidism, and cartilage degeneration.[79] The long-term use of CPN and small bowel resection can lead to selenium deficiency.[114] Several studies have confirmed lower levels of selenium in both UC and CD patients compared with the general population.[115-120]

Zinc

Zinc deficiency can develop in patients with severe diarrhea, high output ostomies, and long-term corticosteroid or CPN use.[121] Zinc is required for the metabolism of vitamin A, including the oxidative conversion of retinol to retinal and vitamin A transport.[122] Measuring the overall zinc status in the body is challenging; however, many use the levels of zinc in RBCs to reflect intracellular status.[79] Supplementation with 220 mg of zinc sulfate once or twice daily is recommended in patients with draining fistulae, recent surgery, or active and severe diarrhea.[79] Zinc repletion should be provided with vigilance because excess zinc interferes with the absorption of iron and copper.[88] Copper deficiency with profound neurological manifestations has been described with high-dose supplementation of zinc because these two micronutrients compete for binding to metallothionine.

Non-Vitamin-Mineral Supplements

Fish Oils or Fatty Acids

There are two major types of essential fatty acids (EFAs): omega-3 and omega-6 polyunsaturated fatty acids

(PUFA). These are considered essential because the body is unable to synthesize them, thereby necessitating dietary intake. Omega-3 has been shown to have beneficial health effects, including antiinflammatory properties, whereas excess omega-6 has been associated with proinflammatory and prothrombotic states. The ratio of omega-6 to omega-3 consumed should be approximately 4:1, but a Western diet has a ratio closer to 10:1 and some experts believe this imbalance contributes, in part, to the development of IBD and or its recalcitrance to medical therapy.[123] Omega-3 supplementation decreases inflammatory cytokines, including TNF-α, IL-1β, and NF-κB, as well as improves the functioning of the immune system.[124,125] Fish oil is an excellent source of omega-3 fats. Up to a quarter of IBD patients have some level of EFA deficiency.[126] Diets high in omega-3 fatty acids are associated with a reduced risk of ulcerative colitis.[127] Several animal studies have suggested a benefit to dietary fish oil supplementation and rectal fish oil treatment in chemically-induced colitis.[128-133] There are no randomized trials investigating omega-3 fatty acids for the induction of remission in Crohn's patients, but maintenance studies have been reported. The Epanova Program in Crohn's study (EPIC) 1 and 2 was a randomized, controlled, multicenter, parallel design study that reported no benefit of fish oil in the maintenance of CD.[134] Subsequently, a second Cochrane review of six studies investigating the role of fish oil on Crohn's disease maintenance found high heterogeneity with slightly improved outcomes in patients on fish oil (RR = 0.77, 95% CI 0.61–0.98). When the studies with high risk of bias and heterogeneity were excluded, there was no longer a benefit to fish oil over placebo.[135] A smaller study reported a benefit of fish oil with concomitant mesalamine use.[136] Another study suggested that fish oil may be more efficacious in Crohn's colitis than in small bowel enteritis.[45]

In contrast to CD, studies on the role of fish oil in the treatment of active ulcerative colitis have shown more promising results.[137-139] Supplementation with fish oil in active UC has been shown to improve clinical disease activity scores,[137] decrease the need for prescription therapy,[137] promote weight gain,[138] and reduce proinflammatory leukotriene B4 levels.[138] A novel nutritional approach using fish oil in a nutrition supplement was consumed by patients with active UC who were corticosteroid dependent. UC patients who consumed a solution containing fish oil, fructooligosaccharides, gum arabic, and antioxidants were more likely to taper prednisone over 6 months compared to placebo (P < 0.001).[140] Interestingly, the same principal investigator conducted a similar study in CD and reported a benefit of this solution in lowering the CD activity index and improving vitamin D status.[141] Only one study has compared mesalamine (sulfasalazine 2 g daily) to omega-3 fatty acids (5.4 g daily) in patients with active UC, with sulfasalazine treatment found to be superior to treatment with omega-3 fatty acids.[142] Therefore, fish oil should be considered as an adjuvant therapy to standard therapies. Of note, a case report has described a woman with distal UC who was brought into clinical and endoscopic remission with daily enemas of 3 g of omega-3 fatty acid.[143] This

is of particular interest given the aforementioned animal studies whereby rectal instillation of fish oils prevented and mitigated chemically induced colitis.

Glutamine

Glutamine is a nonessential amino acid but can be conditionally essential in catabolic conditions. It is the main energy source for small intestine enterocytes.[144,145] Animals provided a glutamine-deficient diet developed increased gut permeability and decreased functioning of the mucosa.[146,147] Supplementation of glutamine is beneficial in patients on TPN as it preserves villous health and prevents disruptions in intestinal permeability.[148,149] A small study investigating the role of glutamine on intestinal permeability in CD found no improvement following supplementation with 7-g glutamine three times daily.[150] The majority of alternative practitioners provide a dose escalating program starting with 5 g tid to a maximum of 30 g daily. In a pediatric CD study, 18 children with active CD were provided either a glutamine-enriched diet or a low-glutamine diet, and no differences were found in the remission rate, weight, or lab values.[151] Two rodent studies have reported harmful effects, with the use of glutamine causing worsening colitis or increased oxidative stress.[152] Currently, glutamine is contraindicated in colitis until further studies can shed light on the efficacy of glutamine in IBD. Glutamine has been recently reported to have favorable effects on the gut microbiome, which may be one reason why many practitioners continue to use this supplement for IBD patients. There is a theoretical concern that glutamine could be converted to glutamate, which is an excitatory neurotransmitter.[153]

N-Acetylcysteine

Glutathione is considered one of the most important antioxidant defenses in the body. N-acetylcysteine (NAC) replenishes glutathione rendered inactive by oxidation within the liver and has been shown to have antiinflammatory effects.[154] Animal models have demonstrated promise in using NAC as a treatment for colitis.[155-158] Only one human study of UC demonstrated clinical improvement with the use of NAC; however, rates of remission did not reach clinical significance (P = 0.19).[159]

Phosphatidylcholine

Phosphatidylcholine (PC) is an important component of the mucosal layer of the colon and acts as a surfactant within the mucus to create a hydrophobic surface to prevent bacterial penetrance. PC levels have been found to be reduced in the colon of UC patients compared to controls.[160,161] Without adequate PC in the mucosa, the intestinal barrier is permeable to colonic bacteria, leading to chronic intestinal inflammation and barrier defects.[161-164] Four human trials have been performed to determine the efficacy of PC in the treatment of UC. Two studies on patients with chronic active UC have reported clinical, endoscopic, and histological improvements.[165,166] Steroid-refractory UC patients were more successful in weaning off steroids when treated with PC compared to placebo (P < 0.01).[167] A double-blinded, randomized, placebo-controlled, multicenter study found that 3.2 g daily of PC improved clinical activity scores, histological remission, and relapse rates without any significant adverse events.[168]

Melatonin

Melatonin is synthesized from the amino acid tryptophan and is important for the circadian rhythm. It is known to induce Th1 lymphocytes and worsen the clinical course of UC and CD. As such, this supplement is contraindicated in IBD patients.[169-171]

Dehydroepiandrosterone

Dehydroepiandrosterone (DHEA) is one of the most abundant endogenous circulating steroid hormones produced mainly within the adrenal cortex. DHEA may inhibit the activation of NF-κB and secretion of IL-6 and IL-12.[172] One study found lower levels of DHEA-S (the sulfated form) in the blood and intestines of IBD patients,[173] although this may have been secondary to the use of corticosteroids.[174] A pilot trial by Andus et al. demonstrated an improvement in clinical activity indices in 20 IBD patients treated with 200 mg of DHEA orally for 8 weeks.[172] A case report suggests that DHEA may also be useful in the treatment of pouchitis.[175]

Probiotic and Prebiotic Supplements in IBD

Probiotics are defined as "live microorganisms which, when administered in adequate amounts, confer a health benefit on the host." To be labeled a probiotic, a number of criteria must be met.[176] Each probiotic must be strictly specified at the genus, species, and strain levels. Probiotics, by definition, contain live cultures when administered and should be shown to be viable prior to consumption, during intestinal transit, and be able to successfully colonize the intestines. There should be human-controlled trials evaluating the health benefits of probiotics. Probiotics are considered safe for their intended use.[177]

VSL#3

VSL #3 is a commercial product containing three genera of bacteria and a total of eight different species: Lactobacilli (*L. casei, L. plantarum, L. acidophilus,* and *L. delbrueckii*), Bifidobacteria (*B. longum, B. breve,* and *B. infantis*), and Streptococcus (*S. salivarius*). VSL#3 has been shown to restore the gut flora, attenuate inflammation, and decrease bacterial translocation.[178-182] It has been studied for CD, UC, and pouchitis, with the most compelling evidence for treatment of pouchitis. Regarding CD, several meta-analyses have failed to demonstrate a benefit of probiotics, although these trials were all quite heterogeneous.[183-186] Several studies have demonstrated a benefit of VSL#3 in the treatment of active UC.[187-191]

A systematic review with meta-analysis concluded that VSL#3 at a dose of 3.6×10^{12} CFU/day is superior when added to standard therapy compared to standard therapy alone in achieving response and remission in mild to moderate UC. This report noted that VSL#3 appears to be an adjuvant therapy and not a therapy that has been shown to be efficacious as monotherapy for active UC. Two trials[192,193] have provided evidence for the use of VSL#3 in the maintenance of remission of UC, and the American recommendations for probiotic use from 2011 strongly recommend VSL #3 for UC maintenance.[194] The most common side effect noted was symptomatic bloating without any serious adverse events reported.[195] The best data for VSL#3 is in UC patients who have undergone ileal pouch anal anastomosis with pouchitis, which is a common complication of total colectomy with ileal pouch anal anastomosis in these patients. Although exact mechanisms are still unknown, mucosal ischemia, genetic factors, and bacteria dysbiosis are thought to contribute to the pathogenesis of UC. Antibiotics temporarily alleviate the symptoms, but they rapidly return after treatment cessation due to gut microbial dysbiosis.[176] Clinical guidelines suggest the use of VSL#3 for the maintenance of remission of pouchitis and prevention of recurrent pouchitis; however, there is insufficient evidence to recommend VSL#3 for the treatment of acute pouchitis.[196]

Lactobacillus GG

Lactobacillus rhamnosus GG (LGG) was first isolated in 1983 and is known to have a strong avidity for human intestinal cells and can survive acid and bile environments. It is considered one of the most studied probiotics, with research showing that it could alleviate rotavirus diarrhea in children,[197] prevent atopic dermatitis,[198] protect against urinary tract infections,[199,200] and improve symptoms of irritable bowel syndrome.[201-203] LGG appears to be safe and effective in prolonging remission in UC patients.[204-207] LGG has also been studied in CD, but found to be no better than placebo.[208,209]

Saccharomyces boulardii

Saccharomyces boulardii (SBC) is a tropical, nonpathogenic strain of yeast, which has been successfully used as a probiotic for alleviating traveler's diarrhea,[210] HIV-induced diarrhea,[211] antibiotic-associated diarrhea,[212] and even in the prevention of *Clostridium difficile* relapses.[213] Animal models have shown hope for the use of SBC in the treatment of IBD.[214-217] A pilot study has demonstrated the efficacy of SBC in treatment of mild to moderate UC.[218] A case series of six patients with left-sided UC who were intolerant to mesalamine reported that patients responded to *S. boulardii* 500 mg plus rifaximin 400 mg.[219] In CD, SBC has been shown to decrease the frequency of bowel movements.[220] The addition of *S. boulardii* to mesalamine has demonstrated utility in maintaining remission of CD.[221] Interestingly, in one study, SBC has been shown to improve intestinal permeability among patients with CD.[222] The largest prospective, randomized, placebo-controlled trial of 165 Crohn's patients in remission who were followed for 1 year found that SBC was no better than placebo in preventing relapse.

Prebiotics

Prebiotics are defined as nondigestible fibrous products that selectively promote the growth or activity of beneficial bacteria and improve the well-being of the host. Prebiotics generally are not digested and absorbed into the intestines and instead provide nutrition to the beneficial bacteria (*Lactobacillus* and *Bifidobacterium*) in the distal small bowel and colon. Some examples of prebiotics include bran, psyllium husk, inulin, fructooligosaccharides (FOS), and galactooligosaccharides (GOS). Prebiotics are commonly used to regulate the bowels both in constipation, where they increase fecal water content, and diarrhea, where they add bulk to the stool. *Plantago ovata*, also known as psyllium, has been studied in the treatment of ulcerative colitis. One small study reported that a 4-month treatment with *Plantago ovata* improved symptoms in UC patients in remission.[223] An open-label trial in 105 patients with quiescent UC who were randomized to one of three groups: 10 g twice daily of *Plantago ovata*, 500 mg three times daily of mesalamine, or *Plantago ovata* plus mesalamine reported similar rates of continued remission.[224] Inulin (12 g daily) has been shown to decrease levels of fecal calprotectin in active UC patients and to be well tolerated.[225] In a mouse model of UC, inulin decreased the amount of nitric oxide in the colon and the severity of the colitis, indicating that inulin may be helpful in the treatment of active UC.[226] Inulin has also shown promise in the treatment of pouchitis.[227] An open-label trial of fructooligosaccharides (FOS, 15 g daily for three weeks) was performed in 10 active CD patients with active ileocolonic disease with clinical improvement.[228] In contrast, a controlled trial of 103 patients found no difference in clinical response, but patients treated with FOS had higher drop-out rates. There are several rodent studies demonstrating a decrease in intestinal inflammation and improvement in colonic bacterial composition after FOS treatment[229-231]; therefore, further studies are required to investigate the potential efficacy of FOS in IBD.

Germinated barley foodstuff (GBF) was initially discovered to attenuate colitis in animal models by increasing luminal short-chain fatty acid production.[232,233] In a pilot study, 10 patients with active UC received 30 g of GBF for 4 weeks and were found to have an improvement in clinical activity and endoscopic scores and an increase in stool butyrate levels.[234] A study by Kanauchi et al. of 18 UC patients found that 20–30 g daily of GBF improved clinical scores and increased *Bifidobacterium* numbers.[235] A follow-up, open label study of 21 UC patients by Kanauchi et al. again demonstrated improved symptomatic scores, a decrease in rectal bleeding, and lower rates of nocturnal diarrhea.[236] To investigate the efficacy of GBF in maintaining remission in UC, 59 patients were administered either GBF (20 g daily) plus standard therapy or placebo plus standard therapy for 12 months. Improved clinical activity index scores were observed in

the GBF group at each time point with lower recurrence rates.[237] In a study investigating the mechanism of action of GBF, Faghfoori et al. demonstrated that GBF reduced levels of serum TNF-α, IL-6, and IL-8. The most recent clinical study of GBF reported a reduction in CRP levels, abdominal pain, and cramping compared to placebo.[238] A rodent model has also shown GBF may prevent the development of colitis-associated neoplasia,[239] although this decreased risk of neoplasia may simply be due to the decrease in inflammation and not necessarily a chemopreventive effect.

> Prebiotics must be used with caution in CD patients with stricturing disease because high fiber loads can lead to obstruction. Additionally, prebiotics are known to cause gas and bloating when commenced, and starting at lower doses may help alleviate these GI effects.

Synbiotics

Synbiotics are a combination of prebiotics and probiotics that are believed to have a synergistic effect by inhibiting the growth of pathogenic bacteria and enhancing the growth of beneficial organisms.[240,241] One study found that synbiotic therapy (*Bifidobacterium longum* plus psyllium) was superior to either therapy alone in improving IBD questionnaire scores and C-reactive protein (CRP) levels.[242] The synbiotic Synergy 1 (FOS/inulin mix) and *Bifidobacterium longum* reportedly improved active UC according to sigmoidoscopy scores and inflammatory markers.[243] A synbiotic containing 10^9 CFU of the *Bifidobacterium breve* strain Yakult and 5.5 g of galactooligosaccharide (GOS) was shown to improve colonoscopic findings and fecal concentrations of *Bacteroidaceae*.[244] In a small study, 10 patients with active CD refractory to mesalamine and steroids were administered a synbiotic containing 75 billion CFU of either *Bifidobacterium* or *Lactobacillus* and 9.9 g of psyllium and were allowed to adjust the consumption of prebiotic and probiotic as needed. Six patients were able to decrease or stop other therapies for CD, including prednisone. Despite the clinical improvement, no improvements were observed in serum inflammatory markers.[245] A randomized, double-blind, placebo-controlled trial of 35 CD patients found that the synbiotic Synergy 1 plus *B. longum* improved CDAI scores (P = 0.02) and histological scores (P = 0.018).[246] In a study investigating the role of synbiotics in the prevention of postoperative recurrence in CD, 30 patients were randomized to either Synbiotic 2000 or placebo in a 2:1 ratio. Synbiotic 2000 consists of four lactic acid bacteria and four fermentable fibers. After 24 months of postoperative follow-up, no effect of Synbiotic 2000 on postoperative recurrence was observed based on symptomatic, endoscopic, laboratory, and histological criteria.[247]

Bovine Colostrum

Colostrum is a form of milk produced in the mammary glands just before giving birth. It contains high levels of antibodies and protein as well as growth factors and antimicrobial factors that help provide passive immunity and stimulate development of the GI tract in newborns.[248-250] Several animal studies have found colostrum prevents or alleviates colitis.[251-253] A study of 14 patients with distal colitis reported improvements in symptoms and histology after 100 mL of 10% bovine colostrum solution enema was given for 4 weeks.[254]

Herbal Therapies in IBD

Aloe Vera

Aloe vera has been shown to have dose-dependent antiinflammatory properties in vitro by inhibiting the production of reactive oxygen metabolites, eicosanoids, and IL-8.[255] A double-blind, randomized, placebo-controlled trial of 44 patients with active UC found that 100 mg of oral aloe vera was superior to placebo in improving clinical and histological disease activity. Additionally, no significant adverse events were observed, indicating that aloe vera may be a safe and efficacious treatment for active UC.[256] To date, there are no trials evaluating the effects of aloe vera on CD.

Andrographis paniculata Extract (HMPL-004)

Herbal treatment with *Andrographis paniculata* has been used in Asian countries to treat inflammatory diseases. An extract *of A. paniculata*, HMPL-004, was found to inhibit the development of chronic colitis in rodent models.[257] HMPL-004 1200 mg/day was found to have equivalent efficacy to mesalamine 4500 mg/day in terms of clinical remission, response, and endoscopic remission in 125 patients from China with active UC.[258] In a larger placebo-controlled trial of 224 patients with mild to moderate active UC, patients were randomized to HMPL-004 at a dose of 1800 mg/day, and a significantly higher rate of clinical response was observed compared to placebo.[259]

Boswellia serrata

Boswellia serrata has been used for hundreds of years in Indian herbal treatments for multiple inflammatory conditions. *Boswellia* is believed to act via inhibition of 5-lipoxygenase, thereby decreasing leukotriene biosynthesis and resulting in diminished proinflammatory cytokine release.[260] A small trial of active UC patients found that *Boswellia* 350 mg three times a day was as effective as sulfasalazine 1000 mg three times a day in decreasing symptoms and laboratory indicators.[261] A second similar study of 30 active UC patients again found *Boswellia* to be as effective as sulfasalazine, with remission rates of 82% and 75%, respectively.[262] *Boswellia* has also been tested in Crohn patients for initiating[263] and maintaining remission.[264] Gerhardt et al. performed a randomized, double-blinded study of 102 patients comparing H15, a proprietary *Boswellia serrata* extract, to mesalazine and found a similar decrease in CDAI in both groups, showing that *Boswellia* is noninferior to mesalamine for treatment of CD.[263] Holtmeier et al. evaluated *Boswellia* versus placebo for maintenance of remission in CD and

found no significant difference, but did confirm excellent tolerability and minimal adverse effects.[264]

Bromelain

Bromelain is a concentrate of proteolytic enzymes derived from the stem of the pineapple fruit and is believed to have antiinflammatory properties. Rodent models of colitis reportedly improved after treatment with bromelain.[265] A case series described two chronic UC patients who achieved clinical and endoscopic remission after treatment with bromelain supplementation.[266] Larger trials are required to further explore the potential for this novel therapy.

Cannabis sativa

Cannabis sativa, or marijuana, is frequently used for both recreation due to its psychoactive properties and medicinal use due to its effects on pain, nausea, and perhaps inflammation. Cannabis contains more than 60 cannabinoid compounds, with tetrahydrocannabinol (THC) being one of the main active components that act on CB1 and CB2 receptors in the body.[267] New findings show that there are endogenous endocannabinoids that also act on these receptors and may play a role in limiting intestinal inflammation.[268,269] Numerous basic and clinical studies have shown that cannabis use has positive effects on pain, specifically that originating within the GI tract, and inflammation.[269-276] Cannabinoids have also been shown to prevent or ameliorate colitis in animal models.[277-281]

A retrospective observational study reported that 21 of 30 patients improved clinically after cannabis treatment. Additionally, the need for other CD therapies and the number of surgeries both decreased.[282] A prospective, placebo-controlled study of cannabis in the treatment of refractory CD showed benefit (P = 0.028), with clinical remission (CDAI < 150) achieved in 45% in cannabis group versus 10% in placebo group (P = 0.43).[283] A recent study investigating the effects of cannabis on IBD reported an association between more severe disease and higher risk of surgery among cannabis users, although causality could not be determined based on this study design.[284]

Marijuana use is most common amongst IBD patients with a history of abdominal surgery and worse symptom scores.[285] Cannabinoids have been shown to inhibit intestinal secretion and may help with diarrheal symptoms.[268,269,286] Severe IBD patients also suffer with a loss of appetite, and cannabis is known to enhance appetite.[287] Notably, cannabis is not without side effects. Almost a third of patients reported paranoia and anxiety,[285] and there are known long-term mental health consequences of chronic cannabis use.[288] Palpitations and cardiac effects have been reported in cannabis users.[289]

Curcumin and Turmeric (Curcuma longa)

Curcumin is a naturally occurring substance from the plant *Curcuma longa* and is an active phytochemical contained within turmeric.[290] Curcumin has been shown to possess antioxidant, antiinflammatory, and anticarcinogenic properties.[291-293] By inhibiting the synthesis of IL-2, TNF-α, and IFN-γ, curcumin also acts as an immunosuppressant.[292,294] The antiinflammatory effects of curcumin on the colonic tissue have been shown to be at least in part due to inhibition of chemokine expression and direct inhibition of neutrophil chemotaxis and chemokinesis.[295] The poor systemic absorption of curcumin maintains the active compound within the intestines, where it has antiinflammatory properties.[294] Preliminary studies in rodents have reported that curcumin is able to prevent and treat chemically induced colitis.[296-300]

Several human studies have reported promising results and an excellent safety profile for the use of curcumin in IBD patients. An initial open-label study of 10 IBD patients (5 UC, 5 CD) found symptomatic improvement in 90% of patients.[301] Hanai et al. conducted a randomized, double-blind, placebo-controlled trial of 89 UC patients with quiescent disease on stable doses of baseline mesalamine therapy. Two grams daily of oral curcumin was associated with reduced symptoms, UC flares, and endoscopic inflammation compared to placebo.[302] A recent multicenter, randomized, double-blind, placebo-controlled study by Lang et al. reported that the combination of mesalamine and curcumin may have a synergistic effect in mild to moderately active UC. Oral curcumin at a dose of 3 g daily was administered to 26 UC patients on optimized mesalamine therapy and compared to placebo plus mesalamine administered to 24 patients. Clinical remission was achieved in 54% of patients receiving curcumin compare to 0% of patients receiving placebo. Additionally, clinical improvement, endoscopic remission, and endoscopic improvement were significantly improved in the curcumin group compared to the placebo group. Importantly, no difference in rates of adverse events were observed between the two groups, again demonstrating curcumin as a safe and well-tolerated treatment in UC.[303] Curcumin has also been shown to be antineoplastic and has proven to decrease polyp growth in familial polyposis syndrome.[293] Due to these known chemopreventive effects against colon cancer, curcumin may be an excellent choice for IBD patients who have a known increased risk of colorectal cancer. Curcumin definitely appears to have promise in the treatment of UC and possibly CD, although further studies are required.

Wormwood (Artemisia absinthium)

Wormwood is a fragrant herb traditionally used to treat various digestive disorders with favorable effects on the gut microbiome, leading to resolution of gut microbial dysbiosis.[304] Two human studies have evaluated the efficacy of wormwood in CD. In an initial study of 40 patients with CD receiving 40 mg of prednisone daily, participants were administered 1500 mg of wormwood or placebo daily for 10 weeks. More patients receiving wormwood compared to placebo were able to successfully taper the steroids.[305] The second study of 20 CD patients administered either 2250 mg of wormwood or placebo daily. Patients receiving wormwood had a decrease in serum TNF-α levels after 6 weeks.

Additionally, patients treated with wormwood had reduced CDAI and overall mood scores (Hamilton's Depression Scale).[306]

Wheat grass juice (Triticum aestivum/Poaceae)

Wheat grass juice is made from the pulp of the common wheat plant *Triticum aestivum*, which is a subspecies of the family Poaceae. Antioxidant properties have been exhibited by wheat grass extracts due to radical scavenging and antiinflammatory activity.[307,308] In a study of 23 patients with UC, patients were administered either 100 cc of wheat grass juice or placebo daily for 1 month. Those who received active treatment had significantly reduced overall disease activity (P = 0.031) and rectal bleeding severity (P = 0.025) without any serious side effects.[309] Due to the concurrence of IBD and celiac disease, patients should be certain they do not have celiac disease before using wheat grass juice.

Xilei-san

Xilei-san (XLS) is a mixture of herbs used in Chinese medicine for inflammatory or ulcerative diseases, such as oral ulcers, gastritis, and peptic ulcer disease.[310] XLS consists of a fixed combination of eight natural herbs/minerals.[310] Animals treated with XLS enemas were shown to have less severe colitis.[310] XLS suppositories 0.1 g daily were used for refractory ulcerative proctitis patients who improved clinically and endoscopically compared to placebo.[311] A second human study was performed on 35 patients with ulcerative proctitis where the researchers compared XLS to dexamethasone enemas. After 12 weeks, XLS was found to be equivalent to dexamethasone in terms of clinical, endoscopic, and histological grading scores. No adverse events were noted with XLS, and it was found to be well tolerated overall. XLS may be considered as an adjuvant or alternative therapy for patients with ulcerative proctitis.

Pharmaceuticals and Helminths

Antimicrobial Drugs

Because studies have suggested that infectious agents may be the cause or exacerbating factor in IBD, antibiotics have been frequently used in the treatment of IBD. The data is sparse, and there is no clear benefit in UC, a small benefit in CD, and the most benefit in pouchitis.[312-315] Antibiotics are mainly used to treat the complications of IBD, such as abscesses, perforations, or wound infections. Antibiotics have common side effects that limit their use, and the most significant risk is *Clostridium difficile* infection, to which IBD patients are more susceptible.[316-319] Additionally, antibiotics are only effective in the short term, with no long-term data currently available. The available evidence indicates a moderate benefit with the use of metronidazole 10–20 mg/kg/day or the combination metronidazole plus ciprofloxacin 500 mg twice daily for colonic CD, but not isolated small bowel CD.[320] A meta-analysis from 2011 reported that antibiotics were superior to placebo in inducing and maintaining remission in CD and reducing fistula drainage.[321] There is some emerging data on the benefits of rifaximin, a non-absorbable antibiotic, in the treatment of CD[322-324]; however, further studies are required.

> Metronidazole is a frequently used antibiotic for IBD patients but has significant adverse effects, including irreversible peripheral neuropathy, which should be discussed with the patient prior to prescribing. Metronidazole causes severe GI upset in some patients leading to nausea, vomiting, abdominal cramping, and diarrhea, which can be difficult to discern between a disease flare or medication side effect.

Naltrexone

Naltrexone is a nonselective opioid receptor antagonist that acts on the three opioid receptor subtypes μ, κ, and δ. Endogenous opioids are believed to play a role in immune system modulation.[325,326] Narcotics are considered to be proinflammatory, with several studies reporting an association between narcotic use and worsened IBD.[327,328] Opioid antagonists appear to promote tissue growth, repair, and healing. Naltrexone has been shown to reverse chemically induced rodent colitis by reducing levels of the proinflammatory cytokines IL-6 and IL-12. Naltrexone has predominantly been studied for the treatment of CD in humans. In an open label study, 17 patients with active CD were treated with 4.5 mg of naltrexone daily. After 12 weeks, 89% had a clinical response, and 67% achieved clinical remission.[329] A case report noted a child with duodenal CD that was treated successfully with low dose naltrexone.[330] The first double-blind, placebo-controlled study of 40 active CD patients treated with 4.5 mg of naltrexone demonstrated a significant response clinically (P = 0.009) and endoscopically (P = 0.008) compared to placebo.[331] The most recent study evaluated naltrexone (0.1 mg/kg) use in children with active CD in an open label trial. There were no serious adverse outcomes. Remission was achieved in 25% of patients treated with naltrexone, and 67% had clinical improvement based on disease activity indices.[332]

Helminths

Industrialization and improved sanitation have led to the eradication of many infectious parasites. The prevalence of helminth infections in developed Western countries has significantly decreased to less than 2%.[333] Based on the hygiene hypothesis contributing to the development of IBD, the disappearance of helminth infections may predispose developed nations to an increased risk of developing IBD[334] and other autoimmune diseases. In response to helminthic infections, the Th2 immune response is invoked, leading to suppression of Th1 and Th17 effector cells, which promote chronic inflammation in IBD.[335-342] A number of IBD animal models have indicated that helminth infection may be a promising treatment for colitis.[343-346] Summers et al. conducted three clinical studies investigating the pig whipworm, *Trichuris*

suis (*T. suis*), as a treatment for IBD. An open label trial in seven IBD patients showed significant clinical improvement, although patients required repeated doses to maintain efficacy.[347] In the second study, 29 CD patients were administered 2500 *T. suis* orally every 3 weeks for 24 weeks, resulting in remission and response in 72% and 79% of patients, respectively.[348] A randomized, double-blind, placebo-controlled study of 54 UC patients administered 2500 *T. suis* every 2 weeks for 12 weeks reported improvement in 43% of treated patients compared to 17% in the placebo group (P = 0.04).[349] The most recent study investigated the safety and tolerability of *T. suis* at three doses (500, 2500, or 7500 parasites) compared to placebo. There were no significant differences in patient-reported symptoms, and there were no dose-dependent side effects.[350] A small study investigating the hookworm *Necator ameriacanus* in nine CD patients observed an improvement in CDAI scores.[351] The data thus far show that helminths do attenuate chronic inflammation in IBD and other autoimmune diseases, but long-term safety still has to be evaluated as the potential for migration of the helminths is a possibility. This treatment is only available through clinical trials that are ongoing.

5-Aminosalicylic Acid (Mesalamine)

There are multiple formulations of mesalamines currently on the market, including sulfasalazine, asacol, delzicol, lialda, pentasa, and apriso. Mesalamines are also available in suppositories and enemas to treat distal colitis. Mesalamines are effective for inducing and maintaining remission in ulcerative colitis patients with mild to moderate colitis. The exact mechanism is still unknown, but they act topically on the colonic mucosa as antiinflammatory agents. Sulfasalazine is a prodrug composed of 5-aminosalicylic acid (5-ASA) and sulfapyridine. 5-ASA is the active drug, whereas sulfapyridine can cause allergic reactions in patients with sulfa allergies, folate deficiency, agranulocytosis, and anemia and azoospermia in men. Other mesalamine products only contain 5-ASA, which is poorly absorbed and has a low risk of side effects. A paradoxical reaction with mesalamines may cause worsening of colitis in approximately 3% of patients. This is considered an allergy, and other mesalamines should not be used. Mesalamines are the mainstay of therapy for mild to moderate ulcerative colitis. In left-sided only colitis, enemas alone may be effective, although oral plus rectal therapy is recommended. Proctitis, inflammation confined to the rectum, can be managed with suppositories and/or enemas. Pancolitis is best managed with oral and rectal mesalamine therapy. Because CD is characterized by transmural inflammation, mesalamines are not as effective. There is some evidence to suggest that mesalamine therapy may provide some benefit in mild Crohn colitis, although typically, immunosuppressive medications may be required. Mesalamines have the least toxic side effect profile of the pharmaceutical agents approved for IBD.

Glucocorticoids

Steroids were previously the only therapy available for IBD patients. They are potent antiinflammatory agents and reduce intestinal inflammation rapidly and effectively. Steroids have been shown to bring both UC and CD into remission, although there is no benefit of maintaining remission for either disease. The use of steroids has tremendous risks, including the development of diabetes, hypertension, weight gain, gastritis, growth failure, osteoporosis, poor wound healing, and severe infections. Aseptic necrosis of the femoral head is a commonly feared adverse effect. Steroids have been shown to decrease intestinal absorption of calcium, phosphorus, and zinc.[79] The use of steroids in CD has become more controversial, and data are emerging that the risks of steroids in CD far outweigh the benefits. Expert opinions currently suggest that steroids can increase the risk of abscesses, fistulas, and need for surgery. Therefore, CD therapy is shying away from the use of steroids if possible, especially in children.[352]

Immunosuppressants

6-mercaptopurine and its prodrug azathioprine (thiopurines) are immunosuppressant medications that have shown benefit in the maintenance of remission in both CD and UC. These drugs do not induce remission and can take up to 3 months to have their full effect. Multiple studies have shown excellent efficacy of thiopurines in maintaining steroid-free remission in IBD.[353,354] Thiopurines may help heal Crohn fistulas and prevent postoperative recurrence of CD.[355] Once thiopurine treatment is discontinued, the risk of CD flare is high.[356] The major risk of thiopurines is bone marrow suppression, which can lead to life-threatening cytopenias. It is therefore recommended to monitor blood counts frequently. There is an increased risk of lymphoma and nonmelanoma skin cancers with the use of thiopurines. Yearly dermatology visits are recommended for full skin exams. Cyclosporine is another immunosuppressant agent previously used in the treatment of UC. Although it has fallen out of favor with the advent of tumor necrosis factor blockers (described in the subsequent text), it is still occasionally used for the induction of remission of steroid refractory UC. Cyclosporine is a fast-acting immunosuppressant that decreases T-cell activity and the subsequent immune response. Cyclosporine has a narrow therapeutic window, with elevated levels resulting in nephrotoxicities, neurotoxicities, seizures, and GI upset.

> Patients receiving thiopurine medication are required to undergo frequent blood monitoring of white and red blood cell counts because life-threatening pancytopenia uncommonly may occur. Liver function tests should also be performed as there is a potential for hepatotoxicity.

Tumor Necrosis Factor-α Blockade

The first tumor necrosis factor-α (TNF-α) inhibitor, infliximab, was approved for use in CD and UC in 1998. Since that time, adalimumab, certolizumab pegol, and golimumab have been approved as TNF-α inhibitors for the treatment of IBD. Infliximab is administered as an intravenous infusion, while the others are self-injectables. TNF inhibitors have revolutionized the treatment of IBD because they are fast-acting and potent inhibitors of proinflammatory cytokines. They have been shown to be effective in inducing and maintaining remission in CD and UC. TNF inhibitors can heal fistulas in CD patients, decrease relapse rates of IBD, and promote mucosal healing. These are steroid-sparing agents and are used as first-line agents in severe UC and moderate to severe CD. As immunosuppressants, TNF inhibitors increase the risk of serious infections, such as reactive hepatitis B and latent tuberculosis (TB). Prior to initiating therapy with these agents, a purified protein derivative (PPD) or Quantiferon Gold serum test is required to confirm a negative TB status. Hepatitis B serologies should be performed to ensure that hepatitis B is not present, and vaccination should be offered. There is a possible increased risk of lymphoma and skin cancers with the use of TNF inhibitors, although this may only occur in combination with thiopurine therapy.

Surgery

The goal of medical therapy in IBD is to prevent the need for surgery. In UC, severe colitis refractory to medical therapy can develop and require a complete colectomy. After the initial operation, there are two options: a permanent ileostomy or an ileal pouch anal anastomosis (IPAA). A total colectomy is seen as a "cure" for ulcerative colitis and, after struggling with refractory colitis for many years, patients typically feel significantly better. Although there is no further colitis, the ileostomy can be difficult to manage, can leak, and may develop a hernia around the stoma. If an ileal pouch is created, patients should anticipate having six to seven loose BMs daily, including possible nocturnal BMs and chance of seepage. There is also the risk of pouchitis, inflammation of the pouch, requiring antibiotic therapy. VSL#3 has shown to be protective against the development of pouchitis and recurring pouchitis. IPAA can cause infertility in females. More-so than in ulcerative colitis, surgery is strongly avoided in CD. As CD can affect the entire GI tract from mouth to anus, frequent surgeries can lead to short gut syndrome and severe malabsorption. CD is also known to recur at the site of previous surgical anastomosis. Surgery for CD is required when stricturing disease occurs that causes bowel obstruction and inability to tolerate oral intake. There are ongoing studies investigating endoscopic dilation and stent placement of Crohn strictures in an attempt to delay if not avoid surgery.

Mind-Body Medicine

Inflammatory Bowel Disease and Stress

Perceived stress is a significant predictor for flaring in ulcerative colitis (UC), and the risk of experiencing exacerbation is multiplied by prolonged exposure to stress.[357] Up to 70% of patients with inflammatory bowel disease (IBD) regard stress as a modifying factor for their disease,

TABLE 50.1 Randomized Trials of Stress-Reducing Therapies in IBD

Authors	Disease	Patients	Design	Intervention	Control	Duration	Outcome
Berrill et al.[361]	IBD	66, 2 groups	RCT	Multiconvergent Therapy (MCT); 6 × 40-min sessions over 16 weeks	Standard care (SC)	4, 8, 12 months	No difference in outcomes (IBDQ, perceived stress, coping)
Langhorst et al.[360]	UC	60, 2 groups	RCT	Lifestyle modification (MBSR)	Wait list control (WLC)	3, 12 months	Improved SF-36 (3 months in MBSR—reduction of BSI anxiety (3 months in MBSR) compared with WL
Mizrahi et al.[365]	IBD	56, 2 groups	RCT	Relaxation training (RT)	WLC, SC	5 weeks	Stress, mood, pain, anxiety, QOL, depression improved by RT
Milne et al.[364]	IBD	80, 2 groups	RCT	Stress management techniques	SC	4, 8, 12 months	Improvement within the treatment group, but not control group for all time points, CDAI
Keefer et al.[363]	UC	54, 2 groups	RCT	Gut-directed hypnotherapy	Attention control (AC)	52 weeks	More patients in remission in hypnotherapy vs. control, more days to clinical relapse in hypnotherapy
Jedel et al.[362]	UC	55, 2 groups	RCT	MBSR	AC	2, 6, 12 months	Sig. group difference in bowel subscale and systemic subscale
Elsenbruch et al.[359]	UC	30, 2 groups	RCT	MBSR	WLC	2, 4, 6, 8, 10 weeks	Improved SF-36 mental health scale, Psychological Health Sum Score and IBDQ after 10 weeks in MBSR vs. WL

and 85% regard stress coping as having a positive impact on their course of disease.[358] A number of studies (Table 50.1) have evaluated the effects of different interventions targeting stress and psychological well-being on the course of IBD.

Lifestyle Modification

Two studies investigated the effect of lifestyle modification programs on disease activity, quality of life, psychological parameters, and laboratory profiles in 30[359] and 60[360] patients with UC. Both studies applied a randomized wait-list controlled study design. Results showed significant improvements in psychological quality of life after 10 weeks[359] and 3 months[360] as well as significant reduction of anxiety after 3 months.[360] Neither medication nor laboratory profiles showed any change. The risk of bias was low in both studies.

Mindfulness-Based Interventions

There are two studies which have investigated the effects of mindfulness-based interventions on IBD. The first involved 66 patients with inactive IBD,[361] which compared one-to-one multiconvergent therapy (MCT) plus standard care (SC) to standard care alone. The other study involved 55 patients with inactive UC and compared mindfulness-based stress reduction (MBSR) courses to time/attention control courses.[362] Neither study showed significant group differences regarding disease activity,

relapse, or psychological variables in the main analysis. However, significant improvements in quality of life (QOL) were observed in inactive IBD patients with additional irritable bowel syndrome-type symptoms.[361] The risk of bias was low.[361] MBSR was found to mitigate the effects of stress and C-reactive protein in UC patients who flared during the course of the study, which was noted to have a high risk of bias.[362]

Hypnotherapy

Keefer et al.[363] investigated the effects of gut-directed hypnotherapy, a program that was developed for irritable bowel syndrome. Patients received seven weekly sessions of hypnotherapy compared to an attention control (AC) group. After 52 weeks, patients were significantly better regarding the probability to flare; however, no effects were found on quality of life or other psychological measures. The risk of bias of the trial was low.

Relaxation Training

A study by Mizrahi et al. involving 56 subjects investigated the effects of relaxation training in patients with IBD in general.[365] Study subjects were randomized into three sessions and subsequent home practice of relaxation or a usual care group. The authors found significant improvements in pain, anxiety, depression, mood, stress, and quality of life, including bowel symptoms within the relaxation group, but not the usual care group. Risk of bias was high in this study as it failed to report a random allocation procedure and no attempt was made to blind patients or outcome assessors.

Traditional Chinese Medicine (TCM)

Acupuncture is an ancient tradition of healing that prevents and mitigates illness by balancing the flow of energy (chi) in energy circuits (meridians). Acupuncture can modulate neuroenteric circuits, inflammation, and many physiological processes that influence the gastrointestinal tract.[366] There are studies to support the use of acupuncture for treating gastrointestinal pain and other symptoms. Acupuncture has been shown to benefit patients with gastroparesis, nausea (postoperative, chemotherapy), irritable bowel syndrome, constipation, functional dyspepsia, gastroparesis, and possibly more.[367-370] Joos et al. evaluated the potential role of acupuncture in the management of IBD and were the first to report a therapeutic effect upon IBD with regard to disease activity scores, but not to quality of life questionnaires or symptom scores, in active CD as well as UC.[371,372] A recent meta-analysis by Ji et al. included 43 studies of which 37 are in the Chinese literature.[373] Among the 43 included trials, 10 trials compared oral sulphasalazine (SASP) with acupuncture and/or moxibustion treatments for induction of remission and demonstrated the superiority of acupuncture and moxibustion therapy.[373] However, use of the Jadad scale to assess the methodological quality of these studies demonstrated a score of 1 or 2 (scale of 1–5 in ascending order of quality) in a total of 39 studies, demonstrating low methodical standards including insufficient description of endpoints and randomization process, and missing power calculations. Lee et al. conducted a meta-analysis of the effect of moxibustion/acupuncture on ulcerative colitis including five RCTs published in the Chinese literature.[374] The studies compared the effects of moxibustion/acupuncture with conventional IBD drug therapy (sulfasalazine alone or with other drugs). The results showed favorable effects of moxibustion on response rates compared to conventional drug therapy but with a high-risk bias (n = 407; risk ratio = 1.24, 95% CI = 1.11 to 1.38; P < 0.0001; heterogeneity: I2 = 16%). The authors concluded that there is insufficient evidence to show that moxibustion/acupuncture is an effective treatment of UC. Further high-quality research is mandatory to provide higher levels of evidence in the field of acupuncture and TCM.

The pathogenesis of IBD involves a multifactorial process, which includes genetic predisposition, immune dysregulation, barrier dysfunction, and altered microbial flora as well as environmental and lifestyle factors. Thus, it seems plausible that subgroups of patients may benefit from a tailored therapy with emphasis on individually different modalities. In particular, mind-body medicine widens the spectrum and adds a resource-orientated salutogenetic dimension to introduce a multimodal integrative treatment program. Future high-quality designs in health research are warranted.

PREVENTION PRESCRIPTION

PRIMARY PREVENTION

- Minimize exposure to antibiotics in childhood and beyond, particularly the tetracycline family of antibiotics.
- Eating a diet high in fiber-rich fruits and vegetables while minimizing Western-based diets (red meats, fried foods, refined sugars, and grains).
- Encourage probiotic and prebiotic foods to promote gut microbial diversity.

SECONDARY PREVENTION

- Curcumin 1000 mg twice daily (UC).
- Fish oils 4000–5000 mg daily (CD).
- Mind-body relaxation techniques.
- Germinated barley foodstuff (GBF) 20 g daily (UC).
- VSL#3 three sachets daily (UC, pouchitis).

THERAPEUTIC REVIEW

Inflammatory bowel disease (IBD) is a chronic autoimmune disease without a "cure" that has the potential for numerous complications, including gastrointestinal cancer. Thus all patients should be under the care of a gastroenterologist for regular screening colonoscopy and ongoing medical therapy. The integrative practitioner can provide personalized lifestyle and dietary guidance to achieve improved quality of life.

LABORATORY TESTS

A number of laboratory tests are available for disease monitoring and nutritional guidance. Patients with IBD should have annual testing with a complete blood count, complete metabolic profile, and C-reactive protein. Nutritional markers for IBD patients with chronic diarrhea should include red blood cell (RBC), zinc, serum homocysteine, RBC magnesium, serum iron, and 25-OH vitamin D. In steroid-treated patients with refractory disease, serum de- hydroepiandrosterone sulfate (DHEA-S), 25-OH vitamin D, and an essential acid profile may be useful. Patients with recent onset, relapse, or exacerbation of IBD—especially those with diarrhea—should undergo stool testing for parasites, pathogenic bacteria, *Clostridium difficile* toxins, and yeast. The potential role of more advanced stool testing using genetic analysis and metabolomics for stool pathogens is controversial; however, integrative gut experts and functional medicine practitioners have anecdotally reported intriguing benefits.

SELF-MANAGEMENT

Patients are oftentimes in need of health coaching to manage their medical care, which can become overwhelming and interfere with QOL and productivity at work. Encouraging a support network to help maintain good mental health and resources in the midst of a flare are helpful adjuncts to good integrative care.

Continued

NUTRITION

- Overarching recommendation is to maintain a balanced macro and micronutrient rich diet with ample antiinflammatory nutrients, minimize fiber for fibrostenosing CD, and limit sucrose and symptom-provoking foods.
- Lactose intolerance is common in patients with IBD and should be avoided only in those who are intolerant because dairy contains calcium which is important for bone health.
- Provide prebiotic soluble fiber-rich foods for ulcerative colitis (UC) to maintain remission.
- Consider an elimination diet for symptoms relief and control.
- The specific carbohydrate diet has some evidence to suggest benefit for symptom control but is no substitute for recommended medical therapy.
- An enteral formula diet may help improve symptoms and may help induce or maintain remission in children with CD.

SUPPLEMENTS

- Patients taking mesalamine (5-ASA) medications or sulfasalazine, or those who have high homocysteine not due to low B12 status, should consider taking folate 1 mg/day and should get tested to confirm sufficiency. Consider genetic testing for methylene tetrahydrofolate reductase (MTHFR) homozygosity if sufficient serum folate levels are difficult to achieve.
- Vitamin B_{12}: 1 mg/month for patients with ileitis or previous ileal resection A1, receiving folic acid, or with high homocysteine.
- Vitamin B_6: 10 to 20 mg/day, especially for patients with high homocysteine or taking high-dose folic acid or with urolithiasis.
- Vitamin D_3: 1000 units/day or more to maintain levels of 25-OH vitamin D at 40 ng/mL
- Calcium: 1000 mg/day for patients taking steroids or with low dietary calcium
- Chromium: Up to 600 mcg/day for patients with steroid-induced glycemia or as part of micronutrient mix on central parenteral nutrition
- Zinc sulfate: 220–440 mg/day recommended in patients with draining fistula, recent surgery, or active, severe diarrhea.
- Fish oils supplying 4000 to 5000 mg/day of omega-3 fatty acids (eicosapentaenoic acid and docosahexaenoic acid) for patients with active UC and to maintain remission for CD, more effective in Crohn colitis than enteritis. Fish oils may cause burping and bloating.
- Prebiotic oligosaccharides: approximately 10 g/day for UC. They can cause distention and flatulence.
- Germinated barley foodstuff: 20–30 g/day has been shown to maintain remission in UC patients when added to standard medical therapy. Side effects include bloating and flatulence.
- HMPL-004: 1200–1800 mg/day improves clinical scores in active UC patients. A higher incidence of rash was reported compared to placebo.

BIOLOGICAL AGENTS

- VSL-3: one sachet twice to three times a day for patients with mild-to-moderate UC who are not sensitive to corn, the growth medium used as an adjunct to medical care, to maintain remission for pouchitis or to maintain remission for UC. Any probiotic may aggravate bowel symptoms in patients with IBD.
- DHEA: 200 mg/day for patients with refractory disease and low DHEA-S .

BOTANICALS

- *Boswellia serrata* gum resin: 350 mg three times daily for patients with UC who are intolerant of 5-ASA derivatives. No adverse effects reported to date.
- Curcumin: 1000 mg twice daily with meals to maintain remission in UC as an adjunct with mesalamines.

PHARMACEUTICALS

- 5-ASA derivatives for induction of remission in mild-to-moderate colitis and for maintenance of remission.
- Antibiotics for acute exacerbations of CD or perianal disease.
- Glucocorticoids for induction of remission in severe disease.
- 6-Mercaptopurine or azathioprine for steroid-dependent IBD or for maintenance of remission when 5-ASA derivatives fail. Consult GI.
- TNF-α blockers. For patients with severe CD, initiating pharmaceutical therapy with immunosuppressants and TNF-α blockers (step-down therapy) produces superior long-term results to initiating therapy with steroids and 5-ASA derivatives (step-up therapy). None of these studies included dietary interventions, which are of proven value in CD. Consult GI.

SURGICAL RESECTION

- For patients with colonic dysplasia or for those who fail to respond to medical management.
- Postsurgical recurrence is high for CD, and pouchitis is a frequent complication of ileal pouch–anal anastomosis for UC.

THERAPIES TO CONSIDER

- Phosphatidylcholine: 3.2 g daily improved clinical activity scores, histological remission, and relapse rates in UC patients without any significant adverse events.
- Inulin may be efficacious in treating active UC.
- Fructooligosaccharides 15 g daily improves clinical active CD.
- Aloe vera gel: 100 mL bid for patients with UC. Aloe may cause diarrhea. Use latex-free inner leaf extract formulations.
- Cannabis may have beneficial effects in the treatment of IBD with appetite stimulation and modulation of pain; however, due to its effects on the central nervous system, further studies are needed.
- Woodworm has been shown to improve active CD in small studies.
- Xilei-san was found to improve ulcerative proctitis in two studies.
- Antibiotics may have a role in the maintenance of CD in a subset of patients that have yet to be well defined.
- Naltrexone has shown promising results in Crohn's patients, but further studies are needed.
- Helminth therapy decreases mucosal inflammation, but long-term effects are still unknown.

Key Web Resources

Crohn's and Colitis Foundation: This website provides information about improving quality of life and ongoing research into inflammatory bowel disease.	http://www.ccfa.org
Specific Carbohydrate Diet: This site contains a description of the specific carbohydrate diet (SCD) and details about its implementation.	http://www.breakingtheviciouscycle.info
Digestive Wellness: This online store is for patients using the SCD.	http://www.digestivewellness.com
Ovamed: This website is a source of information related to helminth therapy of IBD.	http://www.ovamed.org

REFERENCES

References are available online at ExpertConsult.com.

SECTION X

OBSTETRICS/GYNECOLOGY

SECTION OUTLINE

51 PRECONCEPTION COUNSELING AND FERTILITY

52 LABOR PAIN MANAGEMENT

53 POSTDATES PREGNANCY

54 NAUSEA AND VOMITING IN PREGNANCY

55 MANAGING MENOPAUSAL SYMPTOMS

56 PREMENSTRUAL SYNDROME

57 DYSMENORRHEA

58 UTERINE FIBROIDS (LEIOMYOMATA)

59 VAGINAL DRYNESS

CHAPTER 51

PRECONCEPTION COUNSELING AND FERTILITY

Victoria Maizes, MD

OVERVIEW

From childhood, we play with dolls and imagine becoming parents. Our ability to conceive and bear a child is often assumed; when it does not occur with ease, or at all, it can be a source of great suffering. Most religions consider bearing children a blessing, and traditional societies often embrace elaborate preparations for conception. In our society, up to 50% of pregnancies are unplanned. Simultaneously, we are faced with increasing numbers of children who suffer from chronic diseases, such as autism and ADHD, obesity, and diabetes, some of which might be prevented through preparation for pregnancy and the adoption of healthier lifestyles. Sadly, we are not doing a good job at preconception counseling. Only 7% of primary care physicians prescribe preconception folic acid, and only 20% of obstetricians query their pregnant patients about environmental chemical exposures.[1] Given the fetal origins hypothesis, which suggests that the seeds of both childhood and adult diseases are planted in the womb, preconception counseling may be the most important preventive care we provide. This chapter outlines preconception advice that enhances the likelihood of conception as well as giving birth to a healthy child.

INTRODUCTION

The 1960s brought reliable contraception and, for the first time in human history, the ability to reliably control reproduction. It conferred new freedoms and increased the average age of first childbirth in the United States from 21 to 26 years. Within conventional medicine, tremendous advances in assisted reproductive technologies (ART) have helped couples that struggle to become pregnant. The best-known treatment, in vitro fertilization (IVF), has made it possible for couples who may never have conceived to become parents. Recognizing this fact, the 2010 Nobel Prize was awarded to Sir Robert Edwards, PhD, who developed IVF.

The success of high-tech solutions, including IVF, has reduced the emphasis in our culture on the simpler, more natural, less invasive, lower cost, and lower risk strategies that are the strength of integrative medicine. While assisted reproductive technologies can be miraculous, the cost and higher risks to mother and baby should make them a second-line approach except under special circumstances.

Causes of Infertility

Approximately 15% of couples in the United States struggle to conceive. Infertility is defined, somewhat arbitrarily, as an inability to conceive despite 12 months of unprotected intercourse. Of the couples deemed infertile, 43%–63% of women younger than 40 years will conceive naturally within the second year of trying.[2]

Male Infertility

Male infertility can be due to a variety of diseases (diabetes, cystic fibrosis, and varicoceles), behaviors (smoking, use of marijuana, testosterone or other anabolic steroid supplementation, alcoholism, and hot tub use), trauma, infection, chemotherapy, or radiation therapy. Infertility may also result from environmental exposures, such as pesticides, lead, and electromagnetic fields. It has been postulated that decreasing male sperm counts may be due to environmental toxins. Male infertility is usually evaluated with a semen analysis during which the number, movement, and morphology of the sperm are evaluated.

Female Infertility

Women need functional ovaries, fallopian tubes, and uterus as well as a perfectly tuned endocrine system to conceive. The most common reason women struggle to become pregnant is advanced age. All the oocytes a woman will ever have are formed when she is a fetus. As women age, so do their oocytes, thereby reducing the likelihood of conception somewhat after 30 and significantly after 40 years of age. Yet, media portrayals of celebrities conceiving and bearing children in their late 40s has created a cultural message that modern medicine has all but obliterated the significance of women's biological clocks. This prevalent myth suggests that women can wait until they are ready, and then if they need help, ART will fix the problem. As will be explained later in the chapter, this is a false message that integrative clinicians can help dispel.

Ovulatory infertility is the next most common cause of female infertility and includes polycystic ovarian syndrome, luteal phase dysfunction, hypothalamic problems, and stress-induced infertility. Anatomical causes of infertility include blocked tubes (often due to infection), endometriosis, and congenital or acquired uterine anomalies. Trauma, infection, chemotherapy, or radiation therapy may also cause infertility in women.

INTEGRATIVE THERAPY

Lifestyle

Nutrition

Abundant research supports the role of a healthy diet in conception.[3] An optimal fertility diet is made up of freshly prepared whole food and includes substantial vegetables and fruits, sufficient omega-3 fatty acids, and vegetable sources of protein. The diet should also be low in processed foods, meats, and rapidly digesting, high–glycemic load carbohydrates.

> Mediterranean diet has been studied and is associated with a 44% lower risk of infertility in women attempting to conceive naturally and a 40% greater likelihood of conception in couples using IVF to conceive.[4,5]

The Nurse's Health Study II (NHS II) used food frequency questionnaires to examine the macro and micronutrients that impact ovulatory infertility. The researchers found that carbohydrates, protein, and fats, as well as micronutrient intake, all influenced female fertility.

Increased ovulatory infertility occurred in women who ate high glycemic index (GI) carbohydrates: breakfast cereals nearly doubled the risk.[6] Flour, a high GI carbohydrate, is the first ingredient in most breakfast cereals; it is rapidly metabolized, elevating blood sugar, which leads to spikes in insulin levels and subsequent inflammation. Higher levels of insulin reduce sex-hormone-binding globulin (SHBG) and increase free testosterone, which can reduce fertility. Soda, another high GI carbohydrate, has also been associated with a longer time to conception[7,8] (see Chapter 87).

The type of protein the nurses ate was also related to the risk of ovulatory infertility in the NHS II.[9] Women aged more than 32 years were most affected, with each additional daily serving of red meat, chicken, or turkey increasing the risk of ovulatory infertility by nearly one-third. Fish and eggs had no effect, and vegetable protein reduced the risk by 50%.

With respect to fat, trans fats were found to increase the risk of ovulatory infertility by 73%.[10] More surprising was the NHS II finding that full fat dairy was associated with enhanced fertility as compared with nonfat or low fat dairy foods.[11] Women who ate two or more daily servings of low fat dairy had almost double the risk of ovulatory infertility when compared with women who ate one or less servings per week. A 27% reduction in risk was found when women ate one or more servings of full fat dairy per day compared to less than one per week. Milk is centrifuged to create varying fat concentrations; an unintended consequence is differing hormonal concentrations. Estrogens are lipophilic and are found in higher proportions in full fat than reduced fat dairy products. In contrast, prolactin and insulin-like growth factor 1, both of which reduce fertility, are lipophobic and are proportionally more abundant in lower fat dairy products. In 2014, the FDA/EPA revised their recommendations to pregnant women and women of childbearing age regarding fish consumption.[12] Evidence had shown that in

response to the 2004 warning, 90% of women were consuming less than the FDA-recommended amount of fish, placing themselves and their babies at risk of insufficient levels of omega-3 fatty acids. The new draft guidelines recommend that women eat a minimum of 8–12 ounces of low mercury fish each week.[13] The agencies continued to advise against eating high-mercury containing fish (shark, swordfish, king mackerel, and tilefish) and advise limiting albacore tuna to six ounces or less per week.

Male fertility is also impacted by diet. While fewer studies exist, we know that a father's diet plays an important role in the health of his sperm and his offspring. Oxidative stress is a leading cause of male subfertility, yet 80% of men in the United States do not consume the recommended five servings of fruits and vegetables per day that are the source of dietary antioxidants.

Fat intake impacts sperm quality and quantity. A study of military recruits in Denmark found that men who ate the most saturated fats had a 38% lower sperm concentration and 41% lower sperm counts than those who ate the least fat.[14] A similar result was found in semen analyses of men attending a U.S. infertility clinic.[15]

> Eating more monounsaturated fat may protect sperm health; when 2.5 ounces a day of walnuts were added to the Western-style diet of healthy young men, sperm vitality, motility, and morphology were increased.[16]

Some women will do well to experiment with an elimination diet (see Chapter 86). Common food sensitivities that can cause inflammation and in turn reduce fertility include gluten, dairy, soy, corn, eggs, and citrus. One prospective trial found previously undiagnosed celiac disease to be the root cause of unexplained infertility in 5.9% of women.[17]

Physical Activity

As health professionals, we generally counsel people to be more physically active. During preconception counseling, however, we sometimes find ourselves asking women to cut back on their activity. Up to 44% of athletic women experience intermittent or regular amenorrhea; an even higher percentage will have intermittent luteal phase dysfunction.[18] Vigorous exercise, more frequent exercise, or exercising to exhaustion significantly increased time to conception in a prospective Norwegian population study of 3887 women.[19] The exception is overweight or obese women in whom exercise reduces the time required to conceive.[20] Limiting exercise to less than 4 hours per week may be prudent advice for women of normal weight who struggle to conceive, as is encouraging walking and gentle forms of yoga in place of running, cycling, and vigorous yoga.

Spirituality

The mystical perspective holds that it takes three parties to create a new life: a woman, a man, and God. Some adults will resonate with this spiritual point of view and may seek out religious or secular preconception ceremonies. Indeed, every religion has special prayers that are used to beseech God's intervention to be blessed with a child. Both Judaism and Hinduism advise a period of abstinence prior to conception; the former then advises immersion in the waters of the Mikveh, and the latter meditation practices, special foods, and adaptogens. Ceremonies can be created to help women prepare to become a vessel that bears a newly forming life. They may also be designed to help women and men acknowledge their longing for a child, their frustration at not conceiving with ease, the loss of a child to miscarriage, or the loss of the dream of bearing children.

Struggling to conceive can lead to a crisis of spirit. Couples may wrestle with existential questions and the inherent unfairness of life. "Why is this happening to me?" may be the unspoken question in the exam room. Religious traditions can be of great help to some couples grappling with these questions and can pose conflicts for others when infertility is experienced as a punishment from God or when reproductive treatments are prohibited. Examples of practices forbidden by some religious traditions include IVF, use of a third party donor or surrogate, and embryo wastage.

Environmental Chemicals

The environmental chemical exposures we face as individuals and as a society are unprecedented. Yearly, we release more and more industrial chemicals into the environment while rarely testing their risks. A fetus or young child is uniquely susceptible because its neurological and immune systems are still developing and its detoxification systems have not fully matured, thereby rendering them less able to metabolize harmful chemicals.

Shockingly, studies of umbilical cord blood reveal that babies have an average of 232 chemicals in their bodies at the time of birth.[21] These environmental chemicals can potentially increase a child's risk of ADHD, autism spectrum disorders (ASD), and leukemia; later in life they increase the risk of diabetes and heart disease.[22] A 2014 review of 37 trials of environmental toxicant exposure and ASD in preconception, pregnancy, or early childhood found a positive association in 34 of the studies. The strongest evidence was found for air pollutants and pesticides, and phthalates, polychlorinated biphenyls (PCBs), solvents, and toxic waste sites were also implicated.[23]

> Studies of umbilical cord blood have revealed that babies have an average of 232 chemicals in their bodies at the time of birth.[24]

Awareness is the first important step towards behavior change. Lifestyle modification can reduce exposures to toxic chemicals in parents, thereby reducing the risk to the fetus.[25,31] For example, exposure to air pollution can be reduced by avoiding idling one's car or standing near a vehicle's exhaust, and by turning on the "recirculate" function when driving in traffic. Purchasing organic food can minimize pesticide levels. Indeed for most people, food and beverages are the most significant source of environmental toxin exposure. Choosing

organic meat, poultry, pork, and produce, whenever possible, is the best way to avoid pesticides and genetically modified organisms (GMO). When the cost of organic food is prohibitive, shoppers can selectively purchase the least contaminated conventionally grown vegetables and fruits by using the Environmental Working Group's updated list (www.ewg.org). The EWG has calculated that you can reduce your pesticide exposure by 92% when you eat from the "clean fifteen" rather than the "dirty dozen."[27] Packaging introduces other forms of industrial chemicals. Frozen vegetables are a better choice than canned as the liners of most cans contain bisphenol A (BPA). Avoiding storing and microwaving food in plastic containers reduces BPA and phthalate exposure.

Many excellent online resources are available to help guide choice of food, water, cleaning, and personal care products.[28] The fish with the least amount of mercury, PCBs, and other environmental toxins can be identified by using the Monterey Bay Aquarium website (www.montereybayaquarium.org/cr/seafoodwatch). Skin deep (www.cosmeticsdatabase.com) reviews personal care products for carcinogenic, reproductive toxicant, and allergenic ingredients. Flame retardant exposure from mattresses, computers, TVs, carpeting, and furniture can be minimized by exploring and purchasing products listed at www.saferproducts.gov. Websites such as www.treehugger.com list companies that package in BPA free cans. In response to consumers' desire for green products, newer packaging made from glass or cardboard is increasingly available.

Adopting new behaviors can significantly reduce the body burden of many, but not all, environmental toxins. For example, a 2011 San Francisco study revealed that adults dropped their urinary BPA levels by two-thirds in 3 days when they were provided with fresh, catered meals that avoided canned foods and the use of plastic containers[29-31] (see Chapter 108).

In response to the pervasive presence of environmental chemicals, the Royal College of Obstetricians and Gynecologists published a scientific impact paper titled "Chemical Exposures During Pregnancy: Dealing with Potential, but Unproven, Risks to Child Health." Specifically, the following recommendations were made for pregnant and lactating women[32]:

- Use fresh food rather than processed foods whenever possible
- Reduce the use of foods and beverages in cans and/or plastic containers, including their use for food storage
- Minimize the use of personal care products, such as moisturizers, cosmetics, shower gels, and fragrances
- Minimize the purchase of newly produced household furniture, fabrics, nonstick frying pans, and cars whilst pregnant or nursing
- Avoid the use of garden, household, pet, pesticides, or fungicides (such as fly sprays or strips, rose sprays, flea powders) and avoid paint fumes
- Only take over-the-counter analgesics or painkillers when necessary
- Do not assume the safety of products based on the absence of "harmful" chemicals in their ingredients list or the presence of a tag "natural" (herbal or otherwise)

Micronutrients

Vitamins

The American Academy of Pediatrics, the American College of Obstetrics and Gynecology, the American Academy of Family Physicians, and the United States Preventive Services Task Force all recommend that women of childbearing age take a multivitamin with folic acid. When taken prior to conception and throughout the first trimester of pregnancy, these supplements reduce the risk of neural tube defects, heart defects, musculoskeletal defects, and orofacial defects.[33] Multivitamins and folic acid have benefits beyond reducing birth defects. The NHS II found that multivitamins made it easier for women to conceive and decreased the risk of miscarriage.[34] Three large studies have revealed a 40% lower risk of autism in women who took folic acid in the 3 months prior to conception and the first trimester of pregnancy.[35-37]

Yet, the 2011 National Health and Nutrition Examination Survey (NHANES) revealed that only 34% of women between the ages of 20 and 39 consume the recommended amount of supplemental folic acid. One study revealed that women who received preconception counseling from their primary care physician were five times more likely to take folic acid before conception.[38] However, data from the CDC's National Ambulatory Medical Care Survey and the National Hospital Ambulatory Medical Care Survey reveal that folic acid or a multivitamin with folic acid is prescribed at only 7.2% of primary care visits in women of reproductive age.[39]

Prenatal multivitamins can contain very different ingredients. Iodine, for example, is only present in 51% of prenatal multivitamins.[40] In the UK, where salt is not routinely iodized, mild iodine insufficiency is thought to contribute to lower cognitive function in children.[41] Some women require higher doses than the 400–800 mcg of folic acid found in most prenatal vitamins. This includes women with inflammatory bowel disease, diabetes, a body mass index > 35, or a personal or family history of having a child with a neural tube defect. Higher doses are also indicated for women who take anticonvulsant medications, folate antagonists, (e.g., methotrexate, sulfonamides), smoke cigarettes, or belong to higher-risk ethnic groups (Sikh, Celtic, Northern Chinese).[42] While some advocate the use of 5-methyltetrahydrofolate to address single nucleotide polymorphisms (SNPs), to date, no studies have been carried out.[43]

> ## PRECONCEPTION MULTIVITAMIN INGREDIENTS
>
> - Vitamin A: the current recommended dietary allowance (RDA) of preformed vitamin A is 700 retinol activity equivalents (RAEs) or 2300 IU per day, with a tolerable upper intake level for pregnancy of 3000 RAEs/day or 10,000 IU/day.[44] Most experts recommend no more than 5000 IU per day should be preformed since we also get vitamin A in our food and through food fortification. (The RDA during pregnancy is 2567 IU/day preformed vitamin A and 4300 IU/day for lactating women.)

> - Iron: 18 mg (once pregnant, 27 mg and 9 mg when lactating).[45]
> - Iodine: 150 mcg (once pregnant, the iodine RDA is 220 mcg/day from all sources and 290 mcg/day for lactating women).[46]
> - Folic acid: 400 mcg or more (once pregnant 600 mcg or more).[47]
> - Vitamin D: 600 IU[48] (or more depending on vitamin D level). Both vitamins D2 and D3 are effective.
> - Vitamin B12: 2.4 mcg (once pregnant, 2.6 mcg).
> - Vitamin E: the RDA is 22.4 IU/day for women aged more than 14 years including while pregnant and 28.4 while lactating.[49]
> - Calcium: the Food and Nutrition Board at the Institute of Medicine recommends total calcium from food and supplements of 1000 mg for women aged more than 19 years and 1300 mg a day for girls aged 9–18 years.[50]
> - Trace minerals: small amounts of copper, zinc, magnesium, and potassium.

Subfertile men also benefit from taking multivitamins. A Cochrane review of 34 studies found that men who received supplements were four times more likely to impregnate their partner and almost five times as likely to have a live birth.[51] A wide variety of antioxidant supplements were used across the 34 studies including vitamins C and E, folate, zinc, selenium, omega-3, and N-acetylcysteine.

Supplements

Omega-3

Women who consume less than the recommended 12 ounces of fish per week may benefit from supplementation with omega-3 fatty acids.

> ### DOSAGE
>
> A consensus statement from the World Association of Perinatal Medicine recommends a dose of at least 200 mg of DHA during pregnancy.[52] A consensus was not formed for the dose of EPA; however, the group noted that intakes of up to 1 g/day of DHA or 2.7 g/day of total omega-3 have been safely used in randomized clinical trials.[53] Subfertile men may benefit from omega-3 supplementation as well. One study reported higher sperm counts and more normal morphology in men who received 1.1 g of EPA and 700 mg of DHA.[54]

Fertility Blend

Two randomized controlled studies of Fertility Blend (a supplement formula containing chaste tree berry; green tea extracts; L-arginine; vitamins E, B6, B12, and folate; iron; magnesium; zinc; and selenium) were conducted in women. The first pilot study followed 30 women who had been unsuccessful conceiving for 6–36 months. Participants were administered Fertility Blend or a placebo for three cycles. Five women in the treatment group conceived compared with zero in the control group.[55] The second study randomized 93 women; at 6 months, 17 women in the treatment group had conceived compared with 10 women in the control group.[56] A male Fertility Blend formulation has also been developed but has not been clinically studied.

Vitamin C

Vitamin C has also been shown to enhance fertility in women with luteal phase dysfunction. In a randomized controlled trial of 150 women, vitamin C supplementation was associated with significantly higher progesterone levels and higher pregnancy rates after 6 months (25% vs. 11%; p = .045).

> **DOSAGE**
> The dose used was 750 mg/day.[57]
>
> **PRECAUTIONS**
> High doses of vitamin C may cause diarrhea.

Herbal medicine
Chasteberry (Vitex agnus-castus)

Herbal medicines have a long tradition of use in women's health, including for supporting fertility. One of the best-known herbs, *Vitex agnus-castus* has been studied for premenstrual syndrome, cyclic mastalgia, and infertility as part of a mixed herbal formulation called Mastodynon. Vitex has been shown to reduce levels of follicle-stimulating hormone and increase luteinizing hormone, thereby reducing estrogen and increasing progesterone levels. At higher doses, Vitex inhibits prolactin production. Thus, it can be particularly helpful in women who have luteal phase disorders.[58]

> **DOSAGE**
> The dose is Mastodynon 60 drops/day (32.4 mg of chasteberry extract).

Shatavari root (Asparagus racemosus) and Damiana (Turnera aphrodisiaca)

Less well studied, but highly esteemed for their use in fertility, are the Indian adaptogenic herb, Shatavari root (*Asparagus racemosus*), and the southwestern herb, damiana (*Turnera aphrodisiaca*).

> **DOSAGE**
> Damiana can be prepared by steeping 2–4 g of the dried leaf in one cup of boiling water, straining, and drinking three times daily. A traditional Shatavari dose is 1–2 g/day.

Detoxifying Prior to Conception

Herbs are also used at times to help women cleanse or detoxify before pregnancy. Schisandra (*Schisandra chinensis*) fruit is said to tonify and strengthen the hypothalamus, pituitary gland, ovaries, and adrenals.[59] Milk thistle (*Silybum marianum*) is another safe choice; it is thought to maximize the ability of the liver to detoxify chemical pollutants. The dose of Schisandra is variable depending on the strength of the extract. Milk thistle is commonly prescribed as an extract containing 70%–80% silymarin at a dose of 140 mg three times daily.

Herbal medicines can also act as abortifacients and should be prescribed by knowledgeable practitioners. In addition to western herbal preparations, Chinese medicine, Ayurveda, and other traditional systems have their favored herbal preparations.

Mind-Body Therapies

Our ability to conceive can be affected by stress. Elevated cortisol levels signal receptors on the ovaries, testes, pituitary, and hypothalamus to tone down reproductive capacity. From an evolutionary biology perspective this makes perfect sense. Our body's clear message is, "Bad timing! Focus on survival, not reproduction."

Infertility can take a huge toll on our well-being. A survey of 121 couples with infertility revealed depression in 32% of the women (19% moderate depression and 13% severe depression). In addition, 26% were at high risk for sexual dysfunction.[60]

Mind-body therapies have been found to help normalize reproductive function and reduce the stress of infertility. One small study examined the use of hypnosis in twelve women with functional hypothalamic amenorrhea; each woman had one hypnotherapy session and was followed for 12 weeks. Nine of the twelve participants resumed menstruating and all twelve described improvements in well-being and confidence. While this was a very small sample, it is notable that one hypnotherapy session led to three-fourths of women resuming menstruation, with broad salutogenic effects observed in all participants[61] (see Chapter 95).

Another small study evaluated cognitive behavioral therapy (CBT) for functional hypothalamic amenorrhea. Fifteen women were enrolled and followed for 20 weeks. Six of the eight women randomized to CBT resumed ovulating; the remaining two women had partial recovery of ovarian function. In contrast, only two of the women in the control group experienced renewed ovarian activity.[62]

Mind-body groups are commonly designed as multiple-session, skill-building classes. They typically include a wide range of practices including yoga, guided imagery, breath work, mindfulness, journaling, body scanning, and cognitive restructuring.[63] The goal is for participants to find one or more practices that resonate and that they will continue to use once the class ends. A meta-analysis of psychological interventions for infertility showed that skill-building groups are more effective than educational programs or individual therapy.[64] A second meta-analysis showed that mind-body groups lasting six or more sessions were more effective than those with fewer sessions[65] (see Chapter 94).

Acupuncture

Traditional Chinese medicine (TCM) includes acupuncture, herbs, tui na, moxibustion, dietary advice, and more. A retrospective chart review of 1069 fresh, nondonor IVF cycles was recently conducted. This study evaluated whole systems TCM compared with acupuncture at the time of IVF or routine IVF (without acupuncture) and revealed live birth rates of 61.3% in the whole systems TCM compared to 50.8% in the acupuncture at embryo transfer and 48.3% in the routine IVF group.[66]

Acupuncture is the modality most commonly studied for its impact on fertility. Most studies examine the impact of acupuncture before and after embryo transfer during IVF. While many individual trials have demonstrated benefit, eight meta-analyses have been published with contradictory findings. It has been suggested that this discrepancy may be attributed to the use of a non-validated acupuncture protocol (the Craig protocol.)[67] Another possible reason lies with the challenge of finding an appropriate sham for acupuncture. Some researchers have suggested that noninsertive needling at true acupoints is an active treatment. Acupuncture has also been studied in subfertile men and shown to significantly increase the fertility index of sperm.[68]

Ayurveda

Ayurveda has even fewer studies than TCM examining its impact on fertility. Ayurveda has a rich set of traditional practices including panchakarma (detoxification practices), abstinence before attempting conception, meditation practices, herbs, and specific foods. The most commonly recommended herb for female fertility is Shatavari (*Asparagus racemosus*). In Sanskrit, Shatavari means "she who possesses a hundred husbands," suggesting its ability to promote fertility and vitality. Male fertility is often enhanced with the adaptogenic herb Ashwagandha (*Withania somnifera*).

Conventional Medicine

Conventional medicine has a wide range of recommendations in the preconception period. A healthy diet and discontinuation of hazardous behaviors, including the use of alcohol, cigarette smoking, and illicit drugs, are universally recommended. A review of prescribed and over-the-counter medications that may pose harm to a fetus is suggested for men and women. Assessment of immunization status is recommended for measles, mumps, rubella, varicella, and, for high-risk women, hepatitis B. Prenatal supplementation with multivitamin containing folic acid is recommended.

Inquiring about future interest in childbearing during regular well-women visits can serve to educate and address misconceptions regarding the relationship between age and fertility. Egg freezing is the newest option available to preserve fertility in women. Accordingly, it is especially important to discuss in women of childbearing age who have a cancer diagnoses for which

treatment may impede future fertility. While it is being suggested as insurance policy for women in their early thirties who are delaying childbearing, egg freezing may provide "insufficient coverage." Current statistics suggest that egg freezing resulted in successful pregnancies in 18.8% of women who were less than 30 years of age when their eggs were frozen and only 10.3% of women who were more than 40.[69]

Clomid and N-Acetylcysteine

For women who struggle with infertility, conventional medicine provides more options than ever. Clomid is frequently used for ovulation induction, sometimes in combination with metformin, in women with polycystic ovarian disorder (PCOS). Several studies suggest that integrative medicine approaches can enhance the effectiveness of conventional treatment alone. N-acetylcysteine (NAC) has been studied in combination with Clomid in women aged 18–39 years with Clomid-resistant PCOS. Women who took the combination reportedly had a 49% ovulation rate and a 21% pregnancy rate compared with 1% ovulation and 0% pregnancy with Clomid alone. The dose used was 1200 mg of NAC plus 100 mg Clomid.[70] A prospective study randomized 56 subfertile women receiving Clomid for ovulation induction to receive either folic acid alone or a multivitamin multimineral supplement. The women who received the multivitamin had statistically significant higher pregnancy rates (67% vs. 39%; p = .013) and became pregnant more quickly.[71]

In Vitro Fertilization

In vitro fertilization has become an important option for women who cannot conceive naturally. Overriding a woman's normal cycle with gonadotropins leads to the production of multiple eggs that are removed in an office-based surgical procedure. The eggs are fertilized and used fresh or frozen. Fifteen states require insurance coverage for IVF, while the remainder do not require insurance coverage.[72] The procedure is costly and less likely to be successful than many women imagine. According to the CDC, the overall success rate of IVF using fresh nondonated embryos in 2012 was 36%.[73] Success rates of IVF are significantly higher for women under the age of 35 (42% live birth rate) than women aged 41–42 years (26% live birth rate).[74] Particularly surprising to many is that women aged more than 44 years have a 2% live birth rate when using IVF with their own eggs.[75]

In vitro fertilization also poses potential risks to mother and baby. A rare but serious risk is ovarian hyperstimulation syndrome. There is some research that links IVF to an increased risk of ovarian and breast cancer,[76,77] and IVF is associated with a higher rate of twins and multiple births, which poses risk to both mother and child. Finally, there is evidence of a higher rate of birth defects in children born as a result of IVF.[78]

Natural Procreative Technologies

Natural procreative technologies (NPT) are based on the Creighton Model FertilityCare System, which helps women identify ovulation through daily observations of cervical fluid. It was developed in response to the Catholic Church's prohibition against IVF. Pre- and postovulatory estradiol and progesterone levels are sometimes assessed to diagnose hormonal deficiencies and, when needed, medications are prescribed to enhance cervical mucus production (such as vitamin B6, guaifenesin, or antibiotics) or to increase luteal hormones (oral, vaginal, or transbuccal progesterone or human chorionic gonadotropin injections). NPT has been studied in Ireland and Canada and has been shown to significantly increase birthrates over a 2-year period.[79,80]

PREVENTION PRESCRIPTION

While living a healthy lifestyle is always of value, evidence points most strongly to the 3- to 4-month window prior to conception; this is the time it takes both the oocyte and sperm to fully mature. This interval can be used for physical, emotional, mental, and spiritual preparation. Changes in lifestyle, environmental chemical avoidance, and detoxification can be practiced. The fetal origins theory affirms the critical importance of the uterine environment and its influence on an individual's health over the course of a lifetime.[81] It is a compelling reason to follow a healthy lifestyle when trying to conceive as well as during pregnancy.

PRECONCEPTION COUNSELING

- Counsel all women about the impact of age on fertility. Explain that IVF success rates are markedly affected by age.
- Discuss the physical signs of fertility and set appropriate expectations for the time it will take to conceive.
- Consider the need for genetic counseling and refer as needed.
- Discuss discontinuation of dangerous behaviors (e.g., smoking, illicit drugs, and alcohol).
- Discuss a healthy fertility diet.
- Discuss avoidance of environmental toxin exposures.
- Assess immunizations: recommended vaccines include MMR, varicella, DPT, and influenza.
- Recommend an appropriate multivitamin with 400–800 mcg of folic acid.
- Review prescribed and OTC medications and supplements carefully and make a plan to discontinue any that present risk or are not absolutely necessary.

THERAPEUTIC REVIEW

NUTRITION
- Encourage a Mediterranean-type diet that is rich in vegetables, fruit, and essential fatty acids in the form of nuts and 8–12 oz of low mercury fish per week. Encourage a low–glycemic index diet. Avoid trans fats and soda.

EXERCISE
- Maintain moderate physical activity. Aim for 4 hours or less of physical activity per week unless you are overweight or obese.

MIND-BODY
- Recommend mind-body groups that build skills and last six or more sessions.

TOXIC EXPOSURE
- Avoid environmental toxins to the extent you are able. Avoid canned beverages and foods that contain bisphenol A; avoid exhaust fumes; and choose to eat organic foods or those with minimal pesticides.

SUPPLEMENTS
- Take a multivitamin with at least 400 mcg of folic acid daily.

- If unable to eat low mercury fish, consider supplementing with 1 g of fish oil that contains 200 mg of DHA. Do not exceed 2.7 g/day of total EPA + DHA.

ACUPUNCTURE
- Consider acupuncture for infertility.

SPIRITUALITY
- Consider recommending a ceremony based on patients' beliefs to create positive expectation in preparation for a healthy conception.
- Refer to spiritual counselor if there is anger or angst towards a higher power in relation to infertility.

PHARMACEUTICALS
- Clomid (dose to be selected and monitored by OB-GYN or reproductive endocrinologist).
- Clomid and N-acetyl cysteine for those with polycystic ovarian syndrome. 1200 mg of NAC plus 100 mg Clomid.

SURGERY
- In vitro fertilization

Key Web Resources

Environmentally safer products	http://www.ewg.org/
	http://www.saferproducts.gov
Safer skin care products	http://www.ewg.org/skindeep/www.nomoredirtylooks.com
Fish with the fewest environmental toxins	http://www.montereybayaquarium.org/conservation-and-science/our-programs/seafood-watch
	http://www.seafoodwatch.org/seafood-recommendations/consumer-guides
Sustainable and organic agriculture information	http://www.cornucopia.org
Dietary supplement fact sheets	http://ods.od.nih.gov/
Exposure history forms	http://prhe.ucsf.edu/prhe/clinical_resources.html
Companies that use BPA-free cans	http://www.treehugger.com
CDC Fertility Clinic Results	http://cdc.gov/artdata/index.html
General fertility and environmental recommendations	http://www.victoriamaizesmd.com

REFERENCES

References are available online at ExpertConsult.com.

SUGGESTED RESOURCES

Maizes V: *Be fruitful: the essential guide to maximizing fertility and giving birth to a healthy child*, New York, 2013, Scribner.

Wechsler T: *Taking charge of your fertility*, 10th Anniversary Edition. New York, 2006, Collins.

Domar A: *Conquering infertility*, New York, 2004, Penguin.

Indichova J: *Inconceivable: a woman's triumph over despair and statistics*, New York, 2001, Three Rivers Press.

CHAPTER 52

LABOR PAIN MANAGEMENT

Michelle J. Mertz, MD • Connie J. Earl, DO, ABIHM

After a period of heavily medicated birth in the United States during the midtwentieth century, a backlash against the medical model arose, and women began to demand the right to choose their own childbirth experience. Today, women are much more at liberty to influence these experiences. This chapter explores the birthing woman's many options for pain management.

PHYSIOLOGY

Labor is separated into three stages. The first stage involves dilation of the cervix and the beginning descent of the fetus into the pelvis. The second stage is full dilation and birthing of the fetus, and the third stage is passage of the placenta.

Pain in the first stage is primarily visceral, resulting from the mechanical dilation of the cervix and lower uterus. Nociceptive information is carried back on sympathetic fibers to the posterior nerve root ganglia at T10 through L1, as well as on parasympathetic fibers from the pelvic splanchnic nerves (S2 through S4).[2] The T10–L1 segmental levels also receive nociceptive information from the skin of the back.[2] This last mechanism may explain why many women feel contractions in their back. Pressure on the pelvic nerves may explain why labor pain can radiate to the thighs or buttocks as well. In some cases of fetal malposition, such as occiput posterior or occiput transverse, the woman may experience more severe back labor resulting from a relative increase in diameter of the head passing through the pelvis in these positions. However, back labor is not isolated to the occiput posterior or occiput transverse position.

During the second stage of labor, pain primarily stems from mechanical stretching and distention of the perineum and pelvic floor musculature. This is somatic pain, carried to the central nervous system on the pudendal nerve fibers (S2 through S4).[2] It is often described as being sharp. Many women report a sensation of rectal pressure during descent of the fetus. As the presenting part begins to stretch the perineum, many women describe a classic "ring of fire" sensation.

Pain Relief in Labor

Any acute pain, including labor pain, has two main physiological components: the transmission of the physical pain stimulus to the brain and the interpretation of the information that is filtered through the hypothalamic and limbic systems. Thus, the experience of pain is influenced by emotions and memories.[3] Whereas pharmaceutical agents are typically geared toward relief of physical pain, many of the nonpharmacological methods do not attempt to remove the sensation, but instead target the perception of the pain stimulus. One mechanism proposed for many of the therapies discussed in this chapter is the *gate control theory*: sensations such as pressure, vibration, pain, or temperature stimulate superficial tactile nerve endings, and this stimulation leads to inhibition of the pain signal transmission from the organs and deeper tissues at that segmental level.[4]

INTEGRATIVE THERAPY

Continuous Labor Support or Doula

Historically, women have long provided continuous labor support to other women in labor. In the twentieth century, a break in that tradition occurred as birth moved from an out-of-hospital midwifery model of care to a more institutionalized model. Since the 1980s, resurgence in labor support has attempted to integrate the two models. Research in this area typically focuses on the labor "doula," a person present solely to support the birthing woman and her family.[5] Doulas have no medical role in the labor or birth and are often hired in the second or third trimester of pregnancy to form a relationship with the birthing family before labor begins.

A large Cochrane Review demonstrated a significant decrease in pain medication required, length of labor, and incidence of cesarean delivery and operative delivery with continuous labor support by a doula.[6] This benefit was most pronounced when doula support was initiated in early labor.[6] The most important factor appears to be the continuous presence of labor support.[7] An earlier study demonstrated that even the continuous presence of a silent female observer had a positive effect on the foregoing outcomes, although the greatest benefit was observed when a trained doula was present.[8] Continuous support is most efficacious when the provider is not a member of the hospital staff.[9,10] Given the benefits, all women in labor should be offered a doula. Several states in the United States are exploring Medicaid reimbursement for doula care in an effort to reduce medical costs. Indeed, a study in Minnesota, which demonstrated a decreased incidence of Cesarean births in Medicaid patients supported by doulas, used multivariate regression to estimate impacts of doula care nationwide and predicted significant obstetrical cost savings with provision of a paid doula support to Medicaid recipients.[11]

Childbirth Preparation

Half of the women in the United States are estimated to attend some sort of childbirth education class during pregnancy.[12] Many approaches are used, but most classes aim to prepare women and their partners for childbirth and parenthood. Some of these classes introduce women and their partners to various pain relief techniques reviewed in this chapter. Data on pain during labor in relation to childbirth education are sparse. Although individual studies have demonstrated benefits of prenatal education besides pain relief, a systematic review of the literature found the study methods too diverse to clearly comment on the benefits.[13,14] A large randomized controlled trial (RCT) found no difference in the epidural rate or pain level rated retrospectively with one form of childbirth education.[15] Given the popularity of antenatal education, more research is needed to determine its best use.

Lifestyle

Exercise

Research suggests that regular aerobic exercise during pregnancy is associated with decreased pain scores in labor.[16,17] Moderate-intensity exercise in labor has also been observed to lower pain scores, even after the exercise ends.[18] No known risks to the fetus are associated with moderate exercise, though some increased uterine activity occurs with exercise at term.[18,19] Women should be encouraged to exercise regularly during pregnancy.

Biomechanical Therapy

Positions During Labor and Ambulation

Western medicine long ago adopted the lithotomy position as the position of choice for childbirth, mostly for ease of the practitioner. In contrast, historically around the world, women have employed an upright position in the first and second stages of labor.[20]

Ambulation, use of a birth ball, and an upright position during the first stage of labor are associated with a decreased length of the first stage, a decreased use of epidural anesthesia, and no difference in adverse maternal or neonatal outcomes.[21-23] Additionally, in women with a fetal malpresentation associated with back labor, the hand and knees position during labor appears to decrease back pain.[24]

The use of an upright or side-lying position in the second stage of labor is associated with a decreased length of the second stage. It was also associated with a decreased report of severe pain in a systematic review of 23 RCTs.[25] A small but significant increase in the incidence of blood loss greater than 500 mL was reported, but without adverse maternal or fetal outcomes. Unless medically contraindicated, all women should be allowed to ambulate and choose the positions they assume in labor and birth.

Water Immersion

Originally relegated to home birth and out-of-hospital birthing centers, water birth and water immersion in labor are now options in many hospital labor and delivery units. Laboring in water has many purported advantages, including ease of position change with the decreased effects of gravity, relaxation, decreased sensation of pain, and greater control for the laboring woman over her personal space.

A Cochrane Review of water immersion demonstrated a significant reduction in use of pain medication with water immersion in the first stage of labor and no difference in adverse maternal or neonatal outcomes.[26] Two of these RCTs also demonstrated increased maternal satisfaction with water immersion in the second stage of labor,[26] with no difference in mode of delivery or adverse maternal or neonatal outcomes.[26,27] A small RCT found an increased incidence of normal vaginal delivery in water birth compared with land birth.[28]

In 2014, the American College of Obstetrics and Gynecology (ACOG) released a committee opinion on immersion in water during labor and birth, questioning its safety as a result of one small study, excluded from the previously mentioned Cochrane Review,[6] that reported increased NICU admission of newborns following water immersion in labor.[29,30] Of note, this study was designed to investigate water immersion and expectant management versus pitocin augmentation in nulliparous women diagnosed with labor dystocia; the multiple variables in these study groups complicates analysis for causality.[30] While most research has demonstrated maternal and fetal safety for water immersion in labor, perhaps more research on its use in protracted labor would yield different results.

More research is needed to evaluate water immersion in labor and birth. Water immersion in labor does not appear to increase the risk of chorioamnionitis or endometritis, even in women with ruptured membranes.[31]

> The temperature of the water should be no more than 99°F to avoid raising maternal core temperature in labor.[26]

Chiropractic, Osteopathic, and Manual Therapy

Back pain is a common phenomenon in pregnancy because the body changes shape, joints relax from hormonal effects, and the spine and frame are required to support added weight. Some data suggest that back pain in pregnancy may be associated with increased back pain in labor.[32] One small retrospective study demonstrated that women who received prenatal chiropractic manual therapy reported less pain in labor than those who did not.[32] Manual therapy is an option for the management of musculoskeletal back pain in pregnancy, and it may lead to less pain in labor for women who receive regular treatments during pregnancy. Further study in this area is needed. No adverse events have been reported with the use of manual therapy in pregnancy.[33]

Massage

Although research is limited, intrapartum massage has been shown to reduce pain perception[34-38] and decrease anxiety[34-36] in the first stage of labor.[39] No evidence indicates that it decreases the use of pain medication in labor. Regardless of the paucity of research on this topic, clinicians generally accept that massage can promote relaxation and enhance the quality of women's birth experiences.

Sterile Water Injections

Nearly 30% of women have severe continuous back pain in labor that persists between contractions. Sterile water injections in the low back can be used to relieve this pain. In contrast to isotonic saline, the salt-free water causes irritation as well as physical distention of the skin. The underlying mechanism of pain inhibition is not fully understood. Many investigators refer to the process of counterirritation,[40,41] in which one type of pain masks another, or to the gate control theory.

Several studies demonstrated that intracutaneous or subcutaneous sterile water injections provided good pain relief in the first stage of labor, particularly for low back pain.[42-48] The effect lasted for up to 2 hours.[42-47] These injections are simple to administer, inexpensive, and carry no known risks. They were not shown to reduce the use of pain medication in these studies. Administration can be quite painful, but the pain is transient, and subcutaneous injection may be less painful than the intracutaneous route.[49] The precise location of the points does not appear critical to the success of the procedure.[50]

Technique

Palpate the posterior superior iliac spines, and mark them with a pen. From these sites, measure 3 cm inferiorly and 2 cm medially. Mark these two spots, and swab all four spots (two on the left and two on the right) with alcohol.[50] During a contraction, inject 0.1–0.5 mL of sterile water subcutaneously or intracutaneously with a fine needle, thus forming a small white bleb, as during a tuberculin skin test. Repeat at the remaining three sites as quickly as possible. It may help for two providers to inject simultaneously. Repeat as necessary.

Bioenergetics

Transcutaneous Electrical Nerve Stimulation

Transcutaneous electrical nerve stimulation (TENS) emits low-voltage electrical impulses through electrodes, with operator-controlled variation in frequency and intensity. TENS units are portable, battery operated, and relatively inexpensive. TENS has typically been used to treat musculoskeletal and neuropathic pain, although its efficacy is controversial. The mechanism of action most often proposed is the gate control theory. Application of the electrodes is not standardized in labor. Although electrodes are typically applied paraspinally at T10 and S2, many studies also describe acupoints and cranial placement.[51]

A Cochrane Review of studies with notably heterogeneous methods demonstrated little evidence of significant

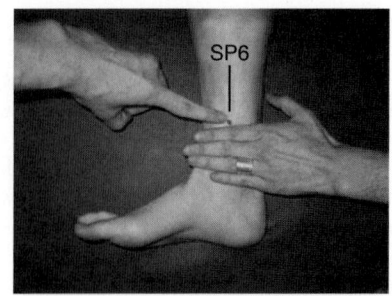

FIG. 52.1 ■ Acupressure to SP6.

pain relief in labor from the use of TENS. Despite this finding, fewer women reported severe pain with the use of TENS, and women who had true TENS were more likely to want to use it in a future labor than those who received sham TENS.[51] The trials that applied TENS to known acupoints more consistently demonstrated pain relief.[52,53] Application can be intermittent or continuous, although continuous TENS may be more effective in active labor.[53]

The application of transcutaneous electrical nerve stimulation may interfere with electronic fetal monitoring.

Acupuncture

In obstetrics, acupuncture has been used to promote version in a breech presentation, decrease nausea, induce or augment contractions, and provide pain relief.[54] It has also been used for pain management during perineal suture repair. Spleen 6 (SP6) and large intestine 4 (LI4) are the most commonly used acupoints in labor (Figs. 52.1 and 52.2).

The considerable heterogeneity among the study designs, treatment protocols, and outcome measures of studies in the literature make it challenging to comfortably draw conclusions about the effect of acupuncture on labor pain. Early data of a systematic review drawing from three trials of acupuncture for labor pain was quite hopeful,[55] and newer data is still optimistic, but the studies draw conflicting conclusions. One recent study[56] of 303 women concluded that acupuncture does not reduce women's experience of labor pain; however, fewer women in the electroacupuncture group used epidural analgesia compared with those receiving standard treatment. Another recent trial[57] found that electroacupuncture reduced pain and shortened the active phase of labor. The most recent Cochrane systematic review[58] included nine trials of acupuncture. Pain scores were not significantly reduced overall using acupuncture; however, there was a significant reduction in the use of pharmacological analgesia in the acupuncture group compared with placebo and standard care. Length of labor was reduced and satisfaction with pain relief was increased when compared with placebo. Compared with standard care, women receiving acupuncture reported greater relaxation. When acupuncture was compared with no treatment for pain, there was reduced pain intensity reported by the acupuncture

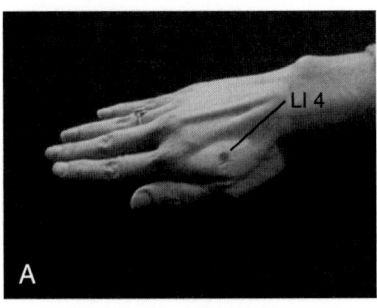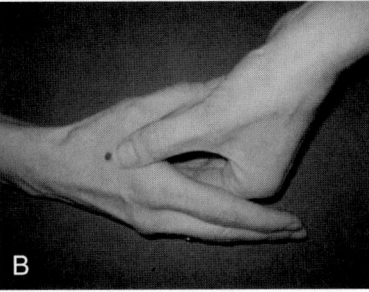

FIG. 52.2 ■ A and B, Acupressure to LI4.

group. An earlier review[59] of 10 trials and 2038 women (some overlapping with the previously mentioned review) did not support the use of acupuncture for controlling labor pain, but the acupuncture group showed a significant reduction in the requirement for all forms of analgesia, including epidural. Women in the acupuncture group had a significantly shorter duration of labor, were more satisfied with their pain relief, and were more relaxed.

When reviewing the literature, we acknowledge that the heterogeneity among the studies may have contributed to conflicting conclusions. An additional consideration is that a nonsignificant or equal score among those receiving acupuncture and those receiving conventional analgesia may actually suggest that acupuncture is equivalent to conventional analgesia. We agree with the authors of a recent narrative literature review[60] who concluded that the benefit of acupuncture may lie largely in the capacity to help women avoid pharmacological medication.

> SP6 and LI4 are purported to cause uterine contractions and should therefore not be used if labor is not desired.[61]

Acupressure

Acupressure is a variation of acupuncture involving the application of a constant pressure on specific acupoints. Like acupuncture, it is frequently used to enhance labor, manage labor pain, and shorten the time to delivery.[62] Because the needles are replaced by pressure, this technique is noninvasive, requires no equipment, and can easily be taught to partners or support staff. Two recent relatively small trials[63,64] measured the effect of acupressure on pain scores at several intervals during labor and found that the women in the control group perceived pain as more severe at nearly each phase of labor compared with the acupressure group. These results are consistent with a prior study.[65] Additionally, labor duration has been shown to be shorter in the acupressure group.[64] A 2011 Cochrane Database Review[58] included four separate studies looking at acupressure with more than 400 women. It revealed a significant reduction in pain scores, reduced length of labor, and decrease in anxiety among women using acupressure during labor compared with controls. The authors ultimately concluded that acupressure may be beneficial in reducing pain, but stated that the risk of bias was high in the studies, and there was need for more research.

> Find SP6: Located one handbreadth (four finger widths based on the proximal interphalangeal joints) above the prominence of the medial malleus, in a depression just medial to the border of the tibia (see Fig. 52.1).[61]
> Find LI4: Ask the patient to squeeze the thumb against the base of the index finger (see Fig. 52.2A). LI4 is on the dorsum of the hand, at the height of the muscle bulge, level with the end of the crease. It is between the first and second metacarpal bones (see Fig. 52.2B).[61]

Mind-Body Therapy

Hypnotherapy

Hypnosis is a state of focused concentration in which the patient is relatively unaware, but not completely blind to her surroundings.[54] *Hypnotherapy* refers to the clinical use of suggestions under hypnosis to achieve specific therapeutic goals.[66] During labor, these suggestions focus on the diminished awareness of pain, fear, and anxiety, thus leading to a decreased perception of each. Generally, this technique requires practice before the onset of labor.

Multiple small, heterogeneous studies have demonstrated decreased use of pain medications,[67] higher pain thresholds,[67] shorter hospital stays,[68] less surgical intervention,[68] fewer complications,[68] and a more satisfying birth experience[66] in hypnotized women. A 2012 systematic review[69] of seven studies, including many of the above, concluded that while there is a positive trend for pain relief in labor using hypnosis techniques, the difference is not statistically significant. Further research with more consistent study design is needed to truly assess its efficacy.

Yoga

Yoga uses the breath to focus on the interconnectedness between the mind and the body. It is thought to bring the individual toward a state of greater relaxation, increased self-awareness, and increased emotional well-being. Yoga also promotes muscle strength and flexibility.[70] Although yoga has been linked to improved birth weight[71,72] and decrease in labor duration,[71] preterm labor, intrauterine growth restriction, and emergency cesarean rate,[72] few studies have focused on maternal comfort in labor. While two of these studies failed to demonstrate a decrease in the use of pain medication in labor, both demonstrated that regular yoga practice in pregnancy was associated with higher levels of maternal comfort during labor and 2 hours afterward and a shorter duration of first stage and total time of labor.[70,73] In addition, investigators noted that the yoga group remained "in control" despite intensifying labor. One small RCT demonstrated a significant decrease in the visual analog scale-rated pain during labor with a regular prenatal yoga practice in women who became pregnant by in vitro fertilization.[74] A nonrandomized controlled trial demonstrated[66] that women who participated in a prenatal yoga program had significantly fewer pregnancy discomforts and increased childbirth self-efficacy. Participants also felt more in control and had lower pain levels that allowed them to be more active in their childbirth experience. Yoga is considered safe in pregnancy because all poses can be modified for the pregnant woman.

Music and Audioanalgesia

The use of music as adjunct therapy has been shown to reduce pain significantly in patients with chronic, postoperative, and cancer pain. Music has also been shown to decrease anxiety during colposcopy and in cardiac patients.[75-77] Many people have extrapolated the analgesic effects of music to labor as well. In the limited available studies, music therapy indeed appears to be mildly effective in reducing both labor pain and distress from that pain.[78,79] Music should be offered to women in labor if they desire.

Biofeedback

With biofeedback, physiological information such as pulse or blood pressure is recorded through electrodes and shown in real time on a monitor while the patient adjusts her behavior or thoughts to control physiological functions that were previously considered involuntary. Patients like biofeedback because it puts them in control and allows them to learn by trial and error.[54] Results are equivocal regarding the efficacy of biofeedback in labor.[80-83] The technique is risk free; however, it does require practice to master during pregnancy.

Biochemical Therapy: Aromatherapy

Aromatherapy is a natural healing art that uses essential oils extracted from aromatic botanical sources. These oils can also be used in the bath water, rubbed on clothing or towels for use as a compress, mixed with oil and applied, or kept available in small vials to open and smell. Examples of essential oils used in labor are lavender, chamomile, mandarin, clary sage, ginger, frankincense, eucalyptus, jasmine, lemon, and peppermint. In one large observational study, women consistently reported aromatherapy to be a helpful adjunct to their labor experience. Incidentally, a substantial overall reduction was noted in the use of systemic opioids in the hospital during the 8 years of the study. Frankincense was rated most highly for pain relief, followed by lavender. Rose and lavender were rated most highly for anxiety reduction. One percent of patients noted mild adverse reactions, such as nausea, itchy rash, and headache.[84] One small underpowered RCT demonstrated a positive trend for decreased pain perception with aromatherapy,[85] and a retrospective study of aromatherapy and massage together demonstrated a decreased use of intrapartum anesthesia.[86] A systematic review[87] of aromatherapy use in labor identified only two studies that met their criteria, and the authors were unable to include any of the data related to pain management because of the way the data was reported. Although more research is required, aromatherapy shows promise for pain relief in labor.

Botanicals

Raspberry Leaf

Raspberry leaf is commonly used as a uterine tonic.[88] As many as 25% of women in the United States use raspberry leaf in pregnancy,[89,90] and up to one-third of U.S. nurse midwives use raspberry leaf to stimulate labor.[90] A review of the existing studies demonstrated a positive trend toward decreases in the length of first and second stage of labor and operative vaginal delivery.[91] No data are available on pain in labor with prenatal raspberry leaf. None of the studies have evaluated raspberry leaf in the form of tea, although this is typically how it is used.

> **DOSAGE**
> The dose is 1.2 g orally twice daily,[92] starting in the third trimester.

Motherwort, Cramp Bark, and Black Cohosh

These botanicals are used by some herbalists to relieve back pain and spastic uterine contractions during labor.[88] No human studies have evaluated the efficacy of these botanicals. Black cohosh may be linked to hepatotoxicity and should be used with caution until more data on its use are available.[88]

Pharmaceuticals

Maternal discomfort in labor is multifactorial. A few common combinations of pharmaceuticals are often given together in labor to address the pain, nausea, anxiety, and extreme fatigue that often accompany this process. Pharmaceuticals can be divided into two main categories: systemic and regional.

Systemic Agents

Essentially all analgesic agents cross the placenta.[95-98] Because of the complexity of fetal circulation, only a small percentage of the drug may reach the fetal brain.[99] Therefore the mother may be affected by a certain concentration of drug without affecting the fetus. Providers should anticipate that beat-to-beat variability of the fetal heart rate may be reduced markedly with the use of these agents, but this may not necessarily affect the clinical status of the newborn. Systemic agents can be divided into three types: opioids, inhaled analgesics, sedatives, and antiemetics (the last two are not completely discussed here).

Opioid Analgesia. Parenteral opioids are frequently used for pain relief in labor, although a large meta-analysis demonstrated that the efficacy is mild to moderate at best, and maternal satisfaction is moderate as well.[100] Whether one opioid is superior to the others remains unclear.[100] Institutional preference often dictates the choice. All opioids are associated with maternal and neonatal respiratory depression, delayed gastric emptying, and nausea and vomiting, which may increase the risk of aspiration if general anesthesia becomes necessary. Some centers use patient-controlled intravenous infusion pumps programmed to give a predetermined amount of drug at the patient's request. Please see Table 52.1 for a comprehensive list of parenteral opioids and their profiles.

Inhaled Analgesics. Inhaled analgesia was introduced in the mid-1800s as one of the first forms of systemic pain control for labor, and is still used widely around the world, although not often in the United States. It can be self-administered after simple instruction, and therefore requires less effort by labor attendants than that required for other forms of analgesia/anesthesia. The agents used primarily for labor pain are nitrous oxide and fluorine derivatives, selected because of their rapid uptake/washout rate, which allows rapid onset of the analgesia. It can be used only during contractions or continuously in labor. There has been some controversy about the risks of nitrous oxide, as it has been associated with decreased fertility and increased spontaneous abortions in maternity professionals, possibly via inactivation of methionine synthase.[101] The precise mechanism of action is unknown, but a systematic review of inhaled analgesia for labor pain in the first stage of labor[87] revealed that there were fewer reports

TABLE 52.1 Parenteral and Inhaled Analgesia

Drug	Dose	Pros	Cons	Comments
Morphine Opioid	2–5 mg IV Onset less than 5 min Lasts 1.5–2 h 10 mg IM Onset 10–20 min Lasts 2.5–4 h	Long-acting when given IM	Nausea and vomiting[99] Urinary retention[99] Orthostatic hypotension[99]	Used primarily for therapeutic rest during early prodromal labor[99]
Meperidine (Demerol) Opioid agonist	25–50 mg IV every 1–2 h Onset 5 min 50–100 mg IM every 2–4 h Onset 30–45 min	Less respiratory depression than with morphine[99] Slightly less urinary retention than with morphine[90]	Active metabolites accumulate in fetal tissue after first hour[90] Active metabolites may cause dose-dependent neurobehavioral depression demonstrated up to 3 days[104] Neonatal risk if delivery occurs within 1–4 h[99] Nausea and vomiting[99] Delay in gastric emptying	Losing favor in pain management
Fentanyl Opioid	50–100 mcg IV every h Onset 1 min Can load up to 200 mcg	Rapid pharmacokinetics No active metabolites Less neonatal neurobehavioral depression[99]	Requires frequent redosing May cause transient benign sinusoidal fetal heart tracing[104]	
Butorphanol (Stadol) Opioid agonist-antagonist	1–2 mg IV every 4 h Onset 1–2 min 1–2 mg IM every 4 h Onset 10–30 min	Ceiling effect for respiratory depression[99] Nausea and vomiting less common[99]	Somnolence[99] Dysphoria[99] Dizziness[99]	May cause increased blood pressure; avoided in hypertension or preeclampsia[104] Opioid antagonist effect may promote opioid withdrawal in opioid-dependent women[99]
Nalbuphine (Nubain) Opioid agonist-antagonist	10 mg IV Onset 2–3 min 10 mg IM every 3 h Onset 15 min Maximum dose 160 mg over 24 h	Ceiling effect for respiratory depression[104] Nausea and vomiting less common than with meperidine[104]	Maternal sedation[104] Dizziness[99] May cause benign transient sinusoidal fetal heart tracing[104]	Potency similar to morphine[99] Opioid antagonist effect may promote opioid withdrawal in opioid-dependent women[99]
Inhaled nitrous oxide[87]	50% nitrous oxide (N_2O) and 50% oxygen[87]	Safely self-administered with simple instruction Decreased drowsiness[87]	Increased nausea, vomiting[87]	Most commonly used inhaled analgesia
Inhaled flurane derivatives[87]	Dosed by anesthesia technician	Decreased nausea vs nitrous oxide Increased pain relief vs nitrous oxide[87]	Increased drowsiness[87] Requires medical provider be present	Typically delivered by anesthesia technicians due to risk of oversedation

75 mg meperidine = 10 mg morphine = 0.1 mg fentanyl = 10 mg nalbuphine.[95]
IM, intramuscularly; *IV,* intravenously.

of pain, as well as decreased pain intensity, with the use of inhaled analgesia using fluorine derivatives or nitrous oxide. Both analgesic agents were associated with side effects such as nausea, vomiting, drowsiness, and dizziness. There was no evidence of short-term harm to the neonate, but because of the significant heterogeneity of this research, more research is required to assess the efficacy and safety of inhaled analgesia in labor.

Sedatives. Sedatives do not possess any analgesic qualities. They are often used in early labor to reduce anxiety, augment the analgesic effects of narcotics, and decrease the nausea often associated with narcotics. Barbiturates, phenothiazines, and benzodiazepines are examples. The last two classes are not commonly used because of their many maternal and neonatal risks.[102-104] Promethazine (Phenergan) is an antiemetic and is the most widely used sedative in labor. It rapidly crosses the placenta and has no known antagonist. In large or small doses combined with opioids, promethazine can depress the fetus for long periods of time. When used carefully with an opioid such as morphine in prodromal labor, however, promethazine may promote therapeutic rest for the patient. In some institutions, zolpidem, a sleep aid, is alternately given for therapeutic rest.

Local and Regional Anesthesia

Because local and regional analgesia methods do not depress the central nervous system, the birthing woman remains awake and able to participate actively, and the neonate is alert on delivery. Regional anesthesia provides the most effective form of pain relief in obstetrics, and the term refers to partial or complete loss of sensation below the T8–T10 level.[104] Depending on the agent used, motor blockade may also be present. Examples of regional anesthesia include spinal anesthesia and epidural anesthesia. Several options for more localized anesthesia also are available, such as the pudendal block, paracervical block, and perineal block. Please refer to Tables 52.2

and 52.3 for detailed information regarding local and regional blocks, respectively.[105,106]

Therapies to Consider

Hot or Cold Application

Although the use of hot or cold application for pain relief in labor is common practice among doulas and labor support staff, no RCTs have evaluated this therapy. Easy to initiate, the use of heat or ice should depend on the desires of the laboring woman. Typically, heat is applied to the back, neck, shoulders, or abdomen by using warm compresses, microwaveable rice-filled pillows, or electric heating pads. Caution should be taken to avoid burns; the heat should never be painful. Cold is typically applied to the forehead, back, or neck using a cool washcloth, ice-filled sacs, a glove, or ice pack. Cold soda cans, which can double as massage tools on the lower back, can also be used. One study demonstrated a decrease in pain scores with ice massage to the acupoint LI4 during contractions.[107]

Homeopathy

Although many birth attendants administer homeopathy for pain, anxiety, and labor management, the use of these remedies is largely driven by traditional homeopathic literature. Currently, no data are available on homeopathy in labor and birth; however, research indicates that homeopathy is a very safe form of therapy with minimal side effects.[108] If a woman is interested in using homeopathy, consult a homeopath or homeopathic literature to find appropriate remedies.

Reflexology

Reflexology focuses on zones in the hands and feet that are believed to correspond to specific areas of the body.[109] The practitioner applies manual pressure in

TABLE 52.2	**Other Analgesia**			
Type	**Description**	**Precautions**	**Indications**	**Technique**
Local perineal analgesia	Direct perineal infiltration with rapidly acting agent Local analgesia lasting 20–40 min[99]	Intravascular injection can rarely cause seizures, hypotension, and cardiac arrhythmias. Avoid injecting into the fetal scalp.	Used before episiotomies, outlet forceps, and laceration repair	Use 1%–2% lidocaine without epinephrine or 2-chloroprocaine. Aspirate for blood before injecting. Use as little as possible to avoid toxicity.
Paracervical block	Simple, effective Duration of analgesia dependent on type of anesthesia used	Fetal bradycardia, which can be associated with fetal acidosis.[104] Do not use in mothers with fetuses with acute or chronic distress.[99]	Pain relief for cervical dilation Administration limited to first stage of labor	Inject 5–6 mL of local anesthetic without epinephrine into lateral fornices of cervix (4 and 8 o'clock or 3 and 9 o'clock).
Pudendal nerve block	Safe Variably effective	Risk of injecting directly into large vessels that lie in close proximity to injection site Hematoma[104] Infection[104]	Pain relief in second stage Spontaneous vaginal delivery, episiotomy, some outlet and low forceps, or to supplement epidural block	Inject 5–10 mL of local anesthetic slightly below the ischial spines bilaterally. Aspirate before injection to reduce the risk of local anesthetic toxicity.

these zones to achieve therapeutic benefits in the target organ, gland, or body part. One small RCT in Iran[110] demonstrated a significant decrease in reported pain throughout the entire first stage of labor after reflexology treatment in early labor, compared to either routine care or routine care plus labor support. The session addressed the areas associated with the pituitary gland, diaphragm, uterus, and genital area, as well as lumbar and sacral spine. The mechanism for reflexology is unclear and has been controversial. Further study is required to assess its efficacy on labor pain, but this study showed promise.

TABLE 52.3 Regional Blocks

Type	Description	Indications/Effects	Precautions
Spinal block	A single-shot, long-acting local anesthetic is often used with or without an opioid agonist.	This is used for the second stage of labor and short procedures such as cesarean delivery.	Hypotension, which may lead to decreased uterine perfusion[104] Pruritus (when opioids are added)[104] Blunting of the pressure sensation during the second stage of labor Impaired ability to push if the motor block is too dense Increased risk for operative vaginal delivery[104] Prolongation of labor[104] Fever,[107] periodically leading to suspicion of infection and subsequent interventions Transient fetal heart rate deceleration[104] Increased need for oxytocin (Pitocin) augmentation[104] Headache[104] Transient painful sensation in legs or buttocks (with spinal)[104] Epidural or spinal hematoma (rare)[104] Abscess (rare)[104] High spinal anesthesia, resulting in paralysis of the respiratory muscles (rare)[104] Neurotoxicity (rare)[104]
Combined spinal–epidural block	This combines the rapid onset of spinal analgesia with the ability for continuous infusion of analgesic though the epidural catheter.[a]	This widely used block provides immediate pain relief during the second stage of labor. It can convert to anesthesia adequate for cesarean section. It continues to provide postcesarean pain relief.	
Epidural anesthesia	Local anesthetic and opioid are injected through a catheter into epidural space, to allow for continuous infusion. The dose can be titrated over the course of labor.	The same catheter can be used for labor, vaginal delivery, and cesarean section. The block is usually not initiated until active labor is established.	
"Walking" epidural anesthesia	This epidural block preserves motor strength for more effective pushing. Most women are not able to walk or support their weight.		

[a]Maternal satisfaction, obstetric outcomes, and neonatal outcomes do not appear to differ between the combined spinal–epidural block and the epidural block.[106]

PREVENTION PRESCRIPTION

- Cultivate the patient-provider relationship prenatally when possible.
- Discuss the woman's expectations about labor prenatally.
- Discuss preferences for labor pain management before labor begins.
- Involve the laboring woman in decision making.
- Recommend that women arrange for continuous labor support.
- Recommend regular moderate exercise or yoga practice during pregnancy.

THERAPEUTIC REVIEW

A laboring woman has many options for pain control. Individually, many of these therapies are quite effective in reducing pain, but nearly all may be used in combination. No research has evaluated the synergistic effect, but we recommend offering multiple options to women.

- Plan for continuous labor support. Consider hiring a trained doula.   A₁
- Consider childbirth education classes to prepare for labor and birth.   C₁

LIFESTYLE

- Regular prenatal exercise   B₁
- Moderate exercise or movement during labor   B₁

BIOMECHANICAL THERAPY

- Ambulation or upright position during first stage of labor   A₁
- Upright or side-lying position during second stage of labor   A₁
- Hands and knees position for back labor   B₁
- Water immersion,
  - First stage   A₁
  - Second stage   B₁
- Massage during labor   B₁
- Regular chiropractic, osteopathic, or manual treatment in pregnancy   B₁
- Sterile water injections for back labor   A₁
- Hot or cold application   B₁
- Reflexology   C₁

BIOENERGETICS

- Transcutaneous electrical nerve stimulation in labor, with possible focus on acupoints   B₁

- Acupuncture during labor   B₁
- Acupressure during labor   A₁
- Homeopathy   C₁

MIND-BODY THERAPY

- Regular yoga practice in pregnancy   B₁
- Hypnotherapy techniques prenatally to prepare for labor   B₁
- Music/audioanalgesia during labor   B₁
- Biofeedback techniques during pregnancy to prepare for labor   B₁

BIOCHEMICAL: AROMATHERAPY

- Aromatherapy during labor (e.g., frankincense, lavender, rose)   B₁

BOTANICALS

- Raspberry leaf to shorten labor: 1.2 mg twice daily in the last trimester   B₁
- Motherwort or skullcap may have a calming effect for anxiety   C₁
- Black cohosh   C₂

PHARMACEUTICALS

- Parenteral opioids for mild to moderate pain relief. Choice of medication and dose is often institutionally driven   A₂
  - See Table 52.1 for options and doses
- Promethazine: 12.5–25 mg, orally or intravenously, every 4–6 hours as needed for sedation and nausea   C₂
- Local anesthesia   A₂
  - See Table 52.2 for technique and details
- Regional anesthesia or epidural anesthesia   A₃
  - See Table 52.3 for options and details

Key Web Resources

DONA International: Find a doula, and learn about doulas.

Betts D. Natural Pain Relief Techniques for Childbirth Using Acupressure: Locate acupressure points, and find further information on acupressure in labor.

Hypnobabies and Hypnobirthing: Locate resources for using hypnosis during labor and childbirth.

Kaiser Permanente guided imagery: Listen to a free downloadable guided imagery session to help prepare for labor. This website also includes other guided imagery downloads for pregnancy and childbirth.

http://www.dona.org

http://acupuncture.rhizome.net.nz/downloads/Acupressure.pdf

http://www.hypnobabies.com
https://us.hypnobirthing.com/

https://www.healthjourneys.com/kaiser/download/download_healthyPregnancy.asp

REFERENCES

References are available online at ExpertConsult.com.

CHAPTER 53

POSTDATES PREGNANCY

D. Jill Mallory, MD

PATHOPHYSIOLOGY

Postdates or postterm pregnancy is defined as a pregnancy that extends to or beyond 42 weeks of gestation (294 days or estimated date of delivery [EDD] plus 14 days). A normal pregnancy lasts approximately 40 weeks from the start of a woman's last menstrual period, but any pregnancy that lasts between 37 and 42 weeks is considered normal. Approximately 4%–7% of all singleton pregnancies extend to 42 weeks or 14 days beyond the EDD.[1]

Postterm pregnancy is associated with a higher perinatal mortality rate (stillbirth and newborn death within the first week) and a higher risk for complications during delivery, such as an emergency cesarean delivery, shoulder dystocia, postpartum hemorrhage, birth asphyxia, meconium aspiration syndrome, and neonatal birth injury.[2] Current research suggests that the lowest infant mortality rate is achieved when pregnant women have completed at least 41 weeks of gestation before labor is induced and when induction occurs before or at 42 weeks of gestation, although the absolute risk for problems from delivering beyond 42 weeks is low.[2] The overall risk for perinatal death is estimated at 0.4% in women who deliver beyond 42 weeks of gestation and 0.3% for women who deliver between 37 and 42 weeks of gestation.[3]

Because of this small increase in perinatal mortality, the induction of labor is widely practiced at or before 42 weeks of gestation, and postterm pregnancy has become the most common reason for induction.[4] Unfortunately, labor induction itself is not without risks. Obstetric problems associated with induction of labor in postterm pregnancy include cesarean section, prolonged labor, postpartum hemorrhage, and traumatic birth. These problems are more likely to result from induction when the uterus and cervix are not ready for labor.[2] Furthermore, induction of labor brings with it increased risks of uterine rupture, uterine hyperstimulation, fetal distress, and instrumentation.[5]

Very few studies have considered women's experiences and opinions when it comes to the timing of inducing labor, and for women seeking a natural, unmedicated labor and birth, induction poses many philosophical challenges. Accurate dating is obviously important for reducing the need of induction, and studies have shown that early ultrasound is associated with a reduced incidence of pregnancies misclassified as postterm.[6] When women have accurate pregnancy dating and are approaching 41 weeks of gestation, many may seek nonpharmaceutical measures of cervical ripening and labor induction. One small study of 50 women showed that many were opposed to medical induction of labor, yet they used self-help measures to stimulate labor at home.[7] More research is needed in the realm of nonpharmaceutical cervical ripening and labor induction options for women who have postdate pregnancies.

INTEGRATIVE THERAPY

Nutrition

Pineapple

Pineapple (Ananas comosus), which contains the compound bromelain, has historical medicinal use both as a whole food and in extract form. Bromelain has been proposed as the active ingredient, and it is present only in the fresh fruit because the canning process destroys it. Bromelain has been used to elicit uterine contractions as a means of shortening labor. Some animal model research suggests that instead of increasing cervical prostaglandins, bromelain may actually inhibit them.[8] No research is available on the possible effectiveness of bromelain for induction of human uterine contractions, although this use is widely suggested in lay pregnancy resources. Some investigators suggest that pineapple's effects on labor may result from gastrointestinal stimulation by fiber and sugar, thus affecting local neural pathways.[9] No known risks are associated with pineapple use in pregnancy.

Supplements

Castor Oil

Castor oil, derived from the bean of the castor plant (Ricinus communis), has a very rich history of use for labor stimulation that dates back to ancient Egypt. One survey completed in 1999 found that 93% of U.S. midwives reported using castor oil to induce labor.[10] Despite this prevalence, research into the use of castor oil has been limited. A recent study in mice found that the castor oil metabolite ricinoleic acid activated intestinal and uterine smooth muscle cells via prostaglandin E2 receptor 3 (EP3) prostanoid receptors.[11] This may explain its mechanism of action in humans. Three trials were included in a recent Cochrane review looking at castor oil for labor induction.[12] It included 233 women at term and compared ingestion of castor oil with no treatment/placebo. Outcomes evaluated included cesarean section rate, meconium staining of amniotic fluid, instrumental delivery, and Apgar scores. All women who ingested castor oil had nausea; otherwise, outcomes were not significantly different from those in women who did not ingest castor oil. A retrospective observational study done in Thailand of 612 women looked at the timing of delivery, fetal distress, meconium-stained amniotic fluid, tachysystole of the uterus, uterine rupture, abnormal maternal blood pressure during labor, Apgar scores, neonatal resuscitation, stillbirth, postpartum hemorrhage, severe diarrhea, and maternal death.[13] No differences were seen in outcomes between the women who ingested castor oil and the women who did not. This finding suggests that castor oil is safe to use but may not be helpful. Prospective randomized controlled trials are needed.

Evening Primrose Oil

Evening primrose oil (*Oenothera biennis*) is often used for several health conditions of women, including breast pain (mastalgia), menopausal and premenstrual symptoms, and labor induction or augmentation. It contains the amino acid tryptophan and an unusually high content of essential fatty acids, especially cis-linoleic acid (CLA) and gamma-linoleic acid (GLA).[10] These fatty acids are prostaglandin precursors, which may explain traditional use of the oil for stimulating cervical ripening.[10] This supplement is used widely during the last month of pregnancy by midwives in the United States both for cervical ripening and to decrease the incidence of postdates pregnancy.[10] Evening primrose oil is traditionally administered as one to two capsules intravaginally at bedtime, starting after 37 completed weeks of pregnancy. There has been one case report of an infant born with petechiae and ecchymosis after its mother took primrose oil a week before giving birth.[14] One study investigated oral administration and showed that this route was not effective.[15] Furthermore, the oral use of evening primrose oil during pregnancy may also be associated with more prolonged labor and an increased risk for premature rupture of membranes, arrest of descent, oxytocin use, and vacuum extraction.[15] This finding is not surprising because oral administration during pregnancy was never a traditional use. Larger trials assessing the efficacy of vaginal administration are needed.

Homeopathy

Homeopathy is a safe choice for pregnant women and babies because the remedies used in this system of healing have no pharmacological action.[16] In the United States, the use of homeopathic remedies has increased, and a survey among nurse-midwives in North Carolina reported that 30% recommend homeopathic substances for use during pregnancy.

The two most common homeopathic remedies used for labor induction are cimicifuga (homeopathic black cohosh) and caulophyllum (homeopathic blue cohosh), which are believed to act directly on the uterus and cervix. These remedies have a long history of use around the world for labor stimulation, especially in Europe and India.[17] Caulophyllum is used either to induce labor or augment labor if uterine contractions are short and irregular or when uterine contractions stop. Caulophyllum and cimicifuga are both indicated for dysfunctional uterine contractions and are thought to help initiate a coordinated and effective contraction pattern. Cimicifuga is used specifically to ease the fear of labor and delivery in women who have a history of traumatic childbirth, miscarriage, or abortion.[18] Cimicifuga alone is administered as a single dose of 30 C or 200 C potency every 30 minutes for at least 2 hours or together with

caulophyllum 200 C, alternating doses of the two remedies for a total of six doses in 24 hours. Other remedies that are commonly used for labor induction include aconite, arsenicum, gelsemium, phosphorus, and pulsatilla. These are all given in 200 C potency as a single dose (two pellets).[19]

A 2003 Cochrane review examined the use of caulophyllum, cimicifuga, and some of these other homeopathic remedies.[16] The review assessed only two studies comparing homeopathy and placebo for cervical ripening or labor induction and found that small sample sizes and insufficient detail in the research made it impossible to draw any meaningful clinical conclusions. More research needs to be conducted to determine whether homeopathy is a potentially viable alternative to oxytocin and prostaglandins for labor induction. Furthermore, studies should be designed to incorporate individualized homeopathic treatments, prescribed by a trained homeopath, to account for the individualized nature of this modality.

> For labor induction, caulophyllum and cimicifuga homeopathic remedies are as follows: 30 C or 200 C given every 30 minutes, 1 pellet of each remedy, for a total of six doses in 24 hours. No remedy is given the next day. Repeat the same protocol on day 3 if needed. Other remedies to consider are gelsemium for fear of birth and pulsatilla when contractions come and go, but labor never becomes established.

Botanicals

Red Raspberry Leaf

Red raspberry leaf (*Rubus idaeus, Rubus occidentalis*) has been used as a uterine tonic and general pregnancy tea for at least two centuries. Although this botanical is often mistakenly recommended to induce labor, its actual role is to increase blood flow to the uterus and aid the uterine muscle fibers in more organized contraction. Studies indicate that some of the plant components, such as fragrine, an alkaloid, do act directly on smooth muscle.[20] Animal studies show conflicting data in terms of the herb's effect on uterine muscle. Some studies show a contractile effect, whereas others show a relaxing effect. Historical uses include prevention of miscarriage, prevention of postdates pregnancy, decrease of discomfort in prodromal labor, and decrease of morning sickness. Red raspberry leaf was also probably consumed for nutritional support because the plant contains many nutrients, including vitamins A, C, and E, as well as calcium, iron, and potassium. Overall, the herb does seem to reduce the risk for postdates pregnancy and appears safe for general use.[21] One randomized controlled trial of 192 women showed no adverse effects to mother or baby, a shorter second stage of labor (a mean difference of 10 minutes), and a lower rate of forceps use.[19] One retrospective, observational study of more than 150 women also found that red raspberry leaf reduced the risk for postdates pregnancy, but more conclusive data are needed.[16]

Black Cohosh

This herb (*Actaea racemosa*) also has a long history of use. Native Americans mixed it with chamomile, ginger, and raspberry tea to induce menses and labor. The active compounds in black cohosh include terpene glycoside fractions, such as actein and cimifugoside, which have been associated with an estrogenic effect and are thought to reduce levels of pituitary luteinizing hormone, thus decreasing ovarian production of progesterone.[18] This effect may contribute to the initiation of uterine contractions because the relaxing effect of the high levels of progesterone on the uterine muscle decreases before the initiation of labor. However, a systematic review on the use of black cohosh in labor found no evidence of efficacy.[22]

One of its alkaloids, caulosaponin, causes coronary blood vessel constriction and direct myocardial toxicity in a dose-dependent manner. This poses challenges to practitioners because the doses present in over-the-counter products may be difficult to verify. At least one case report has been published of toxicity in an infant whose mother was given an unknown dose of black cohosh at term.[23] At this time, the German Commission E, an expert committee established by the German Ministry of Health that evaluates herbal products, does not recommend the use of black cohosh in pregnancy.[24]

Blue Cohosh

The herb blue cohosh (*Caulophyllum thalictroides*) also has a long tradition of use as a uterine tonic. It was traditionally used by Native Americans during 2–3 weeks before the onset of labor.[22] Between 1882 and 1905, blue cohosh was listed in the *United States Pharmacopoeia* for labor induction.[22] Over-the-counter preparations of blue cohosh contain varying amounts of triterpene glycosides, which have documented oxytocic effects.[25] No studies are available on efficacy.

Three case reports are available that demonstrate possible adverse neonatal effects, such as fetal hypoxia, myocardial infarction, and congestive cardiac failure.[26] Whether these effects resulted from the herb itself is not known, given that herbs are often used in combination with other plants, and adulteration and contamination problems can occur. Until further research on this plant is done, it is best avoided for labor induction.

At this time, the use of blue and black cohosh is best avoided in pregnant women because of safety concerns.

Biomechanical Therapy

Breast Stimulation

Breast stimulation has historically been used to induce or augment labor since as early as the eighteenth century.[27] Stimulation of the breast is thought to increase the production of endogenous oxytocin in pregnant and nonpregnant women. The most commonly used protocol for breast stimulation involves using either a manual or electric breast pump, manual massage around the areola of the nipple, or rolling the base of the nipple. Typical hospital protocols recommend stimulating each breast individually for 10 minutes each, with a 10-minute rest period following, for a total of four cycles.

The Cochrane Collaboration performed a systematic review of six trials with a total of 719 participants that compared breast stimulation with no intervention to induce labor in women at term.[28] The review found that compared with no intervention, breast stimulation significantly reduced the number of women who had not gone into labor at 72 hours.[28] This difference was not significant in women with an unfavorable cervix. Breast stimulation also reduced the risk for postpartum hemorrhage by 84%.[28] It did not seem to have an effect on cesarean section rates. No incidences of uterine hyperstimulation were noted.

Breast stimulation for labor induction allows women's participation in the induction process and has the advantage of being a low-cost and nonpharmaceutical means of labor induction. Observational studies, however, have shown a link between bilateral breast stimulation and uterine hyperstimulation.[29] For this reason, unilateral stimulation is typically recommended. Concerns have been raised regarding possible adverse effects on placental perfusion; however, the incidences of abnormal fetal heart rate tracings are similar to those found with oxytocin use.[30] Continuous electronic fetal monitoring is typically used with breast stimulation in the hospital setting. A common protocol used by women in their homes at term is unilateral breast stimulation done for 1 hour per day for 3 consecutive days. Until safety issues have been more thoroughly evaluated, this technique should not be used in high-risk populations.

Shiatsu

Shiatsu is an ancient form of massage based on Chinese acupuncture theory that often includes the use of breathing and stretching. Shiatsu can be done through the clothes or on bare skin and uses static pressure, which can vary from light holding to deep physical pressure applied with the palm of the hand or thumb. Shiatsu lends itself well to maternity settings because specific shiatsu techniques can be taught to birth partners or practitioners. It has historically been used in midwifery practices to induce or augment labor.[31]

One small pilot study evaluated shiatsu for induction and augmentation of postterm labor.[32] Sixty-six women with postterm pregnancies were studied in a hospital-based midwifery practice. Pregnant women were taught to massage three acupuncture points in conjunction with breathing techniques and exercises. The controls attended the same clinic, but they were not taught the techniques. The investigators found that the women with postterm pregnancies who used shiatsu were significantly more likely to have spontaneous labor than were the study participants who did not use shiatsu.

Bioenergetics

Acupuncture

As part of the ancient system of medicine, known as traditional Chinese medicine, acupuncture has been used in pregnancy for thousands of years. Modern studies have evaluated the insertion of fine needles into specific points on the body, as well as the use of mild electrical currents through these needles, known as electroacupuncture. A 2013 Cochrane Systematic Review evaluated acupuncture for inducing labor.[33] The investigators identified 14 trials that included 2220 women for review. Acupuncture was compared with sham acupuncture or usual cases. Most of the trials were undertaken in Western countries. No trial reported on the achievement of vaginal delivery in 24 hours or uterine hyperstimulation. The use of acupuncture did not seem to affect cesarean section rates or neonatal seizure rates. Acupuncture did seem to increase cervical ripening; however, it did not seem to shorten labor. There were no other statistically significant differences between the groups, including no differences in neonatal morbidity or maternal mortality. Overall, the limited studies to date suggest that acupuncture appears safe for inducing labor, has no known adverse effects on the fetus, and may be effective. The inherent difficulties in blinding for acupuncture treatment make the study of this technique challenging. Given its safety profile, it may be worth trying in patients who wish to avoid pharmaceutical induction of labor. Table 53.1 provides acupuncture points that patients can massage at home to stimulate labor.

Lifestyle

Sexual Intercourse

Unprotected sexual intercourse is thought to encourage the onset of labor by two means. One is the release of endogenous oxytocin in the mother, and the other is cervical ripening caused by seminal prostaglandins. A Cochrane review looked at an observational study of 28 women at term. Unprotected intercourse for three consecutive nights neither significantly changed Bishop scores (1.0 with coitus vs. 0.5 controls; $P > .05$) nor increased the number of women who went into labor at the end of 3 days (relative risk, 0.99; 95% confidence interval, 0.45–2.20).[34] Sexual intercourse in pregnancy is considered safe, provided the absence of placenta previa, rupture of membranes, or active genital infection.[30] Larger studies are needed to determine whether sexual intercourse has any significant effect on reducing the risk for postdates pregnancy.

Pharmaceuticals

Misoprostol

Misoprostol is a prostaglandin E_1 analog widely used for off-label indications such as induction of labor in postdates pregnancy. This hormone is given by insertion through the vagina or rectum or by mouth to ripen the cervix and elicit uterine contractions. A Cochrane review looked at 121 trials and found that small doses (25 mcg every 4 hours) of misoprostol vaginally were as effective as other methods of labor induction.[35] Larger doses of misoprostol were found to be more effective than prostaglandins for labor induction, and larger doses also reduced the need for additional oxytocin. Another Cochrane review found that the oral route of administration may be preferable to the vaginal route.[36] Compared with the vaginal route, oral route of administration was associated with a lower rate of babies born with low Apgar scores and a lower rate of postpartum hemorrhage but with a higher rate of meconium-stained amniotic fluid. A third Cochrane review has looked at buccal or sublingual administration.[37] Data on these routes of administration are more limited; however, there was a trend toward a lower cesarean section rate, a reduced need for oxytocin augmentation, and an increased rate of vaginal delivery in 24 hours. More studies are needed to establish the optimal buccal/sublingual dosage. The main risk for misoprostol use is hyperstimulation of the uterus, and this risk seems to increase with increasing dose. At this time, misoprostol is not approved by the Food and Drug Administration (FDA) for induction of labor.

TABLE 53.1   Acupressure Points for Induction of Labor

1. Midway along the top of the trapezius muscles, if you were to draw a line from the acromion to C7
2. The motion sickness point at the angle between the first and second metacarpals
3. In the semicircle around the distal medial and lateral malleoli
4. The little toe, all over

Massage these points for at least 2–3 minutes each.

From Mallory J. Integrative care of the mother-infant dyad. *Prim Care.* 2010;37:149–163.

DOSAGE

The most common dose used in the United States is 25 mcg intravaginally every 4 hours (maximum, 50 mcg). Wait for more than 4 hours after the last dose before adding oxytocin. The most common oral dose used is 50 mcg. Misoprostol comes in 100- and 200-mcg tablet formulations.

PRECAUTIONS

Uterine hyperstimulation, uterine rupture, diarrhea, nausea, vomiting, headache

Although misoprostol is commonly used for labor induction in the United States, it has not been approved by the FDA for this use.

Oxytocin

Oxytocin is the most common induction agent used worldwide. It is used alone, in combination with amniotomy, or following cervical ripening with other pharmacological or nonpharmacological methods. Oxytocin is a synthetic analog of the natural labor hormone by the same name. It binds to oxytocin receptors in the uterine myometrium, increases intracellular calcium, and stimulates uterine contractions. A Cochrane review of more than 61 studies concluded that it is safe and effective.[38] A black box warning placed on the drug by the FDA states that oxytocin is not to be used for elective labor induction.

DOSAGE

Start with 0.5–2 milliunits/minute and increase by 1–2 milliunits/minute every 15–40 minutes until the uterine contraction pattern is established. The maximum for induction is 40 milliunits/minute. Oxytocin is available in intravenous and intramuscular preparations.

PRECAUTIONS

Increased use of epidural anesthesia, uterine hyperstimulation, uterine rupture, abruptio placentae, fetal distress, nausea, vomiting

Vaginal Prostaglandins (PGE₂ and PGF₂ₐₗₚₕₐ)

Prostaglandins have been used for the induction of labor since the 1960s. These drugs are synthetic analogs of the body's naturally occurring prostaglandins, which function to ripen the cervix and bring about contractions. A Cochrane review looked at 70 randomized controlled studies of various forms of prostaglandins and found them to be a safe and effective means of labor induction.[39] Prostaglandin E_2 is the most commonly used type, and it increases the likelihood of vaginal birth in 24 hours and may reduce the risk for cesarean section by 10%.[39]

DOSAGE

The dose is one 10-mg pessary intravaginally. The insert releases 0.3 mg/hour over 12 hours. Remove at 12 hours, at the onset of active labor, or if uterine hyperstimulation occurs. The agent is available as a 10-mg sustained-release insert. It is also available as an intravaginal tablet or gel.

PRECAUTIONS

Uterine hyperstimulation, fetal distress, uterine rupture, bronchospasm, abdominal cramps, headache, nausea, diarrhea

Mechanical Methods

Potential advantages of mechanical methods, compared with pharmacological methods, for the induction of labor in postdates pregnancy include simplicity of use, lower cost, and reduction of side effects, such as uterine hyperstimulation and fetal distress. However, special attention should be paid to contraindications such as a low-lying placenta, risk for infection, and maternal discomfort.

Amniotomy

The deliberate rupture of membranes may be sufficient to bring about labor without the use of pharmaceuticals. This approach has the advantage of being cheap, but it may be uncomfortable for some women. If the time between amniotomy and delivery of the baby is long, infection may occur. The risk for umbilical cord prolapse is also increased, especially if the fetal head is ballotable at the time of membrane rupture. Anecdotal reports note that amniotomy may be less beneficial in nulliparous women. More evidence is needed regarding effectiveness compared with placebo or compared with other methods of induction of labor.[40]

Membrane Sweeping

Sweeping of the membranes, also known as *membrane stripping*, is a simple manual technique usually done in the outpatient setting. The technique involves inserting a finger into the cervical os during a sterile vaginal examination and sweeping the finger in a circular motion to detach the membranes from the lower uterine segment. This method sometimes works to initiate labor by increasing the local production of prostaglandins. A Cochrane review of 72 studies found that sweeping of the membranes performed routinely for women at term was associated with a reduced frequency of pregnancy extending beyond 41 weeks.[41] This method is considered safe and reduces the need for pharmaceutical means of induction of labor in postdates pregnancy.[41] There was no increased risk for cesarean section or maternal or neonatal infection. Adverse effects include maternal discomfort, vaginal bleeding, and irregular contractions.

Transcervical Foley Catheter or Cook Catheter Insertion

This approach involves placing a 30-mL Foley catheter bulb or an inflatable Cook catheter transcervically, inflating it with sterile saline solution, and applying maintenance traction or simply leaving it in place (Fig. 53.1).

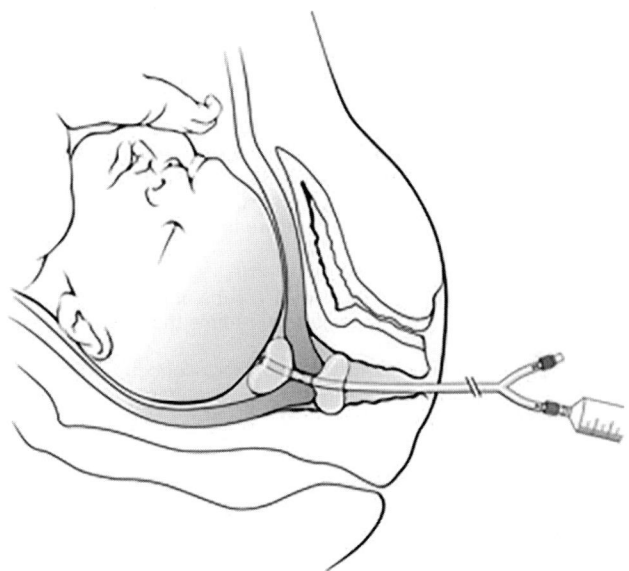

FIG. 53.1 ■ Cook cervical ripening balloon. (© 2012; Lisa Clark, courtesy Cook Medical.)

A Cochrane review looked at 71 studies and concluded that induction of labor with mechanical methods resulted in a similar rate of cesarean section as prostaglandins with equal efficacy of achieving vaginal delivery in 24 hours and a lower risk for uterine hyperstimulation.[42] When compared with oxytocin alone, the rate of cesarean section is lower with mechanical methods. Complications include acute febrile reaction, pain, vaginal bleeding, and altered fetal presentation.

PREVENTION PRESCRIPTION

- Women can be encouraged in the preconception period to track their menstrual cycles and sexual activity closely to aid in accurate pregnancy dating. When women are unsure of their pregnancy dates, first-trimester ultrasound reduces the number of women later incorrectly classified as having postdates pregnancies.
- Good self-care in pregnancy, including aromatherapy, good nutrition, massage, sexual intercourse, spiritual practices, chiropractic, and yoga during the latter weeks of pregnancy may serve to relax the mother and allow the natural rise of oxytocin and reduction of stress hormones, thus resulting in a greater likelihood of spontaneous onset of labor.[43-45]
- Membrane sweeping, done routinely at 39 weeks, may also reduce the risk for a pregnancy that continues beyond 41 weeks.

THERAPEUTIC REVIEW

These therapeutic options for prevention of postdates pregnancy and induction of labor in postdates pregnancy may be considered in the healthy, term patient with no medical complications that would make delivery urgent.

NUTRITION

- Pineapple consumption is commonly recommended for labor induction. Although pineapple has no proven benefit, the risks of this intervention are low.

SUPPLEMENTS

- Castor oil has a long history of use for labor induction. It is considered safe, but it has not been proven effective. Side effects include nausea. Doses are not standardized.
- Evening primrose oil use lacks data on efficacy. The dose is two capsules intravaginally at bedtime, starting at 38 weeks of pregnancy. This supplement should not be used orally in pregnancy.
- The homeopathic remedies caulophyllum and cimicifuga can be dosed at 200 C potency by alternating 1 pellet of each remedy every 30 minutes for a total of six doses in 24 hours to help stimulate labor. The benefit is unknown, and risks are minimal.

BOTANICALS

- Red raspberry leaf, taken as 1–3 cups of tea daily during the third trimester, may reduce the risk for postdates pregnancy.
- Despite a strong history of use, black cohosh and blue cohosh should be avoided in pregnancy because of safety concerns until more data are available.

BIOMECHANICAL THERAPY

- Unilateral breast stimulation can be done for 1 hour per day for 3 consecutive days to induce labor at term.

- Shiatsu may reduce the risk for postdates pregnancy.

ACUPUNCTURE

- Evidence is mixed on the effectiveness of acupuncture to reduce the risk for postdates pregnancy, for cervical ripening, and for labor induction. Acupuncture is considered safe.

LIFESTYLE

- Sexual intercourse may not be effective for reducing the risk for postdates pregnancy.

PHARMACEUTICALS

- Misoprostol is commonly used for cervical ripening and labor induction, despite a lack of approval by the FDA for this indication. See the doses and precautions discussed in the text.
- Oxytocin may be used to induce uterine contractions in postdates pregnancy when cervical conditions are favorable. See the doses and precautions discussed in the text.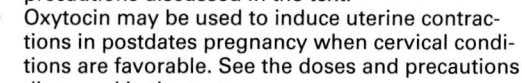
- Vaginal prostaglandins may be used for cervical ripening and labor induction, and they are a good choice for postdates pregnancy in patients with unfavorable cervical conditions. See the doses and precautions discussed in the text.

MECHANICAL THERAPY

- Amniotomy may be used to induce or augment labor, and it may be more beneficial in multiparous women.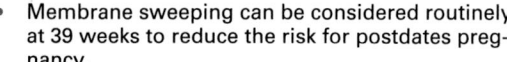
- Membrane sweeping can be considered routinely at 39 weeks to reduce the risk for postdates pregnancy.
- Transcervical Foley catheter insertion or Cook catheter insertion can be done for cervical ripening in postdates pregnancy, and it may have lower risks than pharmaceutical ripening agents.

Key Web Resources

American College of Obstetricians and Gynecologists: Patient hand-out on postdates pregnancy	http://www.acog.org/Patients/FAQs/What-to-Expect-After-Your-Due-Date
American College of Nurse-Midwives: Consumer information on pregnancy and midwifery	http://www.mymidwife.org/
ACOG Guidelines: Management of late-term and postterm pregnancies	http://contemporaryobgyn.modernmedicine.com/contemporary-obgyn/news/acog-guidelines-management-late-term-and-postterm-pregnancies?page=full

REFERENCES

References are available online at ExpertConsult.com.

CHAPTER 54

NAUSEA AND VOMITING IN PREGNANCY

Andrea Gordon, MD • Abigail Love, MD, MPH

PATHOPHYSIOLOGY

Nausea and vomiting in pregnancy (NVP) represent a conundrum for the pregnant woman. On the positive side, NVP are correlated with better fetal outcomes than the absence of these symptoms,[1] but at the other extreme, NVP can interfere with nutrition and hydration for the mother and developing fetus. Symptoms may range from occasional mild nausea to multiple episodes of daily vomiting resulting in weight loss and electrolyte abnormalities. This severe manifestation is often referred to as hyperemesis gravidarum. Definitions of hyperemesis gravidarum vary, but commonly accepted criteria include weight loss (often more than 5% of prepregnancy weight), electrolyte disturbances, and ketonuria.

Usually appearing before the ninth week of pregnancy, NVP will affect up to 85% of normal pregnancies, with symptoms generally remitting by the fourteenth week. Initial presentation of symptoms after the ninth week should prompt a workup to determine an alternative cause. NVP may be mild, but up to 20% of women find their symptoms so significant that they cannot continue to work.[2] The reported incidence of hyperemesis gravidarum, the most severe end of the spectrum, varies from 0.5% to 2%. This severely debilitating condition is the most common reason for hospital admission in the first trimester and the second most common problem for which pregnant women are admitted to the hospital, after preterm labor.[3]

Even at the milder end of the symptom continuum, NVP can lead to a decreased quality of life and missed time from work. The aptly named Motherisk Pregnancy-Unique Quantification of Emesis and Nausea (PUQE) index has been shown to demonstrate a significant correlation between the presence and severity of NVP and poorer quality of life.[4,5] This effect on quality of life and the economic impact of missed work emphasize the need to control these symptoms. Mild or moderate vomiting does not appear to have any significant effects on the fetus. Among women with severe hyperemesis, the reported incidence of low birth weight is higher, but increased reporting of birth defects has not been noted.[6] In fact, several investigators suggested that NVP represent an evolutionary adaptation that helps protect the developing fetus from exposure to foods that may contain potential toxins.[7,8]

The cause of NVP is unknown. Both biological and psychological factors have been proposed. Human chorionic gonadotropin (HCG) and estrogen have been studied as triggers for these symptoms. Suggestive evidence includes the finding that pregnant women with higher levels of HCG, which occur in molar pregnancies and multiple gestations, have significantly more episodes of vomiting and higher rates of hyperemesis gravidarum. This theory is also supported by the observations that nonpregnant women who experience nausea and vomiting after exposure to estrogens are more likely to experience NVP. Cigarette smoking is known to reduce both estrogen and HCG levels, and pregnant smokers are less likely to experience hyperemesis gravidarum.[9]

No controlled studies support the theory that NVP comprise a conversion disorder or an inability to respond to life stress.[10,11] The association of high levels of HCG and estradiol with increasingly severe episodes of vomiting in pregnancy indicates a physiological origin, as do epidemiological factors. Daughters and sisters of women who had hyperemesis are more likely to have NVP as well. Other risk factors include a previous pregnancy affected by hyperemesis, a female fetus, and a history of motion sickness or migraines.[12]

INTEGRATIVE THERAPY

When treatment is considered, risks and benefits must be clearly explained to the pregnant woman. Minimizing the risks of any treatment is desirable, but the presence of a developing fetus makes it more urgent to decrease any unnecessary exposures. This is an ideal time to use integrative approaches because drugs generally represent more risk than other modalities. In addition, some of the behavior modifications such as exercise are beneficial in and of themselves.

Lifestyle

Although the efficacy of lifestyle modifications has not been studied, these interventions are safe and have been anecdotally reported to be useful.[13]

Avoid Odors

Some women report that NVP are triggered by strong odors such as foods, cigarette smoke, or perfume. This is supported by a small study showing that women with congenital anosmia were less likely to develop NVP.[14]

Avoiding these stimuli may be helpful. Women should be supported in doing so, for example, by passing off cooking duties to someone else, avoiding tasks with strong odors such as feeding the dog, or politely asking coworkers not to wear perfume for a few weeks.

Increase Rest

Sleep requirements increase in early pregnancy.[15] Women frequently report nausea in association with feelings of exhaustion. Caregivers should educate pregnant patients that fatigue is common and support them in trying to obtain the additional rest they need.

Exercise

Light to moderate aerobic exercise is associated with fewer NVP symptoms. Women who exercised at least three times a week for 20 minutes or more reported fewer symptoms of pregnancy, including nausea.[16] Women who have already been exercising can remain active during uncomplicated pregnancies. Previously inactive women may benefit from gentle exercise but should be evaluated on an individual basis before recommendations for physical activity are made.[17]

Nutrition

Low blood glucose levels seem to trigger nausea and subsequently vomiting in many women; thus small, frequent, high-protein, high-fiber meals are often recommended.[18] A potentially helpful approach is to decrease simple carbohydrates that rapidly raise blood glucose and thus stimulate insulin secretion, which can cause rapidly falling blood glucose (see Chapter 87). However, this includes foods such as pasta, white rice, potatoes, and white bread, whose blandness seems desirable when patients are nauseated, so education is key. Some patients find that eating something as soon as they wake up and then every 2 hours can suppress nausea. Each pregnant woman may have specific foods she avoids because of a taste or smell that triggers nausea, but it may also be necessary to avoid spicy or fatty foods because they can exacerbate symptoms. Little published evidence exists on the efficacy of dietary changes, but benefit clearly outweighs harm. In one international survey, dietary interventions seemed to help 22% of women with hyperemesis gravidarum.[19]

Two studies found that taking a multivitamin before pregnancy or before 6 weeks of gestation was associated with a decreased incidence of NVP. Although this approach would not help a woman already suffering with symptoms, it could be helpful for women at risk for symptoms in their next pregnancy.[20,21]

Botanicals

Ginger Root (Zingiber officinale)

Historically, ginger has been effectively and safely used to treat nausea, including that of pregnancy. Randomized controlled trials have shown that ginger is effective for treating NVP,[22] and it is the most thoroughly studied herb for this indication. Some trials have shown ginger to be not only more effective than placebo[23] but also

comparable to or better than vitamin B6[24,25] and comparable to dimenhydrinate.[26] It will reduce overall nausea symptoms but not the number of vomiting episodes significantly.[27]

Patients should be advised that it may take longer for ginger to work: up to 3 days, rather than 1 day for dimenhydrinate. The U.S. Food and Drug Administration (FDA) has listed ginger as a food supplement that is generally recognized as safe,[28] and studies have not shown any increased incidence of malformations in children of mothers using ginger.[29]

Ginger seems to work primarily in the gastrointestinal tract on serotonin receptors in the ileum, the same receptors affected by some antiemetics, such as ondansetron. Some evidence indicates that ginger constituents may also have some action in the central nervous system.[30] No toxicity has been demonstrated, although ginger can cause abdominal discomfort or heartburn when it is taken in large doses, especially on an empty stomach.

DOSAGE

Most of the studies have used 1000 mg daily, in two or four divided doses.[23,26,28,31] A higher dose of 650 mg three times daily has also been used,[32] but total doses of less than 1500 mg a day are more effective.[34] Ginger is available in a variety of forms, and an evaluation of products purchased in pharmacies and health food stores found a wide variation in the amount of active ingredients and suggested serving sizes.[35] Women may prefer one form over another, so approximate equivalents can be calculated. In general, 1 g of standardized extract is equivalent to 1 teaspoon of fresh grated ginger root, two droppers (2 mL) of liquid extract, four 8-oz cups of prepackaged ginger tea, four 8-oz cups of tea made with 0.5 teaspoon of grated ginger steeped for 5–10 minutes, 8 oz of ginger ale (made with real ginger—most commercial ginger ales are not effective), two pieces of crystallized ginger (1 inch square, 0.25 inches thick), or two teaspoons (10 mL) of ginger syrup.[36] Capsules of ginger come in various dosages, ranging from 100 to 1000 mg, and chewable tablets may contain 67 to 500 mg, so attention to the dosing of the product used is advisable, with the goal a total of less than 1500 mg a day.

Using ginger throughout the day is also helpful. Patients can incorporate ginger into their diet by sprinkling dried or candied ginger in oatmeal, having some ginger tea, and adding fresh ginger to soup or stir-fries.

PRECAUTIONS

There is a theoretical risk for bleeding as ginger inhibits thromboxane synthetase and may inhibit platelet function. This has not been demonstrated, but precaution should be taken when ginger is used concomitantly with anticoagulants.

Chamomile (Matricaria chamomilla)

Chamomile is a flowering plant that is often used for various types of gastrointestinal upset, including travel sickness, colic, and inflammatory diseases of the bowel. It is commonly used for NVP,[37-39] although no research on this application has been published. Chamomile appears to be safe and well tolerated, however, and the FDA labels it as safe.[40]

DOSAGE

Prepare it as a tea, allowing it to steep for 5–7 minutes while covered, so it will retain the volatile active constituents, and sip as needed.

PRECAUTIONS

Chamomile should be used with caution in patients who are allergic to the Asteraceae/Compositae family, which includes ragweed, daisies, and many other flowers. Some erroneous concern exists about teratogenicity, but that concern is based on a study with alpha-bisabolol at high doses that could not be achieved by someone drinking tea.[41]

Peppermint Leaf (Mentha piperita)

Peppermint is another herb often used in pregnancy.[42,43] The active parts are the stems, leaves, and flowers, as well as the peppermint oil that is distilled from these plant parts. Studies have shown peppermint oil to be effective for reducing bowel spasms in irritable bowel syndrome and for patients receiving barium enemas, but peppermint oil has not been studied in pregnancy.[44] Its mechanism of action is reduction of spasm in smooth muscle, and it may help with NVP by reducing esophageal dysmotility. However, this effect can also reduce lower esophageal sphincter pressure, resulting in reflux. Theoretical concerns exist with using the essential oil in pregnancy because it may cross the placental barrier, but the amount of peppermint ingested in tea or food seems to be safe.[41] Peppermint has been rated as safe by the FDA.[40]

DOSAGE

The dose is two to three cups of tea daily. Many women find peppermint candies or gum to be effective in squelching nausea. A dose of 0.2 mL in 2 mL of isotonic saline solution used as aromatherapy has been used for postoperative nausea and can be tried if teas or foods containing peppermint are not tolerated.[45]

PRECAUTIONS

Peppermint can aggravate reflux by decreasing the lower esophageal sphincter tone.

Bioenergetics

Acupressure: Stimulation of the P6 Neiguan Point

Acupressure of the pericardium 6 (P6) Neiguan (meridian) point, which is located on the inner wrist, may be beneficial. Several small studies have found this to be effective, including a Korean trial, which found significantly less NVP in a group of women with hyperemesis gravidarum,[46] and another that demonstrated self-administered nerve stimulation therapy over using a commercial device.[47] However, a 2014 Cochrane analysis did not find P6 acupuncture or acupressure wristbands to be significantly more effective than placebo. Other studies using a crossover design, which were not included in the Cochrane analysis, also showed benefit to using acupressure at the P6 point,[46,48] and another trial revealed decreased nausea with P6 stimulation, but no change in the frequency of vomiting.[49] Patients should be made aware of this mixed evidence; patients are willing to try acupressure because it is inexpensive and has no significant side effects.

Patients can be taught to find the P6 point and treat themselves with either manual pressure or the application of "Sea-Bands" (Fig. 54.1). These elastic bands with attached plastic disks were originally used for motion sickness. Patients can create their own version of such bands by placing a small, round object such as a bead over the point and securing it with tape and then massaging the bead. This therapy has no known negative side effects.

To have a patient accurately locate the P6 point, have her lay one hand palm up, with the other hand placed palm down at right angles to the upturned arm. The first three fingers of the palm-down hand are held close together, and the edge of the ring finger is placed at the crease of the wrist closest to the palm in alignment with the middle finger of the upturned hand. The P6 point, between the palmaris longus and flexor radialis tendons, is now readily palpable under the tip of the index finger of the examining hand (see Fig. 54.1A). This point is often tender, a characteristic that aids in its location. Many patients use this acupressure in conjunction with other interventions because it has no known side effects or interactions.

Patients can stimulate the P6 point at any time, but they should be cautioned against using any other acupressure points without consulting a trained practitioner. Some commonly used points, such as the Ho-Ku point that is located between first and second metacarpals (often used for headaches), can stimulate contractions.

Patients must be instructed to press on the point when feeling nausea, as just wearing the bands may not provide significant relief.

Mind-Body Therapy

Hypnosis

Hypnosis has been studied as a treatment for hyperemesis gravidarum. A review of six studies showed encouraging effects, but methodological problems did not allow a definitive recommendation.[50] This intervention is safe, however, and some women may want to try it for all levels of NVP. One approach has been to suggest to a woman that the "nausea center" in her brain is very sensitive to the hormones of pregnancy and that she is able to "turn down" that sensitivity as one would a thermostat.[51] Another approach is to link the muscle tension in the stomach and throat or the nausea as a hypnotic cue to pleasant imagery.[52] This imagery may be helpful for patients to use when nausea strikes.

NVP may have an element of conditioned response, as noted with chemotherapy-associated vomiting. Some uncontrolled studies showed that hypnosis can reduce vomiting and anticipatory vomiting in patients

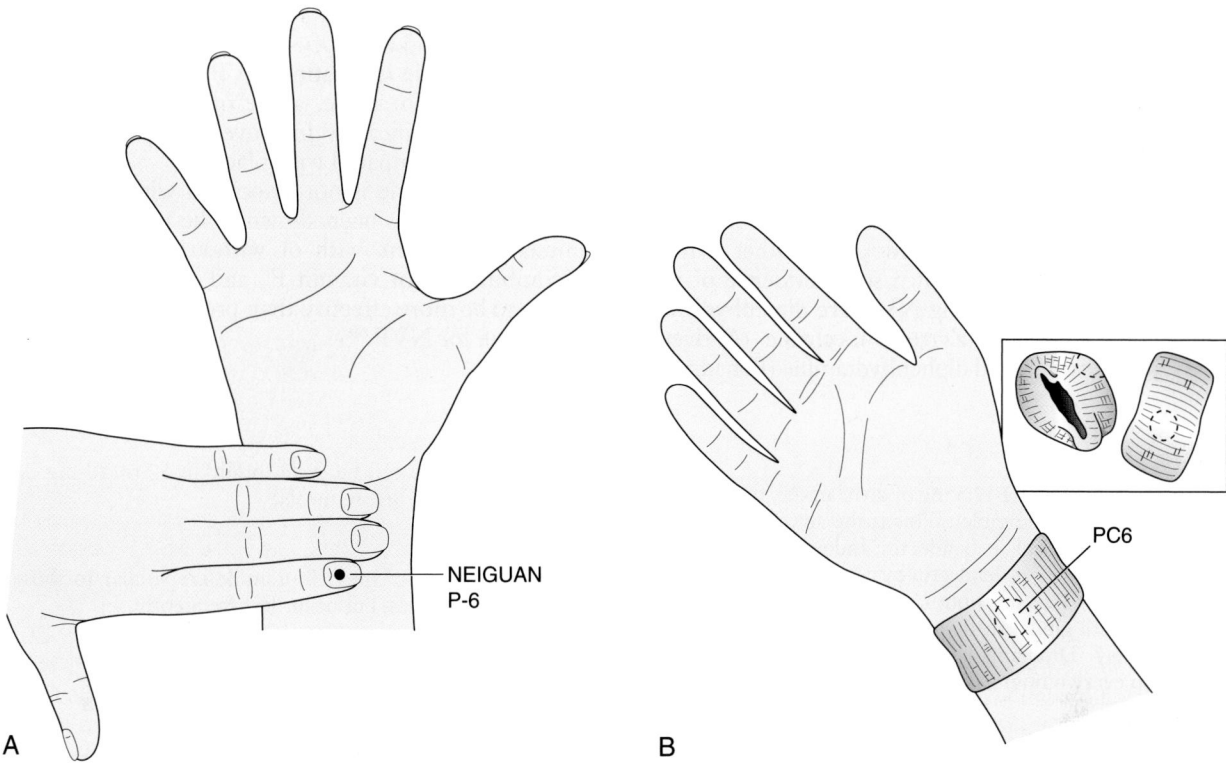

FIG. 54.1 ■ A, The P6 Neiguan acupressure point is located on the volar aspect of the forearm by placing the examining hand three fingerbreadths below the wrist crease. The patient's finger widths should be used for measurement. The P6 point is essentially in the midline between the tendons of the palmaris longus and flexor radialis muscles. B, Location of this point. *PC*, pericardium

undergoing chemotherapy,[10] so the potential exists for hypnosis to work for NVP. Because this treatment may require several sessions of training, the time and expense may be prohibitive for some patients.

Counseling and Psychotherapy

Although the general consensus is that NVP does not represent a conversion disorder and is not caused by emotional responses to the pregnancy,[10] evidence indicates that women with NVP may be under more stress. Two investigators stated that NVP "could subject any normal expectant mother to stress sufficient to trigger adjustment disorders, generalized anxiety, or even depressive episodes."[10] In recognition of this extraordinary stress, counseling or psychotherapy may be helpful in coping with the symptoms and their effects on a woman's life.

Supplements

Vitamin B6 (Pyridoxine)

Vitamin B6 is a water-soluble vitamin that is an effective treatment for nausea in pregnancy. The benefit in reducing vomiting episodes is less clear.[53,54] The mechanism of action of pyridoxine remains unknown, but extensive analysis for teratogenicity has shown no negative effects on pregnancy outcome.[55]

Patients can expect a significant reduction of nausea with few side effects if they take vitamin B6, so this should be used as a first-line treatment of NVP.[56]

A popular medication for nausea and vomiting, known as Bendectin in the United States and Diclectin in Canada, contained pyridoxine and doxylamine. Bendectin was withdrawn from the United States market in 1983 out of safety concerns about teratogenicity, but no studies validated this possibility. Diclectin remains available in Canada and is one of the most widely studied and used medications in pregnancy today. Following removal of Bendectin from the market, no reduction in birth defects was reported, but hospitalization rates for NVP doubled.[57]

Diclectin, a combination of doxylamine 10 mg and pyridoxine 10 mg, is available in Canada and can be purchased online (www.canadadrugs.com). It is expensive, at more than a dollar a pill. A recommended and less expensive alternative is to combine Unisom (contains 25 mg doxylamine), one-half tablet at bedtime, with 25 mg of pyridoxine, as the combination reduces symptoms by 70%.[56] [Category C]

DOSAGE

The most effective dosage of B6 appears to be 30–75 mg daily in three divided doses. Studies performed with the higher end of the dosing range have shown effectiveness against vomiting as well as nausea.[53,54] When vitamin B_6 alone is not effective, it may be combined with doxylamine to obtain relief from NVP.

PRECAUTIONS

Pyridoxine can cause sensory neuropathy, which is related to the daily dose and duration of intake. Doses exceeding 1000 mg daily or total doses of 1000 g or more pose the most risk, so the doses that have been used for NVP appear generally to be safe.[58]

Pharmaceuticals

Antihistamines

Several histamine (H1) receptor antagonists have been studied for the treatment of NVP. The most frequently studied and used is doxylamine (Unisom, an over-the-counter sleep aid). An extensive review of safety data revealed no adverse pregnancy outcomes from the use of doxylamine alone or in combination with pyridoxine.[59] Other drugs in this group, which all have shown some evidence of efficacy and safety for controlling NVP, are dimenhydrinate (Dramamine), cetirizine (Zyrtec), meclizine (Antivert), hydroxyzine (Vistaril), and diphenhydramine (Benadryl).[60]

> **DOSAGE**
>
> Most patients should use 12.5 mg of doxylamine, the amount in one-half of a scored tablet. This is the amount of doxylamine that was present in Bendectin. Indeed, many women try to "make" a form of Bendectin by combining doxylamine with vitamin B6. This safe option can be suggested if vitamin B6 alone or with ginger or P6 point stimulation is not working adequately. Diphenhydramine, given in 25- to 50-mg doses up to every 6 hours, is also safe and easily obtained.
>
> **PRECAUTIONS**
>
> All antihistamines can cause drowsiness.

Phenothiazines

The phenothiazines used to treat NVP include promethazine (Phenergan), prochlorperazine (Compazine), chlorpromazine (Thorazine), and perphenazine (Trilafon). Only promethazine has randomized controlled study data supporting its efficacy and safety.[60,61] However, some evidence indicates that all medications in this group have some efficacy in the treatment of NVP.[55] These medications may be used in the outpatient setting, but therapy is often not started until hospital admission for treatment of dehydration or intractable vomiting. The variable dosing forms are advantageous for NVP: these drugs can be self-administered orally or rectally or given intramuscularly by medical personnel if needed.

> **DOSAGE**
>
> For promethazine, begin with 12.5 mg per rectum or by mouth and progress to 25 mg every 4 hours as needed.
>
> **PRECAUTIONS**
>
> Side effects of promethazine include sedation, hypotension, dystonia, and extrapyramidal symptoms. If needed, diphenhydramine 25 mg can be given orally every 6 hours to treat dystonia or extrapyramidal side effects.

Dopamine Antagonists

Two dopamine antagonists have been studied for the treatment of NVP: trimethobenzamide (Tigan) and metoclopramide (Reglan). Trimethobenzamide has been shown to be safe,[62] but it has been largely studied for nausea in other settings such as chemotherapy.[63] Only one double-blind trial focused on the effectiveness of trimethobenzamide in treating NVP.[64] This study showed that trimethobenzamide, alone or in combination with pyridoxine, significantly improved symptoms of nausea and vomiting compared with placebo.[64]

Metoclopramide is not associated with malformation risk,[65,66] and it has been shown to be effective in hyperemesis gravidarum, with or without promethazine.[67,68] A combination of vitamin B6 and metoclopramide was shown to be more effective than prochlorperazine or promethazine for NVP.[69]

> **DOSAGE**
>
> Metoclopramide can be given orally in 5- to 10-mg doses three times daily before meals.
>
> **PRECAUTIONS**
>
> The side effects of metoclopramide are similar to those of the phenothiazines, but occur less frequently.

5-Hydroxytryptamine₃ Receptor Agonists

Ondansetron (Zofran), a 5-hydroxytryptamine$_3$ receptor agonist, is a potent antiemetic originally used for treatment of chemotherapy-induced nausea and vomiting. Data on NVP are limited, but several small studies have found it to be as effective as promethazine,[70] or as effective as metoclopramide in women with hyperemesis gravidarum.[71] Another trial, which more accurately reflects what is often used in practice, demonstrated ondansetron to be superior to the combination of pyridoxine and doxylamine.[72]

> **DOSAGE**
>
> Ondansetron is given orally or intravenously, 4–8 mg up to every 8 hours. Ondansetron is available in an orally disintegrating tablet. This can be useful if one becomes too nauseated to swallow any medication.
>
> **PRECAUTIONS**
>
> Adverse reactions to ondansetron include headache, fever, and bowel dysfunction, although this agent has been reported to be better tolerated by patients than promethazine, with no dystonic or extrapyramidal side effects.
>
> Two recent studies found no significant increase in major fetal malformations or outcomes,[73,74] and the FDA has labeled ondansetron Pregnancy Category B. However, patients do need to be informed that there is a demonstrated association with an increased risk of cardiac septum defects, mainly atrial septal defect and ventricular septal defect.[74,75]
>
> In light of this evidence, as well as cost considerations, it is prudent to try the other measures and medications discussed previously prior to considering the use of ondansetron, and then discussing the risks with patients.
>
> "No statistically significantly increased risk for a major malformation was found with ondansetron. The risks for a cardiovascular defect and notably a cardiac septum defect were increased and statistically significant (OR = 1.62, 95% CI 1.04–2.14, and RR 2.05, 95% CI 1.19–3.28, respectively). The teratogenic risk with ondansetron is low but an increased risk for a cardiac septum defect is likely."[74]

Corticosteroids

Several small studies have evaluated corticosteroids, primarily methylprednisolone, for efficacy in reducing NVP and hyperemesis. Methylprednisolone reduced symptoms of NVP along with hospital readmission rates for hyperemesis.[76] Another trial found that promethazine worked more rapidly than prednisolone, but after a week both medications worked equally well, and the prednisolone group had fewer side effects.[77] Various oral and intravenous dosages have been studied, but the most common regimen is 16 mg of methylprednisolone 3 times daily, with attempts to taper after 3 days. Most patients respond within 3 days, so if no improvement has been seen by that time, longer treatment is generally not indicated. Methylprednisolone may be continued for up to 6 weeks, but longer use may result in adverse maternal effects related to prolonged steroid exposure.[76,78] Evidence also indicates that a shorter course of hydrocortisone is effective for treating intractable hyperemesis.[79] A meta-analysis found an increased risk of oral clefts associated with prednisone use.[80]

DOSAGE

The dose of methylprednisolone is 16 mg orally or intravenously every 8 hours for up to 2 weeks (tapered course to avoid adrenal suppression). The dose of hydrocortisone is 300 mg intravenously daily for 3 days, then tapered over one week.

PRECAUTIONS

Avoid corticosteroid use before 10 weeks of gestation if possible. Avoid prolonged use for more than 6 weeks to reduce the risk of maternal side effects.

Intravenous Fluids

Intravenous fluids have not been specifically studied for the treatment of hyperemesis, but they are often coadministered with other medications in the hospital setting for the treatment of dehydration. Intravenous fluid is generally recommended when patients fail to tolerate oral fluids for a prolonged period or show electrolyte abnormalities indicating dehydration.

Dextrose and intravenous thiamine can be added to fluids when vomiting has been prolonged and persistent.[12,81]

Extreme Measures for Intractable Nausea and Vomiting in Pregnancy

Enteral or Parenteral Feedings

Evidence to support enteral or parenteral feedings comes from case reports and small series.[82,83] In general, the prudent approach is to start with enteral feedings and move on to peripheral parental nutrition and finally to total parental nutrition if all other methods fail. Serious and even life-threatening complications have been reported with parenteral nutrition, so it is used only as a last resort.[84]

Therapeutic Abortion

With current medical interventions such as intravenous hydration and medications, it is rare for NVP to be so severe as to be life threatening. This was not the case in the early twentieth century, when severe NVP represented an important cause of maternal deaths.[85] However, maternal morbidity in the form of Wernicke encephalopathy caused by vitamin B1 deficiency, esophageal rupture, acute tubular necrosis, and splenic avulsion have all been reported to be caused by intractable vomiting of pregnancy.[1] When the maternal condition is deteriorating as a consequence of hyperemesis gravidarum despite aggressive medical intervention, pregnancy termination may be indicated (Fig. 54.2). Fortunately, symptoms usually subside rapidly as HCG levels fall.

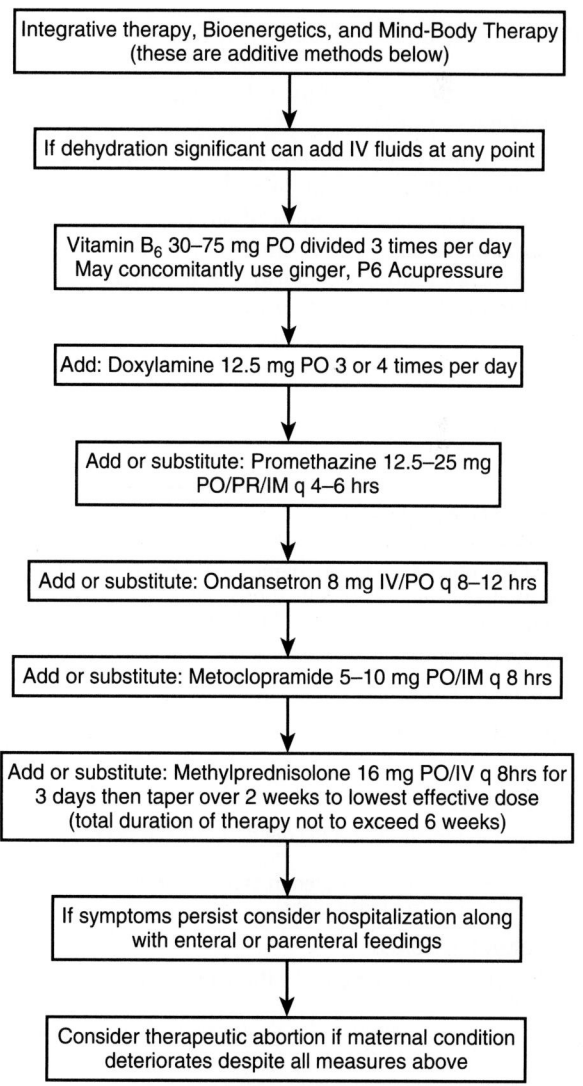

FIG. 54.2 ■ Integrative therapy, bioenergetics, and mind-body therapy algorithm. *IM*, intramuscularly; *IV*, intravenous; *PO*, orally; *PR*, per rectum; *q*, every.

Therapies to Consider

Homeopathy

No studies have evaluated the efficacy of homeopathic remedies in the treatment of NVP. Practitioners cite anecdotal evidence of homeopathy use, but choosing the correct remedy can be complex because many subtle differences in symptoms are taken into account. Some of the remedies commonly used include nux vomica, sepia, and ipecac.[86] Because homeopathic preparations are extensively diluted, they should be safe for pregnant women and unlikely to have any adverse effects if they are not helpful. Some investigators recommend avoiding any remedies with potencies (dilutions) greater than 12C.[87]

Traditional Chinese Medicine

Practitioners of traditional Chinese medicine (TCM) may recommend acupuncture, acupressure, and herbs,

but they also use certain foods such as umeboshi plums (a very salty preserved fruit) to combat nausea. In addition, these clinicians may use practices such as moxibustion, cupping, or massage. The TCM views of health and the body's function are different from those in Western medicine, and different patterns of symptoms lead to different treatments,[88] so a certified TCM practitioner should advise about the use of these approaches.[89] Information about training and accreditation of TCM practitioners can be found at the National Certification Center for Acupuncture and Oriental Medicine (www.nccaom.org).

Umeboshi plums can be found in most Asian grocery stores. If the plum itself is too salty, some women obtain relief from nausea by sucking on the pit only. Another option is to use one-fourth to one-half a plum at a time.

PREVENTION PRESCRIPTION

- Take a multivitamin prior to pregnancy or before 6 weeks of gestation.[20,21]
- Eat frequent, small meals that are high in protein to avoid low blood glucose levels.
- Avoid overconsumption of simple carbohydrates such as cakes, candy, and starchy foods because they may lead to rebound low glucose levels, which could stimulate more nausea.
- Consider trying more salty foods and tart liquids because these are reported by some women to be better tolerated.
- Avoid triggers such as pungent odors or unpleasant visual stimuli that may worsen nausea.
- Increase rest as needed early in pregnancy.
- Do light to moderate exercise for 20 minutes three times a week.

THERAPEUTIC REVIEW

Lifestyle, botanical, bioenergetic, and mind-body therapies are additive to all the other methods listed here. If dehydration is significant, add intravenous fluids at any point.

BIOENERGETICS
- Acupuncture (P6) — B, 1

MIND-BODY THERAPY
- Hypnotherapy — B, 1

SUPPLEMENTS
- Vitamin B6: 30–75 mg PO divided three times per day — A, 1
- Ginger: 250 mg powdered in capsules four times daily or 500 mg twice daily — B, 1

PHARMACEUTICALS
- Doxylamine: 12.5 mg orally three to four times daily — A, 2

- Add or substitute promethazine: 12.5–25 mg orally, rectally, or intramuscularly every 4–6 hours B, 2
- Add or substitute ondansetron: 8 mg intravenously or orally every 8–12 hours  A, 3
- Add or substitute metoclopramide: 5–10 mg orally or intramuscularly every 8 hours B, 2
- Add methylprednisolone: 16 mg orally or intravenously every 8 hours for 3 days then taper over 2 weeks to the lowest effective dose (total duration of therapy not to exceed 6 weeks) B, 2
- If symptoms persist, consider hospitalization along with enteral or parenteral feedings. C, 3

SURGERY
- Consider therapeutic abortion if the maternal condition deteriorates despite all the measures described here and in Fig. 54.2. C, 3

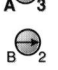

Key Web Resources

Motherisk morning sickness information: This website contains a treatment algorithm for hyperemesis gravidarum.	http://www.motherisk.org/prof/morningSickness.jsp
Evidence-Based Approaches to Managing Nausea and Vomiting in Early Pregnancy: This article provides an overview of NVP and treatment options. It also contains the PUQE index. Registration is required to access this website.	http://www.medscape.com/viewarticle/712662_3
BMJ Clinical Evidence: A systematic review of treatments for NVP. Registration is required to access this website.	http://clinicalevidence.bmj.com/ceweb/conditions/pac/1405/1405.jsp

REFERENCES

References are available online at ExpertConsult.com.

CHAPTER 55

MANAGING MENOPAUSAL SYMPTOMS

Marcia Klein-Patel, MD, PhD • Katherine Gergen-Barnett, MD • Judith Balk, MD, MPH

INTRODUCTION

Since antiquity, menopause has been a marker of transition in a woman's life. Despite all the changes that have occurred in modernity, very little has moved the age at which menopause occurs. Our mothers, grandmothers, and great grandmothers all experienced menopause at the average age of 51 years, as women do today. However, women are now living to the average age of 81 years, spending roughly one-third of their lives after the cessation of menses. The impact of this duration of time, which includes the transition leading up to menopause, can be enormous both physiologically and psychologically. While there are many bothersome symptoms that women may experience during the perimenopausal and menopausal stages of their lives, this is also a time of enormous opportunity for wellness. In this chapter, we will be looking at the physiology and symptomatology of perimenopause and menopause, treatment options to mitigate some of the most bothersome symptoms of menopause, and finally, basic strategies for supporting wellness among women during this rich, reflective time in their lives.

PHYSIOLOGY OF THE FEMALE REPRODUCTIVE LIFE CYCLE

At 20 weeks of gestation, female fetuses have the maximum number of oocytes they can have. From birth until menopause, these oocytes decrease, either through atresia or ovulation, until the final follicles diminish and menopause begins. However, there is a long journey from this 20-week-old fetus to the menopausal woman, and much of this journey is dictated by the dance of a few key hormones.

At puberty, the long dormant follicles are recruited through the cyclic release of the follicle stimulating hormone (FSH) and luteinizing hormone (LH). FSH stimulates the ovary to recruit a follicle from the ovaries, and as this follicle develops, it secretes estrogen. This estrogen serves many roles, including the thickening of the uterine lining, maintaining vaginal blood flow and lubrication, and skin thickness and elasticity. As a dominant follicle develops, estrogen levels increase, and through a negative feedback loop on the pituitary, there is a surge in FSH and LH. This surge is the signal to ovulate. The remaining corpus luteal cells produce progesterone, which in turn further thickens and prepares the lining of the uterus for a possible fertilization. If the egg is not fertilized in the window of ovulation, progesterone will fall and a woman will menstruate. This pathway is called the *hypothalamic-pituitary-ovary axis*.

While there has long been nomenclature to define a woman's transition from regular menstruation to the more irregular (perimenopause) and ultimately cessation of menstruation (menopause), there has been much study over the last decade to clarify the exact physiology in each of these stages as well as work on further characterization of each of these transitions. In 2001, the first group of scientists came together to apply some of this knowledge toward menopause and created a set of standards called STRAW (Stages of Reproductive Aging Workshop), and this had been considered the gold standard for the characterization of reproductive aging through menopause (Fig. 55.1). In 2011, scientists from five different countries and a variety of backgrounds gathered to review data from a cohort of midlife women and evaluated changes in menstrual, endocrine, and ovarian markers of reproductive aging including antimullerian hormone (AMH), inhibin B, FSH, and antral follicle count (AFC).[1] STRAW-10, as this summit was called, was important at a number of levels as it not only helped stratify perimenopause and menopause into seven discrete categories but also revisited important population health questions that had not been addressed 10 years prior.

The STRAW-10 staging, though granular in its definition of each stage, was developed to promote the ability of future researchers and clinicians to determine exactly where a woman may be in her menstrual arc, as well as the sequelae at each stage. The hormonal shifts in each of these stages also bear clinical significance for the rest of the health and wellness of a woman. The original STRAW explicitly recommended against applying the criteria of reproductive aging to smokers, women with a body mass index (BMI) > 30 kg/m², women who had undergone hysterectomy, women engaged in heavy aerobic exercise, women with chronic menstrual cycle irregularities, and women with uterine or ovarian abnormalities. However, these groups are included in STRAW-10.

As already mentioned, as a woman ages through late reproductive age, the number of follicles diminish. In early and peak reproductive years (stages −5 and −4 by STRAW-10), a woman continues to have sufficient follicles for recruitment and her menstrual flow appears regular. However, in the late reproductive stages (−3a and b), a

Stage	−5	−4	−3b	−3a	−2	−1	+1a	+1b	+1c	+2
Terminology	Reproductive				Menopausal transition		Postmenopause			
	Early	Peak	Late		Early	Late	Early			Late
					Perimenopause					
Duration	Variable				Variable	1–3 years	2 years (1+1)	3–6 years		Remaining lifespan
Principal criteria										
Menstrual cycle	Variable to regular	Regular	Regular	Subtle changes in flow/ length	Variable length persistent ≥7–day difference in length of consecutive cycles	Interval of amenorrhea of ≥60 days				
Supportive criteria										
Endocrine										
FSH			Low	Variable	↑ Variable	↑ >25 IU/L**	↑ Variable	Stabilizes		
AMH			Low	Low	Low	Low	Low	Very low		
Inhibin B			Low	Low	Low	Low	Low	Very low		
Antral follicle count			Low	Low	Low	Low	Very low	Very low		
Descriptive characteristics										
Symptoms					Vasomotor symptoms *likely*	Vasomotor symptoms *most likely*				Increasing symptoms of urogenital atrophy

* Blood draw on cycle days 2–5   ↑ = elevated
** Approximate expected level based on assays using current international pituitary standard[67–69]

FIG. 55.1 ■ STRAW stages of reproduction.

woman may note that her cycles are becoming shorter in their length or frequency. This is because, as the follicle supply diminishes and less follicles are recruited, there is less inhibin-B, which in turn has a decreased negative feedback on the hypothalamic–pituitary axis, causing a surge in FSH (as it works to recruit more follicles for stimulation), earlier follicle recruitment, and shorter cycles. This increased number of follicles leads to the increased secretion of estrogen, which can in turn increase the heaviness of the flow and exacerbate estrogen-dominant symptoms, such as increased PMS-like symptoms and agitation. The early phases of the menopause transition are characterized by relative hyperestrogenism and hypoprogesteronism, whereas hypoestrogenism dominates later phases.

In early menopausal transition, estrogen levels increase and progesterone decreases. This can result in heavier and longer menstrual flow, mood changes, and agitation due to estrogen dominance.

There is no particular amount of time for which a woman remains in this late reproductive stage where the rate of follicular release is increased (it can be up to 10 years), but all women will note that their cycles become increasingly varied in length; when their cycles are persistently greater than or equal to a 7-day change in the length of consecutive cycles, women are considered to have entered into early menopausal transition. This stage is characterized by a reduced number of follicles to recruit and thus a decrease in the amount of circulating estrogen, inhibin-B, and AMH. As the follicles continue to decrease, there is decreased ovulation and progesterone production, which in turn leads to lighter and more infrequent bleeds (often with > 35 days between cycles). The length of time between the bleeding can grow longer and longer, and eventually, at the average age of 51, a woman has her final menstrual period (FMP). At this stage, follicles are no longer being released and very little estrogen is produced (Fig. 55.2). After 1 year without menstruation, the patient has officially entered stage 1+ or menopause.

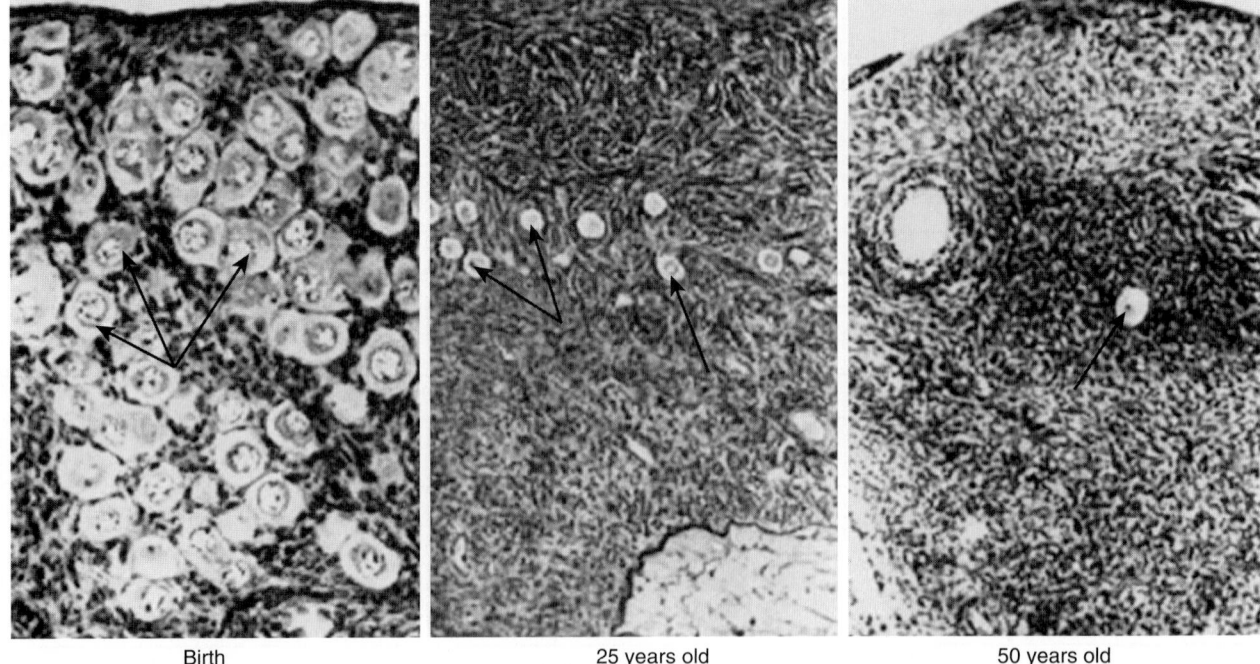

Birth   25 years old   50 years old

FIG. 55.2 ■ Progressive decrease in the number of primordial follicles (shown by *arrow*) with aging. (From Erickson G. An analysis of follicle development and ovum maturation. *Semin Reprod Endocrinol.* 1986;4:233-254.)

Vasomotor Symptoms in Menopause and the Menopausal Transition

The variable secretion of estrogen as well as the overall declining amount being produced in this menopausal transition (stages −2 and −1, +1) cause many of the first, and often most bothersome, symptoms of the menopausal transition: hot flushes and night sweats. These symptoms are caused by the fluctuations in estrogen and the variable dilation of the blood vessels, resulting in unexpected and sudden increases of blood flow, often to the chest, face, and neck, which in turn can produce profuse sweating, heart palpitations, anxiety, and flushing. These symptoms can last anywhere from 1 to 5 minutes and can occur at night. These "night sweats" often lead to poor and disrupted sleep patterns and can lead to downstream consequences of being overtired and more prone to depression.

While vasomotor symptoms (VMS) vary greatly in their frequency and intensity among menopausal transition women, symptoms typically are most debilitating for 1–2 years. However, for some women symptoms may last as long as 14 years. Risk factors for VMS include obesity, smoking, depression/anxiety, and low socioeconomic status. Interestingly, there also may be ethnic and genetic predispositions for VMS. According to the results of the SWAN study (Study of Women's Health Across the Nation), which assessed menopausal symptoms in 14,906 women with diverse ethnic backgrounds aged 40–55 years in the United States, African American women are most likely to report having VMS and Asian women (Japanese and Chinese) are the least likely to report these symptoms.

Nonvasomotor Symptoms in Menopause

Without circulating estrogen, VMS can be accompanied by increased vaginal dryness and atrophy, weight gain, bone loss, increased risk of osteoporosis, increased risk of heart disease, skin dryness and wrinkles, and increased risk for bladder infections. VMS can also create a domino effect. Hot flushes and night sweats can lead to sleep disruption, which then leads to many other changes—from weight gain to decreased sexual function and desire, to mood changes such as depression and anxiety.

Well-Being in the Menopausal Transition

Despite these physiological changes, this can also be a time for many women to reach what Jung characterized as "individuation," a time to bring the "consciousness into a working relationship with our inner *terra incognita* or our unknown inner terrain."[2] In other words, a time to integrate the experiences of their lives into a well-functioning whole. How, in our role as providers for women in the menopausal transition, can we support this change with health, growth, and well-being?

Supporting this journey is part of our role as medical providers. It is our role to be knowledgeable and able to provide patients an array of treatments for perimenopause and menopause, including pharmacological treatments, such as hormones and nonhormonal medications, and integrative approaches. Each visit is an opportunity to provide insight and knowledge into the menopausal transition, understand the patient's expectations and desires for treatment, and determine which treatment is most suited to her. Thus, we discuss each approach, with its risks, benefits, research evidence, and typical use. In each section, we primarily target commonly used modalities for hot flushes.

INTEGRATIVE THERAPY

Pharmaceuticals

After an in-depth discussion about the causes and likely duration of VMS, it is paramount to establish the level of burden of these symptoms on the patient's quality of life and well-being. All medications and supplements have side effects, and it is important for a woman to decide which risks and side effects she is willing to accept to reduce her VMS. Additionally, it is important to discern if there is a pattern to when her symptoms are most troublesome and if her symptoms could be caused by any other disease processes.

Evaluation of the Literature for Management of Vasomotor Symptoms

As with many trials to address patient symptoms, evaluation of effectiveness of an intervention in menopause has several limitations. The first is that there is a high placebo response rate for any intervention, with improvement rates reported to be as high as 50%. Second, the natural course of hot flushes is variable, and in general, over many years, hot flushes will improve. Therefore it is difficult to obtain adequate power. Last, there is no perfect way to measure hot flushes. The diary is most commonly used, but it may be cumbersome for participants and inexact in reporting. Additional research difficulties specific to modality are addressed where appropriate.

Estrogen

Without debate, the most effective therapy for hot flushes is estrogen. By increasing circulating estrogen, the thermoneutral zone is restored. The current recommendation remains "to use the lowest effective dose for the shortest duration" for the woman who decides that the benefits of therapy outweigh the risks. In general, patients should be started on a lower dose of estrogen and titrated upwards until the desired reduction in symptoms is achieved. There are multiple routes and formulations available in the United States and Canada. The transdermal route, which is available in patches, gels, and sprays, is preferred as it avoids the hepatic first-pass metabolism and may decrease venous thromboembolism risk. In our experience, these modes of delivery are highly acceptable to patients. Additionally, with the vast array of doses and delivery systems available, an acceptable method can be found by most women. The newer FDA-approved oral 0.0625 mg of conjugated estrogen with 20 mg bazedoxifene, which is a selected estrogen receptor modulator with antagonistic action on the endometrium, was designed to eliminate the need for progestogen. Awaiting further benefits, the limitation of this medication is its oral route, single available dose, and additional side effects of muscle spasm, nausea, and diarrhea.

The discussion of "bioidentical" hormone therapy is often confusing for our patients, as it is primarily a marketing term used to describe hormone therapy that has been compounded for each patient. The primary estrogen, estradiol, is the same as in the previously reviewed FDA-approved transdermal medications, although oral routes may use conjugated estrogens. There is no evidence at this time that compounded medications are safer. We do use compounded therapy when necessary for patients with allergies. Additional concerns about compounded medications include dosage variation and the common use of transdermal progesterone, which may be inadequate for endometrial protection.

Estriol is a weak estrogen, and some favor its use for vaginal atrophy. Whereas some research suggests that it may be less stimulating to the breast and endometrium, other research suggests that at effective dosages, the risk of endometrial and breast stimulation is present. More research is necessary on whether estriol is advantageous over other vaginal estrogen products.

DOSAGE

A common recommendation is to use the lowest dosage of estrogen for the shortest duration of time. For recently postmenopausal women, we typically start with estradiol transdermal patches at 0.025 mg and increase it based on symptoms. We may also check serum levels if we have increased the dosage and patients are still symptomatic. For recent surgically menopausal patients, such as a premenopausal patient with bilateral oophorectomy, we typically start with a higher dosage such as 0.1 mg estradiol patch.

PRECAUTIONS

The major side effects to be discussed with the patient are the increase in cerebral vascular and thromboembolic events, increase in breast cancer risk, and a possible increase in risk of ovarian cancer with prolonged use.

Progestogen/Progesterone

Progestogen refers to the class of both natural progesterone and the synthetic hormones usually derived from testosterone that mimic progesterone. Progestogen is a necessary adjuvant treatment for endometrial protection when the patient retains her uterus or has a history of endometriosis and is using estrogen. In order to prevent growth of the endometrial lining that can lead to endometrial hyperplasia and cancer, a minimum of 10–14 days of progestogen therapy should be given per month. Additionally, there is evidence that a more extended cycle of 14 days every 3 months can be used and that the levonorgestrel-intrauterine device (IUD) may be effective.

DOSAGE

Our preferred progestogen is oral micronized progesterone at 200 mg 14 days per month. Alternately, if the patient is unable to comply with cyclic progesterone, 100 mg nightly can be used.

PRECAUTIONS

We do not use progesterone for women with breast cancer. The most common side effect of progesterone is sedation, and patients are recommended to take it at night. For some women, progesterone is too sedating and some notice depressive symptoms and low energy. For women with these symptoms, we change to a different progestin or consider a levonorgestrel IUD.

Nonhormonal Medications

Selective Serotonin Reuptake Inhibitors (SSRIs)/ Selective Norepinephrine Reuptake Inhibitors (SNRIs). For those patients in whom there is a contraindication for estrogen containing therapy or the risks outweigh the benefits, consideration should be given for selective serotonin reuptake inhibitors (SSRI) or selective norepinephrine reuptake inhibitors (SNRI). While their mechanism of action is not completely understood, they may widen the thermoneutral zone. The current theory is that as estrogen levels decline, norepinephrine levels increase, which results in an increase in hypothalamic serotonin receptors, further narrowing the thermoregulatory zone (Fig. 55.3).[3] Many SSRI and SNRI have been studied for use in the management of menopausal hot flushes. Because there is an increased prevalence of comorbid psychiatric illness in the menopausal transition, they are particularly useful in the patient who has VMS and endorses mood changes. Many SSRIs and SNRIs have been studied to date and have been generally well tolerated. The SSRIs studied include paroxetine, fluoxetine, citalopram, and sertraline.

DOSAGE

Sertraline at starting doses of 25 mg is the most easily tolerated. Both venlafaxine and desvenlafaxine have been proven useful. The only FDA-approved nonhormonal medication at this time is low dose (7.5 mg) paroxetine.

PRECAUTIONS

For patients with a history of breast cancer on tamoxifen, SNRIs are preferred as they do not increase the CYP2D6 metabolism system.

Gabapentin. Gabapentin, a medication used primarily as an anticonvulsant, has also been shown to decrease VMS. Its mechanism is also unknown. In our experience, this medication is most useful in patients who wish to avoid estrogen therapy and whose primary bothersome symptoms are night sweats. A randomized trial found nonsuperiority of gabapentin 2400 mg with conjugated equine estrogens, but at this dosage the side effects can become limiting.[4]

DOSAGE

While less effective than hormone therapy, gabapentin starting at 300 mg three times a day is well tolerated.

PRECAUTIONS

Its major side effects are sedation, headache, and edema.

Clonidine. Clonidine is an antihypertensive, which was previously used for VMS management in the 1970s for patients with breast cancer. It is a centrally acting α-agonist, which has been theorized to work through raising the thermoneutral threshold by reducing norepinephrine release.

DOSAGE

Dosage for clonidine is 0.1 mg per day as a patch or 0.05 mg orally every 12 hours. Titrate up to a maximum of 0.4 mg every 12 hours.

PRECAUTIONS

It is not used frequently now secondary to modest improvements in hot flush symptoms with a large symptom burden including mouth dryness, constipation, itchiness, drowsiness, and difficulty sleeping.

Bioenergetics

Acupuncture

Acupuncture is effective for hot flushes. The exact mechanism of acupuncture improving hot flushes is unknown. Acupuncture changes levels of beta-endorphins and other neurotransmitters potentially affecting the thermoregulatory center in the hypothalamus. Traditional Chinese Medicine (TCM) colleges in China and nationally accredited acupuncture schools in the United States teach differential diagnosis and treatment strategies for menopausal symptoms. According to the TCM theory, the main cause of menopausal symptoms is a decline in kidney essence, leading to a yin/yang imbalance. A recent meta-analysis of acupuncture showed improvement in both severity and frequency in hot flushes, with effects up to 3 months.[5] Twelve studies with 869 participants were included. Acupuncture significantly reduced the frequency and severity of hot flushes and improved psychological, somatic, and urogenital subscale scores. Long-term effects, up to 3 months, were found. While the authors did not report an analysis of the acupuncture points used, commonly used points include St-36, Sp-6, CV-4, LI4, PC-6, GV-20, Lr-3, and Ht-6. In our clinical practice as well, these are the points most commonly used, although we individualize each session.

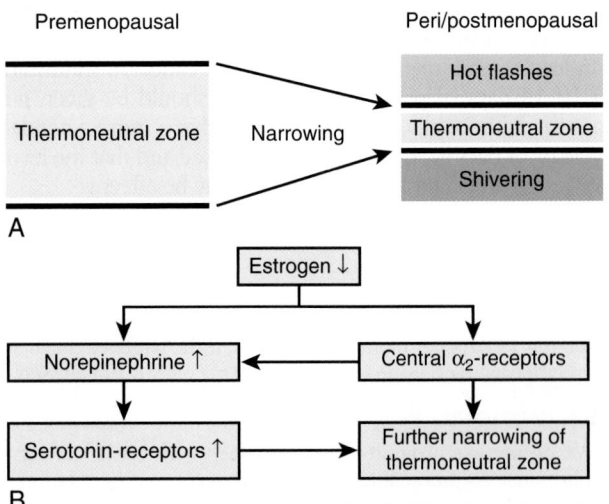

FIG. 55.3 ■ **Mechanism of Decreased Thermoregulatory Zone.** The changes associated with menopausal narrowing of the thermoneutral zone (A) and the presumed neurotransmitter mechanism (B). (From Krause MS, Nakajima ST. Hormonal and nonhormonal treatment of vasomotor symptoms. *Obstet Gynecol Clin N Am.* 2015;42:163-179.)

Acupuncture for VMS is best given weekly or biweekly. The patient generally notices improvement in intensity before a reduction in frequency and often undergoes at least two to three sessions to have an effect.

Hot flush and acupuncture trials are challenging to conduct because of several factors ubiquitous to all acupuncture trials. The first is the lack of a valid, inactive placebo, and studies that use "sham" acupuncture are likely actually receiving an active procedure. If the skin is penetrated, physiological changes occur. The second limitation is that acupuncture treatments are typically individualized making research with a standard approach not actually representative of clinical care. This may be one cause of the variations in effectiveness seen in these trials.

Avis et al.[6] compared true acupuncture to "sham" acupuncture (superficial needling in "nontherapeutic" sites) and to usual care in a pilot trial involving 56 perimenopausal and postmenopausal women. Patients received a standard true acupuncture regimen including the points CV-4, Ki-3, Sp-6, Bl-23, Ht-6, and Ki-7. Additional points were also needled depending on clinical judgment. The intervention occurred twice weekly for 8 weeks. The primary outcome variable was a hot flush score calculated from a daily diary. True and sham acupuncture were not statistically different from each other and both were superior to usual care.

The ACUFLUSH study by Borud et al.[7] was also a randomized controlled trial. This was a multicenter, pragmatic trial including postmenopausal women with at least seven hot flushes per day. The intervention group received up to 10 acupuncture sessions over a 12-week period, and the treatments were individualized. The intervention group also received advice on self-care, and the control group received only advice on self-care. Among the 134 women in the acupuncture group, hot flush frequency decreased by almost 6 per day, and almost 4 per day in the 133 women in the control group. This difference of 2.1 per day was statistically significant. Hot flush intensity was also statistically significantly better in the acupuncture group. The acupuncture group also had statistically significant improvements in vasomotor, sleep, and somatic symptoms.

Most recently, Chiu et al.[5] published a meta-analysis of randomized controlled trials on acupuncture for menopause-related symptoms and quality of life in women with natural menopause. Twelve studies with 869 participants were included. Acupuncture significantly reduced the frequency and severity of hot flushes as well as improved psychological, somatic, and urogenital subscale scores. Long-term effects, up to 3 months, were found.

Yoga

Similar to acupuncture, yoga is difficult to adequately control because it is impossible to mask the treatment arm to the subject, although the hypothesis could be kept from the patient and the researcher conducting the outcome measures could be masked to the treatment group. Also similar to acupuncture, there is a long practice of yoga for menopausal symptoms, with the initial reports being case series and then progressing to randomized controlled trials.

Joshi et al.[8] randomized 200 women to either a yoga group or to a nonyoga group for 90 days. The Menopause Rating Scale was the primary outcome variable. The groups were similar at baseline, but only the yoga group significantly improved by the end of the study period, and the improvement was in the total score and each of the subscales. Yoga occurred daily in this study, which might be difficult to replicate in the United States.

Chattha et al.[9] conducted an 8-week trial comparing yoga therapy (physical movement in the form of sun salutations, breathing, and meditation) to simple physical exercises under supervision in 120 participants. Outcomes were the Greene Climacteric Scale, Perceived Stress Scale, and the Eysenck's Personality Inventory before and after the interventions. VMS statistically and significantly improved in the yoga group, as did perceived stress scores and neuroticism. Other changes were not statistically significant. Thus it may not be merely physical exercise that helps women with hot flushes, as the control group was doing physical exercise. Yoga's effect on perceived stress, thus lowering sympathetic output, may be responsible for effects on hot flushes. Paced respiration, as studied by Freedman and Woodward,[10] significantly reduces hot flush frequency. Breathing techniques are common in yoga.

Available research suggests that yoga therapy has the greatest effect on psychological symptoms of menopause.

In 2012, a meta-analysis of randomized controlled trials found moderate evidence for short-term effectiveness of yoga for psychological symptoms but not for somatic symptoms, VMS, or urogenital symptoms.[11] Improving psychological symptoms is important, and we do recommend yoga for our patients. In our practice, we commonly refer women to hatha yoga because no evidence suggests that it is detrimental for hot flushes, has other health benefits, and women tend to enjoy it. One word of caution: while we do not know of research specifically for "hot" yoga, where yoga is done in a hot room, we do know that high ambient temperatures increase hot flushes. We suggest avoiding "hot" yoga.

Botanicals

Many different botanical regimens have been recommended for the management of hot flushes, such as black cohosh, isoflavones, and multibotanical preparations. One overall concern that we have with botanicals is the lack of oversight and quality control on the products. When recommending supplements of any type, we recommend specific brands that have rigorous quality standards; however, patients are free to choose other brands and may choose ones that are not of high quality and maybe exceedingly expensive.

Black Cohosh

One important study of botanical supplements compared black cohosh alone to four parallel arms: a multibotanical including black cohosh and nine other ingredients, a multibotanical plus dietary soy counseling, hormone therapy with estrogen/progestogen, and to placebo.[12] The botanical regimen did not differ from placebo with one exception, where the botanical was worse than placebo. As expected, hormone therapy improved symptoms. The authors note that differences between treatment groups smaller than 1.5 VMS per day cannot be ruled out. As previously mentioned, due to the variable nature of hot flushes, studies may be underpowered to show a difference. Other studies have also failed to show improvement compared with placebo for black cohosh, red clover, the Chinese herbal preparation Dang Gui Buxue Tang, or in any combinations of these therapies. In our experience, herbal remedies with black cohosh appear to help with mild symptoms for short periods of time; the appearance of improvement may be due to placebo, to the natural course of hot flushes, or to a true effect.

DOSAGE

The dosage of black cohosh extract used in the majority of clinical studies has been based upon the level of a key marker, 27-deoxyactein. For instance, for menopause, the dosage is 1 mg daily of 27-deoxyactein. There is 1 mg of 27-deoxyactein in one 20-mg tablet in the most common studied brand, *Remifemin*. The dose is 20 mg one to two times daily.

PRECAUTIONS

It is important to be mindful that it remains unclear if botanicals affect estrogen receptors and that long-term usage should be discouraged.

Rheum rhaponticum

Another botanical studied for hot flushes is the special extract ERr 731 from the roots of *Rheum rhaponticum* that has been recently studied for the treatment of VMS.[13] In a prospective multicenter, double-blind, placebo-controlled study of perimenopausal women with climacteric complaints over the course of 12 weeks, menopausal symptoms significantly decreased in the ERr 731 group compared to the placebo group. This also showed an increase in quality of life.

DOSAGE

The dosage used in the abovementioned investigation used enteric-coated tablets (250 mg) containing 4 mg of *R. rhaponticum* dry extract.

PRECAUTIONS

From this limited data, it appears to be safe and well tolerated.

St. John's Wort

St. John's wort can be used in menopause.[14] As previously discussed, antidepressants such as SSRIs can reduce hot flushes. It is postulated that if St. John's wort has a similar mechanism, it is possible that it could help with hot flushes too.

DOSAGE

Dosage in the previously mentioned study used drops that included 0.2 mg/mL hypericin, 20 drops three times per day. A common dosage recommendation for both depression and seasonal affective disorder is 300 mg three times daily capsule/tablet, oral: standardized extract (0.3% hypericin content).

PRECAUTIONS

We tend not to recommend this due to the number of drug interactions that St. John's wort has, including drug–herb interactions and concern over a serotonin effect.

Mind-Body

Relaxation Exercise

The early research on the use of mind-body medicine included case studies and case series. Similar to yoga and acupuncture, this research is challenging to blind, as study participants know if they are meditating or having hypnosis. However, participants can be hypothesis blind, and good evidence is possible. Stress triggers hot flushes and stress reduction may reduce hot flushes. The mechanisms of action for mind-body approaches are likely similar to those of yoga and acupuncture, with decreasing sympathetic output playing a role.

In 1990, Swartzman, Edelberg, and Kemmann[15] studied the impact of stress on objectively recorded hot flushes and flush report bias, asking if women under stress were more likely to report hot flushes than women not under stress. The findings were consistent with what many women experiencing hot flushes know: significantly more flushes occur during the stress session compared to the nonstress session, and there was no bias to reporting more hot flushes. We counsel patients that this study showed that lab stress increases hot flushes. We can predict that the effects of "real life" stress may be even more substantial than lab stressors, and anecdotally, patients certainly report stress as a trigger for hot flushes.

One of the first controlled studies investigated relaxation training on menopausal symptoms. Irvin et al., in 1996, randomized women to relaxation response training, reading, or a control group.[16] Participants listened to a 20-minute relaxation audio tape daily, and the reading group read for 20 minutes daily. Hot flush intensity, tension-anxiety, and depression were significantly reduced in the relaxation training group, whereas trait-anxiety and confusion-bewilderment were decreased in the reading group. The control group had no changes. The relaxation training group showed a trend towards decrease in all scores, but the sample size was small and may be underpowered. The authors postulate that the reading group may have chosen to take action and get control over their symptoms and may have read about menopause. This is possible, but it is also possible that relaxing for 20 minutes while reading leisure material is also a form of relaxation training (see Chapter 94).

Hypnosis

Hypnosis now has a solid research backing, thanks to Dr. Gary Elkins and his team at Baylor University. Elkins et al. have studied a hypnosis intervention first in breast cancer survivors (2008) and then in women without breast cancer (2012).[17,18] In breast cancer survivors, hypnosis decreased hot flush scores by 68% from baseline, with significant improvements in anxiety, depression, interference of hot flushes on daily activities, and sleep compared to the no treatment control group. The subjects received a standardized hypnosis intervention. In 2012, Elkins et al.[18] published a large study that included 187 postmenopausal women with at least seven hot flushes per day at baseline. The hypnosis intervention included specific suggestions for mental imagery for coolness, safe place imagery, and relaxation. They had five weekly sessions with home self-hypnosis practice. The control group was structured attention control, which matched the hypnosis intervention in all ways except the actual hypnosis, and also met weekly for 5 weeks with the therapist discussing symptoms and encouraging the subject. No specific cooling suggestions were made. Hot flush frequency reduced 74% in the hypnosis group compared to 17% in the control group. Hot flush score decreased 80% compared to 15% for the control group. Hot flush interference, sleep quality, and treatment satisfaction all improved in the hypnosis group. Finding a local hypnotherapist is helpful for patients, and reaching out to mental health colleagues may be a good way to find a trusted professional to provide hypnosis for hot flushes (see Chapter 95).

Mindfulness

Mindfulness-based stress reduction (MBSR) may reduce the bothersomeness and distress due to hot flushes. MBSR is an approach that allows a nonreactive awareness to an experience. For instance, some women may react to a hot flush with a sense of despair and concern that the hot flushes will never stop and that they will never get a good night's sleep again. The mindfulness approach would halt that thought process and allow a woman to label the hot flush just as a hot flush, something temporary and while it may be uncomfortable, it will go away. It would make sense then, for the mindfulness training to reduce the distress and bothersomeness of hot flushes. Carmody et al.[19] randomized 110 women with hot flushes to either an MBSR intervention or to a waitlist control. The MBSR arm significantly improved in hot flushes, quality of life, sleep quality, anxiety, and perceived stress. Improvements were not only maintained at 3 months, but the hot flush score continued to improve postintervention. Mindfulness-based stress reduction is a learned skill and the effects of it continued to work even when the classes were over (see Chapter 100).

Cognitive Behavior Therapy

Cognitive behavior therapy (CBT) is not traditionally considered an integrative modality; it is a well-known therapeutic technique. However, CBT is much less well known for its effects on menopausal symptoms. Much like MBSR that can decrease the bothersomeness of hot flushes by decreasing the reaction to the hot flush, CBT can also decrease symptomatology by moderating the emotional reactions, negative beliefs, and catastrophic thoughts that can occur with hot flushes. Ayers et al.[20] compared CBT, delivered as a group intervention, to self-help CBT, to a no-treatment control group. Both forms of CBT significantly improved hot flush problem rating, mood, quality of life, and emotional and physical functioning. Learning a different way to think about and react to hot flushes may allow women to gain control over the symptoms. A self-help CBT for menopause workbook is commercially available, and parts of this book may be helpful for both patients and providers to help reframe the menopause experience.

Nutrition

Calcium

As the concentration of the protective hormone of estrogen declines, a woman's bones are more at risk for decreased bone density, making a diet rich in calcium perhaps more important than ever. Calcium is found in abundance in dark leafy greens such as spinach, broccoli, kale, Brussel sprouts, and dandelion greens to name a few. These greens are also high in vitamins A, C, and K, which further serve to strengthen the body and bones. Other traditional sources of calcium such as dairy (milk, cheese, ice cream) can be continued during this time, but search for dairy that has no added hormones. We recommend that a woman lean on vegetable sources or fish such as sardines to supply her with most of her food-derived calcium.

Fiber

A woman's chance for cardiac disease starts to rise after she goes through menopause. Fiber has been well studied for its role in lowering "bad cholesterol" (LDL), improving insulin resistance, decreasing inflammation, and protecting against heart disease. The Institute of Medicine recommends that women over age 50 get 21 g or more of fiber a day. Excellent fiber sources are vegetables, fruits, beans (all kinds), nuts, bran, bulgur, whole-wheat flour, prunes, peas, barley, and potato skins.

Healthy Fats

To further improve cardiac health, decrease inflammation, and potentially improve mood, foods rich in omega-3s are highly recommended. Foods such as almonds, walnuts, flax seeds, chia seeds, cold-water fish such as mackerel, wild coho or Alaskan salmon, sardines, and herring are all excellent sources of omega-3 fatty acids. Food sources are a more reliable source of nutrients, but if needed, a supplement of fish or flax seed oil can be taken.

Fluids

As the body is moving through shifts in temperature and fluid regulations, it is best to treat the body kindly with decreased caffeine intake, moderate alcohol, teas, and plenty of room temperature water. Alcohol, though known to protect against heart disease in moderate amounts, has been less studied in women, and when used in amounts of larger than one drink per day has been shown to increase the risk of breast cancer. Coffee often increases symptoms of hot flushes in menopausal women. Black tea, however, is linked to a decreased risk of osteoporosis and green tea with its antioxidants and vitamin K can help protect against breast cancer. We advise patients that hot beverages can exacerbate hot flushes, so drink when cooled.

Exercise/Movement

Regular and vigorous exercise such as walking, jogging, biking, and swimming are all highly encouraged. The benefits of regular cardiac exercise (at least 30 minutes 5 days per week) and weight-bearing exercises two to three times a week can help protect against heart disease, osteoporosis, insulin resistance, breast cancer, and memory impairment, as well as keep women feeling more alert and well in the day. Movement can bring them back to their bodies and help them feel more at home in their changing bodies (see Chapter 91).

Spiritual Exploration

As a woman is no longer riding the waves of hormone cycles and likely no longer responsible for the continuous needs of children, she may find that she has more space to start focusing on her mind and the larger things that give her meaning. As Dr. Gaudet so beautifully illustrates in her "Consciously Female" guide for women,[2a] this is a time to start asking questions such as *"What are my expectations? Who are my role models? What do I love? What have I accomplished so far with my life, personally as well as professionally? What have I not been able to accomplish yet?"* She urges us to dream big, zero in on ideas, take action, and re-reflect. These questions can be answered alone, explored with communities, or brought to a place of worship. It is noted that while having an opportunity to ask these questions may connote a place of privilege, all women have been granted the opportunity to mark this time of profound change and use it as grist for their future wisdom.

We tell patients: this time is an invitation. Go forth and flourish.

PREVENTION PRESCRIPTION

We find that the cornerstones of a healthy menopause overlap with the cornerstones of a healthy life, and that the menopause transition is much easier for healthy women. The cornerstones are coping with stress, eating appropriate portions of real food, sleeping at night, moving the body, social support, and finding meaning in life.

THERAPEUTIC REVIEW

LIFESTYLE

- Nutrition: vegetables, lean proteins, fiber, and fluids C_1
- Maintain active lifestyle for 30 minutes five times per week C_1

BIOENERGETIC

- Acupuncture: one to two sessions per week A_1
- Yoga B_1

MIND-BODY

- Hypnosis B_1
- Mindfulness-Based Stress Reduction B_1
- Cognitive-Based Therapy, group or self-help B_1

PHARMACEUTICALS

- Hormone therapy, start 0.025 mg estradiol transdermal patch, and titrate to control symptoms. Add micronized progesterone 100 mg nightly or 200 mg for 14 days of the month. A_2
- SSRIs, start low dose SSRI (sertraline 25 mg daily) or low dose SNRI (venlafaxine 75 mg daily) and titrate to effect A_2
- Gabapentin 300 mg three times daily. Titrate to effect B_2

BOTANICALS

- Black cohosh 20 mg one to two times daily B_2
- *Rheum rhaponticum*, one enteric-coated tablet (250 mg) containing 4 mg of dry extract daily    B_2

*Note: For more information on treating vaginal dryness, see Chapter 59.

Key Web Resources

ObGyn.net. Website that provides an overview of managing VMS	http://www.obgyn.net/menopause/managing-menopause-part-1-vasomotor-symptoms
The North American Menopause Society. A site for both patients and clinicians regarding menopause	http://www.menopause.org
Menopro. An app from the North American Menopause Society that guides therapeutic decision making for menopausal symptoms	http://www.menopause.org/for-women/-i-menopro-i-mobile-app/
Information on evidence-based guideline from the National Center for Complementary and Integrative Health	https://nccih.nih.gov/health/menopause

REFERENCES

References are available online at ExpertConsult.com.

CHAPTER 56

PREMENSTRUAL SYNDROME

Tieraona Low Dog, MD

PATHOPHYSIOLOGY

Premenstrual syndrome (PMS) is defined as a recurrent, cyclic set of physical and behavioral symptoms that occurs 7–14 days before the menstrual cycle and is troublesome enough to interfere with some aspects of a woman's life. PMS is estimated to affect up to 40% of menstruating women, and the most severe cases occur in 2%–5% of women who are between 26 and 35 years of age.[1] PMS has been recognized as a medical disorder for many years; however, its cause remains a mystery (Table 56.1). The complex relationships that exist among hormones may offer insight into why some women suffer more than others. For instance, mild elevations of prolactin, a hormone that is primarily involved in regulating the development of the breast during pregnancy, have been associated with PMS, menstrual irregularities, and breast tenderness, whereas low levels of thyroid hormone can contribute to depression, fatigue, and heavy menses.

Hormonal Influences

A deficiency of progesterone or an abnormally high estrogen-to-progesterone ratio during the luteal phase has been a popular theory of the origin of PMS for many years, although studies comparing hormone levels in women with PMS with those in women without the disorder have failed to support this hypothesis.[2] In the 1950s, Dr. Katherina Dalton was the first to postulate this theory. Dr. Dalton administered natural progesterone in the form of injection, suppositories, or subcutaneous pellets; 83% of women in the study reported complete relief of PMS symptoms.[3] Because of the strict inclusion criteria of the study, however, only 18% of women with PMS appeared to be suitable candidates for this therapy. Due to insufficient data, a Cochrane review of two eligible clinical trials was unable to determine if progesterone is beneficial for PMS.[4]

Prolactin

Prolactin levels peak at ovulation and generally remain elevated during the luteal phase of the menstrual cycle. Prolactin excess is associated with menstrual irregularities, diminished libido, depression, and hostility.[5] Some authorities suggested that up to 62% of women with menstrual disorders have some elevation of prolactin.[6] Prolactin plays a role in breast stimulation and may be related to premenstrual breast tenderness. However, no consistent abnormalities have been found in women with PMS.[2]

Aldosterone

Aldosterone levels normally rise at ovulation and remain elevated during the luteal phase of the menstrual cycle. This elevation of aldosterone may be responsible for the congestive symptoms of PMS, such as edema, breast swelling, abdominal bloating, weight gain, and headaches. However, differences in absolute levels of aldosterone between symptomatic and asymptomatic women have not been noted in the literature.[7]

Endogenous Opiates

Some researchers, who have observed an increase in beta-endorphin levels after ovulation, hypothesized that women with PMS may have a lower level of these circulating endogenous opiates or a more sudden withdrawal that causes them to experience greater sensitivity to pain and depression in the luteal phase of the menstrual cycle.[8]

Hypoglycemia

The body appears to be more sensitive to insulin in the luteal phase of the menstrual cycle, a finding that has led some researchers to hypothesize that transient hypoglycemia may account for some PMS symptoms.

Prostaglandins

Prostaglandins are associated with breast pain, fluid retention, abdominal cramping, headaches, irritability, and depression.[9] Patients with physical premenstrual complaints and dysmenorrhea have been shown to respond to prostaglandin inhibitors.

Psychosocial Theory

Emotional and physical stressors have been found to influence the menstrual cycle. Travel, illness, stress, weather changes, and other environmental factors may affect ovulation, length of menstrual cycle, and the severity of PMS.[10] Cultural, societal, and personal attitudes toward menstruation also appear to play a role in the presence and severity of PMS. The dynamic interplay of environment, spirit, and physiology demands an integrated biopsychosocial approach to treatment.

Symptoms

More than 150 symptoms have been associated with PMS; the most common are listed in Table 56.2.

TABLE 56.1	**Proposed Causes of Premenstrual Syndrome**
Hormonal factors	Estrogen deficiency
	Estrogen excess
	High estrogen-to-progesterone ratio
	Progesterone deficiency
	Prolactin excess
	Beta-endorphin deficiency
Fluid and electrolytes	Aldosterone excess
	Vasopressin excess
	High sodium-to-potassium ratio
	Renin-angiotensin abnormalities
Neurotransmitters	Serotonin deficiency
	Cortisol excess
	Hypoglycemia
	Reduced glucose tolerance
	Thyroid abnormalities
	Adrenal insufficiency
Prostaglandins	Prostaglandin excess
	Prostaglandin deficiency
	Essential fatty acid deficiencies
Vitamins and minerals	Pyridoxine deficiency
	Vitamin A deficiency
	Vitamin E deficiency
	Magnesium deficiency
	Calcium excess
	Calcium deficiency
	Potassium deficiency
	Trace mineral deficiency
	Zinc deficiency
	Dopamine deficiency
	Norepinephrine deficiency
	Low platelet monoamine oxidase activity
Hereditary	Genetic risk
Psychological factors	Beliefs about menstrual cycle
	Coexisting psychiatric disorders
	Poor coping skills
	Poor self-esteem
Social factors	Current marital and sexual relationships
	Former marital and sexual relationships
	Social stress
	Psychosexual experiences
	Cultural attitudes about PMS
	Societal attitudes about PMS
	Poor social network

PMS, premenstrual syndrome.

TABLE 56.2	**Symptoms of Premenstrual Syndrome**	
Abdominal bloating		Insomnia
Acne		Irritability
Anxiety		Joint pain
Back pain		Lethargy
Change in appetite		Low libido
Clumsiness		Low self-esteem
Constipation		Mood swings
Depression		Nervousness
Diarrhea		Social isolation
Dizziness		Sugar cravings
Fatigue		Tender breasts
Headache		Water retention

The American Psychiatric Association (APA) defined the diagnostic criteria for premenstrual dysphoric disorder (PMDD), a more severe form of PMS. To be diagnosed with PMDD, a woman must have at least five of the following symptoms, and they must occur cyclically and be serious enough to interfere with her normal activities:

1. Feeling of sadness or hopelessness; possible suicidal thoughts
2. Feelings of tension or anxiety
3. Mood swings marked by periods of teariness
4. Persistent irritability or anger
5. Disinterest in daily activities and relationships
6. Trouble concentrating
7. Fatigue or low energy
8. Food cravings or binging
9. Sleep disturbances
10. Feeling out of control
11. Physical symptoms such as bloating, breast tenderness, headaches, and joint or muscle pain

Although this addition to the fourth edition of the APA's *Diagnostic and Statistical Manual of Mental Disorders,* published in 1994 (DSM-IV), is useful for recognizing PMDD as a valid disorder, it is disturbing that behavioral aspects comprise the primary focus of the disorder. With the vast numbers of physiological and hormonal interactions taking place in a woman's body, a multitude of explanations would seem to exist for the variety of symptoms. Thus assuming that numerous therapies may help and that not all remedies are universally effective is reasonable.

Clinical Evaluation

A complete physical examination, including pelvic evaluation and laboratory tests, should be performed to rule out anemia and hypothyroidism. A prolactin test may be included. An extremely useful approach is for a woman to record her symptoms on a daily basis for at least two complete menstrual cycles to allow the clinician to see just what her symptoms are and how they are related to her menses.

The clinician must address any other underlying medical conditions that may masquerade as PMS. One report found that 75% of women receiving care for PMS at specialized clinics had another diagnosis that accounted for many of their symptoms, primarily major depression and other mood disorders.[11]

INTEGRATIVE THERAPY

Once the diagnosis has been established, an integrative approach should be considered. Therapies to be explored include exercise, dietary manipulation, dietary supplements, mind-body approaches, acupuncture, traditional Chinese medicine, counseling, and conventional medications.

Exercise

Exercise remains understudied in the scientific world because it does not fit well into the double-blind, placebo-controlled, study design. The few studies that have been conducted on the role of exercise in PMS have clearly shown that women who engage in regular physical exercise have fewer symptoms of PMS than women who do not. Women who exercise regularly note improvement in all symptoms of PMS.[12] The frequency, rather than the intensity, of exercise appears to diminish the negative mood and physical symptoms that occur during the premenstrual period.[13] Exercise may reduce symptoms by reducing estrogen levels, decreasing circulating catecholamines, improving glucose tolerance, and raising endorphin levels.[14] Aerobic activity appears to be most beneficial; however, yoga and tai chi are probably equally effective if they are performed at least three times per week.

Diet and Nutrition

Many people in the United States fail to eat a healthy diet, but some researchers have found this observation to be even more accurate for women with PMS. A 1983 report noted that women with PMS consumed 275% more refined sugar, 79% more dairy products, 78% more sodium, 62% more refined carbohydrates, 77% less manganese, and 53% less iron than women without PMS.[15] These dietary excesses and deficiencies may explain some of the symptoms women experience during their premenstrual period. Dairy products are high in sodium and interfere with magnesium absorption. Refined sugars increase the urinary excretion of magnesium.[16] Heavy intake of sugar also increases sodium and water retention owing to the rapid release of insulin. Dietary salt may exacerbate swelling. Consumption of caffeine-containing beverages can increase irritability. Women experiencing irritability or difficulty sleeping during the premenstrual period should be encouraged to try a caffeine holiday for a couple of cycles to see if they notice a difference (Table 56.3).

TABLE 56.3 Caffeine Amounts in Common Foods and Beverages

Serving Size (oz)	Caffeine (mg)
Coffee, instant (6–8)	65–100
Coffee, percolated (6–8)	85–135
Coffee, filtered (6–8)	115–175
Coffee, decaffeinated (6–8)	1–5
Tea, instant (6–8)	35–70
Tea, brewed (6–8)	28–150
Tea, iced (6–8)	40–45
Chocolate, dark semisweet (1)	5–35
Chocolate, milk (1)	1–15
Cola beverage (8)	25–30

From Thys-Jacobs S, Starkey P, Bernstein D, et al. Calcium carbonate and the premenstrual syndrome: effects on premenstrual and menstrual symptoms. Premenstrual Syndrome Study Group. *Am J Obstet Gynecol.* 1998;179:444-452.

Fiber-rich, low-fat diets suppress the ability of fecal bacteria to deconjugate estrogen and thereby enhance fecal estrogen excretion.

Dietary Fat

Fiber-rich, low-fat diets may be beneficial for women with PMS because these diets reduce blood levels of estrogen. Estrogen is conjugated in the liver and sent to the small intestine for elimination in the feces. Certain intestinal bacteria are able to deconjugate estrogen, allowing it to be reabsorbed into the body.

Several studies have shown that reducing fat (less than 20% of total calories) and increasing fiber for only 3 months can lower a woman's serum estrogen level.[17] If one accepts the theory that elevations of estrogen can worsen PMS symptoms, then consuming a diet high in fruits, vegetables, and whole grains and low in saturated fat may be wise. Four to six small meals should be consumed throughout the day to ease both food cravings and mood swings. Alcohol consumption should be limited because it can worsen PMS symptoms.

No food-based strategy has been adequately tested to determine its effects on PMS. However, recommendations such as eating a high-fiber diet, limiting caffeine, and cutting back on high-sugar foods have few drawbacks and numerous health benefits.

Supplements

Calcium

Ovarian hormones influence calcium, magnesium, and vitamin D metabolism. Estrogen is involved in calcium metabolism, calcium absorption, and parathyroid gene expression and secretion. Clinical trials in women with

PMS have found that calcium supplementation improves several mood and somatic symptoms.

A prospective randomized, double-blind, placebo-controlled, parallel-group multicenter clinical trial was conducted to evaluate the effectiveness of calcium carbonate for PMS. Healthy premenopausal women were recruited nationally at 12 outpatient centers and screened for moderate to severe, cyclically recurring premenstrual symptoms. Symptoms were prospectively documented over two menstrual cycles with a daily rating scale that included 17 core symptoms and 4 symptom factors (negative affect, water retention, food cravings, and pain). Of the 720 women screened for the trial, 497 were enrolled and results for 466 were valid for the efficacy analysis. Women were randomly allocated to receive either 1200 mg calcium carbonate or placebo daily for three menstrual cycles. Routine blood chemistry analysis, complete blood cell count, and urinalysis data were obtained for all participants. Each participant kept a daily diary to document symptoms, adverse effects, and compliance with therapy. The primary outcome measure was a 17-parameter symptom complex score. No differences in age, weight, height, use of oral contraceptives, or menstrual cycle length were reported between the treatment and control groups. No differences existed between the groups in the mean screening symptom complex score of the luteal phase (p = .659), menstrual phase (p = .818), or intermenstrual phase (p = .726) of the menstrual cycle. During the luteal phase of the treatment cycle, a significantly lower mean symptom complex score was noted in the calcium-treated group by the third month (p < .001). The researchers concluded, "Calcium supplementation is a simple and effective treatment for premenstrual syndrome, resulting in a major reduction in overall luteal phase symptoms."[18]

A review of studies focusing on calcium for the management of premenstrual symptoms was published in the *Annals of Pharmacotherapy*.[19] On the basis of the medical literature, the reviewer concluded, "Calcium supplementation of 1200–1600 mg/day, unless contraindicated, should be considered a sound treatment option in women who experience premenstrual syndrome." Given that many women, especially adolescents, do not meet the adequate intake recommendations for dietary calcium, a clinical trial seems reasonable.

DOSAGE

The dose used in the clinical trials was generally 600 mg twice per day of calcium carbonate or citrate.

PRECAUTIONS

Calcium products made from oyster shell, dolomite, or bone meal occasionally contain lead.[20] Labels containing the letters "USP" indicate that the product meets the purity and dissolution standards established by the U.S. Pharmacopeia; however, this is a voluntary standard, and many products do not bear USP on their labels. Calcium supplements should not be taken at the same time as tetracycline, iron supplements, thyroid hormones, or corticosteroids because calcium binds to these substances and interferes with their effectiveness and its own absorption. Iron absorption can be reduced by as much as 50% by many forms of calcium supplementation.

Magnesium

Women with PMS have been shown to have low levels of magnesium in their red blood cells. Magnesium deficiency produces fatigue, irritability, mental confusion, PMS, menstrual cramps, insomnia, muscle cramps, and symptoms of heart disturbances. A 2002 Cochrane Review found that magnesium was superior to placebo for relieving dysmenorrhea, likely through inhibition of prostaglandin $F_{2\alpha}$.[21] One small, short-term randomized controlled trial did show that 200 mg of magnesium per day was better than placebo at alleviating the bloating symptoms of PMS.[22] Two small trials found that the combination of 200 mg of magnesium plus 50 mg of vitamin B6 was beneficial for alleviating PMS symptoms.[23]

Magnesium may be beneficial for women with significant bloating and cramping associated with their menstrual cycles and for women with menstrual migraines. Dietary sources of magnesium include green leafy vegetables, tofu, legumes, nuts, seeds, and whole grains.

DOSAGE

The dose is 200–400 mg/day of magnesium as chelate, citrate, or glycinate. Doses of 600 mg per day might be necessary for women with PMS and also migraines.

PRECAUTIONS

Adverse effects of magnesium excess include abdominal cramping and diarrhea. Signs of magnesium toxicity are hypotension, irregular heartbeat, muscle weakness, nausea, diarrhea, and change in mental status. The kidneys excrete magnesium, so women with renal insufficiency must be cautious with magnesium supplementation.

Vitamin B6

Pyridoxine is a water-soluble B vitamin that serves as a cofactor in more than 100 enzyme reactions, many of which are related to the production and metabolism of neurotransmitters. The use of pyridoxine (vitamin B6) to alleviate PMS symptoms has been evaluated in more than 28 trials since 1975. This research was inspired by the work of Adams et al.,[24] who first reported that vitamin B6 successfully alleviated the depression associated with use of oral contraceptives. Wyatt et al.[25] performed a systematic review of these studies. Ten randomized placebo-controlled, double-blind, parallel or crossover studies were examined. Studies of cyclic mastalgia and multivitamin preparations with at least 50 mg of vitamin B6 were also included. Only three of these trials scored higher than 3 on the Jadad scale for methodological quality. Most trials were small (fewer than 60 women). One of the largest studies included women who were also taking oral contraceptives, analgesics, diuretics, and psychotropic medications, thus making the effects of vitamin B6 difficult to ascertain. None of the trials included power calculations. Using a random effects model, Wyatt et al.[25] found the overall odds ratio in favor of pyridoxine to be 1.57 (95% confidence interval [CI], 1.40–1.77). When the researchers looked at the effects on depressive symptoms in five trials, they found the overall odds ratio in favor of pyridoxine to be 2.12 (95% CI, 1.80–2.48).

Current thinking postulates that pyridoxine may ease symptoms of PMS through its ability to increase the synthesis of serotonin, dopamine, norepinephrine, histamine, and taurine.[26] Serotonin is important for the regulation of sleep and appetite and the prevention of depression. Low levels of serotonin and dopamine may play a role in premenstrual symptoms.[27] Trials have used doses ranging from 50–500 mg/day. For most women, the prudent approach is probably to limit single doses of vitamin B6 to 50 mg and not to exceed 100 mg/day. Research suggests that the liver cannot process more than a 50-mg dose of pyridoxine at one time.[28] Conversion of pyridoxine to its active form depends on other nutrients, such as magnesium and riboflavin. Taking vitamin B6 as part of a multiple-vitamin supplement or using the active form, pyridoxal-5-phosphate, is advisable.

DOSAGE

The dose is 50–100 mg/day of pyridoxal-5-phosphate.

PRECAUTIONS

Although pyridoxine is a water-soluble vitamin, it can be associated with toxicity when it is taken in moderate to large doses over time. A few reports have noted nerve damage occurring with prolonged ingestion of 150 mg/day.[29] Toxicity may occur if large doses of pyridoxine overwhelm the liver's ability to add a phosphate group to form pyridoxal-5-phosphate, the active form of vitamin B6.

Combining chaste tree with vitamin B6 may be a beneficial first step in the treatment of premenstrual syndrome.

Botanicals

Chaste Tree (Vitex agnus-castus)

Dioscorides, the Greek physician, described the dried ripe fruits of the chaste tree (Vitex agnus-castus) some 2000 years ago. The Latin name agnus castus means "chaste lamb," in reference to the belief that the seeds reduce sexual desire. From this belief stemmed the other common name of the herb, monk's pepper. Many herbalists consider V. agnus-castus one of the primary herbs for alleviating PMS, a use that is supported by randomized human trials. The most rigorous study to date of chaste tree for PMS was a 3-month, double-blinded, placebo-controlled trial by Schellenberg[30] that randomized 170 women diagnosed with PMS to receive either 20 mg of fruit extract (Ze 440: 60% ethanol mass/mass [m/m], extract ratio, 6 to 12:1; standardized for casticin) or placebo. Five of six self-assessment items indicated significant superiority for chaste tree (irritability, mood alteration, anger, headache, and breast fullness). Other symptoms, including bloating, were unaffected by treatment. Overall, the reduction in symptoms was 52% for the active versus 24% for the placebo group (p < 0.001). The trial investigators concluded: "Agnus castus is a well-tolerated and effective treatment

for premenstrual syndrome, the effects being confirmed by physicians and patients alike."

Two studies conducted in Chinese women also reported favorable results. A randomized, double-blinded, placebo-controlled multicenter 16-week study of 217 women with moderate to severe PMS found that 40 mg of chaste tree extract was superior to placebo, as measured by the PMS diary 17-item daily rating scale (p < .0001).[31] No serious adverse events were reported. A smaller, randomized, placebo-controlled 3-month study of 64 Chinese women with moderate to severe PMS also found that 40-mg/day chaste tree extract significantly reduced symptoms in the PMS diary 17-item daily rating scale (p < .05).[32]

One study evaluated the use of chaste tree in PMDD. A single-blind, rater-blinded study of 41 women (age 25–45 years) who were diagnosed with PMDD and who had regular menstrual cycles failed to note any significant difference between fluoxetine and chaste tree with respect to the Hamilton Depression Rating Scale (HAM-D), the Clinical Global Impression Scale-Severity of Illness (CGI-SI), or the Clinical Global Impression-Improvement (CGI-I).[33] Unfortunately, the investigators did not provide any details regarding the chaste tree product (e.g., extraction method, extract strength).

One comparative trial found chaste tree to be as effective as pyridoxine for relieving PMS symptoms,[34] whereas a pilot study using the combination of St. John's wort (Hypericum perforatum) and chaste tree found the combination highly effective for relieving PMS symptoms in perimenopausal women.[35]

The chaste tree preparation is known to act, in part, by reducing prolactin, increasing progesterone, and binding opiate receptors.[36] Binding of opioid receptors may be the primary mechanism involved in PMS, given that symptoms such as anxiety, food cravings, and physical discomfort are directly and inversely proportional to the decline of beta-endorphin levels. Vitex has an inhibitory action on prolactin because of its dopamine agonist properties. Women with hyperprolactinemia often experience menstrual dysfunction. Some researchers postulate that the correction of hyperprolactinemia causes the reversal of luteinizing hormone suppression and results in full development of the corpus luteum during the luteal phase of the cycle.[37] Studies in both animals and humans have demonstrated prolactin inhibition with Vitex. The German health authorities approved the use of chaste tree fruit for irregularities of the menstrual cycle, premenstrual complaints, and mastodynia.[38]

DOSAGE

The dose varies according to the preparation used in trials. Generally, practitioners recommend 250–500 mg/day of dried fruit or 20–40 mg/day of chaste berry extract.

PRECAUTIONS

Chaste tree has been rarely associated with gastrointestinal reactions, alopecia, headaches, tiredness, dry mouth, and increased menstrual flow.

Binding of opioid receptors may be the primary mechanism of action of chaste tree. As beta-endorphin levels decline, so do common premenstrual syndrome symptoms such as anxiety, food cravings, and physical discomfort.

Black Cohosh (Actaea racemosa, Cimicifuga racemosa)

The Eclectics (early physicians who used botanical medicines extensively) used black cohosh for restlessness, nervous excitement, breast pain, and menstrual headaches.[39] Although most research has focused on black cohosh for the alleviation of menopausal complaints, a study of 135 women found a standardized extract of black cohosh to be effective in reducing the symptoms of anxiety, tension, and depression in women with PMS.[40] Researchers found that compounds in black cohosh bind 5-HT7 receptors, a characteristic that could partially explain the positive effects of this botanical on mood.[41] The German health authorities endorsed the use of black cohosh for premenstrual discomfort and dysmenorrhea.[42]

DOSAGE

The dose is 20–40 mg of the standardized extract twice daily (generally standardized to triterpene glycosides as a marker compound) or 150–300 mg of the crude herb equivalent twice daily.

PRECAUTIONS

The most common complaint is gastrointestinal disturbance. Other potential adverse effects are headache, heaviness of the legs, and weight gain. Two safety reviews concluded that black cohosh is relatively safe when it is used appropriately; since these reviews, however, case reports suggesting a possible link between black cohosh use and liver damage have been published in the medical literature. After an extensive review of the literature, the U.S. Pharmacopeia Dietary Supplements Expert Information Committee recommended that women who have, or who are at risk for, liver disease check with their health care provider before they use black cohosh.[43]

Ginkgo (Ginkgo biloba)

If women experience primarily congestive symptoms in the premenstrual period (fluid retention, breast tenderness, and weight gain), a trial of ginkgo may offer some relief. A double-blind, placebo-controlled trial of ginkgo was conducted in a cohort of 165 women complaining of premenstrual symptoms. Participants received placebo or a standardized extract of ginkgo (EGb761 24% ginkgo flavones and 6% terpenes; Dr. Willmar Schwabe GmbH & Co., Karlsruhe, Germany), 80 mg twice daily, from day 16 of one menstrual cycle through day 5 of the next cycle. Evaluations by patient and physician found ginkgo to be effective for alleviation of breast pain and tenderness and fluid retention.[44] Ginkgo is known to augment venous tone and reduce capillary fragility.

A single-blind, randomized, placebo-controlled trial of 90 women with PMS (85 completed the trial) found that ginkgo was superior to placebo in reducing physical and psychological symptoms when administered at a dose of 40 mg of the standardized leaf extract three times per day from the 16th day of the cycle to the 5th day of the next cycle.[45] The mechanism of action is not completely understood.

DOSAGE

The dose is 80 mg of a standardized extract twice daily or 40 mg three times daily from day 16 of one menstrual cycle through day 5 of the next cycle.

PRECAUTIONS

Ginkgo may cause gastrointestinal symptoms, headache, dizziness, palpitations, and allergic skin reactions.

CAUTION

Patients should be carefully supervised if ginkgo is used with anticoagulant medications; however, bleeding risk is probably quite low in otherwise healthy individuals taking ginkgo. A randomized, double-blind, placebo-controlled, crossover study found no change in coagulation factors, platelet aggregation, or bleeding times in 50 healthy male volunteers who took 240-mg ginkgo extract (EGb761).[46]

Evening Primrose Oil (Oenothera biennis)

Evening primrose oil is extracted from the seeds of the evening primrose plant, a wildflower native to North America and introduced to Europe in the early 1600s. The seed oil has been studied for medicinal effects for decades because it is a rich source of linoleic acid and gamma-linolenic acid. Some researchers reported that women with PMS have impaired conversion of linoleic acid to gamma-linolenic acid, thus leading to the investigation of gamma-linolenic supplementation for symptom alleviation. However, a systematic review identified seven placebo-controlled trials of evening primrose oil and reported that all suffered from methodological flaws.[47] The two highest-quality studies failed to show any beneficial effects of evening primrose oil in PMS, although the sample sizes were small in both trials.

DOSAGE

Evening primrose oil products are generally standardized to specific amounts of gamma-linoleic acid. Capsules typically contain 320–360 mg linoleic acid and 40 mg gamma-linolenic, although levels vary among manufacturers. Vitamin E is often added to prevent rancidity. The range of doses used in clinical studies is 1–6 g/day.

PRECAUTIONS

Evening primrose oil is extremely well tolerated. Minor gastrointestinal symptoms have been occasionally reported in the literature.

St. John's Wort (Hypericum perforatum)

Clinical trials using selective serotonin reuptake inhibitor (SSRI) medications have shown that approximately 60% of women with severe PMS obtain significant relief with use of these drugs. This finding is interesting, given that some herbalists recommend the popular herbal antidepressant St. John's wort *(Hypericum perforatum)* for women reporting depression and irritability during the premenstrual period.

A randomized, double-blind, placebo-controlled, cross-over study in the UK evaluated 36 women (ages 18–45 years) with PMS. After a two-cycle placebo run-in phase, the women were randomized to receive St. John's wort 900 mg/day (standardized to 0.18% hypericin; 3.38% hyperforin) or identical placebo tablets for two menstrual cycles. St. John's wort was found to be statistically superior to placebo in improving physical and behavioral symptoms of PMS (p < 0.05) but not mood or pain.[48]

DOSAGE

The dose generally used for depression is 300–600 mg of St. John's wort, standardized to contain 3%–5% hyperforin or 0.3% hypericin, three times per day.

PRECAUTIONS

Women taking medications that increase photosensitivity, protease inhibitors (for human immunodeficiency virus), cyclosporine, or other medications that are metabolized by the cytochrome P-450 CYP3A4 system or P-glycoprotein should avoid St. John's wort.

Kava (Piper methysticum)

Physicians sometimes prescribe alprazolam, a benzodiazepine, for the treatment of PMS. Because of the risk of habituation and side effects, practitioners have looked for other anxiolytics that could be of benefit. Numerous practitioners have recommended the South Pacific herb, kava, for this purpose. A meta-analysis concluded that kava is an effective treatment for anxiety when compared with placebo, although no studies of kava for the treatment of PMS are available for review.

Concerns have been raised about the safety of kava, however. Approximately 30 cases of hepatotoxicity potentially related to the use of kava products have been reported in the literature. Numerous countries have banned the sale of kava, including Germany, Switzerland, Ireland, Canada, Australia, and the United Kingdom. The U.S. Food and Drug Administration (FDA) issued a cautionary statement, but the herb is still sold in the United States. Until the safety issue is further elucidated, looking for other approaches to help alleviate troublesome symptoms of PMS seems wise. A better option for women reporting irritability and difficulty sleeping during the premenstrual period may be valerian (discussed in the following section).

Valerian (Valeriana officinalis)

Valerian is a common ingredient in over-the-counter relaxants and sleep aid products in both Europe and the United States. It is often included in herbal formulations for PMS with a dominant profile of anxiety or irritability. The herb is sold as a single ingredient but is often found in combination with other relaxant herbs such as hops (Humulus lupulus), passionflower (Passiflora incarnata), or lemon balm (Melissa officinalis). The German Commission E endorses valerian for restlessness and sleeping

disorders caused by nervous conditions,[49] and the World Health Organization recognizes it as a "mild sedative, sleep-promoting agent, and milder alternative to or possible substitute for stronger sedatives (e.g., benzodiazepines) and for treatment of nervous excitation and sleep disturbances induced by anxiety."[50] No clinical trials have evaluated the use of valerian for PMS, but this botanical is often included in formulations on the basis of its mild anxiolytic effects and ability to promote sleep.

DOSAGE

The crude herb is usually taken at a dose of 2–3 g (equivalent to 10–15 mL of tincture [1:5 strength]) approximately 1 hour before bedtime. Smaller doses are often used during the day for relieving mild irritability and anxiety. Standardized extracts are also widely available and should be taken as directed on the label.

PRECAUTIONS

Valerian is generally safe when taken appropriately and is not considered habit-forming. The World Health Organization noted that the use of valerian is contraindicated during pregnancy and lactation because of the lack of studies in this area.

Mind-Body Therapy

Mind-body therapies are approaches grounded in the emerging scientific understanding that thoughts and feelings affect physiology and physical health. Mind-body therapies for PMS include psychotherapy (cognitive-behavioral therapy and group therapy), relaxation techniques and training, body work (massage and reflexology), hypnotherapy, biofeedback, guided imagery, yoga, and qigong. An emerging body of evidence shows that when women are given psychological support and taught self-regulatory techniques, their quality of life and PMS symptom severity significantly improve.[51]

Acupuncture

Acupuncture is only one tool used in traditional Chinese medicine (TCM) for the treatment of disease and promotion of health. Traditional Chinese medicine has a long history of treating what would be called PMS in conventional medicine. Although many women report benefit, a systematic review of clinical trials using acupuncture for the relief of PMS found the data inconclusive.[52] Given the overall safety of acupuncture and its potential benefits, clinicians should not dissuade women who choose to explore traditional Chinese medicine or acupuncture for relief of their symptoms.

Pharmaceuticals
Selective Serotonin Reuptake Inhibitors

In addition to the numerous lifestyle recommendations already mentioned, growing numbers of physicians are prescribing SSRIs for the treatment of PMS and PMDD.

A Cochrane Review of 31 trials that evaluated the efficacy of SSRIs in the management of PMS reported that these medications are highly effective for improving both behavioral and physical symptoms. However, adverse effects are relatively frequent, the most common being nausea and asthenia.[53] SSRIs should be considered for women with severe forms of PMS, and particularly PMDD, that do not respond to lifestyle, mind-body, or supplement approaches.

PREVENTION PRESCRIPTION

Preventive strategies should be directed at those that improve overall health and seem appropriate based on our current understanding of PMS:

- Limit alcohol consumption and avoid drugs of abuse.
- Exercise at least three times per week for a minimum of 30 minutes.
- Limit consumption of salt, sugar, and caffeine, especially 10 days before the onset of menses.
- Eat a well-balanced diet that is rich in fiber and low in saturated fat.
- Take a multivitamin every day that includes pyridoxal-5-phosphate (active vitamin B6).
- Ensure the diet provides 1000–1200 mg of calcium and 320–400 mg magnesium every day; use supplements to make up for any dietary shortcomings.

THERAPEUTIC [REVIEW]

[Handwritten note: PMS — All except SSRIs @ end of list]

LIFESTYLE

- Learn strateg[ies to] obtain adequ[ate] cise routine. [...] breathing tec[hniques]

NUTRITION

- Eat a well-bal[anced] fat.
- Limit intake o[f salt and] sugar product[s]

SUPPLEMENTS

- Calcium: 500–[...]
- Vitamin B6 as [...] day
- Magnesium: 2[...]

BOTANICALS

- Chaste tree *(Vitex):* 250–1000 mg crude herb or 20–40 mg/day of a standardized extract

Treatment for Specific Symptoms

- Breast tenderness
  - Caffeine restriction
  - Chaste tree *(Vitex):* 250–500 mg crude herb or 20–40 mg/day of a standardized extract
  - Evening primrose oil: 1.5 g twice daily (continuous)
  - *Ginkgo biloba:* 80 mg standardized extract twice daily (ovulation through menses)
- Anxiety and mood swings
  - Black cohosh: 20–40 mg standardized extract twice daily or 150–300 mg crude herb equivalent (continuous therapy)
  - Calcium: 500–600 mg twice daily
  - Chaste tree *(Vitex):* 250–500 mg crude herb or standardized extract daily
  - St. John's wort: 300–600 mg standardized extract three times daily (continuous therapy)
  - Valerian root: 2–3 g crude herb or standardized extract 45 minutes before bed
  - Kava root: up to 210 mg kavalactones in standardized extract daily
  - [Dep]ression
    - St. John's wort: 300–600 mg standardized extract three times daily (continuous therapy)
    - Vitamin B6: 50 mg once or twice daily
  - [Cra]mps
    - Magnesium: 200–600 mg/day
  - Insomnia
    - Valerian root: 2–3 g crude herb or standardized extract before bed
- Severe PMS or PMDD
  - Chaste tree *(Vitex):* 250–1000 mg crude herb or 20–40 mg/day of a standardized extract
  - St. John's wort: 300–600 mg standardized extract three times per day (continuous therapy)
  - Serotonin reuptake inhibitors. Low doses often are effective.
  - Fluoxetine: 10–20 mg
  - Sertraline: 50–75 mg
  - Paroxetine: 10–20 mg
  - Citalopram: 10–20 mg

Key Web Resources

U.S. Department of Health and Human Services Office on Women's Health: This website has numerous resources on women's health, including premenstrual disorder.	http://www.womenshealth.gov
PMS Symptom Tracker: This form allows patients to record their symptoms throughout the month.	https://www.womenshealth.gov/files/assets/docs/charts-check-lists-guides/pms-symptom-tracker.pdf
American College of Obstetrics and Gynecology handout on premenstrual syndrome: Patient handout on the condition.	http://www.acog.org/Patients/FAQs/Premenstrual-Syndrome-PMS
National Women's Health Network: This website is an online resource on women's health issues.	http://www.nwhn.org

REFERENCES

References are available online at ExpertConsult.com.

CHAPTER 57

DYSMENORRHEA

Greta J. Kuphal, MD

Dysmenorrhea refers to painful uterine cramping associated with menses. In addition to lower pelvic discomfort, women may also experience low back pain, radiation of pain to the anterior thighs, nausea, vomiting, diarrhea, headache, and various other symptoms starting 1 to 3 days before the onset of menses and typically lasting through the first few days of bleeding. *Primary dysmenorrhea* refers to pain that is not associated with other, obvious pelvic disease and typically begins with the onset of ovulatory cycles just after menarche. *Secondary dysmenorrhea* is associated with another diagnosis (e.g., cervical stenosis, endometriosis) and typically has a later onset, usually after the age of 20 years. This discussion focuses on primary dysmenorrhea because treatment for secondary dysmenorrhea is determined by the underlying cause.

Estimates of the percentage of women affected by dysmenorrhea range from 16% to 90%. Some investigators claim the most reliable estimate to be approximately 75%, based on a large Swedish study of 19-year-old women. Most of these women's symptoms were mild, but 23% and 15% reported suffering from moderate and severe pain, respectively.[1] In addition to the discomfort endured by affected women, dysmenorrhea also results in significant missed school and work as well as a decreased quality of life.[2]

Dysmenorrhea seems to be more significant in women with an earlier age at menarche and in those with longer episodes of bleeding. Being overweight appears to significantly affect the likelihood and duration of painful cramping. Smoking has been associated with prolonged pain, and although alcohol consumption does not increase the probability of painful cramping, it seems to increase the duration and severity of cramping in women with dysmenorrhea.[3] Other predisposing factors include age less than 30 years, low body mass index, longer menstrual cycles, heavy menstrual bleeding, nulliparity, clinically suspected pelvic inflammatory disease, history of sexual abuse, psychological symptoms, chronic exposure to stress, and exposure to secondhand smoke.[4-7]

PATHOPHYSIOLOGY

The pathogenesis of primary dysmenorrhea seems to involve elevated levels of prostaglandins in response to the rise and fall of progesterone that occur after ovulation. As progesterone production decreases by the corpus luteum, lysosomes in the endometrial cells break down and release phospholipase A2, which converts cell membrane fatty acids into arachidonic acid, the precursor to prostaglandins. In women with dysmenorrhea, excessive elevation of prostaglandins, specifically prostaglandin F2α and prostaglandin E2α, leads to uterine hypercontractility; painful cramping; and other prostaglandin-related symptoms such as nausea, vomiting, and diarrhea. These contractions decrease blood flow to the uterus and cause ischemia, which sensitizes nerve fibers to the inflammatory prostaglandins and endoperoxides.[8,9] Elevated levels of vasopressin have also been found in women with dysmenorrhea. This hormone increases uterine contractility, thereby contributing to cramping and ischemia.[10]

INTEGRATIVE THERAPY

Lifestyle

Exercise

Evidence for exercise as a treatment modality for dysmenorrhea has been mixed and limited in quality.[11] Early studies indicated that the type of exercise was less important than the desire to alleviate symptoms with exercise.[12] However, evidence has supported the use of both aerobic and stretching exercise regimens.[13] A 20-minute yoga regimen of Cobra, Cat, and Fish poses combined with yogic breathing decreased intensity and duration of menstrual pain when done for 14 days per month during the luteal phase of the cycle.[14] Given that chronic stress seems to increase perimenstrual symptoms,[5] and exercise is certainly a valid tool for managing stress and overall health, discussing regular exercise with patients suffering from dysmenorrhea certainly has a place.

Substance Use

Tobacco and alcohol use have been associated with worse symptoms of dysmenorrhea. Patients should be counseled on this and supported in addressing unhealthy use of these substances.

Nutrition

Omega-3 Fatty Acids

The release of arachidonic acid from the membranes of cells of the endometrium leads to an increase in proinflammatory prostaglandins. Omega-6 fatty acids are precursors to arachidonic acid, and our consumption of omega-6 compared with omega-3 fatty acids has greatly increased over the past century. The antiinflammatory diet (see Chapter 88) can change the ratio of omega-6 to omega-3 polyunsaturated fatty acids in our bodies and may thereby modulate the levels of prostaglandins, inflammation, and painful uterine contractions

TABLE 57.1 **Dietary Sources of Nutrients Found to Decrease Pain of Dysmenorrhea**

OMEGA-3 Fatty Acids	Magnesium	Vitamin B1	Vitamin B6	Vitamin E
Cold-water fish (e.g., salmon, herring, sardines) Leafy green vegetables Flaxseeds (ground) Walnuts	Halibut Almonds, dry roasted Cashews, dry roasted Soybeans Spinach	Fortified grains (breads, cereals, pasta, wheat germ) Lean pork Fish Dried beans Peas Soybeans	Fortified cereals Potatoes with skin Bananas Garbanzo beans (chickpeas) Chicken breast Pork loin, lean only	Vegetable oils (wheat germ, sunflower, safflower) Almonds Sunflower seeds Spinach Broccoli Fortified cereals, juices, and spreads

Data from MedlinePlus. *Thiamin.* http://www.nlm.nih.gov/medlineplus/ency/article/002401.htm Accessed 24.02.11; Office of Dietary Supplements, National Institutes of Health. *Dietary Supplement Fact Sheets.* http://ods.od.nih.gov/factsheets/ Accessed 20.02.11.

produced. Studies have shown that higher a consumption of omega-3 polyunsaturated fatty acids (either through supplementation or diet) leads to a decrease in painful menses and decreased need for NSAIDs.[15-17,18] Table 57.1 lists dietary sources of omega-3 polyunsaturated fatty acids, as well as other nutrients described in the following section that have been found to be helpful in the treatment of primary dysmenorrhea.[19,20]

DOSAGE

If supplementing with omega-3 fish oil capsules, the dose is 1500–2000 mg daily of docosahexaenoic acid and eicosapentaenoic acid or two to three servings of cold-water fish per week.

Supplements

Magnesium

Magnesium has been found to be beneficial in the treatment of arrhythmias, severe asthma, migraine, dyspepsia, and constipation. Its role in dysmenorrhea may be related to its effect on intracellular calcium concentration,[21] a reduction in prostaglandin synthesis,[22] or its muscle relaxant properties. A Cochrane Review found three studies showing that magnesium was more effective than placebo in decreasing menstrual pain and the use of analgesic medications. The studies were small, but the results are encouraging.[23]

The form of magnesium is important because some forms are more likely to cause diarrhea (see the section on dosage). Foods rich in magnesium include fish, nuts, leafy greens, whole grain cereals, and baked potatoes with the skin.[20] Magnesium is a largely intracellular cation, so red blood cell magnesium may be a more accurate measure of nutrient status than the typically used serum magnesium.

DOSAGE

Unless constipation is present, consider doses of 200–600 mg daily of forms of magnesium less likely to cause loose stools: magnesium glycinate (chelated magnesium), magnesium gluconate, or magnesium chloride. See Table 57.1 for dietary sources of magnesium.

PRECAUTIONS

Use magnesium with caution in individuals who have impaired renal function. If diarrhea develops, decrease the dose until this condition is relieved because diarrhea is one of the first signs of magnesium toxicity.

Vitamin B6 (Pyridoxine)

A series of small studies (n = 21 to 24) in 1988 compared various permutations of vitamin B6 versus magnesium versus vitamin B6 and magnesium versus placebo. The results revealed that vitamin B6 was better than placebo and a combination of vitamin B6 and magnesium at decreasing visual analogue pain scores and the number of ibuprofen tablets used.[23] A mechanism offered to explain the possible beneficial effect of vitamin B6 is its role in increasing the influx of magnesium into the cells, thereby supporting the effects of magnesium described earlier.

DOSAGE

The dose is 100 mg daily. If a higher dose is used, close monitoring is needed. See Table 57.1 for dietary sources of vitamin B6.

PRECAUTIONS

Vitamin B6 toxicity typically manifests as neuropathy that reverses with decreased intake.[20] Doses described were 100 mg twice daily; however, the Institute of Medicine established the upper tolerable intake level for vitamin B6 as 100 mg daily for adults.

Vitamin B6 and magnesium may work synergistically because vitamin B6 increases the influx of magnesium into the muscle cells.[24]

Vitamin B1 (Thiamine)

One of the largest double-blind, placebo-controlled studies investigating the effect of a nutritional supplement on dysmenorrhea was a trial of vitamin B1. This crossover trial involved 556 Indian adolescents who were randomized to receive either 100 mg of vitamin B1 daily for 90 days, followed by placebo for 60 days or placebo for 60 days, followed by 100 mg of vitamin B1 daily. In both groups, complete resolution or significant improvement in pain did not occur until the participants had received thiamine for at least 30 days. "Cure" rates by the end of the trial were approximately 90% in both groups.[25] This overwhelming success at "curing" dysmenorrhea certainly raises the question of whether the results could be confirmed with another study in a different population. The mechanism by which this treatment works may simply be reversal of a deficiency that can manifest with decreased pain tolerance, muscle cramping, and fatigue, which are symptoms similar to those of premenstrual syndrome.[22]

DOSAGE

The dose is 100 mg daily for 90 days. Consider continuing treatment if symptoms recur after initial improvement. See Table 57.1 for dietary sources of thiamine.

PRECAUTIONS

Orally, thiamine is usually well tolerated. It rarely causes dermatitis or a hypersensitivity reaction.[26]

Vitamin E

Vitamin E has been proposed to provide relief from dysmenorrhea through antiinflammatory action and through induction of a marked rise in beta-endorphin levels.[27,28] Several randomized, placebo-controlled studies, including a total of 383 women 15–21 years old, showed a significant decrease in the severity and duration of pain with the intake of vitamin E compared with placebo. The doses used varied from 150 to 500 units daily for either 2 days before and 3 days after or for 10 days before and 4 days after the onset of menses.[29-31] The tolerable upper intake level in healthy people is 1000 mg/day, equivalent to 1100 units of synthetic vitamin E (D-L-alpha-tocopherol or alpha- tocopherol or SRR-tocopherol) or to 1500 units of natural vitamin E (D-alpha tocopherol or RRR-tocopherol).[32,33]

DOSAGE

The dose is 400 units daily for a few days before and a few days after the onset of menses. See Table 57.1 for dietary sources of vitamin E.

PRECAUTIONS

Doses higher than 400 units of vitamin E have higher potential for adverse effects in unhealthy individuals.

Botanicals

French Maritime Pine Bark Extract (*Pinus pinaster*)

Pycnogenol is the trade name for this extract of French maritime pine bark. It has numerous active constituents such as flavonoids, procyanidins, and phenolic acids; the list of indications ranges from asthma, chronic venous insufficiency, and hypertension to coronary artery disease and diabetes. In dysmenorrhea, it may have antispasmodic effects and inhibit uterine contractions through its components ferulic acid and caffeic acid. A study of 116 women with low menstrual pain (did not require analgesic medication) or dysmenorrhea were monitored for two cycles and then treated with either 30 mg twice daily of Pycnogenol or placebo through another two menstrual cycles. Although no difference was noted in the treatment group compared with placebo in the women with low menstrual pain, a significant decrease in pain scores and in analgesic use was reported in women with dysmenorrhea, and the effect seemed to persist for at least 1 month after cessation of the extract.[34]

DOSAGE

The dose is 30 mg twice daily for 2 months. The effect may last for at least 1 month after cessation.

PRECAUTIONS

Pycnogenol is generally well tolerated. Side effects may be limited to gastrointestinal problems, dizziness, and vertigo but have possibly included headache and mouth ulceration.[35]

Fennel (*Foeniculum vulgare*)

Fennel essential oil has been found to be comparable to the nonsteroidal antiinflammatory (NSAID) medication, mefenamic acid.[36,37] The mechanism seems to involve the inhibition of uterine contraction induced by prostaglandin E2 and oxytocin.[38]

DOSAGE

The dose is 30 drops of fennel extract at the onset of menses and then continuously every 6 hours for the first 3 days of menses.

PRECAUTIONS

Fennel has a Generally Recognized as Safe (GRAS) status in the United States, but there have been case reports of neurotoxicity in two breastfeeding infants whose mothers drank an herbal combination tea containing fennel.[39] Fennel supplements should be avoided during pregnancy because in vitro studies have shown some toxic effects on fetal cells.[40]

SCA by Gol Daro Herbal Medicine (Saffron [*Crocus sativus*], Celery Seed [*Apium graveolens*], Anise or Fennel [*Foeniculum vulgare*])

An Iranian blend of highly purified extracts of saffron, celery seed, and anise (SCA by Gol Daro Herbal Medicine) was compared with mefenamic acid and placebo for effectiveness in alleviating symptoms of dysmenorrhea in 163 women 18–30 years old. SCA, at 500 mg three times daily, was found to be more effective than placebo and the NSAID, at 250 mg three times daily, in decreasing menstrual pain intensity and duration. All agents were taken for 3 days at the start of the menstrual cycle. No side effects were noted.[41]

DOSAGE

The dose of SCA is 500 mg three times daily for 3 days, starting at the onset of pain or bleeding.

PRECAUTIONS

Saffron is generally well tolerated and has a GRAS rating unless it is taken at high doses. Taking 5 g or more of saffron can cause severe side effects, and doses of 12–20 g can be lethal.[42] Celery seed also has a GRAS rating but may cause an allergic reaction (especially in individuals sensitive to mugwort, birch, dandelion, or wild carrot); large amounts should be avoided during pregnancy because of the potential abortifacient effects.[43]

Willow Bark Extract (*Salix cortex*)

The major active ingredient of willow bark, salicin, was the original source of aspirin. It appears to inhibit the cyclooxygenase-2 pathway. Other components of willow bark may have other antiinflammatory properties. Willow bark seems to inhibit platelet aggregation, but not as much as aspirin.

DOSAGE

The dosage is 240 mg daily of salicin, in divided doses. This is roughly equivalent to 87 mg of aspirin. Willow bark extract may work better if it is started the day before expected symptoms.[44]

PRECAUTIONS

Willow bark extract is generally safe, but avoid it in children with viral infections, given a theoretical risk of Reye syndrome. It can cause gastrointestinal side effects but less than those seen with NSAIDs. Avoid in patients with kidney disease and in patients allergic to aspirin.

Cramp Bark (*Viburnum opulus*) *and Black Haw* (*Viburnum prunifolium*)

Traditionally, these herbs have been used as uterine relaxants. Very few data are available regarding their efficacy. The root bark and stem bark of black haw contain certain active ingredients, including scopoletin and oxalic acid. Scopoletin may be a uterine relaxant. Because of the presence of oxalic acid, black haw should be avoided in patients with a history of renal stones. Black haw also contains salicylates that could

trigger an allergic reaction in patients sensitive to aspirin.[45]

DOSAGE

The dose of black haw is 2–3 mL of a tincture made in 1:3 proportion every 2 hours or as needed; or 4–8 mL of fluid extract (1:1) three or four times daily; or simmer one tablespoon of bark in 12 oz of water for 15 minutes and drink one-third cup every 2–3 hours as needed.[46]

PRECAUTIONS

Avoid black haw in persons with a history of renal stones or aspirin allergy.

Other Herbs

Many other herbs used traditionally by herbalists can be effective in easing the pain of dysmenorrhea, but scientific trials are lacking. Table 57.2 summarizes other herbs from which patients may benefit.

Pharmaceuticals

Nonsteroidal Antiinflammatory Drugs

As inhibitors of prostaglandin formation, NSAIDs such as naproxen, ibuprofen, and mefenamic acid have been shown to be quite effective for the treatment of dysmenorrhea when compared with placebo or acetaminophen. These medications are used and tolerated by a great number of women and bring relief from painful menstrual cramping. NSAIDs are not effective in approximately 20% of cases, however, and they can be associated with significant side effects. Gastrointestinal symptoms such as nausea and indigestion seem to be especially common with naproxen. Overall, NSAIDs are associated with a higher risk than placebo of such mild neurological adverse effects as headache, drowsiness, dizziness, and dryness of the mouth. Naproxen and indomethacin seem to be more likely to produce these types of symptoms.[47]

Hormonal Treatments

Combined oral contraceptive pills have been shown to reduce menstrual pain significantly. A meta-analysis of nearly 500 women showed decreased pain with both low-dose and medium-dose estrogen formulations. The type of progesterone does not seem to matter. Side effects noted were nausea, headache, and weight gain.[48] More serious side effects of oral contraceptive pills include thromboembolic and cardiovascular events; the risks of these adverse effects rise greatly with age and cigarette smoking.

Levonorgestrel-containing intrauterine devices have been reported to be equal or superior to oral progestins or oral contraceptives in their ability to decrease menstrual cramping in women of all reproductive ages,[49] perhaps by

TABLE 57.2 Other Herbs That May Be of Benefit for Easing Menstrual Pain

Herb	Dose	Comment
Black cohosh *Actaea racemosa*	Tea: 2 tsp dried root steeped in two cups boiling water for 10 minutes. Drink one-fourth cup two to three times daily Capsule: 40–200 mg dried rhizome daily in divided doses Tincture: 1–2 mL three times daily Standardized extract: 20–40 mg twice daily	Popularly used as an herb for menopausal symptoms. Seems to have antiinflammatory and antidepressant activity that can reduce experience of and sensitivity to pain. Few, rare reports suggested potential of liver damage—use with caution in those at risk.
Dong quai *Angelica sinensis*	Tea: Steep 1–2 tsp root in one cup water for 5–7 minutes. Drink one cup two to three times daily. Capsules: 1 g two to three times daily Tincture: 3–5 mL, two to three times daily	May cause photosensitivity. May increase bleeding risk in those on anticoagulants or with bleeding disorders. May increase heaviness of menstrual bleeding.
Shatavari *Asparagus racemosus*	Tea: Steep 1 tsp dried root in one cup water for 15 minutes. Drink one to two cups daily Capsules: 500 mg one to two times daily Tincture: per manufacturer's dosing	Well tolerated and safe.
Chamomile *Matricaria recutita*	Tea: Steep 1 tsp flowers in one cup water for 5–7 minutes or longer	Use with caution in those with severe ragweed allergies. May be especially helpful in those with menstrual cramps and gastrointestinal discomfort.
Hops *Humulus lupulus*	Tea: Steep 1 tsp female flowers in one cup water for 5–7 minutes Capsules: 500 mg one to three times daily Tincture: 2 mL, one to three times daily	Can be sedating. Potential for hormonal activity; avoid in women at risk for breast cancer.[a]
Bee balm (Oswego tea) *Monarda didyma*	Tea: Steep 1 tsp powdered herb in one cup water for 7–10 minutes. Take one to three cups daily	Avoid in pregnancy as it may stimulate menstrual flow. Also used for flatulence and as a diuretic, which may help other symptoms uncomfortable menstrual-related symptoms.[b]

[a]Source: Johnson R, Foster S, Low Dog T, Kiefer, D. *National Geographic guide to medicinal herbs*. Washington D.C.: National Geographic;2010.
[b]Source: http://naturaldatabase.therapeuticresearch.com/nd/Search.aspx?cs=CEPDA&s=ND&pt=100&id=169&fs=ND&searchid=54575942. Accessed 12/15/15.

inhibiting buildup of the endometrium and thus reducing the total prostaglandin load. Such devices also frequently reduce menstrual flow, which may be desirable in some cases. Uterine perforation, one of the more serious risks of placement of an intrauterine device, occurs at a rate of approximately 2 in 1000 women. The expulsion rate is approximately 5% in the first year. These devices have the advantage of providing contraception for up to 5 years before they must be replaced.

Mind-Body Therapy

A comprehensive health plan for any individual with chronic pain often involves recognition of the component of the experience of the pain that is influenced by the perception of that experience. Chronic pain is frequently accompanied by mood disturbances such as depression and anxiety. At times, distinguishing whether mood affects pain or the other way around may be difficult; the relationship is likely bidirectional. Given the risk factors listed previously of a history of sexual abuse and psychological symptoms, it is easy to see that a significant mind-body relationship may play a role in some cases of dysmenorrhea.

A 2007 Cochrane Review (reprinted in 2010) included five studies that evaluated behavioral interventions such as biofeedback, relaxation techniques, and pain management training. An overall benefit was apparent, but the studies were small, and some had relatively poor methodology.[50] A small 2014 study compared as needed use of NSAIDs to hypnosis for dysmenorrhea and found that both were effective for decreasing pain while being actively employed. However, only the hypnosis seemed to have a lasting effect of at least 3 months after cessation of treatment on the decrease of nonpain symptoms such as nausea, vomiting, diarrhea, headache, and dizziness.[51]

In areas such as this, the relationship between the provider and the individual is very important. Listening to and understanding the individual on a deeper level allows the provider to determine more appropriately whether, for example, referral to a counselor or health psychologist may be beneficial. Providers skilled in relaxation techniques or guided imagery may be able to strengthen their therapeutic relationship with patients by employing those skills for symptoms of dysmenorrhea. More research is needed in this area to develop protocols for techniques that can be easily taught to patients for their use during times when they are symptomatic.

Bioenergetic Therapy

Heat Therapy

Patients may report that they have tried using heating pads or microwavable bean bags, with some relief of symptoms. Studies have shown that heat does indeed decrease pain and, when combined with NSAIDs, reduces the time until noticeable pain relief is achieved.[52,53] Recommend heat of approximately 39°C (102°F) for up to 8–12 hours on the lower abdomen or back.

> **PRECAUTIONS**
>
> Ensure that the heat is not so high that it causes burns or is applied to areas of decreased sensation because an injury may not be recognized.

Magnet Therapy

A study of 35 women in London found a significant decrease in pain over one menstrual cycle by using a 2700-gauss magnet that attached to the underwear over the suprapubic area. The noncompletion rate in this study was significant, but the investigators reported that this was a pilot study for a much larger study using the same device. The manufacturer of the device was involved in the funding of the study.[54] The device is sold in England and on the Internet for approximately $40 U.S. A Korean study using 800- to 1299-gauss magnets over the suprapubic area, lower back, and medial lower leg revealed similar results.[55]

Transcutaneous Electrical Nerve Stimulation

By delivering electrical currents and various frequencies through the skin, transcutaneous electrical nerve stimulation (TENS) machines appear to affect the body's ability to receive and understand pain signals. TENS devices are used quite commonly for musculoskeletal pain, including low back pain; they are portable, thus making them available for home and clinic use. A 2010 Cochrane Review found seven small studies covering a total of 164 women suffering with dysmenorrhea that compared high- or low-frequency TENS therapy or TENS therapy with placebo TENS, a placebo pill, or medical treatment (NSAIDs). The results of the meta-analysis showed that high-frequency TENS (using 50–100 Hz) was significantly more effective than placebo for the relief of dysmenorrhea. The effect of low-frequency TENS (1–4 Hz) was not significant, but trended toward benefit over placebo. Neither was as effective as medical therapy.[56] Consideration of the long-term effects of electromagnetic radiation to the pelvis, especially in young women, may be wise.

Acupuncture

Acupuncture is becoming more and more widely accepted in the Western world as a treatment modality for various indications, pain being among the most common. Investigating efficacy can be difficult, however, in that control arms for acupuncture studies are challenging to design because even sham acupuncture may indeed have some therapeutic benefit. A 2009 systematic review of 27 trials showed that only 9 trial groups adequately described their randomization methods, and none described their allocation and concealment methods. However, the results of the studies included did support significant benefit of acupuncture over pharmaceutical or herbal interventions. Two of the studies did not show a benefit of acupuncture over sham acupuncture.[57] A 2011 Cochrane Review found 34 trials that studied acupuncture and acupressure for dysmenorrhea.[58] Ten trials were included in the review: six involving acupuncture and four involving acupressure. Of the 24 trials not used, nearly all were excluded because of either details around randomization or the use of multiple interventions (e.g., Chinese herbs, moxibustion). Meta-analysis of the 6 included acupuncture trials (n = 673) did indeed show significant benefit of acupuncture for dysmenorrhea compared with control, NSAIDs, and Chinese herbs. Acupuncture was also shown to have a positive impact on other menstrual symptoms (e.g., headache, nausea) and quality of life.[58] Several reviews[59,60] pointed to a methodologically sound trial of 48 women randomized to acupuncture, sham acupuncture, no treatment control, or visitation control (office visits only without treatment). This study found a significant decrease in the number of patients who had "improved" symptoms (greater than 50% reduction in pain scores) with true acupuncture compared with controls.[61] There is also some evidence that acupuncture may be more beneficial after osteopathic manipulation.[62] A larger study of a similar design would certainly be beneficial in securing acupuncture's role in the treatment of dysmenorrhea.

The World Health Organization lists primary dysmenorrhea as one of the indications "for which acupuncture has been proved—through controlled trials—to be an effective treatment."[63] Dysmenorrhea was also on the National Institute of Health's 1997 list of indications for which acupuncture was deemed potentially useful.[64]

Acupressure

Acupressure has an advantage over acupuncture in that it can be performed on oneself, or with simple devices, and is therefore practically and financially more accessible to greater numbers of women with primary dysmenorrhea.

A 2010 review of randomized controlled trials of acupressure alone as treatment for primary dysmenorrhea, trials that used outcome measures of pain relief and adverse effects, found four that met inclusion criteria (total n = 458; range, 61–216). Although considerable deficits were noted in descriptions of the randomization and allocation concealment methods, acupressure treatments did seem to bring about an overall significant reduction in menstrual pain.[65] The acupressure points used varied in each study. One study that showed benefit used a "cotton Lycra panty brief with a fixed number of lower abdominal and lower back latex foam 'acupads' that provide pressure" on specific acupressure points and that was worn for as long as comfortable.[66] The 2011 Cochrane Review of acupuncture and acupressure for primary dysmenorrhea also included four acupressure studies (n = 271).[58] Meta-analysis of these studies showed a significant decrease in pain with acupressure compared with placebo. Two of the four studies in this review used auricular acupressure,[67,68] which may decrease the accessibility of treatment.

> Simple regimens described have used the acupressure points spleen 6 (SP6) and large intestine 4 (LI4).[69,70] Figs. 57.1 and 57.2 illustrate the locations of these points. Consider alternating between 6 seconds of pressure and 2 seconds off, for a total of approximately 5 minutes. Pressure should initially be relatively light (just shy of "really hurting") but increase as the treatment continues. Work on each point on both sides of the body for a total treatment time of approximately 20 minutes. To decrease the treatment time required, if performing on oneself, consider acupressure on the right SP6 with the left hand while pressing on the left LI4 with the right hand for 5 minutes and then reversing for another 5 minutes.

Biomechanical Therapy

Spinal Manipulation Therapy

Therapies such as osteopathic or chiropractic manipulation of the spine may increase spinal mobility and blood flow to the pelvis and lead to improvement in symptoms of dysmenorrhea. A 2006 Cochrane Review concluded that spinal manipulation therapy showed no benefit over sham manipulation in improvement of symptoms of dysmenorrhea, although both interventions decreased pain.[65] The investigators acknowledged, however, that significant challenges exist with the control arm in such studies in that, similar to acupuncture, sham manipulation may actually have some clinical benefit.[71] One of the studies included in the review also measured pretreatment and posttreatment serum levels of a prostaglandin F2α metabolite. Both pain and the metabolite were decreased in both spinal manipulation therapy and sham manipulation groups.[72] This finding may indicate that spinal manipulative therapies do indeed have a role

in the treatment of dysmenorrhea, but the evidence is challenged by the inability to find a true placebo.

Surgery

Laparoscopic presacral neurectomy and laparoscopic uterine nerve ablation (LUNA) are surgical approaches to relieving dysmenorrhea. A 2010 update of a 2005 Cochrane Review found two studies with a total of 68 women that showed decreased menstrual pain after LUNA compared with diagnostic laparoscopy at 12 months, but not at 6 months, postoperatively. A third trial in the review found that laparoscopic presacral neurectomy resulted in significantly better relief scores compared with LUNA at 12 months, but not at 3 months, after surgery.[73]

Therapies to Consider

Aromatherapy with Massage

A study of 57 Korean college women with dysmenorrhea compared abdominal massage with aromatherapy (a mixture of two drops of lavender, one drop of clary sage, and one drop of rose in 5 mL of almond oil), abdominal massage with almond oil only, and no intervention. The aromatherapy group showed a significant decrease in menstrual discomfort based on scoring using a visual analogue scale compared with massage alone or no treatment. Massages in the study took place for approximately 15 minutes daily for 1 week before the start of menses. No side effects were reported.[74]

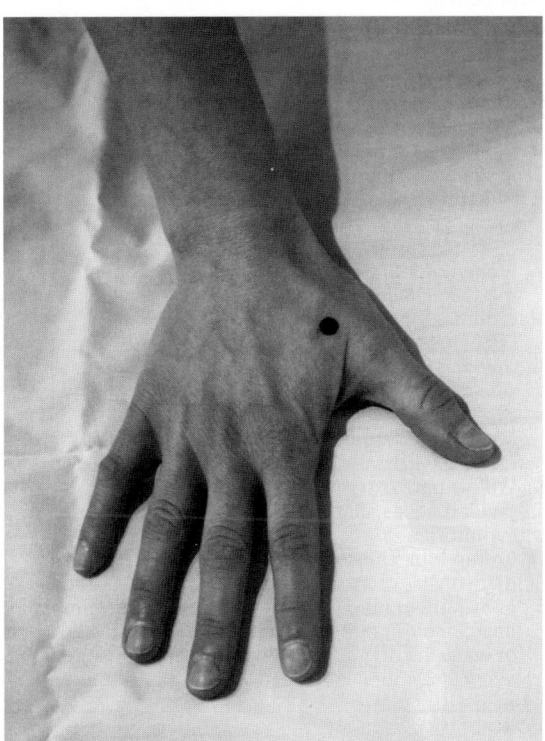

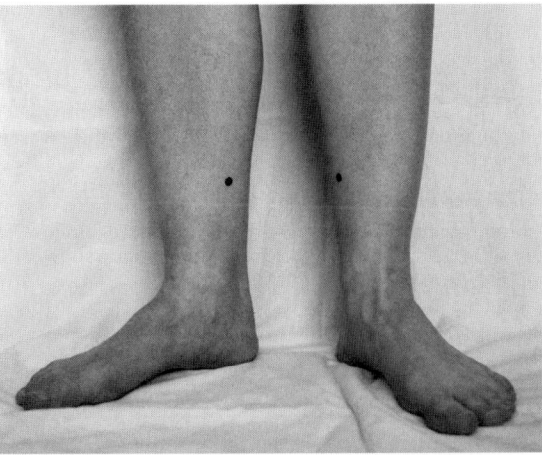

FIG. 57.1 ■ Spleen 6 (Sanyinjiao): Four finger widths superior to the prominence of the medial malleolus posterior to the medial margin of the tibia. When a patient is experiencing dysmenorrhea, the point may be very tender.

FIG. 57.2 ■ Large intestine 4 (Hegu): On the dorsum of the hand midway between the first and second metacarpals at the level of the midpoint of the shaft of the second metacarpal. When a patient is experiencing dysmenorrhea, the point may be very tender.

AROMATHERAPY MASSAGE FOR DYSMENORRHEA

Use slow, smooth, and continuous strokes with mild to moderate pressure and a mixture of lavender, clary sage, and rose oils in almond oil (see previous section). The strokes should start with the masseur's left hand on top of the right in the right lower quadrant of the abdomen, go up to the ribs, and then across the abdomen to the left lower quadrant. The masseur can then provide gentle kneading of the left and right lower abdomen, followed by stroking across the abdomen. This sequence can be repeated for a total of 15 minutes and performed daily for 1 week before the expected onset of menses.

PREVENTION PRESCRIPTION

- Maintain a healthy weight.
- Follow an antiinflammatory diet.
- Participate in regular, moderate-intensity aerobic exercise.
- Avoid use of tobacco.
- Avoid alcohol in excess.
- Employ effective stress management techniques.

THERAPEUTIC REVIEW

EXERCISE

- The benefits of exercise on stress reduction and maintenance of a healthy weight may reduce risk factors for dysmenorrhea. $\quad$ C 1

NUTRITION

- Diets rich in omega-3 fatty acids can reduce menstrual pain. Supplement with 1500–2000 mg daily of docosahexaenoic acid and eicosapentaenoic acid. Through diet, omega-3 fatty acids can be obtained with two to three servings of cold-water fish weekly and other, plant-based sources. $\quad$ B 1

SUPPLEMENTS

- Magnesium (glycinate, gluconate, or chloride): 600 mg daily, decreased if diarrhea develops. Use with caution in patients with kidney disease. $\quad$ B 2
- Vitamin B6 (pyridoxine): 100 mg daily (may work better with magnesium) $\quad$ B 2
- Vitamin B1 (thiamine): 100 mg daily for 90 days, or longer if symptoms recur after cessation $\quad$ B 1
- Vitamin E: 400 units daily $\quad$ B 1

BOTANICALS

- French maritime pine bark extract/Pycnogenol: 30 mg twice daily. The effect may last for at least 1 month after cessation. $\quad$ B 1
- Fennel: 30 drops of extract at the onset of menses, then every 6 hours for the first 3 days of menses. Avoid during pregnancy or lactation. $\quad$ B 1
- SCA (saffron, celery, and anise, by Gol Daro Herbal Medicine): 500 mg three times daily for 3 days, starting with onset of pain or bleeding. $\quad$ B 2
- Willow bark extract: 240 mg daily of salicin in divided doses, starting on the day before expected symptoms. $\quad$ C 2
- Cramp bark and black haw: 2–3 mL of a tincture made in 1:3 proportion every 2 hours or as needed; or 4–8 mL of fluid extract (1:1) three or four times daily; or simmer one tablespoon of bark in 12 oz of water for 15 minutes, one-third cup consumed every 2–3 hours as needed. $\quad$ C 2

- Other herbs per Table 57.2. $\quad$ C 2

PHARMACEUTICALS

- Nonsteroidal antiinflammatory drugs such as ibuprofen, 400–600 mg with food every 6 hours, starting the day before symptoms expected to occur until symptoms cease $\quad$ A 2
- Combined contraceptive pills $\quad$ B 2
- Levonorgestrel-containing intrauterine device $\quad$ C 2

MIND-BODY THERAPY

- Consider counseling or health psychology referral for relaxation techniques, biofeedback, or pain management training, for example, if determined relevant given the individual's history. $\quad$ C 1

BIOENERGETIC THERAPY

- Use a heating pad or microwavable bean bag on the low back or abdomen for up to 8–12 hours. $\quad$ B 1
- Consider purchasing a magnet therapy device (e.g., mn8; see Key Web Resources). $\quad$ B 1
- Consider using a transcutaneous electrical nerve stimulation unit. $\quad$ B 2
- Consider acupuncture. $\quad$ B 2
- Consider acupressure. $\quad$ B 1

BIOMECHANICAL THERAPY

- Consider spinal manipulation therapy (chiropractic or osteopathic treatment). $\quad$ B 2
- As a last resort, laparoscopic presacral neurectomy may be more effective than laparoscopic uterine nerve ablation. $\quad$ B 3

OTHER THERAPIES TO CONSIDER

- Aromatherapy with abdominal massage using a mixture of two drops of lavender, one drop of clary sage, and one drop of rose in 5 mL of almond oil $\quad$ B 1

Key Web Resources

mn8: Website for purchase of magnet devices for dysmenorrhea that insert into underwear	http://www.mn8.uk.com/about.php
Environmental Defense Fund Seafood Selector: Guide for safe fish consumption	http://www.edf.org/page.cfm?tagID=1521
AcuMedico: Acupuncture points database describing how to locate acupuncture points	http://www.acumedico.com/acupoints.htm

REFERENCES

References are available online at ExpertConsult.com.

CHAPTER 58

UTERINE FIBROIDS (LEIOMYOMATA)

Allan Warshowsky, MD, FACOG, ABIHM

PATHOPHYSIOLOGY

Prevalence and Etiology of Uterine Fibroids

Uterine fibroids affect 5.4%–77% of women, depending on the method of diagnosis.[1] Fibroid tumors can be small and difficult to feel, especially in obese women. These benign tumors have been known to grow to the size of a watermelon. Most gynecologists do not consider fibroid tumors to be a surgical problem until they reach the size of a 12-week pregnancy. At that size, it becomes difficult to feel small ovarian tumors. Ultrasonography and other imaging techniques make size less of a concern. Now, larger fibroid tumors allow for evaluation of ovaries through sonography, magnetic resonance imaging (MRI), and computed tomography (CT) scan. Reasons for considering surgery include symptoms such as menorrhagia and dysmenorrhea. Historically, hysterectomy has been the procedure of choice for patients with large fibroid tumors. Approximately 300,000 hysterectomies are performed per year for these benign tumors. Hysterectomy is an invasive procedure; in 1975, 1700 deaths occurred among 787,000 hysterectomies performed.[2] More recent studies have confirmed the morbidity of these invasive procedures.[3,4] Conventional medicine has little else to offer other than a "watch and wait" attitude to women who suffer from small fibroids. However, if these small fibroids are approached from an integrative holistic perspective when they are initially observed, much of the disability and invasive surgical procedures can be avoided.

The second edition of the American College of Obstetrics and Gynecology's *Guideline for Women's Health Care* suggests the following: "As benign neoplasms, uterine leiomyomata (fibroids) usually require treatment only when they cause symptoms."[5] An integrative, holistic approach that eliminates symptoms and stops the growth of these benign fibroid tumors can help women to avoid invasive surgery and disability.

Hormonal Changes in the Normal Ovulatory Menstrual Cycle

The healthy menstrual cycle is a marvel. In the first part of the well-orchestrated cycle, follicular cells of the ovary produce estradiol. This follicular phase lasts from 7 to 21 days. During this part of the cycle, follicle-stimulating hormone (FSH) and luteinizing hormone (LH) are produced and secreted by the anterior pituitary gland in the brain.

The necessary midfollicular phase peak of estradiol affects an LH surge during this part of the cycle.

Ovulation occurs after the LH surge. Only after ovulation is progesterone produced and secreted by the corpus luteum of the ovary.

LH and FSH are in an inhibitory feedback loop relationship with the main ovarian hormone, estradiol. The anterior pituitary gland is also under the control of the hypothalamus through the secretion of gonadotropin-releasing hormone (GnRH). The limbic system, which contains the amygdala and hippocampus, encircles the hypothalamus and pituitary gland and is the known repository of emotions in the body. The limbic system and thus our emotions and perceptions affect the production and secretion of GnRH. The physiology of this is not clear, but all clinicians know that women become menopausal after a significant stressor in their lives.

We must also consider the association of ovarian hormones with the thyroid and adrenal glands. Alterations of thyroid function are invariably associated with menstrual irregularities. Low progesterone-to-estradiol (P/E_2) ratios are associated with reduced conversion of less active thyroxin (T_4) to more active triiodothyronine (T_3). Therefore, hypothyroidism with normal levels of T_4 and low levels of T_3 can be an indicator of sex hormone imbalance and estrogen dominance. Adrenal gland function also affects sex hormone production and metabolism and must be evaluated along with the thyroid and ovarian hormones.

The origin of fibroids is not well understood. Some evidence indicates that chromosomal abnormalities may play a role. Chromosomal translocations, deletions, inversions, and breakpoints have been shown to be associated with familial patterns of fibroid growth.[6] The fibroids in these affected families tend to be quite large.

The incidence of uterine fibroids seems to be higher in African-American, obese, nonsmoking, and perimenopausal women than in other women. Fibroid tumors are associated with high estrogen levels or estrogen dominance. Obesity and the perimenopausal state are often associated with higher estrogen levels. Studies have shown that estrogen levels are actually higher in perimenopausal women. With obesity, adipocytes act as endocrine organs that produce estrone, another strong estrogen. The inflammatory mediators interleukin-2 (IL-2), IL-6, tumor necrosis factor-alpha (TNF-alpha), and leukotriene B_4 (LTB$_4$) are also produced in adipocytes and contribute to fibroid formation.[7]

Vitamin D research has begun to shed light on the higher incidence of fibroids in African-American and other dark-skinned women.[8] Low vitamin D (measured as 25-hydroxyvitamin D_3) levels are associated with increased inflammatory cytokines and have been shown to be associated with higher incidences of epithelial cancers such as those of the breast, colon, and prostate.[9] Vitamin

D is necessary for healthy cell apoptosis, or regulated cell death, and also has profound effects on glucose metabolism. Later discussion explains how unhealthy glucose metabolism can contribute to fibroid growth through the development of insulin resistance.[10] The form of vitamin that circulates to all the cells of the body is 25-hydroxyvitamin D_3, and it is a good measure of the total body reserve of vitamin D_3. The optimal range of 25-hydroxyvitamin D_3 is between 40 and 80 ng/mL.[11] Low levels are treated with vitamin D_3 in the range of 50,000 units/week for 12 weeks, at which time the measurement should be repeated.[12]

Studies by Dr. Elizabeth Stewart et al.[13] in Boston support the connection between systemic inflammation and fibroid growth. She showed that various growth factors, such as fibroblast growth factor, vascular endothelial growth factor, and transforming growth factor, which are concentrated in fibroid cells, are responsive to inflammatory mediators. These stimulated growth factors increase blood vessel growth or angiogenesis in the fibroid and thereby stimulate and support growth. All successful tumors, whether benign or malignant, increase their own blood supply through this process of angiogenesis and enable growth. Controlling vascularity with antiangiogenesis factors, as shown by the work of Dr. Judah Folkmann,[14] can reduce the growth of the tumor or fibroid by decreasing its blood supply and supporting shrinkage.

The "gut connection" to fibroid growth concerns bacterial imbalance or intestinal dysbiosis and a "leaky gut." A dysbiotic intestinal environment produces gut-associated inflammatory mediators. These inflammatory mediators include IL-2, IL-6, TNF-alpha, and other leukotrienes and cytokines. They surround the pelvis, where nature's fertilizer, estradiol, stimulates the growth of atypical cells that develop into autonomously growing leiomyomata or fibroids. Intestinal dysbiosis with associated bacterial and yeast overgrowth also contributes to estrogen dominance through the estrogenic effects of bacterial toxins and yeast mycotoxins. Associated constipation can also increase serum estrogens by breaking down the estrogen–glucuronic acid bond by the action of the enzyme beta-glucuronidase, which is produced in this dysbiotic environment.[15]

Estrogen Dominance

Estrogen dominance is a term coined by the late Dr. John Lee (Fig. 58.1).[16] It applies to conditions associated with stronger estrogen effects than can be balanced with existing progesterone. Estrogen dominance can also manifest through imbalanced estrogen metabolism, as discussed later. Fibroids are just one condition associated with estrogen dominance (Table 58.1). Others are as follows:
- Autoimmune diseases: Hashimoto thyroiditis, systemic lupus erythematosus, rheumatoid arthritis, multiple sclerosis, ulcerative colitis, scleroderma, Sjögren syndrome, and others
- Fibrocystic breast problems
- Gallbladder disease
- Cervical dysplasias and other hormone-dependent cancers (breast, uterine, and ovarian)
- Endometriosis
- Infertility

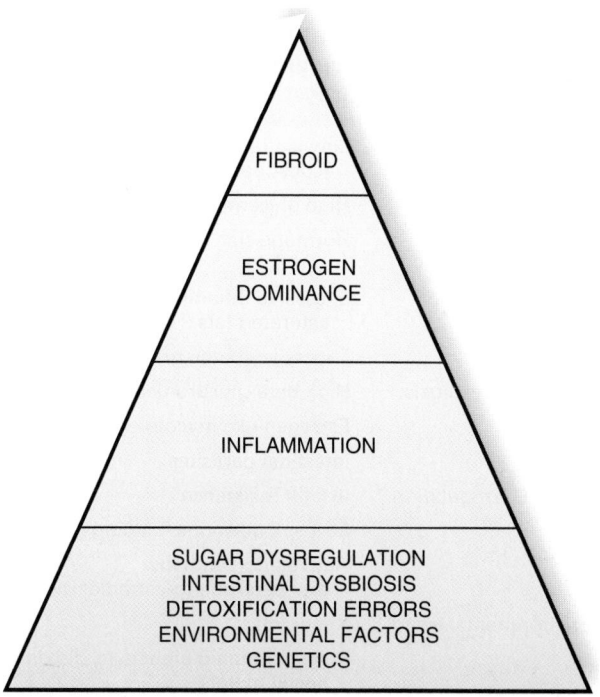

FIG. 58.1 ■ The fibroid that can be felt and measured is the physical manifestation of estrogen dominance and inflammation. Estrogen dominance and inflammation in the body are created and supported by underlying sugar dysregulation, intestinal dysbiosis, detoxification errors, environmental factors, and genetics.

- Menstrual irregularities of all kinds
- Polycystic ovary syndrome
- Premenstrual syndrome

Effects of Diet, Digestion, Absorption, and the Intestinal Environment on Hormone Balance

Hormone imbalance and estrogen dominance are often associated with intestinal dysbiosis. Intestinal dysbiosis designates an unhealthy gut environment often associated with increased intestinal permeability or a "leaky gut." Signs and symptoms of dysbiosis include digestive issues, such as bad breath, body odor, bloating, gas, nausea, and constipation. The concept of a leaky gut describes a condition in which, instead of normal protein digestion into amino acids that are actively transported through the intestinal cells, large peptides and proteins are absorbed intact through or in between intestinal mucosa cells in the intestinal wall and stimulate inflammatory reactions due to an overstimulated and out-of-balance immune system.

Intestinal dysbiosis can be caused by antacid abuse and resultant hypochlorhydria, antibiotics, chronic stress, eating practices that do not enhance digestion and absorption ("eating on the run"), intestinal infection, and birth control pills.

Intestinal dysbiosis can contribute to estrogen dominance through several mechanisms. Beta-glucuronidase is an enzyme produced by pathogenic gut bacteria.[17] It cleaves the glucuronic acid molecule conjugated to estradiol that would enable its excretion and thus allows the estradiol to be reabsorbed into the body. The result is

TABLE 58.1 **Factors That Promote Estrogen Dominance and Subsequent Fibroid Growth**

Poor Dietary Choices*	Low-isoflavone, low-fiber foods (constipation)
	High glycemic index foods
	Hormone-rich meats, poultry, and dairy
	Excessive inflammation–causing saturated fats
	Excessive gluten grains
Intestinal Dysbiosis	High beta-glucuronidase levels†
	Estrogen-like mycotoxins
	Intestinal parasites
Sugar Dysregulation	Insulin resistance
	Low sex hormone–binding globulin
	Anovulation with low progesterone-to-estradiol ratios
Environmental Issues‡	Xenobiotics
	Polychlorinated biphenyls, dioxins, heavy metals
	Birth control pills and hormone replacement therapy§
	Violence and sex effects on the limbic system
Stress	High cortisol levels contribute to low progesterone
Reduced Estrogen Detoxification	Leading to estrogen dominance

*Data from Goldin BR, Adlercreutz H, Gorbach SL, et al. Estrogen excretion patterns and plasma levels in vegetarian and omnivorous women. *N Engl J Med.* 1982;307:1542–1547.
†Data from Minton JP, Walaszek Z, Hanausek-Walaszek M, et al. β-Glucuronidase levels in patients with fibrocystic breast disease. *Breast Cancer Res Treat.* 1986;8:217–222.
‡Data from Wolff MS, Toniolo PG, Lee EW, et al. Blood levels of organochlorine residues and risk of breast cancer. *J Natl Cancer Inst.* 1993;85:648–652.
§Data from Gruber CJ, Tschugguel W, Schneeberger C, et al. Production and actions of estrogens. *N Engl J Med.* 2002;346:340.

an elevation of total body estrogen that puts more stress on the liver and its detoxification capacities. Pathogenic intestinal bacteria and pathogenic yeasts can also produce bacterial toxins and mycotoxins having strong estrogenic effects. Concomitant inflammation can increase estrogen production and the growth factors that reside in the fibroid tissue thus supporting angiogenesis.

Intestinal dysbiosis can be diagnosed with the proprietary Comprehensive Digestive Stool Analysis (Genova Diagnostics; see Key Web Resources). Elevations of the organic acid indican can indicate poor protein digestion and suggest intestinal dysbiosis (Organix test; Genova, see Key Web Resources). Greater intestinal permeability is evaluated using the lactulose-mannitol test. In this test, the variable absorption of the two sugars lactulose and mannitol determines whether permeability in the intestines is increased. The larger sugar lactulose should not find its way into the urine, unlike the smaller sugar mannitol. Finding abnormal ratios of these two sugars in the urine after oral ingestion indicates increased intestinal permeability or dysbiosis.

Intestinal dysbiosis is treated with an intestinal restoration program such as the 4-R program described by Jeffrey Bland.[18] The four Rs are as follows:
- Remove irritants affecting the gut. This includes microorganisms, food allergens, and other toxins.
- Replace betaine hydrochloride, enzymes, bile salts, and fiber.
- Reinoculate with prebiotics (inulin) and probiotics.
- Repair, which is done with gut restorative nutrients, including zinc, glutamine, N-acetylcysteine, N-acetylglucosamine, *Boswellia*, cat's claw, licorice root, and curcumin.

For further information, see Chapter 86.

For a woman to have symptomatic fibroids and not to have functional intestinal dysfunction and associated dysbiosis would be unusual and uncommon.

Effects of Insulin Resistance on Hormone Balance and Estrogen Dominance

Elevations of insulin and insulin-like growth factor-I can also contribute to estrogen dominance and fibroid growth. Metabolic syndrome (prediabetes) is a disorder of elevated insulin related to increasing insulin resistance.[19] The syndrome is defined by a constellation of signs and symptoms including abdominal obesity with a waist-to-hip ratio greater than 0.8:1 (waist circumference larger than 35 inches in women), a high level of triglycerides with a low level of high-density lipoprotein cholesterol and a high level of low-density lipoprotein cholesterol, hypertension, impaired glucose tolerance, increasing hypoglycemia, and a higher incidence of adult-onset diabetes. Metabolic syndrome is associated with these laboratory markers:
- Elevation of fasting insulin and blood glucose
- Elevation of fasting fructosamine
- High hemoglobin A1c measurement (greater than 5.6%)
- Increased inflammatory mediators: IL-2, IL-6, TNF-alpha, LTB_4
- Increased levels of the prostaglandin-2 series thus increasing inflammation
- Strong estrogen produced in adipocytes as estrone (E_1)
- Estrogen dominance, most apparent in polycystic ovary syndrome, which is highly associated with insulin resistance
- Decreased sex hormone–binding globulin (SHBG) increases the amount of free estradiol available at the cellular level[20]
- Increased aromatase enzyme activity, increasing conversion of testosterone and androstenedione (testosterone precursor) to estradiol and estrone, and increasing estrogen dominance

Insulin sensitivity can be improved by various methods, all thoroughly discussed in Chapter 32.

Liver Detoxification and Estrogen Dominance

Metabolic detoxification consists of three phases that need to be in balance. In phase one, lipid-soluble substances—toxins, hormones, or drugs—are transformed into intermediate substances, which are more water soluble, by the cytochrome P450 set of enzymes.[21] This enzyme system can be upregulated or downregulated by various drugs, stressors (e.g., alcohol, cigarette smoke, smoke from charred meat), and herbs. An example in the world of estrogen dominance and uterine fibroids is the effect of gluten grains on estrogen metabolism. Gluten, the active protein in wheat, rye, and barley, reduces the cytochrome P450 isoenzyme 3A4 and leads to reduced estrogen metabolism and subsequent estrogen dominance.

The intermediate substances that are formed in phase one must be made more water soluble, enabling excretion from the body. In phase two of the detoxification process, these intermediates are conjugated with amino acids and peptides such as glucuronic acid, glutathione, and glycine, or they undergo conjugation processes such as methylation, sulfation, acetylation, and sulfoxidation.[22] These now water-soluble substances can be excreted in stool, urine, or sweat or as water vapor through the lungs.

In phase three, the now ready for excretion estradiol–glucuronic acid molecule previously discussed is eliminated through the bile into the intestines. This molecule is cleaved in the dysbiotic gut by elevated amounts of the enzyme beta-glucuronidase, which is produced by imbalanced gut bacteria. This allows estradiol to be reabsorbed into the circulation.

Phase one and phase two detoxification errors cannot be determined by conventional aspartate aminotransferase and alanine aminotransferase (AST/ALT liver function tests) enzyme levels, which are indicators only of hepatocyte breakdown (see Chapter 106). More integrative and functional assessments of detoxification can be made through organic acid testing or functional detoxification tests that evaluate the phase one cytochrome P450 enzyme system and phase two conjugation factors. Estrogen metabolites and their intermediaries consist of catechol (hydroxy) estrogens and methyl-estrogens. The anticarcinogenic estrogen modulator 2-hydroxyestrone (2OH-E_1) comes from naturally produced ovarian estrogens; high levels of this substance because 2-methoxyestrone reduce the risk for breast cancer. Higher amounts of 4-hydroxyestrone (4OH-E_1) occur with metabolism of conjugated estrogens (Premarin) to form DNA-damaging quinones.

Recent studies confirm that the 2-methoxyestrogens are protective against hormone-dependent cancers while the 4- and 16-hydroxyestrogens are most carcinogenic.[23]

Epigallocatechin gallate (the main polyphenol in green tea) and other antioxidants, such as vitamins A, C, and E; selenium; N-acetylcysteine; and lipoic acid, convert damaging quinones into mercapturates. This process occurs through the production of glutathione. The 16alpha-hydroxyestrone (16OH-E_1) forms a very strong bond with the estrogen receptor, is a strong estrogen, and has carcinogenic potential. These estrogen metabolites are not all good or bad. Like everything else in nature, they need to be in balance.

Appropriate levels of 16alpha-hydroxyestrone support good bone density.[24] The ratio of the three hydroxyestrogens and their methylated end products, which can be measured in urine or blood (Genova Diagnostics), can help evaluate risk in estrogen dominance conditions. In menstruating women, the ratio of 2OH-E_1 to 16OH-E_1 should be evaluated during the luteal (late) phase of the cycle. The following factors increase either this ratio or the level of 2OH-E_1:

- A diet rich in cooked cruciferous vegetables (broccoli, Brussels sprouts, kale, cabbage, cauliflower, etc.)
- Indole-3-carbinol (I-3-C) from cruciferous vegetables (broccoli, Brussels sprouts, cabbage, kale): 200–800 mg/day
- Diindolylmethane (I-3-C activated by stomach acid), used alone or in conjunction with I-3-C
- Epigallocatechin gallate (green tea polyphenol)
- Isoflavones, including soy, flaxseed, and kudzu[25]
- Omega-3 fatty acids
- Vigorous exercise, a minimum of 30 minutes three times/week

The ratio of 2OH-E_1 to 16OH-E_1 can be reduced, with an increased proportion of 16OH-E_1, by the following conditions:

- Obesity
- Hypothyroidism
- Xenoestrogens: any estrogenic substances, including dioxins and polychlorinated biphenyls
- Cimetidine (Tagamet) and other drugs that interfere with the cytochrome P450 system[26]
- Estriol: Although in most people, estriol is a metabolic end product, concern exists that as a stereoisomer it can revert to the 16alphaOH-E_1 from which it was formed; this is more of a concern when estriol is prescribed as part of a bioidentical hormone replacement therapy program. Regular monitoring of hormone levels can prevent problems from these imbalances.

Most of the studies of hormone imbalance and fibroid tumors of the uterus have concerned themselves with estrogen dominance, although mifepristone studies create some controversy and doubt.[28] Mifepristone is also known as RU-486, the "abortion pill." It functions as a progesterone receptor antagonist. Long-term use of mifepristone has been associated with fibroid regression.[28] As a progesterone receptor antagonist, mifepristone's action would suggest that progesterone also stimulates fibroid growth. The answer may not be that simple because progesterone also increases blood vessel support in the endometrium in anticipation of a fertilized egg. My opinion is that some fibroids may take advantage of the increased progesterone-supported blood supply and increase in size because of it. Studies also show that there are two isoforms of progesterone receptors: A and B (PRA and PRB). If PRA is stimulated, there will be increased inflammation. Stimulating PRB will reduce inflammation.[29]

The negative effects associated with long-term mifepristone use are bone loss and endometrial hyperplasia, conditions indicating that more complicated mechanisms concerning PRA and PRB are at work.

Determining Whether a Fibroid Has Malignant Potential

The malignant potential (sarcomatous change) of fibroids or leiomyomata is less than 1%. Recent complications of minimally invasive surgery for fibroid tumors have created controversy related to the malignant fibroid and the process of intraabdominal morcellation of the fibroids.

The American College of Obstetricians and Gynecologists (ACOG) estimates of malignant fibroids are approximately 1/325 fibroid tumors. The morcellation procedure allows for removal of large fibroids through small incisions, but it does increase the risk for spreading malignant cells throughout the abdominal cavity. The results of this can be disastrous, causing a rapidly growing, widely disseminated malignant sarcoma.[31,32]

Whether a fibroid changes from benign to malignant or is malignant to begin with is not well established. One sign that can indicate a malignant fibroid or leiomyosarcoma is rapid growth. Unfortunately, the only conventional way to confirm malignancy is to remove the fibroid and examine a sample for the number of mitotic events per high-power field; more than 20 mitoses per high-power field would indicate a sarcoma. Table 58.2 lists tests that should be considered in evaluating a patient with fibroid tumors of the uterus.

INTEGRATIVE THERAPY

Nutrition

The patient should begin a hormone-balancing diet that involves foods with low inflammation effects, low acidity, and low glycemic load.

Foods That Increase Estrogen Dominance

Acidic and inflammatory foods, such as commercial red meats, poultry, and dairy products, are sources of arachidonic acid, which increases inflammatory prostaglandins and other inflammatory mediators that help to support fibroid growth through the process of angiogenesis. Avoiding commercial meat products also reduces exposure to added hormones and pesticide residues in these products.[33] Small amounts of organic grass–fed meats can be added back as inflammation subsides (see Chapter 88).

Sweets and other foods with a high glycemic index are potentially stressful and can increase insulin resistance, increase estrogen dominance, and support fibroid growth. Eating a breakfast that contains good-quality protein, fats, and carbohydrates in combination is imperative to avoid hypoglycemic stress–induced cortisol and norepinephrine elevations, which deplete lean muscle and increase the tendency for insulin resistance through gluconeogenesis (see Chapter 87).

Gluten grains, especially wheat, rye, barley, and spelt, contain genetically engineered gluten that is much stronger than that found in the more ancient gluten grains such as spelt. These newer grains can increase estrogens by inhibition of the cytochrome P450 3A4 enzyme system and can also affect thyroid hormones. Because all the wheat in this country is now genetically modified to be glyphosate ready (Roundup) and all the corn and soy in this country are now genetically modified to be 2,4-D-ready (a component of Agent Orange), it would be best to avoid these when trying to lower inflammation.[34]

Alcohol is not a problem if it is consumed in moderation. Studies show that women consuming more than five alcoholic drinks per week have a higher risk for breast cancer. This increase probably results from the effect of alcohol on the detoxification of estrogens. Organic coffee in moderation (1–2 cups per day) is also safe. Artificial ingredients, colorings, flavorings, and preservatives should be eliminated. Margarines and other sources of trans-fatty acids and hydrogenated oils are also unhealthy and must be avoided.

TABLE 58.2	Tests to Consider for Evaluation of a Patient With Fibroid Tumors of the Uterus
25-Hydroxyvitamin D measurement*	Low levels increase fibroid growth by several mechanisms (see text)
Vitamin A measurement†	Low levels have been shown to increase menorrhagia
Iron or total iron-binding capacity measurement, ferritin measurement	Low iron stores reduce myometrial contractility and increase menstrual blood loss
Progesterone/estradiol ratio (100–300:1) Luteal phase progesterone measurement	Low luteal phase progesterone level supports estrogen dominance and fibroid growth
Thyroid function testing	Hypothyroidism is associated with menstrual dysfunction
MTHFR polymorphism	35% weakness in methylation, increased estrogen dominance
Comprehensive digestive stool analysis	Intestinal dysbiosis is a cause of estrogen dominance through several mechanisms (see text)
Phase one and phase two detoxification evaluation	Unhealthy estrogen metabolism contributes to estrogen dominance
Transvaginal and abdominal ultrasonography	To determine the sizes and locations of fibroids and rule out ovarian tumors
Testing for celiac disease (antigliadin antibodies)	Gluten grain sensitivity is common in fibroid tumor sufferers and can lead to further estrogen dominance

*Data from Chiu KC, Chu A, Vay LWG, et al. Hypovitaminosis D is associated with insulin resistance and beta cell dysfunction. *Am J Clin Nutr.* 2004;79:820–825.
†Data from Lithgow DM, Politzer WM. Vitamin A in the treatment of menorrhagia. *S Afr Med J.* 1977;51:191–199.

Foods That Reduce Estrogen Dominance

Deep sea, cold-water fish, such as wild Pacific salmon, sardines, mackerel, and cod, have large quantities of omega-3 oils (eicosapentaenoic acid [EPA] and docosahexaenoic acid [DHA]).[35] Because heavy metals, such as mercury, contribute to estrogen dominance, I recommend eating fish with lower levels of mercury. These are fish at the lower end of the food chain. The larger game fish, such as swordfish, tuna, and bass, concentrate the contaminants from eating smaller fish. Krill, small crustaceans, are a good source of noncontaminated EPA and DHA. Algae sources of DHA are also available.

Seeds and nuts, especially flaxseed, hemp seed, and chia seed, contain isoflavones.[36] These are hormone-balancing. I recommend 2–4 tablespoons per day added to a yellow pea-rice protein powder shake first thing in the morning. Coconut oil (1 tbsp) would be another good addition to this morning shake.

Other seeds and nuts, such as pumpkin seeds, sunflower seeds, and walnuts, are also good sources of omega-3 oils.[37]

Cooked cruciferous vegetables, such as broccoli, Brussels sprouts, cabbage, and cauliflower, support healthy estrogen metabolism (Fig. 58.2). Legumes, such as adzuki beans, peas, lentils, and edamame, all have hormone-modulating flavonoids and can safely be eaten.[38]

> A head of cabbage contains approximately 1200 mg of I-3-C. Eating one-fourth of a cabbage daily would provide 300 mg of I-3-C daily. Cabbage should be cooked and not raw to avoid goitrogens.

I have been consistently impressed by the reduction of symptoms related to estrogen dominance by the elimination of milk casein, high-glycemic index carbohydrates, and gluten grains. The symptoms that seem to be most affected are gastrointestinal symptoms, headache, dermatologic rashes, fatigue, insomnia, and mood issues.

Lifestyle

Exercise

Aerobic exercise consumes oxygen and helps "burn" carbohydrates (glucose). Oxygen-consuming exercises are exemplified by running, fast walking, and swimming. Because carbohydrates are consumed during aerobic exercise, this form of exercise is associated with improvements in insulin resistance and sugar use.

Anaerobic exercise classically uses fats (triglycerides) as an energy source. Weight trainers consume medium-chain triglycerides during their workouts to enhance energy and "fat burning." Weight training also helps stabilize hormones such as growth hormone and testosterone. Because fat cells (adipocytes) are hormone factories that produce inflammatory mediators and estrone, limiting adipose tissue also reduces estrogen dominance. A regimen of 30 minutes of regular exercise three times per week has also been shown to lower the incidences of breast and colon cancer.

Botanicals

Botanical therapies can be very useful in reducing fibroid growth and decreasing fibroid symptoms.[39] Recent studies indicate that curcumin from the spice turmeric and green tea extracts are effective in reducing angiogenesis by supporting peroxisome proliferator–activated receptor (PPAR) activation.[40]

Botanicals for Liver and Detoxification Support

Healthy estrogen metabolism must be reestablished to reverse estrogen dominance. By obtaining functional liver detoxification studies performed by laboratories such as Genova Diagnostics and Doctor's Data, the clinician can determine in which specific aspects of the detoxification pathway the patient is lacking and provide the appropriate nutritional support. Many botanicals and nutraceuticals can be helpful in restoring and maintaining healthy detoxification.

Epigallocatechin Gallate from Green Tea

Epigallocatechin gallate reduces the DNA-damaging effects of 4OH-E$_1$. It may also be an antiangiogenesis factor.

> **DOSAGE**
>
> The dose is 600 mg two times/day with 60% polyphenols.
>
> **PRECAUTIONS**
>
> These agents can cause insomnia if caffeine is consumed in large amounts.

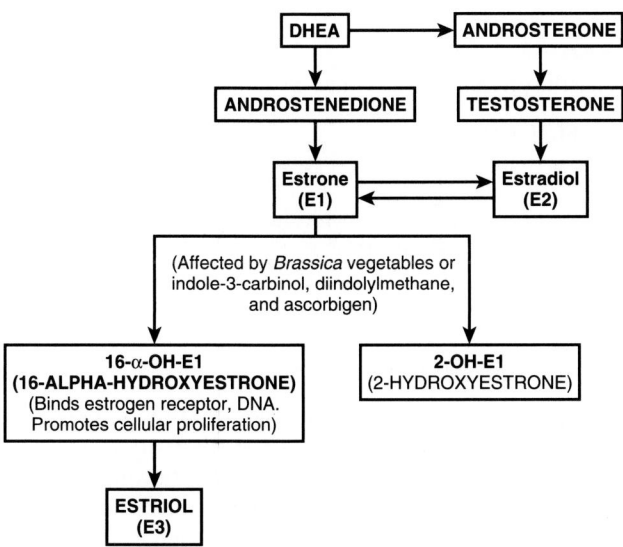

METABOLISM OF SELECTED ESTROGENS

FIG. 58.2 ■ Metabolism of selected estrogens. DHEA, dehydroepiandrosterone.

Indole-3-Carbinol or the Stomach-Activated Diindolylmethane

I-3-C increases the production of estrogen-modulating $2OH\text{-}E_1$.[41]

> **DOSAGE**
> The dose is 200–400 mg/day.
>
> **PRECAUTIONS**
> I-3-C is generally free of side effects.

Milk Thistle (Silybum marianum)

Milk thistle is a general liver antioxidant that supports healthy detoxification and estrogen metabolism.

> **DOSAGE**
> The dose is 280–420 mg of milk thistle per day standardized to 70%–80% silymarin content.
>
> **PRECAUTIONS**
> This agent is virtually devoid of negative effects.

Botanicals to Modulate Pelvic Lymphatic Drainage

These botanical formulas are used in combination to modulate pelvic lymphatic drainage. Scudder's alterative (a combination herbal product containing corydalis, alder root, mayapple root, figwort, and yellow dock) modulates cellular metabolism. Echinacea/red root compound modulates toxin elimination, immune system, and inflammatory mediators.

> **DOSAGE**
> The dose is 30 drops of Scudder's alterative combined with echinacea/red root compound as a tea twice/day for 3 months. This is followed by 2 weeks without this treatment.
>
> **PRECAUTIONS**
> This combination of formulas has no known negative effects.
>   Anecdotally, the technique of dry skin brushing has also been used to support healthy lymphatic drainage.

Botanical Therapies for Specific Symptoms

Menorrhagia

Heavy menstrual bleeding (menorrhagia) due to fibroids is the symptom that brings most women to the operating room. Menorrhagia is defined as blood loss of more than 80 mL per menses. Controlling heavy bleeding, or menorrhagia, is probably the most important first step in the fibroid healing program. Severe iron deficiency anemia is one of the most common symptoms of problematic fibroids and a main reason for surgery. Combinations of botanicals that act differently within the uterus can be very effective in reducing blood loss and keeping women out of the operating room. Use of a combination of the following herbal types can significantly reduce menstrual bleeding.

Uterotonics: these include red raspberry, false unicorn root, and black cohosh.
Astringents: these include yarrow, lady's mantle, beth root, and cinnamon.
Oxytocics: I have only used shepherd's purse for its oxytocic (contracting) effect. It has a long history of use among midwives to help control postpartum bleeding.

These botanicals are also used in combination. A combination botanical preparation consisting of tinctures of a tonic such as red raspberry and an astringent such as yarrow can be used at a dose of 30 drops each twice a day for 2 weeks before the period. This protocol supports healthy uterine contractions during menses. The result is a more normal menstrual flow and nonspasmodic uterine contractions. When bleeding begins, add 30 drops of an oxytocic tincture such as shepherd's purse. The combination of all three herbal tinctures can be taken every 30 minutes for up to six doses. No scientific reason exists for using six doses as an arbitrary cutoff. I believe that if the patient is still hemorrhaging after 3 hours of using these herbs, something else needs to be considered. However, this protocol has been extremely useful in reducing menorrhagia and reversing iron deficiency anemia. Other herbs in the same categories can be substituted if the patient has a reaction to one of the herbs or if the effect is less than desired. Several botanical companies such as Gaia and Herbpharm create standardized herbal tinctures (see Key Web Resources, later).

> **DOSAGE**
> See the preceding protocol.
>
> **PRECAUTIONS**
> These herbs have minor gastrointestinal effects. Yarrow rarely causes rash or sun sensitivity. Shepherd's purse in large doses may interfere with thyroid function. Follow-up with thyroid function testing is suggested.

Antiinflammatory Botanicals

Inflammatory prostanoids, cytokines, and leukotrienes increase the cellular growth factors that support vascularization and neoangiogenesis of the fibroid. Specific botanicals can reduce this inflammation. Botanicals are often found in combination products, such as those containing *Boswellia* (400 mg), ginger (200 mg), turmeric (300 mg), and cayenne (50 mg) in every two tablets.

DOSAGE

One to two tablets are taken three times/day. The patient may take one to two tablets every 2 hours as needed.

PRECAUTIONS

Taking such a combination product on an empty stomach can cause abdominal pain in sensitive individuals. These botanicals can be taken with food.

Systemic Enzymes

Elimination of excessive inflammation with potent (serratiopeptidase-containing) systemic enzyme formulations may reduce the size of fibroids by limiting vascularization of fibroids and by enzymatic myolysis of the fibroid.[44] Such systemic enzymes are Neprinol, Wobenzym, Vitalzyme, and bromelain (from pineapple stems).[45] Other preparations of proteases can also be used. Neprinol[46] has the following ingredients: SEBkinase, Peptizyme SP, serratiopeptidase, lipase, protease, amla, papain, NattoSEB, nattokinase, bromelain, rutin, coenzyme Q10, and magnesium.

DOSAGE

These enzyme formulations should be taken on an empty stomach to avoid action on food rather than on the protein of the fibroid. The dose is gradually built up from one tablet three times/day to 15 tablets per day in divided doses.

PRECAUTIONS

As with any antiinflammatory agent taken on an empty stomach, the clinician must caution the patient about stomach pain. Such enzyme preparations must be used with caution in patients with gastritis and a history of gastric ulcer, as well as in patients who take blood thinners.

Antiangiogenesis Factors

The work by Judah Folkman[14] in cancer therapy illustrates the effect of antiangiogenesis on reducing tumor growth. The convolvulus product and other antiangiogenesis factors are used to reduce blood flow to the fibroids.[47] *Convolvulus arvensis* (bindweed) works as an antiangiogenesis factor.[48] Green tea catechins and polyphenols also have antiangiogenic effects.

DOSAGE

The dose of *Convolvulus arvensis* (bindweed) is two tablets three times/day, slowly increased from one tablet twice/day.

PRECAUTIONS

Headaches are a side effect if the dosage is increased too rapidly. Increase slowly to avoid headaches.

Nutraceuticals

Vitamin C and the Citrus Bioflavonoids (Rutin and Hesperidin)

Vitamin C strengthens capillary desmosomes and can also be helpful in reducing menorrhagia.[49] Citrus bioflavonoids such as rutin and hesperidin enhance this vitamin C effect and are also mildly estrogenic, and as such, can have a tonic effect by reducing the effects of estrogen dominance.

DOSAGE

The dose is 1000–2000 mg/day, but the dosage can be increased up to 75% of bowel tolerance.

PRECAUTIONS

Vitamin C has been known to cause diarrhea. This is what has been referred to as *bowel tolerance*. Reducing the dosage to 75% of the amount that causes diarrhea may be the most appropriate individualized approach. Some question exists about the use of vitamin C in patients with a history of kidney stones.

B Vitamins

Vitamins B_1, B_2, B_3, B_5, and B_6 are important for sugar, fat, and neurotransmitter metabolism, hormone balance, and healthy cortisol production from the adrenal glands.[50] Vitamin B_3 in the form of niacinamide is also a potent antiinflammatory agent. Niacin can be used to reduce menstrual cramping often associated with fibroids.[51] Other B vitamins, such as choline and inositol, support healthy liver function. Vitamins B_2, B_6, B_{12}, and folic acid support the process of methylation, which is necessary for healthy hormone metabolism and for DNA repair. Vitamins B_5 and B_6 also support adrenal function, which is important in healthy hormone balance.

DOSAGE

A 50-mg B-complex vitamin can supply basic vitamin B needs. Separate additional B vitamins may be necessary. The recommended dose of vitamin B_{12} is 2000 units/day.

The dose of folic acid is 800 mcg or more per day. Doses up to 5–10 mg/day have been used for cervical dysplasias. Approximately 35% of the population is estimated to have a mutation of the *MTHFR* gene that decreases their ability to methylate. Most laboratories check for the *MTHFR* C677T and the A1298C gene mutations. I recommend this test, and if a patient is heterozygous or homozygous for the mutations, supplementation, at least in part, with methylfolate or methylcobalamin seems wise. A reasonable dose of methylfolic acid is 5 mg/day.

Methylcobalamin doses are in the 2000–5000 mcg/day range and are best as intramuscular (IM) injections or buccal lozenges.

PRECAUTIONS

When high doses of folic acid are used, attention must be taken to supplying vitamin B_{12} in addition to avoid masking the signs of pernicious anemia. Peripheral neuropathies have been reported with vitamin B_6 dosages larger than 200 mg/day. Practicing caution when dosing and educating patients to report any tingling in their fingers and toes are important.

For treatment of menstrual cramps, consider having the patient take niacin, 100 mg twice/day throughout the month, then 100 mg every 2 hours while having cramps.

Vitamin D

Vitamin D is very important for the healthy functioning of every cell in the body. Because of fear of sun exposure and resultant skin cancer, most people use ultraviolet-B–blocking, sun protective factor (SPF) 30 or higher sunblock.[52] This situation has created almost an epidemic of low levels of vitamin D. Measuring 25-hydroxyvitamin D levels and restoring them to at least 40 ng/dL are imperative. Investigators have estimated that 32 ng/dL will be required to prevent rickets in children. Restoration of vitamin D levels can be accomplished by using 50,000 units/week of vitamin D_2 for 12 weeks and then reassessing. Supply 600 mg/day of calcium in supplements to a patient being treated with vitamin D.[53]

DOSAGE

If the 25-hydroxyvitamin D blood level is low, give 50,000 units of vitamin D_2 once a week for 12 weeks; then recheck the 25-hydroxyvitamin D level.

PRECAUTIONS

As with any fat-soluble vitamin, excessive amounts of vitamin D can be toxic. Measuring blood levels again after 12 weeks of supplementation is necessary. Supplying at least 600 mg/day of calcium in the diet and 600 mg as a supplement can prevent loss of calcium from bone. Evaluation of parathyroid hormone levels screens for hyperparathyroidism and is important before supplementing. Evidence indicates that supplementation with the other fat-soluble vitamins A, E, and K may be necessary for optimal absorption.

It has been shown in many studies that vitamin K_2 (menatetrenone) either as the MK-7 (recommended dose is 45 mcg/day) or the MK-4 (recommended dose is 45 mg/day) form aids vitamin D_3 in supporting calcium mineralization of bones. It makes good sense to use a vitamin D_3 supplement that also includes vitamin K_2.[54]

Calcium D Glucarate

Calcium D glucarate reduces the activity of the enzyme beta-glucuronidase, which is produced in patients with intestinal dysbiosis. This enzyme, which is produced by dysbiotic intestinal bacteria, cleaves the glucuronic acid–estrogen bond on estrogens meant for excretion in the stool and instead reabsorbs the estrogens back into the circulation. By the action of beta-glucuronidase, estrogen dominance increases and adds more stress to the already stressed detoxification system.[55]

DOSAGE

The dose is 500 mg twice/day.

PRECAUTIONS

No precautions are reported.

Iron

Women with fibroids tend to have heavy menses, or menorrhagia, which is defined as losing more than 80 mL of blood during menstruation. This greater iron loss associated with the blood loss sets up a vicious circle.[56] Low iron levels cause weak myometrial muscle cell contraction thus contributing to more menstrual blood loss. Evaluation and treatment of low iron stores by measurement of iron levels, total iron-binding capacity, and serum ferritin levels help guide restoration of iron levels and maintain healthy myometrial contractility. A boggy, noncontractile uterus bleeds more than a healthy, iron-rich, well-toned uterus.

DOSAGE

The dose is 325 mg/day of ferrous sulfate or its equivalent. Double doses may be needed during menses.

PRECAUTIONS

Measuring serum iron levels during supplementation prevents iron overload. Some iron formulas can be constipating.

Selenium

Selenium is a potent antioxidant that supports the action of vitamin E and other antioxidants. It also is used in the production of the antioxidant glutathione. Selenium is necessary for the formation of thyroid hormones.

DOSAGES

The dose is 200–500 mcg/day.

PRECAUTIONS

Dosages exceeding 1000 mcg/day can precipitate skin and nail changes. "Garlic breath" may be an early sign of too much selenium.

Magnesium and Zinc

Important for hormone support, magnesium and zinc are responsible for catalyzing approximately 500 different reactions in the body. These minerals are estimated to be deficient in 50%–75% of the population. One theory for the craving of chocolate in the premenstrual period is the need for magnesium[55]; chocolate is rich in this mineral.

DOSAGES

The dose of magnesium is 400–600 mg/day, and the dose of zinc is 15–30 mg/day.

PRECAUTIONS

Taking too much magnesium can increase diarrhea. Magnesium can also compete with calcium for absorption; if this problem is suspected, magnesium should be taken separately from calcium. Zinc may interfere with copper absorption, and supplementation requires that 2 mg copper be added to the protocol. Red blood cell levels should be checked.

Women who crave chocolate (a rich source of magnesium) before their period may benefit from magnesium replacement therapy.

Omega-3 Fatty Acids (Eicosapentaenoic Acid and Docosahexaenoic Acid)

The omega-3 essential fatty acids (EPA and DHA) help maintain the fluidity of all cell membranes, reduce inflammatory cytokines and leukotrienes, and are building blocks for hormones. These essential fatty acids are not synthesized by the body and must therefore be consumed.

DOSAGE

The dose is 3–6 g/day of EPA and DHA (fish oil).

PRECAUTIONS

Caution is recommended when prescribing more than 3–4 g/day of omega-3 acids to diabetic patients. Reports have noted elevations of blood glucose. Also use caution with patients on blood thinners.

Mind–Body Therapy

Encourage patients to create emotional flexibility by "staying in the moment." Stretching and yoga exercises not only help maintain physical flexibility but also promote emotional flexibility. When we live in the present moment,[57] we can modulate stress effects from worrying about a possible future that may never come and from fretting about the past that cannot be changed. This chronic stress, which raises cortisol levels and lowers dehydroepiandrosterone (DHEA) levels, contributes to estrogen dominance by "stealing" or shunting progesterone and pregnenolone to produce more cortisol.

Body awareness exercises, such as tai chi and qi gong, and meditation and visualization exercises help to reduce blood flow to fibroids and lessen their impact and growth. Moving and other meditation exercises help to mobilize stagnated energy, as do acupuncture, deep tissue massage, craniosacral work, and psychotherapeutic techniques such as bioenergetics.

Exercise of all kinds has been shown to reduce the harmful effects of stress. Meditation also helps reduce cortisol levels.[58] Techniques that focus the chakras or energy centers that correspond to anatomical nerve plexuses and glands of the endocrine system help to promote balance. One such technique is Freeze Frame, developed by the HeartMath Institute: the patient is taught to focus on heart energy or the fourth chakra while "breathing in through the energy of the heart." Thoughts that are stressful are not internalized but are instead blown out while exhaling. This is a simple but powerful way of staying in the moment and is effective in reducing the inflammatory effects of stress on the body (see Chapter 96).

Journaling is a technique used for ridding the body of stored emotional energy.[59] Removing this stagnating energy is like cleaning out the closet and getting rid of all the clutter in your life. Energy moves again. This might be similar to acupuncture's effects on "needling the meridians."

While meditating and performing visualization exercises, the patient is instructed to be aware of second chakra issues—relationships, creative blocks, and abuse issues. Journaling has been shown to help reduce the negative effects of these stored emotions (see Chapter 98).

Another powerful technique that supports meditation and stress reduction and thereby alleviates symptoms of fibroids and reduces their growth is visualization of the desired results and the intent of bringing healing energy into the area to be healed. The Freeze Frame technique allows for a new perspective about the fibroid. It is no longer loathed or feared. Instead, feelings of gratitude are expressed as the message of the fibroid, an imbalance of some kind, has been received and now the fibroid can "leave."

Pharmaceuticals: Gonadotropin Receptor Agonists

The following GnRH receptor agonists may be used.

Leuprolide Acetate

Leuprolide acetate (Lupron) is used to shrink fibroids before surgery to enable easier tumor removal.[60] This drug can effect a 30%–60% reduction in fibroid size. Surgeons sometimes complain that using leuprolide decreases their ability to enucleate fibroids easily during myomectomy.

DOSAGE

The dose is 3.75–7.5 mg/month that is intramuscularly administered for 1–6 months.

PRECAUTIONS

Unfortunately, if nothing else is done to prevent regrowth, many fibroids rapidly achieve the same sizes as they were before treatment. This agent causes chemical castration, menopausal symptoms, and osteoporosis.

Danazol

Danazol (Danocrine), which suppresses LH and FSH, can also be used to shrink fibroids.

DOSAGE

The dose is 600–800 mg/day.

PRECAUTIONS

Precautions are the same as those listed for leuprolide acetate, but they are more intense.

Agents for Menorrhagia Associated With Fibroids

Norethindrone Acetate

Norethindrone acetate is used for menorrhagia associated with fibroids.

> **DOSAGE**
>
> A dose of 5–15 mg/day has been effective in slowing bleeding.
>
> **PRECAUTIONS**
>
> The risks for blood clots, fluid retention, breast tenderness, nausea, insomnia, and depression are increased.

Progesterone-Containing Intrauterine Devices

Studies have shown that progesterone-containing intrauterine devices (Mirena, Skyla, Progestasert) reduce menstrual flow.[61]

> **PRECAUTIONS**
>
> An intrauterine device may be difficult to insert in a woman who has not experienced vaginal delivery, and it may not be effective for a submucous fibroid.

Birth Control Pills

Birth control pills have been shown to reduce menstrual flow.

> **DOSAGE**
>
> Either daily dosing or the newer 3-month (seasonal) dosing is effective.
>
> **PRECAUTIONS**
>
> All the precautions considered when the pill is prescribed for contraception are relevant here.

Nonsteroidal Antiinflammatory Drugs

Studies have shown that nonsteroidal antiinflammatory drugs (NSAIDs), such as ibuprofen and naproxen (Aleve), reduce menorrhagia by 20%–50%.

> **DOSAGE**
>
> The dose of naproxen is one to two 220-mg tablets or capsules every 12 hours. The dose of ibuprofen is 400 mg every 4–6 hours.
>
> **PRECAUTIONS**
>
> All NSAIDs can increase gastric discomfort and the risk for gastrointestinal bleeding.

Tranexamic Acid (an Antifibrinolytic Agent)

Tranexamic acid (TA; Lysteda) is a U.S. Food and Drug Administration (FDA)–approved medication for menorrhagia. TA is an antifibrinolytic agent such as Amicar, which is used in dental procedures to prevent bleeding after dental procedures. It is very effective at 1300 mg three times/day, during days of heavy bleeding only, in slowing menstrual flow by prevention of clot breakdown. This leads to the theoretical concern of peripheral thrombosis. In almost 30 years of using TA, I have not seen any negative effects other than the occasional stomachache.

> **DOSAGE**
>
> A dose of 650 mg three times daily during menses.
>
> **PRECAUTIONS**
>
> The most common side effects include headache and sinus congestion.

Natural Hormones

Dehydroepiandrosterone

DHEA reduces IL-6, a potent inflammatory cytokine that can promote the production of estrogens in the body. DHEA stimulates the PPAR-gamma receptor thus reducing inflammation, increasing insulin sensitivity, and reducing estrogen levels by maintaining healthy sugar metabolism and normal insulin levels. It also helps balance the effects of stress on the body by being in equilibrium with cortisol.

> **DOSAGE**
>
> The dose of DHEA is 5–10 mg once or twice/day. The dose of 7-keto DHEA is 25–50 mg/day.
>
> **PRECAUTIONS**
>
> DHEA can convert to estradiol. Use of the 7-keto form may obviate this issue. Following hormone levels is always necessary when supplementing.

Surgical Treatment

The conventional approach to dealing with uterine fibroids remains largely surgical.[1] Total abdominal hysterectomy—removal of the uterus with the cervix, ovaries, and fallopian tubes—is the most common procedure recommended. Subtotal procedures are also performed. These procedures may leave the cervix (supracervical hysterectomy) or the ovaries and fallopian tubes. Hysterectomy can also be performed by a vaginal or laparoscopic route. Robotic-assisted laparoscopies are now performed.

Hysterectomy and other invasive procedures are not without consequences. Postoperative recovery can take up to 4–6 weeks. Infectious complications can affect 10% of women. Major injuries to the bladder, bowel, ovaries, and ureters happen approximately 1% of the time.

Myomectomy involves removal of the fibroid only, thereby preserving the uterus. Myomectomy can also be performed abdominally or laparoscopically.

These "mini-surgeries" have evolved into robotically assisted operations. These high-tech surgeries allow for very large fibroids to be removed through small and easily healed abdominal incisions.

The morcellation (removing in small pieces) technique that allows for this process to be successful has recently been called into question because of its effect in disseminating previously unknown leiomyosarcoma (malignant fibroid). Performing the procedure within an intraabdominal bag may be an answer, but will make a difficult procedure more difficult.[65]

Myolysis techniques require the use of an energy source, which is applied to the fibroid through various instrumentation methods. The energy used may be ultrasound, laser, or electrical. The interior of the fibroid is destroyed, and the fibroid shrinks. The U.S. FDA has approved a myolysis[66] procedure using magnetic resonance imaging guidance and ultrasound as an energy source (ExAblate).

Uterine artery embolization is another procedure that effectively reduces blood flow to the fibroid and hastens shrinkage. Inert polyvinyl alcohol particles are placed in the uterine artery through an artery in the upper thigh.

Except for total hysterectomy, all these procedures have one thing in common: the fibroids grow back. Complications of the procedures include infections, pain, and injuries to major organs in the area, such as the ureters, bowel, and bladder.

Other Therapies to Consider

Castor Oil Packs

Castor oil packs are hot packs made with wool flannel and hexane-free castor oil. Evidence suggests that they work through the lymphatic system and reduce inflammation. The castor oil pack is applied over the fibroid for 20–60 minutes per session. This device is a very effective meditation and visualization tool. The patient meditates on her uterus and visualizes the fibroid shrinking. She also visualizes the blood supply to the fibroids as pipes with turnoff valves, and while doing the meditation, visualizes turning off the valves thus shutting down the blood supply to the fibroids. The spiritual aspects of healing come into play here.[67]

Through meditation and visualizing the healing of their fibroids, patients are instructed to be aware of any thoughts, feelings, or memories that can be associated with stagnation of second chakra energy and subsequent growth of the fibroid. The classic second chakra issues include relationship issues, not only with people but also with jobs, money, control, and the outside world. Creativity issues may also be expressed here. Abuse issues may come up also and can be related to physical, emotional, or sexual abuse. The idea is to remove these blockages to the healthy flow of energy from the pelvis, where they are creating stagnation and the growth of the fibroid. The release of these issues can be ritualized by having the patient journal everything that comes up and then put the pages into a bowl and burn them—letting them go.

Acupuncture and Deep Pelvic Massage

Acupuncture and deep pelvic massage (Mayan massage is one technique) are other ways of moving or restoring pelvic energy. These modalities are all complementary with the other approaches presented here.

Homeopathy

The following homeopathic remedies can be effective in reducing symptoms, as specified:
- *Aurum muriaticum*: to reduce the size of fibroids
- Belladonna: for heavy, red bleeding
- *Hydrastinum muriaticum*: for large anterior wall fibroids with bladder symptoms
- Ignatia: for grief associated with fibroids
- Medorrhinum 200C: fibroids; for benign tumors
- Phosphorus 6C, 200C: for bright red bleeding with no clots
- Sabina: for bright red bleeding with clots and for severe cramps
- Secale: for almost black blood and for profuse bleeding
- Sepia: for pressure and anger
- Silicea 6C: for heavy bleeding; for cold, thin, and fatigued patients
- Thlaspi bursa pastoris 6C (shepherd's purse): for frequent, heavy, dark bleeding
  See Chapter 115.

PREVENTION PRESCRIPTION

- Consume a hormone-balancing, vegetarian-style, low saturated fat diet, including organic non-genetically modified soy, green tea, ground flaxseed, omega-3 fatty acid, and cruciferous vegetables.
- Follow a moderate exercise program (4–5 hours/week).
- Reduce xenobiotic (hormone-like) exposures such as pesticides, atrazine (herbicide), and polycyclic aromatic hydrocarbons (found in diesel exhaust), and avoid petroleum-based cosmetics.

- Maintain an appropriate weight.
- Practice stress modification techniques.
- Take a high-potency multivitamin and multimineral supplement.
- Foster healthy digestion and elimination.
- Maintain healthy relationships and have a sense of purpose in life.

THERAPEUTIC REVIEW

This integrative, holistic approach to healing fibroid tumors of the uterus can avoid some of the invasive therapies offered. It is effective in reducing the symptoms associated with these benign tumors. I ask patients to commit to a 3-month trial period, during which they will do as much of the protocol as possible.

At the end of these first 3–4 months, we assess symptoms, such as menorrhagia and dysmenorrhea, and any growth or shrinkage of the fibroids. The protocol is considered successful if the patient perceives a reduction in symptoms and no further fibroid growth has occurred. We then continue the program for 3–4 month periods while continuing to monitor symptoms and uterine size. If at any time symptoms recur or worsen or the fibroids begin to grow, other more aggressive measures must be considered, including surgery.

LIFESTYLE

* Maintain an appropriate weight.
* Avoid xenoestrogens (dioxins, polychlorinated biphenyls) by eating local, in-season, and organic foods as much as possible.
* Obtain regular aerobic exercise.

NUTRITION

* Follow a hormone-balancing diet. The patient should consume a diet that reduces inflammation, acidity, and hormone, pesticide, and antibiotic residues; these foods may encourage the growth of fibroids. High glycemic index foods similarly should be avoided because of their effects on insulin and sex hormones. Gluten grains that increase estrogens through action of the phase one cytochrome P450 enzyme 3A4 must be limited. There is evidence that fibroid cells concentrate the cytochrome P450 enzyme 1B1. The 1B1 enzyme converts estrogens into the potentially carcinogenic 4-OH estrogens. This may become another therapeutic target for nonsurgical treatment.
* The patient should add foods that will be hormone-balancing, such as non-genetically modified organic soy and flaxseed. She should approximate the Asian diet, with 30–70 mg/day of isoflavones (genistein and daidzein) and 2 tablespoons of ground flaxseed per day. Omega-3 fatty acids, found in foods such as wild Pacific salmon and sardines, should be consumed at approximately 2–4 g/day and are also antiinflammatory.
* Reduce intake of unhealthy saturated fats and trans-fatty acids (feedlot red meat, dairy, fried foods).
* Increase intake of omega-3 fatty acids (vegetables, nuts, flaxseed, cold-water fish).
* Eat a low glycemic index diet.
* Avoid gluten as much as possible and completely if gluten sensitive.
* Eat cooked cruciferous vegetables (broccoli, cabbage, cauliflower, Brussels sprouts).
* Drink 3 cups of green tea daily.

GUT AND DETOXIFICATION RESTORATION

* The clinician should restore the hormone balance and remove sources of inflammation by looking for and healing intestinal dysbiosis and supporting liver detoxification.
* Search for and treat hidden reasons for intestinal dysbioses, such as heavy metal overload, parasites, and food sensitivities.

SUPPLEMENTS

Add nutrients to support hormone metabolism:

* A B-50 complex vitamin daily.
* Magnesium salts are taken at 400–600 mg/day.
* Maintain vitamin D$_3$ levels in the range of 40–100 ng/mL.
* Support normal levels of vitamin A to reduce menorrhagia.
* Citrus bioflavonoids, 1000 mg once or twice/day, can also reduce menorrhagia.
* Zinc needs to be at an optimal level; consider supplementing if low.
* I-3-C or diindolylmethane is taken at 200–800 mg/day to reduce estrogen dominance.
* Calcium D glucarate is taken at 500 mg twice/day to reduce increased enterohepatic recirculation of estrogens.

HORMONES

* Insufficiencies in adrenal or thyroid hormones have been shown to increase symptoms related to fibroids. Assess and treat low thyroid levels and adrenal insufficiency.
* DHEA has important implications related to the immune system, sugar metabolism, and stress modification. If the DHEA level is low, add 5–20 mg of DHEA/day. Watch for conversion to estrogens.

BOTANICALS

* Add botanicals to reduce heavy bleeding. Red raspberry leaf and yarrow are used for 2 weeks before the period at 30 drops each; once the period starts, add 30 drops of shepherd's purse.
* Botanicals to support lymphatic drainage from the pelvis are also added. These consist of Gaia herbal combinations such as Scudder's alterative and echinacea/red root formulas. They are taken twice/day at 30 drops each.
* Antiangiogenesis factors such as *Convolvulus* and green tea extract may reduce blood flow to the fibroids.
* To reduce inflammation, add antiinflammatory systemic enzymes (Wobenzyme, Vitalzyme, Neprinol) up to 15 tablets/day in divided doses taken on an empty stomach.

MIND-BODY THERAPIES

* Meditation and visualization exercises using castor oil packs help restore health to the pelvic organs by allowing for the free flow of energy in the meridians of the second chakra. These activities also help identify stored emotional issues in these energy areas of the body and their impact on the fibroid.

CONVENTIONAL THERAPIES

* Should the less invasive and more natural approaches fail to reduce the symptoms or growth of the fibroid, one can resort to the time-tested, more invasive conventional approaches. These powerful tools should be considered when necessary. The integrative holistic approach can still be used to help prevent any further growth of fibroids after the conventional treatment is performed.
* Surgery (hysterectomy)
* Strong pharmaceuticals: leuprolide acetate (Lupron), 3.75 mg intramuscularly once a month for up to 6 months
* Interventional radiographic procedures

Key Web Resources

Genova Diagnostics: Source for the Comprehensive Digestive Stool	http://www.gdx.net
Gaia Herb: Source for the Organix test of protein digestion	http://www.gaiaherbs.com
Herbpharm: Analysis used to diagnose intestinal dysbiosis	http://www.herb-pharm.com
Doctor's Data: Source for essential and toxic elemental testing and standardized herbal tinctures	http://www.doctorsdata.com

REFERENCES

References are available online at ExpertConsult.com.

CHAPTER 59

VAGINAL DRYNESS

Myrtle Wilhite, MD, MS

DESCRIPTION AND PREVALENCE

Vaginal dryness is defined as a reduction of physiological lubrication of the luminal surface of the female vagina. Vaginal dryness can:

- Occur at any age, with prevalence ranging from 13% to 31%,[1] although rates are significantly higher for postmenopausal women (50%)[2] and women treated for breast cancer (63%).[3]
- Cause discomfort singularly, or be accompanied by other symptoms, such as itch or dyspareunia.
- Occur subsequent to a change or alteration of serum estradiol levels. For risk factors, see Table 59.1, but the leading causes are as follows:
  - *Premenopausal women*: hormonal contraceptives, anticholinergic or chemotherapeutic medications, postpartum/breastfeeding, inflammatory conditions, or unwise health behaviors.
  - *Peri- and postmenopausal women*: menopausal decline in estrogen production, anticholinergic or chemotherapeutic medications, metabolic and inflammatory conditions, or unwise health behaviors.
- Progress to other conditions such as vulvovaginal atrophy (VVA, also known as atrophic vaginitis or urogenital atrophy). VVA is a tissue-altering inflammation of the vagina (and the distal urinary tract) caused by decreased blood flow.[4] With chronic progression, VVA leads to dry, thin, friable tissue with poor capacity for blood flow or lubrication.[5] Prevalence of vaginal atrophy in postmenopausal women is 43% in the United States but varies by nation.[6]

PHYSIOLOGY OF VAGINAL LUBRICATION

Vaginal lubrication is reliant upon healthy blood flow because vaginal lubrication is ultrafiltrated blood.

- The vagina contains no glands.
- Blood pressure pushes fluid from the capillaries through intracellular gap junctions between vaginal epithelial cells.[7] The resultant vaginal transudate is mainly composed of water and very small proteins, which combine at the vaginal surface with dead epithelial cells.
- Sufficient pelvic blood flow is dependent on the bioavailability of nitric oxide (NO).[4] Gaseous NO is produced in capillary endothelia in response to shear stress or vibration or in response to sexual arousal via parasympathetic nitrergic nerves.[9] Once produced, NO induces vasodilation through a cyclic guanosine monophosphate (cGMP) cascade, which diminishes as phosphodiesterase enzymes subdue the effect.

- Therefore, vaginal lubrication production depends upon the synthesis, enzymatic facilitation, and bioavailability of NO (Table 59.2). The enzymatic function of NO synthase is enhanced by steroid hormones, most notably estrogen in a rapid-action nongenomic effect.[10]
- Importantly, the presence of NO is not sufficient for its effect. Many biological feedback mechanisms exist to suppress the production of NO as high production of NO in an inflammatory environment can lead to irreversible free radical production.[11] Metabolic conditions of low inflammation are supportive to the bioavailability of NO in facilitating vaginal lubrication.

TABLE 59.1 Risk Factors for Vaginal Dryness

Reduced Estrogen Availability

Postpartum, breastfeeding

Menopausal transition

Premature ovarian failure

Oophorectomy

Pelvic radiotherapy

Other Medical Conditions

Untreated hypertension

Diabetes (Types 1 and 2), metabolic syndrome

Pituitary disorders

Neuropathies, especially autonomic neuropathy

Dermatoses (psoriasis, lichen sclerosis, Sjögren syndrome)

Prescription Medications

Antihistamines and decongestants

Antidepressants (SSRI, atypical TCAs)

Antiestrogen therapy for chemoprophylaxis

Antiestrogen therapy for endometriosis/fibroids

Chemotherapy

Diuretics

Progesterone predominant oral contraceptives

Unwise Behaviors

Dehydration, including alcohol use

Use of douches, extremely hot baths, and/or strong detergents and dehydrating soaps

Use of highly absorptive tampons

Use of male condoms with insufficient external lubricant

Lack of sufficient arousal before vaginal penetration

Smoking

SSRI, selective serotonin reuptake inhibitors; TCA, tricyclic antidepressants.

The vagina's lubrication does not come from glands but from a transudative fluid expressed through vaginal epithelial cells from filtered blood that requires adequate perfusion and NO.

PATHOPHYSIOLOGY OF VAGINAL EPITHELIUM

Mature vaginal epithelial cells produce and store glycogen, which is released during normal cell death and provides nutritional support for *Lactobacillus sp. Lactobacilli* uniquely release hydrogen peroxide during metabolism, thereby acidifying the luminal vaginal pH. Vaginal maturation index (VMI)[12] correlates strongly with pH of noninfected, noninflamed vagina,[13] and both can be used to assess the health of vaginal tissue.

Changes to the tissue and function of the vagina during the menopausal transition (perimenopause) are highly influenced by declining levels of sex hormones. Waning estrogen causes a decrease in cellular maturation (VMI decreases; pH increases), mitotic activity of the basement membrane (reduced cellular renewal), decreased collagen

TABLE 59.2 Manipulation of Nitric Oxide Function

Production of Nitric Oxide

Mediterranean diet: sufficient L-arginine intake
- Nuts: peanuts, almonds, walnut, hazelnuts
- Fruits: berries, chocolate
- Beans
- Some meats: fish, chicken
- Some seeds: sunflower, flaxseed

Sufficient dietary calcium

Facilitation of Enzyme Activity of Nitric Oxide Synthase

Hormones
- Estriol or estradiol: rapid action, nongenomic effect
- Estradiol, soy phytoestrogens, testosterone(s): genomic effect

Medications, vitamins, and supplements
- Niacin (recouples eNOS)
- Angiotensin-converting enzyme inhibitors (ACE-i)
- Ginseng (increases eNOS, inhibits iNOS)

Other
- Reduce hyperglycemia

Prolonged Activity of Nitric Oxide

PDE-5 inhibitors (sildenafil, tadalafil, vardenafil)

Improve Bioavailability of Nitric Oxide (preventing free radical formation)

Medications, vitamins, and supplements
- Aspirin (reduces iNOS)
- Vitamin D_3 (decreases iNOS)
- Ginseng, American (decreases iNOS, increases eNOS)

Behaviors
- Routine moderate aerobic exercise

synthesis (weaker dermal structure), and thickened dermoepidermal junctions (making it harder for capillary fluid to move through to the surface).[14] All of these factors lead to a dry, immature, weakened cellular structure, which is more susceptible to friction damage and decreased repair capacity.

Antiestrogen therapy can lead to moderate-to-severe vaginal atrophy.[15] Selective estrogen receptor modulators, such as tamoxifen, increase mucin production and maturity of vaginal epithelium[16] while simultaneously reducing blood flow to vaginal tissues in experimental models.[17] Aromatase inhibitors cause severe vaginal dryness due to estrogen production suppression.[18]

INTEGRATIVE THERAPY

Topical Vaginal Lubricants

Sexual lubricants applied topically and intravaginally are highly effective at addressing vaginal dryness,[19] as effective as topical estrogen treatment,[20] easy to use, readily available, and inexpensive. However, because the vagina is a biologically active organ, sexual lubricants are not without risk of harm, and the United States Food and Drug Administration (FDA) has made major changes to the classification and testing of products intended for sexual use inside the body.

Sexual Lubricant Safety

Prior to 2014, sexual lubricants had been minimally regulated by FDA as cosmetics (e.g., class I device) because it was felt that the use of sexual lubricants had little associated health risk. Serious consequences began appearing in clinical trials, however, as vaginal lubricants were used as drug delivery mechanisms:
- Spermicidal detergents such as nonoxynol 9 were shown in 2002 to increase transmission of HIV.[21]
- In 2010, sexual lubricants with high osmolality increased transmission of herpes type 2.[22] Osmolality (a physical property of liquids whereby fluid is drawn out of cells) weakening the cell and damaging the protective function of skin cells impacts infection transmission.

This data led the FDA to conclude that sexual lubricants are not harmless cosmetics but substances that deserve scientific attention prior to their release into the public marketplace. The FDA now considers sexual lubricants to be class II medical devices subject to formulation testing and rigorous manufacturing standards.
- All lubricants sold for sexual penetration are now considered FDA class II medical devices.
  - This is true whether the lubricant is used with a partner or solo, with a latex barrier (condom) or without, and whether it is applied inside the vagina or anus.
  - Products from both international and domestic manufacturers without FDA class II approval are being forced off the U.S. market.

- An unfortunate aspect of this regulation is that not all approved class II devices are equivalent or *necessarily* safe.
  - For example, some manufacturers conducted and registered products as class II devices years before these issues arose. Neither in past or at present have there been any published FDA manufacturing standards to use that if met suggest a low level of biological risk. Some FDA class II lubricant devices have received approval even though current testing procedures are more complicated than those that were originally accepted. Other products have been class II approved but were withdrawn from the market due to safety concerns.

Choosing Vaginal Lubricant(s)

Generally, the most effective sexual lubricants have the following properties:
- Incorporate *both* moisturizing and moisture-sealing qualities,
- Have a pH compatible with vaginal pH (between 4.4 and 5.5),
- Do not have allergenic, sensitizing, or contact-irritant botanical components, and
- Meet the physical slip and cushion needs of the user.

A successful outcome lies in knowing how to choose the right lubricant, and this task has become difficult. The chemical ingredients,[23] physical properties,[24] and the comfort in use determine both the degree of client acceptance and long-term compliance. **All** sexual lubricants should **reduce** friction with skin-to-skin rubbing and evaporation. Other considerations include the following:

- **Moisturizing**, thinner, water-based lubricants are generally low in osmolality, so they are less likely to draw moisture from the skin and instead add more moisture to the skin and vagina. Hyaluronic acid improves vaginal dryness in women with severe dryness.[25]
- **To seal** moisture in place, silicone-based lubricants have, generally, the highest tolerance for use during sexual play. This is compared with other organic oils, butters, and petroleum-based (mineral oil) lubricants.

Many people use **both** types of lubricants (watery, moisturizing lubricant plus silicone-based lubricants) during sexual play. Experimentation is highly encouraged as the specific needs of an individual might not be easily ascertained without home trials. See Table 59.3[26-29] for properties of commonly available sexual lubricants. Each of the following recommended OTC lubricants have a different formulation. Remember that formulations and availability change quickly, so check for availability locally or by Internet.

Evaluate Different Lubricants

Encourage experimentation with samples of different sexual lubricants available OTC. Product availability is highly variable as manufacturers comply with FDA standards. Suggested lubricants are listed in Table 59.3.

TABLE 59.3	**Features of Over-the-Counter Lubricants and Food-Grade Oils**						
Product	**Preferred?**	**Base**	**pH**	**Moisture**	**Seals**	**Ideal Use**	**Comments**
Oasis Silk	Yes	Water + silicone	4.8	**Yes**	**Yes**	Hybrid; both	Paraben-free
Sliquid Organics Silk	Yes	Water + silicone	6.5	**Yes**	**Yes**	Hybrid; both	Aloe; very thin for sexual use. Paraben-free
Aloe Cadabra	Yes	Water	4.0	Yes	No	Moisturizer	Aloe
Good Clean Love	Yes	Water	4.8	Yes	No	Moisturizer	Aloe; best as moisturizer as is very sticky in sexual use
KY Silk-E	Yes	Water	3.8	Yes	No	Moisturizer	Aloe
Liquid Assets	Yes	Water	4.8	Yes	No	Both	Aloe; hyaluronic acid; very thin for sexual use
Swiss Navy, water	Yes	Water	4.4	Yes	No	Both	Aloe
Femani Smooth	Yes	Silicone	4.4	No	Yes	Seals; sexual use	Excellent for sexual use
Uberlube	Yes	Silicone	4.0	No	Yes	Seals; sexual use	Excellent for sexual use
Coconut Oil[28]	Perhaps	Fruit oil	–	No	Yes	Seals only	Difficult to remove; coconut smell
Astroglide	No	Water	6.5	No	No		Glycerin/high osmolality
KY Jelly	No	Water	4.5	No	No		Glycerin/high osmolality/chlorhexidine
Pre~	No	Water	7.0	Yes	No	Pregnancy	Sperm friendly
Replens	No	Petroleum oil	2.8	No	Yes		Med-hi osmol; stings in use
Olive Oil[26,27]	No	Fruit oil	–	No	Yes	Exfoliant	Desquamates skin

DOSAGE

1–3 mL applied to the antecubital fossa (inside elbow). Wait for 1 hour and then check for redness or irritation. Check again in 24 hours to evaluate for delayed sensitivity.

PRECAUTIONS

Because sexual lubricants are complicated substances (pH, osmolality, biological interactions, ingredient variability, and base variability), irritating reactions can occur to specific ingredients (propylene glycol,[30] aloe,[31] and glycerin[32]) or specific percentage composition in the formulation. Due to this complexity, users might tolerate/prefer different type(s) of lubricant(s) for different behaviors or at different times of their lives. *One* product will never be suitable for *every* person.

To Moisturize

Self-massage moisturizing lubricant on vulva or in vagina.

DOSAGE

1–3 mL massaged on vulva qhs or after showers. If internal vaginal application is desired, suggest a 1–3 mL needleless syringe and apply pv qhs or as needed. Titrate dose depending on need.

PRECAUTIONS

Users may use one product for moisturizing and a different product for sexual use as some moisturizers are too thin to reduce friction adequately.

Vaginal Renewal Program

The Vaginal Renewal (VR) program helps women recondition the health and flexibility of the skin of the vulva and vagina by reducing friction tearing of vulvar skin as well as increasing blood flow to the vulva and vaginal canal. VR is indicated for those just beginning to feel the effects of hormonal changes, women who have completed pelvic radiotherapy,[33] as well as women with vaginal atrophy who experience skin tearing and pain while penetration is being attempted. Dilation is not the goal, blood flow is. Because of this, static dilators (nonvibrating dilators) have not been found to be as useful for improving function as vibrating wands, and dilators with soft, textured, or adhesive surfaces tear fragile vaginal epithelium too easily.

VR is compatible with topical estrogen therapies, and the combination can be more effective and faster acting than estrogen alone or VR alone. Many women gain enough improvement from the combination of estrogen therapy and VR and are able to discontinue the use of estrogen completely. However, the VR program does not require the use of estrogen and is preferred by clients and clinicians for circumstances where topical estrogen is contraindicated.

PRECAUTION

Because comfortable penetration depends on the flexibility of both the skin and pelvic floor muscles, some women recondition their vaginal skin only to experience uncomfortable penetration because their pelvic floor muscles are inflexible. Referral to a pelvic floor physical therapist is indicated before continuing VR, and no further vaginal penetration should be attempted until pelvic floor muscle evaluation is completed.

For women with vaginal dryness which causes daily discomfort:
- Choose a moisturizing lubricant and place it by the toilet and/or shower.
- Dispense a nickel-to-quarter-sized amount on the fingers.
- Use a press-release motion over the entire vulva.
- Dispense another nickel-to-quarter-sized amount on the fingers.
- Use a press-release and rolling motion to apply on the introitus.
- Repeat 1–2× per day as needed.
- If dryness is felt internally, use 1-cc lubricant in the vaginal applicator qhs.

For women with rehabilitation of the vaginal canal needing lubrication and dilation:
- Follow instructions for daily moisturizing.
- Help the client choose an appropriately sized vibrating wand.
  - The diameter of the wand is the most important criteria; choose one that can be inserted comfortably during pelvic examination. A smaller diameter is always better. The client can graduate to a larger size when a finger can be placed beside the wand comfortably during vaginal penetration.
  - Low-hertz vibration is more effective than high hertz.
- Instruct the following:
  - At home, the client is to lubricate the wand.
  - Insert it into the vagina to the deepest comfortable depth.
  - Turn on the vibration.
  - Lie back and let the wand vibrate for 5–10 minutes.
  - Remove the wand.
  - Repeat 3× weekly as needed.

For women with dryness-related dyspareunia:
- Follow instructions for moisturizing and vibrating the wand, as previous.
- Lubricate partner (penis, fingers, glass, or steel dildo) with silicone-based lubricant prior to penetration.
- If the object of penetration is made of silicone, cover the object with a nonlubricated condom and apply silicone to outside of the condom.

Behaviors

Regular Vaginal Penetration Through Sexual Activity

This has been associated with enhanced sexual function in postmenopausal women.[34]

DOSAGE

Vaginal penetration once per week appears sufficient when symptoms are absent.

PRECAUTIONS

It is easier to maintain function than it is to rehabilitate, so asymptomatic women should be encouraged to continue routine vaginal penetration, with or without a partner, even if the goal is for comfortable routine pelvic examinations.

Utilize Vibrating Wand Massage to Create Shear Stress

This stress on the endothelial capillaries increases blood flow and vaginal lubrication.

Habitual Physical Exercise

It is an effective way to combat vascular aging[35] and enhance the function of small vessel blood flow,[36] including vaginal perfusion.[37] Aerobic exercise positively affects NO[38] and is linked to improved endothelial and cardiovascular health[39] as well as improved sexual arousal in women taking antidepressants.[40]

DOSAGE

Walking once per day, 30–60 minutes to the level of gentle sweat. Walking prior to anticipated sexual activity improves vaginal lubrication as well as subjective symptoms of arousal (see Chapter 91).

PRECAUTIONS

Vigorous exercise is not indicated, but exercising to the level of gentle sweat is sufficient. Walking is ideal.

Nutrition

Dietary reduction in inflammation assists endothelial function[41] by improving nitric oxide–dependent blood flow.[42] For example, despite the increased incidence of sexual dysfunction in women with diabetes,[43] adherence to a Mediterranean diet is associated with a lower prevalence of sexual dysfunction in diabetic women.[44]

Mediterranean Diet

A low-glycemic, low-carbohydrate Mediterranean diet positively manipulates endothelial health and NO bioavailability. There is benefit of increasing NO bioavailability *prior* to NO production because increasing NO in the presence of inflammatory/oxidized conditions worsens NO bioavailability and damages endothelia directly.
- First, focus consumption on initially increasing both lipid- and water-based antioxidants and reduce high-glycemic index foods that spike blood glucose levels and increase insulin resistance (see Chapter 87).
- Second, increase food consumption that targets protein levels of L-arginine (See Table 59.2). Fortunately, these foods are beneficial to satiety, and many incorporate both antioxidants and L-arginine simultaneously.
- Finally, consider whether soy phytoestrogens might be of benefit. Experimentally, fermented soy may also function as a free radical scavenger.[45]

DOSAGE

Strict adherence to a Mediterranean diet with small meal portions with mid-meal grazing on nuts + dried berries/cherries (see Chapter 88).

PRECAUTIONS

Soy consumption (90 mg isoflavone/day) has shown positive effect on vaginal dryness,[46] but the safety is in question,[47] particularly for western populations.[48]

Vitamins and Supplements

Although there is a slim positive evidence of supplements supporting sexual function, there is data on vitamin and supplement effect on endothelial function. Because endothelial function underlies the physiological mechanism for vaginal health and lubrication, recommendations are included here.

Vitamin D$_3$

Vitamin D receptors are present in all layers of the vaginal epithelium.[49] Vitamin D$_3$ plays an important role in absorbing dietary calcium, manipulating calcium at neural membranes, and in the calmodulin-cofactor[50] required for NO production and protects endothelial cells from glucotoxicity.[51] Studies support the use of oral supplementation[52] and intravaginal application.[53]

ORAL DOSAGE

Begin at Vitamin D$_3$ 2000 IU po qd taken with fish oil and calcium citrate. After 1 month, check blood levels of 25(OH)D and aim for serum level of at least 50 ng/mL. In women who are more symptomatic for menopausal symptoms, aim at serum level of 60 ng/mL.

INTRAVAGINAL DOSAGE

Vitamin D$_3$ 1000 IU per suppository qd × 8 weeks.

PRECAUTIONS

Calcium metabolism and kidney disorders as well as some inflammatory disorders (sarcoidosis, tuberculosis) are worsened with vitamin D therapy.

Fish Oil (Highly Purified Omega 3)

Omega 3 oils assist absorption of vitamin D and act as lipid-based antioxidants helping endothelial and neural function.[54]

DOSAGE

2–3 g po qd taken with vitamin D and calcium.

PRECAUTIONS

Fish oil/omega-3s act as anticoagulants, so the dosage needs to be modified in those taking heparin, Coumadin, SSRIs, aspirin, ginkgo, high-dose garlic, or other potentially blood-thinning regimens.

L-Arginine

Take as a supplement. It acts as the protein substrate for NO production.

DOSAGE

500 mg po qd.

PRECAUTIONS

Dietary supplementation is more strongly suggested than direct supplementation and may cause hyperglycemia, hypotension, and nausea; it is contraindicated in kidney disease. High serum levels of L-arginine and L-citrulline (production byproduct) also act as feedback inhibitors of NO production.

Sea Buckthorn Oil

Oral supplementation with sea buckthorn oil, an antiinflammatory phytosterol, has been shown to improve vaginal epithelium parameters but not significantly improve subjective symptoms of vaginal dryness.[55] Topical applications improve barrier function of full thickness skin[56] but have not been studied for vulvovaginal use.

DOSAGE

3 g po qd × 3 months.

PRECAUTIONS

Sea buckthorn can act as a blood thinner and may lower blood sugar in diabetics taking hypoglycemic medication. They also may interfere in heart, gastrointestinal, cancer, or autoimmune treatments.

Niacin

Reversal of endothelial dysfunction is responsive to niacin therapy.[57]

DOSAGE

500–1000 mg bid.

PRECAUTIONS

Warning about flushing and prolonged incremental increase beginning at 100 mg/day is most successful. It may make vulvar dermatoses initially worse[58] as recoupling of NO production will temporarily advance inflammation.

Botanicals

American ginseng (Panax quinquefolius)

Improves blood flow related to NO bioavailability, reduces inflammatory NO release from macrophages,[59] facilitates endothelial NO release, and acts as a potent antioxidant.[60]

DOSAGE

500 mg capsule bid or 2 g root tea infusion, tid.

PRECAUTIONS

May cause insomnia or hypoglycemia if taken in conjunction with diabetes medications.

Ginkgo Biloba

Ginkgo acts on NO vasodilation in several different ways.[61] It modulates NO second messenger action, scavenges excess NO, inhibits NO production under inflammatory conditions, and inhibits platelet activation. Ginkgo supplementation has been shown to improve sexual function,[62] although the data is conflicting.[63]

DOSAGE

Ginkgo biloba extract 50:1 60 mg bid; may be advanced to 120 mg bid.

PRECAUTIONS

Do not use with anticoagulants, nonsteroidal antiinflammatory drugs, aspirin, or high consumption of garlic.

Not Recommended

Attempts to reverse vaginal dryness with oral black cohosh[64] and topical genistein[65] or red ginseng (*Panax ginseng*)[66] have been unsuccessful. Damiana (*Turnera diffusa*) blocks progesterone receptors without receptor activation but may boost unopposed estrogen activity.

Pharmaceuticals

Estriol Gel

Two weeks of vaginal daily estriol gel improves vaginal dryness[67] and may be indicated as initial therapy in severe cases of vaginal atrophy.

DOSAGE

Estriol cream (0.005%) 50 mcg intravaginally qd × 2 wks. Taper to 3×/wk for 2 months, then D/C.

PRECAUTIONS

Estriol causes measurable systemic changes suggestive of estrogen effect in breast cancer survivors taking aromatase inhibitors.[68]

Estriol is the main estrogen of pregnancy, which helps prepare the vagina for delivery. However, estriol does stimulate breast cell proliferation (although less than estradiol) and should only be used as very short-term therapy in cases of severe dysfunction. (See Vaginal Renewal, previously described, for nonhormonal therapy.)

Estriol–Lactobacilli Combination (Gynoflor) Vaginal Tablet

Intravaginal tablets with a low-dose estriol/*Lactobacilli* combination improved sexual activity in women experiencing VVA due to breast cancer treatment.[69]

DOSAGE

Estriol cream (0.03 mg + *Lactobacilli*) intravaginally qd × 4 weeks. Taper to 3×/wk for 2 months, then D/C.

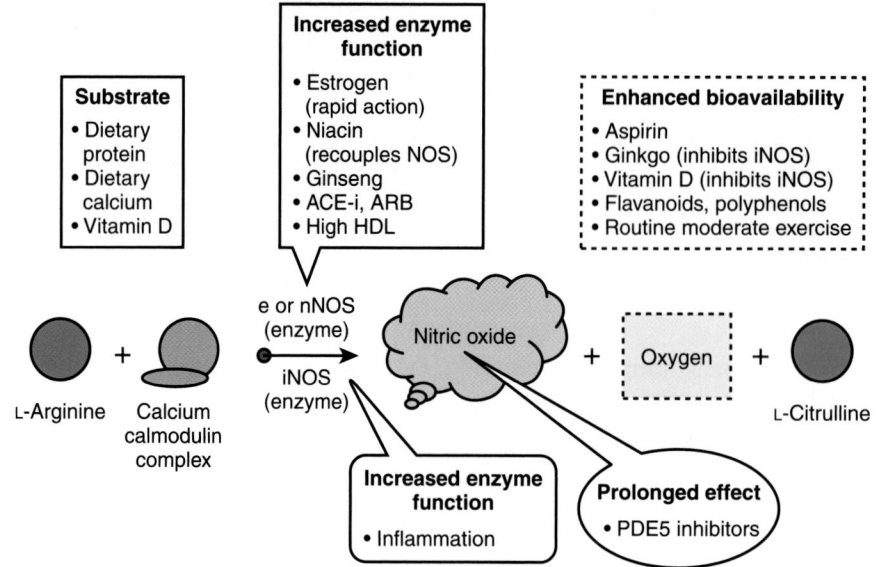

FIG. 59.1 ■ Nitric oxide interventions. *ACE-I,* Angiotensin-converting enzyme inhibitor; *ARB,* angiotensin II receptor blocker; *eNOS,* endothelial nitric oxide synthase; *iNOS,* inducible nitric oxide synthase; *nNOS,* neuronal nitric oxide synthase; *PDE5,* phosphodiesterase-5.

PRECAUTIONS

Estriol causes measurable systemic changes suggestive of estrogen effect in breast cancer survivors taking aromatase inhibitors.[68]

Sildenafil [Phosphodiesterase-5 (PDE5) Inhibitors]

Physiologically, PDE5 inhibitors reduce insulin resistance in endothelial capillaries[71] in addition to prolonging cGMP vasodilatory effect and show beneficial genital perfusion effect in women[72] as well as sexual function improvements among women taking antidepressants.[73]

DOSAGE

12.5–50 mg qd. May be taken qhs to reduce hypotension symptoms. Client should experiment whether timing prior to sexual intimacy improves vaginal lubrication.

PRECAUTIONS

It may cause nausea, headache, nasal congestion, renal or hepatic impairment, hypotension, change in vision, and ototoxicity. They are contraindicated with nitrates and α_1-blockers.

Not Recommended

Oral raloxifene[74] or low-dose topical estradiol cream. The efficacy of topical local estradiol treatment is high,[75] but women are generally reluctant to use the therapy because of perceived risks,[76] including DVT, CVA, and breast cancer risk. Serum levels of estrone and estradiol increase in response to vulvovaginal topical treatment with estradiol after 1 week of therapy.[77]

PREVENTION PRESCRIPTION

- Maintain regular exercise and movement to enhance blood perfusion to the vulva and vagina.
- Encourage a Mediterranean diet that is rich in berry fruits, nuts, vegetables, and whole grains and low in red meat and processed carbohydrates. Focus on foods with high L-arginine levels. Encourage beverage choices of tea (black, green, red, or white), coffee, or water.
- Experiment to find a topical sexual lubricant that is comfortable and moisturizes the vulva and vagina.
- Maintain vaginal penetration (once a week) to stimulate vaginal lubrication and elasticity. Consider intermittent VR therapy if not interested in self sexuality or partner is not available.
- Check vitamin D levels and supplement to maintain levels above 50 ng/mL.
- Avoid tobacco products.

THERAPEUTIC REVIEW

There are three main strategies for resolving vaginal dryness without the use of hormones that are most effective when combined: topical vulvovaginal application of a suitable moisturizer, VR, and lifestyle improvements in NO-related blood flow.

SEXUAL BEHAVIOR

*   Have the client experiment with a client-matched topical moisturizing lubricant. B₂

*   Utilize massage and vibration (VR) to create sheer stress on the endothelial capillaries, increasing blood flow and vaginal lubrication. C₁

    When addressing a comprehensive lifestyle solution, holistically address diet and lifestyle issues that help facilitate the production and bioavailability of NO (see Table 59.2 and Fig. 59.1). B₁

NUTRITION

*   First reduce overall metabolic inflammation with strict adherence to a Mediterranean diet with daily exercise. This enhances bioavailability and decreases inflammatory free radical production. B₁

*   Then, focus the diet more specifically on foods high in L-arginine and selectively strip high-glycemic foods from the diet. Address satiety with proteins. C₁

SUPPLEMENTS

*   Consider adding L-arginine 500 mg daily to enhance NO production; B₂

*   Vitamin D₃ 2000 IU qd; achieving serum levels of 50 ng/mL; omega 3 fish oil 2–4 g qd B₁

BOTANICALS

*   P. quinquefolius 500 mg–1 g bid. B₁
*   Sea buckthorn 3 g po qd B₁

MEDICATIONS

*   Use an angiotensin converting enzyme inhibitor (instead of a β-blocker or diuretic) B₁

*   For severe cases, apply estriol cream 0.005% ointment to the vulva and intravaginally daily ×2 weeks, then reduce to 3×/week for 2 months and then DC. B₂

*   Or estriol 0.03 mg + Lactobacilli suppository intravaginally qd ×4 weeks. Taper to 3×/week for 2 months, then DC.  B₂

*   Consider whether PDE5 inhibitors (sildenafil 12.5–50 mg daily) may facilitate daily genital perfusion to increase genital blood flow and vaginal lubrication. B₂

REFERENCES

References are available online at ExpertConsult.com.

SECTION XI

UROLOGY

SECTION OUTLINE

60 BENIGN PROSTATIC HYPERPLASIA

61 UROLITHIASIS (KIDNEY AND BLADDER STONES)

62 CHRONIC PROSTATITIS/CHRONIC PELVIC PAIN SYNDROME

63 ERECTILE DYSFUNCTION

64 TESTOSTERONE DEFICIENCY

CHAPTER 60

BENIGN PROSTATIC HYPERPLASIA

David Rakel, MD

PATHOPHYSIOLOGY

Even though benign prostatic hyperplasia (BPH) is one of the most common diseases of aging men, its etiology remains relatively unknown. From our current understanding, BPH appears to be related to age, androgens (dihydrotestosterone [DHT]), estrogens, and detrusor dysfunction of the bladder neck. An accumulation of DHT inhibits prostatic cell death, promotes cell proliferation, and thus increases the size of the gland (Fig. 60.1).

As a man passes his fifth decade of life, serum testosterone levels decrease and estrogen (as well as prolactin, luteinizing hormone, and follicle-stimulating hormone) levels rise. Estrogen increases the number of androgen (DHT) receptors in the prostate and inhibits androgen metabolism by interfering with hydroxylation. As urinary outflow obstruction develops, the detrusor muscles of the bladder try to compensate by increasing pressure to expel urine, a process that leads to instability of the muscle and worsening symptoms. In summary, factors that promote the accumulation of DHT and estrogens lead to symptoms of BPH and obstruction of the lower urinary tract that, in turn, cause detrusor muscle dysfunction. Stimulation of the alpha-adrenergic system leads to contraction of the smooth muscle fiber that further restricts flow in an enlarged prostate gland. Finally, there is reason to believe that prostaglandins, leukotrienes, and insulin resistance play roles in the inflammatory process of the prostate.

Components of the metabolic syndrome have been shown to cause prostatic enlargement.[1,2] Insulin resistance and truncal obesity appear to be the main culprits.[3] Elevated insulin levels increase sympathetic nerve activity and also bind to insulin-like growth factor (IGF) receptors that stimulate prostate cell growth.[4] Excessive amounts of visceral fat also increase the circulation of estradiol and further stimulate prostate cell growth by increasing DHT levels (Fig. 60.2). Obesity, metabolic syndrome, and insulin resistance also increase systemic inflammation, which is also correlated with the incidence of BPH.[5]

Light to moderate alcohol consumption has been associated with a protective effect on BPH and lower urinary tract symptoms. The association of light to moderate alcohol consumption with an improvement in insulin sensitivity[6] and a decrease in testosterone concentrations[7] may help explain the beneficial influence of alcohol. However, this positive effect is not seen in men with high alcohol consumption.[8] Consuming seven or more alcoholic drinks per week is associated with worsening symptoms.[9]

INTEGRATIVE THERAPY

Table 60.1 gives the mechanism of action of common pharmaceuticals, botanicals, and supplements used for BPH, and Table 60.2 gives information on botanicals and hormones that may worsen symptoms of BPH.

Nutrition

Soy

Soy is thought to work in two ways. It is an inhibitor of 5-alpha-reductase and a low-potency estrogen. Soy may block the receptor sites that the stronger estrogens use to increase the accumulation of DHT. Consumption of nonfermented soy products (tofu, soy milk, edamame) has also been found to result in a decreased incidence of prostate cancer.[10,11]

Beta-sitosterol (a major phytosterol found in soy) was found to increase urinary flow and decrease residual volume in the bladder in a double-blind, placebo-controlled study using a 20-mg dose.[12] A 3.5-oz serving of soybeans, tofu, or another soy food preparation provides approximately 90 mg of beta-sitosterol.[13] A 1-oz preparation (which is a portion approximately the size of the palm of the hand) equals approximately 25 mg.

Cholesterol

Cholesterol has been associated not only with BPH but also with prostate cancer. Cholesterol metabolites (epoxycholesterols) have been found to accumulate in the hyperplastic and cancerous prostate gland. For this reason, hypocholesterolemic drugs (3-hydroxy-3-methylglutaryl–coenzyme A reductase inhibitors or "statins") have been associated with a lower risk of BPH and prostate cancer.[14,35] In addition, treating the dyslipidemia of metabolic syndrome (high triglyceride and low high-density lipoprotein levels) with exercise and a low–glycemic index/load diet (see Chapter 87) may also prove beneficial because of the association of BPH with metabolic syndrome. Foods high in cholesterol and saturated fat are rich in arachidonic acid as well, which is the main precursor of inflammation. Reducing consumption of these foods can benefit BPH patients by reducing inflammatory triggers.

Omega-3 Fatty Acids

A diet rich in omega-3 fatty acids helps reduce the influence of prostaglandins and leukotrienes on the inflammatory component of BPH (see Chapter 88). Recommend foods rich in omega-3 fatty acids such as

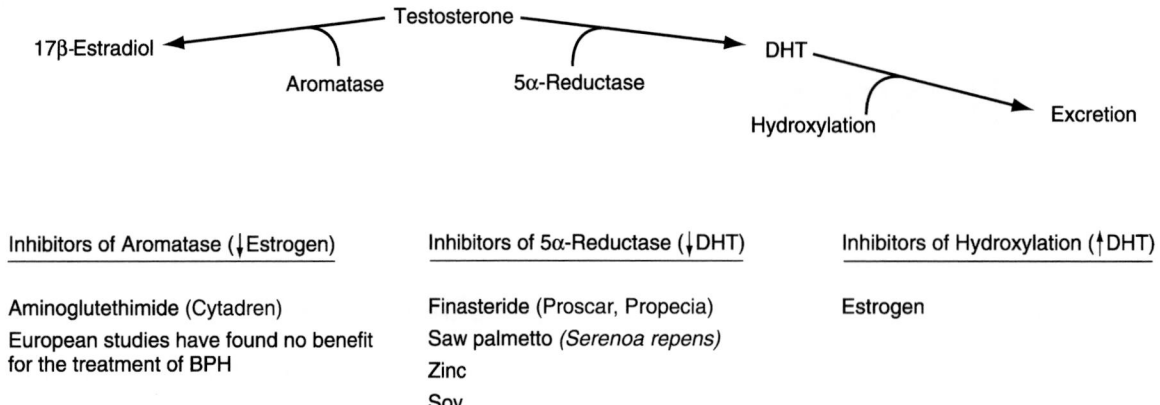

FIG. 60.1 ■ Inhibitors of aromatase, 5-alpha-reductase, and hydroxylation. *BPH*, benign prostatic hyperplasia; *DHT*, dihydrotestosterone.

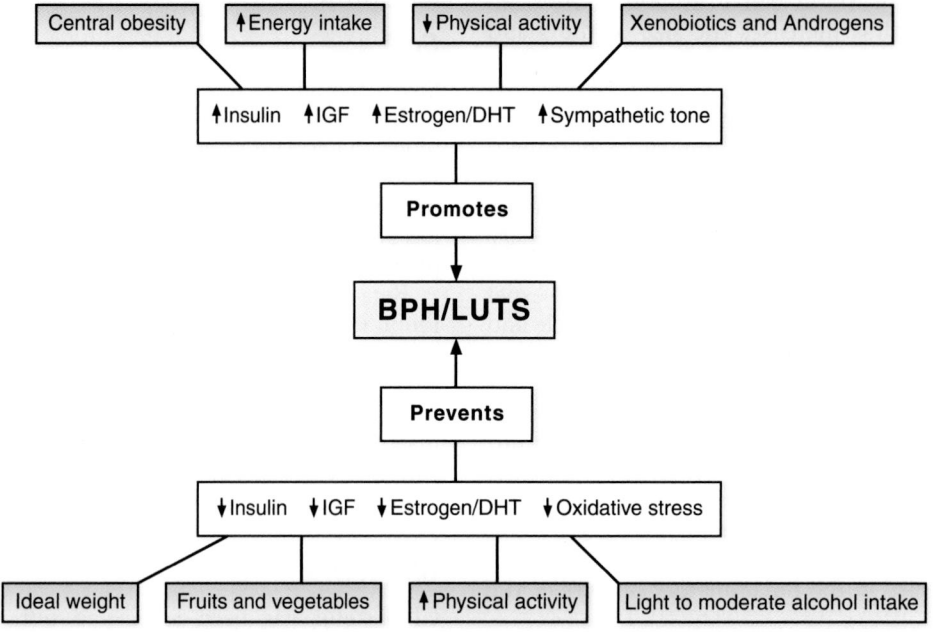

FIG. 60.2 ■ Influences affecting the promotion and prevention of benign prostatic hypertrophy (BPH) and lower urinary tract symptoms (LUTS). *DHT*, dihydrotestosterone; *IGF*, insulin-like growth factor.

cold-water fish (salmon, mackerel, and sardines), vegetables, and ground flaxseed or flaxseed oil. Flaxseed oil can be taken in capsule form. Recommend lignan-rich flaxseed oil, two to four 500-mg capsules twice a day. Patients can also buy whole flaxseeds, grind two tablespoons (approximately 30 g) of the seeds, and sprinkle the ground flaxseed on salads or yogurt or add it to a smoothie. Flaxseed has the added benefit of lignan fiber, which helps bind estrogen in the gut and thus promotes estrogen removal.

Supplements

Beta-Sitosterol

Beta-sitosterol is a sterol found in almost all plants. It is one of the main subcomponents of a group of plant sterols known as phytosterols that are very similar in composition to cholesterol. These plant sterols are the active ingredients in popular margarine spreads (Take Control, Benecol) used to lower cholesterol. Beta-sitosterol is found in rice bran, wheat germ, peanuts, corn oils, and soybeans. High levels are also found in botanicals such as saw palmetto, rye grass pollen, pygeum, and stinging nettles, which have been found to be beneficial for BPH. Unlike cholesterol, beta-sitosterol cannot be converted to testosterone. It also inhibits aromatase and 5-alpha-reductase. Beta-sitosterol is likely one of the many reasons that eating vegetables is good for health. Encourage adequate consumption of these plants in the diet.

Two randomized studies showed a benefit of beta-sitosterol in treating BPH, with little potential harm.[15,16] This benefit persisted for up to 18 months of use.[17] A Cochrane Review found beta-sitosterol to improve

TABLE 60.1 Mechanism of Action of Common Pharmaceuticals, Botanicals, and Supplements Used for Benign Prostatic Hyperplasia

Mechanism of Action	Therapy
Alpha₁-adrenergic blockade	Nonselective: Terazosin (Hytrin) Doxazosin (Cardura) Selective: Tamsulosin (Flomax) Alfuzosin (Uroxatral) Silodosin (Rapaflo)
5-Alpha-reductase inhibition	Finasteride (Proscar) Dutasteride (Avodart) Saw palmetto (*Serenoa repens*)
Phosphodiesterase-5 inhibitors	Tadalafil (Cialis)
Antiproliferative action	African wild potato (*Hypoxis hemerocallidea*) Beta-sitosterol Lycopene Pumpkin seed (*Cucurbita pepo*) Pygeum (*Prunus africana*) Red clover (*Trifolium pratense*) Soy Stinging nettle root (*Urtica dioica*)
Antiinflammatory action	Rye grass pollen (*Secale cereale*) (Cernilton)

Modified from http://naturaldatabase.com.

TABLE 60.2 Products That Can Worsen Symptoms of Benign Prostatic Hyperplasia

Mechanism of Action	Product
Sympathetic stimulation: Increases tone of prostatic stroma, causes constriction of urethra, and can also stimulate bladder spasm	Bitter orange Caffeine, gotu kola Ephedra (commonly found in over-the-counter cold remedies) Country mallow Yohimbe
Anticholinergic stimulation: Makes urination more difficult by inhibiting bladder contraction and causing urinary retention	Henbane Scopolia Jimson weed Wild lettuce Many pharmaceuticals (tricyclics, antispasmodics, etc.)
Hormonal stimulation: Accelerates growth of the prostate	Androstenediol Dehydroepiandrosterone (DHEA) Androstenedione Pregnenolone

Adapted from Lee M. Management of benign prostatic hyperplasia. In: *Pharmacotherapy: a pathophysiological approach.* 5th ed. New York, 1999, McGraw-Hill.

urinary symptoms and flow measures. This supplement does not appear to reduce the size of the prostate gland.[18]

DOSAGE

The dose is 60 mg twice daily. This dose can be reduced to 30 mg twice daily after symptoms improve.

PRECAUTIONS

In general, beta-sitosterol is well tolerated. Gastrointestinal side effects are the most common. This supplement can enhance the cholesterol-lowering effects of antihyperlipidemic medications.

Zinc

Intestinal uptake of zinc is inhibited by estrogen. Because aging men have increased estrogen levels, men with BPH may have low zinc levels. In fact, marginal zinc deficiency is common in older adults, and in men, it may worsen the symptoms of BPH. In the 1970s, research showed that supplementing with zinc resulted in a reduction in the size of the prostate gland and in symptoms of BPH.[19] Further research showed that zinc inhibits 5-alpha-reductase,[20] and it also inhibits the binding of androgens to their receptors in the prostate.[21] This effect on androgens is thought to result from zinc's ability to inhibit prolactin, which, like estrogen, increases the receptors for DHT in the prostate. Therefore, zinc not only decreases the production of DHT but also inhibits DHT binding to its receptors.

Coffee can decrease zinc absorption by 50%. Because caffeine stimulates the adrenergic nervous system (smooth muscles of the prostate), encourage patients with BPH to limit their intake.

Prescription drugs that can result in low serum zinc levels include angiotensin converting enzyme inhibitors (ACE), thiazide diuretics, steroids, methotrexate, tetracyclines, and fluoroquinolones. Consider zinc supplementation in patients with BPH who are taking these medications. Do not give zinc to patients taking tetracycline or fluoroquinolone antibiotics; however, because zinc can affect the absorption of these drugs. Pumpkin seeds are a rich source of zinc, and this may explain their potential therapeutic benefit for BPH.

DOSAGE

The dose of zinc is 30 mg per day.

PRECAUTIONS

When prescribing zinc supplements, be aware that zinc competes with copper, calcium, and iron absorption. Make sure that the patient does not take more than the recommended dose and does not take calcium and iron supplements with zinc.

Botanicals

Saw Palmetto (Serenoa repens)

Saw palmetto has been found to be a weak inhibitor of 5-alpha-reductase, but it may have a more active role in reducing the number of estrogen and androgen (DHT) receptors, as well as an antiinflammatory effect on the prostate. Saw palmetto inhibits fibroblast growth factor and epidermal growth factor and stimulates apoptosis, thus further slowing prostate cell proliferation. Its principle ingredient, beta-sitosterol, is also found in soy products (see earlier), as well as in other herbs used to treat diseases of the prostate including pygeum bark, stinging nettle root, and pumpkin seed extract.

Saw palmetto reduces the inner prostatic epithelium but does not reduce the size of the gland. Nonetheless, saw palmetto has been found to improve symptom scores, nocturia, residual urine volume, and urinary flow in patients with BPH. It does not affect prostate-specific antigen (PSA) levels.[22] In a large randomized study, saw palmetto was found to be as effective as finasteride (Proscar), but without the drug's side effects, and the International Prostate Symptom Score (IPSS) was reduced by 37%.[23] However, a more complete evaluation of 32 randomized trials by a 2012 Cochrane Review of 5666 subjects, concluded that no significant difference existed between *Serenoa repens* (saw palmetto) and placebo for the treatment of urinary symptoms related to BPH.[24]

Although the evidence for BPH improvement is marginal, saw palmetto has three positive influences on the prostate gland: it is antiandrogenic, antiproliferative, and antiinflammatory.

DOSAGE

The recommended dose is 160 mg twice daily. Allow 8 weeks before seeing therapeutic benefit.

PRECAUTIONS

Mild adverse effects include headache, nausea, diarrhea, and dizziness. Saw palmetto does not influence the cytochrome P-450 enzyme system of the liver, and drug interactions are rare.

Accumulative data suggest that saw palmetto has little benefit over placebo. Like pygeum, it can be used for its beneficial influence on prostate health that includes being rich in plant sterols. However, if LUTS symptoms are significantly affecting a man's quality of life, using an alpha-blocker will result in a quicker, more effective therapeutic outcome.

Rye Grass Pollen (Secale cereale)

Rye grass pollen is also known as *grass pollen* and *grass pollen extract*. Clinical studies used a form called Cernilton (flower pollen), a brand manufactured by Cernitin. This has been bought by the company Graminex and is now marketed under the name of PollenAid.

This extract has been used in Europe for BPH since the 1970s. Double-blind clinical studies found it to be effective, with an overall response rate near 70%.[25] Rye grass contains a substance that has been found to inhibit prostatic cell growth[26] and reduce inflammation of the prostate by inhibiting prostaglandins and leukotrienes.[27]

Studies have shown the greatest improvement in nocturia, urinary frequency, and residual urine volume.[28] Rye grass and flower pollen are also used for symptomatic relief of prostatitis and prostatodynia.

DOSAGE

The typical dose of rye grass pollen is 126 mg three times daily. A standardized extract 20:1 of *Secale cereale* can be obtained through the following companies: Graminex PollenAid, 500 mg three times daily, or Pure Encapsulations ProstaFlo, 320 mg three to five capsules per day in divided doses.

PRECAUTIONS

Abdominal distention, heartburn, and nausea may occur. This product is not likely to cause allergy because allergenic proteins are removed in the manufacturing process.

Pygeum africanum (*synonym:* Prunus africana)

Pygeum is obtained from the bark of the African plum tree. As with saw palmetto, its benefits are thought to come from fatty acids (sterols) that reduce inflammation through the inhibition of prostaglandins, as well as prostatic cholesterol levels that are precursors to testosterone production. Pygeum also increases prostatic and seminal fluid secretions.

A meta-analysis revealed that men taking pygeum had a 19% reduction in nocturia and a 24% reduction in residual urine volume. Peak urine flow was increased by 23%, and side effects were mild and similar to those reported with placebo.[29] The TRIUMPH study included treatment outcomes of BPH from six European countries. After 1 year of therapy, participants who received either *Pygeum africanum* or *Serenoa repens* (saw palmetto) showed a 43% improvement in IPSS scores and improvement in quality of life compared with no treatment.[30]

Pygeum is more expensive than saw palmetto, and overharvesting of the bark is threatening the survival of the species.

DOSAGE

The recommended dose is 100 to 200 mg per day.

PRECAUTIONS

Nausea and abdominal pain may occur.

Cranberry

The phenols found in cranberry and other dark colored grapes and berries may also prove beneficial for the symptoms of LUTS. In a small study 21 men were given 500 mg of dried cranberry powder three times daily (1500 mg a day) for 6 months versus control. The cranberry group had a greater improvement in their IPSS, quality of life, and urinary flow measurements than the control group.[31]

DOSAGE

Dried cranberry powder, 500 mg three times daily.

PRECAUTIONS

Well tolerated. High doses can cause gastrointestinal intolerance.

Pharmaceuticals

Alpha-Adrenergic Blocking Agents

The TRIUMPH study mentioned earlier followed 2351 men with BPH.[30] After 1 year, the therapies that showed the most benefit in IPSS scores were, in descending order, alpha blockers (68%), finasteride (57%), and *Serenoa repens* or *Pygeum africanum* (43%) compared with watchful waiting. Of the therapies discussed, the alpha blockers are likely to give the most subjective improvement. Blocking the alpha-adrenergic system results in relaxation of the smooth muscle fibers of the prostate gland, with reduction of symptoms and improved urinary flow. The response is rapid (within hours), and studies have shown long-term efficacy.

The most common nonselective alpha blockers, terazosin (Hytrin) and doxazosin (Cardura), require dose titration to avoid postural hypotension. The newer and more expensive selective $alpha_{1a}$-adrenergic antagonists include tamsulosin (Flomax), alfuzosin (Uroxatral), and silodosin (Rapaflo). These are more specific for the prostatic tissue, thus reducing the incidence of hypotension and the need to titrate the dose.

DOSAGE

For terazosin (Hytrin), start at 1 mg nightly and titrate every week to effect, up to a maximum of 20 mg. Terazosin is available in 1-, 2-, 5-, and 10-mg formulations. For doxazosin (Cardura), start at 1 mg nightly and titrate every week to effect, up to a maximum of 8 mg. Doxazosin comes in 1-, 2-, 4-, and 8-mg formulations. The recommended dose of tamsulosin (Flomax) is 0.4 mg 30 minutes after a meal every day, up to a maximum of 0.8 mg per day. Tamsulosin is available in a 0.4-mg formulation. Alfuzosin is available in a 10-mg formulation only and silodosin is available in 8 mg only.

PRECAUTIONS

Postural hypotension, dizziness, fatigue, headache, nasal stuffiness, and retrograde ejaculation may occur. This class of drugs should be avoided prior to cataract surgery as they may increase the risk of floppy iris syndrome. Tamsulosin has the greatest risk of this.

5-Alpha-Reductase Inhibition

Finasteride prevents the conversion of testosterone to DHT and lowers DHT serum levels. This drug can take as long as 6 months to work, but it appears to halt the progression of prostate growth. In terms of patient satisfaction and symptom reduction, finasteride is not a great drug unless the goal includes treatment of male-pattern baldness. Finasteride causes a 50% reduction of PSA.

DOSAGE

The recommended dose of finasteride is 5 mg once a day, and it comes in 5-mg tablets. The recommended dose of dutasteride is 0.5 mg once daily, and it is available in 0.5-mg tablets.

PRECAUTIONS

Side effects such as decreased ejaculatory volume (2.8%), impotence (3.7%), and decreased libido (3.3%) have been reported. These drugs can take up to 6 months to show benefits.

Phosphodiesterase-5 Enzyme Inhibitors

Studies have shown that although urodynamic testing (detrusor pressure, bladder outlet obstruction, and maximum urinary flow rate) did not show improvement compared to placebo, the subjective quality of life did improve with improvement in the IPSS.[32,33] Consider this therapy in men who have both LUTS and erectile dysfunction.

DOSAGE

Tadalafil (Cialis), 5 mg daily

PRECAUTIONS

Headache, myalgia, and upper respiratory tract infection and irritation are the most common side effects. This is also an expensive drug compared to previously discussed treatments.

Anticholinergics

Occasionally anticholinergic agents are used in men with irritative triggers that result in worsening symptoms related to bladder neck contraction. These medicines (tolterodine and others) should not be used in those with a large postvoid residual bladder (>250 mL), as anticholinergics can worsen dilation of the bladder. Long-term use of anticholinergic medicines has also been found to increase the risk of dementia due to the reduction of acetylcholine.[34]

Surgery

When severe symptoms are not controlled with the previously discussed therapies, consider urological referral for minimally invasive therapy or surgical resection, as follows:
- Transurethral microwave thermotherapy (TUMT) uses a microwave antenna that generates heat in the transition zone and results in coagulation necrosis. This procedure is performed on an outpatient basis.
- Transurethral needle ablation (TUNA) involves the placement of small needles in the prostate via cystoscopy that emit radiofrequency energy resulting in necrosis of prostatic tissue.

The minimally invasive procedures described here have a lower morbidity compared with transurethral resection of the prostate; however, they are not as effective in reducing symptoms, and no tissue is obtained for pathological evaluation.

- Transurethral resection of the prostate (TURP) is the gold standard and will likely result in the greatest symptomatic improvement (95% of patients reported improved symptoms). Complications, such as incontinence (1%), blood transfusion (3% to 5%), retrograde ejaculation (20% to 75%), and stricture formation (5%) are becoming less severe with the use of laser prostatectomy that reduces bleeding. TURP is the most invasive procedure (except for open prostatectomy) and requires a hospital stay.

- Transurethral incision of the prostate (TUIP) involves endoscopic placement of one to two incisions along the prostatic capsule to reduce urethral constriction. This procedure has been found to be effective (83% of patients have improved symptoms) and safe for men with smaller glands (smaller than 30 g) who may not need TURP.

PREVENTION PRESCRIPTION

- Avoid excessive amounts of saturated fats, such as those found in red meat, fried foods, and dairy.
- Consume omega-3–rich fats found in cold-water fish, nuts, greens, and ground flaxseed.
- Consider light to moderate (one glass or less daily) alcohol consumption.
- Eat plenty of natural plants, particularly those rich in beta-sitosterol, such as green leafy vegetables, rice bran, wheat germ, peanuts, corn oils, nuts, and soybeans.
- Encourage soy-based foods such as soy milk, edamame, soy nuts, and tofu. Try to eat 1–2 oz per day, and consider substituting soy milk for dairy milk.

- Avoid dietary supplements or environmental exposures that may increase circulating hormone levels such as pesticides, herbicides, and recombinant bovine growth hormone (rBGH)-rich dairy products. Also avoid drugs that include dehydroepiandrosterone (DHEA), androstenedione, testosterone, and human growth hormone.
- Maintain appropriate weight and perform regular aerobic exercise.
- Treat metabolic syndrome with exercise, weight loss, and a low–glycemic index/load diet to reduce inflammation of the prostate (see Chapters 32 and 87).

THERAPEUTIC REVIEW

This is a summary of therapeutic options for benign prostatic hyperplasia (BPH). A patient presenting with severe symptoms (BPH Symptom Index Score or International Prostate Symptom Score [IPSS] greater than 19) will benefit by jumping ahead to a more aggressive therapy such as alpha blockers or referral to a surgeon. For the patient who has mild to moderate symptoms, however, this ladder approach is appropriate.

REMOVAL OF EXACERBATING FACTORS

- Ask the patient to stop taking over-the-counter cold remedies or diet aids (phenylpropanolamine [PPA]), nasal decongestants (pseudoephedrine), herbs (ma huang, Ephedra), or caffeinated products that contain sympathomimetics, which increase prostatic muscle tone.
- Consider asking the patient to stop taking pharmaceutical products that have anticholinergic effects leading to urinary retention. These agents include antihistamines, bowel antispasmodics, bladder antispasmodics, tricyclic antidepressants, and antipsychotics.
- Avoid excessive water consumption before bed.

NUTRITION

- Increase soy-rich foods in diet. A 1-oz serving each day (approximately the size of the palm of the hand) provides approximately 25 mg. B₁
- Encourage a diet that is low in saturated fat from red meat and dairy. B₁
- Encourage foods rich in omega-3 fatty acids (salmon, nuts, or flax), or take one tablespoon of lignan-rich flaxseed oil twice daily or one to two tablespoons of ground flaxseed twice daily. B₁

SUPPLEMENTS

- Beta-sitosterol: 60 mg twice daily A₁
- Zinc: 30–40 mg daily B₂

BOTANICALS

- Consider pygeum: 100 to 200 mg twice daily or saw palmetto: 160 mg twice daily B₁
- If no improvement after 8 weeks, consider adding rye grass pollen: 126 mg three times daily. Rye grass pollen has more of an antiinflammatory effect, which may act synergistically with saw palmetto or pygeum. B₁
- Other herbal products that have potential benefit include stinging nettles and pumpkin seed extract and cranberry.

PHARMACEUTICALS

- If no improvement occurs with the use of botanicals, discontinue them and start an alpha-adrenergic blocker (see text for doses). A₂
- If the patient is unable to tolerate an alpha blocker or if a greater response is desired, consider finasteride, at 5 mg daily. A₂
- For those with both erectile dysfunction and symptoms of BPH, consider a PDE-5 inhibitor such as tadalafil, 5 mg daily. B₂

SURGICAL THERAPY

- If the patient's symptoms persist or worsen despite the foregoing measures, refer for urological evaluation and treatment, with the following options: B₂
- Transurethral microwave thermotherapy (TUMT)
- Transurethral incision of the prostate (TUIP) B₂
- Transurethral resection of the prostate (TURP) A₃

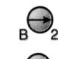
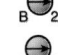

Key Web Resources

PDF of American Urologic Association (AUA) symptom score: Handout you can give to patients to fill out and score to judge severity of symptoms. This is also known as the International Prostate Symptom Score (IPSS)	http://urologyhealthteam.com/auass-qol.pdf
AUA (American Urological Association) Foundation: Management of Benign Prostatic Hyperplasia: Patient education on BPH	http://www.urologyhealth.org/urology/index.cfm?article=144
Prostate Pal: A smartphone app developed by Dr. Ronald Yap that allows patients to monitor their AUA scores in relation to their fluid intake and urinary output	Android devices: https://play.google.com/store/apps/details?id=com.quarkstudios.prostatepal&hl=en IOS devices: https://itunes.apple.com/us/app/prostate-pal-3/id732970382?mt=8

REFERENCES

References are available online at ExpertConsult.com.

CHAPTER 61

UROLITHIASIS (KIDNEY AND BLADDER STONES)

Jimmy Wu, MD, MPH

PATHOPHYSIOLOGY

Over the past few decades, an increasing percentage of Americans has had the misfortune of experiencing the disabling pain that accompanies urolithiasis. A recent National Health and Nutrition Examination Survey (NHANES) in 2007 reported that about 1 in 11 Americans will have experienced at least one symptomatic stone in their lifetime.[1] Notable epidemiological risks include being white, male, obese, insulin resistant, and living in hot, arid regions.[2] As evidenced by Hippocrates' reference to "...persons laboring under the stone,..." in his famous oath, this common medical problem has challenged even history's most renown healers.[3]

In addition to being responsible for so much morbidity in the individual patient, kidney stones were estimated by several recent studies to cost between $4.5 and $5.3 billion in lost work hours and direct health care costs.[4,5] Because most patients with idiopathic kidney stones have some underlying urine metabolic abnormality, there is a recurrence risk of 40% at 5 years and 75% at 20 years.[6] This tendency for urological stones to recur within the same people presents an opportunity for health care providers to promote a preventive and integrative approach in protecting against stone recurrence.

There are data that demonstrate certain epidemiological disparities in gender, geographic location, and race. For reasons that are still unclear, men consistently have a higher risk of developing kidney stones. Geographically, the "stone belt," consisting of the southeastern U.S. region, also tends to have higher prevalence of renal lithiasis; this is likely due to its hotter climate. Finally, black Americans appear to suffer less from this disease than their white counterparts.[7]

Increased research on the consequences of the growing obesity epidemic is also demonstrating that obesity is an independent contributing factor for kidney stone formation. There are several theories behind this including the idea that the increased adiposity leads to an altered thermogenesis situation which produces a dehydrated state (thereby predisposing the body to supersaturation of stone ingredients). Obese individuals also tend to experience hyperuricemia and hypocitraturia, which are known risk factors for kidney stones.[2]

To provide the most appropriate counseling, it is important to understand how kidney stones form and what elements are commonly present in stones. Kidney stones are a product of normally soluble material (i.e., calcium, oxalate, etc.) that supersaturate in urine to a level that facilitates crystallization of that very material (Fig. 61.1).[8] With this etiology in mind, any approach that discourages urinary crystallization or promotes crystallization inhibition forms the basis for the following preventive recommendations.

> Individuals with recurrent kidney stones or with urolithiasis before age 30 should get a 24-hour urine test done to check for high levels of calcium, oxalate, and uric acid or for low levels of citrate. See Table 61.1 for recommendations based on the test results.

More than 80% of kidney stones primarily consist of calcium, with most being calcium oxalate. These oxalate stones can also contain phosphate or uric acid. The remainder kidney stones can be divided into uric acid, struvite (magnesium ammonium phosphate or infection stone), and cystine as their primary constituents. Most calcium stone formers possess some sort of urinary metabolic abnormality that can be detected with a 24-hour urine sample[8] (see Table 61.1).

The majority of patients (33%–66%) who suffer from calcium-based kidney stones have hypercalciuria, which is mostly idiopathic but can be familial as well. The urine is supersaturated, with a high enough level of calcium that calcium renal calculi begin to form. It is important to note that if there is accompanying hypercalcemia, other disorders must be ruled out (i.e., hyperparathyroidism, sarcoidosis, cancer, etc.).[9]

Similarly, patients who are found to have high urinary oxalate levels are predisposed to passing calcium oxalate stones. Hyperoxaluria is due to two main causes. There is a rare primary form that is inherited in an autosomal recessive fashion. There is also a more common acquired form that involves increased oxalate absorption secondary to ileal compromise and fat malabsorption (enteric fat does not get absorbed and subsequently binds to dietary calcium, which results in higher levels of absorbed oxalate).[10]

The third metabolic disorder found in patients with calcium stones is hypocitraturia. Citrate serves as a protective factor against calcium stone formation because it can chelate calcium in urine, thereby forming a soluble complex that is harmlessly excreted. Therefore people with low levels of citrate in their urine are at risk for calcium stone formation.[10]

Of the stones that are not composed of calcium, primary uric acid nephrolithiasis is the next most common (10%). Any factor that acidifies the urine pH (i.e., protein intake, insulin resistance) creates an environment that is more susceptible to stone formation. The other two factors that contribute to uric acid stone formation include low urinary volume (i.e., dehydration, diarrhea) and hyperuricosuria (i.e., enzymatic deficiency syndromes, drugs, gout, etc.).[11]

Struvite stones typically form in patients who have chronic urinary tract infections due to urease-producing bacteria such as *Proteus* or *Klebsiella*. These patients classically develop staghorn calculi that are found in the renal pelvis. The stones consist of multiple magnesium ammonium phosphate crystals and calcium carbonate-apatite.[12]

Finally, cystine stones (1%) are the result of cystinuria, which is a rare genetic autosomal-recessive metabolic disorder. Cystine stones should be considered in patients who present with their first stone during early childhood (median age = 12 years).[13]

INTEGRATIVE THERAPY

Nutrition

Any dietary recommendation that limits lithogenic ingredients and promotes lithoprotective factors serves as the basis for the following nutritional and supplemental suggestions (Tables 61.1 and 61.2). There is an abundance of literature regarding the role of nutrition and supplements in kidney stone prevention, but there is a relative lack of solid evidence to support the following dietary recommendations.

Weight

As mentioned previously, obese people who develop qualities of metabolic syndrome are at increased risk

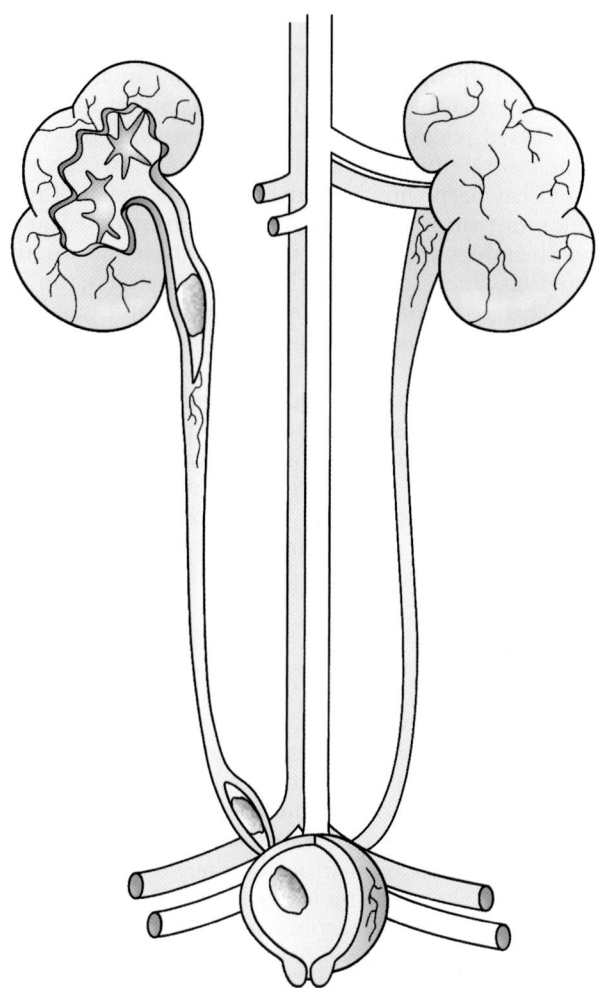

FIG. 61.1 ■ Kidney stones in the kidney, ureter, and bladder. (From National Kidney and Urologic Diseases Information Clearinghouse: http://kidney.niddk.nih.gov/kudiseases/pubs/stonesadults/index.htm).

TABLE 61.1	Lithogenic Values of Urinary Biochemical Factors With Dietary Prescription	
Urine Factor	**24-Hour Urine Value**	**Dietary Prescription**
Fluid volume	<2 L/24 hours	Maintain total fluid intake > 2 L/day Reduce caffeine Stay more hydrated if strenuous physical activity
Calcium	Female >250 mg/24 hours Male >300 mg/24 hours	Maintain adequate dietary calcium intake Reduce sodium and animal protein intake Reduce calcium supplements Reduce carbohydrate intake
Oxalate	>40 mg/24 hours	Maintain adequate dietary calcium intake Reduce dietary oxalate intake Avoid vitamin C supplements Increase magnesium-rich foods
Citrate	Female <550 mg/24 hours Male <450 mg/24 hours	Increase fruit and vegetable intake Reduce sodium and animal protein
Uric Acid	Female >600 mg/24 hours Male >800 mg/24 hours	Reduce purine-high foods Reduce animal protein intake Reduce alcohol intake

Adapted from Graces F, Costa-Bauza A, Prieto RM. Renal lithiasis and nutrition. *Nutr J.* 2006;5:1-7 and Taylor EN, Curhan GC. Diet and fluid prescription in stone disease. *Kidney Int.* 2006;70:835-839.

for stone formation. There is no research that directly studies the potential protective impact of weight loss on the development of kidney stones. However, it has been well established that the risk for stones increases with BMI[14]; therefore one can reasonably infer that weight loss in individuals with unhealthy BMIs should decrease their risk for nephrolithiasis. This underlines the overall importance of promoting healthy nutrition and physical activity in the prevention of kidney stones.[15-17]

Water

Increasing fluid intake is a dietary recommendation that possesses strong scientific support for its role in preventing recurrent renal lithiasis. Several observational studies dating to 1966 have postulated that increased fluid intake is beneficial; results from one randomized control trial in 1996 showed that fluid intake achieving a urinary volume of 2 liters reduced stone recurrence rate from 27% to 12%.[18-21]

A safe recommendation would be to ask patients to drink 2–3 liters of water per day. One approach is to tailor the fluid recommendation with the calculated urine volume from the 24-hour urine test. For example, if the 24-hour urine volume were 1.5 liters, it would be best to advise the patient to drink two more 8-ounce (2×240 = 480 mL) cups of water to achieve a total of 2 liters.[22] There is no evidence for the following, but some doctors recommend their patients maintain urine at a very light color. Some have also advocated drinking water at bedtime because urinary concentration usually occurs during sleep.[22] It is especially important for endurance athletes with stones to be aware of their fluid loss through sweat. Furthermore, mineral water should be ingested with some caution because it may contain calcium or other lithogenic material.

Beverages

There is a smattering of studies that have examined the efficacy of encouraging or discouraging intake of different types of beverages for the prevention of stones. Fruit-based juices have especially been studied because of their citrate (lithoprotective) content. However, vitamin C has been shown to increase urine oxalate (lithogenic); not surprisingly, evidence for fruit-based juices is still ambiguous.[15] Several studies have shown that grapefruit juice increases the risk for stones; on the other hand, lemon juice, orange juice, and cranberry juice have mostly been viewed as protective against renal stones.[7,15,23-26]

Not much is discussed about the role of soft drinks in stone formation, but the general recommendation would be to limit consumption, possibly because of their high fructose content.[27] However, sodas with higher citrate content may theoretically neutralize any lithogenic effect.[24] The effects of caffeinated beverages such as coffee and tea (especially black) on stone formation are quite mixed.[26-27]

Sodium

Studies have shown that increase in dietary sodium results in an increased urinary excretion of calcium and a decreased urinary excretion of citrate. This combination effect makes high sodium intake a potential risk factor for higher stone recurrence; such intake is associated with a 50%–61% increase in risk of kidney stones.[28] Recent studies have shown that a low-salt diet could reduce calcium excretion.[27] It is recommended that sodium intake be restricted to less than 3–6 grams per day, especially for patients with hypercalciuria.[7,15,20]

Protein

Increased protein intake appears to increase urinary calcium and uric acid and decrease urinary citrate levels.[7,15,20] Therefore, reducing protein intake may also benefit individuals with calcium and uric acid stones. There have been some studies that have examined combination diets, and those that consisted of a low-protein component had a lower stone recurrence rate.[29]

Carbohydrates

Some postulate that a possible relationship between higher intake of carbohydrates/refined sugar and increased urinary calcium is partially responsible for why wealthier countries have higher rates of kidney stones.[7] However, the association is too weak to recommend carbohydrate cessation as a form of protection against stone recurrence.

Omega-3 Fatty Acids

Increased intake of dietary omega-3 fatty acids does not reduce the risk for kidney stone formation. However, there is promise that fish oil supplements may have a role in preventing stone formation because small studies have

TABLE 61.2	Foods High in Bioelements Related to Calcium Oxalate Stone Formation	
Lithoprotective		
Calcium (dietary)	**Magnesium**	**Citrate**
Milk	Almonds	Orange
Yogurt	Cashews	Lemon
Cheese	Soybean	Cranberry
Broccoli	Potato	Pineapple
Salmon	Nuts	High-citrate juices and sodas
Lithogenic		
Sodium	**Oxalate**	**Purine**
Potato chips	Rhubarb	Legumes
Canned foods	Spinach	Spinach
Frozen dinners	Chocolate	Red meat
Soy sauce	Peanuts	Alcohol
Table salt	Cashews	Sardines

Adapted from http://ods.od.nih.gov/factsheets/list-all/ and Graces F, Costa-Bauza A, Prieto RM. Renal lithiasis and nutrition. *Nutr J.* 2006;5:1-7.

shown that it reduces the urinary excretion of calcium and oxalate.[30-32]

Purines

People with uric acid stones are generally advised to avoid a high-purine diet. Purine-containing foods include organ meats, legumes, mushrooms, spinach, alcoholic, sardines, and poultry.[11]

Oxalate

Despite several studies, there is currently no consensus regarding the effect of dietary oxalate on stone formation, even in those with hyperoxaluria.[15,27] Dietary oxalate may not be readily absorbed due to its low bioavailability.[7,20] Therefore, there is no firm recommendation about limiting dietary oxalate; however, there is also little harm in such advice. Oxalate-rich foods include nuts (almonds, peanuts, pecans, walnuts, cashews), vegetables (rhubarb, spinach), and chocolate.[15,20]

Calcium (Dietary and Supplemental)

Contrary to conventional wisdom, it is not recommended to limit dietary intake of calcium. This conclusion has been proven several times with strong evidence. Two prospective observational studies from the 1990s concluded that kidney stone formation was inversely associated with dietary calcium intake.[30,33,34] In addition, a 5-year randomized control trial comparing groups that differed by the calcium load in their diet showed that decreasing dietary calcium was a risk factor for symptomatic stone recurrence.[30,35]

The theory behind this conclusion is that dietary calcium protects against stone formation by binding with oxalate, thereby reducing urinary oxalate levels. It takes a smaller increase of urinary oxalate, than of urinary calcium, to precipitate stone formation, which makes a high urinary oxalate level a larger risk factor in calcium oxalate stone formation. This finding explains why dietary calcium is actually lithoprotective.[33]

Supplements

Calcium

Contrary to dietary calcium, it has been suggested that calcium supplements increases risk of urolithiasis. A 1997 study showed that women using calcium supplements had a higher risk of calcium stone formation. This finding was explained by the fact that the supplements were not taken with food, thereby nullifying calcium's function in reducing dietary oxalate absorption. However, other data have shown a neutral effect of calcium supplements for men and younger women.[20,30,34,36]

Vitamin C

Vitamin C can be metabolized to oxalate and therefore could theoretically increase the risk of stone formation. A trial has shown that supplemental vitamin C increases urinary oxalate excretion; however, there has been no evidence that it actually causes an increase in symptomatic stone formation. Therefore, recurrent stone formers should not be instructed to limit their dietary vitamin C intake, especially since foods high in vitamin C are also high in citrate. However, it is reasonable to suggest limited intake of supplemental vitamin C.[7,15,20,37]

Vitamin D

Recently, increased vitamin D intake has been encouraged as sound general health advice. However, due to its role in calcium absorption, there is a theoretical possibility of increased vitamin D being a risk factor for calcium stones. On the contrary, several studies have shown that high serum vitamin D levels are not associated with a high prevalence of kidney stone disease.[27,38]

Zinc

High dietary zinc intake has also been shown to increase the risk of kidney stone formation. This may partially explain why animal protein intake also possesses strong lithogenic properties.[39]

Magnesium

In theory, magnesium binds to oxalate, potentially decreasing one's risk for calcium oxalate stones. There is sparse data suggesting that dietary and supplemental magnesium can lower risk of stone formation in men.[28,40] Dietary magnesium can be mostly found in dairy products, meat, seafood, avocados, dark green vegetables, and cocoa.[15]

Botanicals and Other Herbal Medicines

There are many studies that have examined the potential use of various botanicals and herbs for prevention of stone formation. However, most studies have used in vitro or animal models. There are only a few that have demonstrated some promise within human models.[41]

Phyllanthus niruri (i.e., Stonebreaker, Chanca Piedra, etc.) is a plant that has been studied and used in Brazil; it has been studied in the human population and has shown efficacy in preventing stone recurrence.[41] Other studied herbals include *Andrographis paniculata*, *Hibiscus sabdariffa*, and *Orthosiphon grandiflorus*.[41] Most of these are frequently consumed as teas.

> *Phyllanthus niruri* may potentiate insulin and other antidiabetic medications, as well as antihypertensive medications. Do not take during pregnancy.

Probiotics

Oxalobacter formigenes is an anaerobic bacterium responsible for degrading oxalate in our body. It has been postulated that a probiotic containing this species would be useful for preventing stone formation in those with hyperoxaluria. Results from a study that evaluated some probiotic products on the market showed that they did not contain any *Oxalobacter formigenes* and therefore would be unlikely to benefit patients with calcium oxalate stones.[42] There have not been many studies that have shown actual benefit in decreasing symptomatic stone incidents, but several have demonstrated its physiological significance in decreasing urinary oxalate levels.[27,43,44]

Traditional Chinese Medicine

Acupuncture

There is a paucity of data in the literature about acupuncture as a preventive measure for kidney stones, but it has been used extensively as an analgesic for both the acute renal colic presentation and for those who are receiving a planned extracorporeal shock wave lithotripsy (ESWL) procedure.[45]

There is some anecdotal evidence that acupuncture utilizing techniques that facilitate energy manipulation of the kidney and bladder organs may help with acute stone-related pain and with stone recurrence.[46]

Herbals

There is limited data from the Kampo traditional Japanese herbal medicine tradition indicating that some herbal mixtures, including chorei-to, wullingsan, jin qian cao, and niao shi mixture, have been helpful mostly as diuretics in stone prevention.[45,47]

Ayurvedic Medicine

Including *P. niruri*, as described previously, there have been several other ayurvedic medicines commonly used for nephrolithiasis management including *Tribulus terrestris*, *Orthosiphon stamineus/grandiflorus* (java tea), and *Dolichos biflorus* (horse gram).[47] One of the more studied ayurvedic products is known as Cystone. It contains several ingredients that have been claimed to decrease urinary supersaturation. There has been one good study on the Cystone that does not support its efficacy.[48]

Pharmaceuticals

The following text contains a discussion on medicines that have demonstrated efficacy for the prevention of stone recurrence. Management of acute nephrolithiasis-related symptoms (i.e., pain, nausea, etc.) will not be discussed in this chapter.

Alkalinizers

This class of drugs primarily works by increasing urine pH. Because uric acid stones tend to supersaturate in acidic urine, alkalinizers such as potassium citrate and sodium bicarbonate are mostly used to prevent documented uric acid stones. Potassium citrate is preferred because it can also reduce urinary calcium and provide citrate as a lithoprotective element.[49]

Potassium Citrate

DOSAGE

10 mEq three times a day (if $U_{citrate}$ > 150 mg/day) or 20 mEq three times a day (if $U_{citrate}$ < 150 mg/day) with meals, up to 100 mEq/day. Comes in 5- and 10-mEq pills.

PRECAUTIONS

Nausea, hyperkalemia (especially when taken with other medicines that may cause hyperkalemia).

Sodium Bicarbonate

DOSAGE

650 mg three times a day. Comes in 325 and 650 mg tablets. Also in powder form.

PRECAUTIONS

Bloating.

Calcium-Channel Blockers

Data indicate that this class of medicines acts as an "expulsive" medicine that assists with stone passage. It works as an antispasmodic on the ureter, eliminating the fast, uncoordinated components of ureteral smooth muscle contraction. Most studies have examined its use in conjunction with a steroid (25 mg/day of methylprednisolone) and results have demonstrated a higher stone-expulsion rate, shorter expulsion time, and a reduced need for analgesia.[49]

Nifedipine

DOSAGE

30 mg daily extended release (ER) for 20–30 days. Comes in 30 mg ER tablets.

PRECAUTIONS

Flushing, peripheral edema, lightheadedness/dizziness, headache, gastrointestinal upset.

Alpha-1 Channel Blockers

Alpha-1 channel blockers also work as antispasmodics, especially on the distal ureter. Several studies, especially for distal ureteral stones, have demonstrated a higher stone-expulsion rate with their use.[49]

Tamsulosin, Doxazosin, Alfuzosin

DOSAGE

- *Doxazosin*: Start 1 mg at night and titrate every week to effect. Maximum dose is 8 mg/day. Comes in 1, 2, 4, and 8 mg tablets.
- *Tamsulosin*: Take 0.4 mg, 30 minutes after a meal each day. Maximum dose is 0.8 mg daily. Comes in 0.4 mg tablets.
- *Alfuzosin ER*: 10 mg daily. Comes in 10 mg ER tablets only.

PRECAUTIONS

Postural hypotension, dizziness, fatigue, headache, nasal stuffiness, and retrograde ejaculation.

Recommendation is that medical expulsive therapy can be used for stones up to 10 mm. Alpha channel blockers appear to perform better with stones 5–10 mm.[50]

Thiazide Diuretics

Thiazides can lower calcium excretion by as much as 50% and therefore benefit patients with recurrent stones due to hypercalciuria. Thiazides should be considered if recurrence of stones persists despite appropriate dietary changes. Studies have shown a 90% reduction in incidence of new stones with the use of thiazides. Chlorthalidone can be given just once a day because of its lower half life. However, be weary of hypokalemia because low potassium can reduce urinary citrate excretion. To avoid hypokalemia, it is advisable to add potassium citrate.[49]

Hydrochlorothiazide, Chlorthalidone

DOSAGE

- *Hydrochlorothiazide*: 25 mg daily, but higher doses may be needed to achieve adequate calcium-lowering effect. Comes in 12.5, 25, and 50 mg tablets.
- *Chlorthalidone*: 25 mg daily. Comes in 25 mg tablets.

PRECAUTIONS

Hypokalemia, hyperuricemia, hyponatremia, dizziness, and headache.

Xanthine Inhibitors

Frequently used in patients with gout, these medicines can also be used for management of stone formers with hyperuricosuria (with either uric acid or calcium stones). It interferes with the conversion of xanthine into uric acid.[11]

Allopurinol.

DOSAGE

200–300 mg per day divided once daily to three times a day.

PRECAUTIONS

Use with caution in patients with renal failure.

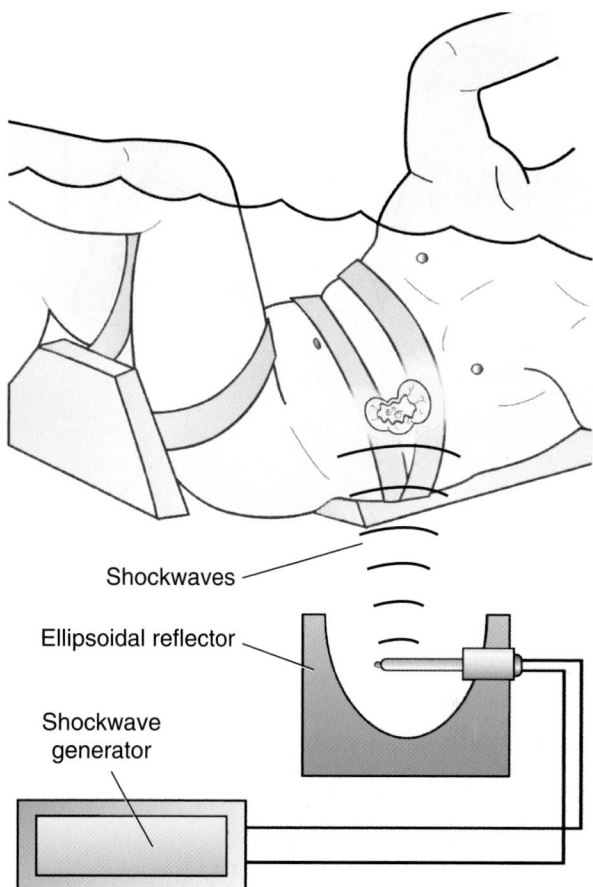

FIG. 61.2 ■ Extracorporeal shockwave lithotripsy. (From National Kidney and Urologic Diseases Information Clearinghouse: http://kidney.niddk.nih.gov/kudiseases/pubs/stonesadults/index.htm).

Surgery

Most stones smaller than 4 mm are generally watched conservatively and felt to have a 90% chance of passing by themselves, especially if they are located in the distal ureter. Stones between 4 and 6 mm have a dramatically lesser chance of passing (50%), whereas stones between 7 and 10 mm have only a 20% chance of spontaneously passing. Besides those of a larger size, stones that are more proximally located in the ureter have greater difficulty for spontaneous resolution.[51]

Surgery is considered for kidney stones that are felt to have a low chance of self-resolution. This includes lithotripsy, ureteroscopy, and percutaneous nephrostomy—choice of therapy depends on several factors including the position and size of the stone.

Extracorporeal Shockwave Lithotripsy

Of the three surgical options, extracorporeal shockwave lithotripsy (ESWL) is the least invasive and considered to be first-line therapy for the appropriate context. Lithotripsy has been considered to be just as effective as ureteroscopy for stones that are smaller than 10 mm (86% vs. 90% stone free rate, respectively), regardless of location in the ureter. If the stone is large, lithotripsy may have to be performed several times (Fig. 61.2).[52]

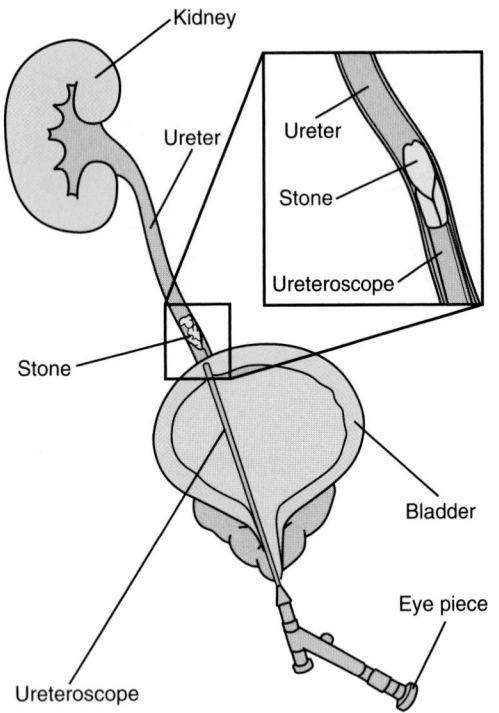

FIG. 61.3 ■ Ureteroscopic stone removal. (From National Kidney and Urologic Diseases Information Clearinghouse: http://kidney. niddk.nih.gov/kudiseases/pubs/stonesadults/index.htm).

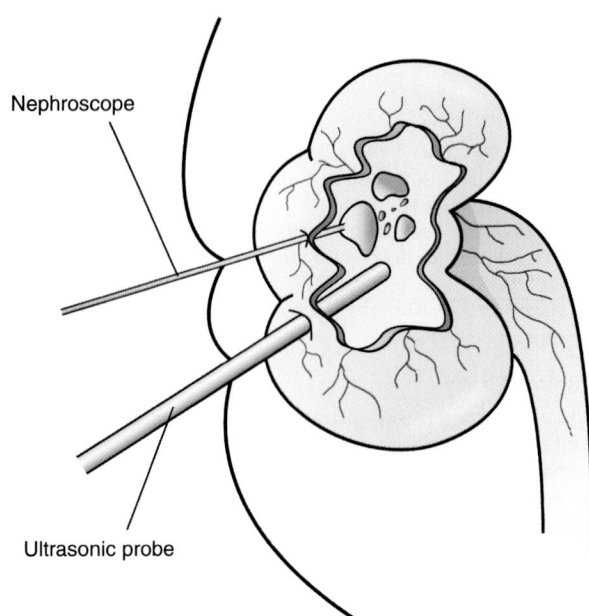

FIG. 61.4 ■ Percutaneous nephrolithotomy. (From National Kidney and Urologic Diseases Information Clearinghouse: http://kidney. niddk.nih.gov/kudiseases/pubs/stonesadults/index.htm).

Serious complications of ESWL are not common, but the procedure can cause transient pain, hematuria, nausea, and vomiting. More life-threatening complications have been common in patients who have required multiple treatments for larger stones. Pregnancy, uncontrolled hypertension, uncontrolled coagulopathy, and distal obstruction to stone are absolute contraindications.[52]

Rigid and Flexible Ureteroscopy

In stones that are larger than 10 mm, while ESWL can still be considered, ureteroscopy has been reported to have better success (67% vs. 73%, respectively). This technique involves passing a scope through the ureter to physically remove the stone, sometimes with the help of laser (Fig. 61.3). This technique is preferred, especially for larger, proximal, and impacted stones. In patients who have absolute contraindications to ESWL therapy, ureteroscopy is an acceptable alternative.[52-53] Especially with the development of more advanced technology (flexible and smaller caliber scopes) and techniques, complications such as ureteral perforation or stricture formation have become much less common.[52-53]

Percutaneous Nephrolithotomy

Because of a larger side-effect profile, this is reserved for treatment of renal calculi (especially staghorn struvite stones) and large impacted proximal ureteral stones. Stones that have failed ureteroscopy are also candidates for percutaneous nephrolithotomy. This procedure involves inserting a needle through the skin into the kidney's collecting system and dilating the tract to 1 cm, which allows the urologist to break up and remove the stones (Fig. 61.4). Just like any other invasive procedure, percutaneous nephrolithotomy has complications such as bleeding, injury to other organs, or infection.[52-53]

PREVENTION PRESCRIPTION

- Maintain a daily fluid intake of 2–3 L (~8–10 glasses of water). Try to limit situations that would exacerbate dehydration (i.e., hot weather, endurance exercise, etc.).
- Do NOT limit your dietary calcium intake (strive for 1000–1200 mg/day).
- A low sodium, low protein diet can be helpful.
- Drink lemonade, orange juice, and cranberry juice, but limit grapefruit juice and sodas.
- Develop a healthy lifestyle that maintains a normal body mass index.
- For those with hyperoxaluria, limit intake of foods with high oxalate levels, including nuts (almonds, peanuts, pecans, walnuts, cashews), vegetables (rhubarb, spinach), and chocolate.

THERAPEUTIC REVIEW

Following is the summary of therapeutic options for kidney stones. The purpose behind these suggestions is to prevent recurrence of symptomatic stones. Regardless of composition, all patients with kidney stones should be advised to increase their water intake. Depending on the type of stone and results of the metabolic evaluation, additional dietary, supplemental, and medical recommendations can also be made. Surgery is reserved for large stones, recalcitrant disease, obstructing disease, and for stones located in certain difficult-to-access positions along the urological tract.

REMOVE EXACERBATING FACTORS

- Avoid excessive exposure to any environment or activity that promotes dehydration (warmer climates or strenuous physical activity).
- Maintain general healthy eating and physical activity habits that prevent development of metabolic syndrome conditions (obesity, hypertension, hyperlipidemia, etc.).

NUTRITION

- Drink lots of water. Two to three liters per day is recommended (8–10 glasses of water).
- Do not limit dietary calcium intake.
- Limit caffeine, soda, grapefruit juice, protein, carbohydrate, and salt intake (<2.5 g daily).
- Drink lemonade, orange juice, and cranberry juice.
- Decrease consumption of oxalate-containing foods, especially in those with hyperoxaluria. These include nuts (almonds, peanuts, pecans, walnuts, cashews), vegetables (rhubarb, spinach), and chocolate.
- Decrease intake of purine-rich foods, especially in those with uric acid stones.
- Tailor your diet based on type of metabolic abnormality.

SUPPLEMENTS

- Limit supplemental calcium, but if needed for bone fortification, take with food.
- Limit supplemental vitamin C.

- Take supplemental omega-3 fatty acids.
- Take supplemental magnesium.
- Probiotics containing *Oxalobacter formigenes* can be used, especially for those with hyperoxaluria.

BOTANICALS

- *Phyllanthus niruri* (a.k.a. Stonebreaker, Chanca Piedra)—take 250 mg daily to twice a day before meals.
- Other Chinese herbs can be tried (chorei-to, wulling-san, jin qian cao, and niao shi).
- Other herbs frequently used in Ayurvedic medicine (*Tribulus terrestris, Orthosiphon stamineus/grandiflorus* (java tea), and *Dolichos biflorus)* can be considered.

ENERGY MEDICINE

- Acupuncture can be used for post-ESWL pain and possibly as a kidney/bladder energy modifying treatment.

PHARMACEUTICALS

- Diuretics, especially thiazides, can be used for their hypocalciuric effects.
- Potassium citrate is useful as an alkalinizer and citrate promoter.
- Alpha-1 blockers and calcium channel blockers can facilitate stone expulsion.
- Allopurinol can help prevent uric acid stones.

SURGICAL THERAPY

- ESWL is very successful for smaller stones (<1 cm) located in the distal ureter.
- Ureteroscopy can be utilized for larger stones that are located more proximally or are impacted.
- Percutaneous nephrolithotomy is reserved for recalcitrant stones and for staghorn calculi.

National Kidney & Urologic Diseases Info Clearinghouse	http://kidney.niddk.nih.gov/kudiseases/topics/stones.asp
Interactive patient module on Kidney Stones	https://medlineplus.gov/kidneystones.html
Prevention for kidney stones	http://www.webmd.com/kidney-stones/kidney-stones-prevention

REFERENCES

References are available online at ExpertConsult.com.

CHAPTER 62

CHRONIC PROSTATITIS/CHRONIC PELVIC PAIN SYNDROME

Myles Spar, MD, MPH

PATHOPHYSIOLOGY

Chronic prostatitis affects an estimated 9% of men in the United States.[1] The name is misleading as no infectious or causative agent is identified in the majority of cases. In fact, among specialists and researchers, this condition has come to be more accurately termed as chronic prostatitis/chronic pelvic pain syndrome (CP/CPPS) because most men with the condition describe symptoms of intermittent pelvic or urethral discomfort or pain. Patients often have other symptoms, similar to women with CPPS, including fatigue, depression, and irritative voiding symptoms; these symptoms are similar to those of benign prostatic hypertrophy (BPH). Sexual dysfunction, including erectile dysfunction and premature ejaculation, has also been shown to be strongly correlated with CPPS symptoms.[2,3]

The exact etiology of CP/CPPS is unknown, and there is no single established course of treatment. However, the condition is not only prevalent but also the impact of CPPS on quality of life is sizeable—comparable to that of Crohn's disease or myocardial infarction.[4]

> The impact of CPPS on quality of life is sizeable—comparable to that of Crohn's disease or myocardial infarction.

DIAGNOSIS

The diagnosis of CP/CPPS is made by screening for infectious causes of symptoms by looking for leukocytes in prostatic secretions using expressed prostatic secretions (EPS) or by postdigital rectal exam urinalysis (post-DRE U/A). Postprostatic massage urinalysis has been shown to correlate well with expressible prostatic secretions.[5]

The National Institute of Diabetes and Digestive and Kidney Diseases (NIDDK), which is the institute within the National Institutes of Health that oversees research devoted to CP/CPPS, recognizes five categories of prostatitis syndromes, with type III (CP/CPPS) being by far the most common, comprising 90% of all cases of symptomatic prostatitis[6] (Table 62.1). This chapter focuses on type IIIB, which is the most prevalent as well as the most challenging to treat.

Risk factors for CP/CPPS have not been clearly identified, and traditional risk factors for many diseases, such as smoking, obesity, or alcohol consumption, were not associated with CP/CPPS risk as assessed from the longitudinal Health Professionals Follow-Up Study (HPFS),[7] although higher leisure-time physical activity has been shown to be associated with a lower risk of CP/CPPS.[8]

The intensity of CP/CPPS symptoms can be measured using the National Institutes of Health Chronic Prostatitis Symptom Index (NIH-CPSI), which is a self-administered questionnaire that focuses on location, quality, and severity of pain; irritative and obstructive urinary symptoms; and overall quality of life (Fig. 62.1). The NIH-CPSI reports subscores for pain (0–21), urinary symptoms (0–10), and quality of life (0–12), as well as a total score (0–43).[9]

Since the NIH-CPSI was validated in 1999, the recognition of CP/CPPS as a heterogeneous disorder with multiple causes and various presenting symptomology has explained why clinical treatments have, in general, largely failed to have a substantial impact. This has led to other approaches for categorizing the disorder so that treatment can be better studied for each type of presentation. Thus, the urinary, psychosocial, organ-specific, infection, neurological/systemic, and tenderness (UPOINT) phenotype system has been validated as an effective phenotype system in classifying patients with CP/CPPS.[10] The identification of which phenotype a patient presents with helps guiding the course of treatment.

With the UPOINT system, history review, physical examination, urine cultures, and EPS or post-DRE urine results lead to a yes/no classification for each of the six UPOINT domains:
- Urinary is positive if the patient has bothersome urinary symptoms or high postvoid residual.
- Psychosocial is positive in the presence of clinical depression or catastrophizing.
- Organ-specific is positive if there is specific prostate tenderness on examination, leukocytosis on microscopic examination of prostatic fluid or post-DRE U/A, or presence of hematospermia.
- Infection is positive (in the absence of a current or previous urinary tract infection) if gram-negative bacilli or enterococci are found in prostatic fluid or if urine is positive for ureaplasma.
- Neurological/systemic is positive if there is pain outside the abdomen and pelvis or a concurrent diagnosis of fibromyalgia, chronic fatigue syndrome, or irritable bowel syndrome.
- Tenderness is positive if there are palpable muscle spasms or trigger points in the abdomen or pelvic floor.

TABLE 62.1	**National Institute of Diabetes and Digestive and Kidney Diseases (NIDDK)–Recognized Prostatitis Syndromes**

Type I: Acute bacterial prostatitis
Type II: Chronic bacterial prostatitis (bacteria can be cultured from semen or post-DRE urine)
Type III: Chronic abacterial prostatitis, chronic pelvic pain syndrome (CPPS)
 Type IIIA: Inflammatory CPPS (Leukocytes > 10/hpf in EPS/post-DRE urine)
 Type IIIB: Noninflammatory CPPS (Leukocytes < 10/hpf in EPS/post-DRE urine)
Type IV: Asymptomatic inflammatory prostatitis

DRE, digital rectal exam; *hpf,* high-power field.

The most common presenting phenotypes are urinary, organ specific, and tenderness.

The most appropriate diagnostic approach in a patient suspected of having CP/CPPS may be the use of the self-administered NIH-CPSI and then identification of the particular phenotype through history, physical examination, and lab analysis to decide on the best course of treatment. Then NIH-CPSI can be used to monitor the impact of treatment over time.

INTEGRATIVE THERAPY

There are several interventions that have been shown to be helpful in studies grouping all phenotypes of CP/CPPS together. One meta-analysis of randomized controlled trials of all interventions from 1947 through 2011 included 35 controlled trials for CP/CPPS treatment.[11] Symptom improvement was observed with several therapies, including some medications not approved in the United States (mepartricin and a muscle relaxant, thiocolchicoside), with each showing benefit in one study. Urinary symptom improvement was demonstrated with percutaneous tibial nerve stimulation, especially when combined with acupuncture. Interestingly, across all studies, placebo administration resulted in symptom improvement over time for all outcomes, indicating a strong mind-body component of CP/CPPS symptoms and/or a natural waning of symptoms over time.

Pharmaceuticals

The previously mentioned analysis showed no therapeutic effect of alpha-blockers or antibiotics, either alone or in combination. However, another review looked at the effectiveness of the following: alpha-blockers, antiinflammatories, antibiotics, finasteride, phytotherapy, gabapentin, glycosaminoglycans, and placebo.[12] The authors concluded that alpha-blockers, antibiotics, and a combination of both appeared to improve symptoms compared with placebo, while antiinflammatory drugs, finasteride, and phytotherapies (pollen extract or Quercetin) also had a measurable effect on symptoms. The authors noted that publication bias and small-study effects may have accounted for the positive findings, especially regarding

alpha-blockers and antiinflammatories. A further systematic review failed to demonstrate the effectiveness of pregabalin in improving overall symptom scores.[13]

Alpha-Blockers

Alpha-adrenergic blockers relax the smooth muscle in the prostatic urethra and bladder neck.

DOSAGE

Doxazosin and terazosin must be titrated up from a starting dose of 1 mg, usually taken at bedtime, to 8 mg maximum for doxazosin and 10 mg maximum for terazosin. The typical dosage for alfuzosin is 10 mg; for silodosin is 8 mg, and for tamsulosin is 0.4 mg, all to be taken with food.

PRECAUTIONS

All of the alpha-blockers can cause dizziness, postural hypotension, retrograde ejaculation, and nasal congestion. Rarely, alpha-blockers can cause syncope. Alfuzosin and silodosin should not be taken by men with severe hepatic or renal insufficiency.

Antibiotics

The most commonly studied and used antibiotics for CPPS are the quinolones, including ciprofloxacin and levofloxacin. These may help reduce inflammation, explaining the improvement observed in some studies, even among men with abacterial prostatitis.

Trimethoprim-sulfamethoxazole represents an alternative treatment for CPPS.

DOSAGE

Ciprofloxacin is dosed at 500 mg twice a day and levofloxacin at 500 mg once a day. Both are used for 4 weeks. Trimethoprim-sulfamethoxazole is used at double strength (160/800 mg) twice daily for 4 weeks.

PRECAUTIONS

Excessive use of antibiotics can lead to resistant infections, as well as dysbiosis of the gut. Specific precautions with the fluoroquinolones include risk of tendon rupture and aortic aneurysm. Trimethoprim-sulfamethoxazole can cause photosensitivity and possible severe allergic reactions in those sensitive to sulfa drugs.

Lifestyle

Because of the paucity of good evidence on the use of pharmaceuticals for CPPS, it is recommended to consider nutrition and exercise recommendations as these can make significant impacts on symptoms.

Nutrition

Herati and Moldwin published a systematic review of studies of the following therapies for CP/CPPS: diet and lifestyle modifications, phytotherapy, acupuncture,

Pelvic Pain Questionnaire

Male NIH Symptom Index (NIH-CPSI)

Name: _____   Date: _____

Pain or Discomfort

1. In the last week, have you experienced any pain or discomfort in the following areas:

		Yes	No
a.	Area between rectum and testicles (perineum)	1	0
b.	Testicles	1	0
c.	Tip of the penis (not related to urination)	1	0
d.	Below your waist, in your pubic or bladder area	1	0

2. In the last week, have you experienced:

		Yes	No
a.	Pain or burning during urination	1	0
b.	Pain or discomfort during or after sexual climax (ejaculation)	1	0

3. How often have you had pain or discomfort in any of these areas over the last week?

0 Never
1 Rarely
2 Sometimes
3 Often
4 Usually
5 Always

4. Which number best describes your AVERAGE pain or discomfort on the days that you had it, over the last week?

0 1 2 3 4 5 6 7 8 9 10
NO PAIN   PAIN AS BAD AS YOU CAN IMAGINE

Urination

5. How often have you had a sensation of not emptying your bladder completely after you finished urinating, over the last week?

0 Not at all
1 Less than 1 time in 5
2 Less than half the time
3 About half the time
4 More than half the time
5 Almost Always

FIG. 62.1 ■ Pelvic pain questionnaire. (Adapted from Litwin M, McNaughton-Collins M, Fowler FJ, et al. The National Institutes of Health chronic prostatitis symptom index: development and validation of a new outcome measure. *J Urol* 1999;162(2):369-375).

6.   How often have you had to urinate again less than two hours after you finished urinating, over the last week?

    0 Not at all

    1 Less than 1 time in 5

    2 Less than half the time

    3 About half the time

    4 More than half the time

    5 Almost Always

Impact of Symptoms

7.   How much have your symptoms keep you from doing the kinds of things you would usually do, over the last week?

    0 None

    1 Only a little

    2 Some

    3 A lot

8.   How much did you think about your symptoms, over the last week?

    0 None

    1 Only a little

    2 Some

    3 A lot

Quality of Life

9.   If you were to spend the rest of your life with your symptoms just the way they have been during the last week, how would you feel about that?

    0 Delighted

    1 Pleased

    2 Mostly satisfied

    3 Mixed (about equally satisfied and dissatisfied)

    4 Mostly dissatisfied

    5 Unhappy

    6 Terrible

Scoring the NIH-Chronic Prostatitis Symptom Index Domains

Pain: Total of items 1a, 1b, 1c, 1d, 2a, 2b, 3, and 4 ____

Urinary Symptoms: Total of items 5 and 6 _____

Quality of Life & Impact: Total of items 7, 8, and 9 _____

FIG. 62.1, cont'd

myofascial physical therapy, and stress management/ cognitive behavioral therapy.[14] They found that dietary modification frequently helps in alleviation of symptoms, with the most common aggravating foods being spicy foods and caffeine. The most common alleviating consumables were water and fiber supplements.

> The most powerful dietary recommendations would be increasing water and fiber intake and decreasing intake of spicy foods and caffeine.

Exercise

Exercise has definitively been shown to be helpful in the treatment of CPPS. One randomized controlled trial, in particular, with excellent methods and analysis reported significant improvements in NIH-CPSI scores as well as VAS pain and quality of life scores in the group that performed aerobic exercises for 18 weeks compared with the group that performed stretching only. Pain initially increased at 4 weeks in the aerobic exercise group (to a tolerable level) but then decreased significantly.[15]

Supplements

Rye Grass Pollen Extract

The Herati review included several studies reporting statistically significant improvements with pollen extract. Pollen therapy is thought to exert smooth muscle spasmogenic and spasmolytic effects as well as antiinflammatory effects specifically in prostate tissue.

Specifically, Elist et al. performed a randomized controlled trial demonstrating improvements in pain, sexual function, and lower urinary tract symptoms with pollen extract; 73% of extract users reported improvements compared with 36% in the control group. One brand that is widely available is called Pollen-Aid.[16] Saw palmetto was not found to be helpful in studies on its use in treating CP/CPPS.

> **Dosage**
> Pollen-Aid (*Secale cereale*); one to two capsules three times daily before meals.
>
> **Precautions**
> Rarely can cause digestive symptoms such as mild nausea.

Quercitin

A study reporting beneficial effects with quercetin was included in the two previously mentioned reviews. Quercetin, a bioflavonoid, has antioxidant and antiinflammatory properties. Quercetin was shown to significantly improve symptoms in a double-blind, placebo-controlled trial by Shoskes et al. When a subgroup was given a special preparation, including quercetin as well as bromelain and papain, symptoms improved even more dramatically.[17]

> **Dosage**
> 250–500 mg on an empty stomach three times daily. Bromelain improves the absorption of quercetin, so it is best to take an equal amount of bromelain along with quercetin.
>
> **Precautions**
> Quercetin is well tolerated, but does interact with some pharmaceuticals. It can increase blood levels of digoxin, cyclosporine, estrogen, and doxorubicin. Quercetin should not be taken along with the chemotherapy drug cisplatin.

Cannabis

A survey of 342 men regarding cannabis use for CP/CPPS published in the Canadian Urological Association Journal showed that more than 50% reported using cannabis, with more than half reporting improvement of symptoms with regard to mood, pain, muscle spasms, and sleep but not weakness, fatigue, numbness, or urination.[18]

Acupuncture

Acupuncture has also been shown to help with CPPS symptoms. In a randomized controlled trial of acupuncture versus antibiotics and nonsteroidal antiinflammatory drugs (NSAIDs), acupuncture was shown to be better at improving pain, urinary symptoms, quality of life, and NIH-CPSI scores among 54 participants.[19] Lee et al. published a summary of clinical trials on acupuncture in treating CP/CPPS, including pilot studies, randomized trials, and nonrandomized trials. Although they did not perform a systematic review or meta-analysis, they described many studies reporting overall improvements in most CP/CPPS symptoms with acupuncture treatments with or without electrical stimulation or moxibustion.[20]

> Acupuncture has been shown to be better than antibiotics or NSAIDS at improving pain and quality of life.

Physical Therapy

There is a vicious cycle of pain with urination, leading to straining and pelvic floor tightening, which worsens symptoms in many men with CP/CPPS. Myofascial physical therapy, including trigger point physiotherapy and relaxation techniques such as biofeedback, manual manipulation, and teaching self-use of a trigger-point "wand," have been shown to be helpful.[14] It can be difficult to find practitioners with expertise in treating trigger points, which are often located at the puborectalis and/or pubococcygeus muscles and which cause pain directly in the area when manipulated or referred pain to the prostate or penis. This referral pattern of pain is a frequent complaint among men with CP/CPPS and can be elicited by any pressure, including bicycle riding or long periods of sitting, in the puboanal area.

Mind-Body Therapy

Mind-body approaches can be a powerful intervention for men with CPPS.

Cognitive Behavioral Therapy

Cognitive behavioral therapy (CBT) and stress management have been shown to be helpful, given the comorbidity of depression, anxiety, and panic disorder that is common in men with this condition. Stress has been shown to worsen symptoms, and CBT can help teach men how to cope with the debilitating nature of their symptoms, making symptoms feel less intense or less bothersome.

Matching the Therapy to the Clinical Presentation

There is some benefit to individualizing therapy according to which clinical symptoms predominate. Of course, most patients will have overlapping symptomatology but many will present with a preponderance of one or two symptoms.

Lower Urinary Tract Symptoms

For example, men with mostly lower urinary tract symptoms similar to those of BPH complain of straining with urination and a feeling of constantly needing to void. For this population, similar treatments used for BPH, including alpha-blockers or antimuscarinics, may be helpful.[21] Pollen extract and acupuncture, as previously noted, are especially useful in men with a preponderance of lower urinary tract symptoms.[22]

Tenderness and Pain

Patients who predominantly present with tenderness on perineal or anal palpation and complaints of trigger point pain (perhaps elicited by sexual activity or bicycle riding) may respond best with expert physical therapy that includes biofeedback as well as antiinflammatory supplements, including quercetin along with bromelain and papain, and mind-body techniques, including CBT and stress management training.

Neurological/Systemic Symptoms

A man with primarily neurological/systemic symptoms has a presentation similar to those with tenderness but also has generalized symptoms such as fatigue, irritable bowel, or generalized pain. He may have leukocytes in his post-DRE U/A without bacteria. Such men may respond to potent antiinflammatories as previously described, perhaps adding curcumins or prescription NSAIDs. Herbalists may use *Eryngium yuccafolium* (rattlesnake master root), corn silk, or *Pulsatilla occidentalis* (western pasque flower); however, trials with these herbs have yet to be published. For these men, urinary symptoms may be relatively minor. Mind-body therapies and adaptogens

are useful, with therapies focusing on the fatigue or gut symptoms.[23]

Psychological Phenotypes

Patients with psychosocial phenotypes present with anxiety and/or depression, perhaps with a history of abuse. Mind-body therapies and antianxiety or antidepressant modalities and herbs, supplements, or medications are most appropriate for these men.

Infectious

Men with the infection phenotype may have bacteria in their post-DRE U/A, but often do not respond to antibiotics. Unless systemic signs of infection are present or greater than 100,000 colonies of specific bacteria are identified, antibiotics are unlikely to be useful. These men should be treated using the previously described therapies depending on their specific symptoms.

Treating Intestinal Permeability

Even those men who do not describe gastrointestinal symptoms may benefit from treatment for presumed leaky gut. CP/CPPS is an inflammatory condition, and we know that stimulation of gut-associated lymphoid tissue can be a large factor in upregulating the inflammatory system. A traditional leaky-gut 4R treatment approach (see Chapter 41) may be very helpful in men with CP/CPPS (Table 62.2). This would include an elimination diet and the use of glutamine and probiotics along with antiinflammatory herbs or supplements in an attempt to heal leaky gut and overstimulation of the immune and inflammatory systems.

TABLE 62.2 **Chronic Prostatitis/Chronic Pelvic Pain Syndrome (CP/CPPS) Treatment by UPOINT Phenotype**

Urinary	Alpha-blockers Pollen extract Acupuncture
Psychosocial	Mindfulness classes CBT Stress management Antidepression treatment
Organ specific	Herbal remedies Antiinflammatory approach
Infection	Antibiotics if > 100,000 colonies Pollen extract Acupuncture
Neurological/systemic	Antiinflammatories Curcumin, quercetin, bromelain Leaky gut 4R approach Elimination diet
Tenderness	Physical therapy Trigger point treatment Biofeedback Quercetin, bromelain, papain

CBT, cognitive behavioral therapy; *UPOINT*, urinary, psychosocial, organ specific, infection, neurological/systemic, and tenderness.

PREVENTION PRESCRIPTION

- Engage in a daily stress management practice, such as meditation, yoga, or journaling
- Exercise aerobically at least 4 days a week for 30 minutes
- Drink plenty of water every day, enough to keep urine fairly clear (more lemonade than apple juice in appearance)
- Eat five to nine servings a day of various colored fruits and vegetables

THERAPEUTIC REVIEW

CP/CPPS is a relatively common and tremendously impactful problem with no specific cause. As it is considered inflammatory in nature, most treatment regimens should start with an antiinflammatory approach including mind-body and leaky gut treatments. Beyond those, treatment may include diet, exercise, supplements, and/or use of acupuncture or physical therapy, but it should be based on the specific symptoms reported by the sufferer as the condition is heterogeneous and best treated using a symptom-targeted individualized approach.

LIFESTYLE

- Exercise aerobically at least four times per week at moderate intensity for at least 30 minutes B 1

NUTRITION

- Add fiber to the diet
- Eat five to nine servings of fruits and vegetables every day
- Avoid spicy foods, caffeine, and alcohol C 1

SUPPLEMENTS

- A 6-week trial of supplements may be helpful

- Quercetin: 500 mg tid with equal amounts Bromelain  B 2
- Rye grass pollen (Pollen-Aid): two capsules tid B 2
- Consider cannabis in states where medicinal use is allowed C 2

PHYSICAL THERAPY

- Consider physical therapy or prostatic massage by a well-trained practitioner, especially focusing on pelvic floor release and trigger-point treatment B 2

MIND-BODY THERAPY

- Cognitive-behavioral therapy B 1
- Meditation or biofeedback B 1
- Encourage stress management C 1

ACUPUNCTURE

- Acupuncture by a trained practitioner B 2

ANY OTHERS YOU WANT TO INCLUDE

- Treatment for leaky gut using a 4R approach C 1

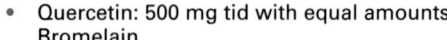

Key Web Resources

Patient-oriented information from the American Urological Association	https://www.auanet.org/education/modules/pathology/prostate-neoplastic/prostatitis.cfm
Recommendations on CPPS from the AAFP	http://www.aafp.org/afp/2010/0815/p397.html
Easy guide to 4R approach to leaky gut	http://www.mindbodygreen.com/0-6172/How-to-Heal-Your-Gut-and-Heal-Yourself.html

REFERENCES

References are available online at ExpertConsult.com.

CHAPTER 63

ERECTILE DYSFUNCTION

Luke Fortney, MD, FAAFP

PATHOPHYSIOLOGY

Erectile dysfunction (ED), the most common sexual problem among men, affects up to one-third of men at some point in their lives. ED is defined as the inability to achieve or maintain a sufficient erection for satisfactory sex. The prevalence of ED increases with age,[1] and it is most commonly associated with poor cardiovascular health, psychosocial factors, hormonal disorders, recreational drug abuse, and adverse effects from prescribed medications. Less common are anatomic, traumatic, or infectious causes.[2] Normally, an erection is stimulated by a combination of neurovascular, hormonal, and environmental factors beginning with sexual interest and desire (which is mediated predominantly by testosterone). Through parasympathetic activation, nitric oxide (NO) synthase (NOS) in endothelial cells is activated to produce NO from the precursor amino acid l-arginine. With NO present, the corpus cavernosum is engorged with arterial blood as a result of smooth muscle endothelial relaxation while venous return is simultaneously restricted.[3]

Evaluation

The World Health Organization and the American Urological Association recommend an initial limited evaluation for ED symptoms,[4] starting with the simplified five-item International Index of Erectile Function Questionnaire (IIEF-5) (Table 63.1).[5,6] A careful review of medications that contribute to ED (Table 63.2) is recommended in addition to substance abuse screening for alcohol, tobacco, marijuana, and other drugs.[7]

Cardiovascular risk factors should be assessed in all patients presenting with ED (Box 63.1).[8,9] Blood pressure and body mass index (BMI) scores are quick, but useful, initial assessments of cardiovascular health, which is the most important risk factor for ED.[10,11] Testicular, prostate, penis, and breast inspection should also be considered to rule out endocrine abnormalities such as hypogonadism, mammary hypertrophy, genitourinary masses, and Peyronie's disease.[12]

Nocturnal penile tumescence can be assessed by patient self-report or use of the "stamp test,"[13] Rigiscan, or Snap-Gauge cuff testing.[8,14] However, advanced imaging such as penile duplex ultrasonography is not recommended or necessary for the diagnosis of ED.[8,15] Typically the presence of nocturnal erections in a patient with ED suggests a psychogenic origin such as stress, fatigue, or mood disorders.[8,16]

Additional ED evaluation should also include the following laboratory tests: fasting glucose and lipid panel, thyroid-stimulating hormone, complete blood count, prostate-specific antigen, urinalysis, creatinine, electrolytes, and liver function panel.[4,8] Serum total testosterone level should be considered for men older than 50 years as well as younger men with signs of hypogonadism, which can be a sign of other comorbidities.[17] In addition to positive physical examination findings, hypogonadism is defined as a morning serum total testosterone level less than 300 ng/dL (10.4 nmol/L).[2,4,8,18] The prevalence of hypogonadism in men ranges from 5% to 15% with age-related increases.[19,20]

> Presentation of erectile dysfunction provides a window of opportunity to improve health and reverse the development of cardiovascular disease.

INTEGRATIVE THERAPY

Pharmaceuticals

Phosphodiesterase Inhibitors

Phosphodiesterase type 5 (PDE5) inhibitors (Table 63.3) such as sildenafil, vardenafil, and tadalafil remain first-line therapy options for ED.[8,21] These drugs are very effective, used as needed, and generally well tolerated and safe.[22,23] Common side effects can include headache, nasal congestion, flushing, abnormal vision, and gastrointestinal upset. Evidence supports equal effectiveness of these agents.[24-26] However, approximately one-third of men do not respond to PDE5 inhibitors. Additionally, these agents are not considered effective for improving libido, which is more a function of testosterone.[27] That being said, it is worth noting that testosterone does indirectly influence PDE5 activity. For example, research shows that administration of finasteride (which inhibits 5-alpha-reductase, the enzyme responsible for converting testosterone to its more potent form dihydrotestosterone, or DHT) increases the severity of erectile dysfunction and decreases testosterone levels in men.[28]

> **DOSAGE**
> Doses are provided in Table 63.3.

Testosterone

Testosterone supplementation in hypotestosteronism and hypogonadism is superior to placebo in improving erections, sexual function, and libido.[19,29,30] Close supervision with clinic follow-up and laboratory tests are needed every 2 weeks with initiation of a new testosterone

TABLE 63.1   **International Index of Erectile Function Questionnaire (IIEF-5)**

Over the Past 6 Months:	Score				
	1	2	3	4	5
1. How do you rate your **confidence** that you could get and keep an erection?	Very low	Low	Moderate	High	Very high
2. When you had erections with sexual stimulation, **how often** were your erections hard enough for penetration?	Almost never/never	A few times (much less than half the time)	Sometimes (about half the time)	Most times (much more than half the time)	Almost always/always
3. During sexual intercourse, **how often** were you able to maintain your erection after you had penetrated (entered) your partner?	Almost never/never	A few times (much less than half the time)	Sometimes (about half the time)	Most times (much more than half the time)	Almost always/always
4. During sexual intercourse, **how difficult** was it to maintain your erection to completion of intercourse?	Extremely difficult	Very difficult	Difficult	Slightly difficult	Not difficult
5. When you attempted sexual intercourse, **how often** was it satisfactory for you?	Almost never/never	A few times (much less than half the time)	Sometimes (about half the time)	Most times (much more than half the time)	Almost always/always

IIEF-5 Scoring:
The IIEF-5 score is the sum of the ordinal responses to the five items.

22–25: No erectile dysfunction

17–21: Mild erectile dysfunction

12–16: Mild to moderate erectile dysfunction

8–11: Moderate erectile dysfunction

5–7: Severe erectile dysfunction

From Rosen RC, Cappelleri JC, Smith MD, et al. Development and evaluation of an abridged, 5-item version of the International Index of Erectile Function (IIEF-5) as a diagnostic tool for erectile dysfunction. *Int J Impot Res*. 1999;11:319-326.

supplementation until satisfactory subjective and objective results are achieved. However, testosterone supplementation, with either compounded bioidentical testosterone or pharmaceutical brands, should continue to be monitored every 6 months over time with the following laboratory tests: morning serum testosterone level, complete blood count, liver function panel, and prostate-specific antigen.[31]

DOSAGE

Pharmaceutical testosterone (e.g., Androderm, AndroGel, Striant, and Testim) is prescribed at 12.5 to 100 mg applied topically every morning and titrated to normal serum total testosterone laboratory levels.[31] Compounded bioidentical testosterone preparations are available through reputable compounding pharmacies[32] (see Chapter 64).

Prostaglandin E₁ Injection

The prostaglandin E_1 agent alprostadil is self-administered as an intracavernosal injection (e.g., Caverject, Edex) or urethral suppository (e.g., Muse). Alprostadil is considered the gold standard of ED therapy, but is still second-line therapy behind oral PDE5 inhibitors.[8,33,34] Furthermore, alprostadil in either formulation requires training and patient education for self-administration; it can be uncomfortable or inconvenient for some men. Dosing for alprostadil intracavernosal injection ranges from 2.5 to 7.5 mcg three times a week as needed. Alprostadil intraurethral suppository treatment ranges from 125 to 1000 mcg daily as needed.

TABLE 63.2 **Medications That May Contribute to Erectile Dysfunction**

Medication Class	Examples
Alcohol and drugs of abuse	Alcohol, amphetamines, barbiturates, cocaine, heroin, marijuana, tobacco
Analgesics	Opiates
Anticholinergics	Tricyclic antidepressants
Anticonvulsants	Phenytoin, phenobarbital
Antidepressants	Lithium, monoamine oxidase inhibitors, selective serotonin reuptake inhibitors, tricyclic antidepressants
Antihistamines	Dimenhydrinate, diphenhydramine, hydroxyzine, meclizine, promethazine
Antihypertensives	Alpha blockers, beta-blockers, calcium channel blockers, clonidine, methyldopa, reserpine
Antiparkinsonian agents	Bromocriptine, levodopa, trihexyphenidyl
Cardiovascular agents	Digoxin, disopyramide, gemfibrozil
Cytotoxic agents	Methotrexate
Diuretics	Spironolactone, thiazides
Hormones	5-Alpha-reductase inhibitors, corticosteroids, estrogens, LH-releasing hormone agonists, progesterone
Immunomodulators	Interferon-alfa
Sedatives	Benzodiazepines, butyrophenones, phenothiazines

Data from references 2, 6, and 7.

BOX 63.1 | **Risk Factors for Erectile Dysfunction**

- Advancing age
- Alcohol abuse or alcoholism
- Cardiovascular disease
- Diabetes mellitus
- Drug abuse (e.g., marijuana, cocaine, methamphetamine)
- Dyslipidemia or hypercholesterolemia
- History of pelvic/prostate irradiation or surgery
- Hormonal disorders (e.g., hypogonadism, hypothyroidism, hyperprolactinemia)
- Hypertension
- Medications (e.g., cardiovascular and antihypertensive medications, antihistamines, benzodiazepines, selective serotonin reuptake inhibitors)
- Neurologic disorders (e.g., dementia, multiple sclerosis, parkinsonism, paraplegia or quadriplegia, stroke)
- Obesity
- Penile venous leakage
- Peyronie's disease
- Psychological conditions (e.g., anxiety, depression, guilt, history of sexual abuse, marital or relationship strain, stress)
- Sedentary lifestyle
- Tobacco use

Data from references 2, 4, and 7.

Vacuum Erection or Constriction Device

For men who are comfortable, motivated, and open-minded, vacuum erection or constriction devices (e.g., Erec-Tech, Firma) have shown promise for ED due to postsurgical, structural (e.g., Peyronie's disease), and prostate cancer radiation rehabilitation.[35-37] Satisfaction rates are higher than 80%, but these devices should be avoided in men with sickle cell disease or other bleeding disorders.[38,39] Patients should be counseled by a health care worker experienced with these devices.

Nutraceuticals

In general, supplements have proven to be much less effective than pharmaceutical options in treating ED.[40] In 2009, the U.S. Food and Drug Administration reissued a statement warning consumers to avoid ED supplements.[41] Patients should be counseled to avoid email promotions and internet advertisements for these and other products that falsely claim to enhance male libido and sexual function. Furthermore, most of these products are contaminated or adulterated,[42] and they are not considered reliable or safe for use (Box 63.2). Recent developments in quality testing have revealed rampant adulteration of "natural" supplements with PDE-5 inhibitor analogues (dimethylsildenafil, thiodimethylsildenafil, and thiomethisosildenafil).[43,44] Other products may be commonly used but are ineffective (Box 63.3).[40,45,46] However, some evidence indicates that the judicious use of some high-quality nutraceuticals may be considered in appropriate situations (Table 63.4).[47-68]

Manual Therapies and Bioenergetics

Evidence is generally lacking for acupuncture and massage in treating ED.[69] Further, massage therapy may be socially inappropriate in this context. Evidence is also lacking for osteopathic and chiropractic manipulation.[45] Furthermore, evidence for yoga, energy medicine, physical therapy, and the Alexander technique for the specific treatment of ED is insufficient.[45]

Mind-Body Therapy

Sexual desire, arousal, and climax are mediated through complex psychoneurological mechanisms. In general, sexual problems are highly prevalent among patients with psychiatric disorders, stemming from both adverse effects of medication and primary underlying psychopathology.[70]

TABLE 63.3	Phosphodiesterase Type 5 Inhibitors for Erectile Dysfunction				
Medication	**Dose**	**Onset**	**Duration**	**Precautions**	**SOR/HARM**
Sildenafil (Viagra)	25–100 mg	15–60 min	4 hr	Avoid with nitrates and alpha blockers	A⊘₂
Vardenafil (Levitra)	5–20 mg	30 min	4 hr	Avoid with nitrates and alpha blockers	A⊘₂
Tadalafil (Cialis)	5–20 mg	15–45 min	36 hr	Avoid with nitrates and alpha blockers	A⊘₂

SOR, strength of recommendation.
Data from Brant WO, Bella AJ, Lue TF. Treatment options for erectile dysfunction. *Endocrinol Metab Clin North Am.* 2007;36:465-479 and Palit V, Eardley I. An update on new oral PDE5 inhibitors for the treatment of erectile dysfunction. *Nat Rev Urol.* 2010;7:603-609.

BOX 63.2	Food and Drug Administration Statement: Hidden Risks of Erectile Dysfunction "Treatments"[42]

Since 2004, the FDA has identified several unsafe products that have been advertised as treatments for erectile dysfunction and/or to enhance sexual performance. These products have contained potentially harmful and undeclared ingredients:

- Actra-Sx
- Actra-Rx
- Libidus
- Nasutra
- Neophase
- Vigor-25
- Yilishen
- Zimaxx
- 4EVERON
- Liviro3
- Lycium Barbarum L.
- Adam Free
- Rhino V Max
- V.Max
- True Man
- Energy Max
- HS Joy of Love
- NaturalUp
- Blue Steel
- Erextra
- Super Shangai
- Strong Testis
- Shangai Ultra
- Shangai Ultra X
- Lady Shangai
- Shangai Regular, also marketed as Shangai Chaoji-mengnan
- Hero
- Naturalë Super Plus
- Xiadafil VIP tablets (Lots 6K029 and 6K209-SEI only)

Data from U.S. Food and Drug Administration (FDA). *Hidden risks of erectile dysfunction "treatments" sold online:* http://www.fda.gov/ForConsumers/ConsumerUpdates/ucm048386.htm (accessed 15/08/15).

BOX 63.3	Supplements With Insufficient Evidence

- 5-Hydroxytryptophan (5-HTP)
- Ambra grisea (ambrein)
- Androstenediol
- Ashwagandha
- Brazilian wandering spider venom (peptide Tx2-6)
- *Bufo* toad (bufotenine, Chan Su)
- *Butea superba*
- Chaste tree berry
- Clove
- Coleus
- Creatine
- Deer velvet
- Ephedra
- Horny goat weed
- Maca (*Lepidium meyenii*)
- Melatonin
- *Muira puama* (potency wood)
- Niacin
- Pomegranate
- Pygeum
- Rhinoceros horn
- Rhodiola
- Saffron
- Saw palmetto
- Spanish fly (cantharides)
- *Tribulus terrestris* (TT)
- Wild yam

Data from references 38, 42, and 43.

Lifestyle

A very strong association exists between lifestyle-associated chronic diseases and ED (see Box 63.1). Most importantly, research shows that ED is predominantly the result of advancing cardiovascular disease.[77-79] One study found that ED symptoms manifest, on average, 2–3 years earlier than symptoms of CAD.[80,10] Conversely, blood pressure control with lifestyle change is associated with a lower prevalence of ED, particularly in older patients.[81] However, antihypertensives such as thiazide diuretics, aldosterone-blockers, and beta-blockers are also known to aggravate ED in men with hypertension that is uncontrolled by lifestyle change alone.[82]

Metabolic syndrome plays an important role in the pathogenesis of ED.[83-85] For men diagnosed with

---

Psychological interventions have a strength of recommendation taxonomy category 1B for ED resulting from anxiety, depression, posttraumatic stress disorder, guilt, sex abuse history, relationship strain, performance anxiety, postsurgical adjustment disorder, and general stress.[8,45,71-76] There is insufficient evidence to recommend art therapy, hypnosis, aromatherapy, meditation, or guided imagery.[45]

TABLE 63.4 Common Supplements for Erectile Dysfunction

Supplement/Herb	Mechanism	Dose	Precautions	Tip	SOR/Harm
Panax ginseng[41,50-52]	Ginsenosides, increased NO	900 mg tid	Insomnia, mania, dysrhythmias	SS-cream[51] may help premature ejaculation	B 1
Yohimbine[41,55-58] (Yocon)	MAO inhibition, calcium and alpha blockade, NO	5–10 mg tid	HTN, CAD, DM, mood disorders, renal/liver disease, BPH	Use very cautiously, monitor closely	B 2
L-Arginine[59,60] (Prelox, Sargenor, R-Gene-10 Solution)	Precursor to NO	1000–2000 mg tid	Gout, asthma, GI upset	Additive effect with pycnogenol[59]	B 1
Pycnogenol[59,61] (Prelox, Sargenor)	Pine bark extract, activates NO synthase	40 mg tid	GI upset, vertigo, warfarin use	Alone may take up to 12 wk; additive effect with 500 mg L-arginine tid	B 1
Propionyl-L-carnitine[62,63]	Antiinflammatory, mediates NO	1000 mg bid	GI upset	Improves sildenafil effectiveness after prostate surgery and DM	C 1
Ginkgo biloba[67,68]	Flavonoids, terpenoids	60–120 mg bid	ASA, warfarin use, GI upset	May help ED caused by SSRIs	B 2

ASA, acetylsalicylic acid; *bid*, twice daily; *BPH*, benign prostatic hyperplasia; *CAD*, coronary artery disease; *DM*, diabetes mellitus; *ED*, erectile dysfunction; *GI*, gastrointestinal; *HTN*, hypertension; *MAO*, monoamine oxidase; *NO*, nitric oxide; *PDE5*, phosphodiesterase type 5; *SOR*, strength of recommendation; *SSRIs*, selective serotonin reuptake inhibitors; *tid*, three times daily.
From Natural Medicines Comprehensive Database. *Erectile dysfunction.* http://naturaldatabase.therapeuticresearch.com/nd/Search.aspx?cs; Accessed 22.03.11 (subscription required).

diabetes mellitus, the prevalence of ED is as high as 89%[80,81] while obesity (BMI > 30) nearly doubles the risk of ED.[1,84] The risk of ED is also nearly double in men who smoke.[86] Alcohol abuse is known to adversely affect sexual function.[86] New data also suggests that the severity and extend of periodontal disease may be a significant risk factor for ED, sperm motility, and time to conception.[87,88]

ED therefore presents a window of opportunity to identify early cardiovascular disease and recommend lifestyle modifications.[10,84] One study found that men who seek treatment for ED may prefer alternatives to pharmaceutical intervention, such as lifestyle change.[73] As such, comprehensive treatment should include counseling for weight loss, healthy nutrition, stress management, and regular exercise (see Prevention Prescription in the following text).[2,7,8,77,83]

> The most important recommendation to prevent and treat erectile dysfunction is to encourage overall healthy behaviors that reduce the incidence and severity of cardiovascular disease.

No particular exercise or nutrition regimen is specifically designed to treat ED. However, exercise and nutrition should be tailored to each patient's specific needs, with special emphasis on adopting a Mediterranean-style diet that has been shown to improve cardiovascular function in patients with ED.[89] Interestingly, analysis of the National Health and Nutrition Examination Survey (NHANES) of 3724 men found that two to three cups of caffeinated coffee per day reduced the odds of prevalent ED, even among obese and hypertensive men.[90] Other lifestyle recommendations include regular dental care, which may be beneficial for both cardiovascular disease and ED.[91] In addition, prolonged or frequent bicycle riding may inhibit neurovascular flow to the perineum and thereby negatively influence ED. In these patients, a trial of rest, change in exercise routine, or cycling adaptations (e.g., split seat or recumbent posture) can be tried.

Therapies to Consider

Emerging Therapies

Novel approaches for ED target inhibition of arginase, an enzyme that competes with NOS for l-arginine. Excessive arginase activity and expression in the corpora cavernosa has been implicated in ED, while inhibition of arginase has been shown to increase blood flow in penile circulation.[92] Ongoing investigation into gene therapies that target arginase include *RhoA/Rho-kinase (ROCK)* and *p38-MAPK*, among others. Another example is the Maxi-K protein gene *(MKPG)* that is expressed as a potassium channel whose function is needed to initiate and sustain an erection. Local injections of a plasmid containing the *MKPG* gene appears to be safe, but it is invasive, relatively new, expensive, often not covered by insurance, unavailable in many locations, and the long-term effects have not been well established. Advantages include enabling sexual spontaneity, twice-yearly injection therapy, synergistic activity with PDE5 inhibitor medications, and it can be used by men taking nitrates.[8,93-95]

PREVENTION PRESCRIPTION

- Exercise in any capacity for at least 150 minutes a week.
- Follow a healthy calorie-controlled Mediterranean diet rich in phytonutrients and antioxidants (organic fruits and vegetables), omega-3 fatty acids, whole grains, nuts, seeds, and legumes.
- Reduce stress through exercise, rest, vacation, retreats, meditation, breathing exercises, yoga, journaling, or various manual therapies.
- Maintain healthy sexual relationships, good communication, and regular erections and ejaculations (three times/week).

- Avoid tobacco, marijuana, and other illegal or recreational drugs.
- Be moderate with alcohol consumption (one to two drinks or less per day).
- Avoid highly processed foods that contain high amounts of "antinutrients" (e.g., high-fructose corn syrup, trans fats, and artificial sweeteners/colors/preservatives).
- Avoid overexposure to pesticides, herbicides, and overuse of chemical or cleaning products.
- Avoid heating or storing food in plastics (e.g., endocrine and hormone disruptors such as bisphenol-A).

THERAPEUTIC REVIEW

WORKUP AND EVALUATION

- History with International Index of Erectile Function-5 (IIEF-5) short survey and medication review.
- Physical examination with blood pressure, body mass index, and genitourinary examination.
- Laboratory tests (complete blood count, fasting glucose and lipids, electrolytes, creatinine, liver function tests, thyroid-stimulating hormone, prostate-specific antigen, and morning total serum testosterone).

LIFESTYLE

- Mediterranean diet
- Weight loss (goal BMI < 30)
- Regular exercise > 150 minutes per week
- Stress reduction
- Smoking cessation[90]
- Alcohol reduction
- Two to three cups of coffee per day

FIRST-LINE PHARMACEUTICALS

- Trial of phosphodiesterase type 5 inhibitor
- Sildenafil (Viagra): 25–100 mg orally daily as needed, or
- Vardenafil (Levitra, Staxyn): 5–20 mg orally daily as needed, or
- Tadalafil (Cialis): 5–20 mg orally every 72 hours as needed

NUTRACEUTICALS

- Yohimbine: 5–10 mg three times daily
- *Panax ginseng:* 900 mg three times daily
- Pycnogenol: 40 mg three times daily with or without 500–1000 mg of L-arginine three times daily

- L-Arginine: 1000–2000 mg three times daily
- Propionyl-L-carnitine: 1000 mg twice daily (to improve sildenafil response)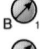

MIND-BODY THERAPY

- Psychotherapy for patients with mood disorder, posttraumatic stress disorder, sex abuse history, relationship strain, or performance anxiety
- Stress reduction through yoga, meditation, breathing, massage, journaling, psychotherapy, and rest

SECOND- AND THIRD-LINE THERAPIES

- Vacuum erection or constriction devices with training, or
- Alprostadil (Muse) urethral suppositories: 125–1000 mcg pellet intraurethrally daily as needed, or
- Alprostadil (Caverject) injections: 2.5- to 7.5-mcg intracavernosal injection three times weekly as needed

HORMONE REPLACEMENT

- Hypogonadism or testosterone deficiency, low total serum testosterone less than 300 ng/dL.
- Topical testosterone: 12.5–100 mg every morning titrated to normal laboratory levels checked every 4 weeks until stable
- Compounded bioidentical testosterone
- Serum total testosterone laboratory test every 2 weeks until stable and then every 6–12 months
- Initial and annual serum total testosterone, complete blood count, liver function tests, and prostate-specific antigen laboratory tests with genitourinary examination

Key Web Resources

Cornell University Medical College: Academic resource for the evaluation of erectile dysfunction (ED)	http://urology.weillcornell.org/erectile-dysfunction
Titan Healthcare: Information on vacuum erection devices and options for purchase	http://titanhealthcare.co.uk
MedlinePlus, National Institutes of Health: Patient education tutorial on ED	http://www.nlm.nih.gov/medlineplus/erectiledysfunction.html
American Association of Sexuality Educators, Counselors, and Therapists: Information and resource to help find a certified therapist	http://www.aasect.org
Mayo Clinic: Patient information for herbal ED treatments	http://www.mayoclinic.org/diseases-conditions/erectile-dysfunction/in-depth/erectile-dysfunction-herbs/art-20044394
Penn Medicine, University of Pennsylvania: Information about ED and the "stamp test"	http://www.pennmedicine.org/encyclopedia/em_DisplayArticle.aspx?gcid=003164&ptid=1

REFERENCES

References are available online at ExpertConsult.com.

CHAPTER 64

Testosterone Deficiency

Robert Z. Edwards, MD

PATHOPHYSIOLOGY

The most important human androgen is testosterone. Testosterone is a steroid hormone composed of 19 carbons (Fig. 64.1). Another prominent androgen is dehydroepiandrosterone (DHEA), which belongs to a group of prohormones collectively referred to as 17-ketosteroids. In adult males, the testes produce approximately 7 mg of testosterone per day.[1] In females, the daily rate of testosterone production is approximately 0.25–0.3 mg.[2] In males, an additional 0.25 mg of testosterone is produced per day in the adrenal glands, but the amount can vary depending on the patient.[3] In females, the adrenal glands contribute to approximately 25% of daily testosterone production or about 50–75 mcg/day, the ovarian contribution is 25%, and the remaining 50% of daily testosterone production is from peripheral conversion.[2] The rest of the discussion will be directed toward testosterone deficiency (TD) in men and the mechanisms of control related to male physiology.

Testosterone is regulated by luteinizing hormone (LH) from the anterior lobe of the pituitary gland. LH stimulates the release of testosterone from the Leydig cells in the testes. Sperm production is under the influence of follicle-stimulating hormone (FSH), also released from the anterior lobe of the pituitary gland. Testosterone inhibits the secretion of LH by negative feedback.[1] Testosterone plasma levels follow a circadian rhythm, with the highest peak in the early morning around 7:00 a.m. and another, smaller peak in the afternoon around 4:00 p.m.[4] However, the peak and nadir of testosterone are not as dramatic as those of cortisol.

Testosterone is generally found in the body bound to proteins, most specifically to the sex hormone–binding globulin (SHBG). Testosterone bound to SHBG is measured as total testosterone (TT). SHBG production in the liver is controlled by a number of hormones. Liver disease, estrogen, and thyroid hormones increase SHBG. SHBG decreases in response to androgens, insulin resistance and diabetes, and in the presence of hypothyroidism.[5] Plasma SHBG levels tend to increase with increasing age. The fraction of testosterone bound to SHBG in the serum is proportional to the SHBG level.[5] This helps explain the faster rate of reduction of free testosterone (free T) compared with TT (2%–3% per year decline compared with 1%–2%, respectively) after 40 years of age.

> Diabetes, metabolic syndrome/insulin resistance, obesity, and hypothyroidism can lead to falsely low TT despite normal free T levels. Checking free T is a more accurate test in these individuals.

Testosterone can be converted to estradiol by aromatase, especially in adipose tissue, and to dihydrotestosterone (DHT) by 5-alpha reductase in specialized tissues such as sebaceous glands, hair follicles, and prostate tissues (Fig. 64.2). Testosterone governs the development of secondary sex characteristics in the male. Sufficient testosterone is essential for normal libido, fertility, and potency of the male. It can also influence erythropoiesis. Testosterone exerts anabolic effects on muscularity and can affect behavior and aggressiveness. Testosterone is metabolized in the liver and primarily excreted in the urine.[1]

There are many clinical manifestations of TD, thereby making diagnosis challenging. Physical symptoms include decreased bone mineral density, decreased muscle mass and strength, increased body fat or body mass index (BMI), gynecomastia, anemia, axillary/genital hair loss, and fatigue. Psychological symptoms may include depressed mood, diminished energy/sense of vitality or wellbeing, decreased self-confidence, and impaired cognition/memory. Many times, however, men will present with a chief complaint of sexual dysfunction. Sexual symptoms include diminished libido, erectile dysfunction, difficulty in achieving orgasm, decreased morning erections, and decreased sexual performance[6] (Box 64.1).

While there is debate regarding what level of TT constitutes deficiency, most experts agree that a healthy range for TT is 300–1050 ng/dL when considering testosterone replacement therapy.[7,8] Data suggest that levels <440 ng/dL are associated with elevated 10-year cardiovascular risk in middle-aged and elderly men.[8a] There is general agreement that free T or bioavailable T (free T plus albumin-bound T) would provide a better estimation of T status; however, there is concern about the reliability of these assays and a general lack of research using these measures. There is evidence of an excellent correlation between saliva testosterone levels and free T levels obtained simultaneously.[9] This may prove to be a reliable alternative to serum testing; however, some of the same concerns mentioned previously remain. A single low AM testosterone level should be repeated to confirm the diagnosis of TD.

Much of our current data on the normal changes in adult testosterone levels related to aging are from the Massachusetts Male Aging Study (MMAS). This study followed men over 3 decades. At the beginning of the study in 1987, there were 1667 participants, and by the end of the study in 2004, there were 584 participants remaining. Longitudinal data revealed an average of 1%–2% TT decline per year, with a more rapid decline in free T due to the increases in SHBG with aging as discussed previously.[5,10] Interestingly, there was variability in the rate of decline with some subjects' TT levels not declining over time and a few participants had increases with age. The mean TT level at 45 years old was approximately 540 ng/dL, while it dropped down to approximately 440 ng/dL by 70 years old.[5] The prevalence

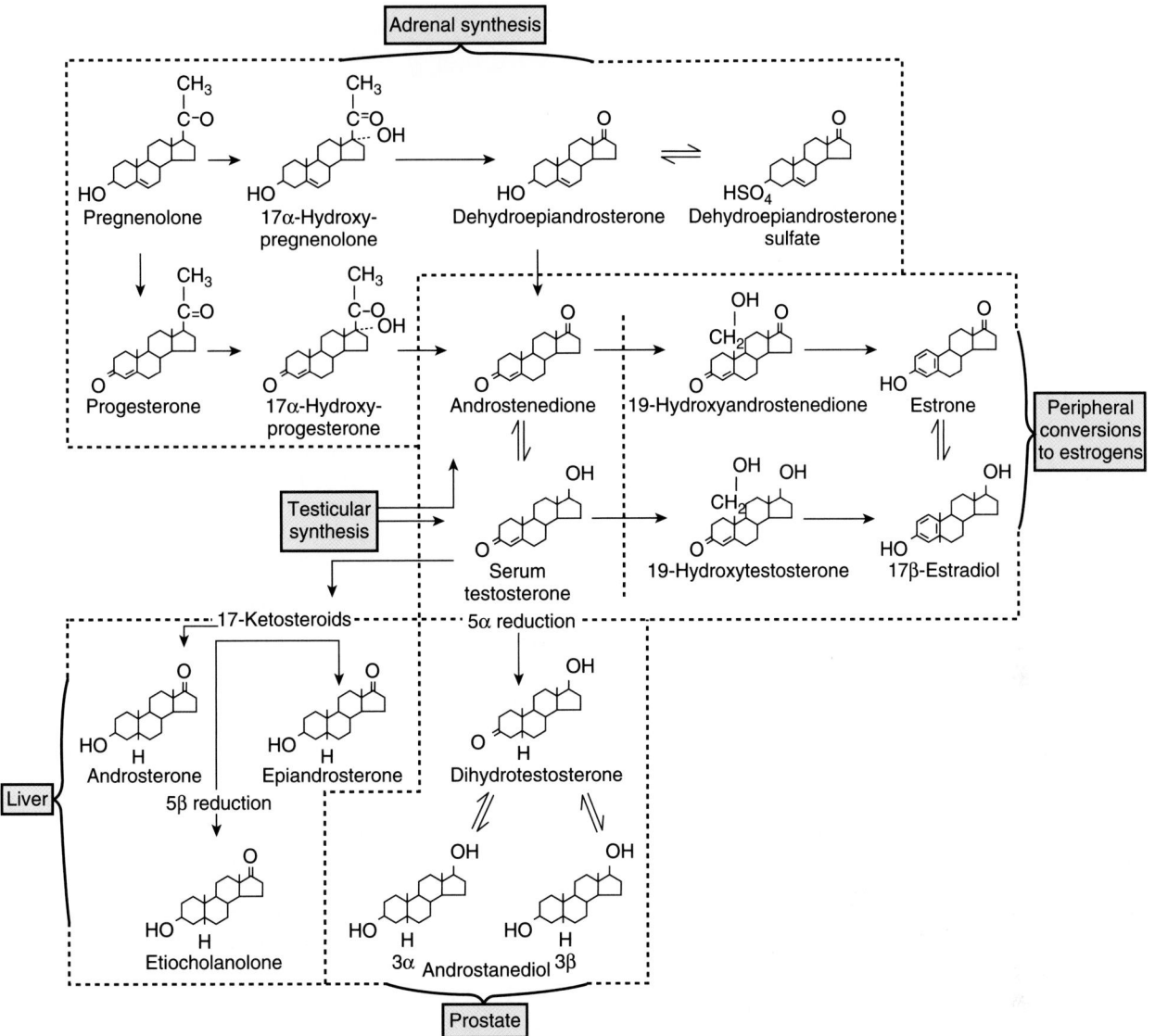

FIG. 64.1 ▓ Overview of the synthesis and metabolism of testosterone in four main body compartments: adrenal synthesis of androstenedione, peripheral conversion of androgens (androstenedione and testosterone) to estrogens, formation of active androgen (DHT) within the prostate, and inactivation in the liver of testosterone to three types of 17-ketosteroids. (From Ross AE. Development, molecular biology, and physiology of the prostate. In: Wein et al., eds. *Campbell-Walsh urology*/Elsevier; 2016:2393–2424.e9.)

of TD is estimated to be about 6%–12% in the general primary care population.[11] One other interesting trend from the MMAS was an age-independent decline in testosterone levels over the past 3 decades. The analyses indicate a 1% per year decrease in TT.[5] Put another way, the mean TT of a 60-year-old man in 1988 was 500 ng/dL compared to approximately 440 ng/dL in 2003. This seems to be consistent with other observations of population-level declines in sperm counts and other reproductive disorders in men.[12,13]

INTEGRATIVE THERAPY

Nutrition

Most of the focus here can be on reducing metabolic syndrome and diabetes.[14,15] Many of the same guidelines used to promote cardiovascular health and prevent cardiovascular disease (CVD) apply to reducing the risk for TD and sexual dysfunction.[15] Thus, reducing refined carbohydrates and educating men on the concepts of glycemic index and glycemic load are worthwhile (see Chapter 87).

In addition, promoting diets higher in vegetables and fruits while reducing animal-based foods makes sense on many fronts. Fruits and vegetables are high in flavonoids, which, along with isoflavones from soybean, have been studied as aromatase inhibitors and 5-alpha reductase inhibitors.[16-18] The polyphenol epigallocatechin gallate (EGCG), the most abundant catechin found in tea (white, green, and black), has been studied as a 5-alpha reductase inhibitor and aromatase inhibitor as well.[16-18] Reducing consumption of animal products reduces exposure to toxins that can bioaccumulate up the food chain. We will discuss endocrine disruptors in more detail later.

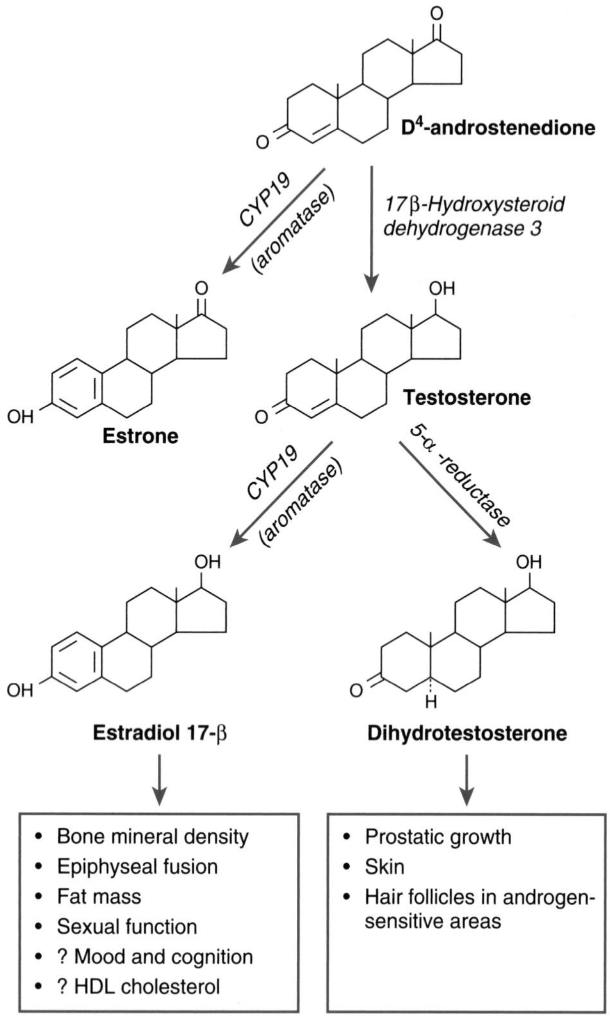

FIG. 64.2 Active metabolism of testosterone. Testosterone may be converted to the potent estrogen, 17beta-estradiol, by the enzyme aromatase (CYP19) or to the more potent androgen, dihydrotestosterone (DHT), by the enzyme 5alpha-reductase. The effects of testosterone on prostatic growth, skin, and hair follicles in androgen-sensitive areas require 5alpha-reduction of testosterone to DHT. The effects of testosterone that require aromatization to estradiol are prevention of bone resorption, increase in bone mineral density, epiphyseal fusion, decrease in fat mass, sexual differentiation of the brain, sexual function, and possibly some aspects of cognitive function, mood, and plasma lipids (high-density lipoprotein [HDL] cholesterol). (Modified from Bhasin S. Testicular disorders. In: Kronenberg HM, Melmed S, Polonsky KS, et al., eds. *Williams textbook of endocrinology.* 11th ed. Philadelphia: Elsevier; 2008:645–698; Matsumoto AM. Testicular disorders. In: Kronenberg HM, Melmed S, Polonsky KS, et al., eds. *Williams textbook of endocrinology*, Elsevier; 2016:694–784.)

> Aromatase promotes the conversion of testosterone to estrogen. Inhibiting aromatase by eating vegetables, fruit, and drinking green tea raises levels of testosterone while reducing estrogen. Estrogen (more than testosterone) is the main trigger of benign prostatic hyperplasia.

Exercise

In a study by Khoo et al. in 2013, improvements in TT levels were documented with moderate and high levels of exercise. The moderate-level exercise group exercised for 90–150 minutes per week at 55%–70% of the maximum heart rate (HR). The high-intensity group exercised for 200–300 minutes per week at a similar HR intensity. Both groups were encouraged to eat approximately 400 kcals less per day. After 24 weeks, the high-intensity exercise group had a statistically significant increase in both TT and FT. Both groups had improvement in erectile dysfunction measures.[19]

BOX 64.1 Signs and Symptoms of Testosterone Deficiency

Unexplainable weight gain with muscle loss
- Osteoporosis/osteopenia
- Fatigue
- Anemia
- Depressed mood
- Loss of self-confidence
- Impaired cognition
- Loss of libido
- Erectile dysfunction
- Diminished sexual performance

Mind–Body

Can posing make a difference in testosterone levels? It appears a "high-power pose," in which there is expression of expansiveness and openness of the limbs held for 2 minutes, can lead to an increase in testosterone levels and decrease in cortisol levels measured in the saliva.[20] Over time, practicing power poses may improve a person's general health and wellbeing. It is a very simple practice that also has a very low risk. Many yoga poses possess qualities of high-power poses. Pursuing training in yoga would be another reasonable recommendation for men with TD.

The loss of a spouse can dramatically affect TT, equaling 10 years of aging decline.[21] The effects of psychological stress have often been underappreciated in the field of endocrinology and generally are not discussed in treatment protocols. It is important to take a social history to fully understand in what context TD is being diagnosed in terms of a man's life. If appropriate, suggesting psychological counseling, helping identify local social support, and serving as a healing, mindful presence can be extremely important for a patient recently diagnosed with TD.

Toxins

Opioids

Opioid-induced androgen deficiency (OPIAD) is often underrecognized in clinical practice. OPIAD is inappropriately low levels of gonadotropins (FSH, LH) in the face of low plasma testosterone levels. OPIAD can be seen for months to years while being treated with morphine. Levels can drop as quickly as a few hours after starting opioids. Once morphine therapy is interrupted, levels can recover within a few hours to days. Less is known about long-term opioid use and hypothalamus/pituitary suppression. In one case-control study on 40 cancer patients receiving opioids, 90% were hypogonadal compared with 40% of the controls. In women, DHEA and

BOX 64.2	Recycling Symbols on Plastic
Avoid	**Safer for use**
3 (PVC/phthalates)	2
6 (polystyrene foam)	4
7 (BPA)	5
	7 PLA (polylactide biodegradable corn)

BPA, bisphenol A; PVC, polyvinyl chloride.

DHEA sulfate levels have been found to be suppressed, thus indicating adrenal androgen suppression as well. It appears that the higher the dose of opioids, the higher the risk for hypogonadism. One can anticipate OPIAD when the range of oral morphine equivalence exceeds 100–200 mg/day. An additional risk is being on opioids for more than 1 month.[22] Even with that level of exposure, OPIAD should be reversible after opioid cessation. Given this information, health care providers are responsible for providing full consent regarding the risk for developing an endocrinopathy prior to starting opioids.

Endocrine Disruptors

There is increasing awareness that chemicals commonly encountered in our environment can interrupt normal endocrine function. These have been classified as endocrine disruptors by researchers. Two of the best studied and most commonly encountered of these are phthalates and bisphenol A (BPA). They are both chemicals used in the manufacturing of plastics that impart various favorable qualities to plastic products. Phthalates provide soft, flexible plastics, are a major component of polyvinyl chlorides (PVCs), and are common in personal care products. BPA is used to create hard plastics and epoxy resins used to line food and beverage cans to prevent corrosion. Human studies on phthalates have demonstrated decreased free T levels in infants exposed to phthalates in breast milk and abnormal sperm morphology and sperm DNA damage in adult males.[23] Human studies on BPA reveal that humans are exposed to concentrations similar to or higher than doses that have been found to increase the risk for precancerous cells in animal prostate tissue.[24] There is also evidence of increased risk for obesity with BPA exposure.[25] BPA acts as a weak estrogen in mammals as well. Taken together, these last two facts make BPA exposure a risk factor for developing symptomatic TD.

The best advice is to avoid exposure to these chemicals when possible. Do not heat or microwave food or beverages in plastic. Do not heat or microwave plastic wraps. Avoid placing plastics in the dishwasher. If using hard plastic containers, do not use them for warm or hot foods or liquids. Avoid canned food and beverages when possible, unless verifying that they are BPA-free. Use a washable fabric shower curtain as opposed to plastic/vinyl. The new car smell, which is at least in part from PVC off-gassing phthalates, can increase exposure through inspiration. Plastic containers with the recycling symbol 1 on the bottom are generally safe but made for one-time use. Look for alternatives to plastic for repeated use containers such as glass and stainless steel. Avoid plastics with the symbols 3 (PVC/phthalates), 6 (polystyrene foam), and 7

(BPA) on the bottom of the container. Recycling symbols of 2, 4, 5, and 7 (polylactide [PLA] biodegradable corn) are safer options (Box 64.2) (see Chapter 108).

Supplements

Zinc

Zinc is a cofactor in numerous metabolic processes in the human body. There is evidence of a significant positive correlation between zinc supplementation and serum testosterone levels in elderly men.[26] A 2010 systematic review of randomized controlled trials on sexual dysfunction and chronic kidney disease identified zinc deficiency as a reversible cause of sexual dysfunction and TD in this high-risk population.[27] Zinc citrate, zinc acetate, or zinc picolinate may be best absorbed, although zinc sulfate is less expensive. Consider checking the zinc level in men with TD.

DOSAGE

The dose is 25–50 mg PO daily.

PRECAUTIONS

Zinc taken orally seldom causes any immediate side effects other than an occasional stomach upset, usually when it is taken on an empty stomach. Some forms do have an unpleasant metallic taste. Use of zinc nasal gel, however, has been associated with anosmia (loss of sense of smell). Long-term use of oral zinc at dosages of 100 mg or more daily can cause a number of toxic effects, including severe copper deficiency, impaired immunity, heart problems, and anemia.[28]

Dehydroepiandrosterone

DHEA is an androgen prohormone that has been shown to decrease dramatically with age, and its decline is believed, by some, to accelerate the aging process. It is manufactured synthetically from soybean precursors. DHEA has shown some promise for improving erectile dysfunction in men who have low DHEA blood levels.[29] DHEA serum levels should also be checked in those with TD.

DOSAGE

The recommended dose is 5–50 mg PO 1–2×/day. I usually start men on 25 mg PO BID and titrate as needed.

PRECAUTIONS

DHEA appears to be safe when taken in therapeutic doses, at least for a short term. Women may experience adrenergic side effects such as acne and unwanted hair growth. I would recommend similar precautions and contraindications for using DHEA, as described later for testosterone replacement therapy (TRT).

Botanicals

Quercetin

Quercetin may reduce aromatase activity, thereby increasing available testosterone (Box 64.3).

DOSAGE

The dose is 400 mg PO 1–2×/day.

PRECAUTIONS

Quercetin may increase homovanillic acid on urine and serum tests, leading to false-positive tests for neuroblastoma.[30]

Resveratrol/Grape Seed Extract

Resveratrol/grape seed extract has been found to modestly improve glycemic and hypertension (HTN) control in type 2 diabetes mellitus (T2DM).[31] They may also reduce aromatase activity.

DOSAGE

The dose is 100–300 mg PO 1–2×/day.

PRECAUTIONS

It is well tolerated in short-term studies. There are concerns that resveratrol specifically may have mild estrogenic activity. In addition, it may have antiplatelet activity, so it should be cautiously used with other blood thinners.

Pycnogenol

Pycnogenol supplementation improves health risk factors in subjects with metabolic syndrome. Men's waist circumference decreased from 106 cm to 98 cm in 6 months with supplementation.[32] Decreasing abdominal fat should decrease conversion of testosterone to estradiol.

DOSAGE

The recommended dose is 50 mg PO TID.

PRECAUTIONS

Appears to be safe and is generally well tolerated, although a low incidence of adverse effects, including gastrointestinal symptoms, dizziness, and vertigo, have been reported.

Saw Palmetto

Saw palmetto (*Serenoa repens*) is a weak inhibitor of 5-alpha reductase (Box 64.4). It may also have a role in reducing the number of estrogen and DHT receptors.[33]

BOX 64.3	Aromatase Inhibitors

Anastrozole (Arimidex)
    Letrozole (Femara)
    Quercetin
    Resveratrol/grape seed extract
    Zinc
    Progesterone

DOSAGE

The dose is 160 mg PO 2×/day or 320 mg PO daily.

PRECAUTIONS

Saw palmetto is thought to be essentially nontoxic. In addition, in clinical trials, it has shown little to no adverse effects. There is one report of excessive bleeding during surgery related to saw palmetto ingestion. Caution is recommended when adding to other blood thinners.

Maca

Maca (*Lepidium meyenii*) has been found to increase testosterone levels in some animal studies, but not all studies show this effect. Human studies have revealed subjective improvements in sexual function.[34]

DOSAGE

The dose is 500–1000 mg PO up to 3×/day.

PRECAUTIONS

In reported human clinical trials, use of maca has not led to any serious adverse effects.

Pharmaceuticals

Testosterone replacement in men with TD provides significant improvements in lipid profiles, decreases body fat, increases lean muscle mass, and decreases fasting glucose.[35] A well-publicized study by Basaria et al. in 2010 revealed an increased risk for cardiovascular adverse events with 100 mg of testosterone in a transdermal gel compared with placebo in elderly men with limited mobility and a high prevalence of chronic disease.[36] When looking at all-cause mortality, it appears men treated with testosterone for TD have decreased mortality in observational studies.[37] Calof et al. performed a meta-analysis of 19 randomized studies and did not find a statistically significantly greater risk for prostate cancer in men on TRT versus placebo. However, there was greater detection of prostate events (elevated prostate-specific antigen [PSA] and prostate biopsies) and hematocrit (HCT) greater than 50% in men on TRT.[38] Similar to female hormone replacement therapy (HRT) before the Women's Health Initiative (WHI), we will likely not have consensus on the long-term safety of TRT until large, long-term studies are completed. Until then, decisions to start HRT will need to be based on the clinical severity of TD and informed consent on the part of the patient.

BOX 64.4	5-Alpha Reductase Inhibitors

Finasteride
    Dutasteride
    Zinc
    Progesterone
    Saw palmetto
    L-Lysine
    Epigallocatechin gallate (ECGC)
    Linolenic acid

Testosterone replacement does not appear to increase the risk for prostate cancer, but there is concern that it may increase the risk for cardiovascular events.

At a minimum, baseline labs should include AM free and TT, PSA, and a complete blood count (CBC; hemoglobin [HGB]/HCT). A digital rectal exam should also be performed. Additional labs to consider are thyroid-stimulating hormone (TSH) and free T4, DHEA sulfate, LH, fasting glucose, HGB A1c, lipids, and liver function. In selected cases, SHBG, estradiol, prolactin (if LH/FSH are low), and zinc levels may be helpful. If LH is elevated in the face of low serum testosterone levels, consider Klinefelter syndrome, alcoholism, and heavy metal poisoning as the cause of primary hypogonadism. If there is confusion, consider requesting an endocrinology consult. My experience is that LH is rarely elevated with low testosterone levels related to aging or obesity (Box 64.5).

Contraindications to treatment are active prostate cancer (but not previously treated prostate cancer with a Gleason score of 7 or less), breast cancer, prostate nodule, unexplained PSA elevation, HCT of >50%, unstable congestive heart failure (CHF) or coronary artery disease (CAD), and severe obstructive sleep apnea (OSA) (Box 64.6).

Monitoring treatment should include a follow-up office visit to discuss symptoms and potential side effects (acne, behavior changes, and edema) and dose adjustments 1–3 months after starting treatment. TT and FT can be checked 2–4 weeks after starting TRT. The timing of the serum levels should be 3–12 hours after application of gels and creams, and about halfway between testosterone injections. Advise patients using topical preparations to be mindful of exposure to children and women. Also avoiding hairy areas and scrotal application is recommended to reduce conversion to DHT by 5-alpha reductase. Men should be followed every 3–4 months for the first year with testosterone levels, PSA, CBC, and digital rectal exam (DRE). Annual monitoring after that is acceptable if stable. Some authors recommend a target TT level of 400–700 ng/dL (possibly > 350 for elderly men).

Testosterone Cypionate Injections

DOSAGE

The recommended dose is 50–200 mg IM q1–2 weeks or 30–50 SQ 1–2×/week.

PRECAUTIONS

As with all testosterone, it is a controlled substance. Self-administration can lead to misuse and overdosing, injection site reactions, and infections. Men should be warned of the potential for infertility related to any form of testosterone replacement.

Testosterone Creams (Compounding Pharmacy)

DOSAGE

The dose is 10–200 mg topically daily. I usually start with 40–50 mg daily (qhs or qAM).

PRECAUTIONS

The most common adverse reaction is local skin reactions, which can include redness. As with any of the topical hormone preparations, men need to be mindful to avoid exposure to women, children, and pets after application.

Testosterone Gels and Patches (Available Commercially)

DOSAGE

Depends on the formulation
- 1% gel: 50 mg testosterone = four pump actuations = one 5-g pkt. 50–100 mg qAM
- 1.62% gel: 40.5 mg testosterone = two pump actuations = one 2.5-g pkt. 40.5–81 mg qAM
- 2 mg and 4 mg/24 hour patch. Apply 1–2 patches qhs. Adjust based on serum testosterone levels.

PRECAUTIONS

The most common adverse reaction is local skin reactions, which can include redness. As with any of the topical hormone preparations, men need to be mindful to avoid exposure to women, children, and pets after administration.

Methyltestosterone

DOSAGE

The dose is 10–50 mg PO daily divided qd–qid.

PRECAUTIONS

Generally not used because of concerns about liver toxicity. Studies reveal hepatotoxicity is extremely rare, but concerns with oral use persist, especially at higher doses required by some men.[39]

BOX 64.5	**Recommended Baseline Laboratory Testing for Testosterone Deficiency**

AM free and total testosterone–serum
    PSA
    CBC
    TSH
    Fasting glucose
    Also consider DHEA sulfate, zinc, LH, fasting glucose/hemoglobin A1c, lipids, and liver function tests.

BOX 64.6	**Contraindications to Testosterone Hormone Replacement**

- Active prostate cancer (not previously treated prostate cancer if the Gleason score is 7 or less)
- Breast cancer
- Prostate nodule
- Unexplained PSA elevation
- Polycythemia (caution if HCT > 50%)
- Unstable CHF or CAD
- Severe OSA

CAD, coronary artery disease; CHF, congestive heart failure; OSA, obstructive sleep apnea.

PREVENTION PRESCRIPTION

- Maintain a healthy weight and especially avoid obesity (BMI > 30). There is evidence that maintaining a waist circumference less than 40 inches (approx. 102 cm) can reduce erectile dysfunction.
- Reduce the risk for diabetes and metabolic syndrome by eating foods with a lower glycemic index and with a low-to-moderate glycemic load.
- Eat a diet rich in fruits and vegetables.
- Exercise regularly to help maintain a healthy weight and physical fitness. Exercising 200–300 minutes per week has been shown to increase testosterone levels.
- Consider developing a yoga practice and embrace posing in a powerful way to naturally boost testosterone levels and lower cortisol.

- Establish and nurture strong social bonds throughout life to avoid social isolation during stressful and painful events such as the loss of a spouse.
- Avoid opioid medications if at all possible for chronic pain. If they must be used, try to use the lowest effective dose for the shortest amount of time.
- Avoid plastics and personal care products made with phthalates and BPA. Eliminate eating or drinking from containers made from plastics or cans unless you can verify they are BPA/phthalate free. Replace plastic stamped with the recycling symbols 3, 6, and 7 with ceramic, glass, or stainless steel.

THERAPEUTIC REVIEW

NUTRITION

- Reduce metabolic syndrome and diabetes   A①₁
- Reduce refined carbohydrates   A①₁
- Increase a plant-based diet and reduce consumption of animal products   A①₁

EXERCISE

- Encourage moderate-to-high levels of exercise and weight loss   B⊘₁

MIND-BODY

- Practice "power posing" on a daily basis   B⊘₁
- Encourage finding resources and help to support men dealing with difficult psychological problems and concerns   C→₁

TOXINS

- If exposure to opioids is causing TD, try to limit exposure if possible   B⊘₁
- Avoid food and drink contamination from plastic products made from phthalates and BPA   A①₁

SUPPLEMENTS

- Zinc 25–50 mg PO daily
- DHEA 5–50 mg PO 1–2×/day
- Quercetin 400 mg PO 1–2×/day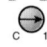

BOTANICALS

- Grape seed extract 100–300 mg PO 1–2×/day
- Pycnogenol 50 mg 3×/day
- Saw palmetto 160 mg PO 2×/day
- Maca 500–1000 mg PO 3×/day

PHARMACEUTICALS

- Testosterone cypionate 50–200 mg IM q1–2 weeks
- Testosterone cream 10–200 mg topically daily   C⊘₂
- Testosterone gel 25–100 mg topically daily

Key Web Resources

American Urological Society
This organization, founded in 1902, is the premier professional association for the advancement of urological patient care. It works to ensure that its more than 17,000 members are current on the latest research and practices in urology. If you search "testosterone" on the website, you gain access to articles and other information.

http://www.auanet.org

Environmental Working Group
This organization's mission is to use the power of public information to protect public health and the environment. The group specializes in providing useful resources to consumers while simultaneously pushing for national policy change.

http://www.EWG.org

Endocrine Society
Founded in 1916, this group is the world's oldest, largest, and most active organization devoted to research on hormones and the clinical practice of endocrinology. Members of the Endocrine Society represent the full range of disciplines associated with endocrinologists: clinicians, researchers, educators, fellows and students, industry professionals, and health professionals who are involved in the field of endocrinology.

http://www.endo-society.org

REFERENCES

References are available online at ExpertConsult.com.

SECTION XII

MUSCULOSKELETAL

SECTION OUTLINE

65 OSTEOARTHRITIS

66 MYOFASCIAL PAIN SYNDROME

67 CHRONIC LOW BACK PAIN

68 NECK PAIN

69 GOUT

70 CARPAL TUNNEL SYNDROME

71 EPICONDYLOSIS

CHAPTER 65

OSTEOARTHRITIS

Adam I. Perlman, MD, MPH • Lisa Rosenberger, ND, LAc • Ather Ali, ND, MPH, MHS

Osteoarthritis (OA) is a slowly progressive degenerative disease of the joints that afflicts approximately 27 million Americans.[1,2-7] OA is already the most frequently reported chronic condition in the elderly, and with the aging of the baby boomer population and increased rates of obesity, it is estimated that by 2030, more than 67 million Americans (25% of the population) will have OA.[7-9] The costs of OA in terms of human suffering are extremely high, with increased all-cause mortality in adults with OA compared to those without OA.[10]

Conventional therapies for OA have limited effectiveness, and toxicities associated with suitable drugs often limit utilization, leaving many facing surgery or chronic pain, muscle weakness, lack of stamina, and/or loss of function.[3,11-17] OA of the hip or knee is particularly disabling because it limits ambulation, but OA also strikes the hands, spine, feet, and other joints with the same destructive process.[2,4,13-15] The endpoint of the OA disease process is total loss of joint cartilage in the affected area and the need for joint replacement.[14,15] Fig. 65.1 illustrates degenerative findings in the knee joint.

OA is a disease of multiple etiologies and should be considered not a consequence of wear and tear but rather a breakdown in normal physiological pathways that manifests as progressive damage of articular cartilage as well as bone remodeling or new bone formation.[18] However, ultimately the whole joint is affected in OA, with pathological changes in not only the bone and cartilage but also synovium and ligaments.[19,20] Imbalances within the joint occur between metabolic and degradative processes facilitated by cytokines, inflammatory mediators, and chondrocyte activity.[19-21] OA is broadly broken down into two categories: primary (idiopathic) OA, in which no specific risk factors, except for age, can be identified, and secondary OA, in which changes can be related to systemic and/or local factors.[22] Fig. 65.2 shows the systemic and local factors that increase susceptibility to OA.

PATHOPHYSIOLOGY

Normal Joints

The major constituents of cartilage are water, proteoglycans (composed of protein cores plus chondroitin sulfate and keratin sulfate side chains), and collagen (predominantly type II). Collectively, they form the extracellular matrix (ECM). Chondrocytes are metabolically active cells that are responsible for synthesis of the ECM. Proteoglycans provide elasticity of cartilage, and collagen provides tensile strength. Muscles and ligaments provide support and protection, while nerve endings provide proprioceptive information. Cartilage health and function depends on compression (pumping fluid from the cartilage into the joint space and into capillaries and venules) and release (allowing cartilage to reexpand, hyperhydrate, and absorb nutrients).

Early Changes of Osteoarthritis

The articular cartilage surface becomes irregular with superficial clefts in the tissue with increased chondrocyte proliferation and cluster formation.[20] Increased hydration of the ECM leads to a failure of the elastic restraint of collagen (i.e., weakening of the collagen network) and also alters the proteoglycan distribution.[19,20] Progression leads to a net decrease in proteoglycans and an increase in the permeability of water. Loss of elasticity and greater permeability of water lead to higher chondrocyte stress and more exposure to degradative enzymes. As the process continues, the articular cartilage has deepening of the clefts and irregularities, eventually resulting in ulceration and exposure of the bone.[19-21]

Late Changes of Osteoarthritis

Subchondral osteoblasts increase bone formation, leading to stiffer and less compliant bones. This in turn results in microfractures, followed by callus formation, more stiffness, and more microfractures. Osteophytes (outgrowths of bone) are formed, the hallmark of OA. They ultimately cause restricted motion. Subchondral cysts are formed in an attempt to equalize pressure. Gross ulceration of articular cartilage will have focal and then diffuse areas of complete loss of cartilage. In later stages, proteoglycan and keratan sulfate levels in the ECM decrease, as does the length of chondroitin sulfate chains. These changes in concentrations of components within the ECM lead to cartilage resembling the composition of immature cartilage.[20] Soft tissues around the joint are also affected, leading to inflammatory infiltrates in the synovium, greater laxity of ligaments, and weakened muscles.

Other factors involved in inflammatory and destructive processes in the joint include the matrix metalloproteinase (MMP) family of proteinases, which degrade proteoglycans and collagen,[20,21] as well as cytokines, IL-1, and TNF-α, which upregulate MMP gene expression, facilitate damage to the joint, and inhibit reparative pathways that would restore joint integrity.[23] Other cytokines involved in OA processes include the proinflammatory cytokines IL-6, IL-8, IL-11, IL-17, and leukemia inhibitory factor (LIF), as well as antiinflammatory cytokines IL-4, IL-10, and IL-13.[23]

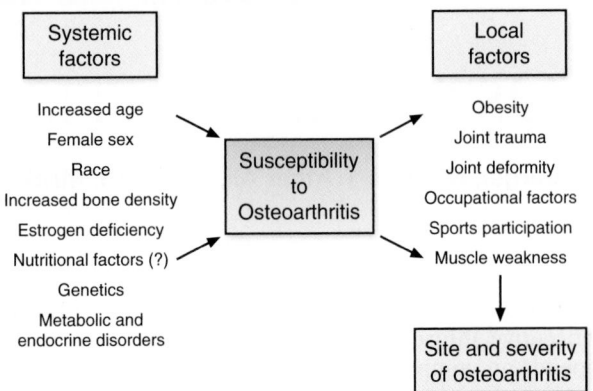

FIG. 65.1 ■ Systemic and local factors that increase susceptibility to arthritis. (Modified from Dieppe P. The classification and diagnosis of arthritis. In: Kuettner K, Goldberg V, eds. *Osteoarthritic disorders.* Rosemont, IL: American Academy of Orthopaedic Surgeons; 1995:7.)

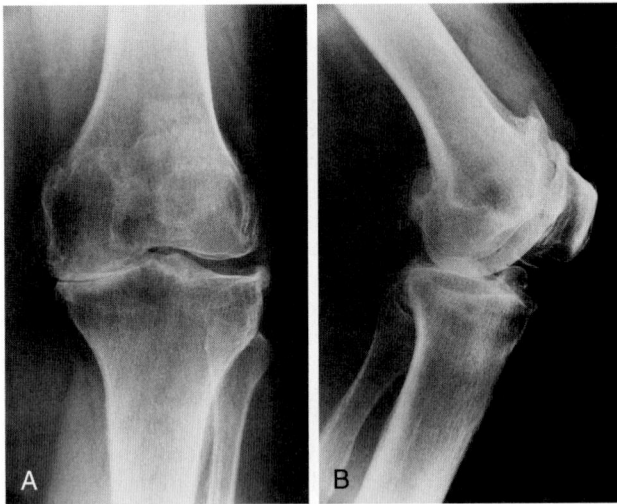

FIG. 65.2 ■ Degenerative joint disease. Anteroposterior (A) and lateral (B) views of the knee show the characteristic finding of osteoarthritis. Joint space narrowing and osteophyte formation at the medial and patellofemoral compartments with varus alignment at the knee are visible. A large suprapatellar joint effusion is also apparent. (From Scott NW. *Insall and Scott Surgery of the Knee.* 4th ed. Philadelphia: Churchill Livingstone; 2005.)

INTEGRATIVE APPROACHES

Integrative therapy in OA is aimed at reducing pain, improving joint functionality, and reducing the further progression of osteoarthritis. Some complementary therapies have potential disease-modifying effects, such as glucosamine and chondroitin sulfates, while others provide symptomatic relief.

Lifestyle

Antiinflammatory Diet

An antiinflammatory diet is characterized by emphasizing omega-3 fatty acids (found primarily in deep-water fish), minimizing omega-6 fatty acids, with an emphasis on unprocessed whole grains, beans, and fruits and vegetables. Fish oil, especially EPA, is often added as a supplementary measure. There is significant overlap between the antiinflammatory diet and the Mediterranean diet that can reduce the risk of cardiovascular disease.[24,25] A diet high in fruits and vegetables, independent of lifestyle effects and BMI, is likely to be protective against radiographic hip OA.[26]

Antiinflammatory diets have demonstrated clinical benefits in persons with inflammatory diseases such as rheumatoid arthritis.[24,27-30] Studies have largely demonstrated a reduction in number of tender joints and the duration of morning stiffness.[30] Fish oil supplements may reduce the need for nonsteroidal antiinflammatory drugs (NSAIDs).[30,31]

Arachidonic acid, found only in animal foods, is eliminated from the diet in strict vegetarians; vegetarianism has been associated with symptomatic relief in rheumatoid arthritis.[32-34] Other studies report symptomatic relief of rheumatoid arthritis symptoms with gluten-free vegan diets[35] (see Chapter 88).

Weight Loss

Dietary Measures

Weight is directly related to the development of OA; therefore, weight management is an important element in both the prevention and management of OA of the knees and hips.[36-39] Rapid, substantial weight loss through dietary restriction may have significant benefits on symptoms and functionality in overweight patients.[38] Messier et al.[40] found that the combination of dietary weight loss plus exercise (compared to either alone, or a control group receiving educational materials) resulted in significant long-term symptomatic improvement in obese sedentary people with OA. In a 2010 study, it was found that a 10% weight loss in obese and overweight patients with OA had a reduction in biomechanical pathology of OA of the knee by reduction in lower knee joint compressive loads during walking compared with low to no weight loss groups[41] (see Chapter 37).

Exercise

A 2015 Cochrane Review of 54 randomized controlled trials found that land-based exercise provided short-term benefit for OA patients that is sustained for 2–6 months following treatment. Exercise can result in reduced knee pain and improves physical function in persons with knee OA.[42] Furthermore, exercise programs can help prevent disability from OA.[43] Exercise programs may be more useful for knee OA compared to hip OA.

Although multiple guidelines with varying recommendations on the physical management of OA exist, exercise is an important strategy in the management of this condition.[44] Three types of exercise should be incorporated into a program for OA sufferers: aerobic training, resistance training with muscle strengthening, and flexibility or range of motion. Both group- and home-based programs may be effective, making patient preference an important consideration.[45] In addition, some evidence supports water-based exercise as an option for patients with OA.[46] Aerobic training can also reduce risk of cardiovascular disease and diabetes, thereby improving overall health status. Recommended exercises are walking, biking, swimming, aerobic dance, and aerobic pool exercises. For patients with symptomatic hip OA, aquatic exercises can be effective.[47,48]

> Exercise is an effective nonpharmacological treatment for reducing pain and improving function. Although formal guidelines vary, some form of physical activity should be done on most days, with a more formal exercise routine at least three days per week for a total of at least 150 minutes, or 75 minutes if more vigorous.[49]

Muscles are important shock absorbers and help stabilize the joint; therefore, periarticular muscle weakness may result in progression of structural damage to the joint in OA. In addition, insufficient loading of a joint will lead to atrophy of both articular cartilage and subchondral bone.[50] In general, strength training helps offset the loss in muscle mass and strength typically associated with normal aging. Strength training has been found to be beneficial for older adults, but especially beneficial for those older adults with OA because it not only improves muscle strength but also function and pain reduction.[51] Reassure patients with OA that strengthening exercises will not exacerbate their symptoms if done in the appropriate manner and dose.[51]

Flexibility is a general term that encompasses the range of motion of single or multiple joints and the ability to perform certain tasks. The range of motion of a given joint depends primarily on the structure and function of bone, muscle, and connective tissue. Cartilage needs regular compression and decompression to enable it to remodel and repair damage and receive appropriate nutrients. OA affects the structure of these tissues, such that range of motion and flexibility are reduced. The basis for exercise interventions to improve flexibility is that the muscle and connective tissue properties can be improved, thereby enhancing function.[52]

Dosing. Although the optimal exercise prescription and dosage is unclear, patients should consider following the guidelines for active adults or active older adults recommended by the Centers for Disease Control and Prevention.[49] These guidelines include a goal of a minimum of 150 minutes of moderate intensity or 75 minutes of more vigorous intensity aerobic exercise per week, with muscle strengthening activities at least 2 days per week. More benefits may be seen with increased time and/or intensity.

Another option is to consider 20 minutes of exercise three times a week, building up to at least 180 minutes of mild to moderate exercise per week. Better adherence to exercise regimens occurs in supervised settings in comparison to unsupervised settings.[53] In the following section are some exercise recommendations based on studies assessing exercise for the treatment of OA. These regimens are only guidelines and should be modified according to patient's current health status and severity

of OA. These regimens can also be appropriate for those attempting a weight loss program.

Aerobic Exercise

Aerobic exercise consists of three phases: (1) the warm-up phase (slow walking, calisthenics: arm circles, trunk rotation, shoulder and chest stretches, and side stretches) for approximately 10 min, (2) the stimulus phase (walking at 50%–70% of heart rate reserve) for up to 40 min, and (3) the cool down phase (slow walking, flexibility exercises, shoulder stretches, hamstring stretches, and lower back stretches) for 10 min.

Aerobic interventions: 1 hour per session, three times a week.[54]

Dosing. The optimal exercise prescription and dosage remains unclear; however, patients should consider building up to exercising for 1 hour per session, three times weekly[32,55] (see Chapter 91).

Resistance Training/Muscle Strengthening

A strength training program that provides progressive overload to maintain intensity throughout the exercise program has been found to be most beneficial for improvements in strength, function, and pain reduction in older adults with OA.[51]

A resistance program also consists of three phases: (1) warm-up phase, 10 min, (2) stimulus phase, 40 min, and (3) cool down phase, 10 min. During the stimulus phase, employ exercises that improve the overall muscular fitness of the person and strengthen major muscle groups of the both the upper and lower extremities. Each exercise should be done in two sets of 12 repetitions. Exercises can include leg extensions, leg curl, step up, heel raise, chest fly, upright row, military press, biceps curl, and pelvic tilt. These exercises can be performed using dumbbells, cuff weights, and/or resistance machines.[54]

Dosing. The optimal exercise prescription and dosage remains unclear; however, patients should consider building up to exercising for 1 hour per session, three times weekly, with at least two sessions per week of resistance training.[32,55]

Flexibility/Range of Motion

Exercises that develop and improve range of motion, also aid in maintaining flexibility. These exercises involve static movements and maintained stretching of the major muscle groups. These exercises should be performed two to three times per week and should be of moderate intensity (intensity of 5–6/10, with 10 being the most intense).[52,56]

Dosing. When beginning a resistance/strength training program, one should start with the lowest possible resistance (1.3 kg for the upper body and 1.1 kg for the lower body). Weight should be increased in a step-wise fashion and based on patient tolerance. If a patient is able to complete 2 sets of 10 repetitions then the weight is tolerable. If a patient establishes a plateau in weight tolerance, then it is appropriate to increase the amount of weight when the patient is able to perform 2 sets of 12 repetitions for 3 consecutive days.[54]

Precaution. Two precautions should be considered before implementation of an exercise program in patients with OA: (1) exercise of an acutely inflamed or swollen joint should be deferred until the acute process subsides and (2) an exercise stress test should be performed to identify cardiac disease in those at risk.[57]

Mind-Body Therapies

Telemedicine Interventions

Interactive programs utilizing computers and web-based interactions with patients have been shown to have a benefit for patients with OA following arthroplasty as well as with those needing chronic pain management.[58-60]

Telephone-based strategies can be an integral part of the management of chronic disease. A randomized controlled trial evaluated whether telephone-based or office-based interventions, or both, improved the functional status of patients with OA.[61] Subjects in the intervention groups were contacted monthly by telephone or scheduled clinic visits by trained people who were not health care professionals. At each contact, the following items were discussed: (1) joint pain, (2) medications, (3) gastrointestinal and other medication-related symptoms, (4) date of the next scheduled outpatient visit, (5) an established mechanism through which patients could telephonically contact a physician during weekends and evenings, and (6) barriers to keeping appointments. At 1-year follow-up, in comparison with the control group, persons receiving telephone calls reported less physical disability and pain and tended to have better psychological status.[62] Smartphone and Internet-based interventions are ubiquitous and can be adapted to large populations.

DOSAGE

Telephone calls (or possibly text messages) are typically made to patients biweekly[61] or monthly.[62]

PRECAUTIONS

A good patient–provider relationship ensuring effective communication and the ability to understand and implement medical guidance over the telephone should exist before patients are counseled by telephone.

Group Programs

The Arthritis Self-Management Program (ASMP) is a community-taught, peer-led intervention, in which patients gain the confidence and the necessary tools to manage their disease. Participants attend 2-hour weekly sessions for 6 weeks. These sessions include education about pathophysiology and pharmacotherapy, as well as the design of individualized exercise and relaxation programs, appropriate use of injured joints, aspects of patient–physician communications, and methods for solving problems that arise from illness. The sessions are taught from an interactive model, which promotes individual participation and self-management techniques.[63] A 4-year follow-up study found that participants had reduced pain and fewer physician visits, and they spent fewer days in the hospital.[63]

DOSAGE

Patients attend a group course with an experienced teacher twice weekly for at least 12 weeks.

PRECAUTIONS

This approach may not work for patients who need more attention or individual face-to-face

Yoga

Yoga, a traditional Indian practice of a physical and mental nature, involves the use of postures or *asanas*, breathing techniques or *pranayama*, and mental concentration/meditation or *dhyana*. All of these are focused on the intention of promoting relaxation, *savasana*. As stress, physical dysfunction, and lack of exercise are confounders for OA and worsening of the disease, a therapy that can address all of these areas is ideal. Yoga has been studied as a complementary (adjunct therapy to conventional care) and an alternative therapy (tried instead of a conventional therapy, such as pharmaceuticals, injections, and/or surgery). A 2012 review assessing tai chi and yoga as complementary therapies in rheumatological conditions noted that most studies in knee OA were small and uncontrolled. Yoga was found to improve pain and functionality compared to control interventions in several randomized trials.[64] A 2013 review noted general safety and feasibility for yoga interventions in OA and at least short-term benefit.[65] More research on the various types of yoga practice as well as the specific joints affected by OA needs to be further studied. Long-term effects and benefit, as well as comparison to other OA interventions, both conventional and complementary, in different age groups should also be further studied.[65]

DOSAGE

Although the dose is variable, patients should consider Hatha yoga at 1 hour per week for 8 weeks. Yoga can be done in conjunction with other physical therapy modalities.

PRECAUTIONS

Several types of yoga practices exist; it is important to begin with gentle, easy exercises.

Tai Chi

Tai chi is also an effective exercise strategy for OA that has the benefit of not only improving pain and function, but also balance.[66] Tai chi has been noted to be particularly effective in improving pain, stiffness, and overall function in knee OA.[67]

Physical Modalities

Reduction of Joint Loading

Patients with OA of the knee or hip should avoid prolonged periods of standing, kneeling, or squatting. In patients with unilateral OA of the hip or knee, a cane, when held in the contralateral hand, may diminish joint pain by reducing joint contact force. Bilateral disease may necessitate the use of crutches or a walker.[68] A Cochrane Review on the use of braces or orthoses for knee OA indicated only limited evidence to support the effectiveness of these devices.[69] However, the trials that have been undertaken indicate good symptom relief from the use of wedged insoles in patients with OA of the medial knee compartment.[70] The 2008 Osteoarthritis Research Society International (OARSI) guidelines indicated that patients with knee OA and mild to moderate varus or valgus instability may benefit from knee bracing because it can reduce pain, improve stability, and reduce the risk of falling.[47]

Heat Therapy

Application of heat can raise the pain threshold and produce muscle relaxation. Moist heat produces greater elevation of the subcutaneous temperature than dry heat and is often preferable for relief of pain. A randomized, placebo-controlled, double-blind clinical trial examining the effects of local hyperthermia induced by 433.92-MHz microwave diathermy in OA of the knee found that three 30-minutes sessions per week for 4 weeks produced significant improvements in pain reduction and physical function.[71]

Superficial heat penetrates the skin only a few millimeters and does not reach deeper joints such as the hip and knee. In contrast, a heat mitten may raise the temperature of the small joints of the hand.[72]

DOSAGE

For commercial hot packs (temperature, 165–170°F), treatment time is 15–30 minutes, and the temperature is adjusted to the patient's tolerance by using commercial covers or increasing towel thickness between the patient and the hot pack. For diathermy, patients undergo 30-minute sessions three times weekly for 4 weeks.

PRECAUTIONS

The risk of thermal injury is higher in patients with poor circulation or impaired sensation.[68] Use heat therapy with caution in patients who have reduced peripheral circulation or severe cardiac insufficiency. Be aware of superficial metal implants and open or closed wounds in the skin.

Cold Therapy

Cold applications are often recommended after strenuous exercise to relieve muscle aching. They may be delivered by ice packs, ice massage, or local spray. Superficial cooling can decrease muscle spasms and raise the pain threshold. A Cochrane Review of three randomized controlled trials showed that ice treatment may improve the range of motion and reduce edema in knee OA.[73]

DOSAGE

Most cold applications are for 20–30 minutes and are reapplied in 2 hours. Rewarming times should be at least twice as long as cooling times, to avoid excessive cooling.

A classic ice pack (23–32°F) is a mixture of crushed ice and cold water wrapped in terry cloth or enclosed in a plastic bag. These packs usually maintain a surface temperature above freezing and thus do not require an insulator between the patient's skin and the pack.

Cold packs (33–50°F) are a mixture of water and antifreeze that forms a gel mixture in a vinyl cover. These gel packs may induce frostbite because of their low temperature, so a layer between the skin and the pack is warranted. Treatment should be limited to less than 30 minutes with these cold packs.

PRECAUTIONS

Cold applications should not be used in patients with Raynaud's phenomenon, cold hypersensitivity, cryoglobulinemia, or paroxysmal cold hemoglobinuria.[68]

Transcutaneous Electrical Nerve Stimulation

Transcutaneous electrical nerve stimulation (TENS) has been considered as a treatment modality for OA of the knee or hip. It can help with short-term pain relief, and no serious side effects have been reported.[47]

DOSAGE

For conventional TENS, the frequency is 85 pps and the pulse width is 75 μsec. The intensity is sensory, with placement of pads over the target tissue, dermatome, or nerve distribution. The duration of application is 15–30 minutes to 4 hours (until relief is obtained). The frequency of application is one to six times daily, depending on the patient's response and the intensity of pain. A review study noted that TENS has increased benefit when the highest intensity tolerated by the patient is applied, and when pads are placed at acupoint locations rather than nonacupoint locations.[73a]

PRECAUTIONS

Use TENS with caution in patients who have cardiac pacemakers, implanted cardioverter defibrillators, electrocardiography monitors, other electronic implants, skin allergic reactions, and impaired skin sensation, as well as in patients who drive or operate hazardous machinery and are currently taking pain medications.

Stimulation over the intercostal muscles should be avoided or closely monitored because, in one case report of a patient with cardiac disease, this stimulation led to respiratory failure. In addition, caffeine intake higher than 200 mg/day (approximately three cups of coffee per day) decreased the ability of the TENS to modulate pain.[74]

Massage

Massage may lead to improvement in pain and function. A randomized controlled trial of Swedish massage therapy in patients with OA found significant improvements in pain, stiffness and physical function, pain perception, knee range of motion, and time to walk 50 ft.[75] Research to replicate these findings and further define the role of massage in the treatment of OA of the knee is ongoing; however, a 2012 study identified an "optimal practical dose."[76] Research evaluating the role of massage in the treatment of other joints afflicted with OA is also needed.

DOSAGE

The dose of Swedish massage is 60 minutes per week for 8 weeks.

PRECAUTIONS

Although the risk of local pain from excessive pressure or bruising does exist, massage is commonly performed and is generally not harmful. Massage likely has no serious risks.

Acupuncture

Acupuncture-associated analgesia is believed to work through the release of opioid peptides.[77] Numerous randomized controlled trials have been undertaken to assess the efficacy of acupuncture for treatment of pain associated with OA. In a 1975 study, 40 patients were randomly allocated to receive acupuncture either at standard points or at placebo or sham points.[20] Analysis before and after treatment showed a statistically significant improvement in tenderness and subjective report of pain in both groups.[78] In a 1982 study, 32 patients with OA of the hip, knee, or humeroscapular joint were randomly allocated either to receive weekly acupuncture or to take piroxicam, with checkup visits at 2, 4, 6, 12, and 16 weeks. The extent of improvement was equal in both groups at 2 weeks (30%); after that, however, the acupuncture group showed greater pain relief than the piroxicam group.[79] A systematic review of 11 randomized controlled trials of acupuncture for OA concluded that the most rigorously conducted studies showed that acupuncture is not superior to sham needling in reducing pain from OA.[80] The most recent Cochrane Review of acupuncture reported that although sham-controlled trials do have statistically significant benefits, the benefits do not meet the predefined thresholds for clinical relevance and the benefits are small.[81] The investigators also noted that the benefits are likely the result of a placebo effect or participant expectations.[81]

Another randomized controlled trial, however, suggested that acupuncture may indeed provide relief for OA pain, unlike sham acupuncture.[82] In this trial, 570 patients with knee OA were randomly allocated to receive 23 sessions of either true or sham acupuncture over 26 weeks or to participate in six 2-hour education sessions over 12 weeks (controls). Persons in the true acupuncture group showed an improvement in function at 8 weeks and a significant improvement in pain at 26 weeks compared with the sham and control groups, as evidenced by scores on the Western Ontario and McMaster Universities Arthritis Index (WOMAC).[82]

Acupuncture may serve as an adjunct to a conventional medical regimen by allowing a reduction in dosage of nonsteroidal antiinflammatory drugs (NSAIDs) and therefore potentially reducing the side effects occasionally seen with long-term NSAID use.[83] Each state has its own requirements for acupuncture licensure and certification. Patients should be referred only to a licensed or certified practitioner.

The 2008 OARSI recommendations for managing OA of the knee noted that acupuncture may be of symptomatic benefit in patients with knee OA.[47] In addition, although multiple sham-controlled trials showed minimal benefit over sham, acupuncture may still provide symptomatic relief for patients with OA who are wary of or unable to use pharmaceutical interventions.[84]

DOSAGE

Acupuncture treatments vary depending on the patient's underlining conditions, the severity and location of pain, and the practitioner's assessment. However, most acupuncture treatments last between 15 and 30 minutes, with needles inserted. A common acupuncture regimen consists of treatment once to three times weekly.

PRECAUTIONS

Acupuncture may cause bleeding or bruising at the site of needle insertion. Therefore, patients taking blood thinning medications may have a higher incidence of this side effect.

Acupuncture has been shown to improve both pain and function in osteoarthritis of the knee. Six or more treatments are often required before efficacy can truly be assessed.

Supplements
Glucosamine Sulfate and Chondroitin Sulfate

Glucosamine's primary role is as a substrate for glycosaminoglycans and the hyaluronic acid backbone used in the formation of proteoglycans found in the structural matrix of joints.[85] Chondroitins are the main glycosaminoglycans in human joints and connective tissue, and they play a role in cartilage formation through the stimulation of chondrocyte metabolism and synthesis of collagen and proteoglycans.[86] Destructive synovial enzymes are inhibited by chondroitin.[87] Unlike other therapies used as symptom modifiers, such as NSAIDs, these supplements are potentially structure modifying.[47] Glucosamine sulfate and chondroitin sulfate are sulfate derivatives of glucosamine and chondroitin, and doubts regarding their absorption and metabolic fate have fueled skepticism about their therapeutic potential.[88] This dilemma has stimulated numerous studies.

In a 2001 double-blinded, randomized controlled trial,[89] 212 patients with knee OA were randomly assigned to receive either 1500 mg of glucosamine sulfate or placebo once daily for 3 years. Seventy-one of 106 patients who received placebo completed the trial, and radiographs of their knees showed progressive joint space narrowing. Sixty-eight of 106 patients who received glucosamine sulfate completed the trial, and they had no radiographic evidence of joint space narrowing. This study concluded that oral administration of glucosamine sulfate over the long term could prevent joint structure changes in patients with OA of the knee as well as improve symptoms.[89]

Two randomized controlled trials looked at the effectiveness of chondroitin sulfate in OA.[90,91] In one trial, 300 patients with knee OA were randomly assigned to receive either 800 mg of chondroitin or placebo once daily for 2 years.[90] Although the study found no significant symptomatic effect, results suggested that long-term chondroitin sulfate use may retard radiographic progression of the disease. A 2004 study of 120 patients receiving either the same dosage of chondroitin sulfate or placebo for 1 year provided some evidence that chondroitin sulfate may reduce pain and improve function associated with knee OA.[91]

To evaluate the benefit of glucosamine sulfate and chondroitin sulfate for OA, a meta-analysis combined with systematic quality assessment was performed.[92] Fifteen double-blind, randomized, placebo-controlled trials were included in the analysis. The knee was the joint studied in all the trials, and in one study the hip was also evaluated. Glucosamine or chondroitin sulfate was taken orally in 12 of the studies, intramuscularly in 2 of the studies, and intraarterially in 1 of the studies. Glucosamine sulfate or chondroitin sulfate demonstrated a moderate to large effect on OA symptoms. However, methodological problems may have led to exaggerated estimates of benefit. Overall, these compounds do appear to have efficacy in treating OA symptoms, and they are safe.[92] Glucosamine may not be as effective in patients who are obese compared with patients of normal weight.

The Glucosamine/Chondroitin Arthritis Intervention Trial (GAIT) compared 1500 mg of glucosamine hydrochloride alone and in combination with chondroitin in 1500 people with mild knee pain from OA. Using an end point of 20% reduction in pain, no significant benefit of each supplement individually or in combination was noted. Those individuals with more severe symptoms (moderate to severe OA) reported a 22% reduction in pain. Glucosamine hydrochloride was used in this trial. Most over-the-counter products contain glucosamine sulfate.[93]

> Glucosamine is believed to work, in part, by retaining fluid content within the joint cartilage, while chondroitin works, in part, by increasing the viscosity of the synovial fluid.

Glucosamine and chondroitin are sold as dietary supplements in most health food stores and in many pharmacies. They are often sold in combination; however, it is unclear whether the combination is superior to either treatment alone.[94] In December 1999 and January 2000, a health consultant firm purchased 25 brands of glucosamine, chondroitin, and combination products to test whether the products contained the amounts listed on their respective labels. Nearly one-third of the products did not contain the stated amounts of the supplements.[95] According to Vangsness et al.,[96]

glucosamine and chondroitin sulfate have shown inconsistent but overall positive efficacy in decreasing OA pain and improving joint function. The safety of these compounds was equivalent to that of placebo. In addition, although the literature suggests that individual use of glucosamine sulfate, chondroitin sulfate, or glucosamine hydrochloride has therapeutic value, the effectiveness of monotherapy with these agents has not been proven.[96]

DOSAGE

The dose of glucosamine sulfate is 500 mg three times daily, or 1500 mg/day. The dose for chondroitin sulfate is 400 mg two to three times daily, or 800-1200 mg/day. Both are used for a minimum of 6 months to show benefit.

PRECAUTIONS

Potential adverse effects include dyspepsia, nausea, and headache.

S-Adenosylmethionine

S-Adenosylmethionine (SAMe) is a physiological molecule formed in the body from the essential amino acid methionine. It functions in a wide variety of anabolic and catabolic reactions in all living cells. Although the mechanism of action on the symptoms of OA is not fully understood, it may be related to the agent's ability to stimulate proteoglycan synthesis in OA cartilage.[97] The US Food and Drug Administration approved SAMe for sale as a dietary supplement in 1999; however, it has been used since the mid-1970s, primarily in Europe to treat depression and arthritis.[98]

> To encourage production of S-adenosylmethionine in the body, patients with osteoarthritis who have low folic acid levels should consider increasing these levels through higher consumption of dark green leafy vegetables or supplementation.

A 1987 double-blind, randomized controlled trial compared 1200 mg of SAMe with 1200 mg of ibuprofen taken by 36 patients with OA of the knee, hip, or spine, or a combination, for 4 weeks.[99] Morning stiffness, pain at rest and during motion, crepitus, swelling, and limitation of motion in the affected joints were assessed before and after treatment. The study found that both treatments were well tolerated and equally effective in lessening symptoms. The investigators thus concluded that SAMe exerted a beneficial effect on the symptoms of OA.[99] Similar results were found in a trial comparing 1200 mg of SAMe and 150 mg of indomethacin; SAMe was better tolerated.[100] A later randomized, double-blind, crossover study comparing celecoxib with SAMe in 56 patients with knee OA suggested that SAMe may be as effective as celecoxib at reducing symptoms but may have a slower onset of action.[101] *The Arthritis Foundation's Guide to Alternative Therapies* noted that SAMe is a promising treatment worth trying for pain relief, but that more scientific evidence is needed to prove that it supports cartilage repair.[102]

DOSAGE

The dose is 400–1600 mg daily; a common regimen is 600 mg twice daily.

PRECAUTIONS

Watch for nausea and gastrointestinal distress. Ensure adequate intake of vitamin B_{12} and folate through diet (green leafy vegetables) or supplementation to optimize SAMe supplementation.[103,104] Do not take close to bedtime because of the risk of insomnia.

Methylsulfonylmethane

Methylsulfonylmethane (MSM) is a dietary supplement commonly sold for the treatment of OA. The MSM metabolite dimethyl sulfoxide is found naturally in the human body. Because sulfur is necessary for the formation of connective tissue, MSM is thought to be useful in the treatment of OA. Animal studies have suggested that MSM may help decrease inflammatory joint disease,[105] but unfortunately, no published human trials are available. Overall, the literature on the sulfur-containing compounds SAMe and MSM in OA appears to be limited. However, the literature shows a trend toward decreased pain and increased function with the consistent use of these compounds. The therapeutic benefit and safety of these compounds for long- and short-term use needs to be further researched, especially through randomized clinical trials.[96,106]

DOSAGE

The dose is 1000–3000 mg three times daily.

PRECAUTIONS

Watch for nausea, diarrhea, and headache. Although MSM is promoted as being nontoxic, clinical data are lacking, and further scientific study is needed to define the efficacy and safety of this supplement.

Pharmaceuticals: Nonopioid Analgesics

Acetaminophen

Acetaminophen acts by inhibiting prostaglandin synthesis in the central nervous system. It may relieve mild to moderate joint pain and may be used as initial therapy on the basis of its overall cost, efficacy, and toxicity profile.[107]

DOSAGE

The dose is 325–1000 mg every 4–6 hours, up to a maximum of 4 g/day.

PRECAUTIONS

Reactions are uncommon with normal therapeutic doses of acetaminophen but include nausea, rash, and minor

allergic reactions, a transient drop in white blood cell count, liver toxicity, and prolongation of the half-life of warfarin. Patients with hepatic impairment or active hepatic disease must be monitored when acetaminophen is prescribed for the long term. Patients with viral hepatitis, alcoholism, or alcoholic hepatic disease are at greater risk for acetaminophen-induced hepatotoxicity.[108] Long-term acetaminophen use should be avoided in patients with underlying renal disease. Tobacco smoking may also potentially increase the risk for acetaminophen-induced hepatotoxicity.[108]

Tramadol

Tramadol is a synthetic opioid agonist that inhibits reuptake of norepinephrine and serotonin. It should be considered for patients with moderate to severe pain in whom acetaminophen therapy has failed and who have contraindications to NSAIDs.[99]

DOSAGE

The dose is 50–100 mg every 4–6 hours, up to a maximum of 400 mg/day.

PRECAUTIONS

Watch for nausea, constipation, drowsiness, and, rarely, seizures.

Pharmaceuticals: Nonsteroidal Antiinflammatory Drugs

Nonsteroidal Antiinflammatory Drugs

Nonselective NSAIDs are a group of chemically dissimilar agents that act primarily by inhibiting the cyclooxygenase (COX) enzymes and thus inhibit the production of prostaglandins in peripheral tissues. Examples are aspirin, ibuprofen, naproxen, indomethacin, sulindac, and piroxicam.

DOSAGE

- Aspirin: 2.6–5.4 g in divided doses daily
- Ibuprofen: 300–800 mg three or four times daily; maximum, 3200 mg/day
- Naproxen: 250–500 mg twice daily; maximum, 1500 mg/day
- Indomethacin: 25 mg two or three times daily; maximum, 200 mg/day
- Sulindac: 150–200 mg twice daily; maximum, 400 mg/day
- Piroxicam: 20 mg daily or 10 mg twice daily

Cyclooxygenase-2 Inhibitor

COX-2–specific inhibitors act in the same manner as nonselective COX inhibitors, but their action is confined to inflamed tissues. Celecoxib (Celebrex) is the only COX-2 inhibitor currently available on the market.

DOSAGE

The dose of celecoxib (Celebrex) is 200 mg daily or 100 mg twice daily.

PRECAUTIONS FOR ALL NONSTEROIDAL ANTIINFLAMMATORY DRUGS

Precautions vary with specific agent and include epigastric distress, nausea, vomiting, gastrointestinal bleeding (nonselective NSAIDs more than COX-2 inhibitors), prolonged bleeding (aspirin), headache, dizziness, and renal toxicity. Epidemiological studies have shown that COX-2 inhibitors may increase the risk of myocardial infarction.[109]

The choice between nonselective NSAIDs and COX-2–specific NSAIDs should be based on the risk of upper gastrointestinal bleeding.

Data from epidemiological studies demonstrate that among persons aged 65 years and older, 20%–30% of all hospitalizations and deaths resulting from peptic ulcer disease are attributable to NSAID use.[110]

Persons at increased risk of gastrointestinal bleeding are those aged 65 years or older, as well as those with a history of peptic ulcer disease, previous upper gastrointestinal bleeding, concomitant use of oral corticosteroids or anticoagulants, and, possibly, smoking and alcohol consumption.[111] Patients in this category may benefit from a COX-2–specific inhibitor or a nonselective NSAID with gastroprotective therapy (e.g., misoprostol, omeprazole, or high-dose famotidine).

Pharmaceuticals: Opioid Analgesics

Patients with OA who have tried acetaminophen, tramadol, and NSAIDs without success may consider opiates. Opiates bind to receptors in the central nervous system to produce effects that mimic the action of endogenous peptide neurotransmitters, specifically, the relief of intense pain. These agents should usually be avoided for long-term use, but their short-term use helps in the treatment of acute exacerbations of pain.[112] Commonly used opiates are fentanyl, meperidine, propoxyphene, acetaminophen plus propoxyphene, hydromorphone, long-acting morphine, oxycodone plus acetaminophen, and acetaminophen plus hydrocodone.

DOSAGE

Doses and routes vary.

PRECAUTIONS

In addition to the potential for addiction to these agents, side effects include constipation, nausea, vomiting, sedation, urinary retention, and respiratory depression.

Pharmaceuticals: Topical Analgesics

In patients with OA of the hands or knees, topical analgesics may relieve mild to moderate pain.[113] A cream may be used alone or in combination with an oral agent.

Capsaicin Cream

Capsaicin cream (Zostrix) is a commonly used topical agent. It exerts its pharmacological effect by depleting local sensory nerve endings of substance P, a neuropeptide mediator of pain.

DOSAGE

A thin film of capsaicin cream (0.025%, 0.075%) should be applied to the symptomatic joint four times daily.

PRECAUTIONS

A local burning sensation is common but rarely leads to the discontinuation of therapy.

Diclofenac

Aside from capsaicin cream, diclofenac sodium is available as a topical solution. This product (Pennsaid) combines diclofenac with dimethylsulfoxide (DMSO). Pennsaid is indicated for the treatment of signs and symptoms of OA of the knee. Most studies have shown topical diclofenac to be equivalent to oral diclofenac in the treatment of OA of the knee.[114-118] Pennsaid, in particular, has also shown similar effectiveness in treatment of OA of the knee, although further studies to compare Pennsaid with other formulations of diclofenac have yet to be done.[114]

DOSAGE

Diclofenac topical (Pennsaid 1.5% topical solution plus DMSO, Solaraze 3% gel, Voltaren topical 1% gel) is applied to the knee four times daily. It may also be used for other areas of body or joint pain. The Flector patch is applied directly to the area of pain. The skin patch can be worn for up to 12 hours and then removed. Apply a new patch at that time if pain continues. Do not wear a skin patch while taking a bath or shower or while swimming.

PRECAUTIONS

Although diclofenac is applied topically, it is absorbed systemically and has possible side effects. Aside from local irritation at the site of application, diclofenac topical solutions, like other NSAIDS, may increase the risk of serious cardiovascular thrombotic events, myocardial infarction, and stroke or increased gastrointestinal events such as bleeding, ulceration, and perforation of stomach or intestines.

Intraarticular Steroid Injections

Injections are useful in treating a joint effusion or local inflammation that is limited to a few joints. Injections should be limited to three or four per year because of concern about the possible development of progressive cartilage damage through repeated injections in weight-bearing joints.[119]

Other Pharmaceuticals: Diacerein

Diacerein (INN), also known as diacetylrhein, is a drug used in the treatment of OA. It works by inhibiting IL-1. A 2006 Cochrane Review found no significant difference between diacerein and NSAIDS.[120] Although diacerein may have a better risk-to-benefit ratio compared with NSAIDS, it also has an important side effect of diarrhea.

In addition, diacerein may have a mild effect on the symptoms of OA and structure-modifying effects in patients with symptomatic OA of the hip, and further research is necessary to confirm the short- and long-term effectiveness and toxicity.[47,120]

DOSAGE

The dose is 50 mg twice daily.

PRECAUTIONS

Diacerein may cause diarrhea. It is also a long-acting drug with symptomatic effects appearing 4 weeks after beginning treatment.[120]

Surgery

Surgical treatment is usually considered only after failure of nonsurgical treatments. The two categories of surgery are nonbiological and biological.[113]

Nonbiological Approaches

- Osteotomy: This conservative approach may provide effective pain relief and slow disease progression. Its greatest benefit is in patients with only moderately advanced disease.
- Arthroscopy: Removal of loose cartilage fragments can prevent locking and relieve pain. When joint space narrowing is substantial, this type of surgical procedure is of limited benefit.
- Arthrodesis or joint fusion: This alleviates pain and is most commonly performed in the spine and in small joints of the hand and foot. In the hip and knee, it is reserved for very young patients with unilateral disease.
- Arthroplasty or total joint replacement: This is the mainstay of surgical treatment of the hip, knee, and shoulder. It is the most effective of all medical interventions and can restore patients to near-normal function. It is limited in durability in persons with life expectancies exceeding 20 years and in those who wish to participate in high-demand activities.

Biological Approaches

- Biological restoration of articular cartilage uses resident hyaline cartilage, which is stimulated to repair its own defects.
- Biological restoration of articular cartilage is performed using one of three types of cartilage transplantation: osteochondral autografting, osteochondral allografting, and tissue engineering.

Therapies to Consider

Omega-3 Fatty Acids

Omega-3 fatty acids, the precursors for antiinflammatory prostaglandin production in the body, can be very supportive in the treatment of patients with OA. Multiple studies have shown efficacy of increased omega-3 fatty acids in the diet or by supplementation for reducing or alleviating symptoms of rheumatoid arthritis.[121-124] In different animal (dog) studies, investigators found that dietary supplementation with omega-3 fatty acids from fish oil led to an increase in weight-bearing tolerance and a reduction in the need for the NSAID carprofen.[125,126] An in vitro study showed that omega-3 fatty acids caused a reduction in the levels of mRNA for a disintegrin and metalloproteinase with thrombospondin motifs (ADAMTS)-4, ADAMTS-5, matrix MMP-3, MMP-13, COX-2 (but not COX-1), IL-1alpha, IL-1beta, and TNF-alpha, which are key contributors to the pathological process of OA. Investigators also found that eicosapentaenoic acid was most effective, followed by docosahexaenoic acid, and finally by alpha-linoleic acid. Arachidonic acid, an omega-6 fatty acid, had no effect.[127]

Curcumin

Curcumin is the active ingredient in the spice turmeric. It has been used in various cultures around the world, particularly in India and Asia. Research on curcumin has found that it has many properties, which may explain the diversity of its traditional uses. These properties include anticancer, antiinflammatory, antioxidant, and hypolipidemic effects.[128] Curcumin has been researched for benefits in the treatment and management of cardiovascular disease, hypercholesterolemia, diabetes mellitus, insulin resistance, weight loss, and inflammatory conditions.[128] This supplement may be most beneficial for those with OA with other concomitant conditions, such as obesity, diabetes, heart disease, or autoimmune conditions.

In 2009, an in vitro study using articular chondrocytes found that curcumin acted as a strong inhibitor of inflammatory and catabolic mediators, nitric oxide stimulated by IL-1beta, prostaglandin E2, IL-6, IL-8, and MMP-3, produced by chondrocytes.[129]

Avocado Soybean Unsaponifiables

Avocado soybean unsaponifiables (ASU) are extracts of unsaponifiable fractions from one-third avocado oil and two-thirds soybean oil.[130] In multiple animal and human in vitro studies, investigators found that ASU extract had an effect on various cytokines in articular chondrocytes and monocyte/macrophages.[131] In a multicenter, randomized controlled trial, persons taking ASU had slightly lower need for NSAIDs and an improvement in functional disability. Improvement was greatest in patients with hip OA.[130] Most of the in vitro and in vivo studies have used an ASU product that is patented and sold in Europe (Piascledine 1300, Laboratoires Expanscience, France). Because this formulation is unique, the data obtained from its use cannot be extrapolated to all ASU extracts, and thus further studies examining various ASU extracts from multiple manufacturers and processes of extraction are needed.[131]

Boswellia serrata

Boswellia serrata, also known as H15 or indish incense, is a botanical used in traditional Ayurvedic medicine; in vitro, it decreases leukotriene synthesis.[132] A double-blind pilot study evaluated the efficacy of H15 in 37 patients with rheumatoid arthritis. Treatment with H15 showed no measurable efficacy.[132] A double-blind, randomized controlled trial found that *Boswellia* improved symptoms of knee OA. Treatment included a combination of herbs, rather than *Boswellia* alone.[133] A single-blind, randomized controlled trial in which *Boswellia* was taken along with *Withania, Curcuma,* and a zinc complex found that this combination led to improvement in pain and disability in OA.[134]

Although the literature on this agent is promising, it is insufficient to support the use of *Boswellia* for OA. Taken in combination with other herbs, *Boswellia* may improve pain and function.

Ginger

Ginger root is an herb used extensively as a spice in many world cuisines. More recently, attention has focused on the possible medical benefits of ginger, including reduction of nausea and analgesic effects. One study suggested that ginger may be moderately effective in reducing pain from knee OA.[135] This 6-week multicenter, randomized controlled trial evaluated the effect of a highly concentrated standardized ginger extract in 261 patients in comparison with placebo. A moderate reduction of pain was observed in the ginger-treated group. Some mild adverse gastrointestinal effects were also observed in the ginger group, but the overall safety profile was good.

Magnet Therapy

A popular therapy for the treatment of various medical conditions is the application of a magnetic field. The biological effects of low-level magnetic fields have been studied since the 1500s. Explanations of these effects include increased circulation and decreased inflammation.[136] One double-blind, randomized controlled study[137] evaluated bipolar magnets for the treatment of chronic low back pain. The researchers concluded that the application of magnets had no effect on patients' pain.[137] However, a later randomized controlled trial suggested that standard-strength magnetic bracelets may be effective in decreasing pain from OA of the knee and hip.[138] Although magnet therapy does appear to be harmless, its therapeutic use remains questionable. According to the OARSI guidelines for the management of hip and knee OA, five placebo-controlled, randomized controlled trials showed that improvement in function was small and efficacy for reduction in pain was not significant with pulsed electromagnetic field therapy.[139]

Therapeutic Touch

In a 6-week, single-blinded, randomized controlled trial, therapeutic touch was evaluated for effectiveness in the treatment of OA of the knee. Thirty-one participants were enrolled and randomized to therapeutic touch, mock therapeutic touch, or standard care. The main outcome measures were pain and its impact, general well-being, and health status measured by standardized validated instruments, as well as the qualitative measurement of a depth interview. Twenty-five participants completed the study. The findings were that participants receiving therapeutic touch had significant improvements in pain, function, and general health status compared with both placebo and control groups.[140] Further studies with a larger sample size and further evaluation into treatment time and time for course of treatment are required.

PREVENTION PRESCRIPTION

- Maintain appropriate weight.
- Exercise regularly with a combination of aerobics, resistance training, and stretching.
- Consider glucosamine and chondroitin sulfate if at high risk for osteoarthritis.
- Avoid excessive trauma to the joints.

THERAPEUTIC REVIEW

THERAPEUTIC MODALITY

Nutrition

- Antiinflammatory diet: individualized
- Weight loss: individualized program

Exercise

- Aerobic exercise: Three times weekly
- Resistance training/muscle strengthening: 1-hour sessions, three times weekly
- Flexibility exercise: Two to three times weekly

Mind-Body Therapy

- Telephone interventions: Twice weekly for 6 months
- Group programs: Group course with experienced teacher twice weekly for at least 12 weeks
- Yoga: 1 hour weekly for 8 weeks

PHYSICAL MODALITIES

- Knee bracing: as needed
- Heat applications: as needed
- Cold applications: 20–30 minutes, reapplied every 2 hours
- Transcutaneous electrical nerve stimulation: 15-minute to 4-hour session, once daily to six times daily
- Swedish massage therapy: 60 minutes weekly
- Acupuncture: 15–30 minute sessions, once weekly to three times weekly

SUPPLEMENTS

- Glucosamine sulfate and chondroitin sulfate: Glucosamine sulfate, 500 mg three times daily; and chondroitin sulfate, 400 mg three times daily, both for a minimum of 6 months
- S-Adenosylmethionine: 400–1600 mg daily; common regimen, 600 mg twice daily
- Methylsulfonylmethane: 1000–3000 mg three times per day

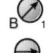
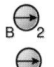
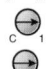
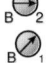
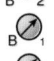
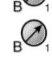

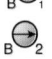
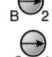

PHARMACEUTICALS

- Acetaminophen: 325–1000 mg every 4–6 hours; maximum, 4 g/day
- Tramadol: 50–100 mg every 4–6 hours; maximum, 400 mg/day
- Nonsteroidal antiinflammatory drugs: Dose variable by drug
- Opioid analgesics: Doses and routes variable
- Capsaicin cream (topical): Thin film of cream (0.025%, 0.075%) applied to the symptomatic joint four times daily
- Diacerein: 50 mg twice daily

INJECTIONS

- Intraarticular steroid injections

SURGERY

- Knee replacement

Key Web Resources

Center for Disease Control and Prevention. Leading national public health institute of the United States	http://www.cdc.gov/
Johns Hopkins University Arthritis Center. Information for clinicians on exercise in osteoarthritis	http://www.hopkins-arthritis.org/patient-corner/disease-management/exercise.html
Johns Hopkins University Arthritis Center. Information for clinicians on yoga for arthritis	http://www.hopkins-arthritis.org/patient-corner/disease-management/yoga.html
Arthritis Today. Online magazine with information on arthritis for patients	http://www.arthritistoday.org/index.php
National Center for Complementary and Integrative Health. Information for clinicians and patients on acupuncture	https://nccih.nih.gov/health/acupuncture
The Brace Shop. Resource for braces for arthritis	http://www.braceshop.com/

REFERENCES

References are available online at ExpertConsult.com.

CHAPTER 66

MYOFASCIAL PAIN SYNDROME

Robert Alan Bonakdar, MD

EPIDEMIOLOGY

Myofascial pain syndrome (MPS) and similar terms (Box 66.1) refer to pain and associated sequelae developing from and aggravated by myofascial trigger points (TrPs). The actual prevalence of MPS varies, based on terminology and diagnostic criteria. However, myofascial pain is considered to be a leading cause of musculoskeletal pain, affecting up to 85% of the population at some point during their lives.[1] The prevalence of MPS also appears to be related to age and gender. Persons aged 30–60 years appear to a have a 37% (male) and 65% (female) prevalence, whereas those older than 65 years have a prevalence rate higher than 80%.[2,3]

Even with a high prevalence rate, MPS is often refractory and clinicians often characterize available treatment options as insufficient. In a recent survey of clinicians, the authors concluded:

> Despite a variety of commonly prescribed treatments, the moderate effectiveness ratings and the frequent characterizations of the available treatments as insufficient suggest an urgent need for clinical research to establish evidence-based guidelines for the treatment of myofascial pain syndrome.[4]

DIAGNOSIS

There are currently no definite criteria for the diagnosis of MPS. Classic criteria include those developed by Simons and Travell as noted in Box 66.2.[6] More recently an international survey of pain management providers was undertaken to create a preliminary set of diagnostic criteria.[7] These are listed in Box 66.3 and are similar to the initial criteria while noting the importance of stress as well as coexisting diagnosis. Due to issues with interrater reliability of palpatory diagnosis, some researchers have suggested the incorporation of imaging techniques, such as use of sonography, to aid in the objective diagnosis of MPS.[8] However, routine imaging, including the use of techniques such as whole-body 18F-FDG positron emission tomography/computed tomography (PET/CT), has not been found to be consistently helpful in the diagnostic process.[9]

PATHOPHYSIOLOGY

The actual mechanism for initiation of a TrP is not completely understood, but it likely arises from both local and central changes.[10] Locally, leakage of factors such as acetylcholine, which cause neurogenic inflammation, interact with dysfunctional motor end plates, promoting shortening of sarcomeres and formation of precursor taut muscular bands. These bands, which are found commonly in the latent state in asymptomatic individuals, may become activated in response to predisposing factors (Table 66.1). These factors are believed to be the exclusive causes of active TrPs (thereby making MPS a secondary phenomenon). Once activated, TrPs are associated with multisystem dysfunction, especially vascular and neurological. Doppler ultrasound examination of active TrPs demonstrates constricted vascular beds and enlarged vascular volumes that create higher peak systolic velocities and negative diastolic velocities as compared with latent myofascial TrPs and normal muscle sites.[5]

Subsequent to sensitization of motor end plates, TrP activation appears to be further propagated neurologically

---

BOX 66.1 Synonyms for Myofascial Pain Syndrome

- Myofascial pain and dysfunction
- Trigger points syndrome
- Localized fibromyalgia
- Fibromyositis
- Muscular rheumatism
- Soft tissue syndrome
- Somatic dysfunction
- Tension myalgia

BOX 66.2 Classic and Confirmatory Signs of Active Trigger Points in Myofascial Pain Syndrome

- Palpable, taut muscular band containing a nodular structure
- Tenderness to palpation locally or in referred pattern replicating patient complaints
- Visual or tactile identification of local twitch response produced with needling or snapping ("guitar string") palpation
- Decreased range of movement of the involved muscle
- Increased spontaneous electrical activity on electromyography
- Low skin resistance points found over trigger points, unlike in surrounding tissue (skin resistance may normalize after treatment of trigger points)
- Imaging of local twitch response induced by needle penetration of tender nodule
- Characteristic referred pattern of pain for specific muscles involved (as described by Simmons and Travell[6])

BOX 66.3	Proposed Set of Diagnostic Criteria for Myofascial Pain Syndrome Based on International Survey

Myofascial pain syndrome can be diagnosed when the following criteria have been met[a]:
- A tender spot is found with palpation, with or without referral of pain ("trigger point")
- Recognition of symptoms by patient during palpation of tender spot

AND at least three of the following[b]:
- Muscle stiffness or spasm
- Limited range of motion of an associated joint
- Pain worsens with stress
- Palpation of taut band and/or nodule associated with tender spot

Considerations:
- It is important to rule out other conditions that may manifest as local muscle tenderness.

[a]These items were judged by more than 50% of respondents as "essential" to the diagnosis.

[b]These items from palpatory findings and signs and symptoms were judged by more than 80% of respondents as "essential" or "associated with" the diagnosis. Items with conceptual redundancy were combined.

Rivers WE, Garrigues D, Graciosa J, Harden RN. Signs and symptoms of myofascial pain: an international survey of pain management providers and proposed preliminary set of diagnostic criteria. *Pain Med.* 2015;16:1794-1805.

by activation of mechanosensitive afferents, as well as their connection at the dorsal horn of the spinal cord. Once established, this process may have cortical ramifications such as thalamic asymmetry, which may create spontaneous or stimuli-generated tissue hypersensitivity in a progressive process known as *central sensitization.* Because of cortical sensitization, patients with MPS may exhibit phenomena including allodynia and spontaneous contralateral sensitivity initiated from a unilateral TrP.[11] The hypothesized mechanism for MPS generation is illustrated in Fig. 66.1.

Once initiated, MPS has classic features, typically linked to active TrPs that allow physical and electrophysiological identification and differentiation from other pain conditions, including fibromyalgia (see Box 66.2). In addition to physical signs, differentiation is sometimes possible between MPS and fibromyalgia on the basis of comorbidities seen in patients with fibromyalgia, including greater fatigue, sleep dysfunction, mood disturbance, headaches, and irritable bowel syndrome.[12] Although differentiating between these two entities is advantageous, coexistence of MPS with fibromyalgia is quite common, thus making distinct classification often difficult, and in some cases not possible.[13] MPS is believed to be a secondary phenomenon, so in addition to proper diagnosis, initiating and propagating factors must be investigated and, if possible, corrected. Of key importance is the appreciation by the treating clinician of the possible and likely psychological and lifestyle triggers of MPS. Therefore, the contributing factors in MPS are quite broad and require a biopsychosocial assessment to determine proper treatment. Some of the more common

TABLE 66.1	Predisposing and Coexisting Conditions Requiring Identification in Myofascial Pain Syndrome
Skeletal and soft tissue abnormalities	Trauma Repetitive stress injury Muscular strain or tear Ligamentous sprains Joint instability (spondylolisthesis) Osteoarthritis Facet joint abnormality Local inflammatory conditions (e.g., tendinitis or bursitis, epicondylitis, costochondritis) Craniofacial or temporomandibular joint (TMJ) dysfunction (e.g., TMJ syndrome, headaches of various origin) Leg-length discrepancies
Functional asymmetry	Postural and ergonomic dysfunction Pelvic girdle dysfunction? Prolonged immobility
Neurologically Mediated Reflex Sympathetic Dystrophy Syndrome	Neurologically mediated reflex sympathetic dystrophy Spinal and peripheral nerve entrapment: Cervical and lumbar radiculopathy Sciatic nerve, median nerve (carpal tunnel syndrome), others
Other rheumatological disorders	Polymyalgia rheumatica Polymyositis
Metabolic deficiencies	Calcium Magnesium Potassium Iron Vitamins C, B_1, B_6, and B_{12}
Medical conditions	Anemia Hypothyroidism Hyperuricemia Hypoglycemia Celiac disease Chronic infections Visceral diseases
Psychological disorders	Chronic stress Sleep deprivation and dysfunction Depression Anxiety Somatization disorders

medical and psychological triggers of MPS are listed in Table 66.1.

INTEGRATIVE THERAPY

As previously discussed, lifestyle factors can play a significant role in the initiation and propagation of MPS. Although prescription and interventional approaches can provide immediate relief, patient education on the importance of lifestyle and self-care approaches should be emphasized early in the process of creating a treatment plan. Shared decision making and motivational interviewing, as discussed elsewhere in the book, should be utilized to create an individualized treatment plan with

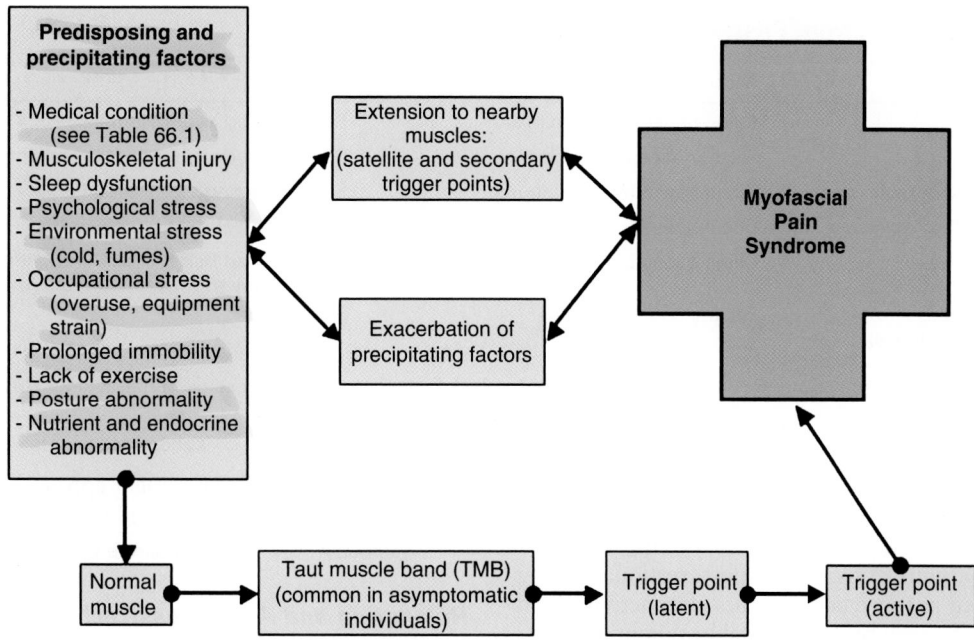

FIG. 66.1 ■ Integrated mechanism for development of myofascial pain syndrome.

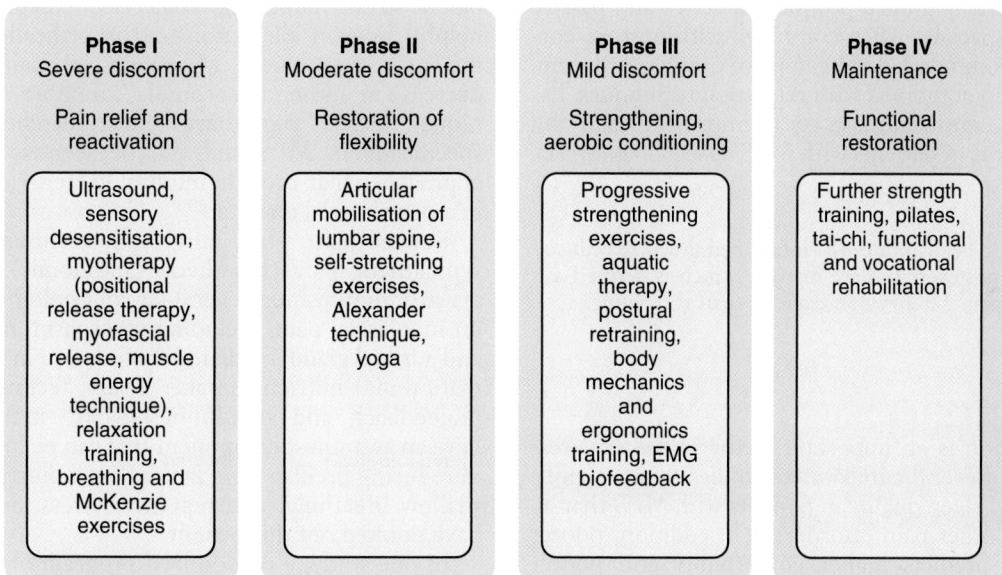

FIG. 66.2 ■ Example protocol of integration and transition of physical therapies for myofascial pain syndrome treatment. (From Sharan D, Rajkumar JS, Mohandoss M, Ranganathan R. Myofascial low back pain treatment. *Curr Pain Headache Rep.* 2014;18:1-8.)

steady transition from passive to active self-management approaches. This has also been borne out in the literature. Chan et al. compared 6 weeks of clinic-based physical therapy alone or in combination with home exercise and self-massage.[14] All parameters, including pain, neck disability, patient-specific functional scales (PSFS), and autonomic tone (heart rate variability), improved more significantly in the home treatment group, leading the researchers to note: "Treatment with physical modalities plus combination of self-massage and home exercise is more effective than the physical modalities alone." This general adage can be applied to most of therapies

discussed in the following text. An example of this type of plan with focus on nonpharmacological approaches is illustrated in Fig. 66.2.[15] In addition, examples of the transition from passive to active modalities are shown in Table 66.2.

Exercise

Low physical activity level has been linked to the development and progression of MPS. Conversely, exercise is essential in myofascial rehabilitation through its physiological effect on tissues including improvement in tissue

TABLE 66.2 **Transition from Passive to Active Modalities**

Modality	Passive	Active
Acupuncture	Clinic based acupuncture	Self-directed acupressure
Yoga/yoga nidra	Facility based yoga classes	Self-directed with video, exercising
Nonallopathic chiropractic care	Clinic based manipulations	Self-correcting exercises
Therapeutic medical massage	Clinic based treatments	Partner or self-treatment
Biofeedback	Clinic based biofeedback techniques	Self-directed biofeedback with video, heart rate variability monitors, meditative practices
Mind-body therapies (meditation, mindfulness)	Facility based classes	Self-directed

Adapted from Office of The Army Surgeon General Pain Management Task Force May 2010. Access on September 25, 2015 at http://www.dvcipm.org/files/reports/pain-task-force-final-report-may-2010.pdf

oxygenation, sensitivity, and range of motion, as well as cortical effects including modulation of neurochemicals, such as endorphins and serotonin. Exercises must be chosen carefully to diminish significant postexertional flaring (typically defined as more pain 2 hours after activity than at baseline). Flaring can be detrimental by potentially promoting both central sensitization and activity avoidance. To maximize the benefit of an activity regimen, a progressive and preferably guided program of active and passive movement, especially when combined with posture correction, is recommended. This type of exercise program, especially when combined with relaxation techniques, has demonstrated significant success in improving pain and functional status in patients with MPS[16] (see Chapter 91).

> Exercise should be introduced or intensified slowly to reduce the risk of a postexercise flare in pain, which is defined as having more pain 2 hours after exercise than at baseline.

Sleep

Sleep regulation is an important factor in the progression of MPS. Several comparative studies found significantly reduced sleep quality in patients with MPS than in patients with other pain disorders.[17] In addition, poorer sleep quality predicts higher comorbidity and poorer response to planned therapy. Even in patients without a pain condition who are placed in an experimental setting of frequently disrupted sleep for several nights, investigators report a significant drop in pain threshold and a rise in musculoskeletal discomfort and fatigue.[18] The clinician should discuss sleep difficulties with patients who have MPS and describe strategies to correct sleep as a paramount goal in the treatment plan, such as stress management, sleep hygiene, and biochemical interventions (see Chapter 9).

Mind-Body Therapy

The clinician should assess past or ongoing psychosocial stresses or traumas that may be related to MPS. Several questionnaires (e.g., Perceived Stress Scale [PSS]) can help identify stresses or psychogenic attitudes that may be higher in MPS, including premorbid pessimism, future despair, and somatic anxiety.[19] Treatment approaches can be effectively based on the symptoms and patient's preference. Several choices of mind-body therapy are described here.

Relaxation and Awareness Techniques

Relaxation techniques—breathing techniques (see Chapter 92), guided imagery (see Chapter 97), mindfulness-based stress reduction, yoga (see Chapter 100)—are helpful in pain alleviation and, specifically, the stress-mediated component of myofascial pain through a decrease in autonomic arousal. A number of these techniques, such as yoga, have been researched for benefit specifically in MPS and can be seen as combination approaches that provide mindful exercise and relaxation in a coordinated manner.[20]

Beyond pain relief, mind-body techniques influence sympathetic–parasympathetic (autonomic) balance and assist in diminishing several key physiological influences on myofascial pain, including vasospasm, muscle spasm, and adrenal gland–mediated dysfunction in tissue inflammation and nutrient uptake. Lastly, techniques such as biofeedback and mindfulness-based stress reduction, have an awareness component that can be highly effective in reducing predisposing factors, including poor posture, shallow breathing, and repetitive stress. Several studies have pointed out this benefit.

In one study, a randomized program of physical self-regulation with training in breathing, postural relaxation, and proprioceptive reeducation was taught to 44 patients with myofascial facial pain and compared with standard care. At 26-week follow-up, the two-time, 50-minute intervention demonstrated a significant reduction in pain (p < .04), as well as affective distress, somatization, obsessive-compulsive symptoms, tender point sensitivity, and sleep dysfunction.[21]

> A useful question to ask patients with myofascial pain syndrome is where in the body they carry their stress (neck, back, stomach, or head). Have patients use this sign of stress as a "red flag" that, when it appears, encourages them to step back and see what in their life may be exacerbating their pain. Once the subconscious stressor enters the consciousness, the pain often improves because the body no longer needs to sympathize.

In addition to being highly effective in decreasing the pain and sequelae of MPS, mind-body techniques can also be cost effective. In another study, a biofeedback-based program implemented in a primary care setting for functional disorders including MPS was measured against standard care (n = 70). Implementation of the program brought about significantly lower frequency and severity of symptoms, as well as lower medical costs, for the 6 months after the intervention (p < .001).[22] The clinician should reinforce the importance of mind-body techniques in overcoming MPS, a condition that the patient may understand on mainly physical terms. In addition, various techniques should be reviewed to locate those most suitable for the particular patient's needs (see Chapters 94 and 102).

Biomechanical Therapy

Posture Correction

Any active treatment regimen must discuss, train for, and reinforce active postural correction.[23] Dysfunctional posture both at rest and during work activities increases tissue strain and asymmetry. If not corrected, poor posture is theorized as a leading factor in the development and maintenance of MPS. Evaluation by a well-trained clinician (including but not limited to physician, physical or occupational therapist, or body mechanics specialist, such as a Feldenkrais or yoga practitioner) can provide invaluable information on the presence and severity of such dysfunction. Baseline and follow-up evaluations by a biofeedback therapist can also be helpful in demonstrating physiological progress to the patient. Ongoing correction and monitoring can help patients with MPS realize the preventive capabilities of this often overlooked intervention. Tools that help reinforce postural correction, such as kinesiotaping and behavioral techniques, can successfully reduce the severity of MPS.[24,25]

Massage Therapy, Manual Therapy, and Myofascial Release Techniques

Massage therapy and manual therapy (MT) have been shown to change several important components of MPS. In general, MT has demonstrated upregulation of modulatory neurochemicals, including oxytocin, serotonin, and dopamine. Locally, MT has been shown to improve circulation near TrPs, allowing for improved oxygenation and substrate/metabolite exchange.[26]

The efficacy of practitioner-provided MT in MPS has been demonstrated in several trials. The strongest evidence appears to be with compression type MT directly at TrPs, which has shown improved outcomes versus superficial massage or compression at non-TrPs.[27] In addition to local effects as noted, compression at MTrPs induces an increase in parasympathetic activity.[28]

Several schools of myofascial release techniques have developed to address the key features of MPS with training resources and courses noted as in the resources section. Many of these techniques are based on Simmons and Travell's foundational work, *Myofascial Pain and Dysfunction: The Trigger Point Manual.*[6] Myofascial release, as well as spray and stretch techniques, should be considered as a first-line approach to MPS[29] (see Chapter 109). As noted in the introduction, providing instructions on identification and home MT of TrPs has been shown to have an added benefit in improving TrP sensitivity and pain intensity. Providing passive and active MT works well with other active treatments (thermotherapy and topical therapy) in improving awareness and self-management of MPS.[30]

Low-Level Laser Therapy

Low-level laser therapy (LLLT) has been used for several decades in Europe for pain management, and soft tissue conditions are among the conditions most effectively treated with this technique. The mechanism of action of LLLT is not completely elucidated, but it may be related to improvements in microcirculation, inflammatory response, and adenosine triphosphate production.[31,32] In addition, direct laser treatment of TrPs is believed to increase serotonin production, and trials demonstrated increased excretion of serotonin byproducts after treatment.[33] One 4-week trial (n = 60) comparing LLLT with dry needling and placebo laser demonstrated a significant improvement in pain at rest and with activity, as well as a rise in pain threshold in the laser-treated group.[34] LLLT has the advantage of being noninvasive and thus well tolerated, especially in patients with high tissue sensitivity. The treatment regimen and device specifications vary widely; clinicians should review the available research on the efficacy of the lasers they are considering incorporating into their practices.

Peripheral Biostimulation

Similar to LLLT, more conventional avenues of biostimulation (e.g., electrical stimulation and ultrasound) have been applied to MPS because of their ability to increase tissue microcirculation and help correct the myofascial contraction-relaxation cycle. The mechanism of such techniques includes improvement in circulation, local analgesic effects, and correction of electrical disturbances found in TrP. Namely, TrPs typically demonstrate lower resistance and microvoltage abnormalities compared with surrounding tissue. In addition, electrostimulation has been shown to be partially inhibited by the use of naloxone, and thus its benefit is likely related in part to endorphin upregulation at the spinal cord and higher centers. Use of these techniques, including transcutaneous electrical nerve stimulation (TENS) and interferential and neuromuscular stimulation (NMS), has provided patient-dependent improvements in pain threshold and range of motion in several studies.[29,35]

Definitive conclusions regarding parameters cannot be drawn from the literature due to variability in protocols and outcomes.[36] However, trends in the literature suggest that continuous ultrasound (3 MHz, $1W/cm^2$) may be more effective that pulsed treatment.[37]

Also, for TENS as little as 10 minutes of treatment directly over TrPs, typically using a burst mode (pulse width, 200 μs; frequency, 100 Hz; and burst frequency, 2 Hz) at an intensity that is felt but which does not induce visible muscle contraction, has been shown to improve pain parameters in placebo-controlled trials.[38-40]

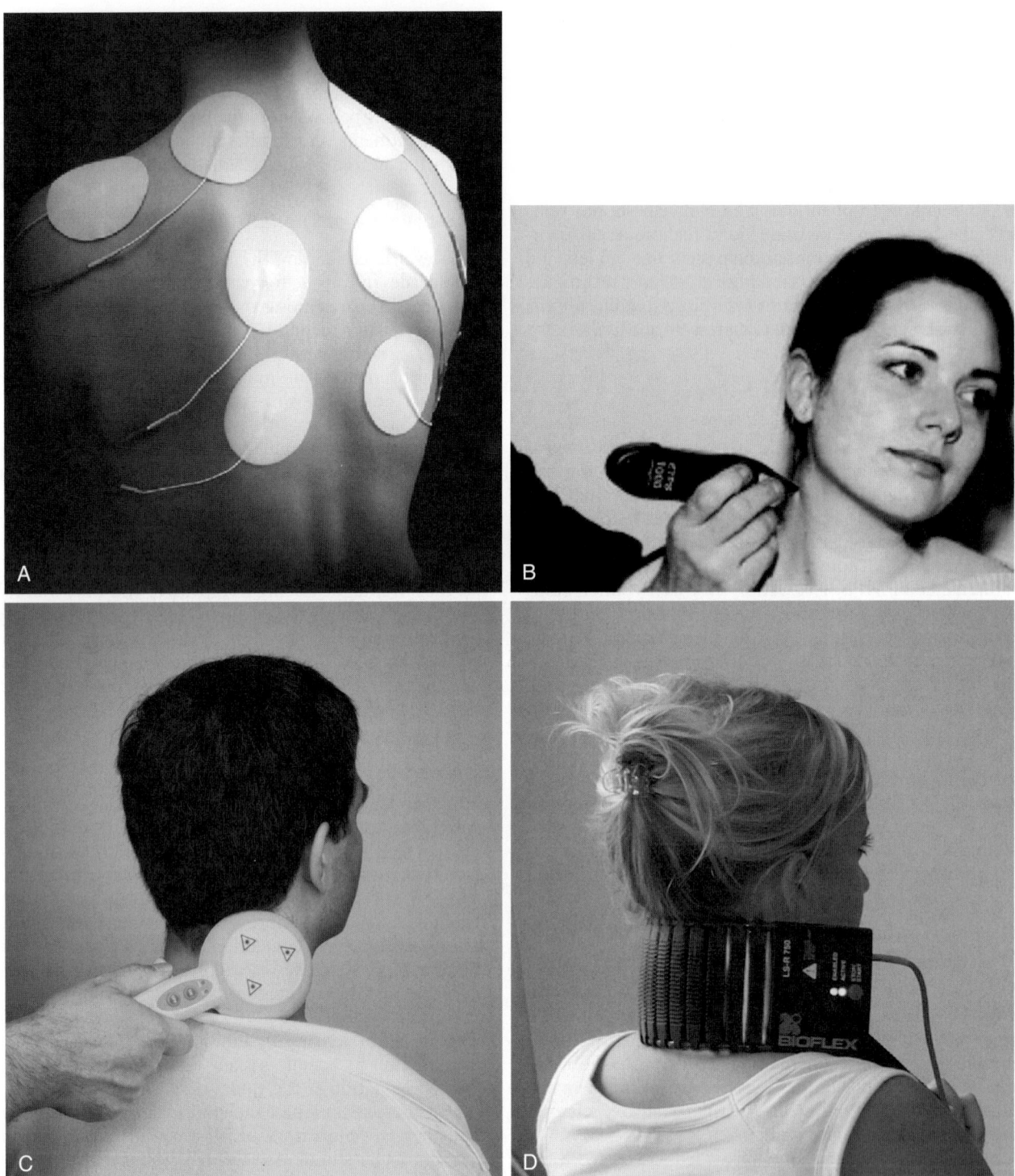

FIG. 66.3 ■ Application of various types of biostimulation in myofascial pain syndrome. A, Interferential and neuromuscular stimulation. B, Individual trigger point electrostimulation. C and D, Low-level laser therapy. (A, RS 4i unit courtesy RS Medical, Vancouver, Wash. B, Electrotherapeutic point stimulation unit courtesy Acumed Medical Supplies, Toronto. C, Courtesy Theralase, Markham, Ontario, Canada. D, Courtesy Meditech International, Toronto.)

Several biostimulation modalities should be considered in the clinic setting to assess response. Many are cost effective and or covered by insurance, such as TENS. If one technique is successful, the patient should be transitioned to home use. These include TENS as well as electrotherapeutic point stimulation (ETPS) devices. Fig. 66.3 demonstrates the application of various types of biostimulation

techniques that can help patients identify and locally address TrPs.

Central Biostimulation

Several recent pilot trials have utilized brain stimulation protocols in the setting of MPS. The rationale for this includes the potential ability to reduce central sensitization as well as modulation of neurochemicals related to MPS including brain-derived neurotrophic factor (BDNF). Two randomized, placebo-controlled trials found that five 20-minute treatments daily at 1 to 2 mA with anodal transcranial direct-current stimulation (tDCS) over the motor cortex (M1) or the dorsolateral prefrontal cortex (DLPFC) improved pain intensity versus usual care or TPI.[41,42] A third placebo-controlled trial using 10 treatments with repetitive transcranial magnetic stimulation (rTMS) at 10 Hz also demonstrated reduced pain scores of 30% as well as higher levels of BDNF.[43] At this point, central stimulation is still evolving, with further research required to elucidate optimal parameters and areas of stimulation.

Hydrotherapy and Thermotherapy

As discussed earlier, the tissue of patients with MPS tends to have abnormal microcirculation, which can have negative ramifications, including buildup of inflammatory markers and a drop in tissue temperature and effective range of motion. The application of short-term intense heat (heating pad, diathermy, or warm hydrotherapy) and long-term use of low-intensity heat pads can help alter the thermal dysregulation and muscle spasm seen in MPS. Similarly, water immersion, by removing weight from the joints, facilitates reduction in muscle spasm and joint stiffness and thereby facilitates functional mobility. Because of the benign nature of these interventions, patients with MPS should undergo thermotherapy and hydrotherapy when available and, if possible, in combination with other therapies.[29]

Biochemical Therapy

Topical and Transdermal Applications

Topical and transdermal medications can be a useful adjunct because of their ability to disrupt hypersensitive signaling from the myofascial focus to the spinal cord and higher centers. Lidocaine in various topical formulations (cream, transdermal patch) is believed to block sodium channels that may increase pain signaling. Lidocaine 5% patches were tested in a 1-month, open-label trial in 27 patients with myofascial pain.[44] By the end of the trial, several key parameters, including average pain intensity, mood, sleep, walking ability, and enjoyment of life, were significantly improved. These results have been replicated in a larger randomized, placebo-controlled trial as well as in a trial noting that lidocaine patches demonstrated benefit similar to bupivacaine injections, with improved tolerability.[45,46]

Antiinflammatory preparations (e.g., diclofenac patch) have also been shown to be helpful in MPS and related conditions, such as delayed-onset muscle soreness.[47] In a placebo-controlled study of 300 subjects with MPS of the upper trapezius, diclofenac patch demonstrated improved pain, cervical active range of motion, and neck disability at the end of 1 week.[48] Moreover, topical applications of diclofenac have demonstrated efficacy similar to that of oral administration with fewer adverse effects.[49]

Botanical and nonprescription applications, including capsaicin and menthol, appear to have local pain-modulatory activity.[50,51] Specifically, capsaicin can deplete sensory C-fibers of substance P, the principal neurotransmitter of nociceptive impulses, and thus potentially decrease central sensitization. Another popular topical agent is magnesium, which in some studies has been found to reduce local myofascial pain.[52] Application of topical agents also provides active patient feedback on the location and sensitivity of myofascial pain. For patients without contraindications, such as allergies to the agents, a trial of standardized or compounded prescription topicals should be considered. For compounded formulations, local clinicians should contact local pharmacies (see resources) to help coordinate appropriate formulas.

DOSAGE
Lidocaine

Patients can apply up to three lidocaine 5% (Lidoderm) patches for up to 12 hours, or over-the-counter 4% patches for up to 12 hours. Patches can be cut to size, and they come in a carton of 30 patches.

Capsaicin

Patients can apply capsaicin in 0.025%, 0.035%, 0.05%, 0.075%, 0.1%, and 0.25% patch, cream, gel, and lotion formulation) to the painful area two to four times daily for 3–4 consecutive weeks to reduce pain sensitivity. As most patients will experience burning with use, it is recommended that over-the-counter or prescription lidocaine be placed on the area prior to capsaicin application. Patients should thoroughly wash hands after application and avoid contact with their eyes.

NSAIDs

All topical NSAIDs are currently approved for osteoarthritis. The diclofenac (Flector) patch is indicated for osteoarthritis and contains 180 mg of diclofenac; one patch is applied to the painful areas twice daily. Other FDA-approved antiinflammatory topical formulations include diclofenac sodium 1% gel (Voltaren) and diclofenac sodium topical liquid solution 1.5% w/w dimethyl sulfoxide (Pennsaid).

Compounded Products

Compounding pharmacies can prepare creams and gels with various NSAIDs combined with other agents (e.g., lidocaine, cyclobenzaprine, and capsaicin). A dime-sized amount of gel (approximately 1 g) is rubbed into the painful area two to four times per day based on the patient. A typical starting formulation could be ketoprofen 10%, lidocaine 5%, and cyclobenzaprine 2%. Patients should attempt a formula for several weeks before reassessing and considering switching or adding other agents.

Trigger Point Needling or Injection

Various needling and injection techniques have been endorsed for treatment of myofascial pain. The mechanistic rationale for the use of these techniques is based on several lines of evidence. The simplest technique, dry needling of primary TrPs, has demonstrated reversal of spontaneous electrical activity, one of the hallmark abnormalities noted in MPS.[53] Dry needle-evoked inactivation of a primary TrP in the shoulder region also improves pain sensitivity of satellite TrPs as well as range of motion in the zone of pain referral.[54] Additionally, certain types of dry needling may activate muscle afferents more effectively than superficial needling to produce segmental analgesia.[55-59]

Injection techniques that involve introduction of sterile water, saline solution, or various pharmaceutical agents (often termed "wet" needling) are conjectured to provide adjunctive benefit to needling, based on both the properties of the injected agent and the tissue pressure effects created by the volume of agent introduced. The superiority of various techniques, including dry needling and the injection of saline, anesthetics, corticosteroids, and botulinum toxin type A have not been clarified in the research because of variation in trial size and methodology.[60,61] Several trials found no distinct advantage for TrP injection over dry needling.[62,63] Furthermore, studies have both demonstrated and refuted the advantage of injection of active drug (e.g., lidocaine, botulinum toxin) over saline injection.[64,65] The most recent systematic review of 20 randomized controlled trials involving 839 patients noted that both dry and wet needling can be recommended for short-term relief of TrP pain in the neck and shoulders, with wet needling appearing to be more effective in the medium-term.[66]

Without a clear advantage of needling interventions, dry needling and acupuncture (see the following text) are initially recommended to evaluate their efficacy and patient tolerance. Injection of saline and other active agents should be reserved for more advanced or refractory cases and administered by clinicians with the proper understanding of the role of these agents in comprehensive management. Although injection therapy is potentially effective in short-term TrP management, it is often pursued without regard to the global needs of patients with MPS. To minimize a repetitive cycle of passive interventions, clinicians are admonished to address triggers and active treatment options for MPS (e.g., posture correction, home stretching, mind-body therapies) that are pursued in conjunction with injection therapy. All needle interventions with potential benefit are based on the experience of the practitioner in isolating TrPs. Adverse effects may be related to incorrect needle placement, reaction to the injected agent, or improper use of aseptic technique.

Pharmaceuticals

Currently, there are no FDA-approved medications indicated specifically for the treatment of MPS. Overall, when looking at their efficacy in the setting of temporomandibular disorder–associated MPS, one review noted that "…evidence in support of the effectiveness of these drugs is lacking."[67] However, certain over-the-counter (OTC) and prescription agents, including NSAIDs, corticosteroids, muscle relaxants, antidepressants, anticonvulsants, anxiolytics, and opiates, are utilized off-label in the treatment of MPS to provide symptomatic relief. In addition, several of these agents may provide improvement in common comorbidities including depression, headache, and insomnia. As some patients with MPS fail initial medication attempts, lack of response or tolerability to one agent, it is important to keep in mind that this may not imply the same for other agents. For example, in an elegant, stepped

pharmacotherapy trial of patients with MPS, 43% showed ≥ 50% reduction in pain intensity (mean doses of amitriptyline = 16 mg and nortriptyline = 25 mg). Nonresponse was predicted by higher age, comorbid medical illness, and more widespread pain spread. Subsequently, 36.8% of nonresponders demonstrated ≥ 50% reduction in pain intensity with gabapentin therapy at a mean daily dose of 975 mg. Overall, 54.8% of all treated patients reported a significant pain reduction.[68]

Muscle Relaxants

Evidence for the effectiveness of muscle relaxants (e.g., tizanidine hydrochloride, cyclobenzaprine) and medication with muscle relaxation properties, including benzodiazepines and tricyclic antidepressants, is variable in MPS.[69] A Cochrane Review examining the use of cyclobenzaprine in MPS found that based on the minimal available published research in this area and the difficulty in estimating risk versus benefit, evidence was insufficient to support the use of this drug in the treatment of MPS.[70] Although not routinely endorsed, muscle relaxants may be worth a short-term trial to assess improvement while initiating a multimodality program. In a randomized trial of temporomandibular disorder, cyclobenzaprine (10 mg/night) was compared with clonazepam (0.5 mg/night). Cyclobenzaprine was better than placebo and clonazepam when incorporated into a self-care and education program for the management of jaw pain. Unfortunately, no significant improvement in sleep was noted.[71]

DOSAGE

Cyclobenzaprine, 10 mg at bedtime taken for a limited course, may provide some pain relief for temporomandibular disorder.

PRECAUTIONS

This drug is structurally related to tricyclic antidepressants. As with all tricyclics, caution should be used when utilizing this agent, especially in individuals with a cardiovascular history.

Nonsteroidal Antiinflammatory Drugs

The use of NSAIDs may be justified in the short-term treatment of acute myofascial strain. In one study, ibuprofen appeared to work as well without the addition of a muscle relaxant (800 mg of ibuprofen three times per day, with or without the use of cyclobenzaprine 10 mg three times per day).[72] However, with the lack of long-term evidence and the potential increased toxicity of oral NSAIDS based on length of use, utilization on a regular basis should be avoided.

DOSAGE

Ibuprofen, 800 mg three times daily with meals for short periods of time, can help reduce the pain of myofascial strain.

Antidepressants

Antidepressants are often considered in the setting MPS because of their potential benefits in common mood and sleep comorbidities. The benefit of these agents for primary MPS in nondepressed individuals may not be significant, however, with the possible exception of amitriptyline and duloxetine. Amitriptyline was tested (at 75 mg/day) in a small (n = 31), 32-week placebo-controlled, double-blind, three-way crossover study trial versus the highly selective serotonin reuptake inhibitor citalopram (at 20 mg/day). Study participants taking amitriptyline had significantly reduced myofascial tenderness and headache intensity than participants taking placebo (p = .01 and p = .04, respectively). The researchers concluded that amitriptyline may elicit its analgesic effect in myofascial pain by reducing transmission of painful stimuli from myofascial tissue, as opposed to reducing overall pain sensitivity: "We suggest that this effect is caused by a segmental reduction of central sensitization in combination with a peripheral antinociceptive action."[73] Similarly, duloxetine, which is a serotonin-norepinephrine reuptake inhibitor (SNRI), has been noted to have benefit in the setting of a number of chronic musculoskeletal pain disorders and may be worth considering in the setting of MPS.[74]

DOSAGE

Amitriptyline, 75 mg at bedtime, can reduce myofascial pain and headaches.

Duloxetine, 60 to 120 mg/day can reduce chronic musculoskeletal pain and comorbid depression.

Other Agents

As previously noted, anticonvulsants such as gabapentin can often be helpful when other first-line prescription agents have not been helpful. Other agents, such as opioids, ketamine, and memantine, do not demonstrate clear benefit for MPS and in some cases may be detrimental to reducing disability.[75]

DOSAGE

Gabapentin at 300–1800 mg/day, titrated gradually for refractory myofascial pain. Dose in the evening to reduce daytime drowsiness.

Diet and Dietary Supplements

Diet can have a significant effect on pain in general as well as myofascial pain syndrome.[76] There are numerous ways this can happen including proinflammatory or highly processed diets inducing changes at the microbiome and cellular level to increase inflammation and muscle spasm. A poor diet can add to the prooxidant status present in some cases of MPS. For example, research has noted that total antioxidant capacity (TAC), total oxidative stress (TOS), and oxidative stress index (OSI) values are impaired in those with MPS versus matched controls, implying that MPS may be partially related to increased oxidative stress.[77]

In addition, specific nutrient deficiencies, which may be linked to background diet, have been implicated in the progression of MPS. Specifically, deficiencies of minerals (e.g., magnesium, calcium, and zinc) and vitamins or enzymes (e.g., vitamin D, vitamin B_{12}, and coenzyme Q10) have been reported in some studies of those with MPS.[78] These deficiencies, such as with vitamin D, have been noted to increase pain sensitivity in general and may contribute to the overall burden of MPS.[79]

The level and type of deficiency, however, have not been consistently elucidated. In one trial, significant deficiencies in zinc levels in patients with MPS versus controls were noted without similar deficiencies in other nutrients such as magnesium or folic acid. These results may have reflected the type of testing done, including traditional extracellular versus intracellular testing. Although typical electrolyte analyses ("panels") may rule out gross abnormalities, levels of these electrolytes are usually normal in MPS. Clinicians should be aware of specialized testing, such as ionized or intracellular testing methods (e.g., NutraEval by Genova Diagnostic, SpectraCell by SpectraCell Laboratories) that may identify more occult deficiencies. The response to replacement of nutrients (e.g., magnesium in the setting of migraine) appears to be more highly correlated with intracellular or ionized fraction level, but not with total serum levels.[80-82] On the basis of identified or suspected nutrient abnormalities, clinicians should use focused dietary and nutrient supplementation with careful patient monitoring of symptoms.

Consider checking serum levels of vitamin B_{12}, 25-hydroxyvitamin D, coenzyme Q10, and electrolytes, as well as red blood cell magnesium levels in patients with myofascial pain syndrome.

Recommendations on the use of dietary supplements in MPS suffer from inconsistencies, as noted previously.[83] Especially in patients with refractory cases of MPS unresponsive to lifestyle change, clinicians should proceed with supplements that may possess properties beneficial for pain and comorbid symptoms. A stepwise approach in which dietary supplements are incorporated and evaluated on a 2- to 3-month trial basis (i.e., a therapeutic trial) is suggested. These supplements may include those helpful for muscle function (e.g., magnesium, malic acid, calcium, vitamin D, and coenzyme Q10), antiinflammatory action (e.g., essential fatty acids, white willow bark, and *Boswellia*), or comorbidities such as sleep or mood dysfunction (e.g., St. John's wort, *S*-adenyl-L-methionine [SAMe], valerian, and melatonin). As with prescription medications, the use of dietary supplements should be monitored on a regular basis to ensure benefit and to minimize adverse reactions.

Bioenergetics

Traditional Chinese Medicine

The use of traditional Chinese medicine, specifically acupuncture, was one of the earliest attempted treatments of MPS. More recently, investigators have speculated about the correlation between acupuncture and myofascial TrPs. In 1977, Melzack et al.[84] postulated an approximately 70% correlation between these two entities, although this correlation has been disputed.[85] Because of the likely coexistence of these entities, a separate discussion of dry needling and localized acupuncture appears somewhat arbitrary. However, acupuncture offers treatment avenues based on meridian and energetic dysfunction, which may entail treatment at distal or reflex points (auricular therapy) and thereby provide additional therapeutic options.[86] The global assessment of the patient that is undertaken in Chinese medicine is especially helpful in MPS because of likely comorbidities that must be considered in the formulation of a treatment plan.

The specific type of acupuncture that should be pursued in MPS has not been elucidated. Several reports argue that deep needling may be more effective in decreasing MPS than superficial needling, although the two terms have not been well defined.[57,58] Conversely, Japanese acupuncture treatment, which typically uses superficial needling, was also shown to be effective in MPS in controlled trials.[87] The depth, frequency, and duration of treatments should be tailored to the patient; treatments typically should take place one or more times per week initially, followed by a gradual decrease with functional improvement.

PREVENTION PRESCRIPTION

- Encourage posture awareness with frequent repositioning and adaptive stretching to reduce strain.
- Consider an ergonomic evaluation if patients remain in one position for prolonged periods at work.
- Incorporate stress management techniques to identify and reduce stress buildup. Ask patients to pay attention to where they carry stress in the body and use this to learn from the body's symptoms.

- Incorporate a regular exercise and movement program. At a minimum, patients should exercise three times/week for 30 minutes each session while stimulating movement, range of motion, and tone in all muscle groups.
- Encourage adequate quantity and quality of sleep.
- Encourage the consumption of a healthy diet rich in fruits and vegetables with adequate fluid content to ensure perfusion to muscles.
- Encourage maintenance of an ideal weight.

THERAPEUTIC REVIEW

Myofascial pain syndrome (MPS) is a disorder that affects up to 85% of the general population at some point and is primarily characterized by local and referred pain, as well as comorbidities affecting mood, sleep, energy, and functional status. Although numerous treatment options are available, no widely accepted treatment guidelines exist. Clinically, MPS is a condition that is often difficult to treat, and physicians often characterize available treatments as insufficient.[4] Based on its complex nature, MPS is a condition that requires a biopsychosocial evaluation and incorporation of individualized, preferably active, treatment options geared at underlying propagating factors with a focus on long-term neurobehavioral and functional rehabilitation.

EXCLUSION AND TREATMENT OF CONDITIONS THAT MIMIC OR CONTRIBUTE TO MYOFASCIAL PAIN SYNDROME

- See Table 66.1.
- Symptom-focused laboratory testing should be considered, including 25-OH vitamin D_3, coenzyme Q10, carnitine, vitamin B_{12}, folate, methylmalonic acid, and, as appropriate, baseline thyroid-stimulating hormone, creatine phosphokinase, alkaline phosphatase, and complete blood count and electrolytes with intracellular magnesium to rule out modifiable causes of MPS and associated symptoms.

REMOVAL OF EXACERBATING FACTORS

- Take measures to correct sleep dysfunction, including sleep hygiene and other interventions.
- Increase awareness of stress and environmental triggers (poor posture, repetitive stress) by using periodic daily cues.

LIFESTYLE MEASURES

- Incorporate stress management techniques
- Biofeedback, preferred for baseline myofascial and autonomic measures and retraining efforts
- Guided imagery, meditation
- Exercise to decrease deconditioning and improve myofascial biomechanics. Mindful exercise (e.g., yoga, tai chi) is especially helpful in improving MPS.

BIOMECHANICAL INTERVENTIONS

- Posture evaluation and correction: Consider ongoing optimization with yoga, Feldenkrais, and physical therapy.
- Manual and manipulative techniques, including massage, myofascial release, and spray and stretch: These should be considered in areas of distinct trigger points. Osteopathic manipulation is desired when functional skeletal asymmetry is provoking MPS. Refer to Simmons and Travell[6] for detailed instructions. Several techniques can be taught to and successfully incorporated by the patient (e.g., compression massage with stretch).
- Biostimulation: Low-level laser therapy, electrostimulation, hydrotherapy, and thermotherapy are  recommended on a regular basis to assess reduction in symptoms, especially pain, with transition to home therapy.

BIOENERGETIC INTERVENTIONS

- Acupuncture is used to release trigger points and decrease autonomic arousal.
- Other energetic treatments (e.g., healing touch, Reiki) should be used to assess for and treat energy imbalance.

NUTRITION

- Have patients increase their intake of fruits and vegetables, with a focus on appropriate levels of vitamins and minerals essential for musculoskeletal function.
- Consider a trial of an antiinflammatory diet or elimination diet (see Chapters 86 and 88).

SUPPLEMENTS

- Consider an 8- to 12-week trial of supplements for correction of myofascial pain and comorbid conditions (including identified deficiencies):Magnesium: starting with a chelated form if available for increased gastrointestinal tolerance; magnesium glycinate, 100–200 mg twice daily, advance as tolerated (other formulation doses vary; typically, starting at a low dose and advanced based on gastrointestinal tolerance)
- Malic acid: 600 mg, one to two capsules daily
- Carnitine: 2000 mg/day
- D-Ribose: 5 g twice daily
- Coenzyme Q10: 100–300 mg/day (dose increased based on response and serum levels)
- B vitamins typically used: 50–100 mg of thiamine (vitamin B_1) and pyridoxine (vitamin B_6), 0.5–2 mg of folic acid and vitamin B_{12}
- Vitamin D_3: baseline 800–1000 units/day and based on individual level to maintain adequacy

PHARMACEUTICALS

- Topical pharmaceuticals/compounded creams with ingredients based on patient presentation are applied to affected areas three times/day. Patients should be warned that some topical agents cause localized burning or rare allergic reactions. Systemic absorption negligible if these agents are used as directed.
  - Ketoprofen 10%–20%
  - Lidocaine 5%
  - Capsaicin 0.025%–0.075%
  - Cyclobenzaprine 5%
- Oral pharmaceutical
  - If the response to other interventions is unsatisfactory, consider a trial of amitriptyline (up to 75 mg/day) for long-term treatment, as well as a trial of short-term antiinflammatory agents for acute exacerbations.
- Needle-based injection therapy
  - If the patient's symptoms persist or worsen despite the preceding measures, consider needle-based intervention in a stepwise approach.
  - Acupuncture or dry needling
  - Saline injection
  - Anesthetic injection (e.g., a combination of 2% lidocaine and 0.05% bupivacaine in a 1:3 ratio up to a total of 8 mL)
  - Botox injection

All treatments should be well integrated, with the goal of improving patient awareness of biomechanical and stress triggers. Treatments should gradually move from passive (practitioner directed and supervised) to active (patient initiated), with improving awareness of the patient's ability to address and diminish the myofascial pain cycle.

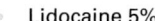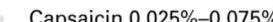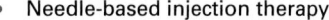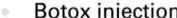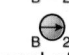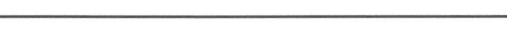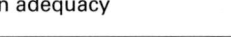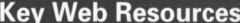

Key Web Resources

Mayo Clinic: Myofascial Pain Syndrome: Handout on myofascial pain syndrome for patients — http://www.mayoclinic.com/health/myofascial-painsyndrome/DS01042/METHOD=print

Academy of Integrative Pain Management: Integrative pain management organization with listing of providers, and CME resources in the area of myofascial pain — http://www.AAPainManage.org

University of New Mexico Myofascial Pain Syndrome, Trigger Point Diagnosis and Treatment: CME course with lecture and hands-on learning in conjunction with the American Academy of Pain Management — http://som.unm.edu/cme search: "myofascial"

Professional Compounding Centers of America: Website provide locator for local accredited compounding pharmacies — http://www.pccarx.com/

Mayo Clinic: Stress Management — http://www.mayoclinic.com/health/relaxation-technique/SR00007

University of Wisconsin Health Services: Stress and Sleep Stress management and relaxation tools. Resources for stress and sleep management — http://www.uhs.wisc.edu/services/wellness/stress.shtml

UCLA Ergonomics: Exercise, posture and stretching guides that can be done at home — http://ergonomics.ucla.edu/exercises.html

Arthritis Foundation — http://www.arthritis.org
YMCA — http://www.ymca.net/
Organizations offering exercise and stretching classes, including aquatic therapy

REFERENCES

References are available online at ExpertConsult.com.

CHAPTER 67

CHRONIC LOW BACK PAIN

Russell Lemmon, DO • Eric J. Roseen, DC

INTRODUCTION

Low back pain (LBP) is a tremendously common condition challenging patients, clinicians, and health care systems worldwide. The lifetime prevalence of LBP is reportedly as high as 84%; therefore, most adults will experience at least one episode.[1,2] Back pain is the fifth most common reason to visit one's primary care physician and is the single most common reason adults in United States use complementary and integrative medicine (CIM).[3,4]

Over the last several decades, the management of back pain has been associated with increased expense and disability.[5] In 2008, annual direct costs of LBP were estimated at $86 billion, similar to the costs associated with arthritis, diabetes, or cancer.[6] Total direct and indirect costs (e.g., absenteeism, lower productivity) for LBP are thought to be even higher, an estimated $625 billion in the United States alone.[7] In 2012, the World Health Organization (WHO) published the Global Burden of Disease Report, which ranked LBP as the 6th most burdensome condition in 2010, a notable increase from 1990 when it was ranked 11th.[8] Additionally, the WHO's report also determined back pain to be the top cause of morbidity in the United States and worldwide.[9] The societal problems associated with increased opioid use are also closely linked to chronic low back pain (CLBP), as it is the leading cause of opioid prescriptions for noncancer pain.[10,11]

Despite its high prevalence and substantial global impact, back pain remains poorly understood. Effective management of acute back pain in the primary care setting is perhaps the most important factor to prevent progression to chronic back pain. Multiple evidence-based guidelines for the management of acute and chronic back pain are readily available to guide providers; however, adherence to such recommendations remains low.[12-19] LBP patients increasingly utilize high-cost, invasive interventions despite their risks and questionable benefits.[20,21] A conservative approach, using a personalized combination of evidence-based conventional and complementary therapies, is consistent with current guidelines and is cost effective and safer. Using these therapies in the context of the patient's psychosocial picture, preferences, and values are also vital and often overlooked components of effective treatment plans. This integrative approach is ideally suited to address the costly and complex condition of CLBP.

PATHOPHYSIOLOGY

Acute low back pain (ALBP) is defined as pain in the lumbosacral region, with or without leg pain, which has been present less than 6 weeks.[22] The condition is considered subacute when it has been present between 6 and 12 weeks. By extension CLBP is often defined as pain persisting for more than 12 weeks.

A recent National Institutes of Health (NIH) task force defined CLBP as pain persisting greater than 3 months and bothering at least half the days in the past 6 months.[23]

A precise diagnosis for acute, subacute, or CLBP is often not possible, causing significant frustration for patients and providers alike. The vast majority of patients with ALBP can expect a favorable prognosis and a significant improvement within 6 weeks, regardless of the treatment given. However, recurrence rates are high (20%–35%), and approximately 5%–20% of patients will go on to develop CLBP.[24-26] Intriguingly, a growing literature base is suggesting that the majority of back-related pain persists at a mild or fluctuating intensity after an acute episode.[27-29] This evidence may help inform patient expectations and support longitudinal conservative management of patients experiencing recurrent or persistent LBP symptoms.

LBP origins and perpetuating factors vary tremendously among patients. Given that identifiable pathological causes are relatively uncommon, a broad biopsychosocial approach to back pain is more appropriate for understanding useful approaches to the treatment of "nonspecific" LBP than a traditional biomedical paradigm (Fig. 67.1).[22,23,30] If specific pathology is unlikely, origins of pain may be linked to a neuromusculoskeletal dysfunction (e.g., tissue irritation, weakness, or imbalance) from one or many sources. However, pain may persist long after an injured tissue has healed. A chronic, recurring back pain experience is perhaps common, although associated pain and disability are rarely progressive. Contributing psychosocial factors (e.g., anxiety, depression, or work dissatisfaction) may perpetuate the pain experience and should be identified early.

Specific Pathology

Definitive causes of LBP include disk herniation with suspected radiculopathy or spinal stenosis (5%), osteoporotic compression fracture (4%), and inflammatory arthropathies (3%) (Table 67.1). Other specific organic causes of LBP are cancer and infection (1%), cauda equina syndrome (<1%), and visceral pathologies (<2%) such as aortic aneurysm, pelvic, gastrointestinal, and renal pathology.[12,22,31] These definitive causes are uncommon, and the vast majority of patients presenting with back

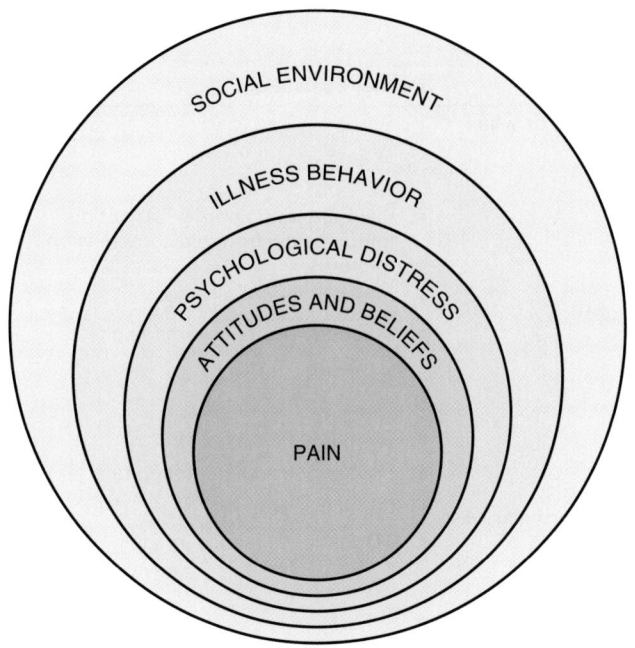

FIG. 67.1 ■ Biopsychosocial model of pain. (From Main CJ, Williams AC. ABC of psychological medicine: musculoskeletal pain, *BMJ* 325:534-537, 2002.)

pain will have nonspecific LBP of a less clearly understood origin.

Neuromusculoskeletal Dysfunction

An estimated 80%–90% of all back pain is nonspecific and may emanate from ligaments, facet joints, muscle, fascia, nerve roots, the vertebral periosteum, or the outer portion of the disk.[31] Despite sophisticated systems for evaluating these other causes of back pain, successful identification of a pain generator is often not consistent among or between providers who commonly evaluate back pain. Joint irritation, maladaptive movement patterns, muscle stiffness, spasm, and weakness commonly contribute to back pain and are often identified on examination. Peripheral and central neurophysiological mechanisms also play important roles in acute and chronic pain. Unfortunately, providers can rarely agree on the cause of one's back pain, and systems of identifying neuromusculoskeletal dysfunction (NMS) often have uncertain clinical relevance.

Psychosocial Factors

Psychological and social factors play a very important role in the prognosis of musculoskeletal conditions.[32,33]

TABLE 67.1 Specific Conditions Causing Low Back Pain

Syndrome	Red Flags	Further Evaluation
Cauda equina syndrome	• Widespread neurological symptoms	• Medical emergency: immediate magnetic resonance imaging and neurosurgical referral
	• Fecal incontinence or urinary retention	
	• Weakness in limbs and/or gait abnormality	
	• Saddle numbness	
Lumbar radiculopathy	• Severe lower extremity pain	• If no improvement with conservative treatment after 6 weeks, magnetic resonance imaging considered
	• Significant neurological deficits indicative of nerve root compression	
	• Sensory impairment, weakness, or diminished deep tendon reflexes consistent with nerve root distribution	
	• Significant neurological deficits indicative of nerve root compression	
Spinal canal stenosis	• Pain, sensory loss, or weakness in one or both legs	• Magnetic resonance imaging
	• Pain worse with walking or standing	
	• Pain relieved with sitting or lumbar flexion	
Spondyloarthropathy	• Presence of four or more of the following:	• HLA-B27
	• Age younger than 40 years	• Erythrocyte sedimentation rate
	• Insidious onset	• C-reactive protein
	• Improvement with exercise	
	• No improvement with rest	
	• Pain at night (with improvement on arising or walking)	
Cancer	• History of cancer	• Erythrocyte sedimentation rate
	• Age older than 50 years	• Plain film radiographs
	• Failure to improve with treatment	• Magnetic resonance imaging

Continued

TABLE 67.1   Specific Conditions Causing Low Back Pain—cont'd

Syndrome	Red Flags	Further Evaluation
	• Worsening pain especially at night, at rest, or when lying down	
	• Urinary retention	
Fracture	• Age older than 50 years	• Plain film radiographs (cannot distinguish new from old compression fractures)
	• Osteoporosis	• Computed tomography
	• Significant trauma	• Magnetic resonance imaging
	• Steroid use	
	• Structural deformity	
Infection	• Fever	• Complete blood count
	• Immunosuppression	• Erythrocyte sedimentation rate
	• Intravenous drug use	• C-reactive protein
	• Multiple comorbidities	• Magnetic resonance imaging
	• Trauma	

Comorbid stress, anxiety, and depression have been linked with risk of chronicity. "Fear avoidance beliefs" and catastrophizing may cause maladaptive movement patterns or activity avoidance that may cause spinal muscle deconditioning. The purpose of the biopsychosocial evaluation shifts from the characterization of a causative agent to the identification of inappropriate attitudes and beliefs, high levels of distress, and fear-avoidance behaviors that can impede recovery of function and place the patient at higher risk for developing chronic LBP. To effectively manage back pain, providers must address identifiable causes and perpetuating factors (see Chapter 102).

EVALUATION

A thorough history and physical exam can guide care for patients with acute and chronic back pain. Applying three conceptual frameworks may be helpful for the evaluation and successful management: (1) rule out specific pathology, (2) differentiate patients with nonspecific LBP, and (3) identify psychosocial factors. Understanding these categories can help providers better understand a patient's pain and prognosis and help inform and individualize treatment.

HISTORY

While taking a patient history, it is helpful to think in terms of three basic diagnostic categories: nonspecific LBP, back pain with suspected radiculopathy or spinal stenosis, or back pain that is a result of a specific pathology.[12] A thorough history is helpful for identifying red flag symptoms of serious, albeit rare, causes of LBP, such as cancer, infection, and abdominal aortic aneurysm.[34,35] Other definitive causes of LBP include disk herniation with radiculopathy, spinal stenosis, compression fractures, and inflammatory arthropathies.

The history should begin with a description of the primary complaint in order to identify pain severity and functional limitations. The patient should be questioned about the pattern and nature of any lower extremity symptoms, as well as the presence of significant neurological deficits, gait abnormalities, or bowel or bladder dysfunction. Attention to any history of trauma, immunosuppression, constitutional symptoms, substance use, comorbidities, and previous history of back troubles including spinal surgery is important. In addition, postures or spinal loading strategies (e.g., flexion, extension) that aggravate or palliate the patient's lumbar spine and/or extremity symptoms should be explored. Because most patients will benefit from conservative care and the incorporation of one or more integrative therapies, history is also very important for matching a treatment to a patient.

PHYSICAL EXAMINATION

During physical examination, emphasis should be placed on the observation of posture and gait, back inspection, palpation, range-of-motion testing, orthopedic maneuvers, and a comprehensive neurological evaluation. Observing transitional movements is informative; for example, a reverse lumbopelvic rhythm (bending knees to return from flexed position) suggests dynamic lumbar instability, which may benefit from stabilization exercises.[36] Active and passive range-of-motion testing, especially active repetitive flexion and extension, can help determine which tissues are pain generating. Particular attention should be paid to repetitive movements that centralize the pain or cause it to move from a more peripheral location (e.g., buttocks) to a more central location (midline of the lumbar spine). Orthopedic tests are particularly meaningful when they recreate a patient's chief complaint pain. For example, a series of six orthopedic tests are very reliable for identifying sacroiliac joint pain when three or more provoke familiar pain.[37,38] Nerve tension tests, such as the straight leg raise and slump test, apply tension

TABLE 67.2 **Common Radiculopathies**

Level of Disk Herniation	Nerve Root Involved	Muscle to Be Tested	Area of Sensory Loss	Reflex
L3–4	L4	Tibialis anterior	Medial calf	Patellar
L4–5	L5	Extensor hallucis longus	Lateral calf	None
L5–S1	S1	Gastroc-soleus	Lateral foot	Achilles
Cauda equina syndrome	S2–S3–S4	External anal sphincter	Perirectal	None

to the sciatic nerve and may recreate the chief complaint of leg pain in patients with nerve root irritation.[39] The neurological examination should focus on the L4, L5, and S1 levels by evaluating myotomes (including heel and toe walking), dermatomes (light touch or pin prick sensation), and deep tendon reflexes (knee and ankle).[12,15,17,18] Distribution of myotomes, dermatomes, and deep tendon reflexes are outlined in Table 67.2.

RED FLAGS

Roughly 10% of patients will have examination findings suggesting a specific underlying cause, some of which warrant immediate further evaluation. Observing absence or presence of such red flag signs is an important part of an evaluation and can help identify rare causes of back pain, including cauda equina syndrome, cancer, fracture, or infection. Table 67.3 lists constellations of red flags concerning specific LBP pathologies and recommendations for further evaluation and referral.[12,15,17,18,40] The minority of patients with LBP (2%) will have one of these serious underlying causes of back pain. The majority of specific LBP cases involve lumbar stenosis and disk herniation with correlating radiculopathy type leg pain. For most patients with suspected radiculopathy or spinal stenosis, conservative management aimed at alleviating pain and improving function is recommended, unless they present with progressive neurological symptoms. However, if the patient demonstrates persistent leg pain or neurological findings after 6 weeks of conservative care, surgical referral should be considered.[31]

YELLOW FLAGS

Yellow flags are key patient characteristics that are linked with poor prognosis.[33,41] Yellow flags have significant prognostic importance, and their presence should influence a patient's course of treatment. Table 67.4 describes common yellow flags such as comorbid anxiety, depression, and stress. The presence of nonorganic signs (Table 67.5) is a very strong predictor for chronicity.[33] Additionally, patients who fear reinjury may avoid movements or exercise and consider activity harmful (i.e., fear-avoidance beliefs). Such patients also have an increased likelihood of developing chronic back pain. Providers should choose words carefully for back pain patients and provide clear, concise patient education to patients with yellow flags. For example, such terms as *stenosis* and *disk degeneration* should

TABLE 67.3 **Historical Red Flags**

Fever, weight loss, nausea	History of intravenous drug use
Saddle anesthesia	History of cancer
Recent trauma	History of immune suppression
Bowel/bladder incontinence/ retention	History of chronic steroid use
Recent urinary tract infections	History of tuberculosis

always be coupled with thoughtful patient education and reassurance to avoid any strong, potentially negative, association a patient may have regarding their prognosis. Encouraging patients to participate in a healthy framing of back pain is key because the vast majority of patients will experience relief of pain and back-related disability.

SUBGROUPING

The broadly defined category of nonspecific back pain does not represent a uniform population of patients. Given the heterogeneous nature of nonspecific LBP, employing a "one size fits all" treatment approach is paradoxical and has led to unsatisfactory results.[42] Attempts to subgroup patients with nonspecific back pain has been a research priority since the 1990s.[43] Several strategies have linked back pain subgroups to more specific treatments with the goal of improving clinical outcomes.[44]

Developing subgrouping systems involves stratifying patients based on key individual patient characteristics such as prognostic factors, likely response to specific treatment, or suspected underlying causal mechanism, all of which can help tailor treatment. The subgrouping process is thought to result in better, more efficient care.[45] Three important examples of subgrouping strategies include (1) the Keele STarTback tool (prognostic factors), (2) treatment-based classification (TBC; likely responders) systems, and (3) the McKenzie method of mechanical treatment and diagnosis (MTD; underlying causal mechanisms).[44,46,47]

Keele STarTback Tool

Capturing a patient's biopsychosocial profile is tremendously important in the primary care setting, but is often

TABLE 67.4 Yellow Flags: Risk Factors for Disability and Chronic Low Back Pain

Psychosocial Factors	Occupational Factors	Interview Questions
• Inappropriate attitudes and beliefs	• Work status	• What do you believe is causing your back pain?
• Poor or maladaptive coping strategies	• Low job satisfaction	• What do you think will help your back pain?
• High levels of emotional distress	• High physical job demands	• Do you think your pain will ever get better?
• Fear-avoidance behavior	• Inability to modify work	• How do you deal or cope with your back pain?
• Depressed mood and social isolation	• High levels of job stress	• Have you been feeling worried, down, or blue?
• Resistance to change	• Working conditions	• How do your family, friends, and coworkers respond when you have pain?
• Family reinforcement of illness behavior	• Worker's compensation claim or litigation • Health benefits and insurance	• Have you had time off work because of your back pain? • When do you think you will return to work?

TABLE 67.5 Waddell's Nonorganic Signs[a]

Sign	Description
Superficial or nonanatomical tenderness	Pain with light or superficial palpation of the skin, or widespread deep tenderness that is not localized to one skeletal or neuromuscular structure, does not follow an anatomic distribution, and often extends to the thoracic spine, sacrum, or pelvis
Pain on axial loading or simulated rotation	Pain with downward pressure applied to the top of the patient's head when standing, or back pain when the shoulders and pelvis are passively rotated as a unit with the patient standing relaxed with the feet together
Nonreproducibility of pain when patient is distracted	A positive physical finding elicited during the examination that is not present later in the examination when the patient is distracted and the finding is checked again (e.g., pain with a standard straight leg raise test, but not when the examiner passively extends the leg of a seated patient)
Regional weakness or sensory change	Regional, nonanatomical sensory change (stocking sensory loss, or sensory loss in an entire extremity or side of the body) or regional weakness (weakness that is jerky, with intermittent resistance such as cogwheeling or catching)
Overreaction	An exaggerated painful response to a stimulus that is not reproduced when the same stimulus is given later, or an exaggerated response to a stimulus that should not cause back pain (e.g., gently pinching the skin on the back in the area of pain)

[a]Elicitation of one or more of these signs on physical examination suggests a nonorganic or psychological component to the patient's back pain.

Adapted from Chou R, Shekelle P. Will this patient develop persistent disabling low back pain? *JAMA.* 2010;303:1295-1302.

neglected in the evaluation of back pain. The Keele STarTback Tool is a brief (nine-item) questionnaire that separates patients into low, medium, and high risk for developing back pain disability. It measures, in part, the patient's amount of worry and lack of hope toward improvement. Patients in the moderate or high-risk groups have been shown to have better outcomes if treatment is augmented by a cognitive behavioral intervention[48] (see Key Web Resources).

Treatment-Based Classification (Fig. 67.2)

The TBC subgrouping strategy uses clinical prediction rules, which are specific clusters of signs and symptoms, to match patients to a particular treatment that they are more likely to respond favorably to. Essentially, TBC classifies patients into categories that help guide decision making when considering the many treatments available for back pain. Currently, TBC categories include specific

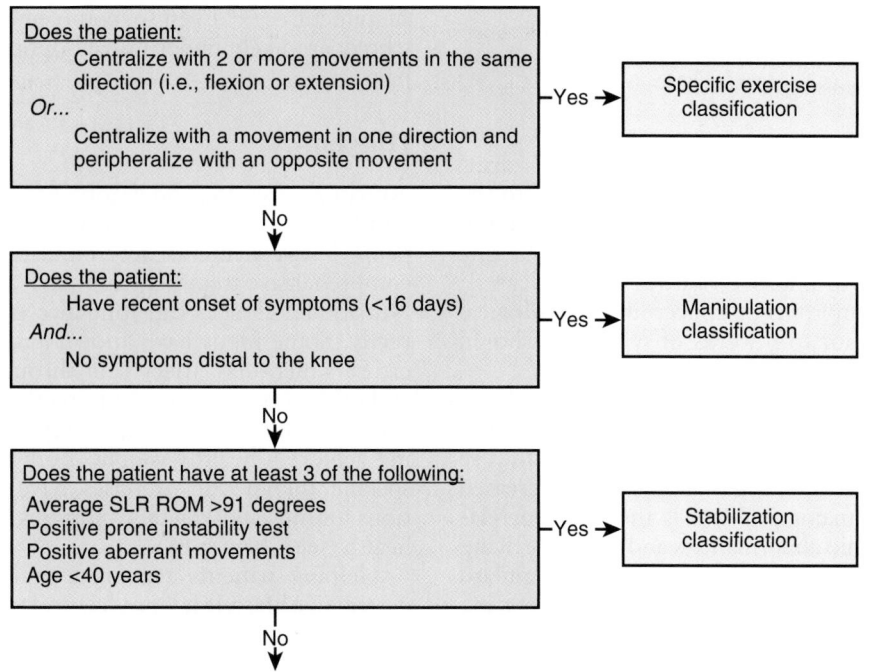

FIG. 67.2 ■ Treatment-based classification. (From Brennan, Fritz JM, Hunter SJ, Thackeray A, Delitto A, Erhard RE. Identifying subgroups of patients with acute/subacute "nonspecific" low back pain. *Spine* 31:623-631, 2006.)

therapeutic exercise (flexion, extension, and lateral shift patterns of bias), stabilization exercises, and spinal manipulation. Unfortunately, TBC does not include therapies where the specific characteristics of "treatment responders" are unknown (e.g., acupuncture, yoga). TBC's clinical predication rules have been incorporated into a variety of clinical settings and have shown better clinical and cost outcomes when compared to usual care.[44]

McKenzie Method

The McKenzie method describes three syndromes: postural (end-range stress of normal structures), dysfunction (end-range stress of shortened structures possibly due to scarring, fibrosis, or nerve root adhesion), and derangement (anatomical disruption or displacement within the spinal segment). Each distinct syndrome is addressed with specific static physical postures and repetitive movements.[47] A specific set of therapeutic interventions is suggested for each of these categories.

The MTD classifies patients by evaluating the cause and effect relationship between a patient's historical pain behavior and their pain response to repeated test movements, positions, and activities.[47] This classification approach is most commonly used by physical therapists.

IMAGING

A history and physical exam is adequate for making a diagnosis and determining a treatment plan for the vast majority of patients with LBP. The potential benefits of imaging in spinal pain are to advance the diagnosis, exclude urgent medical and surgical pathology, or guide evidence-based treatment. In most cases, imaging does not add useful information or value. Despite this, use of magnetic resonance imaging (MRI) in lower back pain increased by 307% from 1994 to 2005, with no evidence of improved outcomes.[49]

Early imaging in acute back pain has not been shown to improve either short- or long-term outcomes and is not recommended by several clinical guidelines.[10,50]

Imaging has been shown to be costly, can be harmful, and findings most commonly do not correlate to the clinical course of LBP.[50] Avoiding the use of imaging in the early evaluation of LBP has been identified as one of the top five ways to improve value in primary care.[51] Without red flag symptoms or concerning neurological findings, imaging prior to 6 weeks of symptoms should be discouraged.

Even after the acute period, patients should undergo imaging only if it may reasonably guide treatment decisions. There are several limitations associated with the use of radiographic and MRI testing that can lead to increased risks to patients. A major problem is the poor correlation between anatomic abnormalities and the underlying source of pain. For example, there is no known standard to identify diskogenic pain as the primary pain generating tissue. Simply identifying a disk herniation on an MRI is not well correlated with the disk being the source of pain. Also, MRI findings of degenerative changes in lumbar facet joints are not predictive of a patient benefiting from a facet joint injection.[49] The same is true of degenerative changes in the sacroiliac joints. This makes interpreting imaging studies difficult and may overestimate their importance when trying to correlate information to the patient presentation. Potential harms of advanced imaging include unnecessary subsequent procedures and "labeling" a patient with a condition, such as degenerative disk disease, which may ultimately have no bearing on the course of their clinical symptoms. In some patients this labeling may cause avoidance of helpful activities out of fear that the activity will cause further damage.[52] Direct harms related to radiation exposure are unlikely because computed tomography (CT) scans are seldom used in back pain evaluations, but worth considering for patients who receive repeated imaging studies. If the decision is made to proceed with imaging in LBP, plain radiographs are recommended initially. If there is a specific neurological concern or the patient is considering interventional treatments, an MRI may help guide treatment.

INTEGRATIVE THERAPY

Current "usual care" approaches to the diagnosis and treatment of chronic back pain are costly and often ineffective, leaving significant room for improvement. A 2009 study on cost of LBP noted, "National expenditures on spinal pain...increased 82% from 1997 to 2006. Paradoxically, mental health and physical functioning worsened for patients with spinal pain over this time frame."[53] Patients are frustrated with treatment options and outcomes, and turn to complementary treatments for pain more often than for any other diagnosis.[54] LBP is an area where an integrative approach is clearly needed.

A wide range of treatments is available for LBP. Some complementary modalities are featured prominently in guidelines, such as exercise, spinal manipulation, and acupuncture.[12,18] Even so, complementary therapies, as a whole, are likely underutilized options in treating spinal pain.

Lifestyle

Nutrition, exercise, and ergonomic awareness are important behaviors that may contribute to or perpetuate back pain. These elements are foundational in providing a comprehensive treatment approach to chronic back pain. Nutritional choices can influence pain directly or indirectly. Some foods have known antiinflammatory properties, which may affect pain through altering cytokine and oxidant production.[55] Indirectly, food can affect pain through improving mood, energy level, sleep, and helping achieve a healthy weight. Both general exercise and specific therapeutic exercises have important implications for musculoskeletal conditions as well as for general health (see Chapter 88).

Helping patients recognize and change potentially destructive lifestyle habits is central to an integrative treatment approach. A tool that can be useful in this process is the concept of SMART goals (Table 67.6). This approach can help patients develop attainable goals related to their treatment, and these goals can be monitored at future office visits, allowing for focused discussion.

Self-Care Strategies

Education and self-management are cornerstones of widely used guidelines on the treatment of chronic back pain.[12,18] Both the American College of Physicians (ACP) and National Institute for Health and Care Excellence (NICE) guidelines recommend advising patients to stay active and giving information to support self-care.[12,18] A 2012 systematic review concluded that moderate evidence exists that self-care provides a mild benefit in chronic back pain.[56] Self-care strategies are inclusive of patients taking an active role in the management of their pain, which is a vital step in effective treatment plans.

Self-management differs philosophically from traditional patient education. Goals of self-management programs include building self-efficacy, goal setting, and self-tailoring of information.[57] In addition to educating about a topic, self-management strategies give patients

---

TABLE 67.6   SMART Goals (Using the Example of Wanting to Increase Exercise)

Specific: Walk 15 minutes every day before breakfast (avoid generic goals such as "exercise more").

Measurable: Track time spent walking on kitchen calendar for the next month.

Attainable: I currently am able to walk 15 minutes, but do so sporadically. Physically I am able to do this, and it is realistic to wake up 15 minutes earlier.

Relevant: Increasing exercise is a vital part of my pain treatment plan.

Time-sensitive: I will find my tennis shoes today and start walking tomorrow.

practical tools. Self-management education regarding LBP often includes information on acceptance of pain, staying active, activity pacing, and tools on how to effectively manage pain flares.

Biomechanical Interventions

Exercise Therapy

Regular routine exercise can help maintain good back health. Furthermore, physical exercise is one of the few proven treatments for CLBP, albeit with modest effects. Patients should choose activities they enjoy; no specific type of exercise has been shown to be clearly superior to reduce pain or improve back related function.[58,59] Regular exercise supports general fitness and may successfully address perpetuating factors contributing to back pain such as sedentary lifestyle, obesity, and lumbopelvic instability.

Patients may benefit from professional guidance with exercise when experiencing back pain. Exercise therapy refers to a broad range of techniques designed to improve strength, coordination, flexibility, range of motion, endurance, and aerobic capacity. These techniques can vary according to frequency, intensity, and duration. Exercise therapy is the most widely used nonpharmaceutical intervention for LBP. Exercise therapy is primarily provided by physical therapists although chiropractors and physicians frequently prescribe it.[58]

The benefit of exercise therapy for acute LBP remains unclear. However, there is strong evidence that exercise therapy provides a small but significant benefit for short and long term pain compared to usual care in the CLBP population.[58-60] Exercise is effective as a stand-alone or conjunctive therapy for LBP. Studies comparing different forms of exercises to one another in the CLBP population have not found clinically meaningful differences.[58] Individually designed, supervised, high intensity programs are recommended as they have been found to achieve better pain reduction and functional improvements than standardized group or home programs.[59] Adverse events associated with back exercise programs are rare.[58] If home programs are used, frequent patient follow-up to encourage compliance is needed because adherence is typically poor.[58,61]

There may be subgroups of patients with LBP that respond differently to various types of exercise therapy.[58] A common component of the TBC and the McKenzie methods of classification is the identification of patients whose symptoms "centralize" in response to specific postures or movements. The centralization phenomenon, which occurs when movement in a specific direction, such as lumbar flexion or extension, causes the patient's pain to rapidly decrease or move from a peripheral location to a more central location in the axial spine.[62] Likewise, movement in the opposite direction may peripheralize the pain or reverse the effect. Indications in the patient's history that these movement patterns should be explored include constant pain that varies in intensity; pain often in seated positions; and movement restrictions are usually asymmetrical.

TBC also utilizes a clinical prediction rule by Hicks et al. to identify patients likely to benefit from lumbopelvic or core stabilization exercises.[36] Criteria that are supportive of benefit from core exercises include age < 40 years, passive straight leg raise range of motion > 90 degrees, aberrant movement pattern during trunk flexion, and a positive prone instability test.[36] Exercises target the transversus abdominus, erector spinae/multifidus, quadratus lumborum, and oblique abdominal musculature.

The major clinical practice guidelines recommend offering exercise therapy according to patient preference for CLBP. In addition, insights from the TBC and MTD may be helpful in identifying patients who are likely to benefit from specific forms of exercise (see Chapter 93).

Spinal Manipulation

Spinal manipulative therapy (SMT) involves high-velocity low-amplitude (HVLA) forces to spinal segments and supporting soft tissues. The result is thought to have local biomechanical effects (e.g., facet joint gapping, stretching of soft tissues) that stimulate a cascade of peripheral and central events resulting in pain relief and improved spine related function. The exact mechanism of action of spinal manipulation is unclear, although multiple potential mechanisms have been observed. The clinical effect is the likely sum of improved joint biomechanics and multiple peripheral and central nervous system mechanisms.[63,64] In the United States, spinal manipulation is primarily performed by chiropractic and osteopathic physicians, although physical therapists and physicians may also provide SMT.[65] Specific manipulative techniques differ slightly within and between professions although mechanisms and clinical effectiveness appear to be similar across providers who are properly trained and regularly perform SMT.

More than 100 randomized controlled trials have evaluated spinal manipulation for LBP, making it one of the most studied interventions for back pain.[66] Spinal manipulation is the only nonpharmacological therapy recommended for ALBP by the practice guidelines from the American Pain Society and ACP.[12] Additionally, all major international guidelines recommend spinal manipulation as a treatment option for subacute and CLBP.[12,15,17,18] Spinal manipulation is likely effective in improving function and pain in both acute and chronic low back pain compared to sham manipulation, analgesic medications, or exercise therapy.[60,66] Evidence suggests that spinal manipulation is as effective, but not more effective, than other nonpharmacological therapies.[67] Serious adverse events (e.g., disk herniation, cauda equina syndrome) associated with lumbar spine manipulation are very rare with an estimated risk of less than 1 in 1,000,000 manipulations.[68] Spinal manipulation is likely most effective when provided in addition to standard medical care or as part of a set of guideline-recommended care.[69]

The TBC system uses a clinical prediction rule to identify patients who are most likely to be manipulation responders. The prediction rule has been validated for use in patients with ALBP or an acute exacerbation of CLBP.[70,71] The five criteria in the prediction rule are (1) duration of current episode < 16 days, (2) extremity symptoms not distal to the knee, (3) low fear-avoidance score (<19) as determined by the Fear Avoidance Beliefs

Questionnaire work subscale, (4) palpation of ≥1 hypomobile lumbar segment, and (5) one or both hips with internal rotation range of motion > 35 degrees.[70] Patients who met four out of five criteria and received manipulation had more than a 90% likelihood of a successful outcome, defined by a 50% improvement in Oswestry Disability Questionnaire scores at 1 week.[70] In this subpopulation, the clinical benefit was also maintained at 4 weeks and 6 months.

LBP patients most likely to respond to manipulation:
1. Duration of current episode < 16 days
2. Extremity symptoms not distal to the knee
3. Low fear-avoidance
4. Palpation of ≥1 hypomobile lumbar segments
5. One or both hips with internal rotation range of motion > 35 degrees.

Clinical practice guidelines recommend that spinal manipulation be offered according to patient preference or when they have failed to improve with a short-course of advice and self-care. In addition, the clinical prediction rule is a useful decision support mechanism for identifying patients who are more likely to benefit from spinal manipulation. For individual patients who would prefer an alternative to HVLA manipulation a number of nonthrust manual therapies may be more appropriate.

Nonthrust Manual Therapy

Nonthrust manual therapies include a number of common techniques directed at the joints and soft tissues. Commonly, joint mobilization is a stretching of the joint without the presence of HVLA thrust. Nonthrust manual therapies also include passive procedures such as flexion distraction, strain-counter strain (see Chapter 109), myofascial release, instrument assisted soft tissue manipulation, and craniosacral therapy. Active nonthrust therapies include muscle energy techniques. Chiropractors, physical therapists, and osteopathic physicians commonly perform nonthrust therapies.

A meta-analysis by Licciardone looked at six randomized controlled trials in subacute and chronic low back pain populations which used a combination of nonthrust manual therapies, all described under the umbrella of osteopathic manipulative therapy.[72] In some of the trials HVLA spinal manipulation was also used. The authors concluded that these combined therapies significantly reduced LBP versus active treatments, sham, and no treatment control. Furthermore, these pain reductions were observed across short, intermediate, and long-term end points. Spinal mobilization provides better pain relief and greater increase in range of motion when compared to no treatment but is not significantly different from placebo.[73,74] There is also moderate evidence to show that spinal mobilization produces benefits in both acute and chronic back pain populations.[66] Nonthrust manual therapies may be offered according to patient preference or when patients have failed to improve with a short-course of advice and self-care.

Massage

Massage refers to a broad range of techniques where a therapist will press, rub, and otherwise manipulate a body's soft tissues. Massage is typically performed in the outpatient setting, often in private community-based clinics. Massages are often of longer duration, lasting between 30 and 90 minutes and covering a range of body areas.

Clinical guidelines recommend massage for subacute and chronic back pain patients.[15,60] A 2008 Cochrane Review of massage in CLBP patients found similar improvement in pain and function when compared to exercise therapy. In addition, the review concluded massage provides better short-term outcomes when compared to several other common therapies, including spinal mobilization, relaxation therapy, physical therapy, acupuncture, and self-care education.[75] This evidence is mixed, as other reviews have concluded that there is not one superior physical modality in the treatment of CLBP.[74] In addition to short-term benefits, one clinical trial found massage provided long-term beneficial effects when compared to acupuncture and self-care in CLBP patients.[75] Patients with acute LBP have also shown short-term benefits from massage.[74]

There is evidence to show that acupressure massage (gently pressing healing points) produces better results than Swedish massage (effleurage, petrissage, and tapotement) and that Swedish and Thai (stretching and deep massage) massage are equivalent.[75] It should be noted that minor pain or discomfort is experienced in a small percentage (<15%) of patients during or shortly after receiving massage.[76] It is important to work with an experienced and/or licensed massage therapist.

Mind-Body Interventions

The link between mind-body interventions and chronic pain is important to consider given the adaptive changes of the central nervous system in chronic pain. Using mind-body interventions directly addresses this component of central-mediated pain.[77] In addition, therapies targeted at a patient's psychosocial experience could be hypothesized to affect both pain perception and related psychological symptoms, such as depression or anxiety. Overall, this is an important category of therapies to discuss with patients as it may improve not only pain, but also mood-related symptoms, stress management, and illness-related coping skills.

Psychotherapy, meditation, relaxation, imagery, hypnosis, and biofeedback are among the modalities included within mind-body therapies. Collectively these modalities have been studied in many pain conditions, including LBP. A Cochrane Review on behavioral therapies in CLBP concluded that strong evidence exists for a moderate effect on pain relief and mild improvement in functional status with behavioral therapies.[78] A meta-analysis of cognitive behavioral therapy found improved pain and coping skills in patients with chronic pain.[79] There is evidence that mindfulness meditation can decrease pain intensity and stress levels[80,81] (see Chapter 100).

Yoga

In the West, yoga is often conceived as a form of physical exercise; a set of postures (*asanas*) with variable difficulty connected by potentially rigorous transitions. However, yoga practice often incorporates additional components such as meditation (*dhyana*) and breathing (*pranayama*) and is commonly classified as a mind-body intervention by clinicians and researchers. Additional components may include yogic philosophy, diet, and lifestyle. This multifaceted practice allows yoga to address multiple interrelated domains (i.e., physical, mental, emotional, social, cultural, spiritual), which may be important in managing CLBP. The multimodal nature of yoga parallels the biopsychosocial model. Yoga can be modified to an individual's fitness level and is therefore accessible to most individuals. Certain styles such as Iyengar yoga utilize props (e.g., straps, blocks) to facilitate postures and in some instances to augment the stretching experience. While the specific mechanisms by which yoga helps back pain are uncertain, several are plausible. Increased physical activity, enhanced body awareness, reduced maladaptive movements, correction of postural strain, and relief of physical and mental stress are all possible. Specific conceptual models have suggested how these multiple therapeutic mechanisms may overlay and synergistically enhance the therapeutic effect.[82]

Current evidence for yoga strongly suggest that yoga has an important role to play in the management of back problems for adults who are willing to practice it. There is good evidence that yoga is moderately effective for CLBP, based on the relatively large number of high-quality trials and their broadly consistent findings of reducing pain and improving back function.[83] Moreover, yoga for back pain appears to be a safe intervention in the context of clinical trials with carefully selected postures and well-trained instructors with the most common adverse event being a temporary increase in musculoskeletal pain. Trials of yoga have used various different styles of yoga. In addition, they have used a variety of postures. Across studies, the postures have overlapped but have not been identical. Although no study has directly compared different styles of yoga for back pain or different sets of postures, the evidence suggests that a variety of styles and postures may be helpful for patients with nonspecific CLBP.

Tai Chi

Similar to yoga, tai chi is a low-impact exercise therapy potentially augmented by important mind-body components. Participants complete a series of whole body movements with focus and attention to movement patterns and quality.

Recent literature suggests tai chi may be beneficial for back pain, although it has not been included in clinical guidelines as a recommended therapy for CLBP. One trial of tai chi found reductions in pain and back-related disability when compared to usual care.[84] Tai chi is generally considered safe for a wide range of individuals and may be an appropriate option for sedentary or elderly individuals.[85] Additionally, tai chi has been shown to improve balance, which may be important for some patients with back pain.

First-Line Pharmaceuticals

Acetaminophen and nonsteroidal antiinflammatory drugs (NSAIDs) are the initially recommended medications in treating CLBP.[12,18] These medications are recommended as initial choices for pain by the WHO. Acetaminophen is generally considered to be the analgesic option with the fewest side effects, although it is not benign. In excess, it can cause hepatic failure. NSAIDs have been found to be effective in the short-term treatment of lower back pain, although the effect is thought to be small.[86] NSAIDs may cause gastrointestinal ulcers/bleeding, interfere with platelet aggregation, worsen renal function, and increase risk of cardiovascular events.[87] However they carry less risk than second-line medication choices, such as muscle relaxants or opioid medications.[86]

Second-Line Pharmaceuticals

Tricyclic Antidepressants

Tricyclic antidepressant medications are recommended as adjunctive treatments for both nociceptive and neuropathic pain.[87] They are recommended as adjunctive agents for CLBP in the NICE guidelines.[18] An additional benefit in some patients may be an aid in sleeping. As such, a common side effect is sedation. It is recommended to use tricyclics with caution in elderly patients.[88]

Skeletal Muscle Relaxants

Muscle relaxant medications affect muscle spasm indirectly by acting on the central nervous system. The specific mechanism varies depending on the agent.[89] An older systematic review found muscle relaxants were effective for short-term pain relief with a high likelihood of adverse effects.[90] There was no evidence of effectiveness for CLBP. Muscle relaxants have similarities with benzodiazepine medications, including similar side effects, most notably dizziness and sedation.

Opioid Medications

The use of opioids is a source of increasing tension among physicians treating patients with chronic musculoskeletal pain. Effectiveness of opioids has been questioned when used in the setting of treating chronic, nonmalignant pain. The medications come with a long list of potential side effects, and the list continues to grow. In addition, opioid abuse and overdose has become a societal burden with increasing publicity and scrutiny of prescribing physicians. Although problematic, opioids may be indicated in the treatment of select patients due to few effective pharmacological options.

The NICE guidelines currently list weak opioids (codeine) as a second-line medication, especially in the short term.[18] A 2010 Cochrane Review evaluated long-term opioid use for chronic pain. They found weak evidence of pain relief; however, an inconclusive effect on function was found.[91]

A systematic review on opioids for several types of chronic pain concluded that, on average, opioids result in a small magnitude of pain relief, but actually less functional improvement than other analgesics.[92]

There are many adverse effects and precautions of opioids. They commonly cause constipation, dizziness, and sedation. These side effects are so common that they cause large numbers of patients in clinical trials to withdraw due to medication intolerance.[93] In some patients they can actually cause hyperalgesia, worsening the pain syndrome.[94] Opioids lower testosterone levels in men.[95] Importantly, they carry a high risk of addiction and misuse.

Botanicals and Supplements

Devil's Claw

Devil's claw comes from the roots of the *Harpagophytum* species, a perennial plant native to southern Africa. Its healing properties have been known for centuries and have been traditionally used for a variety of symptoms. Currently, its most common use is in the treatment of pain. A 2007 review of the evidence found five systematic reviews on devil's claw, with strong evidence of effectiveness in LBP and osteoarthritis pain of the knee and hip.[96] This effect was not inferior to NSAIDs. The review concluded by stating "since there is strong evidence for devil's claw...the possible place in the treatment schedule before NSAIDs should be considered."[96]

DOSAGE
Doses should be at least 50 mg of the harpagoside and effects are dose dependent.

PRECAUTIONS
These are generally well tolerated, with few side effects. The most common side effect in trials is diarrhea. It is recommended to use cautiously in combination with anticoagulant medications.

Willow Bark

Willow bark is an herb containing salicin, which is related to aspirin. It has been used for centuries to relieve pain.[97] The mechanism of action is thought to be through the combined antiinflammatory effects of salicin and flavonoids, without affecting the gastrointestinal (GI) mucosa or blood clotting as seen with aspirin.[98] There is evidence of efficacy in CLBP similar to that seen in rofecoxib 12.5 mg.[97] Evidence of its efficacy in osteoarthritis is mixed.[97]

DOSAGE
The effect is dose dependent, and the willow bark dosage used in studies was standardized to 240 mg of salicin.

PRECAUTIONS
Willow bark has precautions similar to those using aspirin. Avoid use if a patient is allergic to aspirin. It can cause GI upset, headache, and can impair platelet function, but less so than aspirin. Caution should be used in patients with kidney disease.

Topical Capsaicin

Capsaicin is widely available a cream in various doses. It is useful as a short-term analgesic, and a review has shown that it is superior to placebo for acute episodes of CLBP.[99] Side effects can include a burning or stinging to the skin after it is applied, which tends to improve with repeated use. It is important to advise patients to wash their hands after using capsaicin to avoid inadvertently getting the product in their eyes, which can result in irritation and discomfort.

Vitamin D

The relationship between vitamin D deficiency and chronic back pain is intriguing, but not yet clear. Epidemiological studies have correlated low vitamin D levels and chronic musculoskeletal pain, with prevalence in one study exceeding 90%.[100,101] Vitamin D deficiency is known to cause osteomalacia and a resultant dull, achy pain, which can be either localized or widespread.[102] Despite the high correlation and a plausible mechanism of contributing to pain states, a recent Cochrane Review found poor evidence to support vitamin D supplementation in chronic pain.[103] This finding was based on four studies, three of which were deemed of low quality. A smaller study, published since the Cochrane review on vitamin D supplementation, in veterans showed improved pain, sleep, and quality of life.[104] Clearly more research is needed in this area to guide future recommendations. At this time it seems reasonable to test vitamin D levels in patients with chronic musculoskeletal pain and institute a trial of supplementation with low levels given the safety of supplementation and the potential to have a positive impact on other aspects of health.

Acupuncture

Acupuncture stems from traditional Chinese medicine (TCM), with a history of more than 2000 years of use. TCM is holistic system encompassing acupuncture, herbal medicine, nutrition, meditative practices (qi gong), and movement (tai chi). Acupuncture stimulates points on the body, usually with needles, altering the flow of qi attempting to achieve this balance. Even though acupuncture represents one piece of TCM, it is often practiced as an independent therapy.

Recommending acupuncture may be uneasy for some physicians because the theoretical basis of yin, yang, and qi does not relate to a modern understanding of human physiology or pathology. However, basic science research has uncovered multiple mechanisms of action that likely contribute to acupuncture's physiological effect, especially in the treatment of pain. Needling an acupuncture point stimulates the natural endorphin system, altering the pain sensation.[105] This endorphin stimulation is reversible with naloxone.[106] Serotoninergic systems also seem to be involved centrally. Multiple chemicals released peripherally appear to influence acupuncture analgesia, including interleukins, substance P and adenosine.[105] A local anesthetic injected around a peripheral nerve at an acupoint blocks acupuncture's analgesic effect.[107] The gate control theory is also believed to play a role, with modulation of sensory input at the level of the dorsal horn of the spinal cord.[105] Taken together, acupuncture likely has mechanisms of action in the brain, spinal cord and at the periphery, making it a unique therapeutic modality. It remains controversial how these mechanisms interact and how they could have persisting effects on chronic pain.

While the WHO lists more than 40 disorders effectively treated with acupuncture, pain is the most common reason acupuncture is used.[107] There is a growing literature base and multiple reviews supportive of using acupuncture for these multiple indications. From 1991 to 2009, nearly 4000 acupuncture research studies were published, with pain accounting for 41%.[107] Cochrane Reviews showing effectiveness of acupuncture have been published for L, as well as neck pain, headaches and osteoarthritis.[108] Several other literature reviews support the use of acupuncture in the treatment of CLBP.[109-111] The NICE low back pain treatment guidelines list acupuncture as a primary therapeutic option.[18]

Injections

Patients who have persistent back pain after medications and physical therapy are frequently referred for injection therapies. The most common injections are epidural steroid injections, but others include facet joint injections, sacroiliac joint injections, and prolotherapy. Injection therapies are common, and their use is growing in popularity. More than 1.5 million epidural procedures were performed in Medicare patients alone in 2006, more than double the amount 10 years prior.[20] The rate of facet joint injections has increased by 543%.[20] Despite the rapid rise in their use, injections therapies as a whole have very limited evidence of effectiveness. A 2008 Cochrane Review concluded that "no strong evidence exists to support any injection therapy."[112]

Among the injection therapies, epidural injections have been the most studied. Patients with lumbosacral radicular pain are the most likely to have some benefit from epidural injections. Several systematic reviews have found low quality or fair evidence of short-term relief of radicular symptoms with epidural injections.[113-117] This benefit is no longer seen after 6 weeks.[116] Injections do not seem to impact the need for subsequent surgical intervention.[117] For LBP patients without radiating leg pain, there is no evidence of benefit from an epidural injection. A 2013 review gives the following summary: "the evidence for epidural injections ranges from nil to possible based on the cause of chronic back pain. There is no evidence of efficacy…for long-term relief of back pain of any etiology."[116] Adverse effects are relatively uncommon with epidural procedures, but as noted in two systematic reviews, these are not well reported in trials.[113,117] The possibility of significant morbidity is real, however. This was highlighted by the widely publicized case reports of Aspergillus meningitis associated with contaminated epidural injection medications in 2012.[118] Overall, epidural injections remain an option for patients with refractory radicular pain. In light that the relief will likely be short-lived, the treatment can be viewed as a bridge allowing for a patient to start rehabilitation-based therapies.

> A randomized trial of epidural steroid injections for spinal stenosis found no difference in outcomes between the xylocaine alone and the xylocaine plus steroid groups. However, both groups showed improvement. The needle insertion alone may hold the therapeutic potential.[119]

Facet joint injections are sometimes performed on patients with perceived facet joint-mediated LBP. An inherent problem with the treatment is determining which patients are likely to benefit from the procedure. Finding facet joint degenerative changes on MRI is not predictive of benefiting from a facet joint injection.[49] This leads to varied definitions and inclusion criteria in trials that test facet joint injections. That said, high-quality reviews to this point have not shown facet joint injections more effective than placebo interventions.[112-114,117] Very few studies have evaluated sacroiliac joint injections, and to at this point there is no evidence of effectiveness.[117]

Prolotherapy

Prolotherapy is an injection therapy for painful ligaments, tendons, and joints. It involves the injections of an irritant solution, most commonly a solution containing dextrose. The goal of the treatment is to induce an inflammatory response in the affected tissues, and therefore stimulate the body's natural healing response. Prolotherapy is a promising therapy for certain musculoskeletal conditions, especially knee osteoarthritis.[120] Cochrane reviewed prolotherapy injections for CLBP, and did not find them effective when used as a standalone therapy.[121] When combined with other therapies such as exercise and spinal manipulation, there is evidence of some pain relief from prolotherapy[121,122] (see Chapter 112).

Surgery

Much like injection therapies, surgical therapies are also on the rise to treat CLBP in the United States. Spinal fusion rates more than doubled from 1998 to 2008.[21] During the same time period, charges for spinal fusion more than tripled, outpacing many other surgical procedures in cost escalation.[21] There is also significant geographic variation, as surgical therapy for LBP is more common in the United States than anywhere else in the world.[123]

The evidence base regarding surgical therapies for LBP can effectively be divided into three clinical groups: those with radicular symptoms and a concordant herniated disk on imaging, those with severe neurogenic claudication from lumbar spinal stenosis, or those with nonspecific back pain, often with associated degenerative changes. Patients with radicular symptoms and an associated herniated disk seem to benefit from discectomy in the short term. A 2007 Cochrane Review and a subsequent systematic review concluded that good evidence exists for symptomatic improvement compared to nonsurgical treatment for up to 3 months.[124,125] Long-term follow-up studies have shown inconsistent results, and there does not appear to be a benefit to surgery past 1 year.[125]

Patients with severe neurogenic claudication from spinal stenosis may also benefit from surgical treatment. In patients with severe symptoms, conservative care is effective approximately 33% of the time, in contrast to 80% effectiveness of surgical decompression.[126] A challenging part of evaluating a patient with symptoms suspicious for spinal stenosis is correlating the symptoms to imaging findings. Although there are objective measures to determine the severity of spinal canal narrowing, the degree of severity has not been shown to correlate to any clinical measure. Specifically, there is poor correlation between MRI assessment of stenosis and walking distance, degree of disability, patient-reported pain, and the physician's clinical impression.[126] The best approach would be to not obtain MRI studies in patients with mild–moderate symptoms as the findings would not alter the initial treatment options.

For patients with chronic nonradicular LBP, surgical treatment is often performed in the United States, but not often indicated. Trials assessing spinal fusion for patients with CLBP presumably due to degenerative changes have revealed inconsistent results. However, spinal fusion has not been shown to have better results than intensive physical therapy or cognitive-behavioral programs.[125] Despite this, degenerative CLBP continues to be the most common reason for spinal fusion.[21] As a general rule of thumb, patients with primarily radicular symptoms are more likely to benefit from surgery or injection therapies than patient with primarily axial back pain. This clinical pearl can help guide imaging decisions as well. Patients who have nonradicular LBP without red flag symptoms are unlikely to benefit from interventional procedures, so results of an MRI are unlikely to provide clinical benefit.

PREVENTION PRESCRIPTION

- Maintain a healthy weight.
- Stay active and physically fit.
- Reassurance. Nearly everyone experiences acute back pain at some point, but associated pain and functional limitations typically improve quickly.

- Encourage graded return to physical activity following an episode of acute back pain.
- Improve mental health resilience by practicing some form of stress reduction on a regular basis.

THERAPEUTIC REVIEW

EVALUATION

- Red flag findings help identify serious, albeit rare, causes of back pain.
- Yellow flag findings help identify patients with acute back pain with an elevated risk of developing chronic back pain.
- Avoid imaging in patients with acute or subacute symptoms when red flag symptoms are not present.
- For nonspecific back pain, consider patients' preferences and clinical subgrouping strategies in treatment planning.

EDUCATION AND SELF-MANAGEMENT

- Educate patients on the multiple facets of chronic pain and the need for patient engagement in treatment. A_1
- Provide resources to aid patients in starting a general exercise program or staying active. A_1
- Reassure patients of favorable outcomes and address psychosocial risk factors for chronic back pain (e.g., catastrophizing, fear-avoidance beliefs). A_1
- Provide resources for patients to improve self-management of pain flares. A_1

MIND-BODY INTERVENTIONS

- Consider a referral to a health psychologist with experience in improving pain-related coping skills, especially if yellow flag symptoms are present.
- Consider a referral for cognitive-behavioral therapy, especially if yellow flag symptoms are present. A_1
- Encourage patients to develop a stress management practice, such as relaxation breathing or meditation. C_1
- Encourage patients to try yoga through a program specifically tailored for those with back pain. B_1

PHARMACEUTICALS

- Acetaminophen, 500–1000 mg, three to four times daily, up to a maximum of 3000 mg/day B_1
- Nonsteroidal antiinflammatory medications  A_2
  - Ibuprofen, 600–800 mg up to three times daily
  - Naproxen, 500 mg two times daily

BOTANICALS

- Devil's claw, 400 mg supplements, two capsules three times daily. Most are standardized to 1.5% harpogoside. A_2
- Willow bark, 240 mg of salicin, one to two times daily. B_2

BIOMECHANICAL MODALITIES

- Spinal manipulation is recommended for acute, subacute and chronic low back pain; it is likely most effective when combined with therapeutic exercise. One to two times per week for 4 weeks. B_1
- Exercise therapy is recommended for subacute and chronic low back pain, two to three times per week for 4 weeks. A_1
- Consider massage therapy for four to eight visits for acute or chronic LBP. B_1

BIOENERGETIC MODALITIES

- Consider acupuncture as an adjunctive treatment, 6–12 treatment sessions. B_1

INTERVENTIONAL TREATMENTS

- For patients with persistent radicular symptoms despite a minimum of 8 weeks of integrative therapy, consider further imaging with an MRI to evaluate for primary discogenic pain. If disc disease correlates to the persistent radicular leg pain, consider further evaluation for an epidural injection.
- Advise against interventional injection therapies or surgery for patients without radicular pain.

Key Web Resources	
University of Wisconsin Integrative Medicine patient handouts: Information for clinicians and patient handouts on integrative and comprehensive management of chronic low back pain	http://www.fammed.wisc.edu/integrative/modules/low-back-pain
Pain Toolkit: A practical, patient-designed chronic pain self-management guide	http://www.paintoolkit.org
Low back pain exercise guide	http://orthoinfo.aaos.org/topic.cfm?topic=a00302
Books for starting meditation "Wherever You Go, There You Are," by Jon Kabat-Zinn "Mindfulness-Based Stress Reduction Workbook," by Bob Stahl and Elisha Goldstein	http://www.amazon.com/Wherever-You-Go-There-Are/dp/1401307787/ref=sr_1_1?s=books&ie=UTF8&qid=1432225458&sr=1-1&keywords=wherever+you+go+there+you+are http://www.amazon.com/Mindfulness-Based-Stress-Reduction-Workbook/dp/1572247088/ref=sr_1_1?s=books&ie=UTF8&qid=1432225584&sr=1-1&keywords=mindfulness+based+stress+reduction+workbook
Keele STarTback Tool	http://www.keele.ac.uk/sbst/startbacktool/
SOAPP opioid risk assessment tool	http://www.painedu.org/soapp.asp

REFERENCES

References are available online at ExpertConsult.com.

CHAPTER 68

NECK PAIN

Alexandra Ilkevitch, MD • Taryn Lawler, DO • J. Adam Rindfleisch, MPhil, MD

In many Eastern traditions, the neck is considered our center of communication, self-expression, and creativity. Metaphors related to the neck tell us something about its association with vulnerability. Something frustrating is "a pain in the neck," and something depressing gives one a "lump in my throat." We "stick our necks out for others" when we are being brave, and we "go for the throat" when we are being aggressive.

The neck houses our voice, our capacity to swallow, and the major blood vessels that are the lifelines between the heart and head. It has 37 separate joints and moves an average of 600 times per hour. It has evolved to be simultaneously rigid and flexible, and it houses separate flexor and extensor muscles for the head and cervical spine. It contains our cervical spinal cord, multiple nerve roots and joint facets, and the atlantoaxial joint. The neck is indeed a vulnerable part of the body. At any given year, 30%–50% of people in the United States are experiencing neck pain,[1] and two-thirds of people have neck pain sometime during their lives.[2] Not surprisingly, neck pain is one of the most common complaints primary care providers encounter.[3] Even with a full biomedical course of treatment, neck pain often recurs.[4] An individualized, relationship-centered, and holistic integrative approach can markedly improve outcomes.

PATHOPHYSIOLOGY

Pinpointing the exact anatomical source of neck pain is often difficult. Most neck pain is the result of cervical paraspinal muscle spasm or other musculoskeletal factors, but clinicians must rule out various other causes, as noted in Box 68.1.[2,3,5] Most neck pain is localized to the posterior or lateral aspects of the neck, over the suboccipital region, cervical spine, or attachment points of such structures as the trapezius muscles; that said, however, there are certainly some anterior neck pain sufferers. Due to lack of available research and evidence-based therapies for anterior neck pain, this chapter will focus on more common lateral and posterior neck pain.

Musculoskeletal neck pain can be traumatic or nontraumatic in origin.[1] Traumatic neck pain is most commonly associated with hyperextension syndrome (whiplash). As many as 40% of whiplash injuries are estimated to result in long-term symptoms.[6] In countries where litigation for whiplash is uncommon, long-term sequelae of whiplash are almost unheard of, a situation that leads one to wonder about the role of mind-body and economic influences on pain outcomes.[7]

Nontraumatic neck pain, which is more common, can be related to a structural or degenerative disorder, but more commonly it is caused by soft tissue disorders. Twin studies revealed a link between genetics and a predisposition to development of nontraumatic neck pain.[8] Common causes of soft tissue pain include poor posture, repetitive activity, and sports injuries. A strong connection exists between soft tissue neck pain and emotional or mental states, such as anxiety and depression.[9] Myofascial trigger points—clusters of muscle fibers locked in a contractile state—are commonly present in soft tissue pain.

The pathophysiological basis of neck pain is complex, and our knowledge of the multitude of chemical and structural processes involved is far from complete. Pain begins with tissue irritation, which may be caused by infection, disk or joint deterioration, sustained use (or sustained immobility), psychological stress, or trauma. Irritation activates nociception. Muscle spasms often occur as the neck is voluntarily or involuntarily repositioned to avoid pain. Inflammation follows, and a vicious positive-feedback circle arises as inflammation leads to even more pain. As edema, structural changes, and harmful metabolites accumulate, they can cause ischemia of the tissues. If these alterations are not interrupted or reversed in time, long-term changes in neck structure may arise, and disability can result.

INTEGRATIVE THERAPY

The goals of an integrative approach to neck pain are three-fold:[10]
1. Understand the pain in a broader context. Move beyond an exclusively physiological perspective to explore how emotions, occupation, social issues, relationships, past trauma, and other factors contribute. What burdens is a person "carrying" on his or her shoulders? Asking people their views on why they have pain can offer interesting insights.
2. Explore where the cycle of pathophysiology may be interrupted and how that could best be done. Identify the initial insult or insults causing the pain. Supplements or diet may help to lessen inflammation. A mind-body approach may alter the tendency to fear or avoid the pain and/or maintain tension. Manual therapy, acupuncture, or exercise may help patients alleviate any structural dysfunction and diminish the pain, as they learn to carry themselves differently. The key is to collaborate on a plan of action, with care taken not to overwhelm people with too many options. Trust your intuition as a provider.
3. Remain mindful of therapeutic complications and factors likely to cause pain recurrences. Pain can often be a powerful teacher. Why is this signal arising, and what changes are needed so that the signal will no

BOX 68.1	Key Points to Remember in the Evaluation of Neck Pain

- Keep in mind that severe neck pain associated with fever is meningitis until proven otherwise.
- Consider a tumor or other mass lesion in a patient who has pain at night or whose pain does not improve when the body is supine, an elevated erythrocyte sedimentation rate, or lytic lesions found on imaging.
- Neck pain with associated neurological symptoms (e.g., dizziness, paresthesias, weakness, and/or bowel/bladder dysfunction) merits diagnostic imaging studies, most commonly computed tomography or magnetic resonance imaging of the neck.
- If neck pain is associated with joint pain in other areas, rule out a systemic rheumatic disorder, such as osteoarthritis, rheumatoid arthritis, ankylosing spondylitis, or gout. Lyme disease should also be considered.
- Neck pain can be referred from a source in the head or arms. Consider dental disorders, temporomandibular joint disorders, and rotator cuff injuries. For example, cervical spine disorders may lead to patient descriptions of the eyes being "pulled" or "pushed" if the sympathetic nerve plexuses that surround the arteries of the neck and innervate the eyes are irritated.
- Referred neck pain can arise from nearly any organ system. In addition to nervous and musculoskeletal causes, myocardial ischemia, gastrointestinal ulcers or hiatal hernias, and pancreatic inflammation are all in the differential diagnosis. Referred diaphragmatic pain and tumors of the apical lung must also be considered.
- Keep in mind that uncommon local sources of neck pain can include the carotid arteries, vertebral arteries, lymph nodes, and the thyroid.

Data from references 1–3 and 174.

BOX 68.2	Risk Factors for Neck Pain

- Depression
- Drug abuse
- Increasing age
- Heavy physical work, manual labor
- High job demands
- History of headaches
- Lack of control-over-work situation
- Low job satisfaction
- Work with exposure to repetitive vibration or unusual postures
- Obesity
- Smoking (and frequent coughing)

Data from Devereaux MW. Neck pain. *Med Clin North Am* 93: 273-284, 2009; Teets RY, Dahmer S, Scott E. Integrative medicine approach to chronic pain. *Prim Care* 37:407-421, 2010; and Christensen JO, Knardahl S. Work and neck pain: a prospective study of psychological, social, and mechanical risk factors. *Pain* 151:162-173, 2010.

longer be necessary? It is easy for a pattern to arise if the pain is masked, rather than truly treated. Some therapies (e.g., long-term narcotics) can lead to long-term problems and should be used cautiously, if at all.

Lifestyle

Box 68.2 lists some of the risk factors for neck pain.[2,10,11] Smoking, obesity, work activities, and substance abuse should all be given attention in an integrative visit.

Exercise and Movement

To assume that exercise for musculoskeletal neck pain would be beneficial seems logical. Patients with chronic neck pain demonstrate altered muscle activation patterns during the performance of tasks that may influence how rapidly their muscles become fatigued.[12] There are many therapeutic disciplines that can help teach patients healthier movement patterns.

Physical Therapy

A good starting point for many neck pain patients is a course of physical therapy (PT), preferably done by a provider who specializes in spine care. A randomized controlled trial (RCT) by Tunwattanapong discovered

that office workers had an improvement in chronic neck and shoulder pain as well as quality of life and function when they participated in a stretching program.[13] However, in a 2015 Cochrane Review, Gross and colleagues found that stretching alone did not provide benefit for mechanical neck pain.[14] In fact, O'Riordan et al. concluded that multimodal approach may be best when it comes to PT for chronic neck pain with particular emphasis placed on active strengthening. Adding aerobic exercise and stretching provided further improvement in positive outcomes.[15] More studies are needed.[16]

If PT does not provide satisfactory relief, many other movement-based disciplines are available. Some of the most common ones are described in the following text.

Alexander Technique, Feldenkrais, Pilates

Medical research continues to be limited regarding the potential benefits of the Alexander technique, Feldenkrais, and Pilates for neck pain, but these therapies are increasingly popular with patients with chronic pain, are effective for other musculoskeletal complaints, and tend to be safe.[17-19] A 2013 pilot study showed preliminary evidence in favor of Pilates in reducing disability and pain related to neck pain.[20] A 2015 RCT found that patients practicing the Alexander technique for 5 weeks scored higher on physical function and general health measures, as well as satisfaction, with this modality compared to the other two intervention groups (local heat and guided imagery). There was no difference between the three groups in disability, analgesic requirements, or pain levels.[21]

Yoga

A 2014 systematic review found that supervised Qigong, Iyengar yoga, and combined programs involving stretching, range of motion, and strengthening were all similarly efficacious for the patients with chronic neck pain (i.e., there was no superiority of one exercise modality over the other).[22] However, Crow and colleagues conducted a systematic review in 2015 and concluded that Iyengar

TABLE 68.1 **Examples of Various Osteopathic Manipulative Techniques**

High-velocity low-amplitude (HVLA)	The physician uses an HVLA thrust to push through a joint in order to restore the range of motion of that joint.
Springing	The physician repetitively gently rocks or pulses against the restriction of a joint to restore the range of motion of that joint.
Muscle energy	The physician asks the patient to push or pull against the physician's resistance, in order to rebalance the muscles around a dysfunctional joint or increase range of motion.
Soft tissue techniques	The physician kneads, stretches, or applies inhibitory pressure to relax the soft tissues.[75]
Functional techniques	The physician monitors the soft tissues while small motions are applied to the joint to decrease resistance. These techniques often use the patient's breathing to cause the restriction in the joint to "release."
Strain-counterstrain	These techniques involve palpating tender points, and utilizing various body positions to take away the palpatory pain of these points. This position is held until the restriction releases (approximately 90 seconds).[76]
Myofascial release	In these techniques, the joint or tissue is taken to the position of most comfort. It is then held until the physician palpates a tissue tension release.
Facilitated positional release	In these techniques, the joint or tissue is taken to the position of most comfort. Traction or compression is applied to facilitate an immediate release of the tissue tension.
Still technique	This technique, thought to be developed by osteopathy's founder Dr. A.T. Still, is set up like facilitated positional release, but after traction or compression is applied, the joint is moved into the joint's restriction and is then returned to neutral. The goal is increased range of motion and restored joint function.
Cranial OMT	This gentle, manual technique emphasizes balancing of the primary respiratory mechanism, as well as the tensions of the cranial bones, dura, and overlying tissues.[162,163]
Lymphatic techniques	Gentle techniques aimed at promoting the movement of the lymphatic fluid are used to promote healing of several conditions.

Data from Chila AG, executive ed. *Foundations of osteopathic medicine.* 3rd ed. Baltimore, MD, 2011, Lippincott Williams & Wilkins, pp 513-527.

yoga was more effective compared to control interventions for short-term relief of chronic neck and low back pain.[23] The control interventions varied and included no treatment, educational materials on self-treatment, standard medical care, and home-based exercise.[23]

Moreover, participants of a 9-week weekly Iyengar yoga sessions appeared to have more body awareness, manifested as improved coping, decreased pain, and increased sense of control over and acceptance of pain.[24] In a randomized controlled trial studying the same population, yoga was more effective than a home exercise program in several measures, including improvement in neck pain severity and related disability and life quality.[25]

Cervical Support

Early mobilization was found to be superior to cervical collar use in the treatment of neck pain.[26] In another study of patients with an acute cervical radiculopathy, a semi-hard cervical collar combined with rest was comparable to physical therapy and superior to watchful waiting.[27] One small randomized controlled trial from Sweden found that cervical pillows could be useful for both neck pain and poor sleep.[28] Proper neck positioning during sleep is important. Prolonged flexion of the neck should be avoided; maintenance of the neck's natural lordotic curve is preferable. Cervical spine pillows may be useful. Evidence on whether traction is beneficial is insufficient.[29]

Repetitive Strain

Certain movements and activities can put the musculoskeletal structures of the neck under chronic stress and tension. Examples are holding a phone between the shoulder and the ear (administrative work), carrying a heavy purse or backpack on one shoulder, staring at a computer monitor for long periods of time, and looking over the shoulder (farming, mechanical work). Bifocals may lead to awkward flexion of the neck as well. The effects of such postures should be brought to patients' attention. Many people "carry their stress" in their neck and shoulder muscles. Chronic stress can result in a constant readiness to duck or to dodge danger, and many people chronically tense the muscles used for these actions without realizing it.

Nutrition

Increase Essential Fatty Acids

Increasing intake of omega-3 fatty acids and reducing consumption of omega-6 fatty acids lower the levels of prostaglandins and leukotrienes that cause inflammation and can worsen pain[30,31] (see Chapter 88). Several months may pass before patients derive a benefit from using an antiinflammatory diet, and diet changes are most likely to be beneficial when neck pain has been chronic.

Increase Antioxidants

Elevations of serum free radicals can occur as a result of poor nutrition, excessive stress, and toxic environmental exposure. Foods rich in antioxidants, such as fruits and vegetables, seem to play a role in reducing pain by removing free radicals.[32] Eating a combination of green, yellow, red, purple, and orange produce will guarantee that numerous beneficial antioxidants are consumed. High doses of supplemental antioxidants, such as vitamin E, have been the subject of some controversy and may be inadvisable in patients with heart disease or other chronic conditions.[33]

Decrease Saturated Fats

Eating saturated fats, which come primarily from animal products such as red meat and dairy foods, can also contribute to inflammation and pain.[34] A transition to a vegetarian diet, or at least toward a significant reduction in saturated fat consumption, is worth recommending. Some patients may benefit from a trial of an elimination diet, specifically avoiding dairy and meat products (see Chapter 86).

> Take care not to underestimate the impact of mental health on the course of neck pain. Encourage the use of at least one of the many mind-body therapies that may offer benefit.

Mind-Body Therapy

Pain perception does not necessarily correlate with the severity of an injury. Some people with structural neck abnormalities develop chronic pain, whereas others do not. Numerous landmark studies have shown magnetic resonance imaging (MRI) examinations of *asymptomatic* individuals indicating that up to 52% had one or more bulging disks, and the number went up to 80% in subjects aged more than 60.[35] Similarly, nearly everyone who is older than 70 years has some degree of cervical spondylosis, but not everyone in that age group has neck pain.[2] Pain is often centrally mediated, with abnormal intensification of sensation noted in the portions of the brain that govern a chronically painful part of the body.[10] Fortunately, the brain's plasticity allows for the possibility for "rewiring" the brain; sensory processing may be changed to someone's advantage. The key is to discern how to help someone with pain make that happen, and this is where mind-body approaches can come into play.[36]

Emotions and Neck Pain

Emotional well-being plays an important role in whether pain arises.[37] A Stanford University study that evaluated both symptomatic and asymptomatic patients with abnormal MRI findings concluded that the severity of the MRI lesions did not predict the presence of pain; rather, pain severity correlated with whether patients had underlying psychological issues.[38] Pain is more likely to become chronic in people who tend to catastrophize,[39] or somaticize,[40] or feel a lack of control in decision making.[41] Stress also plays a role. A British study of 12,907 people concluded that the association between perceived neck pain and mental stress was much stronger than the association between neck pain and repetitive occupational activities.[42]

In his book, *The Mindbody Prescription: Healing the Body, Healing the Pain*, John E. Sarno, MD, suggested that unexpressed emotions are responsible for neck, back, and limb pain in most patients.[43] Sarno held that unexpressed anger, accumulated as a result of internal and external pressures, is of particular significance. After physical concerns have been appropriately ruled out, the following elements can be used to help people markedly decrease pain:

- *Learn about pain and its relationship to one's feelings.* Patients attend a series of lectures describing the relationship between pain and emotions.
- *Focus on emotions when pain strikes.* When patients become aware of the pain, they practice consciously shifting their focus toward the psychological, as opposed to physical, causes of their discomfort.
- *Maintain physical activity.* Patients must overcome fears that physical activity will worsen the underlying condition. This step is implemented after the pain has been decreased through exploration of emotional issues.
- *Discontinue physical or physiological treatments.* Sarno contended that focusing on physical causes of pain distracts the mind from the unexpressed emotions that are the pain's true cause. Medications are used sparingly for episodes of severe pain only.
- *Consider counseling.* Patients are encouraged to seek help from a counselor in moving through the various emotional issues they encounter during the program.

Although outcomes research on the efficacy of Sarno's program is limited, the program has proved helpful for many people with chronic neck pain. Once potentially dangerous causes of pain have been ruled out, the risk of harm from participating in such a program is minimal. Many health care institutions offer pain management and coping groups, which may be similarly helpful (see Chapter 102).

Journaling

By writing about stressful events, patients may be able to reduce pain and inflammation. One study found that symptoms of asthma and rheumatoid arthritis improved significantly in people who wrote about stressful life events in a journal for just 20 minutes for 3 consecutive days.[44] To assume that other disorders may also respond to this approach is reasonable (see Chapter 98).

Hypnosis

Hypnosis has been found to be useful in helping patients manage chronic pain.[45,46] In one study, 25 patients with head and neck pain were treated with acupuncture. After a washout period, they were treated with hypnosis. Both interventions were found to be helpful, but hypnosis scored slightly better, with an average reduction of 4.8 points on a 10-point symptom scale, compared with 4.2 points for acupuncture. Acupuncture was more appropriate for acute pain, whereas hypnosis appeared to work better for psychogenic pain. Subjects who also received healing suggestions through audiotape experienced less pain than those who did not[47] (see Chapter 95).

Interactive Guided Imagery

Interactive guided imagery (IGI) is based on the philosophy that insight and knowledge gained from the creation of internal images can be used to improve symptoms. One interactive guided imagery technique is to have a patient visualize an image representing a particular symptom. The patient is asked to have a dialogue with the image that arises and to explore why it is present and what it would "need" for healing to occur. The image can serve as a means by which the conscious mind can access the subconscious[48] (see Chapter 97).

Phillips found that that 78% of chronic pain patients reported an emotionally charged "index image." Recalling this image increased negative emotional response and pain levels.[49] Also, catastrophizing was found to be a predictor of higher future pain levels in patients who suffered from whiplash associated disorder.[50] Although further research is necessary, this may have important implications for techniques that help rewrite the image, such as IGI, hypnosis, neurolinguistic programming, motivational interviewing, and cognitive behavioral therapy.[49]

Relaxation Exercises

Relaxation exercises, such as breathing techniques and progressive muscle relaxation, can reduce sympathetic stimulation, a potential contributor to muscle tension and pain. One study comparing relaxation, exercise, and ordinary activity for neck pain treatment did not find a benefit from either intervention in comparison with placebo.[51] Nevertheless, perhaps these techniques can serve as a safe and potentially useful way to empower patients to decrease their neck pain (see Chapter 94). Autonomous sensory meridian response is an emerging relaxation modality in which heightened bodily sensations arise and are usually accompanied by a state of deep relaxation as well as temporary reduction in pain. More research is required.[52]

Biofeedback

Biofeedback uses technology or instrumentation to help people gain awareness of and control over various body processes.[53] Functional MRI studies indicated that biofeedback training can allow people with pain to alter pain perception by controlling activation of the rostral anterior cingulate cortex and other brain locations.[54,55] Severe chronic pain can be decreased. For example, sensors placed over the trapezius muscle can be used to train a patient to relax more efficiently. A small study of older patients with trapezius pain showed a 70% reduction in pain with biofeedback-assisted relaxation.[56] Another small pilot study found that a 10-week heart rate variability biofeedback training course for patients with chronic neck pain was correlated with improved perception of health.[57] Biofeedback is worth considering in patients with neck pain.

Bioenergetic Therapies

Acupuncture

The principle that energy flows through or over the surface of the body is common to several healing systems worldwide. Acupuncture, a 3000-year-old therapy based on the idea that the body contains multiple energy channels or meridians, maps out more than 350 major points. Needles are inserted at those points to improve the flow of energy (known in China as *qi*). Many of these points are located within or in close proximity to the neck.[58,59]

Evaluations of acupuncture as a treatment for chronic neck pain show promise. A 2008 review by the Task Force on Neck Pain and Associated Disorders noted that acupuncture was superior to sham treatment, no treatment, and many other modalities for chronic neck pain.[60] A 2012 systematic review and meta-analysis by Furlan et al. had the following findings:[61]

- Acupuncture was better than no intervention for myofascial neck pain of unknown duration.
- Acupuncture was no better than sham acupuncture for posttreatment pain in individuals who had neck pain of both known and unknown etiology.
- Multiple studies compared acupuncture to pain medications for instant and short-term posttreatment pain relief and results were inconsistent. The same was true for acupuncture compared to manipulations. No difference in efficacy was found between acupuncture and mobilization or laser therapy for short-term neck pain relief after the treatment.

A 2015 systematic review and meta-analysis by Yuan and colleagues found moderate evidence in favor of acupuncture for treatment of chronic neck pain when compared to sham acupuncture. Pain was measured by visual analogue scale immediately after the treatment.[16]

Less evidence is available at this time to indicate whether acupuncture is useful for acute neck problems.[62] Evidence regarding electroacupuncture and auricular acupuncture is also limited.[16]

Acupuncture has been found to be extremely safe when it is offered by a well-trained provider.[63]

Other Energy Medicine Modalities

Many Eastern traditions hold that the neck houses the throat chakra, a wheel of energy that extends anterior and posterior to the body at the level of the thyroid. Although therapies that purport to balance the human energy field, such as therapeutic touch and reiki, require further study, some interesting findings are beginning to emerge,[64,65] especially regarding emotional responses to illness.

Authors of a 2014 review of nontouch human biofield modalities found that most of the evidence reviewed demonstrated a statistically significant improvement in at least one primary outcome. However, the preliminary nature and small size of the currently available trials warrants further investigation.[66] Harm is minimal, provided that patients do not defer potentially lifesaving biomedical therapies to focus on receiving energy medicine treatments. For more information about energetic therapies, see Chapter 116.

Other Therapies

Practitioners are encouraged to look beyond the immediate sources of pain to see where the imbalance causing the pain originates. Awareness and appreciation of the body's fascial network, myofascial meridians, and the deep front lines (DFL) (myofascial connections that originate at the sole of the foot and extend all the way up to the prevertebral fascia, which attaches at the base of the occiput; psoas muscle is one of the many important muscles comprising DFL[76]) may offer additional insight into the origins of neck pain.[67] These concepts can help illustrate how imbalances in lower parts of the body can contribute to neck discomfort.

Additionally, although currently there is no supporting evidence, the correlation between tight cervical myofascial structures and the function of the glands that are housed in the neck, specifically thyroid and parathyroid glands, may be a potential future subject worthy of investigation.

It is also important to mention the recent rise of interest in using therapeutic neurogenic tremors for various conditions including posttraumatic stress disorder and chronic pain, in a technique known as trauma and tension release exercise, or TRE, as described by Dr. David Berceli, Ph.D. in his book, *The Revolutionary Trauma Release Process. Transcend Your Toughest Times.*[68] Although the research is currently very limited, the subject definitely warrants further investigation given the low cost, ease of learning and utilizing the therapeutic tremor, and the potential to improve the patients' quality of life.[69]

Manual Therapies

Manual medicine is another common approach to neck pain. Manual techniques are performed by various health professionals, including some osteopathic physicians, physical therapists, massage therapists, manual therapists, some specially trained occupational therapists, and chiropractors.[70] Spinal manipulation performed by chiropractors, in fact, is the most common complementary and alternative therapy provided in the United States.[71]

The nomenclature of biomechanical therapies can be confusing. Chiropractic and physical therapy manual techniques are typically broken into two groups. Manipulation refers to a technique that uses a high-velocity, low-amplitude (HVLA) thrust.[72-74] Mobilization refers to techniques that incorporate lower-velocity, passive movements to the joints.[72] Osteopathic providers use the term manipulation to describe more than 100 different techniques including but not limited to HVLA.[74] Osteopathic manipulation is categorized into several groups of techniques, as outlined in Table 68.1.[75-77] In this chapter, manipulation refers to the term as defined by chiropractors and physical therapists, and osteopathic manipulative treatment (OMT) refers to manipulation as defined by the osteopathic profession.

Safety

The safety of manipulation of the cervical spine has been questioned in the past. Most of these potential risks occur because of the rapid thrust, and therefore the safety of high-velocity manipulation techniques has been studied much more than mobilization or non-HVLA techniques. Common transient effects of cervical manipulation include local pain, headache, tiredness (fatigue), and

BOX 68.3	Contraindications to Manipulation (High-Velocity Manipulation or HVLA Osteopathic Manipulative Treatment) of the Neck

- Aneurysm or other vertebral artery structural anomaly
- Bone tumor
- Carotid or vertebrobasilar disease
- History of pathological fractures
- Vertebral infection
- Acute vertebral fracture
- Ligament rupture and instability
- Metastatic carcinoma
- Osteopenia or osteoporosis
- Anticoagulation therapy
- Previous surgery involving neck joints
- Rheumatoid arthritis of the cervical spine
- Unstable odontoid peg

Data from references 82–89.

radiating pain.[78,79] Transient effects occur in 30%–61% of patients, begin within 4 hours of spinal manipulation, and usually resolve within 24 hours.[78,79]

Substantive reversible risks of manipulation are much less common. Worsening disk disease can occur with manipulation, but it occurs in fewer than 1 in 3.7 million patients,[78] though this adverse effect is more common with manipulation of the low back than in cervical manipulation. Because of this risk, manipulation is relatively contraindicated in patients with signs or symptoms of disk herniation until this disorder has been ruled out radiographically.[80]

The most concerning risks of cervical manipulation are those that are nonreversible. The most common of these is iatrogenic stroke, although vertebral artery dissection can also occur. These complications are quite rare, and in a review of injuries caused by manipulative therapy between 1925 and 1993, only 185 cases of serious injury were reported.[81]

As noted in Box 68.3,[82-85] however, few contraindications exist, and manipulation seems to be significantly safer than other modalities (including antiinflammatory medications) commonly used for musculoskeletal conditions.[86-89] A study by Rubinstein et al.[90] showed that the "benefits of chiropractic care for neck pain seem to outweigh the potential risks," and recent study by Ekhardt et al. showed no change in vertebral artery blood flow after high velocity thrust, in healthy subjects, when done by trained physical therapists.[89]

Research in Manual Therapies for Neck Pain

Chiropractors and physical therapists have performed more manual therapy studies than other health professionals, and this is true when it comes to studies of neck pain as well.[91] Whether study findings are generalizable from one type of therapy to another is difficult to know because of the differences in categorization of the various types of manual therapies, the difficulties in creating sham manipulation, and the use of osteopathic manual manipulation (in the United States) as adjuvant therapy.[92]

Chiropractic and Physical Therapy Studies

Neck pain is the second most common reason (behind low back problems) for a patient to visit a chiropractor. Approximately 24% of visits to a chiropractor are for neck pain.[93] Chronic neck pain has been studied by chiropractors more than acute neck pain, and Gross et al. summarized the findings in multiple Cochrane Review meta-analyses. In these reviews, Gross et al. assessed whether manipulation or mobilization improved pain, function or disability, patient satisfaction, quality of life, and perceived effect in patients with neck pain (with or without headache or radicular symptoms). The 2004 meta-analysis of 33 trials showed that combined mobilization, manipulation, and exercise achieved clinically important improvements in pain, global perceived effect, and patient satisfaction in subacute and chronic neck disorders with or without headache.[94] A more recent review of 27 trials found only immediate- or short-term pain relief with a course of cervical manipulation or mobilization alone; however, a multimodal approach, including manipulation, seems to have the best long-term benefit.[95]

Less literature is available on the use of manipulation and mobilization for acute neck pain.[74,96] A small pilot study of 36 patients showed less pain intensity (p < .05) and a greater range of motion (p < .05) immediately following a single manipulation to patients with acute neck pain.[97]

Some research showed that manipulation of the thoracic spine results in immediate improvement in neck pain,[72] and a follow-up study showed that using thrust manipulation techniques in the thoracic spine resulted in greater short-term reductions in pain and disability than nonthrust mobilization in patients with neck pain. No additional side effects were noted in the thrust-treated group.[98] Previous studies had also shown significant improvements in patients with whiplash-associated disorders after thoracic mobilization was used.[99] Investigators proposed that techniques performed in the thoracic back may be an even safer option in patients with neck pain. However, further research must be done to assess long-term effects and to determine whether thoracic manipulation is most beneficial in isolation or in combination with some form of neck manipulation for the treatment of neck pain.[72]

Osteopathy. There are few studies are available in the osteopathic literature to assess the effects of OMT on patients with chronic neck pain. In one study, 17 patients with chronic neck pain were recruited. These patients were treated with OMT for a total of 4 weeks (twice weekly for 2 weeks and once weekly for the final 2 weeks). They were analyzed before treatment, at 2 weeks, and at 4 weeks for changes in pain and disability. Significant improvements were found in pain (p < .001) and disability (p < .001) over the treatment course in the group receiving OMT. Improvements in pain and disability were found to be significant in patients with chronic pain and in those with subchronic pain. Further follow-up was not done.[100]

In a second, slightly larger study, 41 patients with nonspecific neck pain were divided into two groups. One group of 17 patients received ultrasound therapy only (every week for an average of 10 weeks), whereas a second group received ultrasound (every week for an average of 10 weeks) and OMT (every other week for an average of

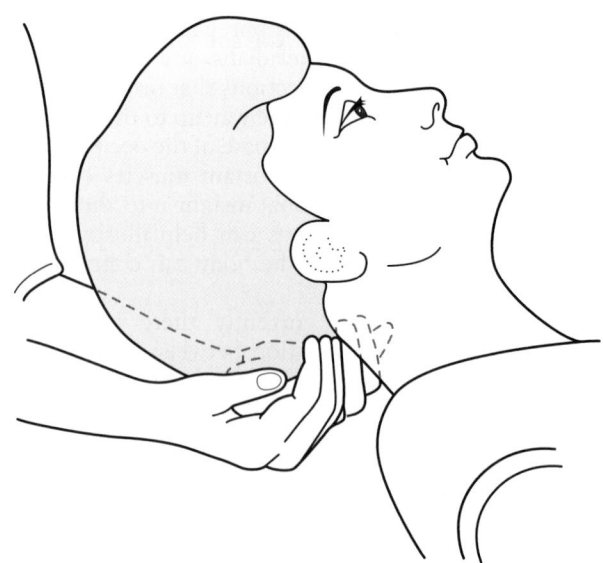

FIG. 68.1 ■ Hand positions for suboccipital release. See Box 68.4 for explanation of technique. (From Chaitow L. *Cranial manipulation theory and practice: osseous and soft tissue approaches*, New York, 1999, Churchill Livingstone, 119.)

10 weeks). Pain was measured at each of the treatments, 1 week after the treatments, and 3 months after the last treatment. The OMT used a combination of various techniques. Pain intensity decreased in both groups, with more improvement noted in the group receiving OMT (p = .02). No long-term follow-up was done.[101]

Another study looked at OMT in patients with acute neck pain, in which 58 patients were randomized to receive either OMT (HVLA, muscle energy, and soft tissue techniques) or 30 mg intramuscular ketorolac (a known effective nonsteroidal antiinflammatory drug for musculoskeletal pain). Both groups showed a significant reduction in pain intensity (p < .01 for both groups), but patients receiving OMT reported a significantly greater decrease in pain intensity (p = .02).[74]

A systematic review done in 2015 found OMT to be an effective treatment for chronic, nonspecific neck pain, in spite of the small sample sizes in the reviewed studies.[102]

Gua Sha

A traditionally East Asian technique called gua sha, which involves the use of a smooth-edged spoon or other object to rub over the skin, resulting in petechial rash, has also been studied in relation to its efficacy for treatment of neck pain. One small RCT showed that a single gua sha treatment offered significantly more pain relief and functional improvement (95% confidence interval -43.3; -16.6 mm on visual analogue scale; p < .001) after 1 week than localized heating pad therapy.[103]

In summary, the available literature indicates that manual therapies hold promise and are worth considering in the management of neck pain.

Strain-Counterstrain and the Suboccipital Release

Two techniques that the primary care provider can incorporate into his or her practice for the manual therapy of

| BOX 68.4 | Suboccipital Release |

The suboccipital release (also known as the cranial base release) is a manual soft tissue technique that can be incorporated into your daily practice. It is most useful for patients with cervical myofascial tension that has led to suboccipital neuralgia and headache. If you find it helpful, consider referring the patient to a cranial osteopathic practitioner.

The suboccipital release loosens soft tissues that attach to the base of the cranium. If hypertrophic and inflamed, these tissues can restrict cervical and cranial range of motion and cause pain.

- See Fig. 68.1. The patient is supine on the table. Seat yourself at the head of the table with your arms resting on and supported by it.
- Rest the backs of your hands on the table. The pads of your fingertips, which are bent toward the patient's posterior neck, are positioned at the base of the occiput in the suboccipital sulcus.
- Your fingertips serve as a fulcrum for the patient's occiput. The patient should allow the full weight of the head to rest in your hands. The resultant pressure will induce tissue release in the suboccipital space, under your fingertips.
- As relaxation proceeds and your fingers sink deeper into the soft tissues, apply gentle cephalic traction with your fingertips for a few minutes. This movement allows the arch of the atlas to disengage from the occiput. This portion of the technique is also known as an occipitoatlantal decompression. Cephalic traction should be started only after you are a few minutes into the technique, to allow for initial relaxation.
- This "release" of deep structures of the upper neck reduces tension, improves drainage of the sinuses, lymphatic and venous structures of the head and neck, increases circulation to the head, and helps reduce intracranial congestion.

Data from Chila AG, executive ed. *Foundations of osteopathic medicine.* 3rd ed. Baltimore, MD, 2011, Lippincott Williams & Wilkins, pp 513-527; and from Chaitow L. *Cranial manipulation therapy and practice: osseous and soft tissue approaches.* New York, 1999, Churchill Livingstone, pp 113-114.

neck pain are strain-counterstrain and the suboccipital release (Fig. 68.1 and Box 68.4). Strain-counterstrain is helpful for relieving trigger points and muscle spasms (see Chapter 109). The suboccipital cranial base release is beneficial for patients with suboccipital neuralgia and tension headaches. For challenging cases, appropriate referral is indicated. See Table 68.1 for a detailed list of commonly used osteopathic techniques.

Injections

1. Trigger point injections (TPIs): Although definitive evidence is lacking, some studies suggest that TPIs may help with the neck and shoulder pain regardless of medication injected. They can also be used as an adjunct therapy.[104] It is important to be aware of diagnostic criteria for trigger points and the less invasive strategies of treating them, such as stretching and massage.[105] Needling may be an important part of the TPI's therapeutic effect.[104] Providing ischemic compression to the trigger points postinjection for at least 30 seconds resulted in greater improvement in symptoms than with trigger points alone.[106]

2. Botulinum toxin A: There is some favorable evidence for injection for treatment of musculoskeletal and myofascial neck pain.[107,108] However, a 2011 systematic review did not find any evidence in favor of botulinum toxin A injections for chronic neck pain.[109] Larger, higher quality studies are necessary.[110]

3. Regenerative medicine: A growing field of medicine. There is currently no strong evidence to support the use of prolotherapy or platelet rich plasma injections for patients with neck pain in the literature, but that may change with time. Please see the Chapter 112 for an in-depth discussion.

4. Epidural steroid injections (ESIs): If noninvasive measures fail to relieve neck pain and improve daily function, ESIs may be considered in carefully selected candidates. There is good evidence that interlaminar ESIs may be helpful for patients with chronic neck and arm pain stemming from cervical disk herniation. Evidence is not as strong for diskogenic, axial, spinal stenosis, or postsurgical pain.[111] A 2015 systematic review by Manchikanti revealed positive evidence in favor of interlaminar ESIs for all of the neck pain etiologies listed previously.[112] Patients need to be aware of significant potential risks of ESIs.[113]

5. Facet joint injections: There is limited evidence, but fair evidence for medial branch blocks or radiofrequency neurotomy for patients with chronic neck pain.[114]

Surgery

Considering surgery, such as cervical fusion, is reasonable when patients have symptoms of radiculopathy, progressive myelopathy, neurological deficits that do not improve with other forms of treatment, or imaging-confirmed operable conditions.[115] However, according to a 2010 Cochrane Review, the evidence supporting the use of surgery for chronic neck pain, resulting from degeneration radiculopathy, is not conclusive.[116] The review found no benefit at 1 year postoperatively for patients with mild symptoms preoperatively, and the reviewers noted that additional research is required to confirm when surgery is most appropriate.

A 2015 meta-analysis by Wu found that in appropriate surgical candidates cervical disk arthroplasty yielded better outcomes compared to fusion in multiple parameters, including but not limited to neck disability index, visual analogue scale of neck and arm pain, and physical quality of life measures.[117]

Pharmaceuticals

Western medical therapy goes to great lengths to suppress inflammation and nociception. Steroids, cyclooxygenase-2 inhibitors, NSAIDs, and other medications are effective largely because they interfere with the inflammatory cascade. Muscle relaxants, opioids, and antidepressants are used to alter nervous system signaling at various levels.

Table 68.2 lists medications commonly used in the treatment of neck pain, along with recommended doses and precautions regarding their use.[118-121,121a] In addition to the medications listed in the table, second-line medications such as antiepileptics (gabapentin,[122] pregabalin),[123,124] selective serotonin reuptake inhibitors (SSRIs), serotonin norepinephrine reuptake inhibitors (SNRIs) (duloxetine), and topical medications (lidocaine, diclofenac, magnesium, capsaicin,[125] compounded topicals, and essential oils) may also be considered separately or as adjunct treatments, although the overall evidence for the use of most of these remedies specifically for neck pain is limited.[124] Intravenous lidocaine infusion therapy may provide hours to weeks of relief and may also be considered for treatment of chronic pain refractory to more conservative measures, but more research is needed and no studies have yet looked at the neck pain population specifically.[126] Screening electrocardiogram is required.

Clinicians must also be vigilant about possible drug interactions with use of multiple agents (e.g., when combining opioids and SNRIs).[127]

A 2007 Cochrane Review concluded that, for mechanical neck disorders, "Muscle relaxants, analgesics, and NSAIDs had limited evidence and unclear benefits."[128]

Between 1997 and 2004, the use of opioids for treating spinal disorders increased by 108%, but pain, poor quality of life, and percentages of disability claims did not show improvement.[120] Long-term narcotic administration downregulates endorphin receptors, which are partially responsible for the pain relief conferred by mind-body therapies such as hypnosis and guided imagery. In other words, long-term narcotic use can impede the symptomatic relief that comes from these therapies.

Use of inhaled or ingested cannabinoids for painful conditions is a highly controversial topic, is associated with significant side effects, and has not been investigated specifically in the neck pain population.[129]

> Pharmaceuticals should be considered only as stopgap approaches, to be used on a short-term basis as the root causes of pain are being sought. Research on long-term opioid use is becoming less supportive of chronic pain medication use.

TABLE 68.2   Pharmaceuticals Commonly Used to Treat Neck Pain

Medication	Example(s) and Dosage	Comments/Precautions
Tricyclic antidepressants (TCAs)	Amitryptiline: 10–25 mg at bedtime, titrated up by 10–25 mg every 3–7 days as tolerated to a maximum of 150 mg/day. Nortriptyline: 10–25 mg at bedtime, titrated up by 10–25 mg every 3–7 days as tolerated to a maximum of 150 mg/day.	- Modulation of ascending and descending pathways - Can give for 2–4 wk for pain reduction - Decrease dose if excess sedation or anticholinergic effects - Sedating - Consider checking serum levels if high doses used for long periods - Taper dose when stopping therapy
Muscle relaxants	Cyclobenzaprine: 5–10 mg at bedtime or three times/day	- Anticholinergic side effects - May cause anxiety and restlessness - Do not give with TCAs - More effective than placebo in back and neck pain[118]
	Tizanidine: 2 mg every 4–6 h as needed up to 3 times daily, titrated by 2–4 mg per dose every 1–4 days; give consistently with food or on empty stomach, up to 36 mg/day.	- Alpha-2 agonist - Centrally acting muscle relaxant - Sedation - Dry mouth - Hypotension - Effective compared to placebo in the patients with acute neck pain[118] - Taper dose when stopping therapy[121]
Other muscle relaxants	Baclofen, dantrolene, carisoprodol (Soma), chlorzoxazone, methocarbamol, metaxalone (Skelaxin)	- Data is inconsistent or limited for musculoskeletal conditions[118] - Carisoprodol has a high abuse potential[121]
Nonsteroidal antiinflammatory drugs (NSAIDs)	Ibuprofen: 200–800 mg with food up to every 6 h to a maximum of 3200 mg Naproxen: Typically no more than 1000 mg per day in divided doses. Contraindicated in the setting of coronary artery bypass graft (CABG) surgery Many other NSAIDs available	- Can cause gastrointestinal bleeding, anticoagulation - No one NSAID known to be better than others.[119] Black box warnings include increased risk of serious cardiovascular thrombotic effects, including myocardial infarction and stroke, and serious gastrointestinal bleeding, ulceration, and perforation
Acetaminophen	325–650 mg every 4–6 h as needed to a maximum of 3000 mg/day	- Use caution in liver disease - Comparable to NSAIDs for arthritis pain
Opioids	Hydrocodone 5 mg/acetaminophen 325 mg (other doses available): one to two tablets every 4–6 h as needed Acetaminophen 300 mg/codeine 30 mg; one to two tablets every 4–6 hours as needed	- Best to use short term only - Significant addictive potential - Constipation common - Use caution with alcohol or sedatives - No clear benefits long term for quality of life, pain level, or disability[120]
Topical agents	Lidocaine patches or gel, diclofenac gel (NSAID class), OTC capsaicin, OTC essential oils—apply to the painful area, follow manufacturers' directions with regard to duration of use.	- Localized allergic reaction may occur

Supplements

Omega-3 Fatty Acids

Ideally, as with any nutrients, essential fatty acids should be obtained through a healthy and varied diet, but this often proves difficult. Not many foods contain omega-3 fats in large amounts. Fish oil supplements decrease inflammation for many conditions, and although studies of its use specifically for neck pain are few, a reasonable approach is to give these supplements a try (see Chapter 88).

DOSAGE

The dose is 1–8 g fish oil daily, as tolerated.[130]

PRECAUTIONS

Doses of more than 3 g of fish oil a day may have an anticoagulant effect and should be used with caution in patients who are prone to bleeding disorders or who are taking anticoagulant or antiplatelet medications.[130]

Phytoantiinflammatory Agents

Few studies have focused specifically on the role of herbal remedies in treating musculoskeletal neck pain. However, several trials have evaluated the overall antiinflammatory properties of herbal remedies and the use of these remedies for pain in general,[10,62,131] as well as for conditions such as osteoarthritis,[132,133] rheumatoid arthritis,[132] and low back pain.[133] Overall, these supplements are quite safe and well tolerated. Most of them work by altering levels of one or more compounds involved in the inflammatory cascade, including cyclooxygenase-2, lipoxygenase, nitric oxide, tumor necrosis factor-alpha, interleukin-1 and interleukin-6, and prostaglandin E_2.[130] For mild to moderate chronic pain, phytoantiinflammatory agents are worth considering, with the intent of decreasing pharmaceutical use and reducing the risk of adverse effects. As with conventional medications, these agents would ideally be used only in the short term while other approaches are used to reveal the root of the neck pain. Table 68.3 lists some of the most commonly used phytoantiinflammatory agents, their dosage, evidence of their efficacy, and precautions related to their use.[62,125-150]

TABLE 68.3   Herbal Antiinflammatory Agents[a] (Please refer to Chapter 65 as well)

Botanical and Dose	Efficacy Evidence	Precautions
Avocado (*Persea americana*)/Soy unsaponifiables[62,131,150] 300–600 mg/day	Decreased NSAID intake in people with knee and hip OA Stimulated collagen growth A 2014 Cochrane Review found a small improvement in OA symptoms and function.[150]	Seems to take 2 mo to reach full effect, and effects linger for 2 mo after patients stop taking them Do not use in people with banana or chestnut allergies
Boswellia[132,135,130] (*Boswellia serrata*, Indian frankincense) Extract: 300 or 333 mg three times/day	Rated as possibly effective for osteoarthritis by Natural Standard, a producer of good-quality, evidence-based monograph Conflicting research regarding efficacy for RA A small 2014 study found benefit for pain threshold and tolerance.[151] Patients who were treated for 90 days with 100 mg of *Boswellia serrata* had a significant improvement in OA symptoms.[150]	No evidence of harm from any preparation Rare GI effects
Cat's claw[130,136-139,152] (*Uncaria guianensis* or *Uncaria tomentosa*) *U. tomentosa* most common in United States (dosing varies with species) Capsules: 350–500 mg once or twice/day Tincture: 1–2 mL, two or three times/day Freeze-dried aqueous extract: 100 mg/day Oxindole alkaloid-free extract: 20 mg three times/day	Rated as possibly effective for OA by Natural Standard Freeze-dried extract decreased knee pain with activity in OA Modest improvement with some forms in RA Decreased need for drugs in OA May also have antioxidant and immune-stimulating properties	Studies have not shown harmful effects May lower blood pressure May inhibit CYP 3A4 May interfere with immunosuppressants May work better if oxindole alkaloids removed May increase bleeding risk Avoid in pregnancy Not for children younger than 3 yrs
Devil's claw[130,131,136,138,140-142,152,153] (*Harpagophytum procumbens*) Dried root: 1800–2400 mg in aqueous solution three times/day Tincture: 0.2–1.0 mL (1:5) in 25% alcohol three times/day	Rated by Natural Standard as having "good" (level B) scientific evidence for therapeutic use Effective for back pain and osteoarthritis A small observational study found pain relief in OA patients who took combination product containing Devil's claw, turmeric, and bromelain.[153]	Rated as safer than analgesic medications; side effects rare May alter GI tract acid levels; avoid in duodenal ulcer disease May lower blood glucose and increase bleeding risk

Continued

TABLE 68.3 **Herbal Antiinflammatory Agents[a] (Please refer to Chapter 65 as well)—cont'd**

Botanical and Dose	Efficacy Evidence	Precautions
Ginger (*Zingiber officinale*)[130,135,138,143,144,154] Powdered root: 500 mg–1 g twice or three times/day Tincture (1 g:5 mL): 1.25–5 mL, three times/day	Rated as possibly effective for OA by Natural Standard A 2015 meta-analysis found reduction in OA pain and disability compared to placebo.[154]	Occasional mild GI effects Whole root consumption may increase stomach acid; theoretical increase in anticoagulation (no evidence in humans)
Phytodolor[131,138,149] Mixture of aspen (*Populus tremula*), common ash (*Fraxinus excelsior*), and goldenrod (*Solidago virgarea*) Tincture: 20–40 drops tincture three times/day in a beverage, taken for 2–4 wk to reach full therapeutic benefit	Rich in salicylates Studies of more than 300 subjects showed reduced drug dosing in rheumatological disease Improved grip in OA Comparable to diclofenac in one OA study A 2011 reanalysis and meta-analysis concluded that Phytodolor was better than placebo for pain in musculoskeletal disorders and was as effective as NSAIDs.[155]	No adverse effects noted in trials Theoretical side effects similar to aspirin; avoid in patients with salicylate allergy No drug interactions known Should be avoided in pregnancy
Rose hips (from *Rosa canina* subspecies)[130,131] Rosehip powder or seeds: 5 g/day	Rated as possibly effective for OA by Natural Standard	No contraindications
Turmeric(*Curcuma longa*)[130,136,137,145,146] Root: 1.5–3 g/day, divided into several doses (can be made into tea; one heaping teaspoon is 4 g)	Rated as possibly effective for OA by Natural Standard Many mechanisms of action, including alteration of arachidonic acid metabolism Improved swelling, stiffness and walking time in RA Improved OA pain and disability but not other clinical parameters May lower LDL and raise HDL	Generally recognized as safe in doses of 8 g/ day or less Can be taken in place of an NSAID Seems to protect stomach against NSAIDs
Willow bark[130,136,148] (*Salicis* cortex) Powdered bark: 1–3 g three to five times/ day	Rated as possibly effective for back pain by Natural Standard Studies indicated benefit for mild pain Best evidence was for dose-dependent effect in 191 patients with back pain Antiinflammatory effect was largely related to salicylate content	Theoretically, may have similar side effects to aspirin, but this has not been found Occasional nausea, rash, and wheezing Caution with use in asthmatic patients
Other herbal antiinflammatory agents found possible effective by natural standard for OA or RA	Borage seed oil (RA) Stinging nettle (OA) Thunder god vine (*Tripterygium wildfordii*) (RA)	Please consult a reference for detailed side effect and safety profiles

CYP, cytochrome; *GI*, gastrointestinal; *HDL*, high-density lipoprotein; *HIV*, human immunodeficiency virus; *LDL*, low-density lipoprotein; *NSAIDs*, nonsteroidal antiinflammatory drugs; *OA*, osteoarthritis; *RA*, rheumatoid arthritis.

Evidence regarding the use supplements containing gamma-linolenic acid (GLA), such as evening primrose oil, black currant seed oil, and borage seed oil, for pain has been less convincing. Of the three, borage oil has the highest GLA content and should be tried first at a dose of 500–1000 mg twice/day.[130] Other promising supplements include stinging nettle, green-lipped mussel extract, *Geranium robertianum*, *Tripterygium wilfordii* (Hook F), and green tea.[130,131]

[a]Efficacy data are based primarily on studies of symptom control in RA, OA, or back pain. No studies focusing specifically on the treatment of neck pain were found.

Aromatherapy/Essential Oils

New and favorable evidence is emerging regarding the use of essential oils and aromatherapy for neck pain specifically (using a blend of peppermint, black pepper, marjoram, and lavender)[156] as well as other painful and nonpainful conditions. This holds true especially in the populations that are at high risk for side effects with pharmaceutical or invasive interventions such as the elderly.[156-160]

- Avoid tobacco and other substance use.
- Maintain a healthy body weight.
- Exercise regularly, and include exercises that strengthen the neck muscles.
- Ensure that the normal curve of the neck is maintained when sleeping.
- Take measures at work to minimize the risk of pain:
  Avoid heavy lifting, or be sure to do it safely.
  Try to cultivate a sense of control in the work environment, as neck pain is less likely when someone has higher job satisfaction.
- Pay close attention to posture.
  Frequent backpack use can increase neck pain.
  Make sure that posture is good when reading or using a computer.

Use a headset rather than holding a phone between the ear and shoulder.
- Eat a diet that will prevent or reduce inflammation.
  Increase dietary intake of omega-3 fatty acids or supplement with fish oil or flaxseed oil.
  Increase fruit and vegetable intake to 8–10 servings a day.
  Avoid foods high in saturated fats.
- Maintain a healthy social support network.
- Decrease stress levels. Use stress-reduction techniques regularly, such as meditation, progressive muscle relaxation, journaling, and any others that prove helpful.
- Treat anxiety or depression, if they are present.

THERAPEUTIC REVIEW

LIFESTYLE MODIFICATIONS INCLUDING EXERCISE

- Exercise should be encouraged to prevent and treat soft tissue neck pain. B1
- Postural therapies, such as Alexander technique, Feldenkrais, and Pilates therapy, can improve cervical muscle support. Iyengar yoga may help. C1
- Preserve the normal lordotic curve of the neck during sleep; cervical spine pillows may help. B1
- Avoid repetitive strain (holding telephone on the shoulder, leaning over a desk, carrying heavy over-the-shoulder bags, looking over the shoulder). C1
- Avoid smoking and use of tobacco products. C1
- Work to maintain a sense of control in your work environment. B1
- If your neck has been injured, avoid prolonged use of a cervical collar and instead work to regain full range of motion as early as possible. B1

NUTRITION

- Increase intake of foods high in omega-3 fatty acids (cold-water fish, flaxseed products, nuts, green leafy vegetables). B1
- Decrease intake of foods rich in omega-6 and trans-fatty acids (hydrogenated vegetable oils, margarine, processed foods). A1
- Decrease saturated fat intake. C1
- Eat foods rich in antioxidants, including a combination of colorful (green, yellow, red, purple, and orange) produce. B1

MIND-BODY THERAPY

- Address underlying emotional issues that may be causing or exacerbating pain and spasm. A1
- Reduce chronic stress and watch for indications of psychological causes of neck pain, such as depression and anxiety. B1
- Journaling, self-hypnosis, biofeedback, and guided imagery are worth exploring, and hypnosis (with recorded guidance or when done by a trained therapist) may be more effective than acupuncture for neck pain. B1

BIOENERGETIC THERAPIES

- Acupuncture is a well-studied, potentially beneficial, and safe adjunctive treatment if performed by a trained professional. A1
- Therapeutic touch and other "hands-on" healing techniques are of potential benefit and quite safe. C1

BIOMECHANICAL THERAPIES

- Consider manipulative therapies:
  - A multimodal approach that includes manipulation and/or mobilization has good evidence of benefit, especially in patients with whiplash injury. A2
  - Be cautious with high-velocity, low-amplitude manipulation because it may have some sequelae. B2
  - Soft tissue manipulation and massage are other possibilities. B1
- Suboccipital release and strain-counterstrain are useful techniques that can be easily performed in the office environment. C1
- Invasive interventions (such as various injections or surgery) should be considered only in carefully selected patient populations, for example if there was no improvement with noninvasive options, or when there is a known nerve root or spinal cord disorder. B3

SUPPLEMENTS

- Taking 1–8 g/day as tolerated of omega-3–rich oil capsules can help reduce inflammation. The risk of gastrointestinal upset and prolonged bleeding time increases with higher doses. A1

PHARMACEUTICALS

- For chronic pain, if other approaches not effective, consider a tricyclic antidepressant (TCA), such as amitriptyline (10–25 mg at night, or a serotonin-specific reuptake inhibitor, such as fluoxetine (10–20 mg in the morning). Doses of these agents may be gradually increased as needed.  B2
- Consider prescribing a muscle relaxant for 2–3 weeks. Cyclobenzaprine (5–10 mg at bedtime) is a reasonable choice if the patient is not already taking a TCA. B2
- Provide a nonsteroidal antiinflammatory drug, such as ibuprofen (200–800 mg every 6 hours) with food. B2
- Consider the use of narcotics for severe pain on a short-term basis only: hydrocodone 5 mg/acetaminophen 325 mg tablets, one to two every 4–5 hours as needed. B2

BOTANICALS

- Consider a phytoantiinflammatory agent to complement or replace pharmaceutical therapy (see Table 68.3). B2

AROMATHERAPY

- Consider adding aromatherapy to your treatment plan. B1

Key Web Resources

University of Wisconsin School of Medicine suboccipital release technique: Video showing how to perform a suboccipital release or cranial base release for neck pain and suboccipital neuralgia and tension headaches	http://www.fammed.wisc.edu/our-department/media/618/sub-occipital-release
American Osteopathic Association: Information on osteopathy and how to find a DO in your area	http://www.osteopathic.org/osteopathic-health/Pages/default.aspx
Back and Body Care neck pain information: Patient-created site with information for patients on neck pain	http://backandbodycare.com/neck-pain/
Everyday Health alternative treatments for neck pain: Patient-oriented site with numerous neck pain–specific articles on an array of approaches to neck pain	http://www.everydayhealth.com/pain-management/neck-pain/alternative-and-complementary-therapies.aspx
Continuum Center for Health and Healing: New approaches to chronic pain: Patient-oriented site designed to teach various approaches for dealing with chronic pain	http://www.healingchronicdisease.org/en/chronic_pain/index.html
Mayo Clinic neck pain information: Patient information on complementary medicine and neck pain; searchable site for exercises for various types of pain	http://www.mayoclinic.com/health/neck-pain/DS00542/DSECTION=alternative-medicine
Dr. Howard Schubiner's Mind Body Program: Site focusing on the mind-body factor as it relates to chronic pain	http://unlearnyourpain.com/
Tension and Trauma Release Exercise/TRE: TRE is a series of exercises that help release muscle patterns of stress, tension and trauma, which include shaking or vibrating that in order to calm the nervous system.	http://traumaprevention.com/

REFERENCES

References are available online at ExpertConsult.com.

CHAPTER 69

GOUT

Fasih A. Hameed, MD, ABIHM

PATHOGENESIS AND HISTORY

Gout is a painful deposition of uric acid crystals in the synovial tissues of the body. Acute attacks usually manifest as a painful monoarticular inflammatory arthritis, classically of the first metatarsophalangeal joint, although other joints as well as the kidneys may be affected. A polyarticular presentation is more common with increasing age and length of disease (Fig. 69.1).

Purines are ubiquitous in the body and in nature. As adenine and guanine, they form part of the "building blocks" of DNA and RNA. Uric acid is the product of purine metabolism by the enzyme xanthine oxidase. Uric acid is excreted primarily by the kidneys, but also excreted by the small bowel. The build up of uric acid crystals can result from overproduction, underexcretion, or a combination of the two. A 24-hour urine assay with >800 mg of uric acid supports the diagnosis of overproduction, whereas a value of <600 mg suggests underexcretion.[1]

Due to the numerous diseases with a similar presentation, confirmation of the diagnosis should be made via aspiration of synovial fluid, examination of which will reveal needle-shaped monosodium urate crystals with negative birefringence. Care should be taken not to miss potentially devastating mimics, most notably septic arthritis.

Gout has been recognized since ancient times, with mentions by the Egyptians dating as early as 2640 BC. In the fifth century BC, Hippocrates referred to gout as "the unwalkable disease." It has also been called "the disease of kings" due to the association with the intake of heavy foods and alcohol, apparently common in members of the ruling class. The name "gout" is derived from the Latin "gutta," meaning "drop"—a reference to a drop of one of the four medieval "humors" once believed to rule our health or lack thereof.[2]

New Clinical Significance

Though gout is often considered solely in terms of its presentation as an acute inflammatory arthritis, it is truly a systemic disease with significant associated metabolic comorbidities. Gout is linked to obesity, hypertension, dyslipidemia, insulin resistance, hyperglycemia, and coronary artery disease.[3] Data from the National Health and Nutrition Examination Survey (NHANES III) demonstrated that metabolic syndrome was present in 62.8% of persons with gout but only 25.4% of those without gout.[4] The Framingham study demonstrated an *independent* 60% increased risk of coronary artery disease in men with gout after controlling for other factors.[5] The 12-year prospective Health Professionals Follow-up Study of 51,529 men showed those with gout had 55% increased

risk of fatal myocardial infarction, 28% increased risk of *all-cause mortality*, and 38% increased risk of death from cardiovascular disease.[6] These strong associations were independent of age, body mass index, smoking, family history, diabetes, hyperlipidemia, and hypertension. The implications of these data cannot be overstated. Gout is an independent risk factor for death from *all* causes.

One proposed mechanism of this relationship may involve a renal-mediated increase in blood pressure caused by hyperuricemia. In a rat model of gout, elevated uric acid caused increased blood pressure through activation of the renin-angiotensin system and inhibition of neuronal nitric oxide synthase. Blood pressure normalized with appropriate pharmacological management and reduction in uric acid levels. This causal relationship may warrant early administration of urate-lowering therapies in patients with gout and hypertension.[7]

Perhaps the most surprising development surrounding gout is the emerging data, which suggest it may be

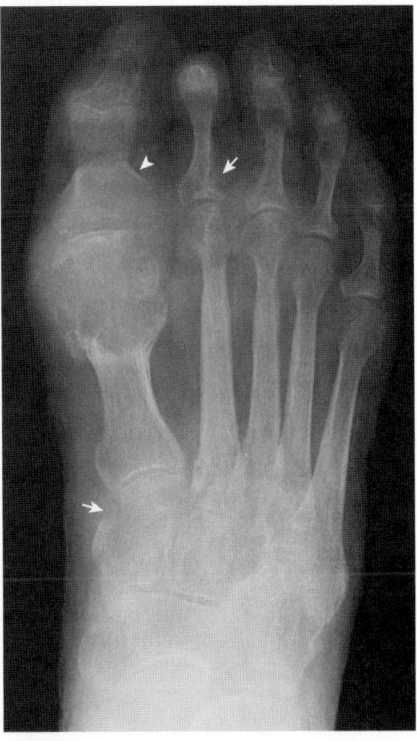

FIG. 69.1 ■ Radiographic forefoot abnormalities in tophaceous gout. Extensive bone destruction is seen at the great toe metatarsophalangeal joint with overhanging edges *(arrowhead)* and soft tissue swelling. Smaller erosions are present involving the first tarsometatarsal and second metatarsophalangeal joints *(arrows).* (From Firestein G: *Kelley's textbook of rheumatology.* 8th ed. Philadelphia, 2008, Saunders.)

inversely associated with Alzheimer's disease.[8] Further studies to clarify the potential neuroprotective role of elevated uric acid levels are needed.

> Hyperuricemia can *cause* hypertension. Recent evidence supports early treatment of gout because elevated uric acid can be a risk factor for heart disease.

The association of gout with numerous metabolic diseases warrants aggressive lifestyle counseling and screening to prevent long-term morbidity (Fig. 69.2). All persons with gout should thus receive extensive education regarding the health implications of this disease. Comorbidities, once identified, should be promptly managed, and the patient should be made aware of the interconnectedness of his/her various diseases. These preventable diseases of "lifestyle" may result in significant health consequences even with prompt identification and treatment. It is therefore imperative that the patient be encouraged, through appropriate use of behavioral change models, such as appreciative inquiry and/or motivational interviewing, and empowered to make positive changes in his/her life.

> Gout is a metabolic disease, which independently increases risk of all-cause and cardiovascular mortality. Like other metabolic diseases (e.g., diabetes), gout warrants aggressive lifestyle counseling and modification.

INTEGRATIVE THERAPY

Lifestyle

Understanding gout as a complex metabolic process, which independently increases the risk of all-cause mortality, underscores the need for a holistic lifestyle prescription as the primary treatment of gout in all patients.

Weight Loss

Encourage weight loss and maintenance of a healthy body mass index. Adiposity is associated with hyperuricemia, whereas weight loss leads to reductions in gout incidence.[9] Weight loss will also have the greatest benefit on mediating the numerous comorbidities associated with gout. All patients with gout should be encouraged to control weight through exercise and diet modification. Emphasis should be placed on the associated increased risk of cardiovascular and all-cause mortality in persons with gout.[10]

Nutrition

Decrease consumption of red meat and most seafood. Persons consuming higher amounts of beef, pork, and lamb have a 41% increased risk of gout. Those consuming higher amounts of seafood have a 51% increased risk of gout.[11]

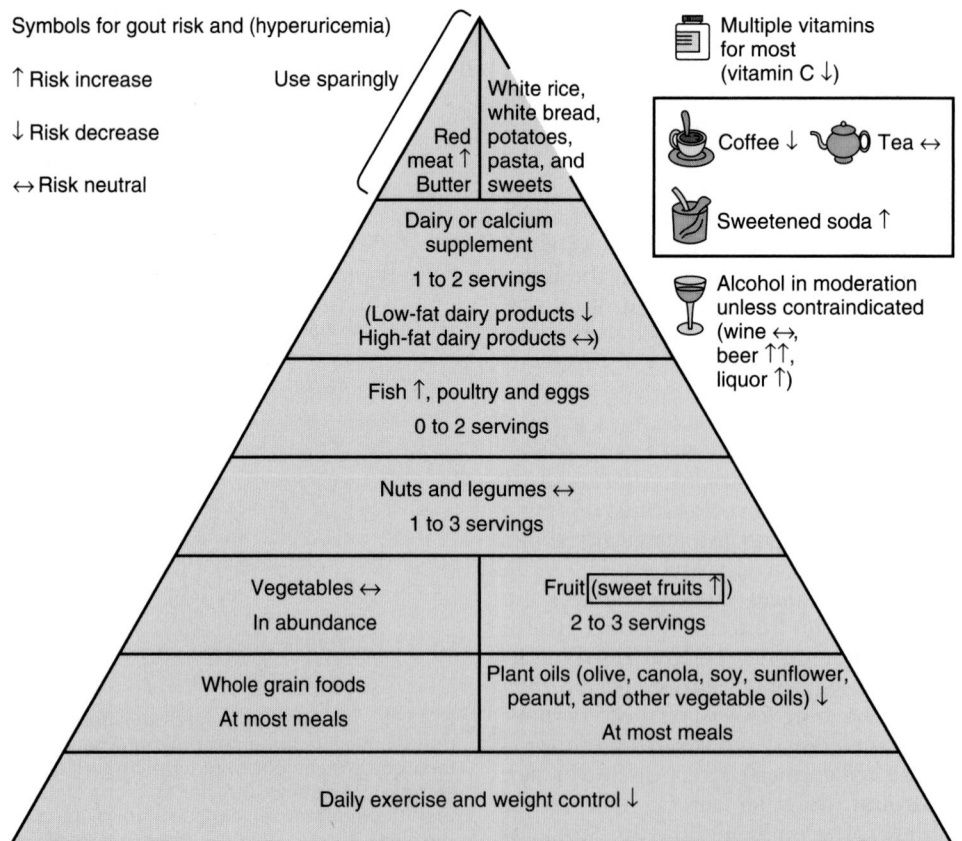

GOUT RISK AND A HEALTHY EATING PYRAMID

FIG. 69.2 ■ Gout pyramid. (From Choi HK. A prescription for lifestyle change in patients with hyperuricemia and gout, *Curr Opin Rheumatol* 22:165–172, 2010.)

Given the potential cardiovascular benefits of omega-3 fatty acids found in oily fish, patients can be counseled and may consider moderate intake of small, sustainably caught, cold-water fish (e.g., sardines). The low purine diet is generally no longer recommended.

Increase intake of omega-3 fatty acids. Patients wishing to absolutely avoid the purines associated with fish should be encouraged to increase dietary intake of plant sources of omega-3s such as flax, purslane, walnuts, and leafy greens. Supplementation may also be encouraged (see the following section, Omega-3 Fatty Acids).

Increase intake of vegetables, legumes, nuts, and vegetable proteins. Purine-rich vegetables, which were once thought to contribute to gout, are now understood to have no impact on the incidence of gout.[11] Furthermore, increased intake of vegetable protein was actually associated with up to 27% lower incidence of gout.[11] Additionally, there are numerous cardiovascular and metabolic benefits associated with the aforementioned foods, which are particularly relevant given the negative impact of gout on these conditions.

> Due to new evidence, experts are no longer advocating the avoidance of purine-rich vegetables or an overall purine-restricted diet. Avoidance of animal meat seems to have a larger impact than purine intake.

Decrease intake of sugar-containing beverages and fructose. Sugar intake was independently associated with elevated uric acid levels in men.[12] Additionally, there is a direct relationship between intake of fructose-containing soft drinks and hyperuricemia as well as gout.[13,14]

Diet soft drinks do not appear to affect uric acid levels, but their use should be discouraged due to an association with metabolic syndrome.[15] Sweet fruits may increase uric acid levels, but the health benefits of these foods outweigh the associated risks, which can easily be countered through numerous other dietary modifications (i.e., less meat, alcohol, refined sugars).

Limit alcohol to no more than one to two drinks per day, and drink wine rather than beer or liquor. Alcohol intake has been positively correlated with gout. Beer has the strongest association—each 12-ounce beer consumed increases the risk of gout by 50% compared to non–beer-drinkers. Distilled spirits have a smaller but still significant association, whereas wine does not appear to be strongly associated with increased risk of gout.[16] Numerous studies have demonstrated the health benefits of moderate alcohol consumption.[17] Nonetheless, it is probably not advisable to recommend intake of alcohol to those currently abstinent. Persons wishing to imbibe should consider wine the healthiest option.

Increase intake of low-fat dairy, up to two servings per day. Low-fat dairy intake, specifically milk and yogurt, appears to have a protective effect on the incidence of gout.[11] Interestingly, a randomized controlled trial (RCT) of milk confirmed its urate-lowering effect.[18] The mechanism is likely related to the milk proteins casein and lactalbumin.[19] Low-fat dairy also has the advantage of protecting against metabolic syndrome.[15]

Drink water. Though there are no studies to quantify or confirm the effect, adequate hydration is often considered a mainstay of treatment and prevention. The rationale is that a dehydrated state will concentrate uric acid and lead to precipitation. Patients should be advised to drink a minimum of 48 ounces of water per day.[20]

Consider coffee. Coffee appears to reduce uric acid levels by a mechanism not linked to caffeine content.[21] Modest intake of coffee may be considered as part of a therapeutic prevention program. Abrupt increases in consumption may trigger an acute gouty attack and should therefore be discouraged.

Alkalinize urine. A study of an acidic versus alkaline diet found a direct correlation between urine pH and uric acid excretion. This occurred despite the lower purine content of the acidic diet.[22] Patients may therefore be encouraged to follow an alkalinizing diet, low in animal protein and rich in vegetables.

Supplements

Vitamin C and Bioflavonoids

Vitamin C supplementation was once thought to exacerbate gout. Recent data, however, have reversed that belief. Vitamin C most likely decreases serum uric acid levels through competitive binding of proximal tubule uric acid reuptake channels and may also increase uric acid clearance through a modest improvement in global glomerular filtration.[23] Recent studies show an inverse relationship between vitamin C intake and uric acid levels.[24] A double-blind RCT showed supplementation with 500 mg per day of vitamin C significantly lowered uric acid levels compared to placebo, although a later study had conflicting results.[25,26] A 20-year, large prospective study in the *Annals of Internal Medicine* confirmed an inverse relationship between vitamin C intake and the incidence of gout, with as much as a 45% reduced incidence in those ingesting >1500 mg of vitamin C per day.[27]

While it is probable that vitamin C can prevent and aide in the treatment of gout by reducing uric acid levels, there may be an additional benefit conferred by increasing intake of citrus foods and by taking supplements with the citrus bioflavonoid hesperidin. Hesperidin is found in citrus foods as well as plants from the family *Lamiaceae* (mint family), such as the common herb rosemary. An extract of rosemary demonstrated antinociceptive effects in an animal model of gout and hesperidin was identified as a chief contributor to this effect.[28]

> **DOSAGE**
>
> It is recommended that all patients increase their intake of citrus foods. Patients may also consider increasing intake of herbs from the family *Lamiaceae*, especially rosemary. Interested patients should also take 500 to 1500 mg of a high-quality vitamin C with citrus bioflavonoids including hesperidin.
>
> Vitamin C is likely *protective* against gout, though supplementing may not have a dramatic effect on uric acid levels.

Eicosapentaenoic Acid and Gamma-Linolenic Acid

Though purine-rich seafood has been shown to increase uric acid levels and gout,[11] eicosapentaenoic acid (EPA), found in certain fatty fish, and gamma-linolenic acid (GLA) have been shown to suppress inflammation in monosodium urate-induced arthropathies such as gout.[29] EPA and GLA appear to work via complementary mechanisms. Besides decreasing the inflammation of acute gouty arthropathy, omega-3 fatty acids have also demonstrated cardiovascular benefits.[30] This is significant given the association of gout with cardiovascular mortality. In those wishing to avoid the purine intake associated with fish, supplementation with EPA and/or GLA may be encouraged. GLA is an omega-6 fatty acid found in evening primrose oil, borage oil, and black currant seed oil.

DOSAGE

Though the ideal dosing has not been determined, consider supplementing with 500 mg of EPA and/or 3000 mg of evening primrose oil (GLA).

Cherry

Consumption of cherries and cherry juice should be encouraged. Studies indicate that intake of 280 g (two servings) of Bing sweet cherries lowers plasma urate levels and increases urine urate levels in healthy volunteers.[31] There is also a trend toward decreased C-reactive protein and nitric oxide with cherry intake, which suggests that cherries may help inhibit inflammation. Indeed, a double-blind, placebo-controlled trial of cherry juice in long-distance runners showed that those who ingested cherry juice seven days before running reported less postrun pain than those who ingested placebo juice.[32]

DOSAGE

Approximately half-pound of cherries or an equivalent amount of cherry juice consumed daily.

Quercetin

In addition to displaying antiinflammatory properties, the flavonoid quercetin inhibits xanthine oxidase.[33] Quercetin can also play a role in the treatment and prevention of cardiovascular diseases by reducing blood pressure and oxidized low-density lipoprotein.[34] Quercetin may thus be of some clinical use in patients with gout. No human clinical trials have been performed to date, though a study in animals showed a positive effect.[35]

DOSAGE

Food sources of quercetin include onions, apples, berries, grapes, green and black tea, citrus fruits, capers, tomatoes, broccoli, and leafy greens. Encourage adequate intake of these foods. Consider supplementation with up to 500 mg twice daily.

Bromelain

Use of a proprietary bromelain-containing product was clinically equivalent to diclofenac in a double-blind RCT of patients with acute pain from osteoarthritis of the hip.[36] Similar benefits may be conferred to persons with gout, though no studies have yet been performed.

DOSAGE

Encourage daily consumption of pineapple, which is the source of bromelain. Alternatively, supplementation with 500 mg once or twice daily may be considered.

Botanicals

Hibiscus (*H. sabdariffa*)

Hibiscus calyx has mounting evidence demonstrating blood pressure lowering qualities, which are believed to be due to and ACE-inhibitor-like effect.[37] Hibiscus tea increased uric acid excretion and clearance in healthy volunteers but did not affect serum uric acid levels.[38]

DOSAGE

Patients with gout and borderline hypertension may wish to try hibiscus 1.5-g calyx as tea taken two to three times daily. This can be purchased in the bulk herb section of most progressive grocery stores. Hibiscus tea is also readily available in Mexican grocery stores where it is known as "Jamaica."

Physical Medicine

Acupuncture

Acupuncture alone appears to be an effective treatment for acute gouty attacks. A trial of acupuncture versus western treatment with allopurinol and indomethacin found acupuncture to be superior (93% vs. 80% effective, $p < .01$). The acupuncture group also had greater reductions in serum uric acid and fewer adverse effects.[39] This trial was limited due to its small size ($n = 60$) and use of allopurinol during acute attack—a practice which is generally not employed by Western physicians, but is not necessarily contraindicated. Nonetheless, the outcomes were impressive, and given the lack of significant side-effects, acupuncture can be recommended as a viable option for management of acute gouty attacks. Physicians trained in acupuncture may want to try the daily surround treatment, which is similar to the Tendinomuscular meridian treatment described by Dr. Joseph Helms.[40] Referral to a licensed practitioner of traditional Chinese medicine (TCM) may also be considered.

Ice

In contrast to most arthritides, application of ice to inflamed gouty joints causes significant pain relief. Though most arthritic conditions benefit from heat application, patients with gout prefer ice.[41] Frequent use of topical ice during painful attacks should be encouraged. This difference may also help distinguish gout from other inflammatory mimics (e.g., rheumatoid arthritis) and thus help aid in diagnosis.

Response to therapeutic application of ice may help distinguish gout from other inflammatory arthritides.

Rest

Patients will inevitably resist movement of a painful joint, and this should be allowed within reason until symptoms are resolving.

Traditional Chinese Medicine

There are numerous trials of TCM demonstrating clinical effectiveness. A small trial (n = 67) of blood-letting cupping plus Chinese herbs versus a control group of diclofenac found both treatments to be effective in improving acute gouty arthropathy.[42]

The traditional Chinese herbal formulation "Simiao pill" or "Si Miao," which is a combination of herbs commonly used in the treatment of gout, was clinically superior to Western medicine control in a randomized trial of three distinct formulations.[43] Simiao pill traditionally consists of a specific blend of the following individual herbs: *Phellodendron chinense*, *Atractylodes lancea*, *Achyranthes bidentata*, and *Coix lacryma-jobi*. This formulation of Simiao pill was also found to have in vivo uricosuric and nephroprotective effects in hyperuricemic rats.[44]

> **DOSAGE**
>
> Based on specific formulation, generally between three and seven tablets taken three times daily.

Pharmaceuticals: Acute Treatment

Nonsteroidal Antiinflammatory Drugs

Despite the relative lack of high-quality large randomized control trials, nonsteroidal antiinflammatory drugs (NSAIDs) are considered the first-line agents for an acute gouty episode. Indomethacin has historically been favored, but given the lack of data or rationale for its use, any high-dose regimen should suffice.[45]

> **DOSAGE**
>
> Indomethacin 50 mg three times daily, naproxen 500 mg twice daily, or ibuprofen 600 mg three times daily as needed for 5–10 days.
>
> **PRECAUTIONS**
>
> Standard NSAID precautions should be reviewed, and therapy should be tapered as soon as clinical improvement is noted. Aspirin should be avoided due to the potential uric acid raising effect of salicylates.

Colchicine

Alexander of Tralles, a sixth-century Byzantine physician, was the first to use *Colchicum autumnale* for the treatment of gout. Though this plant, autumn crocus, is no longer recommended due to significant toxicity, its active derivative colchicine is still widely used for acute gout attacks, though no head-to-head studies have been conducted to show it offers benefit over any other acute method of treatment. The older methods of hourly high-dose treatments and intravenous colchicine are no longer recommended due to risk of toxicity and unnecessary side effects as well as lack of significant benefit over oral dosing.

> **DOSAGE**
>
> Oral colchicine 1.2 mg followed by 0.6 mg 1 hour later (total dose 1.8 mg), initiated as soon as possible in gouty flair.[46] Some patients may wish to use daily colchicine 0.6 mg for suppression, though use of the other preventive methods should be preferentially encouraged as colchicine has no effect on uric acid.
>
> **PRECAUTIONS**
>
> Do not use in cases of end-stage renal disease. Potentially severe drug–drug interactions do exist. Check specific interactions before prescribing.

Glucocorticoids

Oral, intravenous, or intraarticular steroids may be useful in cases where NSAIDs or colchicine are contraindicated.

> **DOSAGE**
>
> Oral prednisolone 35 mg was equivalent to twice-daily naproxen 500 mg in a double-blind RCT.[47] This dose can be tapered over 7–10 days as clinical improvement ensues. In monoarticular cases, intraarticular injection of 10–40 mg triamcinolone can be effective, although data is limited.[48] Intravenous glucocorticoids can be used in patients unable to take oral prednisone or in polyarticular crisis.
>
> **PRECAUTIONS**
>
> Standard steroid precautions should be observed. Take oral steroids with food as early in the day as possible. If split doses are used, advise taking second dose with lunch rather than dinner to avoid insomnia.

Pharmaceuticals: Prevention

New guidelines were published by the European League Against Rheumatism (EULAR) in 2016. The EULAR guidelines suggest treating to a uric acid target of <5 for severe gout. Otherwise, the goal of treatment should be <6 (Figure 69.3). The American College of Physicians' gout guidelines do not recommend treating to uric acid levels, but simply treating to reduce recurrent flares.[48a,48b]

ACE Inhibitors Versus Diuretics

Although diuretics have been blamed for precipitating many a gouty crisis, their negative effect is actually less than that of hypertension itself.[49] At low doses, thiazide diuretics have a relatively small effect on the serum uric acid levels and addition of an ACE inhibitor or ARB can offset this increase. That being said, the uric

2016 EULAR RECOMMENDATION FOR THE MANAGEMENT OF HYPERURICEMIA IN PATIENTS WITH GOUT

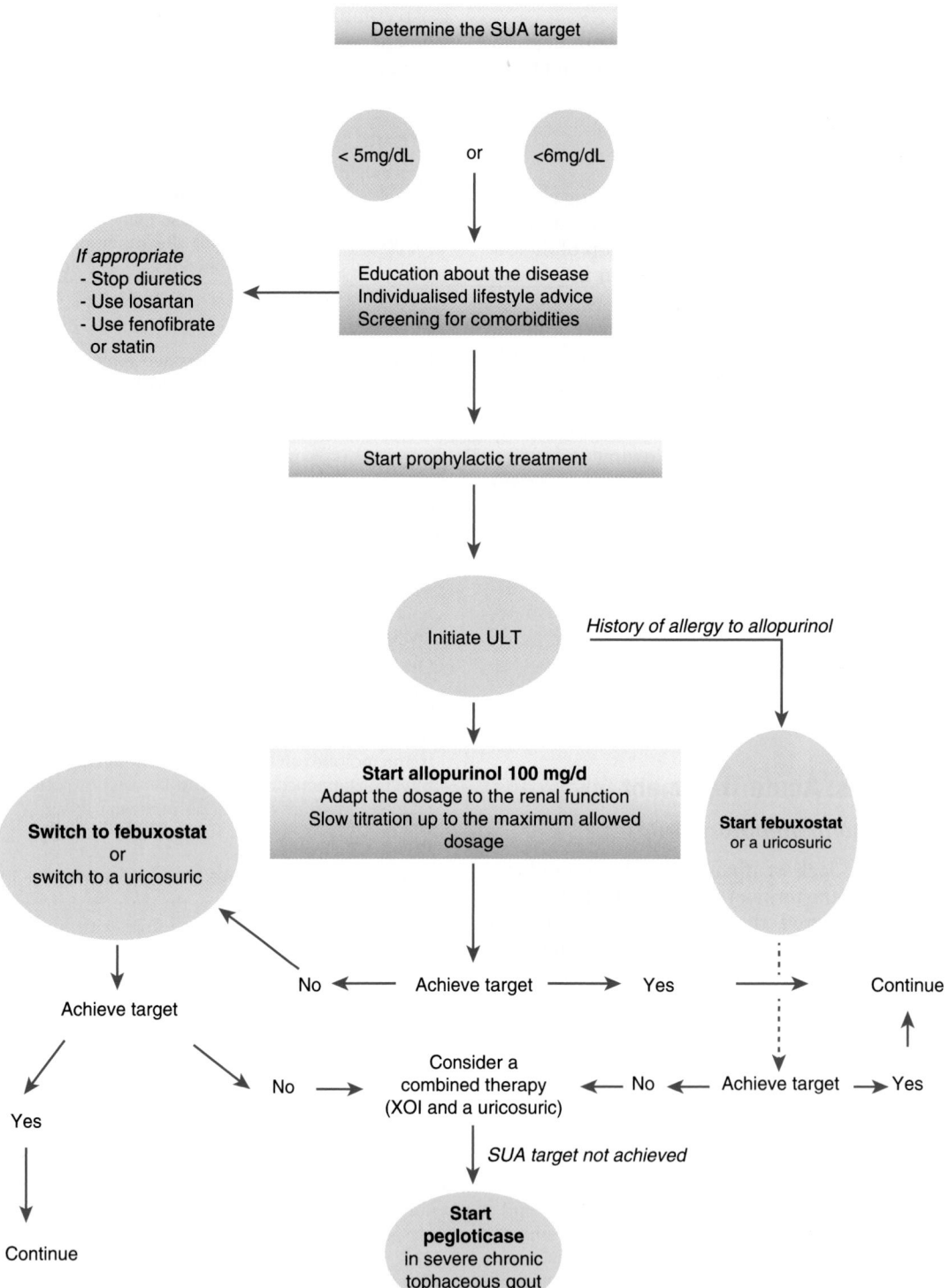

FIG. 69.3 ■ Management of hyperuricaemia in patients with gout according to the European League Against Rheumatism recommendations. At this stage, combined allopurinol and a uricosuric is also recommended. SUA, serum uric acid; ULT, urate-lowering therapy; XOI, xanthine oxidase inhibitor. (From Richette P, et al.: 2016 updated EULAR evidence-based recommendations for the management of gout, *Ann Rheum Dis* 0:1-14, 2016.)

acid–lowering effects of ACE inhibitors may warrant consideration of these as first-line agents for hypertension in patients with gout.

Probenecid

Probenecid is a uricosuric drug and therefore helpful in cases of underexcretion. It is the "gold standard" in elderly patients on thiazide diuretics.[1] Uricosuric agents should be avoided in persons susceptible to nephrolithiasis such as those with tophaceous disease or urate overproduction.

DOSAGE

Starting dose of prebenecid is 250 mg twice daily. Titrate up to effective dose, usually 500–1000 mg twice daily.

PRECAUTIONS

Probenecid is less effective at glomerular filtration rates less than 60 mL/min. Avoid use in persons prone to nephrolithiasis and in those with cystinuria.

Allopurinol

Allopurinol inhibits xanthine oxidase activity. Unlike probenecid, it is useful in all causes of hyperuricemia. Due to theoretical risk, allopurinol is generally not started during an acute attack. Patients on allopurinol should not, however, stop the medicine if an acute attack does occur.

DOSAGE

Allopurinol can be started 100–300 mg daily and titrated up until normal uric acid levels are achieved. Most patients can be adequately treated with 300 mg daily, although the maximum daily dose is 900 mg, and treatment should be titrated to achieve a uric acid level less than 6.[50] To reduce the risk of precipitating a gouty attack, low-dose colchicine may be started simultaneously.[51]

PRECAUTIONS

Up to 5% of patients will experience side effects including rash, leukopenia, thrombocytopenia, diarrhea, or drug fever. The allopurinol hypersensitivity syndrome (AHS) is a rare (less than 0.1% of patients) but potentially fatal adverse reaction consisting of erythematous rash, fever, hepatitis, eosinophilia, and acute renal failure.

Alternatives. Febuxostat is a newer xanthine-oxidase inhibitor that may be used in place of allopurinol.[50] At starting doses, it may be more effective than allopurinol at reducing uric acid levels.[52] However, it is significantly more expensive and does not confer additional benefit if allopurinol is titrated to doses sufficient to achieve target serum uric acid levels.

Titrate urate-lowering therapies to achieve serum uric acid levels less than 6.

Therapies to Consider

Botanicals

There are numerous new ethnobotanical studies of traditional antigout agents, many of which are yielding promising results and confirming the wisdom of indigenous healing systems.

In mice, in vivo trials of the Ayurvedic gout treatments *Coccinia grandis* (Ivy gourd) and *Vitex negundo* (five-leaved chaste tree) demonstrated significant decreases in serum uric acid levels. Impressively, Coccinia grandis in particular showed urate reductions nearly equivalent to those of allopurinol (3.90 +/– 0.07 mg/dL vs. 3.89 +/– 0.07 mg/dL).[53]

Polynesians used noni (*Morinda citrifolia*) juice for treatment of a variety of ailments, including gout. Noni was found to have in vitro inhibition of xanthine oxidase,[54] but no clinical trials have been performed to date.

Populus nigra (black poplar) and *Betula pendula* (Silver Birch) were found to have the highest level of xanthine oxidase inhibition in a study of traditional Czech herbal folk remedies for gout.[55]

In a similar study of 120 traditional Chinese antigout treatments, the following herbs demonstrated the most pronounce xanthine oxidase inhibition: *Cinnamomum cassia* (Chinese cinnamon), *Chrysanthemum indicum*, leaves of *Lycopus europaeus* (bugleweed, gypsywort), and the rhizome of *Polygonum cuspidatum* (Japanese knotweed).[56]

Supplements

In vitro studies have shown folic acid is a weak inhibitor of xanthine oxidase.[57] More potent effects on

---

PREVENTION PRESCRIPTION

- Encourage weight loss and maintenance of a healthy body mass index.
- Decrease consumption of red meat and excessive seafood.
- Increase intake of vegetables, legumes, nuts, and vegetable proteins.
- Decrease intake of sugar-containing beverages and fructose.
- Limit alcohol to no more than one to two drinks per day and drink wine rather than beer or liquor.
- Increase intake of low-fat dairy, up to two servings per day.
- Maintain adequate hydration.
- Consider drinking coffee, one to two cups a day.
- Increase food intake of vitamin C and consider supplementing with 500 mg per day.
- Increase intake of cherries; half-pound per day should be adequate.
- Increase intake of omega-3 fatty acids or take a supplement.

THERAPEUTIC REVIEW

LIFESTYLE MODIFICATION

- Encourage weight loss
- Maintain hydration
- Limit intake of beer and liquor

NUTRITION

- Decrease consumption of red meat and most seafood
- Increase intake of vegetables, legumes, nuts, and vegetable proteins
- Decrease intake of sugar-containing beverages and fructose
- Increase intake of low-fat dairy, up to two servings per day
- Consider coffee, one to two cups a day

SUPPLEMENTS

- Increase intake of vitamin C through foods; consider supplementing with 500 mg daily
- Eat more cherries: up to half-pound daily
- Supplement with EPA and/or GLA: EPA 500 mg daily and/or evening primrose oil 3000 mg daily
- Eat more pineapple or take bromelain supplements 500 mg daily
- Eat more apples, grapes, onions, and tea or take quercetin supplements 500 mg twice daily

BOTANICALS

- Hibiscus tea can be used for borderline blood pressure and may lower uric acid levels

PHYSICAL MEDICINE

- Acupuncture can help relieve a gouty attack
- Ice and rest painful joints

PHARMACEUTICALS

Acute Treatment

- Use NSAIDS for first-line treatment unless contraindications exist
- Consider colchicine, but use only a low-dose regimen: 1.8 mg divided over 1 hour
- Use glucocorticoids in patients unable to take NSAIDs or colchicine

Prevention

- Use probenecid for inadequate uric acid excretion. Start 250 mg twice daily
- Use allopurinol for all causes of uric acid excess. Start 100–300 mg daily
- Titrate urate-lowering therapies to achieve serum uric acid levels less than 6.0

---

inhibition have been traced to the activity of a common folate contaminant pterin aldehyde.[58] Nonetheless, few in vivo trials have been conducted. Daily doses of folate 1000 mcg failed to lower serum uric acid concentrations in five hyperuricemic subjects.[59]

Therefore, we do not recommend that folate be prescribed for gout unless stronger evidence emerges to support its usefulness.

Niacin has a small uric acid-raising effect, which is doubtful to be of negative clinical significance.[60]

Key Web Resources

Good information for both patients and clinicians on the new approach to gout

http://gouteducation.org/

REFERENCES

References are available online at ExpertConsult.com.

CHAPTER 70

CARPAL TUNNEL SYNDROME

Gautam J. Desai, DO, FACOFP • Dennis J. Dowling, DO • Joshua W. Harbaugh, OMSIV

PATHOPHYSIOLOGY

Carpal tunnel syndrome (CTS) is a compressive neuropathy of the median nerve that affects women roughly three times as often as men and usually develops after the age of 30 years.[1,2] Symptoms typically include pain, numbness, tingling, weakness of the thumb and first finger, and involvement of the palm and other fingers except the fifth. Wasting of the thenar eminence may be visible. Activities that may precipitate CTS include repetitive stress activities involving the wrist such as mechanical work, gardening, house painting, meat wrapping, and typing.[3] Trauma, both recent and remote, should be explored, and one of the "keystone" bones of the carpal floor, the lunate, has been implicated in ventral compression of the median nerve against the flexor retinaculum when it is subluxed or displaced.[4] CTS is also commonly seen in persons involved in the occupations listed in Table 70.1.[5,6]

The carpal tunnel contains nine flexor tendons and the median nerve. The tunnel is created by the three sides of the carpal bones and the flexor retinaculum.[7] Any development that leads to tunnel narrowing or increased pressure within the limited space may cause CTS. These conditions may include edema, bony overgrowth, or inflammation of the tendons. The pressure compresses the median nerve and the small blood vessels that feed the nerve, with resulting ischemia and decreased nerve conduction. Initially, the compression and ischemia result in pain, numbness, and tingling. Chronic compression may result in more prolonged symptoms and signs such as weakness and wasting of the thenar eminence.[8,9] Some conditions that may be associated with CTS are listed in Table 70.2.[10,11] At times, the origin may be multifactorial, both functional (overuse) and structural (osteoarthritis).

Clinical Manifestations and Diagnosis

Patients typically present with sensory or motor changes along the distribution of the median nerve, which includes the thumb, index finger, middle finger, and radial half of the ring finger.[8] Sparing of pain and numbness in the thenar eminence is usually seen in CTS as the palmar branch of the median nerve, innervating this region, diverges proximal to the carpal tunnel and travels over the flexor retinaculum, although there are reported cases of concurrent compression of this nerve in CTS.[12,13] Patients may experience greater pain at night or after sleeping. Some patients find relief of symptoms by shaking their hands, which may temporarily relieve ischemia.[14] Pathognomonic physical findings may be absent early in the course of CTS; as pressure increases

within the carpal tunnel, however, patients may demonstrate weakness of the thumb, which causes difficulty with writing or holding objects. Thenar eminence atrophy may be present on physical examination in advanced CTS.[15] Other nerve and vascular compressive syndromes that can cause the same or similar symptoms and signs should also be explored. These disorders can occur separately or concomitantly with CTS in what are known as double-crush and triple-crush syndromes. These syndromes can include cervical root impingement, thoracic outlet syndrome, cubital tunnel syndrome, ulnar neuropathy, pronator syndrome, median nerve neuropathy of the forearm, brachial plexopathy, anterior interosseous nerve syndrome, and Raynaud phenomenom.[16]

The National Institute of Occupational Safety and Health defines CTS as having two or more of the following criteria:

- One or more of the following symptoms affecting at least part of the nerve distribution of the hand: paresthesia, hyperesthesia, pain, and numbness
- One or more of the following symptoms: physical findings of median nerve compression including a positive Hoffman-Tinel sign or a positive Phalen test result, diminished sensation to pinprick in the median nerve distribution, and electrodiagnostic findings indicating median nerve dysfunction across the carpal tunnel.[17]

> The exact location of nerve entrapment can be diagnosed with electrodiagnostic studies; however, results of nerve conduction studies may be normal in clinically symptomatic patients.[18]

INTEGRATIVE THERAPY

Lifestyle

Behavior Modification

Elimination of aggravating factors and repetitive motions may help reduce symptoms of CTS, but many patients do not have the opportunity to change occupations. Patients may obtain some relief by using their hands less forcefully, taking frequent breaks, and performing stretching and strengthening exercises. The practitioner should query the patient about hobbies that require repetitive motion as well, because patients may not associate those hobbies with their symptoms. A wrist splint worn during waking hours may provide additional symptom relief, but most patients cannot tolerate daytime splinting. Occasional use of the same splints while sleeping may also bring about

TABLE 70.1 Occupations Associated With Carpal Tunnel Syndrome

- Food processing
- Manufacturing
- Logging
- Construction work
- Poultry work
- Use of vibratory tools (machine operators)

Data from Bernard B, ed. *Musculoskeletal disorders and work-place factors: a critical review of epidemiologic evidence for work-related musculoskeletal disorders of the neck, upper extremity, and low back.* DHHS (NIOSH) publication no. 97-141. Cincinnati: National Institute for Occupational Safety and Health; 1997. Updated June 6, 2014; Kothari M. *Etiology of carpal tunnel syndrome.* <www.UpToDate.com>; 2014 Accessed May 4, 2015; and Dale AM, Zeringue A, Harris-Adamson C, et al. General population job exposure matrix applied to a pooled study of prevalent carpal tunnel syndrome. *Am J Epidemiol.* 181:431-439, 2015.

TABLE 70.2 Causes of Carpal Tunnel Syndrome

Endocrine	Use of corticosteroids or estrogen
	Myxedema from hypothyroidism
	Amyloidosis
	Gout
	Diabetes mellitus
	Acromegaly
	Obesity
Musculoskeletal	Acute trauma
	Fractures
	Overuse injury
	Inflammatory/rheumatoid arthritis
Pulmonary	Tuberculosis
Reproductive	Pregnancy

Data from Solomon D, Katz J, Bahn R, et al. Nonoccupational risk factors for carpal tunnel syndrome. *J Gen Intern Med.* 14:310-314, 1999; and Stevens J, Beard C, O'Fallon W, et al. Conditions associated with carpal tunnel syndrome. *Mayo Clin Proc.* 67:541-548, 1992.

some relief during the waking hours.[19,20] Splints should be individually adjusted (most have a metal stay within a sleeve on the volar surface) to maintain an angle of the wrist that avoids excessive flexion or extension. One study looked at wrist positioning and resultant pressure within the carpal tunnel, finding that the lowest pressure was in slight extension (2 +/– 9 degrees) and ulnar deviation (2 +/– 6 degrees).[21] Many braces available off the shelf place the wrist into too high a degree of extension.

Exercise

A 10-month aerobic exercise program demonstrated a reduction in symptoms of CTS, but whether these results were related to the natural course of the disease or to the therapy is unclear.[22] Although performing aerobic activity for cardiovascular health is certainly in the patient's best interests, such exercise has not been proven to be of benefit for CTS treatment, so no evidence supports its

use. Stretching of the flexor tendons, the major occupants of the tunnel, may have some benefit in reducing compression of the median nerve (see Fig. 70.2).

Ergonomic Keyboards

Results of studies comparing the use of ergonomic keyboards for amelioration of symptoms of CTS have been mixed.[23,24] One small study (*N* = 37) confirmed swelling and changes in the median nerve after 30 minutes and 60 minutes of typing; however, the changes resolved after a period of rest, thus only offering speculation of a link between keyboarding and CTS while also not addressing long-term symptoms.[25] If a patient believes that using such a keyboard will help, it may be worth the higher price to try the device to determine if it has no adverse effects. No evidence exists for its use. The position in which patients place their hands may have more to do with effectiveness than the keyboards themselves. Patients should avoid resting their wrists on the surface while extending their wrists to reach their fingers to the keyboard. Pianists and touch typists classically hover their hands above their respective keyboards.

Pharmaceuticals

Acetaminophen

Acetaminophen has a limited role in CTS owing to a lack of its antiinflammatory properties. Acetaminophen appears to display analgesic and antipyretic effects by inhibiting the isoenzymes cyclooxygenase-1 (COX-1) and cyclooxygenase-2 (COX-2) in the central nervous system. This inhibition does not seem to extend into the periphery, thereby eliminating any antiinflammatory properties.[26] However, because it has a relatively safe profile, acetaminophen remains a good choice for relief of mild to moderate pain in CTS, especially in patients who have concomitant osteoarthritis.

DOSAGE (ADULT)

The recommended dose of acetaminophen (Tylenol) is 500 mg every 4–6 hours; the maximum dose is 3000 mg/day.[27]

PRECAUTIONS

Acetaminophen should be used with caution in patients with a history of liver disease and in patients who consume more than three alcoholic beverages daily.[28] In addition, consideration should be given to the appropriate dosage of acetaminophen when patients are taking other concomitant medications that are similarly metabolized by the liver. At recommended dosages, acetaminophen is considered safe in pregnancy.

Nonsteroidal Antiinflammatory Drugs

Median nerve compression caused by inflammation of the flexor tenosynovium can cause patients a great deal of pain.[29] Nonsteroidal antiinflammatory drugs (NSAIDs) exert pain-relieving and antiinflammatory properties through prostaglandin inhibition

TABLE 70.3 **Common Nonsteroidal Antiinflammatory Drugs Used for Pain Relief**

Generic Name	Brand Name[a]	Recommended Adult Dose	Route	Maximum Daily Dose
Aspirin	Bayer Aspirin	325–650 mg every 4–6 h	Oral or rectal	3600 mg
Salsalate	Salflex	500–1000 mg every 8–12 h	Oral	3000 mg
Ibuprofen	Motrin and Advil	200–400 mg every 4–6 h	Oral	2400 mg
Diflunisal	Dolobid	500–1000 mg every 12 h	Oral	1500 mg
Choline magnesium	Tricosal	500–1000 mg every 8–12 h	Oral	3000 mg salicylate
Naproxen sodium	Aleve and Anaprox	220–550 mg every 8–12 h	Oral	1500 mg
Naproxen	Naprosyn	250–500 mg every 12 h	Oral	1500 mg
Ketoprofen	Orudis KT	12.5 mg every 6–8 h; second dose may be taken after 1 h if needed	Oral	75 mg
Fenoprofen	Nalfon	300–600 mg every 6–8 h	Oral	3200 mg
Flurbiprofen	Ansaid	200–300 mg in 2–4 divided doses	Oral	300 mg
Oxaprozin	Daypro	600–1200 mg/day	Oral	1800 mg
Indomethacin	Indocin and Indocin SR	25–50 mg, 2–3 times/day	Oral	200 mg
Diclofenac	Voltaren	50 mg every 8 hours; 75 mg every 12 h	Oral	150 mg
Etodolac	Lodine	200–400 mg every 6–8 h	Oral	1200 mg
Nabumetone	Relafen	500–1000 mg, 1–2 times/day	Oral	2000 mg
Meloxicam	Mobic	7.5 mg/day	Oral	15 mg
Piroxicam	Feldene	10–20 mg/day	Oral	20 mg

[a]More than one brand may exist for an agent.
Data from references 18, 19, and 22.

by inhibition of COX-1 and COX-2 isoenzymes.[28] In general, all NSAIDs have similar efficacy regarding analgesia and antiinflammatory effects. However, these effects remain to be proven adequate for control of symptoms of CTS, despite common use of NSAIDs in the treatment of this condition. In a study comparing the efficacy of NSAIDs, oral steroids, diuretics, and placebo, only steroids achieved a significant improvement in signs and symptoms of CTS.[30]

DOSAGE

Common NSAIDs and dosages are listed in Table 70.3.

PRECAUTIONS

NSAIDs must be used with caution in patients with a history of gastrointestinal bleeding, ulcers or perforation, hypertension or other cardiac disorders aggravated by fluid retention, asthma, renal insufficiency, or coagulation defects, as well as in pregnant patients.[26,28,31]

Diuretics

A rise in tissue pressure in the carpal tunnel is theorized to lead to perineural edema.[32] Diuretic therapy has been employed in efforts to rid the body of excess fluid accumulation and ameliorate CTS. Although case reports exist regarding successful use of furosemide to alleviate symptoms of CTS associated with iatrogenic fluid administration, larger comparative studies refute the

benefit of diuretic use in CTS.[33] In a study comparing bendrofluazide (a thiazide diuretic not available in the United States) with placebo, no improvements in CTS symptoms were seen.[23] Diuretics should not be used in treatment of CTS.

Corticosteroids

The human body endogenously produces glucocorticoids. At supraphysiological doses of exogenous corticosteroids, an antiinflammatory response is seen. Modified cellular transcription and protein synthesis lead to local inhibition of leukotriene penetration, suppression of the humoral response, and a reduction in lipocortins, thus diminishing the inflammatory response.[28] In CTS, corticosteroids may offer relief and can be given orally or directly injected into the carpal canal.[9] Short-term oral steroid therapy with conventional treatment, such as splinting, has reduced symptoms in patients with CTS. In a study comparing the use of NSAIDs, diuretics, oral steroids, and placebo, only the group receiving oral prednisolone demonstrated significant relief of CTS symptoms.[30]

Corticosteroid injection, administered on the radial side of the palmaris longus tendon, has shown short-term efficacy in providing CTS symptom relief.[34,35] In a study comparing surgical decompression with local steroid injection, patients receiving steroid injections had better symptom relief 3 months after treatment than patients who had undergone surgery. At 6 months and 12 months, however, the percentage of patients in whom relief of symptoms was maintained after injection began to decline, whereas the level of relief in the surgically treated group remained constant.[35] Steroid injections are most beneficial to patients with mild to moderate CTS, thus delaying the need for surgery. Injection may be repeated 3 weeks after the initial dose, but the need for a third dose in less than 1 year indicates a need for surgical treatment.[34]

DOSAGE

A standard dosage for oral steroids in CTS has not been determined. A study comparing two prednisolone regimens—2 weeks of 20 mg/day followed by 2 weeks of 10 mg/day versus 2 weeks of 20 mg/day followed by 2 weeks of placebo—for long-term improvement found no difference in treatment response with respect to the duration of steroid therapy.[36] Hence, the lower dosage should be used to minimize adverse effects.

Injection therapy consists of methylprednisolone acetate, 40 to 80 mg mixed with 1 mL of 1% lidocaine,[37] or 6 mg of betamethasone combined with 1% lidocaine.[35]

PRECAUTIONS

Long-term oral steroid use has been associated with immunosuppression, hyperglycemia, hypertension, Cushing syndrome, osteoporosis, and electrolyte disturbances. Injection of steroids must be performed by a skilled practitioner trained in CTS injection to avoid nerve atrophy and necrosis, which may be created by entry of corticosteroid into the median nerve sheath.[28,31,34] The use of corticosteroids in pregnancy is controversial. Although drug monographs indicate corticosteroids to be relatively safe in pregnancy (safety category B), animal studies have indicated possible long-term developmental abnormalities. More research using corticosteroids during pregnancy is needed.[38]

Botanicals

Patients using dietary supplements should be advised to choose brands that have been certified for content and purity. Testing for content and purity is not a mandatory requirement for dietary supplements. Trusted organizations that voluntarily test product purity are the United States Pharmacopeia (USP), the Association of Analytical Communities (AOAC), and Consumer Labs (consumerlabs.com). Table 70.4 provides a list of sample USP-verified brands.[41]

TABLE 70.4	United States Pharmacopeia–Verified Brands

- Berkley & Jensen
- Kirkland Signature
- Nature Made
- Tru Nature

Data from United States Pharmacopeia. *USP-verified dietary supplements.* <http://www.usp.org/USPVerified/dietarySupplements/supplements.html/>; Accessed May 4, 2015.

Ginger *(Zingiber officinale)*

Ginger, also known as *African ginger*, *black ginger*, *cochin ginger*, and *imber*, is a mixture of several compounds, which include gingeroles, beta-carotene, capsaicin, caffeine, curcumin, and salicylate.[42] However, these chemical entities seem to vary according to the form of the herb. Ginger is most often used for relief of nausea, vomiting, motion sickness, dyspepsia, flatulence, migraine headache, rheumatoid arthritis, osteoarthritis, and pain. Although the exact mechanism remains unknown, investigators have speculated that some of the constituents in ginger may inhibit COX-1, COX-2, lipoxygenase pathways, tumor necrosis factor-alpha, prostaglandin E2, and thromboxane B2.[43] Each of these inhibited mechanisms plays a role in inflammation. A randomized, placebo-controlled, crossover study was conducted comparing the efficacy of ginger, ibuprofen, and placebo in patients with osteoarthritis. Although ibuprofen was found to be the most effective at treating pain, both ibuprofen and ginger had a significant pain-rating reduction in comparison with placebo.[44] Ginger may be of benefit in patients who have both CTS and osteoarthritis. Patients with nausea and vomiting of pregnancy and CTS may benefit from the antinausea properties of ginger as well.

DOSAGE

In osteoarthritis management, Eurovita Extract 33, a specific ginger extract, is often used. The dosage of this formulation is 170 mg orally three times daily or 255 mg twice daily.[43]

PRECAUTIONS

Because of possible inhibition of platelet aggregation, ginger should be used with caution in patients who are concurrently undergoing anticoagulant therapy or have coagulation disorders. Common adverse reactions with ginger are gastrointestinal discomfort, heartburn, and diarrhea. The use of ginger during pregnancy is relatively safe when it is orally ingested for medicinal purposes. Although some concerns have been expressed about ginger and its involvement in altering fetal sex hormones, and one case report of a spontaneous abortion exists, the overall risk of fetal malformation does not appear to be higher than the baseline (1%–3%).[43]

Willow Bark *(Salix alba)*

Willow bark, also known as white willow bark, brittle willow, and simply willow, is a dietary supplement from the Salicaceae family. It is most often used by patients to treat headache or pain caused by osteoarthritis, myalgia, gout, and dysmenorrhea. Although components of willow bark include flavonoids and tannins, its pain-relieving properties are attributed to the salicin glycosides present in the compound. After ingestion of willow bark, the salicin glycosides are converted in the intestine to saligenin, which is then metabolized to produce salicylic acid. At this point, elimination becomes the same as for aspirin (acetylsalicylic acid).[43] As with aspirin, willow bark demonstrates analgesic, antipyretic, and antiinflammatory properties. Platelet aggregation may be inhibited by willow bark, but to a lesser extent than by aspirin. Studies comparing willow bark, diclofenac, and placebo in patients with osteoarthritis and rheumatoid arthritis found willow bark to be no better than placebo for pain relief.[45] Although no studies have evaluated willow bark use for CTS, this substance can be regarded as having efficacy similar to that of aspirin and other NSAIDs in pain management.

DOSAGE

Willow bark should be dosed according to the salicin content in the supplement: salicin, 120–240 mg orally in two to three divided doses daily.[43]

PRECAUTIONS

Safety concerns about using willow bark are similar to those for salicylate therapy. Willow bark may cause gastric irritation, nausea, vomiting, and bloody stools. It should be used with caution in patients who are also taking antiplatelet medications or other salicylate-containing products. Insufficient evidence exists for using willow bark in pregnancy. Pregnant women are advised to avoid it.

Arnica (Arnica montana)

Also known as arnica flower, leopard's bane, and mountain tobacco, arnica is used to treat inflammation and as an immune system stimulant. The boost in immune response is thought to decrease healing time in bruises, aches, and sprains. The primary active constituents in arnica are sesquiterpene lactones.[43] Although the exact mechanisms are not completely understood, the antiinflammatory effects seen with arnica seem to differ mechanistically from those of NSAIDs. A specific sesquiterpene lactone, helenalin (which is implicated in inflammation), inhibits nuclear transcription factor NF-kappaB.[46] Helenalin has also been shown to inhibit platelet function. In a randomized, placebo-controlled study using arnica to control pain and swelling in patients who had undergone surgical repair of CTS, no difference in swelling was seen in patients receiving arnica and in those receiving placebo. However, a significant reduction in pain was seen 2 weeks after surgery in patients receiving arnica.[47] Arnica may be useful in patients who have undergone surgical treatment for CTS, but the potential side effects and toxicity, as well as the difficulty in obtaining standardized doses, may be obstacles to its use.

DOSAGE

Unless diluted, arnica is toxic when taken by mouth. Although no standard or well-studied doses or arnica preparations are available, the usual homeopathic preparations are diluted to 1:10 and 1:100 strengths. Serial dilutions continue until the desired strength is reached. For example, a 1:100 solution that is diluted 30 times is said to be 30C potency.[47] Caution should be exercised because of the difficulty in obtaining a standardized dose and the possible side effects.

PRECAUTIONS

Arnica in homeopathic doses is generally safe.

Arnica belongs to the Asteraceae/Compositae family. Patients allergic to other members of this family will also be allergic to arnica. Additional members of the Asteraceae/Compositae family include ragweed, chrysanthemums, marigolds, daisies, and many other herbs.[43]

Supplements

Vitamin B₆ (Pyridoxine)

Vitamin B_6 is required by the body for many functions, including metabolism of amino acids, carbohydrates, and lipids. Vitamin B_6 is also a coenzyme in various metabolic reactions, such as transamination of amino acids, conversion of tryptophan to niacin, synthesis of gamma-aminobutyric acid, metabolism of serotonin, norepinephrine, and dopamine, and the production of heme for hemoglobin. It is also required in myelin sheath formation.[43] Clinically, vitamin B_6 is used to offset neuropathy caused by certain medications, such as isoniazid. Vitamin B_6 was first thought to be an effective treatment in CTS on the basis of low tissue levels seen in deceased patients with CTS. Investigators now know, however, that pyridoxine levels decline in deceased or infarcted tissue.[43] Two studies involving a total of 50 subjects with CTS demonstrated no benefit for vitamin B_6 in comparison with placebo.[48]

Mild deficiencies in vitamin B_6 are relatively common. Sources of this vitamin include potatoes, milk, cheese, eggs, fish, carrots, spinach, and peas. Vitamin B_6 is useful in treating general deficiency and neuritis. Patients with CTS receiving benefit from pyridoxine therapy are thought to have an underlying deficiency or neuropathy. More studies are needed to assess the effectiveness of vitamin B_6 in CTS, but the supplement may be useful in patients with an underlying deficiency.

DOSAGE

For vitamin B_6 deficiency, 2.5–25 mg/day orally is taken for 3 weeks, with a maintenance dose of 1.5–2.5 mg/day thereafter. For neuritis, the dose is 10–50 mg/day orally.[43]

The U.S. Recommended Dietary Allowance (RDA) values for vitamin B_6 are as follows:
- Men: 19–50 years old, 1.3 mg; 51 years old and older, 1.7 mg
- Women: 19–50 years old, 1.3 mg; 51 years old and older, 1.5 mg. Some researchers think that the RDA for women 19–50 years old should be increased to 1.5–1.7 mg.
- Pregnant women: 1.9 mg; lactating women: 2 mg.[43]

PRECAUTIONS

Adverse reactions associated with vitamin B_6 therapy include abdominal pain, nausea, vomiting, increased serum aspartate aminotransferase values, and decreased serum folic acid concentrations. This vitamin has been shown to cause sensory neuropathy at doses exceeding 1000 mg. It should be used with caution in patients concurrently taking phenytoin, phenobarbital, or levodopa. Pyridoxine may increase the metabolism of these drugs and thereby reduce the plasma levels of phenytoin, phenobarbital, or levodopa.

Biomechanical Therapy

Massage Therapy

A small study ($N = 16$) showed a short-term benefit of pain reduction and functionality improvement in patients treated with four weekly massages by a therapist (not further defined) as well as daily self-massage.[49] The type of massage described resembled pétrissage and effleurage-type stroking and was focused on the hand and forearm. No group received sham massage, so whether the benefits resulted from direct action of the massage on the carpal tunnel and surrounding tissues to mobilize fluid or from neurotransmitter release in the central nervous system is unclear. Because teaching a patient to massage his or her own hand and forearm has minimal cost, a trial of this modality may be of benefit.

Yoga

In another small study, a group of patients taking part in a highly individualized and methodical yoga program (Iyengar approach) demonstrated significant reduction in pain and significant improvement in grip strength compared with a control group offered a wrist splint in addition to continuation of the current treatment.[50] No significant difference was reported in the median nerve motor and sensory conduction time between the two groups. The yoga regimen, for which the group met twice weekly for 8 weeks, was designed to focus on improving strength and balance in each joint in the upper body, and it also covered a relaxation technique. Although a larger study with long-term follow-up is needed, yoga may be an option for patients who are able to afford such a program, as well as for those who may be unable or unwilling to use other approaches or treatment options for CTS.

Physical Therapy and Occupational Therapy Modalities

Wrist Splinting. Splints that prevent excessive flexion or extension of the wrist are inexpensive options shown to be moderately effective in the treatment of CTS and should be a first-line choice for most patients with mild to moderate CTS.[51,52] Although full-time splint use may produce better results, most patients generally do not tolerate daytime use of the appliance, thus nighttime splinting is recommended. Splints that keep the wrist in a neutral position may be more beneficial than those placing the wrist in extension. Patients should try a noncustom orthotic first, which is less expensive than the custom-fitted counterpart. Generally, negative effects are not associated with splint use, other than the initial discomfort of wearing a new appliance. Splinting may be used in combination with other therapies. Commonly splints, along with stretches, are utilized, and one study revealed a 4-week trial of a nighttime cock-up splint along with lumbrical intensive stretches improved symptoms and function in CTS compared to other splinting and stretching regimens.[53] Another study demonstrated splinting to be superior to steroid injection of the carpal tunnel in patients with mild and moderate CTS, in terms of both symptomatic relief and

improvements in sensory and motor nerve conduction velocities.[54] These results were obtained with near-nightly use of the splint for 1 year, a regularity and duration that may be more difficult to obtain in a nonstudy patient population. Patients in whom CTS is unresponsive to this therapy after 3 weeks of use must be reexamined; in addition, patients with thenar wasting on initial presentation may benefit from another treatment modality. Pregnant patients may be especially good candidates for splinting.

Ultrasound Therapy. Ultrasound therapy may benefit patients with mild to moderate CTS, although the cost and frequency of treatments may be a barrier. One study demonstrated an improvement in symptoms and motor distal latency in wrists receiving ultrasound treatment that was not seen in wrists receiving sham ultrasound.[55] The investigators postulated that the antiinflammatory and tissue-stimulating effects of ultrasound could be responsible for the results. However, studies are limited and more research is required.[56] Long-term benefits of ultrasound therapy are unknown.

Osteopathic Manipulative Treatment

Randomized controlled studies of osteopathic manipulative treatment (OMT) for the treatment of CTS are scarce. Palpatory examination was noted to be 92% sensitive, but only 75% specific, when compared with electrodiagnostic studies for determining CTS.[58] However, cadaver studies demonstrated an elongation of the transverse carpal ligament after treatment with OMT (nonthrust techniques designed to stretch the transverse carpal ligament) directed at the wrist, in conjunction with static loading (weights).[59,60] Whether these results may be applied to living patients remains to be seen, although animal studies have shown minimal change in postmortem biomechanical properties of ligaments after freezing.[61,62] Thus, these findings may possibly be relevant. The female cadaver wrists tended to be smaller and had greater elongation of the transverse carpal ligament, especially when OMT was done first, followed by static loading.

Osteopathic physicians practice many specialties, and many serve as primary care physicians and can easily perform OMT in the office, as shown in Fig. 70.1, during the first presentation of the complaint. The patient can be instructed in self-stretching exercises (shown in Fig. 70.2), which can be done at home at no cost and often with increasing relief of symptoms. One small study ($N = 16$ wrists) demonstrated a reduction in symptoms with OMT,[63] and another reported magnetic resonance imaging evidence that OMT and self-stretching enlarged transverse and anteroposterior dimensions of the carpal canal.[64] However, three of the four patients undergoing this treatment had symptoms of CTS after trauma, which may respond differently than CTS from other causes, such as repetitive motion. A quasi-single blinded pilot study revealed statistically significant improvements in symptoms and function on a self-reported pain scale specific to CTS, the Boston Carpal Tunnel Syndrome Questionnaire

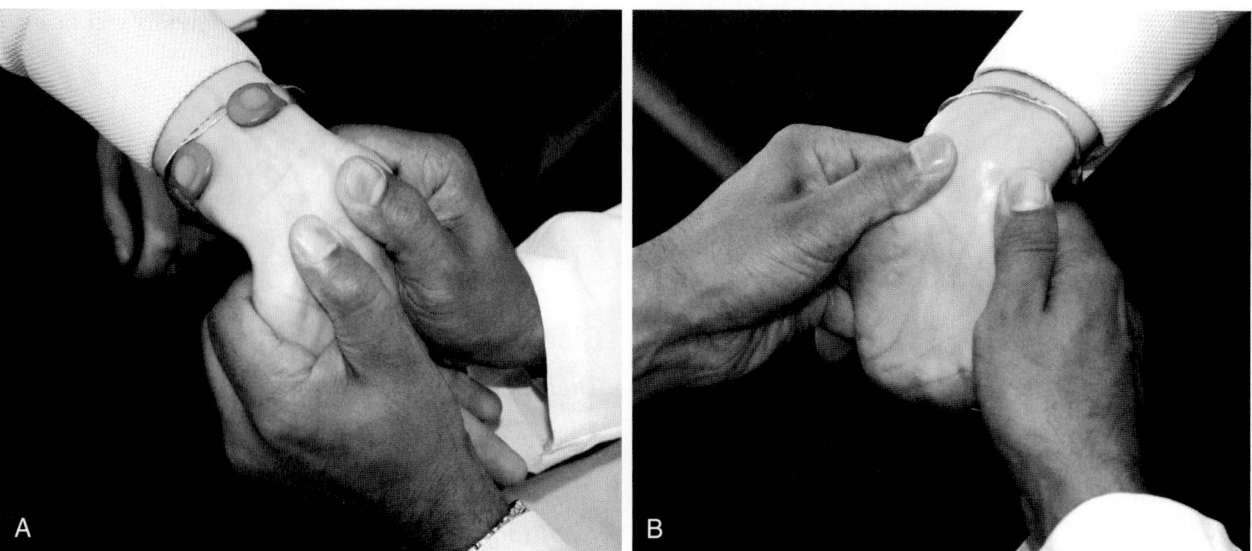

FIG. 70.1 ■ A, The physician's thumbs apply pressure away from the center of the wrist, while the fingers below simultaneously apply an upward force to create a spreading effect. B, Once an initial stretch has been achieved and held, the physician can then gently extend the patient's wrist farther (by pushing patient's fingers with his or her knee) and create more of a spread by moving his or her thumbs farther away from the center of the wrist. The goal is to increase the length of the transverse carpal ligament and widen the carpal canal, thereby reducing the amount of pressure on the median nerve. (From Sucher BM. Myofascial release of carpal tunnel syndrome. *J Am Osteopath Assoc.* 93:92-101, 1993.)

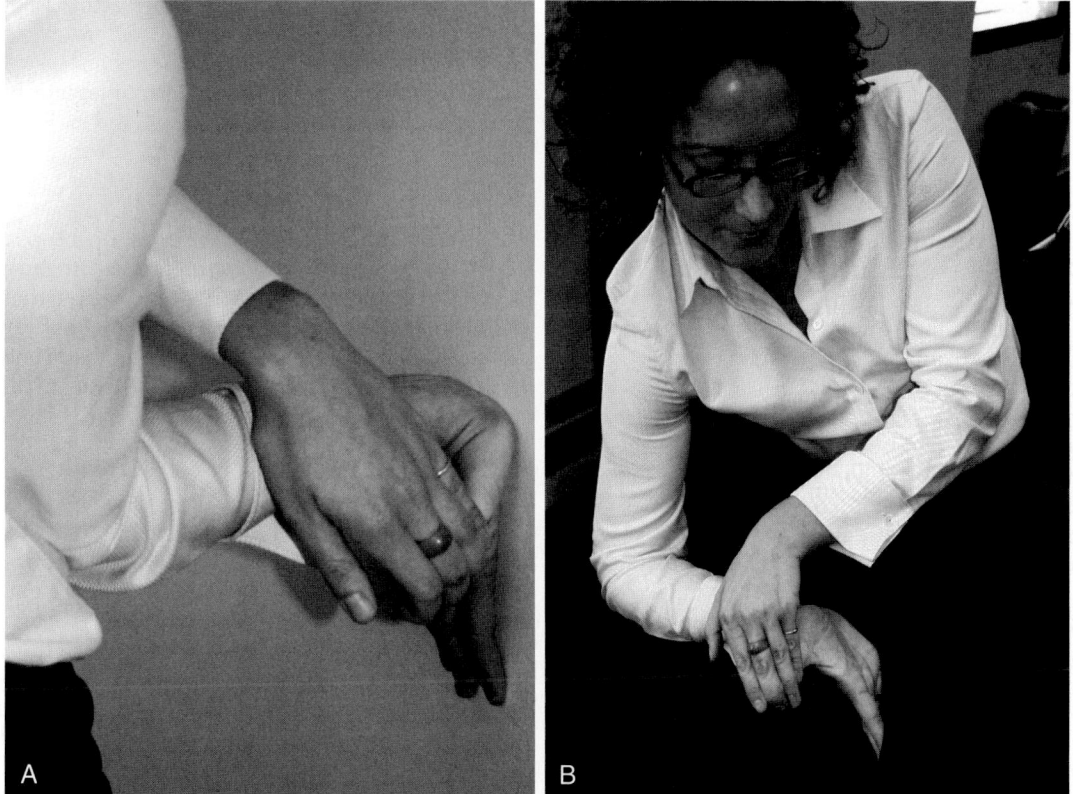

FIG. 70.2 ■ A, The patient is instructed to stand near a wall, place the affected hand's palm flat against the wall (fingertips down), and, with the other hand, add a downward force to the thumb of the affected hand. With this maneuver, the elbow is compressed by pressure from the iliac crest, and the pressure can be gently increased as stretching occurs. B, The patient can also perform a similar technique while seated, by placing the palm (fingertips down) on the inside of one thigh and the olecranon process on the other side and then bringing the legs together as the free hand exerts downward pressure on the thumb. The patient should be taught this stretching maneuver in the office and should perform it 5 to 10 times a day. (Adapted from Sucher B. Myofascial manipulative release of carpal tunnel syndrome: documentation with magnetic resonance imaging. *J Am Osteopath Assoc.* 93:1273-1278, 1993.)

(BCTQ), after 6 weeks of OMT (F = 11.0; p = .004). The improvements tended to be more pronounced on the treated side. There was also a decrease in symptom-specific diagramming scores after 6 weeks of treatment, and this was also statistically significant (F = 4.19; p = .0002). The patient estimate of overall improvement of symptoms was statistically significant for the treated side. No statistically significant changes in electrophysiological function of the median nerve, cross-sectional area of the median nerve, or transverse carpal ligament bowing were observed. The transverse carpal ligament length was increased in length following the treatment period and was also statistically significant, but no side-to-side difference was detected. The authors concluded that OMT resulted in patient-perceived improvement in symptoms and functions associated with CTS. However, median nerve function as measured by electrophysiological studies and the morphology at the carpal tunnel did not change, possibly indicating a different mechanism by which OMT had been effective.[65] Large randomized trials including sham OMT are needed before OMT can be clearly stated as being beneficial for CTS. However, given the low risk of adverse events with OMT, as well as the low cost, a patient can be treated by a combination of approaches, including self-stretching and wrist splints. Before more invasive approaches (i.e., injection, surgery) are considered, a trial of OMT may be of benefit. Additionally, the holistic philosophy of osteopathic medicine mandates taking into account the person as a whole, considers other potential aggravating factors, and seeks ways to reduce or remove these factors.

Surgery

The three basic types of surgical procedures for carpal tunnel release, all of which attempt to visualize and cut the transverse carpal ligament, are as follows:
- Traditional open (approximately a 5-cm incision)
- Mini-open (approximately a 2.5-cm incision)
- Endoscopic (one or two portals)

Relief of symptoms is similar with all three types, but patients undergoing endoscopic surgery performed by an experienced surgeon will likely return to work sooner than those undergoing traditional open surgery.[8] A 2005 randomized controlled trial demonstrated open surgery to be superior in terms of symptom relief, but not grip strength, compared with a single steroid injection for CTS over a 20-week period.[66] Although most patients report satisfaction with surgical outcomes, some caveats apply:
- Hand strength may take months to recover.
- The surgical scar site may be tender for up to a year after the operation.
- Attorney involvement (in cases of Workers' Compensation) may predict a worse surgical outcome.[67]

Before considering surgical intervention, one must carefully rule out reversible causes of CTS, and referral to a specialist to be certain of the diagnosis may be warranted. Patients with mild CTS symptoms should especially be made aware of the risks and benefits of surgery. Pregnant patients should not be considered candidates for CTS surgery because their symptoms will probably improve after delivery.

> If surgical intervention is being considered, the patient should be referred to a surgeon experienced in carpal tunnel syndrome and should undergo electromyography before the surgical procedure to be certain of the diagnosis.

Bioenergetics

Therapeutic Touch

Therapeutic touch has not been shown to be better than sham therapeutic touch in the treatment of CTS.[68]

Traditional Acupuncture

Although the National Institutes of Health issued a consensus statement supporting the use of acupuncture in the treatment of CTS,[69] randomized controlled trials are required.[70] In 2004, the modality was approved as a treatment for CTS in Massachusetts for Workers' Compensation cases. Acupuncture may be regarded as an adjunct to other therapies or as an alternative to surgery for mild cases of CTS. One barrier is the cost of acupuncture.

Laser Acupuncture

Laser acupuncture is probably not of benefit in the treatment of CTS.[23]

Traditional Chinese Medicine

A retrospective, single-case series of 11 patients with CTS who were treated with jackyakamcho-tang (shaoyaogancao-tang), an herbal formulation that has been used for spasmodic muscles and pain in Eastern countries, demonstrated an analgesic effectiveness of approximately 72%.[70] However, this study had many limitations, and approximately 11% of the patients treated also had adverse effects.

Therapies to Consider

Many models of health care outside the traditional Western model likely offer beneficial treatments for many ailments of the Western world, such as CTS. Some involve a detailed and highly individualized assessment of the patient, and treatment is often multifaceted, with a combination of products (traditional Chinese medicine) that are not easily found or identified in the United States without some advanced knowledge. Ayurvedic medicine, for example, takes into account a balance of the life energies as well as the constitution of the individual, and the treatment offered varies from patient to patient, thus making it difficult to perform randomized controlled trials to study its effects. As we continue a push toward evidence-based medicine, potential therapies for CTS treatment and other disorders will emerge.

PREVENTION PRESCRIPTION

- Avoid repetitive hand motions, especially those with forceful thrusting.
- Avoid prolonged gripping.
- Avoid prolonged positioning of the wrist in extremes of flexion or extension.
- Avoid gripping vibrating workplace tools for a prolonged time.

- Avoid isolated finger motions, such as typing, for a prolonged time.
- Schedule rest and stretching breaks every 1–2 hours.

THERAPEUTIC REVIEW

If a patient presents with mild to moderate symptoms of carpal tunnel syndrome (CTS), has no thenar flattening, and has had symptoms for less than 1 year, a stepwise approach is appropriate. Most therapies can be combined with nighttime splinting. If a patient has unrelenting numbness or pain or a history of symptoms lasting longer than 1 year, a thorough examination should be conducted to ensure a correct diagnosis, and then referral to a surgeon specializing in CTS release may be the most appropriate therapy.

If a patient presents with thenar atrophy, this indicates long-standing neurological compromise, so more aggressive diagnostic and therapeutic options should be given priority.

LIFESTYLE CHANGES

- Have the patient reduce activities that bring on symptoms.
- Take frequent breaks to rest hands.
- Perform stretching or strengthening exercises for the hands (see Fig. 70.2).

SPLINT THERAPY

- The patient should wear a splint as often as possible, even during the day if tolerated.
- Start with a rigid over-the-counter appliance first, ensuring proper fit and prevention of wrist flexion.
- Better results may be achieved with the wrist held in neutral position rather than extended.
- Reconsider therapy if no benefit is seen after 3 weeks.

YOGA

- A patient who is willing to try yoga, despite the cost of an individualized program, may see some benefit from it.

GINGER

- The dose of eurovita extract 33 is 170 mg three times daily or 255 mg twice daily.
- Ginger may be of benefit in patients with both osteoarthritis and CTS, as well as in pregnant patients with CTS and nausea or vomiting.
- Ginger should be used with caution in patients taking anticoagulants.

OSTEOPATHIC MANIPULATIVE TREATMENT

- Osteopathic manipulative treatment (OMT) can be done in combination with other therapies.

- In addition to OMT in the office (see Fig. 70.1), patients can do self-stretching exercises at home (see Fig. 70.2) 5 to 10 times daily until symptom resolution or for 2–3 weeks, at which point reassessment is warranted if no improvement has occurred.

ORAL STEROIDS

- Prednisolone is taken at 20 mg/day for 2 weeks.
- The use of steroids in pregnancy is controversial.

STEROID INJECTION

- Injection of methylprednisolone acetate, 40 mg mixed with 1 mL of 1% lidocaine, into the carpal canal by a physician trained in this procedure may offer some relief of symptoms. It may also delay the need for surgery.
- Use of more than three doses in 1 year suggests a need for surgical intervention.

ULTRASOUND

- Although costly and time consuming, ultrasound may be beneficial in patients with mild to moderate CTS. It can be combined with splint therapy, OMT, or medications.

TRADITIONAL ACUPUNCTURE

- Acupuncture can be used as a possible alternative to surgery for mild CTS.
- It may be costly and is usually not covered by medical insurance.

SURGERY

- Surgery is likely most useful for patients with unrelenting pain or numbness, thenar atrophy, or treatment failure with other modalities.
- The clinician must be certain of the diagnosis and must choose a surgeon who has performed many CTS procedures.
- Referral to a CTS specialist for evaluation is recommended before surgery is suggested to the patient.
- Surgery is not advised for pregnant patients with CTS, which will probably resolve with delivery.
- Indications for surgery are unrelenting pain, thenar eminence atrophy, loss of motor function with diminished finger strength, and failure of other treatments.

Key Web Resources

National Institute of Neurological Disorders and Stroke, National Institutes of Health carpal tunnel syndrome (CTS) fact sheet: Fact sheet and information page touching on diagnoses, etiology, and treatments	http://www.ninds.nih.gov/disorders/carpal_tunnel/detail_carpal_tunnel.htm
MedicineNet article on CTS: A comprehensive and patient-friendly site referencing and explaining CTS	http://www.medicinenet.com/carpal_tunnel_syndrome/article.htm
American Society of Surgery for the Hand information on CTS: Information on surgical treatment of CTS	http://www.assh.org/handcare/hand-arm-conditions/carpal-tunnel/

REFERENCES

References are available online at ExpertConsult.com.

CHAPTER 71

EPICONDYLOSIS

David Rabago, MD • Sarah James, DO • Aleksandra Zgierska, MD, PhD

PATHOPHYSIOLOGY

Lateral epicondylosis (LE) and medial epicondylosis (ME) are common, painful, debilitating soft tissue disorders. LE (tennis elbow) involves primarily the extensor carpi radialis brevis and common extensor tendon at its proximal insertion; pain is experienced over the lateral epicondyle. LE affects up to 7 out of 1000 persons per year in general medical practices.[1,2] Both conditions are well known as sport-related injuries, but they have their greatest effect on workers who perform repetitive stressful hand tasks.[3] The prevalence of LE among industrial workers is up to 30%; auto industry workers have a chronic lateral epicondylosis (CLE) prevalence of 16%.[4] ME (golfer's elbow) is much less common and is associated with less functional impairment.[2] The most common causes of LE and ME may be low-load, high-repetition activities such as keyboarding, although formal data are lacking.[5] The cost of time away from work attributed to these disorders is significant.

The understanding of the pathophysiology underlying LE and ME is evolving and remains controversial. Both LE and ME were traditionally seen as inflammatory conditions. The terms *lateral epicondylitis* and *medial epicondylitis* are often used indiscriminately to refer to both acute injury and chronic overuse elbow injury. However, most overuse tendon injuries, including LE and ME, show minimal histopathological evidence of inflammatory cells.[6-9] Rather, they are chronic degenerative conditions. Therefore, *epicondylosis* is the preferred term.[10,11] The current understanding identifies overuse of or trauma to elbow extensor or flexor tendons, microtearing, and failed tendon healing as the key mechanisms of injury. The result is weakened, fibrosed, and, finally, calcified and necrotic tendon insertions at the lateral or medial epicondyle.[7,12] Although inflammation may be present early in the disease process, biopsy studies have shown an absence of inflammatory mediators and cells, as well as dramatically disorganized collagen (Figs. 71.1 and 71.2). However, tenocyte hyperplasia and hypertrophy provide indirect evidence of upregulated inflammatory mediators in the long term suggest that elements of the inflammatory response may still play a role in the progression or continuation of tendon disrepair. Tendinopathy has been used as a general term for this class of injury.[12,13] LE and ME are clinical diagnoses. Exam findings for LE include pain with gripping and resisted extension of the wrist with the elbow extended, and reduced grip strength.[14,15] Tenderness if often elicited just distal and anterior to the lateral epicondyle but can also be present at the lateral supracondylar ridge, over the annular and radial collateral ligaments related to the radial head and the muscle bellies of the wrist extensors just distal to these ligaments.

However, these tests have not been validated.[16] Exam findings for ME include pain and tenderness near the origin of the wrist flexors on the medial epicondyle of the humerus, and sometimes on the ulnar side of the forearm, radiating to the wrist and occasionally to the fingers.

> Lateral epicondylosis and medial epicondylosis are examples of overuse tendinopathies, which often require 3 to 12 months for complete healing.

INTEGRATIVE THERAPY

The treatment of epicondylosis has been assessed in more than 100 randomized controlled trials (RCTs) and in critical reviews, most addressing LE. The results of these reviews can be disheartening, given that no therapy was found to be definitively better than conservative treatment, in the long term. Existing studies often suffer from limitations such as small sample size, poor evaluation over longer periods (12 to 24 months), and inconsistency of diagnostic criteria, treatment protocols, and outcome measures. Key issues, such as quality of life, the cost and benefit of various therapies, and return to work parameters, have not been studied. Very few studies compare a given intervention with either watchful waiting or physical therapy designed specifically for epicondylosis; this is a critical issue given that up to 90% of patients will fully recover by 1 year with a combination of time, relative rest, and conservative therapy. Although better research is sorely needed, recommendations can be made based on both clinical trial data and clinical experience.

Lifestyle

Healing Context

An integrative approach for the treatment of LE and ME focuses on pain relief, preservation of movement, muscle conditioning, and prevention. Most patients respond well to conservative treatment. The clinician should explain the pathophysiology of epicondylosis to the patient and should establish realistic expectations about treatment and expected time to full recovery. Many patients are surprised by both the nature of the condition (noninflammatory) and the lengthy period often required for complete healing. Most patients attain complete recovery in 3 to 6 months regardless of treatment.[7] However, some patients with LE and ME suffer from symptoms that are

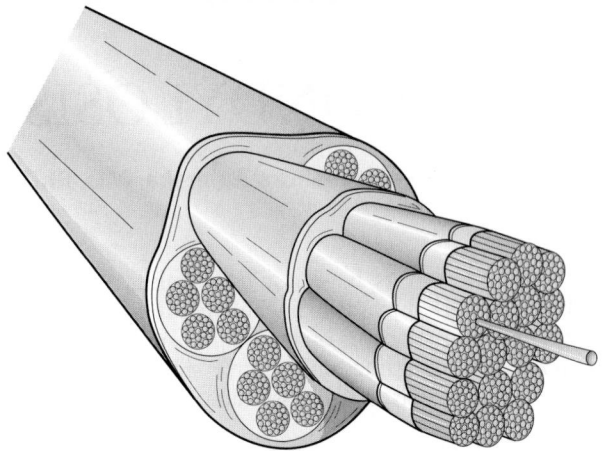

FIG. 71.1 ■ Histology of a normal tendon. (From Wilson JJ, Best TM. Common overuse tendon problems: a review and recommendations for treatment. *Am Fam Physician.* 72:811-818, 2005. Copyright 2005 American Academy of Family Physicians.)

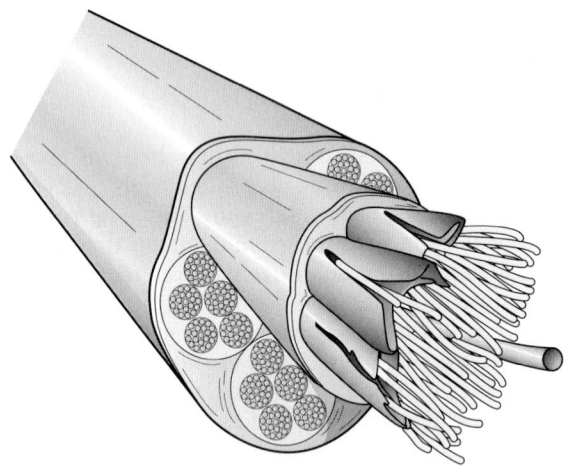

FIG. 71.2 ■ Histology of a damaged tendon. Note the collagen disorientation and separation. (From Wilson JJ, Best TM. Common overuse tendon problems: a review and recommendations for treatment. *Am Fam Physician.* 72:811-818, 2005. Copyright 2005 American Academy of Family Physicians.)

refractory to initial therapy. In a general practice trial of watchful waiting, 20% of patients who had elbow pain for more than 4 weeks did not experience resolution of the pain and disability within 1 year.[17]

Relative Rest

The pain of LE and ME is likely caused, and is certainly exacerbated, by activities that overuse the extensor and flexor tendons (Fig. 71.3). Pain from LE can be decreased by limiting wrist extension; ME-related pain can be decreased by limiting wrist flexion and pronation.

Patients whose work activity necessarily exacerbates pain should be transferred to more benign tasks, lighter or shorter duty, or should be given medical leave. Because relative rest makes good clinical sense, but is unstudied, the duration and extent of rest or leave, as well as the effect of short breaks, should be monitored clinically.

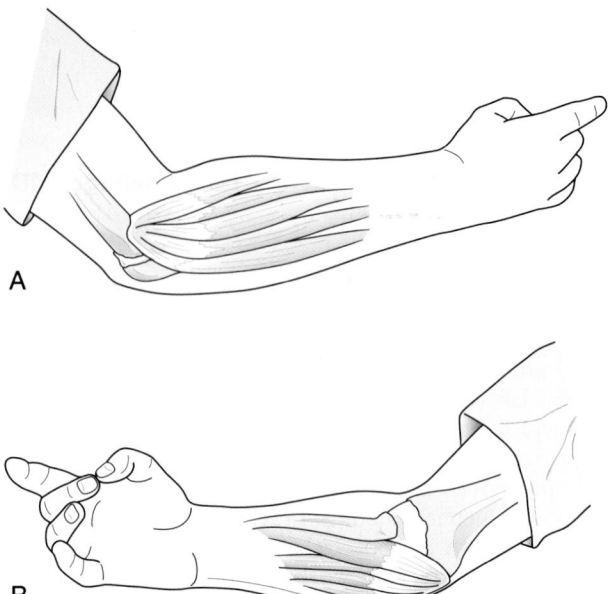

FIG. 71.3 ■ A, Lateral epicondylosis. B, Medial epicondylosis.

Ice

Because the role of inflammation in tendinopathies is unclear, the importance of icing, a traditional antiinflammatory technique, is also uncertain. However, cryotherapy is probably effective in the acute phase (first 7 days), especially in the setting of trauma. Results from a systematic review performed in 2004, evaluating icing treatment for soft tissue injury, showed that application of ice through a wet towel for 10 minutes every 4 to 6 hours was effective.[18]

Mind-Body Therapy

Psychosocial Stress

The severity of epicondylosis has been found to be related to the intensity of work environment stress.[3] Patient education about stress relief techniques, and workplace assessment to reduce psychosocial stressors, may affect the level of pain of LE and ME. It may also help prevent further tendinopathy when these measures are combined with other therapies.

Evidence suggests that acupuncture alleviates lateral epicondylosis pain in the short term.

Bioenergetic Therapy

Acupuncture

Acupuncture is based on the idea that patterns of energy flow (qi) through the body are essential for health. Disruptions of this flow are believed to be responsible for disease.

Acupuncture may alleviate or reduce epicondylar pain through activation of endogenous opioids.[19] Reviews and RCTs have shown that needle acupuncture is significantly more effective than sham acupuncture for the treatment of LE,[20] acupuncture may increase the duration of pain relief and the proportion of people with at least 50% pain reduction after only one treatment,[21] and that acupuncture increased the proportion of subjects who reported good or excellent result from treatment (22 out of 44 with acupuncture compared with 8 out of 38 without acupuncture).[22] Acupuncture is a reasonable therapeutic option if pain and disability are refractory to more conservative treatment.

PRECAUTIONS

Acupuncture must be performed by a trained specialist. Only one study reported harm resulting from needle acupuncture.[23] The investigators noted that one patient withdrew from the study because of needle pain. Given that needle acupuncture has provided pain relief in the short term period and is a very low risk procedure, it is a reasonable treatment option for patients in whom more conservative management has failed.

Pharmaceuticals

Nonsteroidal Antiinflammatory Drugs

Nonsteroidal antiinflammatory drugs (NSAIDs) target the inflammatory process thought to play a role in the early stage of LE and ME. A systematic review of the use of topical NSAIDs (diclofenac and benzydamine) for lateral elbow pain in adults found that pain was significantly improved after 4 weeks of NSAID use in comparison with placebo.[24] However, no differences in grip strength or range of motion were reported. Another study noted significant improvements in pain and function after iontophoresis and diclofenac.[25] A systematic review of oral NSAIDs found that diclofenac significantly reduced short-term pain compared with placebo, but the studies reviewed did not assess function or long-term pain.[26]

> Nonsteroidal antiinflammatory drugs and corticosteroid injections have been shown to relieve acute epicondylar pain, but not improve long-term outcomes.

Although beneficial in the short term, use of NSAIDs is controversial because the role of inflammation is not fully understood; inflammation may have an efficacious role in soft tissue healing. In addition, studies have assessed the use of NSAIDs in the acute phase, when spontaneous healing is most likely. Acetaminophen has not been studied, but it may provide relief of mild to moderate pain without gastrointestinal risk.

DOSAGE

Topical diclofenac 3% gel is applied twice daily for 1 to 2 weeks. The regimen for topical diclofenac with iontophoresis is as follows: 3% gel, 150 mg using a 4- to 8-mA intensity for 20 sessions of 25 to 30 minutes each.

The dose of oral diclofenac is 75 mg twice daily for 1 to 2 weeks. The dose of oral ibuprofen is 600 mg every 6 hours for 1 to 2 weeks.

PRECAUTIONS

Topical NSAIDs may cause skin irritation. Oral NSAIDs may cause abdominal pain and diarrhea, and patients have an increased risk of gastrointestinal complaints (relative risk, 3.0 to 5.0).[27]

Corticosteroid Injections

Corticosteroid injections also target inflammation and have traditionally been a mainstay of conventional therapy for LE and ME. Clinical trial data support their use on a limited basis for pain and disability from LE and ME, although the effects may be relatively short lived; clinical trial and systematic review data suggest that the effectiveness of these injections is limited to 6 months or less. One review concluded that steroid injections were effective on a short term basis (2 to 6 weeks) compared with placebo, elbow strapping, physical therapy, and NSAIDs, but not in the long term.[26] A methodologically strong study compared steroid injections with physical therapy and watchful waiting; at 6 weeks, the injection-treated group was most improved, but at 1 year, the other two groups experienced a higher rate of complete symptom relief.[28] A systematic review and clinical trial both reported that corticosteroid injection use was associated with limited effectiveness at 1 year and even overall long term negative effect in the intermediate (13–26 weeks) and long terms (≥52 weeks).[29,30] Corticosteroid injections may have a role in a small set of patients whose work or sport activity requires rapid, short-acting relief of pain, and who are clearly informed of potential lesser long term effects, or harm, compared to other therapies. Patients can be reinjected at 4 to 6 weeks, to a maximum of three injections.[24]

DOSAGE

The dose is 1 mL of 40 mg/mL methylprednisolone in 2 to 3 mL of 1% lidocaine.

PRECAUTIONS

One systematic review found that 17% to 27% of patients in two RCTs suffered some skin atrophy. A more common adverse event is postinjection pain, experienced by approximately half of patients.[31] The theoretical outcome of tendon rupture was not reported in two separate reviews, and this complication seems to be rare.[26]

Other Injection Therapies

Two other injection-based therapies, prolotherapy and platelet-rich plasma (PRP), directly address the hypothesis that tendinopathic pain and functional loss result from degenerative effects. Both have received attention in small but well done RCTs. In both cases, patients had a therapeutic solution injected at the attachment of the common extensor tendon with optional injection of surrounding ligamentous attachments. A peppering injection technique is often employed. Although the precise mechanism of action for both techniques is not well known, both purport to heal damaged, degenerative tendons at the tissue level. As such, both therapies attempt to address the contemporary understanding of LE and ME as degenerative conditions, and have been categorized as "regenerative" therapies, although their mechanisms of action are not well understood.

PRP is a concentrated solution of autologous platelets that delivers growth factors directly to areas of degeneration and is hypothesized to enhance tissue healing.[32,33] Autologous blood is drawn and is centrifuged at the point of care to separate the portion with the greatest abundance of platelets. Studies reported that PRP for LE could result in improved quality of life through decreased pain and function, and PRP could modify the disease course at the level of the damaged tendons.[30,34] Promising early clinical trial and anecdotal evidence have resulted in increasingly common use of PRP in clinical practice.[32,33] One RCT showed that at 52 weeks, subjects with LE who received PRP injection reported a 66% effect size compared to baseline values, whereas study participants who received steroid injections reported only a 17% improvement ($P < .05$) in disease-specific quality of life.[30] However, a recent controversial systematic review has challenged the positive conclusions of several positive PRP studies[35] and has drawn sharp criticism.[36]

The efficacy of prolotherapy, an injection-based therapy reported to enlarge and strengthen ligaments, has been evaluated in systematic and descriptive reports.[37,38] Prolotherapy is used for the treatment of various soft tissue conditions including LE and ME. While the mechanism of action is not well understood, it is thought to involve inflammation, which initiates a local physiological reaction favoring anabolic processes, recruitment of growth factors, and direct sensorineural effects.[39] The net effect is hypothesized to strengthen and revitalize tendon and ligament tissue at the bony insertion. Injectants include hypertonic dextrose and morrhuate sodium. In one RCT, subjects with severe refractory LE responded well to three prolotherapy treatments. Compared with participants receiving blinded saline injections, subjects treated with prolotherapy experienced pain reduction (absolute effect size between groups of 68%; $P < .01$) and improved isometric strength ($P < .05$) compared with control saline injections by 16 weeks, and these effects were maintained at 52 weeks.[40] A more rigorous study confirmed these findings using hypertonic dextrose alone.[41] Both were of a small sample size; a larger study is under way (see Chapter 112).

Both prolotherapy and PRP injection appear to be safe when performed by an experienced injector and are reasonable treatment options for patients in whom more conservative management has failed. Neither therapy is typically covered by third-party payers; costs for each vary considerably.

DOSAGE AND PRECAUTIONS

There is currently no formal dosing for either PRP or prolotherapy. Both therapies require specific injection techniques. Obtaining these services is best done in consultation with physicians who are experienced at performing these procedures. Both procedures are performed in an outpatient setting without significant analgesia, similar to corticosteroid injections. Both solutions are injected at tender points at the attachments of the common extensor tendon and radial collateral ligament. PRP injection therapy is performed in a single treatment session, whereas prolotherapy is more typically performed in a minimum series of three treatment sessions that are separated by approximately 4 weeks each.

Biomechanical Medicine

Physical Therapy

Exercise and physical therapy make sense clinically and are well accepted. Eccentric exercises preferentially load tendons and promote the formation of new collagen. These exercises were reported to be beneficial in one small RCT comparing exercise for epicondylar pain at 8 weeks with ultrasound and friction massage,[26] as well as in other tendinopathies.[42,43]

Exercise and physical therapy are reasonable conservative modalities, although their overall long-term efficacy is unclear.

One review and one well-done RCT reported that exercise, stretch, and mobilization were effective therapies and yielded significant improvement compared with wait-and-see, placebo, and ultrasound approaches.[44,45] Unfortunately, the physical therapy protocols vary, and studies do not describe them in detail. Examples of exercises and recommendations for their use are shown in Fig. 71.4.

Osteopathic Manipulation

Practitioners of osteopathic medicine understand the human body as a coherent unit of mind and body that is capable of self-regulation and self-healing. Structure and function are assumed to reciprocally interrelated[51]; achievement of normal body mechanics is viewed as being central to maintaining good health.[47] Osteopathic manipulative treatment (OMT) is aimed at improving the body's physiological and homeostatic processes that have been inhibited by a somatic dysfunction, which can be myofascial, vascular, neurological, cartilaginous, or bone-related. The osteopathic view of LE and ME is that they may be not only be a tendon enthesopathy but also include articular, myofascial, and/or vascular/lymphatic elements leading to pain at the lateral or medial elbow. The goal of osteopathic OMT is to remove joint and muscle restriction, as well as to address any associated tissue texture changes. Treatment is usually directed at the affected extremity[48] but can include manipulation of

Lateral Epicondylosis Physical Therapy

Start exercises with set **A** and proceed slowly through the set. Advance to exercises with weights when pain begins to decrease, usually after 7-10 days.

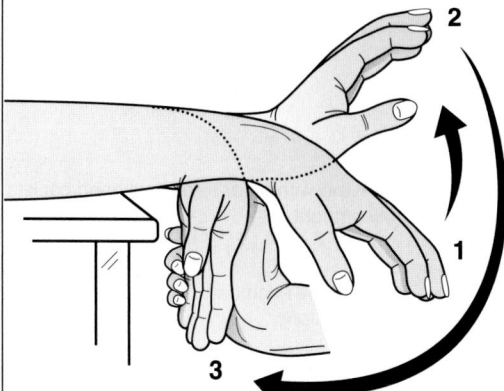

A. Active range of motion and strengthening

1. Place forearm on table with hand off edge of table, palm down.
2. Move hand upward.

Hold position for 15 seconds.
Return to starting position.
Perform 1 repetition every 4 seconds.
Perform 1 set of 12 repetitions twice per day.

After 7-10 days, or as range of motion improves and pain diminishes, advance to step **3**:

3. With other hand, grasp at thumb side of hand and bend wrist downward gently.
Perform 1 set of 4 repetitions twice per day.

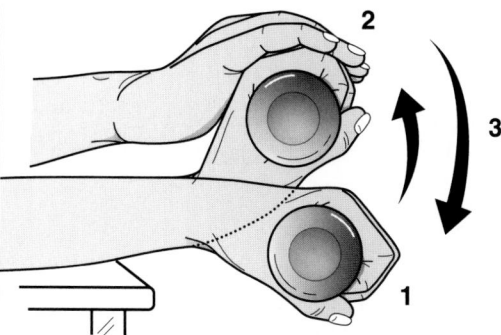

B. Exercise with weight

1. Place forearm on table, palm down, weight in hand.
2. Use other hand to raise wrist fully upward.
3. Release wrist and slowly lower weight.

Start with 1/2-lb weight, advance to 1-lb weight.
Perform 1 repetition every 4 seconds.
Perform 3 sets of 10 repetitions once every other day.
Rest 1 minute between sets.

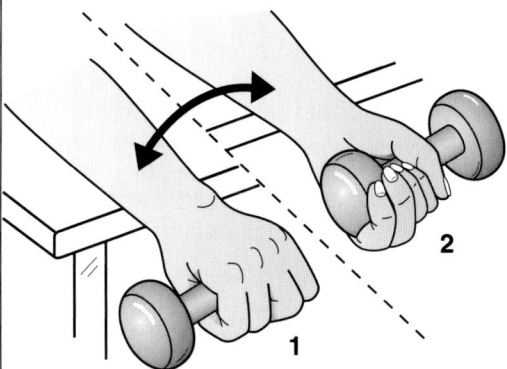

C. Exercise with weight

1. Support forearm on table or armchair, hand palm down holding weight.
2. Rotate hand to thumb up.
Return to starting position.

Start with 1/2-lb weight, advance to 1-lb weight.
Perform 1 repetition every 4 seconds.
Perform 3 sets of 10 repetitions once every other day.
Rest 1 minute between sets.

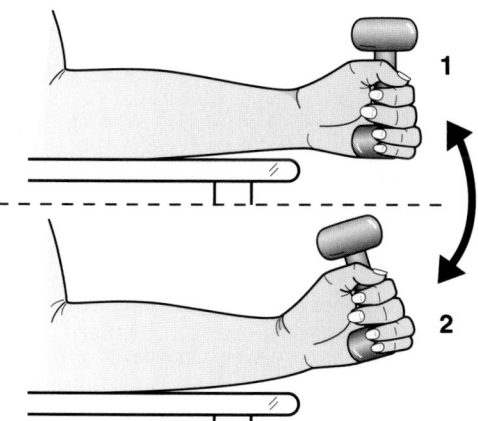

D. Exercise with weight

1. Support forearm on table or knee.
Hold weight in hand, thumb up.
2. Lift weight upward.
Return to starting position and repeat.

Start with 1/2-lb weight, advance to 1-lb weight.
Perform 1 repetition every 4 seconds.
Perform 3 sets of 10 repetitions once every other day.
Rest 1 minute between sets.

FIG. 71.4 ■ Physical therapy for lateral epicondylosis.

Continued

Medial Epicondylosis Physical Therapy

Start exercises with set **A** and proceed slowly through the set. Advance to exercises with weights when pain begins to decrease, usually after 7-10 days.

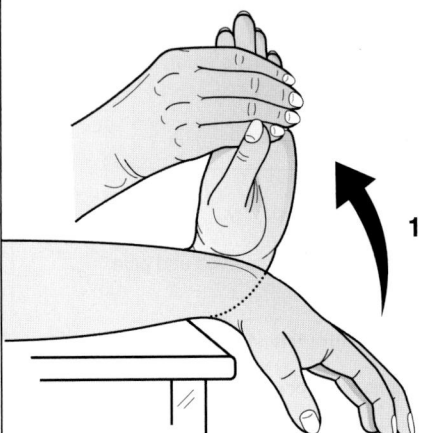

A. Stretch exercise

1. Grasping fingers of one hand with other hand, pull hand back gently. Keep injured elbow straight.

Hold position for 15 seconds.
Perform 1 set of 4 repetitions twice each day.
Rest 30 seconds between repetitions.

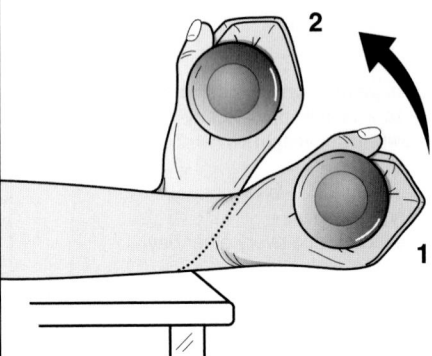

B. Exercise with weight

1. Grasp weight with hand.
Place forearm on table with hand off edge of table, palm up as shown.
2. Move wrist upward.
Return to starting position.

Start with 1/2-lb weight, advance to 1-lb weight.
Perform 1 repetition every 4 seconds.
Perform 3 sets of 10 repetitions once every other day.
Rest 1 minute between sets.

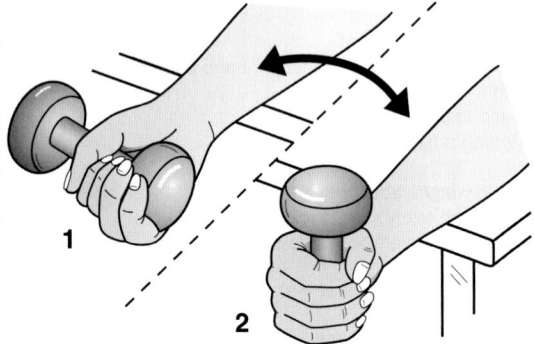

C. Exercise with weight

1. Support forearm on table or armchair.
Position hand palm up with weight in hand as shown.
2. Rotate hand to thumb up.
Return to starting position.

Start with 1/2-lb weight, advance to 1-lb weight.
Perform 1 repetition every 4 seconds.
Perform 3 sets of 10 repetitions once every other day.
Rest 1 minute between sets.

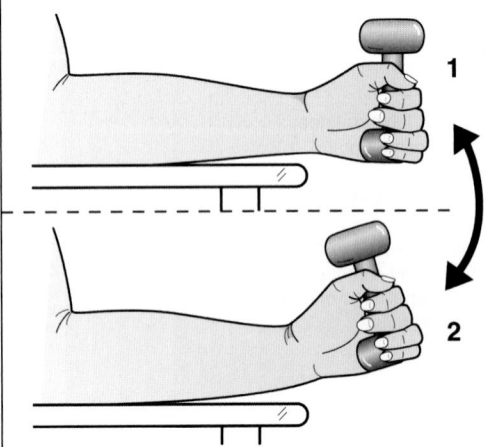

D. Exercise with weight

1. Support forearm on table or knee.
Hold weight in hand, thumb up.
2. Lift weight upward.
Return to starting position and repeat.

Start with 1/2-lb weight, advance to 1-lb weight.
Perform 1 repetition every 4 seconds.
Perform 3 sets of 10 repetitions once every other day.
Rest 1 minute between sets.

FIG. 71.4, cont'd

the ipsilateral cervical and thoracic spines and ribs.[49,50] Treatment of the radial head, interosseous membrane, or ulnar somatic dysfunction has been reported to improve lateral elbow pain and function.[51] Limited objective and descriptive data suggest that OMT alone is effective for epicondylosis, as well as in combination with routine care.[52,53]

PRECAUTIONS

OMT is typically performed by osteopathic physicians (doctor of osteopathy [DO]) or MDs who have received additional osteopathic training. Obtaining these services is best done in consultation with physicians who are experienced with these procedures. OMT is performed in an outpatient setting without analgesia. The patient should be made aware that following treatment, muscle soreness or increased localized pain may occur for 24 to 72 hours. However, the pain usually decreases rapidly with maintenance of function and overall pain improvement.[54]

Orthoses (Braces)

Orthotic devices (e.g., brace, splint, cast, or strap) are thought to decrease the pain of LE or ME by removing the damaging load from the lateral and medical epicondylar tendon attachments. A systematic review of five RCTs assessing various orthotic devices was unable to provide a general recommendation for their use.[55] However, the notion of reducing stress and strain at the tendon insertion makes sense and is generally accepted; clinically, many patients respond well to a simple and inexpensive elbow strap or wrist splint combined with relative rest. Complete immobilization with any orthotic device should be avoided because of the risks of deconditioning and muscular atrophy.

PRECAUTIONS

Local deconditioning should be avoided.

Surgery

A 2005 review found no RCTs that evaluated surgical intervention for LE or ME.[26] However, data from case series have demonstrated the efficacy of surgery in patients with symptoms refractory to more conservative therapy. The goal of surgery is to excise abnormal tissue or release the affected portions of the extensor or flexor tendons. Findings from one case series, consisting of 1300 patients that underwent surgery for refractory epicondylar pain (1000 for LE and 300 for ME), showed that 85% of patients experienced complete pain relief and strength return, 12% had partial improvement, and 3% had no improvement.[12] Surgery is a reasonable option for patients with significant pain for whom more conservative therapy has failed.

PRECAUTIONS

Precautions include postoperative concerns such as infection and nerve damage. In the study cited previously, however, reported complications were rare.[12]

PREVENTION PRESCRIPTION

LIFESTYLE
- Stop smoking.
- Reduce stress.

AVOID EXACERBATING ACTIVITIES
- Reduce or avoid the lifting of objects with the arm extended.
- Reduce repetitive gripping.
- Decrease overall tension of gripping.
- Avoid extremes of wrist bending and full extension.
- Work or train with the elbow in a partially flexed position.
- Use wrist supports when weight training.
- Enlarge the gripping surface of tools or rackets with gloves or padding, use a hammer with extra padding to reduce tensions and impact, and hold heavy tools with two hands.

ERGONOMIC EVALUATION
- Evaluate repetitive motion activity, duties, equipment, and techniques, especially in work situations.
- More complete information on ergonomic evaluation of computer, laboratory, and industrial settings is available through the Centers for Disease Control and Prevention (see Key Web Resources).

EXERCISE
- Use stretching and strengthening exercises once daily, along with frequent periods of short rest.

THERAPEUTIC REVIEW

LIFESTYLE

- Prevention: Most of the techniques listed in the Prevention Prescription box also off-load affected tendons and may speed healing.
- Establish a time course of healing; most patients recover in weeks to months, but recovery may take up to 1 year or longer.
- Relative rest: Remove or reduce repetitive, heavy activity affecting wrist flexors or extensors.
- Use ice during the first 2 to 4 weeks of pain.

MIND-BODY THERAPY

- Stress reduction techniques and workplace evaluation are recommended.

BIOENERGETIC THERAPY

- Needle acupuncture may be used.

PHARMACEUTICALS

- Nonsteroidal antiinflammatory drugs and corticosteroid injections have good efficacy for pain control in the early stages of lateral epicondylosis and medial epicondylosis, but they do not change outcomes in the long term.
- Topical diclofenac, 3% gel, may be applied twice daily for a duration of 1 to 2 weeks.
  Topical diclofenac may be applied with iontophoresis, using 150 mg at 4 to 8 mA for 25 to 30 minutes, for 20 sessions.
- Oral ibuprofen, 600 mg, may be taken every 6 hours for no more than 2 weeks.

- Injection: Methylprednisone, 40 mg in 1 mL of lidocaine, may be injected weekly for up to four treatments.

PHYSICAL THERAPY AND PREVENTIVE EXERCISE

- Various exercises may be performed in sets of repetitions with and without weights from twice daily to every other day (see Fig. 71.4).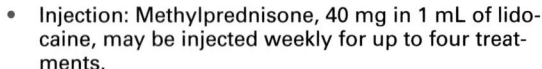

ORTHOTICS

- Simple wrist splints and elbow straps may be used in conjunction with relative rest.

PROLOTHERAPY

- Prolotherapy appears to be safe when performed by an experienced injector and is a reasonable treatment option for patients in whom more conservative management has failed.

PLATELET-RICH PLASMA

- Platelet-rich plasma injection appears to be safe when performed by an experienced injector and is a reasonable treatment option for patients in whom more conservative management has failed.

SURGERY

- Surgery is a reasonable option for patients with severe pain that is refractory to conservative care.

Key Web Resources

Mayo Clinic information on tennis elbow: This site is a basic but helpful patient-oriented online tool.	http://www.mayoclinic.org/diseases-conditions/tennis-elbow/home/ovc-20206011
Centers for Disease Control and Prevention information on ergonomics: This site provides information on ergonomic evaluation of computer, laboratory, and industrial settings.	http://www.cdc.gov/niosh/topics/ergonomics/
Hackett-Hemwall-Patterson Foundation, and American Association of Orthopaedic Medicine: These nonprofit organizations provide information and educational programs on comprehensive nonsurgical musculoskeletal treatment including prolotherapy and PRP. These searchable sites list members who perform prolotherapy.	http://www.hackethemwall.org/WELCOME.html http://www.aaomed.org
This is the home Website of the American Osteopathic Association	http://www.osteopathic.org/Pages/default.aspx

---

REFERENCES

References are available online at ExpertConsult.com.

SECTION XIII

DERMATOLOGY

SECTION OUTLINE

72 ATOPIC DERMATITIS

73 PSORIASIS

74 URTICARIA

75 APHTHOUS STOMATITIS

76 SEBORRHEIC DERMATITIS

77 ACNE VULGARIS AND ACNE ROSACEA

CHAPTER 72

ATOPIC DERMATITIS

Amanda J. Kaufman, MD, ABIHM

Atopic dermatitis (AD) is a pruritic, hereditary skin disease affecting 15%–25% of children; in 30% or more, it will persist into adulthood.[1] The heavy impact of atopic dermatitis on quality of life and medical care costs has led to an explosion of basic science and clinical research. Great strides have been made to understand the pathophysiology of the disease and study the impact of treatment modalities. Causes stem from genetic mutations that impair the skin barrier, which allow greater permeability for allergens and pathogens, enhancing Th2 immunity. Atopic dermatitis is also an outward manifestation of inner imbalances including nutrient deficiencies, food allergies, and other intestinal dysbiosis. It is essential to take the time for a thorough history and examination to best guide each individual on their treatment options. Interest in the integrative approach stems from seeking to address the underlying causes rather than suppressing the immune system enough to overcome the symptoms.

PATHOPHYSIOLOGY AND DIAGNOSIS

The diagnosis of atopic dermatitis requires three major and three minor features.[1] Major features are as follows:
- Pruritus
- Typical morphology and distribution
- Flexural lichenification in adults
- Facial and extensor involvement in infants and children
- Chronic or chronically relapsing dermatitis
- Personal or family history of atopy (asthma, allergic rhinitis, atopic dermatitis)

The 22 minor features in the following list illustrate the varying degrees, extent, and distress that patients endure:
- Itch caused by sweating
- Xerosis
- Eczema (perifollicular accentuation)
- Recurrent conjunctivitis
- Wool intolerance
- Keratosis pilaris
- Palmar hyperlinearity
- Pityriasis alba
- White dermatographism
- Susceptibility to cutaneous infection (*Staphylococcus aureus*, herpes simplex virus, and other viruses)
- Nipple dermatitis
- Dennie-Morgan lines
- Elevated immunoglobulin E (IgE)
- Immediate (type I) skin test reactivity
- Food intolerance
- Cataracts (anterior-subcapsular)
- Cheilitis
- Facial pallor or erythema
- Hand dermatitis
- Ichthyosis
- Keratoconus
- Orbital darkening

Genetic, immunologic, and environmental risks collide to influence the course of disease and provide opportunities to mediate the clinical course. The stratum corneum permeability barrier is made up of the cornified envelope, fatty acids such as ceramides, and keratin proteins tightly bound by filaggrin (FLG). FLG mutations and/or impaired ceramide levels result in abnormal permeability and poor water retention. This abnormal skin barrier allows penetration of allergens and microbes that trigger an inflammatory cascade as they stimulate proinflammatory type 2 helper T (Th2) cells excessively.[1] Epidermal cells communicate to sensory neurons through cytokine thymic stromal lymphopoietin (TSLP) to promote itching.[2] This cytokine also promotes Th2 cells and the "atopic march" from AD to asthma and allergic rhinitis.

Among environmental exposures, Phthalates also stimulate TSLP; higher exposure in utero and in early life confers additional risk of AD.[3,4]

> Improving the skin barrier is essential in treatment and prevention. Emollient use has been shown to cut AD risk in half among high-risk infants.

Light stimuli and contact irritants such as sweating, wool, and detergents cause itching. Skin damage caused by scratching releases inflammatory cytokines and further stimulates itch. Reduced barrier function allows entry of *S. aureus*, *Malassezia* yeasts, *Candida* organisms, and *Trichophyton* dermatophytes, thereby inducing local inflammation. Herpes simplex virus (HSV) can cause eczema herpeticum, with vesicles throughout vulnerable skin, usually with a bacterial superinfection. During a flare, the skin of patients with atopic dermatitis has reduced microbiome diversity with predominance of pathogenic bacteria, especially in the skin areas most often affected.[5] During recovery, the microbiome diversity is restored.

Food allergies, especially to eggs, soy, milk, wheat, fish, shellfish, and peanuts, are implicated in one-third to one-half of children with AD. Aeroallergens can also increase peripheral eosinophilia and serum IgE levels, which lead to an increased release of histamine and vascular mediators. These features induce edema and urticaria and thus cause persistence of the cycle of itch, scratch, and rash.

Food allergies, especially to eggs, soy, milk, wheat, fish, shellfish, and peanuts, are implicated in one-third to one-half of children with atopic dermatitis.

The relationship between psychological stress and atopic disorders is bidirectional.[6] Psychosocial stressors increase both self-reported and objective measures. The lack of sleep and physical suffering cause irritability and worsen mood disorders. Self-reporting of itch severity is increased when depression scores are elevated, similar to the relationship with pain scores.

INTEGRATIVE THERAPY

Atopic dermatitis is improved through an integrative approach focusing on improving the barrier function and reducing the itch-scratch cycle. Least invasive therapies are presented first, followed by those with a greater potential for harm. Outcomes are better when time is taken for education and self-determination of the great variety of available treatment options.[7] Akin to asthma therapies, developing an eczema action plan (Fig. 72.1) where the regimen can be amped up to provide control and then relaxed as the flare resolves reduces use of pharmaceuticals and improves patient satisfaction.[8]

LIFESTYLE AND SUPPORTIVE CARE

Hydration

Rehydration of the stratum corneum improves barrier function and reduces the effects of irritants and allergens. Soaking in a lukewarm bath for 10–20 minutes daily is ideal, or lukewarm showers may be taken. If even plain water is irritating during acute flares, one cup of salt or baking soda added to the water will reduce the sting.

Bleach Baths

Evidence is growing that all atopic dermatitis treatments improve skin microbiome diversity and reduce the dominance of *S. aureus*. Dilute bleach baths have been used successfully with this goal in mind and have improved symptom control.[9] In the original study, 31 children aged 6 months–17 years were treated with cephalexin, 50 mg/kg (maximum 2 g daily) divided three times daily for 14 days, and were then randomized to bathing in a dilute bleach solution (approximately one-half cup to a bathtub of water) twice weekly for at least 5 minutes (then rinsing off) and applying mupirocin ointment intranasally for the patient and for all household members twice daily for the first 5 consecutive days of each month or placebo. The mean Eczema Area and Severity Score (EASI) of 19.7 was reduced by 10.4 points at 1

ECZEMA ACTION PLAN

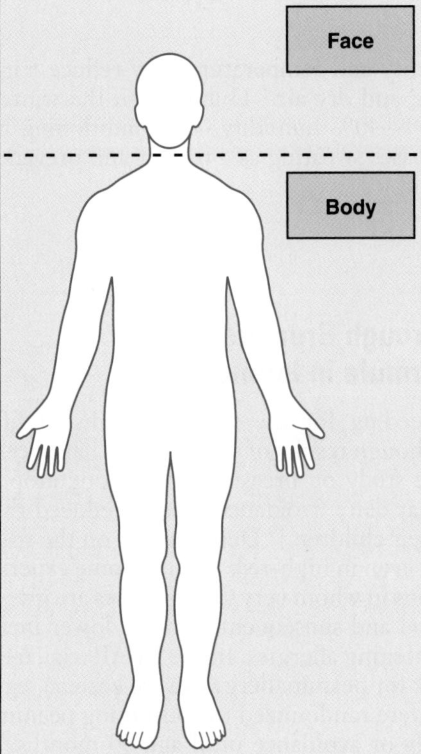

		Clear	Mild-mod	Severe
Face	AM	Moisturizer*	Moisturizer*	Moisturizer*
	PM	Moisturizer*	Moisturizer*	Moisturizer*
Body		Moisturizer*	Moisturizer*	Moisturizer*
	AM			Call your doctor if not improving after 2 weeks
	PM	Moisturizer*	Moisturizer*	Moisturizer*
				Call your doctor if not improving after 2 weeks

A moisturizer is extremely important. We recommend applying the moisturizer at least twice per day for any patient with eczema.

FIG. 72.1 ■ Eczema action plan.

month and by 15.3 points at 3 months compared with 2.5 and 3.2 points in the placebo group. These reductions were in exposed areas, but not in head and neck lesions, although the head and neck can also be carefully exposed to the bleach solution. Follow-up studies have demonstrated equal effectiveness to baths only and have validated the ease of use.[10]

Mild Soap or Soap Substitutes

Use mild, neutral-pH soap (Dove, Aveeno, Basis) minimally if needed for the face, axillae, and groin. Alternatively, hydrophobic lotions or creams such as Cetaphil can be applied without water, rubbed until foaming, and wiped away with a soft cloth. Even use of the emollient itself can be effective for washing. Other guidelines include avoiding sodium laurel sulfate and bath oils or additives; use shampoo only on hair; avoid baby wipes as much as possible.[11] Invite new parents to leave the protective vernix on newborn skin.

Moisturizers Following Bathing

Follow bathing by lightly patting the skin with a towel and immediately applying an occlusive emollient over the entire skin surface to retain moisture. Application within 3 minutes improves hydration, whereas beyond 3 minutes, the surface dries due to evaporation. Emollient use from birth prevents AD. One hundred twenty-six high-risk infants were randomized to daily emollient use or none; emollient use resulted in a 50% risk reduction at age 6 months.[11] Parents in the United Kingdom were given a choice of sunflower seed oil with a high linoleic:oleic acid ratio, double base gel (Dermal laboratories), or liquid paraffin 50% in soft white paraffin. Parents in the United States were given a choice of sunflower seed oil, Cetaphil cream, or Aquaphor ointment. Virgin coconut oil had excellent effects of reduced TEWL; it additionally reduces colonization with *S. aureus* and thus provides an added benefit.[12] Ceramide-containing emollients are effective. One formulation (EpiCeram) showed improvement nearly equal to that with fluticasone cream after 28 days of use.[13] Urea, alpha-hydroxy acid, and lactic acid products have long been used for their exfoliation and moisturizing properties. However, studies are limited.[14]

Wet Dressings

Wet dressings are useful for severely affected skin. The constant moisture is therapeutic, the cooling sensation with evaporation reduces itching, and the mechanical barrier prevents scratching. Additional use of very dilute steroids such as 1:3 mometasone furoate 0.1% ointment for body and 1:19 mometasone furoate 0.1% ointment for the face under a mask are effective with less use of steroids.[15] Two recent reviews discuss how effective this can be for the most severely affected patients.[16,17] Apply a wet cloth with either plain water or Burow solution to recalcitrant lesions, and periodically rewet the compress. Wet dressings increase penetration of corticosteroids. Burow solution can be made 1:40 by dissolving one Domeboro packet or tablet in a pint of lukewarm water. Children can wear cotton pajamas dampened in the affected areas with other clothing worn over them to prevent them from getting too cold. The eczema company (see online resources) carries a variety of clothing and wet wrap products.

Wet dressings are highly effective and well tolerated, especially in severe disease. Hospital care can be replicated at home by using wet dressings as much as possible on the weekends.

Avoidance of Allergens

Eliminate known allergens. Eliminate smoke exposure for children with allergies. Dust mite control measures may be helpful in patients with documented sensitivity to dust mites. In children with animal allergies, consider removing animals from the home. A dog living in the home at the time of birth is associated with a 50% decrease in the incidence of atopic dermatitis at age 3 years.[18] However, parents caring for a dog are less likely to be severely allergic to dog dander.

Loose-Fitting Clothing

Wear loose-fitting clothing made of cotton, silk, or other natural, smooth fibers. Avoid wool. Launder new clothes before wearing to remove formaldehyde and other chemicals. Use liquid detergent, ideally without fabric softeners or optical brighteners, and consider an extra rinse cycle to more completely remove detergent.

Humidity

Controlled humidity and temperature may reduce triggers of cold, heat, and dry air.[1] Humidify in the winter with a goal of 30%–40% humidity. Air conditioning in the summer decreases sweating as a trigger and prevents the growth of mold.

NUTRITION

Prevention Through Breastfeeding or Hydrolyzed Formula in Infancy

Exclusive breastfeeding for the first 6 months of life reduces atopy, although results of some studies have been inconclusive. One study on breastfeeding among atopic mothers noted that dairy avoidance greatly reduced the risk of atopy in their children.[19] Debate exists on the role of food avoidance even in high-risk infants. Some experts point to populations in whom very young babies are given tastes of adult food and subsequently have a lower incidence of life-threatening allergies. In the LEAP trial, 640 babies at high-risk for peanut allergy (severe eczema, egg allergy, or both) were randomized to consuming peanuts three times weekly or avoidance until age 60 months.[20] They were also tested by pin-prick testing for peanut protein allergy prior to randomization. Among the 530 with negative prior testing, 13.7% among controls developed peanut allergy versus 1.9% in the consumption group ($p <$ .001). Among the 98 participants with positive prior testing, 35.3% of controls developed peanut allergy versus 10.6% in the consumption group ($p = .004$). There were no significant differences in adverse events. The theory is that when we are first exposed to a protein through the healthy gut, versus first seeing it topically, we are less likely to develop an allergy. This is even more important in those with AD as their impaired skin barrier is more likely to be sensitized from peanut antigen in house dust.[21]

For those infants who cannot breastfeed, hydrolyzed formulas have been found effective for the prevention of atopic dermatitis. A 6-year follow-up to a study of 2252 newborns with a familial history of atopy, who were randomized to various hydrolyzed formulas versus standard cow's milk formula when breastfeeding was insufficient, revealed a significant risk reduction for allergic disease.[22] The relative risk of development of atopic eczema was 0.79 for partially hydrolyzed whey formula, 0.92 for extensively hydrolyzed whey formula, and 0.71 for extensively hydrolyzed casein formula. A meta-analysis and a more recent study also found that partially hydrolyzed whey formulas appear to be as good at preventing atopic disease as extensively hydrolyzed formulas, and they cost less.[23,24]

Allergy Elimination Diet

A study attempting to show a benefit to an allergy elimination diet in a broad sample of children with atopic dermatitis found a benefit only to an egg-free diet in infants with suspected egg allergy positive for specific IgE to eggs.[25] By the age of 5 years, many of these food allergies resolve. The most common foods causing positive oral challenges are egg, soy, milk, wheat, fish, shellfish, and peanuts. Elimination diets can be stressful on parents, especially exhausted breastfeeding mothers. However, many parents will become aware of their own allergies through the process. Parents often desire testing to guide them; however, testing is not as reliable as a clinical response. The skin in atopic dermatitis can develop a wheal with a needle prick alone.[1] Serum-specific IgE/IgG tests have significant false-positive rates.[26] For example, in the LEAP study, all consumers of peanut had increases in their peanut IgG. The gold standard for diagnosis is a placebo-controlled, double-blind oral food challenge because history, prick tests, and specific IgE do not correlate well with clinical reactivity, especially in delayed eczematous skin reactions.[1,26] Diagnostic elimination diets, such as those described in this text (see Chapter 86), should be used. A review of the serum radioallergosorbent test (RAST) and enzyme-linked immunosorbent assay (ELISA) and their inherent challenges provides further detailed guidance.[27]

Oolong Tea

With consuming Oolong tea three times a day (made from five tea bags daily), 63% of patients had significant objective improvement, and the response persisted at 6 months in 54% of patients.[28] The antiallergenic properties of polyphenols are thought to produce the effect. Consuming five to six cups of green tea or green tea extract, at 200–300 mg three times daily, may provide similar results.

> The main difference among green, oolong, and dark tea (all *Camellia sinensis*) is the length of fermentation of the leaf. Green is the shortest and dark the longest.

Mind-Body Therapy

Psychosocial stressors trigger flares of atopic dermatitis, and this connection prompted studies on the effectiveness of mind-body interventions. A Cochrane Review states that at least some patients may benefit from biofeedback, massage therapy, and hypnosis.[29] A study on the benefits of support groups found improved quality of life scores, especially personal relationships and leisure scores.[30] A study of a structured education program on coping skills in children with atopic dermatitis and their parents showed that the intervention improved psychological scores beyond what would be expected with disease improvement.[31] Dr. Ted Grossbart, a Harvard Medical School (Boston) psychologist, created a mind-body program for skin disorders, and his e-book is available for free (see Key Web Resources). Many therapies with known effectiveness in similar conditions have not been studied. Given the low risk of side effects and the known benefits of mind-body therapies for other measures of well-being, these approaches are worth exploring.

Supplements

Vitamins

Vitamin D and E supplementation with vitamin D_3 (1600 units) and vitamin E (600 units synthetic all-rac-alpha-tocopherol) were compared to placebo for 60 days, reducing objective scoring measures by 64.3% ($p = .004$).[32] In various studies, vitamin D supplementation had a greater effect in the winter in those with darker skin and in those with higher BMIs.[33] Higher serum vitamin D levels are correlated to milder disease and lowers IgE to microbial antigens.[34] Higher cord blood levels of vitamin D reduced risk of AD in children followed to age 5 years.[35]

> **DOSAGE**
> Vitamin D_3 2000–5000 IU daily (consider testing for adequacy) and vitamin E 400 IU as mixed tocopherols. Many practitioners recommend supplementation with antiinflammatory supplements such as 5000 IU of vitamin A daily and 20 mg of zinc per daily. Vitamin B_{12} cream, 0.07% used twice daily, was found to be effective and well tolerated in adults and children with eczema in small studies.[36]

Essential Fatty Acids

Linoleic acid is a precursor to ceramide. Docosahexaenoic acid (DHA) and eicosapentaenoic acid (EPA) primarily function through their antiinflammatory effects.

The primary sources of DHA and EPA are salmon and other cold-water fish. Good sources of gamma-linolenic acid (GLA) include borage oil (23% GLA), black currant seed oil (17% GLA), and evening primrose oil (8%–10% GLA).[37]

Supplementing DHA/EPA, or getting breastmilk with adequate levels, prevents AD and improves objective measures.[38] An 8-week study of 53 adults randomized to DHA (5.4 g daily) or isoenergetic saturated fatty acids revealed significant improvement in the DHA-treated group.[39] Another small study of evening primrose oil with 2 g of linoleic acid and 250 mg of GLA for 3 months showed significantly improved inflammation in AD.[40]

DOSAGE

For children, a combined total of 2000 mg of DHA, EPA, and GLA is likely effective compared with the doses recommended in single-agent trials. For adults, use 2–4 g daily of EPA/DHA and/or borage oil 500 mg–1 g daily or evening primrose oil 1–2 g daily.

PRECAUTIONS

Adverse effects of supplements are few, and they are primarily gastrointestinal.

Probiotics

A lack of microbiome diversity in the gut is associated with a myriad of illnesses. Greater diversity with known beneficial flora on the skin such as lactobacilli and *Bifidobacterium species* prevents and improves symptoms in AD. Vaginal birth, breast-feeding, and a greater number of siblings increases rates of colonization with lactobacilli, and decreased rates of clostridia.[41] The opposing conditions are associated with more clostridia and an increased risk of AD. Prenatal and postnatal use of *Lactobacillus rhamnosus* GG among atopic mothers reduces the prevalence of atopic dermatitis in their infants by 50%, with a number needed to treat of 4.5.[42] To prevent atopic dermatitis, women with a history of atopy should consider supplementation with *L. rhamnosus* when they are pregnant and breast-feeding. Supplementation after diagnosis also provides improvement.

DOSAGE

For adults, the dose is 20–50 billion CFUs daily of a combination probiotic containing *L. rhamnosus*. For infants and children, the dose is 5–10 billion CFUs daily.

PRECAUTIONS

Patients with extreme immune compromise or those with indwelling catheters should use caution with regard to taking these live organisms.

Encouraging the presence of lactobacilli and a diverse microbiome, either through lifestyle circumstances or supplementation, improves outcomes.

Botanicals

Much of the long heritage of herbal treatment of atopic dermatitis has not been studied, although several compounds have had small, successful trials, and no safety concerns exist. Ensuring the quality of the compound used is essential to achieve these treatment effects.

Glycyrrhetinic Acid

Derived from licorice root, glycyrrhetinic acid has antiinflammatory actions when it is used topically. Two percent glycyrrhetinic acid cream used in a 5-week study noted significant improvements in objective disease scores and itch.[43] Atopiclair is a hydrophilic cream containing hyaluronic acid, telmesteine, *Vitis vinifera* (grape), and 2% glycyrrhetinic acid. Two vehicle-controlled, randomized studies of 218 adults and 142 children with mild to moderate atopic dermatitis found highly significant response rates.[44,45] Atopiclair cream is available by prescription (100-g tube) and over the counter.

DOSAGE

These products are applied to effected area two to three times daily as needed.

PRECAUTIONS

Atopiclair cream contains a nut oil and thus should not be used in patients with a nut allergy.

Other Botanicals

Studies demonstrate the effectiveness of an extract of St. John's wort (*Hypericum perforatum*). This botanical has antimicrobial activity and may have beneficial immunological effects. A study of 28 patients found significant clinical improvement when this extract was applied as a cream compared with its vehicle.[46] Oregon grape root (*Mahonia aquifolium*) has antimicrobial properties and inhibits proinflammatory cytokines.[47] A 10% cream used in 42 adult patients three times daily over 12 weeks demonstrated significant clinical improvement. Twenty-one patients with mild atopic dermatitis who were 5–28 years old were randomized to 0.3% *rosmarinic acid* emulsion twice daily or vehicle.[48] These patients had significantly reduced erythema and transepidermal water loss. Honey has been used to reduce inflammation and promote healing; small studies have shown it is helpful.[49] Chamomile is regarded as gentle and safe, and it has antiinflammatory and antibacterial properties. Cold, wet packs with chamomile tea are traditionally used for bacterial superinfections.[50] Herbavate, a topical preparation that contains the oil extracts of *Calotropis gigantea, Curcuma longa, Pongamia glabra, and Solanum xanthocarpum* in a cream base, showed promise in an open-label 4-week pilot study.[51] These extracts have been used in Indian traditional medicine and Ayurveda.

It is easy to find combination products online or in health food stores. One example is Four Elements Herbals' product Look No X E Ma!, which contains almond oil, calendula, chamomile, licorice and comfrey root decoction, beeswax, shea butter, borax, evening primrose oil, and vitamin E (www.fourelementsherbals.com).

> Familiarize yourself with the products available from your local herbalist or compounding pharmacist. Use of more than two topical products can be cumbersome for patients, although many products can be compounded together for ease of use. Many commercially available products contain several agents in combination.

Conventional Modalities

Coal Tar

Coal tar preparations have antipruritic and antiinflammatory effects and were used before the development of topical corticosteroids. Research shows coal tar activates the aryl hydrocarbon receptor (AHR), restoring filaggrin expression to wild-type levels.[52] They work well on chronic and lichenified lesions.[1] Tar shampoos can be used for scalp involvement. Adverse effects include contact dermatitis, folliculitis, and photosensitivity. One review found that most studies reported favorable profiles of effectiveness with few side effects (including staining and odor) and also noted that these preparations are cost effective.[53]

Immunotherapy

Allergen immunotherapy is typically indicated for patients with allergic rhinitis or allergic asthma, although it has shown promise for atopic dermatitis. A meta-analysis of eight small, heterogeneous trials (385 subjects) was encouraging.[54] These included studies targeting house dust mites (8), animal dander (2), molds (1), and pollen (2). Clinically, there are some pediatric allergists performing peanut immunotherapy.

Immunization and Childhood Diseases

Concerns have been raised about the effect of immunizations on atopic dermatitis. Analyses concluded that both natural infection and immunization protect against childhood atopic dermatitis.[55] With varicella, infection has a decreased odds ratio of 0.55 for development of atopic dermatitis.[56] Children who are infected with wild-type varicella zoster infection, as opposed to vaccine, who develop atopic dermatitis have fewer doctor visits for atopic dermatitis (odds ratio, 0.17). In a study of 2184 infants with atopic dermatitis and a family history of atopy, exposure to vaccines (diphtheria, tetanus, pertussis, polio, *Haemophilus influenzae* type b, hepatitis B, mumps, measles, rubella, varicella, bacille Calmette-Guérin, meningococci, and pneumococci) was not associated with an increased risk of allergic sensitization to food or aeroallergens.[57] On the contrary, immunizations against varicella and pertussis and cumulative numbers of vaccine doses were inversely associated with eczema severity.

Ultraviolet Light

Ultraviolet (UV) light may be helpful for some patients, although this technique is less popular because of the acceleration of photoaging and increased risk of skin cancer. Many small studies and its popularity among patients support the use of sun and sea-water bathing.[58] A study of narrow-band UVB showed a statistically significant advantage when light therapy was accompanied by synchronous bathing in a 10% Dead Sea salt solution.[59] In one study, narrow-band UVB and medium-dose UVA1 dosed three times a week were equally effective.[60]

Pharmaceuticals

Antimicrobials

Despite the role of bacteria in AD, use of antibiotics has not been found effective as treatment for atopic dermatitis.[61] This reflects that it is not the eradication of the infection that is effective but the return of a diverse microbiome. Lesions that are not responsive to corticosteroids may need treatment for subclinical bacterial superinfection.[62] Also consider testing for HSV with a smear or culture. Dermatophyte infections can contribute to head and neck lesions.[63]

> **DOSAGE**
> • Mupirocin or bacitracin ointment twice daily for 7–10 days; cephalexin, 250 mg four times daily for 7 days; or dicloxacillin, 250 mg four times daily for 7 days.
> • For HSV, acyclovir 800 mg orally five times daily for 7–10 days.
> • For *Candida albicans* or *Malassezia furfur*, ketoconazole used topically or taken orally 200 mg twice daily for 10 days.

Antihistamines

Antihistamines may be useful to reduce scratching. Oral antihistamines may be mostly useful for their sedative properties.[1] Doxepin cream can cause sedation if it is used over large areas of the body.

> **DOSAGE**
> • Doxepin cream 5%, a thin layer applied up to four times daily
> • Diphenhydramine, 12.5–50 mg orally every 6 hours
> • Hydroxyzine, 10–50 mg orally every 6 hours; or loratadine, 10 mg orally daily

Topical Corticosteroids

The standard medical treatment of atopic dermatitis consists of topical corticosteroids. Interestingly, measured effects of topical steroids and topical calcineurin inhibitors (discussed in the following section) are reduction of transepidermal water loss and improved barrier function.[64] These drugs are typically used twice daily for up to 2 weeks during an acute flare and then once to twice daily on weekends to maintain remission. Because this disease is more common in young children, concerns arise that long-term use may suppress the hypothalamic-pituitary-adrenal (HPA) axis, cause growth retardation, and have other side effects. Despite these concerns, no other medication is as effective during an acute flare, and its use only during these times does not appear to pose a risk.

For quick control of flares, consider using a higher-potency product and then reducing the strength for maintenance or switching down to an herbal preparation. Use only class IV and V corticosteroids on the face, axilla, groin, and intertriginous areas.[1] For children, use class III agents when a more potent agent is desired and titrate downward. For the eyelids, use a class V or VI agent for 5–7 days. Apply a thin layer directly after bathing, followed by emollient use. Ointments are generally recommended, although not in warm, humid climates, in which their occlusiveness can cause sweat retention dermatitis and acne. Gels can be used for weeping lesions and on the scalp and bearded skin. A full list of potencies of topical steroids is available in Chapter 73.

DOSAGE

- Class I (superpotent): clobetasol ointment 0.05% twice daily (also available as a gel)
- Class III (upper midstrength): triamcinolone 0.1% ointment twice daily
- Class IV (midstrength): hydrocortisone valerate 0.2% ointment twice daily
- Class V (lower midstrength): desonide 0.05% ointment twice daily
- Class VI (mild): hydrocortisone 1% ointment twice daily

PRECAUTIONS

Prolonged use of steroid creams can cause skin atrophy or acne, and prolonged use of potent steroids carries a risk of growth retardation in children.

If systemic steroids are warranted, use in conjunction with an aggressive topical regimen and give as a 14-day taper to avoid a rebound flare.

Topical Immunomodulators

Tacrolimus ointment and pimecrolimus cream, inhibitors of calcineurin, are additional nonsteroidal options for treatment of atopic dermatitis. These agents decrease T-cell activation and cytokine release while inhibiting mast cell and basophil degranulation. They have been studied largely as steroid-sparing agents for use after control of an acute flare to maintain remission. Investigators and clinicians were hopeful to find an agent to provide control without the risks of skin thinning and effects on the HPA axis.

After case reports of skin cancer and lymphoma with use of these agents appeared, the U.S. Food and Drug Administration issued a black box warning noting that although a causal relationship had not been established, these agents should be used with caution. Continued study has not demonstrated an increased risk of malignancy.[65] Patients with atopic dermatitis have an increased risk of lymphoma, and this risk increases with severity of disease. Experts comment mistaking cutaneous T-cell lymphoma for severe AD might account for the increased risk in these patients. Avoid the use of topical immunomodulators in immunocompromised patients or in those with a known neoplasm. If AD does not respond to usual treatments, perform a biopsy to rule out (CTCL) or other causes. Encourage sun protection to reduce photocarcinogenesis.

A meta-analysis of tacrolimus use in children found it safe and effective, with no statistical difference between tacrolimus 0.03% and 0.1% preparations and a good response compared with vehicle, 1% hydrocortisone acetate, and 1% pimecrolimus (odds ratio: 4.56, 3.92, and 1.58, respectively).[66] Use creams as infrequently as possible to maintain remission. Use only on lesional skin and without occlusive dressings. Use only in children who are older than 2 years old. Adverse effects include burning on application and photosensitivity.

DOSAGE

Tacrolimus 0.03% ointment is applied twice daily in patients older than 2 years, including adults with mild disease. For adults, tacrolimus 0.1% ointment is applied twice daily, or pimecrolimus 1% cream is applied twice daily. Typical use is twice daily for no longer than 6 weeks and then reduce to daily or every other day use. Tacrolimus used three times weekly has been proven effective in children to maintain remission.[67]

Other Immunomodulators

Cyclosporine can be used, but only by a provider experienced in its use. *Leukotriene inhibitors* (e.g., montelukast) are not effective monotherapy for atopic dermatitis, but they may reduce itching.

Therapies to Consider

Traditional Chinese Medicine

Several trials of traditional Chinese medicine herbal blends for atopic dermatitis have shown promising results. A Cochrane Review concluded that although the studies were small, they showed some evidence of effectiveness.[68] A five-herb concoction was studied in children with moderate to severe disease for 12 weeks, and although no significant difference was noted in clinical severity scores, the treatment group used one-third less corticosteroid and had significantly improved quality of life index scores at the end of treatment and 4 weeks later.[69]

Traditional Japanese Medicine (Kampo)

A case report on treatment with kampo, traditional Japanese medicine, had color pictures showing resolution of flexural lichenification and provided an excellent review of the likely immunomodulatory effects of this therapy.[70] A trial of shiunko, an herbal mixture commonly used in kampo for atopic dermatitis, lowered bacterial counts in the areas treated in four of seven patients.[71] A trial involving 95 patients using kampo showed promise, with a moderate to marked effect in more than half and no effect in just 4 patients.[72]

Homeopathy

Homeopathic studies have largely not shown an effect of this therapy in atopic dermatitis, although results from one small study in children were promising. An open-label trial of 27 children using a homeopathic cream of Oregon grape root (*M. aquifolium*), pansy (*Viola tricolor hortensis*), and gotu kola (*Centella asiatica*) revealed complete resolution in 6 children and marked improvement in 16.[73]

PREVENTION PRESCRIPTION

- Moisturize the skin. Apply emollients daily to newborn skin for the first 3 months of life, especially if at high risk for atopic dermatitis.
- Bathe in lukewarm water up to every day; if the water is irritating, add one cup of baking soda or salt to the water. Consider bathing in dilute bleach water (half cup per tubful) twice weekly for 5–10 minutes, then rinse off.
- Barely pat dry and the apply emollients to lock in moisture. Good choices include sunflower seed oil, virgin coconut oil, Cetaphil cream, Aquaphor ointment, paraffin, and creams containing creamed.
- Prevent break down of the skin barrier. Use soap minimally; when needed, use a mild, pH-balanced soap such as Dove, Aveeno, or Basis. Avoid sodium laurel sulfate and baby wipes when possible.
- Wet dressings using dilute corticosteroids such as such as 1:3 mometasone furoate 0.1% ointment for body and 1:19 mometasone furoate 0.1% ointment for the face can quickly gain control of recalcitrant lesions.
- Do not scratch! Pat, firmly press, or grasp the skin.
- Avoid triggers. Eliminate cigarette smoke exposure. Wear smooth, natural fibers that do not rub the skin. Avoid wool.
- Avoid fabric softeners and other chemicals in laundry detergent, use liquid detergent, and consider an extra rinse cycle.
- Humidify air in the winter. Dehumidify air in the summer.
- Reduce exposure to dust mites if sensitive; avoid rugs in bedrooms, wet mop floors, use mattress covers, and launder bed clothes weekly in hot water.
- Consider an allergy elimination diet if a food allergy is suspected.
- Discover ways to control emotional stress. Seek low-stress work environments. Mindfulness meditation, massage, or learning self-hypnosis may be helpful. Consider reading *Skin Deep* on www.grossbart.com.
- Pursue an antiinflammatory diet with frequent sources of omega-3 fatty acids such as cold-water fish, walnuts, and flaxseed. Drink green or oolong tea.
- Consider essential fatty acid supplementation, adding docosahexaenoic acid and eicosapentaenoic acid 2 g daily if your fish intake is inadequate and gamma-linolenic acid in the form of borage oil, 500 mg daily, or evening primrose oil, 1–2 g daily.
- Consider vitamin D_3 2000 IU daily and vitamin E 400 IU daily for adults and half that for children aged less than 8 years.
- Pregnant women with strong history of atopy should consider taking *Lactobacillus rhamnosus* GG prenatally and while breastfeeding. Continue giving it to the infant until age 2 years. Other conditions where lactobacilli colonization may need encouragement include birth by C-section, bottle feeding, and antibiotics use. Others may also find this useful. Dosage is 25–50 billion CFU for adults, 5–10 billion CFU for children.
- Encourage a diverse microbiome. Avoid antibacterial products, avoid antibiotics in animal products, and consume fermented foods and beverages.
- If you cannot breastfeed, consider hydrolyzed formulas for atopy prevention for at least the first 4 months of life.
- Natural chickenpox (varicella) infection and childhood immunizations have been shown to reduce AD.
- Moderate amounts of sunshine may be useful and allow you to obtain vitamin D.
- Reduce exposure to plastics, food packaged in plastics, and topical skin care products containing phthalates.

THERAPEUTIC REVIEW

AVOIDANCE OF TRIGGERS

- Reduce exposure to known allergens.
- Wear smooth, comfortable, breathable clothing.
- Use liquid detergents and fully rinse clothing to avoid disturbance of barrier function.

IMPROVEMENT IN BARRIER FUNCTION

- Hydrate by bathing daily and applying an emollient such as sunflower oil, virgin coconut oil, Cetaphil cream, Aquaphor ointment, double base gel (Dermal Laboratories, Hitchin UK), or liquid paraffin 50% in soft white paraffin. This can prevent half of AD in infants.
- Bathing with one-half cup of bleach added significantly reduces AD.
- Wet dressings with very dilute corticosteroids are effective for severe disease. Apply a 1:3 of their typical corticosteroid, use bandages or clothing over, and keep damp.
- Ceramide-containing creams, such as *EpiCeram* or *TriCeram,* may have added benefit over other emollients.
- Virgin coconut oil reduces *Staphylococcus aureus* colonization.

NUTRITION

- Avoid known food allergies. (The most common foods triggers of atopic dermatitis are egg, soy, milk, wheat, fish, shellfish, and peanut.)
- When breastfeeding atopic mothers avoid dairy it prevents AD in their babies.
- Infants at high risk who cannot exclusively breastfeed should use hydrolyzed formula (broken down proteins) in the first 4 months of life. Examples of hydrolyzed formulas include Nutramigen LIPIL, Pregestimil, and Alimentum Advance.
- Infants with AD or egg allergy benefit from beginning peanut ingestion three times weekly after age 4–6 months to prevent peanut allergy.
- Drink three cups of strong oolong tea daily.

MIND-BODY THERAPY

- Support groups
- Coping skill educational program
- Psychotherapy

SUPPLEMENTS

- Vitamin D_3: 2000 daily for adults, 1000 IU daily for children aged less than 8 years, or consider supplementing to keep normal serum levels
- Vitamin E: 600 IU daily
- Docosahexaenoic acid/eicosapentaenoic acid: 2–4 g daily

- Gamma-linolenic acid: such as borage oil 500 mg daily
- *Lactobacillus rhamnosus:* 20 billion CFUs daily for an atopic mother prenatally and postnatally for prevention of atopic dermatitis in the infant

BOTANICALS

- 2% glycyrrhetinic acid (Atopiclair or others) applied three times daily
- Topical formulations of *Hypericum perforatum* (St. John's wort), Oregon grape root, rosmarinic acid, honey, or chamomile applied twice daily

OTHER CREAMS

- Vitamin B_{12}: 0.07% cream used twice daily
- Coal tar preparations applied twice daily to chronic or lichenified lesions

PHARMACEUTICALS

Antihistamines

- Doxepin cream: twice daily to affected areas
- Diphenhydramine: 12.5–50 mg orally every 6 hours
- Hydroxyzine: 10–50 mg orally every 6 hours
- Loratadine: 10 mg orally daily

Antimicrobials

- Consider ketoconazole, 200 mg twice daily for 10 days, for head or neck involvement.
- Consider skin culture or smear for herpes or empirical antibacterial treatment for recalcitrant lesions.

Corticosteroids

- Triamcinolone 0.1% ointment: twice daily for up to 2 weeks for flares, then up to twice daily on weekends to maintain remission.
- Hydrocortisone 1% ointment: used on thin skin at higher risk for adverse events (face, neck, axilla).

Topical Immunomodulators

- Tacrolimus 0.03% ointment: twice-daily short-term use for patients older than 2 years.
- Tacrolimus 0.03% ointment: three times weekly to maintain remission in patients older than 2 years.
- Tacrolimus 0.1% ointment: twice-daily short-term use in patients older than 15 years.
- Pimecrolimus 1% cream: twice daily for short-term use.

Key Web Resources

Eczema and Sensitive-Skin Education: Patient education and support	http://www.easeeczema.org
The Eczema Company: Central resource for eczema products. Especially has a great selection of wet wrap products and clothing	http://www.eczemacompany.com/
Eczema Awareness, Support, and Education (EASE) program: Clear information and downloadable brochures in multiple languages including, "But It Itches So Much!" (for children) and "Eczema: It's Time to Take Control"	http://www.eczemacanada.ca
Skin Deep: Home of Skin Deep, Dr. Ted Grossbart's mind-body program for healthy skin that is available by free e-book	http://www.grossbart.com
iHerb.com, Vitacost: Online sources for difficult to find over-the-counter products at prices often lower than suggested retail price	http://www.iherb.com http://www.vitacost.com

REFERENCES

References are available online at ExpertConsult.com.

CHAPTER 73

PSORIASIS

Apple A. Bodemer, MD

PATHOPHYSIOLOGY AND CLINICAL BACKGROUND

Psoriasis is a chronic inflammatory skin disease characterized by abnormal differentiation and hyperproliferation of the epidermis. Its most common clinical presentation is as thick bright red to pink plaques with silvery scale (Figs. 73.1 and 73.2). Psoriasis is fairly common, affecting approximately 2% of the general population. It has a bimodal age distribution, with peak onsets between 20 and 30 years and 50 and 60 years.

Psoriasis is generally regarded as a disorder of the immune system that is driven by abnormally activated T helper cells that stimulate proinflammatory cytokine production and overproduction and abnormal maturation of the outer layer of skin cells. Activation of these T cells can occur through specific interactions with antigen-presenting cells (APCs) or nonspecific super-antigen interactions (guttate psoriasis triggered by streptococcal antigens). APC activation requires costimulatory signals. Once activated, psoriatic T cells produce a type 1 helper T cell (Th1)–dominant cytokine profile that includes interleukin-2 (IL-2), tumor necrosis factor-alpha (TNF-alpha), interferon (IFN)-gamma, and IL-8. These cytokines attract and activate neutrophils, which are responsible for much of the inflammation seen in psoriasis.

While genetics play an important role in the development of psoriasis, behavioral and environmental factors clearly influence the course of the disease. A family history can usually (but not always) be elicited. If one parent has psoriasis, the risk for having the disorder is approximately 14%. This figure increases to 41% if both parents have psoriasis. Several genetic foci and human leukocyte antigens (HLAs; histocompatibility antigens) have been identified to be linked to the development of psoriasis.

Environmental factors implicated in triggering psoriasis or psoriatic flares include physical trauma (isomorphic or Koebner phenomenon), infections (e.g., streptococcal pharyngitis), hypocalcemia, stress, and medications (lithium, beta-blockers, antimalarials, IFNs, rapid tapers of systemic corticosteroids). Paradoxically, psoriasis and psoriatic lesions have been described to develop in patients treated with anti-TNF drugs for inflammatory bowel disease.[1] The effect of pregnancy on psoriasis is not consistent; half of the women with psoriasis worsen during pregnancy, while the other half improve. Patients infected with human immunodeficiency virus (HIV) tend to have a more severe disease. Other factors associated with psoriasis include rapid weight changes, higher body mass index, alcohol consumption, vitamin D deficiency, and tobacco use. Smoking has been clearly implicated in the onset and severity of psoriasis, with the incidence of psoriasis decreasing after successful smoking cessation.[2] Additionally, people with psoriasis are at a greater risk for developing coronary artery disease (CAD) and metabolic syndrome.

> The Koebner phenomenon occurs when skin trauma or irritation triggers a skin reaction such as a psoriatic plaque. Treatment of itching is important because scratching can trigger flares through this mechanism.

Clinically, psoriasis may manifest in several ways (Table 73.1). In addition to skin findings, nail abnormalities are often present. These include pits, oil slicks, subungual hyperkeratosis, and onycholysis. The incidence of nail psoriasis is not known, but it does occur in the majority of people with the disorder at some point and is more common in people who also have psoriatic arthritis.[3]

The incidence of psoriatic arthritis effects is not clear and estimates vary widely. Generally, skin lesions precede the joint disease by up to 10–20 years; however, the joint disease may be the first manifestation 10%–15% of the time. The five classifications of psoriatic arthritis are summarized in Table 73.2. Psoriatic arthritis can be extremely disabling and thus warrants more aggressive systemic treatments, such as methotrexate or newer biological immune response modifiers (see later discussion of systemic pharmaceuticals).

INTEGRATIVE THERAPY

Skin Care

Gentle skin care can help minimize pruritus and skin trauma and can thus prevent the Koebnerization of psoriatic lesions. It can be helpful to bathe in cool-to-tepid water using only gentle cleansers (e.g., Cetaphil soapless cleanser, Aquanil). Additionally, frequent and regular application of thick emollients—especially while the skin is still damp—will help keep psoriatic skin hydrated and more manageable. Natural oils such as coconut oil, avocado oil, almond oil, or olive oil can be very helpful and soothing. Colloidal oatmeal in the form of an emollient or bath (e.g., Aveeno) may also help soothe itching and irritation associated with psoriasis.

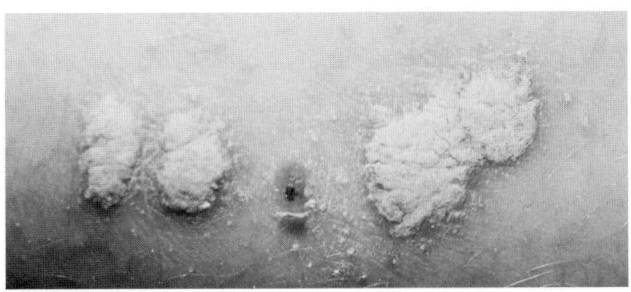

FIG. 73.1 ■ Auspitz sign. Pinpoint bleeding areas where scale was lifted from psoriatic plaque. (From Weston WL, Lane AT, Morelli JG. *Color textbook of pediatric dermatology.* 4th ed. Philadelphia: Mosby; 2007.)

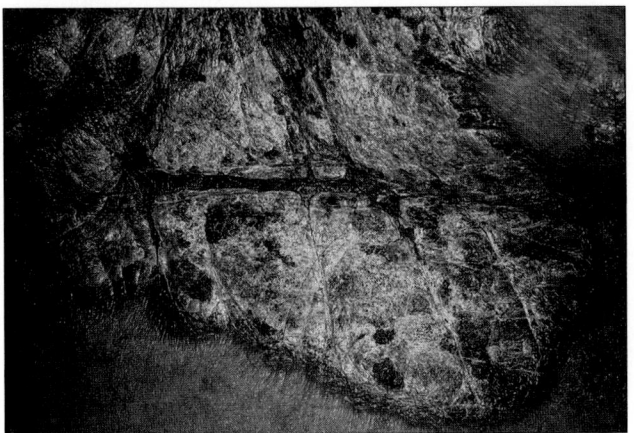

FIG. 73.2 ■ Psoriatic plaque. Note the sharp demarcation and silvery scale. (From van de Kerkhof PCM, Schalkwijk J. Psoriasis. In: Bolognia JL, Jorizzo JL, Rapini RP, eds. *Dermatology.* 2nd ed. Philadelphia: Mosby; 2008.)

Oatmeal baths can be made by placing whole oats in a blender and grinding them into a fine powder. Add water to a half cup of the oat flour to make a loose slurry that can be poured into a bath. A thicker paste can be made and patted onto psoriatic lesions as a poultice.

Ultraviolet Radiation

Psoriasis typically improves during the summer months, when there is more exposure to ultraviolet radiation (UVR). People have been taking advantage of this response to UVR for many years in many forms. Well-controlled clinical exposure in the form of phototherapy offers more predictable clinical results and will be discussed in the pharmaceutical section.

Climatotherapy and Balneophototherapy

Climatotherapy means to relocate to a climate more favorable for treatment of a condition. *Balneophototherapy* is treatment with water and sun, usually in a spa setting. Dead Sea climatotherapy has long been touted as beneficial for patients with psoriasis. Patients visit resorts at the Dead Sea for 2–4 weeks and expose themselves to both the water and sun. One study of 740 German patients treated at the Dead Sea found a 70% complete clearance of symptoms after 4 weeks at one of the clinics.[4] Several reviews have found this to be effective from a clinical as well as a cost standpoint and have found improved quality of life for patients with psoriasis

TABLE 73.1 Subtypes of Psoriasis

Subtype	Characteristics	Associations
Chronic Plaque	Erythematous plaques with silvery scale Typically involving the scalp, knees, elbows, low back, umbilicus, and gluteal cleft Pruritus variable Nail findings common	Most common; accounting for approximately 90% of all cases of psoriasis
Guttate	Diffuse salmon-to-red "drop-like" papules and plaques with fine scale Typically involving the trunk and extremities	Second most common type (2%) Most common in children and young adults Affecting children and young adults Associated with group A *Streptococcus* infections Tends to resolve with eradication of the infection Possibly persistent in "strep" carriers Best prognosis for remission
Inverse	Affecting predominantly the axillae, groin, and submammary area Less scale than in other types	Prone to secondary bacterial or yeast infections
Erythrodermic	Erythema with scaling over more than 80% of the body surface area	Potential complications include high-output cardiac failure, renal failure, and sepsis
Pustular	Confluent pustules on an erythematous base von Zumbusch type: generalized with acute fever, chills, nausea, headache, and joint problems Annular type: subacute or chronic; systemic symptoms possible Acrodermatitis continua of Hallopeau: distal fingers; fingernails possibly floating away on lakes of pus and permanent nail destruction common	Life-threatening Potential complications include high-output cardiac failure, sepsis, and hypercalcemia Systemic symptoms are less common than with the Hallopeau type
Palmoplantar Pustulosis	Pustules of the palms and soles with yellow-brown macules	Commonly associated with sterile inflammatory bone lesions

TABLE 73.2 **Classification of Psoriatic Arthritis**

Type	Characteristics	Associations
Asymmetric Oligoarticular	Digits of the hands and feet are affected first Inflammation of the flexor tendon and synovium occurring simultaneously Usually affecting fewer than five digits	"Sausage digit" (involvement of both the DIP and PIP of one digit)
Symmetric Polyarthritis	Clinically identical to rheumatoid arthritis Possibly affecting the hands, wrists, ankles, and feet Involvement of the DIP Rheumatoid factor negative	Erosive changes seen on radiographs
DIP Arthropathy	Unique to psoriasis Affecting only 5%–10% More prominent in men	Nail involvement with chronic paronychia
Arthritis Mutilans	Osteolysis leading to telescoping of the finger with an "opera-glass" hand More common in early-onset disease More common in men	Osteolysis (dissolution of the joint) "Pencil-in-cup" deformity on radiographs
Spondylitis With or Without Sacroiliitis	Occurring in 5% of patients with psoriatic arthritis More common in male patients Asymmetric involvement of vertebrae	Morning stiffness of the lower back is the most characteristic symptom

DIP, distal interphalangeal joint; PIP, proximal interphalangeal joint.
Data from Hammadi AA, Gorevic PD. *Psoriatic arthritis.* www.emedicine.com/med/topic1954.htm. Accessed 28.08.06.

as well.[4-6] One proposed explanation for the success of this approach is that the elevation of 400 m below sea level and the thick haze present in the area increase the thickness of the atmosphere. This could attenuate shorter ultraviolet B (UVB) wavelengths and allow a larger proportion of longer-wave UVB to reach the patients' skin. Additionally, the water has a high mineral content. In vitro studies indicated that Dead Sea water had an antiproliferative effect on exposed cells.[7] These clinics and solariums offer patients an extended retreat from stressful lives; the relaxation likely plays a role in the outcomes as well.

Studies looking at the safety of this type of therapy have found increased actinic damage but not an increase in skin cancers compared to patients with psoriasis treated by other means.[8,9] Nevertheless, recommending protection of exposed, noninvolved skin is prudent.

Nutrition

Antiinflammatory Diet

Healthy dietary choices are important for overall health. Antiinflammatory or Mediterranean-style dietary approaches have been found to enhance many aspects of health—especially in the setting of inflammatory diseases. A recent study asked 62 patients with mild-to-severe psoriasis to complete questionnaires that were created to assess their adherence to a Mediterranean-style diet. The Psoriasis Area Severity Index (PASI—a well-established tool for evaluating the severity of psoriasis with higher numbers indicating more severe disease) and C-reactive protein (CRP) levels (a general marker of systemic inflammation) were found to be negatively correlated with consumption of extra virgin olive oil (EVOO), vegetables, fruit, legumes, fish, and nuts and positively correlated with the consumption of red meat. The strongest negative correlations were with EVOO and fish.[10] More

information about these dietary approaches can be found in Chapter 88.

Elimination Diet/Gluten-Free Diet

Some patients with psoriasis have experienced improvement on a gluten-free diet.[11] Elevated markers for celiac disease (immunoglobulin A [IgA] antibodies to gliadin, tissue transglutaminase, and endomysium) have been found in some patients with psoriasis, and in those people, disease severity appears to correlate with circulating levels of these markers.[12-14] A positive family history of celiac disease/gluten sensitivity or presence of gastrointestinal (GI) symptoms may suggest sensitivity to gluten. Testing for markers of gluten intolerance may help identify those patients who are most likely to benefit from a gluten-free diet. Please find more information about how to eliminate gluten from the diet in Chapters 31 and 86.

Weight Loss

Low-calorie diets that promote weight loss have been found to be beneficial in overweight and obese patients with psoriasis.[15,16,18] Naldi et al. conducted an intervention study that looked at over 300 obese people with psoriasis who were unresponsive to systemic therapies. They were randomized to either a 20-week qualitative and quantitative dietary and exercise program focused on weight loss or to an informational session about the importance of weight loss for control of psoriasis. At the end of the 20 weeks, there were significant improvements in PASI scores in the intervention group as compared with the control group.[18] There is also evidence that bariatric surgery in obese patients with psoriasis results in improvement of psoriasis—at least in the short term—which also supports that weight loss can benefit psoriasis.[19,20] Additionally, it appears that weight loss can improve responses to systemic medications.[21,22] It is important to work closely with obese patients toward weight loss goals and to help them find the support they might need. An emphasis should be placed on long-term dietary and exercise patterns to improve overall health and minimize not only the skin and joint effects of psoriasis but also cardiovascular and metabolic risks as well.

Supplements

Fish Oil

Rates of psoriasis and other inflammatory conditions are low in populations that consume high levels of fish oils that are rich in omega-3 fatty acids such as eicosapentaenoic acid (EPA) and docosahexaenoic acid (DHA). In vitro evidence supports the theory that omega-3 fatty acids improve psoriasis by inhibiting the inflammatory cytokines IL-6 and TNF-alpha, as well as by decreasing levels of leukotrienes.[23] Collier et al. examined the effect of consumption of oily fish on chronic plaque psoriasis compared with whitefish. These investigators found that people who ate oily fish (6 oz/day for 6 weeks) had significant improvement in their PASI score.[24]

Bittiner et al. conducted a double-blinded placebo-controlled study of patients supplemented with 10 fish oil capsules (1.5 g EPA each) compared with 10 olive oil capsules for 12 weeks and found significantly less itching, scaling, and erythema in the group treated with fish oil.[25]

Other randomized and double-blinded studies that investigated dietary intake of omega-3 fatty acids have not found significant benefit.[26,27]

Some evidence indicates that fish oils can minimize side effects of other systemic therapies. Fish oils may help decrease triglyceride levels and improve cholesterol profiles in patients treated with retinoids.[28] Additionally, fish oils may help reduce the risk for nephrotoxicity associated with cyclosporine.[29,30]

DOSAGE

Doses vary depending on the source. Flaxseed; walnuts; and cold-water fish, such as mackerel, lake trout, herring, sardines, albacore tuna, and salmon, are all rich natural sources of omega-3 fatty acids. Supplements that contain 1000–4000 mg EPA and DHA should be provided daily.

PRECAUTIONS

Some types of fish may contain high levels of mercury, polychlorinated biphenyls (PCBs), dioxins, and other environmental contaminants. Fish listed by the American Heart Association as having the highest mercury levels are shark, swordfish, tilefish, and king mackerel. PCBs are found in high concentrations in farmed salmon. Choosing wild-caught salmon, trimming fat before cooking, and avoiding over-grilling can help decrease exposure to PCBs. Though there has been concern about the risk for blood thinning with fish oil supplementations, studies have shown that there was no significant increase in bleeding incidents with up to 4 g/day EPA + DHA.[31] Nevertheless, it is prudent to be cautious in patients already taking blood thinners.

Curcumin

Curcumin is the active component of turmeric. It has been shown to inhibit proinflammatory molecules and pathways important in psoriasis, including TNF, proinflammatory ILs (IL-1beta, IL-6, IL-8, and IL-12), and the nuclear factor (NF)-kappaB signaling pathways.[33,34] Studies evaluating clinical use are limited, but clinical studies have found it to be safe at doses up to 8–12 g/day, with the only side effects being reversible GI problems (nausea and diarrhea).[35]

DOSAGE

The dose is 1500 mg three times a day.[36]

Vitamins and Minerals

Vitamin D. The role of vitamin D in the development or exacerbation of psoriatic flares is not yet clear, but it appears that there may be an inverse correlation between vitamin D levels and severity of chronic plaque psoriasis.[37] There is one study that found benefit with high-dose vitamin D supplementation for 6 months in patients with psoriasis and vitiligo who were also vitamin D deficient. The doses were very high (35,000 IU of cholecalciferol [D_3]), and participants were required to be on a low-calcium diet with a minimum of 2.5 liters of oral fluids daily. Serum 25-hydroxyvitamin [25(OH)] D_3, parathyroid hormone (PTH), total calcium, ionized calcium, urea, and creatinine were carefully monitored, and PASI scores were followed. Significant clinical improvement was seen in all nine patients with psoriasis.[38] While this protocol may be extreme and further studies need to be conducted to better understand the potential utility of this treatment, determining the vitamin D level and moderate supplementation of vitamin D deficiencies is prudent.

DOSAGE

The dose is 600 IU/day for supplemental uses.[39]

Administer 1000–2000 IU/day for treating vitamin D deficiency and titrate on the basis of serum levels.

PRECAUTIONS

Recent research suggests that doses up to 10,000 IU/day are safe.[40] Higher than 10,000 IU/day, a person should be under the care of a physician and should be monitored for signs of vitamin D toxicity from hypercalcemia (headache, nausea, vomiting, abdominal pain, increased urination, and thirst).

Zinc. Zinc is a cofactor in many reactions important for skin health and immune function and has also been shown to have antiinflammatory properties. Some investigators have suggested that patients with psoriasis have decreased epidermal zinc levels.[41] One group compared plasma levels of zinc in 35 patients with psoriasis with those in age- and sex-matched controls. No significant differences in zinc levels were found, but they did note a trend toward lower plasma zinc levels, independent of serum albumin and alkaline phosphatase levels, in patients with more extensive psoriasis.[42] Subsequent studies have not reproduced this finding, and most clinical studies examining zinc supplementation for treatment of psoriasis have not shown benefit.[43] However, some clinicians who use zinc supplements for patients with psoriasis strongly believe that it can be beneficial.

The formulation of zinc may influence biological activity and may partly explain some of the conflicting results in the literature. Effervescent preparations of zinc, zinc picolinate, and methionine-bound zinc are more bioactive than other formulations such as zinc gluconate and zinc sulfate.

DOSAGE

The dose is 30–50 mg of elemental zinc per day.[44]

Foods rich in zinc include oysters, beef, poultry (dark meat), pork, beans, and nuts.

PRECAUTIONS

Minor side effects include nausea, vomiting, and a metallic taste in the mouth. At even higher doses, zinc toxicity can manifest as watery diarrhea, irritation and erosion of the GI tract, acute renal tubular necrosis, interstitial nephritis, and a flulike syndrome.

*At doses higher than 30 mg/day, zinc can induce a copper deficiency. Furthermore, 2 mg of copper should be added for every additional 30 mg of elemental zinc.

Inositol. Lithium is known to worsen psoriasis and depletion of inositol is known to occur in people taking lithium. Inositol supplementation for people taking lithium has been shown to reduce some of the side effects of lithium without diminishing its clinical usefulness. In 2004, Allan et al. conducted a randomized placebo-controlled crossover study and found that PASI scores were improved when patients taking lithium (300–1200 g/day) also took inositol (6 g/day) for 10 weeks. These investigators did not see a worsening of bipolar disorder, but this outcome was not formally evaluated in this study.[45]

DOSAGE

The dose is 6 g/day.

PRECAUTIONS

Inositol appears to be safe. However, patients who have bipolar disorder should undergo close monitoring of their psychiatric state during inositol supplementation.

Topical Botanicals

Indigo Naturalis *Extract*

Indigo naturalis (qing dai) is used by traditional Chinese medicine (TCM) healers to treat various inflammatory skin conditions. It has been used orally for psoriasis in

TCM, but long-term use is associated with GI side effects and risk for liver damage.[46] Topical *Indigo naturalis* extract has shown promise in clinical studies evaluating its usefulness in both chronic plaque psoriasis and in nail psoriasis with no significant side effects.[46-48] *Indigo naturalis* has been shown to have antiproliferative effects, to inhibit TNF-alpha-dependent inflammatory pathways, and to downregulate inflammatory markers seen in psoriatic skin.[46,49,50]

DOSAGE

Apply 3%–5% oil, ointment, or cream once to twice a day.

PRECAUTIONS

People may experience mild itching at the beginning of treatment, but that should go away after a few days. Contact sensitization could theoretically occur.

Capsaicin

Itching is a common complaint in psoriasis. The neuropeptide substance P has been shown to be elevated in psoriatic skin[51] and is known to elicit itching when it is applied to normal skin.[52] This compound also upregulates the expression of adhesion molecules important in the activation and recruitment of leukocytes.[53] Capsaicin is an extract of chili peppers that acts by depleting substance P locally in the skin. A double-blinded placebo-controlled study looking at the potential use of capsaicin four times daily for 6 weeks found that the treatment group tended to have better global improvement, greater pruritus relief, and reductions in psoriasis severity scores; however, none of the differences reached statistical significance.[54]

DOSAGE

Apply 0.025% or 0.075% capsaicin cream three or four times/day.

PRECAUTIONS

Patients typically experience burning during initial applications. The burning disappears with consistent use. Patients must be careful to wash their hands after application and to avoid rubbing capsaicin into their eyes.

Aloe Vera

Aloe vera is a succulent plant whose thick leaves contain an inner pulpy mucilaginous gel. Compounds in aloe vera have been found to have antiinflammatory and antiitch properties, as well as pain reduction and wound healing effects. Although results from controlled studies have been variable, topical aloe extract seems to reduce the desquamation, erythema, and infiltration associated with psoriatic plaques. One small study of patients with mild psoriasis compared the application of a 0.5% extract in a hydrophilic cream three times a day for 4 weeks with a placebo and found improvement of psoriatic plaques in the treatment group.[55] Another double-blinded placebo-controlled study with right-left comparisons in 40 patients found a slightly better response in the placebo group.[56] Although aloe is very safe, topical sensitization can occur.

Glycyrrhetinic Acid (Licorice)

Cortisol is inactivated by the enzyme 11beta-hydroxysteroid dehydrogenase. This enzyme is inhibited by glycyrrhetinic acid, a compound found in licorice. Through this mechanism, topical glycyrrhetinic acid has been shown to potentiate the action of hydrocortisone.[57] Glycyrrhetinic acid is available in 1% and 2% formulations and appears to be safe when it is used topically. No studies have specifically investigated the use of this compound in psoriasis.

Systemic Botanicals

Milk Thistle (Silybum marianum)

Although milk thistle has not been suggested to play a role in psoriasis treatment, this botanical has been purported to protect against methotrexate-induced hepatotoxicity. Milk thistle has been shown to act as an antioxidant by scavenging free radicals and inhibiting lipid peroxidation. Investigators have also suggested that it may protect against DNA injury and increase hepatocyte protein synthesis.[58]

> **DOSAGE**
>
> The dose is 140 mg (70% silymarin) two or three times/day.
>
> **PRECAUTIONS**
>
> Diabetic patients taking silymarin require careful monitoring of blood glucose because this botanical may cause hypoglycemia secondary to increased insulin sensitivity.[59]

Topical Pharmaceuticals

Keratolytics

Keratolytics are compounds that break down the outer layers of the skin and can decrease the thickness of psoriatic plaques. This class of compounds includes salicylic acid (2%–10%), urea (20%–40%), and alpha-hydroxy acids (glycolic and lactic acids). Along with providing added comfort, thinner plaques allow for enhanced penetration of other topical medications. Keratolytics can be applied once to several times a day as long as they do not cause irritation.

> **PRECAUTIONS**
>
> Salicylic acid should not be applied extensively on the body, especially in children. Systemic absorption can lead to salicylism, which is characterized by tinnitus, nausea, and vomiting.

Topical Steroids

Corticosteroids are considered first-line therapy for mild-to-moderate psoriasis. They have antiinflammatory, immunosuppressive, and antiproliferative properties. These activities are mediated by alterations in gene transcription. The efficacy of an individual topical corticosteroid is related to its potency and its ability to be absorbed into the skin.[60]

> **DOSAGE**
>
> Table 73.3 provides information on potencies of different topical steroids.
>
> **PRECAUTIONS**
>
> Topical corticosteroids are associated with tachyphylaxis—decreased efficacy with continued use. Intermittent treatment schedules and combination with other topical medications minimize this problem. Local side effects are more common with higher potency and include skin atrophy, acne, and localized hypertrichosis. Systemic absorption can occur with frequent or long-term use over large areas and can cause side effects similar to those of oral steroids (e.g., hyperglycemia, adrenal suppression, mood changes, weight gain).

Calcipotriene (Dovonex)

Vitamin D receptors are present on many different cells, including keratinocytes and Langerhans cells. The bioactive form (1,25-dihydroxycholecalciferol) has been shown to inhibit keratinocyte proliferation and promote keratinocyte differentiation.[61] Calcipotriene is a synthetic analog of the naturally active form of vitamin D. It is locally metabolized very rapidly thus leading to less interference with calcium metabolism.[61] It can safely be combined with other topical and systemic treatments.

> **DOSAGE**
>
> Apply 0.005% cream, ointment, or lotion once or twice daily.
>
> **PRECAUTIONS**
>
> Self-limited irritant dermatitis is the most common complaint and can be minimized by combination with topical steroids. Photosensitivity can develop in patients who receive UVB after calcipotriene is applied, so calcipotriene should be used after phototherapy sessions. Hypercalcemia is the most significant potential risk, but this is not a problem as long as the dose is kept at less than the recommended 100 g/week.[62]

Tazarotene Gel

Tazarotene is a topical retinoid (vitamin A derivative) that decreases epidermal proliferation and increases keratinocyte differentiation.

TABLE 73.3 Potencies of Topical Steroids

Class	Brand Name	Generic Name
1: Superpotent	Clobex lotion, 0.05%	Clobetasol propionate
	Cormax cream/solution, 0.05%	Clobetasol propionate
	Diprolene gel/ointment, 0.05%	Betamethasone dipropionate
	Olux foam, 0.05%	Clobetasol propionate
	Psorcon ointment, 0.05%	Diflorasone diacetate
	Temovate cream/ointment/solution, 0.05%	Clobetasol propionate
	Ultravate cream/ointment, 0.05%	Halobetasol propionate
2: Potent	Cyclocort ointment, 0.1%	Amcinonide
	Diprolene cream AF, 0.05%	Betamethasone dipropionate
	Diprosone ointment, 0.05%	Betamethasone dipropionate
	Elocon ointment, 0.1%	Mometasone furoate
	Florone ointment, 0.05%	Diflorasone diacetate
	Halog ointment/cream, 0.1%	Halcinonide
	Lidex cream/gel/ointment, 0.05%	Fluocinonide
	Maxiflor ointment, 0.05%	Diflorasone diacetate
	Maxivate ointment, 0.05%	Betamethasone dipropionate
	Psorcon cream, 0.05%	Diflorasone diacetate
	Topicort cream/ointment, 0.25%	Desoximetasone
	Topicort gel, 0.05%	Desoximetasone
3: Upper Midstrength	Aristocort A ointment, 0.1%	Triamcinolone acetonide
	Cutivate ointment, 0.005%	Fluticasone propionate
	Cyclocort cream/lotion, 0.1%	Amcinonide
	Diprosone cream, 0.05%	Betamethasone dipropionate
	Florone cream, 0.05%	Diflorasone diacetate
	Lidex-E cream, 0.05%	Fluocinonide
	Luxiq foam, 0.12%	Betamethasone valerate
	Maxiflor cream, 0.05%	Diflorasone diacetate
	Maxivate cream/lotion, 0.05%	Betamethasone dipropionate
	Topicort cream, 0.05%	Desoximetasone
	Valisone ointment, 0.1%	Betamethasone valerate
4: Midstrength	Aristocort cream, 0.1%	Triamcinolone acetonide
	Cordran ointment, 0.05%	Flurandrenolide
	Derma-Smoothe/FS oil, 0.01%	Fluocinolone acetonide
	Elocon cream, 0.1%	Mometasone furoate
	Kenalog cream/ointment/spray, 0.1%	Triamcinolone acetonide
	Synalar ointment, 0.025%	Fluocinolone acetonide
	Uticort gel, 0.025%	Betamethasone benzoate
	Westcort ointment, 0.2%	Hydrocortisone valerate
5: Lower Midstrength	Cordran cream/lotion/tape, 0.05%	Flurandrenolide
	Cutivate cream, 0.05%	Fluticasone propionate
	Dermatop cream, 0.1%	Prednicarbate
	DesOwen ointment, 0.05%	Desonide
	Diprosone lotion, 0.05%	Betamethasone dipropionate
	Kenalog lotion, 0.1%	Triamcinolone acetonide
	Locoid cream, 0.1%	Hydrocortisone
	Pandel cream, 0.1%	Hydrocortisone
	Synalar cream, 0.025%	Fluocinolone acetonide
	Uticort cream/lotion, 0.025%	Betamethasone benzoate
	Valisone cream/ointment, 0.1%	Betamethasone valerate

TABLE 73.3   Potencies of Topical Steroids—cont'd

Class	Brand Name	Generic Name
6: Mild	Westcort cream, 0.2%	Hydrocortisone valerate
	Aclovate cream/ointment, 0.05%	Alclometasone dipropionate
	DesOwen cream, 0.05%	Desonide
	Synalar cream/solution, 0.01%	Fluocinolone acetonide
	Tridesilon cream, 0.05%	Desonide
	Valisone lotion, 0.1%	Betamethasone valerate
7: Lowest Potency	Hydrocortisone	
	Dexamethasone	
	Methylprednisolone	
	Prednisolone	

From The National Psoriasis Foundation: *Potencies of topical steroids.* www.psoriasis.org/treatment/psoriasis/steriods/potency.php. Copyright 2006 National Psoriasis Foundation/USA.

DOSAGE

The dose is 0.05% or 0.1% gel.

PRECAUTIONS

Local skin irritation and pruritus are common side effects, so concomitant use with topical steroids is common.[60] Tazarotene may be teratogenic, so it should be used extremely carefully by women of childbearing age.

Tar

Tar-based products are either derived from coal or wood (pine, birch). A precise mechanism of action is difficult to determine because of the large number of compounds present, but tar has antiinflammatory, antiproliferative, and antiitch properties.

DOSAGE

The dose is 1%–5% crude tar or 10%–20% tar extract (LCD; liquor carbonis detergens).[63]

PRECAUTIONS

Side effects are infrequent and include local irritation or allergic reactions, folliculitis or acne-like eruptions, and increased photosensitivity. Prolonged use of high concentrations in sun-exposed areas may result in an increased risk for skin cancer. If the formulation is too strong or irritating, it can worsen psoriasis via Koebnerization.

Anthralin

Anthralin is a synthetic derivative of chrysarobin from the bark of the araroba tree of South America. The mechanism of action is not well understood, but it has been shown to inhibit cell growth and promote cell differentiation.[60]

DOSAGE

A 0.5%–1% preparation is applied for 10–30 minutes and is then washed off. Repeat once or twice daily.

PRECAUTIONS

Irritation to normal skin can be minimized by protection with petrolatum or zinc oxide paste around psoriatic plaques. Anthralin is messy and can stain hair, skin, nails, clothing, and bedding a brownish-to-purplish color. The hair discoloration can be minimized by using neutral henna powder to coat the hair.

Phototherapy

Ultraviolet B

UVB consists of radiation and includes wavelengths between 290 and 320 nm. UVB is known to decrease DNA synthesis and to have immunosuppressive effects. Langerhans cells (the main APCs in the epidermis) are extremely sensitive to UVB, and exposure limits antigen presentation to T lymphocytes. UVB also stimulates keratinocytes to secrete various cytokines that can further alter the immune response and limit inflammation.[64] Narrow-band UVB (nb-UVB), with wavelengths between 308 and 313 nm, has proven to be much more effective than full-spectrum UVB in the treatment of psoriasis.[65,66] The 308-nm excimer laser offers an additional option for limited plaque psoriasis. This has been found to be effective and safe and may require fewer treatments than other phototherapy options.[67]

DOSAGE

Treatment protocols are based on determining a minimal erythema dose (MED)—the dose of UVB that elicits barely perceptible erythema. Once an MED is defined, treatments are started at approximately 70%–75% of the MED and are given three times a week with the goal of maintaining minimally perceptible erythema. Once the skin is clear, some practitioners simply stop phototherapy, but others recommend tapering. There are no defined guidelines for accomplishing a UVB taper, and some people may require a maintenance dose.

PRECAUTIONS

Potential short-term side effects of UVB include erythema, xerosis, pruritus, and higher frequency of herpes simplex outbreaks. Longer-term side effects consist of photoaging and possibly increased risks for skin cancers. The carcinogenetic risk for UVB appears to be much less than that associated with ultraviolet A (UVA) combined with psoralen (PUVA; see next section). One small study examining people who had had more than 100 treatments with UVB showed an increase in skin cancer in this group.[68] Other larger studies have not found this association.[69] Additionally, a study specifically examining the correlation between nb-UVB and skin cancer found no significant association.[70]

Ultraviolet A and Psoralen

Information on this topic can be found online at ExpertConsult.com.

Systemic Pharmaceuticals

Methotrexate

Methotrexate is a folic acid antagonist that blocks dihydrofolate reductase—an enzyme necessary for making building blocks for DNA synthesis—and leads to cell cycle arrest. It also has immunosuppressive effects and acts as a potent antiinflammatory as well.[73] Methotrexate is particularly useful in patients with psoriatic arthritis.

DOSAGE

Methotrexate is available as a 2.5-mg pill or as solutions of 2.5 or 25.0 mg/mL. Typically, a 5- to 10-mg test dose is given, and complete blood count and liver function values are measured 7 days later. A dose of 10–15 mg/week is usually enough to control psoriasis. Methotrexate is given weekly either as a single dose or divided into three doses given 12 hours apart.[73]

PRECAUTIONS

Multiple side effects are associated with methotrexate. The most common is gastrointestinal upset, and the most dangerous is pancytopenia. Both can be decreased by adding 1 mg of folic acid daily. Other significant concerns are hepatotoxicity, pulmonary fibrosis, induction of malignancy, and teratogenicity. The concern for induction of malignancy is much greater when methotrexate is combined with PUVA; the risks for skin cancer and lymphoma appear to be increased (see the earlier section on PUVA). These potential complications require frequent monitoring with a complete blood count as well as renal and liver function tests. Liver biopsy to evaluate for fibrosis is indicated after a cumulative dose of 1.5–2.0 g. Additionally, the dose needs to be adjusted if the creatinine clearance value is less than 50 mL/minute.

Cyclosporine

Cyclosporine was initially isolated from the soil fungus *Tolypocladium inflatum*. It inhibits IL-2 gene transcription and leads to decreased T-cell proliferation and activation. Cyclosporine also inhibits the transcription of various proinflammatory cytokines.[74] It is useful in all types of psoriasis, but because of its rapid effect, cyclosporine is particularly useful in widespread pustular or erythrodermic psoriasis. Rebound typically occurs when cyclosporine is discontinued, and bridging with another medication can be helpful when weaning off of this medication.[73]

DOSAGE

Treatment should start at 5.0 mg/kg per day and slowly taper by 0.5 mg/kg per day, until the minimum dose required to prevent recurrences is achieved (typical doses range from 2 to 4 mg/kg per day).

PRECAUTIONS

Potential side effects include renal dysfunction, hypertension, hypertrichosis, gingival hyperplasia, gastrointestinal upset, neurological effects (headache, tremor, paresthesias), electrolyte imbalances, sleep disturbances, acneiform eruptions, hypertriglyceridemia, decreased seizure threshold, and bone marrow suppression. Monitoring consists of measurements of blood pressure; renal function parameters, including urinalysis, complete blood count, liver function tests; and blood chemistry analyses, including magnesium, potassium, and uric acid.

Because cyclosporine is metabolized by the cytochrome P450 3A4 enzyme system, it has many potential drug interactions. The clinician should review a complete medication and herbal list with each patient before cyclosporine therapy is initiated.

Acitretin

Acitretin is an oral retinoid with antiproliferative and antiinflammatory effects. It can reduce lymphocyte proliferation and decrease arachidonic acid metabolism, thus leading to decreased neutrophil activation and inflammatory mediators. Acitretin has been especially useful for rapid control of pustular psoriasis.

DOSAGE

The dose is 10, 25, or 50 mg/day and is taken orally with food.

PRECAUTIONS

Acitretin, like all retinoids, is highly teratogenic. It can cause drying of the skin and mucous membranes, which some investigators have suggested to be improved by adding 800 units of vitamin E daily.[75] Decreased night vision may occur, as well as pseudotumor cerebri, especially if acitretin is given with tetracycline antibiotics. Arthralgias, myalgias, bony changes (hyperostosis), poor wound healing, and gastrointestinal symptoms are all potential side effects. Serum cholesterol and triglyceride values may be elevated in 25%–50% of patients, and lipids must be monitored throughout therapy. Liver transaminase values may be elevated in up to 33% of patients, but toxic hepatitis is very rare.[76]

Monitoring should include pregnancy tests, fasting lipid panels, liver function tests, complete blood count with platelets, renal function tests, and creatine phosphokinase concentrations.

Biological Immune Response Modifiers

Biological immune response modifiers are directed specifically at neutralizing cytokines and blocking costimulatory messages important for the activation of T cells. There are a number of these medicines, including adalimumab (Humira), certolizumab pegol (Cimzia), golimumab (Simponi), infliximab (Remicade), and ustekinumab (Stelara).

All of the biological immune response modifiers require a thorough baseline evaluation. This includes history and physical examination (with special attention to hepatic, neurological, or cardiac disease, infection, and malignancy), complete blood count, chemistry screen with liver function tests, viral hepatitis screening, and screening for latent tuberculosis. Patients require annual tuberculosis screening and blood chemistry with liver function testing every 2–6 months. Patients are generally advised to have any necessary vaccinations before they begin treatment with biological immune response modifiers.[77]

Phosphodiesterase 4 Inhibitor

Apremilast (Otezla) is a new oral option for treating psoriasis. It acts by inhibiting phosphodiesterase 4 (PDE4) within the cell to block inflammation. The dose must be titrated over several days to 30 mg twice a day. Some GI upset with loose stool/mild diarrhea can occur for the first couple of weeks but resolves with continued treatment. Although this is a very new drug, it appears to be very safe, and unlike other biologics, no laboratory monitoring is required.[78]

Mind–Body Therapy

It is well understood that patients with psoriasis experience greater stress as a consequence of their disease. A large survey study including members of the National Psoriasis Foundation documented that psoriasis had profound emotional, social, and physical effects on quality of life.[79] Additionally, emotional factors—particularly stress—have been shown to have a strong correlation with the onset and exacerbation of psoriasis.[80]

How stress affects psoriasis is beginning to be understood more clearly. Garg et al. showed that injury to the epidermis promotes higher levels of keratinocyte growth stimulators, such as substance P and vasoactive intestinal peptide, and increases neural proliferation, which stimulates Langerhans cell activity. These researchers suggest that psychological stress may change the level of tolerance for physical insult or may prolong epidermal recovery time. This effect could lower the threshold for disease initiation and/or interfere with treatment.

Fortune et al. examined 112 patients with psoriasis before they started PUVA phototherapy and compared the stress level with the time to clearance of symptoms. These investigators found that high-level worry was the only significant predictor of the time taken for PUVA to clear psoriasis. Patients in the high-level worry group cleared 19 days later (1.8 times slower) than patients in the low-level worry group. Severity of disease, rates of positive family history, and levels of

alcohol intake at the onset of the study were not significantly different between the two groups.[81] This suggests that improving stress levels may enhance results from more conservative or traditional therapies. Other studies looking at various psychogenic interventions support this as well.[82,83]

> Improving stress levels may enhance results from more conservative or traditional therapies.

Meditation

A small study found that patients who listened to a mindfulness meditation–based stress reduction tape during PUVA or UVB therapy for psoriasis cleared 1 month earlier in the UVB plus relaxation tape group compared with the UVB only group and 6 weeks earlier in the PUVA plus relaxation tape group compared with the PUVA only group.[84] Another small study looked at symptoms of psoriasis as rated by dermatologists after treatment with 12 weeks of meditation (*n* = 5) or meditation plus imagery (*n* = 4) compared with controls (*n* = 9). A significant difference was noted between the treatment groups and the control group, but imagery did not yield more improvement than meditation alone.[85] The study was very small and had flaws; nevertheless, the results suggested that some patients may be able to decrease symptoms of psoriasis with meditation (see Chapter 100).

Hypnosis

A 3-month randomized blinded controlled trial looked at the efficacy of active (suggestion of disease improvement) versus neutral (no mention of disease) hypnosis for the treatment of psoriasis in patients classified as highly or moderately hypnotizable. Although the groups were very small, highly hypnotizable patients showed significantly greater improvement regardless of their assigned treatment group.[86] This observation suggests that patients who are highly hypnotizable may benefit from adding hypnosis to their treatment plan (see Chapter 95).

Therapies to Consider

Traditional Chinese Medicine

According to TCM, the main cause of papulosquamous skin disorders is an inadequate supply of nutrients to the skin. The inadequacies include external pathogenic wind-heat and wind-cold, accumulation of blood-heat resulting from dietary or emotional influences, qi stagnation and blood stasis from retention of pathogenic wind, damp, and heat, and yin deficiency of the liver and kidneys.

Topical Preparations. Xu Yihou discusses topical therapies only briefly in his text *Dermatology in Traditional*

Chinese Medicine.[87] He recommended combinations that emphasize gentle, nonirritating ointments used to decrease the scale and thickness of psoriatic plaques. An abundance of combination topical TCM preparations are available. Many actually contain corticosteroids, which would explain their efficacy.[88] Additionally, reports exist of contamination with heavy metals, toxins, and other pharmaceuticals. Such contamination can have significant adverse effects, as exemplified by the report of salicylate toxicity after the use of an herbal preparation containing oil of wintergreen over a large body area with occlusion.[89]

Systemic Herbs. A full description of all the Chinese herbs and combinations that can be useful for patients with psoriasis is beyond the scope of this chapter. Tse reviewed clinical trials in both the English and Chinese literature that pertained to the use of Chinese herbal medicines for psoriasis from 1966–2001. He found only seven poorly performed controlled trials but was also able to gain information from the 20 noncontrolled trials he identified. Of the 174 different herbs used in these trials, Tse specified 10 herbs that were commonly encountered and discussed their potential mechanisms of action. They were *Rehmannia glutinosa* (dried root), *Angelica sinensis* (root), *Salvia miltiorrhiza* (root), *Dictamnus dasycarpus* (root cortex), *Smilax glabra* (underground stem), *Oldenlandia diffusa* (whole plant), *Lithospermum erythrorhizon* (root), *Paeonia lactiflora* (root), *Carthamus tinctorius* (flower), and *Glycyrrhiza uralensis* (root).[90]

PRECAUTIONS

Many herbal preparations are not well regulated, and the risk for hepatotoxicity can be significant, either from the herbal components themselves or from contaminants.[91]

Acupuncture

As with the prescription of herbs, the acupuncture points used depend on the individual patient's pattern of psoriasis. The main points discussed by Xi Yihou focused on correcting blood-heat (BL18, BL23, BL12, and BL15) and wind-dryness from blood deficiency (BL17, BL19, BL12, BL13, and BL20). He also provided guidance on selecting points on the basis of the location of the disease: LI4, LI11, TB6, and GB20 are useful for the scalp and arms; SP6, SP10, and GB34 treat the trunk, buttocks, or genital area; SP6, SP10, and ST36 treat the lower limbs; and GV14, LI11, SP6, and SP10 are good for generalized lesions.[87]

In one case series, 61 patients with psoriasis not responsive to more conventional therapies were treated with acupuncture. After an average of nine sessions (range, 1–15), 30 patients experienced complete or almost complete clearance of the skin lesions, 14 had two-thirds clearance, eight experienced one-third clearance, and nine had minimal or no improvement.[92]

PRECAUTIONS

Acupuncture is quite safe, but because the needles are inserted into the skin, the Koebner phenomenon could potentially occur. Clearly, more work is needed in this area if we are to gain a better understanding of its usefulness in the treatment of psoriasis.

Assessment of TCM as a system is very difficult within a Western framework. The classification of disease in TCM is based on a different point of view, and because each patient is evaluated and treated individually with various combinations of herbs and acupuncture, creating standardized protocols to measure treatment outcomes is difficult.

Homeopathy

Like TCM, the system of homeopathy looks at psoriasis as the local expression of a systemic disturbance. Each patient is evaluated individually, and treatments are given on the basis of a constitutional approach. Because each patient is viewed as having a unique imbalance, the specific remedy chosen depends greatly on the patient. Though research is limited, homeopathy can be effective for treating psoriasis.[93] The practitioner must be well trained and have a deep understanding of homeopathy. Certification is not uniformly required, so one should look for practitioners who are accredited by one of the following organizations: Council for Homeopathic Certification (CHC), American Board of Homeotherapeutics (ABHt), Homeopathic Academy of Naturopathic Physicians (HANP), and North American Society of Homeopaths (NASH).

PRECAUTIONS

With homeopathic treatments, patients may experience an exacerbation of symptoms before resolution. This exacerbation is known as a healing crisis.

PREVENTION PRESCRIPTION

We currently do not have a way to prevent psoriasis. Although some situations are known to exacerbate psoriasis, flares are often unpredictable. Some choices patients and clinicians can address include the following:

• Maintain a balanced lifestyle.
• Minimize stress.
• Maintain a stable weight.
• Avoid alcohol overuse.
• Avoid tobacco.
• Eat a well-balanced diet.
• Keep your skin well hydrated.
• Treat skin infections early.
• Avoid medications known to exacerbate psoriasis (i.e., lithium, beta-blockers, antimalarials, IFN, and rapid tapering of systemic corticosteroid dosage).

THERAPEUTIC REVIEW

GENERAL MEASURES

- Gentle skin care: avoid hot water for bathing and use gentle cleansers and thick emollients and colloidal oatmeal
- UV exposure—climatotherapy and balneophototherapy

NUTRITION AND SUPPLEMENTS

- Antiinflammatory diet: see Chapter 88
- Low caloric diet for weight loss
- Fish oil or oily fish: this is also useful as an adjuvant to decrease side effects of systemic retinoids and cyclosporine. Consider 2–3 g/day of DHA + EPA.
- Curcumin: 150 mg three times a day
- Zinc: no good evidence has indicated a benefit in psoriasis; however, some clinicians do report a benefit. The dose is 15–30 mg/day.
- Inositol: this may be useful in patients with lithium-induced psoriasis. The dose is 6 g/day, with monitoring of psychiatric disease in patients with bipolar disorder.

TOPICAL BOTANICALS

- *Indigo naturalis* extract: 3%–7% oil, ointment or cream once to twice a day.
- Capsaicin for itching: 0.025% or 0.075% cream applied three or four times/day. Patients may experience stinging or burning during initial applications.
- Aloe vera: 0.5% extract in a lipophilic cream may help decrease scaling and redness.
- Glycyrrhetinic acid 1%–2% formulation: this may enhance the effect of topical steroids by inhibiting their degradation.

SYSTEMIC BOTANICALS

- Milk thistle: 140 mg (70% silymarin) two to three times/day
  Best used as a hepatoprotective agent in patients taking hepatotoxic medications such as methotrexate

TOPICAL PHARMACEUTICALS

- Keratolytics, to decrease scale and plaque thickness:
  - Salicylic acid (2%–10%) twice daily
  - Urea (up to 40%) twice daily
  - Alpha-hydroxy acids (glycolic and lactic acids) twice daily
- Topical steroids: see Table 73.3. The clinician should pay attention to the location treated and watch for side effects.

- Calcipotriene (Dovonex): 0.005% cream, lotion, or ointment twice daily, limited to no more than 100 g/week
- Tazarotene gel (Tazorac): 0.05%–1% gel applied at bedtime
- Tar: 2%–20% preparations
- Anthralin: 0.5%–1% preparation applied for 10–30 minutes once or twice daily, to protect normal skin from irritation

PHOTOTHERAPY

- nb-UVB or UVB

SYSTEMIC PHARMACEUTICALS

- Methotrexate: 10–15 mg/week; a single weekly dose or divided into three doses given 12 hours apart
- Cyclosporine: started at 5.0 mg/kg per day, with dosage tapered by 0.5 mg/kg per day to the lowest required dose
- Acitretin (Soriatane): 10, 25, or 50 mg daily
- Biological immune response modifiers:
  - Adalimumab (Humira): 40 mg/subcutaneously every other week
  - Certolizumab pegol (Cimzia): 400 mg/week subcutaneously once a month
  - Etanercept (Enbrel): 50 mg once or twice a week subcutaneously
  - Golimumab (Simponi): 50 mg subcutaneously once a month
  - Infliximab (Remicade): 5 mg/kg over 2–3 hours intravenously on weeks 0, 2, and 6 and then every 8 weeks thereafter
  - Ustekinumab (Stelara): 45 or 90 mg as a subcutaneous injection on weeks 0 and 4 and then every 12 weeks thereafter
- Oral PDE4 inhibitor:
  - Apremilast (Otezla): 30 mg orally twice a day
    This is a very new drug, and though safety and efficacy studies are very promising, there is not as much experience with this type of drug.

MIND–BODY THERAPIES

- Meditation: great for stress reduction or minimization
- Hypnosis: most potential benefit for hypnotizable patients

THERAPIES TO CONSIDER

- TCM
- Homeopathy

Key Web Resources

General Websites for Psoriasis	
National Psoriasis Foundation	http://www.psoriasis.org
Mayo Clinic	http://www.mayoclinic.com/health/psoriasis/DS00193
American Academy of Dermatology	http://aad.org/public/diseases/scaly-skin/psoriasis

Information about Traditional Chinese Medicine Practitioners	
National Certification Commission for Acupuncture and Oriental Medicine	http://www.nccaom.org
American Academy of Medical Acupuncture	http://www.medicalacupuncture.org

Information about Homeopathic Practitioners	
Council for Homeopathic Certification (CHC)	http://www.homeopathicdirectory.com
National Center for Homeopathy	http://www.homeopathycenter.org
Homeopathic Academy of Naturopathic Physicians (HANP)	http://www.hanp.net
North American Society of Homeopaths (NASH)	http://www.homeopathy.org

REFERENCES

References are available online at ExpertConsult.com.

CHAPTER 74

URTICARIA

Apple A. Bodemer, MD

PATHOPHYSIOLOGY

Urticaria, also known as hives, is a common problem affecting approximately 20% of people at some point in their lives. It is characterized by wheals—discrete areas of swelling, erythema, and pruritus that are often surrounded by a pale halo. Individual lesions typically wax and wane over the course of 24 hours, but recurrent crops can appear for weeks. *Acute urticaria* refers to outbreaks of wheals occurring for at least 2 days a week for up to 6 consecutive weeks. When the process lasts for 6 weeks or longer, it is considered *chronic urticaria*. Patients who have less frequent outbreaks are classified as having *recurrent urticaria*.[1] The skin findings and symptoms of urticaria are the result of increased inflammatory and vasoactive mediators such as histamine, prostaglandins, leukotrienes, proteases, and cytokines. These mediators are primarily found in mast cells and basophils. Although the main physiological event is mast cell degranulation, any mechanism that elevates these mediators can result in urticaria.

Mast cell degranulation can occur through both immunological and nonimmunological pathways. Immunological mechanisms include allergic mast cell degranulation, which is a type I hypersensitivity process initiated by antigen-mediated cross-linking of immunoglobulin E (IgE) receptors. Additionally, autoantibodies either to IgE or to the high-affinity IgE receptor (FcεRI) can bind to mast cells and result in degranulation.

Nonimmunological processes cause degranulation without interacting with the IgE receptor. This category involves compounds that can directly bind to mast cells to elicit degranulation, such as opiates and radio contrast media, as well as other compounds that can induce the production of factors that bind to other receptors on the mast cell to cause degranulation. C1 esterase inhibitor deficiency can lead to higher levels of inflammatory and vasoactive mediators that are important in urticaria. This deficiency causes uninhibited activation of the complement system that leads to an increase in bradykinin—a vasoactive inflammatory mediator.[2] Some compounds, such as aspirin, can alter the balance of prostaglandin and leukotriene synthesis and others, including nettle plants, can directly implant vasoactive mediators into the skin.[3]

Determining the causative factor for urticaria is often very frustrating. No specific cause is ever identified in 50%–80% of patients. The most commonly implicated causes of acute urticaria are infections (especially viral infections of the upper respiratory tract), drugs (such as penicillins, sulfonamides, salicylates, nonsteroidal antiinflammatory drugs, and opiates), and foods (particularly shellfish, fish, eggs, cheese, chocolate, nuts, berries, and tomatoes) or food additives (including annatto—a yellow dye, as well as other colorants, butylated hydroxyanisole [BHA], and butylated hydroxytoluene [BHT]). Chronic urticaria can be caused by these same agents but is more likely to be secondary to physical stimuli (e.g., dermatographism, pressure, vibration, heat, cold, exercise, sun, and water), stress, autoimmune diseases (most commonly thyroid disorders), and other chronic medical diseases, such as connective tissue disease, cryoglobulinemia or cryofibrinogenemia, rheumatoid arthritis, amyloidosis, or cancer (Table 74.1).[1,4,5]

The most important factor in a good evaluation is the medical history. Particular attention should be given to coexisting physical symptoms such as fever, unexplained weight changes, nausea/vomiting, weakness, fatigue, arthralgias/arthritis, etc. Thorough questioning about events surrounding urticarial flares may help patients recognize associations between stimuli and symptoms. Detailed diaries of a patient's activities, exposures, and ingestants can be invaluable in helping identify factors associated with urticarial outbreaks. Random screening laboratory tests have been proved to be of little value,[6] but for selected patients, laboratory investigations directed by the history and physical findings should be considered. Tests may include complete blood count with differential, urinalysis, liver function tests, erythrocyte sedimentation rate, stool examination for ova and parasites, antinuclear antibody titer, screening for hepatitis B and C, thyroid function, thyroid antibody titer, and age-directed screen for malignant disease.[7]

Interestingly, there have been a few case studies and case series that demonstrate resolution of urticaria that either did not respond or only partially responded to conventional antihistamine therapy when low vitamin D levels were treated.[8,9] It has been suggested that the effects of vitamin D in urticarial and other inflammatory conditions is mediated by cathelicidin—a vitamin D responsive antimicrobial peptide that also plays a role in regulating inflammation.[10] While more and better studies will hopefully clarify this issue in the future, it seems clear that testing for low vitamin D levels and supplementing when appropriate is warranted in people who have chronic urticaria.

Understanding the difference between urticaria and urticarial vasculitis is important. Urticarial vasculitis looks identical to other forms of urticaria, but individual lesions typically last for more than 24 hours and may be purpuric. Patients often complain more of burning sensation than itching.[11] Additionally, systemic symptoms such as arthralgia, gastrointestinal pain or digestive disturbance, pulmonary obstructive disease, or renal disease may be present.[12] Urticarial vasculitis has been associated

TABLE 74.1	Histamine-Rich and Histamine-Releasing Foods
Histamine-Rich Foods	Avocados
	Fermented drinks
	Cheese
	• Emmenthal
	• Harzer
	• Gouda
	• Roquefort
	• Tilsiter
	• Camembert
	• Cheddar
	Fish
	• Anchovies
	• Mackerel
	• Herring
	• Sardines
	• Tuna
	Processed meat
	• Ham
	• Salami
	• Sausage
	Jams and preserves
	Sauerkraut
	Sour cream
	Spinach
	Tomatoes
	Vinegar
	Yeast extract
	Yogurt
Histamine-Releasing Foods	Alcohol
	Bananas
	Chocolate
	Eggs
	Milk
	Some nuts
	Papaya
	Shellfish
	Strawberries
	Tomatoes

Data from Wantke F, Gotz M, Jarisch R. Histamine-free diet: treatment of choice for histamine-induced food intolerance and supporting treatment for chronic headaches. *Clin Exp Allergy.* 23:982-985, 1993.

with connective tissue diseases (most commonly systemic lupus erythematosus), infections (viral hepatitis), and, rarely, with medications or hematological disorders. The evaluation and treatment of urticarial vasculitis are beyond the scope of this chapter.

INTEGRATIVE THERAPY

General Principles

When a cause of urticaria is recognized, treatment can be as simple as avoiding the causative agent. In many cases of urticaria, however, the trigger is never identified. Even if the trigger is known, some patients may be unable to avoid the exposure. In these situations, many options are available for the management of urticaria.

The patient must be educated that a causative agent may never be found and that urticaria can be a chronic disease. He or she should understand that the skin reaction itself is not dangerous but is often very frustrating and difficult to live with. Chronic idiopathic urticaria can

be a very unsatisfying disorder to manage, and the health care practitioner may become easily frustrated with the patient. Practitioners must not let this happen and should be open and supportive of the patient, with the recognition that urticaria is most frustrating for those who live with it.

General conservative measures can increase comfort during an exacerbation. They include staying in a cool, calm environment, wearing loose, comfortable clothing, and taking lukewarm to cool baths with added baking soda, cornstarch, or colloidal oatmeal (Aveeno). Many topical preparations can help calm the itching associated with urticaria, including menthol-containing products, aloe, and topical steroids.

Nutrition

Dietary Limitations

In the setting of acute urticaria without a clear trigger after ingestant and activity diaries have been analyzed, an elimination diet may be useful (see Chapter 86). Although food is a rare cause of chronic urticaria (approximately 1% of all cases), it may still be helpful to try eliminating histamine-rich and otherwise antigenic foods from the patient's diet (see Table 74.1).[13-15] Magerl et al. conducted a prospective trial, in which 140 people with difficult to control chronic urticaria were put on a pseudoallergen free diet. (A pseudoallergen is a compound that elicits an inflammatory reaction without activating an antigen-specific immune response). Thirty-nine people had a strong to partial response to the diet after 3 weeks, and an additional nine were able to substantially reduce their medication without worsening of their condition.[16] The diet prescribed eliminated all processed foods, artificial additives, dyes, antibiotics, preservatives, phenols, and foods naturally rich in aromatic compounds (such as tomatoes, artichokes, peas, mushrooms, spinach, rhubarb, and olives).

Antiinflammatory Diet

Research on the role of an antiinflammatory diet in patients with urticaria is lacking. Intuitively, it seems that if general inflammation can be minimized, urticaria—which is driven by inflammatory mediators—should improve. However, many antiinflammatory diets focus on foods rich in omega-3 fatty acid, including fish and nuts, which are known to cause or exacerbate urticaria in some patients. This type of diet should be tried only in patients who have already determined that their urticaria is not exacerbated by the recommended foods (see Chapter 88).

Botanicals

Many different botanicals have been reported to be useful for the treatment of urticaria. They vary with sources, including canthaxanthin, field scabious, Japanese mint, kudzu, peppermint, alfalfa, bilberry extract, cat's claw, chamomile, echinacea, ginseng, licorice, nettle, yellow dock, and sarsaparilla. Many of these remedies have no evidence of efficacy from controlled studies. This section focuses only on the botanicals for which at least some in vitro evidence supports potential mechanisms of action to explain their possible benefit for patients with urticaria.[17]

Quercetin

The bioflavonoid quercetin can be found in many foods, including red wine, black tea, green tea, onions, apples, berries, citrus fruit, and brassica vegetables. Its antiinflammatory effects are thought to be mediated by inhibition of leukotriene and prostaglandin synthesis, as well as by inhibition of histamine release from mast cells and basophils.[17,18] Although theoretically, quercetin should help ameliorate symptoms of urticaria, no studies looking specifically at its use in urticaria could be found.

DOSAGE
The dose is 500 mg by mouth twice daily before meals.

PRECAUTIONS
None are known.

Quercetin works by stabilizing mast cells, and butterbur inhibits histamine and leukotrienes. These botanicals may work synergistically on the allergic type of reaction seen in urticaria.

Butterbur (Petasites hybridus)

Butterbur lowers serum levels of histamine and leukotrienes.[19] It also decreases priming of mast cells in response to contact with allergens.[20] One study found butterbur to be as effective as cetirizine (Zyrtec) for allergic rhinitis, without associated sedation.[21] No studies have been conducted specifically on the use of butterbur for treatment of urticaria. However, because of its positive mechanism of action on the mediators of this condition, butterbur should be considered for patients who are intolerant of the sedating side effects of antihistamines.

DOSAGE
The dose is 50 to 100 mg of extract twice daily with meals (extract should be standardized to contain a minimum of 7.5 mg of petasin and isopetasin).

PRECAUTIONS
The major concern with butterbur is its hepatotoxic pyrrolizidine alkaloid content. Any formulation used should be labeled as free of pyrrolizidine alkaloids. This herb should not be used in patients with liver disease, and liver function parameters should be monitored in any patient who uses it over a long period.

Sarsaparilla

The sarsaparilla root contains quercetin. Please refer to the earlier section on quercetin for more details.

DOSAGE
The dose of dried root is 1–4 g, or one cup of tea, three times/day. The dose of liquid extract (1:1 in 20% alcohol or 10% glycerol) is 8–15 mL, three times/day.

PRECAUTIONS
Gastrointestinal irritation or temporary kidney impairment may occur when sarsaparilla is used in excessive doses.

To prepare sarsaparilla tea, simmer 1–4 g of dried sarsaparilla in 8–12 oz of water for 5–10 minutes.

Stinging Nettle (Urtica dioica)

The leaves of the stinging nettle contain flavonoids, including quercetin, rutin, and kaempferol. Please refer to the earlier section on quercetin for more details.

DOSAGE
The dose is 300 mg three times/day (up to seven times/day).

PRECAUTIONS
Possible side effects include gastrointestinal complaints, sweating, diarrhea, and rash. Stinging nettle may worsen glucose control in patients with diabetes, lower blood pressure, and act as a diuretic.[22]

Peppermint

Luteolin-7-orutinoside from the peppermint leaf may inhibit histamine.[23] Additionally, menthol volatile oil, found in peppermint, is useful as a soothing topical preparation for itchy skin.

DOSAGE
The dose of peppermint oil is 0.2–0.4 mL three times/day between meals. Enteric-coated tablets are available.

PRECAUTIONS
Topical use of peppermint oil can cause contact dermatitis and hives. Oral peppermint can relax the gastroesophageal sphincter and possibly worsen symptoms of gastroesophageal reflux disease. Some people have peppermint sensitivity leading to burning mouth syndrome or pruritus ani. Other side effects of peppermint that may be seen at very high doses include cramping, diarrhea, drowsiness, tremor, muscle pain, slow heart rate, and coma. Additionally, peppermint oil appears to inhibit several cytochrome P-450 enzymes, thus resulting in several potential drug interactions. Pure menthol is toxic and should never be ingested.

<table>
<tr><td>

Menthol-Containing Products for Topical Use

- Aveeno Skin Relief Moisturizing Lotion: menthol and colloidal oatmeal
- Sarna Anti-Itch Lotion: 0.5% menthol and 0.5% calamine
- Gold Bond Medicated Body Lotion: 0.15% menthol (Extra Strength has 0.5% menthol)
- PrameGel: 0.5% menthol and 1% pramoxine
- Watkins Menthol Camphor Ointment: 2.8% menthol and 5.3% camphor
- Eucerin Itch-Relief Spray: 0.15% menthol

</td></tr>
</table>

Ginkgo biloba

Ginkgo biloba contains ginkgolides, which are strong inhibitors of platelet-activating factors. Some early evidence indicates that platelet-activating factor may be implicated in some cases of cold-induced urticaria.[24] No studies have looked at the use of *Ginkgo biloba* in urticaria, but this botanical may be useful in some patients with cold-induced urticaria.

DOSAGE

The dose is 120 mg/day of standardized extract.

PRECAUTIONS

Because of its antiplatelet activity, *Ginkgo biloba* may potentiate other anticoagulants and concomitant use requires extreme caution. Other side effects may include gastrointestinal upset and dizziness.

Valerian Root

Valerian has long been used as an anxiolytic and may be useful in patients in whom urticaria is induced by high levels of emotional stress. No studies have specifically evaluated its use for the treatment of urticaria.

DOSAGE

The dose is 200 to 300 mg/day for generalized anxiety.

PRECAUTIONS

No known contraindications exist. Possible side effects may include upset stomach, headache, and itching.

Pharmaceuticals

Antihistamines

The four known histamine receptor subtypes are H_1, H_2, H_3, and H_4. H_1 receptors are found throughout the body and are involved in evoking pain and pruritus, vascular dilatation, vascular permeability, bronchoconstriction, and stimulation of cough receptors. H_2 receptors are widely distributed as well and have functions similar to those of the H_1 receptors, with increased activity in the gastrointestinal system leading to higher secretion of gastric acid and mucus. In allergic processes, H_2 receptors act indirectly by altering the cytokine milieu. H_3 and H_4 receptors have been described, and their expression appears to be limited to neural and hematopoietic tissues, respectively.[25]

Antihistamines are the mainstays of treatment for patients with urticaria. Pharmacological control is typically initiated with H_1-receptor antagonists. These agents can be broken down into the first-generation, more sedating drugs (chlorpheniramine, diphenhydramine, hydroxyzine, and promethazine) and the newer, less sedating medications (fexofenadine, cetirizine, levocetirizine, loratadine, and desloratadine). Because additional factors are involved in the development of urticaria, antihistamines may not completely control symptoms, but they can be expected to improve symptoms in most patients. Antihistamines should be used on a regular basis, rather than as needed, to reduce inflammation and prevent symptom development.[26]

Many studies on various antihistamine medications have shown that efficacy is equivalent for the sedating and nonsedating classes.[27] No specific drug works consistently better, but some patients may have a better response to one than to another. If one agent does not adequately control symptoms, switching medications or adding a second antihistamine is appropriate. In fact, combining two nonsedating agents is not an uncommon practice and can be very useful. Additionally, some patients may have good response to a combination of H_1 and H_2 antagonists.[28,29] Histamine-2 receptor blockers include ranitidine, cimetidine, famotidine, and nizatidine.

The tricyclic antidepressant doxepin has potent antihistamine properties that make it useful for patients with chronic urticaria.[30] Doxepin is very sedating and therefore is best used either in patients who have symptoms primarily at night or in combination with nonsedating antihistamines during the day.[31]

Dosage of First-Generation H1-Receptor Antagonists. The dose of hydroxyzine is 50 mg at bedtime or up to four times per day. The dose of diphenhydramine is 25–50 mg every 6–8 hours. The dose of chlorpheniramine is 4 mg every six hours. The dose of promethazine is 12.5–25 mg every 6–8 hours.

Dosage of Second-Generation H1-Receptor Antagonists. The dose of loratadine (Claritin) is 10 mg once or twice daily. The dose of desloratadine (Clarinex) is 5 mg once or twice daily. The dose of cetirizine (Zyrtec) is 10 mg daily or twice daily. The dose of levocetirizine is 5 mg once or twice daily. The dose of fexofenadine (Allegra) is 60–180 mg once or twice daily.

There is some evidence that desloratadine and levocetirizine can be used up to four times the recommended daily use without harm and with increasing benefit.[32]

Dosage of H2-Receptor Antagonists. The dose of ranitidine (Zantac) is 150–300 mg twice daily. For famotidine (Pepcid), the dose is 20–40 mg one or twice daily. The dose of cimetidine (Tagamet) is 200–400 mg once or twice daily.

DOSAGE OF DOXEPIN

The dose of doxepin is 10–75 mg, taken at bedtime.

PRECAUTIONS

The possible side effects of first-generation H_1-receptor antagonists include central nervous system depression, cardiac arrhythmias, electrolyte imbalance, dry mouth, constipation, blurred vision, dysuria, and drug interactions.

Second-generation H_1-receptor antagonists have no significant adverse effects. Loratadine may interact with some antidepressant medications.

The side effects of H_2-receptor antagonists are generally mild and reversible. Common side effects include constipation, diarrhea, fatigue, headache, insomnia, muscle pain, nausea, and vomiting. Cimetidine has some antiandrogenic activity, and high doses may rarely lead to breast enlargement in men or impotence. Cimetidine is an H_2 blocker that is typically used to block stomach acid production, but it can be used for patients with recalcitrant urticaria. Its use in patients with urticaria is considered "off-label."

Doxepin is extremely sedating and has the potential for causing significant drug interactions. Other possible side effects are cardiac conduction disturbances (QT prolongation), orthostatic hypotension, and anticholinergic effects (dry mouth, blurry vision, constipation, urinary retention).

The tricyclic antidepressant doxepin has potent antihistamine properties that make it useful for patients with chronic urticaria.

Leukotriene Inhibitors

Leukotrienes are secondary inflammatory mediators in the pathogenesis of urticaria. Inhibitors of these compounds include zafirlukast, montelukast, and zileuton. These agents are used successfully in patients with asthma and, theoretically, should work for patients with chronic urticaria as well. While case reports have shown somewhat mixed results,[33,34] these medications appear to be especially helpful for NSAID-exacerbated urticaria.[35,36] These agents are most useful when they are combined with traditional histamine receptor antagonists.[31]

DOSAGE

The dose of zafirlukast (Accolate) is 20 mg twice daily. For montelukast (Singulair), it is 10 mg daily. The dose of zileuton (Zyflo) is 600 mg up to four times/day.

PRECAUTIONS

Use these agents cautiously in patients with liver disease and consider potential drug interactions.

Corticosteroids

Corticosteroids are very effective for rapid resolution of urticarial symptoms. Because side effects can be significant, the use of these drugs should be limited to occasional short, tapering dosages for severe exacerbations. These agents should be used cautiously and sparingly, with reliance on other therapies for maintenance control. Short, rapidly tapered dosages of corticosteroids are generally safe and well tolerated, but repetitive tapered dosages or long-term use can lead to significant side effects and complications.

DOSAGE

The dose of prednisone is 40–60 mg/day for 2–3 days, then tapered over 1–2 weeks. Some patients may need longer, slower tapers.

PRECAUTIONS

Common side effects include euphoria or depression, gastrointestinal distress, hypertension, sodium and fluid retention, impaired wound healing, higher risk of infection, osteoporosis, and skin atrophy. Growth retardation may occur in children. More serious side effects include adrenocortical insufficiency, cataracts, glaucoma, Cushing syndrome, hyperglycemia, and tuberculosis reactivation.

Cyclosporine

Cyclosporine is a strong immune suppressant that can be useful for patients with severe debilitating urticaria that has been recalcitrant to other therapies. It blocks the transcription of interleukin-2, which is required for T-cell activation. Among other effects, cyclosporine blocks the release of histamine from mast cells. Side effects are severe and significant, so appropriate monitoring is essential. Long-term treatment with cyclosporine is not ideal, although some patients may require long-term, low-dose therapy. Fortunately, many patients experience a period of improvement, or even remission, after 4–12 weeks of treatment.[37]

DOSAGE

Many dosage regimens have been described. All use cyclosporine at doses at or less than 5 mg/kg/day for various durations. One regimen described specifically for chronic and debilitating urticaria is as follows: 3 mg/kg/day divided into two doses for 6 weeks, followed by 2 mg/kg/day divided into two doses for 3 weeks, followed by 1 mg/kg/day divided into two doses for 3 weeks.[38]

PRECAUTIONS

Cyclosporine is contraindicated in patients with uncontrolled hypertension, severe renal disease, serious infections, or a current or prior history of malignant disease.

Potential side effects include renal dysfunction, hypertension, hypertrichosis, gingival hyperplasia, gastrointestinal upset, neurological effects (headache, tremor, paresthesias), electrolyte imbalances, acneiform eruptions, hypertriglyceridemia, bone marrow suppression, and sleep disturbances. Monitoring includes urinalysis, complete blood count, liver function tests, and blood chemistry analysis including magnesium, potassium, and uric acid.

Because cyclosporine is metabolized by the cytochrome P-450 CYP3A4 enzyme system, it has many potential drug interactions. The clinician should review a complete medication and herb list with each patient before initiating cyclosporine therapy.[39]

Omalizumab (Xolair)

Omalizumab was approved in 2014 for treatment of chronic urticaria in people aged 12 years and older. This humanized anti-IgE monoclonal antibody binds to free IgE, blocking it from interacting with IgE receptors on mast cells and basophils, which effectively blocks degranulation of these cells. This decrease in the blood level of free IgE also leads to downregulation of IgE receptors, further decreasing opportunity for degranulation and thus symptoms of urticaria.[40] Typically, people see benefits within the first month of treatment, if not in the first week.

Dosage

The typical initial dose is 300 mg via subcutaneous injection every 4 weeks. If a person responds, tapering to 150 mg every 4 weeks and monitoring for recurrence of symptoms is suggested.

Precautions

This medication appears to be very safe. Resistance rates appear to be low, and there is no laboratory monitoring required. As with any of the biological medications, hypersensitivity reactions can occur including anaphylaxis, injection site reaction, and, ironically, hives.

Mind-Body Techniques

Background

Several studies have shown that psychological stress can trigger or exacerbate flares of urticaria.[41,42] Up to 81% of people with chronic urticaria report stress as an aggravating factor.[43] Additionally, people with chronic urticaria have been found to have a higher incidence of depression and anxiety.[44-46] Additionally, people with chronic urticaria are more likely than controls to suffer from posttraumatic stress disorder (PTSD).[47] Although the mechanism is not well understood, the release of neuropeptides is thought ultimately to lead to elevations of histamine or greater sensitivity to histamine.[48] Human skin mast cells have been shown to release histamine in response to stimulation from various neuropeptides, including substance P, vasoactive intestinal polypeptide, and somatostatin.[49] Much more work needs to be done before we have a clear understanding of the relationship between the neural impact of stress on inflammation and urticaria. Though quality studies are lacking for the usefulness of most mind-body approaches for this condition, it does seem clear that stress management should be addressed in people who suffer from chronic urticaria, and their treatment plan should address stress and overall psychological health.

Hypnosis

Most information on the effectiveness of hypnosis is in the form of case reports. The flare reaction to histamine prick testing has been shown to be significantly reduced with hypnosis.[50,51] One study evaluating the use of relaxation techniques among patients who were classified as hypnotizable and unhypnotizable found that both groups experienced improvement in symptoms; however, only patients classified as hypnotizable had fewer clinical lesions.[52] In spite of the limited evidence, hypnotherapy may be a beneficial alternative—either alone or in combination with other therapies—for some patients with urticaria.

> Hypnosis is a therapy that should be encouraged for treatment of chronic urticaria. The evidence is promising, and the potential for side effects is minimal.

Traditional Chinese Medicine

Within the framework of traditional Chinese medicine (TCM), urticaria is thought to be caused primarily by wind-heat, which obstructs energy channels and networks and causes red inflammation on the skin. When excess wind is present in the body, it can wander through the skin and cause itching. Wind-heat can arise through several different mechanisms. Invasion of pathogenic wind is often combined with pathogenic cold or heat. Emotional disturbances and irritability cause heat accumulation in the heart and blood that makes one more susceptible to invasive wind. Damage to the spleen and stomach (resulting from a diet that is unhygienic or heavy in fish, seafood, or spicy foods) impairs the function of these organs and leads to increased dampness. When dampness accumulates internally, it can be transformed into wind-heat.

Each situation leading to the accumulation of wind-heat can be specifically treated with various herbal concoctions that are beyond the scope of this chapter. Acupuncture can also be used alone or in combination with cupping and/or herbal remedies. The main general acupuncture points used for urticaria vary according to the source, but generally include PC6 Neiguan, GB20 Fengchi, and ST36 Zusanli[53] or LI11 Quchi, SP10 Xuehai, SP6 Sanyinjiao, and S36 Zusanli.[54] Because TCM treatments are highly individualized for each patient and vary based on the specific symptoms, the general acupuncture points may differ significantly from patient to patient. Cupping involves placing a cup filled with warm air on the surface of the skin. As the cup cools, skin is drawn in and suction is created, which theoretically removes stagnant blood and wind thought to contribute to chronic urticaria. This can be done at specific acupuncture points. The assistance of a well-trained TCM physician should be sought, especially if one is interested in pursuing TCM herbal therapies.

Wide variation exists from state to state regarding certification, so when choosing an oriental medical doctor (OMD), one should ask whether the person has passed the National Certification Commission for Acupuncture and Oriental Medicine herbal examination. If someone is interested in acupuncture alone, the American Academy of Medical Acupuncture is a good additional source of well-trained practitioners.

Homeopathy

Like TCM, homeopathy views urticaria as the local expression of a systemic disturbance. Each patient is evaluated individually, and treatments are given on the basis of the constitutional approach. Because each patient is viewed as having a unique imbalance, the specific remedy chosen depends greatly on the patient. Two patients with urticaria may be successfully treated with vastly different therapies. Approximately 20 remedies are commonly employed to help patients with urticaria, including natrum muriaticum (a derivative of sodium chloride), apis mellifica (derived from the honey bee), urtica urens (derived from the stinging nettle plant), silica, kali carbonicum (derived from potassium carbonate), pulsatilla (from the pasqueflower), sulphus (sulfur), sepia (cuttlefish), and byronia (wild hopps).

To give a patient an appropriate cure, a practitioner must be well trained and have a deep understanding of homeopathy. Certification is not uniformly required, so one should look for practitioners who are accredited by one of the following organizations: the Council for Homeopathic Certification (CHC), the American Board of Homeotherapeutics (ABHt), the Homeopathic

Academy of Naturopathic Physicians (HANP), and the North American Society of Homeopaths (NASH).

PRECAUTIONS

With homeopathic treatments, patients may experience an exacerbation of symptoms before resolution; this exacerbation is known as a healing crisis.

PREVENTION PRESCRIPTION

If a cause is identified in a particular patient, recurrences can be limited by having the patient

- Avoid exposure to known triggers.
- Limit stress.
- Eat a healthy, balanced diet with a low-histamine content.

THERAPEUTIC REVIEW

This is a summary of therapeutic options for urticaria. Laboratory investigation should be directed by the patient's medical history and physical findings. Particular attention to associations with systemic disease is warranted in patients with chronic urticaria.

GENERAL MEASURES

- Identify and avoid any precipitating factors, if possible. Activity and ingestant diaries may be particularly useful in this endeavor. **A** ⬆ 1
- Use topical measures, including a cool, calm environment, loosely fitting, comfortable clothes, baths with cornstarch, colloidal oatmeal (Aveeno), or baking powder. **B** ➚ 1

NUTRITION

- Avoid allergenic foods, pseudoallergens, and foods high in histamine (see Table 74.1). **B** ➚ 1
- Consider an elimination diet (see Chapter 86). **C** → 1

BOTANICALS AND SUPPLEMENTS

- Quercetin: 400 mg orally twice daily before meals **C** → 1
- Butterbur (Petadolex): 75 mg orally twice daily **C** ⊘ 2
- Sarsaparilla: 1–4 g as dried root or tea three times daily; liquid extract (1:1 in 20% alcohol or 10% glycerol): 8–15 mL three times daily **C** ⊘ 2
- Stinging nettle: 300 mg three times daily **C** ⊘ 2
- Peppermint: 0.2–0.4 mL oil three times daily between meals or equivalent in enteric-coated tablets **C** ⊘ 2
- Ginkgo biloba for cold-induced urticaria: 120 mg per day standardized extract **C** ⊘ 2
- Valerian root for stress-related urticaria: 200–300 mg per day **C** ⊘ 2

PHARMACEUTICALS

- Antihistamines: H₁-receptor blockers alone or in combination with H₂-receptor blockers **A** ➚ 2
- First generation
  - Hydroxyzine: 50 mg one to four times daily
  - Diphenhydramine: 25–50 mg every 6–8 hours
  - Chlorpheniramine: 4 mg every 6 hours
  - Promethazine: 12.5–25 mg every 6–8 hours

- Second generation
  - Loratadine (Claritin): 10 mg once or twice daily
  - Desloratadine (Clarinex): 5 mg once or twice daily up to 20 mg a day
  - Cetirizine (Zyrtec): 10 mg once or twice daily
  - Levocetirizine: 5 mg once or twice daily up to 20 mg a day
  - Fexofenadine (Allegra): 60 to 180 mg once or twice daily
- H₂-receptor antagonists
  - Ranitidine (Zantac): 150–300 mg twice daily
  - Famotidine (Pepcid): 20–40 mg one to twice daily
  - Cimetidine (Tagamet): 200–400 mg one to four times daily
  - Doxepin: 10–75 mg before bed **B** ➚ 2
- Leukotriene inhibitors
  - Zafirlukast (Accolate): 20 mg twice daily
  - Montelukast (Singulair): 10 mg daily
  - Zileuton (Zyflo): 600 mg up to four times daily
- Corticosteroids: 40–60 mg/day for 2–3 days, then tapered over 1–2 weeks **A** ➚ 2
- Cyclosporine: 3 mg/kg/day for 6 weeks, 2 mg/kg/day for 3 weeks, and 1 mg/kg/day for 3 weeks. Appropriate monitoring is essential. **B** ⊘ 3
- Omalizumab (Xolair): 300 mg subcutaneous injection once every 4 weeks **B** ➚ 2

MIND-BODY THERAPY

- Relaxation and stress management: Good for everyone! **C** → 1
- Hypnosis, especially for people classified as hypnotizable **B** ➚ 1

TRADITIONAL CHINESE MEDICINE

- Please refer to the text Dermatology in Traditional Chinese Medicine, by Xu Yihou,[35] for more detailed and complete information on and understanding of TCM.
- Please also refer to Key Web Resources for websites listing traditional Chinese medicine practitioners.

HOMEOPATHY

- Work with a well-trained credentialed homoeopathist.
- See Key Web Resources

Key Web Resources

General Overview of Disease and Treatment

American Academy of Dermatology	https://www.aad.org/dermatology-a-to-z/diseases-and-treatments/e---h/hives
Mayo Clinic	http://www.mayoclinic.com/health/chronic-hives/DS00980

Websites for Information about Traditional Chinese Medicine Practitioners

National Certification Commission for Acupuncture and Oriental Medicine	http://www.nccaom.org
American Academy of Medical Acupuncture	http://www.medicalacupuncture.org

Websites for Information about Homeopathy Practitioners

Council for Homeopathic Certification (CHC)	http://www.homeopathicdirectory.com
National Center for Homeopathy	http://www.homeopathycenter.org
Homeopathic Academy of Naturopathic Physicians (HANP)	http://www.hanp.net
North American Society of Homeopaths (NASH)	https://homeopathy.org/

REFERENCES

References are available online at ExpertConsult.com.

CHAPTER 75

APHTHOUS STOMATITIS

David Rakel, MD

Recurrent aphthous ulcers (RAUs), also called aphthous stomatitis and canker sores, are the most common oral mucosal lesions, affecting 20% of the population in North America. They appear as recurrent ulcers with circumscribed margins with erythematous halos and gray or yellowish floors (Fig. 75.1).

RAUs affect the nonkeratinized or poorly keratinized mucosa of the mouth and oropharynx. No specific test is available for RAUs, and diagnosis is made from the patient's history and clinical findings.

PATHOPHYSIOLOGY

RAUs appear to be multifactorial in origin, with a strong component of immune mediation. Histologically, there is an increase in immunoglobulin (Ig)E–bearing lymphocytes along with an increase in the number of mast cells and tumor necrosis factor-alpha (TNF-alpha) in the prodromal stages.[1] Cytotoxic action of lymphocytes and monocytes seem to cause the ulceration, but the exact trigger is not clear.

The three main clinical variations are as follows[2]:

- Minor aphthous ulcers: Commonly less than 5 mm in diameter, these are the most common form (80%). Typically one to five ulcers may be present at any one time, and they usually heal without scarring in 7 to 14 days.
- Major aphthous ulcers: These ulcers, which are less common, are larger and deeper than minor aphthous ulcers, tend to have irregular edges, and are more

painful. They affect the lips, soft palate, and oropharynx and can take up to 6 weeks to heal, often leaving a considerable scar. Major and minor RAUs can be associated with Behçet's syndrome and human immunodeficiency virus (HIV) infection.

- Herpetiform RAUs: Measuring 1 to 3 mm in diameter, herpetiform RAUs often occur in groups of 10 to 100 that commonly coalesce to form large, irregular areas of ulceration. These are not as deep as major aphthous ulcers. They heal without scarring in 7 to 14 days and, despite their name, are not associated with the herpes or any other virus.

Minor and major RAUs usually begin in childhood or early adolescence and have a tendency to resolve naturally later in life. Herpetiform RAUs appear later in life compared to minor and major RAUs, usually in the third decade (Box 75.1).

INTEGRATIVE THERAPY

Lifestyle

Toothpaste

Sodium lauryl sulfate is a common detergent used in toothpastes that has been shown to precipitate RAUs.[21] Other ingredients may also affect RAUs, so a good question to ask patients with newly developed RAUs is whether they have recently changed toothpaste. *CloSYS*, *Tom's of Maine*, *The Natural Dentist*, *Burt's Bees*, and *Squigle* are examples of brands of toothpaste that do not contain sodium lauryl sulfate.

Nutrition

Several nutritional deficiencies have been associated with RAUs. Vitamin B_{12}, iron, and folic acid have been the most studied nutrients and have been found to be commonly deficient in patients with RAUs.[3] Laboratory evaluations for red cell folate, serum vitamin B_{12}, and ferritin levels should be included in any evaluation of RAUs.

Vitamins B_1,[4] B_2, B_6, and B_{12} have also been found to be deficient in some patients with RAUs.[5]

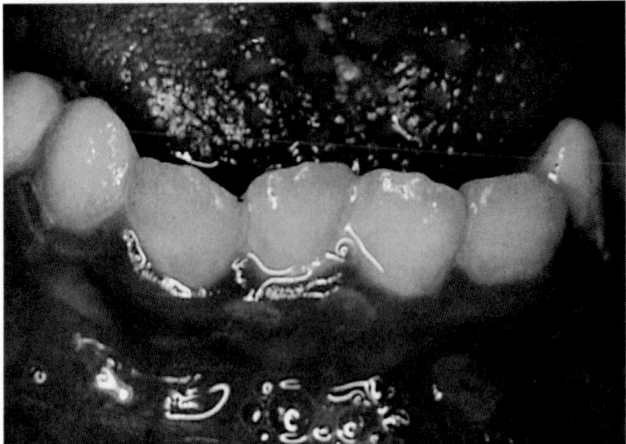

FIG. 75.1 ■ Recurrent aphthous ulcers. The ulceration seen on the labial mucosa is surrounded by a characteristic erythematous halo. (From Zitelli BJ, Davis HW. *Atlas of pediatric physical diagnosis.* 5th ed. St. Louis, 2007, Mosby.)

Laboratory evaluation for red cell folate, serum vitamin B_{12}, and ferritin levels, as well as a complete blood count, should be ordered in the evaluation of recurrent aphthous ulceration. HIV infection should be considered if the patient is at risk for this infection.

BOX 75.1 | **Etiology of Recurrent Aphthous Ulceration**

The origin of recurrent aphthous ulceration seems to be multifactorial and can include one or several of the following factors:
- Familial and genetic basis
- Nutritional deficiencies: vitamins B_1, B_2, B_6, and B_{12}, folic acid, iron
- Stress
- Stopping smoking
- Menstruation
- Food allergies (cow's milk and gluten most common)
- Sensitivities to toothpastes (sodium lauryl sulfate)
- Medications
  Antineoplastic (methotrexate, daunorubicin, doxorubicin, hydroxyurea)
  Angiotensin-converting enzyme inhibitors (captopril most common)
  Antimicrobials
  Metformin
  Barbiturates
  Griseofulvin
  Nonsteroidal antiinflammatory drugs (NSAIDs)
  Sulfonamides
  Quinidine
  Penicillamine
- Physical trauma
- Systemic conditions
  Celiac disease
  Crohn's disease
  Human immunodeficiency virus infection
  Neutropenia and other immune deficiencies
  Neumann bipolar aphthosis
  Behçet's syndrome
  MAGIC (mouth and genital ulcers with inflamed cartilage)

Diet

A few patients with RAUs have gluten-sensitive enteropathy and improve considerably with a gluten-free diet.[6] The diagnosis is usually made by jejunal biopsy or by assay of tissue transglutaminase IgA with a positive antiendomysial antibody. Although no evidence in the literature shows that gluten-free diets help patients with RAUs who do not have gluten sensitivity,[7] anecdotal observations indicate that some patients without gluten sensitivity may benefit from a gluten-free diet.[8] For the patient with recurring ulcers, a 2- to 4-week therapeutic trial of gluten avoidance is a reasonable option to assess effect.

The role of food allergies in the pathogenesis of RAUs is controversial. Several foods—milk, chocolate, coffee, nuts, strawberries, pineapple, citrus fruits, tomatoes, azo dyes—and food additives—monosodium glutamate (MSG), benzoic acid, tartrazine (yellow dye no. 5), and cinnamaldehyde—have all been suggested as a cause of RAUs[9,10] (see Chapter 86).

Honey

Honey has been found to be helpful in healing stasis ulcers of the legs as well as preventing mouth ulcers in patients receiving radiation therapy. In 40 patients with head and neck cancer who were receiving radiation, those who took 20 mL of honey 15 minutes before therapy and

at 15 minute intervals at the time of therapy, and then again 6 hours after therapy, developed significantly fewer mouth ulcers than the saline treated control group.[11]

Supplements

Glutamine

Glutamine, the most abundant amino acid in the body, is essential for maintaining intestinal function, immune response, and amino acid homeostasis during times of severe stress. Glutamine supplementation has been found to improve nutritional and immunologic status and reduce complications in critically ill patients.[12] However, not everyone benefits from supplementation. Those who have the greatest nutritional deficiency are thought to have the best clinical response.[13] Supplementation with glutamine is beneficial during times of skeletal muscle wasting because most of glutamine is produced in skeletal muscle, and glutamine depletion raises the incidence of oral and gastrointestinal ulcerations. This amino acid has been found to reduce the duration and severity of oral stomatitis in patients undergoing chemotherapy.[14]

DOSAGE

Glutamine can be purchased in powder form. The patient should mix 4 g of powder in water, swish in the mouth, and swallow four times daily. If glutamine is used with chemotherapy, it should be taken on the day of chemotherapy and then used for 4 days after completion of each treatment.

PRECAUTIONS

Grittiness of the oral solution may be unpleasant. Glutamine is otherwise well tolerated. It may cause mania in patients with bipolar disease.

Vitamin B_{12}

A randomized, double-blind trial using 1000 mcg of sublingual vitamin B_{12} taken daily before sleep for 6 months in 58 patients with RAU showed that those in the treatment arm of the trial had significant reduction in ulcer formation, and 74% (compared with 32% in the placebo group) reported "no aphthous ulcer status" after 6 months. The response was not predicted by the baseline serum vitamin B_{12} levels; study subjects with normal B_{12} levels still responded to therapy.[15] Metformin can cause B-vitamin deficiency. Consider supplementing if patients on this medicine have RAU.[30]

DOSAGE

The dose of vitamin B_{12} is 1000 mcg sublingually daily for ulcer prevention.

PRECAUTIONS

Vitamin B_{12} therapy is safe. The body excretes any excess into the urine, with the resulting classic bright yellow coloration seen with vitamin B supplementation.

Botanicals

German Chamomile (Matricaria recutita)

Chamomile is used for its antiinflammatory properties in the treatment of dyspepsia, leg ulcers, and oral mucositis. When used as a mouthwash, it has been found to prevent oral mucositis associated with radiation therapy and chemotherapy.[16]

DOSAGE

Make an oral rinse with 10 to 15 drops of German chamomile liquid extract in 100 mL warm water, and use three times daily.

PRECAUTIONS

The plant has allergic potential but is otherwise safe.

Licorice (Glycyrrhiza)

Licorice, which has antiinflammatory action, has been used as a mouthwash and is available in oral disks.[17] A randomized, double-blind study using a *Glycyrrhiza* oral patch compared with placebo patch showed significantly faster resolution of ulcers in the *Glycyrrhiza*-treated group at 8 days.[18]

DOSAGE

To use licorice as a mouthwash, mix half of a teaspoon of licorice extract with a quarter cup of water, swish, gargle, and expel the mouthwash four times daily for symptomatic aphthous ulcers.

A product called CankerMelt contains 30-mg *Glycyrrhiza* extract. The disk is applied to the ulcer and allowed to dissolve over time; then a new disk is applied every 6 hours.

PRECAUTIONS

If the mouthwash is not swallowed, side effects are rare. Licorice can cause sodium retention and hypokalemia if it is swallowed. Care should be taken with the use of licorice in patients with hypertension because licorice ingestion can worsen the condition.

Although research is limited, many patients find pain relief due to the tannins found in tea leaves (*Camellia sinensis*). A brewed black or green tea bag can be applied to the ulcer as needed.

Homeopathy

Several homeopathic remedies have been used historically to treat RAUs. Unfortunately, all of the evidence for their use is anecdotal. A classical homeopath would look for a constitutional remedy that fits the whole patient. Symptomatic remedies that may help are as follows:

- Mercurius solubilis is indicated if the RAUs are associated with foul breath and increased salivation.
- Borax is indicated if the RAUs are brought on by citrus or acidic foods. The mouth usually feels dry even though some saliva may be present.
- Arsenicum album is indicated in patients with RAUs that are brought on by stress and eased with hot drinks.

DOSAGE

All the preceding remedies are best given initially at a potency of 6X or 6C four times daily (the X and C refer to the potency, which is the extent of dilution of the remedy). They should be discontinued when the RAUs begin to improve (see Chapter 115).

Mind-Body Therapy

Stress, both emotional and physical, triggers RAUs. Emotional and environmental stress may precede 60% of first-time aphthous ulcer cases and be involved in 21% of recurrent episodes.[8] The pathogenesis may involve the known alteration of the immune response from stress, the depletion of B vitamins, or may be unknown.

Meditation and stress reduction techniques, such as guided imagery and hypnosis, have been shown to be useful in the management of RAUs.[19,20]

Pharmaceuticals: Antiinflammatory Agents

Amlexanox

The only prescription medication approved by the U.S. Food and Drug Administration (FDA) for treatment of aphthous stomatitis is amlexanox (Aphthasol) 5% paste. It accelerates healing through an unknown mechanism that inhibits release of inflammatory mediators (histamine and leukotrienes) from mast cells, neutrophils, and mononuclear cells. This agent has no direct analgesic properties.

DOSAGE

Apply 0.5 cm to the sore with fingertip four times daily after meals and at bedtime. Start at the onset of symptoms and stop with resolution. If no resolution has occurred in 7 days, reevaluation is warranted. Amlexanox is dispensed in a 5-g tube.

PRECAUTIONS

This agent may cause minimal burning on application. Rash, diarrhea, nausea, and worsening stomatitis have been reported in less than 1% of cases.

Triamcinolone and Dexamethasone

Steroids such as triamcinolone and dexamethasone reduce inflammatory mediators but do not decrease the frequency of RAU occurrence.

DOSAGE

For triamcinolone acetonide: 0.1% in carboxymethyl cellulose paste (Kenalog in Orabase), apply 0.5 cm to the sore two or three times daily. Start at the onset of symptoms and stop with resolution. If no resolution has occurred in 7 days, reevaluation is warranted. This agent is dispensed in a 5-g tube.

For dexamethasone (Decadron) oral solution: 0.5 mg/5 mL, rinse the mouth with one teaspoon (5 mL) for 2 minutes and spit out, three times daily after meals and once at bedtime.

PRECAUTIONS

Thrush may occur.

Pharmaceuticals: Analgesic Agents

A helpful approach is to avoid spicy, salty, and vinegar containing foods that may irritate and increase pain of the ulcers. The following analgesic agents may also be useful:

Viscous Lidocaine (Xylocaine 2% solution)

This agent provides anesthetic properties that diminish pain while eating.

DOSAGE

To use viscous lidocaine (Xylocaine 2% solution), swish 15 mL and expel, every 3 hours or before meals, as needed for pain relief. Do not use more than eight doses daily. This agent is dispensed in 50-, 100-, and 450-mL bottles.

PRECAUTIONS

Care should be taken not to ingest large amounts of viscous lidocaine because of its potential for cardiotoxicity. Benzocaine gel (10% to 20%) is a safer alternative, particularly for use in children.

Pharmaceuticals: Mouthwashes

Chlorhexidine Gluconate

Chlorhexidine gluconate 0.12% oral solution (Peridex or Periogard oral rinse) is a mouthwash that has been shown to reduce the incidence, duration, and discomfort of RAUs.[22] It does not, however, appear to be as effective as the other pharmaceutical topical agents.[23]

DOSAGE

Swish 15 mL for 30 seconds and expel, twice daily. Chewing sugarless gum after using this mouthwash can help reduce tooth discoloration.

PRECAUTIONS

This agent can cause stinging when it is first used, reversible discoloration of the teeth and tongue after 1 week of use, transient disturbances of taste, and burning sensation of the tongue.

Tetracycline–Fluocinolone Acetonide–Diphenhydramine Mouthwash

For more severe cases, a formula containing tetracycline, fluocinolone acetonide, and diphenhydramine can be used. Tetracycline is thought to work through antimicrobial and antiinflammatory mechanisms. Fluocinolone and diphenhydramine work through antiinflammatory and anesthetic mechanisms. This mixture has been found to be very helpful in severe cases of RAUs resulting from immunosuppressant therapy.

DOSAGE

Mixing this formula requires the help of a pharmacist. Most pharmacies are able to comply with these directions. The following should be mixed together to make a total of 150 mL:
- Tetracycline: At a concentration of 500 mg per 5 mL (which a pharmacist makes by dissolving a 500 mg capsule in 5 mL of water) for a total of 60 mL
- Diphenhydramine syrup (Benadryl): 12.5 mg/5 mL for a total of 60 mL
- Fluocinolone acetonide 0.01% solution (Synalar) for a total of 30 mL
  Swish 10 mL and expel four times daily until the ulcers resolve. Do not use for more than 7 days at a time.

PRECAUTIONS

Tetracycline should not be given to children younger than 9 years because it stains the teeth. Fluocinolone, like most steroids, can cause thrush if it is used for extended periods.

For severe cases, a trial of tetracycline–fluocinolone acetonide–diphenhydramine mouthwash is indicated before using systemic therapy.

Systemic Pharmaceuticals

For cases resistant to topical therapy, consider the following systemic pharmaceuticals, in descending order as discussed in the following.

Colchicine

Colchicine has been used for stomatitis associated with Behçet's disease.[24] It has also been found to be beneficial for RAUs in patients without this disorder and is even more effective when combined with systemic steroids.[25]

DOSAGE

The dose is 0.6 mg orally twice daily. It may be increased to three times daily as tolerated with regard to gastrointestinal side effects.

PRECAUTIONS

The most common side effects are gastrointestinal, consisting of diarrhea, nausea, and cramping. Colchicine can also cause thrombocytopenia and aplastic anemia.

Systemic Steroids

No good studies have been conducted on the use of systemic steroids for RAUs. These agents should be used cautiously in immunocompromised hosts.

DOSAGE

The dose of prednisone is up to 40 to 60 mg/day for 5 days. If longer use is needed, taper the dosage over 10 to 14 days.

PRECAUTIONS

In patients with HIV infection, adverse reactions include cushingoid facies, thrush, reactivation of herpes simplex virus, and accelerated progression of Kaposi sarcoma.[26]

Thalidomide

Thalidomide has efficacy in healing oral aphthae. In two trials involving difficult cases, thalidomide completely healed 48% to 55% of ulcers, compared with 7% to 9% in patients receiving placebo. This effect was temporary, however; many of the patients treated had recurring symptoms.[27]

DOSAGE

The dose is 200 mg/day orally.

PRECAUTIONS

Because of the potential for teratotoxicity and irreversible peripheral neuropathy, this treatment should be used only for the most serious, intractable cases.

Because of the elevation of tumor necrosis factor-alpha (TNF-alpha) in recurrent aphthous ulceration, some people with resistant cases related to autoimmune conditions may benefit from a TNF inhibitor drug such as infliximab, etanercept, or adalimumab. These medications also pose a significant risk resulting from inhibition of immune function.[28]

Cautery With Silver Nitrate

The use of silver nitrate sticks to provide chemical cautery was found to reduce pain significantly compared with placebo, but it did not reduce healing time. The study involved only one application. Clinicians contemplating this therapy should consider pretreating the ulcer with 2% viscous lidocaine and then painting the ulcer with the silver nitrate stick until it turns completely white.[29]

Therapies to Consider

Traditional Chinese Medicine

Chinese medicine views RAU as a condition caused by heat in the stomach; it can also be caused by yin deficiency or toxic heat. Treatment is with topical watermelon frost or internally with formulas that cool stomach heat and clear toxic heat, such as dao chi pian or niu huang jie du pian. Although no reliable studies on the use of traditional Chinese medicine in the treatment of RAUs have been conducted, referral to a Chinese medicine practitioner is a valid approach if other treatments are not indicated or are unsuccessful.

PREVENTION PRESCRIPTION

Have patients:
- Avoid oral trauma from biting, dental procedures, brushing, and eating of rough foods.
- Avoid toothpaste that contains sodium lauryl sulfate.
- Ensure adequate nutrition by consuming seven to nine servings of fruits and vegetables daily.
- Avoid trigger foods; cow's milk protein and wheat (gluten) are most common.

- Consider a B 100 complex vitamin daily for recurring cases.
- Help patients learn how to change their interpretation of stressful information and events to reduce physical consequences (see Chapters 94 and 100).
- Avoid the use of medications associated with recurrent aphthous ulcers (see Box 75.1).

THERAPEUTIC REVIEW

The most important issue in dealing with recurrent aphthous ulcers (RAUs) is to exclude systemic conditions, particularly Behçet's syndrome (mouth, genital, and eye ulcers). Because the origin of RAUs is multifactorial, a simple list of treatments is not applicable; a good history helps focus on the triggers and can lead to a specific treatment plan. The following is a guide to the most common causes and treatments of RAU.

LABORATORY EVALUATION

- Identification of nutritional deficiencies should be the first step in treating RAUs.
- Order laboratory measurements of serum ferritin, red cell folate, and serum vitamin B_{12}. Replace these nutrients if the patient is deficient.
- Giving 250 mg of vitamin C with iron is often helpful to assist with iron absorption.

NUTRITION

- If you suspect celiac disease, assess the patient for tissue transglutaminase immunoglobulin A and anti-endomysial antibodies.
- Identify any foods that trigger the RAUs and consider elimination (see Chapter 86).
- Consider using honey, 20 mL before, during, and after radiation therapy of the head and neck to reduce the severity of mouth ulcerations.

SUPPLEMENTS

- B vitamins (vitamins B_1, B_2, B_6, B_{12})
  - Because the cost and potential harm of B vitamins are low, a 3-month trial of one B 50 complex vitamin pill daily can be used to see whether the frequency of RAUs is reduced. A B 50 complex vitamin contains approximately 50 mcg or mg of each B vitamin.
  - Vitamin B_{12}, 1000 mcg sublingually daily for 6 months, has been found to reduce the incidence of ulcers.
- Glutamine
  - Mix 4 g of powder in water, swish, and swallow four times per day.
  - This is best for RAUs resulting from severe disease or injury or in patients undergoing chemotherapy.

BOTANICALS

- Licorice (*Glycyrrhiza*) mouthwash: Mix half teaspoon of licorice extract in a quarter cup of water; swish and expel four times per day.
- CankerMelt disks contain 30 mg *Glycyrrhiza* extract. The disk is applied to the ulcer and allowed to dissolve over time; then a new disk is applied every 6 hours.

HOMEOPATHY

- Mercurius solubilis is indicated if the RAUs are associated with foul breath and increased salivation. Use 6X or 6C potency four times per day until healing begins.
- Borax is indicated if the RAUs are brought on with citrus or acidic foods. The mouth usually feels dry even though some saliva may be present. Use 6X or 6C potency four times per day until healing begins.
- Arsenicum album is indicated in patients whose RAUs are brought on by stress and eased with hot drinks. Use 6X or 6C potency four times per day until healing begins.

MIND-BODY THERAPY

- Because stress is often a component of RAUs, stress reduction techniques, such as meditation and guided imagery, are usually advisable to include in management (see Chapter 94).

PHARMACEUTICALS

- Topical therapy
  - Amlexanox (Aphthasol) 5% paste: 0.5 cm applied to sore four times daily
  - Triamcinolone acetonide 0.1% in carboxymethyl cellulose paste (Kenalog in Orabase): 0.5 cm applied to the sore three to four times daily
  - Viscous lidocaine (Xylocaine 2% solution): 15 mL swished every 3 hours as needed for pain
  - Chlorhexidine gluconate 0.12% oral solution (Peridex or Periogard oral rinse): 15 mL rinsed and expelled twice daily
  - Tetracycline 500 mg per 5 mL to make 60 mL, fluocinolone acetonide solution (Synalar) 30 mL, and diphenhydramine syrup (Benadryl) 60 mL, mixed together to make 150 mL; 10 mL swished and expelled four times daily
- Systemic Therapy
  - Colchicine: 0.6 mg twice daily, increased to three times daily as tolerated in terms of gastrointestinal side effects
  - Prednisone: 40 to 60 mg per day for 5 days
  - Thalidomide: 200 mg per day; used only for most severe cases

CAUTERY

- Premedicate with 2% viscous lidocaine and paint the ulcer once with silver nitrate stick until it turns white.
- This technique helps reduce pain but not ulcer duration.

Key Web Resources

Dentist.net: This consumer site sells sodium lauryl sulfate–free toothpastes.	http://www.dentist.net/sls-free-toothpaste.asp
OraHealth: This company developed oral adhering disks that allow the medicinal application of specific treatments for recurrent aphthous ulcers.	http://www.orahealth.com/

REFERENCES

References are available online at ExpertConsult.com.

CHAPTER 76

SEBORRHEIC DERMATITIS

Alan M. Dattner, MD

PATHOPHYSIOLOGY

Seborrheic dermatitis (SD) involves a predisposition toward a specific inflammatory desquamative reaction pattern in typically oily areas rich in *Malassezia*. An overabundance of or an inappropriate immune reaction to the common skin and follicular microflora species known as *Malassezia* (formerly *Pityrosporum*) has been both demonstrated and disputed in the literature.[1] Since the identification of seven major strains of *Malassezia* in 1996, studies have begun to demonstrate which species are most predominant in SD in different populations. *Malassezia globosa* and *Malassezia restricta* predominate, according to some reports,[2,3] and various other strains have been reported to be associated with SD as well. Evidence both for and against an association with increased or altered sebum production has been presented, but increased sebum production leading to greater growth of *Malassezia* seems to be a contributor.

Seborrhea is aggravated by Parkinson's disease and by drugs that induce parkinsonism; clinical improvement is obtained with levodopa treatment of Parkinson's disease. Aggravation by emotional stress and changes associated with cases of partial denervation suggest a neurohumoral influence as well. Some drugs have been implicated in inducing SD. Infantile SD, or Leiner disease, has been reported to respond to biotin and essential fatty acids (EFAs). Recent reports have shown a biotinidase deficiency in such infants.[4]

The observation of an increase in both frequency and severity of SD among patients with acquired immunodeficiency syndrome (AIDS) has renewed interest in this otherwise benign disorder. These findings suggest that immune alterations may play some role in SD. *Malassezia* metabolites including free fatty acids released from triglycerides of sebaceous origin are also thought to induce the inflammation seen in SD.[5]

> *Malassezia* is a genus of fungi found to cause seborrhea and skin depigmentation commonly associated with tinea versicolor. It requires fat to grow and thus is common in sebaceous glands.

Because *Malassezia* species are present in most people, one should ask why SD develops in some people and not others. Besides the specific species, sebum production, and particular circumstances just mentioned, reactions initiated by both the keratinocytes and the immune system may account for this difference. Some of the response in SD may be related to direct interactions between *Malassezia* organisms and keratinocytes that generate cytokines such as interleukin-8 (IL-8).[6] Activation of innate immunity through Toll-like receptors (TLRs) also seems to play a role. Keratinocytes infected with *Malassezia furfur* upregulate TLR-2, as shown by RNA analysis.[7]

Another possible explanation of the mechanism of SD may come from the observation that symptomatic *Candida* vulvovaginitis does not develop unless an aggressive response by polymorphonuclear leukocytes occurs.[8] A similar excessive neutrophilic hypersensitivity may play a role in SD because a neutrophilic infiltrate is a characteristic histopathological finding in SD.

My own interpretation of the pathophysiology is that the trigger involves cytokines and TLRs, as described previously, as well as a specific hyperactive cross-reactive immune response to some antigenic component of *Malassezia* that contributes greatly to the inflammation. The cross-reactive stimulation is a hyperactive response to the *Malassezia* organisms resulting from primary stimulation of the lymphocytes by *Candida* and other gut fungal microflora products. Patients with scalp psoriasis and seborrhea have been shown to have elevations of *Candida* organisms in the feces and on the tongue, a finding suggesting higher gut levels.[9,10,11] Elevations of *Candida* in the stool and *Candida* phospholipase A, as well as the improvement of seborrhea with oral nystatin (which tends to remain in the gut), further argue for a role for *Candida* cross-stimulation in SD.[12] This phenomenon of primary stimulation and secondary response has been demonstrated in vitro[13] and in the clinical setting.[14]

I believe that the immune response to the organism is biphasic, leading to both a tolerance to some components (epitopes) of yeast and a hyperactive response to others. Cross-reactivity among *Malassezia*, *Candida*, and other yeasts relative to immunoglobulins has been well demonstrated.[15,16] Such a biphasic response would explain the mixed results in the literature showing both hyporeactivity and hyperreactivity to *Malassezia* antigens in patients with SD. The first component allows some overgrowth of *Malassezia* and related organisms (i.e., yeasts in gut and on skin). The hyperactive response precipitates a cascade of immune-mediated activity leading to the erythema and desquamation characteristic of the disease. Resident microflora (especially *Candida*) and ingested antigens from related microflora (e.g., yeasts and molds and their byproducts) provide the cross-reactive stimulus leading to both the tolerance and the hyperreactivity. Consideration of this etiological hypothesis changes the way one treats chronic SD, described later.

The proinflammatory response disposition comes in part from a metabolic shift toward the production of proinflammatory prostanoids, caused by the common dietary oils rich in arachidonic acid.[17] Antiinflammatory precursors, such as the omega-3 EFAs eicosapentaenoic acid (EPA) and docosahexaenoic acid (DHA), are insufficient. A study of psoriasis, a related skin disease, demonstrated a higher ratio of arachidonic acid to omega-3 EFAs in patients receiving fish oils than in a control group. Supplementing with fish oil reduced arachidonic acid and malondialdehyde (another inflammatory molecule that is a marker of oxidative stress) and was associated with clinical improvement.[18] Arachidonic acid is a precursor to the proinflammatory leukotriene B$_4$ (LTB$_4$), which has been well documented to play a role in the pathogenesis of the psoriatic lesion.

The mixed nature of those findings may result in part from a lack of control of other critical factors influencing both lipid metabolism (e.g., oxidant status of the patient and relative intake of proinflammatory lipid precursors) and biochemical influences on the delta-5 and delta-6 desaturases, which play a key role in the metabolic pathway toward proinflammatory or antiinflammatory prostanoids. An additional key factor is that carbohydrate excess leads to excess insulin release. The excess insulin both inhibits the delta-6 desaturase and causes long-term release of proinflammatory cytokines,[19] thus favoring the inflammatory disease process despite the antiinflammatory effects of ingested EFAs. Most published studies do not address this important variable, which is best managed by encouraging a diet low in simple carbohydrates. In my experience, such a diet leads to positive results in a significant proportion of patients with SD as well as in patients with other inflammatory disorders of the skin (see Chapter 88).

INTEGRATIVE THERAPY

Changing to antiinflammatory oils, controlling yeast on the skin and in the bowel, and calming the nervous system are mainstays in controlling seborrheic dermatitis.

Nutrition

Omega-3 Essential Fatty Acids

Omega-3 unsaturated fatty acids should be substituted for other dietary fats. Saturated, heat-altered, and partially hydrogenated fats should be eliminated from the diet because they lead to production of proinflammatory prostaglandin E2 (PGE2) prostanoids. In addition, they block the delta-6 desaturase that catalyzes the formation of antiinflammatory leukotriene precursors. Extra fats contribute to the unfavorable ratio of proinflammatory lipids in the cell membrane and to weight gain because of their caloric content. Other indicators of a need for omega-3 oils are dry skin in winter, dryness around the nailfold area, a lack of dietary intake of such oils, depression, and a high ratio of arachidonic acid to omega-3 EFAs in the plasma or red blood cell membrane. EPA appears to be the primary antiinflammatory component of omega-3 unsaturated fatty acids.

An excellent source of omega-3 unsaturated EFAs is EFA-enriched fish oil capsules or liquid. Krill oil, cod liver oil, and other cold-water fish oils are also good sources. Eating four to five portions weekly of oily cold-water fish is also recommended. Flaxseed oil, which contains alpha-linolenic acid, is also a potential source, but it must undergo chain elongation involving an extra step requiring the delta-6 desaturase, and some people cannot use this oil effectively. Canola oil and walnut oil are lesser sources of omega-3 unsaturated EFAs.

Oils can be either taken as supplements or worked into the diet as foods. For example, flaxseed oil can be used in making smoothies or salad dressing. These oils should not be heated because the unsaturated bonds that make them useful are unstable on heating. Because of their unsaturated nature, they should be accompanied by vitamin E in the diet. Similarly, other factors contributing to high oxidative stress in the individual patient should be corrected, or counterbalanced with additional antioxidants, to maximize the effectiveness of these oils. Omega-3 fish oil can induce glucose intolerance in diabetic patients. To counter this effect and to reduce the proinflammatory mediators from carbohydrate-stimulated insulin elevation, a proper balance of carbohydrate intake with protein intake and exercise should be achieved.

DOSAGE

The dosage is based on the severity of presentation, a history of inadequate dietary intake of omega-3 EFAs, and a low red blood cell membrane ratio of EPA to arachidonate. Whereas daily intake of five capsules (approximately one teaspoon) of flaxseed oil or EPA-DHA fish oils may be helpful, some patients may need as much as 15 mL (three teaspoons) per day for a short time, mixed into a shake to make it palatable. Vitamin E, 400 units/day, should be taken to protect these unsaturated oils from oxidation. At least 1000 mg of EPA should be present in the product used. Flaxseed oil may not be effective if the individual is unable to chain elongate the 18-carbon alpha linolenic acid.

PRECAUTIONS

Fish oils have been known to prolong bleeding time through the anticoagulant effect of PGE3 for which they are precursors. Use of large doses in pregnant women has also been associated with elevated birth weight of their infants.

Yeast Elimination

For patients who require additional measures to control their seborrhea, a yeast and mold elimination diet should be instituted. The basis of this diet is the elimination of bread, cheese, wine and beer, excessive carbohydrates (especially sugar and simple starches), and other foods containing or produced by yeast or fungus. This diet has been touted as highly effective in the popular literature, and the success of different variations is probably related both to yeast reduction and to relief of different food allergies in patients with yeast sensitivities. Probiotics such as *Lactobacillus acidophilus* and *Bifidobacterium bifidus* should be taken before or during meals to help repopulate the normal flora of the gut. Patients who cannot give up bread should be counseled to eat true sourdough bread, the leavening agent for which is derived from limited cultures of different yeasts captured from the air.

Supplements

Vitamins

Oils, which can be used as either foods or supplements, have already been discussed. Vitamin E, at 400 units/day, should be added as an antioxidant to protect the oils. Adequate levels of magnesium, zinc, vitamin C, and vitamin B6 should be maintained by supplementation if intake of any of these nutrients is insufficient in the diet, to enhance the function of the delta-6 desaturase. Vitamin B6 cream, 50 mg/g, compounded in a water-based cream by a compounding pharmacy, has been used for treatment of SD of the scalp.[20,21]

Biotin is especially useful in infantile SD,[22] and it may have a role in the treatment of adult seborrhea as well. Besides contributing to the generation of antiinflammatory prostanoids through activation of the delta-6 desaturase (as do other vitamins mentioned here), biotin is reputed to retard the formation of the mycelial form of *Candida*. Other B vitamins shown to be helpful in seborrhea are vitamin B6, folate,[23] and vitamin B12.[24]

DOSAGE

One or two tablets per day of a high-potency multivitamin with mineral (even for those with a three- to six-tablet per day recommendation on the bottle label) can be used for vitamin B supplementation in most patients. If clinical improvement is not seen, extra biotin up to 7.5 mg/day and vitamin B6 or pyridoxal 5-phosphate, 20–50 mg/day can be added; zinc picolinate, 25–50 mg/day, and vitamin C, 500 mg one to three times per day, are also useful.

Probiotics

To address the yeast overgrowth, adding probiotic bacteria such as *Lactobacillus acidophilus* and *Bifidobacterium*, or the yeast *Saccharomyces boulardii* to the diet is nearly as important as proper diet in restoring normal gut flora and reducing the yeast population. Caprylic acid can be added to inhibit attachment of the yeast to the intestinal wall.

DOSAGE

GI Flora (Allergy Research Group, Alameda, California) is an economical, effective source of multiple probiotic strains; the dose is one or two capsules with meals. Ultra Flora Balance or the higher-potency Ultra Flora IB, one capsule per day (Metagenics, San Clemente, Calif), are other useful sources. Doses for caprylic acid are begun at one capsule three times per day before meals and are gradually increased to two capsules per meal, if necessary, or augmented by other anti-yeast supplements.

If the patient has known overgrowth of yeast in the gastrointestinal tract, consider Caprystatin (Ecological Formulas, Concord, California), which contains caprylic acid,

a short-chain fatty acid that inhibits *Candida* growth and prevents attachment of yeast to the intestinal wall. Start with one capsule three times per day before meals, and increase the dose as necessary. Some patients, especially those who have associated fatigue or hypersensitivities, may have a die-off reaction and have some symptoms worsen before they improve. Follow these patients closely to ensure that they are not reacting to something in the treatment regimen. Resume the program at a slower rate if symptoms occur.

PRECAUTIONS

The addition of a source of fiber is important to ensure that bowel movements are occurring at least one or more times per day during yeast reduction therapy, so that allergenic moieties are not absorbed from the dying organisms. Fiber also promotes healthy mucosa along the gastrointestinal tract in which bacteria live.

Probiotics should not be given to a patient with a compromised immune system because of the slight risk of infection.

Many companies that produce probiotics claim to offer the absolute best species, combinations, or strains of bacteria. Clinicians are advised to start with an affordable *Lactobacillus acidophilus* or *Bifidobacterium bifidus* preparation and then add others to their personal pharmacopoeia as evaluation of a specific product is found to be convincing and its effects are confirmed to be beneficial. Different patients do better with different probiotic bacteria. *Bifidobacterium bifidus* is thought to be more beneficial initially.

Topical Nicotinamide (Vitamin B3)

Topical nicotinamide cream 4% was found to cause a 75% reduction in SD scores as compared with placebo cream giving a 35% reduction. It was also found to work as well as 1% clindamycin for moderate inflammatory acne.[25]

DOSAGE

Apply 4% cream twice per day after washing.[26]

PRECAUTIONS

Can cause drying of the skin and/or peeling and itching.

Botanicals

For topical treatment, any application that reduces yeast on the skin may be helpful. Various essential oils may be useful for their incorporation in scalp sebaceous lipids and antimicrobial action against *Malassezia*. Tea tree oil, honey, and cinnamic acid have been shown to reduce *Malassezia* and SD.[27] Tea tree oil and cinnamic acid, as well as other essential oils, however, can cause contact dermatitis, especially in inflamed skin, and honey is messy to use on the scalp. *Monarda fistulosa*, a distinctive-smelling herb from the mint family, has also been reported to yield an essential oil that is effective against seborrhea.[28]

Many different antifungal herbs and combination products with probiotics are available on the market today, and a comprehensive evaluation of these products is beyond the scope of this chapter. A few are mentioned here, but most that are effective in significantly reducing the yeast population in the gut will work. The use of fiber products such as psyllium and of other vegetable fiber is essential to maintain rapid passage of treated organisms through the bowel.

Grapefruit seed extract and *Artemisia annua* can also be added to reduce the yeast population. Some newer herbal preparations constituted for this purpose are available. Pau d'arco tea is another product with reported antiyeast activity. Application of aloe has been shown to be useful in seborrhea.[29]

DOSAGES

Tea tree oil may be used in adults on an occasional basis, applied sparingly to the areas of intense scaling after wetting the scalp. Because it is a potent allergen, I do not recommend it for regular, ongoing use. Aloe vera (*Aloe barbadensis*) gel may be applied directly from the cut leaf of the plant. Avocado may contain oils and sugars[30] that are helpful in controlling SD.

Mind-Body Therapy

SD is more prevalent in patients with depression.[31] Perhaps the improvement seen in the summer is the result either of reduced depression or of the effects of increased sunlight on melatonin release.[32] Addressing depression or seasonal affective disorder with light therapy, visits to a sunnier climate, psychotherapy, Bach Flower Remedies, supplements, or medications may be considered in a patient with SD in whom the disease severity varies with his or her affective state.

Pharmaceuticals

Shampoos

The two mainstays of topical treatment of SD are tar shampoos and antiyeast shampoos. Antiyeast shampoos consist, in order of potency, of zinc pyrithione, selenium sulfide 1% (over-the-counter shampoos), selenium sulfide 2.5% (prescription), and ketoconazole shampoos (available over the counter in some countries). Tar shampoos have antiinflammatory and antiyeast activity.

DOSAGE

A more recent treatment for fungal infections is ciclopirox 1% shampoo (Loprox), which is also approved for use in SD. Side effects include pruritus (itching), burning, erythema (redness), seborrhea, and rash. This product comes in a gel and a shampoo. Use the shampoo twice a week for 4 weeks or apply the gel twice daily for 4 weeks.

Tar shampoo (Tegrin, T/Gel) is used three times per week initially and then once per week.

Keratolytic Treatments

Oils are applied to the scalp to loosen scale. Olive oil is particularly useful in this regard, especially in infants with thin hair. Wetting the scalp and applying a warm oil turban for an hour, with 6% salicylic acid mixed into the olive oil, may remove more adherent scale. Patients must remove the oil with dishwashing liquid detergent before they apply a therapeutic shampoo.

Other salicylic acid preparations may also be used for the same purpose when thick, adherent scale is difficult to remove. Urea preparations may be used for the same purpose. These preparations also need time to act and generally require shampoo for removal. After thick scale is removed, a therapeutic agent can be applied to penetrate the scalp more deeply. Keratolytics such as salicylic acid have antifungal properties as well.

DOSAGE

Consider the following treatment to help reduce scaling. Olive oil is compounded with 6% salicylic acid; the oil is applied to a wet scalp under a warm towel turban for 1 hour, and then scales are removed with a soft brush.

Topical Corticosteroids

Topical corticosteroids are another mainstay of conventional treatment of SD. Even 1% hydrocortisone cream brings temporary improvement in SD of the face and nasolabial folds in a previously untreated patient. Liquids, gels, and even a foam vehicle are available, with a more potent fluorinated corticosteroid used to avoid the hair and reach the scalp.

DOSAGE

Patients should apply 1% to 2.5% hydrocortisone cream sparingly once or twice daily for 1–2 weeks. Hydrocortisone cream, Triamcinolone solution or betamethasone valerate foam (Luxiq) once or twice per day can be used to relieve pruritus and inflammation for brief periods of time.

PRECAUTIONS

Frequent or repeated application of corticosteroids results in tachyphylaxis (a progressively diminished response), requiring more potent steroids to obtain the same response. In addition, some patients behave as though they are addicted to the topical steroids. The problem becomes worse, and the corticosteroid is needed increasingly more often in higher strengths to control the redness and scaling. Repeated use on the face, especially of stronger corticosteroids, and even the use of hydrocortisone on the thin tissues of the eyelids, can result in atrophy of the skin with permanent show-through of the underlying capillaries or the development of problematic steroid acne.

Other Creams

Ketoconazole (Nizoral) cream applied sparingly twice daily is extremely helpful for management of SD of the face and hairline. It inhibits the *Malassezia*, gives dramatic clinical improvement, and does not cause the atrophy resulting from prolonged corticosteroid use. Other antifungal creams, including ciclopirox (Loprox) and nystatin cream, are also useful.

DOSAGE
Ketoconazole cream 2% is applied twice daily to affected areas, sparingly.

Lithium Succinate

Lithium succinate 8% ointment has been reported to be helpful in SD. An antiyeast effect has been confirmed in vitro,[33] as well as in patients.[34] The ointment is applied twice daily. The relationship between lithium as a drug for depression, which has been implicated as a cause of seborrhea, and direct application of lithium as a treatment for seborrhea is interesting to contemplate. A common mediator pathway for both disorders may exist.

Oral Antifungals

Oral antifungals should be used only when seborrhea is serious enough to warrant the risk of taking the drug or when the underlying condition of overgrowth has not responded to diet and herbal treatment alone.

Nystatin. Oral nystatin is useful to reduce the *Candida* population in the gut. It has the benefit of being poorly absorbed and therefore remaining in the gut. It works by causing defective yeast cell wall formation, resulting in release of intracellular contents, which has in turn been blamed for the aggravation of symptoms constituting a Herxheimer-type reaction (flulike feeling from the die-off effect of yeast) in some patients after a large dose.

Ketoconazole and Fluconazole. Ketoconazole (Nizoral) is well absorbed, exerts an antiyeast effect in the gut and skin, and is excreted in high concentrations in the sweat. Other oral antifungal agents, such as fluconazole (Diflucan), have also been used for severe cases of seborrhea. An antiyeast regimen should be instituted gradually, starting with diet, *Lactobacillus acidophilus*, and supplements and botanicals before oral pharmaceuticals are used. The first reason is to avoid rapid kill-off of a large number of organisms, which may result in a die-off effect, or Herxheimer-type reaction. The second reason is to reduce the intestinal yeast population less drastically. If the gut ecology is altered to favor a more gradual reduction in yeast population, a rebound growth of yeast resistant to the most powerful agents available is less likely to occur. Although these agents may be effective in the short term, I question whether it is responsible practice to use these agents without initially or simultaneously altering the ecological conditions that favor yeast overgrowth.

DOSAGE
The dose of nystatin for Candida is increased slowly from 500,000 units once daily to 1–2 million units three times daily; this dose is then maintained until the patient's condition is improved. Lesser dosages may be needed if seborrhea is the only manifestation of this issue. Dosing should begin with one capsule (500,000 units) per day of the powder, with addition of an extra capsule every 2 or 3 days until a total

dose of four capsules three times daily (6 million units/day total) is achieved. Doses for the pure powder should begin with 1/8 teaspoon/day increased to 1/2–1 teaspoon/day (3–6 million units/day total, depending on response and severity) in the same gradual manner. This dose should be continued for 1 month or tapered for 1–2 weeks after symptoms clear.

The FDA has warned against using ketoconazole for skin and nail infections, and fluconazole is regarded similarly. Such off-label use is mentioned but not recommended, and should only even be considered when dietary measures have been instituted and all other methods have failed, and the risk of severe side effects or death is less than the risk of not trying the drugs. For fluconazole (Diflucan), the dose is 100–200 mg/day for 10–14 days. (Many drug interactions and cautions are cited in the package insert.) Seborrhea is not a listed indication and should only be used in cases with severe underlying yeast issues.

The dose of ketoconazole (Nizoral) is 100–200 mg/day. Ketoconazole should be used only if other indications exist and liver enzyme values are monitored. In general, this drug should be avoided, or the liver can be protected with silymarin (milk thistle). Seborrhea is not a listed indication and should only be used in cases with severe underlying yeast issues.

PRECAUTIONS
Adverse effects include elevation in liver enzymes, hepatic failure (uncommon with oral ketoconazole and less likely with fluconazole), a Herxheimer-type die-off phenomenon (especially with nystatin), and overgrowth of resistant organisms.

Before an oral antifungal is considered, intestinal yeast growth should be reduced with dietary measures. This will help prevent the growth of resistant strains of yeast and lead to improved response from the oral antifungal.

Therapies to Consider

Homeopathy

A homeopathic dilution of tobacco was reported to clear SD in a patient with tobacco sensitivity. I mention this not to recommend this specific remedy but rather to emphasize the potential benefits of choosing an appropriate homeopathic or other remedy that addresses prominent underlying imbalances in the patient. Other homeopathics, including natrum muriaticum, arsenicum album, and bryonia, may be considered, but homeopathics should be prescribed according to other characteristics of the patient besides local presentation.

Food Allergy

As in patients with atopic dermatitis, addressing food allergies by removing the offending foods from the diet may benefit some patients with recalcitrant SD (see Chapter 86).

Energy-Based Treatments

When addressing a variety of apparent causal factors is not sufficient, the clinician must address ways in which the seborrhea may be an expression of some deeper autonomic or psychological pattern. Psychotherapy may be useful if it is powerful and targeted. Classical homeopathy addressing mental and emotional symptoms may touch this level. Newer forms of treatment that use acupressure meridian activation or tapping to release patterns of sensitivity in the autonomic nervous system, including Lang desensitization and neuromuscular therapy (NMT), may be considered by the practitioner skilled in these techniques.

PREVENTION PRESCRIPTION

- Use a Mediterranean-type diet based on olive oil and fresh vegetables.
- Supplement with omega-3 essential fatty acids from fish oil, northern fish, and flaxseed.
- Reduce the intake of bread, cheese, wine, beer, and yeast.
- Reduce the intake of sugar, refined carbohydrates, and heated oils.
- Shampoo the scalp at least twice a week, with an antidandruff shampoo when necessary.

THERAPEUTIC REVIEW

The following is an outline of therapeutic options for the treatment of seborrheic dermatitis. Determining which factors lead to the disease presentation in a given patient may improve the chances of success of a given therapy. For more severe or resistant cases, a progressive, sequential approach with multiple therapeutic avenues is recommended, with either intensification of treatments or addition of systemic pharmacological agents, as indicated by the clinical response.

ANTIDANDRUFF SHAMPOOS

- Zinc pyrithione, selenium sulfide (Selsun), tar, or ketoconazole (Nizoral) shampoo is used for 5 minutes two or three times/week.
- If the patient has used one type with no clinical improvement, another can be tried.

ANTIYEAST CREAMS

- Ketoconazole cream 2% (Nizoral) or another pharmacological or herbal substitute works well on the face and nonscalp areas.

SUPPLEMENTS

- Eicosapentaenoic acid and docosahexaenoic acid (fish oils) can be added at 1–2 g/day and titrated to clinical improvement.
- Other sources of omega-3 essential fatty acids—oily cold-water fish, such as salmon and sardines, three to five servings per week and flaxseed oil, one teaspoon/day—can be used.
- Vitamin E 400 units/day should be given with the aforementioned oils to prevent oxidation.
- Vitamin B complex, vitamin B6 500 mg, and biotin up to 8 mg/day may be beneficial in patients with resistant cases.

- Caprylic acid is taken at 100–200 mg two to three times per day to reduce the attachment of yeast to the intestinal wall.
- Topical nicotinamide (B3), 4% cream twice per day.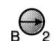

NUTRITION

- A diet low in yeast and simple carbohydrates, especially one that eliminates bread, cheese, wine, beer, fermented foods, and starches, is helpful in patients with persistent cases.
- Some improvement may result from removal of other food allergens.
- Adding probiotic bacteria such as *Lactobacillus acidophilus,* one capsule per meal, or live-culture yogurt may also help.

BOTANICALS

- The antiyeast botanicals grapefruit seed extract and *Artemisia annua* may be used at two to six capsules/day.
- Undecenoic acid, derived from the castor bean, is another antiyeast product (Formula SF 722 [Thorne Research, Sandpoint, Idaho]), used at two to six capsules/day.

PHARMACEUTICALS

- Nystatin is used in slowly increasing doses from 0.5–6 million units/day.
- Hydrocortisone cream, triamcinolone solution or betamethasone valerate foam (Luxiq) once or twice per day can be used short-term to relieve pruritus and inflammation.

Key Web Resources

Holistic Dermatology: Information on alternative treatments for numerous skin conditions, including seborrheic dermatitis

http://www.holisticdermatology.com

Medscape: Conventional medications for seborrhea

http://emedicine.medscape.com/article/1108312-treatment

American Academy of Dermatology EczemaNet: Photographs and a description of conventional treatments for seborrheic dermatitis

http://www.aad.org/public/publications/pamphlets/common_seb_dermatitis.html

Wikipedia: Overview of seborrheic dermatitis, including treatment

http://en.wikipedia.org/wiki/Seborrhoeic_dermatitis

REFERENCES

References are available online at ExpertConsult.com.

CHAPTER 77

ACNE VULGARIS AND ACNE ROSACEA

Hana Grobel, MD • Sarah A. Murphy, MD

ACNE VULGARIS

PATHOPHYSIOLOGY OF ACNE VULGARIS

Acne vulgaris is a common skin condition that affects around 85% of adolescents around the world and can be moderate to severe in 20% of the world's population.[1] It commonly continues into adulthood, affecting 64% of those in their 20s and 43% of those in their 30s. There is a strong genetic component, with 80% of those affected having first degree relatives with similar conditions.[2]

Acne is a condition of the pilosebaceous unit of the skin, which includes the oil glands and hair follicles (Fig. 77.1). Following are the four main factors that contribute to acne formation and are the basis of most treatments[3]:

1. Keratinization of the pilosebaceous unit: The skin consists of pores that contain hair follicles that carry sebum and keratin from dead skin cells to the surface. When sebum and keratin are blocked due to increased proliferation and decreased desquamation of keratinocytes, a microcomedo forms (and later turns into closed or open comedones). This might be influenced by inflammatory cells. The follicle can then rupture and also trigger the inflammatory response.[4]

2. Increased sebum production: During puberty, sebum production increases, in part due to the effects of androgen on the skin. Androgen is not only produced by adrenal glands and gonads but also within the sebaceous glands of the skin. One study investigating men with androgen insensitivity found that they do not develop sebum or acne.[5] This lipid-rich environment of the pilosebaceous unit makes it easier for *Propionibacterium acnes* (*P. acnes*) to multiply and thus might explain the rise of acne formation during the adolescent period.

3. Colonization of sebaceous unit with *P. acnes*: *P. acnes* are anaerobic, gram positive bacteria that are part of the normal skin flora, yet there might be different pathogenic forms of the bacteria that can induce the inflammatory response. The anaerobic nature of the sebaceous follicles creates an environment where these bacteria can thrive and influence the inflammatory response.

4. Inflammatory response: The exact mechanism is unknown, but it is believed that the presence of *P. acnes* triggers the inflammatory cascade, including Toll-like receptors, cytokines, lymphocytes, and interleukins, which cause an inflammatory response in the skin, forming papules, pustules, and nodules.

INTEGRATIVE THERAPY

Hygiene

There has been some speculation that washing the face reduces the development of acne vulgaris. However, a systematic review done in 2005 showed that there is no great evidence that washing the face often helps prevent acne, and it might even harm the skin if done too often.[1,8] Scrubbing the face can remove healthy oils from the skin surface and might trigger an increase in oil production.[1] One study reported less inflammatory lesions in people who used acidic gentle synthetic detergent cleansers (which have a pH of 5.5–7, closer to that of normal skin pH) rather than most alkaline soaps (with a pH of 9–10).[9] The recommendation is to wash the face twice a day with a gentle nonsoap cleanser.

Emotional Stress

Many people who suffer from acne vulgaris and rosacea report stress to be a common trigger and worse than other exacerbating factors. In the United States (US), a small study of Stanford university students that measured acne severity during nonexam and exam times found the severity significantly increased during exam periods, particularly when those students reported an increase in their stress levels (even after controlling for diet and sleep changes during exams).[14]

The pathophysiology of stress contributing to dermatological issues includes the increase in serum cortisol level in people with acne who experience emotional stress.[13,16-18] Another contributing factor is corticotropin-releasing hormone (CRH), a neuropeptide involved in the stress response, specifically the hypothalamic-pituitary-axis. A study by Zouboulis investigated the role of CRH and discussed its influence on lipid synthesis in human sebaceous glands, thus possibly linking the relationship between stress and acne.[19]

Finding techniques that can help alleviate stress may therefore decrease the severity of acne vulgaris and rosacea. One study taught biofeedback-assisted relaxation and cognitive imagery to those with acne vulgaris in 12 sessions over 6 weeks and found a significant reduction in acne severity compared to controls.[21]

Diet

For the past several decades, diet and its relationship to acne was largely refuted by the dermatological community. More recent evidence demonstrates diet does influence acne. The most robust link to increased acne

PATHOGENESIS OF ACNE

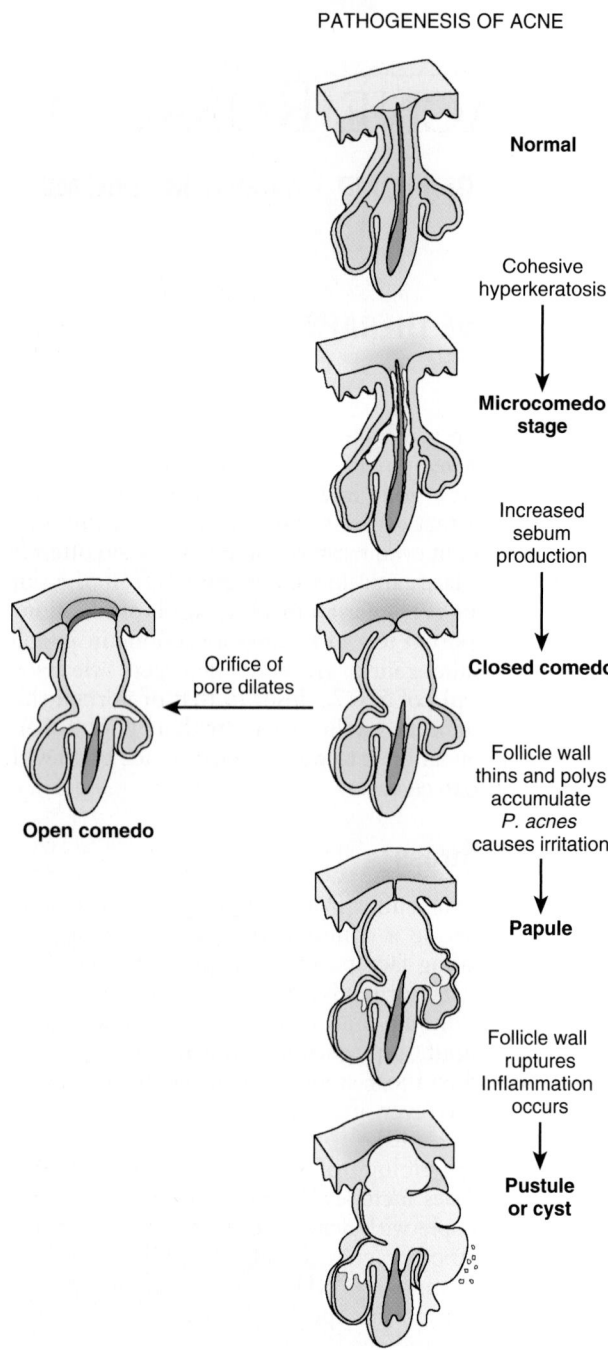

Normal

Cohesive
hyperkeratosis

**Microcomedo
stage**

Increased
sebum
production

Orifice of
pore dilates

Closed comedo

Open comedo

Follicle wall
thins and polys
accumulate
P. acnes
causes irritation

Papule

Follicle wall
ruptures
Inflammation
occurs

**Pustule
or cyst**

FIG. 77.1 ■ The pathogenesis of acne vulgaris. (From Habif TP. Acne, rosacea, and related disorders. In: Habif TP, ed. *Clinical dermatology*. 5th ed. Philadelphia: Saunders; 2009.)

includes diets high in dairy and those with a high glycemic load.

Dairy

There is compelling evidence that diets high in milk and other dairy products can contribute to increased acne.[27] The link between dairy and acne started with a 1949 survey of 1900 subjects with acne. It was found that milk was the food most often implicated in acne flares.[28] More recently, findings from a retrospective, recall-based study

in more than 47,000 adult nurses[29] and a prospective self-assessment study in 6000 teenage girls[30] suggest an association between acne and intake of milk, particularly skim milk and other dairy products. Another prospective study of more than 4200 teenage boys suggested an association with skim milk only.[31] It is hypothesized that milk is hormonally and biochemically active and that these factors might be more bioavailable or present in higher quantities in skim milk.[31] It has also been shown that some dairy products, including milk, have a much higher effect on insulin than expected given their low glycemic index,[32] which may account for some of its effects in a way similar to high-glycemic diets (see the following text).

> In those with acne, encourage a plant-based diet that is low in dairy, rich in omega-3 fatty acids, and has a low glycemic load.

Low–Glycemic Load Diet

Glycemic load takes into account both the quantity of carbohydrates ingested as well as its effect on insulin (see Chapter 87) A well-done randomized controlled trial of 47 male patients showed decreased acne with a low–glycemic load diet (LGLD).[33] It is hypothesized that diets with a high glycemic load increase acne by multiple causes due to increased insulin and insulin like growth factor-1 (IGF-1).[35] Insulin and IGF-1 both increase the synthesis and bioavailability of androgens by inhibiting the synthesis of sex hormone-binding globulin in the liver.[35] Sebum production also increases with increased insulin and IGF-1.[36]

Supplements

Omega-3 Fatty Acids

Omega-3 fatty acids are a group of polyunsaturated fatty acids that have been shown to decrease inflammation in multiple studies.[38] The omega-3s, eicosapentaenoic acid (EPA) and docosahexaenoic acid (DHA), are found in high quantities in fatty fish. The omega-3 alpha-linolenic acids (ALAs) are from mostly plant sources. One recent, small study showed supplementation with 3 g of fish oil daily (930 mg EPA) for 12 weeks decreased acne severity in those with moderate to severe acne at baseline.[39]

The other main polyunsaturated fatty acids are the omega-6s. There is an elevated omega-6 to omega-3 ratio in the Western diet versus more traditional diets, and such ratios are proinflammatory.[41-43] A major dietary omega- fatty acid is arachidonic acid, which is a precursor to the inflammatory signaling molecule leukotriene B4 (LTB4). The importance of decreasing LTB4 action was demonstrated in a study of a novel LTB4 blocker that showed a 70% reduction in inflammatory acne lesions over 3 months.[44] Increased omega-3 intake may decrease the production of LTB4 and other inflammatory signaling molecules.[45] Omega-3 fatty acids have also been shown to decrease IGF-1 levels in healthy men.[46] Therefore, a trial of supplementation with or a diet high in omega-3 fatty acids is recommended for the treatment of acne vulgaris (see Chapter 88).

DOSAGE

Suggested supplementation is with 1–3 g of the EPA plus DHA component of omega-3 fatty acids.

PRECAUTIONS

Fatty fish and fish oil, common sources of omega-3s, can get contaminated with toxins. Purchase supplements that have undergone analysis by independent laboratories. For information on safe fish consumption, see the Monterey Bay Aquarium's Seafood Watch website: http://www.seafoodwatch.org.

High doses of omega-3s may inhibit blood coagulation and increase the risk of bleeding. They are considered safe and commonly used in children, pregnancy, and lactation.[48]

Zinc

Zinc is an essential micronutrient that acts as a cofactor for hundreds of enzymatic reactions in the body and plays an important role in regulating gene expression.[49] It is involved in maintaining the health of many body systems, including immune function, skin health, and smell/taste sensation. Zinc deficiency is rare in developed countries, but conditions that pose the greatest risk include malabsorption syndromes (short bowel syndrome, celiac disease, history of gastric bypass), irritable bowel syndrome, alcoholism, and malnutrition.[49] Dietary zinc can be found in highest levels in red meat, poultry, beans, nuts, and whole grains.[50] In vitro studies using zinc have shown success in inhibiting growth of clindamycin-resistant strains of *P. acnes* as well as decreasing erythromycin-resistant strain development.[52,53] Zinc supplementation has also been found to reduce the number of inflammatory acne pustules.[54]

DOSAGE

Oral zinc gluconate: older than 13 years: 30 mg per day; 9–13 years old: 20 mg per day.[49,61]

PRECAUTIONS

Side effects of oral zinc supplementation can include metallic taste and gastrointestinal (GI) symptoms such as nausea, vomiting, bloating, and diarrhea.[49,62] High doses for long periods of time (>40 mg elemental zinc per day and possibly higher) have been shown to cause sideroblastic anemia and copper deficiency. If taking zinc long term at high doses, we recommend supplementing with 2-mg copper.[63,64]

Likely safe in pregnancy and lactation at aforementioned doses.[60,61]

Brewer's Yeast (Saccharomyces cerevisiae)

Brewer's yeast is an active yeast used to make beer and is a commonly used nutritional supplement as it is a source of protein, B vitamins, chromium, and selenium.[65] One randomized controlled trial investigated the brewer's yeast strain Hansen CBS (*Saccharomyces boulardii*) and showed improvement in acne symptoms with oral supplement over a 5-month duration.[67]

DOSAGE

Recommended dosage is 6 g of freeze dried daily (can take in divided doses: 3 g bid or 2 g tid)

PRECAUTIONS

It is usually well tolerated. Side effects are GI in nature, including bloating and flatulence.[65] Migraine headaches have been reported in some users. Do not administer if patient is on a monoamine oxidase inhibitor (MAOI) as the high levels of tyramine in the brewer's yeast can lead to hypertension with concomitant MAOI use.[68] Caution in Crohn's disease as Brewer's yeast possibly relates to inflammation in Crohn's disease.[69]

Vitamin A

Vitamin A is a fat-soluble vitamin that can be found as preformed retinoids or as provitamin carotenoids (i.e., beta carotene). Retinoids come from animal sources such as liver, kidney, eggs, and dairy. Carotenoids are found in plants such as dark or yellow vegetables, carrots, and tree nuts.[70] The studies on acne have used high doses of preformed vitamin A, which carries a risk of hypervitaminosis as preformed vitamin A is efficiently stored by the liver.[71] There was historical interest in treating acne with vitamin A supplementation starting with articles in the 1940s and 1950s[72,73] that demonstrated some success with treatment at high doses (100,000–300,000 IU/day). Since that time, there have been some studies showing positive[74-76] and some negative[77-79] results at these high doses.

DOSAGE

The tolerable upper intake of vitamin A is 10,000 IU/day for adults.[70] Doses used in the treatment of acne were much higher than this, but we do not recommend use at these doses.

PRECAUTIONS

Symptoms of excess vitamin A without hypervitaminosis A was noted in a 4-month trial using vitamin A 300,000–500,000 IU/day.[80] However, given the short treatment duration, it is likely hypervitaminosis A could develop using these doses for longer courses. Symptoms of excess vitamin A include nausea, vomiting, headache, and dry skin. Symptoms of hypervitaminosis A include hepatotoxicity, teratogenicity, reduced bone mineral density, alopecia, and xerosis.[81]

Botanicals

Tea Tree Oil (Melaleuca alternifolia)

Tea tree oil made from the leaves of the native Australian tree *Melaleuca alternifolia* has been shown to improve acne through its antimicrobial and antiinflammatory properties. It is the most well-studied botanical that has shown to be the most effective for acne vulgaris. Some studies found that topical application of at least 5% tea tree oil used for 4–8 weeks improved mild to moderate acne vulgaris as well as or better than 5% benzoyl peroxide, 2% topical erythromycin, or placebo. Although results took longer for those who used tea tree oil, the adverse side effects were fewer.[82-85]

Green Tea

Green tea, made from unfermented leaves of *Camellia sinensis*, contains a high content of antioxidants called polyphenols (catechins) that help neutralize free radicals. The main polyphenol that has been studied is epigallocatechin-3-gallate (EGCG) and has antiinflammatory, anticancer, and antiandrogen properties that help decrease sebum production, inflammation, and bacterial growth (particularly *P. acnes*) in the skin.[86] Two randomized trials and one other study showed a significant reduction in acne when using topical green tea lotion for treatment of mild to moderate acne vulgaris.[87-89]

Although the sample sizes were small, green tea appears to be promising in the treatment of acne vulgaris and one of the only agents, besides retinoids, that help decrease sebum production.

DOSAGE

- Recommended dosage is green tea lotion 2%–3% applied topically twice a day.
- Recommended daily intake of green tea is two to three cups a day (240–320 mg polyphenols).

PRECAUTIONS

Green tea contains caffeine and can cause caffeine-related side effects.

Use with caution for those taking blood thinning medications because green tea has anticlotting properties. Green tea can increase the effect of some antibiotics and thus the risk of side effects.

Turmeric (Curcuma longa)

Turmeric is a rhizome (root) that comes from the plant of the ginger family (Zingiberaceae) native to India and is used as a spice in cooking. Curcumin is a component of turmeric that has been most studied for its antiinflammatory effects. One study showed decreased Propionibacterium activity in vitro by curcumin-containing, lipid-based vehicles (specifically lauric acid that can be found in coconut oil).[90] Although human studies are lacking specifically for the use of turmeric on acne, it might be a possible remedy for those with inflammatory lesions.

DOSAGE

Used as a topical mixture of turmeric powder with milk or coconut oil and placed on inflammatory lesions daily.

Ingested dose of turmeric is 500 mg two to four times a day.

PRECAUTIONS

Topical turmeric can dye clothes and stain the skin. Side effects when ingested orally are rare but include GI problems (nausea, vomiting, diarrhea, and dyspepsia).

Pharmaceuticals: Topical Preparations

There are a variety of topical therapies for mild to moderate acne vulgaris that are useful for the different patterns of acne (inflammatory versus noninflammatory) and work on different mechanisms. They can be used alone or in combination. If side effects occur, mainly skin irritation, the therapy can be started at a lower dose and gradually increased or the formulation can be changed from alcoholic solutions (that are more drying) to washes or gels to creams or lotions.[1] It takes about 2–3 months of consistent treatment before significant improvement, and therefore patients should be given realistic expectations regarding therapy. Treatment of truncal acne might require oral medications due to the difficulty of reaching a larger area with topical therapy.

Benzoyl Peroxide

Benzoyl peroxide is one of the safest and most effective treatments for inflammatory lesions and is usually used in mild to moderate acne as a first-line therapy. It works as an antimicrobial, against *P. acnes*, although it does not cause bacterial resistance. Some studies have shown that it works better than topical tretinoin for inflammatory acne.[93,94] Most studies have shown that lower doses work just as well as higher doses and cause less irritation, so there is no need to go higher than 5%.[95,96] It has also been shown to improve the effect of antibiotics and decrease the amount of antibiotic resistance, and thus it is recommended to use benzoyl peroxide in combination with topical or oral antibiotics.[97-100]

DOSAGE

Recommended dosage is 2.5%–5% gel, lotion, or cream. Topical application one to two times a day

PRECAUTIONS

Can cause skin irritation, including drying and peeling of skin, pruritis, burning, and redness. It can bleach hair and clothes.

Of note, benzoyl peroxide can inactivate tretinoin and make it less stable and thus should not be used at the same time. It is better to use benzoyl peroxide in the morning and tretinoin at night. There are newer formulations of tretinoin (micronized tretinoin gel, tretinoin gel microsphere) and other types of topical retinoids (adapalene) that are not affected by benzoyl peroxide and thus can be used in combination.[101-103]

Topical Retinoids

Topical retinoids (tretinoin/isoretinoin/adapalene) are vitamin A derivatives that break down keratinocytes and reduce sebum excretion, follicular occlusion, and comedones.[104] They work best for all types of acne (inflammatory and noninflammatory) and can be used to decrease postinflammatory hyperpigmentation.[105] There are two types of topical retinoids available in the United States: tretinoin and adapalene. A meta-analysis of five randomized controlled trials found both to be equally effective, but adapalene was better tolerated.[106] Adapelene also might cause less photosensitivity.[103] Although tretinoin should not be applied in conjunction with benzoyl peroxide (because tretinoin becomes less stable), benzoyl peroxide can be used at the same time as adapelene (and tretinoin gel microsphere and micronized tretinoin gel).[101-103]

DOSAGE
- Tretinoin: creams (0.025%, 0.0375%, 0.05%, and 0.1%), gels (0.01% and 0.025%), microsphere gels (0.04%, 0.08%, and 0.1%), and micronized 0.05% gel (contains fish proteins).
- Adapelene: creams 0.1%, gels (0.15% and 0.3%), and 0.1% lotion.
- Apply a thin layer (pea-sized amount) to the entire affected areas once daily, usually at bedtime.

PRECAUTIONS

Can cause skin irritation including redness, dryness, burning, and soreness. Starting with the lowest dose and applying every third day and slowly increasing the frequency and dose can decrease skin irritation. Might make skin sensitive to ultraviolet light and thus better used at night time before bed; advise patients to wear sunscreen. All retinoids should not be used in pregnancy, and women of childbearing age must use contraception.

Topical Antibiotics

Topical antibiotics are useful against inflammatory acne vulgaris most likely through their action on *P. acnes*. They are not as useful for noninflammatory lesions. The most common topical antibiotics include clindamycin and erythromycin.[1] A newer topical antibiotic used in the treatment of acne vulgaris is dapsone. Two randomized studies showed that dapsone significantly improved inflammatory lesions better than placebo.[107,108]

Due to increasing bacterial resistance, topical antibiotics are not used as monotherapy. Instead, they are used in combination with benzoyl peroxide or topical tretinoins to help reduce bacterial resistance.[97-100]

Due to increasing bacterial resistance, topical and oral antibiotics should not be used alone as monotherapy. Instead, they should be used in combination with benzoyl peroxide or topical tretinoins as both have been shown to improve the effect of antibiotics and decrease the amount of antibiotic resistance.[97-100]

DOSAGE

Applied twice a day:
- Clindamycin: 1% gel, lotion, solution, foam
- Erythromycin: 2% gel, solution
- Dapsone 5% gel

PRECAUTIONS

Can cause skin irritation including erythema, burning, peeling, and pruritis. Bacterial resistance for erythromycin is increasing, making it less effective.[108] Although hemolytic anemia is seen in those taking oral dapsone with glucose-6 phosphate dehydrogenase (G6PD) deficiency, those taking topical dapsone have not been affected. Thus it is not necessary at this time to test for G6PD deficiency before starting therapy.[109,110] Dapsone can also cause temporary yellow discoloration of the skin when applied at the same time as benzoyl peroxide and thus should be applied at separate times of the day.[111]

Salicylic Acid

Salicylic acid is a milder and safer treatment for mild to moderate acne vulgaris, with fewer side effects. It works as an exfoliant and mostly acts against comedonal acne by slowing follicular shedding of cells thus preventing clogging.[1,112] One randomized control trial compared salicylic acid to tretinoin (both in combination with clindamycin) for 12 weeks to assess whether or not salicylic acid is as effective as tretinoin and found both to be equally effective, although tretinoin worked more quickly.[113]

DOSAGE

Recommended dosage is 0.5%–2% creams, gels, solutions, cleansers, soap, and foam. Apply one to three times a day.

PRECAUTIONS

Can cause skin irritation including burning, stinging, and reddening.

Azelaic Acid

Azelaic acid is produced by a yeast (*Malassezia fur fur*, also known as *Pityrosporum ovale*) that is part of normal skin flora. It can help in both acne vulgaris and acne rosacea as an antimicrobial, antiinflammatory, and comedolytic. It can also be used for postinflammatory hyperpigmentation. One study that compared results of European clinical trials showed azelaic acid 20% cream is as effective as tretinoin 0.05%, benzoyl peroxide 5%, and topical erythromycin 2%.[114] It is similar to benzoyl peroxide, but there is less evidence of its usefulness.[115]

DOSAGE

Recommended dosage is 20% cream for acne vulgaris and 15% gel for acne rosacea, both applied one to two times a day.

PRECAUTIONS

Can cause hypopigmentation and some skin irritation but is usually well tolerated.

Pharmaceuticals: Systemic Preparations

Oral Antibiotics

Oral antibiotics are used in moderate to severe inflammatory acne or milder cases of truncal acne where topical application is difficult to reach. Antibiotics work against *P. acnes*, but resistance is increasing, and thus newer recommendations include limiting the use to less than 6 months if possible and using topical benzoyl peroxide or tretinoids in conjunction with antibiotics.[116] One study found an increased incidence in *P. acnes* resistance from 20% in 1978 to 62% in 1996.[117] A trial of 6–8 weeks with the same antibiotic is recommended before switching to a different class. If the antibiotic is discontinued, but was helpful and needs to be restarted, it is better to use the same antibiotic.[116]

Doxycycline: Most frequently used antibiotic due to less resistance and better tolerability. Can be used in smaller doses (20 mg bid) as an antiinflammatory rather than antibiotic.[118]

DOSAGE

- Doxycycline: 50–100 mg bid or 20 mg bid as an antiinflammatory rather than an antimicrobial
- Erythromycin: 500 mg bid
- Azithromycin: Optimum dosing not defined
- Tetracycline: 500 mg bid, take on empty stomach
- Minocycline: 50–100 mg bid
- TMP/SMX: 160/800 mg one to two times a day

PRECAUTIONS

Can cause GI upset or vaginal candidiasis. Can increase occurrence of upper respiratory infections due to bacterial resistance.[120] Tetracycline, doxycycline, and minocycline are prohibited for use in children under 9 years of age or in pregnant/breastfeeding women due to the possibility of tooth discoloration and decreased bone growth. Photosensitivity might occur with doxycycline. Minocycline can cause skin discoloration and lupus-like syndrome. Azithromycin can worsen QT prolongation and should not be given in those with prolonged-QT syndrome.

Hormonal Treatment

Hormonal therapy can be used in postmenarchal women and works primarily to decrease the amount of androgens that are known to increase sebum production. Androgens can stimulate the production of acne and estrogens can inhibit the production. Combined oral contraceptives (estrogens and progesterones) are recommended. Estrogens decrease the production of androgen and increase sex hormone-binding globulin (which then decreases serum free androgen levels).[121] Progesterone-only contraceptives may actually exacerbate acne and thus are not recommended for use in acne treatment. Another potential treatment is spironolactone, which blocks the androgen receptors.

DOSAGE

Any combined oral contraceptive pill (OCP) can be used for the treatment of acne, but three have been more studied than other OCPs[121]:

- All OCPs taken as one tablet daily:
  - Ethinyl estradiol 20/30/35 mcg/norethindrone 1 mg (Estrostep)
  - Ethinyl estradiol 35 mcg/norgestimate 180/215/250 mcg (Ortho Tri-Cyclen)
  - Ethinyl estradiol 20 mcg/drospirenone 3 mg (Yaz)
- Spironolactone 50–200 mg daily

PRECAUTIONS

Combined OCPs can cause nausea, weight gain, and breast tenderness. Combined oral contraceptives are contraindicated in women older than 35 years who smoke due to increased risk of cardiovascular disease and in women with breast cancer, migraine with aura, uncontrolled hypertension, liver cirrhosis or viral hepatitis, history or current stroke, up to 3 weeks postpartum, complicated heart valvular disease, and current or history of deep vein thrombosis.

Spironolactone is contraindicated in pregnancy and can cause GI symptoms, hyperkalemia, orthostatic hypotension, dizziness, and/or headaches.

Oral Isotretinoin

Oral isotretinoin is a vitamin A derivative used for severe nodular acne that is unresponsive to all other therapies. Oral isotretinoin works on all aspects of acne as an antiinflammatory, antimicrobial, comedolytic, and antiscarring agent by reducing the size of the sebaceous gland, thus decreasing the secretion of sebum and reducing the amount of *P. acnes*, which require sebum to survive. It also helps keratinocytes to differentiate.[122]

DOSAGE

Recommended dosage is 0.5 mg/kg per day for the first month, increased to 1 mg/kg per day for a total dose of 120–150 mg/kg for 20 weeks or more.[123]

PRECAUTIONS

Category X in pregnancy—cannot be used in pregnancy, and all childbearing women should be on contraceptive therapy. Causes teratogenicity, including craniofacial, central nervous system, cardiac, and thymic malformations.[124] All childbearing women must be part of the iPLEDGE program, requiring two forms of birth control prior to the start of treatment and monthly pregnancy tests.

Many have debated the relationship between oral isotretinoin and mood disorders and have suggested an association with depression and suicide attempt. However, it is difficult to assess whether or not the medication actually causes increased mood disorders.[125]

Can also cause cheilitis, photosensitivity, dry skin and mucous membranes, and/or pruritus. Other side effects include myalgias, hypertriglyceridemia, and idiopathic intracranial hypertension.

TABLE 77.1 **Therapies With the Most Effective Mechanism of Action for Specific Types of Acne**

	Noninflammatory Acne Vulgaris		Inflammatory Acne Vulgaris	
	KERATINISATION (NONINFLAMMATORY)	SEBUM PRODUCTION (NONINFLAMMATORY)	FOLLICULAR PROPIONIBACTERIUM ACNES (INFLAMMATORY)	INFLAMMATION (INFLAMMATORY)
Benzoyl peroxide	+		+	+
Retinoids	+	+	+	+
Antibiotics			+	+
Azelaic Acid	+		+	+
Salicylic Acid	+			

Adapted from Williams HC. Acne vulgaris. *Lancet*. 2012;379:361-372.

ROSACEA

INTRODUCTION/EPIDEMIOLOGY

Rosacea is a chronic inflammatory skin disorder with varying clinical features including transient or persistent facial erythema, telangiectasias, inflammatory papules and pustules, thickened skin, and ocular changes.[6,7] These features are typically symmetrical on the face, with rare neck, upper trunk, and scalp involvement.[137] Rosacea has a prevalence rate of <1% to 20%, depending on the population studied,[138] with higher rates in women and those of Celtic or Northern European descent.[7] It typically presents in the third to fourth decade of life, with the highest frequency among those more than 50 years old.[139]

CLASSIFICATION OF ROSACEA

There are four subtypes and one variant of rosacea. Patients can have features of multiple subtypes at the same time.[6,7] See Table 77.1 for a summary of how each is treated.

I. Erythematous-telangiectasia—Transient flushing and persistent central facial erythema. Erythema of ears, neck, peripheral face, and upper chest can also occur. Telangiectasias are also commonly seen.
II. Papulopustular—Facial erythema plus transient papules and/or pustules in the central face. Unlike acne vulgaris there are no comedones (unless acne vulgaris occurs with rosacea). Burning or stinging can also occur.
III. Phymatous—Thickened, enlarged and irregular skin in areas with sebaceous glands, most commonly on the nose (rhinophyma), but can occur on the ears, cheeks, forehead, and chin (Fig. 77.2).
IV. Ocular—Eye and eyelid involvement, including foreign body sensation, burning, stinging, dryness, itching, watery or bloodshot eyes, blurry vision, telangiectasias in conjunctiva and lid margin, lid and periocular edema. Furthermore, often observed chronic blepharitis, conjunctivitis, irregular eyelid margins, light sensitivity, chalazion, and styes. Subtype: Granulomatous—Firm, indurated papules and nodules.

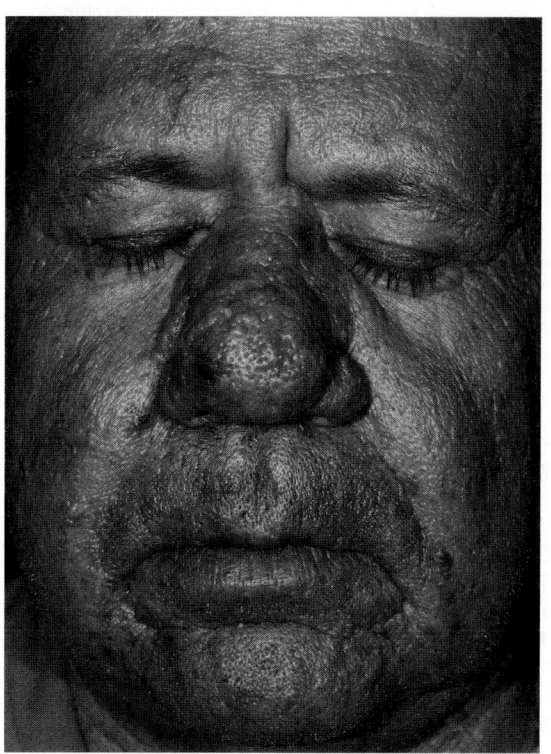

FIG. 77.2 ■ Rhinophyma in phymatous rosacea. (From Habif TP. Acne, rosacea, and related disorders. In: Habif TP, ed. *Clinical dermatology*. 5th ed. Philadelphia: Saunders; 2009.)

PATHOPHYSIOLOGY OF ROSACEA

The exact etiology of rosacea is unclear, but it is thought that a combination of environmental triggers on rosacea-prone skin causes the disease.[6,141,136] Subtypes of rosacea, their characteristics and suggested therapies, can be found in Table 77.2.

Neurovascular Dysregulation

Receptors involved in sensation, vasodilation and inflammatory signaling that are activated by known rosacea triggers (e.g., temperature, spice, heat) are upregulated and found in higher numbers in the skin of patients with rosacea.[6]

TABLE 77.2 **Subtypes of Rosacea With Associated Characteristics and Suggested Therapies**

Subtype	Characteristics	Interventions[a]
I. Erythematotelangiectatic	Flushing and persistent central facial erythema +/− telangectasia	Flushing: trigger avoidance Erythema: topical brimonidine or oxymetazoline. Maintenance treatment with topical metronidazole or azelaic acid or antiinflammatory doxycycline (40 mg) Telangectasia and persistent erythema: devices—pulse dye laser or intense pulsed light therapy
II. Papulopustular	Persistent central facial erythema with transient, central facial papules and/or pustules	First line: topical metronidazole or azelaic acid or topical ivermectin and/or antiinflammatory doxycycline (40 mg) Second line: topical metronidazole or azelaic acid + antimicrobial dose antibiotics (tetracyclines, azithromycin) or low dose isotretinoin
III. Phymatous	Thickened skin, irregular surface nodularities and enlargement; may occur on nose, chin, forehead, cheeks or ears	Oral isotretinoin (will recur when stopped) +/− pulse dye laser or intense pulsed light therapy Advanced: surgical interventions
IV. Ocular	Foreign body sensation in the eye, burning or stinging, dryness, itching, photosensitivity, blurred vision, telangiectasia of the sclera or other parts of the eye, periorbital edema, chronic blepharitis or conjunctivitis, chalazion or styes	Lid hygiene, warm compresses, artificial tears +/− cyclosporine ophthalmic Oral antibiotics: First line—antiinflammatory doxycycline (40 mg) Second line—antimicrobial tetracyclines, azithromycin

[a]All types affecting the skin should include gentle skin care and daily sun protection. Consider use of products containing antioxidant, antiinflammatory, and UV protective botanical.
Adapted from Emer J, Waldorf H, Berson D. Botanicals and antiinflammatories: natural ingredients for rosacea. *Semin Cutan Med Surg.* 2011;30:148-155 and Van Zuuren EJ, Fedorowicz Z, Carter B, van der Linden MMD, Charland L. Interventions for rosacea. *Cochrane Database Syst Rev.* 2015(4): CD003262.

Disordered Innate Immunity

The innate immune system responds to environmental triggers such as microbes, ultraviolet light, and trauma.[141] A triggering event usually leads to a controlled immune response. In rosacea there are disrupted cytokine and antimicrobial peptide (AMP) pathways.[6,141] Triggers for activation of innate immunity in rosacea include UV radiation and microbes. The microbes implicated include those on the skin or in the gastrointestinal tract; see the following text for details.

UV Radiation

UVA light has been shown to cause collagen denaturation,[144] UVB light contributes to hypervascularity via various growth factors,[145] and both increase reactive oxygen species (ROS) in the skin. Those with rosacea have been found to have higher levels of ROS in their skin,[146] which has both vasodilating[147] and proinflammatory[141] effects. Many of the medicines for rosacea act to inhibit ROS formation or have antioxidant effects; see treatment section for details.[141]

Microbes

Skin Microbes

Implicated skin microbes include *Demodex* mites[148,149] or the Gram-negative bacteria associated with them, *Bacillus oleonius*,[150] as well as strains of the colonizing skin bacterium *Staphylococcus epidermidis*.[148,149]

Small Intestinal Bacterial Overgrowth. Small intestinal bacterial overgrowth (SIBO) is a condition where mostly gram-negative aerobic and anaerobic colonic bacteria colonize the small intestine, an area that usually has few bacteria. These bacteria ferment carbohydrates into gas, thought to cause some of the symptoms of SIBO—bloating, diarrhea, flatulence, and abdominal pain that can eventually lead to malabsorption syndromes. One study demonstrated a higher prevalence of SIBO in patients with rosacea (46% vs 5% in controls, *n* = 113) as well as improvement in rosacea when treating SIBO with Rifaximin.[164] Another study did not show higher prevalence of SIBO in rosacea (10% vs 7.8% controls, *n* = 90) but was underpowered to see a difference in rosacea symptoms when SIBO was treated.[157]

INTEGRATIVE THERAPY

Environmental/Hygiene

Rosacea can be worsened or triggered by factors that initiate flushing, including exercise, emotion, menopause, spicy foods, hot liquids, and alcohol.[137,166] In the external environment, sun, heat, wind, and cold can also exacerbate rosacea.[137,167] The first step in care of rosacea is to avoid or limiting exposure to triggers. Proper skin care is also important given the disrupted epidermal barrier. Skin care should include washing with a gentle nonsoap cleanser with a neutral pH one to two times per day, moisturizing, avoiding products such as cosmetics that irritate the skin, and daily use of sunscreen.[167] Examples of gentle nonsoap cleansers include Cetaphil, Dove, Aveeno, and CeraVe.

Diet

Common dietary triggers of rosacea include spicy foods, hot liquids, and alcohol. An elimination diet may be helpful in identifying an individual's specific triggers. Other than avoiding known triggering foods, there are no studies to date that diet effects progression of rosacea. However, based on the role inflammation plays in the pathophysiology of rosacea, a trial of the antiinflammatory diet may be beneficial (see Chapter 88 for details). Diet may also play a role if SIBO is diagnosed. Part of the SIBO treatment protocol usually includes eliminating specific fermentable carbohydrates.

Botanicals

There are few well-studied botanicals used in the treatment of rosacea. However, some botanicals have evidence for exerting dermatological antiinflammatory or antioxidant effects, absorbing UV light, or acting as barrier protection.[168,169] Since these mechanisms are implicated in the pathophysiology of rosacea and many patients prefer to use botanicals, topical products containing the following ingredients may be helpful:

Colloidal Oatmeal

Oats (*Avena sativa*) are often topically used in treatment of atopic dermatitis and were approved by the Food and Drug Administration (FDA) in 2003 as a skin protectant.[170] Well established effects include barrier protection, antiinflammatory, antioxidant, and absorption of UV light.[168,169]

DOSAGE
Varies. Products containing colloidal oatmeal include cleansers, soaps, shampoos, and moisturizers.

PRECAUTIONS
Oat-based products have an excellent safety profile and can be used in children, pregnancy, and in lactation.

Licorice Extract

Extracts from licorice plants *Glycyrrhiza glabra* and *Glycyrrhiza inflata* have antioxidant, antimicrobial, and antiinflammatory properties.[168,169,171]

DOSAGE
Licorice gel 2%, two to three times daily.

PRECAUTIONS
Topical skin irritation, burning, and redness can occur.

Feverfew

Feverfew (*Tanacetum parthenium*) is a flowering herb traditionally used orally to treat fever, migraine headaches,

arthritis, and other conditions.[173] Feverfew has antiinflammatory, antioxidant, antibacterial, and antifungal properties.[168,169,173,174] Topical use should only contain the purified extract form (feverfew PFE). Feverfew PFE does not contain parthenolide, a component that can cause allergic contact dermatitis.[174,175]

DOSAGE
Varies, topical use. Important to obtain products labeled "purified feverfew extract" or "parthenolide free."

PRECAUTIONS
As with most topical products, local skin irritation can occur. There may be cross-allergenicity to those with allergies in the Asteraceae/Compositae family (ragweed, chamomile, daisy, etc.) though parthenolide is one of the main causes of compositae allergy and is removed in the PFE/parthenolide free formulations.[173,175]

Green Tea

Green tea has antiinflammatory and antioxidant activity; it decreases UV-induced erythema and photodamage and may be beneficial in rosacea.[168,169,176] See details under botanical acne vulgaris treatments.

Pharmaceuticals: Topical Treatments

Topical Metronidazole

Metronidazole is a topical antibiotic used for papulopustular rosacea. It comes in cream, gel, and lotion forms. In addition to its antimicrobial action, metronidazole also has antioxidant and antiinflammatory effects.[177] Improvements tend to appear after 3–6 weeks[141,178] with maximum effect after 8–9 weeks of treatment. Metronidazole often has to be used long term for maintenance therapy due to recurrence when stopped.

DOSAGE
Metronidazole 0.75% cream, gel or lotion once to twice* daily
 OR
 Metronidazole 0.1% cream or gel daily

PRECAUTIONS
With topical metronidazole, the most common adverse effects include itching, skin irritation, and dry skin.
*Once daily use may be as effective as twice daily use.[179]

Sodium Sulfacetamide

Sodium sulfacetamide has been used for years for the erythema and inflammatory lesions of rosacea.[141,182] It acts as an antimicrobial and the sulfur acts as a mild keratolytic.[183] Sodium sulfacetamide 10% plus sulfur 5% is the most common formulation and comes in lotion, cream, foam, cleanser, and cleansing pad forms.

DOSAGE

Sulfacetamide 10% or sulfur 5%, applied twice a day. Topically applied forms may be more effective than cleansers.

PRECAUTIONS

Application site reactions such as dryness, erythema, and pruritus are the most commonly reported adverse events.[141,184] Sulfacetamide should not be used by individuals who have a sensitivity to sulfur or sulfa.

Topical Ivermectin

Topical ivermectin was recently approved by the FDA for papulopustular rosacea. Oral ivermectin has been used in demodicidosis and for treatment of blepharitis.[185] It has both antiinflammatory and antiparasitic properties and decreases the *Demodex* mite load.

DOSAGE

Ivermectin, 1% cream (Soolantra), apply once daily. Improvement can be seen after 4 weeks but can take up to 12 weeks.[186]

PRECAUTIONS

The most common adverse events include local irritation and burning.

Alpha Adrenergic Agonists

Alpha adrenergic agonists, including brimonidine and oxymetazoline, are newer treatments that target the background erythema of rosacea.[188-190] They act on muscles surrounding blood vessels in the dermal skin and cause vasoconstriction. Results can be seen within 30 minutes.[191] They do not affect inflammation or telangiectasias, so they should be used in combination with antiinflammatory medications if they occur together.

DOSAGE

- Brimonidine gel 0.33% (Mirvaso)—Apply daily. Can work up to 12 hours after application.
- Oxymetazoline 0.05%—The active ingredient in some decongestant nasal sprays (such as Afrin). Apply daily or twice daily.

PRECAUTIONS

The most common adverse events include local irritation, burning, flushing, pruritis, and allergic contact dermatitis.[189-191] There have been reports of rebound erythema. Theoretically the alpha-blocking action can have systemic effects, but a review of studies found no meaningful changes in intraocular pressure, blood pressure, or heart rate in any of the topical treatments.[141]

Pharmaceuticals: Systemic Treatments

Antibiotics

Antibiotics commonly used in treatment of acne vulgaris have also been used to treat acne rosacea, see earlier in the chapter for details. The most commonly used antibiotics for rosacea include tetracyclines (doxycycline, tetracycline, minocycline), macrolides (azithromycin, clarithromycin) and metronidazole, though other oral antibiotics have been used as well. In addition to antimicrobial effects, the tetracyclines have antiinflammatory activity. In fact, doxycycline at antiinflammatory doses of less than 50 mg per day (vs. antimicrobial at 50–200 mg per day) works just as well with fewer side effects.[192] Macrolides (azithromycin preferred over clarithromycin)[193] or metronidazole can be considered for allergy or other contraindication to tetracyclines.

DOSAGE

Antiinflammatory dosage:
- Doxycycline 20 mg twice per day ($40–80/month retail)
  OR
- Doxycycline 40 mg modified release (30 mg immediate and 10 mg delayed)
  Antimicrobial dosage:
- Doxycycline 50–100 mg twice per day
- Tetracycline 250–500 mg twice per day
- Minocycline 50–100 mg twice per day

PRECAUTIONS

Adverse effects of all antibiotics can include nausea/GI upset, allergic reaction, and vaginal yeast infection. Tetracyclines also cause photosensitivity. Take mineral supplements (iron, calcium, magnesium, etc.) and antacids at least 2 hours after taking tetracyclines to prevent decreased absorption of the medication. Should not be taken in pregnancy or by children younger than 9 years due to staining of teeth and reduced bone growth.

A specific precaution for azithromycin includes QT prolongation. Caution in those with known long QT or if taking other medications that also increase the QT interval (common medications include antiemetics, a complete list can be found at www.QTdrugs.org).

Isotretinoin

For refractory or phymatous rosacea consider off label use of oral isotretinoin. Unlike with acne vulgaris, there will be recurrence when the medication is stopped. One study found oral isotretinoin to be slightly more effective than doxycycline 50–100 mg.[194] However, given its side effect profile, this is not a first line medication.

See isotretinoin under acne vulgaris systemic treatments for details on mechanisms of action.

DOSAGE

Low dose isotretinoin, 0.3 mg/kg per day was found to be effective in rosacea and should be continued for a minimum of 3–6 months.[141,195]

PRECAUTIONS

Patients and physicians need to register at iPLEDGE.org given the teratogenicity of this medication. There are also significant mucocutaneous side effects (cheilitis, dry skin, photosensitivity). Other adverse effects can include myalgias and lipid abnormalities. Concern for use of oral isotretinoin and associations with irritable bowel disease and suicidality have been raised but have not been definitively proven.

Laser and Light Therapy, Surgery

Laser and light based therapies are most effective at targeting telangiectasias in rosacea, though they have also been used in the treatment of background erythema.[126] A large review found pulsed dye laser about equivalent to intense pulse light therapy for treating telangiectasia in rosacea.[127] Rhinophymatous rosacea may require tissue debulking treatments. These include ablative laser and surgical interventions such as scalpel excision, dermabrasion, cryosurgery, and electrocautery.[126,128]

 More information on this topic can be found online at ExpertConsult.com.

PREVENTION PRESCRIPTION FOR ACNE VULGARIS

- Maintain healthy skin care: May wash twice a day with a gentle, synthetic detergent cleanser, but avoid excessive washing or scrubbing because this might reduce healthy oils in the skin.

- Decrease stress levels to protect the skin from developing acne vulgaris.
- Eat a low-glycemic diet and a diet high in omega-3 fatty acids. Maintain a healthy weight. Eliminate or limit the intake of milk and other dairy products.

THERAPEUTIC REVIEW FOR ACNE VULGARIS

MIND-BODY MEDICINE
- Practice stress-reducing techniques such as meditation, guided imagery, hypnosis, or biofeedback to help decrease stress and related acne lesions. C 1

NUTRITION
- Maintain a low glycemic diet. B 1
- Limit the amount of dairy products. B 1

SUPPLEMENTS
- Omega-3 fatty acids: oral supplementation with 1–3 g of the EPA plus DHA components. B 1
- Zinc gluconate 30 mg/day orally (or 20 mg/day for those aged 9–13 years). B 2
- Brewer's yeast 6 g of freeze-dried, daily by mouth (can take in divided doses: 3 g bid or 2 g tid). C 1
- Vitamin A: up to 10,000 IU/day, orally. C 2

BOTANICALS
- Tea tree oil applied topically one to two times daily. B 1
- Green tea lotion 2%–3% applied topically twice a day (recommended daily intake of green tea two to three cups a day, 240–320 mg polyphenols). C 1
- Turmeric powder mixed with milk or coconut oil and placed topically on inflammatory lesions daily. (Ingested doses of turmeric: 500 mg two to four times a day). C 2

PHARMACEUTICAL THERAPY
- Benzoyl peroxide 2.5%–5% gel, lotion, cream, applied topically one to two times a day. A 2
- Topical retinoids: Apply a thin layer (pea-sized amount) to the entire affected areas once daily, usually at bedtime. A 2
- Topical antibiotics (erythromycin, clindamycin, dapsone) applied twice a day, in combination with benzoyl peroxide or topical retinoids to decrease antimicrobial resistance. A 2
- Salicylic acid 0.5%–2% creams, gels, solutions, cleansers, soap, foam. Apply topically one to three times a day. A 2
- Azelaic acid 20% cream, applied topically one to two times a day. B 2
- Oral antibiotics (doxycycline, erythromycin, azithromycin, tetracycline, minocycline, and TMP/SMX) one to two times a day A 2
- Combined oral contraceptive pills once a day B 2
- Spironolactone 50–200 mg daily B 2
- Oral isotretinoin 0.5 mg/kg per day for the first month, and increased to 1 mg/kg per day for a total dose of 120–150 mg/kg for 20 weeks or more. A 3

PREVENTION PRESCRIPTION FOR ACNE ROSACEA

- Skin care should include washing with a gentle nonsoap cleanser with a neutral pH one to two times per day, moisturizing, avoiding products that irritate the skin, and daily use of sunscreen.
- Avoid exposure to environmental triggers such as sun, wind, heat, and cold.

- Avoid dietary triggers such as alcohol and hot, spicy food, and drink. Consider an elimination diet to identify dietary triggers. Consider a trial of an antiinflammatory diet.

THERAPEUTIC REVIEW FOR ACNE ROSACEA

- Gentle skin care $\quad_C \oslash_1$
- Sun protection $\quad_B \oslash_1$
- Avoid environmental triggers $\quad_B \oslash_1$

NUTRITION

- Avoid dietary triggers that flare rosacea $\quad_B \oslash_1$

BOTANICALS

- Colloidal oatmeal: dose in topical products varies $\quad_C \oslash_1$
- Licorice gel: 2% applied topically once or twice daily $\quad_B \oslash_1$
- Feverfew: dose in topical products varies, use products labeled "purified feverfew extract" or "parthenolide free" $\quad_C \oslash_1$

PHARMACEUTICAL PREPARATIONS

- Metronidazole: 0.75% or 1% cream, gel or lotion, applied topically once daily $\quad_A \oslash_2$

- Azelaic acid: 15% gel and 20% cream, applied topically once to twice daily $\quad_A \oslash_2$
- Sulfacetamide 10% sulfur 5%: applied topically twice a day $\quad_B \oslash_2$
- Ivermectin: 1% cream (Soolantra), apply topically once daily $\quad_A \oslash_2$
- For erythema: Brimonidine: 0.33% gel, apply daily OR oxymetazoline: 0.05% liquid, apply topically daily or twice daily $\quad_A \oslash_1$
- Oral antibiotics at antiinflammatory (doxycycline) or antimicrobial doses (doxycycline, tetracycline, minocycline, azithromycin) $\quad_A \oslash_2$
- Isotretinoin: 0.3 mg/kg per day, taken orally once or in two divided doses daily. $\quad_A \oslash_2 - _A \oslash_3$

SURGICAL THERAPY

- Laser and light therapy for telangectasia and erythema $\quad_B \oslash_3$
- Various surgical techniques for phymatous rosacea $\quad_C \oslash_3$

Key Web Resources

REFERENCES

References are available online at ExpertConsult.com.

SECTION XIV

CANCER

SECTION OUTLINE

78 Breast Cancer

79 Lung Cancer

80 Prostate Cancer

81 Colorectal Cancer

82 Palliative and End-of-Life Care

CHAPTER 78

BREAST CANCER

Lucille R. Marchand, MD, BSN • James A. Stewart, MD, FACP

Breast cancer involves an interplay of genes with environmental factors (such as food choices, exercise, lifestyle, alcohol consumption, weight control, and postmenopausal estrogen/progestin exposure) and environmental toxins (such as radiation, electrical lighting at night, and pesticides). It is further complicated by genetic vulnerability to environmental factors.[1,2] Integrative medicine emphasizes personal empowerment to make lifestyle choices that can help prevent cancer from occurring and slow its growth once it has occurred or prevent recurrence. Many factors may not be in our control, but many lifestyle choices are. These same healthy choices also limit the development of other chronic illnesses, such as heart disease, diabetes, obesity, and hyperlipidemia.[1]

Breast cancer is currently the most common cancer among women in the United States. In 2015, it was estimated that 29% (231,840 new cases of breast cancer versus 810,170 of total new cases of all cancers) of women diagnosed with cancer had breast cancer. Overall lifetime risk is that one in eight women will be diagnosed with breast cancer, but risk increases with age. In women less than 50 years of age, the risk is 1 in 53 women; age 50–59 years, 1 in 44; age 60–69 years, 1 in 29; and older than 70 years, 1 in 15 women. It is the second most common cancer that causes death in women—15% mortality rate of all cancers estimated for 2015 (highest mortality rates in women are from lung cancer—26%).[3] Five-year survival rates are high in women with early-stage cancers: stage 0, 100%; stages 1 and 2, 98.6% for local invasion and 84.4% for regional invasion; stage 3, 57%; and in women with metastatic breast cancer, 24.3%.[4] The average age of diagnosis is 61 years, and 72% of breast cancer survivors are 60 years or older; 10% are less than 50 years.[4] One percent of breast cancers occur in men.[5]

PATHOPHYSIOLOGY

Breast cancer is generally a hormone-driven cancer; higher lifetime risk is associated with higher estrogen exposure. Seventy percent of breast cancers express receptors for progesterone or estrogen.[6] Exogenous estrogen use, such as with hormone replacement therapy (HRT), pesticides that have an estrogenic effect in our bodies, and hormones from animal and dairy sources, are most concerning. Obesity is an intrinsic factor that increases risk as well, possibly from the increase in estrogen that comes from aromatization in fat tissue. Soy foods (rather than supplements), which are weak plant estrogens, may have a protective effect. Some genetic mutations have a higher likelihood of cancer development, such as *BRCA1*

and *BRCA2* mutations, which are associated with a 60%–80% lifetime risk for breast cancer. These genetic markers are related to mutations that inactivate cancer suppressor genes.[7,8]

E-Table 78.1, which lists risk factors for breast cancer, can be found online at ExpertConsult.com.

RISK FACTORS

Factors that increase the risk of breast cancer include alcohol consumption of more than one serving per day, taking estrogen-containing products such as HRT and birth control pills, increased estrogen lifetime exposure including early menarche and late menopause, low intake of fruits and vegetables, obesity, exposure to radiation, and sedentary lifestyle (see E-Table 78.1, available online at ExpertConsult.com). Aging is a risk factor in that 80% of women with a breast cancer diagnosis are older than 50 years. Family history of breast cancer and certain mutations, such as *BRCA1*, *BRCA2*, and *p53*, increase the risk for breast cancer. Deleterious *BRCA* gene mutations increase the lifetime risk for development of breast cancer from 40% to 85%. Women with a mother, sister, or daughter with breast cancer are twice as likely to develop cancer as is a woman with no family history of breast cancer in female relatives. Both paternal and maternal relatives are important in determining breast cancer risk.[5]

More information on this topic can be found online at ExpertConsult.com.

Risk-reducing surgery in patients with *BRCA1* and *BRCA2* mutations can attenuate risk of breast and ovarian cancer. Risk-reducing mastectomy significantly reduced the risk for development of breast cancer in mutation carriers compared with matched controls by 90%.[10] Salpingooophorectomy reduced the incidence of breast cancer, ovarian cancer, all-cause mortality, and breast and ovarian cancer–specific mortality.[11] In one study assessing 725 *BRCA1* and *BRCA2* carriers, 218 had been diagnosed with breast cancer within a 10-year period. This study assessed level of exercise with development of cancer and found an inverse relationship of greater intensity of exercise with decreased risk for development of cancer in these carriers, but the significance was at the $p = .053$ level.[12]

A study in Sri Lanka identified prolonged breast-feeding (24 months in a lifetime) in significantly reducing risk of breast cancer. The mechanism may be reduction in lifetime estrogen exposure.[13] Another study in Tunisia showed a similar protective effect of prolonged breast-feeding.[14]

Obesity is a significant risk factor for breast cancer occurrence, recurrence, and mortality. Limiting the intake of high-density foods, such as fat and sugars, and increasing plant-based lower density foods, such as fruits, vegetables, and whole grains, can help maintain healthy weight in combination with regular exercise for energy expenditure and glycemic control.[15,16] Limiting portion size is an important weight control strategy.

> Fat from adipose tissue is a major source of estrone (E_1) which is the main stimulatory hormone after menopause. Weight loss can significantly reduce this hormones influence on breast cancer.

Night-shift work and subsequent disruption of the natural circadian rhythm can put women at increased risk for breast cancer. Melatonin levels are suppressed with these disruptions, and low melatonin levels raise estradiol levels and increase risk of breast cancer.[17-20] Modern electrical lighting, which is rich in blue wavelengths, suppresses melatonin more than red or yellow light wavelengths, such as candlelight or firelight. Fluorescent light, television or computer light, and bedside lamps can strongly suppress melatonin in the evening, and suppression has a more carcinogenic effect than just disruption of sleep or poor sleep in a dark room. People who are blind have the lowest incidence of cancer since their melatonin is less likely suppressed. Melatonin disruption rather than sleep–wake cycle contributes more strongly to cancer growth. By sleeping in the dark, cancer can be prevented and growth suppressed after diagnosis.[21]

2-Hydroxyestrone/16-Hydroxyestrone Ratio

In estrogen receptor–positive (ER+) tumors, estrogen metabolism can contribute to risk. Both strong and weak estrogen metabolites are produced from oxidative processes in the body. 2-Hydroxyestrones are weakly estrogenic and may be protective (similar perhaps in action to weak plant estrogens such as soy foods), and 16-hydroxyestrones are more strongly estrogenic. The 16-hydroxyestrones can stimulate estrogen receptors in vulnerable tissue, leading to ER+ tumors, and can disrupt DNA, which produces oncogenes and tumor suppressor genes (Fig. 78.1).[22-24] Dietary measures (decreased alcohol intake, increased oleic acid such as in olive oil), physical activity, phytoestrogens such as flaxseed meal, and cruciferous vegetables can help favor weaker estrogen metabolites.[23,25,26]

> Exercise, weight loss, cruciferous vegetables, and lignan-rich flaxseed can improve the 2-hydroxyestrone/16-hydroxyestrone ratio, reducing the stimulatory effect on breast tissue.

In women receiving postmenopausal HRT, breast cancer risk for hormone receptor–positive cancers and HER2-positive tumors increases. In women taking estrogen and progestin replacement for more than 15 years, the risk of breast cancer increased by 83% compared with estrogen-only HRT, which increased risk by 19%. Risks associated with HRT were found only in women with body mass index (BMI) less than 29.9 kg/m^2, but not in women with a BMI more than 30.[27]

SCREENING

Information on this topic can be found online at ExpertConsult.com.

INTEGRATIVE THERAPIES

Lifestyle

The European Prospective Investigation into Cancer and Nutrition found that four lifestyle measures were critical in reducing risk of cancer as well as chronic illnesses, such as heart disease and diabetes. These measures included not smoking; BMI less than 30; 3.5 hours a week of exercise or more; and eating a healthy diet of fruit, vegetables, and whole grains, with little meat consumption. Having all four lifestyle factors reduced the risk of cancer by 36%.[33] For patients to make informed decisions about nutritional changes, consultation with a person trained in integrative nutrition must be made available.[34]

> Not smoking, having a BMI less than 30, 3.5 hours of exercise or more a week, and a healthy plant-based diet can reduce the risk of cancer by 36%.

The American Cancer Society introduced guidelines for nutrition and exercise for the prevention of cancer and for cancer survivors undergoing cancer treatment based on the recommendations of an expert panel of scientists and clinicians who reviewed all current research on these topics in 2006 with an update in 2012 (refer to resource section). In summary, the guidelines recommend a higher intake of fiber in the form of fruits and vegetables as well as whole grains, maintaining a healthy weight, and regular exercise.[35] In one study of breast cancer survivors, a low-fat diet had no effect on mortality, but a high-fat dairy diet contributed to increased cancer and noncancer mortality.[36]

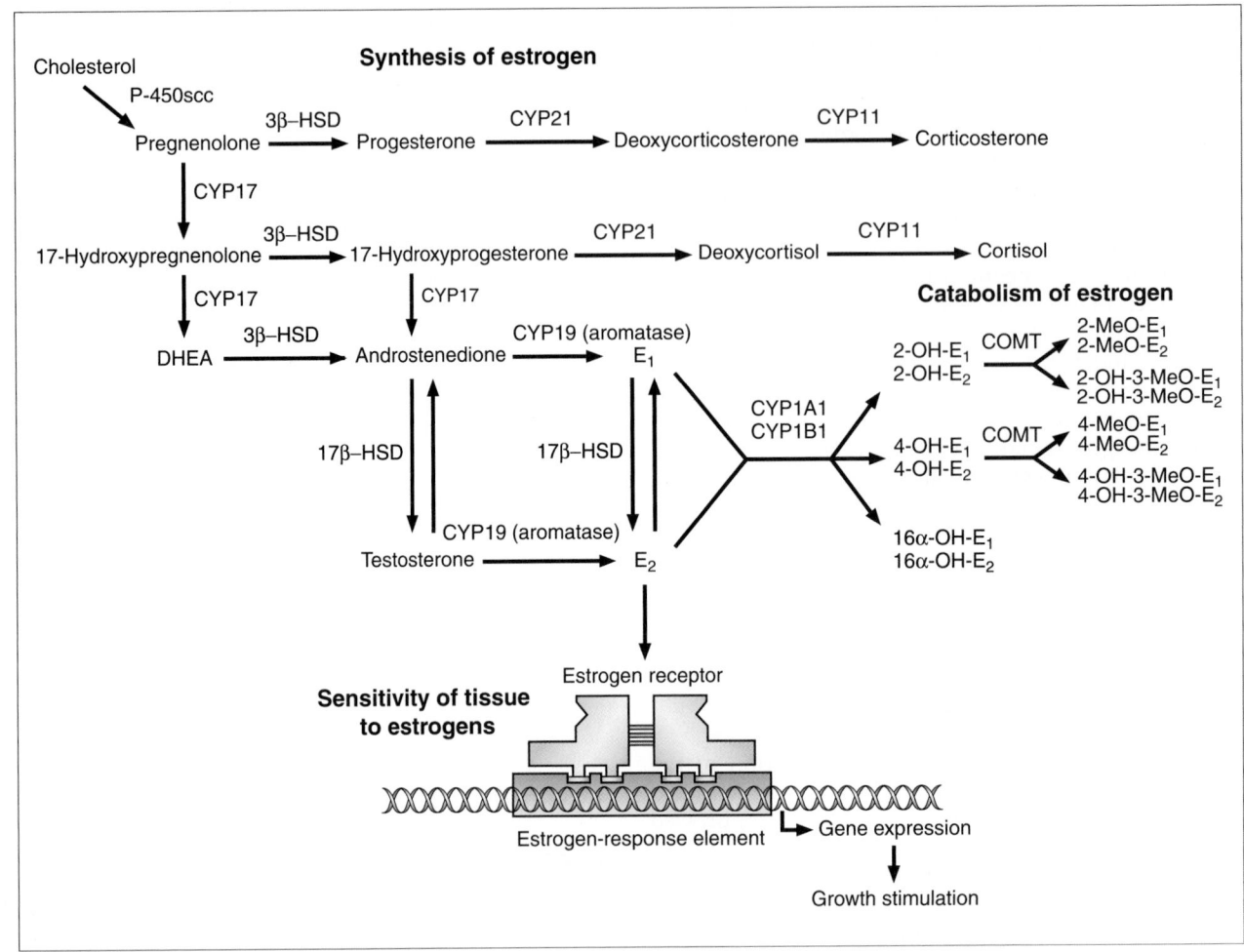

FIG. 78.1 ■ Pathways of estrogen synthesis and catabolism. *2-MeO-E₁*, 2-methoxyestrone; *2-MeO-E₂*, 2-methoxyestradiol; *2-OH-3-MeO-E₁*, 2-hydroxyestrone 3-methyl ether; *2-OH-3-MeO-E₂*, 2-hydroxyestradiol 3-methyl ether; *2-OH-E₁*, 2-hydroxyestrone; *2-OH-E₂*, 2-hydroxyestradiol; *3β-HSD*, 3β-hydroxysteroid dehydrogenase; *4-OH-3-MEO-E₁*, 4-hydroxyestrone 3-methyl ether; *4-OH-3-MeO-E₂*, 4-hydroxyestradiol 3-methyl ether; *4-OH-E₁*, 4-hydroxyestrone; *4-OH-E₂*, 4-hydroxyestradiol; *16α-OH-E₁*, 16α-hydroxyestrone; *16α-OH-E₂*, 16α-hydroxyestradiol; *17β-HSD*, 17β-hydroxysteroid dehydrogenase; *COMT*, catechol O-methyltransferase; *CYP11*, 11β-hydroxylase; *CYP1A1*, cytochrome P-450 1A1; *CYP1B1*, cytochrome P-450 1B1; *CYP17*, 17β-dehydroxylase; *CYP19*, P-450 aromatase; *CYP21*, 21-hydroxylase; *DHEA*, dehydroepiandrosterone; *E₁*, estrone; *E₂*, estradiol; *P-450*, cytochrome P-450; *scc*, side-chain cleavage enzyme. (From Clemons M, Goss P. Estrogen and the risk of breast cancer. *N Engl J Med.* 2001;344:276-285.)

Exercise

Exercise has a role in cancer prevention through weight control, increased muscle strength, and improved immunity and mood control. During and after cancer treatment, exercise can benefit mood, strength, weight control, energy levels, immunity, overall health and well-being, survival, prevention of recurrence, and quality of life (QOL). It allows patients to go through their cancer treatments with increased strength, less fatigue and muscle weakness, better balance, and fewer falls.[37] It can also have beneficial effects on pain, lymphedema, and improved self-image. One study that investigated breast cancer survivors versus controls showed that breast cancer survivors are less likely than non–breast cancer controls to adhere to physical activity recommendations.[39] Unfortunately, what was not assessed was what their health care providers were

recommending for exercise and whether they advised continuing exercise during and after treatment. In a population-based study of breast cancer patients, consistent and long-term, higher activity (more than 3 hours/week) exercisers had lower risk of cancer mortality than did women with low activity levels.[41] In another study of breast cancer survivors, women who had 2–3 hours of walking per week after diagnosis reduced their mortality risk by 45% compared with sedentary women. Women who decreased their activity after diagnosis increased their mortality risk four-fold.[42] In one study, a simple walking intervention reduced pain and maintained cardiorespiratory fitness in patients with breast cancer undergoing radiation therapy and chemotherapy.[43] Physical activity improved mood in yet another study of breast cancer patients which persisted for 60 months postintervention.[44]

In one study, women with breast cancer participated in a tailor-made exercise group. This program increased self-esteem and wellbeing by allowing these women to self-identify more as healthy normal women rather than cancer patients.[45] Pain was significantly reduced in another longitudinal study of breast cancer survivors who exercised regularly and maintained their body weight.[46] Postmastectomy breast cancer survivors studied in a home-based 8-week exercise program experienced reduction of lymphedema and increased QOL[47] (see Chapter 91).

Nutrition

Mediterranean Diet

Diets high in fruits and vegetables, fish, fresh foods, and olive oil and low in animal fat (the Mediterranean diet) reduce the risk of breast cancer and many other cancers.[49] In one large French study of 2381 women with invasive postmenopausal breast cancer, a Western/alcohol-dominant diet was associated with higher risk of breast cancer incidence compared with a healthy Mediterranean diet. The Western diet included meat products, French fries, alcohol, pizza, high-fat foods, and processed foods. The Mediterranean diet included fruits and vegetables, fish, olive and sunflower oils, and nonprocessed fresh foods. This difference was especially significant in women with estrogen-positive, progesterone-negative (ER+/PR-) tumors.[49]

Fiber

Intake of high-fiber foods, as shown by results of the National Institutes of Health–AARP Diet and Health Study, can reduce the risk of breast cancer, especially that of ER-/PR- tumors.[50] In the Malmö Diet and Cancer cohort, intake of high-fiber bread reduced the risk of breast cancer.[51] High-fiber foods are preferable to fiber supplements because of the beneficial nutrients intrinsic to food sources such as fruits, vegetables, beans, nuts and seeds, whole grains, and legumes.[15]

Alcohol

Emerging evidence exists for the role of alcohol increasing risk in breast cancer.[52] In primary prevention, alcohol intake and lower folate levels are associated with an increased risk for breast cancer.[35] In one study of secondary prevention, low to moderate alcohol intake was not associated with increased risk of recurrence or increased mortality.[53] Alcohol (more than one alcoholic drink per day in women) increases circulation of androgens and estrogens, and use of alcohol is associated with lower levels of important nutrients such as folate and B vitamins, with a protective effect noted in women with increased folate intake who drink alcohol.[7] In the Women's Health Initiative study, women who consumed more than seven alcoholic drinks per week doubled their risk of hormone receptor–positive invasive lobular carcinoma. This effect was not seen in ER- tumors or women with ductal breast cancer. Alcohol may have a differing effect on breast cancer risk, depending on the subtype of the breast cancer.[54] Deandrea et al.[55] found increased risk for alcohol and ER+ tumors.

Sugar

High sugar intake increases calories in the diet (sometimes excluding more nutritious food), contributes to weight gain, and increases insulin levels, which can have other deleterious metabolic effects that contribute to cancer cell growth.[15,56] High sugar intake in the form of products with high fructose corn syrup, sugar, honey, and molasses is not recommended.[15]

Polyunsaturated Fatty Acids

Polyunsaturated fatty acids include omega-3 and omega-6 fatty acids. In large quantities and especially if hydrogenated for extended shelf life, omega-6 fatty acids such as sunflower, safflower, soy, sesame, and corn oils can be proinflammatory in the body. Omega-3 fatty acids (eicosapentaenoic acid [EPA] and docosahexaenoic acid [DHA]) are antiinflammatory and are present in fish oil, flaxseed oil, and the oil in walnuts. Omega-3 fatty acids are present in fatty fish (such as salmon, sardines, and mackerel), walnuts, green leafy vegetables, and flaxseed meal. The VITamins And Lifestyle (VITAL) study demonstrated that fish oil reduced the risk of ductal, but not lobular, breast cancers.[57] In a case-controlled study of patients with breast cancer and case controls with no malignant disease, fish omega-3 intake was found to reduce the risk of breast cancer in premenopausal and postmenopausal women, with the greatest reduction in postmenopausal women.[58] Cottet et al.[49] demonstrated in a large cohort study of postmenopausal women that there was a lower risk of invasive breast cancer with a Mediterranean diet (high in fish, fruits, and vegetables) but a higher risk on a Western/alcohol-type diet (high in saturated meat fat and processed foods).

DOSAGE

Approximately 1000 mg of combined DHA and EPA daily in less than 3 g of total high-potency fish oil is recommended. Lignan rich flaxseed oil can be substituted on a vegan diet. If any fishy aftertaste occurs, remember not to take with hot food or drinks and to take before eating; if these measures do not work, freeze fish oil capsules before ingestion.

PRECAUTIONS

If any bleeding occurs, stop fish oil immediately because its action on decreasing adhesiveness of platelets in clotting can increase bleeding. Stop one week before surgery or any invasive procedure. Fish oil is contraindicated with platelet counts of less than 20,000. A more conservative approach is to discontinue fish oil if the platelet count is less than 50,000. Use with caution if the patient is taking any other anticoagulants.

Monounsaturated Fatty Acids

Oleic acid (omega-9 fatty acid) is found in olive oil, avocados, hazelnuts, and cashew nuts. It can help with suppression of HER2 tumor cell growth and can help enhance the action of trastuzumab.[59] Eating these nuts and using olive oil in cooking and as a salad dressing are recommended.

Green Tea

Green tea is a polyphenol that is a natural aromatase inhibitor.[60] Green tea consumption of more than three cups per day may reduce the risk of breast cancer recurrence but no consistent effect could be found on cancer incidence.[60] In a Chinese population, green tea and dietary mushrooms decreased the risk for development of breast cancer.[61]

DOSAGE

Three cups a day is the recommended intake.

Soy

In the recent past, a scarcity of research on soy made this food controversial with estrogen-sensitive tumors because soy is a phytoestrogen and theoretically could stimulate estrogen receptors. Studies in mice using the isoflavone genistein in isolation raised concerns about soy. In mice, genistein stimulated ER+ tumors; but in clinical studies of soy consumption, opposite effects are found.[62] Because they are weak estrogens, however, they might also block receptors from being stimulated by stronger exogenous and intrinsic sources of estrogen. The Shanghai Breast Cancer Survival Study, which included 5042 breast cancer survivors, showed that soy food intake is inversely associated with breast cancer mortality and recurrence. The benefits existed for ER+ and ER- tumors and for both users and nonusers of tamoxifen.[63] In another study of soy food intake, high soy intake reduced the risk of breast cancer recurrence in patients with ER+/PR+ tumors receiving the aromatase inhibitor anastrozole.[64] In another study of soy intake and breast cancer risk, an inverse association was found for high intake to lower risk of breast cancer.[65] In Korean women, soy intake was associated with lower breast cancer risk in postmenopausal women, and the inverse association was marked in women with ER+/PR+ tumors.[66]

In two studies of breast cancer patients, soy food intake reduced mortality and breast cancer recurrence.[67,68] In another study about soy food consumption of greater than 10 mg of isoflavones in U.S. and Chinese breast cancer survivors, mortality was not significantly reduced, but breast cancer recurrence was reduced.[69]

Avoid soy isoflavones in supplements, given concerns in mice; but soy foods do not appear to be contraindicated and indeed seem to be valuable in reducing risk of breast cancer, recurrence, and mortality.

DOSAGE

One to three servings a day, in a balanced diet with other foods, are recommended unless an individual has sensitivity to soy.

Other phytoestrogens, plant lignans, can help reduce risk of breast cancer, especially in postmenopausal women.[70]

Flax

Flax, usually consumed as flaxseed meal or oil, is a rich source of phytoestrogens containing alpha-linoleic acid. It has protective effects by decreasing inflammation in the body as an omega-3 fatty acid, inhibits aromatase activity, binds weakly to estrogen receptors, and increases the weaker 2-hydroxyestrones. It reduces the risk of breast cancer and decreases breast cancer cell growth.[22,23,71]

DOSING

One to two tablespoons a day of the meal can be added to food. Flaxseed meal and oil can become rancid easily and should be kept in an airtight container, refrigerated, and used promptly.

Edible (Medicinal) Mushrooms

Medicinal mushrooms that have an antiinflammatory and immune-enhancing effect include maitake (*Grifola frondosa*), shiitake (*Lentinus edodes*), reishi (*Ganoderma lucidum*), and turkey tail (*Trametes versicolor*).[73] Mushrooms also have a number of other properties, including antifungal, antibacterial, antiviral, and tumor attenuating. Each mushroom has different characteristics. Maitake mushrooms in particular have high antitumor and antiinflammatory activity.[74] In one phase I/II trial of maitake extract, a statistically significant association was found with positive immune response. There was no dose-limiting toxicity.[75] In a review of *T. versicolor* research in Japan and China, Standish et al.[76] discussed data suggesting that this mushroom improves disease-free intervals and overall survival in breast cancer patients by immune modulation. More research is warranted.

DOSING

Mushrooms can be eaten in the diet or taken as a dried supplement.

Whey Protein

Whey protein, which is a byproduct of cheese making, is of the highest protein quality and high in glutamine, which helps prevent mouth sores (stomatitis) in patients receiving chemotherapy. It may be useful in preventing the peripheral neuropathy of certain chemotherapy agents, such as taxanes (Taxol). Glutamine is abundant in whey, and this is the preferred manner of ingesting this nutrient.

DOSAGE

Whey protein powder, 20–30 g twice daily in smoothies, will provide adequate glutamine to prevent these complications of chemotherapy. If whey is not tolerated because of allergy or sensitivity, glutamine can be taken as a supplement, 3–5 g one to three times daily.[77]

Brassica *(Cruciferous) Vegetables*

Cruciferous vegetables include kale, broccoli, cauliflower, Brussels sprouts, and cabbage. Indole-3-carbinol is an important constituent of these vegetables that helps decrease cancer cell proliferation, increase apoptosis, and alter the ratio of weak to strong estrogens (2-hydroxyestrone/16-hydroxyestrone) favorably. Breast cancer risk can be reduced by 20%–40% with one or two servings of cruciferous vegetables daily.[26,78-80] Indole-3-carbinol can interfere with tamoxifen and is safer to eat in vegetable form than in supplement form.[3]

DOSAGE

One or two servings per day is the recommended intake. In supplement form, 400 mg/day of indole-3 carbinol (I3C) is recommended.[23,81,82]

One head of cabbage contains approximately 1200 mg of indole-3-carbinol. Eating of one-third of a head of cabbage daily would equal the common supplemental dose of 400 mg daily and offer the other synergistic properties of the whole plant.

Supplements

Botanicals and supplements can be useful in promoting health; some have an anticancer effect or immunity-enhancing effect, and some are useful in attenuating the side effects of conventional cancer therapies. It is important to consider the interactions of some botanicals and supplements with chemotherapy and radiation therapy that might decrease the effectiveness of these modalities and in some cases increase toxicity. Antioxidants taken in high-dose supplement form can theoretically interfere with radiation therapy and chemotherapy by neutralizing free radical formation key to the effectiveness of these agents. Controversy remains, but most practitioners agree that foods high in antioxidants are safe, given the variety of antioxidants naturally occurring in many foods that act synergistically, are better absorbed, and do not reduce the effectiveness of radiation therapy and chemotherapy because they are in concentrations lower than in supplement forms.

More information on this topic can be found online at ExpertConsult.com.

Multivitamins

Information on this topic is available online at ExpertConsult.com.

Vitamin D

Vitamin D deficiency is common, especially in patients chronically or acutely ill and in northern climates (above 35–40 degrees north or south of the equator). Those individuals with darker skin, who are obese, who have little unprotected sun exposure, who are older than 65 years, and who are taking particular medications such as glucocorticoids or anticonvulsants are also at risk for deficiency. It can express itself as diffuse body aches and can contribute to osteopenia and osteoporosis. It can also be manifested as low-back pain, proximal muscle weakness, and bone pain, especially over the sternum or tibia.[86,87] Vitamin D is also important for immunity and has an anticancer effect. Vitamin D is ingested as vitamin D_2 (ergocalciferol) or vitamin D_3 (cholecalciferol), which is converted in the liver to 25-hydroxyvitamin D (calcidiol), the circulating form of vitamin D. Vitamin D_3 is also formed in the skin when 7-dehydrocholesterol, the skin precursor, is exposed to ultraviolet B light. Calcidiol is converted in the kidney to 1,25-dihydroxyvitamin D (calcitriol), the active metabolite. Calcitriol significantly inhibits cancer cell growth, especially in breast, colon, prostate, and ovarian tissue.[86] In testing for vitamin D deficiency, the 25-hydroxyvitamin D level is most helpful.

Strong evidence exists that vitamin D and calcium intake can help reduce the risk of breast cancer.[88] In a meta-analysis of 36 studies, a 45% lowered risk was found in women whose 25-hydroxyvitamin D levels were in the highest quartile versus the lowest quartile. Decreased cancer risk was also observed in those with the highest quartile of calcium intake.[89] Blackmore et al.[90] found reduced risk of ER+/PR+ breast cancer in women with the highest intake of vitamin D. Nonsignificant positive trends were also seen in women with ER+/PR- and ER-/PR- tumors. Dark-skinned individuals such as African Americans convert less vitamin D in their skin and are more likely to be vitamin D deficient without supplementation. This increases cancer risk, which may help explain why this population group is more at risk for cancer with higher mortality.[91]

Aromatase inhibitors can contribute to myalgias, arthralgias, and loss of bone mass. In combination with other therapies that cause significant side effects and may further prevent meaningful sun exposure, vitamin D deficiency can contribute to these adverse effects of conventional therapy.

Vitamin D–fortified foods contain vitamin D in small and inconsistent amounts. Reliable and potent food sources of vitamin D are oily fish, including salmon, mackerel, and sardines.[92,93] Supplements are usually needed to obtain adequate amounts of vitamin D. In general, a 25-hydroxyvitamin D level of less than 20 ng/mL (50 nmol/L) is deficiency range, and 20–30 ng/mL (50–75 nmol/L) is in the insufficiency range. Treatment of vitamin D deficiency includes oral vitamin D_2 (ergocalciferol) at 50,000 units per week for 8 weeks. After vitamin D levels are normalized, current recommendations are conservative for vitamin D_3 800–1000 units daily.[95] Vitamin D is relatively contraindicated in patients with hypercalcemia, which can occur in metastatic breast cancer with bone involvement.[95]

In an epidemiological projection of optimal serum 25-hydroxyvitamin D levels, Garland et al.[96] estimated prevention of 58,000 cases of breast cancer per year with year-round levels of 40–60 ng/mL (100–150 nmol/L). Abbas et al.[92] found that vitamin D lowered the risk of premenopausal breast cancer. Other studies in Norway and England have found that patients with cancers diagnosed in summer or fall, when vitamin D levels are highest, had longer survival and a milder clinical course than did patients diagnosed in the winter or spring, when vitamin D levels are lowest.[93]

DOSAGE

The recommended dose of vitamin D_3 is 1000–2000 units daily.[95,97,98] Serum levels of 25-hydroxyvitamin D can be used to determine optimal dosing of vitamin D, which can vary from person to person and by time of year, latitude, and degree of sun exposure.

PRECAUTIONS

Signs of vitamin D toxicity include nausea and vomiting, pancreatitis, nephrocalcinosis or vascular calcinosis, metallic taste, and headache.[95]

Melatonin

Melatonin has antioxidant, immune-enhancing, cytotoxic, and estrogen-regulating properties. It is also useful in the treatment of insomnia. Melatonin comes in an immediate preparation for individuals having difficulty in falling asleep and a sustained-release preparation for those having difficulty staying asleep.[99,100] Avoiding melatonin suppression may be more effective than supplementation.[1]

DOSAGE

Doses range from 1–20 mg before bed; a starting dose is 3 mg before bed. Titration occurs to effect, without causing a hangover the next day.

PRECAUTIONS

Melatonin is contraindicated in bipolar illness, and it can worsen depression in some vulnerable individuals. Monitoring for optimal effect with minimal side effects is recommended. Caution must be exercised in use with other sedative medication.

Botanicals

Botanicals can be helpful in the treatment of cancer but must be used carefully during chemotherapy because many botanicals can interfere with the metabolism of the chemotherapy agent by increasing or decreasing its metabolism in the body. For example, certain botanicals can interfere with the metabolism of taxanes, platinum-based drugs, cyclophosphamide, doxorubicin, etoposide, and irinotecan.[5] In general, botanicals do not interfere with radiation therapy. Botanicals such as St. John's wort

can interact with a number of other drugs the patient may be taking through the cytochrome P-450 metabolic pathway.

Spiritual and Emotional Care

Patients who have social support, empowerment, and meaning often have more positive lifestyle behaviors and coping strategies. Those patients with lack of meaning and purpose often have more symptoms from treatment and more difficulty in coping, leading to more negative choices.[101] Small-group psychological interventions for breast cancer patients led by a psychologist and concentrating on stress management and strategies to optimize conventional treatment and to improve mood helped decrease recurrence and mortality.[102] Mindfulness intervention and supportive expressive therapy allowed telomere length to stabilize, rather than shorten, in the control group in a study of woman with breast cancer. Telomere length was not associated with mood or stress.[103]

Emerging evidence on life review and internet-based social networking shows improvement in QOL measures; it is another intervention that is simple yet powerful in cultivating meaning through the challenges of cancer.[104,105] Spiritual and emotional assessment and recommendations for interventions such as support groups, journaling, life review, and psychotherapy with oncology health professionals are reviewed in other chapters (see Chapters 82 and 114).

Conventional Treatment

Of all cancers, breast cancer is one of the most thoroughly studied in terms of clinical trials. From the 1970s on there have been hundreds of randomized controlled trials evaluating surgical, radiation, and medical approaches to treatment. Large trials, often with many hundreds of patients, have incrementally improved treatment with more effective and less toxic strategies.[106,107] A large body of literature documents the evolution of treatment for apparently localized breast cancer, a category that has increased as screening for early breast cancer has become more common.

The move away from mastectomy to breast preservation with lumpectomy and breast irradiation was a major change. An important discovery was that postoperative use of medicine with drugs including cytotoxic chemotherapy and antiestrogen agents such as tamoxifen could favorably influence the natural history of the cancer with greater survival. This occurred by control of apparent microscopic distant disease not detected in the pretreatment period by physical exam, blood tests, or imaging. Much work has been done to better understand the biology of each cancer and with gene expression pattern analysis it has been learned that there are multiple subcategories of breast cancer, each with different behaviors of metastasis and response to treatment.[108,109] Lessons learned in the late 20th century included:

- For appropriate candidates, breast preservation with lumpectomy and radiation to the remaining breast tissue yields survival equivalent to mastectomy.[110]

- Cytotoxic chemotherapy, particularly in premenopausal women, can effectively improve overall outcome in patients with breast cancer that is likely to recur. The amount of benefit, and hence the benefit to toxicity ratio, depends on the risk of recurrence. Greater risk for recurrence is associated with greater absolute benefit from chemotherapy.[106]
- Tamoxifen and other estrogen blocking or reduction agents can improve outcome in women with breast cancers that measure positive for estrogen and/or progesterone receptors (hormone receptor, or HR-positive cancers)[107]
- Anatomic features of the cancer such as the extent of axillary nodal involvement, tumor size, and the histological grade help predict the natural history of the cancer and thus guide the need for postoperative medical therapy.

Surgical Approach

Only a small minority (5%) of patients in the United States diagnosed with breast cancer have identifiable overt distant metastatic disease at the time of diagnosis. Thus, nearly all women will be considered for local therapy (surgery and perhaps radiation) as well as systemic therapy (medicines such as with chemotherapy, antiestrogen therapy, and more recently possible antibody therapy) to optimize recurrence risk reduction.

Lumpectomy is well established as a surgical strategy that when done with postoperative breast irradiation offers excellent long-term control in the breast and survival that is comparable to mastectomy. In the past decade, the major surgical advance has been incorporation of *sentinel node biopsy*, which has replaced axillary dissection for most women.[111] With lymphatic mapping using the sentinel node procedure, a blue dye and or a radionuclide, which can be tracked by a detection device, is injected into the breast. A small incision in the axilla is done to identify the stained or radioactively "hot" node. This is the *sentinel node* (the initial landing site for cancer cells moving to axillary nodes), which can be tested for the histological presence of cancer cells. If none are seen, the patient is deemed to be "node negative" and no further node surgery is needed. Ongoing studies are being done to determine the value of node dissection in patients with positive sentinel nodes. The overall amount of axillary surgery has been reduced significantly with the introduction of the sentinel node procedure.

Breast *conservation* or breast *preservation* are terms that describe removal of the tumor only (lumpectomy) and not the entire breast as with mastectomy. The majority of women diagnosed with invasive breast cancer are candidates for lumpectomy and sentinel node procedure, and this approach became the preferred standard in the early 1990s.[112] Despite the reduction in toxicity with breast preservation and a survival equivalent to mastectomy, some women choose mastectomy or even bilateral mastectomy. A trend for this began in the late 1990s and is perhaps a reflection of fear of recurrence or new breast cancer.[113] Some of this concern is fueled by the fact that

though breast cancer treatments are more effective than ever, many women still die of metastatic breast cancer, and once the disease is metastatic, we cannot offer cure as a realistic goal.

Radiation

Whole-breast radiation to the affected breast is standard after lumpectomy. Despite the lumpectomy being done with clear tissue margins, there is still a significant recurrence rate near the region of the excision. Radiation markedly reduces but does not eliminate risk for recurrence. Traditional schedules have included treatment with external beam radiation for 5–6 weeks, but recent studies in Canada and England suggest that shorter treatment duration, hypofractionated RT, is likely equivalent for disease control as well as short- and long-term toxicity for most patients.[114] It is likely that in the United States shorter course external beam radiation will become the standard, at least for patients with negative nodes. Randomized trials have determined that for elderly women with stage I, HR-positive cancer undergoing lumpectomy radiation is of little value and can often be omitted.

Chemotherapy of Localized Breast Cancer

From the 1970s until recently treatment decisions about adjuvant therapy have been based primarily on anatomic features of the cancer with node positivity and tumor size being the most important predictors of recurrence. Now decision making incorporates protein products and tumor gene patterns and other features that help predict the behavior of the cancer. For example, it was shown in the 1980s that changing the hormonal environment with the antiestrogen tamoxifen could reduce recurrences by half in women with node-negative, hormone receptor–positive tumors.[115] Other studies included node-positive women, and the standard approach of using estrogen blocking or estrogen reduction therapy with or without chemotherapy for women of all ages was established.

Once cytotoxic chemotherapy was shown to change the natural history of node-negative tumors as well, the use of chemotherapy for lower-risk tumors expanded. The result was that much chemotherapy was used for patients who did not need it. Tumor tissue from patients treated in these studies led to development of molecular testing that could allocate node-negative, hormone receptor–positive tumors into higher versus lower recurrence-risk categories. The method also identified tumors that were more or less likely to benefit from chemotherapy. Genomic profiling, e.g., OncotypeDX, have become standard and provide guidance regarding which cancers will not need cytotoxic chemotherapy for optimal care. It is expected that in the future, molecular phenotyping will play a larger role in directing adjuvant therapy for node-positive tumors as well.[116]

Certain categories of breast cancer require different treatments. Fifteen to twenty percent of cancers have overexpression of the epidermal growth factor protein her-2 or amplification of the *HER2* gene. Testing for this is now standard. Without optimal adjuvant treatment, these tumors have a high risk for recurrence. Significant improvement in outcome occurs with the use of trastuzumab, a monoclonal antibody directed at *HER2*, in addition to chemotherapy. This combination treatment has dramatically improved the prognosis for this subtype of breast cancer. Another category, *triple negative* cancer, does not have hormone receptors (estrogen or progesterone receptor) nor overexpression of *HER2*. At present, only cytotoxic chemotherapy is available as adjuvant treatment. These tumors have a worse prognosis.

Chemotherapy of Metastatic Disease

The goal of adjuvant treatment is to prevent disease metastatic to distant organs. Common sites for metastases include bone, liver, lung, skin, and brain. Current goals of treatment for metastatic breast cancer are disease control, not cure, and prevention or treatment of symptoms. For disease that is HR-positive, medical treatment involves sequential use of hormonal strategies such as tamoxifen, aromatase inhibitors for postmenopausal women, ovarian suppression for premenopausal women, and fulvestrant, an estrogen receptor downregulator. Some patients over time respond to several of these agents and control of HR-positive cancer can be achieved for years. At some point, all patients will develop disease that is refractory to hormonal treatment. For disease that is HR negative at the outset or that has progressed despite hormonal therapy, chemotherapy, usually with sequential single agents, is done. For all patients with *HER2*–"positive" disease, a *HER2*-directed agent is used with chemotherapy. It is important to have confidence in the laboratory doing the *HER2* assay. Missing a *HER2*-positive cancer is a major mistake.

It is important to remember that management of metastatic breast cancer can result in good function and a high QOL for many years. In general, there is need for long-term planning with expectations that the patient will receive numerous types of treatment over time, with each sequential treatment ideally offering a good deal of time with disease control. A good working partnership between the physician/nurse team and the patient/family is required. One of the more difficult decisions in patients with metastatic breast cancer is when to stop anticancer therapy. Because there can be periods of success with multiple treatments, there may be a tendency to lose sight of when to stop. Usually performance status and patient preference help determine when symptom management, and not chemotherapy, is the best path. If the patient's performance status is poor (e.g., Eastern Cooperative Oncology Group score 3 or worse, wheelchair-bound, etc.), chemotherapy is generally not well tolerated and not useful.

Summary

Treatment of breast cancer continues to evolve with less surgical morbidity, more effective systemic agents, and better understanding of breast cancer biology all being recent advances. Lessons learned in the early 21st century:

- For some patients with lumpectomy, shorter course radiation (3 weeks) is equivalent to longer treatment periods.
- Genomic profiling tests can identify breast cancers with a relatively good prognosis using adjuvant endocrine therapy only, so that patients can avoid cytotoxic chemotherapy.
- Sentinel node procedures allow the elimination of traditional axillary dissection for the majority of patients.

More information on this topic can be found online at ExpertConsult.com.

INTEGRATIVE MANAGEMENT OF SIDE EFFECTS FROM BREAST CANCER TREATMENT

More information on this topic can be found online at ExpertConsult.com.
See also E-Table 78.2 online at ExpertConsult.com for further reading on integrative oncology.

ACKNOWLEDGMENTS

Thank you to Kelson Okimoto, University of Washington Palliative Care Program (Seattle) operations manager for technical assistance.

TABLE 78.1 Integrative Medicine and Breast Cancer Treatment Symptoms

Symptom	Treatment	Evidence vs. Harm Rating
Fatigue	Exercise	A₁
	Acupuncture	B₁
Postmenopausal symptoms of hot flashes	Medications such as selective serotonin reuptake inhibitors, selective norepinephrine reuptake inhibitors, and gabapentin	A₂
	Acupuncture	A₁
	Exercise	A₁
Nausea and vomiting due to chemotherapy	Acupuncture	A₁
	Ginger	B₁
	Cannabis	B₂
Anxiety, stress, and depression	Acupuncture	B₁
	Mindfulness-based stress reduction	A₁
	Art therapy	B₁
	Exercise	A₁
	Yoga	B₁
	Massage	A₁
	Support groups	A₁
Insomnia	Exercise	A₁
	Melatonin	A₂
	Relaxation techniques	B₁
	Sleep hygiene	A₁
Pain and peripheral neuropathy	Acupuncture	A₁
	Exercise	A₁
	Cannabinoids	A₂
	Massage	A₁
	Mind-body therapies	A₁
Lymphedema	Acupuncture	B₁
	Exercise	A₁
Radiation dermatitis	Calendula cream	B₁

Modified from Deng G, Cassileth BR, Yeung KS. Complementary therapies for cancer-related symptoms. *J Support Oncol.* 2004;2:419-426.

PREVENTION PRESCRIPTION

- Eat primarily a plant-based diet rich in cruciferous vegetables (broccoli, cauliflower, Brussels sprouts, cabbage, and kale). Eat one or two servings of cruciferous vegetables daily.
- Follow an antiinflammatory and Mediterranean diet. This diet avoids saturated fat in dairy and meats; it has no trans-fats and includes increased amounts of omega-3 fatty acids (ocean fish, walnuts, soybeans, greens, flaxseed meal). See Chapter 88.
- Avoid processed foods.
- Organic foods that are not contaminated with pesticides and herbicides. Many organic meats, poultry, and produce can be purchased from local farms or farmers' markets.
- Fatty fish such as herring, mackerel, tuna, salmon, and sardines have high levels of omega-3 fatty acids. Minimize your eating of albacore tuna, shark, swordfish, king mackerel, and tile fish because they can have higher levels of contamination with mercury. You may want to take omega-3 supplements that are detoxified. Fish, however, is an excellent protein source. Eat fish often (three times per week or less) or take fish oil supplements daily. (If you eat fish high in omega-3 content, do not take your fish oil supplements that day.)
- Do not skip meals. If breakfast is a problem, try protein-fortified smoothies in the morning. Whey protein powder is best, and if you are lactose intolerant, buy whey protein powder without lactose.
- Drink lots of water, filtered if possible. Bring it with you everywhere (reuse water bottles). Flavor it with lime or lemon (or cucumber, orange, or any other natural flavor you like).
- Drink green tea, two or three cups a day.
- Moderate alcohol intake if you drink alcohol (no more than one serving per day for women). Do not drink it at all if it makes you feel not well.
- Mushrooms contribute to a healthy diet, especially adding medicinal mushrooms (i.e., maitake, shiitake, reishi, turkey tail) as food or supplement.

- Eat one to three servings of soy food daily. Avoid soy (isoflavone) supplements.
- Eat one or two tablespoons of flaxseed meal daily.
- Consider taking a multivitamin with minerals daily.
- Vitamin D can be obtained from adequate sun exposure or a supplement. For most people, 2000 units/day will maintain adequate levels. I recommend determination of a 25-hydroxyvitamin D level in winter to assess for adequate intake.
- Maintain healthy weight with a BMI of less than 30 and ideally 25 (not overweight).
- Avoid smoking and passive tobacco exposure.
- Exercise for 30–60 minutes at least 5 days a week (more than 3 hours per week is recommended). Combine aerobic activity such as walking with a resistance or strength training program two or three times a week. Nordic walking sticks can increase the overall conditioning of walking while improving posture, balance, and core strengthening. Yoga, tai chi, and qi gong are meditative movement with the benefit of relaxation and exercise. Do exercise that is enjoyable to you.
- Optimize sleep at night. Melatonin can be added if sleeping difficulties are occurring, starting at 3 mg before bed. Sleep in a darkened room at regular hours to improve sleep quality. Do not sleep with a television on in the bedroom.
- Maintain spiritual practices that give meaning and relaxation to your life.
- Maintain a strong support network with family and friends.
- Consider testing for a 2-hydroxyestrone/16-hydroxyestrone ratio, and consider interventions to improve the ratio in favor of weak estrogens.
- Minimize use of estrogen replacement medication. For menopausal symptoms, consider non-hormonal measures first.
- Attend to self-care every day. Make healthy lifestyle choices a part of your routine.

THERAPEUTIC REVIEW

NUTRITION

- The Mediterranean diet can lower the risk of breast cancer and other chronic health conditions, such as heart disease, diabetes, and obesity. This diet is high in omega-3 and omega-9 fatty acids; add five to nine servings of fruit and vegetables per day.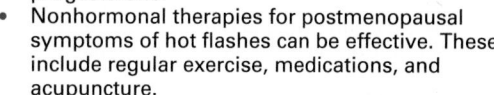

- Cruciferous vegetables are beneficial in a healthy diet to decrease cancer risk.

- In general, antioxidants are preferably obtained in food rather than in supplements.

- Three cups of green tea per day can decrease breast cancer risk.

- Soy foods in moderation are safe and protective for breast cancer. One to three servings of soy foods daily are recommended. Avoid isolated isoflavone supplements.

- Flaxseed meal can lower breast cancer risk.

- Avoid excessive alcohol intake. Drink no more than one alcoholic beverage daily.

- Weight control and gradual weight loss if the patient is obese or very overweight can reduce risk of breast cancer. Weight loss can be achieved with regular exercise, portion control, and eating more fruits and vegetables and fewer calorie-dense foods.

- Vitamin D in supplement form when adequate sun exposure is not available is important for bone health, anticancer effect, immunity, and muscle health. Higher levels of vitamin D are associated with decreased risk of breast cancer. Monitor levels of 25-hydroxyvitamin D in the winter to ensure adequate intake of vitamin D_3.

- Medicinal mushrooms have many potential beneficial effects during cancer treatment and can be part of a healthy diet.

MEDICATION

- Avoid prolonged HRT of both estrogen and progesterone.

- Nonhormonal therapies for postmenopausal symptoms of hot flashes can be effective. These include regular exercise, medications, and acupuncture.

- Tamoxifen is commonly used for ER+ tumors for 5 years after treatment to prevent recurrence. The dose is 20 mg daily.

- Aromatase inhibitors (anastrozole, exemestane, letrozole) are used in postmenopausal treatment of breast cancer to prevent recurrence.

EXERCISE

- Exercising more than 3 hours per week can decrease cancer risk.

LIFESTYLE

- Sleep is important in decreasing cancer risk. Melatonin is implicated in this mechanism of reduced cancer cell proliferation when melatonin levels are high. Suppression of intrinsic melatonin is to be avoided sleeping in a dark room and avoiding exposure to blue wavelength light in the evening after dusk and during the night. Supplemental melatonin can help improve circadian rhythms and quality of sleep. The dose is 1-3 mg at bedtime. Up to 20 mg has been used.

- Psychological interventions can be helpful in cancer care. Those most helpful are psychoeducation and psychotherapy conducted by a psychotherapist individually.

- Mindfulness-based stress reduction programs can enhance well-being and coping and decrease anxiety during and after treatment.

- See Table 77.1.

Key Web Resources

Adjuvant therapy predictor for breast cancer Predicts what chemotherapy and endocrine or targeted therapies might be helpful, given tumor markers and staging	http://www.bmj.com/cgi/content-nw/full/337/jul11_2/a540/ FIG3 (login to *British Medical Journal* required to view)
National Cancer Institute Breast Cancer Risk Assessment Tool Summary of important research studies that inform integrative cancer care International studies are reviewed.	http://www.cancer.gov/bcrisktool/Default.aspx InspireHealth Integrated Cancer Care *Research Updates* To subscribe to newsletters, email: mwiebe@inspirehealth.ca; hard copy or electronic copy Phone: 604-734-7125 #200-1330 West 8th Avenue, Vancouver, BC V6H 4A6
American Cancer Society: Monographs cited in references on the research of exercise and nutrition in the prevention of cancer and during and after cancer treatment	http://www.cancer.org/Cancer/BreastCancer/ index?ssSourceSiteId=null
Susan G. Komen Breast Cancer Foundation: Dedicated to education and research about causes, treatment, and search for a cure	http://ww5.komen.org
Society for Integrative Oncology: International organization of clinicians, researchers, and others interested in evidence-based integrative oncology A monograph is available for integrative oncology practice guidelines. Deng GE, Frenkel M, Cohen L, et al. Evidence-based clinical practice guidelines for integrative oncology: complementary therapies and botanicals. *J Soc Integr Oncol.* 2009;7:85-120.	http://www.integrativeonc.org

Key Web Resources—cont'd

Breast Cancer Recovery: Breast Cancer Recovery's mission is to help women heal mind, body, and spirit after breast cancer. All programs are designed and conducted by survivors for survivors.

http://www.bcrecovery.org

National Institutes of Health National Cancer Institute (NCI) National Center for Complementary and Integrative Health (NCCIH)

http://www.cancer.gov/cancertopics/cam/
https://nccih.nih.gov

Evidence-based information on complementary and alternative medicine and its applications in oncology

National Institutes of Health, Office of Dietary Supplements: Provides information on dietary supplements. The Pub-Med Dietary Supplement Subset succeeds the International Bibliographic Information on Dietary Supplements (IBIDS) database active from 1999-2010.

http://ods.od.nih.gov/research/pubmed_dietary_supplement_subset.aspx

Memorial Sloan-Kettering Cancer Center: A searchable database provides evidence-based information on herbs, botanicals, vitamins, and other supplements. It includes evaluations of alternative or unproven cancer therapies.

http://www.mskcc.org/cancer-care/integrative-medicine/about-herbs-botanicals-other-products

The University of Texas MD Anderson Cancer Center Complementary and Integrative Medicine Educational Resources: Evidence-based review of complementary and alternative medicine and integrative medicine therapies

https://www.mdanderson.org/treatment-options/complementary-and-integrative-medicine

American Society of Clinical Oncology: Patient educational resources that have been physician approved. These resources including podcasts, educational materials, mobile app, blog posts, etc. These resources are available to the public, patients, and clinicians.

http://www.cancer.net

REFERENCES

References are available online at ExpertConsult.com.

CHAPTER 79

LUNG CANCER

Kaushal B. Nanavati, MD, FAAFP, ABIHM • Eric Reed, BA

INTRODUCTION

Lung cancer is the leading cause of cancer-related deaths in the United States, accounting for 26% of cancer-related deaths in women and 28% in men.[1] Lung cancer continues to be the second most common newly diagnosed cancer in both men and women in the United States, accounting for about 13% of all cancer diagnoses. In men, the incidence has been declining since the mid-1980s, but in women, the incidence has only been declining since the mid-2000s.[1] The average age of presentation is 60 years. The lifetime probability of developing lung cancer is 1:13 for men and 1:16 for women. The 5-year survival rate is poor but has improved from 16.4% in 1975 to 21.4% in 2010.[2]

> The lifetime probability of developing lung cancer is 1:13 for men and 1:16 for women.

PATHOPHYSIOLOGY

The classical bifurcation of lung cancer is non-small cell lung cancer (NSCLC), the more common type, and small cell lung cancer (SCLC). SCLC is typically less amenable to surgical resection, whereas NSCLC can more often be treated with surgery. NSCLC can be divided into three major histological subtypes: squamous cell carcinoma, adenocarcinoma, and large cell lung cancer. It is also possible for lung cancers that have mixed features to be identified as mixed small cell/large cell cancers.

Signs and Symptoms

Symptoms do not usually occur until the cancer is advanced and can include persistent cough, hemoptysis, chest pain, voice changes such as hoarseness, worsening shortness of breath, recurrent pneumonia, or bronchitis.[1]

Risk Factors

Smoking and Tobacco Use

Cigarette smoking is by far the most important risk factor for lung cancer, wherein risk increases with both the quantity and duration of smoking.[1] Approximately 90% of lung cancers are the result of tobacco use, and the risk

of a smoker developing lung cancer is 25 times greater than that of a nonsmoker. Smoking is strongly linked with SCLC and squamous cell carcinoma, and adenocarcinoma is the most common type in patients who have never smoked.[3]

> Smoking is strongly linked with SCLC and squamous cell carcinoma. Adenocarcinoma is the most common type in patients who have never smoked.

Environmental Carcinogens

Environmental risk factors that have been implicated in lung cancer include exposure to radon (the second most common cause), secondhand smoke, asbestos, metals (chromium, cadmium), tar exposure, arsenic, certain organic chemicals such as bis(chloromethyl) ether, silica, radiation exposure, air pollution, and diesel exhaust. Certain occupations may increase exposure to lung carcinogens, including rubber manufacturing, paving, roofing, painting, and chimney sweeping. In addition to asbestos exposure, cigarette smoke greatly increases the chances of an asbestos-related lung cancer.[1]

Genetics and Biomarkers

Lung cancer is a complex and heterogeneous disease, not only at the biochemical level (genes, proteins, metabolites) but also at the tissue, organism, and population levels.[4] There are many early detection biomarkers for lung cancer, including both tissue- and biofluid-based biomarkers such as airway epithelium, sputum, blood, and exhaled breath. Mutations in p53 have been seen in chronic smokers before there is evidence of neoplasia, making it a potentially useful predictor of lung cancer. Due to the heterogeneity of lung cancer, detection by one single biomarker remains difficult. Panels of biomarkers can be used, but these frequently have overlap with other diseases, especially other cancers and inflammatory conditions.[5]

> Mutations in p53 have been seen in chronic smokers before there is evidence of neoplasia, making it a potentially useful predictor of lung cancer.

Screening and Detection

Spiral Computed Tomography

Compared with standard chest X-ray (CXR), screening with spiral computed tomography (CT) has been shown to reduce lung cancer–related deaths by 16–20% among adults with a 30 pack-year history who were current smokers or who had quit within the past 15 years.[1] Current American Cancer Society guidelines suggest discussing utilization of low-dose helical CT (LDCT) in current or former smokers aged 55–74 years in good health with at least a 30 pack-year history of smoking. A "pack-year" is the packs of cigarettes smoked a day (1 pack = 20 cigarettes) multiplied by the number of years smoked. "Clinicians with access to high-volume, high-quality lung cancer screening and treatment centers should initiate a discussion about lung cancer screening with apparently healthy patients ages 55–74 who have at least a 30 pack-year smoking history and who currently smoke or have quit within the past 15 years. A process of informed and shared decision making with a clinician related to the potential benefits, limitations, and harms associated with screening for lung cancer with LDCT should occur before any decision is made to initiate lung cancer screening. Smoking cessation counseling remains a high priority for clinical attention in discussions with current smokers, who should be informed of their continuing risk for lung cancer. Screening should not be viewed as an alternative to smoking cessation."[6]

> Low-dose helical CT (LDCT) (Fig. 79.1) is recommended annually starting at age 55 until age 79 in those with a 30 pack-year smoking history. This recommendation continues if a nodule measuring ≤4 mm is found. For nodules that measure 4–6 mm, repeat LDCT in 6 months. If the nodule grows to 6–8 mm or greater, radiology may recommend positron emission tomography (PET)/CT or bronchoscopy based on nodule characteristics.

Chest Radiography

CXR is no longer recommended as a screening technique for lung cancer and is less useful than newer technologies such as LDCT. According to the large Prostate, Lung, Colorectal, and Ovarian cancer screening trial published in 2011, annual screening with chest radiography did not reduce lung cancer mortality when compared with a "usual care" group who did not receive an annual chest radiograph.[7]

Sputum Cytology

This technique is more likely to be helpful in the detection of cancers that start in the major airways, such as squamous cell lung cancers.[8] According to four prospective randomized controlled studies of lung cancer screening using a combination of CXR and sputum cytology,

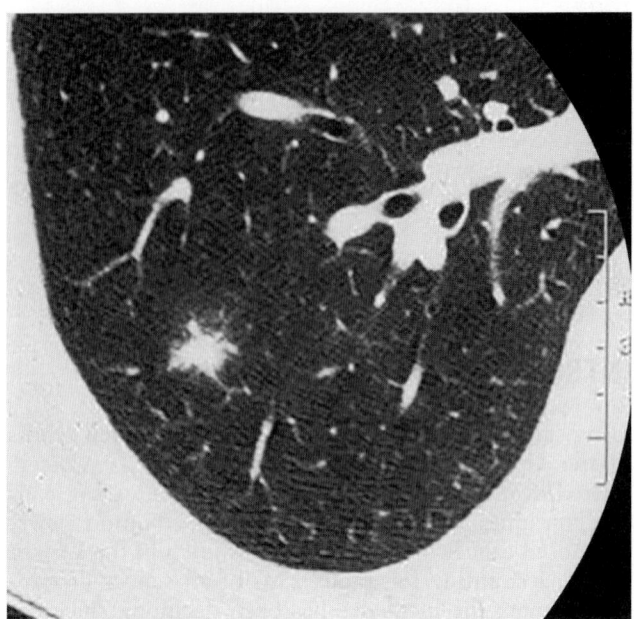

FIG. 79.1 ■ A nodule detected in the right lower lobe with low-dose helical computed tomography (CT) in screening for lung cancer. From Tzung B, Julien PJ. Lung cancer screening. In: Lewis MI, McKenna RJ Jr, et al., eds. *Medical management of the thoracic surgery patient*. Philadelphia: Saunders Elsevier; 2010:197–200.)

there was no significant reduction in lung cancer mortality associated with an invitation to undergo sputum cytology screening.[6]

Positron Emission Tomography

Not all patients with lung cancer will require a PET scan; however, it can be a useful tool for determining cancer staging.[9] It can be effective for determining the level of tissue activity and is more effective than CT in distinguishing between benign and malignant lesions.[10] Glucose uptake alone is nonspecific because it can be increased with inflammatory conditions.

Laser Bronchoscopy

Conventional white–light bronchoscopy (WLB) alone identifies the lesion in only 29% of cases.[11]

INTEGRATIVE THERAPY

Mind–Body Modalities

Patients with lung and other poor-outlook cancers are particularly vulnerable to heavily promoted claims for unproven or disproven "alternatives." Inquiring about patients' uses of these therapies should be routine because these practices may be harmful and can delay or impair treatment. Physician-guided mind–body modalities and massage therapy can reduce anxiety, mood disturbance, and chronic pain. Acupuncture can assist in the control of pain and other side effects and help reduce quantities of pain medication required.[12]

Yoga

Some controlled trials suggest yoga is beneficial for chemotherapy-induced nausea, anticipatory nausea, pain, invigoration, acceptance, fatigue, and appetite loss, and can decrease salivary cortisol levels. Investigators also report a positive dose-response relationship.[13]

Massage

Massage therapy, an effective adjunct to cancer supportive care, can reduce anxiety, depression, and pain. The evidence that supports its effect on anxiety is stronger than that on depression. However, there is a lack of systematic reviews regarding consistent massage methodology and quality for most of the clinical trials.[13]

Exercise-Based Pulmonary Rehabilitation

Overall, the studies published to date suggest that short-term (6–8 weeks), low-intensity, multidisciplinary, exercise-based rehabilitation is potentially feasible and safe for select patients with inoperable NSCLC. The preliminary data further suggest that low-intensity, multidisciplinary, exercise-based rehabilitation is associated with modest improvements in exercise tolerance and functional capacity endpoints in select patients who are able to tolerate and achieve reasonable adherence. Published studies have important methodological limitations, and further carefully designed studies in select populations are warranted[13] (see Chapter 92).

Acupuncture

Acupuncture is a relatively safe and minimally invasive modality that may be useful for treating symptoms of lung cancer and side effects of anticancer treatment. A small case series showed some improvement in both an analog pain scale and well-being score for patients with lung cancer.[14] Overall, there is a lack of data on whether acupuncture could be useful in the treatment of chemotherapy-induced peripheral neuropathy.[13]

Nutrition

Nausea and vomiting are common side effects of chemotherapy treatments. There are numerous methods for treating chemotherapy-related nausea, including corticosteroids, dopamine antagonists, serotonin antagonists, benzodiazepines, aprepitant, and cannabinoids. Ginger can also be recommended for both its antinausea and anticancer benefits.[15] Generally, a diet rich in nonstarchy vegetables and fruits and low in red meat is recommended. B-complex vitamins, tea, and cruciferous vegetable can also be recommended. For patients with weight loss, nutritional supplements may be recommended along with a diet rich in protein while still limiting red meat consumption. In patients with sarcopenia, supplementation with n-3 fatty acids may be beneficial.[13] Oral supplementation of eicosapentaenoic acid (EPA) in patients with NSCLC significantly improves energy, protein intake, and body composition, while decreasing fatigue, neuropathy, and loss of appetite, according to a recent randomized trial.[16]

> In general, a diet rich in nonstarchy vegetables and fruits and low in red meat is recommended.

Curcumin

Curcumin, also called diferuloylmethane, is a hydrophobic polyphenol that is the main curcuminoid of turmeric. "The mechanisms implicated in the inhibition of tumor genesis by curcumin are diverse and appear to involve a combination of antiinflammatory, antioxidant, immunomodulatory, proapoptotic, and anti-angiogenic properties via pleiotropic effects on genes and cell-signaling pathways at multiple levels."[17] Gene inhibition of cyclooxygenase (COX)-2 is thought to be the main antiinflammatory activity of curcumin. Curcumin tends to be well tolerated; however, its systemic bioavailability after oral dosing is poor, which may limit its effectiveness outside the gastrointestinal tract. Piperine, a major component of black pepper, has been shown to increase the bioavailability of curcumin.[18]

> Piperine, a major component of black pepper, has been shown to increase the bioavailability of curcumin.

Smoking Cessation

Smoking cessation continues to be the most important factor in reducing the risk for lung cancer. People who discontinue smoking, even well into middle age, avoid most of their subsequent risk for lung cancer, and discontinuing smoking before middle age avoids more than 90% of the risk attributable to tobacco.[19]

Traditional Treatments

Traditional treatments include surgery, radiofrequency ablation (RFA), radiation therapy, chemotherapies, targeted therapies, and immunotherapy. Palliative therapies may also be used to help with symptoms.

Surgery

Surgery to remove lung cancer may be an option for early stage NSCLC. More advanced lung cancer, especially with metastasis, may not be helped by surgery. If surgery can be done early, it provides the best chance to cure NSCLC. The risk for serious consequences is high.[8] Types of lung surgery include pneumonectomy, lobectomy, and segmentectomy (wedge resection).

Radiofrequency Ablation

RFA may be useful for some small NSCLC tumors that are near the outer edge of the lungs, especially in people who cannot tolerate surgery. In RFA, a thin probe is inserted through the skin and into the tumor. The probe is used to heat the tumor to destroy the cancer cells. This is typically done as an outpatient procedure. Major complications are uncommon but can include a partial collapse of the lung or bleeding into the lung.[8]

> Radiofrequency ablation (RFA) may be useful for some small NSCLC tumors that are near the outer edge of the lungs, especially in people who cannot tolerate surgery.

Chemotherapy

Patients with SCLC are frequently treated with chemotherapy. If the disease is in a limited stage, radiation therapy and rarely surgery may be used for SCLC.[20] The side effects of treatment with chemotherapy for SCLC include hair loss, mouth sores, loss of appetite, nausea, vomiting, diarrhea, constipation, immunodeficiency, easy bruising, and fatigue.[20]

Radiation Therapy

The two major types of radiation therapy include external beam radiation therapy (EBRT) and brachytherapy, a type of internal radiation therapy. The use of EBRT is less common than in the past because there are newer treatments that allow for greater accuracy.[8] When radiation is given with chemotherapy, the side effects are often worse.

Therapies to Consider

Further research is ongoing at various stages with herbal and natural preparations with astragalus, ginseng, pomegranate, rosemary, sage, parsley, oregano, and various combinations of Chinese herbs, although definitively conclusive evidence is not yet apparent.[21,23]

Techniques such as mindfulness-based stress reduction, group visit models for education and clinical evaluation, green space exposure, and engagement are being evaluated and studied further to assess their potential impact on health-related quality of life.

PREVENTION PRESCRIPTION

- Assess patient readiness for smoking cessation and assist them toward quitting smoking.
- Guide patients to avoid smoke-filled areas and secondhand smoke exposure.
- Educate patients on environmental and occupational hazards and provide resources that guide people on appropriate safety measures and precautions to minimize exposure.

- A diet rich in nonstarchy vegetables and fruits and low in red meat is recommended. Processed meats should be avoided.
- Regular physical exercise is recommended. Encourage people to get 150 minutes of moderately intense exercise weekly and 2 days of strength training.

THERAPEUTIC REVIEW

This review is based on the American College of Chest Physician's evidence-based clinical guidelines for complementary therapies and integrative medicine in lung cancer.[22]

NUTRITION

- In people who might develop lung cancer, a diet rich in nonstarchy vegetables and fruits is suggested to reduce the risk for lung cancer.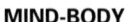
- In people who might develop lung cancer, limiting the consumption of a large amount of red and processed meat is suggested; lower meat consumption may reduce the risk for lung cancer.
- In patients undergoing treatment of lung cancer who have experienced weight loss, the addition of high-calorie and protein supplements (1.5 kcal/mL) as a nutritional adjunct is suggested to achieve weight stabilization.

- In patients with lung cancer who have sarcopenia, oral nutritional supplementation with n-3 fatty acids is suggested in order to improve nutritional status.

MIND-BODY

- Mind–body modalities are suggested as part of a multidisciplinary approach to reduce anxiety, mood disturbance, sleep disturbance, and improve quality of life (QOL).
- Mind–body modalities are suggested as part of a multidisciplinary approach to reduce acute or chronic pain.
- Mind–body modalities are suggested as part of a multidisciplinary approach to reduce anticipatory chemotherapy-induced nausea and vomiting.

ACUPUNCTURE

- In patients with cancer-related pain and peripheral neuropathy, acupuncture is suggested as an adjunct treatment in patients with inadequate control of symptoms.
- In patients having nausea and vomiting from either chemotherapy or radiation therapy, acupuncture or a related technique is suggested as an adjunct treatment option.

MASSAGE

- In lung cancer patients whose anxiety or pain is not adequately controlled by usual care, the addition of massage therapy performed by trained professionals is suggested as part of a multimodality cancer supportive care program.

YOGA

- Yoga, a movement-based mind–body modality, is suggested as part of a multidisciplinary approach to reduce fatigue and sleep disturbance while improving mood and QOL.

PULMONARY REHABILITATION EXERCISES

- In postsurgical lung cancer patients with compromised lung function, supervised exercise-based pulmonary rehabilitation is suggested to improve cardiorespiratory fitness and functional capacity.
- In advanced (inoperable) lung cancer patients receiving palliative anticancer therapy and with compromised lung function, supervised exercise-based pulmonary rehabilitation is suggested to improve cardiorespiratory fitness and functional capacity.

Key Web Resources

Resources for Patients

Lung Cancer Risk Assessment tool	http://aats.org/tools/lung-cancer/
Resource to Quit Smoking	http://www.smokefree.gov
Online Cancer Communities	http://acor.org

Information for Patients and Clinicians

National Cancer Institute	http://www.cancer.gov
American Cancer Society	http://www.cancer.org/cancer/lungcancer/index
National Center for Complementary and Integrative Health	https://nccih.nih.gov

Phone Apps (Apple store)

Tool for Healthcare Providers to Guide Screening	Lung Cancer Screening Guide with Lung-RADS
Resource for Lung Cancer Awareness and Support	Lung Cancer Foundation

REFERENCES

References are available online at ExpertConsult.com.

CHAPTER 80

PROSTATE CANCER

Richard T. Lee, MD

BACKGROUND

Prostate cancer accounts for nearly one-quarter of all newly diagnosed cancers in men and is the most common cancer found in them. It is also currently the second leading cause of cancer-related death among men in the United States.[1] Although approximately one in seven men will be diagnosed with prostate cancer, only a small percentage will die because of it.[2] Among men newly diagnosed with prostate cancer, more than 90% will live for 5 years and even past 10 years.[3] This demonstrates that for the majority of patients with prostate cancer, the disease may prove to be indolent, and they may eventually die of other causes.

The single most important risk factor is age as 95% of all cases occur in men aged 50 years and older.[4] Other risk factors include an African ancestry and family history (Box 80.1). Individuals with a strong family history such as two or more close relatives diagnosed under the age of 55 may want to consider further evaluation with a genetic counselor. Additionally, certain genetic syndromes, such as Lynch syndrome and *BRCA1/2* mutations, have also been linked with increased risk and may be associated with 5%–10% of all cases. Other factors that may change the biology of prostate cancer but not incidence include obesity, a diet high in meat or dairy, and smoking.[5]

BOX 80.1	Risk Factors for Prostate Cancer

Age
Family history
African American race
Obesity

PROSTATE CANCER SCREENING

The main function of the prostate is to produce seminal fluid. Symptoms of localized prostate cancer are similar to those of benign prostatic hyperplasia (BPH)—aka benign enlarged prostate. Men may experience increased urination, including at night, difficulty emptying the bladder, and difficulty starting urination.

Prostate cancer screening remains a controversial topic in the medical community as studies have conflicting data on the survival benefit of screening with a prostate-specific antigen (PSA). The United States Preventive Task Force recommends against routine screening with the PSA test, while the American Cancer Society (ACS) and American Urological Association (AUA) currently recommend the PSA for informed men who wish to be tested and have a life expectancy of at least 10 years. Specifically, the ACS recommends starting the screening at the age of 50 years for the general male population, 45 years for men with increased risk factors, and 40 years for men with a risk for hereditary prostate cancer (several first-degree relatives diagnosed before the age of 65 years). Although the PSA can detect prostate cancer at an early stage, the concern is that it will detect insignificant cancers that will not have an impact on overall survival and may adversely affect quality of life. The counter argument is that the portion of PSA-detected prostate cancers are clinically significant and, if left untreated, will lead to prostate cancer-specific death.[6]

Two large randomized controlled trials were conducted to test the impact of prostate cancer screening on prostate cancer–related mortality. The trials reached different conclusions. At 7 and 10 years, the Prostate, Lung, Colorectal, and Ovarian (PLCO) cancer screening trial failed to show a reduction in prostate cancer–related mortality in men who underwent prostate screening compared with the control arm.[7] Conversely, the European Randomized Study for Prostate Cancer (ERSPC) showed 20% fewer deaths in the screening arm than in the control arm after a mean of 8.8 years.[8] However, to prevent one prostate cancer–related death, 1410 men (or 1068 men who actually participated in screening) would have to be screened (NNS) and an additional 48 men would have to be treated (NNT). A further decrease in prostate cancer–specific mortality was seen among men who had been on the trial for 12 years (36% lower mortality; NNS = 500). The incidence of T3 and T4 tumors was 22% lower, and the incidence of M1 lesions was 41% lower in the screening arm of the ERSPC trial than in the control arm. Fundamental differences between the two studies may account for the divergent conclusions.

The ERSPC trial studied 162,000 men from seven European countries, whereas the PLCO trial studied 76,693 men from a single country. The majority of men (85%) with indications for biopsy in the ERSPC trial accepted a prostate biopsy. In contrast, only 30% of men in the screening arm in the PLCO study with an abnormal PSA level had a prostate biopsy. Moreover, in the PLCO trial, 52% of the men in the control arm underwent PSA screening during the study, which may explain why the incidence of and death rate due to prostate cancer were not significantly different between the screening and control arms.

Some data exist to further help identify patients with increased risk for prostate cancer by incorporating percentage-free PSA and PSA velocity.[6] Percentage-free PSA measures the ratio between total PSA (bound and unbound) and unbound or "free" PSA. This test is most useful for PSA values between 4 and 10 ng/mL. The lower the percentage, the higher the risk of prostate cancer.[9] For example, in men aged 50–64 years, if the percentage-free fraction is more than 25%, there is only a 5% risk of prostate cancer; however, if it is less than 10%, the risk of prostate cancer jumps to 56%. Unlike the total PSA value, the percentage-free PSA is affected by manipulation of the prostate gland. Therefore, the clinician should not order a percentage-free PSA test on the same day as rectal examination or within 24 hours of intercourse. PSA velocity (PSAV) is determined by measuring three PSA values at least 6 months apart. A PSAV of more than 0.75 ng/mL per year in men with PSA values between 4 and 10 ng/mL is associated with an increased risk of prostate cancer.[6] PSAV is also relevant for men with PSA values less than 4 ng/mL in which a PSAV of more than 0.4 ng/mL per year may be associated with adverse pathological features and a two-fold increase in significant prostate cancer.[10] The use of free PSA and PSAV is not considered a standard evaluation for screening of prostate cancer.

Overall, all men should have a discussion with their medical team about the controversy regarding screening that is performed using PSA detailing the risks and benefits. Patients with symptoms and/or a strong family history should consider having this discussion before age 50.

> Unlike the total PSA value, the percentage-free PSA is affected by manipulation of the prostate gland. Therefore the clinician should not order a percentage-free PSA test on the same day as rectal examination or within 24 hours of intercourse.

PROSTATE CANCER DIAGNOSIS AND STAGING

The finding of elevated PSA levels (>4 ng/mL) can be due to noncancerous reasons, such as prostatitis, BPH, and urinary tract infection. A digital rectal exam should also be performed if prostate cancer is suspected and will not affect the general PSA test. An elevated PSA more than 20 ng/mL significantly increases the likelihood of prostate cancer. Regardless of the PSA, the diagnosis of prostate cancer requires a tissue biopsy similar to most other cancers. Normally, a sample of 8–12 needle biopsies will be performed in order to sample different regions of the prostate gland.

The pathologists will examine the biopsy, and if prostate cancer is present, a Gleason scoring system is used to grade the aggressiveness of the histology seen (Table 80.1). The lowest score is 1 and the highest 5, with the pathologist providing two numbers—the most predominant grade seen and the highest grade in the entire sample. For example, a low-grade prostate cancer may be reported as 3+3 in 1 out of 10 cores, while a high-grade sample may have a score of 4+5 in 10 out of 10 cores. For precancerous lesions, the term high-grade prostatic intraepithelial neoplasia (HGPIN) is used, and these may require follow-up biopsies.

Further evaluation studies may be indicated depending on the risk of further spread to other tissues. Individuals with a high PSA (10–20 ng/mL) and a T1–2 or Gleason > 8 or T3–4 should undergo bone scan to search for

---

TABLE 80.1   T Categories (Clinical)

There are four categories for describing the local extent of a prostate tumor, ranging from T1 to T4. Most of these have subcategories as well.

T1	Your doctor cannot feel the tumor or see it with imaging such as transrectal ultrasound.
• T1a	Cancer is found incidentally (by accident) during a transurethral resection of the prostate (TURP) that was done for benign prostatic hyperplasia (BPH). Cancer is in no more than 5% of the tissue removed.
• T1b	Cancer is found during a TURP but is in more than 5% of the tissue removed.
• T1c	Cancer is found by needle biopsy that was done because of an increased PSA.
T2	Your doctor can feel the cancer with a digital rectal exam (DRE) or see it with imaging such as transrectal ultrasound, but it still appears to be confined to the prostate gland.
• T2a	The cancer is in one-half or less of only one side (left or right) of your prostate.
• T2b	The cancer is in more than half of only one side (left or right) of your prostate.
• T2c	The cancer is in both sides of your prostate.
T3	The cancer has grown outside your prostate and may have grown into the seminal vesicles.
• T3a	The cancer extends outside the prostate but not to the seminal vesicles.
• T3b	The cancer has spread to the seminal vesicles.
T4	The cancer has grown into tissues next to your prostate (other than the seminal vesicles), such as the urethral sphincter (muscle that helps control urination), rectum, bladder, and/or the wall of the pelvis.

N Categories

N categories describe whether the cancer has spread to nearby (regional) lymph nodes.

NX	Nearby lymph nodes were not assessed.
N0	The cancer has not spread to any nearby lymph nodes.
N1	The cancer has spread to one or more nearby lymph nodes.

M Categories

M categories describe whether the cancer has spread to distant parts of the body. The most common sites of prostate cancer spread are to the bones and to distant lymph nodes, although it can also spread to other organs such as the lungs and liver.

M0	The cancer has not spread past nearby lymph nodes.
M1	The cancer has spread beyond the nearby lymph nodes.
• M1a	The cancer has spread to distant (outside of the pelvis) lymph nodes.
• M1b	The cancer has spread to the bones.
• M1c	The cancer has spread to other organs such as lungs, liver, or brain (with or without spread to the bones).

bone metastases and/or a computed tomography (CT)/ magnetic resonance imaging (MRI) to search for lymph node involvement. Patients with symptoms consistent with metastases, such as bony pain, should also be considered for further imaging to complete staging evaluation. For patients with a more limited prognosis (<5 years) due to other comorbidities, a discussion should be conducted about whether to pursue further diagnostic tests, especially if these will not result in pursuit of treatment. Once the workup has been completed, staging can be accurately determined. This is critical as the staging will help determine the most appropriate therapy (Table 80.2).

TABLE 80.2 Stage Grouping

Once the T, N, and M categories have been determined, this information is combined, along with the Gleason score and prostate-specific antigen (PSA) level, in a process called *stage grouping*. If the Gleason score or PSA results are not available, the stage can be based on the T, N, and M categories. The overall stage is expressed in Roman numerals from I (the least advanced) to IV (the most advanced). This is done to help determine treatment options and the outlook for survival or cure (prognosis).

Stage I
One of the following applies

T1, N0, M0, Gleason score 6 or less, PSA less than 10
The doctor cannot feel the tumor or see it with an imaging test such as transrectal ultrasound (it was either found during a transurethral resection or diagnosed by needle biopsy done for a high PSA) [T1]. The cancer is still within the prostate and has not spread to nearby lymph nodes [N0] or elsewhere in the body [M0]. The Gleason score is 6 or less, and the PSA level is less than 10.

T2a, N0, M0, Gleason score 6 or less, PSA less than 10
The tumor can be felt by digital rectal exam or seen with imaging such as transrectal ultrasound and is in one-half or less of only one side (left or right) of the prostate [T2a]. The cancer is still within the prostate and has not spread to nearby lymph nodes [N0] or elsewhere in the body [M0]. The Gleason score is 6 or less, and the PSA level is less than 10.

Stage IIA
One of the following applies

T1, N0, M0, Gleason score of 7, PSA less than 20
The doctor cannot feel the tumor or see it with imaging such as transrectal ultrasound (it was either found during a transurethral resection or was diagnosed by needle biopsy done for a high PSA level) [T1]. The cancer has not spread to nearby lymph nodes [N0] or elsewhere in the body [M0]. The tumor has a Gleason score of 7. The PSA level is less than 20.

T1, N0, M0, Gleason score of 6 or less, PSA at least 10 but less than 20
The doctor cannot feel the tumor or see it with imaging such as transrectal ultrasound (it was either found during a transurethral resection or was diagnosed by needle biopsy done for a high PSA) [T1]. The cancer has not spread to nearby lymph nodes [N0] or elsewhere in the body [M0]. The tumor has a Gleason score of 6 or less. The PSA level is at least 10 but less than 20.

T2a or T2b, N0, M0, Gleason score of 7 or less, PSA less than 20
The tumor can be felt by digital rectal exam or seen with imaging such as transrectal ultrasound and is in only one side of the prostate [T2a or T2b]. The cancer has not spread to nearby lymph nodes [N0] or elsewhere in the body [M0]. It has a Gleason score of 7 or less. The PSA level is less than 20.

Stage IIB
One of the following applies

T2c, N0, M0, any Gleason score, any PSA
The tumor can be felt by digital rectal exam or seen with imaging such as transrectal ultrasound and is in both sides of the prostate [T2c]. The cancer has not spread to nearby lymph nodes [N0] or elsewhere in the body [M0]. The tumor can have any Gleason score, and the PSA can be of any value.

T1 or T2, N0, M0, any Gleason score, PSA of 20 or more
The cancer has not yet spread outside the prostate. It may (or may not) be felt by digital rectal exam or seen with imaging such as transrectal ultrasound [T1 or T2]. The cancer has not spread to nearby lymph nodes [N0] or elsewhere in the body [M0]. The tumor can have any Gleason score. The PSA level is at least 20.

T1 or T2, N0, M0, Gleason score of 8 or higher, any PSA
The cancer has not yet spread outside the prostate. It may (or may not) be felt by digital rectal exam or seen with imaging such as transrectal ultrasound [T1 or T2]. The cancer has not spread to nearby lymph nodes [N0] or elsewhere in the body [M0]. The Gleason score, is 8 or higher. The PSA can be of any value.

Stage III

T3, N0, M0, any Gleason score, any PSA
The cancer has grown outside the prostate and may have spread to the seminal vesicles [T3], but it has not spread to nearby lymph nodes [N0] or elsewhere in the body [M0]. The tumor can have any Gleason score, and the PSA can be of any value.

Stage IV
One of the following applies

T4, N0, M0, any Gleason score, any PSA
The cancer has grown into tissues next to the prostate (other than the seminal vesicles), such as the urethral sphincter (muscle that helps control urination), rectum, bladder, and/or the wall of the pelvis [T4]. The cancer has not spread to nearby lymph nodes [N0] or elsewhere in the body [M0]. The tumor can have any Gleason score, and the PSA can be of any value.

Any T, N1, M0, any Gleason score, any PSA
The tumor may or may not be growing into tissues near the prostate [any T]. The cancer has spread to nearby lymph nodes [N1] but has not spread elsewhere in the body [M0]. The tumor can have any Gleason score, and the PSA can be of any value.

Any T, any N, M1, any Gleason score, any PSA
The cancer may or may not be growing into tissues near the prostate [any T] and may or may not have spread to nearby lymph nodes [any N]. It has spread to other more distant sites in the body [M1]. The tumor can have any Gleason score, and the PSA can be of any value.

INTEGRATIVE THERAPY

An integrative approach to prostate cancer aims to enhance care for the patient by implementation of a comprehensive, evidence-based treatment plan that will lead to optimal outcomes both in regards to the treatment of the cancer as well as the health and wellbeing of the patient. At the core remain conventional treatment approaches that continue to lead to improvement in cure and/or disease control for the patient, depending on the stage. Treatment planning should also include consideration of comorbidities and life expectancy. Patients with stage I prostate cancer are often monitored as they may not require surgery, especially if they have other active comorbidities and/or limited life expectancy of less than 10 years. Intermediate stage prostate cancers (stage II–III) are highly curable, and treatment should be discussed unless the patient has a limited life expectancy. Patients with advanced prostate cancers (stage IV) should be offered treatment as the disease is likely to impact survival and quality of life.

Conventional Treatments

Observation

Observation and active surveillance is a reasonable approach for patients with early-stage, low-grade prostate cancer as indicated by a T1 or T2a lesion with a Gleason ≤ 6 and a PSA < 10 ng/mL. This is especially true for patients that have a life expectancy of <10 years due to other comorbidities. These patients are often reevaluated every 6–12 months unless other symptoms arise. Such patients should be encouraged to incorporate other aspects of an integrative approach focusing on optimizing their health and well-being, which may have an impact on disease trajectory.

Definitive Treatment—Surgery and Radiation

Patients with early to intermediate stage prostate cancer (stage I–III) have a very good chance for cure, with overall 5-year survival rates more than 95%. These patients should undergo evaluation for definitive curative therapy with surgery or radiation. Both options have essentially equivalent outcomes in terms of disease control, although they each have their own side-effect profile. Surgery involves a radical prostatectomy (RP) and pelvic lymph node dissection (PLND) that will remove the prostate and local lymph nodes. Patients need to undergo presurgical evaluation to determine if they are good surgical candidates. Radiation therapy is available in two forms—external beam radiotherapy (EBRT) and brachytherapy. The latter involves the placement of radioactive seeds into the prostate. Each of these therapies has its own side-effect profile and involves different short- and long-term risks, with erectile dysfunction, incontinence, gastrointestinal side effects due to EBRT, skin changes, and hematuria being some of the most common. Additionally, some patients may have difficulty undergoing 4–6 weeks of EBRT, while RP + PLND and brachytherapy may only require a shorter treatment period. Most patients should undergo evaluation by both a surgeon and radiation oncologist to help make an informed decision about what option would be best for that individual.

Hormonal Therapy

A varietal of hormonal therapies are used to help reduce the risk of recurrence and control metastatic disease as prostate cancer is very sensitive to changes in testosterone levels. The most common initial therapy is called androgen deprivation therapy (ADT) and typically involves luteinizing hormone–releasing hormone (LHRH) for which there are several agonist/antagonists. These essentially will cause the circulating level of testosterone to go <50 ng/dL (normal: 250–1000 ng/dL) and for almost all patients, lead to disease control. Patients with high-risk, intermediate-stage prostate cancer may be provided LHRH therapy for 4–6 months after EBRT. For patients with metastatic disease (stage IV), LHRH is considered the standard first-line therapy.

Abiraterone is another hormonal therapy that blocks testosterone production by inhibiting the CYP17 enzyme and is commonly used when resistance to an LHRH therapy develops, which is referred to as castrate-resistant prostate cancer (CRPC). Antiandrogens, such as bicalutamide, are often combined with LHRH therapy when CRPC develops. Enzalutamide is a newer agent that is an antiandrogen and blocks signaling of the androgen receptor. Other hormonal therapies include corticosteroids, ketoconazole, and estrogen.

The low levels of testosterone induced by hormonal therapy may cause a variety of side effects, including hot flashes, impotence, decreased libido, osteoporosis, anemia, loss of muscle mass, weight gain, fatigue, and mood changes. Many patients will be on hormonal therapy for months to years and thus are at risk for developing metabolic changes such as obesity, insulin resistance, and elevated triglycerides. Patients may want to consider integrative therapies to help mitigate many of these side effects, and these are discussed later in this chapter.

Chemotherapy

In the past, chemotherapy was usually reserved until after resistance to hormonal therapies, although based on new data, chemotherapy is now often considered much earlier in patients with aggressive metastatic disease.[11] More commonly used chemotherapies include docetaxel, cabazitaxel, and mitoxantrone with prednisone. These are intravenously administered on an every 3-week schedule. As with other chemotherapies, these may lead to fatigue, nausea, vomiting, low blood counts, and hair thinning. A trial of 4–6 cycles is usually provided, followed by restaging studies to determine response to treatment.

Immunotherapy

Sipuleucel-T is a cancer vaccine specific for prostate cancer and has been shown to prolong survival for approximately 4 months. This therapy involves collection of blood from patients, to obtain their white cells, and then shipping it to the laboratory for processing. Several weeks later after the activation of white cells, the patients receive three infusions of their own activated white cells, each 2 weeks apart. Patients may experience side effects similar to those experienced after transfusion, including chills, fevers, and fatigue.

Lifestyle Therapy

A pilot study of men with prostate cancer examining the effects of an intensive integrative program of diet, exercise, and mind-body approaches was able to find biological changes that would impact the progression of prostate cancer.[12-14]

Smoking

Among other carcinogens, tobacco contains cadmium, a heavy metal that may increase prostate cancer risk.[15] Although data for smoking and an increased risk of prostate cancer are conflicting, smoking increases the risk of lung, bladder, and other epithelial cancers, and it may induce a more aggressive form of prostate cancer. According to a meta-analysis of 24 prospective cohort studies, the heaviest smokers had a 24%–30% greater risk of death from prostate cancer compared with nonsmokers.[16]

The message is clear: do not smoke.

Physical Fitness and Obesity

A growing body of research indicates that prostate cancer biology may respond to specific integrative therapies, such as exercise. Additionally, some of the side effects experienced by prostate cancer patients can be treated using nonpharmacological integrative therapies. At a minimum, patients with prostate cancer should focus on guidelines published by the ACS and American Institute for Cancer Research (AICR) to help reduce side effects and improve quality of life.[5,17] A provocative pilot study in 10 men demonstrated that a plant-based diet in the context of mindfulness-based stress reduction delayed PSA doubling time from 6.5 to 17.7 months.[18] Regardless of the food source, excessive calorie intake promotes obesity, which increases premature mortality and overall cancer-related death rates, including prostate cancer.[19,20] This was also shown in a study looking at the role of weight and risk of death after diagnosis showing obese men with prostate cancer had a 34% increase in the risk of death.[21]

Nutrition

The role of nutrition is growing, and several cancers are known to be impacted, both positively and negatively, by certain types of foods. Additionally, specific foods are currently being researched as potential therapies for prostate cancer; however, the research remains preliminary. Thus incorporation of these food groups is recommended rather than pursuing specific processed supplements. In general, the ACS and AICR guidelines focus on several key components of a healthy diet, and these should be followed by every prostate cancer survivor.

Limiting Red Meat. Limit consumption of red meats (such as beef, pork, and lamb) and avoid processed meats. Men in the highest quartile for red meat consumption have a significantly higher risk of being diagnosed with prostate cancer and a 30% increased chance for development of advanced disease. Processing of meat and barbecuing and grilling of meat is also associated with an increased risk of total and advanced prostate cancer.[22]

Limit Consumption of Energy-Dense Foods. Although no known link exists between sugary drinks like sodas and prostate cancer, increased intake of these energy-dense foods may lead to obesity. Thus the AICR recommends reduction of these types of foods to prevent obesity, which is a risk factor for several cancers.

Eat a Variety of Vegetables, Fruits, Whole Grains, and Legumes. Higher vegetable intake, especially cruciferous vegetables, is associated with decreased prostate cancer risk.[23,24] More recent studies show that a classic Western style diet is associated with 2.5× higher risk of prostate cancer–specific death, and similarly, those following a diet high in fruits and vegetables have a 36% lower risk of death.[25] Encourage at least five servings of fruits and vegetables daily.

Soy Protein. Soy protein isoflavones, most notably genistein, inhibit prostate cancer cell growth in vitro and in vivo by promoting apoptosis; by blocking beta-estrogen receptor activity in the prostate; by inhibiting angiogenesis and endothelial cell proliferation; and by blocking 5-α-reductase, aromatase, and tyrosine-specific protein kinase activity.[26-28] Even though the age-adjusted incidence of latent prostate cancer in native Japanese and American men is roughly the same, clinical prostate cancer is 10 times higher in American men. Researchers attribute some of this discrepancy to dietary differences. A typical American diet is high in saturated animal fat but low in fruits, vegetables, fish, and soy protein, whereas a typical Japanese diet is the reverse. Japanese men consume substantially more soy protein and fish but less saturated fat from dairy and red meat than American men.[27] According to one report, Japanese men have isoflavone concentrations 30 times higher in the urine and more than 100 times higher in the blood than Western men.[29] A 16-year-long prospective health study showed that men who consumed several glasses of soy milk daily lowered their risk of prostate cancer by 70%.[30] For men with prostate cancer, higher doses of daily soy consumption may provide additional protection. Researchers found that men taking 100 mg of soy isoflavones twice daily slowed the growth of an aggressive form of prostate cancer called androgen-insensitive prostate cancer by 35% and slowed overall cancer growth by 84%.[31,32] Other studies have found promising, although limited, results in patients with prostate cancer.[33-35]

Replacing cow's milk with soy milk can be an effective strategy to reduce the risk of prostate cancer.

Soy protein is available in a variety of food items including tofu, tempeh, soy milk, soy cheese, textured soy foods, and soy flour. Soy protein yields up to 3 mg of isoflavones per gram and provides five times as much protein as wheat and 25 times as much protein as beef. Patients with prostate cancer should consider incorporating soy into their diet as it may have beneficial effects for prevention and disease control.

Lycopene. Lycopene is a cancer-fighting antioxidant vitamin that gives tomatoes, strawberries, and watermelon their rosy color. Although not all studies have found that lycopene confers a protective effect against prostate cancer,[36] data from a variety of case-control and large prospective studies focusing on dietary assessment show a beneficial effect, especially against advanced prostate cancer.[37-39] According to one report, men who consumed tomato products four times weekly reduced their prostate cancer risk by 20% and those who ate 10 or more helpings weekly reduced their risk by 45%.[40] Studies have also been conducted in men with prostate cancer, with some indicating an ability to impact progression.[41-43]

Lycopene is found within the cells of tomato and should be cooked to help release lycopene and increase bioavailability. Other sources of lycopene include papaya, watermelon, pink guava, and pink grapefruit. Men with prostate cancer should consider incorporating foods with lycopene.

Pomegranate. Pomegranate juice contains polyphenolic compounds, especially ellagic acid, which exert antiproliferative and antimetastatic effects on prostate cancer cells. According to a phase II study of 46 men with recurrent prostate cancer after surgery or radiation therapy, consumption of 8 oz of pomegranate juice daily significantly slowed PSA doubling time from 15.6 months to 54.7 months.[44] Pomegranate extract also inhibits prostate cancer cell growth.[26] Additional follow-up studies have shown mixed results with the randomized placebo-controlled study showing no difference between groups.[45-47]

Men with prostate cancer may want to consider incorporating either the fruit or the juice into their diet. Those with diabetes will need to be cautious due to the sugar content.

Green Tea (*Camellia sinensis*). Green tea contains a variety of antioxidants called catechins that have antitumor activity against prostate cancer cells. In vitro and in vivo studies have shown that green tea can inhibit prostate cancer cell growth by inducing apoptosis, activating tumor suppressor genes, and mitigating the activity of stimulatory messenger molecules. According to preliminary data, the beneficial effect of green tea may be dose related, and it may be more effective against early-stage prostate cancer as opposed to end-stage disease.[26] Sixty men with high-grade prostate intraepithelial neoplasia who took 200 mg three times a day of mixed green tea catechins had an 80% reduction in progression to prostate cancer as compared to the placebo group.[48,49] However, two phase II clinical trials in men with prostate cancer did not find any clinical benefit.[50,51]

Green tea has been found to cause liver toxicity when taken in large, concentrated doses.[52] Additionally, there has been shown to be medication interactions with bortezomib, a chemotherapy for multiple myeloma.[53] Patients with liver disease or multiple myeloma should be cautious about ingesting green tea. Otherwise, drinking green tea in moderation (two to three cups daily) may have benefit for those with HGPIN and for prevention.

Flaxseed. Flaxseed contains a variety of compounds, and lignans and α-linoleic acids are actively being evaluated for potential benefits. Lignans are thought to have antioxidant properties and may alter testosterone levels.[54] A small phase II study examining dietary flaxseed in prostate cancer patients found significant decreases in proliferation rates among men randomized to flaxseed.[55] More studies are needed to understand this potential outcome. Incorporation of natural flaxseed into the diet is reasonable to consider.

Alcohol. Alcohol yields 9 calories per gram, the same as fat. Therefore, excessive alcohol consumption increases energy intake and promotes obesity. Nevertheless, only a few studies have found a direct association between alcohol consumption and prostate cancer risk. According to one study, excessive drinking of alcohol—more than 96 oz of alcohol weekly (about 10 drinks)—tripled the risk for development of prostate cancer.[56] On the other hand, moderate consumption of red wine may confer protection against prostate cancer. Red wine is a rich source of resveratrol, a polyphenol that induces apoptosis and modulates androgen receptor function in prostate cancer cell lines.[57] Researchers reported that men who consumed 4 oz of red wine four times weekly experienced a 50% reduction in prostate cancer and a 60% reduction in the diagnosis of Gleason 8 disease.[58]

If consumed at all, limit alcoholic drinks to two for men and one for women a day.

Limit Salt. Several studies have found that total salt consumption, especially that linked to preserved foods, increases the risk for cancer, specifically gastric cancer.[59] Although no strong link exists with prostate cancer, salt intake should be monitored.

Limit consumption of salty foods and foods processed with salt (sodium).

Physical Activity

Although data are inconclusive, physical activity may reduce prostate cancer risk by lowering body fat concentration and by improving use of insulin-like growth factor 1 (IGF-1).[15] IGF-1 has mitogenic and antiapoptotic effects on normal and malignant prostate cells. In one study, men with the highest quartile of IGF-1 levels had a 4.3-fold greater risk for prostate cancer than those in the lowest quartile.[60] Exercise can also lessen the risk for development of aggressive or advanced prostate cancer. Data from the Health Professionals Follow-Up Study show that men older than 65 years who exercise vigorously at least 3 hours per week in activities such as running, biking, and swimming have a 70% lower risk of being diagnosed with high-grade, advanced, or metastatic prostate cancer.[61] Similarly, a British study of 45,887 men aged 45–79 years showed that men with the highest lifetime physical activity had a 16% overall lower incidence of prostate cancer as well as lower risk of advanced prostate cancer compared with men with the lowest activity. Each 30-minute increment of activity reduced the risk of prostate cancer by 7%.[62] For men with prostate cancer, data is also growing regarding the benefits including survival. Kenfield et al. published a study following 2705 nonmetastatic prostate cancer patients and found those exercising vigorously ≥3 hours had 61% decreased risk of prostate cancer-specific death.[63] Additionally, this same cohort demonstrated improvements in quality of life through increased activity.[64] The ACS and AICR guidelines should be followed.

Men should incorporate moderate-intensity exercise (e.g., walking, jogging, and swimming) for a total time of 150 minutes per week.

Data from the Health Professionals Follow-Up Study show that men older than 65 years who exercise vigorously at least 3 hours per week in activities such as running, biking, and swimming have a 70% lower risk of being diagnosed with high-grade, advanced, or metastatic prostate cancer.[61]

Mind-Body Medicine

Psychosocial interventions can improve the quality of life for cancer patients including simple interventions such as meditation, yoga, and support groups. In a study of men undergoing RP, those randomized to a stress management intervention showed improved emotional and physical symptoms, and a correlative study found that subjects maintained immune function better than those in the control group.[65,66]

Men with prostate cancer should consider utilizing a regular relaxation technique.

Acupuncture

Acupuncture involves the placement of solid, sterile, stainless steel needles into various points on the body to help manage different symptoms. Clinical studies have found acupuncture may help treat nausea caused by chemotherapy drugs and surgical anesthesia and help treat both postoperative and chronic pain in cancer patients.[67] A growing number of clinical trials, both controlled and uncontrolled, suggests that acupuncture is beneficial for hot flashes experienced by men on ADT.[68]

Supplements

Vitamin E (Mixed Tocopherols) and Selenium

Secondary endpoints from several key epidemiological and prospective cohort studies suggested that vitamin E and selenium supplementation could decrease prostate cancer incidence and mortality, especially among smokers.[69,70] Accordingly, the Southwest Oncology Group

in collaboration with others sponsored a phase III randomized, placebo-controlled trial of 35,553 men to determine whether taking selenium (200 mcg/day from L-selenomethionine) and vitamin E (400 units/day of all-rac-tocopheryl acetate), either alone or in combination, to determine if these supplements provided a protective benefit against prostate cancer-the Selenium and Vitamin E Cancer Prevention Trial (SELECT).[71] The study was terminated prematurely after 4 years because of concern about a small but significant increased incidence of prostate cancer in the vitamin E-alone arm and a small but insignificant increase in prostate cancer in the combined vitamin E and selenium arm and the selenium-alone arm. Compared with placebo, the hazard ratios for prostate cancer were 1.13 in the vitamin E-alone cohort, 1.05 in the selenium and vitamin E cohort, and 1.04 in the selenium-alone cohort. There was also a nonsignificant increase in the risk for development of diabetes (relative risk [RR], 1.07) in the selenium-alone arm.

On the basis of these data, supplementation with vitamin E and selenium for the prevention of prostate cancer is not recommended.

Vitamin D

Vitamin D is a steroid hormone that can be acquired from the diet and dietary supplements, or it can be synthesized in the skin from 7-dehydrocholesterol in response to ultraviolet radiation. Ultraviolet irradiation of ergosterol from yeast yields vitamin D_2. Ultraviolet irradiation of 7-dehydrocholesterol from lanolin yields vitamin D_3. Although there is no consensus on the optimal blood level of vitamin D, deficiency is defined as a 25-hydroxyvitamin D level of less than 30 ng/mL. According to several studies, 40%–100% of men and women still living in the community are deficient in vitamin D.[72,73] Both prospective and retrospective epidemiological studies have shown that vitamin D deficiency is associated with an increased risk for development of prostate cancer.[72,74] Vitamin D is involved in the regulation of more than 200 genes, including genes that are responsible for cellular proliferation, differentiation, apoptosis, and angiogenesis. Vitamin D decreases cellular proliferation of normal and cancer cells and promotes their terminal differentiation. It also inhibits prostate cancer invasion and metastasis.[26,72] Vitamin D intoxication is extremely rare, but it can occur with excessive consumption of vitamin D. Oral supplementation with vitamin D should be monitored with periodical laboratory testing for 25-OH vitamin D levels.

Consider checking vitamin D 25-OH level and supplement the diet with sufficient vitamin D_3 to maintain a vitamin D level of at least 30 ng/mL for bone health. Further supplementation may be required if the level remains low. A rough rule of thumb is to add 1000 IU of D_3 to raise serum levels by 8–10 ng/mL.

Multivitamins

Researchers examined a cohort of 1,063,023 adult Americans between the years of 1982 and 1989 and compared the mortality of vitamin nonusers with that of users of multivitamins alone; vitamin A, C, or E alone; and vitamin A, C, or E in combination. Surprisingly, the risk of dying of prostate cancer significantly increased with more than 5 years of multivitamin use (RR, 1.31). Furthermore, male smokers who used vitamins A, E, or C alone or in combination with multivitamins had a greater risk of fatal cancer (RR, 1.44 and RR, 1.58) than that of vitamin nonusers.[75] Data from the National Institutes of Health–American Associations of Retired Persons (AARP) Diet and Health Study showed that men who consumed multivitamins more than seven times per week had a significantly increased risk of advanced or fatal prostate cancer (RR, 1.32 and RR, 1.98).[76] Neither the ACS nor the AICR guidelines recommend any supplements at this time for cancer prevention.

Therefore multivitamin consumption is not recommended for the prevention or treatment of prostate cancer. Aim to receive all vitamins and minerals through food.

Hormone-Altering Medications and Supplements

Injudicious use of dehydroepiandrosterone (DHEA), androstenedione, and human growth hormone may increase the risk for development of prostate cancer or promote the growth of existing prostate cancer by increasing IGF-1 levels.[77,78] Although testosterone has not been proven to cause prostate cancer, testosterone is a potent promoter of benign and malignant prostate cell growth. Chondroitin is used as a marker for prostate cancer as there are higher levels in men with it. There is also limited data showing concern that it may promote metastasis and/or recurrence of prostate cancer.[79]

Therefore, men should avoid taking these supplements or androgen replacement therapy unless it is medically indicated, especially men at increased risk for prostate cancer.

Omega-3 Fatty Acids

Although the relationship is complex and data are conflicting, animal data have shown that excess dietary omega-6 polyunsaturated acids generally stimulate tumor growth, whereas omega-3 polyunsaturated fatty acids, especially from fish, and monounsaturated omega-9 fatty acids from olive oil have the opposite effect.[80-82] More recent epidemiological studies indicate conflicting data on whether or not n-3 fatty acids are beneficial or harmful.[83] Until further research clarifies this relationship, patients should avoid taking concentrated supplements of omega-3 fatty acids.

Pomi-T

A recent study randomized 199 men with localized prostate cancer to a supplement containing pomegranate, green tea, broccoli, and turmeric and demonstrated changes in PSA rise favoring the Pomi-T arm. Further research is needed to determine if this supplement will prove to be beneficial for prostate cancer patients.[83a]

Pharmaceuticals for Prevention

5α-Reductase Inhibitors—Finasteride and Dutasteride

Studies have examined the ability of 5α-reductase inhibitors (finasteride and dutasteride) to prevent prostate cancer. In contrast to finasteride, dutasteride inhibits both type 1 and type 2, 5α-reductase enzymes. Type 1, 5α-reductase enzyme predominates in prostate cancer, whereas type 2 enzyme predominates in normal and hyperplastic prostate tissue. The Prostate Cancer Prevention Trial (PCPT) randomized 18,882 men to a 7-year course of placebo or 5 mg of the 5α-reductase type 2 enzyme inhibitor finasteride daily.[84] The results showed a 24.4% prevalence rate of prostate cancer in the placebo arm (1147/4692) versus an 18.4% prevalence in the finasteride arm (803/4368). Although there were a higher number of high-grade tumors in the finasteride group, researchers attribute this difference to an artifact of trial design. The Reduction by Dutasteride of Prostate Cancer Events (REDUCE) trial was a randomized, double-blind, placebo-controlled phase III trial of 8000 men from 42 different countries between the ages of 50 and 75 years with a PSA level of 2.5–10 ng/mL with normal findings on prestudy prostate biopsy. The REDUCE trial data showed that dutasteride reduced the risk of prostate cancer during 4 years by 23% compared with placebo.[85]

Nonsteroidal Antiinflammatory Drugs

Aspirin reduces inflammation by inhibiting cyclooxygenase-1 (COX-1) and cyclooxygenase-2 (COX-2) enzymes. According to a systematic review of the literature and meta-analysis, long-term consumption of aspirin (5 years or more) was inversely associated with the risk for development of prostate cancer. The risk reduction was more pronounced for advanced prostate cancer (odds ratio [OR] = 0.7) than for total prostate cancer (OR = 0.9).[86] A cohort study of 70,144 men reported similar findings; regular use of nonsteroidal antiinflammatory drugs (NSAIDs) decreased the risk of prostate cancer by 18% and the risk of advanced prostate cancer by 33%.[87] Taking one 81-mg baby aspirin daily may be sufficient to reduce prostate cancer risk.

Suppression of COX-2 activity with COX-2–selective inhibitors may also reduce prostate cancer risk.[88-90] Although rofecoxib was withdrawn because of adverse cardiovascular side effects, high doses of the COX-2 inhibitor celecoxib markedly slowed PSA doubling times in men whose PSA level started to rise after local curative therapy without causing any serious adverse cardiovascular effects.[91]

These medications are still undergoing evaluation and currently not approved for prostate cancer prevention. These should not be taken without further discussion with the patient and entire medical team to review the risks and benefits. Patients with an elevated risk for prostate cancer (e.g., strong family history) may want to discuss the risks or benefits of these medications. Patients taking anticoagulation or antiplatelet medication and those with a history of heart, renal, or gastrointestinal disease should check with their health care provider before taking aspirin or NSAIDs. The side effects from finasteride and dutasteride include decreased libido and gynecomastia.

PREVENTION PRESCRIPTION

- For men at normal risk, discuss the pros and cons of PSA screening at 50 years and provide information on prostate cancer prevention.
- For men at high risk, a careful discussion at 40 years regarding routine screening should include the opposing recommendations from the ACS and United States Preventative Task Force.
- Encourage exercise for 30 minutes or longer at least five times weekly.
- Encourage intake of five to nine servings of fruits and vegetables daily.
- Encourage normal body weight with a goal BMI of 18.5–25.

- Avoid hormone-altering medications such as DHEA, androstenedione, human growth hormone, and testosterone, unless medically indicated.
- Limit meat consumption.
- Limit alcohol intake.
- Emphasize that patients should avoid tobacco products.
- Incorporate soy into the diet.
- Moderate natural dietary intake of soy, green tea, flax seed, lycopene, and pomegranate.
- Incorporate relaxation techniques regularly.

THERAPEUTIC REVIEW

Men with a diagnosis of prostate should focus on a comprehensive approach to their care, incorporating standard treatments along with optimizing their health and minimizing side effects from treatment

NUTRITION

- Follow the ACS and AICR guidelines on nutrition. Focus on increasing fruits and vegetables (minimum five servings per day), limiting red meat, alcohol, and energy-dense foods like sugary drinks. Consider incorporating foods like soy, flaxseed, drinking green tea (two to three cups per day), lycopene from cooked tomatoes, and pomegranates. Refer receptive patients to a qualified dietitian.

EXERCISE

- Exercise for 30 minutes or longer five times weekly.
- Consider referral to a physical trainer or physical therapist, especially for patients with physical impairments or risks such as bone metastases.

SUPPLEMENTS

- Check vitamin D levels, and if <30 ng/mL, consider supplementation with vitamin D_3, especially important for patients with bone metastases.
- Avoid any kind of hormonal supplements like DHEA, human growth hormone, androstenedione, chondroitin sulfate, and supplemental androgens.

MIND-BODY

- Discuss mindfulness-based stress reduction techniques, especially for men with high risk, and refer receptive patients to a qualified professional.

ACUPUNCTURE

- Consider using acupuncture to help with symptoms of pain, nausea, or hot flashes.

TOBACCO

- If currently using any form of tobacco, assess for willingness to quit and consider referral to a tobacco treatment program.

ACKNOWLEDGMENT

The author would like to thank Dr. Mark McClure for providing information from a previous edition of *Integrative Medicine*, which informed this chapter.

Key Web Resources

A comprehensive prostate cancer resource, sponsored by the Prostate Cancer Research Institute	http://www.prostate-cancer.org
Prostate cancer home page of the National Cancer Institute	http://www.cancer.gov/cancertopics/types/prostate
An online resource of cancer information for the patient with cancer	http://www.aicr.org/reduce-your-cancer-risk/recommendations-for-cancer-prevention/
ACS resource regarding prostate cancer and cancer prevention guidelines	http://www.cancer.org/cancer/prostatecancer/index

REFERENCES

References are available online at ExpertConsult.com.

CHAPTER 81

COLORECTAL CANCER

Srivani Sridhar, MD

NATURAL HISTORY

Most colorectal cancers begin as a noncancerous polyp, which can be detected during a routine screening colonoscopy. From the time the first abnormal cells start to grow into polyps, it takes 10 to15 years for them to develop into colorectal cancer. Adenomatous polyps have a higher rate of turning into cancer, while hyperplastic and inflammatory polyps are typically not precancerous.[2] Dysplasia is a type of precancerous condition that is usually seen in people with long-standing ulcerative colitis or Crohn's disease as these conditions cause chronic inflammation of the colon. If cancer forms in a polyp or dysplastic area, it can invade the wall of the colon or rectum locally and progress via lymphatic or hematogenous spread. Patients with oligometastatic disease, where only one or two lesions are present in an organ such as the lung or liver, can still experience long-term disease–free survival after treatment.

INCIDENCE AND PREVALENCE

The lifetime risk for developing colorectal cancer is about 1 in 20 (5%), and it is 60% more common in developed countries. This risk is slightly lower in women than in men, but it is the third leading cause of cancer and second leading cause of cancer-related deaths in the United States.[1] Survival rates have been improving, which is thought to from more consistent screenings, improvement of treatment regimens, and the adoption of healthier eating habits.

SCREENING

Regular screening can detect colorectal cancer early when it is most likely to be curable. In many people, screening can also prevent colorectal cancer altogether because polyps can be found and removed before they have the chance to turn into cancer. Colorectal cancer screening tools include the guaiac-based fecal occult blood test (gFOBT) and fecal immunochemical test (FIT), both of which are used to detect blood in the stool; a stool DNA test to check for polyps and cancer; and sigmoidoscopy, colonoscopy, and computed tomography (CT) colonography, which directly visualize the polyp or cancer. The frequencies of screening are as follows: gFOBT/FIT annually, stool DNA test every 3 years, sigmoidoscopy every 5 years with gFOBT/FIT every 3 years, or colonoscopy every 10 years. One in three adults aged 50–75 years has not been screened for colorectal cancer as recommended by the U.S. Preventive Services Task Force. Symptoms of colorectal cancer are nonspecific and include blood in the stool, persistent abdominal pain, and unexpected weight loss but may often only present late into the disease. It is imperative that clinicians encourage patients to pursue routine colorectal cancer screening.

> The number needed to screen (NNS) to detect one case of colon cancer is 154 for colonoscopy, 166 for stool DNA panel, and 208 for fecal immunochemical testing.[3]

RISK FACTORS

Regular screening and removal of polyps with colonoscopy reduces the risk of developing colorectal cancer by up to 90%. People with a first-degree relative who has had colorectal cancer have two to three times the risk for developing the disease compared with those with no family history. About 20% of all colorectal cancer patients have a close relative who was diagnosed with the disease. About 5% of individuals with colorectal cancer have a genetic syndrome that causes the disease. These individuals should have increased screening frequency based on their risk[4] (Table 81.1).

PRIMARY AND SECONDARY PREVENTION

The modifiable risk factors listed in the following require recommendations to lower risk. However, initiation and maintenance of comprehensive diet and lifestyle changes may not be easy to follow. Clinicians can use motivational interviewing tools to guide people on how to follow sustainable health practices. Up to 70% of colorectal cancers can be prevented by diet and lifestyle changes[11] (Table 81.2).

Integrative Therapy

Nutrition

Part of the reason for the difference in colorectal cancer incidence in other countries compared with that in the United States is the difference in diet. People in other countries, especially Asia, tend to have diets higher in fiber, fish, and vegetables and lower in red meat and processed foods.

TABLE 81.1 Risk Factors

Increase in risk:
- Age older than 50 years
- African-American race
- Personal or family history of adenomatous polyps or colon cancer
- Inflammatory bowel disease (Crohn's or ulcerative colitis)
- Genetic syndromes: familial adenomatous polyposis or hereditary nonpolyposis colon cancer, and others
- Type 2 diabetes
- Obesity[5-7]
- Smoking and high alcohol use
- Red and processed meats[8-10]

TABLE 81.2 Modifiable Lifestyle Factors That Decrease Risk

- High-fiber diet[12-13] consisting of fruits, vegetables (especially cruciferous),[14] and omega-3 fats[15]
- Moderate exercise 150 minutes per week or vigorous exercise 75 minutes per week[16,17]
- Maintenance of a healthy body weight (body mass index [BMI] less than 25)[18]
- Limiting alcohol use no more than the recommended maximum daily allowance
- Avoiding tobacco use
- Maintaining good glycemic control by avoiding hyperinsulinemia

Fiber

A large meta-analysis of prospective studies found that increased fiber in the diet contributes to a lower incidence of colon cancer, with dietary fiber, cereal fiber, and whole grains showing the greatest reductions. A linear inverse relationship indicated that every 10 grams of fiber intake resulted in a 10% risk reduction for colon cancer.[12] Another analysis found no association between fiber intake and rectal cancer incidence.[19] It is recommended that one consume at least 30 grams of dietary fiber a day.

Omega-3 Fatty Acids

Omega-3 fatty acids are found in cold-water oily fish. Their activity against colorectal cancer involves modulation of cyclooxygenase (COX)-2 activity, alteration of cell surface receptor function, an increase in oxidative stress, and the creation of antiinflammatory lipid mediators.[20] Epidemiological studies have shown varied results with regard to the influence of omega-3 fatty acids on colorectal cancer risk. A meta-analysis found up to a 22% nonsignificant reduction in colon cancer risk between the highest and lowest fish consumption groups when the difference was seven fish meals per month.[21] A subsequent meta-analysis found that the colorectal cancer risk reduction from omega-3 fatty acids was only significant in men, with the reduction reaching borderline significance with marine omega-3 intake.[22] Because of the amount of mercury in fish, no more than two to three servings of cold-water fish are recommended per week. Fish high in omega-3 fatty acids are wild salmon, mackerel, sardines, anchovies, black cod, and albacore tuna. The omega-3 fatty acid content of 100 grams of salmon and sardines is between 1 and 2 grams. One may also consider taking 1000 mg of omega-3 fatty acids daily in supplement form.

Soy

Soy foods, which consist of soybeans (edamame), tofu, tempeh, miso, and soy milk, are a common part of the Asian diet. A 2010 meta-analysis did not find a connection between soy consumption and a reduction in risk for colorectal cancer. However, when separating the sexes, soy consumption was associated with a 21% risk reduction in females, but not in males.[23]

Red and Processed Meat

Two large meta-analyses have found that greater consumption of red meat was linked to an increased risk for colorectal cancer, with processed meats contributing to a greater risk.[9,10] There was a 36% increased risk for colorectal cancer for every 100 g/day intake of red meat and a 28% increased risk for every 50 g/day intake of processed meat.[9] Heterocyclic amines and polycyclic aromatic hydrocarbons, which form during frying and barbecuing of meats, are carcinogenic. The heme iron content of meats may contribute to colorectal neoplasia by inducing oxidative DNA damage and by increasing endogenous formation of N-nitroso compounds that are also carcinogens. Red meat intake is associated with a risk for large adenomas.[10] Processed meats include most lunchmeats found at deli counters, anything with a casing or in sausage form, and anything smoked or cured, like bacon. Choosing other sources of protein or baking, boiling, and slow cooking unprocessed meats instead are advisable.

> Processed meat is treated with sodium nitrate to preserve the pink color, which combines with the amino acid amine in the meat to form nitrosamine, which is oncogenic to the colon.

Garlic

Garlic (*Allium sativum*) is characterized by a high content of organosulfur compounds and flavonoids, and can be consumed raw or cooked. The allyl sulfur constituents in garlic, which comprise 1% of its dry weight, are responsible for its health benefits. Its anticancer properties include blockage of cell growth, proliferation, and angiogenesis; apoptosis induction; and inhibition of COX-2 expression. Several studies show that a high consumption of garlic decreases the risk for colorectal cancer by 30%, with a greater protective effect on the distal colon.[24,25]

Glycemic Control

Impaired glycemic control is the result of a diet high in simple carbohydrates (fructose and sucrose), which leads to diabetes and hypertriglyceridemia. A 2012 meta-analysis did not support an independent association between diets high in carbohydrates, glycemic index, or glycemic load and colorectal cancer risk.[26] Another review found that glycemic index, but not glycemic load, was associated with an increased risk for colon cancer.[27] It is advisable to avoid simple carbohydrates and refined sugars because of their associations with many other chronic diseases that can result in heart attack and stroke (see Chapter 87).

Mediterranean Diet

The principal aspects of this diet include proportionally high consumption of olive oil, legumes, unrefined cereals, fruits, and vegetables; moderate-to-high consumption of fish; moderate consumption of dairy products (mostly as cheese and yogurt); moderate wine consumption; and low consumption of meat. A European study found that adherence to the Mediterranean diet was associated with an 8%–11% risk reduction in colorectal cancer. This association was stronger in women and was not affected by alcohol intake[28] (see Chapter 88).

Obesity

Obesity is defined as a body mass index (BMI) of 30 or greater and is a risk factor for many solid tumors and chronic diseases. Abdominal obesity, measured by hip and waist circumference, is closely associated with adverse metabolic profiles such as insulin resistance, dyslipidemia, and systemic inflammation, which contribute to cardiovascular disease, diabetes, and certain types of cancer. Studies show that both general and central obesity were associated with an increased risk for colon cancer, with a stronger association in men.[4,7] Childhood obesity and weight change in adulthood may also be associated with colorectal cancer risk. Patients are advised to maintain BMI between 19 and 25.

Dietary Supplements

Calcium

Two meta-analyses indicated that supplemental calcium was effective for preventing colorectal adenoma recurrence in populations with a history of adenomas but not in populations without any risk.[29,30] Food sources of calcium include dairy, white beans, bone-in sardines, kale, black eyed peas, dried figs, seaweed, tofu, and soy milk.

DOSAGE

The dosage is 1200 mg calcium citrate daily.

Vitamin D

Vitamin D may decrease cancer risk by improving differentiation and apoptosis and decreasing proliferation, invasiveness, metastatic potential, and angiogenesis. There is an inverse association between circulating 25-hydroxyvitamin D (25(OH)D) levels and colorectal cancer, with a stronger association for rectal cancer.[31-33] A 50% lower risk for colorectal cancer was associated with a serum 25(OH)D level greater than or equal to 33 ng/mL compared with less than or equal to 12 ng/mL.[34]

DOSAGE

Target 25(OH)D level is between 50 and 80 ng/mL. Every 1000 IU of vitamin D_3 will increase the level by 8–10 ng/mL.

Folate

Folic acid is a type of vitamin B. It is the synthetic form of folate that is found in supplements and added to fortified foods. Two meta-analyses found that a higher intake of total folate in the diet and supplements were associated with a reduced risk for colorectal cancer,[35,36] whereas another found no association with colorectal cancer occurrence.[37] Two meta-analyses actually found an increased risk for colorectal cancer incidence and recurrence in those supplemented with folate.[38,39] Instead of taking a folic acid supplement, it is advised to obtain folate through the diet. Food sources of folate include lentils, most beans, asparagus, spinach, avocados, broccoli, and oranges.

Vitamin B_6

In the United States, the prevalence of inadequate vitamin B_6 intake among adults older than 50 years is about 20% for men and 40% for women. A meta-analysis found that vitamin B_6 intake and blood pyridoxal 5'-phosphate levels were inversely associated with the risk for colorectal cancer, with a 20% decreased risk when comparing high versus low intake.[40] Overall, the risk for colorectal cancer decreased by 49% for every 100-pmol/mL increase in the blood pyridoxal 5'-phosphate level. Food sources of vitamin B_6 include garlic, tuna, cauliflower, mustard greens, bananas, celery, cabbage, cremini mushrooms, asparagus, broccoli, kale, collard greens, Brussels sprouts, cod, and chard.

DOSAGE

The dosage is 50 mg daily or in a multivitamin.

PRECAUTIONS

Vitamin B_6 can cause neuropathy with supplementation at high doses, generally above 150 mg. Do not exceed 50 mg with supplementation.

Curcumin

Curcumin is a compound extracted from turmeric (*Curcuma longa*), a yellow Indian spice. The bioavailability of curcumin consumed orally increases when it is taken with black pepper (piperine) and a meal containing a healthy fat (i.e., coconut oil, avocado, olive oil, etc.). A small open-label trial showed a 60% reduction in colorectal adenoma number and 50% reduction in size in individuals with familial adenomatous polyposis (FAP) who took 1440 mg of curcumin with quercetin daily for 6 months.[41] Another open-label trial found a 40% reduction in aberrant crypt foci in smokers who took 4 grams as opposed to 2 grams of curcumin daily for 30 days prior to colonoscopy.[42] Curcumin can cause blood thinning, so use it with caution in individuals with a low platelet count, anemia, or using medications or herbs that thin the blood. It may cause gastrointestinal discomfort, so titrate the dose up slowly.

DOSAGE

The dosage is 1.5–4 g/day for antiinflammatory benefits. More research is needed with regard to colorectal cancer prevention.

Coriolus (*Trametes*) versicolor

Over 400 in vitro and animal studies of *Coriolus versicolor* mushroom extract have demonstrated that it stimulates the immune system, inhibits the growth of cancer cells, and acts as a strong antioxidant. Polysaccharide-K (Krestin; PSK) and polysaccharide peptide (PSP) are bioactive extracts of *C. versicolor*. In Japan, PSK is an anticancer drug currently used as a cancer treatment along with surgery, chemotherapy, and radiation therapy. It is used as an adjunctive treatment for esophageal, lung, stomach, breast, and colon cancer. A study found that stage II and III colorectal cancer patients who received conventional therapy along with 3 grams of PSK per day had a greater percentage of 5-year disease-free survival and a decreased relative risk for regional metastases.[43] A meta-analysis of three trials involving 1094 subjects with colorectal cancer confirmed that those who took PSK showed a significant improvement in overall survival and disease-free survival.[44]

DOSAGE

No definite dosing schedule has been established.

Physical Activity

One review found that physical activity reduced the incidence of colon cancer but not rectal cancer. There was a 30%–50% risk reduction in people with the highest level of physical activity, with a stronger reduction in left-sided cancers.[45] Another review discusses that increased physical activity after the diagnosis of stage I–III or advanced colon cancer reduced cancer-related mortality. Additionally, there was a reduction in colon cancer recurrence or death in people with the highest level of physical activity 6 months after chemotherapy. This was independent of other lifestyle factors, and walking at a normal or brisk pace for 30 minutes or more daily is effective.[46] Patients who have received chemotherapy that can affect heart function should take extra precautions and talk to their doctor before starting a vigorous exercise program.

Smoking

In November 2009, the International Agency for Research on Cancer reported that there is sufficient evidence to conclude that tobacco smoking causes colorectal cancer. The association appears to be stronger for rectal cancer than for colon cancer.[47] The latency period between tobacco exposure and colorectal cancer diagnosis is about 30–40 years.

Alcohol

Colorectal cancer has been linked to even moderate alcohol use. Individuals who have a lifetime average of two to four alcoholic drinks per day have a 23% higher risk for colorectal cancer than those who consume less than one drink per day.[48]

MEDICATIONS

Aspirin and Nonsteroidal Antiinflammatory Drugs

The chemopreventive effect of aspirin and NSAIDs has been attributed to their inhibition of COX enzymes. COX-2 is abnormally expressed in many cancer cell lines and implicated in the processes of carcinogenesis, tumor growth, apoptosis, and angiogenesis. Studies indicate that regular aspirin use of 75 mg or more for greater than 5 years leads to a 20%–30% reduction in colon cancer incidence.[49] Meta-analyses confirm that daily aspirin use of 81–325 mg reduced the occurrence of tubular adenomas in those with a history of them.[50,51] However, NSAID use prior to diagnosis does not affect survival in colon cancer patients.[52] An international consensus determined that more studies on aspirin and cancer prevention are needed to define the lowest effective dose, the age at which to initiate therapy, the optimum treatment duration, and the subpopulations for which the benefits of chemoprevention outweigh the risks for adverse side effects.[53] The American Cancer Society does not currently recommend the use of these drugs for colorectal cancer prevention because of the potential side effect of gastrointestinal bleeding.

Postmenopausal Hormone Replacement

There is substantial evidence that women who use postmenopausal hormones have lower rates of colorectal cancer than those who do not.[53] Decreased risk is especially evident in women with long-term hormone use, though the risk returns to that of nonusers within 3 years of cessation.[54,55] However, use of postmenopausal hormones increases the risks for breast and other cancers, as well as cardiovascular disease, so it is not recommended for the prevention of colorectal cancer.

TREATMENT

The mainstay of treatment for colorectal cancer is surgery to remove the tumor. When a section of the colon is removed, the ends can often be reconnected. If not, a temporary (rarely permanent) colostomy may be required in the interim. Chemotherapy and radiation are required if the tumor has invaded beyond the muscle wall of the bowel. Surgery can result in fatigue, changes in bowel consistency, sexual side effects, and pain, which improves with healing. Radiation treatment may cause local skin irritation, nausea, diarrhea, rectal or bladder irritation, tenesmus, fatigue, and sexual problems. Chemotherapy frequently causes gastrointestinal side effects, fatigue, hair loss, low blood counts, and neuropathy, many of which can reverse with time after completion of treatment. Maintenance of physical activity, healthy nutrition, and stress reduction are recommended throughout the entire cancer process.

Supplements for Treatment Support

The conventional treatments for colorectal cancer can cause many side effects, only some of which can be treated with medications. Other side effects take time to resolve after the treatment is complete, but some do not resolve at all. Table 81.3 summarizes the numerous evidence-based integrative therapies and supplementation available to prevent and treat the side effects of conventional treatments and symptoms of cancer.

TABLE 81.3	Complementary Therapies for Colorectal Cancer Treatment[57-91]
Nausea	Acupuncture, peppermint, ginger, astragalus, relaxation techniques, yoga, energy work, music therapy, massage
Fatigue	Energy conservation, aerobic exercise, MBSR, CBT, energy work, acupuncture, relaxation techniques, massage, yoga, L-carnitine
Pain	Music therapy, acupuncture, massage, CBT, relaxation techniques, meditation, energy work
Depression, Anxiety	Counseling, therapy, support groups, meditation, MBSR, music therapy, massage, yoga, energy work, relaxation techniques, hypnosis
Insomnia	CBT, meditation, MBSR, yoga, relaxation techniques
Neuropathy	Acupuncture, L-glutamine, acetyl-L-carnitine
Diarrhea	L-glutamine, probiotics

CBT, cognitive behavioral therapy; MBSR, mindfulness-based stress reduction.
Energy work: reiki, healing touch, therapeutic touch.
Relaxation techniques: hypnosis, progressive muscle relaxation, guided imagery.

SURVIVORSHIP AND TERTIARY PREVENTION

Because of the technological advancement in the early detection and treatment of colorectal cancer, the number of deaths has been decreasing. Millions of people are currently in remission after treatment. The 5-year survival rate for localized colorectal cancer is 90%. Tertiary prevention should focus on the same modifiable risk factors included in primary prevention, especially dietary modifications that can be overseen by a clinician and supported by the family. Compliance with follow-up screening procedures should be emphasized, as a personal history of colorectal cancer increases an individual's risk for the development of new colorectal cancers.

PREVENTION PRESCRIPTION

Screening and early detection should focus on identifying high-risk populations, including those with a genetic condition or a family history of colorectal cancer. Those with a normal risk should undergo screening colonoscopy at the age of 50 years. Primary, secondary, and tertiary prevention of colorectal cancer should include the following:

• A whole-food plant–based diet with five to nine servings of fruits and vegetables daily that is low in processed foods, sugar, and red meat

• Moderate physical activity of 30 or more minutes per day (e.g., brisk walking)

• Maintenance of a BMI between 19 and 25

• Minimal alcohol consumption

• Avoid tobacco use

• Supplementation with omega-3 fats, vitamin D₃, and calcium citrate as appropriate

• Mind–body tools for stress management practiced for 10–15 minutes daily

Consistent reevaluation of this comprehensive approach is necessary for adherence, patient satisfaction, and efficacy and to determine if new tools in each category are indicated.

THERAPEUTIC REVIEW

PRIMARY PREVENTION

- Risk reduction in populations with higher risk

SCREENING AND EARLY DETECTION

- Identify high-risk populations for increased surveillance and early intervention.
- Follow the American Cancer Society (ACS) recommendation for screening average-risk populations with colonoscopy starting at the age of 50 years.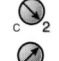

NUTRITION

- A plant-based, high-fiber diet obtained from fruits and vegetables with minimal red meat and sugar
- The diet may include omega-3 fats, unprocessed, preferably fermented soy foods, garlic, and natural sources of calcium.
- Maintain a BMI between 19 and 25.

EXERCISE

- Moderate physical activity of 30 or more minutes per day (e.g., brisk walking)

MIND–BODY

- Mind–body stress reduction to support treatment

SUPPLEMENTS

- Calcium citrate 1200 mg daily for prevention of colorectal adenoma recurrence

- A vitamin D_3 level maintained between 50 and 80 ng/mL, with daily baseline supplementation of 1000 IU/day once that level is achieved, may decrease cancer risk.
- Folate obtained from food sources reduces colorectal cancer risk, whereas supplementation with folic acid increases the incidence.
- Vitamin B_6 50 mg daily reduces cancer risk.
- Curcumin 1.5–4 g/day for antiinflammatory benefits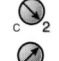
- *Coriolus* PSK improves overall and disease-free survival in individuals with colorectal cancer.

TREATMENT SUPPORT

- Acupuncture and acupressure given prior to, during, or after treatment relieve chemotherapy-induced nausea.
- Ginger root 1 gram daily starting on the first day of chemotherapy and continued for 5 days OR 500 mg every 4 hours starting on the day of chemotherapy and continuing as long as needed relieve chemotherapy-induced nausea.
- Mind–body techniques including meditation, clinical hypnosis, guided imagery, and yoga improve tolerance of, adherence to, and quality of life during treatment.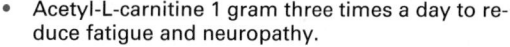
- L-glutamine 10 grams three times a day during the first 7 days of chemotherapy, or 5–10 grams two to three times a day during chemotherapy to reduce neuropathy.
- Acetyl-L-carnitine 1 gram three times a day to reduce fatigue and neuropathy.

Key Web Resources

Colorectal Cancer Risk Assessment Tool	http://www.cancer.gov/colorectalcancerrisk
Fight Colorectal Cancer (patient information)	http://www.fightcolorectalcancer.org
Colon Cancer Alliance (patient information)	http://www.ccalliance.org
American College of Gastroenterology (see patient section)	http://www.gi.org
National Center for Complementary and Alternative Medicine (NCCAM) (information on complementary approaches)	https://nccih.nih.gov/health/cancer
National Cancer Institute Office of Cancer Complementary and Alternative Medicine (OCCAM)	https://cam.cancer.gov/
Society for Integrative Oncology	http://www.integrativeonc.org
Memorial Sloan Kettering Cancer Center (evidence-based information about herbs, botanicals, supplements, and other products)	http://www.mskcc.org/mskcc/html/11570.cfm

REFERENCES

References are available online at ExpertConsult.com.

CHAPTER 82

PALLIATIVE AND END-OF-LIFE CARE

Lucille R. Marchand, MD, BSN

Integrative palliative care (IPC) encompasses whole-person, relationship-centered care using conventional and complementary and alternative modalities (CAM) with an emphasis on health and healing.[1] When delivered at the end of a person's life, palliative care (PC) is usually referred to as hospice care (Fig. 82.1). PC includes evidence-based care directed at the relief of symptoms of advanced serious illness and side effects of treatment as well as communication directed to establishing ever-evolving goals of care based on patient (and family and/or surrogate) preferences. It is appropriate at any stage of the disease trajectory but especially helpful earlier in the course of serious illness so that patients have PC services available throughout the disease trajectory. It occurs together with life-prolonging measures, and with the relief of symptoms and improvement in quality of life (QOL), it may actually prolong life.[2] Goals of care in hospice care and PC include optimization of well-being and QOL, relief of distressing symptoms, empowered decision making, support of caregivers, and effective life closure for peaceful and meaningful dying and death. Bereavement services for family and friends of the person dying are an essential element of care. Grief and loss often begin with the diagnosis of serious diseases. PC incorporates the use of a multi- and interdisciplinary team of health professionals working together to best meet the needs of the patient and family. The team can include the patient's primary and specialty care clinicians and the hospice care and PC clinicians, which may include physicians, nurse practitioners, physician assistants, nurses, certified nurses' aides, chaplains, bereavement counselors, social workers, housekeepers, dietitians, volunteers, occupational and physical therapists, and other integrative practitioners who work in health care settings, including PC outpatient

and inpatient programs and hospice, are affiliated with the hospice, or caring for the patient and family in the community.[3] IPC calls on us to be creative and innovative in the care of seriously ill patients, expanding options to enhance healing, maintain hope, and improve well-being in a unique way for each person.

In a survey of complementary therapy services provided by hospices, 60% of responding organizations offered such therapies. The most common services were massage therapy (83%), music therapy (50%), therapeutic touch (49%), pet therapy (48%), guided imagery (45%), reiki (36%), aromatherapy (30%), harp music (23%), reflexology (20%), art therapy (20%), hypnotherapy (4%), yoga (3%), acupuncture (1%), and humor therapy (1%). Constraints to providing CAM services were lack of funding, lack of staff time, lack of qualified CAM therapists, inadequate knowledge about these services, and patient and staff resistance to CAM therapies. Even in hospices that offered these services, less than 25% of the patients received them.[4] In a 2008 survey of 27 Nevada and Montana hospices using the survey instrument developed by Demmer, it was found that 70.4% of hospices offered CAM services, but less than 25% of hospice patients received them. The most-used CAM therapies included massage and music therapy; 61.1% of hospices had a salaried CAM provider and 88.3% had CAM volunteers. None of the hospices had an assessment tool to determine the patients who might benefit from the CAM services. Barriers to use were the same as those cited for constraints to providing CAM services.[5] Preliminary research outcome data on the program have been favorable.[6] Demmer and Sauer[7] found that patients who received CAM therapies were more satisfied with their hospice services. Sirios[8] compared consumers seeking consultation with CAM practitioners in 1997 and 2005. During that period, consumer motivation changed from the use of CAM due to negative attitudes toward conventional medicine to the use of CAM modalities for their positive effects and a whole-person, empowered approach to health care. In a Canadian hospital PC unit, integration of CAM therapies decreased the severity of pain, restlessness, discomfort, low mood, and anxiety. It also added to a sense of peace.[9]

For patients dying with uncontrolled symptoms, such as pain, the symptoms are often more frightening than death itself. Patients desire pain and symptom control; the ability to prepare for their dying and to have their choices honored; life completion; mental clarity; being touched; being at peace with their God; having clinicians one can trust, who listen, and with whom one is comfortable talking about dying; and being in the presence of loved ones without being a burden.[10] Ira Byock[11]

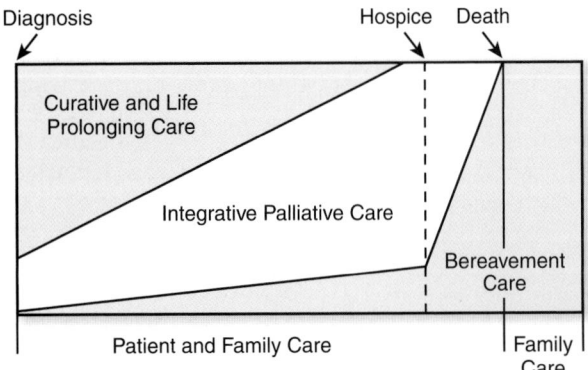

Integrative Palliative Medicine Model

FIG. 82.1 ■ **Model of Integrative Palliative Medicine.**

describes the essential elements of meaningful living as the expression of forgiveness, appreciation, and love. The phrases "Please forgive me," "I forgive you," "Thank you," and "I love you" embody these elements; they can improve relationships at any time in life, particularly at life's closure.[11]

PATHOPHYSIOLOGY

General criteria in patients with advanced chronic illness who are dying are as follows: unintentional weight loss of more than 10% body weight, serum albumin value lower than 2.5 g/dL, spending more than 50% of time in bed (Karnofsky score), inability to perform most activities of daily living, progression of disease, and uncontrolled symptoms despite aggressive treatment of the underlying illness.[12] Physicians tend to be overly optimistic about prognosis, an error that leads to delayed hospice referrals, less time for the patient and family to prepare for death, delay or absence of end-of-life care discussions with informed decision making, lack of preparatory bereavement services, and inappropriate life-prolonging interventions. An important question for clinicians to ask themselves is: "Would I be surprised if this patient died in the next 6 months?" If the answer is no, the patient has reached the end of life; communication about treatment preferences becomes more important and referral to hospice appropriate.[13]

Communication lies at the heart of integrative PC. "Hoping for the best" needs to be balanced with "preparing for the worst."[14] Conversations must be sensitive in eliciting how much a patient wants to know.[15] Goals of care are explored in a patient-centered way, which then serve as guides for further decision making. Armed with knowledge about patient preferences for care, clinicians can avoid unwarranted treatment. Hope is then in keeping with what the patient wants to accomplish in his or her remaining life. Goals and hope will change as the process unfolds. Hope can be viewed as an inner power that moves a person forward in life. Questions that can be helpful in palliative medicine conversations with patients to uncover what will move them forward and inspire hope include the following: "What is your understanding of your situation? How can I be most helpful to you? What worries you most now and for the future? What is important or meaningful to you right now?" When the clinician listens to the answers intently without interruption and with presence, empowerment and a sense of hopefulness can arise in the patient. It allows the patient to heal and to live well in the face of serious illness and end of life. Hope becomes a fluid process of living fully rather than fixed on a particular outcome.[16]

Hope can also help alleviate clinical symptoms and improve well-being.[17] Communicating "bad" or challenging news constitutes an essential skill that is well described by Buckman.[18] It requires deep listening, empathy, presence, and emotional awareness on the part of the clinician (see Chapter 3).

Hope does not lie in a way out, but in a way through.
ROBERT FROST

COMMON ISSUES IN PALLIATIVE CARE

Common symptoms managed in PC are pain; nausea, vomiting, and constipation; dyspnea; depression and anxiety; and delirium. Lancker et al., in a systematic review and meta-analysis of symptoms in older patients with cancer receiving PC, found that more than 50% of patients suffered from pain, incontinence, asthenia, anxiety, constipation, fatigue, and excretory symptoms.[19] Unrelieved physical, emotional, or spiritual discomfort must be treated as a PC emergency, and careful assessment and intensive palliative resources must be applied to prevent unnecessary suffering.[20] Uncontrolled symptoms can lead to the patient's desire for a hastened death.[21] On occasion, physical and psychological symptoms cannot be controlled with conventional and CAM therapies, and palliative sedation must be used to control symptoms such as intractable and intense pain, seizures, and existential psychological suffering. The intention of this therapy is to treat intractable suffering, not to hasten death. Careful guidelines have been developed for its use.[22-26]

Discussing conventional symptom management in detail is beyond the scope of this chapter. Many valuable PC resources are available for this information.[3,27-30]

PAIN MANAGEMENT

Opioids are important in pain management as serious illness, such as cancer, progresses. Pain, however, is a complex phenomenon involving physical, emotional, social, and spiritual aspects that must be addressed for "total pain" management as described by Cicely Saunders, the founder of the modern hospice movement.[31,32] The World Health Organization (WHO) ladder of pain management recommends various levels of pain treatment, depending on pain severity.[27] Physical pain is often a combination of nociceptive and neuropathic pain, and opioids alone are usually not effective in treating the neuropathic component of pain without adjunctive medications, such as antidepressants and anticonvulsant medication.[32]

Methadone is a unique opioid that can effectively treat both components but must be dosed carefully, given its large volume of distribution, and its kinetics differ from those of other opioids. The switch from another opioid to methadone must be done carefully, and it usually requires consultation with a pain or palliative medicine consultant.[33-35] No ceiling dose exists for opioids, but careful titration of the dose to relieve pain is recommended (see Key Web Resources: Fast Facts). Opioid-induced hyperalgesia, noted clinically in some cases of rapid increased titration of opioids, is a condition reported in the literature, but one paper argues that there is little evidence to support this concern.[36] Pain that is unrelieved by opioids can be treated with agents such as ketamine and parenteral lidocaine, nerve blocks, and, in some cases, palliative sedation.[32,37-40]

CAM therapies can be especially helpful in addressing all components of pain. Depression, anxiety, and spiritual distress can all increase the perception of pain intensity, and addressing these components of pain can reduce the need for pain medication.[41,42] A multicontinental WHO study in primary care revealed that persistent pain is associated with greater psychological illness.[43] Lin et al.,[44] in a large randomized controlled trial (RCT), found that amelioration of depressive symptoms decreased pain and improved both functional status and QOL.[44] Because most antidepressants, including St. John's wort, take 2–6 weeks to exert effect, treatment at the end of life depends on the length of life expected. Psychostimulants, such as methylphenidate, may have immediate effects in alleviating depression.[45] Other modalities, such as psychotherapy, energetic medicine, and mind-body, may also have a beneficial effect.

Many integrative modalities for the pain management of chronic conditions are covered in other chapters in this volume and can be applied in PC. Relatively few studies have focused solely on CAM treatments of pain at the end of life.

> Never order opioids without also scheduling a stool softener and/or laxative, such as senna, to prevent constipation that can lead to bowel obstruction (unless the patient is having diarrhea not due to partial large bowel obstruction). A common stool softener is docusate sodium. A laxative is usually needed in conjunction with a stool softener to have a bowel movement every day or every other day as a usual goal.

Botanicals for Pain

Cannabis (Medical Marijuana)

Cannabis can help alleviate pain. Dronabinol (delta-9-tetrahydrocannabinol or delta-9-THC)—a schedule III substance—and nabilone—a schedule II substance—are the oral synthetic forms of cannabis and were licensed and approved in 1986 for chemotherapy-induced nausea and vomiting and the wasting syndrome associated with human immunodeficiency virus (HIV) disease.[48] The medicinal use of cannabis dates back to thousands of years.[49] Other uses of cannabis include its use in treating cancer-related pain, HIV-associated neuropathy, and neuropathic pain. It is a schedule I substance. The cannabis plant has more than 100 different cannabinoids, with delta-9-THC being the most psychoactive component. Cannabidiol (CBD) also has powerful therapeutic effects, but without psychoactive side effects, and can help modulate central nervous system effects of THC. Oral forms of cannabis have low and variable bioavailability, whereas the inhaled form is rapidly absorbed and metabolized for rapid onset and shorter duration of action. It can interact with cytochrome P450 enzymes in the liver, potentially affecting other drugs metabolized via this system. It also has a good safety profile.[49]

Cannabinoid receptors are located in the central and peripheral nervous system (CB1) and the immune system (CB2).[50] Abrams and Guzman summarize the research on the effectiveness of cannabis to relieve neuropathic pain and reduce the dose needed of opioids to relieve cancer pain. Cannabis relieves pain at 10- to 20-mg doses; higher doses have more side effects such as sedation. Abrams and Guzman suggest that cannabis has a potential prominent role in PC as a single agent that can address anorexia, pain, nausea, insomnia, depression, pain, and anxiety.[49]

In 23 states and the District of Columbia, natural cannabis in inhaled or oral form is available as medical marijuana.[49] If legal and available in your state, it can be titrated for effective dosing starting with very small doses as needed. Facilities that are under federal law regulations may not be able to use it.

DOSAGE

Dronabinol is not effective in relieving pain syndromes.[48]

Oral dosing produces milder effects, given its variable bioavailability, and it is available as a tea.

Given variable absorption of oral cannabis, the inhalation route remains the most reliable titration to effect with minimal side effects. Vaporization of cannabis is an alternative to smoking it. The Office of Medicinal Cannabis recommends the inhalation route via vaporization to avoid damage to lungs.[51] In a review of 165 studies on medical marijuana use, less than 7 mg of THC is considered as low dose, 7–18 mg as medium dose, and greater than 18 mg as high dose. Tolerance often occurs in a few days through downregulation of cannabis receptors.[52]

SIDE EFFECTS

Side effects include dizziness, dry mouth, sedation, fatigue, headache, hypotension, irritability, and poor memory or concentration. More serious side effects include paranoia, psychosis, and disorientation.[48]

PRECAUTIONS

Psychoactive side effects are observed in patients with mental illness, dementia, or delirium.

NAUSEA, VOMITING, AND CONSTIPATION

Whenever nausea, vomiting, and constipation symptoms appear, it is important to establish the cause for the antiemetic to be targeted to the responsible mechanism. Common causes are dysmotility, obstruction, side effects of medication such as opioids, metastases in the brain, and vestibular apparatus irritation (sometimes caused by dehydration). Constipation is a common cause of nausea and vomiting. Corticosteroids (such as prednisone and dexamethasone) can reduce nausea and vomiting caused by cerebral edema that occurs due to brain metastases. Laxatives, stool softeners, and enemas can prevent and relieve constipation and bowel obstruction due to severe constipation. The goal is to achieve a bowel movement once daily and at least every other day[56,57] (see Chapter 46). Bulking agents should be avoided in patients consuming insufficient fluids or those on fluid restriction. Metoclopramide can relieve nausea due to dysmotility but can have extrapyramidal side effects, especially in older persons (should be avoided in patients with Parkinson's disease). For dysmotility, promethazine is a potent anticholinergic drug that should not be used for nausea in this situation because it will cause further slowing of gut motility.[58]

Antiemetics represent a variety of drugs with antihistamine, antidopaminergic, antiserotonergic (5-hydroxytryptamine type 3 [5-HT$_3$] receptor antagonists), and anticholinergic effects. They are not interchangeable. Promethazine is an antihistamine with potent anticholinergic and very weak antidopaminergic effects, making it a poor choice for treating the nausea due to opioids. For opioid-induced nausea, metoclopramide can improve motility. Long-acting opioids can prevent drug level peaks that can cause nausea. 5-HT$_3$ antagonists such as ondansetron are expensive second-line agents that are preferred for treating nausea due to chemotherapy or when other agents have failed or are contraindicated, such as metoclopramide in Parkinson's disease.[58] There is evidence that acupuncture as well as other mind-body and energetic therapies can also help relieve nausea. In cases of bowel obstruction, exercise extreme caution with any prokinetic or anticholinergic drugs or laxatives.

Botanicals for Nausea

Ginger (Zingiber officinale)

Ginger can help alleviate nausea. It has been found to be efficacious in nausea of pregnancy, motion sickness, and nausea associated with chemotherapy but not for postoperative nausea.[59,60] Its mechanism of action is unknown, but ginger appears to have a prokinetic effect.[59]

DOSAGE

Take 500–1000 mg of ginger root extract every 4–6 hours as needed, or eat 1 tsp or 5 g of crystallized ginger every 2–3 hours as needed.

PRECAUTIONS

Side effects are rare. Excessive doses can cause heartburn.

Cannabis

Cannabis can help alleviate nausea and improve appetite. In a study of HIV-positive patients, it significantly improved nausea and appetite.[61]

In 1986, it was approved for use in chemotherapy-associated nausea and vomiting.[49]

DOSAGE, PRECAUTIONS, AND SIDE EFFECTS

See the section on cannabis.

DYSPNEA

"Total dyspnea," like the concept of "total pain," encompasses the physical, emotional, social, and spiritual aspects of breathlessness and the suffering it causes.[62] Opioids and oxygen are important palliative treatments of dyspnea. Opioids, such as low-dose oral morphine at 2–4 mg every 3 hours as needed, relieve the sensation of breathlessness and can improve the patient's functional capacity. Diuretics can help relieve dyspnea from fluid overload. Benzodiazepines lack evidence of beneficial effect on breathlessness but can help relieve anxiety that can make breathlessness worse.[62] Optimal treatment of

the underlying condition is essential, but standard conventional interventions may no longer reverse or improve the condition in end-stage disease. Oxygen administered to nonhypoxemic patients has no benefit over inhaled air.[63] Nonpharmacological strategies to help relieve dyspnea include the use of fans for a well-ventilated environment and cool ambient temperature. CAM therapies include mind-body and energetic modalities. Anxiety-reduction training, activity pacing and energy conservation, and use of handheld fans can improve breathlessness.[62]

Scopolamine, glycopyrrolate, atropine, and hyoscyamine are used for drying oral secretions and decreasing the "death rattle."[64,65] Dying is usually marked by progressive dehydration that keeps a patient comfortable by eliminating excessive secretions. Thirst is relieved with small sips of fluids and by keeping the mouth moist with frequent swabbing. Artificial feeding through a gastric tube and artificial intravenous fluids can cause respiratory congestion, pain, nausea, and vomiting. Families and health care professionals who equate caring with feeding can be encouraged to provide caring by other means, such as touch (e.g., hand massage), life review, listening, and expressing love and appreciation to the dying person.[66,67]

Dyspnea is often accompanied by anxiety and is effectively treated using anxiolytics. If carefully titrated, opioids and anxiolytics do not hasten death or cause respiratory depression but make the patient comfortable. Care must be taken in the opioid-naive patient, and initial dosing is low.[64,66]

In a Cochrane review of nonpharmacological interventions that are most effective in relieving malignant and nonmalignant dyspnea, there was strong evidence for the positive role of neuroelectrical muscle stimulation and chest wall vibration, moderate evidence for breathing training and walking aids, weak evidence for the role of acupuncture, and no evidence for the benefit of music therapy. There was insufficient evidence for other modalities, such as relaxation breathing and psychological interventions. Most of the reviewed studies included patients with chronic obstructive pulmonary disease.[68]

ANXIETY AND DEPRESSION

Information on this topic can be found online at ExpertConsult.com.

DELIRIUM

The patient's inability to focus, fluctuating level of consciousness, poor memory, agitation, hallucinations, hyperactivity and restlessness or hypoactivity and somnolence, tangential thinking, insomnia, anxiety, and significant distress characterize delirium. Delirium is often unrecognized and undertreated, especially hypoactive delirium. Even without agitation, delirium can cause great suffering for the patient and family.[75] There are many delirium subtypes.[76] Careful assessment of a delirious patient is essential, and there are many scales that effectively screen for delirium.[76] Delirium should not be reflexively treated using anxiolytics, which can potentially make it worse.[71] Benzodiazepines, however, are the first-line treatment of the delirium associated with alcohol withdrawal or seizures.[77] Medications commonly cause delirium, especially those with anticholinergic side effects, such as tricyclic antidepressants and antihistamines. Opioids can also cause delirium, and decreasing the dose or substituting another opioid with fewer active metabolites—especially in decreased renal clearance—, such as hydromorphone, can help. Steroids can cause delirium as well as hepatic encephalopathy, hypoxia, and hypoglycemia as potential causes. Haloperidol continues to be the first-line medication for initial treatment of acute delirium.

The treatment goal, however, is to treat the underlying cause.[78-81] If delirium cannot be readily reversed, atypical antipsychotics, such as risperidone, olanzapine, and aripiprazole, can be used in scheduled and prn dosing. In a study comparing the efficacy of these agents and haloperidol in treating delirium, all agents were equally effective but differed in side effects. Olanzapine increased sedation (which may be desirable in some patients at bedtime), and extrapyramidal side effects were associated with haloperidol. These agents must be used with great caution in the elderly.[82] All can prolong the QT interval, but this is less of a concern as the patient nears end of life. Palliative sedation (reason for palliative expert consultation) is a possible treatment for refractory delirium with irreversible cause that is leading to severe suffering of the patient.[76,83]

Near-death awareness encompasses a dying person's experience of the dying process. When a patient experiences the presence of a deceased relative, clinicians can interpret this event as delirium with hallucinations and can inappropriately medicate the person with an antipsychotic or anxiolytic agent. The patient, however, may not demonstrate other criteria for delirium. Patients can feel annoyed, frustrated, and isolated in their profound end-of-life experiences. This is a time for clinicians to listen. Patients will attempt to describe these experiences or request something to ensure a peaceful death. They may indicate when they will die. They may use symbolic language to describe their experiences, which can be difficult to interpret. By being curious and appreciative of the experience, clinicians can validate and support the patient, help family members understand the experience, and perhaps learn themselves about the dying process.[84-86]

> Do not treat agitation reflexively using anxiolytics. Careful assessment is needed to determine the cause of agitation, especially in patients with decreased cognitive function such as dementia. Causes can include delirium, near-death awareness, spiritual distress, depression and anxiety, unrelieved pain, and other uncontrolled physical symptoms.

SPIRITUAL CARE

Serious illness and end of life bring questions about life's meaning and purpose. Spiritual and religious concerns often affect decision making.[87] In one study questioning ambulatory outpatients, 66% of respondents said that they would want their physician to ask about their spiritual beliefs if they became gravely ill, and 16% said they would not.[88] In a study of physicians, 81% of 1878 surveyed physicians believed that spiritual distress could worsen physical pain and 88% felt that addressing spiritual distress was just as important as relieving pain.[89] Careful spiritual assessment can help the patient who desires supportive spiritual resources to obtain them. Expressive therapies such as music, art, collage, movement, and writing can facilitate the exploration of spiritual issues.[90] Life review or reminiscence therapy can encourage the discovery of meaning. Chibnall and associates[91] reported that higher levels of death distress in patients correlated with higher levels of physical and psychological symptoms, living alone, lower spiritual well-being, and less physician communication as perceived by the patient. In a study of patients with cancer, Meraviglia[92] found that higher levels of finding meaning in life and greater use of prayer correlated with higher psychological well-being and less physical distress. Use of a spiritual assessment tool can facilitate communication about life's meaning, life closure, and treatment goals and help assess a patient's strengths. It can also be used as a therapeutic tool to increase self-efficacy and well-being.[93-97] Puchalski's model for spiritual assessment with the acronym FICA includes questions related to faith and belief, importance of that faith and belief, spiritual or social community, and how to address those beliefs in PC and end-of-life care (Table 82.1).[94] The clinician can learn how the patient copes with illness, what support systems are in place, and what beliefs the patient may have that could affect decision making.[98] Supporting the dignity of

TABLE 82.1	FICA: Taking a Spiritual History*
Faith and belief	Do you consider yourself spiritual or religious? *or* Do you have spiritual beliefs that help you cope with stress? If the patient responds no, the physician might ask: "What gives your life meaning?" Sometimes patients respond with answers such as family, career, or nature.
Importance	What importance does your faith or belief have in your life? Have your beliefs influenced how you take care of yourself in this illness? What role do your beliefs play in regaining your health?
Community	Are you part of a spiritual or religious community? Is this of support to you? How? Is there a group of people you really love or who are important to you? Communities such as churches, temples, mosques, or a group of like-minded friends can serve as strong support systems for some patients.
Address in care	How would you like me, your health care provider, to address these issues in your health care?

*The acronym FICA can help structure questions for health care professionals taking a spiritual history.
© Christina M. Puchalski, MD, 1996. Modified with permission from Puchalski CM, Romer AL. Taking a spiritual history allows clinicians to understand patients more fully. *J Palliat Med.* 2003;3:129–137.

the patient and his or her "person-ness" is essential in effective spiritual care. Miller et al.[99] demonstrated better spiritual and psychological well-being in patients with life-threatening illnesses who were given supportive-affective group experiences with a spiritual inquiry tool.

Requests from the patient for prayer with the clinician need not compromise the clinician's religious beliefs. A clinician may choose to be with the patient in silence as the patient prays.[98,100] Often, the patient can identify a spiritual mentor, such as a priest, minister, or rabbi, who can guide him or her through the spiritual territory of their illness and dying process. If not, involving the PC or hospice chaplain can provide needed spiritual support. Spiritual support, however, can come from the entire PC and health care team, family, and friends[101] (see Chapter 114).

BEREAVEMENT

The loss of the "healthy or nonseriously ill" self begins at the time of diagnosis of illness. Delivery of "bad" or "important" news requires skill in managing the grief of the patient and family for this loss.[18] Grief is the experience of loss, and bereavement is the process of journeying through grief. Mourning is the public expression of grieving. Grief or bereavement targets the restoration of wholeness and a gradual adjustment to a new reality. Each person journeys through the grief process uniquely, but certain tasks of grieving are universal; they are to gradually accept the reality of the loss, experience the pain of the loss, adjust to a new reality where the deceased is not, and reinvest energy into new relationships and realities.[102,103]

In PC and hospice care, bereavement services are offered to the patient and family before the death (grief can occur for the patient and family before the death) and to the family up to 13 months after the patient's death. Supportive interventions for grief of the patient and family help prevent depression in the patient and complicated grief in the family and significant others left behind by the death. Periyakoil and Hallenbeck[104] suggest psychosocial–spiritual interventions with the acronym RELIEVER: reflect with the patient on emotions, empathize, lead with questions to facilitate grieving, improvise interventions to the unique individual, educate about the grief process and what to expect, validate the experience, and recall the life story and accomplishments of the patient. All health care professionals and bereavement counselors can facilitate this process. As in spiritual exploration, the use of the humanities such as art, music, writing, and collage can help individuals express their grief and work through it one-on-one or in bereavement groups.

Encouragement of healthy grieving can prevent complicated grief, such as delayed grief, absent grief, distorted grief, and chronic grief. When complicated grief occurs, refer to a bereavement counselor, psychiatric consultant, or spiritual counselor. Grief can also be complicated by major depression, anxiety disorder, posttraumatic stress disorder, and, in children, adjustment disorder. Those at risk for complicated grief include mothers after the death of a child, widowers, family members who feel guilt or anger or "unfinished business" with the deceased; survivors of a sudden violent death of a loved one; children and teenagers who have lost a parent; persons with a history of psychiatric illness or substance abuse; and refugees. Patients presenting with somatic or psychiatric symptoms may be experiencing complicated grief, and this should be explored. In a patient interview, the clinician starts a therapeutic intervention by acknowledging the loss and then supporting the patient in the grief process.[105] A study revealed that those who had strong spiritual beliefs were more resilient in the face of grief and had lower incidence of complicated grief.[106]

Depression must be differentiated from grief in the dying patient because depression requires some different interventions for successful treatment. Depression is characterized by flat affect, anhedonia, hopelessness, worthlessness, guilt, and social withdrawal. One must remember that pain can also cause flat affect, anhedonia, and withdrawal. In grief, sadness fluctuates and responds to social support; some activities can be enjoyed, and sadness improves with time. Symptoms such as insomnia and loss of appetite cannot be used to differentiate depression and grief in the dying process. Patients can, at times, sense whether they are depressed or grieving, and asking them if they are feeling depressed can help differentiate between the two states.[107]

INTEGRATIVE THERAPIES

Nutrition

Appetite naturally decreases at the end of life, and progressive dehydration is the rule. Food and fluids optimally are flavorful and of an appropriate consistency to facilitate swallowing. Food is often equated with caring, but forcing the patient to eat and drink is to be avoided. Offering small quantities of food and foods desired by the patient is optimal. Avoid dietary restrictions unless certain foods cause uncomfortable symptoms. In conditions such as congestive heart failure and pneumonia, fluid overload is to be avoided. Cool foods are often better tolerated than warm or hot foods, unless the patient prefers the latter. Fruit-flavored juices, ices, or smoothies can relieve dry mouth and are usually well tolerated. Cancer and its therapies can change taste sensation, and foods that taste good to the patient should be maximized.[108,109]

For patients earlier in the illness trajectory, especially in cancer, nutritious foods can help improve QOL, symptoms of the disease, or treatment and decrease progression of the disease. An authoritative, evidence-based guide to nutrition and exercise in cancer survivors is the American Cancer Society's guidelines.[110] Use of cannabis can also help stimulate appetite.[49]

Movement

A number of studies show that exercise in advanced cancer can help with improvement of fatigue, pain, functional capacity, mood, and QOL. Often, seriously ill patients are discouraged from movement due to concerns that movement will cause them more fatigue. Careful pacing of exercise or any movement modality is essential, and supervision is needed for more exacting exercise such as yoga or resistance training.[2,110,111]

Supplements

Polypharmacy with nutritional supplements is to be avoided, just as polypharmacy with medications in PC and end-of-life (EOL) care can increase the burden on the patient without significant benefit. Only those nutritional supplements essential to the patient's well-being should be continued. In most cases of patients imminently dying, almost all nutritional supplements can be discontinued except for those giving specific symptom relief. Patients and families must be a part of this decision-making process because they may hold strong beliefs about what supplements are essential for their well-being. These supplements can be continued unless the patient is having difficulty swallowing them or if they are contributing to distressing symptoms or contraindicated (e.g., fish oil in a patient with the potential for bleeding or actively bleeding).

Mind-Body Therapies

Mind-body therapies are efficacious in chronic pain, anxiety, depression, and insomnia. In a telephone survey of 2055 Americans, 18.9% had used one mind-body therapy in the past year.[112]

Mindfulness-Based Stress Reduction

In a meta-analytic review of mindfulness-based stress reduction (MBSR), an 8-week program of teaching moment-to-moment awareness of mind-body interactions was significantly correlated with reductions in anxiety, chronic pain, stress, and depression often found in patients at the end of life.[113,114] Practices that can be used in PC include walking, sitting, or lying meditation, depending on the condition of the patient; body scan meditation; gentle Hatha yoga; and breath awareness.[115] MBSR has also been combined with art therapy in patients with cancer, achieving higher quality-of-life measures than in controls as well as diminished psychological distress.[116]

MBSR can increase coping, calmness, and peace and in another study improved mood, QOL, and well-being.[117,118] It can help improve mood including anxiety and depression.[119]

Life Review and Reminiscence Therapy

Life review and reminiscence therapy are techniques used in end-of-life care as therapeutic interventions. Reminiscing is often done in a group setting, focuses on happy memories, and aims to improve socialization and communication skills.[120] It is especially effective in patients with dementia.[121] Life review, in contrast, is performed individually by a health professional who guides the patient in specific recollections to reframe, reexplore, and redefine life events and explore them for meaning. Using Milton Erickson's life-stage approach, life review is a critical developmental task enabling older persons and the dying to achieve ego integrity rather than despair.[122] With the achievement of ego integrity, a person finds meaning in his or her life and dying experience and, it is hoped, fears death less.[123] Chochinov has developed a life review tool to guide patients in looking over their lives for meaning and purpose and to help them maintain their person-ness and dignity in the dying process. The dignity-conserving perspectives fostered by this style of life review include continuity of self, role preservation, maintenance of pride, hopefulness, autonomy and control, generativity and legacy, acceptance, resilience, and fighting spirit. Three personal approaches that enhance dignity are living in the moment, maintaining normalcy, and finding spiritual comfort.[97] More research is needed to document the effects of life review, although many working in PC acknowledged that this tool has significant effects in relieving the existential suffering of patients with advanced illness.[124,125] Wise and Marchand found that in an RCT of life review, a sense of peace was enhanced.[126]

Hypnosis and Guided Imagery

In small trials, hypnosis and guided imagery have been shown to reduce anxiety, pain, and stress and to promote relaxation. Hypnosis creates a state of "focused awareness and attention," which can facilitate improvement in coping, well-being, and acceptance of death.[120] Guided imagery can be facilitated with music to evoke deeper connection.[115,127,128] Hypnosis was found to be efficacious in attenuating nausea and vomiting associated with cancer chemotherapy as well as pain.[129] Hypnosis and guided imagery may be helpful in decreasing pain and increasing relaxation in patients at the end of life, although more research is needed in this area.[130,131] Guided imagery can also be used before death to imagine a person's optimal dying process: who would be with the person, what environment he or she would be in, what he or she would like to hear or say, and so on. Once this process is defined through imagery, family/clinicians can do their best to recreate it (see Chapters 95 and 97).

Music Therapy

Simple music that is relaxing can be provided by anyone, but music therapy is provided by a certified music therapist. In active approaches to music therapy, the patient creates music with voice or instruments as a way of relating or expressing deep feelings. In receptive music therapy, the patient is receptively engaged in listening to music rather than creating it. Some forms of receptive music therapy involve the playing of music while a patient reminisces, paints, relaxes, meditates, or moves gently. Goals of therapy include relief of pain or other discomfort, relaxation, increased energy, better sleep, and relief of depressive symptoms. Music therapy has a clear theoretical framework for its effects. Although a number of studies have examined the use of music therapy for depression, the variety of modalities of music therapy makes it difficult to create a systematic review with strong recommendations.[132]

Music can raise endorphin levels in the brain and lower adrenaline levels.[133,134] The noise level in an intensive care unit (ICU) can exceed 60 dB, engendering anxiety and pain in patients being treated there. Music can help modulate this noisy environment when it is played through earphones, but music therapy need not be continuous, and optimal treatment periods are 25–90 minutes.[135-137] Studies by Chlan[134] and Wong et al.[138] have shown that 30 minutes of music therapy for relaxation is more effective than uninterrupted rest of patients in an ICU undergoing mechanical ventilation, and Zimbardo and Gerrig[139] found that 30 minutes of classical music therapy in an ICU setting equaled the relaxation effects of 10 mg of diazepam. In a 2010 Cochrane review, because of the high risk of bias and a limited number of studies, insufficient evidence was found for beneficial effects of music in end-of-life care to improve QOL.[140] Music therapy can improve mood in depression.[141] This modality reduced the intensity of pain by up to 70% in one study and can decrease opioid requirements.[55]

Music thanatology combines music therapy as medicine and spirituality. Its goals are to relieve suffering and pain and to promote a peaceful and conscious death. The therapy depends on the assessment of the musician and the needs of the patient and is therefore described as prescriptive music. A bedside vigil lasts 45–60 minutes, and caregivers are encouraged to be present. A portable harp produces a polyphonic sound that is described by Therese Schroeder-Sheker,[142] founder of the Chalice of Repose Project in End of Life Care in Oregon and North Carolina, as dissolving, which is well suited to the various environments in which the vigils are held. The tempo of the music is synchronized to the heart and respiratory rate of the patient to produce entrainment to a more relaxed or sleep state.[143] In a study of harp therapy, 77% of patients and families found the therapy to be of great benefit, and 23% found it to be of some benefit. Anxiety was relieved in 84% of patients, fear in 70%, dyspnea in 71%, nausea in 92%, and pain in 63%.[6]

Massage

Massage encompasses many different styles, but in ill patients, gentler forms such as Swedish massage may be better tolerated. Massage is beneficial in treating depression and pain, and it can help alleviate anxiety and promote more restful sleep.[144-153] In a study of 1290 patients with cancer, massage reduced moderate-to-severe symptoms of pain, fatigue, anxiety, and nausea by about 50%.[154] Another study also found this result.[155] A Cochrane review found evidence that massage, especially paired with stress-reduction techniques, improved QOL in patients with HIV/acquired immune deficiency syndrome.[156] Hand massage may be helpful for patients with dementia who are agitated. This modality can promote relaxation.[157] This modality is also combined with aromatherapy at times for a synergistic effect.

Aromatherapy

Aromatherapy is often used together with massage. One RCT showed that massage therapy with or without lavender oil helped promote sleep; massage therapy appeared to be the essential intervention.[158] Lavender oil aromatherapy alone was found to relieve anxiety in two small studies.[159,160] Use of rosemary oil increased alertness and decreased anxiety.[159] In a small study of 20 terminally ill patients with cancer, a regimen of lavender oil aromatherapy, followed by a foot soak with oil and warm water, followed by application of reflexology significantly relieved fatigue.[161] In another small experimental study of 17 hospice patients, inhaled lavender aromatherapy helped relieve anxiety and pain.[162] In a systematic review, aromatherapy massage showed benefit for psychological well-being and anxiety. Limited evidence exists for benefits in nausea, pain, and depression.[163] In one RCT using spearmint and peppermint oils in the treatment of nausea due to chemotherapy, these oils significantly reduced nausea and vomiting without adverse effects. The oils reduced the overall cost of treatment.[164] The species of plant used for the oil and the quality of the essential oil can have an impact on the therapeutic effect.[165] Many essential oil blends exist for specific indications, and the reader is encouraged to read a definitive text on this modality or to seek out the services of a certified aromatherapist.

Energy Medicine

Subtle energies involved in some complementary therapies work on a level of physics that is new to a purely mechanical, materialistic, and chemical view of life, and new discoveries have been slowly accepted in the understanding of biological systems. DNA has been found to have electronic as well as acoustical resonances, in which quantum fluctuations affect DNA expression. Music thanatology, described previously, may very well affect acoustical resonances at a DNA level as well as on a universal healing plane.[166] The emerging understanding that exists today makes the RCT perhaps too insensitive a research tool with which to study these energetic modalities, especially at the end of life, when a person's vibrational energies merge with the energies beyond the human form (see Chapter 116). In a review of biofield therapies for symptom management in PC, the authors found benefit for improving pain and QOL.[167]

Healing or Therapeutic Touch and Reiki Therapy

In small, non-RCT studies, therapeutic touch has been found to reduce anxiety and pain and to improve relaxation. Therapeutic touch is the focused intention to heal on the part of the practitioner; it involves the transfer of energy from the environment through the practitioner to the patient.[168] In a large descriptive study, a hospital evaluated its inpatient therapeutic touch program. The investigators found that it decreased anxiety and pain and increased relaxation.[169] It is challenging to research therapeutic touch with RCTs because it is difficult to have a control group, and the effects cannot be differentiated from a placebo response.[170] Four trials of therapeutic touch for wound healing were variable in effect.[171] A Cochrane review on touch therapies found modest effects on decreasing pain, and positive results seemed to be in part related to the experience of the practitioner.[172]

Reiki therapy balances the bioenergy fields on a deep vibrational level. Its therapeutic goals are to restore balance and resiliency and to promote nonspecific healing. A light touch is used on specific areas of the head and torso. If the patient has lesions, the practitioner's hands can hover a few inches above the patient. Reiki therapy may reduce anxiety and pain.[173] Miles and True[174] reviewed RCTs of Reiki therapy and found inconclusive results.

Acupuncture and Traditional Chinese Medicine

Traditional Chinese medicine has been practiced for thousands of years as a system of healing modalities, including herbs, acupuncture, and qi gong, designed to balance the life energy called *qi*. Acupuncture is an effective modality for breathlessness, nausea and vomiting, and pain.[175-177] One RCT showed a significant decrease in neuropathic pain with acupuncture compared with sham acupuncture.[178] Acupuncture is effective for pain in a number of musculoskeletal pain syndromes, such as

headache, chronic neck and back pain, and osteoarthritis. Adverse reactions are rare.[179-183]

Despite these positive studies for acupuncture use, a Cochrane review of acupuncture for cancer pain did not find sufficient evidence to support its use.[184] A systematic review of acupressure studies showed some efficacy for dyspnea, fatigue, and insomnia.[185]

Therapies to Consider

Art therapy is useful in bereavement groups, especially with children and teens, and with individuals as a means of expressing feelings, communications about the death, and their resulting grief. Pet therapy is increasingly more popular in PC and EOL care. Anyone dying who has a relatively trained pet should be allowed to have the pet present if at all possible. The comfort provided may reduce anxiety.[186] Other modalities to consider in PC are homeopathy, chiropractic care, osteopathic manipulation, and humor therapy. See Key Web Resources for a list of resources for patients and clinicians.

PREVENTION PRESCRIPTION

- Prevention is focused on maximizing comfort, well-being, healing, and life closure rather than on prolonging the dying process.
- Carefully apply and titrate therapeutic interventions to minimize side effects and maximize well-being.
- Avoid skin breakdown with frequent turning and gentle massage.
- Prevent anxiety and spiritual discomfort with supportive and trusting therapeutic relationships, effective symptom management, empowered

decision making by the patient, and bereavement and spiritual care.
- Address grief and loss with effective grief services before and after death.
- Advocate the use of advance directives, educate the patient and family on options in end-of-life care, elicit and honor patient treatment preferences, and deliver PC on the basis of the patient's treatment goals. Doing so will reduce unnecessary and unwanted interventions at the end of life.

THERAPEUTIC REVIEW

A number of therapeutic interventions can be used synergistically to maximize therapeutic effect, in some cases reducing the dose of medication needed for effect and minimizing side effects. In addition to controlling symptoms, many integrative modalities can improve well-being by enhancing psychological and spiritual health as well as by providing physical comfort. In end-of-life care, unnecessary therapies are discontinued and less-invasive modalities are increased in keeping with the needs and goals of the patient, the resources available, and the patient's response to them. Attentive listening, careful assessment, and keen observation are essential in guiding therapeutic choices.

PAIN MANAGEMENT

Pharmaceuticals

- Treat pain as an emergency. Addiction at the end of life is generally a nonissue. Believe the patient's report of pain (suffering), but consider the concept of "whole pain." Treat pain carefully but aggressively. Use a lower starting dose in patients who are opioid naive and in older persons, but increase dosage rapidly and carefully for an adequate response. No ceiling dose exists for opioids.[32]

- For unrelieved severe pain, increase the immediate-acting opioid dose by 50%–100% every 24 hours; for moderate pain, increase the dose by 25%–50%. The dose of short-acting opioids for breakthrough pain should be about 10% of the total 24-hour dose of sustained-release medication and should be given every 2–3 hours as needed. Consider increasing the bedtime dose by 50% or less to avoid administration during the night. Opioid-induced sedation caused by initiation of or increase in the dose of an opioid analgesic usually clears within a few days.[32,187,188]
- Use scheduled dosing of an oral long-acting medication for chronic pain to prevent oversedation and nadirs of pain relief. Adjust dose, generally, every 1–2 days after a steady state is achieved. Increase the dose of immediate-acting opioids for uncontrolled pain. Administer through mouth whenever possible. Avoid intramuscular injections.[32]
- The lowest dose of the fentanyl transdermal patch is 12 mcg/h, which is replaced generally every 3 days. The 25-mcg/h patch is equivalent to approximately 50 mg of oral morphine daily. The patch should be avoided in opioid-naive patients, for whom the starting dose may be too strong.

Most patients can take oral medication, which also costs less. The transdermal patch takes 8–24 hours to achieve the analgesic effect and therefore should not be used alone to treat acute pain. Also, once the patch is removed, the analgesic effect continues for 17–24 hours. Dosage may be usually titrated every 2–3 days. Absorption increases with fever. Subcutaneous fat is needed as a reservoir for the drug. Avoid placing on bony areas. [32,187]

- Decrease dose and intervals of analgesics in patients with reduced hepatic and renal clearance and in those who are dehydrated and oliguric.[32]
- Extended-release tablets cannot be crushed or chewed. Extended-release granules can, however, be mixed with food or fluids or given via a gastric tube.[32]
- Avoid use of meperidine because of its problematic metabolites when used for chronic pain.[187]
- For severe chronic pain, start with extended-release morphine, 15-mg tablet twice daily, with immediate-acting morphine, 10 mg every 3 hours, as needed. Kadian, a long-acting morphine preparation, consists of a capsule containing sprinkles that can be given via a gastric tube or mixed with food.[32]
- Hydromorphone does not have toxic metabolites and is preferred in patients with severe renal insufficiency. Morphine and oxycodone are excreted renally and should be used carefully or avoided in patients with severe renal insufficiency.[32]
- In patients with liver impairment, morphine is preferred. Avoid acetaminophen and tricyclic antidepressants in patients with liver impairment.[32]
- Methadone is useful in the treatment of nociceptive and neuropathic pain; it is inexpensive and can control pain that is not responsive to other opioids.[30] Initiation and titration of methadone therapy are unique, and appropriate resources must be carefully used; alternatively, the clinician can consult with a palliative medicine or pain consultant.[33,35] Conversion to methadone from another opioid is also unique, and guidelines for optimal, safe conversions are available.[32-35,37]
- Always use a gentle laxative when treating a patient with opioids. Stool softeners alone are generally ineffective. They can be used together. Use laxatives liberally; senna at a starting dose of one to two tablets at bedtime works well. The goal is for the patient to have a bowel movement every day or every other day. A stool softener alone is often not effective, and use with a laxative is needed.
- Neuropathic pain often requires the addition of adjuvant medications, such as anticonvulsants (e.g., gabapentin starting at 100 mg three times a day) or antidepressants (e.g., the tricyclic antidepressant nortriptyline starting at 10 mg/day or amitriptyline starting at 25 mg at bedtime), for adequate relief. Opioids alone, except methadone, are usually not adequate to treat neuropathic pain.[32] Use caution in patients with renal or hepatic impairment.

Botanicals and Supplements

- For pain, especially neuropathic pain, cannabis inhaled is most effective. Medical marijuana is only available legally in specific states in the United States and countries worldwide. Check local laws and clinical resources.

Other Modalities

- Consider acupuncture for neuropathic and nociceptive pain, often in conjunction with medication.
- Massage can help relieve pain.

NAUSEA AND VOMITING

Lifestyle

- Target the mechanism of cause and either discontinue the offending medication or treat the underlying cause.

Pharmaceuticals

- Stimulation of chemoreceptor trigger zone (CTZ) in the fourth ventricle of the brain by medications including opioids, hypercalcemia, or uremia commonly causes nausea and vomiting. The CTZ has dopamine and serotonin (5-HT$_3$) receptors. Antidopaminergics such as prochlorperazine and haloperidol and 5-HT$_3$ antagonists such as ondansetron most effectively treat this cause of nausea and vomiting.[58]
    - Prochlorperazine: start at 5 mg every 6 hours as needed orally or 25 mg twice daily as needed via rectal route
    - Haloperidol: start at 0.5 mg orally three times daily as needed; may also be given subcutaneously
- Nausea caused by constipation is relieved with laxatives.[58]
- Nausea caused by infection and inflammation responds well to anticholinergic and antihistamine antiemetics, such as promethazine 12.5–35 mg every 4–6 hours orally and intramuscularly, and 25 mg rectally every 6 hours as needed.[58]
- Nausea caused by dysmotility of the gut, such as in the use of opioids, is relieved best with prokinetic agents such as metoclopramide, starting at 5 mg orally, subcutaneously, or intravenously every 6–8 hours as needed. Anticholinergic drugs make this kind of nausea worse. Avoid this drug in patients with Parkinson's disease and renal failure.[58]
- Vestibular causes of nausea respond best to antihistamine, anticholinergic drugs such as promethazine, and scopolamine; one patch every 72 hours should be administered as needed.[58]

Botanicals

- Ginger: 500–1000 mg of ginger root extract as needed (boiled to make a tea), or eat 1 tsp or 5 g of crystalized ginger as needed for nausea.
- Cannabinoid: Inhalation most effective for nausea and to improve appetite.

DYSPNEA

Pharmaceuticals

- Oxygen therapy can help relieve dyspnea caused by low oxygen saturation.
- Morphine and other opioids can help relieve the sensation of breathlessness.[64] In elderly and opioid-naive patients, consider initially using very low doses of morphine solution in doses of 2–4 mg every 3 hours either as scheduled or as needed. Immediate-release morphine can also be given if the patient must exert himself or herself above baseline activities or if a more strenuous activity causes more dyspnea. The dose is given 30 minutes before the more strenuous activity. If short-acting morphine is needed regularly, consider using long-acting morphine.
- In patients already receiving opioids for pain, the dose of opioid to control breathlessness may need to be 1.5–2.5 times the analgesic dose.[32]
- Drying secretions with glycopyrrolate can help with the sensation of dyspnea at the end of life. Glycopyrrolate does not cross the blood–brain barrier and cause sedation and can be given orally or IV. Avoidance of overhydration is also important.
- Anxiolytics such as lorazepam (Ativan), 0.5–2 mg every 6–8 hours as needed, can help in anxiety associated with breathlessness.

Energy Medicine

- Acupuncture can help relieve dyspnea.

DELIRIUM

- Assess for delirium carefully because the patient can be in a hyperactive/agitated or hypoactive/somnolent delirium state. Do not treat states of agitation reflexively

using anxiolytics, which have a high potential to make delirium worse. Medications (especially with anticholinergic side effects), steroids, benzodiazepines, and opioids are often the culprit, and offending medications must be discontinued or changed, the dose decreased, or the route of administration changed. Treatment is aimed at the underlying cause.[71,78,79]
- Delirium must be differentiated from near-death awareness.[86]

Pharmaceuticals
- Haloperidol is the drug of choice for treatment of acute delirium; dosing starts at 0.5–2 mg orally two or three times a day or 0.5–2 mg intravenously or intramuscularly every 1–4 hours as needed. The dose can be titrated down by 25% daily once the optimal effect is stabilized. It is less sedating and has fewer side effects than other neuroleptics. Side effects are extrapyramidal, consisting of restlessness and tremor.[71,78] Use caution if the QTc interval is prolonged, except in patients at the end of life.
- Benzodiazepines are indicated for delirium caused by seizures and alcohol or sedative withdrawal and in cases not responding to haloperidol.[77,78]

SPIRITUAL CARE
- Indigenous cultural and spiritual practices are important in facilitating healing as well as peaceful, meaningful dying and death. Ritual and ceremony are important in supporting the patient and relieving emotional and spiritual distress, which can have an ameliorating effect on physical symptoms.
- Spiritual inquiry using a spiritual assessment tool, meditation, and prayer can improve spiritual and psychological well-being in the dying process and also relieve physical symptoms.

BEREAVEMENT
- Grief work for the patient can help relieve existential distress, and grief work for the family, friends, and health care staff when needed can help diminish complicated grief after the death.

NUTRITION
- Reducing food and fluid intake is normal in the dying process, and patient discomfort can occur if food or fluids are forced or if given intravenously or via tube feedings. Substitute the nurturing aspects of feeding with touch and other ways to show love and care to the patient. Offer foods in small quantities that the patient enjoys and finds palatable. Swab the mouth frequently to prevent feeling of thirst.

MIND-BODY THERAPIES
- Mindfulness-based stress reduction can decrease anxiety, chronic pain, stress, and depression.
- Music therapy encompasses many modalities. Harp therapy can decrease pain, existential and physical suffering, anxiety, and nausea and can improve sleep.
- Massage therapy also includes many different styles of treatment; it can ameliorate pain, fatigue, anxiety, depression, and nausea as well as promote better sleep.
- Reminiscence therapy can improve cognition in patients with dementia.
- Life review therapy improves depression, spiritual distress, and quality of life and alleviates pain.
- Hypnosis and guided imagery can reduce anxiety, pain, and stress and promote relaxation.

ENERGY THERAPIES
- Aromatherapy massage has been shown to be of benefit for psychological well-being and anxiety. Limited evidence exists for its benefits in nausea, pain, and depression.
- Therapeutic touch may reduce anxiety and pain and promote relaxation. Other benefits are also possible, but this modality is challenging to research.
- Acupuncture is an effective modality for nausea and vomiting and pain.

Key Web Resources

Advance Care Planning

Aging with Dignity Five Wishes	http://www.agingwithdignity.org
Respecting Choices	http://respectingchoices.org/
Partnership for Caring: America's Voices for the Dying	http://www.partnershipforcaring.org
Complementary and alternative medicine integrative pain management	http://www.stoppain.org
Integrative pain assessment and treatment	http://www.HealingChronicPain.org

Palliative Medicine and Hospice

Education in Palliative and End-of-Life Care (EPEC)	http://www.epec.net
End-of-Life Nursing Education Consortium (ELNEC)	http://www.aacn.nche.edu/elnec
Dying Well	http://www.dyingwell.org
National Hospice and Palliative Care Organization	http://www.nhpco.org
Last Acts	http://www.lastacts.org
Palliative Care Network of Wisconsin—Fast Facts	http://www.mypcnow.org/fast-facts
Americans for Better Care of the Dying (ABCD)	http://www.abcd-caring.org
American Academy of Hospice and Palliative Medicine	http://www.AAHPM.org
Society for Integrative Oncology	http://www.integrativeonc.org
Module on grief with patient resources including handouts on coping with grief and tools to help with the grief experience	http://www.fammed.wisc.edu/integrative/modules/grief
Center to Advance Palliative Care	http://www.capc.org

REFERENCES

References are available online at ExpertConsult.com.

SECTION XV

SUBSTANCE ABUSE

SECTION OUTLINE

83 ALCOHOLISM AND SUBSTANCE ABUSE

CHAPTER 83

ALCOHOLISM AND SUBSTANCE ABUSE

Donald Warne, MD, MPH

Alcohol use disorder (AUD) is a medical diagnosis characterized by problem drinking that becomes severe. In the United States, approximately 17 million adults aged 18 and older had an AUD in 2012 (7.2% of adults). Minors can also be diagnosed with an AUD, and approximately 855,000 adolescents aged 12–17 had an AUD in 2012. Diagnostic criteria for AUD are described in the *Diagnostic and Statistical Manual of Mental Disorders* (DSM). According to the DSM-5, anyone meeting two or more of the 11 criteria within a 12-month timeframe is diagnosed with AUD. AUD severity (mild, moderate, or severe) is determined by the number of criteria met.[1]

In addition to alcohol, there are numerous drugs of abuse, including opiates, marijuana, cocaine, methamphetamines, tobacco, and others.[2] See Box 83.1 for a simple three-question screening tool for alcohol disorders (AUDIT-C).

Alcoholism and substance abuse have a negative impact on other chronic diseases managed in the primary care setting due to the direct effects of the substances abused and issues related to compliance and self-care.[3] Acute injury and illness resulting from alcohol and substance abuse are analogous to exacerbations of chronic conditions and therefore constitute issues of extreme importance in the arena of primary care. Unfortunately, many physicians do not routinely address these issues,[4] and few conventional allopathic interventions are easily accessible and efficacious. This chapter examines the treatment options available to the primary care physician and also provides a source of information for appropriate referrals. A multitude of both illicit and prescribed substances are abused; the focus of this chapter is primarily on alcohol, tobacco, opiates, cocaine, and marijuana.

Addiction to drugs and alcohol should be treated as a chronic illness not unlike diabetes mellitus or hypertension.[5] Like these disorders, addiction has behavioral components as well as underlying biochemical mechanisms. Within chronic addiction and recovery, there are also exacerbations of abuse as well as chronic multiorgan system complications.[6] Successful treatment of all chronic diseases requires a good rapport between patients and providers and the use of a nonjudgmental approach.[7,8] Box 83.2 provides simple guidelines to assess the severity of alcohol risk.

PATHOPHYSIOLOGY

Alcoholism and substance abuse have many dimensions, each with unique implications and standards of treatment.

The processes of alcoholism and substance abuse may be divided into broad categories or stages: craving, active abuse, intoxication, withdrawal, detoxification, recovery, and relapse prevention.

A proposed mechanism of addiction for all substances of abuse involves the sudden release of dopamine in the "reward pathway" connecting the midbrain to the prefrontal cortex. This rush of dopamine is believed to cause a sense of euphoria and pleasure that is at the root of drug abuse. With extended drug use, there is a profound alteration in brain chemistry. This neurophysiological change in the central nervous system eventually causes a "switch" in the affected person from a state of drug abuse to one of addiction with uncontrollable cravings and dependence. The exact mechanisms of this process are as yet unknown.[9]

The process of addiction is, of course, not limited to brain chemistry. The effects of environmental, social, cultural, genetic, and behavioral factors are significant in the development of alcoholism and substance abuse.[10] These factors assume varying levels of importance in the development of addiction for each person. Addiction is therefore most accurately viewed as a complex illness with varying degrees of environmental and biochemical features.[11]

INTEGRATIVE THERAPY

Pharmaceuticals

In the last decade, several new and effective pharmacological options have become available to the primary care physician to treat alcoholism and substance abuse. Some of the most effective pharmaceutical agents are available only through licensed intensive outpatient and inpatient programs specializing in the treatment of addictions. However, with the U.S. Food and Drug Administration (FDA) approval of new medications, including acamprosate (Campral) in 2004 and buprenorphine (Subutex) in 2002, primary care physicians have the opportunity to take a more active role in the treatment of addiction to alcohol and opiates.[12,13] For physicians interested in using these medications for their patients with addictions, it is important to remember that these agents are most effective when they are used as part of a comprehensive management program that involves psychosocial support such as counseling and support groups. Table 83.1 provides an overview of pharmaceutical treatments for alcohol and substance abuse. As noted, these treatments may be divided into the broad categories of detoxification/withdrawal and craving/relapse prevention.

Management of Alcohol Withdrawal and Recovery

The most common treatment of acute alcohol withdrawal is administration of diazepam or another benzodiazepine.[14,15] A benefit of benzodiazepine treatment is relief from the anxiety and sleep disturbances experienced during the withdrawal phase. A disadvantage of benzodiazepine therapy is the potential for dependence if the drug is not prescribed appropriately.[16] A benzodiazepine for

detoxification should be prescribed only for a short time in a supervised setting. Phenobarbital or carbamazepine (Tegretol) is occasionally used in managing withdrawal seizures. There is evidence that opioid receptors play a role in the physiological response to alcohol. Naltrexone (ReVia), an opioid antagonist, has been shown to be effective in preventing alcoholic relapse.[17] Disulfiram (Antabuse) inhibits aldehyde dehydrogenase and produces unpleasant effects, such as nausea, vomiting, and dizziness, when alcohol is consumed.

Acamprosate, an amino acid derivative that modulates activity of gamma–aminobutyric acid (GABA) neurotransmission in the brain, appears to be effective in reducing alcohol cravings.[18] As opposed to limiting the "high" sensation of alcohol (as naltrexone does) or producing unpleasant side effects (as disulfiram does), acamprosate can assist in preventing alcohol relapse by reducing the anxiety and sleep disturbances associated with alcohol craving, although its exact mechanism of action is unknown.[19] Pharmacological treatments for alcohol withdrawal generally work well and can potentially be used for outpatient withdrawal management if the primary physician is able to monitor the patient closely. Treatments for relapse prevention generally are not efficacious in the absence of comprehensive follow-up care.[20]

BOX 83.1	AUDIT-C Screening for Alcohol Use Disorders

Instructions: For each question, please check the answer that is correct for you.
1. How often do you have a drink containing alcohol?
Never (0)
Monthly or less (1)
Two to four times a month (2)
Two to three times per week (3)
Four or more times a week (4)
2. How many drinks containing alcohol do you have on a typical day when you are drinking?
1 or 2 (0)
3 or 4 (1)
5 or 6 (2)
7 to 9 (3)
10 or more (4)
3. How often do you have six or more drinks on one occasion?
Never (0)
Less than monthly (1)
Monthly (2)
Two or three times a week (3)
Four or more times a week (4)
Add the numerical value of each answer selected to get your total score.
TOTAL SCORE: _____
The maximum score is 12. A score of ≥4 identifies 86% of men who report drinking above recommended levels or who meet criteria for alcohol use disorders.
A score of >2 identifies 84% of women who report hazardous drinking or alcohol use disorders.

From National Council for Community Behavioural Healthcare. http://www.thenationalcouncil.org/galleries/business-practice%20files/tool_auditc.pdf; Accessed July 5, 2011.

BOX 83.2	Alcohol Risk Terms: Abstinence, Moderate, and Risky or Hazardous

ABSTINENCE
No alcohol use

MODERATE
Men: no more than 2 standard drinks per drinking day
Women and older persons (older than 65 years): no more than 1 standard drink per drinking day

RISKY OR HAZARDOUS
Men
More than 4 standard drinks per drinking day
More than 14 standard drinks per week
Women and older persons (older than 65 years)
More than 3 standard drinks per drinking day
More than 7 standard drinks per drinking week

TABLE 83.1 Pharmaceutical Agents Used for Treatment of Alcoholism and Substance Abuse

Substance of Abuse	Agents Used for Detoxification/Withdrawal	Agents Used for Craving/Relapse Prevention	Agents Used for Other Purposes
Alcohol	Benzodiazepines Phenobarbital	Naltrexone Acamprosate Topiramate	Disulfiram
Tobacco	Nicotine Bupropion	Nicotine Varenicline	Bupropion
Opiates	Methadone Clonidine Buprenorphine	Methadone L-Alpha-acetylmethadol	Naloxone
Cocaine	Selective serotonin reuptake inhibitors Monoamine oxidase inhibitors Amantadine	Tricyclic antidepressants	
Marijuana	N/A	N/A	

N/A, not applicable.

For patients who have not abstained from alcohol, topiramate (Topamax) has been found to reduce heavy drinking and days of any drinking over a 12-week period. It is also cleared through the kidney and thus does not exacerbate toxicity to the liver. It is generally used for 6–12 months as part of a comprehensive treatment program.[21] Research also suggests that topiramate at a mean dose of 200 mg/day may work better to maintain abstinence with reduced cravings than naltrexone at a mean dose of 50 mg/day.[22]

DOSAGE

- Naltrexone 50 mg/day orally reduces the high sensation associated with alcohol.
- For the reduction of the craving of alcohol, acamprosate 333–666 mg three times a day or topiramate titrated from 25 to 300 mg weekly over 8 weeks (Table 83.2) is prescribed.
- Disulfiram 150–500 mg/day creates unpleasant side effects when it is used with alcohol.
- For help with tapering and withdrawal from alcohol, the dosage of benzodiazepine is titrated to achieve a calming effect. High doses may be needed initially. An example is clonazepam (Klonopin) 1 mg three times a day, with a gradual taper over 10–14 days.
- Match the pharmaceutical treatment to the individual's greatest need for successful abstinence.
  - For cravings: use acamprosate or topiramate.
  - For negative feedback and avoidance: use disulfiram.
  - To reduce the high associated with use: use naloxone or topiramate.
  - To reduce symptoms of withdrawal: use a benzodiazepine (diazepam or clonazepam) or clonidine.

Management of Nicotine Withdrawal: Smoking Cessation

Effective outpatient treatment regimens are available for smoking cessation. Tapered nicotine replacement therapy (NRT) is effective in the management of nicotine withdrawal and cravings.[23] Bupropion (Zyban) has been shown to be effective in managing symptoms of anxiety associated with nicotine withdrawal and craving and can be used in combination with NRT.[24] Varenicline (Chantix), a partial nicotine receptor agonist, has been found to help increase smoking cessation more than placebo and as well as bupropion.[25] These medications can be used successfully in the outpatient primary care setting.[26]

DOSAGE

Bupropion 150 mg is administered twice daily for 6 weeks, with a target quit date of 2 weeks after the start of therapy. Varenicline is started 1 week before smoking cessation: 0.5 mg orally for 3 days, 0.5 mg twice daily for 4 days, and then 1 mg twice daily for 11 weeks; the general course of therapy is 12 weeks.

PRECAUTIONS

Varenicline has a black box warning for neuropsychiatric side effects including behavior change, hostility, agitation, depression, and suicidality. These can be exacerbated when it is used long term with nicotine. Adverse events associated with the use of bupropion in clinical trials most commonly included insomnia, headache, dry mouth, nausea, and anxiety.

Management of Opiate Withdrawal and Recovery

Acute opiate withdrawal is commonly treated with methadone, an opioid receptor agonist that can block withdrawal symptoms without producing the euphoria caused by heroin and other opiates. Owing to this effect, methadone is also commonly used in long-term maintenance programs to reduce cravings and relapse. Clonidine has been shown to be effective in lessening opiate withdrawal symptoms and does not foster physiological dependence.[27] L-Alpha-acetylmethadol (LAAM) is derived from methadone and acts in a fashion similar to that noted for methadone.[28] The advantage of LAAM in maintenance therapy is that its effect lasts 72 hours, allowing dosing every other day or three times per week. Naloxone is an opiate antagonist used for treatment of acute opiate overdose.[29]

Perhaps the most significant pharmaceutical development in the management of opioid addiction is the 2002 FDA approval of the use of buprenorphine *(brand name, Suboxone; combines buprenorphine with naloxone)* in the United States. An opiate receptor partial agonist, buprenorphine has shown benefit in managing opioid addiction and preventing relapse.[30] Opioid partial agonists bind to the opioid receptor, but only partially activate the receptor and generate significantly less euphoric sensation than opiate agonists like heroin do.[31] Potential for abuse of buprenorphine is much lower than those of other opiates, and buprenorphine has been shown to be as effective as methadone in weaning clients off this class of drugs.[32]

Buprenorphine requires specific training for prescribing, and referral to an appropriately qualified physician is required. More information is available at the U.S. Department of Health and Human Services Substance Abuse and Mental Health Services Administration (SAMHSA) website (http://buprenorphine.samhsa.gov).

TABLE 83.2	Titration of Topiramate for Treatment of Alcohol Dependence		
Week	Morning Dose (mg)	Afternoon Dose (mg)	Total Daily Dose (mg)
1	0	25	25
2	0	50	50
3	25	50	75
4	50	50	100
5	50	100	150
6	100	100	200
7	100	150	250
8	150	150	300

Management of Cocaine Dependence

Cocaine withdrawal is typically associated with minimal symptoms as compared to other substances of abuse.[33] Several classes of pharmaceutical agents have been studied for their efficacy in treating cocaine dependence and relapse prevention, although none of these are approved by the FDA for this purpose. Extensive abuse of cocaine can cause depression by depleting baseline levels of dopamine.[34] Several antidepressants have been studied for their roles in treating cocaine addiction, including tricyclic antidepressants, selective serotonin reuptake inhibitors, and monoamine oxidase inhibitors; however, results are mixed and inconclusive. Propranolol has been studied for its effectiveness in reducing cocaine withdrawal severity and is showing some promise in mitigating severe symptoms.[35] Amantadine, a dopamine agonist, has been studied for its role in cocaine dependence. In theory, dopamine agonist therapy should cause dopamine restoration and reduce the need for cocaine, but findings of studies have not been convincing.[36] In addition, the results of studies examining the role of buprenorphine in the management of cocaine addiction have been mixed.[37]

Botanicals

Various herbs and combinations of herbs are reported to be effective in reducing cravings, but in general, no studies have proven their effectiveness.

Kudzu

Kudzu, a traditional Chinese herb, has been used as an "antiinebriation" treatment for hundreds of years, although its mechanism of action is not yet known.[38,39]

A small study showed that in heavy drinkers of alcohol, kudzu did result in a reduction of the number of beers consumed after 7 days of treatment.[40] It has not been found to enhance sobriety in chronic alcoholics.[41]

DOSAGE
The recommended dose is 1.2 g twice daily.

PRECAUTIONS
Kudzu is considered safe, with few side effects other than the potential for an allergic reaction to the plant.

Cytisine

In a study comparing cytisine to nicotine replacement, 40% quit on cytisine compared to 31% on nicotine replacement. Cytisine is a plant-based alkaloid found in the seeds of the golden rain tree (*Cytisus laburnum*). It is a partial agonist of nicotine acetylcholine receptors. It works similar to the drug varenicline (Chantix) and has been available in Eastern Europe since the 1960s. The leaves of this plant were smoked by Russian soldiers during World War II when there was a shortage of tobacco. It was known as *false tobacco*.

DOSAGE
Cytisine 1.5 mg (*Tabex*) were used in this study. Patients were told to taper smoking over the first 4 days and quit on the 5th day. The following tapering dose of cytisine was used:
Days 1–3: 1 tablet every 2 hrs, up to 6 tablets a day.
Days 4–12: 1 tablet every 2.5 hrs, up to 5 tablets per day.
Days 13–16: 1 tablet every 3 hrs, up to 4 tablets a day.
Days 17–20: 1 tablet every 4–5 hrs, up to 3 tablets a day.
Days 21–25: 1 tablet every 6 hrs, up to 2 tablets per day.

PRECAUTIONS
The plant *Cytisus laburnum* from which cytisine is derived is traditionally used as an emetic and purgative, so nausea and vomiting is the main side effect. Like verenicline, it can disrupt the sleep cycle and cause nightmares.

Herbal Antidepressants and Anxiolytics

Because people who struggle with alcoholism and substance abuse commonly have coexisting depression and anxiety,[42,43] it is possible that herbal remedies used for these conditions may have a role in recovery and abstinence. Poorly managed anxiety may lead to higher alcohol intake.[44] Herbs that are effective in treating anxiety and insomnia, such as valerian and kava kava, might be helpful in managing anxiety associated with detoxification and cravings. These herbs have been shown to enhance the levels and action of GABA and therefore might also have a role in the control of alcohol cravings and prevention of relapse. Caution should be taken with the use of kava kava in alcoholic patients because it has been associated with liver toxicity.[45] St. John's wort has a mechanism of action similar to that of the selective serotonin reuptake inhibitors and has been shown to be effective in treating depression.[46] Its role in managing depression associated with alcoholism and substance abuse is yet to be determined. The potential uses of herbal antidepressants in addiction recovery warrant further investigation.

Other Herbal Remedies

Lobelia is described as a respiratory stimulant and has been used in homeopathic preparations as an aid to stop smoking.[47] Milk thistle, which has been studied for its hepatoprotective effects, appears to be a promising treatment for alcoholic cirrhosis.[48]

Acupuncture

Acupuncture is perhaps the most extensively studied and most promising integrative treatment of addictions. The practice of acupuncture is documented in Chinese literature as early as the Han dynasty in the second century BC in the *Huang Di Nei Jing (Yellow Emperor's Classic of Medicine)*. In acupuncture terms, the body is seen as having several energy channels, or meridians, that allow the free flow of *qi* (pronounced "chee"), or energy. In a healthy or balanced state, *qi* flows smoothly throughout the body and provides for homeostasis. With disease, injury, or a state of imbalance, the normal movement of *qi* is obstructed or impaired. Acupuncture treatments are designed to unblock obstructions of meridians and to promote the healthy flow of energy.[49]

In 1973, Wen and Cheung[50] reported that opiate-addicted patients who were using electroacupuncture for treatment of postoperative pain described relief from symptoms of withdrawal. Omura brought the treatment protocol to Lincoln Hospital in New York in 1974, and Smith and Kahn[51] developed a five-point auricular acupuncture treatment protocol for addictions that is currently being taught and advocated by the National Acupuncture Detoxification Association (NADA).

In acupuncture terms, substance abuse can be seen as an attempt by the patient to self-treat an imbalance in the flow of *qi*. The "drug of choice" provides temporary relief from energy imbalance, but unfortunately, it also commonly causes further underlying imbalance. As a result, the baseline imbalance slowly worsens, and the need for more drugs slowly increases. The acupuncture treatment therefore provides energy balancing without the need for alcohol or drugs, as well as relaxation and relief from cravings.[52]

> Acupuncture treatments influence the flow of *qi* to achieve energy balancing, relaxation, and reduced cravings for alcohol, tobacco, and illicit drugs.

Another proposed mechanism of action is that the acupuncture needles stimulate peripheral nerves to cause release of endorphins in the brain, thereby resulting in relaxation and a sense of well-being; acupuncture thus can provide direct biochemical treatment for opiate and ethanol craving and withdrawal.[53] The NADA treatment protocol and certification course emphasize the multifaceted nature of this modality and describe treatment benefits in

the biochemical, psychological, and social realms as well as in the traditional Chinese paradigm.

The specific points used in the NADA protocol are shen men (spirit gate), sympathetic nervous system, kidney, liver, and lung (Fig. 83.1). These points have roles in balancing energy and calming as well as in regulating sympathetic nervous system function and specific organ function from the modern and traditional Chinese perspectives of physiology. The kidney, liver, and lung each have specific roles in the generation, regulation, and flow of *qi*. These organ-specific functions are described in acupuncture texts[54] and are beyond the scope of this chapter.

Auricular acupuncture has been studied in the treatment of addiction to various drugs, including alcohol, cocaine, opiates, and marijuana. In 1989, Bullock et al.[55] reported that auricular acupuncture was effective in the treatment of relapsing alcoholics. In this study, 80 relapsing alcoholics who were enrolled in a treatment facility were randomly assigned to receive either the appropriate acupuncture treatment protocol (treatment group) or sham acupuncture points at sites close to the appropriate points (control group). The outcomes measured included completion of the treatment program and self-reported abstinence at 1, 3, and 6 months after the end of the program. Of the 40 subjects in the treatment group, 21 finished the program, whereas only 1 of 40 in the control group completed treatment ($p < .001$). Information about self-reported drinking episodes was collected from all available subjects, including those who did not complete treatment. Fewer treatment group subjects than control group subjects reported drinking episodes at 1-, 3-, and 6-month follow-up evaluations.

In 1998, Shwartz et al. compared residential detoxification programs that used acupuncture with programs that did not. In this retrospective study, 6907 patients completed nonacupuncture programs, and 1104 patients completed programs that used acupuncture as an adjunctive therapy. The study subjects were dependent on alcohol, cocaine, crack, heroin, marijuana, or a combination of these drugs. The primary outcome measured was readmission to a detoxification program in the 6 months after discharge. After controlling for baseline differences among the patients in the study, those who completed programs offering acupuncture were readmitted to detoxification less frequently than those from conventional programs ($p < .02$).[56] A randomized controlled trial of auricular acupuncture for cocaine dependence published in 2000 studied 82 patients who were randomly allocated to receive appropriate acupuncture treatment, sham acupuncture, or relaxation therapy. Thrice-weekly urine screening for cocaine was conducted during an 8-week period. The patients who received the appropriate acupuncture protocol were less likely to test positive for cocaine on urine screening than patients in the sham acupuncture control group ($p = .05$) or the relaxation control group ($p = .01$).[57]

Auricular acupuncture has been shown by these studies to be a useful adjunct in treating alcoholism and substance abuse. Other investigations have found mixed results or little benefit from acupuncture in treating addiction.[58,59] Further investigation in this area is warranted.

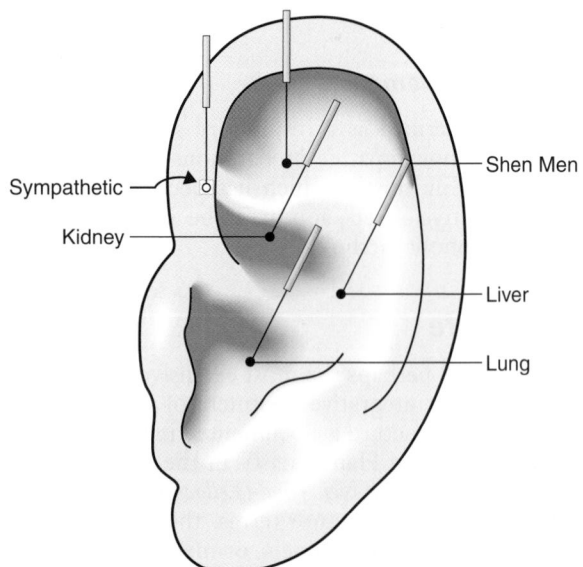

Sympathetic

Kidney

Shen Men

Liver

Lung

FIG. 83.1 ■ Acupuncture points for the National Acupuncture Detoxification Association (NADA) treatment protocol. (Reprinted with permission from Joseph Helms, MD, and Medical Acupuncture Publishers, Berkeley, CA.)

Mind-Body Therapies

As more is learned about the connection between thoughts and physiology, the field of mind-body medicine continues to grow and to gain acceptance. Commonly used therapies classified as mind-body interventions are meditation, biofeedback, hypnosis, guided imagery, yoga, and prayer. Research in this field appears promising for mind-body medicine as an adjunctive intervention for alcoholism and substance abuse.

Meditation

Meditation can be divided into three broad categories: concentrative, mindfulness, and transcendental. Concentrative meditation focuses attention on breathing, imagery, or sounds; mindfulness meditation involves focused awareness on the passage of thoughts and images as they spontaneously appear. Transcendental meditation (TM) is a technique brought to the United States by Maharishi Mahesh Yogi in the 1960s. TM was developed from the ancient East Indian Vedic belief system and helps practitioners of this technique balance the physical, mental, emotional, and spiritual components of health.[60] Within this belief system, prolonged or excessive stress leads to holistic imbalance, which causes illness, including alcoholism and substance abuse. The sense of balancing offered by TM allows optimal function and decreases the need for drugs and alcohol.[61] Several studies and review articles have shown TM to be effective in the treatment of alcoholism and substance abuse; however, most of these studies had flaws in their designs and methods without randomization, blinding, or appropriate control groups.[62] A randomized controlled trial indicated improvement in the number of days of alcohol abstinence with the use of TM or biofeedback compared with electronic neurotherapy and the Alcoholics Anonymous program or counseling.[63] TM has been shown to significantly raise serotonin levels and to decrease cortisol levels in as little as 4 months of practice.[64] This is a possible mechanism for improving senses of balance and well-being and for reducing the effects of stress. In a group of polysubstance abusers, when goal management training was combined with mindfulness-based meditation, there was significant improvement in emotional risks associated with substance use.[65] A study published in 2010 showed effectiveness of Qigong meditation on improved addiction treatment outcomes, particularly among females[66] (see Chapter 100).

> Mind-body therapies, including meditation, biofeedback, hypnosis, guided imagery, yoga, and prayer, use the power of the mind to influence the body. Relaxation and reduced physiological responses to stress are helpful in the recovery process.

Biofeedback

Biofeedback is a technique that uses electronic monitors, including electroencephalography, electromyography, and electrocardiography, as well as cutaneous thermometers and pulse oximeters to teach the patient how to consciously control physiological functions such as respiratory rate, heart rate, skin temperature, and blood pressure. Conscious regulation of these functions is achieved through concentration, meditation, and the use of relaxation techniques. Biofeedback has been shown to be useful in managing stress-related disorders such as hypertension, irritable bowel syndrome, pain, and substance abuse.[67] Electromyographic biofeedback, which focuses on relieving muscle tension, has been shown to be an effective tool in treating alcoholism.[68] Unfortunately, there are only limited studies on the use of this intervention in treating addictions. The mechanism of action and efficacy of biofeedback in managing alcoholism and substance abuse have not yet been determined.

Hypnosis

The German physician Franz Anton Mesmer introduced modern hypnotherapy in the eighteenth century as mesmerism. The American Medical Association recognized hypnosis as a legitimate medical therapy in 1958, and it has been applied by various health care practitioners in the treatment of numerous disorders, including alcoholism and substance abuse. Hypnotherapy involves concentration, mental focusing exercises, relaxation techniques, guided imagery, and suggestion. Studies have shown that hypnosis improves memory and cognitive function[69] and can affect physiological function by reducing sympathetic nervous system activity, heart rate, blood pressure, and oxygen consumption.[70] Many techniques are used in hypnotherapy, making standardization difficult for research purposes; however, there are case reports of positive results of its use in substance abuse treatment and relapse prevention.[71] Controlled trials have not shown long-term benefits in the management of addictions. Some techniques used in hypnosis may be useful as adjunctive modalities in comprehensive recovery programs. One study used self-hypnosis tapes in a residential treatment program for drug and alcohol abuse. Those who listened to the tapes three to five times a week showed the highest levels of self-esteem and serenity and the least amount of anger or impulsivity compared with less frequent users[72] (see Chapter 95).

Guided Imagery

Guided imagery uses the power of the mind to directly affect physiological function. Practitioners of this technique report improved insight into emotional and physical health. Imagery can modulate heart rate, blood pressure, oxygen consumption, and various other physiological measures. Deeper insight into emotions, behaviors, and thoughts can help patients deal with the anxiety and depression associated with the recovery process[73,74] (see Chapter 97).

Yoga

A traditional East Indian healing system, yoga combines specific postures, breathing control, and meditation to reduce stress and to promote balance and a sense of well-being. Yoga, meaning "union," attempts to help its practitioners address and equilibrate the physical, mental, and spiritual forces that coalesce in the process of disease or disharmony. Yoga has been shown to have a beneficial effect on stress-related conditions, including chronic pain, hypertension, and recovery from addiction.[75] There are, however, no randomized controlled trials specifically assessing the efficacy of yoga for management of addictions. The use of this technique has been shown to be beneficial as part of a comprehensive treatment program.[76]

Spirituality

The role of spirituality in medicine and recovery has been steadily gaining acceptance from mainstream health care practitioners.[77] Numerous studies on the role of spirituality in the recovery from addiction have been conducted.[78] Defining spirituality and religion and identifying interventions that exist within these realms are difficult. Spirituality is a subjective concept that can be considered to represent a person's connection with and relationship to a transcendent or higher power.[79] Religion can be defined in terms of a structured value and belief system with its own hierarchy, rituals, and practices.[80]

Commonly described practices in spirituality are prayer and meditation. The field of mind-body medicine often includes prayer with meditation as a synergistic tool to promote wellness and healing. Spirituality is addressed separately here because it transcends mind-body interventions and is not easily defined by objective markers. The role of spirituality—and, to some extent, religion—in the recovery process cannot be ignored. The regular practice of prayer and meditation is strongly correlated with recovery and abstinence from drugs of abuse.[81] Active participation in spiritual practices such as prayer appears to be more important in the recovery process than being prayed for by others.[82]

"Negative spirituality" may be at the root of addictions, and a "spiritual awakening" may be required before an individual can genuinely recover from addiction.[83] Regular church attendance has been associated with negative perceptions of addiction and lower rates of alcoholism, substance abuse,[84] and tobacco use.[85] The extent of family religious practice also has an effect on youth perspectives on substance abuse.[86] Obviously, spirituality cannot be prescribed in the primary care setting, but it is important for the clinician to be aware of the client's spiritual beliefs and value systems when identifying appropriate recovery programs for referral (see Chapter 114).

Twelve-Step Programs

Alcoholics Anonymous (AA) has helped millions of people in their approach to recovery from alcoholism worldwide since it began in 1935. The AA program of recovery is spiritually based, with frequent meetings, mentoring, and social support. The basic spiritual framework is described in the Twelve Steps of AA, presented in Box 83.3.

AA is rooted in spirituality, not religion. The AA preamble, commonly recited at the start of meetings, states that "AA is not allied with any sect, denomination, politics, organization, or institution." The belief in a "higher power" is seen as a point of connection for all AA members, no matter what each calls this higher power. This generalized belief allows a group/mutual connection to a transcendent power that can help in the healing and recovery process without the need for all members to share a common belief system or religion.

Meetings generally begin with reading of the AA preamble and end with reading of the serenity prayer. Meetings may be open, which anyone may attend, or closed, which only alcoholics may attend. AA groups serve specific populations, such as racial or ethnic groups, gays, and lesbians, as well as specific professions, such as doctors, nurses, and other health care providers. Approximately 100,000 AA groups in nearly 150 countries now serve millions of members.

Several concepts used in AA add to the success of the program, including sponsorship, anniversaries, and social support. A new member of AA is mentored by another member, a sponsor, who is usually of the same gender and has been active in AA for a minimum of 1 year. New members are encouraged to contact their sponsors when they are considering drinking or are having difficulties with sobriety. This system of social support and mentoring has been shown to be beneficial both to the new member and to the sponsor. Cross et al.[86] showed that 91% of sponsors had maintained their abstinence from alcohol after 10 years.

BOX 83.3 | **The Twelve Steps of Alcoholics Anonymous**

Reprinted with permission of Alcoholics Anonymous World Service, Inc. Permission to reprint this material does not mean that AA has reviewed or approved the contents of this publication or that AA agrees with the views expressed herein.

We:

Admitted we were powerless over alcohol; that our lives had become unmanageable.

Came to believe that a Power greater than ourselves could restore us to sanity.

Made a decision to turn our will and our lives over to the care of God as we understood Him.

Made a searching and fearless moral inventory of ourselves.

Admitted to God, to ourselves and to another human being the exact nature of our wrongs.

Were entirely ready to have God remove all these defects of character.

Humbly asked Him to remove our shortcomings.

Made a list of all persons we had harmed, and became willing to make amends to them all.

Made direct amends to such people wherever possible, except when to do so would injure them or others.

Continued to take personal inventory and, when we were wrong, promptly admitted it.

Sought through prayer and meditation to improve our conscious contact with God as we understood Him, praying only for knowledge of His will for us and the power to carry that out.

Having had a spiritual experience (awakening) as the result of these steps, we tried to carry this message to alcoholics, and to practice these principles in all our affairs.

Anniversaries of sobriety are emphasized in the AA model. Special events or parties are scheduled to coincide with the individual's anniversary of sobriety. The arrangement encourages members to meet goals of prolonged abstinence and provides another avenue of social support. The social nature of these events also allows members to have fun and to make strong connections with others in the group without consuming alcohol. Primary care physicians should be aware of the AA groups in their geographic area and also should know their patients' sobriety anniversaries to be supportive and to acknowledge their accomplishments in the recovery process.

Several other 12-step programs use models similar to that of AA, including Narcotics Anonymous, Cocaine Anonymous, and Al-Anon. Family support groups like Al-Anon are available to family members and friends of alcoholics and substance abusers for the support of people close to the addicted person who are also deeply affected by substance abuse-related behaviors.

Traditional Native American Interventions

Native American Indians have the highest alcohol-related death rates and the highest prevalence of illicit drug use reported among any racial or ethnic group in the United States. According to Indian Health Service data, the total age-adjusted alcohol-related death rate among Native Americans is over six times greater than that of the U.S. all-races population.[87] SAMHSA reports that 10.6% of Native Americans are illicit drug users. Although alcoholism and substance abuse are common in many Native American communities, there are significant differences between tribes from different regions, and not all tribes are significantly affected by addiction.

Native American people have experienced an immense history of injustice in the past several hundred years. The theft of land, language, culture, and spirituality has created a sense of despair that continues today in many Native American communities. A detailed account of historical events is beyond the scope of this chapter, but it is important to recognize the relatively recent dramatic cultural changes that have occurred. I was fortunate to grow up in a family with many traditional healers and spiritual leaders from the Lakota tribe, and I incorporate this traditional philosophy into my medical practice.

The effect on people of Native American heritage of the loss of their land and culture is recognized by many current traditional leaders. This sense of loss and mourning is at the root of the high rates of depression, alcoholism, substance abuse, and other chronic diseases experienced by Native Americans. As Ed McGaa, Eagle Man, states, "Native American Indians learned how to live with the earth on a deeply spiritual plane."[88] The loss of land resulted in a loss of spiritual tradition. According to *Wounded Warriors*, a book delineating the loss faced by many Native Americans, "We need to understand that the primary reason our people are so afflicted with addiction, poverty, abuse, and strife, is that our way of life was taken from us. Everything was taken. And nothing was replaced."[89] From a traditional perspective, not unlike that previously described for acupuncture and mind-body medicine, the use of alcohol and illicit drugs by some Native Americans fills the void created by the loss of spirituality.

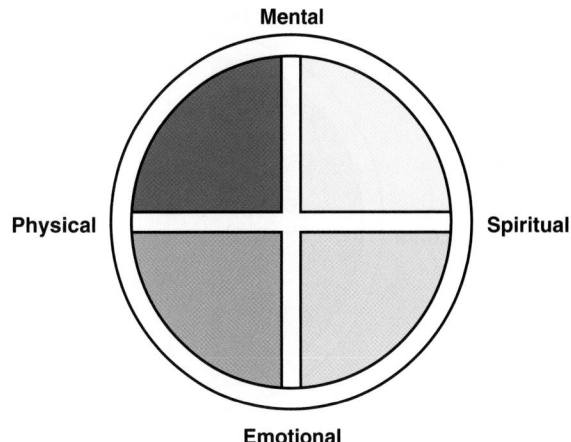

FIG. 83.2 ■ Traditional Lakota Indian medicine wheel.

The medicine wheel is a symbol that has been used by numerous tribes to represent wholeness and balance. To be healthy, each person must achieve a sense of balance among spiritual, mental, physical, and emotional forces (Fig. 83.2). This image provides a visual format for depicting the connection between spirituality and mental, physical, and emotional health. Another interpretation of the medicine wheel shows values, decisions, actions, and reactions as representing the spiritual, mental, physical, and emotional realms, respectively. From a spiritual perspective, in this interpretation, personal values (spiritual) are interpreted into decisions (mental). These decisions are then implemented into actions (physical), and the actions produce reactions (emotional). The emotions then provide feedback to the value system (spiritual). In this way, all decisions, actions, and emotions are rooted in the spiritual realm (Fig. 83.3). When the spiritual realm is weakened or broken, negative emotions such as depression, anger, and low self-esteem have no spiritual basis or value system in which to be processed. As a result, these negative emotions affect decision making and actions. For many Native American people, the sense of a "broken spirit" and emotional despair lead to high rates of alcoholism and substance abuse (Fig. 83.4).

Within this model, health care practitioners can see the importance of addressing the concept of spiritual healing and promoting balance in treating addictions. Clearly, simple allopathic pharmacological interventions are not enough to address addiction in this setting. Comprehensive programs that incorporate traditional cultural perspectives and philosophy with AA and other treatment methods are the most successful in treating substance abuse in Native Americans.

Healing ceremonies such as the sweat lodge and talking circle are commonly used in Native American treatment programs. The sweat lodge is a traditional gathering for prayer, meditation, and purification. The talking circle is analogous to a support group, in which individuals share thoughts, emotions, and prayers in a culturally relevant and sacred manner. Anecdotally, most of my patients who participate in these healing rituals in the treatment of any chronic condition, including alcoholism and substance abuse, find the traditional interventions to promote a sense of balance and wellness

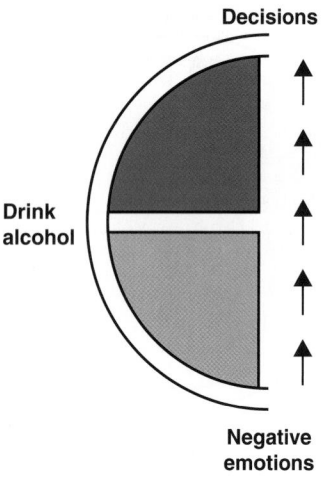

FIG. 83.4 ■ The "broken spirit" factor in alcoholism and substance abuse.

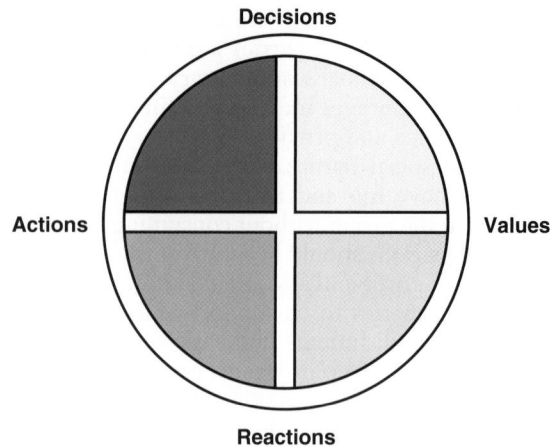

FIG. 83.3 ■ Medicine wheel showing spiritual values in decision making.

more effectively than anything offered by modern allopathic medicine.

Therapies to Consider

Nutrition

There may be a connection between nutritional deficiencies and addiction. Alcoholism is known to cause nutritional deficiencies, but it is not clear whether nutritional disorders lead to addiction. Some studies of nutritional supplements appear promising in maintaining sobriety, reducing depression, and minimizing cravings.[90,91]

Amino acid supplementation may be an effective adjunct in the treatment of alcohol and cocaine addiction.[92]

Homeopathy

Homeopathic remedies have been reported to be helpful in managing addictions, anxiety, and depression. The nature of homeopathy is such that the treatment regimen is formulated to address the patient's specific characteristics and complaints. Therefore, there is no specific "anti-addiction" homeopathic remedy. A skilled homeopath may be able to prescribe remedies for specific patients that can aid in the recovery process.

PREVENTION PRESCRIPTION

- Encourage patients to make a connection with something that gives life deeper meaning and purpose.
- Treat depression and anxiety. Work with a spiritual care provider or other health care providers before symptoms result in self-medication with alcohol or other substances.
- Encourage patients to avoid the use of illicit drugs.
- Be aware of the patient's alcohol intake. If he or she displays any of the following traits, begin an integrative approach for treatment of the addiction:

- Craving: a strong urge to drink alcohol
- Loss of control: being unable to stop drinking once the patient has started
- Physical dependence: symptoms such as sweating, shaking, and anxiety after the patient stops drinking
- Tolerance: the need for greater quantities of alcohol to feel intoxicated

---

THERAPEUTIC REVIEW

The following is a summary of options for treatment of alcoholism and substance abuse. If a patient presents with a history and symptoms consistent with alcohol or substance abuse withdrawal, immediate referral to a detoxification center is warranted.

LABORATORY

Laboratory testing is not helpful in screening, but liver assessment can help in monitoring the toxic effects of heavy drinking and can be a tool in motivating behavior change.

- Alanine aminotransferase (ALT), gamma-glutamyl-transferase (GGT), and carbohydrate-deficient transferrin (CDT): CDT is least affected by nonalcoholic liver disease and thus is a specific indicator of heavy ethanol use. It can be elevated if four or five drinks have been consumed at one time in the previous 2 weeks.
- Consider a complete blood count and determination of levels of B_{12}, folate, electrolytes, magnesium, uric acid, lipase, and prealbumin in chronic alcohol users.

PHARMACEUTICAL AGENTS

Alcohol

- Benzodiazepines are commonly used for detoxification and withdrawal symptoms:
  - Consider clonazepam 1 mg three times daily, with a gradual taper over 10–14 days.
- To reduce the "high" sensation associated with alcohol:
  - Naltrexone (ReVia): 50 mg/day orally
- To reduce the craving for alcohol:
  - Acamprosate (Campral): 333–666 mg three times a day
  - Topiramate (Topamax): titrate 25–300 mg weekly over 8 weeks (see Table 83.2)
- To create unpleasant side effects with use of alcohol:
  - Disulfiram (Antabuse): 250–500 mg/day

Tobacco

- Tapered nicotine replacement: oral, patch, or inhaled over 3–4 weeks
- Cytisine 1.5 mg tablets with a tapering dose over 25 days
- Bupropion (Zyban): 150 mg twice a day × 6 weeks. The patient should set a quit date after taking the medication for 2 weeks. It is effective in managing symptoms of withdrawal and cravings.
- Varenicline (Chantix) is started 7 days before the quit date: days 1–3, 0.5 mg daily; days 4–7, 0.5 mg twice daily; and the subsequent 11 weeks, 1 mg twice daily. It can be used for up to 24 weeks if needed to prevent relapse.

Opiates

- Methadone 15–20 mg/day orally for opiate addiction is the most commonly used pharmaceutical agent for relapse prevention and management of cravings.
- Buprenorphine (Subutex) is an opioid partial agonist that reduces cravings and helps prevent relapses. It also has a lower potential than methadone for dependence. Extra training is required to prescribe it.

Cocaine

- Antidepressant medications (selective serotonin reuptake inhibitors and tricyclic antidepressants)
- Amantadine 100 mg orally twice daily has been used to decrease cravings and to prevent relapse, with varying success.

BOTANICALS

- For anxiety, insomnia, and depression associated with substance abuse, consider the following:
  - Valerian: for anxiety, 300–450 mg three times daily or 400–900 mg 2 hours before sleep. It must be used for 2–3 weeks before an effect can be seen.
  - Kava kava extract standardized to 70% kava-lactones: 100 mg three times a day for anxiety. Avoid in patients with liver disease because of the potential for hepatic toxicity.
  - St. John's wort 300 mg three times daily or 450–600 mg twice daily is used for depression, but its role in alcohol and substance abuse recovery is yet to be determined.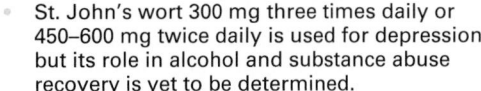
  - Kudzu is a traditional Chinese herb that has been used in alcohol recovery. The recommended dose is 1.2 g twice daily.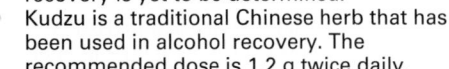

ACUPUNCTURE

- Acupuncture is effective in producing relaxation and minimizing cravings for most substances of abuse.
- Treatment protocols typically involve five needles placed in each ear several times a week and are most effective as part of a comprehensive treatment program.
- Not all treatment facilities offer acupuncture, and referring practitioners should be aware of the treatment options available in their geographic area.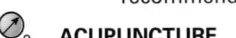

MIND-BODY THERAPIES

Meditation, biofeedback, hypnosis, guided imagery, yoga, and prayer have been shown to be effective adjunctive therapies in treatment programs, but most of the studies conducted to assess them have not been well controlled.

SPIRITUALITY

Numerous studies have shown a benefit in the recovery process in persons who have strong spiritual connections or actively participate in various religious practices. There is no correlation between a specific religion or belief system and recovery; the important factor appears to be the presence of a spiritual connection or practice.

TWELVE-STEP PROGRAMS

- AA has proved to be successful in the alcoholism recovery process. The Twelve Steps are rooted in spirituality and social support.
- Other programs, such as Narcotics Anonymous, Cocaine Anonymous, and Al-Anon, use similar principles and focus on other substances of abuse and their effects on the abuser's family.
- Primary care physicians should be aware of the programs available in their geographic area.

CULTURALLY SPECIFIC INTERVENTIONS

- Various cultural and ethnic groups have been affected by alcoholism and substance abuse to different degrees. In many cultures, including Native American cultures, culture-specific interventions and practices can aid in the recovery process.
- Physicians should be aware of the patient's cultural background and belief system when making referrals to treatment facilities.

Key Web Resources

National Institute of Alcohol Abuse and Alcoholism: Patient education, resources, and helpful links	http://www.niaaa.nih.gov
National Institute of Alcohol Abuse and Alcoholism: Clinical calculators for alcohol, including those used to determine the alcohol content of cocktails, calories in alcohol, financial costs, and blood alcohol concentrations	http://rethinkingdrinking.niaaa.nih.gov/ToolsResources/CalculatorsMain.asp
National Acupuncture Detoxification Association (NADA): Resources for clinicians interested in learning and applying auricular acupuncture in the treatment of substance abuse	http://www.acudetox.com/
Alcoholics Anonymous (AA): Resources for local classes and support for the twelve-step program	http://www.aa.org/
To find AA meetings and times	http://www.aa.org/pages/en_US/find-local-aa
National Institute on Drug Abuse (NIDA): Information on drugs of abuse for clinicians, patients, teachers, and students	http://www.drugabuse.gov/
U.S. Department of Health and Human Services Substance Abuse and Mental Health Services Administration (SAMHSA) website: Information for clinicians interested in establishing prescribing privileges for buprenorphine	http://buprenorphine.samhsa.gov

REFERENCES

References are available online at ExpertConsult.com.

SECTION XVI

OPHTHALMOLOGY

SECTION OUTLINE

84 Cataracts

85 Age-Related Macular Degeneration

CHAPTER 84

CATARACTS

Robert Abel, Jr., MD

PATHOPHYSIOLOGY

The lens is one of the body's most solid tissues, being approximately 36% solid. It is composed of mostly proteins (crystalline fibers and enzymes) and some carbohydrates and polyunsaturated fatty acids. The lens curvature and the alignment of the fibers are designed for the bending of light rays in the visual spectrum and the absorption of radiation above and below that spectrum. A cataract is any opacification of the normally clear crystalline lens of the eye. Oxidation of lens fibers, catalyzed by short, phototoxic ultraviolet (UV) wavelengths of light, destroys the sulfhydryl protein bonds. Breaking of these bonds leads to denaturation and clumping of the protein, with consequent loss of lens clarity.

The eye is a remote outpost that relies on good nutrition, liver function, circulation, and breathing. The lens in particular has no direct vascular or neurological innervations and therefore must rely on the circulation of the small amount of aqueous humor, flowing from the ciliary body out through the trabecular meshwork, for delivery of nutrition and removal of toxins.

The aqueous humor has very high levels of water-soluble compounds, such as ascorbic acid, glutathione, and its key amino acid, cysteine, the major diet-derived antioxidants that protect lens clarity.

However, the eye is not an isolated organ; it is connected to the brain and cardiovascular and digestive systems. It requires protection from bright illumination, which is provided by the lids, lashes, watery tear film, cornea, and iris. Cataract formation is often symptomatic of deeper abnormalities and systemic imbalances. In a common clinical scenario, the ophthalmologist tells the patient that he or she has a cataract, followed by reassurance of its nonacute nature, "Don't worry, I'll see you in 6 months." Six months later, the patient is told, "It's time to operate!" Earlier interventions directed at the disturbances underlying cataract formation can halt or significantly retard this inevitable progression.

There has been evidence to suggest the role of diabetes in the development of cataracts. From a biochemical perspective, the sugar within the bloodstream diffuses into the aqueous humor and, in combination with light, performs photooxidation of the lens proteins.[1] Therefore, it is not unusual for diabetic patients to present with eye complaints related to cataract earlier than one would expect. In fact, Iranian researchers compared patients with type 2 diabetes and a control group to show that the diabetic patients demonstrated visually debilitating cataracts 5 years earlier than the control group.[2]

Cataracts are the leading cause of vision impairment in both developed and developing countries and are the major cause of blindness worldwide.

Vision provides up to 80% of our sensory input and is to be preserved at any cost. This chapter reviews the current evidence correlating antioxidant deficiency with the prevalence of cataract formation as well as the administration of specific antioxidants to reduce the incidence of lens opacification.

SCREENING

Changes in Vision

Subtle cataract development leads to unrecognized loss of color interpretation and fine detail, and to difficulty with contrast and distance vision. In younger patients, fluctuating vision is often related to refractive error, computer use, diminishing accommodation, and even medications. As reported by mature adults, the following visual symptoms may indicate early cataract formation and can serve as the basis for questioning the patient during a general medical history and physical examination:

- Blurred vision
- Difficulty with reading road signs and distance vision
- Trouble reading
- Loss of depth perception
- Difficulty following a golf ball
- Difficulty with night driving
- Glare, especially at night
- Double vision
- Reduced vision

Patients may not volunteer information about decreasing vision because they do not notice the gradual decrement, may fear losing a driver's license, or are anxious about having their eyes examined.

Primary Care Diagnosis

The small-pupil Welch Allyn ophthalmoscope enables primary care physicians to look at the fundus of the eye to detect diabetic and other changes. The device is focused by a simple rotary movement of the thumb. With this instrument, it is possible to assess lens transparency as well as observe the fundus.[3] Patient complaints are the first symptom. Distance vision problems and glare far exceed near-vision disturbances in patients with cataracts; the reverse is true in patients with macular degeneration.

Ophthalmological Referral

The definitive diagnosis of cataract is made by ophthalmological referral and slit-lamp examination. Distance visual acuity, near vision, and depth perception as well as contrast sensitivity and peripheral vision can be evaluated. Glare testing may also approximate real-world conditions and may corroborate functional impairment.

Documentation of Progression

Because cataracts are slowly progressive and phacoemulsification removal with intraocular lens implantation is an elective procedure, most ophthalmologists choose to wait for patients to volunteer information about the level of inconvenience or significant loss of function. The mere appearance of early cataract changes alone rarely warrants surgical intervention. Additional difficulty is posed by lens grading because it requires multiple observers.

> Every year in the United States, cataract surgery is performed in more than 3 million people, engendering more than $2 billion in Medicare costs. Delay of cataracts for 10 years would lead to tremendous cost savings.

EPIDEMIOLOGY

Cataracts are by far the leading cause of blindness worldwide. In fact, cataracts are a major cause of reversible blindness in the United States and Western Europe. The frequency increases with age; modern dogma is that everyone will get cataracts, but the truth is that most will.[4]

RISK FACTORS

The incidence of cataract formation varies with a number of risk factors (Box 84.1). Cataract formation is not inevitable with age. It is not unusual to find men and women in their 80s and 90s with relatively clear lenses who have had healthy lifestyle habits. The following risk factors for cataract formation have been identified:
- Age
- Sunlight exposure

BOX 84.1	Major Stressors to the Eye and Lens

Ultraviolet and blue light (sunlight)
Inadequate nutrition
Lifestyle habits
Stress
Chronic disease

- Stress
- Medications
- Smoking
- Alcohol excess
- Obesity and high body mass index
- Chronic disease
- Malnutrition
- Diet high in saturated fat
- Heredity and genetics
- Trauma
- Congenital disorders
- Inborn errors of metabolism
- Dehydration
- Diabetes
- Vitamin deficiencies
- Low estrogen
- Glass blowing
- Lead exposure
- Long-term aspirin use
- African-American race

INTEGRATIVE THERAPY

Lifestyle Interventions

Ultraviolet Light–Blocking Sunglasses

Increased solar exposure and high altitudes have long been known to raise the frequency of cataracts in all decades of life. UV light, especially in the presence of oxygen, contributes strongly to the denaturation of lens protein, which results in cataract formation; this phenomenon was known to occur even before the deterioration of the ozone layer.

There currently are anecdotal veterinary reports of a higher incidence of cataract in rabbits in Patagonia and in dogs in Australia, both due to thinning of the ozone layer. Beachgoers and sunlamp users must be counseled to always wear adequate eye protection. Parents should encourage their children, including infants, to wear sunglasses and other forms of eye protection. Airline pilots have also been found to have a higher incidence of nuclear cataracts, as have astronauts, who may go into space only once in their lifetime. Part of this risk may be attributable to cosmic radiation and blue light as well as to UV light.

Nevertheless, appropriate protective lenses should also be used in occupations such as welding and ironwork, in which workers experience prolonged exposure to hazardous radiation, even above and below the visual spectrum (400–700 nm). Use of hats and visors has been the recommendation of several long-term epidemiological and longitudinal studies. UVA (also called near-UV) light and UVB (far-UV) light constitute toxic radiation, and their long-term effects are cumulative. Near-UV light penetrates the cornea and is generally absorbed by the lens, whereas far-UV light is more damaging, but is usually absorbed by the cornea, although not entirely. For this reason, astronauts have been known to take large amounts of *N*-acetylcysteine (3000 mg/day), a glutathione booster, while on space missions.

Stress Management

Stress depresses immune function, alters sleep patterns, impairs gastrointestinal absorption, and reduces available antioxidants. Stress also stimulates the sympathetic nervous system, causing vasoconstriction, increasing muscle tension, and, over long periods, decreasing microcirculation through the ophthalmic artery and its tributaries. A direct correlation between stress and cataract formation remains to be proved in humans, but there is ample evidence that stress, smoking, nutritional deficiency, radiation, and corticosteroids increased cataract formation in animal models.

Pharmaceuticals

More than 300 common medications are known to be photosensitizing agents. Many antibiotics, diuretics, antihypertensives, botanicals (St. John's wort), psoralens, and other agents increase the sensitivity of lens protein to UV damage. Therefore, it is important to advise all people taking medicine to wear sunglasses and to ask their pharmacists about whether their medications are photosensitizers. Many medications also require hepatic excretion and may interfere with normal nutritional biochemistry in the liver. For instance, many cholesterol-lowering agents decrease the production of coenzyme Q10 and glutathione in the liver. Glutathione, a sulfur-containing tripeptide, is a major free radical scavenger in the human lens. A recent study has shown that statin use is associated with increased risk of cataract development.[5]

Corticosteroids

Corticosteroids by any route of administration (topical, oral, intranasal, inhaled, or intravenous) are known to raise the incidence of both cataracts and glaucoma in susceptible persons. This adverse effect is most common with topical corticosteroids used in treatment of ocular inflammation and allergies. Therefore, it is advisable for patients who are prescribed ocular steroids for allergies not to have refills without appropriate ophthalmological supervision. There are other ways to treat ocular allergy, such as with topical antihistamines, mast cell stabilizers, and the administration of oral vitamin C (1000 mg/day) and the eucalyptus bioflavonoid preparation quercetin (1000 mg/day).

Often, the patient who sees many physicians develops a polypharmacy, which is perpetuated. Chinese and Ayurvedic healers tend to use a mixture of herbal remedies for a limited time; they then reevaluate the patient within 2 weeks and readjust the formula. This approach is a good one to incorporate into contemporary Western medicine.

Smoking

Smoking not only reduces available ascorbic acid and alpha-tocopherol but also has a direct toxic effect on the lens of the eye. The longitudinal Physicians' Health Study and Nurses' Health Study have shown a significant rise in cataract formation in smokers, with twice the incidence in the male physicians' study and two-third times more cataract surgeries in women who smoked.[6,7] In many pack-a-day smokers, a yellow-brown cast to the nucleus develops during 20 years of smoking.

Alcohol

Excess intake of alcohol is known to raise the incidence of cataract formation, probably by causing loss of some of the B and fat-soluble vitamins as well as through the possible alteration of liver function.

Lack of Exercise

Exercise stimulates breathing and parasympathetic activity. This effect is especially desirable in persons with chronic glaucoma conditions and macular degeneration. A group of University of Oregon investigators[8] found that 30–40 minutes of walking four times weekly lowered intraocular pressure and also reduced stress. Improved aqueous flow is important to the health of the crystalline lens of the eye as well.

Overweight

Obesity or an unfavorable waist-to-hip ratio has been associated with a higher incidence of cataract formation.[9] Chinese researchers noted that there was a higher rate of so-called age-related cataracts in individuals who were deemed overweight and obese by body mass index.[10] This association is yet another reason why it is important to encourage maintenance of ideal body weight and moderation of calorie intake.

Management of General Medical Conditions

Patients with diabetes have three to five times the risk of cataract formation noted in the general population.[11] Effective management of diabetes is important for avoidance of both the highs and lows of serum glucose levels. An elevation in blood glucose concentration causes an influx of fluid into the lens of the eye, significantly changing the refractive error. This change in permeability ultimately enhances protein decomposition and cataract formation through the sorbitol pathway (Fig. 84.1). Quercetin, a preparation of naturally occurring eucalyptus bioflavonoids, inhibits the aldose reductase pathway. Several studies also indicate that hypothyroidism is more common in persons with cataracts. Hypertension and Cushing syndrome are also associated with cataract formation; this is the result of photosensitizing blood pressure medications in the former and elevated steroids in the latter condition.

Female Gender

Some studies have indicated a higher incidence of cataracts in women that cannot be accounted for solely by the slight preponderance of women in the general population older than 65 years. Replacement estrogen therapy is correlated with a protective effect; therefore, the use of natural or synthetic estrogens may be appropriate in patients without contraindications to them.

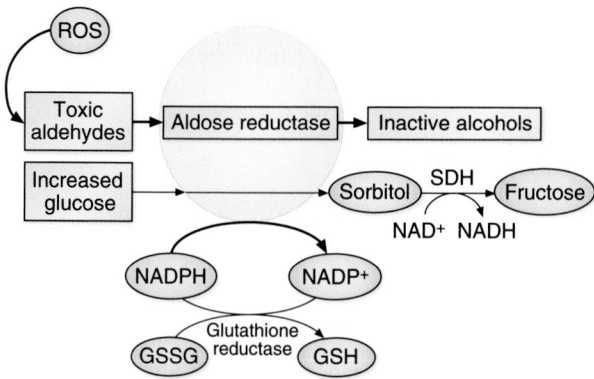

FIG. 84.1 ■ The sorbitol pathway. *GSH*, reduced glutathione; *GSSG*, oxidized glutathione; *NAD⁺*, oxidized form of nicotinamide adenine dinucleotide (NAD); *NADH*, reduced form of NAD; *NADP⁺*, oxidized form of nicotinamide adenine dinucleotide phosphate (NADP); *NADPH*, reduced form of NADP; *ROS*, reactive oxygen species; *SDH*, sorbitol dehydrogenase. (From Brownlee M. Biochemistry and molecular cell biology of diabetic complications. *Nature.* 2001;414:813–820.)

Aging and Longevity

Because the incidence of cataract rises every decade after the age of 45 years, it is important to screen people older than 45 years for general health and driving ability. Several studies in the orthopedic literature have indicated that visual disability is one of the risk factors for hip fracture. The loss of depth perception makes people particularly vulnerable to falls because they assume that they can see well with one eye, yet may be likely to miscalculate steps and distances. Cataract development is seemingly related to overall health and other medical conditions. Several articles point to an inverse relationship between cataract development and lifespan. In fact, Age-Related Eye Disease Study (AREDS) participants with age-related macular degeneration and cataracts had a shorter life expectancy than those without both diseases.[12]

Lack of Sleep

Patients should be advised to get plenty of sleep. Darkness is a time when the eyes, especially the retinae, have a chance to rest, recover, and replenish. The lens and intraocular structures are bombarded by light, with the formation of free radicals, all day; sleep provides an opportunity for the liver and circulation to replenish the necessary antioxidants and minerals to the lens and other ocular tissues.

NUTRITION

Fruits and Vegetables

Ascorbic acid, carotenoids, tocopherol, and glutathione are present in the lens epithelium and lens fibers. Proteolytic enzymes that act to remove damaged protein are also present in the lens and are spared by glutathione and other free radical scavengers. In general, the colored

bioflavonoids and carotenoids are nature's protectors and should be part of a balanced diet. Multiple studies have identified green leafy vegetables as being preventive for cataract as well as age-related macular degeneration.[13] The Australian Blue Mountains Eye Study, which involved 3654 persons, found that subjects consuming a diet high in protein, fiber, vitamin A, niacin, thiamine, and riboflavin had a lower incidence of nuclear cataracts. Persons whose diet had higher levels of polyunsaturated fatty acids had a significantly lower rate of cortical cataract formation.[14] Low serum levels of alpha-tocopherol may not reflect the actual concentration within the lens; interestingly, this may be true for many other nutrients as well.[15] Increased dietary fructose induces cataracts in diabetics and nondiabetics.[16] Dietary total antioxidant capacity reduced the risk of age-related cataract.[17]

Vitamin C

Citrus fruits and many other fruits and vegetables contain high levels of ascorbic acid, which is a major antioxidant in the lens of the eye. The lens and aqueous humor concentrate ascorbic acid in amounts more than 10 times of those found in human plasma. Ascorbate is richer in the cortical fibers than in the older, nuclear fibers. As expected, patients with senile cataracts have a lower serum ascorbate level than that of controls.[18] Higher blood levels of the vitamin seem to confer some protection against cataract. Persons with higher than average vitamin C intake appear to have a lower risk of nuclear cataract, and those younger than 60 years have a lower risk of cortical opacities, with an intake range of 150–300 mg/day.[19]

Lutein-Containing Foods

Spinach, kale, collard greens, guava, and even corn and eggs contain lutein, which has been found to be protective against cataract formation. People who consume high levels of green leafy vegetables and whose serum lutein levels are in the highest quintile have a 20% reduced risk of cataract formation.[20,21] In both the Physicians' Health Study and the Nurses' Health Study, cataract surgery was associated with lower intake of foods such as spinach, which are rich in lutein and zeaxanthin carotenoids rather than beta-carotene.

Avoidance of Saturated Animal Fat

By reducing saturated fats, the patient will find it easier to reach and to maintain an ideal body weight. The change from saturated fat and trans-fatty acids to polyunsaturated fatty acids is protective to the lens and is currently being evaluated in AREDS 2.[22] As an added benefit, the change also helps the patient improve his or her serum lipid profile.

Hydration

The patient should be encouraged to drink plenty of water. The lens of the eye is a dehydrated tissue much

- Adequate hydration can be promoted by drinking six to eight glasses of water daily.
- It is important to remember to blink, especially during work with computers and other tasks requiring visual concentration.
- The beneficial fats in the tear film can be reinforced with supplementation of docosahexaenoic acid (DHA) and fat-soluble nutrients such as vitamin A and lutein. DHA produces significant improvement in comfort within a week. Recommend 800 to 1000 mg/day (or 2 g/day of fish or krill oil).[19a]
- Use of eye drops and ointments as moisturizers is recommended. For example, Tears Again (Cynacon/OCuSOFT, Inc., Rosenberg, TX), a liposomal vitamin A and E spray, can be applied externally on the lid and appears to penetrate the eye quickly, providing relief.
- Mechanical problems with the lower lids should be ruled out, especially in patients who may be sleeping with their eyes open. When observing the patient, the clinician should check to see whether the lower lid moves during routine blinking.
- A humidifier should be kept in the bedroom.
- Periodic evaluation of the patient's medication profile is recommended.

like a fingernail, another avascular ectodermal structure. Drinking six to eight glasses of filtered water a day is an excellent way to increase aqueous humor circulation, which supports lens health. Tips for prevention of dry eyes are presented in Box 84.2.

Sulfur-Containing Foods

Glutathione, a major antioxidant in the lens, is found in such foods as onions, garlic, avocados, cruciferous vegetables, asparagus, and watermelon. Glutathione and its boosters are thiol compounds, which scavenge free radicals. These glutathione boosters include L-cysteine, lipoic acid, and methylsulfonylmethane. Glutathione also spares proteolytic enzymes in the cortical lens fibers. In studies from the late 1960s, extracted mature cataracts were demonstrated to contain very low levels of glutathione and ascorbic acid; this finding was considered to represent a secondary aspect of cataract formation. In retrospect, this deficiency appears to be a preliminary event and one that can be managed nutritionally.

Algae-Eating Fish

Single-cell algae are at the bottom of the food chain. When the early hominids began eating fish, their brains developed further, approaching human dimensions. The traditional Japanese diet appears to protect against cataract formation because of the inclusion of cold-water fish and algae, both of which are rich in docosahexaenoic acid (DHA). (Examples of such fish are tuna, mackerel, salmon, sardines, and cod.) Currently, fish such as salmon are being farm raised.

Because farm-raised fish are fed grain instead of algae, they contain less DHA and provide less benefit to the eyes and body.

SUPPLEMENTS

For a more complete listing of supplements that promote eye health, see Chapter 85.

Lutein and Zeaxanthin

Results of the Physicians' Health Study and Nurses' Health Study have indicated an approximately 20% protection against cataract formation among persons with serum lutein values in the highest quintile.[20,21] Lutein and its isomer, zeaxanthin, are present in high levels in ocular tissues, including the lens. Their importance may lie in the fact that they absorb and reflect the phototoxic blue and UV wavelengths. The carotenoids present in the lens turn out to be lutein and zeaxanthin more than beta-carotene. A daily dose of 2.4 mg of lutein has been shown to double the serum level. Olmedilla et al.[23] showed that lutein had a slowing effect on cataract progression during their 2-year study. In fact, they concluded that visual function improved in patients who received lutein supplementation, suggesting that higher intakes of lutein may enhance vision in spite of cataractous lens changes. Christen et al.[24] found that supplementation with vitamins C and E, lutein, and zeaxanthin significantly lowered the risk of cataracts.

> **Dosage**
> Patients with early cataracts should take 10 mg/day of lutein for the first month, then 6 mg/day as part of their daily regimen.

Vitamin C

Numerous studies have shown that increased vitamin C consumption (60–600 mg/day) over many years protects against cataracts. In one study, the 5-year risk for the development of any cataract was 60% lower among 3634 participants, aged 43–86 years, who had been taking a multivitamin that included vitamin C for 10 years than in participants who had not.[25] Another study showed a 45% protection rate against cataract surgery in women who had consumed vitamin C supplements for 10 years.[26] Jacques et al.[27] found that women with a mean vitamin C intake of 359 mg/day for 10 years had a 77% lower prevalence of earlier lens opacities.

> **Dosage**
> The investigators of the study on vitamin C supplementation recommend approximately 300 mg/day of vitamin C, although I recommend 1000 mg/day.
>
> **Precautions**
> Vitamin C supplementation can cause gastrointestinal disturbance, including cramping and diarrhea.

Vitamin A

Hankinson et al.[26] found a 39% lower incidence of cataract formation in more than 50,000 nurses who had an adequate intake of vitamin A during an 8-year period than in nurses in the study who did not. This association has been reported in other studies as well. However, this finding must be balanced with a study[28] that has described an association between hip fractures and vitamin A supplementation at more than 17,000 units/day in women. This association may be due to competition of vitamin A with vitamin D absorption in some way.

> **DOSAGE**
> Most good multivitamins contain 5000 units of vitamin A or beta-carotene. Additional supplementation is usually not warranted.

Multivitamins

Multivitamin intake has been observed to reduce the risk of cataracts by approximately 20%–60%, depending on the content of ascorbic acid. Vitamin E (*d*-alpha-tocopherol) is also protective, as found by numerous studies. Robertson et al.[29] found that vitamin C (300–600 mg/day) and vitamin E (400 units/day) had a 50% protective effect.

The 10-year randomized AREDS was concluded early. It supported the use of a multivitamin with A, C, E, and zinc in macular degeneration, but did not find a reduction in cataract development. There is not enough scientific evidence to support the notion that a high dose of a single nutrient provides a greater benefit in reducing cataract risk than a daily multivitamin or a healthy diet.[30] One randomized clinical trial showed that one multivitamin preparation prevented the development of cataract but did not stop the progression once it was fully developed.[31] Others found that ascorbate, lutein, and retinol inversely affected the rate of cataract development.[32] Christens and associates found a significant reduction in the risk of cataract formation in middle age and older U.S. males followed for 10 years.[33]

> **DOSAGE**
> Taking a multivitamin is a convenient way to obtain a daily amount of beta-carotene or vitamin A, trace minerals, lutein, and other essential nutrients in two to four capsules, depending on the brand.
>
> **PRECAUTIONS**
> Recent medical reports have indicated an association between copper and an increased risk of memory loss and Alzheimer's disease. Many leading brands of eye vitamins that were created after the AREDS contain very high levels of copper and zinc. The highest recommended daily dose of zinc is 30 mg because higher doses can inhibit the absorption of important minerals including copper, calcium, magnesium, iodine, selenium, and boron. Over time, this loss of minerals can lead to deficiencies in other parts of the body.

Vitamin E

The Lens Opacities Case-Control Study confirmed that alpha-tocopherol is protective against lens opacity.[34] Another study from Linxian, China also found vitamin E to be protective against cataract formation in persons older than 45 years.[35] Results of other studies suggest that vitamin E had no protective effect against cataract formation,[36] but the question remains whether natural (*d*-alpha) or synthetic (*dl*-alpha) vitamin E was administered in these studies.

B Vitamins

The B vitamins, especially riboflavin (3 mg), thiamine (10 mg), and niacin (40 mg), were found to be protective against cataracts in both the Blue Mountains Eye Study in Australia and another study from Linxian, China.[14,35]

Docosahexaenoic Acid

DHA, the end product of omega-3 fatty acid metabolism, is known to protect cell membranes and thiol groups. An important constituent of the retina and brain, DHA has also been found in the lens of the eye. With its presence in all cell membranes and its six double bonds, replenishment of this compound is important. Reduction of DHA stores in women who have experienced pregnancy may be a reason for the gender discrepancy in cataract development. The DHA available in breast milk has been documented to reduce learning disabilities in children and to improve head size and growth in the first year of life. The Mediterranean diet has a 1:1 ratio of omega-3 to omega-6 fatty acids, whereas in the average American diet, the ratio ranges from 1:6 to 1:20.

> **DOSAGE**
> A supplemental regimen of 500–1000 mg/day of DHA is helpful for almost all adults. Amounts up to 6 g/day have not shown any toxicity in volunteers. This supplement, like all fat-soluble vitamins and supplements, should be taken with a meal for enhanced bioavailability.

Carnosine

N-Acetyl-L-carnosine eye drops are appearing everywhere on vitamin store shelves. Toh et al.[37] reviewed the modern treatment of cataracts and stated that the results of clinical trials with carnosine eye drops are encouraging. Marc Babizhayev has found that carnosine eye drops can halt and occasionally reduce early-to-moderate cataracts. My clinical experience has demonstrated a moderate effect.[38] Carnosine is commonly found in antiaging products because of its inhibition of advanced glycosylation end products. Limited human data are available.

BOTANICALS

Numerous herbs are known to improve blood flow to the eye and to strengthen liver function. Bioflavonoids in certain berries have been proved to enhance capillary formation; however, their effect on night vision is inconclusive. Astragalus, milk thistle (silymarin), oleander, turmeric root, garlic bulb in oil, and wheat sprouts are botanicals that strengthen liver function.[39] Some supplements are used to improve and support liver function, such as S-adenosyl-L-methionine (SAMe) and silymarin.

Turmeric

Curcumin, a constituent of turmeric (*Curcuma longa*), is a spice found in Indian curry dishes. This compound is an effective antioxidant known to induce the glutathione-linked detoxification pathways in rats. It significantly reduced the rate of cataract formation in laboratory rats, but human studies have not been performed in the West.[40]

Cineraria

Cineraria maritima, or *Senecio cineraria* (silver ragwort), has been used for centuries as an eye drop preparation for the treatment of conjunctivitis and early cataract. Homeopathic preparations have also been employed, but they have not been subjected to controlled studies.

Bioflavonoids

The eucalyptus bioflavonoid preparation quercetin has been found in multiple laboratory studies to inhibit the formation of cataracts induced by steroids, diabetes, and radiation.

SURGERY

Cataract surgery is the most common surgery performed in the United States today; more than 3 million procedures are performed annually. The subsequent laser treatment of an opacified capsule ranks among the 10 most common surgical procedures. With appropriate history and physical examinations and regular eye examination, early cataract formation can be detected long before functional visual loss develops.

Cataract surgery is performed under sterile conditions with local anesthesia. The procedure involves removal of the cataract by phacoemulsification and insertion of an implant within the lens capsule. The synthetic implant may be silicone, polymer, or acrylic. The complications of cataract surgery include infection, lens dislocation, retinal hemorrhage, and retinal detachment. With modern technology, however, this is one of the safest surgical procedures today. In fact, most patients who undergo cataract surgery in one eye can immediately notice the difference and are satisfied with the results.[41,42]

Untreated poor vision contributes to the progression of dementia. Lerner reported that cognition improved after cataract surgery and Owsley found that the incidence of motor vehicle accidents decreased after cataract procedures.[43-45]

PREVENTION PRESCRIPTION

- Eye examination is recommended every 1–2 years for people older than 50 years and for people at risk. Use of preventive measures is appropriate, even in patients with early cataracts.
- Advise use of sunglasses, with side shields as necessary, as well as hats or visors and sunblock in persons whose occupation or interests dictate spending time outdoors.
- Recommend a balanced diet with five or six servings of fruits and vegetables as well as grains, nuts, berries, and organic eggs for amino acids, with consumption of cold-water fish two or more times per week.
- Recommend lutein-rich foods, such as spinach, three times a week; these foods are especially important for ocular protection.
- Promote adequate hydration with intake of six glasses of filtered water daily, with reduction in intake of soft drinks and artificial sweeteners.

- Recommend a daily multivitamin including taurine, zinc, lutein, an additional 1000–2000 mg of vitamin C, 400 units of vitamin E, and 5000 units of vitamin A palmitate.
- Be certain that there is no copper in your multivitamin because of the risk of memory loss at high levels, and avoid multivitamins with more than 30 mg of zinc.[46]
- Advise the patient to maintain an appropriate body weight and to avoid animal fat in their diet.
- Encourage the healthful lifestyle habits of stretching, exercise, moderate alcohol intake, and a regular sleep pattern, with cessation of smoking.
- Advise the patient to maintain a positive attitude and optimism.
- Periodically review prescription and other medications for ophthalmological effects.
- Encourage regular physical examination and vision testing.

THERAPEUTIC REVIEW

Abundant evidence suggests that we can develop new strategies to maintain our health now, instead of waiting for cataracts to form.

Here is a summary of therapeutic and preventive options for cataracts. If a patient presents with severe symptoms, such as profound visual obstruction, it would be to his or her benefit for the clinician to immediately begin a more aggressive therapy, such as referral for elective surgery. For the patient who has mild-to-moderate symptoms, however, this ladder approach is appropriate.

REMOVE EXACERBATING FACTORS

The patient should be encouraged to
- Stop taking steroid-containing and photosensitizing medications for prolonged durations.
- Stop smoking; have moderate alcohol intake; try to lose weight, if needed, through diet and exercise; and substitute good fats in place of bad fats in the diet.
- Wear sunglasses or transition lenses while outside and a hat or visor with at least a 3-inch brim.

NUTRITION

- Encourage a low-fat, low-cholesterol diet.
- Encourage foods rich in omega-3 fatty acids (wild salmon, nuts, flaxseed) or supplementation with DHA 500–1000 mg/day.

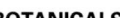

SUPPLEMENTS

- Multivitamins: a daily multivitamin including taurine, zinc, lutein, an additional 1000–2000 mg of vitamin C, 400 units of vitamin E, and 5000 IU of vitamin A palmitate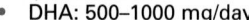
- DHA: 500–1000 mg/day
- Lutein: 6 mg/day for 1 month, then 2 mg/day

BOTANICALS

- Turmeric is a major antiinflammatory agent used throughout Asia; there are many data in the Chinese literature demonstrating its effectiveness in reducing the risk of cataracts.

SURGICAL THERAPY

If the patient's symptoms persist or worsen despite the preceding measures, referral for ophthalmic evaluation and treatment is warranted:
- Cataract extraction by phacoemulsification with intraocular lens insertion (one-step)

Key Web Resources

Dr. Rob Abel's Eye Advisory: This website is devoted to providing the latest options in both traditional and complementary therapies for 21st-century eye care.

http://eyeadvisory.com/

REFERENCES

References are available online at ExpertConsult.com.

CHAPTER 85

AGE-RELATED MACULAR DEGENERATION

Robert Abel, Jr., MD

Nowhere has there been so much scientific documentation about nutritional prevention as in the case of macular degeneration. The irony lies in the fact that this information is often virtually ignored by the very specialists who manage patients with the disease.

PATHOPHYSIOLOGY

Age-related macular degeneration (AMD) is the scourge of the "golden years." People aged 65 years and older constitute the fastest-growing segment of the population in developed countries; the risk for AMD and its impact will only become greater in the future. There is a tremendous need to develop preventive strategies to counter AMD and to arrest early cases before the loss of useful vision.

Retinal photoreceptors are subjected to oxidative stress from the combined exposure to light and oxygen on a daily basis. The body's ability to resupply the photoreceptors and underlying pigment epithelium with essential nutrients is the basis for maintenance of good vision throughout life. Diseases of the retina are the leading cause of blindness throughout the developed countries of the world. Among these diseases, macular degeneration is the most common, and its incidence is rising as the population ages. Population-based studies indicate that approximately 10% of people aged 65–74 years and 30% of those 75 years and older demonstrate early signs of the disease, and 7% already have late signs of the disease.[1]

Free radicals are thought to attack the rod and cone cell membranes; the retinal pigment epithelium (RPE), a monolayer beneath the retina, fails to keep up with the removal of lipid debris, which accumulates as drusen (yellow spots of different sizes). The melanin pigment protects the retina from radiation, but the amount of this pigment diminishes with age, smoking, and low serum lutein levels. When the RPE cells drop out, pigmentary defects can be noted by ophthalmoscopic examination and on retinal photography. Drusen and progressive RPE atrophy characterize the dry form of macular degeneration, which accounts for 90% of cases of AMD (Figs. 85.1 and 85.2).

The other 10% of cases are attributable to the exudative or vascular type of AMD. A hyaline membrane (i.e., Bruch's membrane) separates the choroidal blood supply from the RPE and overlying retina. Degeneration of Bruch's membrane, retinal anoxia, and impairment of choroidal circulation are believed to be factors that induce the vascular ingrowth characteristic of this form

of the disease. These fragile new vessels grow rapidly and may bleed spontaneously.

Most ophthalmologists agree that oxidative stress combined with the failure to fortify the retinal photoreceptors is a major pathophysiological mechanism in this disease, which currently affects 20 million older Americans. Many of these physicians also consider vision loss from macular degeneration to be inevitable, believing that nothing can be done for the dry form and that perhaps only recent interventional therapies are useful for treatment of the wet form of macular degeneration if it is detected in time. Nowak et al.[2] demonstrated significantly higher concentrations of lipid peroxidation products in AMD patients. This finding adds credence to the considerable evidence that nutritional approaches play a major part in prevention and management of this age-related disease. Cumulative photooxidative stress, other systemic diseases, and nutritional deficiencies contribute to the onset and progression of AMD. With aging, the protective cell-derived enzymes—catalase, superoxide dismutase, and glutathione peroxidase—decrease, as does the ability to absorb the diet-derived antioxidants.

SCREENING

Owing to the swelling ranks of the elderly, the number of persons with macular degeneration is growing. Routine dilated-eye examinations are fundamental to early detection and management of AMD. The onset is often so gradual as to go unnoticed.

Use of an Amsler grid, a 4 × 4-inch checkerboard square with a central dot for fixation, is an excellent way to diagnose AMD and allows home monitoring of the condition. This approach to management is especially useful in patients with the slowly progressive, dry form of the disease (Fig. 85.3).

Primary care physicians should know the AMD risk profiles to alert patients about preventive steps and the need for periodic eye examinations. Patients with multiple systemic diseases are at greatest risk. Early detection offers greater flexibility in the use of complementary therapies.

Referral to an ophthalmologist is indicated for dilated funduscopic examination and retinal imaging (photograph, laser tomography, and fluorescein angiography), which can clearly document the stages of AMD. On occasion, retinal specialists are needed for advanced management.

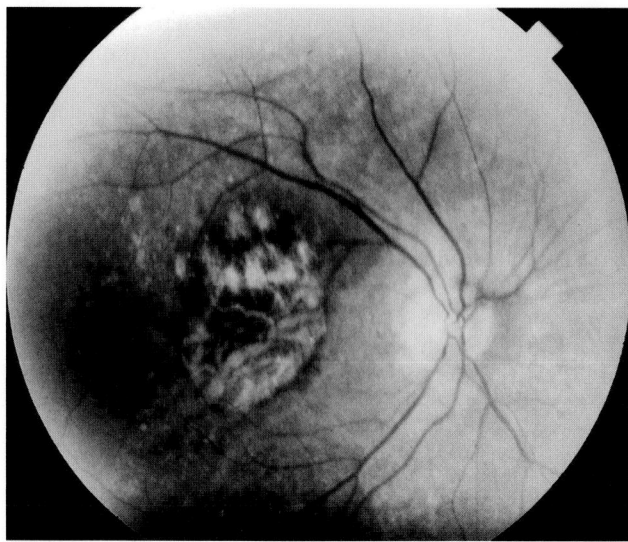

FIG. 85.1 ■ Atrophic (dry) age-related macular degeneration. Geographic atrophy of the retinal pigment epithelium causes loss of central vision. (From Fillit H. *Brocklehurst's textbook of geriatric medicine and gerontology.* 7th ed. Philadelphia: Saunders; 2010.)

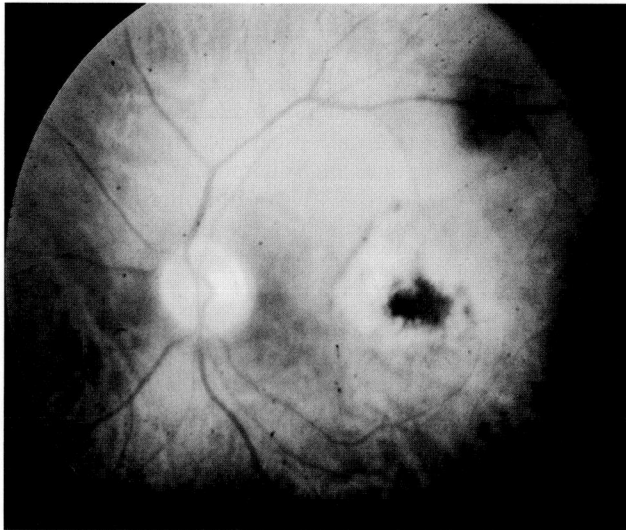

FIG. 85.2 ■ Exudative (wet) age-related macular degeneration. Leakage and scarring from a subretinal neovascular membrane destroy central retinal function. (From Fillit H. *Brocklehurst's textbook of geriatric medicine and gerontology.* 7th ed. Philadelphia: Saunders; 2010.)

Primary care physicians should help patients coordinate the various medicines used in the management of underlying and concurrent diseases. Periodic review of medications is important because polypharmacy may contribute to the risk for AMD.

RISK FACTORS

The following risk factors for AMD have been identified:
- Age
- Sunlight exposure
- Previous cataract surgery
- Light-colored irises, fair complexion

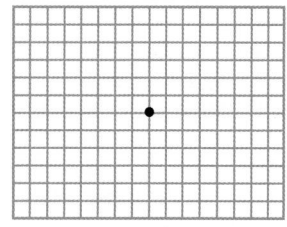

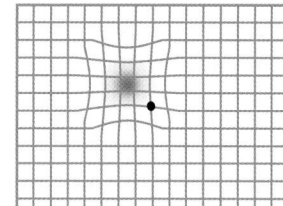

FIG. 85.3 ■ Amsler grid. This checkerboard-patterned square has parallel vertical and horizontal lines. The patient looks at the central dot with one eye covered and notes the pattern of the lines. If any line in any direction is missing or wavy, the patient marks it in with a pencil or makes a note. The Amsler grid can be used to determine whether there is a disorder of the optic nerve or macula; in particular, use of the grid is an excellent way to monitor macular degeneration to determine whether it is stable or progressing.

- Obesity
- Female gender, parity
- Postmenopausal status
- Inflammation
- Smoking
- Physical inactivity
- Elevated serum cholesterol values
- Hypertension
- Nocturnal hypotension
- Poor digestion, use of antacids
- Hypothyroidism, use of thyroid hormones
- Family history
- Low dietary intake of carotenoids, low serum carotenoid levels
- Low macular pigment density
- Low serum zinc levels
- High refractive errors

The National Health and Nutrition Examination Survey demonstrated that for 65- to 70-year-old respondents, the chance for development of AMD was nearly five times that for 45- to 54-year-old respondents.[3]

Sunlight

Reducing exposure to sunlight through the use of hats and sunglasses has been stressed in numerous studies.[4] A University of Wisconsin study of 3684 persons between the ages of 43 and 84 years found a positive correlation between daily sun exposure and the development of AMD. Persons who spent more than 5 hours a day in the sun were twice as likely to have AMD as those with less than 2 hours a day of sun exposure.[5]

Gender

The incidence of AMD is at least three times greater in postmenopausal women than in men of similar age. Two studies have indicated that hormone replacement therapy

(HRT) significantly reduces this risk, although a third study did not find any correlation. Apparently, women require more lutein than men do because it is preferentially deposited in fatty tissue rather than in the retina.[6] Obstetricians and gynecologists should inform their patients about early prevention and participate in decisions about biocompatible HRT when appropriate.

Inflammation

Clemons et al.[7] showed that early or moderate AMD advances with smoking, increasing body mass index, and, probably, with the use of antacid and antiinflammatory medications. Seddon et al.[8] demonstrated that C-reactive protein levels were higher in individuals with advanced AMD.

Smoking and Other Factors

Numerous investigators have determined that current smokers, especially those who smoke one pack a day or more, have a significantly higher risk for development of AMD than nonsmokers and persons who have given up smoking 10 years previously. The Nurses' Health Study revealed that women who smoked 25 or more cigarettes a day were more than twice as likely as nonsmokers to have AMD.[9] The Physicians' Health Study also showed a greater than twofold incidence of AMD in men who smoked 20 or more cigarettes daily.[10] One study indicated an association between smoking, low serum selenium levels, and the development of AMD. Smoking has been shown to contribute to reduced levels of circulating antioxidants as well as of the lutein pigment in the macular area.

The Age-Related Eye Disease Study (AREDS) found that smoking is associated with three of the five stages of macular degeneration.[11] This multicenter, randomized controlled trial also found that hypertension, obesity, hyperopic refractive error, white race, and an increased use of thyroid hormones and antacids were indicators for the most severe stages of the disease.

INTEGRATIVE THERAPY

Lifestyle Interventions

Sunglasses, Hats, and Visors

Everyone's need to wear sunglasses with light protection, hats, and visors should be emphasized as early as childhood. People with dilated pupils, outdoor workers, and people who frequent tanning beds may be at a higher risk for development of macular degeneration. Microscope light during cataract surgery is another source of phototoxicity. Sun exposure is a known causative factor in the progression of the hereditary disorder retinitis pigmentosa.

Stress Management

Hormonal imbalance and lack of sleep contribute to debilitation of retinal health. Depression contributes to food habituation, overeating, and abnormal sleep patterns. Ocular health remains in a sensitive balance between oxidative stress and antioxidant support of cell membranes. Therefore, smoking and inadequate nutrition both tip the scale toward increased or imbalanced free radical activity.

Limiting Alcohol Intake

Excessive alcohol intake has been associated with cardiovascular and liver disorders. The Beaver Dam Eye Study documented an association between beer consumption and risk of RPE degeneration. Two further studies have indicated that one or two glasses of red wine daily may confer a 40%–50% reduction in risk for AMD. However, the Physicians' Health Study and Nurses' Health Study, conducted between 1980 and 1994, could not confirm any significant benefit. Red wine has a protective effect on cardiovascular health and may improve retinal and choroidal blood flow. Apparently, white wine, which lacks the high levels of grape skin bioflavonoids, does not confer as much ocular protection.

Recognition of Medication Effects

Numerous medications, including phenothiazines, hydroxychloroquine, and ethambutol, may negatively affect the RPE. Other agents may alter digestion or liver function. The liver not only filters out all of the nutrients and toxins from the gastrointestinal tract but also stores fat-soluble vitamins, activates the B vitamins, and manufactures glutathione. Chinese and Ayurvedic physicians have known for millennia that the liver is essential to good vision.

> Antacid use has been positively correlated with the development of AMD. The lack of gastric acidity reduces the stimulus for secretion of pancreatic and biliary enzymes into the duodenum. Proton pump inhibition can cause vitamin B_{12}, iron, magnesium, and calcium deficiency.

Hydration

Drinking six or more glasses of filtered water a day hydrates the body, flushes the liver and kidneys, and decreases appetite. Patients should be counseled against excessive consumption of caffeinated soft drinks and artificial sweeteners.

Exercise

Exercise plays a role in cardiovascular health and in stimulating the parasympathetic nervous system. Physical activity also plays a part in relaxation of the mind, decreasing intraocular pressure, and improving ocular blood flow.

Breathing

Deep breathing relaxes the mind, strengthens the diaphragm, and improves blood flow to the eye. Conscious attention to breathing is the foundation of meditation and stress reduction practices.

Whole Body Health

Management of concurrent medical conditions is essential. Regulating blood pressure, maintaining a normal serum cholesterol level, controlling diabetes, supporting necessary weight reduction, and managing cardiovascular health are important to the long-term maintenance of good vision. It is wise to remember that the eye is intimately connected to the rest of the body.

Estrogen

Women are more likely than men to have AMD. Several studies have demonstrated that postmenopausal women who are taking HRT exhibit a lower incidence of macular degeneration, especially the wet form of the disease.[12] However, one study was unable to determine any significant effect of estrogen replacement therapy. Nonetheless, clinicians have observed that more postmenopausal women have AMD than men do.

Sleep

Sleep is crucial to restoration of photoreceptor and ocular health. The eye requires darkness to restore photoreceptor integrity and to replenish nutrients consumed during the daylight hours, when ultraviolet wavelengths and bright light are constantly bombarding the eye.

Attitude

Adopting a positive attitude is the first step in lifestyle modification. The placebo effect is another demonstration of the "power of positive thinking." In one study, 68% of persons who took a multivitamin for 6 months showed an improvement in macular appearance on electroretinograms; however, 32% of the placebo group also showed improvement. Similarly, in an initial study of photodynamic therapy to control retinal bleeding, approximately 50% of subjects receiving the therapy demonstrated some benefit compared with 28% of the placebo group. The placebo effect, which occurred in approximately 30% of subjects and contributed to the cessation of retinal bleeding, is a demonstration of the power of positive thinking.

Nutrition

Box 85.1 lists the foods recommended for the preservation of sight.

Fruits and Vegetables

Fruits and vegetables contain vitamins A, C, and E as well as beta-carotene and lutein. The yellow-orange vegetables, such as carrots and sweet potatoes, are important for daytime vision. Cho et al.[13] found strong evidence of a protective role of fruit against the risk of neovascular AMD or age-related maculopathy.

BOX 85.1	Top 10 Foods for Sight Preservation

- Cold-water fish (sardines, cod, mackerel, and tuna): an excellent source of DHA, which provides structural support to cell membranes and is recommended for dry eyes, treatment of macular degeneration, and sight preservation (see Chapter 86).
- Spinach, kale, and green leafy vegetables: rich in carotenoids, especially lutein and zeaxanthin; lutein, a yellow pigment, protects the macula from sun damage and from blue light.
- Eggs: rich in cysteine, sulfur, lecithin, amino acids, and lutein; sulfur-containing compounds protect the lens of the eye from cataract formation.
- Garlic, onions, shallots, and capers: rich in sulfur, which is necessary for the production of glutathione, an important antioxidant for the lens of the eye and for the whole body.
- Soy: low in fat, rich in protein; has become a staple in vegetarian diets; contains essential fatty acids, phytoestrogens, vitamin E, and natural antiinflammatory agents.
- Fruits and vegetables: contain vitamins A, C, and E, and beta-carotene; the yellow vegetables, such as carrots and squash, are important for daytime vision.
- Blueberries and grapes: contain anthocyanins, which improve night vision; a cupful of blueberries or huckleberry jam or a 100-mg bilberry supplement may improve dark adaptation within 30 minutes.
- Wine: known to exert a cardioprotective effect; has many important nutrients that protect vision, heart, and blood flow (as with any alcohol, moderation is always important).
- Nuts and berries: nature's most concentrated food sources; grains such as flaxseed are high in the beneficial omega-3 fatty acids, which help lower serum cholesterol and stabilize cell membranes.
- Extra-virgin olive oil: a monounsaturated oil and a healthy alternative to butter and margarine.

Lutein-Containing Foods

Spinach, collard greens, kale, guava, and many other green and yellow fruits and vegetables contain lutein and its isomer, zeaxanthin. These two carotenoids are concentrated in the macular pigment; their accumulation depends directly on dietary intake and serum level.

The complete name of the visually sensitive center of the retina is "macula lutea" because of its yellow color (Latin *luteus*, "yellow"). Lutein and zeaxanthin are responsible for the yellow color. The normal retina is capable of concentrating these carotenoids to a level that is several orders of magnitude greater than the serum level. Evidence suggests that the lutein in macular pigment is entirely of dietary origin and is highly protective against AMD.[14]

In one study, persons consuming lutein-rich foods five times a week were eight times less likely to have AMD than those consuming such foods once a month.[15] In addition, persons with serum lutein values in the highest quintile had a 43% lower risk for AMD. Another study demonstrated that consumption of 4–8 oz/day of spinach for 4 months resulted in greater macular pigment density. The vitamin K content in spinach may interfere with blood-thinning agents such as warfarin sodium.

Preliminary data have demonstrated improvement in the visual function of patients with the dry form of AMD whose diet was modified to provide an abundance of dark green vegetables.[16]

There is 44 mg of lutein per cup of cooked kale, 26 mg per cup of cooked spinach, and 3 mg per cup of broccoli.

Avoidance of Saturated Fats

Patients should be advised to decrease their intake of saturated fats. Diets high in saturated fats contribute to the risk of developing AMD, whereas those high in unsaturated fats reduce the risk.[17]

Cold-Water Fish

Docosahexaenoic acid (DHA), found in cold-water, deep-dwelling fish, is an essential nutrient for good brain and retinal function. The flesh of algae-eating fish is high in DHA, which is important in building and protecting photoreceptor membranes. In one study, persons consuming cold-water fish more than once a week were half as likely to experience macular degeneration as those consuming fish less than once a month.[18] The same study found a 2.7-fold greater incidence of AMD in persons consuming high levels of dietary cholesterol. Eating oily fish at least once weekly, compared with less than once weekly, halved the incidence of neovascular AMD.[19]

Wine in Moderation

Most researchers agree that consumption of moderate amounts of red wine reduces the risk of macular degeneration. In addition, many studies have reported that moderate wine consumption is associated with a lengthened life span.

Glutathione

An important study found that glutathione and related precursor amino acids are protective against damage to human RPE cells, which underlie the macula. Foods that contain the tripeptide glutathione are onions, garlic, avocados, asparagus, watermelon, and cruciferous vegetables.

Supplements

Multivitamins

Many studies have demonstrated the protective effect of antioxidants on retinal photoreceptors and the RPE. Some studies have demonstrated an association between vitamin or mineral deficiencies (e.g., zinc, tocopherol, carotenoids, and taurine) and a higher risk of AMD. Ascorbate, as well as lipoic acid, help recycle tocopherol in retinal tissue. Patients with AMD, in general, were found in one study to have a lower intake of tocopherol, magnesium, zinc, pyridoxine, and folic acid. In an important Veterans Affairs study, patients with AMD who were taking an antioxidant capsule (containing 19 ingredients) twice daily maintained better vision than the placebo control group.[20] One review found positive evidence for vitamins A, C, and E as well as for beta-carotene, lutein, zeaxanthin, selenium, and zinc, with the best evidence for vitamins C and E, lutein, and zeaxanthin.[21]

The 10-year randomized-controlled AREDS was concluded 3 years early because of the significant difference in the vitamin groups versus placebo. It demonstrated that the combination of vitamins C and E, beta-carotene, and zinc significantly reduced the progression of macular degeneration.[22] Ophthalmologists regard this as a landmark study acknowledging the effect of supplementation on macular degeneration. This proof of specific benefits of a balanced diet and broader nutrient supplementation has exciting implications.

The National Eye Institute is instituting AREDS II. It will reduce the amounts of zinc and beta-carotene in the study combination and add lutein and DHA.[23] In a 1-year Italian study, a combination of vitamin C, vitamin E, zinc, copper, lutein, and zeaxanthin improved established AMD.[24] The 6-month TOZAL study revealed similar results with a multivitamin including C, E, zinc, beta-carotene, and lutein and recommended prolonged administration.[25]

Multivitamins, which contain high levels of zinc and copper, should be avoided for long-term use. More than 30 mg of zinc will compete with the absorption of calcium, magnesium, selenium, and all other two valance compounds. Copper is an oxidant and has been associated with an increased risk of Alzheimer's.[26]

Lutein

Carotenoids are powerful antioxidants. Lutein and zeaxanthin have been precisely identified at high levels in the retina, particularly in the macular area. They have also been identified at significant concentrations in the iris, choroid, and lens (where they are needed to quench singlet oxygen and to filter out blue light). Greater lutein consumption is directly associated with elevated serum values and an increased macular pigment density. Investigators studying 23 pairs of donor eyes found that the eyes with lower lutein and zeaxanthin levels were the ones with histopathological signs of AMD.[27] Another study evaluated lutein and zeaxanthin levels in 56 donor eyes affected by AMD and 56 donor eyes known to be without the disease. Donor eyes with the highest amounts of lutein and zeaxanthin were 82% less likely to exhibit the signs of macular degeneration.[28]

Lutein and zeaxanthin are associated with improved retinal function in early AMD as well as increased neural processing.[29]

As little as 2.4 mg/day of lutein can double the serum level. A dose of 6 mg/day resulted in a 43% lower prevalence of AMD.[15] The Veterans Lutein Antioxidant Supplementation Trial (LAST) documented improvement in visual function with lutein alone or in combination with other nutrients.[31] With the addition of DHA, lutein buildup in the macular pigment density is even more effective.[32] AREDS II has replaced beta-carotene with lutein and DHA in their current formula. However, high levels of zinc and copper still remain.[33]

Beta-Carotene, Vitamin A, and Other Carotenoids

Investigators have confirmed, in both laboratory and clinical studies, that carotenoids such as vitamin A protect retinal cell membranes from light damage. Vitamin A is required to provide adequate levels of rhodopsin for optimal rod function. Severe vitamin A deficiency causes keratomalacia, xerophthalmia, and visual impairment. Administration of vitamin A has been helpful in patients suffering from retinitis pigmentosa. An early study documented an association between low vitamin A levels and macular degeneration and encouraged the inclusion of yellow fruits and vegetables in the diet.[3] The value of beta-carotene in the management of AMD remains inconclusive.[34,35] Only one study has indicated a specific beneficial effect of the carotenoid lycopene on the macula.

Tocopherols

Tocopherols protect against lipid peroxidation in cell membranes. Multiple studies have shown a powerful protective effect of d-alpha-tocopherol against macular degeneration. Some of these studies indicate a similar protective effect of plasma ascorbic acid and beta-carotene as well. High serum levels of d-alpha-tocopherol have been associated with decreased prevalence of drusen and late macular degeneration. French researchers examining 2500 patients found that those with the highest serum levels of vitamin E had an 82% lower prevalence of AMD.[36] Gamma-tocopherol and tocotrienol may prove to be superior to d-alpha-tocopherol.

Vitamin C

Ascorbic acid reduces the loss of rhodopsin and photoreceptor cell nuclei that occurs on exposure to light. Vitamin C also rejuvenates vitamin E and cell membrane–related enzymes. In several of the major studies that showed a protective effect of multivitamins against AMD, the multivitamin included at least 60 mg of vitamin C. Ocular tissues, especially the lens, contain high levels of vitamin C and glutathione.

Alpha-Lipoic Acid

Alpha-lipoic acid is an important nerve stabilizer that reduces insulin resistance in diabetic patients. It may protect the remaining ganglion cells and nerve fibers in patients with glaucoma. In addition, alpha-lipoic acid helps regenerate the reduced form of ascorbic acid.

B Vitamins

Pyridoxine deficiency has been identified in two observational studies in AMD populations. Folate deficiency has been identified in one of the studies. The B vitamins, in general, are important for nerve conduction, and the methylators (B_4, B_6, and B_{12}) reduce homocysteine levels. Christen et al.[37] reported a reduction in AMD development in 5205 women observed for 7.3 years who were given a supplementation consisting of folate, pyridoxine, and cyanocobalamin. Niacin, a B vitamin used to treat lipid abnormalities, has been shown to increase choroidal blood volume within 30 minutes of administration; however, the perfusion is at a slower rate. Thus, niacin has not been shown to increase total flow to the choroid.[38]

Vitamin D

Vitamin D is the only vitamin that is also a hormone and influences hundreds of genes. Studies have shown that vitamin D deficiency affects the risk of macular degeneration, neurodegenerative disease, and musculoskeletal health.[39] Garland has also reported a relationship between low serum vitamin D levels and all causes of mortality.[40]

Glutathione

Glutathione has been reported to be protective against damage to human RPE cells. Glutathione is manufactured in the liver after ingestion of the appropriate amino acids and sulfur-containing foods. This underappreciated water-soluble compound serves as an antioxidant and regenerator of vitamin E and carotenoids, as well as an intracellular enzyme. Because glutathione is hydrolyzed in the stomach, supplementation with glutathione boosters is recommended. The following have been found to increase glutathione: N-acetylcysteine, 600 mg twice a day; methylsulfonylmethane, 1000 mg once daily; S-adenosylmethionine (SAMe), 200 mg twice daily; and alpha-lipoic acid, 250 mg twice daily.

Bioflavonoids

Studies have shown that quercetin, a preparation of eucalyptus and citrus bioflavonoids, facilitates vitamin E protection of bovine and rat retina from induced lipid peroxidation. It also exerts an antihistaminic effect that may be beneficial for patients with chronic allergies.

Amino Acids

Taurine, the only nonbound circulating amino acid, is a stabilizer of biological membranes that protects the rod's outer segments, supports cardiovascular function, and modulates nerve transmission. Isolated taurine deficiency has been documented to cause retinal degeneration, and taurine administration has been shown to stabilize retinal changes in several studies.[41]

Arginine is one of the most important regulators of ocular perfusion. Intravenous administration of arginine has been shown to increase retinal (and choroidal) blood flow in healthy volunteers. This discovery merits further investigation in the AMD population.[42]

Minerals

Zinc and Copper. Zinc is found in high concentrations in the retina, RPE, and choroid. This trace mineral serves as a cofactor with many important retinal enzymes, including superoxide dismutase, catalase, carbonic anhydrase, retinol dehydrogenase, and protein phosphorylase; it also releases vitamin A from the liver. A 2-year study demonstrated that 100 mg/day of zinc sulfate significantly slowed the progression of AMD compared with the course of the disease in controls.[43] A good multivitamin for long-term use includes 15–30 mg of zinc and no copper. Both copper and zinc are needed to synthesize superoxide dismutase, and both act with other retinal enzymes to scavenge free radicals.

Magnesium. Magnesium has a significant role in nerve conduction and also dilates blood vessels. This mineral is important for maintenance of blood flow to the eye and brain in older persons with macular degeneration or diabetes, whenever blood pressure is decreased because they are lying down. The dose is 400–500 mg at bedtime.

Selenium. Selenium (maximum dose, 200 mcg/day) is a cofactor for vitamin E and glutathione enzymes. Low serum selenium levels and smoking have been associated with AMD.

Docosahexaenoic Acid

The primary source of DHA is algae and the cold-water, deep-dwelling fish that eat them. DHA not only supports retinal health in general but also improves hand-to-eye coordination, sharpens night-driving ability, and stabilizes cell membranes throughout the body. With its six unsaturated double bonds, it comprises 30%–50% of the "good" fat in the outer segments of the retinal photoreceptors. Because people are undersupplied with DHA from infancy, it is important to incorporate DHA capsules in the diet. The suggested supplementation amount is 500–1000 mg/day. One study found that lutein supplementation at 12 mg/day increased macular pigment ocular density (MPOD) in the peripheral macula, whereas the addition of DHA (800 mg/day) increased peripheral and central MPOD.[44] This evidence strengthens the support for supplementing polyunsaturated fatty acids in the diet to raise their concentration in macular photoreceptors. Feher et al.[45] reported that the combination of omega-3 fatty acids, acetyl-L-carnitine, and coenzyme Q10 showed significant stabilization and improvement in vision in a 106-patient study. These three compounds, along with vitamin E, favorably affect mitochondrial lipid metabolism. A 12-year study confirmed

the reduction in neovascular AMD with a high intake of omega-3 fatty acids.[46]

> Alpha-linolenic acid (present in flaxseed oil, among others) is the parent omega-3 fatty acid. It takes 20–30 of the 18-carbon alpha-linoleic acid molecules to make one 22-carbon DHA molecule, which is a building block for every cell membrane in the body.

Botanicals

Ginkgo

The ginkgo tree is the sole survivor of a family of trees that flourished before the Ice Age. *Ginkgo biloba*, which increases cerebral blood flow, has been demonstrated to improve retinal blood flow by 23%[47] and is prescribed regularly by certain glaucoma specialists. For vasodilation, I recommend either 15–60 drops of a ginkgo solution (24% ginkgolides) in water or a 30-mg tablet twice daily. Be sure to check the patient's other medications first for possible blood-thinning influences because ginkgo can exacerbate this effect.

Sage

Sage (*Salvia officinalis*) also improves circulation, but unlike ginkgo, which has an excitatory effect, it has a calming effect.[48] A controlled study from Hunan Medical College in China indicated that *Salvia miltiorrhiza*, as part of a four-herb formula, improved visual field in one-third of a glaucoma population receiving the formula for more than 19 months. Herbalists recommend 1 g orally twice daily. More studies are necessary, however.

Bilberry

Bilberry (*Vaccinium myrtillus*) has been shown to improve night vision; with the exception of one preliminary French study, however, it has not been proven to be effective in stabilizing AMD. Bilberry only improves the effectiveness of rhodopsin, which is necessary for night vision.

Milk Thistle

Silymarin, from the herb milk thistle (*Silybum marianum*), is a major supporter of liver function. The liver is the key organ for maintenance of eye health because the fat-soluble vitamins and glutathione are stored and the B vitamins are activated there. The usual dose of milk thistle is 150 mg two or three times a day. SAMe in a dose of 200 mg twice daily is an alternative.

> The eye is subjected to bright light throughout the day, and the important ingredients for molecular repair are stored in the liver. When the liver is overburdened, eyesight is compromised.

Chinese Herbs

Experienced herbalists report that tien chi root, dang gui root, triphala, lycium fruit, ginseng root, cooked and raw rehmannia, shilajatu, wild asparagus root, and elderberry have been used in ancient formulas to treat vascular disease inside the eye.[42] None of these remedies have been used in controlled studies, although there is ample anecdotal evidence in the Chinese literature of success as measured by nonprogression of disease during 3 years.

Pharmaceuticals

Ranibizumab (Lucentis), bevacizumab (Avastin), and aflibercept (Eylea) are three vascular endothelial growth factor (VEGF) inhibitors that can remarkably reverse leakage into the retina in wet AMD. Ranibizumab has been approved by the U.S. Food and Drug Administration (FDA); bevacizumab, an intravenous therapy for colon cancer, is used off label. Intraocular injections of steroids, pegaptanib sodium (Macugen, an intraocular anti-VEGF), and verteporfin (Visudyne, an intravenous dye that highlights leaky retinal vessels) are relegated to ancillary roles. Dosages are to be determined by the retinal specialist.

Other Therapy

The FDA may soon approve implantable silicone devices that will serve as replacements for damaged retina. Implantable devices and telescopic lenses are also in phase II FDA testing.

Low-vision experts have many optical devices to support people with failing vision.

PREVENTION PRESCRIPTION

- Adoption of a positive attitude and awareness of risk factors and potential medication effects
- Use of sunglasses and other sun protection
- Increased consumption of green leafy vegetables
- Diet rich in polyunsaturated fatty acids and low in saturated fats
- Multivitamins with zinc, taurine, and lutein
- Use of supplements, with attention to overall good dietary nutrition
- Avoidance of long-term use of antacids or gastric acid suppression

- Regular exercise
- Performance of deep-breathing exercises on a regular basis
- Periodic eye examinations with use of the Amsler grid
- Use of low-vision aids for vision loss

Early intervention after recognition of macular degeneration is crucial. The performance of an Amsler grid examination is recommended in all patients (see Fig. 83.3). It is important to remember that the retina can be rebuilt.

THERAPEUTIC REVIEW

If a patient presents with severe symptoms, such as profound visual loss, it would be to his or her benefit for the clinician to immediately begin a more aggressive therapy. For the patient who has mild to moderate symptoms, however, the following nutritional and lifestyle approach is appropriate.

REMOVE EXACERBATING FACTORS
- Encourage smoking cessation, moderate alcohol intake, weight management, and exercise.

NUTRITION
- Encourage foods rich in omega-3 fatty acids (wild salmon, nuts, or flaxseed).
- Increase foods rich in carotenoids, such as lutein and zeaxanthin (dark green leafy vegetables).

SUPPLEMENTS
- Multivitamins have been the focus of many epidemiological studies over the years. It is known that the combination of low-dose antioxidants is supportive of macular function; this fact became evident in the landmark AREDS. The multivitamin should include vitamin C, vitamin E, zinc, selenium, taurine, lutein, and zeaxanthin.
- Incorporate lutein: 6–10 mg/day (6 mg for prevention, 10 mg for treatment).

- DHA supplementation: 500 to 800 mg daily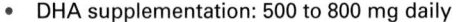
- Vitamin C, 1000 mg/day, has been shown useful in some observational studies to act as an antioxidant and therefore to protect the retinal pigment epithelium from oxidative stressors.

BOTANICALS
- *Ginkgo biloba* has been shown to improve ocular blood flow by 23%; 30 mg twice daily.
- Milk thistle is the primary source of the bioflavonoid silymarin, a major supporter of hepatocyte function, which in turn supports eye health; 150 mg two or three times a day.

CHINESE HERBS
- Although clinical data are lacking, there is an abundance of historical data on the benefits of the use of Chinese herbs for AMD.

PHARMACEUTICAL INJECTION
Antivascular endothelial growth factor (VEGF) therapy
- Intraocular injections of ranibizumab (Lucentis) and bevacizumab (Avastin) have become the best treatment of more advanced disease.

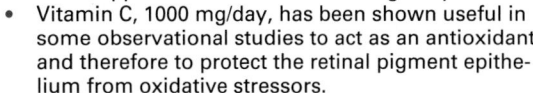

Key Web Resources

The American Academy of Ophthalmology's website provides an updated list of current research and protocols for AMD.	http://www.aao.org/
PDF of the Amsler grid for screening for macular degeneration	http://amslergrid.org/

REFERENCES

References are available online at ExpertConsult.com.

PART III

TOOLS FOR YOUR PRACTICE

PART OUTLINE

SECTION IA	LIFESTYLE: NUTRITION
SECTION IB	LIFESTYLE: EXERCISE
SECTION II	MIND-BODY
SECTION III	BIOCHEMICAL
SECTION IV	BIOMECHANICAL
SECTION V	BIOENERGETICS
SECTION VI	OTHER

SECTION IA

LIFESTYLE: NUTRITION

SECTION OUTLINE

86 THE ELIMINATION DIET

87 GLYCEMIC INDEX AND GLYCEMIC LOAD

88 ANTIINFLAMMATORY DIET

89 THE DASH DIET

90 THE FODMAP DIET

CHAPTER 86

THE ELIMINATION DIET

Suhani Bora, MD • J. Adam Rindfleisch, MPhil, MD

Detecting and eliminating specific antagonistic foods, and designing a nutritionally sound diet to ensure the optimum health of the food-sensitive person, is the ultimate aim in food sensitivity management. This process is often tedious and time consuming, and requires tremendous knowledge, skill, commitment, and dedication...However, when a person who has been chronically sick suddenly feels well for the first time in many years, as so often happens, the rewards for both practitioner and client more than justify the time and effort of the endeavor.

J. V. JONEJA[1]

For centuries, Indian Ayurvedic healing has emphasized the elimination of certain foods and the use of others.[2] In recent years, we have seen a rise in thinking of food as medicine.[3] We have also seen an increase in the prevalence of food allergies[4] and the number of diagnoses of celiac disease and eosinophilic esophagitis[5] for which the mainstay of treatment is elimination of certain foods. Recent dietary trends parallel this with a rise in restrictive diets such as the paleo, gluten-free, and dairy-free diets. Globalization has increased our exposure to traditional, sometimes religiously based, diets that include restrictions such as vegetarianism and veganism. Celebrities and the media have made "detoxing" and "clean eating" mainstream.[6] Pesticide contamination, use of growth hormones and antibiotics in meat production, genetic engineering of food sources, and health risks associated with fast and processed foods as well as food additives, high-fructose corn syrup, sugar, and sugar substitutes are topics of concern that can arise during an integrative medicine visit. An integrative provider must be aware of the potential benefits as well as the limitations and harms of an elimination diet. An in-depth discussion of food allergies and food intolerances is provided in Chapter 31.

Despite controversy surrounding food intolerances in the medical community, many Americans believe they are sensitive to particular foods. A subset of the population may indeed be able to alleviate symptoms, slow the progression of their disease, reduce the use of medications, and have a heightened feeling of control and ownership over often frustrating and incurable diseases or symptoms by eliminating certain foods. Almost one-third of adults in the United States have reportedly decreased their intake of gluten.[7] Most people with irritable bowel syndrome (IBS) believe that certain foods trigger their symptoms,[8] and 30% of patients with fibromyalgia have attempted to change their diet, trying improve their symptoms.[9] Twenty percent of parents believe that their child has a food reaction when only about 5% actually do.[10]

Current evidence indicates that reportedly 35% of the population in developed countries has food hypersensitivities.[11] This does not account for approximately half of U.S. adults who have lactose intolerance.[12] The prevalence of celiac disease is 1 in 160,[13] and the prevalence of nonceliac gluten sensitivity, which has similar symptoms but without enteropathy, is slightly higher.[14] The prevalence of wine intolerance is 7.2%.[15]

Elimination diets may be used for three distinct types of patient encounters: (1) patients who present with multiple symptoms but no clear diagnosis, (2) those who have specific diagnoses for which certain foods have been found to exacerbate symptoms, and (3) for patients who believe they have food intolerances and may have already begun to restrict their diets. This chapter provides an overview of the state of research on elimination diets as a clinical tool, including its potential pitfalls and harms.

A patient handout on elimination diets appears at the end of the chapter.

PATHOPHYSIOLOGY OF NONALLERGIC FOOD INTOLERANCES

A food allergy involves a specific IgE-mediated reaction, usually to a glycoprotein found in a given food. Food intolerance, in contrast, is defined more generally as any adverse physiological response to a food product. This chapter will focus on food intolerances.

PATHOPHYSIOLOGY OF LEAKY GUT SYNDROME: GUT-IMMUNE BARRIER

Increased intestinal permeability, or "leaky gut syndrome," has been proposed as one means by which food or chemical intolerance develops. The epithelial cells of the gastrointestinal tract function as nonprofessional antigen-presenting cells.[16] The gut is constantly sampling various potential antigens, ultimately allowing only 2% of antigens to move into the bloodstream. The epithelial cells, gut dendritic cells, and at least five different T-cell types help regulate intestinal immunity. One of the main T-cell functions is to allow tolerance to develop; that is, the body must be able to minimize allergic reactions to the foreign antigens commonly consumed in foods. In some individuals, this process seems to break down and certain foods begin to elicit symptoms.[17]

The breakdown of the intestinal epithelial tight junction barrier allows antigens and bacterial DNA that are typically too large to cross through the intestinal tract to enter into the bloodstream. The introduction of these foreign proteins elicits a number of negative physiological effects, including initiating and perpetuating inflammatory diseases.[18-20] Permeability is increased by a number of factors, including inflammation, exposure to medications (e.g., nonsteroidal antiinflammatory drugs), shifts in intestinal microflora, micronutrient deficiencies, and the presence of various disease states such as celiac disease and ulcerative colitis[18,21] (Table 86.1, list of factors that increase intestinal permeability). There is increasing evidence that the indigenous intestinal microflora, which is influenced by diet, stress, and disease states, plays a role in altering epithelial and mucosal

TABLE 86.1 Differential Diagnosis of Adverse Food Reactions

Intolerance Category	Description	Comments and Clinical Tips
Food allergy[118-120]	Immune mediated, mainly by IgE, to a food glycoprotein Symptoms arise in minutes to hours. Manifested the same way with every exposure, usually with rash, angioedema, anaphylaxis; GI symptoms may also arise with histamine release	Prevalence increasing (4%–8% in children, 1%–4% in adults). One-fourth of the population claims to have a food allergy. One-third of infants with frequent spitting up respond to oral challenge testing; 10% who react to cow's milk also react to soy; 45% retain a milk allergy past 1 year of age.
Celiac disease[121]	Gliadin, a portion of the grain protein gluten, triggers chronic inflammation through reactive CD4+ T cells in people with the alleles for HLA DQ2 or DQ8. Affects all age groups. Two to three times more common in females than in males. May affect multiple organ systems. 10%–23% may develop neurological symptoms, such as idiopathic ataxia and paresthesias. Grains that can contribute are wheat, rye, barley, spelt, kamut, semolina, triticale, and malt. Oats do not have gluten but are often contaminated with it, so many providers encourage avoidance.	Prevalence 1% and increasing as more testing is being done. 50% of adults with disease present with diarrhea. Increased risk with Down syndrome, Turner syndrome, and type 1 diabetes. 2%–5% do not respond to gluten-free diet and are at risk for T-cell lymphoma. Laboratory results may show decreased calcium and protein as well as increased levels on liver function tests. People with celiac disease have higher risks of iron deficiency and osteoporosis. Best tests are transglutaminase IgA, antiendomysial antibodies, and tissue transglutaminase (an enzyme that reacts with gliadin). These are 90% sensitive, and titers indicate degree of damage.
Cross-allergy[118,122]	Arises when foods with similarities to environmental allergens trigger a response. Often characterized by oral tingling (oral allergy syndrome).	Examples: Birch, alder, and hazelnut can cross-react with apples, pears, cherries, hazelnuts, walnuts, and pistachios. Grass and cereal pollens can be linked to allergy to wheat, rye, and oat flour as well as to tomato, kiwi, and celery. In people with latex allergies, pineapple, kiwi, avocado, potato, banana, and nuts can cause reactions. Feather allergies can mean allergies to hen's eggs, poultry meat, and giblets. House-dust mite allergy can be associated with shellfish allergy.
Pseudoallergies[118,122]	Foods trigger mast cell degranulation without involving IgE antibodies.	Examples: Strawberries, chocolate, tomatoes Salicylates (cause cyclooxygenase-1 inhibition, leading to abnormal prostaglandin levels) used as food preservatives Benzoates (preservatives used in fruit drinks, pickled foods, and alcoholic beverages) Tartrazine (yellow #5)
Eosinophilic esophagogastroenteritis[123]	Eosinophils accumulate in any or all layers of the digestive tract wall. One-half to two-thirds will have elevated serum eosinophil counts with no other explanation.	Affects all ages. Diagnosed by endoscopy and colonoscopy; may be related to chronic acid suppression. Responds to elimination diets and medication. Worth considering in unexplained diarrhea, especially if serum eosinophil counts are inexplicably high.

TABLE 86.1 **Differential Diagnosis of Adverse Food Reactions—cont'd**

Intolerance Category	Description	Comments and Clinical Tips
IgG-related intolerance[20,124]	Intolerances slowly develop hours to days after an exposure as IgG is created by the immune system. IgG may be the pathogen itself, causing increased small intestinal permeability. IgG half-life is 22–96 days, which makes false-positive results possible on testing.	Isolated IgG testing in patients with irritable bowel syndrome is controversial, and no one test is likely to identify all problem foods. Foods that test positive often do not cause symptoms. Tests are not typically covered by insurance.
Physiological reactions[118]	Foods lead to gas production or cause dyspepsia by relaxing the lower esophageal sphincter	Examples of gas-generating foods include legumes, cabbage, bran, and other vegetables and grains. Heartburn and dyspepsia can result from fatty foods, alcohol, mint, chocolate, and citrus.
Pharmacological reactions[118,122]	Some foods have drug-like effects. A common example is histaminergic foods, which influence the histamine pathways in the stomach and other GI tract organs. Sulfites, monosodium glutamate (Chinese restaurant syndrome), and biogenic amines may also cause symptoms through drug-like actions.	Histamine intolerance: Is present in 1% of Europeans Is more common in middle-aged women Can be associated with other histamine-caused symptoms, such as nasal congestion, dyspnea, skin reactions, and headache; dysmenorrhea may also occur Leads to opposite effects for histamine-blocking drugs, such as ranitidine
Toxin mediated[118,122]	A specific toxin is present in a food.	Examples include food poisoning, mycotoxins, perhaps herbicides, and pesticides.
Enzymatic[125-127]	Deficiency of an enzyme, such as lactase, leads to poor digestion. GI symptoms result. Lactose intolerance arises as cells lose their ability to make lactase. Symptoms occur 30–120 minutes after lactose is consumed. Other sugar intolerances, such as to fructose, sorbitol, mannitol, and xylitol, are less common.	Lactose intolerance: Has lowest prevalence in Northern Europeans, highest in Asians, Native Americans, African Americans Is usually not triggered by less than 12 g of lactose (the amount in a cup of milk) Is usually not affected as much by yogurt, especially as it ages Can be triggered by medications; 20% of prescription drugs and 6% of over-the-counter drugs use lactose as a base
Structural[122]	An underlying pathological process leads to intolerance of different foods.	Examples include achalasia, strictures, pancreatitis, inflammatory bowel disease, and abdominal angina.
Infectious[122]	Chronic infections predispose to adverse food reactions.	Examples include lambliasis (Giardia), bacterial overgrowth (especially in immunosuppression, diabetes, or the use of proton pump inhibitors), chronic salmonellosis, Blastocystis infection, and parasites.
Psychogenic[122]	Somatoform disorders, eating disorders, or the discouragement tied to food intolerance itself may lead to food reactions. Note that high norepinephrine levels can trigger histamine release, so stress can cause intolerances through some of the mechanisms previously listed as well.	It is not uncommon in integrative practice to see individuals who become obsessed with their diets. This "orthorexia" can become a pathological process unto itself. Treatment involves working closely with a nutritionist, adding mental health and mind-body approaches to care, and helping them slowly regain their ability to enjoy eating.
Other causes[122]	Mastocytosis, carcinoid and other neuroendocrine tumors, and GI neoplasms may also lead to symptoms.	As always, a careful history and differential diagnosis are mandatory.

GI, gastrointestinal; *Ig*, immunoglobulin.

permeability.[18] Tight junction leakage, enhanced by glucose, salt, emulsifiers, organic solvents, gluten, microbial transglutaminase, and nanoparticles used in the food industry, also increases intestinal permeability. Tight junction dysfunction has been shown to be associated with atopic dermatitis and a variety of autoimmune diseases.[22]

It has been proposed that many cases of food intolerance may be associated with the overall process of toxicant-induced loss of tolerance, which is thought to be precipitated not only by foods but also by inhalants, chemical exposures, and electrical stimuli.[23] As such, any steps that may reduce overall sensitivity may be helpful in treating food intolerances. Examples include exercise, minimizing body inflammation, desensitization, and simple, safe detoxification regimens that include evaluation and reduction of chemicals used in daily cleaning and hygiene. It may be helpful to explore whether an individual with food intolerances is also "reactive" in other ways, physically and emotionally, to his or her environment. Reducing intestinal permeability may allow a person to reintroduce substances that were formerly problematic.

Repairing the gut-immune barrier to reduce intestinal permeability requires a multifaceted approach, one that includes addressing sources of inflammation including diet, lack of adequate physical exercise or sleep, high levels of stress, and unaddressed emotional health including unhealthy relationships.[24] One common approach for treating intestinal permeability is the 4R method, in which foods or substances that could be causing adverse reactions are *removed*, followed by *replacing* digestive enzymes or hydrochloric acid if needed and *repopulation* of the gut flora with prebiotics and probiotics, and finally, *repairing* the intestines with key nutrients and botanicals. Elimination diets are one part, the *removal* part, of an integrative treatment approach.

Aside from certain tests for IgE-mediated food allergies, most tests for adverse food reactions remain controversial. Such tests are more likely to discover clinically insignificant positive results, leading to unnecessary food restrictions, and to miss clinically important reactions. Remember that an elimination diet can serve, in and of itself, as a useful diagnostic tool.

Prescribing an Elimination Diet

A number of disorders are known to be influenced by food (Table 86.2). An elimination diet is, put simply, an eating plan that omits a food or group of foods believed to cause an adverse food reaction. Restrictive diets prescribed for long durations without reintroduction of foods may lead to malnutrition and cause fear or anxiety related to food that, in severe cases, may lead to orthorexia or a fear of food. If you have a patient who presents with multiple chronic symptoms but no clear diagnoses, who has a specific diagnosis that has been shown to be affected by certain foods, or who believe they have a food intolerance, a carefully prescribed elimination diet may be a safe and effective treatment and diagnostic, patient-led tool. In general, four principal steps are followed in prescribing any elimination diet.

Step 1: The Planning Phase

Before recommending an elimination diet, the clinician must take a thorough patient history. For patients with a history of eating disorders, children, and pregnant women, an elimination diet must be approached cautiously, if at all. Children and pregnant women are at risk for nutritional deficiencies and inadequate weight gain. Patients with significant food allergies should be followed in conjunction with an allergist. Ideally, patients should provide a recent diet and symptom log that chronicles food and beverage intake for a least 1 week. Patients should note what symptoms they experience and when these symptoms arise relative to mealtimes and time of day, including alcohol use, supplements, medications, exercise, specific stressors, and sleep quality if those are of concern.[25] Symptoms may range from gastrointestinal complaints and skin changes

TABLE 86.2	**Conditions for Which Elimination Diets Might be Used[1]**
Cardiovascular	Palpitations Tachycardia
Dermatological	Angioedema[a] Atopic dermatitis[a] Contact dermatitis Dermatitis herpetiformis Pruritus[a] Seborrheic dermatitis Urticaria[a,128]
Gastrointestinal	Bloating, belching Celiac disease[a] Cholecystitis, cholelithiasis[a,129] Chronic diarrhea[a,130] Colic[131] Constipation, including laxative resistant in children[132] Cyclic vomiting syndrome[a,133] Encopresis[134] Eosinophilic esophagitis[a,16] Eosinophilic gastroenteritis[a,135] Gastroesophageal reflux[a,136] Irritable bowel syndrome[a] Inflammatory bowel disease[a,137-139] Nausea, vomiting Pruritus ani[140] Recurrent abdominal pain in children with confirmed allergy[a,141]
Genitourinary	Enuresis[a,32,142] Frequency Interstitial cystitis Vulvodynia Chronic pelvic pain
Neurological/ psychological	Attention deficit hyperactivity disorder[a] Autistic spectrum disorders[a] Medication-resistant depression Migraine[a] Other types of headache Seizures (by ketogenic diets)[a,143]
Respiratory/ otolaryngological	Aphthous ulcers (recurrent)[144] Asthma[a,86,145,146] Chronic congestion, rhinitis[a,147] Chronic serous otitis[a] Conjunctivitis Laryngeal edema, hoarseness
Rheumatological	Chronic fatigue[148,149] Gout[33] Rheumatoid arthritis[a] Systemic lupus erythematosus[149] Vasculitis
Miscellaneous	Listlessness, poor concentration Irritability Cold intolerance, low-grade fever Dizziness Excess sweating Pallor

[a]Indicates that at least level B evidence (SORT criteria) exists for treatment of this condition with an elimination diet. Other foods may also be implicated. It is important to tailor therapy to the individual.

to low mood, fatigue, or difficulty with concentration. Free online food tracking apps or websites may be helpful. Table 86.3 lists key issues to address when taking the history of a patient for whom an adverse food reaction is suspected. A sample 1-week dietary log form is included in

TABLE 86.3	**Points to Consider Before Prescribing an Elimination Diet**
Several key questions may reveal which foods should be removed[150]	What foods do you frequently eat? What foods do you crave? What foods make you feel better? What foods would be difficult to give up or go without?
A history should cover several specific topics[1,151,152]	Family history of food intolerance, irritable bowel, headache, and mouth ulcers. Past medical history of respiratory allergies, chronic upper respiratory congestion, asthma, atopic dermatitis, infant colic, gastrointestinal problems (including lactose intolerance or celiac disease), or unusual reactions to medications or foods. History of eating disorders (to avoid risk that an elimination diet may exacerbate these conditions). History of food allergies. Previous laboratory test findings (e.g., results of skin prick testing). Relation of symptoms to exercise (some intolerances are exacerbated with increased activity). Relation of symptoms to substance use, including smoking, alcohol,[a] caffeine, and illicit drugs. Life stressors. Financial resources. Social support. Willingness and ability to make lifestyle changes.[25]

[a]Some clinicians have noted that the development of food intolerance in some patients is preceded by changes in alcohol tolerance. Patients may first note intolerance to red wine and beer and later an inability to drink white wine and spirits.[153] Ultimately, intolerance to other food items is noted.

TABLE 86.4	**Common Food Culprits for Food Allergy and Food Intolerance[1,16]**
Food allergy[a]	Citrus Dairy products Eggs Fish Peanuts Soy Gluten (barley, oats, rye, and wheat) Shellfish Tree nuts (almonds, pecans, and walnuts)

Food intolerance	All of the foods listed for food allergy, plus:
	Beef products
	Corn
	Food additives, including
	   Antioxidants (butylated hydroxyanisole, butylated hydroxytoluene)
	   Aspartame (NutraSweet, an artificial sweetener)
	   Flavor enhancers (monosodium glutamate)
	   Food colors (tartrazine and various other Food Dye and Coloring Act [FD&C] dyes, which are derived from coal tar)
	   Nitrates and nitrites (found in preserved meats)
	   Preservatives (sulfites, benzoates, and sorbates)
	   Thickeners/stabilizers (tragacanth, agar-agar)
	Biogenic amines (histamine, tyramine, octopamine, and phenylethylamine)
	Disaccharides (lactose)
	Foods high in nickel and salicylates (see reference 1 for a complete listing)
	Refined sugars

[a]These foods account for roughly 80% of all food hypersensitivity reactions.

the Patient Handout. Keep in mind that for patients with an unhealthy diet, simply recommending a healthy diet may be more important than an elimination diet. In a UK study[26] of people who believed that they had a food intolerance, 70% were able to improve their symptoms just by following a healthy eating plan for 2 weeks and without any food restrictions. This 2-week healthy eating plan focused on reducing soda, caffeine, and processed foods and eating more whole grains, fruits, and vegetables.

Next, it is important to assess the patient's readiness and motivation to undertake a lifestyle change.[25] Do the patients have upcoming stressful life events? Are they on a limited budget? Do they have resources, energy, and willingness to create new grocery lists and menus and to cook new recipes? Are they able to gather support from family and friends and strategize how to eat at work, in restaurants, at events? Are they committed to tracking what they consume and their symptoms? Do they have adequate stress coping skills? Would another time be better to successfully implement an elimination diet?

After a list of potential problem foods is elicited, the next step is to create a list of foods to avoid. The list should be individualized as much as possible for each patient. Table 86.4 lists the foods most likely to cause adverse food reactions. Table 86.5 lists foods linked to symptoms in various disease states.

Patients often have a sense of which foods are most likely to contribute to their symptoms. The clinician should be sure to explore this issue with them. Trust their "gut feelings." Remember that comfort foods and foods that are often craved can be important culprits.

Step 2: The Avoidance Phase

Elimination diets vary in terms of intensity.[1,24] The type of diet chosen varies according to the number of suspected food culprits, patient preference, likelihood of adherence, and the potential effects on the patient's nutritional status. Patient adherence decreases as diets become more restrictive. The patient handout provides examples of three elimination diets of variable intensity. "Failing" a prescribed elimination diet may cause undue

TABLE 86.5 Foods to Eliminate for Specific Disorders and Synopsis of Key Research

Condition	Foods to Eliminate[a]	Research Summary
Asthma[4,61-69]	Fast food, sulfites (found in commercial foods, soft drinks, beer, wine, commercially prepared lemon and lime juice, vinegar, meat, gelatin, and coconut), tartrazine, MSG, eggs, cow's milk, peanuts, soy, wheat, and fish.	Between 3% and 10% of patients with asthma are allergic to sulfites, and 4%–8% of children with asthma have verifiable food allergies. Consider eliminating common food allergens in children (eggs, cow's milk, peanuts, soy, wheat, and fish) and consulting an allergist if allergies are severe. A low-sodium diet has been shown to improve exercise-induced bronchospasm.
Attention deficit hyperactivity disorder (ADHD)[1,66]	Apples, artificial colors, aspartame (NutraSweet), butylated hydroxyanisole, butylated hydroxytoluene (in packaged cereals), benzoates (chewing gum, margarine, pickles, prunes, tea, raspberries, cinnamon, anise, nutmeg), caffeine, corn, dairy products, nitrates and nitrites (preserved meats like bacon, frankfurters, pepperoni), oranges, propyl gallate, sulfites (dried fruits, mushrooms, potatoes, baked good, canned fish, pickles, relishes), peanuts, tomatoes.	Began with Feingold diet in 1975 but lost favor when research did not show benefit. Food additives such as tartrazine (yellow dye #5), benzoates, and glutamate are known to affect the nervous system, but sugar does not seem to have an effect. A 2010 review concluded that no dietary interventions are helpful with ADHD, except that a small subset of children may benefit from removal of artificial food colors.[67] A 2008 review found moderately good evidence of effect for removal of food additives.[68]
Atopic dermatitis[1,68,69]	Children: dairy, eggs, soy, wheat. Adults: pollen-related foods (fruit, nuts, and vegetables). Other considerations would be artificial colors, benzoates, berries, citrus, currants, fish, legumes, sulfites, tomatoes, and, occasionally, beef, chicken, and pork.	Evidence of an effect of mother's diet when pregnant or breastfeeding is less clear,[70] but breastfeeding itself is preventive.[71] No other dietary interventions were conclusively found to affect atopy in children. A Korean study divided 524 patients into four groups for interferon-gamma treatment, elimination diet, or both. The elimination diet-only group had the most significant decrease in symptom severity.[72] A 1991 study found improvement in 49 of 66 children with eczema, which recurred when cow's milk and tomato were added back.[73] A 1987 study found that 37 of 101 people with eczema reacted to one or more food additives, with 16 reacting to the placebo. Only one-third of the subjects had reproducibility on repeated testing.[74]
Autistic spectrum disorders[4,30,75,76]	Gluten and casein (gluten-free, casein-free [GFCF] diet), food additives, and artificial colors.	Significant numbers of autistic children have relatively high titers of antibodies (IgA, IgG, and IgE) to gluten and casein.[75,76] A 2008 review noted that GFCF diets are "promising" but that current evidence is not conclusive.[30] A 2008 Cochrane review concluded that the current quality of evidence regarding the effect of the GFCF diet is poor.[77] GFCF diets decrease urine peptides, perhaps indicating improved intestinal permeability (after 1 year).[78]
Autoimmune thyroiditis[36]	Dairy products	In one study, 75.9% of patients with Hashimoto's thyroiditis had lactose intolerance. Patients with lactose intolerance who restricted dairy had significant decreases in thyroid stimulating hormone (TSH) levels.
Fibromyalgia[9,33,57-60]	Glutamate, aspartate, MSG, aspartame, food additives, refined and simple sugars, artificial coloring, artificial flavors and sweeteners, caffeinated beverages, gluten, eggs, dairy products, and foods high in arachidonic acid.	Note: While raw vegetarian or vegan diets improved pain, sleep quality, and morning stiffness, they often have poor adherence, likely worsened by decreased functionality (grocery shopping, meal preparation) due to chronic pain, comorbid depression, and chronic fatigue. Aspartame and food additives are excitatory neurotransmitters, which may contribute to central sensitization and play a role in perception of pain in patients with fibromyalgia. It may be prudent to begin with eliminating aspartame, other artificial sweeteners, and additives before trying more restrictive elimination diets; 30% of patients with fibromyalgia have tried dietary changes and 85% have chronic fatigue.
Gout[33]	Meat and fewer sugar-sweetened drinks (including apple and orange juice), alcohol.	

TABLE 86.5 Foods to Eliminate for Specific Disorders and Synopsis of Key Research—cont'd

Condition	Foods to Eliminate[a]	Research Summary
Irritable bowel syndrome (IBS)[1,8,79]	Dairy, eggs, and wheat. Some diets become elaborate, focusing on which starches should and should not be consumed. See reference 1 for a comprehensive IBS diet.	Greater than 60% of IBS sufferers think that specific foods contribute to their symptoms[28] and 50% report that their symptoms arise after eating.[80] A 2010 review found that insufficient data exist to make recommendations about elimination diets and IBS.[81] A 2005 review concluded that "dietary manipulation may result in substantial improvement in IBS symptomatology provided it is individualized to the particular patient."[28] Many IBS sufferers have changes in motility even with the sight or smell of food, which complicates diagnosis.[28] A 1998 review[82] showed a 15%–71% response rate when study data were pooled for IBS and elimination diets. Rule out lactose intolerance in IBS patients.[83]
Migraine[1,7,60,84,85]	Aspartame, beef, chocolate, coffee, corn, eggs, histamine (fish, cheese, wine, and beer), monosodium glutamate (mushrooms, kelp, scallops, preserved meats, Chinese food), nitrates (processed meats), oranges, sugar, tea, tyramine (aged cheeses, some red wines), and yeast. See also www.fammed.wisc.edu/ integrative/modules/headaches for an online "Headache Elimination Diet" handout.	A 2009 review concluded that individualized elimination diets for migraine are a useful therapeutic approach.[86] One study found that 29 of 55 patients had complete symptom resolution with elimination diets and another 21 experienced improvement.[87] A 1979 study found that 85% of a group of 60 became headache free after following a 5-day elimination of an average of 10 different foods. The total number of headaches/month fell from an average of 402 to 6.[88] In a blinded study of aspartame (NutraSweet) compared with placebo, there was a 100% increase in headache frequency during the aspartame consumption phase of the trial.[89] More than 90% of a group of 88 children with severe migraine symptoms had response to a food elimination diet.[90]
Serous otitis media	See the Level 2 diet in the patient handout. Consider removal of dairy foods.	70 of 81 children (aged 1 to 9 years) with documented food allergies had improved tympanometry findings after a 16-week individualized elimination diet.[91] A 1997 trial found a 70%–83% improvement in symptoms of fullness, allergic symptoms, and overall well-being in 151 people with eustachian tube dysfunction and noted to have allergic symptoms.[92] A number of integrative clinicians link dairy and other foods to chronic ear and sinus congestion, and an elimination diet is worth considering in patients with these problems.[93]
Rheumatoid arthritis (RA)	Consider the few foods listed in the patient handout. Corn, dairy, and nightshade vegetables (bell peppers, eggplant, potatoes, and tomatoes) are worth considering.	Interest arose in 1981 when the media described a woman with RA whose 25 years of symptoms resolved with corn elimination.[94] In the 1960s, the nightshade diet, which eliminates eggplant, bell peppers, potatoes, and tomatoes, became popular. There is limited evidence to support the effect of nightshades on RA. A 2009 Cochrane review concluded, "The effects of dietary manipulation, including vegetarian, Mediterranean, elemental and elimination diets, on rheumatoid arthritis are still uncertain due to the included studies being small, single trials with moderate to high risk of bias."[95] One small study of 70 people with RA observed that 19% were able to stay well without medications for 1–5 years after elimination of particular foods.[96]

[a]Other foods may also be implicated. It is important to tailor therapy to the individual.

stress or feelings of failure. Begin with the least restrictive diet.

Level 1: Food Specific Diet: Elimination of One Food or Food Group. The lowest-intensity elimination diets are referred to as *food-specific diets*. In these, just one food, group of foods, or additive (e.g., aspartame) is eliminated. Which food or foods are to be removed is often determined on the basis of both the patient suspicions and their responses to the questions listed in Table 86.3. For some patients, particularly those for whom maintaining healthy nutrition may be a challenge, it is most appropriate to pursue several low-intensity elimination diets, one after another, rather than to remove multiple foods or food groups simultaneously. However, some individuals display intolerance to combinations of foods or food groups; for them, a low-intensity elimination diet may not prove as useful as one in which multiple food groups are removed simultaneously. Given the high prevalence of lactose intolerance, eliminating dairy may be a good way to start.

Level 2: Elimination of Multiple Food Groups. In a moderate-intensity elimination diet, multiple foods or food groups are eliminated. If successfully done, moderate-intensity diets have the potential to serve as useful diagnostic and therapeutic tools. The list of foods eliminated is tailored to the individual patient; examples include a low-fermentable oligosaccharides, disaccharides, monosaccharides, and polyols (FODMaPS) diet for a patient with IBS (see Chapter 90); a six-food elimination diet for eosinophilic esophagitis; a gluten-free, casein-free diet for autism; or a gluten and dairy elimination diet for someone with multiple, nonspecific symptoms. A person with seasonal allergies may have crossover allergies. Disease-specific elimination diets, such as those listed in Table 86.5, are available in the reference materials listed at the end of this chapter. Because moderate-intensity elimination diets are more likely to lead to symptom resolution compared with food-specific elimination diets, they are popular with many integrative clinicians.

Level 3: A "Few Foods" Diet. Finally, for a limited number of patients, a high-intensity or "few-foods" diet may be considered. In this diet, only foods on a specific list may be eaten. Higher levels of supervision are necessary with this type of diet to ensure that nutritional needs are met.[1] The patient handout contains an example of this diet as well.

The patient handout also provides a table of common "foods in disguise." When a specific group of foods is eliminated, some common ingredients that may cause adverse food reactions must also be eliminated. For example, if a patient is to successfully perform a dairy elimination diet, he or she must also avoid anything containing whey, caramel, casein, or semisweet chocolate.

Duration. Patients should follow an elimination diet for at least 2 weeks; most sources suggest 2–4 weeks.[1,16] It is hypothesized that symptoms caused by food intolerance may not arise until a few days after the food has been eaten, so it is important to give food-related symptoms time to "wear off" before foods are reintroduced. A longer duration of 6–12 weeks may be beneficial in some patients. In such cases, it may be necessary to add supplements, such as folate, if gluten is being eliminated and be aware of increasing anxiety surrounding the reintroduction of foods.

> Patients should be warned that with the elimination diet, it is not uncommon for symptoms to worsen before they begin to improve.

Step 3: The Challenge Phase

If symptoms decrease during the avoidance phase, it is likely that the food or foods that were eliminated were, in fact, contributing to the symptoms. However, symptoms of many chronic conditions relapse and remit spontaneously, so it is important to reintroduce eliminated foods or food groups after symptoms have resolved to determine whether they recur. Because symptoms may take a few days to reappear, foods should be introduced back into the diet only every 3 or 4 days. It is best for a patient to consume a small quantity of the reintroduced food on the first day and then to have a larger serving on subsequent days (assuming no untoward effects are experienced with the first serving). In addition to previously experienced chronic symptoms, food-intolerant patients who reintroduce foods may experience lung congestion, increased mucus production, fatigue, concentration difficulties, digestive problems, constipation and diarrhea, bloating, fluid accumulation, mood swings, and drowsiness.[27] The patient handout contains a sample schedule for the elimination and reintroduction of foods in a moderate-intensity elimination diet.

Improvements in symptoms are readily apparent to the patient when they occur during an elimination diet. In fact, many patients are reluctant to attempt the challenge phase because their symptoms have improved so markedly.

Step 4: Creating a Long-Term Diet Plan

Once the initial three phases of the elimination diet are completed, long-term diet planning is necessary. Additional elimination diets may be needed at some point if symptoms are either unchanged or not fully resolved. Many recommendations exist regarding how long a food causing adverse reactions should be avoided. A reasonable approach is to continue the elimination for at least 3–6 months. After that, another challenge with the eliminated food or foods may be attempted. There is some evidence that when a food is reintroduced after a lengthy period, the intolerance may no longer be found. In a study of 10 patients who had chronic urticaria or perennial rhinitis, 38% found their different food intolerances to be resolved at retesting a year or more after the initial evaluation.[28] This finding may be attributable to improvements in the intestinal barrier, including microflora, mucus, and epithelial lining.

Risks of Elimination Diets

Although elimination diets are generally safe, particularly under the supervision of a health care professional, the following potential risks must be acknowledged:

- Elimination diets may activate "latent" eating disorders. The clinician should screen patients for anorexia and bulimia nervosa before initiating an elimination diet. Patients with IBS may be especially vulnerable.[29]
- A food or food group that has led to an anaphylactic reaction should *never* be reintroduced without appropriate supervision by an allergist. In one small study, seven children with fish allergy eliminated fish from their diets. When fish was reintroduced, their hypersensitivity was more florid.[30]
- Malnutrition is a risk if a large number of food groups are eliminated. The clinician must ensure that dieters receive adequate fiber, nutrients (including vitamin D

and calcium when dairy is restricted), and protein. Patients on gluten-elimination diets often become deficient in zinc, selenium, copper, B_6, and B_{12} over time; gluten-free grains lack vitamins B_1, B_2, and B_3 as well as folate and iron. Special caution should be used in the treatment of autistic children, given that they tend to be limited in their diets at baseline.[31]

- The clinician must keep in mind the socioeconomic implications of prescribing an elimination diet because the cost can become prohibitive; for example, various alternatives to gluten-containing grains can be costly or difficult to obtain, and patients following elimination diets have limited ability to eat at restaurants or at other people's homes unless their dietary restrictions are clearly understood by those preparing their meals.[32]
- Enjoyment of eating, an important aspect of general health, may be diminished.
- A fear of food may be created. Some patients have significant symptom improvement with removal of a food. This success can lead to inappropriate association of symptoms with other foods that can snowball toward malnutrition. The goal should be temporary removal of a food, repair of the gastrointestinal ecosystem, and slow reintroduction of the food in the future, if possible, for non-IgE food intolerances.
- The likelihood of patient noncompliance with the diet must always be kept in mind; this can often be quite high, especially for diets prescribed for children.

> The clinician must be mindful of the potential pitfalls of prescribing elimination diets. Patient compliance, nutritional status, and the psychosocial impacts of such a diet must be given consideration. When judiciously used, elimination diets are associated with minimal risk.

SUMMARY OF A PRAGMATIC APPROACH FOR RECOMMENDING AN ELIMINATION DIET

A number of chronic diseases are associated with inflammation and intestinal permeability, indicating that methods of reducing inflammation and intestinal permeability will be beneficial. A multimodal approach that emphasizes mind-body techniques for stress management, physical activity, emotional health, and adequate sleep and nutrition is necessary to reduce sympathetic overdrive and an associated increased inflammatory state. A focused 4R approach to reduce intestinal permeability is an example of a multimodal treatment plan. The goal of the nutrition component is to eliminate or reduce potentially inflammatory foods while encouraging antiinflammatory ones. While specific foods may worsen particular diseases, as noted in the following text, a general approach may be used for any disease with an inflammatory component. An ideal elimination diet eliminates as few healthful foods as possible to achieve improvement in symptoms and overall wellbeing. For many people, simply switching to a more healthy diet will provide adequate symptom relief.[26]

Diseases with an inflammatory component include autoimmune thyroiditis, vitiligo, inflammatory arthritis, lupus, asthma, allergies (food, seasonal, environmental), chronic pain, migraines, diabetes, obesity, coronary artery disease, eczema, fibromyalgia, depression, chronic obstructive pulmonary disease, and cancer.

Step 1

Healthy diet (trial of at least 2 weeks)

Eliminate: high-fructose corn syrup, sugar sweetened beverages, artificial sweeteners (especially aspartame), artificial food dyes, and trans fats

Reduce: alcohol, caffeine, processed foods (with emulsifiers, additives), sugar, saturated fat, and red meat

Encourage: at least five servings of fruits and vegetables daily with a variety of colors, plant-based protein, fatty fish consumption, nuts, legumes, whole grains.

If no improvement, move on to Step 2.

Step 2

A. Diagnosis based elimination (see the following text)
   i. Refer to the following list and eliminate two to three foods eaten most frequently. After 2–4 weeks, reintroduce one food item. On day one, begin with a small amount. On day two, eat a small amount twice during the day. On day three, eat a larger amount. If there is no worsening of symptoms, reintroduce another food item the next day in the same manner and repeat until all eliminated foods have been reintroduced. If symptoms worsen, remove the offending food. Notably, some foods may be tolerated in small amounts but not large amounts, so keeping a close food and symptom diary will be helpful. Repeat until all the listed foods have been eliminated and reintroduced
   ii. If a patient prefers to eliminate ALL listed foods, eliminate for 2–4 weeks and reintroduce in stepwise fashion, every 3 days, as previously mentioned.
   iii. For most patients, begin with the least restrictive diet to maximize adherence.
   OR
A. Elimination of gluten and dairy (trial of 2 weeks) followed by stepwise reintroduction
   i. Consider for people without clear diagnoses; vague symptoms; or limited time, ability, or willingness to adhere to a more complicated elimination diet.

Step 3

If there is no improvement with a disease-specific elimination diet, consider either a more restricted elimination diet (if patient willing and able) or focus on other modalities. If there is no improvement with gluten and dairy restriction, consider a disease-specific elimination diet. Only a few people will be able to adhere to and benefit from a few-foods diet, but it is worth considering.

Summary

Step 1: Encourage a healthy diet (2 weeks)
Step 2: Eliminate foods based on evidence by disease OR eliminate gluten and dairy (2–4 weeks)
Step 3: Reintroduce eliminated foods in a stepwise, graduated manner every 3 days.

Encourage patients to keep a food and symptom diary.

Potential Pitfalls

Poor adherence, initial worsening of symptoms, uncovering of underlying eating disorder, enhancing feeling of failure if unable to adhere to diet, and inadequate calcium intake or B-vitamin intake.

 More information on this topic can be found online at ExpertConsult.com.

Key Web Resources	
Patient education information on food allergies	http://www.aaaai.org/home.aspx
Patient education information about diagnostic testing	http://www.foodallergy.org/diagnosis-and-testing/food-elimination-diet
Patient information about food additives	http://asthmaandallergies.org/food-allergies/adverse-reactions-to-food-additives/
IBS elimination diet	http://www.aboutibs.org/site/treatment/diet/12-week-elimination-diet
United Kingdom Nurses Study evaluating a model of evaluating food intolerances in primary care	http://epubs.surrey.ac.uk/27631/2/The%20development%20and%20evaluation%20of%20a%20nurse%20led%20food%20intolerance%20clinic%20in%20primary%20care.pdf
University of Wisconsin Integrative Medicine Patient Handout	http://www.fammed.wisc.edu/sites/default/files/webfm-uploads/documents/outreach/im/handout_elimination_diet_patient.pdf

Patient Handout: Using an Elimination Diet

An elimination diet can be used to determine whether or not certain foods are contributing to your symptoms. If they are, the diet can also be used as a form of treatment.
There are four main steps to an elimination diet:

Step I: Planning
This step involves working with your provider to make a list of foods that might be causing problems. You may be asked to keep a diet journal for a week, listing the foods you eat and when you have symptoms. To decide what foods might be causing problems, ask yourself these questions:
  • What foods do I eat most often?
  • What foods do I crave?
  • What foods do I eat to "feel better" (comfort foods)?
  • What foods would be hard for me to stop eating?
The answers are foods you should try to eliminate. Other common problematic foods are listed below.

Step II: Avoiding the Foods on Your List
After you have made a list of foods to avoid, you start the elimination diet. You should stop eating the foods on your list for two weeks. If you make a mistake and eat something on the list, you should start over. The foods on the list should be avoided in their whole form and also when they are ingredients in other foods. For example, if you are avoiding all dairy products, you need to check labels for whey, casein, and lactose so you can avoid them as well. Elimination diets take a lot of willpower. You must pay close attention to food labels, and be careful if you are eating out, since you may not know all the ingredients of the foods you eat.

Many people notice that in the first week, especially in the first few days, their symptoms get worse before they get better. If your symptoms become severe or increase for more than a day or two, consult your healthcare provider.

Step III: Add the Foods Back
If your symptoms have not improved in two weeks, you will need to stop the diet and decide whether or not to try it again with a different list of foods. If you feel better after eliminating the foods, the next step is to see if your symptoms come back when you start eating the foods again. As you do this, keep a written record of your symptoms.

A new food or food group should be added every three days. It takes three days to see if your symptoms come back if they are going to. On the day you introduce an eliminated food back into your diet for the first time, start with just a small amount in the morning. If you don't notice any symptoms, eat a larger portion at lunch and dinner. After a day of eating the new food, wait for two days to see if you notice the symptoms. Then add back another eliminated food or food group. Follow the pattern until all foods are added back. If a food doesn't cause symptoms during a challenge, it is unlikely to be a problem food and can be added back into your diet for good. However, don't add the food back until you have tested ALL the other foods on your list.

Step IV: Create Your New, Long-Term Diet
Based on your results, you can plan how to change what you eat so that you'll be most likely to prevent your symptoms. Remember:
  • Some people have problems with more than one food.
  • Sometimes symptoms come and go for other reasons besides what foods we eat, so it can be confusing to tell for certain if a specific food is the cause.
  • Be sure that you are getting adequate nutrition during the elimination diet and as you change your diet for the long-term. For example, if you give up dairy, you must get calcium from other sources.
  • You may need to try several different elimination diets before you identify problematic foods.
  • If a food causes you to have an immediate allergic reaction, or causes you to have throat swelling, a severe rash, or other severe allergy symptoms, it is important to seek the care of an allergist before re-introducing foods that cause problems.

The elimination diet is not a perfect test. A lot of other factors could interfere with the results. Try and keep everything else (the other foods you eat, your stress level, etc.) as constant as possible while you are on the diet.

The Three Levels of Elimination Diets

Level 1: The Simple Diet
Eliminates milk, eggs, and wheat

	FOODS ALLOWED	FOODS ELIMINATED
Animal proteins	Beef, chicken, lamb, pork, turkey	Dairy products Chicken eggs
Grains and starches	Arrowroot, barley, buckwheat, corn, millet, oats, rice, rye, sweet potato, tapioca, white potatoes, yams	Wheat
Oils	Any non-dairy oils	Dairy-based butter and margarines
All fruits, vegetables, salt, spices, sweeteners, and vegetable proteins are allowed		

Level 2: The Stricter Diet
The stricter diet eliminates several foods at once.

	FOODS ALLOWED	FOODS ELIMINATED
Animal proteins	Lamb	All others, including eggs and milk
Vegetable proteins	None	Beans, bean sprouts, lentils, peanuts, peas, soy, all other nuts
Grains and starches	Arrowroot, buckwheat, corn, rice, sweet potato, tapioca, white potato, yams	Barley, millet, oats, rye, wheat
Vegetables	Most allowed	Peas, tomatoes
Fruits	Most allowed	No citrus or strawberries
Sweeteners	Cane or beet sugar, maple syrup, corn syrup	Any others, including aspartame
Oils	Coconut, olive, safflower, sesame	Animal fats (lard), butter, corn, margarine, shortening, soy, peanut, other vegetable oils
Other	Salt, pepper, a minimal number of spices, vanilla, lemon extract	Chocolate, coffee, tea, colas and other soft drinks, alcohol

Level 3: A Few-Foods Diet
Only the foods listed below can be eaten. **All others** are avoided.
• Apples (juice okay)
• Apricots
• Asparagus
• Beets
• Cane or beet sugar
• Carrots
• Chicken
• Cranberries
• Honey
• Lamb
• Lettuce
• Olive oil
• Peaches
• Pears
• Pineapple
• Rice (including rice cakes and cereal)
• Safflower oil
• Salt
• Sweet potatoes
• White vinegar

Modified from Mahan LK, Escot-Stump S: *Krause's food nutrition and diet therapy.* 11th ed. Philadelphia: Saunders; 2004.

A Sample Elimination Diet Calendar

Day Number	Step
1	Begin Elimination Diet
2–7	You may notice symptoms worsen for a day or two
8–14	Symptoms should go away if the right foods have been removed
15	Re-introduce food #1 (for example, dairy)
16–17	Stop food #1 and watch for symptoms*
18	Re-introduce food #2 (for example, wheat)
19–20	Stop food #2 again and watch for symptoms
21	Re-introduce food #3
	...And so on, until all eliminated foods have been re-introduced

*You only re-introduce a new food for one day. Until the diet is over, it is not added back into the diet again.

Some Helpful Tips:
A number of foods can be 'disguised' when you look at food labels.

If You Are Avoiding	Also Avoid
Dairy	Caramel candy, carob candies, casein and caseinates, custard, curds, lactalbumin, goat's milk, milk chocolate, nougat, protein hydrolysate, semisweet chocolate, yogurt, pudding, whey. Also beware of brown sugar flavoring, butter flavoring, caramel flavoring, coconut cream flavoring, "natural flavoring," and Simplesse.
Peanuts	Egg rolls, "high-protein food," hydrolyzed plant protein, hydrolyzed vegetable protein, marzipan, nougat, candy, cheesecake crusts, chili, chocolates, pet feed, sauces.
Egg	Albumin, apovitellin, avidin, béarnaise sauce, eggnog, egg whites, flavoprotein, globulin, hollandaise sauce, imitation egg products, livetin, lysozyme, mayonnaise, meringue, ovalbumin, ovoglycoprotein, ovomucin, ovomucoid, ovomuxoid, Simplesse.
Soy	Chee-fan, ketjap, metiauza, miso, natto, soy flour, soy protein concentrates, soy protein shakes, soy sauce, soybean hydrolysates, soby sprouts, sufu, tao-cho, tao-si, taotjo, tempeh, textured soy protein, textured vegetable protein, tofu, whey-soy drink. Also beware of hydrolyzed plant protein, hydrolyzed soy protein, hydrolyzed vegetable protein, natural flavoring, vegetable broth, vegetable gum, vegetable starch.
Wheat	Atta, bal ahar, bread flour, bulgar, cake flour, cereal extract, couscous, cracked wheat, durum flour, farina, gluten, graham flour, high-gluten flour, high-protein flour, kamut flour, laubina, leche alim, malted cereals, minchin, multi-grain products, puffed wheat, red wheat flakes, rolled wheat, semolina, shredded wheat, soft wheat flour, spelt, superamine, triticale, vital gluten, vitalia macaroni, wheat protein powder, wheat starch, wheat tempeh, white flour, whole-wheat berries. Also beware of gelatinized starch, hydrolyzed vegetable protein, modified food starch, starch, vegetable gum, vegetable starch.

Data from Joneja JV. *Dietary management of food allergy and intolerance.* 2nd ed. Vancouver, BC: Hall Publishing Group, 1998; and Mahan LK, Escot-Stump S: *Krause's food nutrition and diet therapy.* 11th ed. Philadelphia: Saunders; 2004.

A One-Week Food Diary Chart
(Log in foods eaten and times. Note the symptoms you have and what times as well)

	Morning Foods	Morning Symptoms	Afternoon Foods	Afternoon Symptoms	Evening Foods	Evening Symptoms
Day 1						
Day 2						
Day 3						
Day 4						
Day 5						
Day 6						
Day 7						

REFERENCES

References are available online at ExpertConsult.com.

CHAPTER 87

GLYCEMIC INDEX AND GLYCEMIC LOAD

Yue Man Onna Lo, MD, ABIHM

In the past, carbohydrates have been classified as either simple or complex based on the number of simple sugars per molecule. Simple carbohydrates can be categorized as a single sugar (monosaccharides), which include glucose, fructose, and galactose, or double sugars (disaccharides), which include sucrose, lactose, and maltose. Complex carbohydrates, also known as polysaccharides, are starches formed by longer saccharide chains, which means they take longer to break down. It has been assumed that starchy foods cause smaller increases in blood glucose than simple sugars. However, this system is too simplistic and is not predictable because the changes in blood glucose and insulin levels after consuming complex carbohydrates can be very different.[1] For example, complex carbohydrates refer to any starches, including the highly refined starches found in white bread, pastries, and cakes, which induce a very different blood glucose and insulin response than whole grains and starchy vegetables, such as sweet potatoes. As a result, a concept known as the *glycemic index* (GI) was introduced in the early 1980s. It has become a very useful nutritional concept that allows new insight into the relationship between carbohydrate-rich foods and health.[2]

GLYCEMIC INDEX

The GI measures the rises in blood glucose and insulin triggered by a specific food compared with a control food, such as white bread or glucose (Fig. 87.1).

To determine the GI of a specific food, test subjects are given a test food and a control food (white bread or glucose) on separate dates, each food containing 50 g of

available carbohydrates, and changes in blood glucose and insulin are measured every 2 hours. The GI is calculated as the area under the curve of the test food divided by the area under the curve of the control food, then multiplied by 100 to represent a percentage of the control food.[3] For example, a baked potato has a GI of 94 relative to glucose, which means that the blood glucose response to the carbohydrate in a baked potato is 94% of the blood glucose response to the same amount of carbohydrate in pure glucose. In contrast, sweet potato, which is also a complex carbohydrate, has a GI of 44 relative to glucose and induces a much lower blood glucose response in comparison with pure glucose.[2] Therefore, you can say that not all carbohydrates or calories are created equal (Fig. 87.2).

> High-GI foods can stimulate the reward and food craving areas of the brain seen with other addictions. The rebound hypoglycemia (Fig. 87.3) can exacerbate cravings for high-GI foods, which leads to a vicious cycle that can increase insulin, inflammation, and triglyceride levels.[4]

GLYCEMIC LOAD

The concept of glycemic load (GL) was introduced later as an additional tool to more accurately assess the impact of eating carbohydrates on blood sugar. It gives a more complete picture than GI alone because GI only indicates how rapidly a particular carbohydrate turns into sugar, while GL indicates the amount of carbohydrate in a serving.[2] Serving sizes can be different based on cultural and

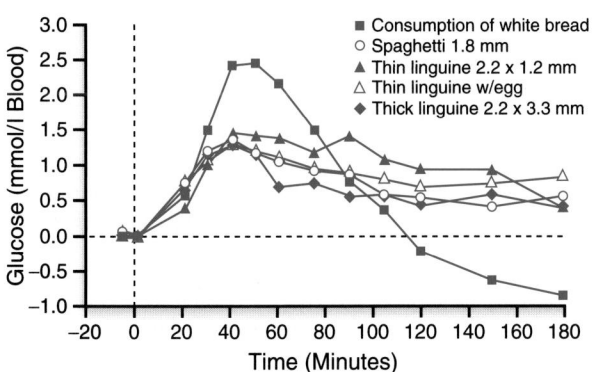

FIG. 87.1 ■ Mean incremental blood glucose responses to different foods in healthy subjects.

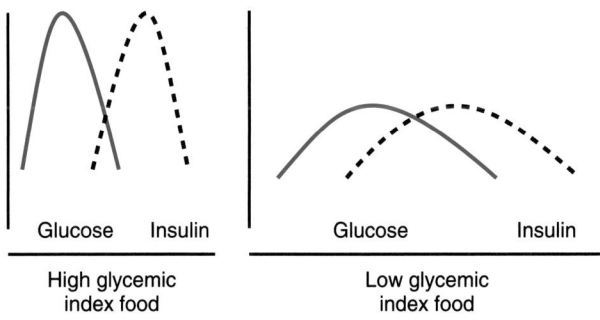

FIG. 87.2 ■ The effect of high glycemic index food versus low glycemic food on glucose and insulin. (From Rakel, D: *Glycemic index and glycemic load*: http://www.fammed.wisc.edu/files/webfm-uploads/documents/outreach/im/handout_glycemic_index_patient.pdf. Accessed 12/25/2016.)

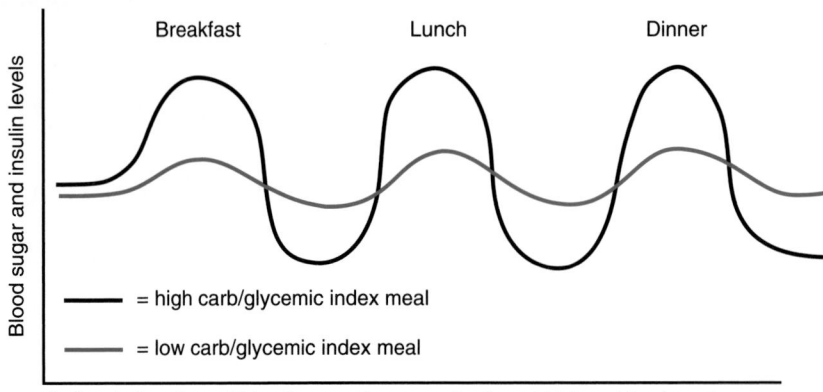

Spikes in insulin and blood sugar trigger production of triglycerides from the liver to help store excess sugar.
Troughs of hypoglycemia is also associated with negative health outcomes.

FIG. 87.3 ■ Blood sugar and insulin levels.

TABLE 87.1 **Calculating Glycemic Load**
Example: Watermelon
Glycemic index (GI) = 72 (high) Glycemic load (GL) = 4 (low) Amount of carbohydrates per serving: 6 g (low)
Calculating Glycemic Load (GL) GL = (GI) × (carbohydrates per serving in grams)/100 GL for watermelon = 72 × 6/100 = 4

TABLE 87.2 How to Interpret Glycemic Index (GI) and Glycemic Load (GL)

Foods that have a low GL almost always have a low GI. Foods with an intermediate or high GL range from a very low to very high GI.[5]

Glycemic Index	Glycemic Load
The smaller the number, the less impact the food has on your blood sugar	The smaller the number, the less impact the food has on your blood sugar per serving size
55 or less = low 56–69 = moderate 70 or higher = high	10 or less = low 11–19 = moderate 20 or more = high

dietary practices. GL helps patients to account for both the quantity and the quality of their carbohydrates at the same time. For example, the GI of watermelon is high; however, most of watermelon is water, and the amount of carbohydrates per serving size is low, which results in a low GL. Therefore, consuming one to two servings of watermelon will not raise blood glucose or insulin significantly when compared with other foods that have a high GI and GL. Table 87.1 shows the calculations for GL.[5]

The GL is calculated by using the amount of available carbohydrates in grams per serving size for a certain food multiplied by the GI value of that food, then divided by 100.[1] The higher the GL, the greater the expected elevation in blood glucose and insulin effect of the food.[2] Table 87.2 shows the interpretation of GI and GL values.

What Can Affect the Glycemic Index in Food?

1. **Ripeness and storage time**—The GI of many fruits such as bananas goes up as they ripen.
2. **Cooking time**—The longer the cooking time for certain grains and starches, like pasta, the higher the GI. Pasta cooked "al dente," where it is slightly undercooked and is more firm, has a lower GI.
3. **Processing method**—The finer a food is chopped, mashed, or juiced, the higher the GI, e.g., whole potatoes versus chopped potatoes.[6]
4. **Combination with other foods or dressings**—Adding fat, fiber, and acid (such as lemon juice or vinegar) lowers the GI since they help slow down the absorption of sugar into the bloodstream. For example, baked potatoes with butter and sourdough bread have lower

GI than just baked potatoes and nonsourdough breads, respectively. Combining high-GI foods with low-GI foods will also decrease blood sugar rise.
5. **Food variety**—Certain varieties of vegetables, grains, and fruits have different GIs than their counterparts, e.g., short grain rice versus long grain rice and russet potatoes versus red potatoes.[7]
6. **An individual's metabolism and digestion**—GI is relative to a person's age, metabolism, and digestive health.[7]

Practical Guidelines
1. Increase consumption of fruits, vegetables, and legumes.
2. Eat multicolored, unprocessed, whole foods.
3. Decrease consumption of "white foods" (e.g., potatoes, fluffy breads, pasta).
4. Consume grain products that are less processed or not overcooked (e.g., steel-cut oats, al dente pasta, stone-ground breads).
5. Always combine your meal with fiber (vegetables and fruits), fats (oils), and proteins (beans and nuts).
6. Eat low-GI foods regularly and high-GI foods rarely and only in small quantities, preferably with a meal.
7. Eat healthy portions. Excessive consumption of low-GI foods can still trigger a hyperglycemic response.[8,9]

DISEASE PREVENTION AND MANAGEMENT

Diabetes and Blood Sugar Control

Medical nutrition therapy is the first line of treatment for the prevention and management of type 2 diabetes and plays an essential part in the management of type 1 diabetes. Although the American Diabetes Association still recommends carbohydrate counting as a main strategy for diabetes management, the Diabetic Associations in Europe, Canada, and Australia have all recommended high-fiber, low-GI foods for individuals with diabetes as a means of improving postprandial glycemia and weight control.[2,10,11] Many studies have shown that low dietary GI and GL is effective in the prevention[12-16] and management of diabetes by improving insulin sensitivity and lowering glycated hemoglobin A1c (HbA1c) levels and fructosamine in diabetic patients.[14,17-19] In a recent cohort study in Hawaii, a high-GL diet showed an increased incidence of diabetes.[13] In a randomized, open-label, crossover study, a low-GI diet for 3 months produced greater weight loss, body fat reduction, and body mass index (BMI) reduction than a standard diabetes diet.[17] There were also fewer reported episodes of hypoglycemia and hyperglycemia in patients on a low-GI diet compared with those on a carbohydrate exchange diet.[19]

Weight Management and Cardiovascular Disease (CVD) Prevention

A low-GL/GI diet has been found to improve weight loss, decrease fat composition, and increase high-density lipoprotein (HDL) cholesterol in obese and overweight subjects.[20] It has also been shown to reduce C-reactive protein (CRP), an emerging CVD risk factor.[21] There are also a number of cohort studies that show a significant association between the consumption of high-GL/GI diets and increased CVD risk in women,[22,23] especially in those with higher fat composition, who are overweight or obese,[24] or have diabetes. However, this association has not been established in men.[21] Increases in dietary GL, but not GI, have also been associated with increased risk of stroke and diabetes in both men and women.[22,21]

Among overweight or obese subjects, dietary GL was associated with increased risk of coronary heart disease (CHD).[22] Among healthy, postmenopausal women, dietary GL has been found to be associated with HDL and triglyceride levels.[26]

Inflammation and Oxidative Stress

Oxidative stress and inflammation have been linked to insulin resistance and cardiometabolic disorders.[9] Postprandial glucose surges correlate directly with an increase in free radicals, resulting in oxidative stress.[27] A blood glucose spike after an excessively high-GL food consumption significantly reduces the mitochondria's capacity for oxidative phosphorylation, driving an increase in free radicals.[8] High-GI foods or meals with a high GL also cause an increase in postprandial inflammatory mediators and markers such as CRP, cytokines, and endothelin-1.[8] On the contrary, minimally processed low-GI foods or meals with a low GL do not result in adverse inflammatory effects.[9] One study showed a strong association between a high dietary GL and elevated CRP levels in 244 middle-aged women where CRP levels almost doubled in the low versus high dietary GL groups.[28] Therefore it is not surprising that most antiinflammatory diets, such as the Mediterranean diet, advocate plant-based, nonprocessed food approaches that are low in GL.

Cancer

A number of prospective cohort studies have shown that diets high in GI and GL are both associated with an increased risk of breast cancer[29,30] and colorectal cancers.[31] The same association was also demonstrated in a case-control study in Italy for ovarian cancer.[32] A positive association has also been noted in studies with dietary GL, but not GI, on gastric cancers[33] and endometrial cancers.[34-36] In a large prospective cohort study in Italy of 47,749 subjects, results showed that a high-GI diet was associated with an increased rate of colorectal cancer, especially in those with a higher waist-to-hip ratio.[31] However, there are currently no strong associations found for pancreatic cancers.[37,38]

Other Conditions

High-carbohydrate diets with a high glycemic response may exacerbate the metabolic consequences of an insulin-resistance syndrome. Two studies have found a positive association between high GI and GL values and symptomatic gallstone disease in men and women.[39,40] This hyperinsulinemia effect also initiates an increase in insulin-like growth factor 1 activity, which is known to stimulate acne pathogenesis,[41] which was confirmed when 43 male acne patients in a randomized controlled trial showed improvement of acne on a 12-week low GI/GL diet when compared to a high GI/GL diet.[42]

CONCLUSION

The consumption of low-GI and low-GL foods is positively associated with the prevention of diabetes, CVD, cancer, gallbladder disease, and acne. More information on the GI/GL diet and its effects on hormones, metabolic responses, and cellular changes is emerging. It is certainly a simple, useful tool to offer our patients facing such health issues. Table 87.3 lists GI and GL values for common foods.

TABLE 87.3 Glycemic Index and Glycemic Load Values for Select Foods

Food Item	Glycemic Index (glucose = 100)	Serving Size (g)	Available Carbohydrates (g/serving)	Glycemic Load (per serving)
Bakery Products				
Angel food cake	67	50	29	19
Pound cake	54	53	28	15
Apple muffin (no sugar)	48 ± 10	60	19	9
Bran muffin	60	57	24	15
Oatmeal	69	50	35	24
Pancakes	67 ± 5	80	58	39
Waffles	76	35	13	10
Beverages				
Coca-Cola	63	250 mL	26	16
Smoothie drink, soy, banana	30 ± 3	250 mL	22	7
Apple juice, pure, cloudy, unsweetened	37 ± 3	250 mL	28	10
Cranberry juice cocktail	68 ± 3	250 mL	36	24
Orange juice	50 ± 4	250 mL	26	13
Tomato juice, canned, no sugar	38 ± 4	250 mL	9	4
Gatorade	78 ± 13	250 mL	15	12
Breads				
Bagel (white)	72	70	35	25
Baguette (white)	95 ± 15	30	15	15
Oat bran bread	44	30	18	8
Rye-kernel bread (whole-grain pumpernickel)	46	30	11	5
Wheat bread (80% intact kernels and 20% white-wheat flour)	52	30	20	10
Wonder enriched white bread	73 ± 2	30	14	10
Healthy Choice Hearty 7-Grain bread	55 ± 6	30	14	8
Breakfast Cereals and Related Products				
All-Bran	38	30	23	9
Cheerios	74	30	20	15
Cornflakes	92	30	26	24
Muesli	66 ± 9	30	24	17
Pop-Tarts, double chocolate	70 ± 2	50	36	25
Raisin Bran	61 ± 5	30	19	12
Special K	69 ± 5	30	21	14
Cereal Grains				
Sweet corn	60	150	33	20
Taco shells, cornmeal	68	20	12	8
White rice, boiled	64 ± 7	150	36	23
Parboiled white rice (high amylose)	35 ± 4	150	39	14
Brown rice, steamed	50	150	33	16
Cracked wheat, bulgur	48 ± 2	150	26	12
Semolina (roasted or steamed)	55 ± 1	150	11	6
Cookies				
Graham wafers	74	25	18	14
Vanilla wafers	77	25	18	14
Crackers				
Breton crackers (wheat)	67	25	14	10
Corn thins	87 ± 10	25	20	18
Rice cakes (low amylose)	91 ± 7	25	21	19
Rye crispbread	63	25	16	10
Stoned wheat thins	67	25	17	12

TABLE 87.3   **Glycemic Index and Glycemic Load Values for Select Foods—cont'd**

Food Item	Glycemic Index (glucose = 100)	Serving Size (g)	Available Carbohydrates (g/serving)	Glycemic Load (per serving)
Dairy Products and Alternatives				
Milk	27 ± 4	250	12	3
Milk, condensed, sweetened	61 ± 6	250	136	83
Ice cream	61 ± 7	50	13	8
Yogurt	36 ± 4	200	9	3
Soy milk	44 ± 5	250	17	8
Tofu-based frozen dessert with high-fructose corn syrup	115 ± 14	50	9	10
Fruit and Fruit Products				
Apple (raw)	40	120	13	6
Apple juice (unsweetened)	40	250 mL	29	12
Banana (ripe)	51	120	25	13
Cranberry juice cocktail	68 ± 3	250 mL	35	24
Fruit cocktail (canned)	55	120	16	9
Grapes (raw)	43	120	17	7
Orange (raw)	48	120	11	5
Orange juice (reconstituted from frozen)	57 ± 6	250 mL	26	15
Pineapple (raw)	39 ± 15	120	12	5
Strawberry (raw)	40 ± 7	120	3	1
Strawberry jam	51 ± 10	30	20	10
Watermelon (raw)	72 ± 13	120	6	4
Legumes				
Black-eyed beans	42 ± 9	150	30	13
Chickpeas (garbanzo beans)	28 ± 6	150	30	8
Kidney beans	28 ± 4	150	25	7
Lentils (green)	22	150	18	4
Lentils (red)	26 ± 4	150	18	5
Mung beans	31	150	17	5
Pigeon peas	22	150	20	4
Pinto beans	39	150	26	10
Soya beans	18 ± 3	150	6	1
Pasta and Noodles				
Fettuccine (egg)	40 ± 8	180	46	18
Linguine (thick, durum wheat)	46 ± 3	180	48	22
Mung bean noodles (Lungkow)	26	180	45	12
Macaroni	47 ± 2	180	48	23
Rice noodles (dried)	61 ± 6	180	39	23
Rice noodles (fresh)	40 ± 4	180	39	15
Rice pasta (brown rice)	92 ± 8	180	38	35
Spaghetti (white)	32	180	48	15
Spaghetti (durum wheat)	64 ± 15	180	43	27
Spaghetti (whole meal)	32	180	44	14
Nuts				
Cashew nuts (salted)	22 ± 5	50	13	3
Peanuts	14 ± 8	50	6	1
Sport Bars				
PowerBar (chocolate)	56 ± 3	65	42	24
Ironman PR Bar (chocolate)	39	65	26	10

Continued

TABLE 87.3 **Glycemic Index and Glycemic Load Values for Select Foods—cont'd**

Food Item	Glycemic Index (glucose = 100)	Serving Size (g)	Available Carbohydrates (g/serving)	Glycemic Load (per serving)
Vegetables				
Beetroot	64 ± 16	80	7	5
Carrots (raw)	16	80	8	1
Corn (sweet, boiled)	60	80	18	11
Green peas	48 ± 5	80	7	3
Parsnips	97 ± 19	80	12	12
Baked potato (in skin)	60	150	30	18
Yam (peeled, boiled)	37 ± 8	150	36	13

Modified from Foster-Powell K, Holt SHA, Brand-Miller JC. International table of glycemic index and glycemic load values: 2002. *Am J Clin Nutr.* 2002;76:5–56.

Key Web Resources

The official website for the glycemic index (GI) and **international GI database,** which is based at the Human Nutrition Unit, School of Molecular Bioscience, University of Sydney The University's GI Group. The Group publishes a monthly e-newsletter with the latest GI research from around the world	http://www.glycemicindex.com
A comprehensive food list with GIs	http://www.mendosa.com/gilists.htm
Patient handout on glycemic index/load from the University of Wisconsin Integrative Medicine	http://www.fammed.wisc.edu/sites/default/files//webfm-uploads/documents/outreach/im/handout_glycemic_index_patient.pdf
International Table of Glycemic Index and Glycemic Load Values from the American Journal of Clinical Nutrition	http://www.ajcn.org/content/76/1/5/T1.expansion

REFERENCES

References are available online at ExpertConsult.com.

CHAPTER 88

ANTIINFLAMMATORY DIET

Wendy Kohatsu, MD • Scott Karpowicz, MD

INTRODUCTION

The rate of chronic disease related to poor diet has risen to staggering proportions in the United States. A recent large meta-analysis indicates dietary factors are currently the leading risk factor for death and disability in the United States, responsible for more than 700,000 deaths and almost 15% of disability-adjusted life years in 2010.[1] These diseases—including cardiovascular disease, diabetes, asthma, metabolic syndrome, depression, arthritis, and others—are characterized by a state of chronic, low-grade inflammation.[2] Medications—nonsteroidal antiinflammatory drugs (NSAIDs), statins, and biological agents—certainly can be used to reduce inflammation;[3] however, we must also help patients tackle the root causes of chronic inflammation created and perpetuated by a lifetime of unhealthy lifestyle habits.

A large and growing body of evidence indicates that dietary modifications can have a significant impact on this chronic, low-grade inflammatory state.[4,5] Americans consume 5.5 pounds of food per day.[6] We can take a more proactive, preventative approach by investing our 5+ pounds of daily food in healthy choices that decrease inflammation and thus chronic disease. To promote health and mitigate inflammation, integrative physicians must promote lifestyle changes and learn to use food as medicine. This chapter provides the most recent data to help integrative physicians tailor an antiinflammatory diet that is effective, acceptable, and delicious to each patient.

Mechanisms and Measurement of Inflammation

Several mechanisms by which food influences inflammation have been studied:

- Modulation of eicosanoid activity. For example, compounds in culinary spices such as turmeric suppress cyclooxygenase-2 (COX-2) expression and in nutmeg, inhibit tumor necrosis factor (TNF)-alpha release in animal studies.[7]
- Pro- and antioxidant effects. Increased antioxidant food intake is correlated with lower C-reactive protein (CRP) levels[8] and with a lower incidence of joint inflammation.[9]
- Insulin and glucose levels. A high dietary glycemic load was associated with elevated CRP concentrations,[10] and elevation in inflammatory markers has been shown to precede type 2 diabetes[11] (see Chapter 87).
- Genetic and intracellular expression. A Mediterranean diet[12] and omega-3 fats have been shown to modulate gene expression related to inflammation.[13]

- Modulation of endothelial function. Mediterranean diets powerfully affect endothelial markers.[14]
- Gastrointestinal dysbiosis. Numerous recent studies support that disruption to the gut microbiome can trigger a host of diverse inflammatory diseases.[15-17] The gut microbiome may indeed be the frontier on which the battle of dietary inflammation is initially fought.

Measuring Inflammation

Current medical practice is better at diagnosing the multitude of illnesses caused by inflammation than catching it early in the disease process. Having validated ways to measure inflammation can enable us to intervene more proactively. CRP is a commonly used biomarker of inflammation, and CRP levels are elevated with both chronic disease and as an acute-phase reactant. High-sensitivity CRP (hs-CRP) is a more sensitive measure to assess basal levels of CRP at the lower range of 0.20–10.0 mg/L; an hs-CRP > 2.0 may signal higher cardiovascular risk.[18] Other markers, such as TNF-alpha, interleukin-6 (IL-6), IL-1 beta, adhesion molecules, and endothelial function tests are used more widely in research to measure inflammation and are starting to emerge for clinical use. Recent studies have examined our food and its relationship with these inflammatory markers directly. A new dietary inflammatory index (DII)[2] has been developed to assess the inflammatory potential of various diets, and a Mediterranean diet score is already in use.[19] We anticipate that these tools will be useful for counseling patients on therapeutic diets in the future.

The Mediterranean Diet Is an Archetype of an Antiinflammatory Diet

The antiinflammatory diet is not one specific diet—indeed, there are many different diets that possess antiinflammatory effects. That being said, the Mediterranean diet is perhaps the most well-researched example of an antiinflammatory diet and serves as an archetypal model to further explore features of an antiinflammatory diet. Multiple studies and a recent meta-analysis have demonstrated the antiinflammatory effects of the Mediterranean diet as measured by serum inflammatory markers and measures of endothelial function.[20-22] The importance of this diet is further underscored by the large and growing body of evidence from both epidemiological studies and randomized controlled trials that demonstrate a significant mortality benefit and reduction in chronic disease with adherence to the Mediterranean diet.[19,24-26]

The Mediterranean diet is rich in vegetables, fruits, and whole grains; emphasizes nuts and olive oil as sources

MEDITERRANEAN DIET PYRAMID
A contemporary approach to delicious, healthy eating

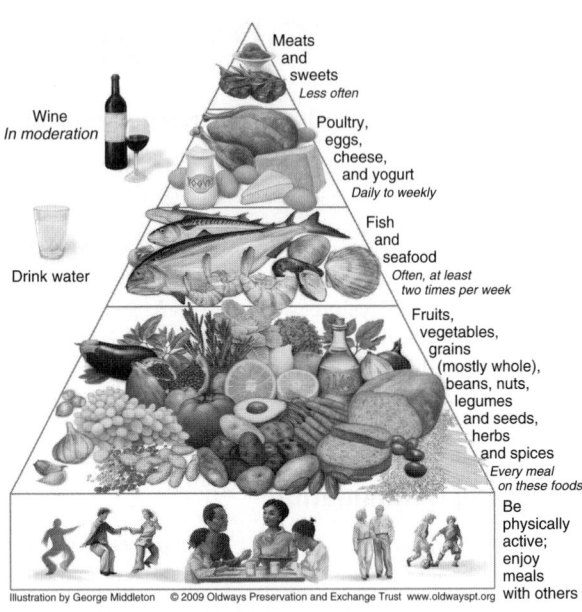

Illustration by George Middleton   © 2009 Oldways Preservation and Exchange Trust www.oldwayspt.org

FIG. 88.1 ■ The Mediterranean diet pyramid.

TABLE 88.1   Original Mediterranean Diet Score[19]

Give yourself 1 point for each "yes" answer and 0 for each "no"

Dietary Component	YES	NO
Vegetables: 4 or more servings a day		
Legumes: 1 or more servings a week		
Fruit: 3 or more servings a day		
Nuts and seeds: 1 or more servings a week		
Whole grains: 1 or more servings a day		
Fish: 4 or more servings a week		
Fats: More unsaturated fats, such as olive oil, than saturated fats, such as butter		
Alcohol: 1/2 to 1 drink a day for women; 1 to 2 for men		
Red and processed meat: Fewer than 2 servings a day for women, fewer than 3 a day for men		
TOTAL:		

Totals of 6 or higher put you in the range of highest benefit. Scores less than 4 mean you are getting little or no protection.

of fat; and gives preference to legumes, lean poultry, and fish rather than red meat (Fig. 88.1 and Table 88.1). Sodas, sweets, and refined baked goods; processed meats; and butter or similar spreadable fats are discouraged. Wine in moderation is an important component of the diet for those who choose to drink alcohol. This diet thus stands in stark contrast to the standard American diet, with its heavy intake of refined carbohydrates, red meat, added sugars, and limited portions of green vegetables, fruits, and whole grains.

It is important to note that the Mediterranean diet is a pattern of eating, not a collection of specific recipes. Thus, while the traditional Mediterranean diet finds its origin in the Mediterranean region, the dietary pattern itself is broadly applicable across other regions, cultures, and food traditions. Multiple studies have demonstrated significant benefits of the Mediterranean diet when taken out of its traditional cultural context, including studies on Nordic,[27] Polish,[28] Indian,[29] and Okinawan[30] diets that follow the overall Mediterranean dietary pattern. Thus, patients whose individual food preferences may not match those of the Mediterranean region should have little difficulty adapting it successfully to their own taste preferences. It is also cost-effective.[31,32]

While it is useful to explore in more detail the individual components of the Mediterranean diet, it is also important to note that the overall benefit of the Mediterranean diet is likely a result of the diet as a whole rather than any specific component. For example, in one of the most important epidemiological studies on the Mediterranean diet, the authors demonstrate that while an increase in a single component of the Mediterranean diet did not result in a significant benefit, an increase in any two components resulted in a statistically significant 25% reduction in overall mortality.[19] Furthermore, data indicate that even relatively small changes can have important health impacts. The PREDIMED trial, a recent large

randomized controlled trial assessing the impact of the Mediterranean diet on cardiovascular disease, showed that patients who were more adherent to the Mediterranean diet by just two of the component items significantly reduced their rate of cardiovascular disease and its associated mortality.[23]

Components of an Antiinflammatory Diet

Fats

Famous for their taste and palatability, antiinflammatory diets, especially the traditional Mediterranean diet, are characterized by their typically higher percentage of calories from fat—usually in the 40%–50% range—which adds both high satiety and flavor. Choosing the *right* fats—both the quantity as well as the quality—is important for reaping the key benefits of an antiinflammatory diet (Table 88.2).

There is a lot of controversy on the amounts of fats in a healthy diet. On one end of the spectrum, the Japanese diet contains only about 7% of its calories from fat, while a Mediterranean diet about 45%. For all types of fats, it is critical to pay attention to the *quality*, not just quantity. Choosing fresh, natural, organic, unrefined oils and fats will ensure protection against rancidity, oxidation, nutrient degradation, and contamination.

The two essential fatty acids—omega-6 and omega-3—need to obtained from the diet as they cannot be synthesized by the body. In general, omega-6 fats lead to more inflammation, and omega-3 metabolism leads to the formation of less-inflammatory or antiinflammatory prostaglandins and leukotrienes. Thus, it is critical to keep a healthy balance between the two.

TABLE 88.2 The Skinny on Fats

Type	Subtype	Metabolite	Food Sources	Notes
Saturated	Long chain TG		Animal fats—meat, butter, cheese	Amount in the diet is controversial, 7%–10% of calories.
	MCT SCT		Tropical oils—coconut, palm	Shorter-chain saturated fats may burn in the body more like carbohydrates.
Monounsaturated			Olive oil Nuts Avocados Peanuts	Higher EVOO intake associated with a reduction in the CVD mortality by half.[55] Reduces LDL and increases HDL.
Polyunsaturated	Omega-6 Essential fatty acid	AA GLA	Corn oil Most vegetable oils Soy[a]	Omega-6 fatty acids are essential fatty acids easily obtainable in the diet; however, usually in gross excess of omega-3s.
	Omega-3 Essential fatty acid	ALA	Flax, hemp, chia, walnuts	ALA conversion to biologically active EPA and DHA is only about 10%–15%.
		EPA DHA	Cold water fish (e.g., salmon), algae	Potent antiinflammatory effects. Eat 2+ fatty fish servings/week.[162]

[a]Soy contains both omega-6 (54%) and omega-3 (7%) fatty acids.

AA, arachidonic acid; *ALA*, alpha linolenic acid; *DHA*, docosahexaenoic acid; *EPA*, eicosapentaenoic acid; *GLA*, gamma linoleic acid, an antiinflammatory omega-6; *MCT*, medium-chain TG; *SCT*, short-chain TG; *TG*, triglyceride.

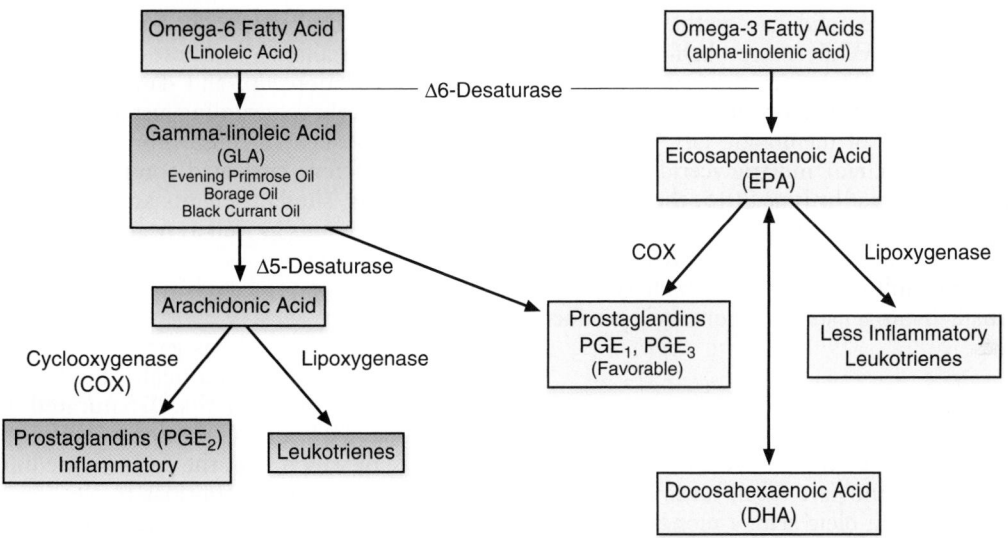

FIG. 88.2 ■ Influence of omega-6 and omega-3 fatty acids on inflammation.

A truly free-range egg has a favorably low omega-6:omega-3 ratio of only 1.3 compared to a conventionally raised egg with a ratio of 19.4.[35]

A few dietary fat dilemmas are as follows:

1. Omega-6 fats are vastly more abundant in the Western diet (usually 15–20×) compared with omega-3s. A ratio of 1:1–4:1 of omega-6 to omega-3 is recommended.[36,37] This means that Americans need to cut down on excessive intake of omega-6 fats and ramp up consumption of omega-3s (Fig. 88.2).
2. Omega-3 and -6 fats compete for the same metabolic enzymes, so high levels of omega-6 fats may suppress the already limited metabolism of omega-3 fats. At low levels of omega-3 intake, omega-6 fats are associated with the highest amount of inflammation.[38]

3. Renewable, plant-based forms of omega-3 fats largely contain alpha-linolenic acid (ALA) rather than eicosapentaenoic acid (EPA) and docosahexaenoic acid (DHA). The body needs to metabolize this ALA into EPA and DHA to exert its antiinflammatory effects, though it is able to do so in only relatively low amounts—only about 10%–15% of ALA is metabolized into EPA and then subsequently into DHA. Cold-water fatty fish, on the other hand, naturally contain higher amounts of preformed EPA and DHA, which exert antiinflammatory effects without the need for further metabolism. However, for environmental, heavy metal contamination, and cost issues, fish consumption is often limited.
4. Fish oil supplements do not seem to yield the same omega-3 benefits as eating fish itself.[39,40] Dose, quality, and human genetic variation may explain these differences.[41]

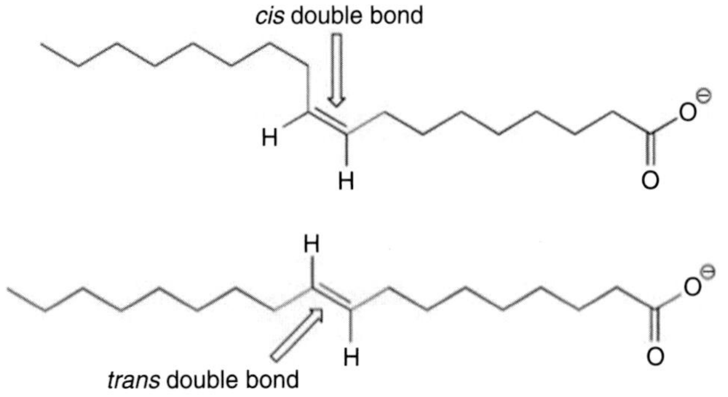

FIG. 88.3 ■ Hydrogenation of polyunsaturated fat.

Remember the acronym S.M.A.S.H. for your best sources of omega-3 EPA and DHA in cold-water fish such as Salmon (wild Pacific), Mackerel (Spanish), Anchovies, Sardines, and Herring.

The Evil of Trans-Fatty Acids. When a naturally liquid polyunsaturated fat is chemically converted via hydrogenation to a more solid fat, synthetic trans-fats are formed (Fig. 88.3). While more shelf-stable, these trans-fats (also known as hydrogenated fats, or partially hydrogenated fats) wreak havoc on the body, disrupting the native cis-alignment of membrane fats,[42] increasing serum levels of lipoprotein(a) and triglycerides,[43] as well as inflammatory mediators. In June 2015, the U.S. Food and Drug Administration (FDA) finally declared that partially hydrogenated oils are not "generally regarded as safe" (GRAS) in human food. Manufacturers have 3 years to remove partially hydrogenated oils from their products.

Olive Oil

Olive oil is a key component of the traditional Mediterranean diet and a growing body of evidence supports its inclusion as an important part of an antiinflammatory diet.[14] Olive oil is rich in oleic acid, a monounsaturated fatty acid. Additionally, virgin and extra virgin olive oils, unrefined versions made by pressing freshly picked olives, have high quantities of polyphenols, which have potent antioxidative properties.[45,46] The benefits of olive oil likely derive from a synergistic relationship between these key components.[47]

Growing evidence from intervention-based trials indicates that olive oil reduces key cardiovascular risk factors. Olive oil, particularly the high-polyphenol virgin or extra virgin varieties, improves lipid profiles and reduces dyslipidemia through an improvement in the quantity and function of high-density lipoprotein (HDL) cholesterol and reduction in low-density lipoprotein (LDL) cholesterol.[23,48,49] Additionally, olive oil has been shown to decrease blood pressure in patients with hypertension, improve endothelial function in patients with atherosclerotic disease, and reduce markers of inflammation.[51,52] Further evidence suggests that regular olive oil consumption, independent of total energy intake, decreases the risk of new-onset diabetes.[53]

Importantly, evidence from both epidemiological and intervention studies demonstrate a mortality benefit from olive oil consumption. The recent PREDIMED randomized controlled trial demonstrated a significant reduction in cardiovascular events and cardiovascular disease-related mortality in patients consuming a Mediterranean diet supplemented with extra virgin olive oil.[23] Further analysis of these data suggests a 10% reduction in cardiovascular disease for every 10 additional grams of extra virgin olive oil consumed per day.[55] These data correspond with multiple epidemiological studies that support a significant inverse correlation between olive oil, particularly the extra virgin variety, and coronary heart disease,[56,57] stroke,[58] and cardiovascular mortality.[59]

Nuts

Nuts are a rich source of monounsaturated and polyunsaturated fats, in addition to providing fiber, minerals, and other important nutrients.[60,61] Increased nut consumption has an important effect on reducing serum inflammatory markers, including CRP and IL-6.[62] More importantly, multiple recent prospective studies indicate that increased nut consumption decreases metabolic syndrome,[63] coronary artery disease,[64] and total mortality in addition to cancer-specific and cardiovascular disease-specific mortality.[65,66] These studies support a dose-response relationship, and data from the PREDIMED trial suggest that consuming just three servings of nuts per week can reduce all-cause mortality by 39%.[66] Despite slightly different fatty acid compositions and nutritional components, similar benefits are observed across a wide range of tree nuts as well as peanuts.[65]

Coconut Oil

Recently, coconut oil has garnered considerable attention in the lay press as a health food with a myriad of purported health benefits.[69] Saturated fat comprises more than 90% of the fat content of coconut oil, the majority of which is in the form of medium-chain fatty acids.[70] However, in contrast to the longer-chain saturated fatty acids more typically found in animal fats, medium-chain fatty acids are more easily metabolized.[71] Recent data from a human trial suggest that coconut oil, at least in daily doses of 30 mL, may not have the same dyslipidemic properties and proinflammatory properties as other saturated fats.[72] In addition, virgin coconut oil contains high concentrations of polyphenols and may therefore have antioxidant as well as antiinflammatory effects, as demonstrated in animal models.[73,74] Nonetheless, there is a dearth of quality evidence from human trials assessing the antiinflammatory or overall health benefits of coconut oil, and additional data are needed before it can be strongly recommended as a component of an antiinflammatory diet.

Carbohydrates

Whole grains contain naturally occurring fiber, lignans, magnesium, zinc, B vitamins, and vitamin E that may help fight inflammation. Actively replacing refined carbs with whole grains in the diet has been shown to reduce inflammatory markers.[75] Prospective studies have shown that higher dietary fiber and whole-grain intake is associated with decreased hs-CRP and IL-6.[76-78] Whole-grain consumption substantially lowers the risk of inflammation-mediated diseases,[79] such as cardiovascular disease, diabetes, cancer, and obesity. One study[80] of 522 diabetic patients showed that including 15 g of dietary fiber for every 1000 calories consumed daily with lifestyle changes (moderate exercise) significantly reduced CRP by 27%.

Perhaps the most important factor that best represents the inflammatory potential of a carbohydrate-containing food is its glycemic load (GL) (see Chapter 87). Excessive consumption of highly processed carbohydrates, e.g., white flour and refined sugars, with high GL, cause abnormal surges in blood glucose and insulin levels, which then overloads mitochondrial capacity thus creating free radicals.[81] Immediate increases in CRP and inflammatory cytokines can be seen with a single meal.[82] One study found a strong link between high dietary GL and elevated CRP concentrations in women; CRP levels were more than doubled (3.7 mg/L) in the group consuming the highest GL compared to the lowest GL (1.6 mg/L).[10] Similarly, higher dietary glycemic index (GI)/GL has been associated with higher levels of TNF-alpha and IL-6.[84] Even with the same amount of calories, choosing higher-quality carbohydrates with low GLs can lower the inflammatory profile.[85] Not surprisingly, diets rich in unprocessed, natural plant foods such as the Okinawan or Mediterranean diets have lower GLs, substantially lower postprandial glucose levels, and are associated with improved cardiovascular health and longevity.[86] Minimally processed low-GL foods—vegetables, fruit, nuts, seeds, and whole grains—do not result in adverse postprandial inflammatory effects, but high-GL foods do.[87]

Other mechanisms besides GL also likely help explain the benefit of whole grains in an antiinflammatory diet. A distinct benefit of whole-grain intake is supporting a more favorable gut microbiome composition that lowers both gut and systemic inflammation.[88-90]

Furthermore, another reason to consume whole grains is that the active phytochemicals are concentrated in bran (fiber) and the germ (carbohydrate); refining wheat with removal of the fiber causes a 200- to 300-fold loss in phytochemicals and increases the speed of sugar absorption (the GI)[91] (Fig. 88.4)!

> **Portion control** is also important! Overconsumption of even healthy, low-GL foods can trigger a hyperglycemic response and inflammation. Excess calories <u>regardless</u> of source also contribute to obesity, which itself produces inflammation.[92]

Vegetables and Fruit

Vegetables and fruit—while often classified under the macronutrient "carbohydrate"—deserve their own stand-alone category due to their natural abundance of nutraceutical benefits! Vegetables contain the highest concentrations of vitamins, minerals, and other protective phytochemicals, with a lower caloric density compared with other foods. Rich in biochemical complexity, whole vegetables and fruit are superior to any single

ANATOMY OF A GRAIN

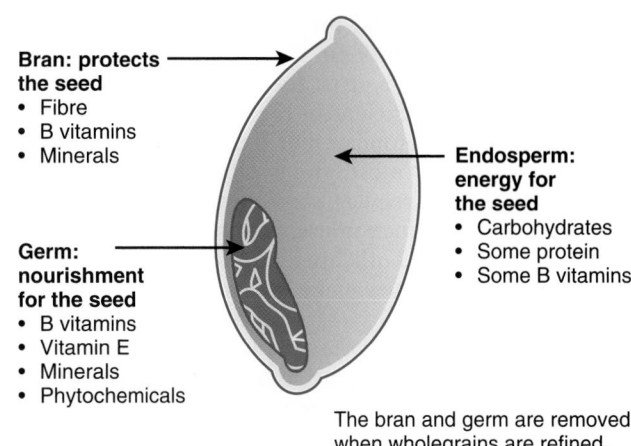

FIG. 88.4 ■ Fiber (bran) helps reduce the speed of sugar (germ) absorption.

isolated nutrient. Citrus fruit, for example, contains not just vitamin C, but some 60 flavonoids, 20 carotenoids, and limonoids. Higher intake of vitamin C from food sources has been associated with lower CRP and tissue plasminogen activator (tPA) levels.[93]

The inadequate consumption of vegetables and fruit in the United States is appalling. It is estimated that Americans only consume 1.6 servings of vegetables per day and only one fruit per day.[94] Fewer than 10% of Americans eat enough fruits and vegetables. Even more concerning is that the largest single contributor to fruit intake was orange juice and that potatoes still dominate vegetable consumption; fried potatoes account for about one-third of the "vegetables" that adolescents consume.[95]

Studies support that people who consume more vegetables and fruit have lower rates of inflammatory disease such as heart disease, insulin resistance, and some cancers.[96-99] High intake of vegetables and fruits, greater than five servings per day, has a significant inverse dose–response association with inflammatory markers such as CRP, IL-6, and adhesion factors.[97,100,101] The more vegetables and fruit one eats, the less inflammation. Estimates from the US Department of Agriculture (USDA) flavonoid databases also show an inverse association between high flavonoid intake (from fruit and vegetables) and lower CRP levels.[103] Flavonoids are responsible for the deep colors of fruits and vegetables and often are a proxy marker for high nutritional quality. In epidemiological studies, higher fruit and vegetable intake was shown to significantly decrease markers of inflammation in adolescents[104] and in adult women.[97] Adding fruits and vegetables to the diet, especially those rich in flavonoids, significantly improved microvascular reactivity and lowered CRP values.[106]

> Watch the sugar! The American Heart Association recommends that women consume no more than 100 calories/day as added sugar. This equals 25 g of sugar or about six teaspoons. For men, the limit is 150 calories, 36 g of sugar, or nine teaspoons per day. Read labels, this adds up quickly! To satisfy your sweet tooth, choose fresh fruit in season.[107]

Proteins

A large body of data supports the health benefits of plant-based proteins, and they are a healthy alternative to animal sources of protein.[108,109] Legumes are high in protein as well as fiber, iron, folic acid, and B vitamins. Most legumes are deficient in the essential amino acids methionine and tryptophan, but these are found in sufficient amounts in most grains. Randomized clinical trials indicate that regular consumption of legumes is associated with a reduction in inflammatory markers and an improvement in both lipid profiles and endothelial function.[110,111] Legumes make up a substantial part of a healthy antiinflammatory diet, can be prepared in many tasty ethnic dishes, and provide the majority of protein for a hungry world. Substituting healthy protein sources like legumes for red meat is associated with a lower mortality risk.[112]

In contrast, diets high in red and processed meats are correlated with increases in inflammatory markers, markers of glucose dysregulation, and dyslipidemia.[113-115] Furthermore, diets higher in red meat, especially in processed forms (e.g., cured meats and sausages, bacon, and processed lunch meats) are associated with higher rates of cardiovascular disease, certain cancers, and all-cause mortality.[116-118] Although it is not entirely clear what component of red meat contributes to its inflammatory effect, several clinical trials suggest that consuming lean meat may not result in the same proinflammatory effect that is observed with the higher fat, more processed red meats typically found in a modern American diet.[119-121] For those who do eat meat, studies support trimming visible fat[122] and avoiding charring the food to lessen the inflammatory impact.[123] In addition to lean meats, animal protein sources from fish[124] and dairy[125,126] are suitable components of an antiinflammatory diet.

Fish

While a source of high-quality protein and healthy fat, fish often swim in waters contaminated with heavy metals such as mercury, cadmium, lead, and other pollutants such as polychlorinated biphenyls (PCBs). These are proinflammatory and impair metabolic function. Even taking this into consideration, one review[127] reports that the health benefits of eating fish exceed the potential risks. Avoid fish highest in methylmercury—shark, swordfish, golden bass (tilefish), and king mackerel. A serving of albacore tuna contains 0.35 ppm methylmercury with 1.0 ppm being the EPA's "allowable" upper limit/day, so limit it to no more than one serving per week.[128] Some of the safest fish are tilapia, anchovies, and wild salmon.

Other Antiinflammatory Foods, Spices, and Supplements

- **Turmeric:** Turmeric is the queen of antiinflammatory spices! Multiple studies have assessed the potential benefits of curcumin, the main component of turmeric (*Curcuma longa*), on a variety of inflammatory conditions. Several recent randomized controlled trials have shown improvements in inflammatory markers and endothelial function with regular administration of curcumin.[129-131] Furthermore, trials have found curcumin equivalent in pain relief to ibuprofen and diclofenac for knee osteoarthritis[132] and rheumatoid arthritis,[133] respectively. Curcumin has shown promise in other inflammatory conditions, including maintenance of remission in ulcerative colitis[134] and improvement in signs and symptoms of oral lichen planus.[135] Especially considering its long track record of culinary use and excellent side effect profile in all the trials in which it has been studied, turmeric represents both a safe and effective addition to any antiinflammatory diet.

- **Wine:** While excessive alcohol consumption is clearly linked to excess morbidity and mortality, a large body of epidemiological data suggests that low-to-moderate alcohol consumption is associated with decreased levels of both cardiovascular and all-cause mortality.[136-139] Wine is of particular interest in the antiinflammatory diet as it is rich in polyphenols, which likely exert numerous antioxidative and antiinflammatory effects.[140,141] Randomized trials have demonstrated a reduction in inflammatory markers[142] and improvement in lipid profiles[143] with regular, moderate consumption of red wine.

- Other spices—ginger, chili pepper, oregano, basil, thyme, and rosemary—also possess antiinflammatory properties[144,145] and add flavor to a wide variety of cuisines.

- **Cocoa:** Cocoa and cocoa-rich products such as dark chocolate contain high quantities of flavonoids, as well as fiber and other important nutrients.[146] Multiple trials demonstrate a reduction in serum inflammatory markers,[147-149] improvement in lipid profiles,[150-152] and enhanced endothelial function[153-155] with consumption of flavonoid-rich cocoa. Furthermore, a recent trial demonstrated improvement in both walking distance and time in patients with peripheral artery disease after consumption of 40 g daily of dark chocolate.[156] Evidence from a meta-analysis of randomized controlled trials indicates a reduction in insulin resistance,[157] and epidemiological data suggests a reduction in diabetes incidence with cocoa consumption.[158] Mortality data are limited, though one epidemiological study indicated an inverse correlation between chocolate consumption and cardiovascular and all-cause mortality.[159] Doses used in trials vary widely from less than 10 g daily to 100 g daily—although the lowest effective dose is not known, 1–2 ounces of dark (at least 70%) chocolate as a tasty and healthy treat is a safe suggestion.

Medical Conditions That May Improve With an Antiinflammatory Diet

Table 88.3 provides a summary of some of the major diseases for which antiinflammatory diet modifications have shown therapeutic promise.

TABLE 88.3   Medical Conditions That May Improve With an Antiinflammatory Diet

Arthritis	Two randomized controlled trials found turmeric extracts to be as good or better than nonsteroidal antiinflammatory drugs (NSAIDs) at controlling symptoms of knee osteoarthritis[132] and rheumatoid arthritis.[133] Doses ranged from 500 mg to 1500 mg daily in these trials. Daily administration of a probiotic for 8 weeks was shown in a randomized controlled trial to reduce symptom severity and inflammatory status in patients with rheumatoid arthritis.[165]
Hypertension	Randomized controlled trials found significant reductions in blood pressure in patients who adopted the traditional Mediterranean diet[166] and the New Nordic Diet, a Mediterranean diet regional variant.[27] Apart from its inclusion in the Mediterranean diet, daily consumption of olive oil results in a clinically significant reduction in blood pressure[168]—olive oil rich in polyphenols, such as extra virgin olive oil, may be more effective at decreasing blood pressure than regular olive oil.[169] Olive oil dosing ranged from 30 mL–60 mL (2–4 tablespoons) daily in these trials.
Asthma	A recent small trial found improvement in spirometry and quality of life scores in patients with asthma who adopted a Mediterranean diet.[170]
COPD	In one randomized controlled trial, patients with COPD showed significant improvement in lung function [increased forced expiratory volume in 1 second (FEV_1)] with greater intake of antioxidant-rich fruits and vegetables.[171]
Diabetes	Data from the PREDIMED trial indicate reduced onset of diabetes with increased adherence to an energy-unrestricted Mediterranean diet.[53,173] In patients with existing diabetes, adherence to an energy-unrestricted Mediterranean diet resulted in a reduction in hemoglobin A1c equivalent to that from mono-drug therapy.[174] A low-carbohydrate Mediterranean diet has also been shown to reduce the need for antiglycemic medications in patients with newly diagnosed diabetes.[175]
Cardiovascular Disease	Large randomized controlled trials have demonstrated the Mediterranean diet as an effective means of both primary[23] and secondary[26,177] prevention of cardiovascular events, including myocardial infarction and stroke. Supplementation with olive oil[55] and nuts[66] likely provides even greater benefit. The effect size of dietary change should not be underestimated—secondary prevention trials indicated risk reductions of nearly two-thirds in those adhering to a Mediterranean-style diet.
Peripheral Artery Disease	The PREDIMED trial suggests that adherence to a Mediterranean diet significantly decreases the rate of new-onset symptomatic peripheral artery disease.[181] In a randomized controlled trial of patients with existing peripheral artery disease, daily administration of 40 g of dark chocolate resulted in a significant improvement in walking autonomy.[156]
Obesity	Adherence to a Mediterranean diet was associated with 51% lower odds of being obese and 59% lower odds of central obesity.[183] A high amount of olive oil consumption was not associated with higher weight gain or a significantly higher risk of becoming overweight or obese.[184] Despite a higher fat content (35% compared to 20%), participants eating a Mediterranean-based diet lost 4.1 kg compared with controls who gained 2.9 kg over 18 months.[185]
Inflammatory Bowel Disease	A randomized controlled trial found that turmeric (*Curcumin*) at daily doses of 2 g given in conjunction with standard therapy significantly reduced rates of relapse and improved endoscopic and symptom-based disease severity scores.[134] A recent case series demonstrated that patients who adhered to a modified antiinflammatory diet showed significant improvement in disease-related symptom scores.[187]
Nonalcoholic Fatty Liver Disease	In adults with nonalcoholic fatty liver disease, data from a randomized controlled trial indicate that patients whose diets are supplemented with olive oil or canola oil at doses up to 20 mg daily showed a reduction in liver span and severity of fatty liver at 6 months.[188] A recent meta-analysis found that daily supplementation with omega-3 fatty acids reduced hepatic steatosis.[189] Daily doses above 800 mg are effective, although the ideal dose is not yet known.
Cancer	A recent meta-analysis found that higher adherence to the Mediterranean diet was associated with a 10% reduction in overall cancer incidence and mortality.[190] This data indicate the effect may be most pronounced in colorectal and prostate cancer, with reductions in incidence of 14% and 4%, respectively, with increased adherence to the Mediterranean diet.
Alzheimer's Disease and Dementia	Adherence to a Mediterranean diet supplemented with olive oil or nuts has been shown to improve cognition and slow age-related cognitive decline.[191,192] In an observational study, higher adherence to a Mediterranean diet was associated with slower cognitive decline as measured by the Mini Mental State Evaluation.[193] A recent small pilot study found that daily supplementation with omega-3 fatty acids and alpha lipoic acid (ALA) reduced the progression of cognitive and functional decline in patients with Alzheimer's disease.[194] Doses used in this study were 1.6 g of omega-3 fatty acids and 600 mg of ALA daily.
Depression	A recent meta-analysis of 19 randomized controlled trials found omega-3 fatty acid supplementation effective in treating patients with both major depressive disorder (MDD) and depressive symptoms without a clear MDD diagnosis.[195] Dosing varied widely across trials but averaged 1.4 g of combined EPA and DHA daily. Additionally, another recent trial found that initiating omega-3 supplementation with a selective serotonin reuptake inhibitor (SSRI) resulted in better reduction in depressive symptoms than the SSRI alone.[196]
Psoriasis	In patients being treated for psoriasis, a randomized controlled trial demonstrated that a hypocaloric, omega-3 rich diet significantly reduced symptom severity at 3 and 6 months.[197]

CONCLUSION

Inflammation is a common pathophysiological mechanism underlying most chronic disease. The antiinflammatory diet is based on evidence-based principles of sound eating to promote health and prevent and reduce inflammation in the body. It is whole food-based nutrition that emphasizes healthy fats, vegetables and fruit, whole grains, legumes, fish, and limited amounts of meat and dairy. It can be recommended as "food as medicine" for a wide variety of common diseases including heart disease, diabetes, obesity, cancer, Alzheimer's disease, chronic obstructive pulmonary disease (COPD), depression, and gastrointestinal (GI) disorders.

Key Web Resources	
Oldways Preservation Trust. Has the original Mediterranean diet pyramid, and also features culturally inclusive Asian, Latino, and African heritage pyramids.	http://oldwayspt.org
Anti-Inflammatory Food Pyramid. Dr. Andrew Weil has published a patient-friendly and illustrative antiinflammatory food pyramid. This plan also features berries, Asian mushrooms, soy, tea, and dark chocolate	http://www.drweil.com and search for "food pyramid."[119]
For data on mercury levels in fish, check out the U.S. Environmental Protection Agency.	http://www.fda.gov/food/foodborneillnesscontaminants/metals/ucm115644.htm
A good website with healthy Mediterranean-style recipes	http://www.eatingwell.com/recipes_menus/collections/healthy_mediterranean_recipes
Check out the "Meatless Monday" campaign online. This international movement encourages all to skip meat once a week and explore healthy and tasty vegetarian options.	http://www.meatlessmonday.com

REFERENCES

References are available online at ExpertConsult.com.

Patient Handout: The Antiinflammatory Diet

Inflammation in the body is known to contribute to chronic disease such as diabetes, heart disease, asthma, inflammatory gut disorders, arthritis, obesity, cancer, and dementia. Eating an antiinflammatory diet may reduce inflammation and decrease chronic disease. Food as medicine is powerful! Here are some simple guidelines:

Antiinflammatory diet guidelines:
1) Choose healthy fats.
   • Substitute extra-virgin olive oil for other vegetable oils, trans-fats, or butter in your cooking for health benefits.
   • Eat two servings (4 ounces each) of fatty fish per week.
   • Reduce use of omega-6 fats (hydrogenated vegetable oils) to keep ratio of omega-6:omega-3 in range of 2:1 – 4:1.

2) Increase vegetable and fruit intake (especially vegetables)
   • Eat at least 5 servings of vegetables and fruit per day, with more than half as vegetables.
   • Color your diet! – deeply-colored fruits and vegetables contain higher amounts of protective phytochemicals.
   • Use the plate method – the biggest portion (half the plate) is where the vegetables go (excluding potatoes).

3) Choose whole grain carbohydrates and limit the portion sizes.
   • Choose carbs that are whole grain (requires chewing!), and aim for at least 25 grams of fiber per day.
   • Rx: double your vegetable intake, and half your intake of refined carbohydrates (anything with flour and/or added sugar)!

4) Get your protein from plant sources such as legumes, nuts and seeds, and/or choose lean, natural animal sources of protein in moderate amounts.

5) Spice it up! Include antiinflammatory herbs and spices such as garlic, turmeric, rosemary, ginger, oregano, cumin, and cayenne in your diet.

6) Eat mindfully
   • Be mindful of your food portions. Quality AND quantity matters. Regardless of how healthy your food choices are, excess calories from any source can increase inflammation and obesity.
   • Chew slowly and savor your food.

7) Adopt the Okinawan philosophy of "*hara hachi bu*" – stopping when nearly 8/10 full and paying attention to your hunger and satiety signals.[22] Remember to focus on the whole diet pattern, not just components. Choose food that is closest to its natural form (i.e., less processed).

8) Best dietary advice in 7 words: "Eat food. Not too much. Mostly plants." [116]

9) Adopt an antiinflammatory LIFESTYLE
   • Incorporate regular exercise that you enjoy into your life.
   • Keep weight under control. It is important to prevent and reduce obesity, especially abdominal obesity, as obesity itself sets up chronic inflammation in the body.[117] [118] Maintain body mass index (BMI) between 18.5 – 24.9.
   • Be aware of, and find healthy ways to reduce stress.

10) Enjoy 1–2 ounces of dark chocolate (at least 70%) as an occasional treat!

Eat more:	Eat less:
Foods high in omega-3 fats • Cold water fish (Salmon, Spanish Mackerel, Anchovies, Sardines, Herring) • Flax seeds, flax oil, chia, or hemp seeds • Walnuts Vegetables • Yellow, orange, and red veggies (peppers, carrots, beets) • Dark leafy greens (spinach, kale, arugula, broccoli) Deeply-colored fruit • Berries, melons, citrus fruit Whole grains • Steel-cut or whole rolled oats • Sprouted-grain breads Antiinflammatory spices • Turmeric • Ginger • Rosemary • Oregano • Cayenne	Foods high in trans- and saturated fats • Processed and red meats • Dairy products • Partially hydrogenated oils Foods high in omega-6 fats (in order to get a better omega 6:3 ratio) • Corn, cottonseed, grapeseed, peanut, soy oils Refined carbohydrates (with a high glycemic load) • White breads or bagels • English muffins • Instant or white rice • Rice and corn cereals • Crackers, cookies, cakes Sodas and juices • Including "diet" drinks

FIG. 88.5 ■ Patient handout: Antiinflammatory diet.

CHAPTER 89

THE DASH DIET

David M. Lessens, MD, MPH • David Rakel, MD

WHAT IS THE DASH DIET?

DASH stands for Dietary Approaches to Stop Hypertension. This eating plan was initially developed to lower blood pressure,[1] but it has since been found to modify several disease risk factors and outcomes, including improvements in cholesterol levels and insulin sensitivity. This diet favors meals that are low in animal and dairy fat and rich in fruits, vegetables, and whole grains. It is a well-balanced diet that can be followed by everyone, including those in low socioeconomic strata,[2] to help lead a healthy lifestyle (Table 89.1). It is similar to the antiinflammatory diet discussed in Chapter 88.

HOW MUCH CAN I EXPECT MY BLOOD PRESSURE TO COME DOWN?

Two sentinel studies have investigated how adherence to the DASH diet can reduce blood pressure. The original study,[1] which took place among four academic health care centers, divided subjects into three groups: one ate a normal American diet, one ate an American diet but with more fruits and vegetables, and one ate the DASH diet. In those eating the DASH diet and with no high blood pressure, the average systolic value dropped by 5.5 mm Hg and the diastolic value by 3 mm Hg. For those who already had high blood pressure, the systolic value dropped by 11.6 mm Hg and the diastolic value by 5.3. Blood pressure also dropped in the group eating more fruits and vegetables, but not as much. Furthermore, these changes occurred after just 2 weeks on the diet.

The second DASH trial[3] examined the effect of a reduced dietary sodium intake (at three separate levels: 3300, 2300, or 1500 mg daily) as participants consumed a normal American diet or followed the DASH eating plan. Results showed that reducing dietary sodium lowered blood pressure for both eating plans, but at each level, blood pressure was lower for those on the DASH eating plan. These studies emphasize and highlight that nutritional features of the DASH diet may play a role in reducing blood pressure, apart from reducing sodium consumption.

> In those with high blood pressure, the DASH diet on an average lowered systolic blood pressure by 11.6 mm Hg and diastolic blood pressure by 5.3 mm Hg.

BESIDES LOWERING SODIUM, BY WHAT OTHER MEANS MIGHT THE DASH DIET BENEFIT HEALTH?

Oxidative stress refers to one's ability to detoxify the products of cellular damage. Much of this damage is caused by inflammation, which plays a foundational role in many chronic diseases, including obesity. In a small study, investigators found that the DASH diet decreased blood pressure and enhanced antioxidant capacity, especially in obese individuals.[4] In another study, researchers found lower levels of proinflammatory markers, including C-reactive protein and interleukin-6, among those consuming this diet.[5]

Researchers have postulated the importance of potassium, magnesium, and fiber in the DASH diet's role in lowering blood pressure. One crossover study, for example, had obese and lean individuals consume a usual diet, the DASH diet, and a usual diet supplemented with specific amounts of potassium, magnesium, and fiber matching those of the DASH diet. Each eating plan was also matched for calcium and sodium. After 3 weeks, only obese individuals adhering to the DASH diet showed an improvement in blood pressure and endothelial function. The study's investigators concluded that nutritional factors other than these five must be contributing to the observed health benefits, and these remain a topic of further investigation.[6]

The DASH diet also contains nitrate-rich root vegetable like beets, carrots, and turnips. Consuming nitrates (NO_3^-) from such sources may increase the body's available nitric oxide (NO), which may lead to vasodilation and decreased blood pressure. Ingested nitrates (NO_3^-) are reduced to nitrites (NO_2^-) by enteral bacteria and then are reabsorbed by the intestines and excreted in the stool (the reason manure is such a good fertilizer, which is rich in nitrites). Nitrites are further reduced in the endothelium to NO (Fig. 89.1).

In a study of 72 hypertensive patients, 36 were given 250 mL of beetroot juice once daily (6.4 mmol nitrate) and 36 were given a nitrate-free beetroot juice placebo. The 24-hour blood pressure monitoring showed sustained reductions of 7.7 mm Hg in systolic pressure and 5.2 mm Hg in diastolic pressure in the treatment group. This is just slightly less than the average blood pressure drop with single antihypertensive drug therapy (9.1 mm Hg/5.5 mm Hg). The nitrate-rich beetroot juice also improved endothelial function by ~20%.[7]

TABLE 89.1   The DASH Diet

Food Group	Daily Servings	Serving Sizes	Examples and Notes	Significance of Each Food Group in the Dash Eating Plan
Grains and grain products	7–8	1 slice bread 1 oz dry cereal* ½ cup cooked rice, pasta, or cereal	Whole wheat bread, English muffin, pita bread, bagel, cereals, grits, oatmeal, crackers, unsalted pretzels, and popcorn	Major sources of energy and fiber
Vegetables	4–5	1 cup raw leafy vegetables ½ cup cooked vegetables 6 oz vegetable juice	Tomatoes, potatoes, carrots, green peas, squash, broccoli, turnip greens, collards, kale, spinach, artichokes, green beans, lima beans, sweet potatoes	Rich sources of potassium, magnesium, and fiber
Fruits	4–5	6 oz fruit juice 1 medium fruit ¼ cup dried fruit ½ cup fresh, frozen, or canned fruit	Apricots, bananas, dates, grapes, oranges, orange juice, grapefruit, grapefruit juice, mangoes, melons, peaches, pineapples, prunes, raisins, strawberries, tangerines	Important sources of potassium, magnesium, and fiber
Low-fat or fat-free dairy foods	2–3	8 oz milk 1 cup yogurt 1.5 oz cheese	Fat-free (skim) or low-fat (1%) milk, fat-free or low-fat buttermilk, fat-free or low-fat regular or frozen yogurt, low-fat and fat-free cheese	Major sources of calcium and protein
Meats, poultry, and fish	2 or less	3 oz cooked meats, poultry, or fish	Select only lean; trim away visible fat; broil, roast, or boil instead of frying; remove skin from poultry	Rich sources of protein and magnesium
Nuts, seeds, and dry beans	4–5 per week	1.5 oz or ⅓ cup nuts ½ oz or 2 tbsp seeds ½ cup cooked dry beans and peas	Almonds, filberts, mixed nuts, peanuts, walnuts, sunflower seeds, kidney beans, lentils	Rich sources of energy, magnesium, potassium, protein, and fiber
Fats and oils†	2–3	1 tsp soft margarine 1 tbsp low-fat mayonnaise 2 tbsp light salad dressing 1 tsp vegetable oil	Soft margarine, low-fat mayonnaise, light salad dressing, vegetable oil (such as olive, corn, canola, or safflower)	DASH has 27% of its calories from fat, including that in or added to foods
Sweets	5 per week	1 tbsp sugar 1 tbsp jelly or jam ½ oz jelly beans 8 oz lemonade	Maple syrup, sugar, jelly, jam, fruit-flavored gelatin, jelly beans, hard candy, fruit punch, sorbet, ices	Sweets should be low in fat

*Equals ½–1¼ cup, depending on cereal type. Check the product's nutrition label. †Fat content changes serving counts for fats and oils. For example, 1 tbsp of regular salad dressing equals one serving; 1 tbsp of a low-fat dressing equals ½ serving; 1 tbsp of a fat-free dressing equals zero servings.

From the Dietary Approaches to Stop Hypertension study, as published by the Joint National Committee on Prevention, Detection, Evaluation, and Treatment of High Blood Pressure and the National High Blood Pressure Education Program Coordination Committee. The sixth report of the Joint National Committee on prevention, detection, evaluation and treatment of high blood pressure. *Arch Intern Med.* 1997;157:2413–2446.

Proton pump inhibitors reduce enzymes (DDAH, ADMA) that are needed to make nitric oxide. Taking this class of medicines may negate the beneficial influence vegetables have on blood pressure and may help explain the increased risk for myocardial infarction seen with long-term use of this class of medicine. H2 blockers do not inhibit these enzymes.

BESIDES LOWERING BLOOD PRESSURE, HOW ELSE DOES THIS DIET AFFECT CARDIOVASCULAR HEALTH?

A study of 116 men and women with metabolic syndrome showed that consuming a DASH diet versus a control diet can reduce most of the metabolic risks, including total cholesterol, low-density lipoprotein, weight, triglycerides, and fasting blood glucose concentration, while raising high-density lipoprotein. Although the magnitude of the effects varied by sex, they were positive in both groups.[8] An investigation of 31 type 2 diabetic individuals also found favorable changes in these parameters, including hemoglobin A1c (decrease of 1.7),[9] and adherence to this diet may actually have the potential to prevent type 2 diabetes.[10] Interestingly, the lipid- and glucose-lowering effects of the DASH diet seem to be independent of sodium intake, which again supports the notion that this eating plan works through several nutritional mechanisms.[9]

In a retrospective analysis using data from the Nurses' Health Study, a DASH score was composed on the basis of foods that individuals had consumed. In comparing the top and bottom 20% on the basis of this score, the investigators found a nearly 50% decrease in

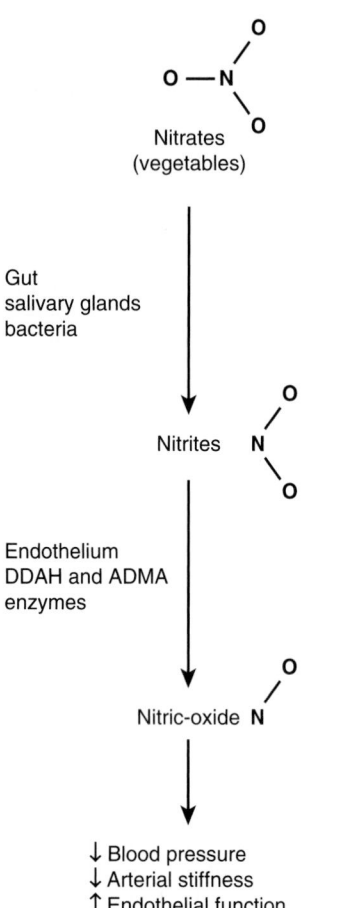

FIG. 89.1 ■ Nitrites are further reduced in the endothelium to nitric oxide (NO). ADMA, asymmetric dimethylarginine; DDAH, dimethylarginine dimethylaminohydrolase.

kidney stones, even in participants with lower calcium intake.[11]

Regarding cardiovascular disease–oriented outcomes, the DASH eating plan has been shown to lower the rates of stroke,[12] heart failure events (including mortality),[13] and coronary artery disease.[14]

DOES THIS DIET REDUCE THE RISK FOR CANCER?

A prospective study assigning a DASH score to more than 100,000 participants showed an 80% reduction in colorectal cancer between the top and bottom 20% of scores during a 26-year period. Those following a Mediterranean diet had no such decrease in their risk.[15] This study was supported by a Canadian study also showing a reduction in colorectal cancer.[16] A review of the available research suggests an overall reduction in the incidence of cancer among those who eat a DASH diet.[17]

HOW DOES THIS DIET AFFECT BONE HEALTH?

Investigators at Duke University found that those who ate a DASH diet had evidence of less bone turnover that over time resulted in a stronger bone structure. This effect was enhanced when the DASH diet group further reduced their intake of sodium.[18]

CAN THE DASH DIET SLOW COGNITIVE DECLINE?

In a sample of 826 older adults with an average age of 81 years, participants filled out a food frequency questionnaire related to both the DASH diet and the Mediterranean diet. Those who ate the most foods in both these dietary plans had the slowest rate of cognitive decline. The DASH diet was rated on a scale of 1–10. For a one-unit higher DASH score, rates of cognitive decline were 0.007 standard units slower, which was equivalent to adults aged at least 4.4 years younger.[19]

WHAT FOODS ARE EMPHASIZED IN THIS DIET, AND HOW DO THEY INFLUENCE ONE'S HEALTH?

To summarize, the diet is:
- High in fruits and vegetables. These are rich in antioxidants (especially those with vibrant colors), are relatively low in calories, and contain significant fiber.
- Low in dairy, animal meat, and saturated fat. These fats increase the risk for atherosclerosis.
- High in nuts, seeds, and beans. These are high in protein and in monounsaturated and polyunsaturated fats, which can decrease inflammation and cardiovascular disease.
- Low in snacks and sweets. Many of these foods contain partially hydrogenated fats that act to preserve shelf life. These types of fats are sources of trans–fatty acids that play a significant role in increasing the risk for heart disease. Many common snacks are also composed of simple carbohydrates, which cause a rapid rise in insulin after they are consumed. Over time, elevations in insulin result in the body becoming less responsive to its effect. In turn, the body will start to produce excessive amounts of insulin, resulting in more inflammation and elevated risk for cardiovascular disease.
- The diet is based on 2000 calories a day. Large portion sizes are a major contributor to rising obesity rates worldwide. Combining this diet with a regular exercise routine can lead to even more dramatic decreases in blood pressure and other chronic diseases.

Key Web Resources

The National Heart, Lung, and Blood Institute (NHLBI). A summary of the DASH diet and its benefits	http://www.nhlbi.nih.gov/health/health-topics/topics/dash
The National Heart, Lung, and Blood Institute (NHLBI). A PDF patient handout explaining the how to use the DASH diet to lower blood pressure	http://www.nhlbi.nih.gov/files/docs/public/heart/dash_brief.pdf

REFERENCES

References are available online at **ExpertConsult.com**.

CHAPTER 90

THE FODMAP DIET

David Rakel, MD

WHAT DOES FODMaP STAND FOR?

Fermentable Oligo-, Di-, and Monosaccharides and Polyol sugars (Table 90.1). See Fig. 90.1 for a description.

WHAT IS THE MECHANISM OF ACTION?

Having high amounts of fermentable sugars in the diet can result in excess gas production, changes in motility, visceral sensations, immune activation, and bowel permeability. This can result in pain, bloating, and altered bowel movements. The sugars are osmotic, pulling fluid into the intestines, worsening diarrhea. Those fruits that have more fructose than glucose are limited. Many patients who respond to the FODMaP diet may be prone to fructose malabsorption. Fructose-rich fruits include pears, apples, and watermelons. Vegetables that contain fructan, a polymeric chain of fructose, are also avoided. These include onions, leeks, asparagus, and artichokes. In a 2-day study where a high FODMaP diet was consumed, there was an increase in the production of hydrogen gas and irritable bowel syndrome (IBS) symptoms in those with IBS, but it only increased flatus production in healthy volunteers without IBS.[1]

TABLE 90.1 **The FODMaP Sugars**

Sugar	Notes
F = Fermentable Sugars	When these sugars come in contact with the gut microbiome, they ferment gas.
O = Oligosaccharides	These are fructans that include wheat, rye, onion, garlic, beans, and some vegetables. This is unfortunate, as many of these are healthy nutrients. Wheat is omitted for its sugar, not for its protein (gluten). But a crossover benefit may occur in those with gluten intolerance.
D = Disaccharides	Lactose in milk and dairy products
M = Monosaccharides	Fructose in high-fructose corn syrup, honey, and some fruits. Maple syrup is OK to use.
a = and	
P = Polyol sweeteners	Any sugar ending in –ol such as xylitol, sorbitol, etc. Be watchful for sugarless chewing gums and any food with artificial sweeteners.

The FODMaP diet's therapeutic benefit is likely mainly related to reducing sugars that stimulate an osmotic shift of fluid into the lumen of the gut while also reducing fermentation that occurs when the sugars interact with the microbiome causing gas, bloating, and distention.

WHAT TYPE OF CONDITION IS FODMaP BEST USED FOR?

The FODMaP diet has been mainly studied for the treatment of IBS. Since it works in part by reducing the osmotic flow of fluid into the intestinal lumen, it has been shown to have a greater effect on diarrhea-dominant IBS (IBS-D). However, a small (n = 30), well-controlled, crossover study of IBS that compared a FODMaP diet to a typical Australian diet found that there was a 50% improvement in symptoms for both diarrhea- and constipation-dominant IBS (IBS-C).[2] Thus although it works best for IBS-D, it may also benefit IBS-C.

WHICH IBS SYMPTOMS ARE REDUCED THE MOST?

In a prospective study of 90 patients with IBS who were followed for almost 16 months, there was statistically significant improvement in abdominal pain, bloating, flatulence, and diarrhea. Seventy-two percent of the patients enrolled were satisfied with the improvement in their symptoms. All patients received hydrogen/methane breath testing and those found to be fructose intolerant (more than lactose intolerant) were most likely to benefit from the FODMaP diet.[3] When the FODMaP diet was compared to a diet that eliminated food triggers in those with IBS-D, both diets improved symptoms by 40%–50% but the FODMaP diet had greater benefit in reducing pain and bloating.[3a]

IS IT THE ELIMINATION OF SUGAR OR FOOD PROTEINS THAT RESULTS IN THE GREATEST BENEFIT?

Since the FODMaP diet also removes foods that contain common food proteins such as gluten and casein, it is difficult to know if the benefits are from eliminating foods where the patient may have sensitivities to food proteins (e.g., non-celiac gluten sensitivity or celiac disease) or by reducing the sugars that are also included in these food groups

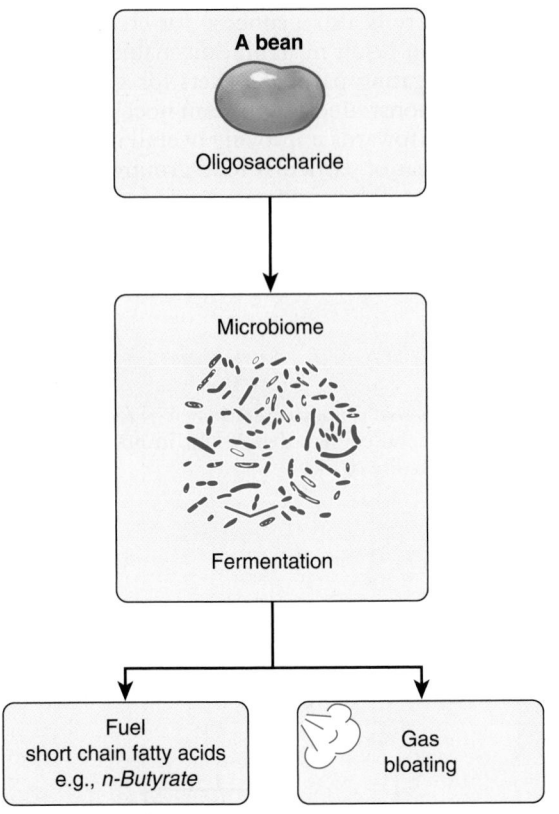

FIG. 90.1 ■ How a bean becomes fuel and gas as it passes through the gastrointestinal tract.

(see Chapter 31). One strategy is similar to what is recommended in the rechallenge phase of an elimination diet (see Chapter 86); after having the patient on a strict FODMaP diet, reintroduce one food group at a time (e.g., gluten or dairy) and see if there is a significant worsening of symptoms. Generally, if there is a food protein sensitivity, there will be a more dramatic return in symptoms compared with adding more sugar. However, this is a subjective assessment.

Polyol sugars are added to foods as sweeteners. They are often found in chewing gum since they are not broken down by bacteria in the mouth and metabolized to acids that can cause tooth decay. Encourage patients to read labels and watch for sugars that end in "-ol." These include maltitol, sorbitol, xylitol, and erythritol. One that does not end in "-ol" is isomalt, which is used to make sugar-free candy.

WHAT TO TELL YOUR PATIENTS WHEN PLACING THEM ON THE FODMaP DIET

The diet is dose-dependent. The fewer fermentable sugars they eat, the more benefit they will achieve. Most will see a benefit in 1 week. Since this is a difficult diet to sustain, it is important to educate patients that most of them do not require long-term strict adherence. Encourage patients to begin with a strict adherence, but then over time, slowly reintroduce foods based on personal

---

TABLE 90.2 **Examples of a High (Top) and Low (Bottom) FODMaP Diet[8]**

FODMaP	Excess Fructose	Lactose	Oligosaccharides (fructans and/or galactans)	Polyols
Problem high-FODMaP food source	*Fruits:* apples, pears, nashi pears, clingstone peaches, mango, sugar snap peas, watermelon, tinned fruit in natural juice *Honey* *Sweeteners:* fructose, high-fructose corn syrup *Large total fructose dose:* concentrated fruit sources; large servings of fruit, dried fruit, fruit juice	*Milk:* cow, goat, and sheep (regular & low-fat), ice cream *Yogurt:* regular & low-fat *Cheeses:* soft & fresh (e.g., ricotta, cottage)	*Vegetables:* artichokes, asparagus, beetroot, Brussels sprouts, broccoli, cabbage, fennel, garlic, leeks, okra, onions, peas, shallots *Cereals:* wheat & rye when eaten in large amounts (e.g., bread, pasta, couscous, crackers, biscuits) *Legumes:* chickpeas, lentils, red kidney beans, baked beans *Fruits:* watermelon, custard apple, white peaches, rambutan, persimmon	*Fruits:* apples, apricots, cherries, longan, lychee, nashi pears, nectarines, pears, peaches, plums, prunes, watermelon *Vegetables:* avocado, cauliflower, mushrooms, snow peas *Sweeteners:* sorbitol (420), mannitol (421), xylitol (967), maltitol (965), isomalt (953), & others ending in '-ol'
Suitable alternative low-FODMaP food source	*Fruit:* banana, blueberry, carambola, durian, grapefruit, grape, honeydew melon, kiwifruit, lemon, lime, mandarin, orange, passionfruit, paw paw, raspberry, rockmelon, strawberry, tangelo *Honey substitutes:* maple syrup, golden syrup *Sweeteners:* any except polyols	*Milk:* lactose-free, rice milk *Cheese:* "hard" cheeses including brie, camembert *Yogurt:* lactose-free *Ice cream substitutes:* gelati, sorbets *Butter*	*Vegetables:* bamboo shoots, bok choy, carrot, celery, capsicum, choko, choy sum, corn, eggplant, green beans, lettuce, chives, parsnip, pumpkin, silverbeet, spring onion (green only), tomato *Onion/garlic substitutes:* garlic-infused oil *Cereals:* gluten-free & spelt bread/cereal products	*Fruits:* banana, blueberry, carambola, durian, grapefruit, grape, honeydew melon, kiwifruit, lemon, lime, mandarin, orange, passionfruit, paw paw, raspberry, rockmelon *Sweeteners:* sugar (sucrose), glucose, other artificial sweeteners not ending in "-ol"

From Gibson PR, Shepherd SJ. Evidence-based dietary management of functional gastrointestinal symptoms: the FODMAP approach. *J Gastroenterol Hepatol.* 2010;25:252-258.

tolerability.[4] Many benefit by simply reducing the total sugar load, which alone can improve quality of life while also reducing enteric inflammatory triggers (Fig. 90.2). Table 90.2 summarizes the foods to avoid (high FODMaP diet) and suitable substitutes (Low FODMaP diet).

WHAT ARE THE LIMITATIONS OF THE FODMaP DIET?

The FODMaP diet runs the risk of significantly reducing the intake of fruits and vegetables, which could have negative long-term health consequences. A deficiency in dietary calcium due to the restriction of lactose and dairy has been reported.[5] The diet may also alter the microbiome by restricting prebiotic (food for bacteria to grow)

sources.[5,6] There is also a concern for creating a fear of food, which can result in significant malnutrition. Many studies investigating particular diets for gastrointestinal symptoms demonstrated a significant nocebo effect.[7] The goal should be towards improving overall nutrition while reducing the fear of particular food groups.

The majority of the positive research for the FODMaP diet comes from one center: Monash University in Australia. A lack of diversity of research sources should always elicit caution because of the risk of institutional research bias.

> The long-term goal is not to create a fear of food, but an improvement in food choices that results in nourishment and an improved quality of life.

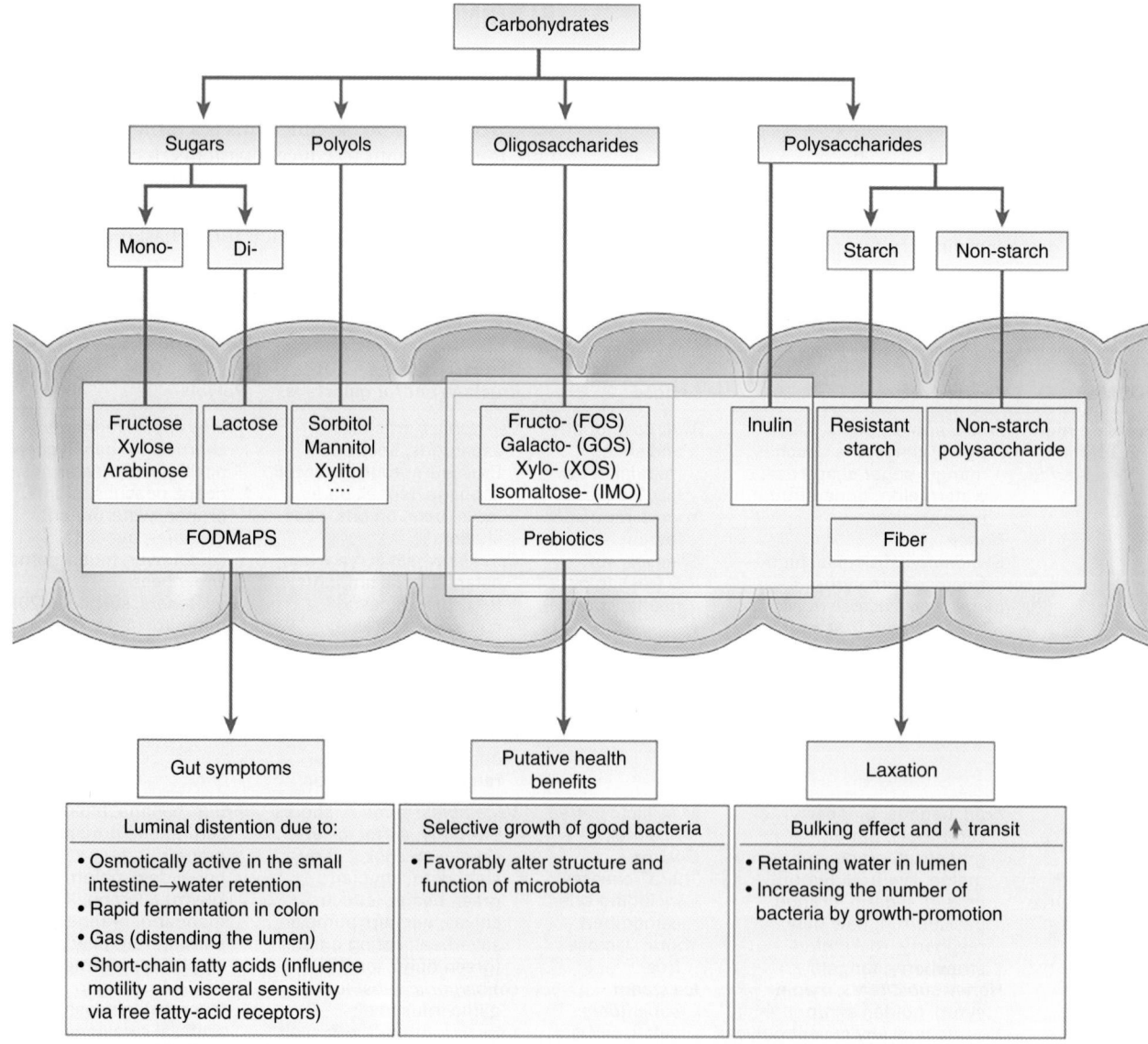

FIG. 90.2 ■ Classification of carbohydrates based on their functional influence on gastrointestinal mechanisms. The FODMaP diet mainly avoids those sugars on the left side of the graphic. (From Gibson PR, Varney J, Malakar S, Muir JG. Food components and irritable bowel syndrome. *Gastroenterology*. 2015;148:1158-1174.e4.)

Notes	URL
A PDF patient handout on a low FODMaP diet from Stanford Hospital and Clinics	http://fodmapliving.com/wp-content/uploads/2013/02/Stanford-University-Low-FODMAP-Diet-Handout.pdf
Monash University website for patient education. Includes recipes, food tips, and clinical direction	http://fodmapmonash.blogspot.com/
Low FODMaP smartphone app from Monash University that provides patient instructions for implementation	http://www.med.monash.edu/cecs/gastro/fodmap/iphone-app.html
IBS Freedom website that contains a nice graphic describing acceptable foods and those to avoid	https://ibsfreedom.wordpress.com/2014/03/18/low-fodmaps-diet-chart/

REFERENCES

References are available online at ExpertConsult.com.

LIFESTYLE: EXERCISE

SECTION OUTLINE

91 WRITING AN EXERCISE PRESCRIPTION

92 THERAPEUTIC BREATHING

93 LOW BACK PAIN EXERCISES

CHAPTER 91

WRITING AN EXERCISE PRESCRIPTION

Michael J. Hewitt, PhD

With the exception of a small number of sessile species, movement is one of the defining characteristics of animals. In humans, regular physical activity, whether it is accomplished through recreation, sport, labor, or participation in a structured exercise program, has been demonstrated to enhance function; to reduce, reverse, and prevent age-related physiological decline; and to lower the risks of a sedentary lifestyle.[1] Most physicians recognize the benefit of exercise, and most medical groups recommend regular physical activity.[2] However, because few medical training programs include even an overview of exercise physiology and few clinical rotations address exercise prescription, it is the rare physician who has experience in the decision-making process associated with recommending physical activity. Prescribing exercise is no different from prescribing medication, surgery, or therapy; it is a thoughtful compromise between the potential benefits of the treatment and its potential adverse effects.[3]

BASIC PRINCIPLES

Two principles form the framework for making exercise recommendations: the overload principle and the concept of specificity of exercise. The overload principle, based on Hans Selye's general adaptation syndrome model, suggests that a body or a physiological system repeatedly exposed to a stressor of appropriate intensity ultimately adapts to that stressor. To scientists who specialize in exercise, this principle underlies the adaptations that occur after cardiorespiratory conditioning or strength training. In general, there is an inverted J-curve relationship between the volume or intensity of the stimulus and the physiological adaptation. Infrequent strength training or work with light resistance brings about only modest increases in muscle strength, but consistent work with heavier loads results in greater strength gains. Too much load and consecutive lifting days, however, are often associated with injury. Cardiorespiratory and flexibility adaptations to exercise training follow similar patterns; some is good, more is usually better, but too much can cause injury.

> The challenge for physicians and their patients is to determine the appropriate exercise frequency and intensity to safely achieve an optimal functional enhancement.

Specificity of exercise refers to the relationship between the type of physiological adaptation and the type of activity performed. It is widely accepted that strength training is beneficial, many believe essential, for enhanced performance in sports. It is an unusual collegiate athletic team that does not have a strength coach. However, if one wishes to become a competitive swimmer or an Alpine skier, strength training alone is woefully inadequate. One must spend time in the pool or on the mountain. For similar reasons, sprinters train differently than middle- or long-distance runners. The implication for physicians is that cardiorespiratory health concerns, weight loss, and osteoporosis prevention all require different modes of exercise therapy.

THE FIVE COMPONENTS OF FITNESS

A useful model for exercise programming is one that addresses five components of fitness: cardiorespiratory or aerobic fitness, muscle strength and endurance, flexibility, body composition, and balance/agility. One could make an argument to include muscle power (i.e., the explosive application of strength), but lack of power is rarely a health limitation. In addition to percentage of body fat and fat-free body mass (FFB), measurement of bone mineral content (BMC) is another important component of body composition assessment. Balance and agility are the most commonly overlooked aspects of physical function, but they have significant implications for fall prevention and mobility and therefore are important for aging patients.[4]

There is typically an age-related decline in each of these components (with the exception of percentage of body fat, which usually increases) that can be attenuated or reversed by appropriate physical activity. In fact, much of the functional decline associated with aging can be more accurately called disuse atrophy.

> The five components of fitness are as follows:
> - Cardiorespiratory fitness (the ability of the heart, lungs, and vascular network to deliver oxygen to the working muscles)
> - Muscle strength (the ability of the musculoskeletal system to move a heavy load) and muscle endurance (the ability to move a moderate load repeatedly)
> - Flexibility (an index of joint range of motion)
> - Body composition (typically, the level of body fat, but a measure of fat-free body mass [FFB] is of equal clinical significance)
> - Balance and agility

Body Composition

Body composition is the one component of fitness that does not require a specific exercise recommendation. Body composition changes as a consequence of cardiorespiratory exercise, strength training, and nutrient intake.[5] However, an initial measure and repeated assessments of body composition are highly useful tools to determine how patients should use their limited exercise time. For instance, a man with more than 25% body fat and a woman with more than 38% body fat are in a group with a statistically greater risk of heart disease, type 2 diabetes mellitus, hyperlipidemia, and hypertension.[6] Exercise programming should attempt to specifically address those risks as well as help reduce the level of body fat.

Quantification of FFB further refines the exercise prescription and can be used to accurately predict resting metabolic rate (RMR).[7] Many adults are at an appropriate weight on the weight-to-height scales or body mass index (BMI; weight in kg/height in m^2) value, but are underlean as indicated by a lower than optimal FFB. In general, cardiorespiratory exercise results in a reduction of percentage body fat but has a limited effect on FFB. In contrast, strength training increases FFB (as well as muscle strength), which will modestly raise RMR, ultimately resulting in a reduction in the percentage body fat. Many obese patients develop adequate FFB simply by transporting themselves and gain only limited benefit from strength training, but their percentage of body fat responds favorably to cardiorespiratory activity. Smaller individuals who have acceptable weight-to-height values despite excess body fat have low FFB and benefit most from combined cardiorespiratory and strength programs.

In addition to the measures of body fat, the determination of BMC (in grams) or bone mineral density (BMD, g/cm^2) further enhances exercise programming. Dual-energy x-ray absorptiometry (DEXA) is considered the new "gold standard" for simultaneous determination of percentage body fat, FFB, and BMC.[6] Its drawbacks are that the technique requires expensive equipment and patients experience a very small x-ray exposure. However, DEXA is fast, accurate, and reliable, and it does not depend on patient skills (as does underwater weighing) or measurer's technique (as does anthropometry). If DEXA is not readily available or is cost-prohibitive and BMD data are not essential, bioelectric impedance analysis (BIA) is a practical alternative. As long as hydration status is controlled, BIA can rapidly and inexpensively provide accurate and repeatable measures of percentage fat and FFB. It eliminates measurement technique and patient cooperation errors and provides significantly more data, as well as a more meaningful assessment of health status, compared with that provided by the ubiquitous determination of BMI. Several other field techniques can be effectively administered in a physician's office; these provide useful body composition data, but each method has limitations. A discussion of body composition assessment methodology is beyond the scope of this text, but interested readers are referred to three excellent summaries.[8-9]

DEXA can determine percentage of body fat, FFB, and BMC.

THE FITT PRINCIPLE FOR EXERCISE PROGRAMMING

For cardiorespiratory conditioning, strength training, flexibility, and balance-agility training, a simple exercise prescription tool is the FITT principle. FITT is an acronym for the following:
- Frequency
- Intensity
- Type
- Time (duration)

These are the four variables that must be considered in exercise programming, and physicians should write a prescription specifically addressing each (Fig. 91.1). For example, individuals with elevated risk for heart disease should be encouraged to improve their cardiorespiratory condition. The type of exercise can be walking, jogging, or running, either outdoors or on a treadmill; bicycling, swimming, or hiking; aerobics and use of any of a variety of aerobic machines (stair climbers, rowing machines, cycle ergometers); or dancing, tennis, and many other possibilities. The choice is affected by geographic concerns (cycling in northern climates during January is difficult) and economic limitations (some patients cannot afford a treadmill or the cost of membership at a fitness center), but the most important factor is usually patient preference. Exercise equipment manufacturers often promote their devices on the basis of efficiency and the effectiveness of the workout they provide. Practically, much of the advantage of one type of exercise device over another is irrelevant when patients miss exercise sessions because they simply do not like the activity. The very best cardiorespiratory exercise is one that the patient will perform. Of course, a patient with knee limitations may not tolerate distance running, and a patient with severe osteoporosis should not be advised to take up ice skating.

In 2011, the American College of Sports Medicine (ACSM) published a position stand on the recommended quantity and quality of exercise that is an excellent reference and should be in the library of any health professional who recommends physical activity.[10] In this position stand, quantity refers to the frequency and duration and quality refer to the intensity of physical activity.

CARDIORESPIRATORY TRAINING

The frequency of cardiorespiratory training is limited more often by patient compliance than by physiology. It is not inappropriate for one to exercise daily, but few people do. The ACSM recommends a duration of 20–60 minutes of continuous or intermittent exercise and a frequency of 3–5 days per week for cardiorespiratory fitness and body composition enhancement. Intermittent exercise is described as a minimum of 10-minute bouts

EXERCISE PRESCRIPTION

Name:_____ Date:_____

COMPONENT OF FITNESS	EXERCISE	FREQUENCY	DURATION	INTENSITY
Cardiorespiratory Fitness	_____ _____ _____	_____ days/week	_____ minutes	_____ beats/minute _____ beats/10 seconds
Strength	Free Weights Machines Elastic bands Floorwork	_____ days/week	_____ minutes _____ sets	_____ repetitions
Flexibility	Static	_____ days/week _____ repetitions	_____ seconds	Hold below pain threshold

Comments/Progression: _____

_____

_____

_____ By:_____
                                              Exercise Physiologist

FIG. 91.1 ▪ Sample of an exercise prescription showing the first three components of fitness, with areas for the prescription to be individualized for the patient.

accumulated throughout the day. The recommended intensity is 65%–90% of maximum heart rate (HR_{max}) in healthy adults and 55%–65% in very unfit individuals. The challenge, of course, is to know one's maximal heart rate. Graded exercise tests rarely continue to exhaustion; therefore, they do not provide a true HR_{max}, and prediction equations for HR_{max} (e.g., 220—age in years) lack sufficient precision to be clinically useful. A maximal or submaximal exercise tolerance test performed by an exercise physiologist, especially if it includes measures of oxygen consumption, can provide a useful estimate of HR_{max} and a target heart range.

Graded exercise stress tests can identify hypertensive responses to activity and clinically significant electrocardiographic abnormalities during exercise and are thereby highly useful for providing a safe and effective cardiorespiratory exercise intensity range for at-risk patients. In healthy adults, heart rate is useful but not essential for monitoring of exercise intensity. The Borg scale has been demonstrated to be an effective tool to assess cardiorespiratory exercise intensity (Table 91.1).[11] Healthy adults should maintain a subjective rating of perceived exertion (RPE) of "moderate" to "heavy" or about 13–15 on the scale. Beginners can improve compliance by limiting intensity to "light" to "moderate" (RPE 11–13). It is not uncommon for athletes to reach "very, very heavy" (RPE 19–20) for short bursts, particularly during interval training such as wind sprints, but there is little reason to recommend these levels for patients. The OMNI RPE scale,

which provides illustrations representing exercise intensity as well as a 0–10 numerical rating scale, may be more appropriate for children or anyone for whom English is not the primary language.[12]

Another approach to recommending appropriate cardiorespiratory exercise intensity is based on the measured energy cost of the activity, reported in metabolic equivalents (METs). One MET, defined as the energy expenditure of sitting quietly,[13] about 1 kcal/kg body weight/hour, requires about 3.5 mL of oxygen/kg body weight/minute. Level walking on a firm surface at 3.5 mph is rated at 3.7 METs, and running at 7 mph (8.6 min per mile) is 11.8 METs. A listing of the MET level of more than 400 recreational and occupational activities has been compiled.[13] This compendium provides a simple comparison of the energy costs of the activities, allowing physicians to suggest several equivalent options. Its utility is further enhanced if a graded exercise test has been performed to quantify the patient's sustainable and maximal MET capacities.

Because cardiorespiratory exercise is a foundation for disease prevention and longevity, any program that increases participation should be welcomed. A 10,000-step program, *Walk to a Healthy Future*, has been endorsed by health providers and is promoted by the International Longevity Center.[14] Requiring only good walking shoes and an inexpensive digital pedometer, this program encourages participants to accumulate 10,000 steps daily, the equivalent of about 5–6 miles. The recommendations

TABLE 91.1	Borg Scale of Perceived Exertion
Number	**Exertion Level**
6	
7	Very, very light
8	
9	Very light
10	
11	Light
12	
13	Moderate
14	
15	Heavy
16	
17	Very heavy
18	
19	Very, very heavy
20	

From Borg GA. Psychophysical bases of perceived exertion. *Med Sci Sports Exerc.* 1982;14:377-381.

are based on research by a Japanese physician, Yoshiro Hatano, who reported that the typical (Japanese) adult takes between 3000 and 5000 steps per day.[15] In contrast, a 7-day study on the walking behavior of an Old Order Amish community in Ontario, Canada, whose members do not use electricity or motorized vehicles, found average daily step totals of 18,425 ± 4685 for adult men and 14,196 ± 4078 steps for adult women.[16] The highest recorded single-day total was 51,514 steps! It is not surprising that rates of obesity (BMI ≥ 30) and overweight (BMI ≥ 25) among Amish adults average only 4% and 26%, respectively; in contrast, these rates are 34.9% and 68.5%, respectively, for the adult U.S. population.[17]

Electronic Activity Monitors

Pedometers continue to be useful tools to monitor physical activity, but are dinosaurs compared to the wearable electronic activity monitoring devices that have been developed in recent years. These sophisticated fitness trackers can be worn on the wrist, clipped to clothing, or incorporated into smartphones. Most utilize an accelerometer to monitor movement, even during sleep, and some versions add GPS technology. Optical sensors for heart rate are common and provide useful data to optimize exercise intensity. Virtually all monitors sync with smartphones or personal computers for tracking and graphic display of physical activity, calorie expenditure, and more. A list of recommended fitness trackers here would be useful to physicians, but development of new devices proceeds much faster than revisions of printed books. However, publications like *PC Magazine* publish online annual reviews of these tools and can provide comparative data for the latest models. It is worth noting that not all activity monitors are water resistant. Like most consumer electronics, function increases and cost decreases almost exponentially each year, so physicians can recommend these devices for patients in all economic groups.

RESISTANCE TRAINING

A nearly universal physiological change associated with aging is sarcopenia, the age- or disuse-related loss of muscle and FFB.[4,18-20] A reduction in FFB typically brings about a proportional drop in metabolic rate. In addition, the decline in FFB negatively influences strength, mobility, and balance, ultimately jeopardizing a person's independence.[20] Clinical rates for sarcopenia are 8%–13% in persons younger than 70 years, about 17.5% in those aged 75 years, and more than 50% in the oldest old.[16,20] Subclinical levels of muscle loss are even more common. As prevalent and as significant as sarcopenia is, few physicians address it, and very few patients have heard the term. Fortunately, sarcopenia is highly preventable, and much of its effects can be reversed with resistance (strength) training. Although cardiorespiratory disease influences morbidity and mortality more than any other factor in our culture and appropriate preventive exercises should be prescribed for it, the prevention of sarcopenia and its long-term effects warrant nearly equivalent attention.

> Sarcopenia, the age- or disuse-related loss of muscle and fat-free body mass, reduces strength, mobility, metabolism, balance, and independence in older adults. Its effects can be attenuated or reversed by resistance training.

Resistance training has also been shown to be effective in combating osteoporosis, the bone loss analogue to sarcopenic loss of muscle. The Bone, Estrogen, Strength Training (BEST) study demonstrated that postmenopausal women, when exposed to a sufficient strength challenge with or without estrogen replacement therapy, could achieve small but significant increases in bone mineral density at the trochanter and lumbar spine (L2–4) sites.[21] Although the increases recorded during the 1-year study were modest (+ 0.77% to + 2.00% for resistance training with estrogen; + 0.02% to + 1.13% for resistance training alone), they were in sharp contrast to the –0.13% and –0.57% losses recorded at the trochanter and L2-4 areas for women in the nonexercise, no-estrogen control group during the same period. The positive outcome in the BEST study can be attributed primarily to the significant and increasing weight challenge (intensity) that participants faced during the study as well as to the frequency, time, and types of strength intervention imposed.

Thus, the FITT principle as suggested for cardiorespiratory programming can also be applied to resistance training. The ACSM suggests that one set of 8–10 weight exercises that work all major muscle groups be performed 2 or 3 days per week. A weight load that causes muscle fatigue in 8–12 repetitions is recommended. Older or frail individuals may find lighter weights that allow 10–15 repetitions before fatigue to be more appropriate.[10,20,22] A second or third set may be advantageous if time and patient interest permit, but the majority of the benefit is derived in the first set.[22] Although many physicians refer patients for an initial session with an exercise physiologist, physical therapist, or personal fitness trainer to learn

TABLE 91.2	Basics of Exercise Prescription			
Exercise/Fitness Component	For Disease Prevention	For Basic Health	For Enhanced Fitness	For Performance-Level Fitness
Cardiovascular exercise	*Accumulate* 30–60 min of physical activity most days	Play or large muscle repetitive activity 20 + min[a] 3 + times/week	Play or aerobic exercise 40–60 + min[a] 4–6 times/week	*Add* interval training or competition
Strength training	Include weight-bearing activity most days	Key Three[b] or equivalent program 1–2 sets two times/week Lift to a "challenge" level in 8–12 or 12–15 repetitions	Balanced whole-body machine or free-weight program 2–3 sets three times/week. Reach "functional failure" in 8–12 repetitions	*Add* muscle endurance or power training *Add* Pilates work *Add* ascending or descending pyramids
Flexibility	Maintain range of motion by bending and stretching in daily activities	Perform 2–4 limitation-specific stretches after activity, 1 repetition Hold about 20–30 s	Perform 6–10 whole-body stretches *after* activity and *before* competition, 1–2 repetitions	*Add* yoga, Pilates work, or facilitated stretches with a partner
Body composition	Men	≥5% ≤25% fat	12%–20% fat	8%–15% fat
		Maintain fat-free (lean) body mass at 125–150 lb. or more		
	Women	≥14% ≤38% fat	20%–30% fat	17%–25% fat
		Maintain fat-free (lean) body mass at 90 to 110 lb. or more		
Balance and agility	—	Act "like a child" Walk a balance line "Don't step on a crack…" Brush teeth while standing on one foot	Recreational sports: tennis, bicycle, tai chi Social dancing Stability ball training	High-level sports: skiing, skating, surfing Yoga Martial arts Performance dancing Agility drills

[a]At a challenging intensity.
[b]Key Three consists of a double-leg press or squat, chest press, and lat pulldown or single-arm row.
Modified from Hewitt MJ. *Basics of exercise prescription.* Tucson, AZ: Canyon Ranch Health Resort; copyright © 2002.

the specifics of a strength training program, a program can be designed on the basis of general advice.[23] Flexibility and balance-agility recommendations should also follow the FITT principle.

LEVELS OF EXERCISE PRESCRIPTION

When prescribing exercise, the health care provider should determine the patient's desired outcome. Strategies exist to help patients overcome their physical and psychological barriers to exercise compliance.[24] Individuals whose primary goal is simply to reduce disease risk may have a level of commitment lower than that of others who seek true physical fitness or athletic performance. Table 91.2 summarizes exercise recommendations for four levels in the cardiorespiratory, strength, flexibility, body composition, and balance-agility areas. General recommendations for body fat and FFB at each level are also reported; however, body composition standards are subject to significant individual variation. A useful approach is to encourage patients to perform at least the recommended activity for the prevention of disease but to strive to consistently exercise at the "basic health" level. When these patterns become habitual, the health care provider can encourage physical activity at the level to achieve "enhanced fitness" (see Table 91.2).[3]

The most effective exercise prescriptions provide guidelines for variety and allow a progression of activity. The programs of long-term participants bear little resemblance to those of new exercisers. Compliance is enhanced if the initial program is broad enough and sufficiently challenging to effect measurable improvement, but compact enough to fit into a patient's busy schedule. An experienced physician or exercise physiologist will develop a small starting program and suggest a progression during a specific time frame. One may start with a 10-minute walking or bicycle ergometer program three times weekly and progress to 20 minutes four times weekly within 2 or 3 months, ultimately striving for 40 minutes or longer on most days.

THE KEY THREE STRENGTH PROGRAM

In strength work, a simple starting program such as the Key Three[20,25] allows a basic whole-body strength workout to be completed in less than 10 minutes (Fig. 91.2). Few patients have an effective argument for why they cannot find 10 minutes for strength work twice a week. The Key Three can be performed using weight machines, inexpensive hand-held dumbbells, or even elastic resistance bands, making equipment and space limitations moot. The three exercises (and the

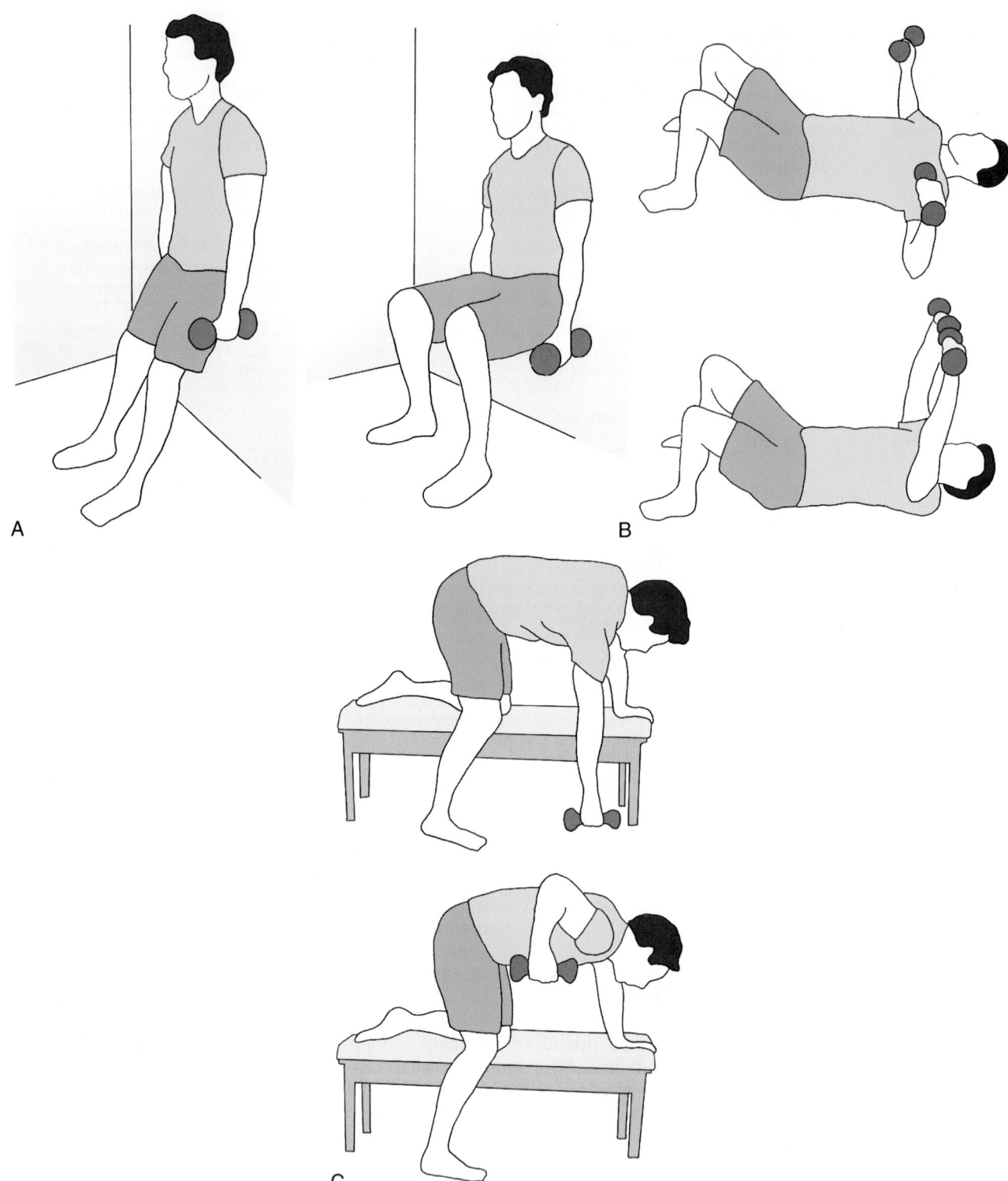

FIG. 91.2 ■ Key Three exercises: A, Dumbbell squat (quadriceps, hamstrings, and gluteals). B, Supine bench press (pectoralis major and minor, anterior deltoid, and triceps). C, Single-arm dumbbell row (trapezius, latissimus dorsi, and biceps). (From Hewitt MJ. *The Key Three strength program.* Tucson, AZ: Canyon Ranch Health Resort; 2002. Illustration by Karen T. Wylie.)

primary muscle groups targeted) are the double-leg press machine or dumbbell squat, which can be performed against the wall for additional support (quadriceps, hamstrings, gluteals); the chest press machine or supine dumbbell bench press (pectoralis major and minor, anterior deltoid, triceps brachii); and either the lat pulldown or seated row machine or the single-arm dumbbell row (trapezius, latissimus dorsi, and biceps brachii). These three exercises challenge approximately 85% of the muscle system. Although bodybuilders might scoff at a basic program such as the Key Three, even smaller series of lifts have been demonstrated to rapidly improve strength, muscle mass, and mobility in older adults,[26-28] and these three core exercises can form the framework for more sophisticated lifting regimens.

FLEXIBILITY VERSUS STABILITY

Traditional thinking among exercise professionals and fitness enthusiasts is that more flexibility is preferable to less. Certainly this is true for dancers, gymnasts, and figure skaters, but it is not always the case for healthy adults. More modern thinking recognizes that optimal control of range of motion (ROM) requires an appropriate balance between limb flexibility and joint stability. Stretching programs have been demonstrated to effectively increase ROM, but physicians should use caution in recommending flexibility training regimens to patients exhibiting hypermobility tendencies (e.g., they can extend the thumb to touch the forearm or can extend the elbows or knees beyond 180 degrees). Hypermobile patients should be encouraged to preferentially participate in strength training to stabilize their joints. Most adults, however, will respond favorably to a modest flexibility program.

Static stretching, in which a joint is moved to a position eliciting mild tension and is held stationary, is the most commonly practiced method to improve joint ROM. There are places where ballistic stretching (incorporating bouncing movements), proprioceptive neuromuscular facilitation (PNF), hold-relax cycles (with a partner or against an immobile object), and dynamic stretching (exaggerated movement mimicking sports-related activity) are indicated, but most patients will see effective adaptations using a compact static stretching program.[29] The scientific evidence is equivocal in support for the common belief that improved flexibility reduces the risk of injury, but enhanced and stable ROM is always desirable. Similarly, recommendations for the optimal time for holding a static stretch vary from as little as 2 or 3 seconds to well above 60 seconds, but most fitness professionals find that patients respond favorably to a hold period of 20–30 seconds.[29] Activities like yoga and pilates also improve joint ROM, although a compact program of two or three static stretches performed daily is often preferable to a larger and more complex program that might be performed only intermittently.

BALANCE AND AGILITY

Balance and agility are the most commonly overlooked components of fitness, yet poor balance and its associated risk of falling are potentially the greatest health concerns for many older adults. Balance and agility require a rapid central nervous system (CNS) response to signals from the inner ears (vestibular signals), eyes (visual signals), postural muscles in the legs and back (proprioceptive signals), and touch (tactile signals). Although some deterioration in the quality of these signals occurs with age, it is primarily a slower rate of integration and response by the CNS that appears to cause the loss of function (disuse atrophy). Function loss is cyclical; low function results in reduced confidence, which leads to avoidance of balance challenges, and further reduction in function follows in a destructive cycle. Even highly skilled athletes lose function rapidly if they become injured or fail to practice.

Balance and agility can be restored by safe challenges to the system with appropriate exercises. Tai chi, dance, and simple balance exercises such as standing on one foot while brushing the teeth or hair provide effective signals to stimulate CNS adaptation.[30] In severe cases, ai chi, a form of tai chi performed in a swimming pool, provides a no-falling-risk stimulus to the balance control system. Sports such as tennis and bicycling are greater challenges and are associated with both higher risk and greater potential to achieve improvement. High-level activities, including skiing, skating, and martial arts, are appropriate for a select group of patients.

THERAPEUTIC REVIEW

The ACSM[4,5,26] provides guidelines that illustrate the standard of care and prove invaluable for clinicians and physiologists who make exercise recommendations. This organization also offers a resource manual to support these guidelines, which includes background summaries in applied anatomy, exercise physiology, exercise testing and programming, emergency procedures, terminology, and more.[31-32]

A comprehensive exercise program has a synergistic effect. Improved strength in the postural muscles is reflected in better balance because those muscles can more effectively respond to signals from the balance centers. Better cardiorespiratory conditioning allows a more challenging strength training program, and improved body composition allows greater range of motion for more effective stretching. Equally important, enhanced function allows greater participation, usually resulting in better compliance. Exercise prescription need not be complicated; virtually any activity has positive effects. The key is to gently challenge each of the physiological systems in such a way to allow patients to experience enhanced function and then encourage them to modestly increase the stimulus.

Key Web Resources

ACSM Position Stands: The American College of Sports Medicine (ACSM) is an international resource for information and certifications for exercise physiologists, sports medicine physicians, physical therapists, and other allied health professionals. The ACSM has published position stands on multiple topics of interest to physicians wanting to optimize exercise prescription for various situations. The list can be viewed at no cost at ACSM.org.	http://www.acsm.org/access-public-information/position-stands
The website for the American Council on Exercise, a not-for-profit organization that trains and certifies health and fitness professionals	https://www.acefitness.org
An issue brief written by this author and published by the International Longevity Center on the basics of a small strength training program for the prevention of sarcopenia. All ILC-USA issue briefs can be reprinted for patients.	http://www.issuelab.org/resources/11921/11921.pdf
Another International Longevity Center issue brief, this one written by Robert N. Butler, MD, Founding Director of the National Institutes on Aging and late CEO and Founder of the ILC. *Walk to a Healthy Future* introduces the 10,000-step program and can be reprinted for patients.	http://www.issuelab.org/resources/12119/12119.pdf
Members of the National Strength and Conditioning Association earn certifications preparing them to be personal trainers and team strength coaches. The NSCA website's publications and education sections provide additional information for readers interested in a deeper understanding of this important component of physical activity.	https://www.nsca-lift.org

REFERENCES

References are available online at ExpertConsult.com.

CHAPTER 92

THERAPEUTIC BREATHING

Vincent J. Minichiello, MD

And the Lord God formed man of the dust of the ground, and breathed into his nostrils the breath of life; and man became a living soul.
GENESIS 2:7, KING JAMES VERSION BIBLE[1]

As long as there is breath in the body, there is life. When breath departs, so too does life. Therefore, regulate the breath.
HATHA YOGA PRADIPIKA, CH. 2[2]

WHAT IS THERAPEUTIC BREATHING?

The importance of breath in the context of health has been understood for millennia. Frequently, the terms used for breath in ancient cultures also carried a broader connotation, implying breath to be a "vital energy": *pneuma* in ancient Greek, *prana* in Sanskrit, *qi* in Chinese, and *ruach* in Hebrew. The tradition of using breath for health and healing has been transmitted from generation to generation through a variety of practices, including religion/prayer, meditation, martial arts, yoga, and qigong, amongst others. These techniques have now become the focus of medical research, with a dramatic rise in the number of publications related to the therapeutic use of breath for multiple disease states over the past 20 years.[3] The purpose of this chapter is to focus on how the physiology of breathing affects the mind-body unit, to provide a framework for broadly classifying specific techniques, and to highlight the strongest evidence for practices that could be utilized in a clinical setting.

> As both voluntary and involuntary processes, breathing is one form of nonpharmacological medicine that can be practiced easily in any setting, at any time of the day.

THE MECHANISM OF BREATHING

While there is perhaps no single "correct" way of breathing, evidence from millennia of practitioners of the healing arts as well as evidence from modern research has shown that there are ways to voluntarily modulate natural breathing to attain better mental and physical health. Typically, respiration involves a continuous cycle of inhalation and exhalation either through the nose or the mouth. On inhalation, the diaphragm contracts and moves downward, creating an increase in negative pressure in the lungs and chest cavity, thus allowing air from the atmosphere to travel down a pressure gradient to fill the lungs. With the help of intercostal and abdominal muscles, the chest wall and/or abdomen will expand

outwards with inhalation. The shoulders may rise. Upon exhalation, the reverse happens—relaxation of the diaphragm decreases the volume of the intrapleural space, air leaves the lungs, chest/abdominal walls contract inwards, and the shoulders fall. At multiple phases of this respiratory mechanism, changes can be made to affect cellular oxygenation, stimulation of the autonomic nervous system, lymphatic flow, and thus total body health and healing (Fig. 92.1).

Many of the techniques used in therapeutic breathing modify this typical breathing cycle. Variations can occur in the following ways and in combinations of the following (Table 92.1):

1. Changing the pace and pattern of breathing
2. Emphasizing different muscles during a breathing cycle
3. Increasing/decreasing airway resistance during therapeutic breathing
4. Linking guided/mental imagery to the breathing process
5. Coordinating breath with movement

Of note, while several studies suggest that breathing modifications will have an immediate effect on the autonomic nervous system, as with other forms of mind-body medicine, the longer the practice period, the more prevalent the positive physiological changes and the more accessible these tools are in settings such as an acute episode of anxiety.

PACED AND PATTERNED BREATHING

First of all, the timing of the respiratory cycle can vary in many ways, and counting can be used to help keep track of this timing. One basic principle for promoting a relaxed state involves simply increasing the length of time spent inhaling and exhaling. This principle comes from the idea that there is a mutual connection between the nervous system and the breath. Shorter breaths or an increased respiratory rate can be the product of an activated nervous system via anxiety, anger, stress, etc. By voluntarily slowing the breathing rate, emotions and stress levels can be more easily stabilized.

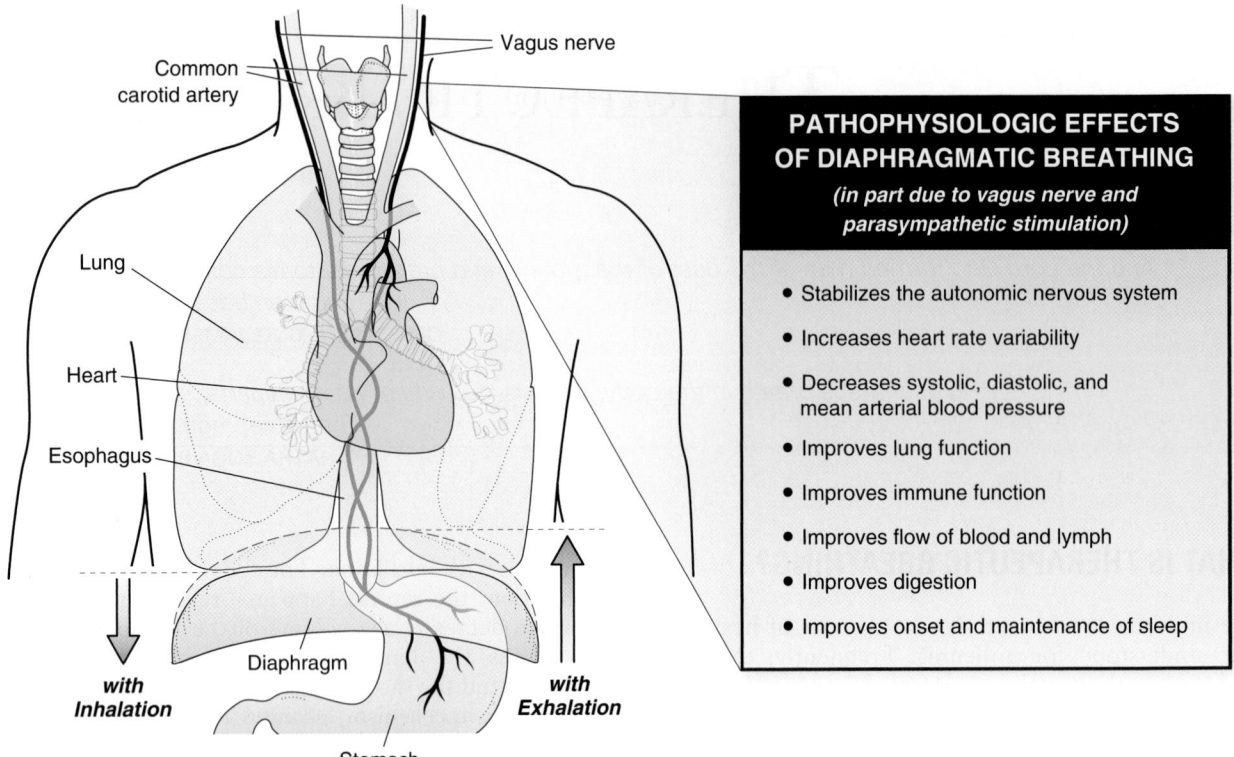

FIG. 92.1 ■ Pathophysiological effects of diaphragmatic breathing.

TABLE 92.1   Techniques Used in Therapeutic Breathing

Categories of Therapeutic Breathing	Examples
Paced or Patterned Breathing	6 breaths/minute, Buteyko method, 1:2 inhalation/exhalation ratio, Kapalabhati breathing, Bellows breathing, "Relaxing Breath"
Body Area/Muscle-Focused Breathing	Thoracic, abdominal/diaphragmatic
Breathing With Increased Airway Resistance	Pursed-lip breathing, alternate-nostril breathing, singing, chanting, vocal prayer, tip of the tongue to roof of the mouth
Imagery Combined With Breathing	Tonglen meditation, 3-Minute Breathing Space, Dan Tian breathing
Movement With Breath Work	Running, yoga, martial arts

It has been suggested that the optimal respiratory rate to enter a state of relaxation is approximately 6 breaths/minute.

Studies have shown that breathing at 6 cycles/minute improves heart rate variability, helps with insomnia,[4] treats hypertension (by increasing baroreflex sensitivity), decreases muscle sympathetic nerve activity,[5] and may help decrease hot flashes in menopausal women[6] (see Chapter 96). The RESPeRATE biofeedback device, which is the only FDA-approved nonpharmacological treatment for hypertension, enhances the benefits of this so-called "paced breathing," or intentionally slowed breathing. RESPeRATE consists of a control box, a respiration sensor, and headphones. The device senses a person's respiratory rate and then produces tones to indicate when to inhale and when to exhale. Over time, the tones sound at longer intervals, ultimately slowing a person's breathing pace to an ideal respiratory rate. The Buteyko method was developed in the 1950s under the principle that biochemical disturbances lead to dysfunctional breathing. This method teaches breath-holding techniques to "normalize" carbon dioxide levels, and research has shown moderate benefit in children with hyperventilation syndrome and in asthmatics.[7]

Another variation on this practice is that by intentionally *increasing* the respiratory rate; an overall increase in the body's parasympathetic tone can also be achieved. Kapalabhati breathing as well as Bellows (Bhastrika) breathing from the yogic tradition function in this manner. Both forms of isolated abdominal breathing work on bringing the respiratory rate to about 1–4 breaths/second. While both practices increase respiratory rate,

Kapalabhati breathing emphasizes sharp exhalations and passive inhalations. These stimulating practices can be used in the short term to help with fatigue, depression, and feeling cold.[8] In the long term, it has been shown that it is possible to decrease baseline heart rate and blood pressure as well as improve heart rate variability,[9] pulmonary function tests,[10] and cognitive function.[11]

> An inhalation-to-exhalation ratio of 1:2 has been shown to promote relaxation.

Some evidence suggests that in addition to modifying respiratory rates, practicing prolonged exhalations activates the parasympathetic nervous system and thus slows the heart rate and produces a relaxation response from the body. Multiple variations on this theme exist based on the particular teacher or tradition that is being practiced. The "Relaxing Breath" or "4-7-8" breathing exercise espoused by Dr. Andrew Weil suggests inhaling for a count of four, holding the breath for a count of seven, and then exhaling for a count of eight. What is most important is not the duration of each inhalation and exhalation, but simply the ratio between the two.[12] Some evidence supports a lower inhalation/exhalation ratio in promoting increased self-reported relaxation and energy as well as improved heart rate variability,[13] although other studies suggest that the breathing rate is more important than the pattern.[14,15]

MUSCLE/BODY EMPHASIS IN BREATH WORK

Most simply, breathing can be categorized as thoracic, abdominal, or diaphragmatic. Although the thorax, abdomen, and diaphragm have a continual interplay in nearly all types of breathing, certain breathing practices emphasize one over the others.

Thoracic breathing typically involves an expansion of the chest wall with inhalation and a contraction of the chest wall with exhalation. In settings of highly emotional states, such as sadness, anxiety, or anger, thoracic breathing often becomes the principal pattern of breathing. Shallow thoracic breathing then perpetuates the stress response by increasing respiratory rate, heart rate, and the overall sympathetic tone of the body. While these are critical functions of the body for survival, to be in a chronic state of activation can have negative health effects on nearly every organ system. It is important to note, however, that sometimes thoracic breathing can be used therapeutically. With complete, deep breathing, the rib cage and chest are intentionally expanded to create increased vital capacity. This may be beneficial for asthmatics.[16]

Abdominal breathing—often used synonymously with the term "diaphragmatic breathing" in published research—allows for a relaxed abdominal wall to expand and contract with every inhalation and exhalation, with minimal movement of the chest wall. This practice is commonly used in relaxation techniques and is often the breathing method used in research protocols. Some studies that have shown benefit from abdominal breathing including using this type of breathing alone or in conjunction with other therapies for the treatment of gastroesophageal reflux disease,[17] anxiety in patients receiving chemotherapy,[18] motion sickness,[19] chronic obstructive pulmonary disease (COPD),[20,21] pediatric functional constipation,[22] quality of life in patients with asthma,[23] and total body oxidative stress.[24]

> Abdominal breathing in most studies is practiced by having the patient either sit or lie supine with one hand on the abdomen and one hand on the chest. Slow, deep breathing is then initiated with careful attention to move the hand resting on the abdomen with each breath while maintaining a stillness in the hand that is on the chest.

AIRWAY RESISTANCE IN BREATH WORK

Intentional modifications to increase the resistance to the normal flow of air in and out of the lungs can be another therapeutic variance in some breathing exercises. These modifications can be either from changes in posturing while breathing or from external sources.

One common practice that has been well studied is that of pursed-lip breathing. Used effectively in people with chronic obstructive pulmonary disease, pursed-lip breathing helps to prop open bronchioles and alveoli by creating an increased pressure behind the lips (and subsequently, down to the lower airways) as air is forced through the smaller opening created by pursed lips. By keeping these lower airways open, more oxygen is able to diffuse through the alveoli to the general circulation and less carbon dioxide accumulates in the body. Hyperventilation and exhaustion from increased respiratory effort are thus diminished. A typical breathing exercise would involve inhaling through the nose with the mouth closed for a count of two, then exhaling through pursed lips for a count of four.[25] Increasing airflow resistance in this manner has been effective in improving exercise tolerance in patients with COPD[26] and treating dyspnea in the setting of COPD[27] as well as treating dyspnea secondary to lung cancer.[28]

Some forms of yogic breathing also incorporate therapeutic resistance; for example, Nadi Shodhana is translated from Sanskrit as "clearing the channels." Specifically, this term is used in reference to alternate-nostril breathing techniques.

> One variation of Nadi Shodhana: Using the right thumb to block the right nostril, inhale through the left nostril. At the end of the inhalation, block the left nostril with the right ring and small fingers and exhale through the right nostril. At the end of the exhalation, inhale again through the right nostril. Once again, use the right thumb to block the right nostril and exhale through the left nostril. Inhale through the left nostril and continue this cycle (http://www.chopra.com/nadi-shodhana-channel-clearing-breath).

A fairly strong evidence base suggests that alternate-nostril breathing has therapeutic effects including decreased systolic blood pressure,[29,30] increased heart rate variability,[29,31] improved metabolic resilience to stress,[32] improved mental attentiveness,[30] and improved coordination.[30]

While pursed-lip breathing and alternate-nostril breathing are two well-researched forms of therapeutic breathing that involve increasing airflow resistance, it is important to note that there are many other disciplines that involve modulating resistance. Singing, chanting, and praying are forms of therapeutic breathing that alter resistance by changing the shape of the vocal cords through which air passes. Some other breathing practices such as those of traditional Chinese medicine will suggest that the tip of the tongue be placed against the inside of the upper teeth. There is limited, if any, literature to explain how this would improve clinical outcomes; however, on a physical level, it does increase the resistance of the outflow of air from the mouth. From a Chinese medicine standpoint, the belief is that by touching the tip of the tongue to the back of the upper teeth, *qi*, or the body's "vital energy," may circulate more smoothly from the anterior *Ren Mai* meridian channel to the posterior *Du Mai* meridian channel, as these two energy channels meet at this location in the mouth.

Internal Imagery Linked to the Breathing Process

In addition to a focus on the timing and mechanics of breath work, imagery used in conjunction with breathing can have an added therapeutic benefit. The following are just a few examples in which breath work and imagery are used together.

Qigong and Zen meditation practices will use Dan Tian-focused (in Chinese) or Tanden-focused (in Japanese) breathing techniques. The Dan Tian (specifically the "lower" Dan Tian) refers to an internal area of the body located between the level of the umbilicus and the pubic symphysis. From a traditional Chinese medicine standpoint, this area is critical to maintaining the body's overall sense of balance and grounding. While there are many variations and traditions, Dan Tian breathing often involves the abdominal or diaphragmatic breathing, previously described, used in conjunction with a visualization of a ball of light located at the Dan Tian. With each inhalation, this focus of light may expand, while the exhalation either stabilizes the light or releases "smoke" or "darkness" from the body. While there is little, if any, research to support the therapeutic benefits of Dan Tian breathing, it is relevant to this discussion in that this practice overlaps to some extent with the realms of both guided imagery (see Chapter 97) and energy/biofield therapies (see Chapter 116), both of which have their own health benefits in the literature.

One of the more researched areas of medicine that incorporates breathing techniques with imagery is the Mindfulness-Based Stress Reduction program (MBSR) as well as the Mindfulness-Based Cognitive Therapy program (MBCT), the latter of which combines the principles of MBSR with cognitive behavioral therapy. These programs have been shown to be effective in treating depression, anxiety, posttraumatic stress disorder (PTSD), pain,

and stress.[33] "Mindful Breathing" is a part of the training program that allows for a present moment awareness of the breath and its physical effects on the body, thoughts, and emotions. One technique taught in MBSR is Tonglen meditation, which comes from Tibetan Buddhist practices and utilizes a combination of breathing exercises and guided imagery. Both techniques are also used in the 3-Minute Breathing Space practiced in MBCT.

TONGLEN MEDITATION:

With inhalation through the nose, visualize breathing in one's own anxiety, stress, and worries or those of the world. Then imagine these feelings/emotions being transformed within the body. With exhalation, visualize compassion and serenity leaving the mouth.

3-MINUTE BREATHING SPACE:

The first minute of this breathing practice involves bringing the attention to the present moment—body sensations, thoughts, and emotions. The second minute involves abdominal breathing and becoming aware of the sensations in the body that arise with this focus. The final minute of this practice involves envisioning/feeling not just the abdominal wall moving with each respiratory cycle but also the rest of the body—all the way to the fingers and toes.

Coordination of Breathing With Movement

One final classification of therapeutic breath work is intentional breathing coordinated with movement. While there are no particular studies showing the direct clinical benefits of well-coordinated breath with physical activity, these two practices need to be synchronized to elicit the most effective level of physical movement. Many examples of this coordination exist. When jogging or running, finding a breathing pattern timed to the footfall is important. Variations based on different coaching styles include inhaling for two to four steps and exhaling for the same number of steps or inhaling for two to four steps and then exhaling for a different number of steps to ensure the start of exhalation on a different foot with each respiratory cycle.[34,35] Either way, the breath is synchronized with the steps. Walking meditation also brings an intention to coordinating footsteps with the respiratory cycle.

As previously described, therapeutic breathing through *pranayama* is essential to the practice of yoga. The word pranayama is explained by B.K.S. Iyengar, who was known for founding the Iyengar style of yoga as well helping to bring the practice of yoga to the Western world: "Prana" means breath, respiration, life, vitality, energy, or strength. When used in the plural, it denotes certain vital breaths or currents of energy. "Ayama" means stretch, extension, expansion, length, breadth, regulation, prolongation, restraint, or control. "Pranayama" thus means the prolongation of breath and its restraint.[2] When combined with the movement practice of yoga, pranayama allows for smooth physical flow and mindful presence between and during the postures.

One last example is the *kiai*, or forceful expulsion of air in conjunction with a loud vocalization, used in martial arts. The term for this yell comes from Japanese traditions; however, it permeates other styles as well. The kiai is often used in synchrony with offensive movements as a way of accentuating the groundedness and power of a particular technique.

RESOURCES FOR PRACTICING THERAPEUTIC BREATHING

A variety of mobile device applications have been developed to assist with the practice of the principles of the previously described therapeutic breathing. One of the original applications developed by a division of the U.S. Department of Defense is called "Breathe2Relax." Adjustments can be made to increase and decrease the pacing of the respiratory cycle. There are also instructional videos that explain how to perform abdominal breathing (although it is referred to as "diaphragmatic breathing" in the application). This particular application does not allow for changing the pattern of the respiratory cycle. Applications such as "Pranayama" and "Breath Pacer" have functionality in adapting pace as well as the pattern of breathing.

Key Web Resources

Some websites that include free access to therapeutic breathing instructions and videos include:

University of Wisconsin, Department of Family Medicine, Integrative Medicine Website with videos demonstrating yogic breathing techniques; the chapter author's video recording of a paced breathing exercise	http://www.fammed.wisc.edu/our-department/media/integrative-medicine; www.youtube.com/watch?v=23K_IFus09w
Andrew Weil, MD: written and video demonstrations of three variations of paced and patterned breathing	http://www.drweil.com/drw/u/ART00521/three-breathing-exercises.html
UCSD Center for Mindfulness: audio file of guided meditation with a breathing awareness exercise	http://health.ucsd.edu/av/mindfulness/Awareness-of-Breath.mp3
Integrative Medicine For the Underserved: written description of therapeutic breathwork connected with imagery and movement; may be used in pediatric populations	http://im4us.org/app/Breathing+Technique+Patient+Handouts?structure=Toolkit
University of Michigan: written breathing exercises focusing on patterned breathing and coordination of breath with movement	http://im4us.org/app/Breathing+Technique+Patient+Handouts?structure=Toolkit

---

REFERENCES

References are available online at ExpertConsult.com.

Patient Handout

A stepwise approach to decreasing sympathetic tone through therapeutic breathing

1) Posture
   Correct posture is a critical component to effective therapeutic breathing. Typically, these techniques are practice in one of three positions – lying supine, sitting, or standing. Below are descriptions of proper posture in these positions.
   Lying supine: lie flat on the back, arms by the side with palms facing upwards. The feet may be separated from each other by several inches. To add comfort and support, a pillow or bolster may be placed under the head and/or under both knees

   Sitting: sit upright in a chair or on a cushion with the sitting bones resting closer to the edge of the chair or cushion. Both feet are flat on the ground, separated by a few inches, if seated in a chair. If sitting on a cushion the legs may be folded and resting on the ground or mat beneath the cushion. The back is straight – without slouching and also without over extending the back. Hands may rest palm down on the top of the knees. Shoulders may relax down and back – paying attention that the shoulders neither slouch forward nor strain backwards too much. Sometimes it is helpful to imagine a string connected to the top of the head gently pulling upwards, allowing the spine's natural curvature to be maintained.

   Standing: similar to sitting, maintaining the integrity of a natural upright posture without straining is important to allowing for effective therapeutic breathing. Feet may be hip-width apart with a very slight bend to the knees. Similar positioning of the back, shoulders and head may be used as with sitting. Arms may rest lightly by the side of the body.

2) Breath awareness
   Once the body has been positioned in a restfully alert way, the attention may shift to the breath. Place the left hand on the lower abdomen and the right hand on the chest. Begin by noticing how the hands move with a normal, unmodified breath. Particularly pay attention to which hand moves and how much that hand moves during each breath.

3) Abdominal breathing
   After taking 5–10 "aware" breaths, shift the focus of the breath to the abdomen. With each inhale, allow the abdomen to expand outwards and with each exhale allow the abdomen to naturally contract inwards. The hand that is resting on the abdomen should be moving almost exclusively, while the hand on the chest has minimal movements. This attention to only moving the abdominal wall allows for cultivation of "abdominal breathing" and ultimately increased relaxation response during this breathing exercise. Of note, placing a book or a sandbag on the lower abdomen during reclining therapeutic breathing may help to provide some direction with regard to how to focus the movement of the breath on the abdomen versus the thoracic cavity.

4) Paced breathing
   The next step is to incorporate a pace or tempo to the breath. The ideal respiratory rate to promote a relaxation response in the body is 6 breaths per minute or one respiratory cycle every ten seconds. Begin with inhalation for a count of two and exhalation for a count of two. Gradually increase to inhaling for a count of five and exhaling for a count of five, as this would result in one breathing cycle in 10 seconds, or 6 breaths per minute.

5) Patterned breathing
   Lastly, to add some variation or pattern to the breath work, the lengths of inhalation and exhalation may be varied. One way to promote a relaxed state is to exhale twice as long as inhale. If breathing at 6 breaths per minute has become comfortable with practice, then inhaling for 3 seconds and exhaling for 7 seconds is an option and a good place to start practicing. Some practices involve varying the length of time that the breath is held between inhalation and exhalation as well as between exhalation and inhalation; however, research does not clearly state how variations in these pauses change the relaxation response.

FIG. 92.2 ■ Patient handout.

CHAPTER 93

LOW BACK PAIN EXERCISES

Brian Degenhardt, DO • Coleen Smith, DO

The management of patients who seek treatment for low back pain can be difficult for any practitioner. The cause of low back pain can be the skin, soft tissue, or skeletal components. Low back pain can be referred from other sources, even visceral structures, or it can be secondary to postural decompensation.

History and physical findings should guide the practitioner to further evaluation and a treatment plan. Multidisciplinary treatment approaches are often necessary to facilitate healing for the patient with low back pain. Understanding of the patient's belief system about his or her low back pain may be an important component of recovery.[1] A treatment plan may include an exercise prescription. Movement, strengthening, and flexibility in patients with chronic lumbar back pain has demonstrated benefit.[2]

The traditional exercise prescription is a written description of the exercise, including the number of repetitions per set, number of sets per session, and frequency of sessions. This format is specific for strength exercises and has been applied to flexibility exercises. Many traditional exercise routines are assigned and performed too literally, without recognition of the subtle changes the patient experiences day to day in a healing exercise program. The goal of any complementary exercise recommendation is to encourage a dynamic interchange between the patient's awareness and the body. With appropriate education, the patient can become more sensitive to information being generated from the body and perform the exercise program in a much more precise, safe, and effective manner. Attention to the body's feedback mechanisms should be encouraged to allow the patient to modify any portion of the exercise prescription. This enables the patient to achieve optimal outcomes from the rehabilitation program. The outcomes of an exercise plan are to enhance flexibility, to minimize or to eliminate pain by reducing muscle tension, and to improve strength, thereby encouraging joint stability. A complementary exercise plan for a person with lumbar back pain should include the following approaches:

- Breathing and relaxation training
- Flexibility training
- Strength training
- Coordination training

The National Institute of Health and Clinical Excellence (NICE) has reviewed the evidence of therapies that have been found to be most useful for low back pain. Of all therapies used for low back pain, the evidence for benefit with least harm supported an exercise program, manual therapy, and acupuncture.[3]

The Patient Handout at the end of this chapter contains examples of the exercises and approaches discussed here.

BREATHING AND RELAXATION TRAINING

Flexibility and relaxation techniques are often great starting points in a patient's exercise prescription. They calm the patient and foster awareness of information from the body that helps guide and individualize the exercise prescription. These exercises enhance diaphragmatic function and improve oxygenation, lymphatic flow, and autonomic nervous system regulation. To begin this component of the exercise prescription, the patient should choose a comfortable position and minimize distraction, perhaps by listening to soothing background music. The patient must use the abdominal diaphragm while taking a slow, deep breath and both the diaphragm and the rib cage as inspiration continues (see Chapter 92, Breathing Exercises). The number of repetitions is likely to vary from day to day because stress and tightness also change daily. The patient needs to learn to recognize when the body is relaxed and ready to move on to other components of the exercise prescription. Once relaxation and focus have been obtained, participants should use deep breathing throughout all cycles of the exercise plan.

FLEXIBILITY TRAINING

The flexibility portion of an exercise plan uses stretching to promote greater range of motion in all planes. Properly performed, stretching allows better neuromusculoskeletal function, promoting less pain and more motion. To stretch properly, the patient must move to the point of tension and then perform deep breaths to gently stretch the tight tissue. It is important to move slowly and gently in and out of stretches. Other models describe how to stretch, but this approach minimizes the chance of exacerbating a patient's back pain by overstretching. Although an outline of a stretch gives the patient a guide to promote flexibility of specific areas of the body, the patient listens each day to the information the body is generating to determine where the tightness is. This approach allows the patient to modify a stretch and to maximize its effectiveness each day. The stretch is considered complete only after the patient appreciates a change in the tension while holding the stretch. This change can occur after only one or two repetitions, or it may need more repetitions, as determined by the patient through attention to the body's feedback system. Patients must stay within their pain limitations to prevent reflex muscle tightening and injury.

In most patients with chronic low back pain, specific instruction is necessary for hip flexors and extensors. For recovery from muscle tightness and to decrease pain, it is also important to achieve greater flexibility as well as a balance of flexibility between the same muscles on the two sides of the body and between reciprocal muscles, particularly with the hamstring, iliopsoas, and piriformis muscles.

STRENGTH TRAINING

Strengthening exercises encourage active use of muscle groups, leading to better muscle tone and greater strength. It is important not to sacrifice flexibility for strength; the two are equally important for proper lumbar mechanics in patients with low back pain. The clinician can evaluate the patient's strength clinically by having the patient perform isometric contractions against the physician's resistance to determine whether there is gross asymmetry of strength. Asymmetry of strength may lead to or be secondary to hypertonicity in one muscle group and weakness in the opposing muscle groups. Once strength asymmetry or weakness has been diagnosed, specific instructions must be given first to stretch the hypertonic muscles and then to motivate the patient to exercise the weakened muscles. Patients are often unaware of this local muscle weakness. In many exercise programs, patients focus on rote repetition of exercises, strengthening hypertonic muscles rather than conditioning weakened muscle groups. It can be beneficial for the patient with hypertonic lumbar extensors to perform abdominal curl-ups to strengthen weakened antagonistic abdominal muscles after stretching the lumbar erector spinae muscles. Both exercises decrease hypertonicity in the lumbar extensor muscle group.

In many cases of lumbar back pain, strengthening activities must start out as isometric exercises instead of the typical isotonic exercises because isometric exercises are safer. Isometric exercises allow the origin and insertion of the involved muscle to remain in constant position while the patient presses against a resisting force that is equal to the patient's force.

An example of an isometric exercise is pushing against a solid wall without moving. Isometric exercises are often useful for patients who have arthritis, in which joint movement causes pain and limitation.

COORDINATION TRAINING

Differences in proprioception exist in individuals with and without back pain. Coordination training in patients with low back pain is based on the observation that the response of a patient's spine to stress causes the postural muscles to tighten and the antagonist muscles to react with inhibition, weakness, and atrophy.[4] Coordination training is imperative for improvement of overall postural balance in the patient with lumbar back pain. Proprioceptive education in patients with low back pain begins with improving ankle, knee, and pelvis coordination, perhaps through the use of a wobble board or fitness ball. The physician must remind the patient of safety precautions at the start of coordination training. Basic coordination exercises can usually be taught in the office and then performed by the patient independently. Advanced proprioceptive training usually requires supervision to ensure correct technique and safety.

Key Web Resources	
The Egoscue technique addresses strengthening and balancing of the whole body unit to reduce back pain. A book that includes back stretching exercises from this method is Escogue P, Gitnes R: *Pain Free: A Revolutionary Method for Stopping Chronic Pain.* New York: Bantam Books; 2000.	http://www.egoscue.com/
Video on how Feldenkrais therapy can be used for low back pain from the University of Wisconsin Integrative Medicine Program.	http://www.fammed.wisc.edu/feldenkrais-low-back-pain/

REFERENCES

References are available online at ExpertConsult.com.

Patient Handout: Exercise Program for Low Back Pain

1. Listen to your body signals; the amount of exercise may vary from day to day. Always stay within pain limitations when performing any exercises.
2. It is important to breathe properly. While performing all aspects of your stretching program, breathe into your abdomen and feel the sides of your rib cage expand.
3. Move slowly and gently during stretching exercises. Do not bounce!
4. If you experience pain during or after a specific exercise, decrease the duration and intensity of the exercise. If the pain reoccurs, eliminate that exercise from your routine and consult with an exercise professional.

Breathing and Relaxation Exercises
Breathing and Body Stretch

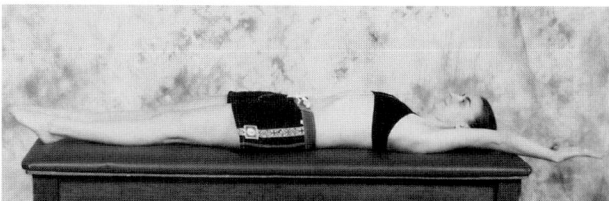

1. Lie on your back. Place your hands on your abdomen. Relax. This is your time to focus on yourself.
2. Breathe deeply into your abdomen so that your hands rise and fall with each breath. Feel the sides of your rib cage expand.
3. Hold your breath in for 3 to 5 seconds, and then exhale slowly.
4. Repeat steps 2 and 3 slowly and gently for 2 minutes.
5. Place your arms above your head and reach upward as you point your toes downward.
6. Hold the stretch for 5 slow, deep breaths.
7. Slowly return to the starting position, and repeat the stretch until the tissue tension experienced during the first stretch has resolved (often 2 times).

Stretching Exercises
Pelvic Tilt Exercise

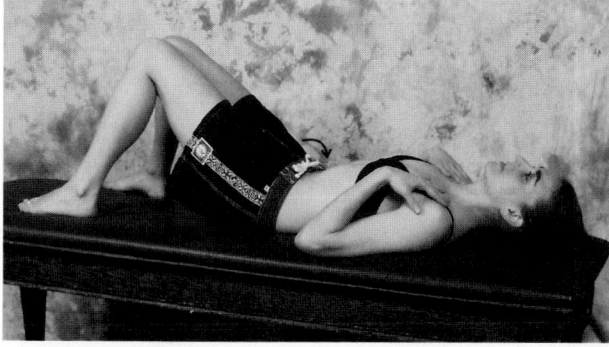

1. Lie on your back. Bend your knees, placing your feet flat on the floor and allowing your knees to touch.
2. Roll your pelvis backward by pushing your belly button toward your spine.
3. Hold this position for 20 to 40 seconds or until fatigued, while breathing slowly and deeply.
4. Release slowly. Repeat.

Low Back Flexion Exercise

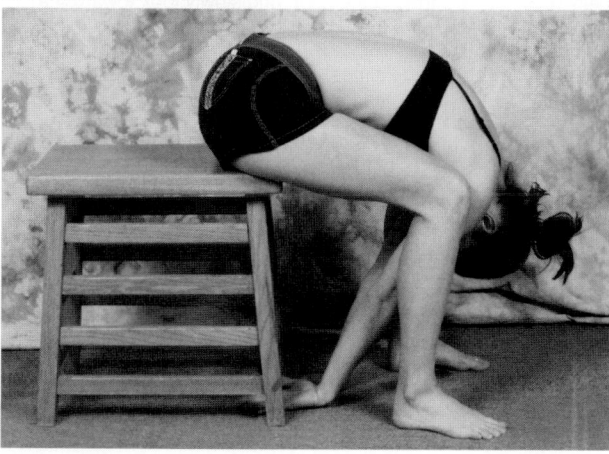

1. Sit. Curl your spine forward one vertebra at a time, from the head, to the neck, chest, and low back. Stop at and hold at any area of muscle tightness.
2. Hold position for 3 deep breaths or until the tissue relaxes.
3. Gently return to a sitting position.
4. Repeat at least 2 times, likely curling farther than the time before, until the tissue tension experienced along the spine has resolved, or if soreness has developed. Be patient with this stretch. It may take weeks before you can easily stretch all the way down the back.

Low Back Extension Exercise

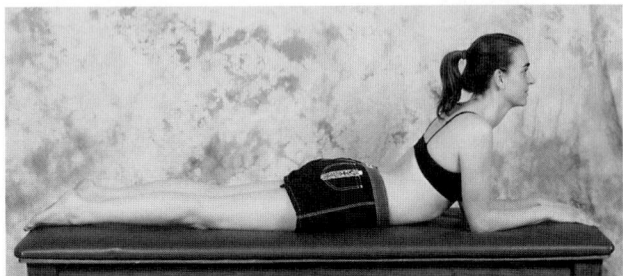

1. Lie on your stomach with your feet shoulder-width apart and your toes pointing downward.
2. Bring your elbows under your shoulders to support your weight.
3. Gently raise your head and slowly arch your back, letting your belly relax forward toward the floor. Go only as far as is painless until your muscles are more flexible.
4. Hold position and breathe into your abdomen for at least 3 deep breaths or until the tightness in your back releases.
5. Repeat until the tissue tension experienced during first stretch has resolved (often 2 times).

Cat/Dog Stretch Exercise

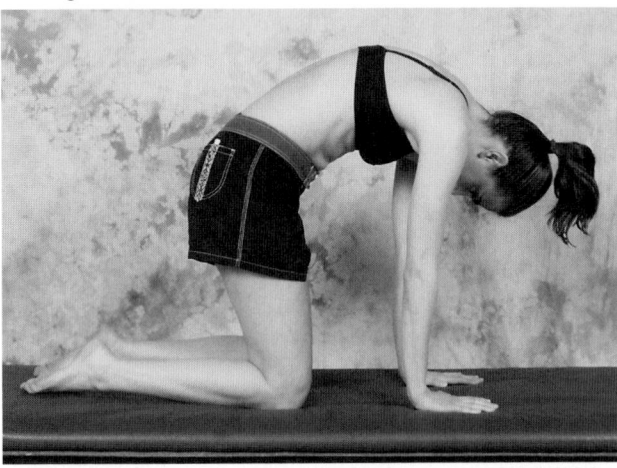

1. Kneel on the floor with your knees hip-width apart. Place your hands on the floor shoulder-width apart and palms down.
2. Slowly arch your back from your tailbone to your upper back like a cat stretches. Allow your head to lower comfortably. Hold position for 3 slow breaths.
3. Slowly release the stretch in the reverse order.
4. Once in the starting position, lift your buttocks upward, let your belly relax forward toward the floor, and slowly look toward the ceiling.
5. Hold this position for 3 breaths and gradually return to the starting position.
6. Repeat until the tissue tension experienced during the first stretch has resolved (often 2 times).

Hip Flexor Stretch Exercise

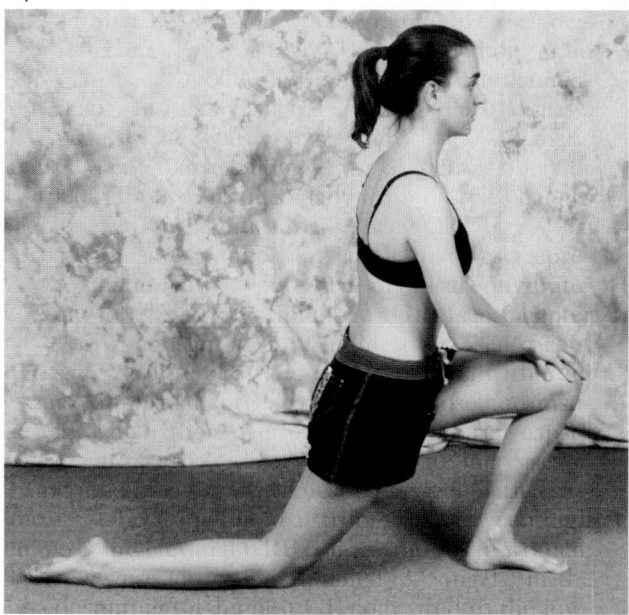

1. Kneel on one knee. Bend your other knee to 90 degrees and place your hands on it for balance.
2. Lean your trunk forward while keeping your low back straight.
3. Hold this position for 3 slow breaths, and then slowly return to the starting position.
4. Repeat until the tissue tension experienced during the first stretch has resolved (often 2 times).

Piriformis Exercise

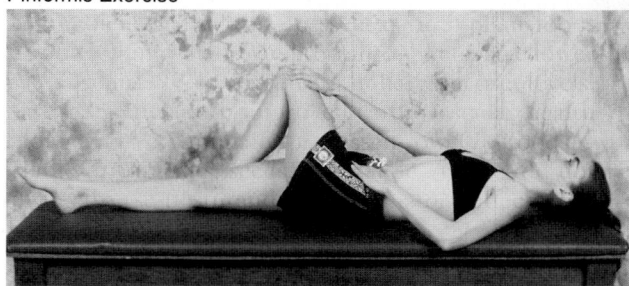

1. Lie on your back with your legs straight. To stretch the left side, bend your left knee and place your left ankle over your right knee with the left foot on floor.
2. Place your left hand on the left side of the pelvis and your right hand on your left knee.
3. Slowly pull your left knee across the right leg, feeling the stretch in your left buttock. Keep your pelvis from rotating off the floor with your left hand.
4. Hold this position for at least 3 slow deep breaths.
5. Slowly and gently return to the resting position.
6. Repeat steps 1 thru 6 until the tissue tension experienced during the first stretch has resolved (often 2 times).
7. Repeat with the right leg.

Hamstring Exercise

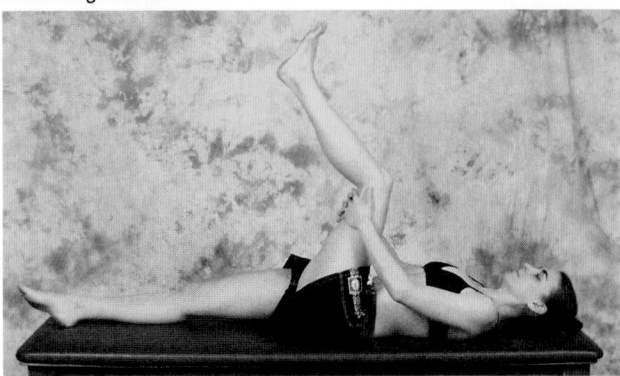

1. Lie on your back with your legs straight.
2. Gently bend one knee and grasp behind the thigh. Do not lift your pelvis or other knee off the floor during this exercise.
3. Straighten your knee. Go only as far as your flexibility will comfortably allow, and hold for 3 slow breaths.
4. Slowly lower your leg to the floor, and repeat for the other leg.
5. Repeat each side until the tissue tension experienced during the first stretch has resolved (often 2 times).

Strength Exercises
Abdominal Curl-Up Exercise

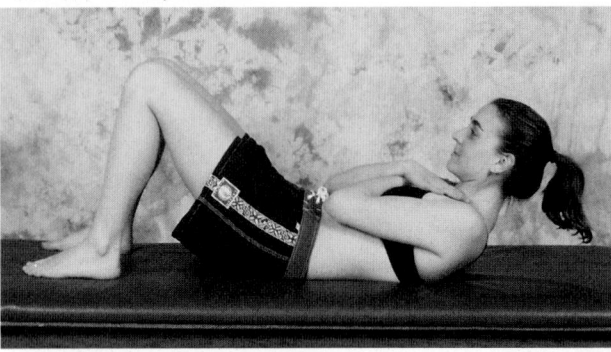

1. Lie on your back with your knees comfortably bent and your arms placed across your chest.
2. Keeping your neck and shoulders relaxed, lift your rib cage from the floor. Move only as far as your body will allow without pain. Hold position for 1 or 2 deep breaths.
3. Slowly and gently return to resting position.
4. Repeat until your abdominal muscles weaken or you notice that you are using your neck and shoulder muscles to perform the exercise.

Gluteus Maximus Exercise

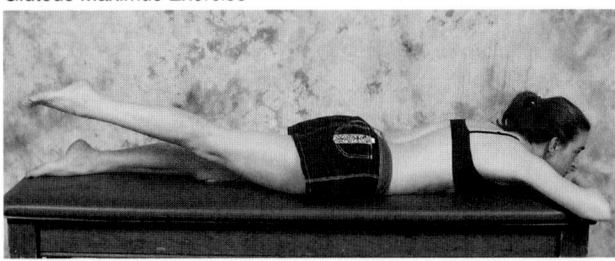

1. Lie on your stomach with your toes pointing downward and your legs straight.
2. Slowly raise one leg as far as is comfortable. Keep your pelvis flat on the floor and the buttock on that side tight.
3. Hold position for 3 deep breaths, or until muscles feel fatigued.
4. Gently return to the resting position. Repeat with the other leg.
5. Repeat with both legs until your muscles feel fatigued.

Gluteus Medius Exercise

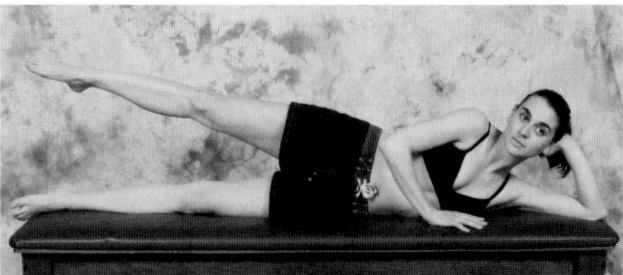

1. Lie on one side, keeping the leg that is on the floor straight or bent at the hip and knee and your top hand on the floor in front of you to maintain stability.
2. Raise your upper leg as far as is comfortable and painless, using your hip muscles only.
3. Hold this position for 3 slow breaths, and slowly return the leg to the resting position.
4. Repeat until fatigued or until you are using other than your hip muscles, and increase repetitions as tolerated.
5. Turn to your other side and repeat steps 1 through 4.

Coordination Exercises
Standing-on-One-Leg Exercise

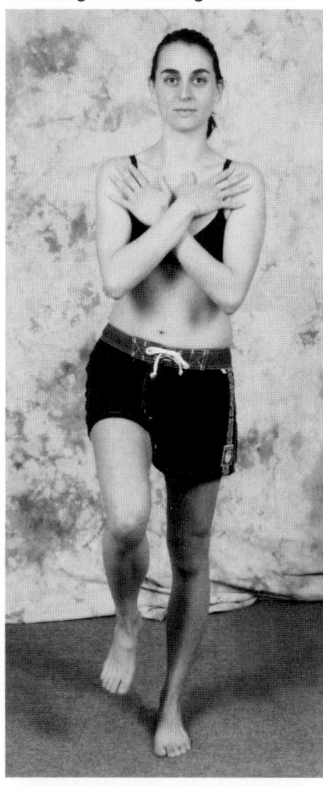

1. Stand on one leg and maintain your balance. Keep your back straight and your arms across your upper chest.
2. Hold this position for 1 minute while continuing slow, deep breaths.
3. Gently return to resting position and repeat 2 times on each leg.
4. After mastering this exercise, perform step 2 with your eyes closed.

SECTION II

MIND-BODY

SECTION OUTLINE

94 RELAXATION TECHNIQUES

95 SELF-HYPNOSIS TECHNIQUES

96 ENHANCING HEART RATE VARIABILITY

97 GUIDED IMAGERY AND INTERACTIVE GUIDED IMAGERY

98 JOURNALING FOR HEALTH

99 FORGIVENESS

100 RECOMMENDING MEDITATION

101 MOTIVATIONAL INTERVIEWING

102 EMOTIONAL AWARENESS FOR PAIN

103 ENERGY PSYCHOLOGY

CHAPTER 94

RELAXATION TECHNIQUES

Vincent J. Minichiello, MD

"... stress, in addition to being itself and the result of itself, is also the cause of itself"
F. ROBERTS, "STRESS AND THE GENERAL ADAPTATION SYNDROME," BRITISH MEDICAL JOURNAL, JULY 8, 1950,
PAGES 104-105, IN AN ATTEMPT TO UNDERSTAND THE NEW TERM "STRESS" AS USED BY DR. HANS SELYE[1]

"... it is not the potential stressor itself but how you perceive it and then how you handle it that will determine whether or not it will lead to stress."
JON KABAT-ZINN, PHD, *FULL CATASTROPHE LIVING*, REVISED EDITION, PAGE 290[2]

"... mind body science has now reached a stage where it should be accepted as the third major treatment and prevention option, standing as an equal alongside drugs and surgery in the clinical medical pantheon."
HERBERT BENSON, MD, *RELAXATION REVOLUTION*, PREFACE.[3]

INTRODUCTION

As suggested by Dr. Benson in the above excerpt, mind-body medicine—within which relaxation techniques play a central role—currently has an adequate foundation in evidence-based medical practices to be an important consideration in the treatment of a vast number of disease states as well as in the maintenance of overall wellbeing. This chapter will briefly review the history and science of stress and its opposite—relaxation. A small sampling of the research in these fields over the past half century will be introduced followed by a discussion of a variety of relaxation techniques, advice about how to prescribe them, and some resources for practice. Using these techniques on a regular basis allows for relaxation to become a habituated response to the stressors of both daily life and chronic disease, ultimately promoting systemic health and healing.

A Brief History of Stress and Relaxation

The concept of stress in relation to the health of human beings spans back to ancient civilizations. Hippocrates is attributed with the statement that disease not only involved *pathos* (suffering) but also *ponos* (toil), suggesting that illness is not purely an organic process.[4] While this understanding may have been inherent in ancient Greece, as Western medicine evolved, a schism developed in the scientific community when René Descartes, the 17th century mathematician, proposed that the mind and body are two distinct "substances" in *The Principles of Philosophy* written in 1644. Not until the early 20th century did this theory come into question. In 1926, Dr. William Cannon wrote an article entitled, "Physiological Regulation of Normal States: Some Tentative Postulates Concerning Biological Homeostatics," in which he discussed what is known today as the fight-or-flight response. He proposed that mammals have the ability to react to outside stimuli that disturb the body's "homeostasis" by increasing levels of hormones such as norepinephrine, which in turn create life-saving physiological changes including increased heart rate, respiratory rate, blood pressure, etc.[5] In 1936, Dr. Hans Selye, a Hungarian endocrinologist, built on Cannon's work, publishing an article in the journal *Nature* that described his research on rats showing that when these animals were exposed to different "stressors," such as cold, surgical injury, or toxic drugs, their bodies all yielded the same pathological changes on both macroscopic and microscopic scales.[6] In his 1956 book *The Stress of Life*, Dr. Selye defined stress as "the nonspecific response of the body to any demand made upon it."[7] Henceforth, "stress" became a part of the international vernacular. As the damaging effects of stress on the body were more and more understood, Dr. Herbert Benson, a cardiologist at Harvard Medical School, discovered the antidote to stress, which he termed the *relaxation response*. In the 1975 book with that title, he described the relaxation response simply as the opposite of the fight-or-flight response. This landmark book discussed research proving that elicitation of a state of relaxation will help decrease blood pressure, heart rate, respiratory rate, and metabolic rate.[8] Since its publication, many other studies have shown the benefits of relaxation in treating various disease states (see the section **The Science of Stress and Relaxation**). Most recently, relaxation research has moved in the direction of epigenetics as studies have begun to show that relaxation training can modify gene expression.

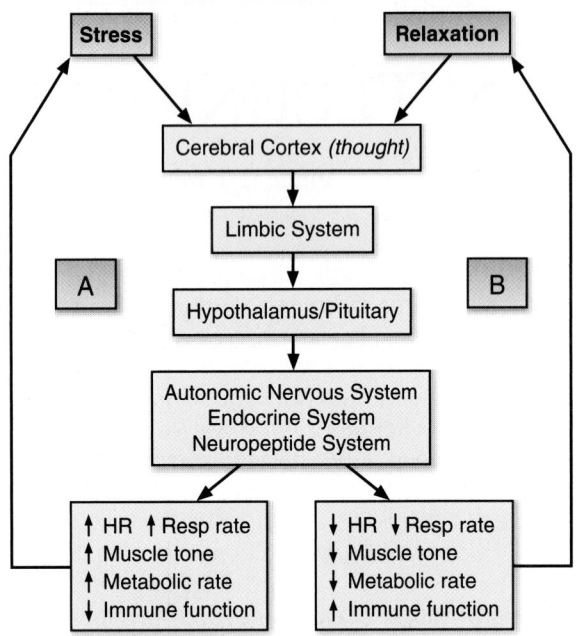

FIG. 94.1 ▪ A simplified chart showing the cyclic mind-body and body-mind influences of stress *(A)* and relaxation *(B)* on health. As our body experiences the physical responses to stress and relaxation, our central nervous system remembers them, thus causing a continuation of the cycle with long-term positive or negative physical consequences. *HR*, heart rate; *Resp*, respiratory.

The Science of Stress and Relaxation

Both the flight-or-fight and relaxation responses involve a complex interplay of endocrine, immune, neurological, and psychological systems (Fig. 94.1). From a neurological standpoint, when a stress response is elicited, the sympathetic nervous system is activated—norepinephrine is released from the locus coeruleus in the brainstem, triggering systemic changes including increased blood pressure, increased heart rate, increased respiratory rate, increased glucose production, and decreased stimulation of the gastrointestinal tract. The hypothalamus in the brain is also triggered as a result of the stress response, allowing for downstream endocrine-related hormonal changes as a part of the hypothalamus-pituitary-adrenal axis. The hypothalamus releases corticotropin-releasing hormone (CRH), which triggers the anterior pituitary gland to release adrenocorticotropic hormone (ACTH), which acts on the adrenal glands and ultimately leads to an increase in systemic cortisol. Cortisol then helps with the redistribution of glucose to vital organs, which is needed to cope with the stress response. The immune system is intricately connected as well because elevated levels of cortisol have an immunosuppressive effect, primarily on T cells, thus leading to an increased potential for infection. Increased cortisol levels inhibit interleukin (IL)-2 (a T-cell growth factor), induce T-cell apoptosis, and impair release of these immune cells from lymphoid tissue.[9] In a healthy system, after the acute stress response is elicited, cortisol will become part of a negative feedback loop, suppressing further release of CRH and ACTH.

While all of these physiological changes are beneficial in the case of acute, short-term stressors, with continually

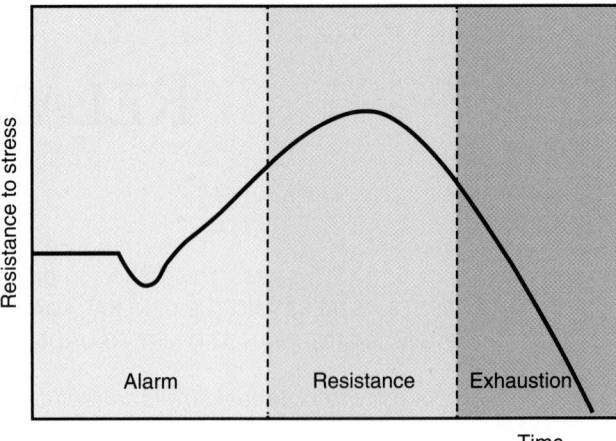

FIG. 94.2 ▪ General adaptation syndrome.

elevated stress levels, a chronic stress syndrome will evolve. Dr. Hans Selye described this progression in what he termed the *general adaptation syndrome* (Fig. 94.2).

> General Adaptation Syndrome: The first phase of this syndrome is the "alarm" response, in which the body is shocked and then attempts to adapt to the stressor. The second "resistance" phase involves further adaptation to the stressful stimulus. As long as the stressor is temporary, this resistance phase will result in a return to the body's homeostasis; however, if the stress continues, the body's resistance will decrease, ultimately resulting in the third phase, which Dr. Selye described as the "exhaustion" phase.

Chronic stress will thus result in more permanent physiological changes, including hypertension, insulin resistance, and chronic immunosuppression, among many other conditions.

So how does relaxation fit in? From a physiological standpoint, the relaxation response—as it is elicited by any of the techniques outlined in Table 94.1—will produce the opposite biochemical and hormonal changes that result from the fight-or-flight response. From the standpoint of the general adaptation syndrome, regular practice of relaxation techniques improves a person's overall resistance to stressors and promotes homeostasis. While the exact mechanism of action is still unclear, over the past 40 years since the realization of the relaxation response, numerous high-quality studies have shown the benefit of relaxation techniques in treating the following conditions: headaches,[10,11] hypertension,[12-14] premature ventricular contractions,[15] anxiety,[16-19] depression,[17-21] premenstrual syndrome,[22] female infertility,[23,24] insomnia,[25] diminished cognition,[26] irritable bowel syndrome (IBS),[27,28] and chronic pain.[29] Two seminal papers in the field of mind-body medicine suggest possible mechanisms by which relaxation produces the previously described effects. One article, published in 2006, suggests that the relaxation response increases fractional exhalation of nitric oxide, an outcome that has been associated with antibacterial, antiviral, and cardioprotective effects on the body.[3,30] Another article published in 2008 showed that the relaxation response can modify gene expression by

TABLE 94.1 **Relaxation Techniques**

Relaxation Technique	Brief Description	Resources
Autogenic Training	Developed by German psychiatrist Johannes Schultz, this technique promotes relaxation by training the body to decrease sympathetic tone via self-suggestions such as "my arms and legs are heavy." Similar to guided imagery and hypnosis, this technique involves visualization, and while it is often self-guided, it may also be facilitated by a trained practitioner.	Script to use for self-guided autogenic training: http://www.stress-relief-tools.com/autogenic-relaxation.html The British Autogenic Society: http://www.autogenic-therapy.org.uk/
Centering Prayer	A contemplative form of prayer originating from Christianity that involves focusing on a "sacred word," acknowledging other thoughts and then letting them go, and in general being more receptive in communication with God. Though its origins come from as early as the 3rd century AD, this practice has been brought to modern religious practice by Fathers William Meninger, M. Basil Pennington, and Abbot Thomas Keating.	A resource for learning about centering prayer and a listing of workshops: http://www.contemplativeoutreach.org/ *Centering Prayer: Renewing an Ancient Christian Prayer Form*, by M Basil Pennington *Open Mind, Open Heart*, by Thomas Keating
Clinical Hypnosis	Similar to the practice of guided imagery in that this technique may be self-guided or guided by an outside source. Typically, hypnosis is individualized and involves an induction phase, the visualization/treatment itself, and then guidance out of the trance state of mind.	See Chapter 95 http://www.healingwithhypnosis.com American Society of Clinical Hypnosis Practitioner Search Engine: http://www.asch.net/Public/MemberReferralSearch.aspx
Exercise	Just as tai chi and yoga are able to elicit a relaxation response, aerobic exercise that involves a focused mind and coordination of physical activity with breathing can also help with stress management.	See Chapter 91 *Beyond the Relaxation Response*, by Herbert Benson
Guided Imagery	A variety of techniques involving visualizations—either self-guided or from an outside source—that can cultivate relaxing thoughts and emotions.	See Chapter 97 http://thehealingmind.org/anxiety-and-stress http://www.healthjourneys.com/kaiser/relieveStress_flash.asp Academy for Guided Imagery Practitioner Search Engine: http://www.healthy.net/scr/PractitionerSearch.aspx?AssocId=8
Meditation	This is a general term that encompasses a great variety of techniques originating from multiple cultures and belief systems, each with their own body of research proving improved health outcomes related to their ability to help manage stress. In general, these techniques promote relaxation by utilizing principles discussed in this chapter, including an active participation in the meditation, a "let-it-be" mind frame, and consistent practice. Some of the commonly practiced forms of meditation include mindfulness meditation, transcendental meditation, and Zen meditation.	See Chapter 100 *Full Catastrophe Living: Using the Wisdom of Your Body and Mind to Face Stress, Pain and Illness*, by Jon Kabat-Zinn (introduction to Mindfulness Meditation) http://www.tm.org (introduction to transcendental meditation [TM] and source for finding local TM practitioners) Zen meditation centers may be searched by city. https://www.headspace.com/meditation-for-beginners (a free website designed to introduce the basic concepts of meditation in general)
Music Therapy	This practice uses music to induce relaxation. Depending on the individual, this type of therapy may be receptive or active and may be practiced alone or with the assistance of a trained music therapist.	American Music Therapy Association Practitioner Search Engine: http://www.musictherapy.org/about/find/
Progressive Muscle Relaxation (PMR)	This technique involves bringing one's attention to various parts of the body followed by tightening then relaxing each part of the body in a progressive fashion. The relaxation portion of this practice is typically coordinated with therapeutic breathing.	Audio files for PMR practice: https://caps.byu.edu/audio-files https://www.dartmouth.edu/~healthed/relax/downloads.html http://www.cmhc.utexas.edu/stressrecess/Level_Two/progressive.html
Tai Chi (Tai Ji Quan)/ Qigong	Tai Chi is a Chinese martial art practiced typically with slower, intentional movements coordinated with breathing. There are traditionally five "families" or styles of tai chi. Qigong, translated as "cultivation of qi," usually involves stationary breathing/movement techniques with a goal towards promoting healthy flow and development of qi, or "vital energy." Tai chi, when practiced well, may be considered a form of qigong.	*The Way of Qigong*, by Kenneth Cohen—an introduction to the history, philosophy, and practice of Qigong *The Harvard Medical School Guide to Tai Chi*, by Peter Wayne Tai Chi and Qigong Teacher Search Engine (not exhaustive, but may provide a starting place): http://www.americantaichi.net/TaiChiQigongClass.asp

Continued

TABLE 94.1 **Relaxation Techniques—cont'd**

Relaxation Technique	Brief Description	Resources
Therapeutic Breathing	As the basis for many of the relaxation techniques described, therapeutic breathing begins by simply bringing an awareness to one's natural respiratory mechanism. A relaxation response may be further elicited by practicing abdominal breathing, changing the respiratory rate to 6 breaths/minute, as well as by breathing with an inhalation:exhalation ratio of 1:2.	See Chapter 92 http://health.ucsd.edu/av/mindfulness/ Awareness-of-Breath.mp3 http://www.drweil.com/drw/u/ART00521/ three-breathing-exercises.html
Yoga	A collection of practices originating from India that involves not only physical postures (*asanas*), but also focuses on breathing, relaxation, diet, and meditation. There are many styles with variations in the way that the asanas are practiced. Yoga therapy is another modality that often involves one-on-one instruction to individualize the yoga practice for a particular condition or medical problem.	*Yoga as Medicine: The Yogic Prescription for Health and Healing*, by Timothy McCall Yoga Alliance Certified Instructor Search Engine: https://www.yogaalliance.org/directory International Association of Yoga Therapists Practitioner Search Engine http://iayt.site-ym.com/search/custom. asp?id=1156

counteracting the cellular changes that occur as a result of chronic stress.[31] Other studies continue to build on this research with some data to suggest that meditation techniques may suppress stress-induced inflammatory responses as well as upregulate mitochondrial function, insulin secretion, and telomerase maintenance.[32,33] More research is necessary to determine these as well as other possible mechanisms by which relaxation techniques have a salutogenic effect on the mind-body unit.

Relaxation Technique Essentials

As outlined in Table 94.1, variety of relaxation techniques have been utilized for millennia with the purpose of promoting overall wellbeing, preventing illness, and treating disease. What are some of the common components of these techniques?

Active Participation

While the word "relaxation" may sound like a person need not do anything and could simply become "flaccid" or "passive" in mind and body, the opposite is in fact true for these relaxation techniques to have a positive health effect. Whether the technique involves movement or not, both the mind and the body are engaged. In practicing tai chi, for example, when there are pauses in the movements, the arms and hands do not become relaxed in the sense that they are flaccid. Instead, there is an intention, awareness, and mindful presence within the still and "relaxed" limbs and entire body. Likewise, when sitting to meditate, the mind remains active even in stillness. Though meditation may sometimes lead to falling asleep, the state of mind during sleep will not elicit the physiological changes produced by practicing with an alert and relaxed mind.

"Let-It-Be" Mindset

This aspect of relaxation techniques is explicitly mentioned in practicing mindfulness meditation as well as in eliciting the relaxation response; however, it is central to other practices as well. As human beings, the mind will naturally wander—for some people more than others. Jon Kabat-Zinn, founder of the Mindfulness-Based Stress Reduction program, describes mindfulness meditation as "paying attention on purpose, in the present moment, and nonjudgmentally, to the unfolding experience moment to moment."[34] A common image used in this particular style of meditation is that of the person meditating being a large mountain—steady and unchanging—as clouds (thoughts) float by, everpresent but not affecting the mountain. Another way to describe this "let-it-be" mindset is "passive concentration,"[8] which, according to Herbert Benson, is one of the most important steps in the practice of the relaxation response.

Duration and Frequency of Practice

One final commonality to the majority of relaxation techniques is the requirement of regular (ideally daily) practice over an extended period of time (months to years). In the short term, practices such as autogenic training or yoga may help decrease stress and overall sympathetic tone; however, with consistent practice, there is a greater possibility of developing increased baseline resistance to stressors as well as increased ability to call upon a relaxed response when faced with an acute stressor. Also, as with any skill, once a person stops practicing a particular relaxation technique, the physiological benefits will also diminish. The importance of this "dose response" of relaxation techniques is described in multiple studies.[35-37]

Prescribing Relaxation Techniques

When recommending relaxation techniques to patients as part of their care plan, it is important to select practices in the context of not only the patients' personal health, but also in relation to their daily lives, families, communities, and belief systems. Following are some questions to raise when discussing relaxation techniques with patients based on these various contexts and recommendations based on the answers.

Context	Questions to Ask	Recommendations
Personal	What is your medical history? Do you prefer being a part of a group or alone? What, if any, relaxation techniques have you tried in the past?	Consider matching a relaxation technique that has evidence for a particular medical condition. Consider tai chi, yoga, qigong, and meditation classes if a group environment is preferred—many of these can also be practiced in private once introductory knowledge is obtained. Be mindful of the patient's positive or negative experiences with certain techniques in the past.
Daily Life	What type of work do you do? Do you prefer waking up early or staying up late?	To help make specific and attainable goals regarding their regular practice of relaxation techniques, consider the structures of patients' day-to-day lives.
Family	How is your relationship with your partner, children, and/or extended family? What are their levels of interest/previous experience with relaxation techniques?	Consider the level of activity or stress in the home environment in determining when to practice relaxation. Involving the family in a regular practice may also be of benefit in maintaining a new relaxation routine.
Community	What schools, studios, and community centers are available where you live? How safe do you feel in your environment?	As a clinician, maintain awareness of the local community and the reputable resources for learning relaxation techniques in the area. In areas that are less safe or where it is harder to find these resources, consider teaching these techniques in the clinic setting and encourage regular home practice.
Belief Systems	What, if any, religious or spiritual beliefs do you have?	Working with a patient's belief system may enhance the relaxation experience, e.g., centering prayer for those with a Christian faith.

Key Web Resources

A nonprofit online resource that includes definitions/descriptions of a variety of relaxation techniques, scripts for practicing these techniques, as well as links to free audio files for meditation, guided imagery, and others. Developed by Jeanne Segal, PhD.	http://www.helpguide.org/articles/stress/relaxation-techniques-for-stress-relief.htm
A website developed by the University of Texas, Austin, to promote student wellness. Includes free access to audio files of relaxation techniques including deep breathing, progressive muscle relaxation, guided imagery, and other meditations.	http://cmhc.utexas.edu/mindbodylab.html
A collection of free audio files and video lectures discussing the keys of mindfulness practice. Multiple guided meditations of varying lengths developed by the University of Wisconsin-Madison Integrative Medicine and Mindfulness Center faculty.	http://www.fammed.wisc.edu/mindfulness
"Headspace" Mobile Application A mobile application that introduces the listener to mindfulness meditation in a step-by-step fashion. A good resource for people with no previous background in contemplative practices. The first 10 recordings are free.	http://www.headspace.com
"Buddhify 2" Mobile Application Designed for the busy mind and constantly on-the-go person, this application has a large selection of guided meditations that help to promote mindfulness in a variety of common daily activities. Costs $2.99.	http://buddhify.com/

REFERENCES

References are available online at ExpertConsult.com.

CHAPTER 95

SELF-HYPNOSIS TECHNIQUES

Steven Gurgevich, PhD

Reviewing the many conceptual and theoretical perspectives that would provide a concise definition of hypnosis is beyond the scope of this chapter. The reader is directed to a special issue of the *American Journal of Clinical Hypnosis*[1] that is devoted entirely to the competing and integration of ideas for a definition of hypnosis. This chapter will simply *describe* hypnosis as a system or collection of methods that allows us to enhance the communication and sharing of information between and within the mind-body. Because the body "hears" everything that enters the subconscious mind, these methods are a way of accessing and influencing subconscious effects on the body. We can do this entirely by ourselves, with the help of others, or through the use of learning materials such as books, videos, and audio programs. Whether someone helps us (such as a trained therapist) or we do it by ourselves, all hypnosis is self-hypnosis.

One of these methods is trance. A hypnotic trance is a state of consciousness in which our focus of awareness allows us to become greatly absorbed in the experience and sensations of our ideas. A daydream is a good example of trance. In a daydream, we are aware of where we are and what we are doing, but at the same time, we are absorbed in the experience and sensations of the daydream—our thoughts, ideas, and images. As a state of absorption, a hypnotic trance and a daydream are very similar; or at least it feels that way to the patient. Although most daydreams might occur spontaneously when we are bored or have too little to actively think about, a hypnotic trance is a state of consciousness we create deliberately. One user-friendly description might be "daydreaming with a purpose" or "an intentional daydream." Learning to use this exquisite tool to enhance mind-body communication for healing, greater performance, comfort, and relaxation is easy and beneficial.

Hypnosis includes many different ways of creating that daydream-like state of mind or focused concentration. Among them are induction techniques; imagery methods; focusing concentration; and forms of passive concentration, relaxation, and meditation. Once we learn them and discover how to achieve the desired results, we own those abilities for as long as we practice them.

What kinds of abilities might we learn this way? A very short list includes overcoming anxiety on an airplane, relaxing the smooth muscle of the intestines for more comfortable digestion, relieving pain, healing skin conditions, improving sleep patterns, changing habits, improving concentration skills, alleviating nausea associated with chemotherapy, improving surgical outcomes, and unlearning physiological stress response patterns. The list of applications where hypnosis can be beneficial is almost endless. Andrew Weil, MD, says, "In general, I believe that no condition is out of bounds for trying hypnotherapy on."

Although there are many different techniques to access subconscious influence on the body, for practicality, this chapter focuses on one process of steps that primary care providers can easily use and teach their patients. This process requires the following six main steps:

- **Educate** to remove preconceived fears and prevailing misconceptions
- **Tailor** to match images, ideas, and hypnotic suggestions to the individual
- **Induce trance**: e.g., eye-fixation, breath technique, thumb-and-finger release technique to trigger trance and staircase technique to help with progressive muscle relaxation and deepening of trance
- **Utilization**: Use trance for a specific purpose (headache, surgery, gastrointestinal disorders, etc.)
- **Re-alert** to guide the patient out of trance
- **Debriefing** to develop insight into what worked and how to implement future techniques

THE SIX MAIN STEPS

Educate

To remove any fear and misunderstanding and to achieve a better clinical response, you must take time to educate your patient about hypnosis. Your first task is to dispel the myths and misconceptions. The most predominant misconceptions and their corrections are as follows.

- That hypnosis is "done to someone." Hypnosis is not done to anyone; it may be guided and taught, as all hypnosis is self-hypnosis.
- The subject loses consciousness and conscious control: At all times, the subject is consciously aware of where he is and what he is doing.
- The subject can be made to do things or to reveal things that she ordinarily would not do in a waking state: The subject is very much aware and is always in control of what she is choosing to experience.
- The subject must be gullible or weak minded to be hypnotized: Again, this concept is false. Research has shown that some of the best subjects are those with greater intellectual capacity, open-mindedness, and creativity.

The next task is to define trance as a heightened state of conscious awareness in which an individual is more prone to suggestion. Emphasize that everyone has experienced trance many times. One example is daydreaming. Another is being absorbed in a good movie, when we are less aware of activities around us and more responsive to suggestions emanating from the screen. We might jump at the sudden appearance of the hideous alien monster or we might cry at the plight of a character. At the same time, we are always in control and can go get popcorn if we want.

Like being absorbed in a good movie, hypnosis involves three factors: absorption, dissociation, and suggestibility. Through an induction technique, the subject becomes fully absorbed in the matter at hand, resulting in dissociation from various distractions. This creates a heightened state of awareness that allows the subject to be more receptive to suggestions that can influence physical and behavioral changes. In addition to these factors, the vital ingredients[2] that enhance therapeutic effectiveness are the patient's motivation, belief, and expectations for success.

> Hypnosis requires three key factors: absorption, dissociation, and suggestibility and requires three vital ingredients: motivation, belief, and expectation.

Tailor

The talented therapist tailors the hypnotic technique to the subject's unique needs and beliefs. The more the technique relates to the subject, the more that person will accept hypnosis and find it useful. In contrast, if you use a technique that encourages an image associated with anger or fear or that is simply foreign to the patient, the process is counterproductive. Think of tailoring as your effort to make the hypnotic experience personally familiar to the subject.

Although there are more complex ways of performing this tailoring, here are a few easily remembered questions or suggestions you can use to help personalize the hypnosis to a patient's beliefs and interests:
- Imagine a favorite place, one that brings comfort and a sense of peace.
- What is your favorite color?
- What are some of your favorite activities and pastimes?
- What kinds of events and activities give you the greatest pleasure?
- What are the times and places where you feel safe and peacefully at ease?

Testing Hypnotic Talent

In familiarizing yourself and your patients with their current level of hypnotic talent, inform them that you would like to explore their present ability for "mind-body communication" with one or both of these simple procedures.

The Hand Clasp
- Clasp your hands together and interlace your fingers. Imagine that your hands are glued together. Feel how tight the glue holds them.
- Now imagine that the glue between your hands has grown even stronger, or you can imagine that your hands are in a vise that keeps them together.
- Continue to concentrate on how firmly your hands are stuck together. Perhaps you have felt how strong superglue is. Keeping the "stuckness" firmly in mind, try

to pull your hands apart while focusing on the image or idea of your hands being stuck together.
- If your hands remain stuck to one another, let yourself play with the idea and how well your body responded to your thoughts.
- Then, imagine your hands free of each other and gently pull them apart.
- If your hands did not remain stuck together, even a little, play some more and see what happens. Sooner or later, your subconscious will accept the idea and image in your mind. The key is to make the image in your mind the dominant idea as you do this.

Ask your patient, were you able to feel as if your hands were stuck together, even momentarily? The greater the ability, the more the hypnotic talent.

Ideosensory Experience. The ideosensory experience refers to the ability or capacity of the mind-body to respond to the idea or imagination of sensory stimuli (idea + sensory = ideosensory), that is, an idea in the mind that produces a sensory response. Proceed by speaking through each step as you help your patient develop the image as fully as possible in the imagination.
- Imagine that you have a freshly picked lemon in your hand. Imagine holding the lemon, feeling its weight, examining the texture of the skin and the color.
- Imagine scraping the skin enough to release some of the oil from the skin. If you are demonstrating this to your patient, squint or act as if lemon oil is squirting from the rind as you scrape it.
- Imagine the smell of the freshly released lemon scent.
- Now imagine that you are placing the lemon on a cutting board and slicing it slowly into two parts.
- See, in your imagination, the lemon juice released as the knife cuts through the lemon.
- Picture the lemon juice on the cutting board as you pick up one half of the freshly cut lemon.
- Imagine bringing the lemon half to your mouth and licking the juicy surface with your tongue.
- If needed or desired, have the patient close the eyes and repeat the instructions.

Ask the patient, could you feel the weight of the lemon? Were you able to smell the lemon? Could you see the oil released when the rind was scraped or the juice released when you cut or squeezed it? Could you taste it? The stronger the sensation, the more the hypnotic talent.

If the patient is not able to experience either of these sensations, that person may not be an ideal candidate for hypnotherapy or will require more time and training with the practitioner.

Induce Trance

The practitioner performs trance induction for the first hypnosis session so that the patient can become familiar with it. It will be helpful if you can walk the patient through this so he or she feels comfortable doing it himself or herself. Children can do this easily, but adults often need a little practice.

In trance induction, it is helpful to use a trigger (i.e., a conditioned response) to tell the body it is time to relax and focus. Each time the individual uses or rehearses hypnosis with that particular method of induction, the procedure signals the associated responses, and the body "learns" and becomes conditioned. This creates a more automatic response to the trigger, and the more it is used, the easier it becomes to induce a trance. It is important to use your voice to convey the message you intend. That is, use inflections, pauses, tone and volume, and accent to emphasize your message. It is also important to embed statements of positive reinforcement during the trance work so patients can develop the ability to do this on their own.

There are many different techniques for trance induction. Four examples are described here.

Thumb-and-Finger Technique. Instruct the patient to gently press the tips of the thumb and index finger together in the OK sign. Then tell him/her that when ready, he/she may close the eyes, take a deep breath, and hold that breath while you count to five. With each increasing number, tell the patient that he/she is deliberately increasing some acceptable anxiety and to make it a physical experience by pressing his thumb and finger more tightly together. Let the patient know that he/she is in control of this form of tension and anxiety, and when you reach five, he/she is to exhale the breath and release and relax the thumb and finger. Tell the patient to continue with the eyes closed and to permit the hand to relax and to allow breathing to become calm and regular. You may say that this acts as a cue or signal for him/her to relax and go into a trance. This technique can be used at any time by the patient for self-hypnosis. Again, with repetition, it creates a conditioned response that facilitates a faster and easier induction.

Imagining a Relaxation Staircase. By imagining a beautiful staircase with 10 steps, the patient can use each step to focus on relaxing a different part of the body as he/she descends to her favorite place. In the brackets in the following passage, insert the patient's preferences that you learned during tailoring, such as a favorite place or color. The relaxation staircase technique, which is also a technique for deepening of the trance, may go something like this:

Imagine a beautiful [favorite color] staircase that has 10 steps. These 10 steps lead to a peaceful and relaxing [favorite place]. In a moment, I am going to start counting backward from 10 to 1. With each step, you can notice your body relaxing more comfortably, allowing you to gently relax deeper and deeper with each step. It will be so very nice to discover which parts of your body relax more quickly and easily, as tension is automatically released.

As you start at the top of the staircase, allow each exhalation to release any tension or strain in your body. Let each breath now be a "relaxing breath."

10…Relax your face and jaw, letting your tongue gently rest on the floor of your mouth.
9…Relax your temples, eyes, and eyelids as we step down to…
8…Relax the back of your neck and shoulders, simply letting go.
7…Relax your arms, knowing that there is nothing for them to do.

And sometimes, you will notice that your body is already getting ahead of my voice and the numbers, and sometimes it feels so comfortable when your body catches up to your relaxation.
6…Relax your chest, with each rise and fall of the breath.
5…Relax your abdomen, setting the muscles free.
4…Relax your pelvis, allowing it to sink into the chair.
Sometimes your body may feel so "heavy" that it feels like you are sinking, and other times you feel so "light" that it may seem that you are floating. Whatever you experience, it is correct for you…let it happen.
3…Relax your legs, giving them the day off with nothing to support.
2…Relax your toes as we arrive at…
1…
And continue past zero as you feel comfortable and at ease with this very relaxed form of concentration.

Eye Fixation and Closure. This technique is helpful for a more reluctant or nervous patient as it begins with their eyes open and involves the common everyday experience of "staring." The instructions may go like this:

While you are sitting upright with your eyes open, select a place or a spot out in front of you above the horizon or midline to let your eyes rest upon. The spot you are seeing is not changing, and it is normal that your eyes would want to wander away. But continue to bring your gaze back to that spot and direct your attention to create "staring." That is, your eyes remain open and you are seeing…but sooner or later…you are not looking at what your eyes are seeing in the same way…you are staring. When you observe that you are staring (seeing but not looking), begin to imagine that your eyelids are becoming comfortably tired and becoming heavier and heavier. You may notice that it is becoming more difficult for your eyes to remain open. Let your eyelids become increasingly and pleasantly heavy and allow them to begin to close by themselves as they become heavier and heavier. If your eyes do not begin closing in 5 minutes, I will count from five down to zero to deepen your experience and close your eyes at zero.

5…sometimes your eyes may flutter as they become comfortably tired.
4…your eyes may even produce some gentle tears to keep them moist.
3…perhaps you can remember how it feels when you want to stay up late to watch a movie, but by the time the movie begins, it would feel so good to let your eyes rest closed.
2…heavier and heavier…allowing them to close.
1…and now as I say "zero," close your eyes and take my voice with you as you begin a very gentle journey to that place or feeling of a place within you where all is well and where you feel safe and peacefully at ease.

Let yourself rest into this place or feeling of comfort for as long as you like, letting go of any "trying."
Tell yourself relaxing suggestions, or picture them as if they are already achieved, and tell yourself that you can return to this level of comfort and relaxation at future sessions.
Now, shift over to bringing yourself to a fully alert, waking state, feeling refreshed and calm as I count from one up to five.

1…you begin orienting yourself to this chair, this room
2…arms and legs begin to feel refreshing energy flowing

3...preparing arms, legs, and hands to move and do activities
4...you bring this refreshment to the front of your mind and at
5...you open your eyes feeling refreshed, alert, and comfortable.

Breathing and Breath Technique. Suggest that your patients adjust their position to be as comfortable as they like, and when ready, to begin to let their eyes close. When they close their eyes you may say:

While sitting, reclining, or lying down with your eyes closed, take three deep breaths, paying attention to any tightness and tension with each inhalation and focusing on comfort and peace with each exhalation. With each of these three deep-breath exhalations, notice the feeling of "letting go."

With each exhaled breath, notice the "letting go" of the breath from your body as a means of releasing tension.

Scan your body from the head to toes or the toes to head and find any places of stored tension or tightness.

Associate each inhaled breath with gathering up some of the tension or tightness and associate each exhaled breath with releasing the tension or tightness. Your breath enters your body to gather up tension, and your breath goes out releasing the tension with it.

Imagine a seashore or something that contains the idea of gathering and releasing.

Each breath is like a wave onto the shore that returns to the sea...each breath rinsing away any tension from your body.

Each breath is now a relaxation breath.

Associate each breath with a deepening of your trance. With each breath, go deeper and deeper into a comfortable relaxation.

Let yourself ease into and rest in this comfort for as long as you like, letting go of any "trying."

Tell yourself relaxing suggestions or picture what you desire as if it has already been achieved. You can return to this level of relaxation whenever you repeat this experience.

When you desire, return to a fully alert, waking state feeling refreshed, alert, calm, and comfortable.

Hypnotic Strategies

We distinguish two hypnotic strategies or approaches in using clinical hypnosis in practice. One strategy is symptomatic, in which the emphasis of the hypnotic work is exclusively directed toward altering or removing symptoms. In most cases, the symptomatic approach is simple and effective. However, when symptoms do not respond to the symptomatic approach, or when "symptom substitution" follows the removal of the original condition (when one symptom resolves but is replaced by another), then we look for a possible underlying or subconscious origin. That is, we look for underlying emotional conflicts that are being expressed by the body. This other strategy is called psychodynamic, and it more specifically addresses the origins or causes of the symptoms. The metaphor for exploring symptoms psychodynamically might best be thought of as the symptoms being "out of mind, but not out of body."

An example to illustrate the two strategies might involve a headache, for which the symptomatic approach relies on relaxation and imagery of comfort to relieve tension. The psychodynamic approach for a headache resilient to the symptomatic approach would address metaphorical questions, such as who is the pain in the neck? or what is the pain in the neck for you? In later examples, we are exploring the possibility of an underlying psychodynamic process in which emotional stresses are being expressed as physical symptoms. For our purposes in this chapter on self-hypnosis techniques, we will limit our examples and exercises to the symptomatic strategy or symptomatic approach. Psychodynamic and interactive approaches are best done with a qualified practitioner.

Utilization

Utilization is the process of focused attention (trance) for a therapeutic purpose, such as symptom relief. This phase is what distinguishes hypnosis from meditation and relaxation exercises. This section describes scenarios that may be used for some common problems seen in the primary care setting.

Gastrointestinal Disorders: Gentle Movement or Healing Color

Hypnosis is an excellent tool for unlearning and relieving gastrointestinal conditions such as irritable bowel syndrome, although the imagery you use can be modified to describe healing comfort from upper gastric distress, constipation, or other gastrointestinal symptoms.

One easy method to use with patients is to have them visualize a soothing color as it travels the entire alimentary canal from the mouth to rectum, calming and healing as it goes. For example, you might speak as follows to your patient:

Recognize that your digestive system and your alimentary canal, from the mouth to rectum, are lined with smooth muscle that functions automatically. Furthermore, throughout the alimentary canal, the smooth muscle produces a gentle, wavelike motion called peristalsis, which moves food through you in the proper direction from swallowing to elimination. Your thoughts and mental images are messages that slow or speed up this gentle wavelike motion so that you are comfortable and can enjoy natural, healthy, and comfortable digestion.

Now imagine that you are swallowing [patient's favorite color] in the form of a gentle light or a soothing liquid that will travel all the way through your digestive system in a comfortable, peaceful, healthy way. Follow that soothing [color] from your mouth and down your esophagus. As the [color] flows downward, let yourself feel a calm inner peace as your digestive tract begins to relax and restore itself so that you can easily digest a wide variety of foods comfortably and easily and with peace of mind. As the soothing [color] gently moves down your esophagus, it comes to your stomach. Visualize the lining of your stomach as healthy and producing exactly the right amount of digestive juices to easily and comfortably digest your food. And as the soothing [color] begins to move into your intestine, you can know that it helps your food move through at the proper rate so your body absorbs all the nutrients from your food to provide you with vitality, energy, and resources for healing.

The beautiful [color] continues to move through your intestines, easily guided by the gentle wavelike motion of peristalsis, as your body remains calm and relaxed and unaware of this motion. Your body is learning from this experience, and now you have the ability to choose a great comfort, a wonderful soothing comfort throughout your stomach, intestines, and colon. Even when your body lets you know there are stresses around you, you can quickly override the bodily stress response by making a conscious decision to give your body the message for comfort as you are doing right now. You can now "let go" of stress, and "let go" is a phrase that will now provide a powerful and soothing message whenever you want to detach from stress around or within you. Let yourself "feel" the calm inner peace and comfort within your digestive tract, the healthy, gentle, calm process by which you easily digest and eliminate your food. Your body has just memorized this experience with you.

Headache: The Cool Breeze Technique

The imagery of cooling the head helps facilitate vasoconstriction. Add the imagery of warming the hands to direct greater circulation to the extremities and to help reduce pressure and pain in the head, particularly for migraines.

This induction technique often also reduces pain by facilitating relaxation. Further time spent on relaxation of the head muscles is warranted because tension is often involved in the pathogenesis of headaches. You might say the following or something similar to your patient:

Feel the muscles in your temples relax, focus your attention on your eyes and forehead, and let them relax with each breath out. With each breath, let the muscles relax more and more. Now follow the muscles through the scalp to the base of the skull and relax this area, exhale, and feel the whole head relax. Imagine walking along a snowy path in the mountains with a cool breeze blowing across your face, cooling your head, your face, and your eyes. Imagine a cool and soothing sensation across your forehead and above each eye. Your hands are tucked in your pockets, so they are warming, and they are warm. Your hands are warm and comfortable, while a cool breeze and cold air make your head feel cooler, soothing and relaxing every muscle, releasing any tightness, any stress. Just feel a calm sensation flow through your eyes and forehead. You are calm and comfortable and relaxed. Just notice the cool breeze of each breath coming in your nose and softly blowing up and into your forehead, and the air warmed by your hands and body now being exhaled. Cool air in, soothing your head…warm air out, relaxing your body.

Repeat if needed.

Hot Flashes

Just as the imagery and suggestion of coolness can be used to relieve headache, it can also be applied to lessen the discomfort of postmenopausal hot flashes. Dr. Gary Elkins[3] has published much research with colleagues on the effectiveness of using hypnosis to relieve hot flashes after menopause and after breast cancer. Begin by asking your patient about the types of cooling ideas and images that they find most pleasant. This may include ideas of a cool mountain stream, a cooling breeze, or even just noticing the cool air that is felt when opening the freezer or refrigerator. Once you know what types of "coolness" are pleasing to your patient, begin a relaxing experience with something like:

With your eyes closed, you can turn on your imagination; in your imagination, you can travel to any place you would enjoy feeling a very pleasant coolness. I might be describing a cool breeze on a mountain trail or putting your hands in a cool mountain stream. But you may be imagining what it feels like as your body begins releasing any excess heat, like opening a faucet that lets heat flow out of your arms, hands, feet, and toes. You can picture yourself walking barefoot in a cool stream or sitting at the shore or edge of a mountain lake and letting your feet rest in the cool water. Sooner or later, the coolness flows from your feet up your legs into your hips, and as the coolness continues you may even imagine that you are even swimming in a cool lake…allowing your body to absorb the coolness. As you imagine the coolness, you can feel the coolness spreading deeply within to quench and quiet your body. Your mind-body is memorizing this experience of coolness right now, so that whenever you need to feel cool you can close your eyes and imagine the scene, the feelings, and all the comforting cooling sensations that can now flow through every part of your body. Each time you practice or mentally rehearse coolness with your self-hypnosis your body is responding with a cooling comfort. You are training your brain, body, and entire endocrine system of hormones to now memorize this experience, and you are able to feel the coolness flow freely throughout your body. When you are ready to bring a comfortable coolness with you to a full alert waking state, allow your eyes to open and enjoy feeling alert and refreshed as the coolness you created remains within you now.

Localized Pain From Injury or Preparation for a Painful Procedure: Glove Anesthesia Technique

The glove anesthesia technique involves creating numbness in one of the patient's hands that then can be transferred from the hand to any part of the body for pain relief. Tailor the technique by asking the patient's favorite color and say something like the following:

Focus your attention on one of your hands. Direct all of your attention on that hand and begin to imagine that hand becoming numb. Recall a time your hand fell asleep and how wooden your hand felt. As you numb your hand, imagine it gradually turning [insert favorite color]. Your hand is turning [favorite color], and as it does, there is a tingling in your fingertips, and warmth flows through your hand. Soon, all the feeling will drain out of your hand as it turns a deeper [favorite color]. Let it go, let the feeling drain from your hand. That hand is feeling so numb, so very numb. That hand feels heavy, and it feels as if it were made of wood. Let all the feeling drain from your hand, so it now begins to glow a beautiful [favorite color]. Let your hand feel numb; let it feel numb as it glows brighter, glows like a beautiful [favorite color] light bulb. Your hand is now completely numb and filled with [favorite color] light.

Now place your numb [favorite color] hand on your [insert part of body…knee, jaw], place your hand on your [body part], and now let the numbness and the [favorite color] light drain into your [body part]. Feel your [body part] become numb, and watch as the numbing [favorite color] light slowly leaves your hand and covers your [body part], making it numb, wooden-like, heavy, numb, numb, thick, as if it were made of wood. When all the [favorite color] light has left your hand numbing your [body part], place your hand back down into a comfortable position [pause]. You can keep your [body part] numb for as long as you need to, as long as you need to. When you have completed

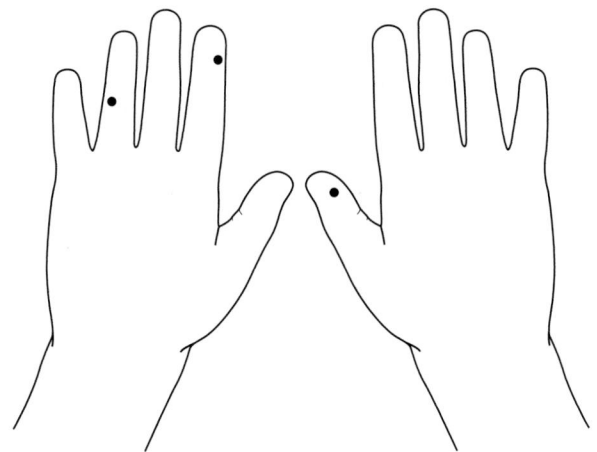

FIG. 95.1 ■ Patient's location of warts on a tracing of the hands.

this process, just let go and feel the numbness and the [favorite color] light drain away, drain away, and your [body part] returns to normal. When you no longer need it to be numb, it returns to normal.

Warts: The Hand Tracing Technique

This technique is best used for children with warts. Proceed as follows:

1. Have the patient trace both hands (or draw other parts of the body that may contain warts) on a piece of paper.
2. Have the patient draw where the warts are located on the tracing (Fig. 95.1).
3. Tailor the technique by asking about his or her favorite place and color.
4. Have the patient go to this favorite place (children are able to do this quickly and easily, but adults may have to use the induction technique discussed previously).

Then say something like the following to the patient:

Imagine that you are miniaturized. Small enough to get in a beautiful [favorite color] spaceship and travel through your body to where your warts are.

Look at the roots of the wart and see what they are like. What would you like to do to prevent the roots from getting any nourishment from your body? Would you like to spray them or paint them with a powerful chemical that only warts can feel? Or would you like to cap them off with a plastic bubble, or cut them off and take them out of your body?

As the patient invents a method to "treat" the roots of the warts, you might give some brief suggestions that reinforce the patient's power to do this from within himself or herself.

Go ahead and do that now and make sure that you treat all your warts.

Do you need more time to work on the warts?

When the patient says that he or she has finished, ask him or her to do "one more thing" to ensure that these warts do not stand a chance.

Your body will continue to work on these warts, even while you are sleeping.

How long do you think it will take your body to remove these warts? I wonder how quickly your body will get the job done for you?

1. Then, have the patient return to normal size and come out of the body. Offer encouragement on how well he or she did, how powerful his or her images seem, and how well his or her body heard everything it needed to do its part of the job.
2. After the patient comes out of the trance, have him or her erase the warts on the tracing created previously.
3. Have the patient perform this technique one more time at home. Success with wart resolution has been found with two or three imagery sessions.

Improving Surgical Outcomes

Much evidence shows that patients can use hypnosis to make surgery a more comfortable experience by lessening pain, blood loss, nausea and vomiting due to anesthesia, and also by speeding up wound healing and overall recovery. Furthermore, studies have shown that hypnotic suggestions to these ends are equally effective if they are delivered by a person or by an audio program.

If at all possible, patients should practice this technique on their own for at least 3 days before surgery. It is not necessary to use or listen to audio devices during surgery. Be sure to emphasize that they are preparing themselves very well for their healing experience by doing so. Postoperatively, they should begin the technique as soon as possible and continue for as long as needed. Overall, the suggestions should indicate that the surgical experience is comfortable and that recovery is rapid, effective, and easy for them.

Before surgery, the following suggestions will be effective:

You are preparing for a wonderful healing experience. Your body and mind are using only your positive words, images, and expectations for a comfortable and effective healing experience. Each time you practice or rehearse with your self-hypnosis, your body and mind are memorizing the positive messages as special instructions for comfortable healing. Any anxiety is easily replaced now by relaxing thoughts and feelings of comfort. You are in control of your inner comfort and can use any sounds or sensations from the environment around you to deepen your comfort.

Whenever you are distracted, you can quickly and easily return to your special place within you, your place of inner peace and confidence that reminds you that you are doing well, all is going well, and that you are preparing for a wonderfully comfortable and effective healing experience. Your body has begun performing its natural function of protecting you from any infection, managing a healthy blood flow, and using the procedure to enhance its inner-healing work. During and after the procedure, you will have all the "comfort control" [spoken with emphasis] that you need to awaken feeling peacefully at ease and comfortable.

The following postoperative suggestions will assist in rapid recovery:

You have done very well, and now your body is concentrating its powerful healing energy to mend the cells and tissues as your immune system maintains a peaceful balance of protection. Your body is releasing an abundance of the natural chemicals of comfort called endorphins, which circulate everywhere within you and concentrate themselves where you need the greatest comfort now. Immediately after the procedure, your body awakens each system and function to continue the healing process. Your intestines and bowels awaken comfortably and gently begin their natural action. Sensations of hunger and thirst awaken gently, and you welcome the nourishment. Your body is healing rapidly and effectively, and you are feeling confidently in control through this rapid recovery time. You recognize how well you have done, and you deserve to take credit for how well you have done.

Re-Alert

Re-alerting the patient out of trance is simply the reversal of the induction technique, such as climbing the staircase with energy coming back into the relaxed muscles, with a suggestion to return to a fully alert, waking state feeling refreshed and at ease. The process of re-alerting involves not only speech but also tone of voice. As you come closer to having the patient open the eyes, the tone of your voice should reflect "refreshment" accordingly. You should reinforce the idea that the patient has done well and can comfortably use this technique as needed in the future.

For re-alerting, say the following or something like it to the patient:

It is now time to shift over and bring yourself to a fully alert, waking state. As we climb the staircase, counting each step, afterward you will be happy that you have done well with this method and proud because you realize that you can revisit this place whenever you need or desire.

As you proceed up the first step, feel the energy awakening your body, starting at your toes…

2…and now allow it to flow up your legs…
3…into your pelvis and lower back…
4…traveling to your abdomen, as you feel your body refreshing itself.
5…Take in this energy with each rise of your chest.

Your voice can become stronger as you return to a more normal pattern of speech.

6…as you feel it travel into your arms…
7…going up to your shoulders and neck….
8…into your temples, eyes, and eyelids.

Your voice should now be normal for the waking state.

9…Feel your tongue, jaw, and the muscles of your face energize and allow your eyes to open when you are ready to feel wonderfully refreshed and energized.

You want to make sure that your patients are out of trance, and that can be done by taking time to engage in conversation, asking them how they are feeling, and ensuring that they are fully reoriented to time, place, and person. The debriefing conversation that follows the trance work is also a good time to make sure that they are fully alert and oriented.

Debrief

After the procedure, when the patients are alert, engage them in a conversation that allows you to assess their experience during the self-hypnosis. You might ask about physical sensations, nature of any resistance, what they liked, what they did not like, and so on. The time to debrief after the hypnotic trance work lets you gain insight not only into what they experienced but also into what you want to remember to use with them in future sessions. The debriefing is an excellent opportunity to provide patients with encouragement about what they achieved and how they will continue to improve these mind-body skills with practice.

HOMEWORK FOR THE PATIENT

Your patients should first undergo induction, use, and re-alerting from a trance with you as a learning experience in a clinical setting so they can see how to do it on their own. Think of it as a rehearsal for what you want your patients to practice by themselves. With the exception of removing warts (which requires only one or two sessions because further sessions may actually hinder the process), it is important to encourage your patients to practice or rehearse their self-hypnosis method to become more proficient with it. For conditions such as pain, there is no limit on the frequency of use.

Educate your patients to use this tool on their own by practicing at home what they experienced with you in the office. Review from the beginning to the end the steps the patients took with you; remind them that the body reacts to everything the patient may say, hear, think, and imagine and that it uses the patient's thoughts and ideas as instructions for the inner work to be achieved. Ask your patients to tell you where they plan to practice at home and what they are going to say or think to themselves to make it happen. Provide instructions as necessary to set them in motion for a positive experience at home. You might even give them a handout containing the words you spoke, along with instructions, or recommend an audio CD or audio program specific to them.

Patient Encouragement and Neuroplasticity

It is very important that your patient practices their self-hypnosis. It is believed that it takes about 21–30 days to create a habit. I like to encourage my patients by helping them see their practice of self-hypnosis as neuroplasticity. That is, I want them to understand that by mentally rehearsing their hypnosis they are exercising neurons such that they create new patterns of learning in the brain, much like creating new circuits. I remind them:

- There are approximately 500 billion neurons in the brain, and each one makes about 5000 connections or synapses to other neurons. This means trillions of connections are created.
- Repetitive stimulation such as their mental rehearsal of self-hypnosis causes neurons to make specific connections consistent with what they are mentally rehearsing. That is, "patterns of learning" or "learned patterns" or new circuits are being created that replace past and undesired patterns.

- Neurons that fire together, wire together[4]
- Think of your self-hypnosis as your self-neuroplasticity

Hypnotic induction and suggestion is an art that takes time and practice, yet simple techniques such as those discussed should be used to enhance care in the primary care setting. For more complicated cases, referral should be made to a licensed practitioner.

WHAT TO LOOK FOR IN A CONSULTANT

When referring your patient for hypnosis, be sure to review the therapist's qualifications to treat the underlying condition. A good rule of thumb: never refer a patient to a practitioner who does not have the qualifications to treat the specific condition without hypnosis.

There are many so-called certified hypnotherapists advertising their services. Frequently, their certification comes from a lay school of hypnosis that teaches them only the techniques of hypnosis, and they do not possess any education in medicine, psychology, social work, or dentistry. Choose a practitioner licensed in a clinical specialty that is certified by the American Society of Clinical Hypnosis (ASCH). This professional organization provides extensive, comprehensive training and requires supervised practice before granting certification. The American Society of Clinical Hypnosis website (www. asch.net) provides referrals to qualified practitioners.

Key Web Resources

National Cancer Institute breast cancer risk calculator	http://www.cancer.gov/bcrisktool/Default.aspx
The American Society of Clinical Hypnosis offers excellent workshops that lead to certification and provides information for finding certified practitioners in clinical hypnosis. Their number is 630-980-4740.	http://www.asch.net
The Society for Clinical and Experimental Hypnosis offers professional training in clinical hypnosis for licensed physicians, psychologists, dentists, clinical social workers, nurses, and counselors. Ample resources are provided for professionals interested in clinical hypnosis.	http://www.sceh.us/
The Milton H. Erickson Foundation is dedicated to promoting and advancing the contributions made to the health sciences by the late Milton H. Erickson, MD, through training of mental health professionals and health professions worldwide.	http://erickson-foundation.org/
International Journal of Clinical and Experimental Hypnosis	http://www.ijceh.com
American Psychological Association, Society of Psychological Hypnosis, Division 30	http://www.apa.org/about/division/div30.aspx
Steven Gurgevich, PhD, Healing with Hypnosis website with more than 50 audio, DVD, and book titles on therapeutic applications of clinical hypnosis, including *Surgery and Recovery, Cancer Support: Chemotherapy and Radiation Therapy, Immune Booster,* and *Healing Mind, Healing Body*	http://www.HealingwithHypnosis.com
The Healing Mind, books and audios on guided imagery by Martin Rossman, MD	http://www.thehealingmind.org/
Health Journeys, guided imagery audios by Belleruth Naparstek	http://www.healthjourneys.com/
The Journal of Mind-Body Regulation. Amir Raz, PhD, McGill University	http://mbr.journalhosting.ucalgary.ca/mbr/index.php/mbr/index

REFERENCES

References are available online at **ExpertConsult.com.**

CHAPTER 96

Enhancing Heart Rate Variability

Malynn L. Utzinger, MD, MA

The healthy human heart does not beat at a steady rate, but rather fluctuates from beat to beat, creating patterns that demonstrate complexity (including a fractal-like variability) and stability over time.[1-4] In medicine, such patterns can be described as regular, as in respiratory sinus arrhythmia, or irregular, as in atrial fibrillation. Collectively, these beat-to-beat changes and larger patterns are called heart rate variability (HRV), which reflects and predicts an organism's degree of healthy functioning in terms of physiological and emotional self-regulatory capacity, adaptability, and resilience.[1,5-10] While in general, high HRV is an indicator of health, there is an optimal range; too much variability is related to instability in a system (e.g., arrhythmias) and inefficient use of energy, whereas too little variability is a predictor of disease.[11,12] This is exemplified by research showing that low baseline measures of HRV are predictive of all-cause mortality[13] and *independently* predict cardiovascular death.[14,15]

HRV reflects sympathovagal balance, which in turn affects inflammatory pathways now understood to be critical and common to many illnesses.[16-24] In fact, research reveals links between HRV and diseases in almost every system of the body, including cardiovascular and metabolic,[11,15,25-40] neurological,[41-52] psychological,[53-68] immune,[17] endocrine,[69-75] rheumatological and autoimmune,[4,23,24,76-88] pulmonary,[89-92] gastroenterological,[23,93-96] and dermatological[97,98] systems. Even cognitive capacities[99-103] and levels of stress[104-106] are associated with HRV. As health care moves toward better systems for disease prediction and early detection, it is important to note that some studies demonstrate significant alterations in the cardiac autonomic modulation capacities of even children of parents with diseases such as hypertension[107] and in first-degree (otherwise healthy) relatives of people with schizophrenia.[65] Despite our growing understanding that healthy HRV appears to be inversely correlated with multiple disease states, not all studies corroborate these associations[108,109] and some show mixed results;[88] thus, greater refinement of our early findings will improve our capacity to establish clinical and lifestyle guidelines.

The ultimate aim of this chapter is to provide clinicians and patients with practical, meaningful, and effective tools to monitor and improve HRV. Preceding this is a review of basic physiology, followed by a discussion of the associations between HRV and health.

BACKGROUND

HRV is driven by a highly dynamic, bidirectional interplay between the heart and the respiratory system, mediated by two branches of the autonomic nervous system (ANS): the sympathetic and parasympathetic nervous systems,[110] the latter of which is under vagal control. A standard explanation for the association between disease states and lowered HRV is that neural damage from disease impairs vagus nerve functioning and thereby lowers parasympathetic tone. One of the most fascinating alternative considerations to emerge from research on inflammatory reflexes is that loss of normal vagal tone may lead to diminished functioning of the cholinergic antiinflammatory pathway that may result in downstream immune dysfunction and exaggerated cytokine release triggered by otherwise harmless stimuli.[18,111] In simple terms, loss of vagal function may *allow* inflammation and disease in the first place.[18] This means that clinicians have a potential opportunity to prevent or slow many conditions by helping people maintain sympathovagal balance.[111]

> Downregulation of vagal function can worsen chronic inflammation by reducing parasympathetic tone and the cholinergic antiinflammatory pathway.

Before exploring HRV physiology, we shall look at the heart itself, which plays a more complex role in health compared with that previously appreciated.[6,99,112-114] The heart not only has novel endocrine roles, such as those of the cardiac receptors for oxytocin (the bonding hormone normally associated with reproduction),[115] but also it has an extensive, intrinsic nervous system that allows it to process and respond to certain emotional and physiological cues even before the brain does.[112,116,117] Moreover, the heart is the body's strongest generator of electrical and magnetic signals, which are 60 times and 5000 times stronger, respectively, than those coming from the brain. These signals can be detected throughout the body by electrocardiography (ECG) or even several feet away by magnetocardiography.[118,119] A theory reviewed and developed by McCraty et al. at the Institute of HeartMath is that the heart is not merely a pump. Rather, it provides an organizing force throughout the body, especially in the brain where synchronization has been observed between R waves on the ECG and alpha waves on the electroencephalogram (EEG).[112,120] Pulsatile signals from the heart travel afferent vagal pathways and arrive in the brainstem and thalamus, where pacemaker cells appear to mediate synchronization of millions of incoming signals from the sensory cortex.[121] In other words, the heart itself may participate in interpreting our experience of the world by synchronizing cortical signals. The positive emotional states and biofeedback tools discussed later appear to increase this synchronization and improve cognitive performance.[53,58,99-101,112,122] In summary, the heart is a pump, a rhythm generator, a sensory organ, and a key node in body-wide communication.

> The heart itself may participate in interpreting our experience of the world by synchronizing cortical signals.

POLYVAGAL THEORY

A brief overview of an elegant theory, developed by Porges,[123-129] deepens our understanding of the mechanisms and pathways through which the heart and vagus nerve serve to shape our physiological and emotional responses to the world. Polyvagal theory holds that there are two vagal circuits: ancient, responsible for defense, and modern, responsible for growth, spontaneous behavior, and social engagement. When a person feels safe, there is an increase in the activity of myelinated (fast) efferent vagal fibers that run to the heart and immediately slow the cardiac pacemaker, inhibit the sympathetic branch responsible for the fight or flight response, lower inflammation through the mediation of cytokines, and dampen the entire stress response of the hypothalamic-pituitary-adrenal axis (e.g., cortisol). All of this allows the body to grow, repair, and restore itself properly. This biological pathway activates a strong social engagement system, seen in the relationship between mothers who sing to and smile at their babies lovingly, thus promoting a physiological and emotional thriving.

On the other hand, when a threat is perceived, in early stages the system gets ready to mobilize in the classical flight or fight response, driven by sympathetic activation and parasympathetic withdrawal to mobilize for high-energy consuming processes. If the level of threat escalates, an even more primitive neural response may kick in, mediated by unmyelinated fibers, which slow the heart, inhibit digestion, and take the organism into a state of complete collapse, a "freeze" response akin to playing dead, meant to protect the organism from harm. For some people, in response to severe trauma, such a response is initiated, causing the person to become all but paralyzed in an extreme attempt to cope.[128] People who suffer from posttraumatic stress may experience this paralysis all too frequently.

A key to treatment in restoring health comes through research and data that suggest that the newer system (the fast, myelinated vagal fibers seen only in mammals) has the power to repress the older, "primitive" vagal defense

circuit. In other words, it is impossible to feel afraid when you are feeling appreciation or love. This idea was first scientifically published by John Hughlings Jackson,[130] who held that the more modern neural circuit could override the earlier pathway, and in fact, it appears to be true. When slow, deep breathing is initiated, for example, or when feelings of appreciation are cultivated, as seen in later sections, the body immediately moves into the "safety, growth, and repair" mode.[6,100,112,117,119,131] Indeed, reviewed in the following text are also studies of the effects of singing a hymn or chanting a mantra,[132,133] all of which might be have some correlation to hearing the voice of one's mother, which instantly triggers the infant that it is okay to relax.

PHYSIOLOGY AND MEASUREMENT OF HEART RATE VARIABILITY

In healthy people, sympathetic tone and parasympathetic tone are finely tuned, each rising and falling as demand changes. Unfortunately, daily stress, which can be felt as threatening, often erroneously triggers increased catecholamines. When this happens on a long-term basis, the body pumps out stress hormones more often than what is healthy or necessary. The ANS may try to compensate by turning up parasympathetic control. Ultimately, sympathetic drive that simmers continuously can deplete the reserve needed to meet true challenges. This depletion usually translates into a feeling of being constantly "on edge," yet sluggish, and lacking vitality.[112]

When the two systems compete inappropriately, the heart's electrical system can become unstable, causing arrhythmias, platelet aggregation, coronary artery constriction, increased stress on the left ventricular wall, and unhealthy remodeling. Reestablishing proper vagal input antagonizes these sympathetic overcompensations and rebalances the system. This happens in part through cardiac baroreceptors or mechanosensory receptors, which are sensitive to stretch and pressure changes and act centrally to restore proper vagal tone and blood pressure.

Baroreceptor sensitivity is a marker of the body's capacity to augment vagal tone reflexively and has a direct link to HRV, observed in respiratory sinus arrhythmia. During inspiration, intrathoracic pressure decreases and the heart rate increases to compensate. During expiration, intrathoracic pressure rises and the heart rate drops. In general, with faster breathing, sympathetic tone increases and the heart rate climbs. With slower breathing, between six and four breaths/minute,[131,132] the balance shifts toward the parasympathetic system and the heart rate slows.

Therefore, the healthy heart does not beat at a steady rate, but rather varies in coordination with the breath and environmental cues. A well-known example of this phenomenon is in obstetrics, in which the fetus is assessed for adequate heart rate accelerations higher than the baseline to ensure a favorable response to the challenges of labor (Fig. 96.1).

A flexible, well-coordinated ANS helps us respond appropriately to stress, and positive emotions seem to cultivate this dynamic synergy. In the state of appreciation,

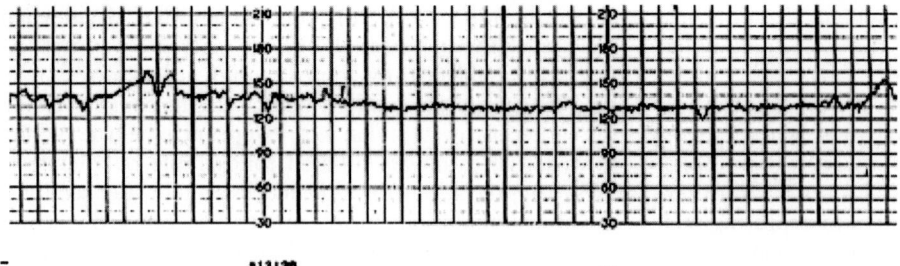

FIG. 96.1 ■ Fetal heart tones. This fetal heart tone strip shows that the baby's heart rate regularly rises higher than the baseline of 130 beats/minute.

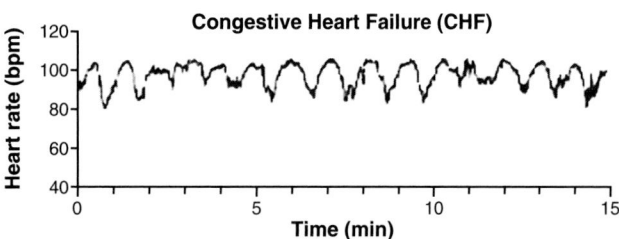

FIG. 96.2 ■ Cheyne-Stokes breathing in congestive heart failure (CHF). Here, the heart rate is regular, but dangerously so. Apparently, some ability to oscillate and respond to bodily cues has been lost in this end stage of CHF.

Changing Heart Rhythms

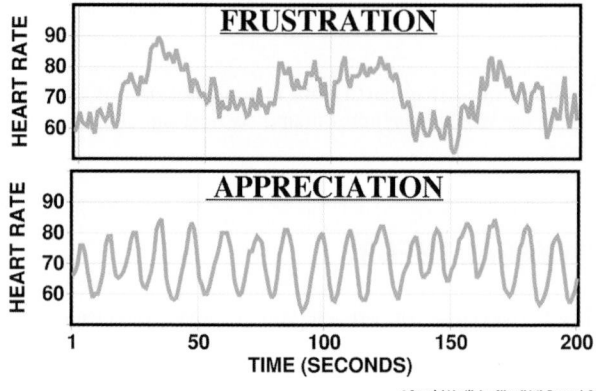

FIG. 96.3 ■ Frustration to appreciation. Here a person's heart rate variability (HRV) goes from erratic and shallow during frustration to smooth, with a more regularly oscillating HRV curve, during appreciation. (From McCraty R, Childre D. *The appreciative heart: the psychophysiology of positive emotions and optimal functioning.* Boulder Creek, CA; Institute of HeartMath; 2000.)

for example, parasympathetic and sympathetic systems both show moderate output, and they oscillate in relative regularity to produce what is known as a coherent HRV pattern, which is a smooth, sine wave–like curve and shows an overall shift toward parasympathetic dominance.[112] In contrast, during stress, anger, or chronic illness, the HRV curve becomes more erratic and shallow thus reflecting the less-coordinated functioning between the two branches of ANS and a shift toward sympathetic drive, as in congestive heart failure, depicted in Fig. 96.2.[117]

Figs. 96.3 and 96.4 are examples of graphed HRV plots. The tachogram in Fig. 96.3, from the Heart-Math Institute, demonstrates the use of a biofeedback technique to shift from frustration, shown with the erratic HRV curve, to appreciation, with a smooth curve. Although both graphs demonstrate similar peak-to-nadir differences in heart rate in beats per minute (bpm) (reflecting the same absolute amount of variability), the patterns of the curves are quite different. Each segment of the frustration tachogram is erratic and shallow, reflecting low coherence. In contrast, the appreciation curve is higher in amplitude, more regularly oscillating, and smoother. This *pattern* of variability, and not absolute amount of variability, determines coherence and optimal ANS output.[61,117]

In Fig. 96.4, three emotional states are compared: anger, relaxation, and appreciation. Tachograms are displayed along with power spectra density (psd) analyses, which plot power (variability) distributed as a function of frequency. Short-term power spectra analyses produce peaks or clusters of data points mostly within three main regions[12]:

1. High frequency (HF), from 0.15 to 0.40 Hz, reflects the activity of the parasympathetic system and efferent vagal flow.
2. Low frequency (LF), from 0.04 to 0.15 Hz, most likely reflects both parasympathetic and sympathetic activity.

3. Very low frequency (VLF), from 0.003 to 0.04 Hz, reflects the sympathetic nervous system and factors possibly including input from chemoreceptors, thermoreceptors, and the renin-angiotensin system.

The Ultralow-frequency region (ULF) is relevant for long-term measurements, such as 24-hour Holter monitor readings.

The *anger* curve demonstrates a disordered pattern with increasing heart rate. The spike in the VLF range demonstrates sympathetic dominance.

In *relaxation*, the tachogram shows an HF, low-amplitude pattern, reflecting an overall *decrease* in ANS outflow. The spike in the HF range correlates with parasympathetic dominance.

In *appreciation*, a smooth, highly ordered (or coherent) sine wave is seen. The large, narrow spike in the LF band at 0.1 Hz is indicative of optimization between the sympathetic and parasympathetic branches of the ANS as well as an entrainment among heart rate, respiration, and blood pressure.[112,134]

Although appreciation and relaxation share a shift toward parasympathetic dominance, appreciation has higher outflow of both parasympathetic and sympathetic drives (higher amplitude), and the two branches are more highly synchronized, shown by the smoothness of the curve and the spike seen at 0.1 Hz in the LF zone of the power spectrum. These qualities define coherence or resonance in HRV.[112,134] Several studies indicated that

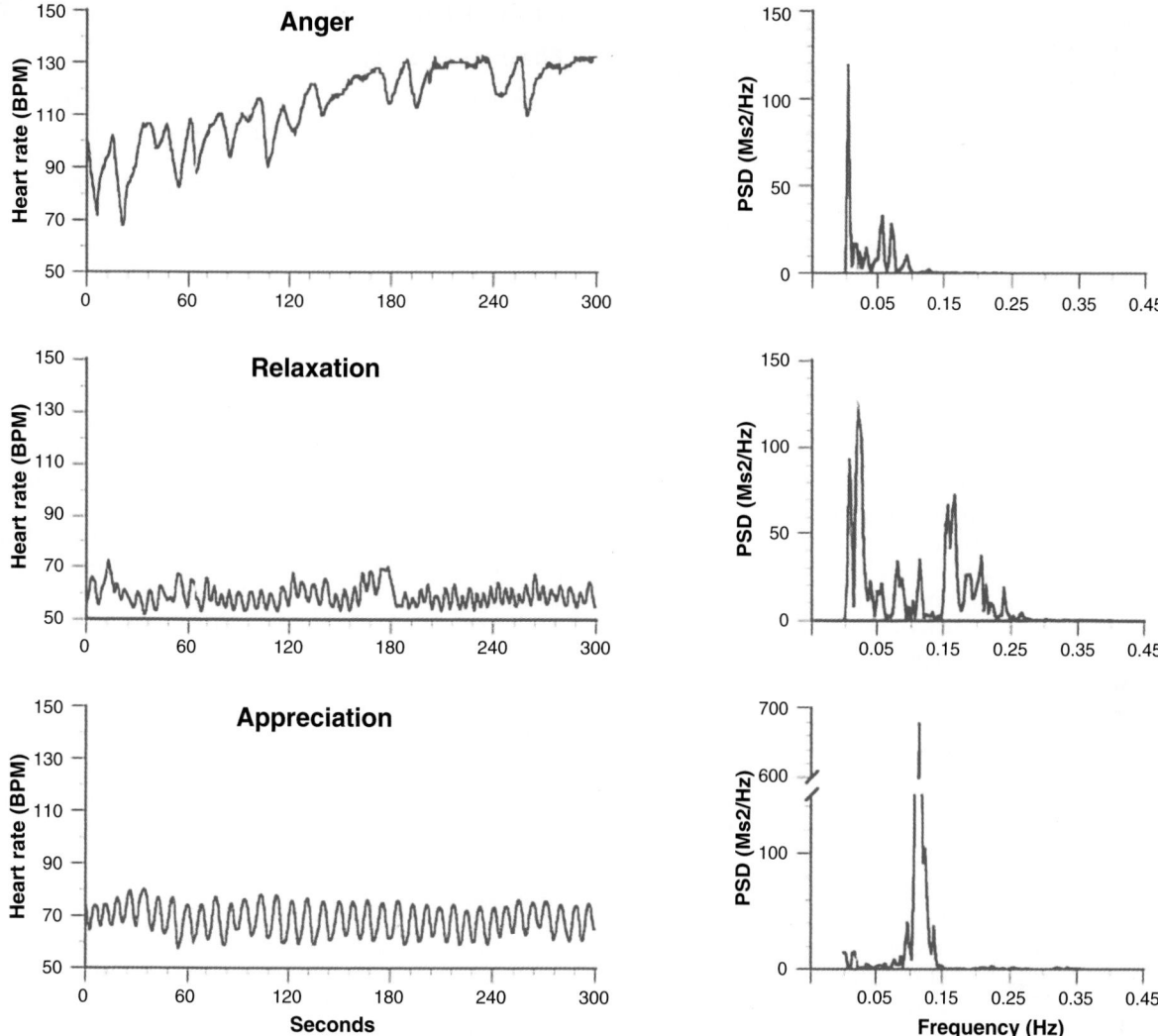

FIG. 96.4 ■ Anger, relaxation, and appreciation. In these three conditions, note the shift from the erratic heart rate variability curve of anger to the somewhat more regular, but low-amplitude, curve of relaxation and finally, into the smooth, sine wave–like curve of appreciation, consistent with "coherence" or good synchronization between sympathetic and parasympathetic systems and the rest of the body-wide network of inputs. BPM, beats per minute; PSD, power spectral density, a form of HRV analysis based on power distribution across given frequencies. (From McCraty R, Childre D. *The appreciative heart: the psychophysiology of positive emotions and optimal functioning.* Boulder Creek, CA; Institute of HeartMath; 2000.)

coherence leads to even greater improvements in health than does relaxation alone.[99,100,112,113,135,136]

In theory, coherence may be achieved at a higher average heart rate (e.g., during light exercise), but obtaining accurate readings is difficult when a subject is moving. Novel technologies including sensors embedded in a T-shirt, a mattress or pillow, using wireless ECG, in a Web cam, or using microwave technology soon will make it possible to track HRV coherence under dynamic conditions.

Some researchers have gathered data to suggest that it is not the mere balance between sympathetic and parasympathetic systems that is important for health, but rather a measure called cardiac autonomic regulation (CAR), reflecting total autonomic control over both branches, which is most predictive of health.[137-139]

HEART RATE VARIABILITY AND HEALTH

Although HRV is linked to system-wide health, an important caveat to the following section is that normative data are still limited, and existing reviews show up to 260,000% individual variation, especially in spectral measures.[140] More research and experience are needed to contextualize test results for individual patients.

Many studies have found that HRV declines with age, potentially as one loses time in deep sleep.[141,142] However, the decline slows after the fifth decade. Parasympathetic function reaches its nadir in the eighth decade and increases in extreme old age, possibly aiding longevity.[143] HRV tends to be lower in postmenopausal women than in girls and younger women,[144] and it has not been shown to improve with hormone replacement therapy.[145] Men have higher sympathetic tone and lower parasympathetic tone than women in general; as women age, however, they appear to lose their parasympathetic dominance more markedly than men do.[141]

In cardiovascular health, low HRV is an independent predictor of future events and mortality, including cardiac-related sudden death from myocardial infarction, fatal arrhythmias, and all-cause mortality in certain populations.[15,17,19,25,29,31] HRV profile stratifies risk for worsening congestive heart failure,[146-148] coronary heart disease,[28] and atherosclerotic plaques, even in young, asymptomatic adults[149-151]; it also stratifies risk for elevated triglycerides.[152] Similarly, HRV correlates with early insulin resistance,[15,39,153] obesity in children and adults,[40,70,152,154-157] multiple metabolic syndrome,[38,158] and hypertension.[156,159-163] Hot flashes are associated with a significant decrease in vagal tone[73] and hence may be a cardiac risk.

Research has verified significant links between HRV and the following conditions: neurological disorders, such as epilepsy, Parkinson disease, restless leg syndrome, migraine, and insomnia;[41-47,49,51,52,164] rheumatological disorders, including fibromyalgia, rheumatoid arthritis, and lupus;[4,76-78,81-88] gastroenterological dysfunctions, including functional dyspepsia and irritable bowel syndrome (IBS);[23,95,96,165,166] and other inflammatory diseases, such as asthma[89,90] and atopic dermatitis.[97,98] In addition, many studies have tracked the effects of HRV on markers of inflammation and immunity.[16-22,111] Innovative researchers are now using HRV to *predict* the onset of infection several days before appearance of symptoms and track its severity.[167-169] Similarly, low HRV can independently predict complicated recovery after abdominal surgery.[170] Conversely, using techniques designed to improve HRV appears to reduce perception of pain.[171]

In mental health, low HRV is linked with depression, anxiety, social isolation, bereavement, posttraumatic stress disorder, and suppressed anger,[37,53-68,172-174] and it may partially mediate the significantly increased risk of cardiac mortality in depressed individuals after myocardial infarction, although even when antidepressants are used to improve symptoms, they do not always improve HRV.[55] Even in otherwise healthy individuals, stress has been demonstrated to change short-term HRV profiles, for example, in teenagers in socially disengaging situations,[105,106] in surgeons performing high-stress operations,[104,170,127] and in physicians during and after a call,[175] to take on too much at a time. Small steps with repeated, intermittent practice may be best.

Environmental and work-related factors also affect HRV. Although results of studies are mixed, most suggest that pollution and tobacco smoke worsen HRV.[176-182] Exposure to factory toxicants, job stress, and shift work diminished HRV,[183] whereas improving workspace and ambient light improved HRV and cortisol rhythms.[184] Disturbingly, a Japanese study showed that people with the provisional tolerable weekly intake (PTWI) of methylmercury (3.4 mcg/kg per week) from bigeye tuna and swordfish for 14 weeks had significant increases in sympathovagal imbalance, which returned to normal 15 weeks later.[185] However, another study on mercury suggests that early-life exposure may cause long-lasting damage to the parasympathetic nervous system, negatively affecting its protective capacities years down the road.[186]

Factors That Improve Heart Rate Variability

Pharmaceuticals

Fortunately, many interventions improve HRV. In the case of lethal arrhythmias, cardiac resynchronization therapy (pacing) is sometimes necessary.[142,187] Other medical procedures, including spinal stimulation,[143,188] vagal nerve stimulation,[66,122,144,145,189,190] and acupuncture (especially points ST36 and PC6),[191,192,146] show positive effects. Among pharmaceuticals and supplements for people with cardiovascular disease (CVD), beta-blockers and some calcium channel blockers appear to be useful,[54,147-150,193-196] and their effect is larger than that of exercise and biopsychological interventions, although both of these nonpharmacologic interventions are useful, showing effect-sizes in the moderate range.[54,196a] Angiotensin-converting enzyme (ACE) inhibitors appear to be less useful than other antihypertensives.[197] In depressed individuals, selective serotonin receptor inhibitors (SSRIs) and cognitive-behavioral therapy improve HRV,[151,152,198-200] whereas tricyclic antidepressants and caffeine lower it.[153,154,201,202] Of note, in the previously mentioned 2012 Blumenthal study on depression in people with CVD, both exercise and sertraline improved depressive symptoms and HRV, but exercise tended to have a larger effect on HRV than did the SSRI. St. John's wort was associated both with improvements and no change in two separate studies,[155,156,203,204] and gamma-aminobutyric acid (GABA)–covered chocolate boosted HRV recovery after stress.[157,205]

Nutrition

Certain foods, including green, leafy vegetables,[158,206] omega-3 polyunsaturated fatty acids in fish and fish oil,[159,160,207-209] and a Mediterranean diet,[161,210] improve HRV. Wine paired with omega-3 fatty acid intake shows some benefit, but whether this benefit exists independently is unclear.[162,211] In fact, separate studies found that both long-term moderate alcohol consumption and alcohol mixed with energy drinks had deleterious effects on HRV.[163,212]

Lifestyle links with clear benefit include smoking cessation, which results in immediate improvements in HRV.[164,165,213]

Exercise

Exercise showed no HRV benefit or mixed results in a minority of studies[83,106,166,214-216] and in two meta-analyses,[217,218] each of which, due to methodological inconsistencies, were able to analyze only two studies. However, the majority of research demonstrates significant exercise-related improvements in HRV parameters in healthy adults;[219,220] the elderly;[156,221,222] fetuses of exercising mothers;[223] and in people with a range of diseases, including cancer,[224] cardiovascular disease,[162,200] obesity, pain and autoimmune disorders, recent surgical procedures, and even congenital disorders.* Research on exercise has even shown improvements in HRV to correlate

---

*85,87,156,157,162,163,166–170,200,215,219-231

with physiological regeneration, such as reversal of cardiac neural remodeling after myocardial infarction[232,171] and crucial clinical outcomes such as improved quality of life.[85] However, it should be noted that some studies of maximal and supramaximal exercise exertion show a prolonged parasympathetic suppression through the recovery phase up to an hour or longer,[233,234] which may represent a period of higher risk for some participants.

Temperature Changes

Entering a hotter or colder ambient temperature also shifts HRV; cold environments acutely (such as a cold lake plunge after a sauna) decrease heart rate and raise HRV temporarily. Whether these conditions result in lasting benefit is unclear. [172,235]

Demonstrating Willpower

Fascinatingly, if people fail to exercise self-control or willpower when faced with a challenge or goal, their HRV goes down, but a host of simple practices discussed in the following text seem to help raise HRV and improve people's ability to exert willpower.

For all people invested in shaping human health behaviors, a most striking finding is that HRV is the strongest known predictor of a person's willpower or reserve of self-control for consciously modifying behavior and achieving goals.[10,101,236,237] For example, hungry research subjects asked to resist eating freshly baked cookies demonstrated a climbing HRV when they successfully held off, but when the next group of research subjects were told that they could go ahead and eat unlimited chocolate chip cookies, their HRV showed no change.[10] Likewise, alcoholics whose HRV goes up when they are tempted with a drink are better able to resist than those whose HRV remain low.[238] Segerstrom et al. have dubbed this successful activation of willpower as the "Pause and Plan Response," a first response of pausing, breathing, and thereby activating the prefrontal cortex (PFC) to help make good executive decisions that override impulses, which can be destructive or self-defeating. Although most people do not equate clear-minded planning with *relaxing*, it turns out that the two have a strong connection. In a relaxed, focused state of mind, there is a lucidity that emerges. The PFC can be trained to respond positively when interfering signals (fear, shame, or panic) from the amygdala arise, which do in everyone, even in expert meditators. Simply by taking a deep breath, or consciously slowing the breath, we increase HRV and activate the PFC, which can return us to a state of greater peace and clarity for healthy planning in our lives.[10]

> HRV increases during time of heightened willpower where the PFC is activated to make decisions that override primitive urges.

In fact, HRV seems to be related to a whole host of behaviors that serve positively in helping people reach their goals. People who can successfully increase their HRV are able to ignore distractions, delay gratification, manage stressful situations (see the examples in this chapter from HRV training among students, cops and correctional officers, and surgeons),[99,100,135] and return to difficult tasks even after they fail.[10] As we have seen, several factors may control HRV, but people who are able to increase their HRV through simple procedures such as lowering their breath rate to four to six breaths/minute for just 1–2 minutes or exercising modestly are better able to increase their self-control or willpower to accomplish goals. However, in an important corollary to this finding, it has also been shown that self-control can be depleted by certain kinds of draining mental or physical tasks, even including practicing unfamiliar relaxation techniques, especially in the context of a draining illness such as chronic pain.[239] Thus for people with pain conditions, learning new techniques to control HRV, it may be important to begin with relaxation-based strategies so as not to drain total mental resources during early learning stages.

Meditation and Prayer

Zen meditators show progressive changes in HRV in advancing stages of practice, likely mediated by change in breath rate.[240,241] Encouragingly, people who have just been introduced to a simple mind-body training technique over 5 days show increased HRV in the short term.[242] Furthermore, the Fiorentini study suggested that 5-year practitioners appeared to maintain increased HRV even during normal daytime periods when they were not practicing special breathing techniques, suggesting that over time, the HRV changes during meditation may become permanent.[241] Practicing conscious slowing of breath even outside of yoga or meditation[139] or chanting a prayer or a mantra strongly affects HRV and baroreceptor sensitivity even in people with advanced congestive heart failure. [68,132,133,173] Prayer in itself, especially centering prayer and prayers of gratitude, can produce high measures of HRV coherence[57,113] as does expressive writing.[174,243] Listening to classical music or meditation music also significantly improves HRV.[175,244]

Biofeedback With Paced Slow Breathing

Biofeedback based on control of breath rate or focus on positive emotion is one of the most highly researched therapies to improve HRV.[176,245] Studies have shown improvements in the following: cortisol and dehydroepiandrosterone levels; symptoms of depression, posttraumatic stress disorder, and mood regulation;[35,57,59,113,177,246] blood pressure;[71,72,135,136] cholesterol levels; aggression levels; and job satisfaction among correctional officers.[84,135] This same technique allowed high school students to perform better in standardized tests and function at a new, higher baseline of HRV coherence after training in biofeedback.[50,99,100] Most of the research has been done on techniques that target four to six breaths/minute, but for practical purposes, any decrease in respiratory rate to slower than 12 breaths/minute is helpful.[131,246] In summary, much evidence indicates that mind-body techniques have a positive effect not only on HRV itself but also on health, emotions, and cognitive performance.

THE BASICS MATTER

In keeping the HRV profile healthy, the most powerful, safe, and reliable measures are the simple ones, namely, learning to develop a positive or appreciative view on life. Acting out these feelings daily in a healthy dose of fun or compassion makes a difference. So be sure to tell your patient that he or she will be practicing good medicine by evaluating life and priorities and by maintaining gratitude and social connectedness.

MAKING RECOMMENDATIONS TO THE PATIENT

Given the foregoing data, you can develop an integrative plan to help patients maintain or enhance their HRV. In making an integrative treatment plan, you should ask the following questions: What are the known effects? What are the risks? What is the evidence? What is the cost or the availability? And, importantly, what does the patient believe or value? As a practitioner, your relationship with the patient and your own experience with a particular approach to healing strongly affect this last point. For this reason, you may want to experiment with several of these approaches yourself before talking to patients about them. Not only will you have the chance to improve your own health and well-being but also you will have a personal experience that allows you to step on a common path with the patient. This kind of mutual and personal teaching honors the spirit of integrative medicine, in which the health and wisdom of both patient and health care practitioners are important, indeed critical, to healing! Luckily, many of the approaches listed here are fun. You may even want to try them with your office staff or at home for your own learning. The Institute of HeartMath offers just such office-based trainings (see Key Web Resources).

STEPS TO ENHANCE HEART RATE VARIABILITY

Remember that patients do not need to attempt all or even most of these therapies immediately. A wise approach is to suggest that patients pick a few therapies that appeal to them first and then modify them as they come to know their own needs.

Step 1: Follow Good Preventive Measures

- Quit smoking.
- Maintain a healthy weight.
- Keep cholesterol levels in check.
- Eat a diet rich in omega-3 fatty acids, either from fish or from fish oils (see Chapter 88).
- Keep alcohol consumption low to moderate.
- Exercise regularly but moderately, with guidance from a physician if heart disease or other significant illness is present.

Step 2: Maintain a Healthy State of Mind

- Keep up social connections or make new ones. Healthy relationships are powerful determinants of heart health.
- Obtain professional help for serious symptoms of depression or anxiety.
- Develop practices that help you feel calm, centered, present, and appreciative (see Chapter 94). Music often makes this easier.

Deep, Slow Breathing

This breathing exercise is cheap, safe, and easy to perform in just a few minutes. The best results are achieved when people maintain six breaths/minute or simply focus on an appreciative or caring emotion that slows the breath and creates coherence automatically.

Meditation

Choose walking meditation, mindfulness meditation, chanting, or any other form that is appealing (see Chapter 100).

Prayer

Pray either on your own or in a group for the social connection.

Journaling

Even writing down a few words and phrases per day can be healing (see Chapter 98).

A SIMPLE BEGINNING

In the office, a simple way to help patients begin enhancing HRV is to teach them a deep-breathing technique.
1. Have the patient place a hand on his or her belly—while you demonstrate!
2. Make sure to have him or her "deep belly breathe" so that the stomach rises on inhalation; on exhalation, the belly falls.
3. In general, have the patient aim to breathe out for twice as long, or whatever he or she can sustain, as compared with the in-breath. A 4–8 count, for example, works well. Imagining exhaling through a straw helps some people to slow down their out-breath.
4. Have the patient repeat this twice a day, morning and night, or whenever stress arises for 3–5 minutes to train the body-mind. If focusing on the breath per se is difficult, focusing on a positive feeling can work just as well.

Biofeedback

Several good computerized tools are on the market to help you learn to use biofeedback.
- www.wilddivine.com. This visually intriguing computerized adventure is driven as you learn skills to

control your bodily rhythms through biofeedback.

- www.heartmath.com. This organization provides literature, handheld devices, and desktop biofeedback software, as well as thorough training for health care professionals and lay people. One limitation is that a person must be still to use these devices, but seeing live feedback is tremendously engaging to many who try it. Music can also be included in the program to assist you. Ultimately, the tools train you to function well without them.

Guided Imagery

Excellent resources for tapes or CDs are as follows:

- www.healthjourneys.com
- www.soundstrue.com

Step 3: Consider Medical Therapies and Supplements

- Beta-blockers, verapamil (and possibly other calcium channel blockers), and antiarrhythmics may improve HRV, but their use must be guided by a physician.
- Regarding depression, tricyclic antidepressants appear to worsen HRV, whereas SSRIs appear to improve it. St. John's wort may be beneficial. GABA appears to help with HRV recovery from stress.

Key Web Resources

HeartMath: This organization provides literature, handheld devices, and desktop biofeedback software, as well as thorough training for health care professionals and lay people. They offer the emWave computer biofeedback system, which costs approximately $300.	http://www.heartmath.com/
Wild Divine: This visually intriguing computerized adventure teaches skills to control your bodily rhythms through biofeedback. The program costs approximately $300.	http://www.wilddivine.com/
FitBit Charge 2: This new product has integrated HRV analysis into its tracking and has included deep breathing exercises designed to improve HRV. A basic unit costs $150. Many other similar products now exist: Ithlete Bioforce Polar HRV monitors	https://www.fitbit.com/charge2 http://www.myithlete.com/ http://www.bioforcehrv.com/ http://www.polar.com/us-en/support/ Heart_Rate_Variability__HRV_

REFERENCES

References are available online at **ExpertConsult.com**.

CHAPTER 97

GUIDED IMAGERY AND INTERACTIVE GUIDED IMAGERY*

Martin L. Rossman, MD

Imagination is more important than knowledge.
ALBERT EINSTEIN

As a physician treating primarily people with chronic and life-threatening illnesses for over 40 years, I have found working with mental imagery, especially in an interactive manner, one of the most useful approaches I have ever encountered.

As doctors, we are trained to diagnose and treat physically observable manifestations of disease and illness. In some instances, we can provide definitive, even life-saving interventions, and both we and our patients are pleased and grateful. In many circumstances, however, our attempts to help do not result in a neat and acceptable result. We may not be able to diagnose the source of our patient's condition (84% of the 15 most common symptoms presented to a primary care doctor never come to be diagnosed as a disease state), or alternatively, we can give the condition a name and perhaps provide some relief but can do little or nothing about much of the suffering that accompanies it. This is especially true for our patients with chronic illness, who often represent the most challenging and time-consuming aspects of our practices.

People with chronic illness need not only excellent medical care but also attention to what we may call the invisible yet important aspects of health care that are accessible only through their own awareness. A skilled clinician with sophisticated imagery skills can help such patients work effectively with their own strengths to help them fare better, whatever their medical condition may be.

WHAT IS GUIDED IMAGERY?

Guided imagery is a term variously used to describe a range of techniques from simple visualization and direct imagery-based suggestion through metaphor and story-telling. Guided imagery is used to help teach psycho-physiological relaxation, to relieve pain and other symptoms, to stimulate healing responses in the body, and to help people tolerate procedures and treatments more easily.

Interactive Guided Imagery (IGI) is a service-marked term coined by the Academy for Guided Imagery for a process in which imagery is used in a highly interactive format to evoke a patient's autonomy. This technique gives patients ways to draw on their own inner resources to support healing, make appropriate adaptations to changes in health, and understand more clearly what their symptoms may be signaling.

Imagery is a natural way that the human nervous system stores, accesses, and processes information. It is the coding system in which memories, fantasies, dreams, daydreams, and expectations are stored. It is a way of thinking with sensory attributes, and in the absence of competing sensory cues, the body tends to respond to imagery as it would to a genuine external experience. The most common and familiar example of this phenomenon is sexual fantasy with its attendant physiological responses.

Imagery has been shown in dozens of research studies to be able to affect almost all major physiological control systems of the body—respiration, heart rate, blood pressure, metabolic rates in cells, gastrointestinal mobility and secretion, sexual function, and even immune responsiveness. Imagery is also a rapid way to access emotional and symbolic information that may affect both physiology and the way that patients care for themselves. For instance, a patient may talk at length about the nature of his or her back pain, yet the clinician may not appreciate it as much as when the patient uses imagery-laden language and says, "It feels like a knife twisting in my back." Not only does this give a graphic, sensory description of the symptom but also it may lead to important psychosocial information involved in the perception of the pain. In this case, respectful questioning about betrayals or related feelings would be appropriate (Box 97.1).

The following personal case history shows how imagery can help us become more aware of the interplay of feelings, physiology, and symptoms.

Case History (Headaches)

A 28-year-old woman with chronic mixed headaches came to my office with a severe migraine. We had worked

---

*Interactive Guided Imagery is a particular approach taught by the Academy for Guided Imagery in Malibu, California, of which Dr. Rossman is a cofounder.

BOX 97.1	Indications for Guided Imagery

- To help reduce acute or chronic stress and anxiety
- To reduce or relieve symptoms once they are diagnosed
- To prepare for a surgical operation or other procedure
- To help reduce or manage side effects of medications or procedures
- To help patients and practitioners better understand symptoms
- To increase coping abilities with chronic illness
- To help fight illness through working with the body's own healing processes
- To help manage anxiety, fear, and pain
- To help people prepare for changes including lifestyle, habits, adaptation to illness, and even death

together before, so I guided her through a simple progressive relaxation technique and asked her to focus directly on her pain and invite an image to come to mind that could tell her something useful about the pain. An image came of a large mynah bird sitting on her head and pecking away in the area of her pain.

"Why's he doing that?" she asked, and I suggested that she ask him and imagine that he could answer in a way she could understand.

To her surprise, the bird answered, "Why not? You let everyone else pick on you!" She started crying and told me that the day before she had accidentally overheard a fellow employee making fun of her in the coffee room. She started to get angry, but then became nauseated and started to feel a migraine aura. She went home for the day, and the migraine developed into the headache that brought her in to see me. In her imagery dialogue, the bird agreed to work with her to understand and prevent her headaches more effectively. She left feeling 90% relieved without any other intervention.

The patient's continuing dialogues with the mynah revealed a long-standing pattern of low self-esteem and lack of assertiveness. The bird told her that the result was holding anger and directing it toward herself, a process that ultimately led to her headaches. I referred her to a good therapist; after 18 months, she was not only relieved of headaches but also much happier and heading in a more successful direction in her life.

APPLICATIONS IN MEDICINE

Because imagery is a natural language of the unconscious and the human nervous system, its potential uses in the healing professions are protean. Guided imagery is essentially a way of working with the patient, rather than of treating particular disease entities, but it is especially effective in the following areas:

- Relaxation training and stress reduction
- Pain relief
- Management of chronic illness and prevention of acute exacerbations
- Preparation for surgery and medical procedures
- Medication compliance and adherence issues

- Cancer treatment and life-threatening illnesses
- Terminal illnesses and end-of-life care
- Fertility, birthing, and delivery
- Grief therapy
- Posttraumatic stress disorder
- Anxiety disorders
- Depression

Guided imagery is a broad term comprising techniques that are applicable in the course of brief medical office visits or in longer counseling or psychotherapy formats. Physicians may practice it themselves or may employ ancillary health professionals to offer longer sessions. Physicians may also teach their patients guided imagery skills for self-care by educating them about it and recommending or prescribing appropriate guided imagery books, compact discs (CDs), and audio downloads (see the later section on resources and the Key Web Resources box).

Is Research Literature Available on Guided Imagery?

A large body of clinical research supports the everyday use of imagery in medicine, and research in this area has significantly increased in the past few years. Of more than 1200 PubMed articles on guided imagery research since 1969, nearly 500 have appeared since 2005, and half of them have been published since 2009. More than 90% of the studies show positive benefits in clinical situations that include stroke rehabilitation, preparing for childbirth, treating anxiety disorders and posttraumatic stress disorder, relieving pain in both children and adults, preparing for surgery and medical procedures, changing eating habits, smoking and drug cessation, and supporting patients during cancer treatment. A summary of the evidence on guided imagery and visualization on immune function is summarized in Box 97.2.

HOW DOES IMAGERY WORK?

Research with functional magnetic resonance imaging indicates that when people visualize things or events, they activate the occipital cortex in the same way they do when they actually see the same things or events. Similarly, the temporal cortex is activated when music or speech is imagined, and the motor or premotor areas of the cortex are activated when a person imagines movement. We believe that this cortical activation sends neural and neurochemical messages to lower centers of the brain that can activate or deactivate stress responses. Neuropeptides can also affect physiology at a distance and can modify physiological states, including blood pressure, clotting mechanisms, and immunity.

Clinically, we have known for many years that when people worry, which is an imaginative function, they can activate stress physiology, which over time can lead to physiological exhaustion, maladaptive behavior, and vulnerability to illness. In the same way, when a patient imagines himself or herself in a beautiful, peaceful, safe

BOX 97.2	Guided Imagery Effects on Immune Function as Summarized by Trakhtenberg

- A relationship exists between immune system functioning and guided imagery and stress/relaxation.
- Guided imagery and relaxation interventions can reduce distress and allow the immune system to function more effectively.
- Changes in immune system functioning are correlated with either an increase or a decrease in white blood cell (WBC) count or with changes in neutrophil adherence.
- Stress/relaxation may account for qualitative (the nature of neutrophil adherence) or quantitative (WBC count) changes in immune system functioning.
- Cell-specific imagery may predict in which WBC category (i.e., type of WBC—neutrophils or lymphocytes) changes in WBC count will occur.
- An active cognitive exercise or process involved in the initial stages of guided imagery is associated with decreases in neutrophil adherence. In contrast, relaxation without an active imagery exercise is associated with increases in neutrophil adherence.
- Decreases in WBC count occur only in the initial stages of exposure to guided imagery or relaxation interventions. After 4–5 weeks of training, however, WBC count increases.
- Increases in WBC count may be caused by an increase in WBC production as a result of enhanced relaxation ensuing from extensive visualization practice, and decreases in WBC count in the initial stage of visualization training are secondary to a decrease in WBC production as a result of possible pressure ensuing from an attempt to learn new training techniques.
- Decreases and increases in WBC count may be caused by the effect of margination. This means that imagery training may change the movement of WBCs and their location within the body, rather than decreasing or increasing production of WBCs.
- The change in WBC count may occur earlier in medical patients with a depressed WBC count and later in physiologically normal, healthy individuals.

Adapted from Trakhtenberg EC. The effects of guided imagery on the immune system: a critical review. *Int J Neurosci.* 2008;118:839-855.

place and concentrates on what he or she imagines seeing, hearing, and feeling there, the patient tends to induce a state of relaxation similar to what he or she would feel if actually in that place. The physiology of the "relaxation response," as described by Benson, takes over, thus allowing a break in the chronic stress state and facilitating certain reparative and restorative processes the body uses for healing. With regular practice, the creation of this state can help reverse some of the effects of chronic stress.

The creation of a relaxed state also allows the patient to experience that he or she has some choice in feelings about and response to stressors, which can lead to greater self-efficacy and changes in lifestyle patterns that affect health. Finally, in a relaxed yet aware state, the body is more responsive to images and suggestions of pain relief, comfort, enhanced or reduced blood flow, and even upregulation of immunity.

Worry is an example of how negative images can trigger stress physiology. Imagery can also be directed toward positive physiological responses.

Imagery is sometimes referred to as a "right brain" type of thinking because it tends to be synthetic, creative, and emotional. This type of thinking contrasts with the "left brain" form of linear, logical thinking with which we are all highly familiar.

These attributions are best considered a shorthand way of referring to modes of thinking that are associated with, but not restricted to, the respective hemispheres of the brain. They may be more accurately termed simultaneous versus sequential information processing. To illustrate the difference between these two types of thinking, let us imagine watching a train go by from two different perspectives. From the left brain or sequential processing perspective, one would observe the train from the level of the track. One would see the engine go by, then the first car, then the next, and the next, and so on—one car at a time, each following the one before. The right brain or simultaneous perspective would place one high above the train, where one could see not only the whole train, but also the tracks for miles ahead and behind, the countryside through which it travels, the place it started, and its next destination. Similarly, the holistic perspective of imagery shows one the forest, whereas the analytic perspective of linear thinking lets one more closely examine the trees; both are useful.

Perhaps the reason that imagery seems so mysteriously powerful is that we have almost systematically ignored it in scientific culture and, as it is rediscovered, its many advantages in mind-body healing make us marvel at its utility. Imagery provides many advantages over analytical thinking when it is applied to personal healing. One is the big-picture perspective that it offers. As the previous case history and the following example illustrate, imagery can often show how life events, emotions, and physical symptoms are connected.

Case History (Lumpy Breasts)

A patient with lumpy breasts was invited to allow an image to come that represented the lumps. She was surprised that she imagined them as pearls. On exploring the pearl image, she realized that pearls are formed in response to something irritating that could eventually turn harmful. Her orientation changed as she considered this idea. "Maybe the lumps are trying to protect me," she said. "They want me to reduce the stress I've been living with and the caffeine I've been using to try to keep up." This understanding led her to stop drinking coffee and change the way she was living to reduce her stress; her fibrocystic lumps soon disappeared.

Another advantage of imagery in mind-body healing is that it is closely related to emotion. Imagery is the basis of the arts and the essence of painting and sculpture as well as of poetry, storytelling, dance, drama, and even music. Imagery moves us and can represent what affects us emotionally. Because unexpressed emotions are often expressed in the body, many common and unexplainable symptoms that doctors see represent patients' feelings that are unrecognized and unattended. Imagery can bring these connections to light and make them available for expression and potential resolution (see Chapter 102).

Imagery is also closely related to physiology. Imagining sucking on a lemon stimulates salivation in most people, whereas imagining frightening events elevates the heart rate and blood pressure. Imagining muscle relaxation produces muscle relaxation, and regular imagining of an activated immune system increases both the number and aggressiveness of natural killer cells. This psychophysiological connection may account for the wide range of syndromes in which imagery has proved useful. These diagnoses include, but are not limited to, asthma, allergic rhinitis, tension and migraine headaches, neck and back pain, irritable bowel syndrome, premenstrual dysphoria, dysmenorrhea, Raynaud syndrome, anxiety, depression, hypertension, angina, and even diabetes. Imagery has also been shown to relieve anxiety and complications of invasive medical and surgical procedures, including endoscopy, colonoscopy, biopsy, and angiography, as well as childbirth.

> Guided imagery acts as a bridge of communication of information between the subconscious and conscious mind that the patient can use to find health.

COMMONLY USED TREATMENT TECHNIQUES

The list of techniques used in guided imagery is quite extensive because this approach has been applied to problems ranging from chronic pain to posttraumatic stress, to stimulating healing responses in the body, to enhancing mind-body awareness, and more. However, some of the more basic techniques are described here.

Mental and Physical Relaxation

Imagery is often the easiest way for many Western patients to learn to relax. Typically, patients are instructed in abdominal breathing and sequential or progressive relaxation suggestions and are then invited simply to daydream themselves to a place of great beauty, safety, or peacefulness or a place that they experience as healing. Patients are guided to notice what they see, hear, feel, and even smell as they imagine themselves in a relaxing place. As they immerse themselves in the imagery in this way, they tend to relax easily and deeply.

Symptom Relief Through Healing Imagery

Symptomatic imagery techniques reduce physical symptoms such as pain, anxiety, and insomnia without concern for the causes. Such techniques are useful alternatives or complements to medications and are particularly helpful when discomfort has a stress-related or functional basis. Many different situations and techniques are used, such as relaxation and then imagining how healing could

happen in an area that is symptomatic. When patients are successful in relieving pain or other symptoms with imagery, they find the experience profoundly therapeutic and empowering.

Interactive Imagery Dialogue

Interactive imagery dialogue can be used with an image that represents anything the client or therapist wants to know more about; in many ways, it is the quintessential insight technique. This method is used to explore an image of a symptom (whether physical, emotional, or behavioral), an image that represents resistance arising anywhere in the process, an image of an inner resource that can help the client deal with the current problem, or an image of the solution.

With interactive imagery, the point is not to analyze the images but to communicate with them as if they are alive (which, of course, they are). This is not to say that the images have an existence apart from the client, but rather that they represent complexes of thoughts, beliefs, attitudes, feelings, body sensations, expectations, and values that at times can function as relatively autonomous aspects of the personality. These constellations were referred to as "subpersonalities" by Roberto Assagioli,[1] the originator of psychosynthesis, and as "ego states" by Watkins and Watkins.[2]

The Inner Advisor

The inner advisor is a specific type of IGI dialogue whereby clients are invited to converse with an imaginary figure that is specified to be both wise and loving or, as characterized in analytic terms, an "ego ideal." This figure can be referred to as the "inner guide," "inner healer," "inner wisdom," "inner helper," "inner physician," "higher self," or any other term that is meaningful to and comfortable for the client. Because the client is invited to imagine a figure that has these qualities, a dialogue with whatever figure arises is usually meaningful and helpful. Specifying the positive qualities offers some safety to clients if they find themselves exploring issues that may be emotionally difficult. When used properly, this is one of the most useful imagery dialogue techniques.

Evocative Imagery

The state-dependent technique called evocative imagery helps clients to shift moods and affective states at will, thus making new behaviors and insights more accessible to consciousness. Through the structured use of memory, fantasy, and sensory recruitment, the client is encouraged to identify a personal quality or qualities that would serve especially well in his or her current situation. For instance, a client may feel the need for more "calmness" or "peace of mind" to deal more effectively with a life issue or a medical illness. The guide then invites the client to relax and recall a time when peace of mind was actually experienced. Through the use of sensory recruitment and present-tense recall, the client is encouraged to imagine that he or she is in that time again now, feeling that peace of mind. Once this peaceful feeling state has been well established and amplified, the patient is invited to let the past images go, but to come back to the present, bringing along the feelings of peace of mind. As the client now becomes aware of the situation while strongly in touch with this feeling, he or she is usually able to tolerate it far more effectively.

Dr. Sheldon Cohen[3] at Carnegie-Mellon University in Pittsburgh researched evocative imagery and found it to be highly effective in shifting affective states. Research aimed at assessing the effects of those altered affective states on subsequent behavior, problem solving, and self-efficacy remains to be done and offers a fertile field for future psychological and behavioral study.

Grounding: Moving From Insight to Action

Grounding is the process by which the insights evoked by imagery are turned into actions and greater awareness and motivations are focused into a specific plan for attitudinal, emotional, or behavioral change. This process of adding the will to the imagination involves clarification of insights, brainstorming, choosing the best option, affirmations, action planning, imagery rehearsal, and constant reformulation of the plan until it actually succeeds. It is often the missing link in insight-oriented therapies because it connects the new awareness to a specific action plan. Grounding is "where the rubber meets the road," and imagery can be used to enhance the process by providing creative options for action; the guide and client can use imagery rehearsal to troubleshoot and anticipate obstacles to success.

HOW TO GET STARTED WITH GUIDED IMAGERY

The first thing the practitioner should do is notice how much imagery-laden language and suggestion are used in daily interactions with patients. Notice the terms patients use when they describe "knife-like" pains or the feeling of a "hot poker in my stomach." The practitioner should notice his or her own uses of imagery, too, such as in describing the mechanisms of a medication or intervention. Simple word pictures are commonly used when we prescribe and try to motivate patients to follow the regimen. Simple descriptions such as "This will relax the little muscles in your blood vessels and that will lower your blood pressure" and "Acupuncture releases brain chemicals that relax your muscles and relieve pain" are very brief forms of what can be called guided imagery. Physicians can sometimes forget this effect when they become caught up in the necessities of informed consent, which tends to focus too much on the negative potential of treatments. Without "overpromising," physicians should accompany any prescription or recommendation with an expectation that it will be of help, and a brief word picture of how that can happen conveys a large amount of information in a concise way.

The practitioner should read books on guided imagery and experiment personally with guided imagery CDs or audios available through mp3 downloads (see Key Web Resources, later). The more personal experience a practitioner has with guided imagery, the easier it will be to teach these skills to patients or simply to recommend or prescribe particular guided imagery exercises, lessons, or techniques. Some physicians recommend that patients listen to guided imagery audios and write about their experiences. The physician then debriefs the experience with the patient at a later time, answers questions, and offers guidance on how to use the technique on a continuing basis.

The physician who wishes to guide patients through imagery experiences but has no experience or training in any form of relaxation, hypnosis, or meditation should pursue such training. Continuing medical education courses or local classes at community colleges or through other local sources are means of becoming familiar with mind-body approaches. Training that is specifically created for physicians or health professionals is more likely to be quickly usable with patients. For example, the Academy for Guided Imagery offers an excellent introductory course in a home study format, "The Fundamentals of Interactive Guided Imagery." This course provides rationale, references, and an introduction to clinical skills that can allow the physician to explore guided imagery safely in practice. I consider such a course the minimum a professional should study before using guided imagery in practice.

THE STRUCTURE OF A TYPICAL INTERACTIVE GUIDED IMAGERY SESSION

At the Academy for Guided Imagery, we refer to the time spent before entering into a formal guided imagery exploration as the "foresight" part of the process. Along with evaluating the appropriateness of using imagery with the client or patient, the guide works with the client to establish the desired goals and objectives for their work together.

As with any medical or psychological situation, goals can be defined in physical, emotional, or behavioral terms, and a reasonable trial period of exploration is agreed on by the client and guide. We often ask patients to have three exploratory sessions and then decide whether this approach seems useful to them, whether they can best use guided imagery as self-care, in a brief, time-limited period of work (10–15 sessions), or whether longer-term work seems to be needed.

The typical processes involved are described here. Not every session uses the same approach; all sessions may use any of a wide variety of processes and methods of exploration drawn from the guide's training and experience (Boxes 97.3 and 97.4).

PRECAUTIONS AND CONTRAINDICATIONS

Although directive guided imagery sessions are generally quite safe, receptive imagery, as used in IGI, can be a powerful tool that can connect people with emotional material very quickly. If patients are emotionally fragile, have a history of psychosis, or have repressed traumatic material, receptive imagery can reveal affective content

---

BOX 97.3 | A Typical Interactive Guided Imagery Session (see also Box 97.4)

1. **Assessment (foresight):**
   a. Ask what symptom, illness, or thoughts the patient would like to explore.
   b. Ask what the patient wants to get out of the session.
   c. Ask the patient to narrow the problem to a short phrase or question.
   d. Formulate a one-sentence summary of goals.
   e. Obtain the patient's consent.
2. **Imagery process (insight):**
   a. Relaxation:
      (1) Ask how the patient best relaxes.
      (2) Use the patient's best method or teach him or her a method.
   b. Imagine a beautiful, safe place:
      (1) "Allow yourself to imagine a comfortable and peaceful place. It may be a place that you have been before or something that's just coming into your imagination now. If you imagine several places coming to mind, allow yourself to pick just one to explore now."
      (2) Ask the patient to describe the place in regard to sensations ("What do you see, hear, smell, feel, and taste? What makes you feel comfortable there?")
      (3) Invite the patient to find a comfortable place to settle down.
   c. Imagery dialogue:
      (1) Invite the patient to form an image that represents the illness, symptom, or issue.
      (2) Ask the patient to describe the image in detail. (Have him or her describe at least three things, such as the appearance, character, and emotions of the image.)
      (3) Ask the patient to describe the qualities that the image portrays.
      (4) What feelings does the patient have about the image?
      (5) Invite the patient to express these feelings to the image, and allow the image to respond.
      (6) "Imagine that it can communicate with you in a way you can easily understand."
      (7) Facilitate the imaginary conversation as needed, using "content-free" questions and suggestions such as the following:
         (a) "Do you have any questions you would like to ask the image?"
         (b) "How does it respond?"
         (c) "Ask the image what it wants from you, and let it respond."
         (d) "What does it want you to know?"
         (e) "What does it need from you?"
         (f) "What does it have in common with you?"
         (g) "What does it have to offer you?"
         (h) "Ask the image what it can tell you about the problem so you can better understand."
         (i) "Ask the image what it can tell you about the solution so you can better understand."
         (j) "Go back to the safe place, and return from the inner place."
   d. When the image communicates, you may ask the patient how he or she feels about that or wants to respond, then encourage the patient to respond, and let the image respond to that. Your role is to facilitate the dialogue, not provide the answers.
   e. If the patient appears frightened, ask whether he or she feels safe; if not, have the patient go back to the safe place or ask what he or she needs to feel safe.
3. **Evaluation (hindsight):**
   a. Ask the patient what he or she felt was interesting or significant about the dialogue.
   b. Ask the patient whether he or she learned anything from or about the image or the symptom.
   c. Ask the patient whether the information changes his or her perspective or how he or she wants to respond.
   d. Ask the patient what he or she would do next with what was learned.

Many physicians, nurses, and therapists work for a defined period of time (6–20 sessions) with patients in a psychoeducational or counseling model, with well-defined symptomatic or behavioral goals, and they refer patients to mental health practitioners if their work becomes psychologically complex. At the same time, we urge mental health practitioners to take precautions to ascertain the medical status of any patient and to ensure that the patient is also aware of the medical options.

At the end of each session, and at the end of the agreed-on period, the goals of the work are reviewed and progress is assessed. After this evaluation, an agreement is made to terminate treatment, to continue for another period, to refer the patient to another practitioner, or to define a period in which the patient will do "ownwork" and then return to report his or her progress.

BOX 97.4 | Common Interactive Guided Imagery Suggestions and Questions

- Allow an image to form.
- What do you notice about it?
- What are you aware of?
- What are you experiencing?
- What would you like to notice yourself having?
- What would you like to say to it?
- What sensations are you aware of?
- Let me know when you are ready to move on.

---

that can be overwhelming. The practitioner should be sufficiently trained in guided imagery skills to be able to recognize potentially problematic situations and to prevent or remedy them when encountered unexpectedly.

Although guided imagery can sometimes help shed light on a puzzling diagnostic situation, it should not be used in lieu of a proper medical diagnosis to avoid overlooking necessary medical treatment. With due attention to this issue and the precautions and contraindications listed in Boxes 97.5 and 97.6, the practitioner can practice guided imagery safely and help patients become more active participants in their own health.

RESOURCES

Training

Simple guided imagery for relaxation and healing is generally safe if the guidelines provided are followed. IGI is a powerful proprietary method of personal and

BOX 97.5	Contraindications to Guided Imagery

- Strong religious beliefs proscribing the use of imagery
- Disorientation, dementia, or impaired cognition in response to pharmacological or other agents
- Inability to hold a train of thought for at least 5–10 minutes
- Potential litigation (guided imagery may be considered a form of hypnosis, which affects the legal status of information obtained with its use)

BOX 97.6	Conditions in Which Guided Imagery Should Be Used With Caution*

- History of physical or sexual abuse
- Active psychosis or a prepsychotic state
- Diffused dissociative disorders
- Posttraumatic stress disorder or anxiety disorders
- Personal history of a suicide attempt or family history of suicide or a suicide attempt
- Unstable medical problems, such as severe asthma, heart disease, and pain

*Practitioners treating people with these conditions/situations should be very well versed in both the treatment of the underlying disorder and the use of guided imagery.

psychological inquiry that can rapidly expose high levels of affect that can be overwhelming to certain patients. Practitioners desiring to use IGI should have an appropriate level of training for the applications they choose. The "Fundamentals of Interactive Guided Imagery" is a 13-hour home study course that will give you a thorough and meaningful introduction to this form of treatment and its roles in medicine, along with several essential skills you can begin to use in your practice. The Academy for Guided Imagery (800-726-2070; see also the Key Web Resources box) also offers in-depth training that leads to certification in IGI.

Guided Imagery Recordings and Self-Study Programs

Audio recordings and self-study programs can be helpful tools to facilitate healing. Some respected resources for imagery tapes and CDs are listed in the Key Web Resources box. These website listings offer disease-specific recordings as well as recordings addressing general topics such as surgical preparation and recovery, immune support, and cancer therapy.

Key Web Resources

The Healing Mind: This website offers many guided imagery CDs and self-study programs by Dr. Martin Rossman and others, based on interactive imagery principles, as well as research, health tracker, interactive opportunities, and other material useful to patients and professionals.

http://www.thehealingmind.org

The Source: Dr. Emmett Miller has spent many years studying and practicing psychophysiological medicine and offers a wide variety of excellent health-oriented guided imagery and hypnosis recordings.

http://www.drmiller.com

Health Journeys: This large selection of excellent guided imagery CDs on many health topics is created by Belleruth Naparstek, LISW.

http://www.healthjourneys.com

Academy for Guided Imagery (AGI): This website provides information, research, resources, and certification in guided imagery.

http://www.acadgi.com

Kaiser Permanente audio library: This audio library contains free downloadable guided visualizations for various health conditions including preparing for surgery.

https://members.kaiserpermanente.org/redirects/listen/?kp_shortcut_referrer=kp.org/listen

Mind Body Sessions: This website-app offers over 500 streaming audio experiences teaching guided imagery, self-hypnosis, mindfulness meditation, and more.

http://www.mindbodysessions.com

REFERENCES

References are available online at ExpertConsult.com.

CHAPTER 98

JOURNALING FOR HEALTH

Adrienne Hampton, MD • David Rakel, MD

I find, by experience, that the mind and the body are more than married, for they are most intimately united; and when one suffers, the other sympathizes.

LORD CHESTERFIELD

The sorrow that hath no vent in tears may make other organs weep.

HENRY MAUDSLEY

PATHOPHYSIOLOGY OF DISCLOSURE

The expression of emotionally upsetting experiences by writing or talking has been found to improve physical health, enhance immune function, and result in fewer visits to medical practitioners.[1]

In attempting to understand the pathophysiology behind the positive clinical effects of disclosure, we can review a study by James Pennebaker,[2] a pioneer in the field. He interviewed polygraphers (operators of lie detectors) who worked for the Federal Bureau of Investigation and Central Intelligence Agency. In performing these tests, the polygraphers would look for changes in parameters of the autonomic nervous system, such as heart rate, blood pressure, respiratory rate, and skin conductance, for clues of validity. Pennebaker described what was called the polygraph confession effect, in which readings in these areas significantly dropped after a person confessed. These changes were consistent with those seen with relaxation. Investigators believe that to inhibit actively one's thoughts, feelings, and behaviors requires physical work that can result in chronic low-grade stress to the autonomic nervous system, which may, in turn, lead to disease. This inhibition can also lead to dysregulation of the hypothalamic-pituitary-adrenal axis and cause hypercortisolemia and immune suppression.[3]

Disclosing stressful events transfers repressed thoughts from the unconscious to the conscious level, at which they can be organized and controlled. This transfer removes the need for chronic low-grade stress to stimulate the autonomic nervous system and the hypothalamic-pituitary-adrenal axis that can lead to disease and somatic symptoms. Disclosing allows the mind to interpret this new information from the subconscious and unlocks emotions that can stimulate positive physical results.

To illustrate how a stressor is stored in the mind, let us consider the money machine that is often an attraction at a county or state fair. The machine consists of an enclosed booth, a pile of paper money, and a fan. A lucky person wins the chance to enter the booth and grab as much money as possible while the fan blows it all around. When the human mind stores a stressful event, the event is not organized and stored as a concrete thought, but rather exists as a chaotic accumulation of a multitude of images, sensations, and emotions, like the money in the booth. Not until we grab the money, hold it in our hand, and count it are we aware of what we have. Disclosing is the process of organizing chaotic thoughts, thus allowing a person to interpret and evaluate the stressor. When this is done, the chronic somatic stress improves because the body no longer needs to sympathize.

When people put their emotional upheavals into words, either through expressive writing or talking, their physical and mental health improves.

JOURNALING AFTER A STRESSFUL EVENT

A review of online journal entries before and after the World Trade Center destruction in New York City on September 11, 2001 (9/11) offers insight into how a community discloses and communicates after a tragic event. If a community opens up and talks about the event, the health of the community improves. After 9/11, the city of New York had fewer visits to health care providers. It appears that this tragic event opened people up and stimulated communication that fostered relationships and a sense of community. The words they used in their writing switched to include less use of the ego-centered "I" to a more communal use of "we." This event brought the community together and reduced social isolation, in part by allowing its members to express their emotions (Box 98.1).[4]

This process happens naturally in the first 2–3 weeks after a tragic event. This period is called the emergency phase, during which people and the media open up and discuss the event openly. Approximately 3 weeks after the event, the amount of discussion significantly declines, even though emotions and thoughts about it remain (Fig. 98.1). At this time, called the inhibition phase, when thoughts of the event remain but no one is talking about it, one may wish to encourage continued emotional expression.

Although seeing how this process unfolds in communities is interesting, how may this process of disclosure help us facilitate better health for individual patients? Let us first explore some key studies that show benefit.

BOX 98.1	How to Journal

1. Find a quiet place where you will not be disturbed.
2. Using pen, pencil, or computer, write about an upsetting or troubling experience in your life, something that has affected you deeply and that you have not discussed at length with others.
3. First, describe the event in detail. Write about the situation, surroundings, and sensations that you remember.
4. Then, describe your deepest feelings about the event. Let go and allow your emotions to run freely in your writing. Describe how you felt about the event then and how you feel now.
5. Write continuously. Do not worry about grammar, spelling, or sentence structure. If you come to a "block," simply repeat what you have already written.
6. Before finishing, write about what you may have learned or how you may have grown from the event.
7. Write for 20 minutes for at least 4 days. You can write about different events or reflect on the same one each day.
8. If the process proves helpful, consider keeping a journal regularly.

Adapted from Rakel DP, Shapiro D. Mind-body medicine. In: Rakel RE, ed. *Textbook of family practice.* 6th ed. Philadelphia: Saunders; 2001.

KEY AREAS OF RESEARCH

Asthma and Rheumatoid Arthritis

Smyth et al.[5] asked 107 patients with asthma or rheumatoid arthritis to write either about the most stressful event of their lives (study group) or about daily events (control group) for just 20 minutes over 3 consecutive days. Four months after journaling, the asthmatic patients in the treatment group showed a 20% improvement in lung function compared with no improvement in the control group. The patients with rheumatoid arthritis who wrote about stressful events showed a 28% reduction in disease severity, whereas the control group showed no change. These are excellent results requiring only paper, pencil, and 60 minutes of a patient's time.

Memory Function

Writing about emotional events may enhance cognitive function and memory. In one study, college freshmen at North Carolina State University who were assigned to write about their thoughts and feelings about coming to school showed better working memory after 7 weeks compared with students who wrote about trivial topics.[6] Another group in the same study who wrote about their negative emotions had not only better memory but also less intrusive thinking; they were better able to focus on their studies. When students wrote about the stress of an upcoming test, they performed better on the examination.[7] Other research has linked such writing to higher grades among college students.[8,9]

Wound Healing

A study of similar design showed that writing about emotional events resulted in quicker wound healing than writing about trivial topics such as time management.[10]

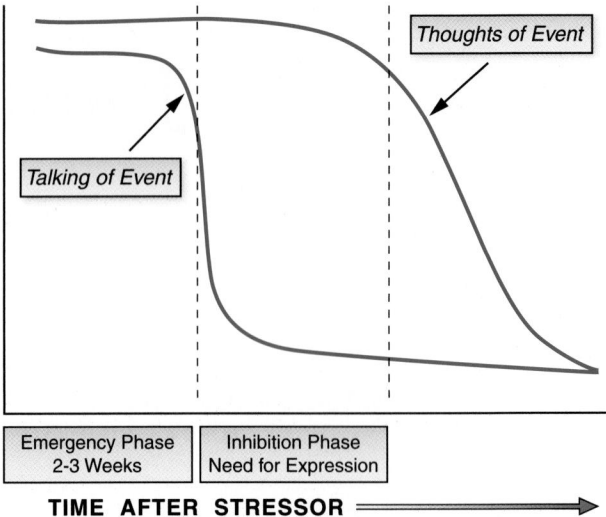

FIG. 98.1 ■ The pattern of talking compared with thinking about a traumatic event. Journaling is most beneficial during the inhibition phase when talking decreases but thoughts remain. (Adapted from Rakel DP. Journaling: the effects of disclosure on health. *Altern Med Alert.* 2004;7:8-11.)

(No noticeable health benefit has been found in control groups who write about managing time in their lives.) In the second week, after writing for 20 minutes a day for 3 days, the subjects underwent a punch biopsy in the upper arm. Those who wrote about traumatic events had significantly smaller wounds 14 days after the puncture than did those who wrote about trivial topics.[10]

Irritable Bowel Syndrome

Of 103 study subjects with irritable bowel syndrome, 82 in the writing group were asked to write for 30 minutes at an online portal for 4 consecutive days about their deepest thoughts, emotions, and beliefs regarding the disease and their perception of its effects. Compared with the nonwriting control group, the expressive writing resulted in improved disease severity and fewer negative thoughts about their irritable bowel syndrome.[11]

Blood Pressure and Infectious Disease

Steffen et al.[12] reported that African-American subjects who had a higher level of perceived racism with the suppression of anger were also found to have higher blood pressure than subjects with lower levels of perceived racism. The first group also had higher blood pressure during sleep, a finding suggesting a baseline elevation in sympathetic tone.

Another study showed a higher incidence of infectious diseases and cancer in homosexual men who concealed their homosexual identity than in those who were open about their sexuality.[13]

Employment

In times of challenging economies and job layoffs, learning how the expression of emotions through writing can enhance the ability to obtain a job can be helpful. A group of senior level engineers who wrote about the emotions of being laid off found new jobs more quickly than did those who did not write. The writing allowed the former group to address the anger, deal with it, and move on. The researchers of the study concluded that this work allowed the first group to have a more positive interview presence when they were looking for a job.[14]

WRITING CHARACTERISTICS ASSOCIATED WITH HEALTH

For therapeutic benefit, the health care practitioner does not need to read what is written. In fact, more harm can come from having patients read their writing to others. The therapeutic benefit comes from the expression of the emotions themselves. In evaluations of such writing, however, the following key characteristics have been most commonly associated with a shift toward improved health:[15,16]

- The writer constructed an evolving story. People who created a story with a beginning, middle, and end did better than those who wrote the same story day after day. Creating a story transforms the event into one that is easier to understand and learn from.
- The writer developed insight and used more causal words (realize, understand).
- The writer developed more optimism, with greater use of positive words and a moderate number of negative words.
- As the story evolved, pronouns changed from the first person singular (I, me, my) to the second person plural (we, us), suggesting that with writing, the person became less isolated and more connected to his or her community.

> The writing topic is less important than the exploration of emotions and thoughts related to a topic.

PRECAUTIONS

The process of disclosure may improve physical but not always mental health.[17] Our minds suppress traumatic events for a reason, and uncovering these events can be difficult for the conscious mind to handle, especially in children. In many cases, patients should work closely with a licensed therapist so they can continue to heal from this expression.

The timing of disclosure is also important. When the mind-body is ready to deal with repressed emotions, it generally has a way of letting us know. The danger comes in encouraging someone to write or express emotions when he or she is not ready to do so. This gives meaning to the old Zen saying, "Don't push the river." Do not encourage writing immediately after a stressful emotional event. Research suggests that this is not helpful and may be harmful.[18] A general recommendation on when to write is to consider expressive writing when the individual finds his or her mind focusing on an event repetitively or ruminating over something.

In helping others explore emotions of past events, one must avoid creating guilt. Little evidence shows that traumatic events in our lives can increase the risk of a disease such as cancer. We must not create this association but simply learn how these events can help us improve our current and future health.

RELATIONSHIP-CENTERED CARE

The primary care practitioner is in an ideal position to help patients heal through disclosure because people are more likely to discuss stressful events with someone who is accepting and whom they trust.[15] This relationship takes time to develop to a point at which a patient feels comfortable with disclosure. It takes an average of 1 month for children to discuss an abusive event with a psychotherapist.[19] The most important aspect of relationship-centered care is that we provide an environment in which the patient feels comfortable exploring issues that allow us to discover the root of what can influence long-term health. In doing this, whatever tool we use, be it journaling or counseling, will work better because our patients have a connection with someone with whom they feel comfortable sharing their deepest and most meaningful stories. Listening with intention and compassion may be our most valuable therapeutic tool.

The Patient Handout at the end of this chapter offers directions for patients on how to journal to improve health.

Key Web Resources

James W. Pennebaker: This website of one of the key researchers in the field includes relevant publications, research tools, and links. — http://homepage.psy.utexas.edu/homepage/Faculty/Pennebaker/Home2000/JWPhome.htm

Dr. Howard Schubiner's Mind Body Program: This program, offered by Howard Schubiner, MD, uses expressive writing to help provide healthy expression of emotions to reduce pain and tension. — http://www.unlearnyourpain.com/index.php

Center for Journal Therapy: The Center for Journal Therapy offers classes and instruction on using journaling for health. — http://www.journaltherapy.com/

My Therapy Journal: This online journal with secure entries provides multiple ways to express oneself. A fee is required. — https://www.mytherapyjournal.com/

REFERENCES

References are available online at ExpertConsult.com.

CHAPTER 99

FORGIVENESS

J. Adam Rindfleisch, MPhil, MD

I forgive you. You took something very precious from me. I will never talk to her again. I will never, ever hold her again. But I forgive you. And have mercy on your soul.
NADINE COLLIER, DAUGHTER OF ETHEL LANCE, WHO WAS KILLED IN THE 2015 CHARLESTON
CHURCH SHOOTINGS, SPEAKING IN COURT TO THE MAN WHO KILLED HER MOTHER[1]

It is estimated that more than 90% of people experience severe trauma at least once in their lives, and recent research confirms what clinicians instinctively know: Traumatic experiences can lead to lasting health effects.[2] A 2010 review found that childhood traumatic events greatly increase the likelihood of several negative outcomes, including tobacco dependence, injection drug use, alcoholism, posttraumatic stress disorder, and other psychiatric issues.[3] Childhood traumatic events are also linked to a decrease in overall quality of life,[4] increased incidence of chronic pain,[5,6] shorter lifespan,[7] and a multitude of other chronic physical problems. Unfortunately, the effects of trauma can even have negative consequences for a traumatized person's descendants as a result of epigenetic and other influences.[8]

Many traumas—violent crime, domestic violence, rape, child abuse, automobile accidents, or the effects of war—are the result of the actions one person or group of people perpetrates on others. Pain inflicted by others, from minor slights and insults to the most horrifying experiences of brutality or betrayal, can have lasting health effects. How can healing occur? For many people, being able to forgive is vital to reclaiming wholeness after traumatic events.

Integrative medicine is built upon empathic, trusting relationships between caregivers and patients. If patients have the time, opportunity, and safety to do so, they may disclose traumatic experiences that they may not have ever shared before. Some people recognize the role of forgiveness in healing the damage caused by traumatic experiences, whereas many others do not. How and when to address issues of forgiveness can be one of the most challenging aspects of caring for those who have been traumatized; however, the potential benefits make it well worth the effort. Indeed, a 2014 study of 148 young adults indicated what was described as a "Stress x Forgiveness Interaction Effect." For people who were more predisposed to forgive, stress had a relatively lower negative impact on their health.[9]

This chapter describes how forgiveness can influence health. It provides an overview of many of the key elements that are part of the forgiveness process and describes ways clinicians can make use of the power forgiveness in their practices. Resources for further learning are provided at the end of the chapter.

THE HEALTH EFFECTS OF FORGIVENESS

In the past several years, increasing numbers of studies have demonstrated that forgiveness favorably influences physiology and a number of physical and mental health outcomes. These effects are described in the following text; however, it should be noted that, as is the case for many therapeutic approaches, one need not have a specific health problem to make good use of forgiveness for supporting overall well-being.

- Longevity. A 2012 review of data from a nationally representative sample of 1232 US adults concluded that "conditional forgiveness of others is associated with [reduced] risk for all-cause mortality, and that the mortality risk of conditional forgiveness may be conferred by its influences on physical health."[10]
- Vital signs. Simply imagining oneself granting forgiveness alters physiology. Blood pressure is lowered, heart rate decreases, and skin conductance changes.[11]
- Immune function. Forgiveness of self is associated with decreased blood viscosity and improved ratios of helper T to cytotoxic T white blood cells.[12]
- Mental and emotional health.[13] People who are more inclined to forgive are less likely to experience symptoms of depression,[14] anxiety,[15,16] and posttraumatic stress.[17] In women suffering from spousal emotional abuse, forgiveness therapy was found to lower depression, anxiety, and posttraumatic stress and to improve self-esteem, emotional mastery, and the ability to find meaning in suffering.[18] Forgiveness improves mental health by decreasing the tendency to ruminate, and probably improves social relationships as well.[12] College students who were able to forgive others had less suicidal ideation than their peers, and those who were more capable of self-forgiveness had lower levels of depression.[19] People with borderline personality[20] and eating disorders[21] are less predisposed to forgive and may benefit from forgiveness training.

A strong relationship exists between traumatic experiences and the emergence of physical and mental health problems. Strong evidence also indicates that forgiveness negates the harmful effects of trauma.

- Chronic pain. A 2005 study of 61 people with chronic low back pain found a direct relationship between an inability to forgive and pain intensity; the more a person could forgive, the less psychological distress and pain he or she experienced.[22]
- Cardiovascular effects. Forgiveness is associated with lower cardiovascular risk, possibly due to decreased anger and hostility.[23] It has even been linked to improvements in lipid measures and has been found to have the opposite effects to anger when it comes to cardiac function measures,[24] with a recent study reporting decreased anger-induced myocardial ischemic events.[25] In a 2015 study, forgiveness was found to provide cardioprotection, at least in part because it decreases aortic blood pressure.[26]
- Substance use disorder. Forgiveness has been shown to decrease anger, depression, anxiety, and vulnerability to drug use in former substance abusers.[27] Forgiveness of self, but not forgiveness of others, has also been found to be linked to lower levels of high-risk alcohol use in college students.[28]
- Oncology and palliative care. A 4-week intervention helped terminally ill older patients with cancer to enhance levels of hope and quality of life.[29] Use of a course entitled "Restore: The Journey Toward Self-Forgiveness" led to significant changes not only in self-forgiveness but in acceptance, self-improvement, and pessimism.[30]
- Other chronic health disorders. Investigators have suggested that forgiveness therapy may hold great potential in the treatment of fibromyalgia and chronic fatigue.[31] A small 2014 pilot study found that a forgiveness intervention decreased fibromyalgia symptoms.[32]
- Miscellaneous benefits. Meta-analyses have also pointed out the benefits of forgiveness for healing intergenerational pain, recovery from sexual abuse and incest, and abortion-related guilt.[33,34]

THE NATURE OF FORGIVENESS

Several different measurement instruments are used to conduct research studies, and many have proven quite useful. Ultimately, however, each person must discern his or her own way of defining forgiveness and knowing when and how it has occurred. Even when people do not actually feel equipped to forgive, they are often able to recognize that forgiving is important. When patients are ready, integrative providers can guide them through the process. As Jack Kornfield, a well-known writer and teacher of Buddhist meditation, noted, "We have all heard stories about the mysterious power of compassion and forgiveness in the lives of others. Each time we are inspired by these accounts, we remember that we, too, can forgive."[35] As is so often the case in integrative practice, trying these approaches ourselves as clinicians before suggesting them for others is likely to be beneficial.

The Nature of Forgiveness

The following perspectives are based in part on the work of Enright and Luskin, as provided in the reference list.

- Forgiveness is a transformation. The key is to release suffering and thereby increase inner peace and understanding.
- Forgiveness is not forgetting. In fact, you have to remember and acknowledge negative emotions and events before forgiveness can occur.
- Forgiveness is not pardoning, excusing, or saying that something will be treated as acceptable behavior in the future.
- Forgiveness is, first and foremost, done for the person doing the forgiving. It is paradoxical in that when you forgive others, you heal yourself.
- Forgiveness is a path to freedom. It frees you from the control of the person who caused the harm. That person loses his or her power to cause you to feel negative emotions.
- Forgiveness can break old patterns that may otherwise interfere when you try to create new relationships.
- Forgiveness can take a long time and much hard work.
- Forgiveness need not require "making up" with the person who caused the harm. It is an internal process. It is primarily for you. The goal is to help you heal, to help you grow.
- Thinking about forgiveness may not be enough. For many, tapping into principles described in various spiritual traditions from around the world is necessary. Meditation, interpersonal dialogues, and intense emotional work may be essential parts of the forgiveness process for many people (see the reference list and Key Web Resources).

GUIDELINES FOR HELPING PEOPLE TO FORGIVE

William Meninger defines the process of forgiveness as follows:

We begin to deal with our wounds by denying or minimizing them. When we finally do face them squarely and recognize the ones who inflicted them, we move on to the next step. This usually involves trying to excuse the perpetrator and blaming ourselves for causing or, at least, not stopping, the original wounds. When we are able to cease the self-blame, we begin to feel sorry for ourselves and to wallow in a mud hole of self-pity, bitterness, and recrimination. The next step is anger. We determine that we will do something about what happened to us and move forward with our lives. We stop rubbing salt in our wounds, and we actively seek healing. This leads us to the final stage, wholeness.[36]

Fig. 99.1 illustrates some of the key steps that occur as a person goes through the forgiveness process. These steps need not always occur in a particular order, and not every person experiences every step before forgiveness occurs.

Stepwise approaches guiding forgiveness have been developed by several authorities, and suggestions derived from several of these are summarized in the patient

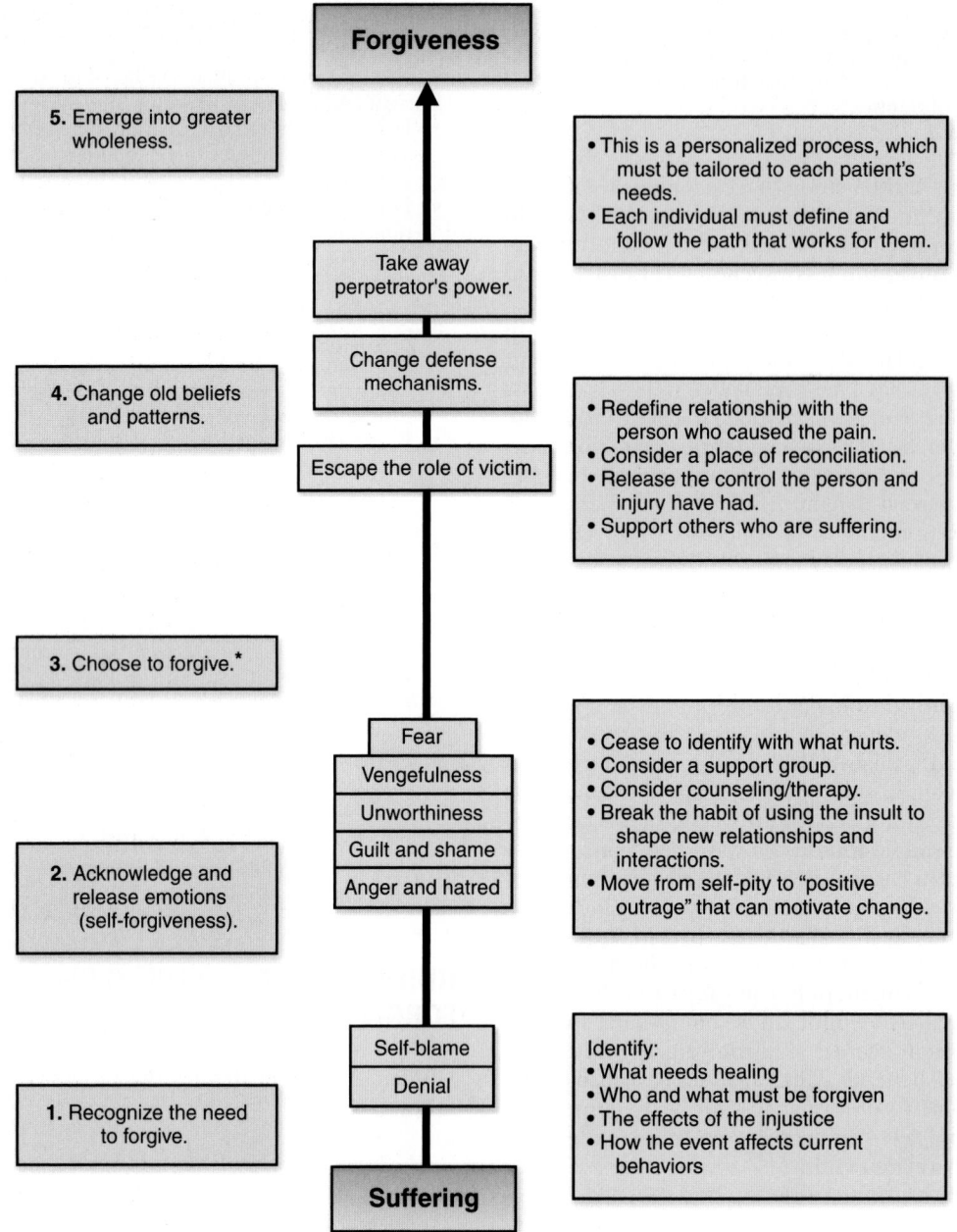

FIG. 99.1 ■ The forgiveness process. General stages in the process are listed in the column on the *left.* Boxes overlying the *arrow* list major obstacles to forgiving. Specific actions are listed on the *right.* More detailed steps are outlined in the resource list in the patient handout at the end of this chapter. *Often the most difficult step.

handout at the end of this chapter. For further information, clinicians are referred to the work of Robert Enright[37,38] at the University of Wisconsin, Madison, and Frederic Luskin,[39,40] coordinator of the Stanford Forgiveness Project in Palo Alto, California. Additional recommended books and websites for both patients and providers are listed in the previously mentioned patient handout.[41-48]

In discussing forgiveness with patients and using the patient handout, keep the following in mind:
• As with counseling for weight loss, substance abuse, or other types of behavioral change, suggesting that people cultivate forgiveness is only likely to be useful if people are "in a place" where they are willing and able to con-

sider doing so. Some people may be offended if they are encouraged to forgive when they are not yet prepared to begin the process. As in motivational interviewing for substance use, the provider must assess readiness for change. Is the patient precontemplative, contemplative, or already taking steps toward forgiveness?
• The provider should emphasize, as noted in the patient handout, that forgiveness is not the same as tolerance, passivity, or forgetting what happened. No expectation exists that the patient must accept the perpetrator's behavior as acceptable or allowable. Forgiveness is done for the person doing the forgiving; the goal is to free him or her as much as possible from the negative consequences of a traumatic experience.

- Moving through the steps described in this chapter may be associated with an intense release of emotions. The provider must carefully assess whether mental health professionals are needed to assist a patient with the forgiveness process.
- Asking a person to forgive may be asking him or her to move away from a pattern of thoughts and feelings that has been present for many years. It is not a simple process for many people. Follow-up is important. The process takes time.
- A person's concept of forgiveness is based on his or her cultural and religious background. The provider should take a spiritual history and be aware of cultural beliefs, to suggest forgiveness as part of an individualized treatment plan that respects these beliefs and encourages appropriate social support.
- Meditation has shown promise in bringing about forgiveness and should be considered.[49]
- Forgiveness is not just a therapeutic intervention, it is an end point—a healthier state of being—unto itself.[50]

> An integrative provider must carefully gauge whether a person is prepared to do forgiveness work. Readiness to change must be carefully assessed.
>
> A spiritual history can be useful in guiding a discussion of forgiveness as a tool for improving health.
>
> Forgiving can be a difficult, emotion-laden, and time-consuming process. Be certain someone has the support he or she needs before beginning the process. Strongly consider requesting assistance from mental health professionals.

Unconditional forgiveness is a different model of forgiveness than the gift with strings. This is forgiveness as a grace, a free gift freely given. In this model, forgiveness frees the person who inflicted the harm from the weight of the victim's whim—what the victim may demand in order to grant forgiveness—and the victim's threat of vengeance. But it also frees the one who forgives. The one who offers forgiveness as a grace is immediately untethered from the yoke that bound him or her to the person who caused the harm. When you forgive, you are free to move on in life, to grow, to no longer be a victim. When you forgive, you slip the yoke, and your future is unshackled from your past.

DESMOND AND MPHO TUTU*

Father William Meninger describes the tale of Sister Catherine, a 55-year-old nun who was informed that a physician had mistakenly injected a lethal medication into her during the brain operation she had just undergone. Her response was to call in her fellow church officials and declare, "There will be no repercussions. No one is to be held at fault…I forgive without reservation anyone who may have been in any way responsible for what has happened." She died 2 hours later.[36]

CONCLUSION

Viktor E. Frankl, a psychiatrist and Holocaust survivor, summarizes the importance of how we deal with traumatic experiences in his work, *Man's Search for Meaning:*

> *We must never forget that we may also find meaning in life even when confronted with a hopeless situation, when facing a fate that cannot be changed. For what then matters is to bear witness to the uniquely human potential at its best, which is to transform a personal tragedy into a triumph, to turn one's predicament into a human achievement.*[52]

Patients continually seek the meaning underlying their illnesses, their suffering, and their terrible losses. As healers, we can help to guide this search. Forgiveness is one tool that may help us all move through tragedy and pain toward greater wholeness.

> *If you want to see the heroic, look at those who can love in return for hatred. If you want to see the brave, look for those who can forgive.*

THE BHAGAVAD-GITA

---

*Tutu D, Tutu M: Why we forgive, *Spirituality and Health*, 2014: http://spiritualityhealth.com/articles/why-we-forgive. Accessed 12/10/2015.

Key Web Resources

World Forgiveness Alliance: This alliance is "dedicated to evoking the healing power of forgiveness worldwide." — http://www.forgivenessday.org/

International Forgiveness Institute: This institute was created by Robert Enright, a well-known forgiveness researcher. This website has information on books and other resources, as well as course offerings through the University of Wisconsin. — http://www.forgiveness-institute.org/

Forgive for Good: This website of Dr. Fred Luskin, who has done extensive forgiveness research, has links to his books, forgiveness tools, and other resources. — http://learningtoforgive.com/

"The Power of Forgiveness": This website for the movie, "The Power of Forgiveness," has resources including a "How Forgiving Are You?" quiz. — http://www.thepowerofforgiveness.com

---

REFERENCES

References are available online at **ExpertConsult.com.**

Patient Handout: Healing Through Forgiveness

To err is human; to forgive, divine.
—*Alexander Pope*

Scientific research has indicated that forgiving past wrongs can be helpful for a variety of health problems, including anxiety, depression, substance abuse, and chronic pain. When we focus on forgiving, our blood pressure drops and our heart rate slows down. Our mood improves. Forgiveness can alter the state of our health.

What follows is a series of steps designed to help you forgive a past wrong. Follow each step, one at a time, and take a moment to write down your answers to each question. You need not share your answers with others. This process should be based on what feels best for you.

1. Think of a person who has wronged you, someone who you have not been able or willing to forgive thus far.
2. Describe the experience or experiences in which this "offender" harmed you or treated you unjustly. Does it help to have the pain and unfairness validated by a trusted person?
3. Describe the emotions you feel as you consider these events. Do you feel anger? Shame? Guilt? How much time do you spend thinking about or reliving what happened? Take as much time as you need to acknowledge your feelings and experiences and put them into words.
4. How has being unable to forgive affected your health? Has it affected your ability to relate to others? Did it change your view of the world? How has being hurt in the past caused you to protect yourself? Does how you defend yourself limit you in any way?
5. Consider what it means to forgive as well as the potential benefits of forgiving.
6. Are you ready and willing to forgive? When you feel that the answer is "yes," continue with the steps described below. Sometimes just deciding to forgive is the most difficult step of all! (Note: The following guidelines/suggestions are inspired by the works listed in the Further Reading section at the end of this chapter. Follow the steps in whatever order works best for you.)
7. Consider a situation in which another person had to forgive you for something. How did you feel? Recognize that everyone is involved in both forgiving and being forgiven. If you put yourself in the position of the person who hurt you, considering his or her life history and current circumstances, can you understand why he or she did this? (Again, understanding helps you to develop empathy for the person; it does not mean you are minimizing, condoning, or excusing what he or she did.)
8. Practice withholding resentment and developing goodwill toward the one who hurt you. You could consider performing an act of kindness toward the person who hurt you, if it is safe and possible to do so, but any attitude of goodwill that honors your decision to forgive is important. Do what respects your inherent worth as a human being as well as the inherent worth of the one who hurt you.
9. Consider that being realistic about the relationship with the person who hurt you can also be an aspect of goodwill. It can be helpful for both you and the person who hurt you to break any harmful patterns or connections.
10. Mourn and release the pain and emotions that the unjust event(s) caused you. Ask for support from friends or family members as you do this. In this way, you will no longer waste energy on this past injury, and you will be able to avoid passing the pain from the injury back to the person who hurt you and to other people around you.
11. Now that you are facing the pain in order to move through it, what virtues will you choose to follow to turn your suffering into triumph? Will you choose courage, compassion, kindness, love… forgiveness itself? What meaning will you discover? What kind of person are you becoming?
12. As you experience meaning and release, offer support to others who are experiencing similar difficulties. Helping others who have been suffering can help you find renewed purpose as a result of your own painful experiences.
13. For additional insight and assistance, consider discussing these issues with a health professional (counselor, psychologist, physician) or referring to the books mentioned in the Further Reading section of this chapter.

CHAPTER 100

RECOMMENDING MEDITATION

Luke Fortney, MD, FAAFP

WHAT IS MEDITATION?

Found in cultures, spiritual traditions, and healing systems throughout the world, meditation is a mind-body practice with many methods and variations. Most are grounded in the silence and stillness of compassionate, present-moment awareness. Although contemplative meditation practices are rooted largely in the world's spiritual traditions, the practice of meditation does not require belief in any particular religious system. In fact, secular familiarization with meditation and increased research within the fields of neuroscience, psychology, and medicine have led to an increased understanding of consciousness and improved treatment for many health conditions.

Mindfulness is one aspect of the meditation experience that reflects a fundamental human capacity to attend to relevant aspects of experience in a nonjudgmental and nonreactive way, which in turn cultivates clear thinking, equanimity, compassion, and open-heartedness. According to University of Massachusetts Center for Mindfulness founder Jon Kabat-Zinn, "Meditation is simplicity itself. It's about stopping and being present. That is all." Stated as simply as possible, *meditation means being present with what is.*

The goal of mindfulness is to maintain fluid awareness in a moment-by-moment experiential process that helps one disengage from strong attachment to beliefs, thoughts, or emotions in a way that generates a greater sense of emotional balance and well-being.[1] This simple yet radical assertion holds the potential for wide-reaching therapeutic benefit for many current health care challenges such as rising costs,[2] chronic diseases of lifestyle,[3] clinician burnout,[4,5,7] patient dissatisfaction,[6] and generalized stress.[8]

> Mindfulness is one aspect of the meditation experience that reflects a fundamental human capacity to attend to relevant aspects of experience in a nonjudgmental and nonreactive way, which in turn cultivates clear thinking, equanimity, compassion, and open-heartedness.

WHY MEDITATE?

Prescribed meditation practice can elicit physical ease and mental stability, which provide a foundation for health and wellness as it directly influences one's ability to meet the challenges that result from stress, burnout, and illness for the patient and clinician alike. For many people, illness can bring out feelings of confusion, anxiety, fear, and anger. Shock, isolation, depression, fear, and helplessness are some common experiences patients face in dealing with chronic disease.[9] Feeling out of control or losing one's grounding can give rise to reactivity of the mind and body that leads to increased pain and suffering. Practicing mindfulness—nonjudgmental present-moment awareness—and experiencing how this process can influence one's relationship with life stressors is an essential part of addressing the epidemic of mind–body afflictions that can include acid reflux, migraine headache, low back pain, restless legs, fibromyalgia, chronic fatigue, and irritable bowel. These and other conditions disproportionately burden the health care system and often do not respond to conventional treatment alone.[2]

Meditation is an inward-orienting, self-empowering practice that can stimulate the healing process and help patients and clinicians navigate unsettling and turbulent experiences. According to Charlotte Joko Beck,[10] "The practice of meditation provides a skill that affords a greater sense of self-determination—the ability to cultivate and draw upon inner resources to help meet all circumstances with equanimity and clarity." To learn the basic elements of mindfulness, see Boxes 100.1–100.3 and Fig. 100.1.

> Prescribed meditation practice can elicit physical ease and mental stability, which provide a foundation for health and wellness because it directly influences one's ability to meet the challenges resulting from stress, burnout, and illness for the patient and clinician alike.

REVIEW OF MEDITATION RESEARCH

Evidence pointing to the medical benefits of meditation is widely documented and continues to increase in quality and quantity. As of 2015, there were more than 1000 scientific articles published on meditation. In particular, the biological correlates of meditation experience have received the most attention in medical research, which is disproportionate to the complete meditative experience that includes both objective external effects and subjective internal experience. However, research continues to elucidate how the mind-body connection affects health in promoting wellness, as well as in preventing disease.

The interplay between the mind and body has been difficult to describe and operationalize from a scientific standpoint. However, many case examples reveal the value in developing clinically oriented mind-body

---

| **BOX 100.1** | **Getting Started With Mindfulness Meditation Practice: SOLAR or SOL Acronym** |

STOP

- Find a quiet place where you will not be interrupted for the next several minutes.
- Set your cell phone alarm to vibrate in 5 or more minutes, and then forget about time altogether. You can adjust the length of your meditation time as you feel is appropriate.
- Sit comfortably in an alert position with a straight and relaxed back. With eyes open or closed, position your hands as you like.
- Allow an intention for this time, such as, "May I allow myself to be present to the simplicity of movements in the body as breathing, feeling, and sensing. May I enjoy the benefits of silence and stillness."

Observe

- Notice the sensations of the body such as posture, feet on the floor, and hips on the chair.
- Allow the breath to flow in and out of the nose at a natural and unforced rate. Avoid manipulating either a slower or faster rate. Just let the body breathe and simply notice the sensations of breathing.
- Moment by moment, allow yourself to take *pause, breathe,* and *feel.*

LET IT BE

- For this time now, *let everything be as it is* without reacting to or trying to change anything. Like a watchful bystander, just witness your experience moment by moment as it happens, whether pleasant or unpleasant.
- If your thoughts drift into stories, fantasies, daydreams, ruminations, or other distractions, simply stop, drop into the sensations of breathing, and allow all sensations and thoughts to roll past the screen of your awareness like moving frames on a filmstrip.

AND...

Return

- Let the breath be your anchor in the present moment. If you become distracted or caught up in any particular *thought, image, emotion,* or *sensation (TIES mnemonic),* just bring your attention back to the breath and *return again and again* to the experience of breathing in a nonjudgmental and self-forgiving way.
- At the end of your meditation period, remain still for a few more moments. Notice how you feel. Be present by taking a moment to *pause, breathe,* and *feel* whatever is happening in any experience at any point in the day.

| **BOX 100.2** | **Practice Suggestions and Getting Started** |

- For "formal practice," find a quiet place to sit, with few distractions. In the beginning, it may be difficult to sit still for even 5 minutes. You may note restless or distracting thoughts. Over time with regular practice, the mind will become more stable and clear.
- Do not meditate too long in the beginning. It may be useful to start with short, guided practices (http://www.fammed.wisc.edu/our-department/media/mindfulness).
- Commit to a set amount of time specifically for meditation. A good intention before you start is, "For this short time now, I have nowhere to go and nothing to do." Having a timer such as a smartphone application (e.g., Insight) can ease any worry of having to keep track of time.
- Sit in a comfortable and alert position with an upright spine. For most people, sitting in a chair with feet flat on the floor is ideal. Other positions can include crossed legs, kneeling on a bench, or straddling a cushion (i.e., Zafu).
- With eyes open or closed, allow the gaze to settle easily ("rest the eyes").
- Be persistent and regular with daily meditation. Progress comes by maintaining a daily practice. In time, try to meditate for 15–20 minutes in the morning just after rising or before going to bed, but any duration and opportunity for meditation is beneficial, even if it is only one breath or 1 minute. The daily commitment of meditation requires a continual nonjudgmental return to the practice itself, over and over again every day (similar to building a muscle). If you miss a day, or a week, or even years, simply return to the practice of meditation without judgment.
- For "informal practice," try to approach everyday activities with the same mindful intention, attitude, attention, and presence as in "formal" meditation. While driving to work, focus on driving. When at work, concentrate on the performance of each task. At home, live and be completely present with others. Keep in mind that meditation is not about withdrawal from the world or responsibilities. It is about living with purpose, awareness, and kindness.
- A deepening of spiritual life or "religious experience" may occur. Although this can be pleasant, it can also be disconcerting early on and may require the reassurance and guidance of an understanding teacher.

---

therapies. As early as 1935, French cardiologist Brosse[11] studied Indian yogis capable of decreasing their heart rates to almost zero as shown on electrocardiography (ECG). In 1961, Bagchi and Wenger[12] found that some expert meditation subjects could produce bidirectional changes in every measurable autonomic variable. The *Lancet* published an account of the voluntary live burial of a yogi who sat cross-legged underground for 62 hours while continuous vital sign recordings revealed

no distress.[13] In 1968, Hoenig[14] witnessed an experiment in which a yogi confined for 9 hours in a small enclosed pit and monitored with electroencephalography and ECG demonstrated a normal waking rhythm for the full 9 hours. He observed that the expert meditator was awake and relaxed throughout the experiment. He also observed a variable heart rate from 40 to 100 beats/minute in recurring cycles on ECG.[14] As in fetal heart monitoring, later research would show that synchronous increases in heart rate variability in adults predict a decrease in cardiovascular mortality,[15,16] which can be reproduced and maintained using meditation practice[17,18] (see Chapter 96).

BOX 100.3	Precautions and Recommendations for Meditation Practice

- Leg and back discomfort are common concerns. Do not strain the body. Sit in an alert and comfortable position. Remember that meditation is about openness and receptivity, not about distorting the body or being uncomfortable.
- In the beginning, intrusive, repetitive, or distracting thoughts may make it difficult to sit still for even 5 minutes. Keep in mind that meditation is not about making things go away. It is simply the nonjudgmental process of staying present with whatever is happening moment-by-moment, pleasant or unpleasant. However, over time and with regular practice, the mind will become more stable.
- In learning meditation, one should be guided by teachers and practices that resonate authentically, are nondivisive, and instill feelings of support and wellbeing. Do not forfeit personal boundaries and safety for any teacher or teaching. Listen to your intuition and reason, and trust that the experience you are having is exactly what you need in this moment.
- Meditation can at times uncover preexisting stressors or traumas, similar to peeling back the layers of an onion, thus revealing unpleasant underlying emotions. A professional mental health therapist familiar with contemplative practice can help facilitate the healthy release of these emotions.
- Be attentive to and honest about your experience. In a compassionate way, attend to realizations and insights that arise from regular meditation practice. This may include journaling, creative expression, and talking with a skilled meditation teacher.
- Include a gentle form of movement, such as contemplative or mindful walking, walking a labyrinth, yoga, Pilates, Nia, tai chi, or qi gong (or swimming, biking, running, hiking, canoeing, or skiing). However, avoid striving and straining.

THE EXPERIENCE (TIES MNEMONIC)

- Talk/thoughts: mental chatter, incessant thinking, storyline, narratives
- Images: mental pictures, imagined scenes, visualized scenarios
- Emotional feelings: love, hate, fear, joy, sadness, anxiety, etc.
- Physical sensations: sound, touch, sight, taste, smell

Benson et al.[19] helped pioneer academic interest in meditation through research on the physiological and neurochemical principles of "the relaxation response," which is defined as a hypometabolic state of parasympathetic activation.[19] Furthermore, many studies have demonstrated that meditation can reduce anxiety and increase positive affect,[20–22] whereas others have shown that mindfulness can help prevent recurrence of depression.[23,24] In a 1985 study by Kabat-Zinn et al.,[25] patients with chronic pain showed a statistically significant reduction in various measures of pain symptoms when they were trained in mindfulness-based stress reduction (MBSR). Meditation can also be helpful for headaches,[26,27] psoriasis,[28] blood pressure,[29–31] hyperlipidemia,[31] smoking cessation,[32–34] alcohol abuse,[35] atherosclerosis,[36] coronary artery disease,[3,37,38] longevity and cognitive function in older adults,[39,40] psychiatric disorders,[19–24,41] excessive worry,[42] overuse of medical services,[43] and medical costs in treating chronic pain.[44] Meta-analyses have found mindfulness training useful for a broad range of chronic disorders that are difficult to treat, such as healthy behavior change,[45] depression and anxiety,[46] attention deficit hyperactivity disorder (ADHD),[47] borderline personality disorder,[48] fibromyalgia, chronic insomnia,[49] cancer, coronary artery disease, chronic pain, obesity, and eating disorders.[50,51] The investigators noted consistent and strong effect sizes across these very different situations, thus indicating the potential wide-reaching benefits for both daily life stress and more complex medical disorders.[50]

In a meta-analysis of brain imaging studies on various meditation styles, Newberg[52] suggested that the neurophysiological effects derived from various meditation practices seem to outline a consistent and reproducible pattern of significant brain activity in key cerebral structures such as the posterior cingulate cortex.[53] Davidson[54] described a positive correlation between meditation practice and left-sided prefrontal cortex activity, which is associated with a positive effect. In this study, mindfulness meditation was associated with increases in antibody titers to influenza vaccine, a finding suggesting correlations among meditation, positive emotional states, localized brain activity, and improved immune function. Corroborating research demonstrates a direct link between immune function and mood, with positive affective states resulting in stronger immune function and decreased incidence of illness.[55–57] Lutz[58] observed increased left-sided prefrontal cortex gamma wave activity and synchronicity in expert Tibetan Buddhist meditators with more than 10,000 hours of meditation experience when compared with novice meditator controls, both at rest and during meditation. In addition, compared with short-term mindfulness practitioners, long-term meditators showed lower frontal theta activity, indicating the ability to limit excessive processing of unnecessary information (discursive thought).[59] These findings reveal that attention and affect are flexible traits that can be improved.

Although ongoing research aims to elucidate the measurable biological correlates of meditation and their significance with regard to health, the experiential knowledge that has arisen from time-tested practices of great spiritual traditions should be acknowledged. Meditation practitioners continue to explore the subtle inner dimensions of the meditative experience using methods and perspectives that, like objective sciences, equally address the human condition.

Mindfulness has potential wide-reaching benefits for both daily life stress and more complex medical disorders.

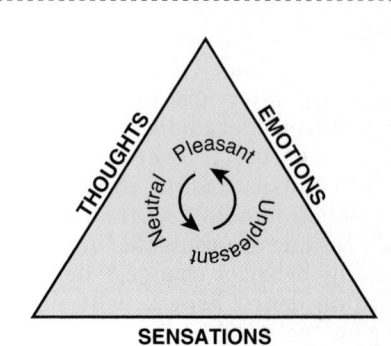

Mindfulness practice (SOAP):

- **Stop:** Pause, notice your breathing, settle into the present moment just as it is...
- **Observe:** Drop into the body, being aware of and feeling whatever is happening in this moment (sensations/feelings/thinking)...
- **Assess:** Without judgment, recognize the pleasant/unpleasant/neutral nature of this experience and let it go...
- **Proceed:** Take a deep breath, and move on...

Triangle of mindful experience:

- **Mental thoughts:** Rumination, thinking, storylines, narratives, mental images, internal conversations, and so on...
- **Emotional feelings:** Love, hate, fear, guilt, anger, joy, sadness, anxiety, and so on...
- **Physical sensations:** Sound, touch, taste, smell, vibration, pressure, and so on...

Intentional kindness practice:

- May I/you/we be well
- May I/you/we be at ease
- May I/you/we be safe and protected
- May I/you/we understand and be understood

FIG. 100.1 ■ Mindfulness "practice as you go" cards (a cutout handout for patients).

MINDFULNESS IN MEDICAL PRACTICE

Practicing health-oriented medicine in a dysfunctional disease-focused system that does little to honor prevention is increasingly difficult.[60] Clinicians are pressured to see more patients, work longer hours, and are incentivized to quickly improve reported quality measures (e.g., A1c values) with medications as opposed to lifestyle changes. Particularly in primary care, clinicians are forced to reduce their restricted time, energy, and attention on laboratory tests, imaging studies, documentation, billing and coding, electronic medical record interfacing, and quick prescriptions at the expense of meaningful time with the patient.[5] For clinicians, maintaining a balance between personal needs and the demands of medical training and practice is often neglected at the cost of their own well-being and health. Sleep, exercise, relaxation, and personal interests take a back seat to increasingly invasive clinical demands that contribute to burnout.[5,61]

Research suggests that mindfulness can help cultivate present-moment awareness that may reduce medical error and improve patient care and health care quality.[62] For example, faulty thinking, such as snap judgments, distracted attention, discursive thought, inadvertent stereotyping, and other cognitive traps can lead to critical mistakes.[59,63] Growing research also shows that clinicians who themselves exhibit healthy habits are more effective in motivating patients to make significant positive changes in their own lives.[64] This is also true of clinicians who themselves practice meditation. In a randomized controlled trial of 124 psychiatric inpatients managed by 18 psychology residents, Grepmair[65] showed that patients of interns who received mindfulness training did significantly better than did patients

treated by interns who did not receive mindfulness training.

The University of Wisconsin Integrative Medicine Program created a collaborative online education module (http://www.fammed.wisc.edu/mindfulness; Box 100.4, first item) to provide ongoing support for mindfulness practice and to help clinicians bring mindfulness into the clinical encounter by using a three-step process: (1) pause, (2) presence, and (3) proceed[66] (see Chapter 3). The first step, *pause*, encourages the clinician to stop and take a momentary pause. The second step, *presence*, encourages the clinician to focus on the present moment and be aware of sensations, emotions, and thoughts that arise without judgment or analysis. The third step, *proceed*, encourages health-oriented action that responds in a skillful and compassionate way by using insight gained from steps one and two. For example, the symptom-focused visit would only result in a medication to abort a migraine headache, but the mindful clinician is more likely to recognize and address the emotional stressors that are triggering the migraines. This approach focuses more on the underlying cause of the pain rather than just the pain symptoms alone. The mindful clinical encounter encourages the clinician to pay attention to and illuminate key healing mechanisms that arise from the patient-clinician interaction.

TYPES OF MEDITATION

Most styles of meditation are influenced by the realizations of a particular teacher or group and should be considered within their historical and cultural context. The vast collection of information, teachings, and practices

BOX 100.4	Resources and Links to Learn Meditation

- http://www.fammed.wisc.edu/mindfulness (online guided practices and resources for mindfulness in medicine from the University of Wisconsin)
- http://www.umassmed.edu/content.aspx?id=41252 (University of Massachusetts Center for Mindfulness)
- https://www.fammed.wisc.edu/aware-medicine/mindfulness (University of Wisconsin Aware Medicine Curriculum)
- http://eomega.org/ (New York/East Coast Omega Institute)
- http://nccam.nih.gov/ (National Center for Complementary and Alternative Medicine)
- http://diydharma.org/about-us (Do It Yourself Dharma)
- http://www.spiritrock.org/ (California/West Coast Spirit Rock Meditation Center)
- http://www.contemplativeoutreach.org/site/PageServer (Contemplative Outreach [Centering Prayer])
- http://www.christinecenter.org (Wisconsin/Midwest Christine Center)
- *Meditation for Beginners*, by Jack Kornfield, PhD (book and CD)
- *Guided Mindfulness Meditation*, by Jon Kabat-Zinn (CD)
- *Full Catastrophe Living*, by Jon Kabat-Zinn (book)
- *Open Mind Open Heart*, by Fr. Thomas Keating, OCSO (book)
- *The Beginner's Guide to Contemplative Prayer*, by James Finley, PhD (CD)

BOX 100.5	Other Popular Meditation Styles, Teachers, and Spiritual Practices

Ram Dass, formerly a Harvard University psychologist and researcher, learned Hindu meditation and chanting from his guru Maharaji. Books: *Be Here Now* and *Still Here.* Website: http://learnoutloud.com/Resources/Authors-and-Narrators/Ram-Dass/392

Eckhart Tolle, formerly an Oxford University research scholar, experienced a spiritual transformation and teaches contemporary spirituality. Book: *The Power of Now.* Website: http://www.eckharttolle.com

Tom Brown, Jr. was mentored by "Grandfather," an Apache Medicine Man and Scout. Book: *The Vision.* School: Nature and Wilderness Survival Schools. Website: http://www.trackerschool.com

Ken Wilber, creator of the unified field theory of consciousness. Book: *A Brief History of Everything.* School: Integral Institute. Websites: http://www.kenwilber.com, https://integrallife.com, http://wilber.shambhala.com

John Main, a Catholic monk, founder of Christian Meditation inbreath mental mantra "MA-RA" and outbreath "NA-THA" Sanskrit for "Come Lord Jesus." Book: *Word into Silence.* Website: http://www.wccm.org

Neale Donald Walsch, author of *Conversations with God* and founder of Re-Creation retreats. Website: http://www.nealedonaldwalsch.com

can seem daunting, and selecting a meditation practice style can be challenging. One way to help is to begin reading about the different styles with an open mind, or by attending an introductory class, or meeting with a meditation teacher to help discern what practice is a good fit. Although the practice styles vary, the insights and realizations that arise from meditation practice have a universal quality. As the common saying goes, "all paths lead to Rome" (see Box 100.4; Box 100.5 and Table 100.1). It is also helpful to keep in mind that, like exercise, any amount of mindfulness practice can be helpful, even brief interventions.[5,67]

"What joy awaits discovery in the silence behind the portals of your mind no human tongue can tell. But you must convince yourself; you must meditate and create that environment."

PARAMAHANSA YOGANANDA

MOVEMENT AS MEDITATION

Often, we think of meditation as sitting on a cushion, folding the legs in a lotus position, closing the eyes, and focusing the attention on something such as a candle, a word, or a chant. These are just a few of the many meditation varieties, but this is not the only way. "Formal" meditation practice typically involves being seated and still in a comfortable and alert position, generally on a supportive chair or meditation cushion on the floor (called a *Zafu*) (Fig. 100.2; meditation postures). In addition, most styles of meditation also incorporate some form of movement such as yoga, contemplative or mindful walking, tai chi, labyrinth walking, dance, and just strolling through nature (including long distance running, biking, hiking, and skiing). Being present and connected with the body and noticing the qualities of the various physical sensations that arise with movement are fundamental to this process. Body sensations are effectively an anchoring force to facilitate grounding and centering in the present moment. Meditation is an inward-orienting, self-empowering mind–body practice that can stimulate the healing process and help patients and clinicians navigate unsettling and turbulent experiences.

TABLE 100.1 Systems of Meditation Table*

	Centering Prayer/ Contemplation	Kabbalah (Qabalah)	Mindfulness Meditation	Ridhwan School Diamond Approach	Self-Realization Fellowship (SRF)	Transcendental Meditation	Tibetan Buddhism	Zen Buddhism/ Ch'an
Traditional Background	Catholic/Christian	Jewish mystical	Vipassana/insight; mindfulness-based stress reduction medical	Sufi Islam, mystical psychology	Hindu Kriya yoga	Vedic Hindu	Various Tibetan lineages	Numerous Chinese and Japanese lineages
Teachers	Thomas Keating; Thomas Merton; Cynthia Bourgeault; M. Basil Pennington; William Meninger	Yehuda Ashlag; David Cooper; Michael Laitman	Jon Kabat-Zinn; Bhante Gunaratana; Sharon Salzberg; Jack Kornfield; Thich Nhat Hanh	A.H. Almaas (Hameed Ali)	Paramahansa Yogananda; Sri Daya Mata	Maharishi Mahesh Yogi (Various)	Fourteenth Dalai Lama; Panchen Lama; Chogyam Trungpa; Seventeenth Karmapa	Bodhidharma; Eisai; Dogan; Huang Po; Charlotte Joko Beck; Claude A. Thomas
Technique	Sacred word; prayer; lectio divina	Kabbalah	Breath/body awareness	Inquiry	Kriya yoga; Hong-Sau; Aum	Personalized mantra	Mantra; visualization; chanting	Zazen
Body/Activity Focus	Contemplative walking	Self-directed	Mindful walking; Hatha yoga; body scan	Breathing exercises	Energization exercises	Self-directed	Rlung-sgom walking; mudras	Martial arts (Kungfu); Zen arts (ceramics, archery, calligraphy)
Readings/Books	*New Seeds of Contemplation* (Merton); *Open Mind Open Heart* (Keating)	*A Beginner's Guide to Kabbalah* (CD); *A Heart of Stillness* (Cooper)	*Mindfulness in Plain English* (Gunaratana); *Full Catastrophe Living* (Kabat-Zinn); *A Path with Heart* (Kornfield)	*Essence; The Diamond Heart Series I–IV; Inner Journey Home* (by Almaas)	*Autobiography of a Yogi; SRF Lessons* (Yogananda)	*Science of Being and Art of Living; Transcendental Meditation* (Maharishi)	*The World of Tibetan Buddhism; Path to Bliss* (Gyatso); *Start Where You Are* (Chodron)	*Zen Mind Beginner's Mind* (Suzuki); *The Three Pillars of Zen* (Kapleau); *Everyday Zen* (Beck)
Coursework	Retreats; contemplative outreach	Tree of Life; Ten Sefirot; Devekut; teacher-directed	Mindfulness-based stress reduction/cognitive therapy	Diamond approach lessons; retreats	Mailed lessons; retreats; guru relationship; interviews with monks	Seven-step coursework; interviews; personal mantra; retreats	Teacher-student; lineage-directed	Teacher-student
Main Sites/ Headquarters	Abbey of Gethsemani, Trappist, KY; Snowmass, CO; multiple/ regional	Multiple	Insight Meditation Society, MA; University of Massachusetts (for mindfulness-based stress reduction); Spirit Rock, CA; Plum Village, France; multiple	Berkeley, CA; Boulder, CO; multiple	Los Angeles; Multiple (see also Yogoda Satsanga Society of India, sister organization to SRF)	Fairfield, IA; multiple; (Transcendental Meditation Independent UK)	Lhasa, Tibet; Dharamsala, India; multiple	Shaolin Temple, China (birthplace); multiple centers

Websites/ Contact Information	www. centeringprayer. com (also see Christian Meditation: www.wccm.org)	www.kabbalah. info; www. kabbalah.com; 1-800-kabbalah	www.dharma. org; www. umassmed. edu/cfm/mbsr; www.eomega. org; www. spiritrock. org; www. plumvillage. org	www. ahalmaas. com; www. ridhwan. org	www.srf- yogananda. org	www.tm.org; www. maharishipeacepalace. org; 1-888-learnTM; (www.tm-meditation. co.uk, independent, less expensive)	www.tibet. com; www. deerparkcenter. org; www. dawnmountain. org; www. drikungtmc.org	www. dharmanet. org; www. tricycle.com
Comments	Contemplation dates back to St. Anthony and the Desert Fathers; revived after Vatican II; in the tradition of Christian saints and mystics	Ancient oral tradition of wisdom and mystery; tells of Light of Creation; Jewish renewal movement	Popularized in the 1980s; from an 8-wk course in a medical/ research setting; many vipassana/ insight sanghas or groups	Founded in the 1970s; called the Work, draws from psychology and integrates a spiritual approach to self- liberation	Founded in 1920; popularized yoga- meditation in the United States; teaches a direct path to self- realization through ancient Kriya yoga	Popularized in the 1960s, expanded meditation in the United States; large corpus of health research at Maharishi Vedic University	Model of nonviolence, loving compassion for sentient beings; ongoing dialogue with neuroscience researchers	Chinese/ Japanese tradition arrived in the United States after World War II; most Zen meditation research is in Japanese

*This table is representative and not exhaustive.

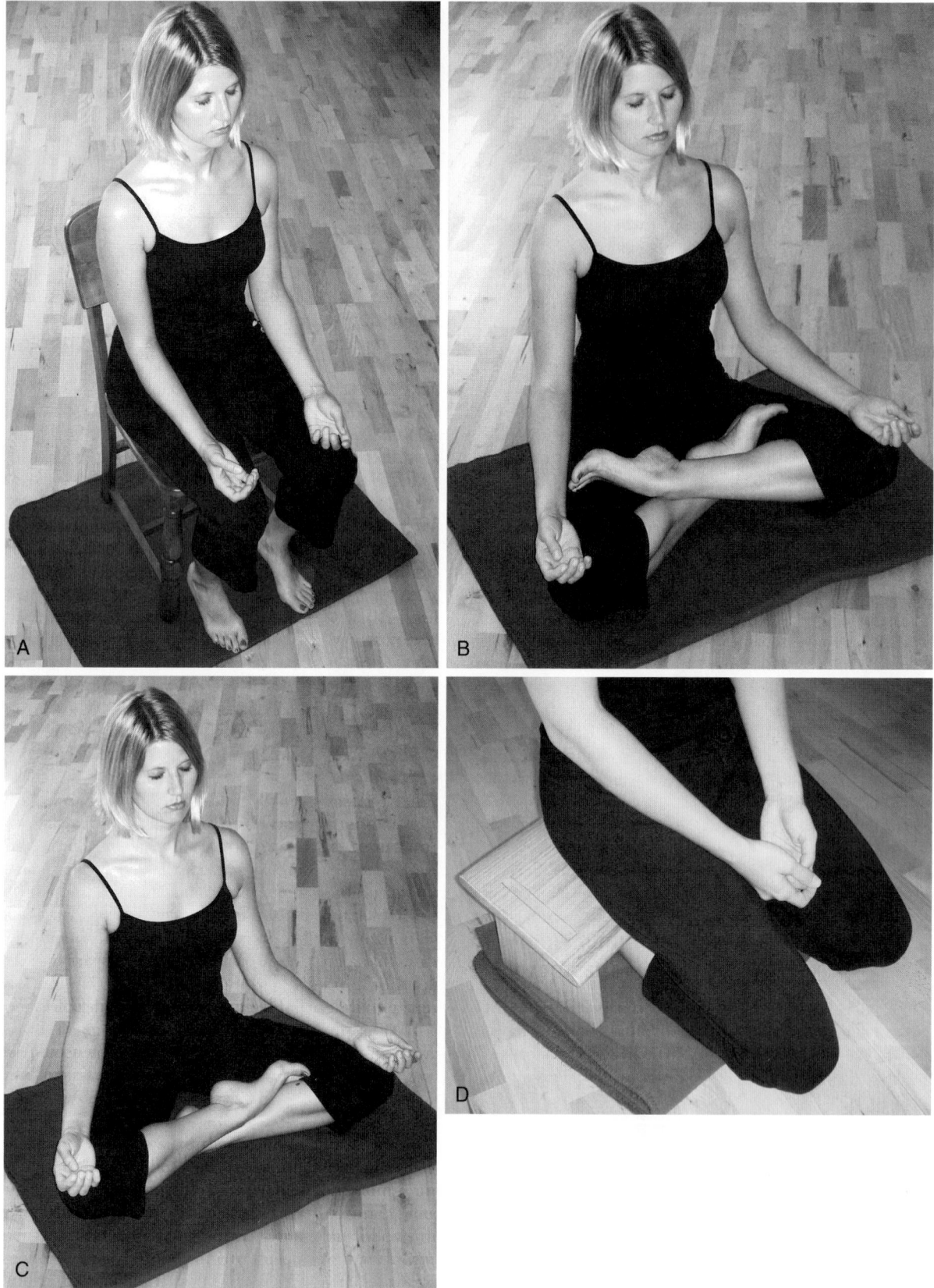

FIG. 100.2 ■ Meditation postures. A, Seated position with a chair. Maintain a straight back. B, Full lotus position. Maintain a straight back. Use of a cushion, shawl, mat, or blanket for comfort may be helpful. C, Half-lotus position. Maintain a straight back. Use of a cushion, shawl, mat, or blanket for comfort may be helpful. D, Kneeling position with a bench. Maintain a straight back. Use of a shawl, mat, or blanket for comfort may be helpful.

Key Web Resources

The University of Wisconsin Integrative Medicine, Mindfulness in Medicine Program: Offers guided practices and resources for mindfulness in medicine.	http://www.fammed.wisc.edu/mindfulness
University of Massachusetts Center for Mindfulness: Mindfulness resources and information on obtaining mindfulness teacher certification.	http://www.umassmed.edu/content.aspx?id=41252
New York/East Coast Omega Institute: A retreat center in the East that offers a variety of meditation and health-oriented experiences.	http://eomega.org/
California/West Coast Spirit Rock Meditation Center: A retreat center on the West Coast that offers a variety of meditation and health-oriented experiences.	http://www.spiritrock.org/
The University of Rochester Mindful Practice: Offers retreats and continuing medical education on a self-reflective mindful approach to clinical practice.	https://www.urmc.rochester.edu/family-medicine/mindful-practice.aspx
Contemplative Outreach: Offers instruction on Centering Prayer, a Christian contemplative meditation practice.	http://www.contemplativeoutreach.org/category/category/centering-prayer
Other Suggested Resources	*Meditation for Beginners,* by Jack Kornfield, PhD (book and CD) *Guided Mindfulness Meditation,* by Jon Kabat-Zinn (CD) *Full Catastrophe Living,* by Jon Kabat-Zinn (book) *Open Mind Open Heart,* by Fr. Thomas Keating, OCSO (book) *The Beginner's Guide to Contemplative Prayer,* by James Finley, PhD (CD)

REFERENCES

References are available online at **ExpertConsult.com**.

CHAPTER 101

MOTIVATIONAL INTERVIEWING

Robert Rhode, PhD

Health care providers often diagnose a patient's condition and recommend health-promoting behaviors (e.g., take this drug as prescribed, exercise, stop smoking, decrease substance use, make appointments for care, follow a diet). Integrative medicine is more than just recommending some alternative or complimentary health-promoting behaviors. It also involves the way in which the health care provider interacts with the client.

THREE HELPING STYLES[1]

Directing

In most health care settings, the health care provider uses a directing helping style, which often includes identifying the health goal or destination and giving clear advice on how to reach that destination. The health care provider is using his or her expertise, identifying the problems to be addressed, and prescribing treatments or prescribing behaviors. The client would do well to heed and follow this well-intended advice. Health care providers with years of experience are familiar with how their accurate advice is not always followed by clients.

Even though a directing helping style may not always facilitate the desired health improvement, it is valuable in health care, and some clients are responsive to it. In some situations, the client's cooperation cannot be solicited, such as during an emergency or when the client is unconscious. At such times, the clinician takes charge, acts unilaterally, and performs the treatment to the client or for the client.

Following

A following helping style is more common in counseling or psychotherapy than in medical settings. There is a goal of developing rapport and staying with the client. Health care providers facilitate healing by being genuinely present and attending to clients with heart and mind. When one choice or another has no obvious risks or benefits (e.g., changing jobs, relationships, or becoming pregnant), the clinician is very likely to use a following helping style to facilitate the client's talking about his or her choices and avoid advocating or emphasizing any particular choice.

Guiding

A guiding helping style is a third way, and may be somewhere between a directing and a following helping style. Motivational interviewing can be considered a specialized version of a guiding helping style that assists clients to access their thoughts, experiences, and emotions to engage in the health-promoting behavior. It may be a style that is most useful when the client is the one who has to implement the health-promoting behavior and the health care provider cannot do it to the client or for the client. Many lifestyle behaviors might be responsive to this helping style because it is the client who has to exercise, eat more nutritiously, engage in meditation, or abstain from smoking.

> Motivational interviewing can be considered a specialized version of a guiding helping style that assists clients to access their own thoughts and experiences to implement the health-promoting behavior.

A guiding helping style involves going toward a destination, and in that way it resembles a directing helping style. It also is client centered, by collaborating with the client and recognizing the client as an expert and the primary decision maker, and in that way it is similar to a following helping style.

A directing helping style has been called a "push technology."[2] The clinician is attempting to install knowledge or motivation as if the client is missing it. A guiding helping style is a "pull technology." The health care provider is attempting to pull the knowledge and motivation from the client's existing resources and experiences. A directing helping style is consistent with the clinician's role as the healer, the one who cures, and the expert. A guiding helping style emphasizes healing rather than the healer, with two experts (the client and the clinician) in the consultation room. In settings where a directing helping style is common, the recipients of care are often called "patients." When a guiding or following helping style is more often used, the care recipients are often called "clients" or even "consumers."

All these styles are helpful, and you might think where in your clinical encounters each style is useful. A trauma surgeon is going to need and use a directing helping style more than a following helping style, but a primary care provider might use a guiding helping style more than a directing helping style, especially for health-promoting behaviors that involve lifestyle changes (eating, exercise, stress management, etc.). This chapter focuses on the guiding helping style and, in particular, on motivational interviewing, not because it is always better but because it is often underused given the common reliance on a directing helping style in health care settings. A guiding helping style may also be more consistent with integrative medicine.

Knowing About Versus Using Motivational Interviewing

Many health care providers have heard about motivational interviewing. However, it is sometimes reduced to "be nice" or "roll with client resistance," which hardly helps the health care provider know what to say during a consult. Less than 18% of primary health care providers report that they are generally or very familiar with motivational interviewing.[3] Even after some formal training, the frequency and quality of the motivational interviewing skills used with actual clients is probably less than what is required to see improvements in client behaviors.[4-6] Motivational interviewing is like other areas of health care: knowing that a surgery can be done is not the same thing as being able to perform that surgery skillfully. William Miller, one of the primary authors in the field, has said that it can take up to 10 years to become really good at using motivational interviewing. Although this may be so, this chapter presents several ways for the health care provider to use it immediately. All of them are consistent with motivational interviewing, although perhaps only the most elegant one is particular to motivational interviewing.

FOUNDATION OR SPIRIT OF MOTIVATIONAL INTERVIEWING

A motivational interviewing approach is built upon four foundational values. Most health care providers, particularly integrative medicine ones, find that these are already part of their consultations or interactions:

1. **Accepting the client.** This includes empathizing with the client and recognizing that the client is valuable and competent regardless of his or her circumstances. It also involves recognizing that it is the client who has to adopt the health-promoting behavior; the health care provider cannot do it to the client or for the client. This also includes demonstrating support for the client's ability to decide to change now, later, or not at all.
2. **Compassion.** Dedication to others' welfare and well-being has often been present in the health care provider's life and values long before formal training and working with clients.
3. **Collaboration.** Involves coming along side, joining up, or looking at the client's life or situation with the client; partnering with the client to consider a difficult situation.
4. **Curiosity.** Instead of trying to instill knowledge or motivation, the health care provider helps the client access his desire and reasons for doing the health-promoting behavior. The health care provider does not lead with his or her expertise but rather solicits and learns what the client knows first.

A directive helping style does not involve a lot of collaboration with the client because the health care provider is adopting an expert role and "driving the bus." Similarly, it is not so important to be curious about the client's experience because the clinician is deciding what needs to be done. An example of this is when the clinician tells the client that he or she is drinking too much, meets the criteria for alcoholism, needs to attend Alcoholics Anonymous meetings, and should abstain from drinking. The client's objection to the diagnosis and treatment recommendation does not change the clinician's directions and is often labeled, very logically, by the clinician as an example of the client's denying reality or the truth ("The patient is in denial.").

> Noncompliance is often used to blame the patient that does not follow a directive helping style. In fact, noncompliance is two people working towards different goals.

When a motivational interviewing style is used, the clinician respects the client as capable and competent, and therefore it makes sense to collaborate with him or her. If the clinician intends to collaborate with the client, it makes sense to respect and support his or her autonomy. The client will literally be the one to implement (or not) the health-promoting behavior. During a stay in the hospital, health care providers may have more control over the patient's diet, activity, and medication. When the client is out of the hospital, he or she decides what to eat, what to do, and what medication to take. Respecting this reality and explicitly recognizing that the client will make these decisions relieves the clinician of the frustrating task of trying to control the client. The clinician is no longer driving the bus but is "on the bus" with the client, looking at health behaviors and decisions with the client. If the client is capable, competent, and believed to be the key person to implement any treatment, then it makes perfect sense to be curious about the client's experience and his or her reasons for embracing or rejecting the health-promoting behaviors.

The client who is drinking too much is approached differently with this mindset. The clinician still maintains a focus on the destination of less drinking or abstaining, but instead of telling the client what the problem is, he or she now asks what the client thinks about the drinking and how it fits with other goals or values. Instead of pushing a treatment, the clinician explores what makes sense to the client. The client's objections to abstaining are not heard as denial but rather as the client's natural ambivalence to giving up something that he or she enjoys or to which he or she is attached. The clinician may help the client find his or her motivation to change this drinking by exploring which of the client's goals or experiences are diminished by the current drinking.

This collaboration with a client who is recognized as capable seems consistent with integrative medicine as described by Andrew Weil:[7] "There is this tremendous innate healing capacity that we all have. When I sit with a person who is sick, always at the back of my mind is the question, *What is blocking healing here? What is preventing it? What can I do from outside that can facilitate that process?*"

Table 101.1 describes some ways to experiment with a helping style that is consistent with motivational interviewing. This can be summarized as, "Don't tell, ask."

TABLE 101.1   One Way to Experiment With a Helping Style That Is Consistent With Motivational Interviewing

Directing Helping Style	Motivational Interviewing Style
These may be methods that a health care provider could use to help a client. These fit with a directing helping style.	Instead of using a directing helping style, a health care provider could use a style consistent with motivational interviewing:
Explaining why the client should engage in the health-promoting behavior.	Listening with the goal of understanding the client's dilemma concerning the health-promoting behavior.
Teaching the client, telling him or her what to do, or giving advice.	Asking what the client knows, then providing some information or advice if necessary, and finally asking how that fits with his or her understanding or experience.
Describing specific benefits that would result from doing the health-promoting behavior.	Asking, "What benefits may there be for you if you engaged in this health-promoting behavior?"
Telling the client how to implement the health-promoting behavior.	Asking, "What are you already doing that would make it possible for you to do this health-promoting behavior?" Or, "How might you do this health-promoting behavior so it fits into your day?"
Emphasizing how important it is for the client to engage in the health-promoting behavior.	Asking, "Why is it important to you to think about or do this health-promoting behavior?"
Telling or inspiring the client to engage in the health-promoting behavior.	Asking, "Why would you want to enhance your health?"

TABLE 101.2   A Second Way to Experiment With a Helping Style That Is Consistent With Motivational Interviewing

1. Would it be OK if I asked you a couple of questions about how you are taking care of your _____ {health, diabetes, asthma, blood pressure, etc.}?
2. What are you doing these days that you think makes a positive contribution or helps with your _____ {health, diabetes, asthma, blood pressure, etc.}? (Spend a minute or two on this. The client is likely to say one or two things. Help the client elaborate about what they are doing and why.)
3. Most of us at one point or another forget to take our medicines or forget our good intentions to follow the advice of a physician or nurse. What are you sometimes forgetting to do or sometimes not getting around to doing that might otherwise help your health?
4. Sometimes we might do things that we might enjoy but others think aren't good for us, like drinking too much alcohol, eating too much fast food, or being too sedentary. What might you put in this category?

A similar way to generate a motivational interviewing consistent approach is for the health care provider to suspend the expert role. He or she will very likely join the client who is facing the challenge of improving well-being or managing a chronic condition. Although "care" today has the connotation of intervening in a beneficial way, another meaning is "to be with." Collaborating includes looking together at the situation. While looking in the same direction, being curious about the client's motivation for the health-promoting behaviors is easier. Table 101.2 outlines four questions that have been used in this manner.

WHAT DIFFERENCE MAY IT MAKE IF A MOTIVATIONAL INTERVIEWING APPROACH IS USED?

Meta-analysis and reviews of the effectiveness of motivational interviewing have been published.[8-13] Much of the initial research was related to health behaviors in the area of substance use. Over the years, more studies have focused on a broader range of health-promoting behaviors (Fig. 101.1). The effect sizes for various health behaviors 3 and 12 months after treatment are shown in Fig. 101.2.

Perhaps the Strength of Recommendation Taxonomy rating for the evidence would be grade A for health behaviors such as substance use and human immunodeficiency virus risk behaviors. For other health behaviors such as nutrition, exercise, and smoking, the rating may be grade B. The rating for potential harm may be grade 1 for all health behaviors.

HELPING CLIENTS FIND AND USE THEIR MOTIVATION

Motivation is not binary, on or off, there or not there. Most clients are ambivalent about engaging in health-promoting behaviors, rather than either being motivated or not motivated. They have some motivation for the health-risky behavior and some for the health-promoting behavior. They enjoy smoking but know they should quit. They have reasons to lose weight but have failed in the past. They want to reduce their blood pressure but have no time to meditate or exercise. When clinicians use a motivational interviewing helping style, they think of this ambivalence as a common human experience rather than an indication of denial or resistance.

A client who is not engaging in some health-promoting behavior can be conceptualized by the health care provider as not having sufficient motivation to do what would be health promoting. Trying to install more motivation either by inspiration or by threat can be seductive. That kind of directing helping style sometimes works. A health care provider who intends to use a motivational interviewing style similarly recognizes that the client does not have sufficient motivation to engage in the health-promoting behavior; in this case, however, the clinician goes looking for what motivation there is and ways that the client may find additional motivation.

> The health care provider can work hard to instill motivation into the client or help the client find his or her already existing experiences, thoughts, and emotions that go with doing the health-promoting behavior.

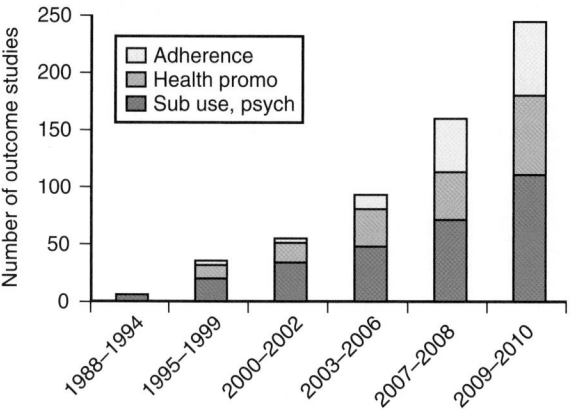

FIG. 101.1 ■ Growth of motivational interviewing studies. *promo*, promotion; *psych*, psychological issues; *sub use*, substance use.

Finding the client's motivation can be easier when the clinician thinks about various aspects of motivation. Researcher Paul Amrhein[14] identified that statements about desire, ability, reasons, and need often come up in conversations with a focus on changing a particular behavior (in motivational interviewing, this particular behavior or goal is called the *target behavior*). Statements the client makes in these categories probably indicate some facet of the client's motivation about doing the health behavior. Two additional categories related to the client's action can also be heard from clients sometimes: already taken steps (past tense) and commitment (future tense). Clients can make statements in any of these six categories in the direction of health (in which case motivational interviewing refers to it as change talk) or in the direction of not engaging in the health-promoting behavior (in which case it is referred to as *sustain talk*, as in maintaining the status quo). Table 101.3 provides additional descriptions of each of these categories.

These categories provide the health care provider with guidance about where to go fishing for the client's motivation. A client who says "I don't have time to meditate" is describing something about ability. The clinician may then focus on a different category to try to solicit a motivation for meditating, "You don't have time to meditate, but it sounds like you wish you did." This statement involves recognizing ability in the sustain direction and fishing for desire in the change direction. If the client complains about following a new cholesterol-lowering diet, the clinician can respond, "You are not finding it fun to follow this diet, so why are you intending to do so?" This question involves recognizing desire in the sustain direction and fishing for reasons in the change direction. Table 101.4 provides examples of each category of motivation in both sustain and change directions for the target behavior of engaging in behaviors that would promote heart health after a heart attack.

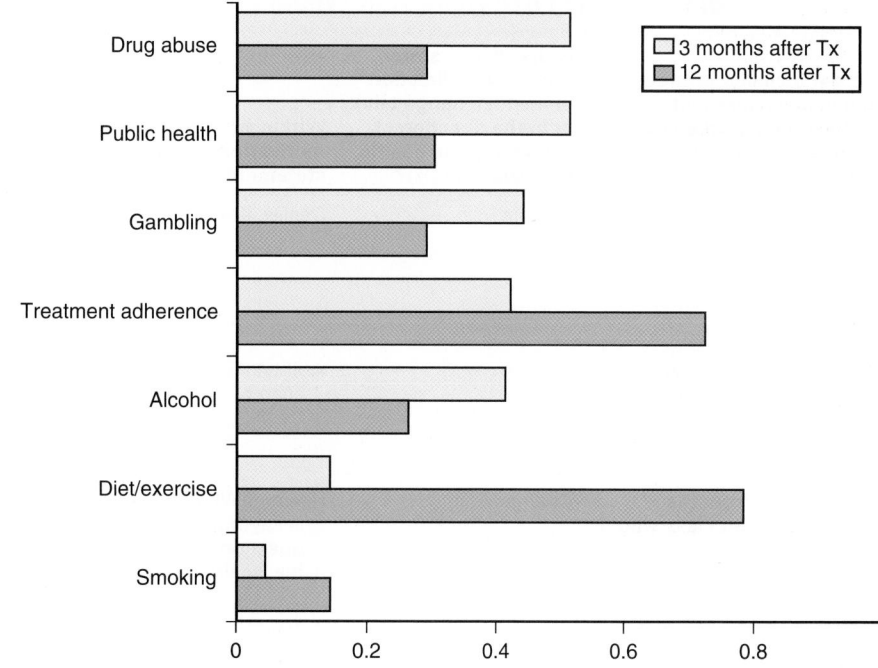

FIG. 101.2 ■ Effect size comparing motivational interviewing to a directing helping style at 3 and 12 months. (From Hettema J, Steele J, Miller W. Motivational interviewing. *Annu Rev Clin Psychol.* 2005;1:91-111.)

TABLE 101.3 **Change Talk and Sustain Talk by the Client**

Category	Client Talks About	Words That May Be Clues That the Client Is Talking About This Aspect of His or Her Motivation	
Desire	What he may enjoy or not enjoy, like or dislike, find as fun or not fun, and want or not want.	I want I would like I enjoy It's fun to...	I don't want I hate, I don't like I wouldn't enjoy It's no fun to..., It's work to...
Ability	What he perceives he is able or unable to do, what is possible or impossible, and what he or she can or cannot do.	I can, I could I'm able It's possible	I can't I'm unable It's impossible
Need	What he thinks he should do, has to do, should not have to do, what is just or unjust, what the "right" or "wrong" thing is to do.	I need to I should I'd better I have to	I don't need to I shouldn't have to It's not important that I... I don't have to
Reasons	The rationale, justification, or motive for doing or not doing the behavior.	Reasons are often preceded by "so," "because," or "so that," and they often follow statements in other categories, particularly need: "I don't need to because..." Reasons answer the question, "Why?" or "Why not?" Desire and Need are two specific reasons. Anything that answers the question, "Why?" or "Why not?" that is neither Desire nor Need might be a Reason.	
Already Taken Steps	Behaviors he has performed (in the recent past) that may be in the direction of change or in the direction of staying the same.	Already Taken Steps are actions that have already occurred and have helped or hindered progress toward the health-promoting behavior.	
Commitment	What the client will or will not do in the future and intentions or agreements about the future. The strength of the commitment can vary, but they are commitment statements because they talk about the future.	I'll try I definitely will I promise to I suppose I might try to I will	I'm not going to try I won't There is no way I will I won't I am not going to

TABLE 101.4 **Categories of Motivation in Both Sustain and Change Directions for the Target Behavior of Engaging in Behaviors That Would Promote Heart Health After a Heart Attack**

Target behavior is engaging in behaviors that would reduce the risk of another heart attack. The client says this:	Is the client's statement in the direction of health (change talk) or in the direction of continuing the health risk (sustain talk)?	Within what category of motivation may the client's statement fit?	Possible response by the health care provider to manage the sustain talk or pull for or reinforce the change talk:
I don't like reduced-salt foods.	Sustain	Desire. Key word is, "like."	"So using a salt substitute is going to be hard to do. Why were you thinking it may be a good idea?" (Demonstrate that the desire in the sustain direction has been heard, and then pull for reasons in the change direction.)
I can't get to that evening Healthy Heart meeting.	Sustain	Ability. Key word is, "can't."	"You aren't able to get there, but it sounds like you have some recognition that it may be useful." (Recognize the sustain talk, and then pull for reasons or need in the change direction.)
The support from the Healthy Heart class would be helpful.	Change	Reason. What the client is saying answers the question of, "Why go to the Healthy Heart class?"	"You may like the class." (Attempt to evoke change talk in an additional category of desire.) Or, "You can imagine some benefits from the class." (Reinforce the change talk in the reason category.)

TABLE 101.4 Categories of Motivation in Both Sustain and Change Directions for the Target Behavior of Engaging in Behaviors That Would Promote Heart Health After a Heart Attack—cont'd

Target behavior is engaging in behaviors that would reduce the risk of another heart attack. The client says this:	Is the client's statement in the direction of health (change talk) or in the direction of continuing the health risk (sustain talk)?	Within what category of motivation may the client's statement fit?	Possible response by the health care provider to manage the sustain talk or pull for or reinforce the change talk:
I shouldn't have to do all this for my heart.	Sustain	Need. Key word is, "shouldn't."	"It's not fair." (Acknowledge the sense of injustice and injury.) Or, "You would prefer that your heart just work." (Recognize how taking care of the heart is not enjoyable, but begin to call attention to the client's desire for the heart to work, which could lead to recognizing the need to take care of the heart.)
I think I may enjoy that support group.	Change	Desire. Key word is, "enjoy."	"You are looking forward to it." (Reinforce the desire change talk.) Or, "What are you hoping to get out of it?" (Attempt to evoke additional change talk in the reason category.)
I got a salt substitute.	Change	Already Taken Step. Key is that the client is talking about some action that he has already taken.	"Good for you." (Affirm the client's action in the change direction.) Or, "What will you do next?" (Pull for more change talk in the commitment category.)
I'm not having any angina anymore, so I figure I don't need to take that medication.	Sustain	Reason. What the client is saying answers the question of, "Why don't you have to take your medication?"	"You're glad your angina is gone." (Stay away from the reason category, go to another category, desire, and hope to find change talk there.)
I gave up on those recipes with less salt.	Sustain	Already Taken Step. Key is that the client is talking about some action that he has already taken.	"Something else makes more sense to you to try than reducing your salt." (Avoid trying to install reasons or motivation to reduce salt, and pull for other things the client may be willing to do.)
I could get a ride to the Heart Health class.	Change	Ability. Key word is, "could."	"Sounds like it is important to you to try it out." (Pull for change talk in the need or reason category.)
I won't be weighing myself every day.	Sustain	Commitment because the client is talking about what he won't be doing in the future.	"It doesn't make sense to you to weigh every day. Why do you think it is so often recommended?" (Avoid arguing about what the client is going to do, and pull for reasons or need in the change direction.)
I probably need to go to a yoga class every day.	Change	Need. Key word is, "need."	"It's something that you think would help." (Pull for change talk in the reasons category.)
I will be going to that exercise class tomorrow.	Change	Commitment because the client is talking about what he will be doing in the future	"You've made up your mind to try it out." (Reinforce the change talk in the commitment category.)

These categories can be used by the health care provider to guess where to go next during the consult. Several research studies found that the goals of the consult where change talk is elicited were associated with the desired behavior change. In one study of clients in treatment for alcohol problems, 16% of the days a client abstained 9–15 months after treatment could be predicted from how much the client was drinking at the start of treatment. A similar amount, 19% of the days a client abstained and 34% of the amount the client consumed alcohol, could be predicted from how much change talk the client said in a single session 9–15 months earlier.[15] Patients that

made two or more change talk statements about taking their antidepressant medications during a consult were almost twice as likely to have filled the prescription over the next 6 months as those patients that said none or only one change talk statement.[16] Change talk during today's consultation may be a good proxy for the actual behavior change in the future.

A client who says things such as those listed in the change talk column of Table 101.5 is rehearsing what he or she literally must think or say after the consultation is over to remind, justify, or motivate himself or herself to engage in behaviors related to managing diabetes.

TABLE 101.5 **Target Behavior Is to Engage in Those Behaviors That Would Manage a Diabetic Condition**

Sustain Talk	Facet of Motivation	Change Talk
I don't like sticking my finger.	Desire	I like keeping a record of my sugars.
I can't take my meter with me during the day.	Ability	I could get that new, smaller meter.
I don't need to do all this checking and changing my diet.	Need	I must learn more about the glycemic index.
I don't follow my diet sometimes because I don't want people to know I have diabetes and have to accommodate my dietary needs.	Reasons	If I lower my sugars, maybe I won't wind up like my mother, who had diabetes and lost her foot.

Similarly, a client who is making statements during the consult such as those in the sustain talk column is probably reducing his or her motivation to engage in health-promoting behaviors. One way that health care providers inadvertently arrange this is by saying the change talk. The client, who is ambivalent, then brings up the sustain talk, and that is what he or she may remember after the consultation. However, a health care provider who says the sustain talk before the client says it may be perceived as very empathic. The client experiences the clinician as someone who understands why it is so difficult to engage in the health-promoting behavior. By saying the sustain talk first, the health care provider alleviates the client from having to say it and decreases the client's reinforcement of the status quo. Having recognized the sustain talk, the health care provider has perhaps increased the client's willingness to consider if there is some change talk.

HELPING THE CLIENT ACCESS HIS OR HER MOTIVATION FOR CHANGE

Helping the client experience and say more change talk can sometimes be as simple as asking the client to describe his or her desires, abilities, needs, or reasons for engaging in the health-promoting behavior.

"What would you *enjoy* about meditation?"
"How might you be *able* to arrange to take your medications reliably?"
"Why do you think you *need* to reduce the salt in your diet?"
"What *reasons* do you have for continuing with your exercises?"
"What are you *already doing* that helps you lose weight?"

Notice these examples are all open questions, which help the client take the lead toward doing the health-promoting behavior, whereas closed questions allow the client to be more passive. Also these questions pull for change talk rather than sustain talk. It is very common when using a directing helping style to ask open or closed questions that pull for sustain talk. Evoking from the client his or her experiences, thoughts, and emotions that support doing the health-promoting behavior is central to using a motivational interviewing helping style. So, these open questions are a third way to implement

TABLE 101.6 **A Third Way to Experiment Using a Motivational Interviewing Helping Style**

Possible Open Question to Ask the Client	Which Pulls or Fishes for This Facet of Motivation
What might you enjoy about _____ {insert the health-promoting behavior}?	Desire
What abilities do you have that would make it possible for you to _____ {insert the health-promoting behavior} if you decided to do it?	Ability
How important is it to you to _____ {insert the health-promoting behavior}?	Need
What, if any, are the important benefits of _____ {insert the health-promoting behavior}?	Reason
What are you already doing that makes it possible to _____ {insert the health-promoting behavior}?	Already Taken Steps

a motivational interviewing helping style. It is not as creative or elegant as you might ultimately be, but you can use the scripted questions shown in Table 101.6. If the client does respond with change talk, providing reinforcement and encouragement through affirmation, paraphrase, or summary can be useful.

Sometimes, change talk can be solicited by having the client envision the future. The health care provider can ask the client to talk about what he or she imagines in the future if changes are made or if changes are not made. Possible examples are: "What do you imagine will happen in the future if you don't lower your blood pressure this year?" or "How do you think this _____ (health-risky behavior) might become worse?" Both these examples pull for reasons to engage in the health-promoting behavior.

Facilitating the client's talking about goals or values and how they fit or do not fit with health behaviors may also evoke change talk. This could sound like: "How does the _____ (health-risky behavior) help or hurt your work?" or "How would taking care of your heart fit with what you want to do with your family?"

These ideas of change and sustain talk, the various facets of motivation, and the range of possible responses creates the steep learning curve for motivational interviewing. A fourth way to implement and approach doing motivational interviewing is just to listen for what you are glad the client is saying. If you are glad to hear the client talk a certain way about his health-promoting behavior, it is probably change talk. As you listen to the client's story, listen in particular for what part you like that the client is explicitly saying or even implying. When you hear it, reinforce it by asking for more explanation, summarizing it, or connecting it with other statements the client has said that you are glad to hear.

Client: I've been in AA for 6 years, but I am having trouble relating to it.
Health care provider possible response 1: Good for you for using that resource.
Health care provider possible response 2: Sounds like you are glad to have created some sobriety but now are looking for something else that will help you continue.
Health care provider possible response 3: You are looking for something to which you can relate better.

Because most clients are ambivalent about engaging in health-promoting behaviors, some sustain talk by the client is normal and to be expected. To help the client increase his or her motivation for the health-promoting behavior, the health care provider should be active in helping the client manage the sustain talk. Often, a first step is to demonstrate to the client that the sustain talk has been heard and understood. This is where the health care provider's skill in expressing empathy through paraphrasing or summarizing is useful and necessary. Sometimes, the client will return to change talk if the health care provider overstates the sustain talk the client has just said. Possible examples are:

Example 1: Client: "I don't really see the ankle swelling as a problem. They just hurt some."
Counselor: "You're not using the ankle swelling to think at all about your heart."
Example 2: Client: "I doubt if there is a problem. I don't have difficulties moving around."
Counselor: "As long as you can move, *everything* is OK."

The health care provider must say these kinds of amplified reflections (called *amplified* because the health care provider is increasing the emphasis or overstating the sustain talk) in a neutral voice tone. A sarcastic or critical tone will very likely increase the client's sustain talk rather than decrease it.

Earlier in this chapter, examples were given of managing sustain talk by first paraphrasing the sustain talk and then focusing on a different category. These double-sided reflections will help manage sustain talk if the first side or phrase is the sustain side and the second side or phrase is the change side. The client is more likely to talk about the side (sustain or change) on which the health

TABLE 101.7	Examples of Providing an Alternative Meaning for the Client's Observation in Sustain Talk
Observation the client has made	I've tried in the past and haven't succeeded (stopping smoking, maintaining my exercise, and improving my diet).
Meaning client may give this observation	I can't do this. Or I'm not successful. (Notice this statement is sustain talk in the ability category.)
Meaning you may want the client to have	This is important to you. You have tried out several ways that have not worked as well as you want. (The past failures are given a new meaning, and attention is called to desire, which is a different category than ability.)

care provider finishes his or her statement. Another way to manage sustain talk is to provide an alternative meaning for the client's observation (Table 101.7).

ENHANCING YOUR MOTIVATIONAL INTERVIEWING SKILLS

Most health care providers use all three helping styles. Although the directing helping style is most frequently used, most health care providers occasionally use a guiding helping style whether or not they have received formal training in it. However, research has demonstrated that reading or attending workshops is probably not sufficient to enhance motivational interviewing skills. Listening to audio recordings of your consultations with clients is very likely helpful.[18] Whether alone, with one or several peers, or with an expert in motivational interviewing, you could listen for the characteristics listed in Box 101.1. A health care provider who practices with as few as six instances (not even hours, just the minutes during the consult where the health care provider was intending to use a motivational interviewing approach) of recordings may significantly enhance his or her motivational interviewing skills.

One perhaps memorable way to remember the approach described here are these clinical pearls:
1. **Quit your job.** Do not be the only expert in the room. Imagine that you do not know, because it will make it easier for you to avoid adopting an expert role and easier for you to be curious about the client's experience.
2. **Get on the bus.** Be with the client, ride with him or her for a while, and look together at his or her life and dilemma of making this change. Respect that the client is going to get off the bus at whatever stop he or she chooses.
3. **Go fishing.** This is easier to do if you give up being the expert and the one who has to solve the problem. Treat the client as competent. Then it makes sense to go looking with the client for his or her motivation and the solutions he or she can create.

BOX 101.1   A Way to Enhance Your Practice

Audiotape a session with a client. By yourself, with a colleague, or a motivational interviewing expert:

- Count the number of open questions and closed questions. You are more likely to be using a motivational interviewing style if at least 50% of your questions are open.
- Count the number of reflections you made. You are more likely to be using a motivational interviewing style if you have at least twice as many reflections as questions and you have at least one reflection every minute. Complex reflections often elicit more change talk than do simple reflections.
- Did you talk less than the client? You are more likely to be using a motivational interviewing style if the client talks approximately twice as much as you.
- Listen for where you did or could have solicited or reinforced any client statements about desire, ability, need, reasons, or already taken steps toward the health-promoting behavior (change talk).

- What did the client say or imply that you were glad to hear the client say? This is very likely change talk. How could you have called more attention to it?
- Identify instances in which the client was saying sustain talk. Now that you have more time to think about your response, how else could you have demonstrated that you understood this sustain talk and called attention to possible change talk? How might an amplified reflection sound or a double-sided reflection or a reframe?
- Look at any instance where you gave the client advice. Did you use an elicit-provide-elicit format or in some other way ask for permission and ask the client to consider how well the advice fits?
- Did you warn the client of any possible consequences, confront the client regarding the behavior, or raise concerns without using elicit-provide-elicit? You are more likely to be using a motivational interviewing style if you avoid warning or confronting the client.

Key Web Resources

Motivational Interviewing: This central resource for trainers of motivational interviewing includes readings, links to other resources, and transcripts of some interviews focused on substance use problems.

http://www.motivationalinterviewing.org/

Change talk and childhood obesity: Interactive exercise using a virtual example of a conversation with a mother and adolescent about his weight.

http://www.kognito.com/changetalk/

Stephen Rollnick: Stephen Rollnick provides resources and a discussion forum for motivational interviewing in medical (rather than substance use) health care settings.

http://www.stephenrollnick.com/

REFERENCES

References are available online at ExpertConsult.com.

CHAPTER 102

EMOTIONAL AWARENESS FOR PAIN

Howard Schubiner, MD

INTRODUCTION

There is an epidemic of chronic pain and related disorders in the United States and around the world.[1-3] It is estimated that there are more than 100 million individuals with chronic pain in the United States, and this number is increasing.[4-6] Back pain, neck pain, fibromyalgia (FM), tension and migraine headaches, temporomandibular joint (TMJ) syndrome, and abdominal and pelvic pain syndromes are among the most common diagnoses made in primary care and consume a significant proportion of medical costs.[7] In addition to these disorders associated with chronic pain, there are a variety of commonly associated disorders such as chronic fatigue, irritable bowel syndrome (IBS), interstitial cystitis (IC), and postural orthostatic tachycardia syndrome (POTS) that are frequently seen by both traditional and integrative practitioners.[8]

The traditional biomedical model attempts to identify an underlying local and structural cause for pain. However, evidence of pathological conditions in this group of disorders has been elusive. Furthermore, treatment of these conditions has proven to be difficult,[9,10] as becomes clear when one considers the number of people who chronically suffer from these conditions. For example, the vast majority of individuals diagnosed with headaches, abdominal and pelvic pain syndromes, and FM have no clear evidence of peripheral nociceptive inputs generating pain. Chronic back pain often occurs in the absence of radicular pain corresponding to an observed nerve root lesion or evidence of nerve root compression, such as altered muscle strength, deep tendon reflexes, or sensation. In these patients, magnetic resonance imaging (MRI) evidence of degenerative disk disease, bulging or herniated disks, spinal stenosis, and other syndromes are assumed to be the cause of pain. However, studies comparing MRI findings of individuals with and without pain show similar findings.[11,12] The assumption that commonly seen MRI findings are the cause of pain in those without objective evidence of structural abnormalities often leads to overtreatment and the resulting increased costs and complications.[13,14] Whiplash is another example of a chronic pain syndrome that has been shown to be unrelated to ongoing injury or a specific disease process in the neck.[15]

For many pain syndromes the etiology is complex with no simple cause and effect. When the mind suffers, the body sympathizes. This chapter addresses this powerful effect.

While central nervous system (CNS) transmitters have been found to be associated with FM and migraine headaches,[16] it is not clear whether they are the cause of these disorders or the result. There are genetic predispositions toward some of these conditions, such as migraine, anxiety, and depression.[17] However, studies have shown that life events are required to trigger these conditions, that is, to cause expression of underlying genetic predispositions.[18] In fact, one study showed that a particular genotype for depression can be activated by a stressful childhood (thus increasing risk for depression) and can be deactivated by an emotionally supportive childhood (thus decreasing depression risk).[19]

Because of the inability to identify and treat the underlying cause for most chronic pain conditions, attention has shifted to pain management. However, biomedical approaches to pain management, including pain medications (including opiates), injection techniques, and surgical and chemical ablations, have also not been shown to be efficacious.[9,10,13-15,20] There is clearly a need for a new understanding and approach to these disorders. Please note that the disorders considered in this article exclude those with objective evidence of structural pathology, such as cancer, fractures, and inflammatory and infectious conditions. This chapter describes a mind-body model in which these disorders are conceptualized to be related to individual reactions to stressful events and unresolved emotions.

THEIR PAIN IS REAL

Neuroscientists have identified areas of the brain that process, accentuate, and reduce pain.[21-24] To appropriately diagnose and treat chronic pain, it is necessary to develop a more nuanced view of the relationship between pain and the brain. Physical injuries do not always result in the experience of pain; and pain (even severe pain) can result in the absence of a physical injury.[25] There is clear evidence that pain can originate in the absence of a tissue disorder in the area where the pain is being felt, as seen in phantom limb syndrome.[26] A study by Derbyshire et al. confirmed that pain initiated by the brain is identical to pain originating in peripheral tissues.[27] This implies that pain is a function of the brain, with inputs from peripheral nociceptors as well as from pain generating/processing centers in the brain and that the resultant pain experiences are indistinguishable. This understanding is important for reassuring patients that all pain is real and will be taken seriously.

The anterior cingulate cortex (ACC) is a key area within the brain that, when activated, augments pain.[22,24]

Pain also activates the amygdala and the autonomic nervous system (ANS).[28,29] Emotional memories are stored in the amygdala, and individuals with adverse childhood experiences are more likely to develop migraine, FM, IC, IBS, and chronic pelvic pain.[30-36] Evidence also indicates that the amygdala, the ACC, and the ANS are activated when emotions are experienced.[37,38] To summarize, these areas are involved in the activation of pain pathways, and these pathways are strongly influenced by thoughts and emotions.[22-24]

Learned pain pathways can develop after an injury (even a mild one) or can be created during times of significant stress and emotional reactions. While most injuries heal within a reasonable amount of time, pain pathways can persist (become "wired"), thus creating intermittent or chronic pain that may be refractory to medical therapies. These pain pathways are often very specific and can involve discrete or large areas of the body. A veteran told me that he was injured in the Vietnam war during an ambush that led to a dangerous Med-evac escape. He had shrapnel wounds to his left leg, resulting in pain and limping. Within a few months, both of these symptoms had completely resolved. Interestingly, he had a recurrence of the pain and limping 20 years later when a helicopter flew overhead.

There are also built in central mechanisms for reducing pain. Notably, activation of the dorsolateral prefrontal cortex (DLPFC) area results in diminished pain.[23] Positive emotional states and reductions in pain are correlated with activation of the DLPFC[39] (Fig. 102.1).

THE PSYCHOLOGY OF PAIN

There are two major components of the mind: conscious and subconscious. We are consciously aware of many of our actions, decisions, thoughts, and feelings. However, the majority of our thoughts and emotions are actually derived from subconscious processes.[40,41] In addition, these subconscious processes are typically the basis for most of our actions. Thus many of our activities are routine and programmed by our subconscious minds, such as walking, talking, eating, driving, as well as reactions to people, places smells, and situations. These activities

and reactions are carried out via sets of learned neural pathways.

Another function of the subconscious mind is to protect us from physical threats, and therefore we continuously monitor our environment for stimuli that might be "dangerous" in some way.[38] Innate neural pathways cause our bodies to react very quickly to a snake, a thrown object, or other physical threats. Our reactions to these threats are immediate and do not involve conscious processing (i.e., we are aware of them after they occur).[38,41] The subconscious mind also notices emotional threats and causes our bodies to react to them in a similar fashion. In fact, Kross and colleagues demonstrated that the same regions of the brain were activated by both peripheral nociceptive stimulation and emotional stimulation.[42] We are all aware that our bodies react to stress with a variety of reactions, including facial flushing, tight stomach muscles, sweaty palms, voice changes, and others. Given the previous, it should not be surprising that during times of significant tension and stress, our bodies can develop physical reactions in a myriad of ways, such as the development of neck or back pain, headache, gastrointestinal or genitourinary symptoms, and many other symptoms. The danger or alarm pathways (fight/flight and freeze/submit) are centered in the amygdala and are necessarily sensitive to relatively small stimuli that are potentially harmful for protective purposes.[38,43]

> A useful question to ask is, "Where do you carry stress in your body?" This often gives insight into how we can learn from these subconscious pathways.

Individuals subjected to adverse childhood events develop a priming of the brain's danger pathways along with a corresponding emotional memory for specific types of threats.[44] These children may develop stomachaches, insomnia, anxiety, headaches, and other disorders.[30,31] Later in life, if new emotional or physical threats occur (especially if they are similar to those that occurred in childhood), neural pathways can be activated causing new symptoms to develop, with musculoskeletal or visceral

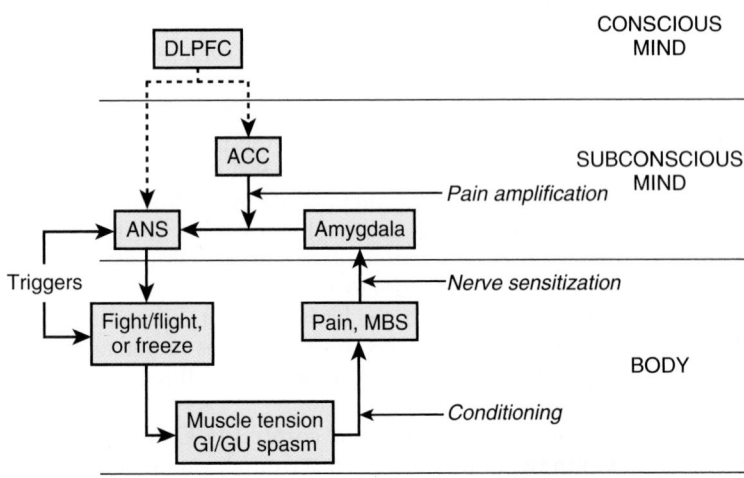

FIG. 102.1 ■ The neurology of psychophysiologic disorders (*thick solid line*, activating; *dashed line*, deactivating). *ACC*, anterior cingulate cortex; *ANS*, autonomic nervous system; *DLPFC*, dorsolateral prefrontal cortex; *GI/GU*, gastrointestinal/genitourinary; *MBS*, mind-body syndrome.

pain syndromes being the most common.[45] In a typical history, a girl who grows up with an emotionally abusive and controlling parent may develop migraine headaches as a teen when she is subjected to a jealous and controlling boyfriend. If she marries an abusive husband in her twenties, she may develop abdominal or pelvic pain. In her thirties, when subjected to a threatening work situation or a motor vehicle accident, she may develop widespread pain that will often be diagnosed as FM, as well as anxiety and/or depression. These symptoms prompt medical attention that usually leads to symptom-based pharmaceutical or physical interventions. If these treatments are ineffective, the persistence of symptoms activates fear, which leads to increases in the danger signal and resulting increases in symptoms. This vicious cycle is common and can explain the fact that pain syndromes often worsen over time in terms of the location, frequency, and severity of pain.

These physical reactions are real, and the pain they cause is real. The source of pain, whether due to nociceptive inputs or created by neural pathways, cannot be distinguished by the quality or severity of pain. Since neural pathways are physiological, rather than pathological, responses (i.e., they do not involve tissue destruction), they can be reversed. These symptoms are created by the subconscious mind in an attempt to warn us or protect us from some threat (for example, a controlling boss, an abusive husband, or an overwhelming set of responsibilities). In essence, pain and other symptoms serve as a "danger" message from the brain. In the case of an arm fracture, the message is "rest and get a cast," while in the situation of stressful life events causing headaches or neck pain, the message should be "you are feeling threatened, take action to alter the situation or respond to it." We are currently using the term "psychophysiologic disorders" (PPDs) to describe these neural pathway symptoms, but they have also been termed psychosomatic or functional disorders, medically unexplained illnesses,[46] tension myositis syndrome,[47] stress-related illness,[48] and mind-body syndrome.[45]

> Psychophysiologic disorders (PPD) is the current term being used to describe this process.

Another observation commonly made about those who develop psychophysiologic reactions is that they tend to have a highly developed conscience.[45,47] Individuals who are affected by this group of disorders (Table 102.1) typically exhibit the following characteristics: being selfless, highly responsible, or self-critical; feeling excessive guilt; lacking assertiveness; being perfectionists; holding themselves to very high standards; caring what others think of them; holding emotions in; and neglecting their own needs. Large international studies have shown that women are more likely than men to display these characteristics (possibly due to higher rates of childhood and adult victimization and gender-based socialization).[49,50] These personality factors may play a role in the higher rates of chronic pain and other PPDs among women.

DIAGNOSIS OF PSYCHOPHYSIOLOGIC DISORDERS

PPD should be suspected in patients who present with symptoms of one or more of the common PPD diagnoses (Table 102.2) and for whom a specific structural condition is not identified. If it is understood that PPD can cause a wide variety of symptoms, the practitioner can suspect it from the beginning of an encounter. There are several clues in a medical history that suggest a PPD. An injury, particularly a mild one, that doesn't follow the usual pattern of gradual diminution of pain over time is likely to be due to PPD. This diagnosis should be considered when symptoms vary significantly with regard to time and place, such as pain that goes away when on vacation or when doing certain activities or pain that occurs only when sitting in some chairs but not in other chairs. Similarly, pain that shifts from one location to another within the body is often due to PPD. I saw a patient who had wrist and hand pain while keyboarding at her job, forcing her to be unable to work. Rest and antiinflammatory medications had not been effective. Her doctors assumed that this was simply a repetitive strain injury. However, further history revealed that the pain also regularly occurred on Sunday evenings when she hadn't done any keyboarding. This suggested that her brain was activating pain in anticipation of stress during the workweek. She had a complete recovery after treatment for a PPD. Of course, a medical workup should be conducted to rule out any structural conditions such as tumors, fractures, infections, or vascular or inflammatory conditions. A physical exam to rule out evidence of nerve root compression is mandatory as those findings would preclude a diagnosis of PPD. Imaging studies of the neck and back are likely to demonstrate degenerative changes because asymptomatic individuals have high rates of such MRI findings. A study from Finland showed that degenerative disk disease and bulging disks were identified in 50% and 25%, respectively, in healthy 21-year-olds.[51] As mentioned, similar

---

TABLE 102.1   Personality Traits Common to Those With Psychophysiologic Disorders (PPDs)

Would you describe yourself as:
1. Having low self-esteem _____
2. Being a perfectionist _____
3. Having high expectations of yourself _____
4. Wanting to be good and/or be liked _____
5. Frequently feeling guilt _____
6. Feeling dependent on others _____
7. Being conscientious _____
8. Being hard on yourself _____
9. Being overly responsible _____
10. Taking on responsibility for others _____
11. Often worrying _____
12. Having difficulty making decisions _____
13. Following rules strictly _____
14. Having difficulty letting go _____
15. Feeling cautious, shy, or reserved _____
16. Tending to hold thoughts and feelings in _____
17. Tending to harbor rage or resentment _____
18. Not standing up for yourself _____

TABLE 102.2	**Syndromes That Are Commonly Caused by Psychophysiologic Disorders (PPDs)**

Chronic Pain Syndromes

Tension headaches
Migraine headaches
Back pain
Neck pain
Whiplash
Fibromyalgia
Temporomandibular joint (TMJ) syndrome
Chronic abdominal and pelvic pain syndromes
Chronic tendonitis
Vulvodynia
Piriformis syndrome
Sciatic pain syndrome
Repetitive stress injury
Foot pain syndromes
Myofascial pain syndrome

Autonomic Nervous System-Related Disorders

Irritable bowel syndrome
Interstitial cystitis (irritable bladder syndrome)
Postural orthostatic tachycardia syndrome
Inappropriate sinus tachycardia
Reflex sympathetic dystrophy (chronic regional pain disorder)
Functional dyspepsia

Other Syndromes

Insomnia
Chronic fatigue syndrome
Paresthesias (numbness, tingling, burning)
Tinnitus
Dizziness
Spasmodic dysphonia
Chronic hives
Anxiety
Depression
Obsessive-compulsive disorder
Posttraumatic stress disorder

degenerative MRI findings are found in the majority of middle-aged adults,[11,12] and physicians should be cautious in attributing back pain to these findings. Similar studies document the presence of abnormal MRI findings of the hips, shoulders, and knees in healthy individuals without pain.[52-55]

Once this is accomplished, the topic of PPD should be broached with the patient. Talking with patients about PPD should be done in a way that emphasizes that their symptoms are real and with empathy toward their situation and frustration in not getting better. The clinician should explain that real symptoms, including severe and chronic pain, can frequently occur in the absence of structural disease processes, and one can use phantom limb syndrome as an example of this phenomenon.[26] Introducing the concept of learned neural pathways helps patients to connect their symptoms to a CNS processes. The practitioner should state that learned neural pathways are simply sets of nerve connections that have developed through experiences, such as the pathways that allow us to ride a bicycle, throw a ball, walk, and talk a certain way. Pain and other symptoms are easily learned, and once these pathways are established, they can continue for several

years and can be reactivated after many years. Reassure the patient that there is no physical and structural disease process and offer hope that the real condition that they suffer from can be reversed. Whether or not a physical injury occurs, stressful situations and powerful subconscious emotions are universal triggers of pain pathways in PPD. These pathways become engrained in the presence of situations and emotions that remain unresolved. In addition, chronic pain frequently leads to frustration about ongoing pain and fear about an underlying physical disease. These reactions further activate pain pathways in the brain by activation of the amygdala, ANS, and ACC.[56,57]

This educational process is extremely important to allay fears of a disease process, explain the reason for the symptoms, and offer hope and the expectation that these symptoms can be resolved. Treatment for PPD in the absence of understanding and accepting the above is typically not effective.

The Diagnostic Interview

Many practitioners are not trained, nor do they have the time, to conduct an in-depth psychological interview that begins in childhood and attempts to elicit the key psychological factors that have created psychophysiologic disorders. However, the author has published a template for this type of assessment that can be used by patients and/or practitioners.[45] A brief description of this interview is provided herein. As previously mentioned, before diagnosing a form of PPD, the practitioner should rule out a pathological medical condition so that the practitioner and patient are comfortable that they are dealing with a form of PPD. Prior to the interview, it is helpful to have the patient complete a checklist of symptoms and syndromes that are commonly caused by PPD (Table 102.3). Five questions form the basis of this interview (Table 102.4).

Begin the interview by gathering data on the patient's family of origin and ask probing questions about their parents, siblings, and any other important individuals in their childhood. Gently inquire about episodes or patterns of emotional, physical, or sexual abuse; of criticism, taunting, teasing, blame, humiliation, or judging; and of overly high expectations or conditional love. Ask about parental alcohol or drug abuse, divorce or extramarital affairs, unequal treatment of siblings, and psychological and physical illnesses among family members. Inquire about sibling relationships with special regard to episodes of cruel behaviors, psychological or physical illness, or acting out behaviors. Synthesize the patient's childhood experiences and reactions to them in an attempt to understand the effects that their upbringing had on their personality and development. Most people with PPD develop a set of personality traits that include having an overly developed conscience (heightened sense of responsibility) and a lack in self-esteem, self-worth, and assertiveness (see Table 102.1). Typically, one finds a set of events and responses that create a priming of the ANS that sets the stage for the development of PPD later in life. Some of the common patterns are those of loss, abandonment,

TABLE 102.3 Common Symptoms of Psychophysiologic Disorders (PPDs)

1. Heartburn, acid reflux _____
2. Abdominal pains _____
3. Irritable bowel syndrome _____
4. Tension headaches _____
5. Migraine headaches _____
6. Unexplained rashes _____
7. Anxiety and/or panic attacks _____
8. Depression _____
9. Obsessive-compulsive thought patterns _____
10. Eating disorders _____
11. Insomnia or trouble sleeping _____
12. Fibromyalgia _____
13. Back pain _____
14. Neck pain _____
15. Shoulder pain _____
16. Repetitive stress injury _____
17. Carpal tunnel syndrome _____
18. Reflex sympathetic dystrophy (RSD) _____
19. Temporomandibular joint syndrome (TMJ) _____
20. Chronic tendonitis _____
21. Facial pain _____
22. Numbness, tingling sensations _____
23. Fatigue or chronic fatigue syndrome _____
24. Palpitations _____
25. Chest pain _____
26. Hyperventilation _____
27. Interstitial cystitis/spastic bladder (irritable bladder syndrome) _____
28. Pelvic pain _____
29. Muscle tenderness _____
30. Postural orthostatic tachycardia syndrome (POTS) _____
31. Tinnitus _____
32. Dizziness _____
33. PTSD _____

TABLE 102.4 Five Questions to Rule in a Psychophysiologic Disorder (PPD)

1. Did you have a stressful childhood? Did you experience neglect, abandonment, loss, criticism, or conditional love?
2. Did you experience traumatic events, such as physical or sexual abuse?
3. How many symptoms/syndromes have you had in your lifetime? See Table 102.2 for a checklist.
4. Were stressful life events occurring at the time of the onset of the symptoms?
5. Do you have several of the personality traits commonly associated with PPD? (See Table 3 for a description.)

TABLE 102.5 Synthesis of the Diagnosis of Psychophysiologic Disorder (PPD) Chart

Age	PPD Symptom	Potential Triggering Events	Emotions That Were Triggered/Core Issues
7	Stomach aches	Parents arguing	Fear of parents separating/loss
16	Irritable bowel syndrome	Parental divorce	Loss of father, mother depressed
28	Migraines	Husband "cheating"	Loss, anger, betrayal
38	Fibromyalgia/fatigue	Divorce/difficult boss	Loss, fear, powerlessness

The next phase of the interview consists of an evaluation of the events that trigger PPD syndromes. A simple approach is to inquire about the onset of each of the PPD syndromes (Table 102.5). Although the onset may coincide with injury or a viral infection, these events create neural pathways that are usually transient. PPD symptoms can become chronic if the danger signals in the brain are activated. This process occurs in two ways. First, the individual may be in a situation where several of the following circumstances are present: there is an inherently stressful situation; the current events trigger emotional memories of stressful events from childhood; the individual experiences guilt, self-criticism, a strong sense of responsibility, or other issues listed in Table 102.1; the individual is unable to express emotions of fear or anger or is unable to escape feeling trapped in the triggering situation. Second, the symptoms are worrisome or severe, are believed to be due to a disease process, and are labeled by health practitioners as something other than a psychophysiologic process. These beliefs lead the patient to develop a significant amount of fear of the symptoms. This fear activates the danger signal and causes increased symptoms often leading to a vicious cycle of pain-fear-pain. Complete this process with each of the PPD symptoms that have occurred in the lifetime of the patient. You will frequently see clear patterns emerge that will help the patient understand that their symptoms are, in fact, caused by PPD and that they are not crazy, incompetent, or weak, but rather someone who has been exposed to a series of events that have created physical or psychological symptoms in response to a particular combination of stressful life events. When this occurs, the patients can be encouraged to see that they are not to blame for the symptoms, are not physically or psychologically damaged, and have the opportunity to overcome these symptoms.

If it is appropriate, the interview may be concluded with the following messages:

"You have a form of PPD, rather than a structural disease process. PPD is caused by learned neural pathways that have been triggered by the particular set of stressors that you have encountered. It is not your fault. Almost everyone gets PPD, and anyone would likely develop these symptoms given the events that occurred. You can get better because learned neural

fear, guilt, resentment, and anger. In many instances, people with PPD have very healthy childhoods, and when they are exposed to stressful situations later in life that belie the values that they learned in childhood, PPD symptoms can develop. I often explain to patients that since they are human, they have a mind and a body, and since those are intimately connected, it is not surprising that physical symptoms occur at times of stress; in fact, it probably happens to most people at some points in their lives.

pathways can be reversed. There is a way to unlearn your pain and other PPD symptoms if you are willing to do the work."

TREATMENT APPROACH

Because PPD is a disorder caused by stress and unresolved emotions, it is possible for everyone with PPD to experience dramatic improvements or remissions. However, it is primarily patient-related factors that determine successful treatment, rather than practitioner-related factors. It is the author's clinical experience that successful patients are those who are convinced that they have PPD rather than a structural disease process, are confident that they can address the issues that created PPD, are willing and able to devote a significant amount of time for psychological interventions, and have adequate resources as well as a lack of overwhelming obstacles in their lives. It is the practitioner's job to help the patient develop the first of these attributes, while it is primarily up to the patient to attain the latter ones.

Research Support

There are two studies that have been conducted documenting the efficacy of the therapeutic approach. The first was a randomized controlled trial for individuals diagnosed with FM.[58] In this small trial, at a 6-month follow-up, those who participated in a 3-week intervention had a mean decrease in pain of 2.5 on a 10-point Likert pain scale. In addition, 45% had a decreased pain level of at least 30% and 25% had a decrease of at least 50%. A second study described the outcomes of patients with a variety of musculoskeletal pain syndromes, including FM, back and neck pain, headache, and other syndromes. Patients had a mean duration of pain of 8.8 years and had even better results. After the month-long intervention, 6-month follow-up pain scores showed that 67% had at least a 30% pain reduction and 53% had at least a 50% pain reduction.[59]

Therapeutic Program

Once a biomedical condition has been ruled out, the interview has demonstrated the linkages between priming and triggering events as well as the onset of PPD symptoms, and the patient has been educated and accepts the diagnosis, the intervention may proceed. The author has developed a comprehensive program designed to empower the patients and guide them toward healing.[45] It consists of a mixture of cognitive-behavioral, mindfulness, and emotional expressive techniques, which is primarily self-guided. It has been shown to increase an internal locus of control, i.e., patients begin to believe that their thoughts and actions are capable of reversing their PPD symptoms.[58,59]

Several authors have developed a variety of expressive and therapeutic writing techniques.[60,61] James Pennebaker and others have conducted research on many of these techniques, which has documented beneficial effects on health and well-being.[60-63] The author

TABLE 102.6	**Expressive and Therapeutic Writing Exercises**

Free writing: uncensored expressive writing about an emotionally charged topic.
Unsent letters: expressing thoughts and feelings fully in a letter format.
Dialogues: creating an imaginary conversation between two entities who discuss a relevant issue.
Gratitude: writing about things for which one is grateful.
Forgiveness: writing to express forgiveness toward oneself or others.
Barriers: writing about potential barriers, both internal and external, that may prevent healing.
Creating new responses: writing how one chooses to respond to potentially difficult situations.
Life narratives: creating an alternative life story that emphasizes overcoming obstacles rather than being victimized.

has incorporated several of these techniques along with others into a program designed to reverse PPD.[45] These techniques are summarized in Table 102.6 and discussed in Chapter 98. One of the keys to the efficacy of expressive writing is the ability of the patient to identify, express, and release emotions. The clinician can help patients recognize that their feelings are justified and valid. Encouraging patients to experience and give voice to feelings of anger or resentment, guilt, and grief is often an important process in recovery. A therapeutic model that emphasizes emotional experiences, intensive short-term dynamic psychotherapy, has been shown to have benefit in patients with somatic disorders.[64]

Meditations and visualizations are useful adjuncts in the treatment of PPD. Mindfulness meditation has been shown to reduce reactivity to emotional issues and thus reduce pain;[65,66] guided imagery is an effective tool to create images of health and well-being, which are essential to this therapeutic model.[67,68] The author has created a CD with meditations designed to help patients reverse PPD,[45] and Chapters 97 and 100 provide practical advice on using these methods.

A key element of the program is to change how one views the symptom and how one responds to it. As mentioned, patients with PPD are often caught in a cycle of pain-fear-pain. To break this cycle, fear of pain must be reduced. Once the symptoms are accepted by the patient as being due to PPD, he or she can begin to stop fearing the pain, separate from it, and take control over it. Consciously choosing to stop monitoring pain and focus more on being active and engaged in living deprives the pain of its fuel, fear. It is remarkable that simple, strong assertions can often reverse pain within minutes when one is convinced of the diagnosis of PPD and of one's power in overcoming it. However, it can take several months of programmatically ignoring the pain to reprogram learned pain pathways. Box 102.1 offers a script for patients to use.

Another key component in healing is to challenge triggers that maintain symptoms. A trigger can be defined as a stimulus that leads to PPD symptoms, yet would not typically cause a symptom in someone else. Typical examples are weather changes, bright lighting, foods, wine or

| BOX 102.1 | Sample Script for Reducing Psychophysiologic Disorder (PPD) Symptoms |

When pain or other symptoms occur, stop and take a deep breath. Then take a moment to remind yourself that there is nothing seriously wrong with your body. You are healthy, and the mind-body syndrome (MBS) symptoms will subside soon. Tell your mind that you realize that the symptoms are just a way of warning you about underlying feelings of fear, guilt, anger, anxiety, shame, inadequacy, or other emotions. Tell your mind to stop producing the symptoms immediately. Do this with force and conviction, either out loud or silently. Separate from the pain or other neural pathway symptoms and reframe them as sensations that are not harming you. Take a few deep breaths, and focus on things that you need to do in your life. Congratulate yourself on the steps you are taking to bring about recovery, even if symptoms persist for the time being.

| BOX 102.2 | Sample Script for Reducing Psychophysiologic Disorder (PPD) Triggers |

When you notice you are encountering or are about to encounter any triggers to the symptoms or any stressful situations, immediately stop and take a deep breath. Take a moment to remind your mind that this activity or trigger will NOT cause any symptoms or problems any more. For example, if you are lifting an object, remind yourself, "This will not cause any back problems. My back is healthy and strong, and I can do this without worrying about hurting myself." It is important to have a deep understanding that your body is healthy and that you can get better by using these methods. Keep reminding yourself that you will not be allowing your mind to produce symptoms at these times. Relax and breathe in order to decrease fear. Repeat positive phrases about yourself, your body, and your recovery when you encounter any of your triggers until your brain unlearns unwanted neural pathways.

other alcoholic drinks, family gatherings, visiting certain people, places, movements, driving, and many others. Triggers become activated by subconscious processes in a similar way that Pavlovian responses develop (i.e., operant conditioning). Therefore, triggers cause symptoms because they activate learned neural pathways, and they can be attenuated by understanding this process and by actively challenging them. Avoiding triggers allows them to exert even greater effects, so patients should be encouraged to seek out these triggers and expose themselves to them in order to overcome them. It requires significant courage to begin to engage in exercise despite pain or the anticipation of pain. See Box 102.2 for a script regarding eliminating triggers.

As previously mentioned, many patients with PPD have personality traits of being overly responsible, self-critical, and unassertive. Individuals with PPD often find themselves in situations in which they feel trapped or conflicted. They may be caring for an ailing parent who was abusive, work for a boss who is controlling and manipulative, or have a spouse or child who continually takes advantage of them. In these situations, it is often necessary to take action. Pain is often dramatically reduced when a difficult situation is resolved or ameliorated to a significant degree. It is often necessary to encourage patients and help them find assertive, yet civil, methods for dealing with these situations.

Finally, individuals who have endured significant childhood and adult stressors and who have suffered with chronic pain often have a negative view of themselves and low levels of self-esteem and self-efficacy. Therefore, an overarching theme for guiding individuals with PPD to health is the development of love and compassion toward themselves. This can be accomplished by positive affirmations, meditations and visualizations, and encouraging them to stand up for themselves and take time for themselves. There are some excellent resources for helping patients achieve compassion for themselves.[69,70]

CONCLUSION

A significant proportion of people with chronic pain do not have a structural cause for this pain and are actually suffering from PPD. Biomedical approaches to PPD often lead to an endless cycle of pain and ineffective interventions. When a biomedical condition is ruled out, a careful interview will usually identify the priming and triggering events leading to the onset of pain. Education about PPD will help the patient discard the biomedical explanation for their pain and empower the patient to take control of their symptoms and their lives. Reversing PPD often takes time and a variety of cognitive, behavioral, and emotional interventions. However, it can be gratifying to help patients realize that their pain, even if it has persisted for many years, can be reversed or reduced.

Key Web Resources

Unlearn Your Pain: The website of Dr. Howard Schubiner	http://unlearnyourpain.com
Dr. John Sarno: The official website of John Sarno, MD	http://johnesarnomd.com
Stress Illness: The website of Dr. David Clarke	http://stressillness.com/
Dr. David Schechter: The website of Dr. David Schechter	http://www.schechtermd.com/
PPD/TMS Peer Network: A participant-oriented information site on psychophysiologic disorders, including a list of practitioners who practice in this area and an active forum	http://tmswiki.org
RSI-Back Pain: A patient-run information site for people suffering with chronic painful conditions	http://rsi-backpain.co.uk/
Pain Psychology Center: Counseling center specializing in PPD therapy via phone and Skype	http://www.painpsychologycenter.com
Defined Organized Comprehensive Care (DOCC) Project: Website of Dr. David Hanscom, a spine surgeon's program that incorporates PPD	http://www.backincontrol.com/

REFERENCES

References are available online at ExpertConsult.com.

CHAPTER 103

ENERGY PSYCHOLOGY

Larry Stoler, PhD, MSSA

The cell is a machine driven by energy. It can thus be approached by studying matter, or by studying energy. In every culture and in every medical tradition before ours, healing was accomplished by moving energy.

ALBERT SZENT-GYORGYI, NOBEL LAUREATE IN MEDICINE

CASE STUDY 1: FEAR OF A FLU SHOT

A female patient enters your office, and you recommend that she receive a flu shot. However, this patient is terrified of needles. You learn that because of this fear, the patient has never had a flu shot, despite being at risk. You explain to the patient that you can help her overcome this fear of needles by teaching her how to calm herself using a simple technique. You obtain her consent, and then you ask her to rate her fear of needles from 0 to 10, where 0 means she has no fear at all and 10 is the worst imaginable fear. She says that her fear at that moment, while just thinking about getting the flu shot, is a 9. This is her Subjective Units of Distress (SUDS) rating. Then you instruct her to tap on several acupuncture points on her hand, face, and chest. The procedure takes a couple of minutes. Immediately following this intervention, you observe that she has become calmer: her breathing has slowed down, she is smiling, and her body posture is softer. You ask her how high her fear rating is now. She pauses briefly, has a somewhat confused expression on her face, and reports that the fear is hardly there. She reports that her SUDS rating is now 3. You ask her what the fear is based on now. She says that it is the image of the nurse preparing the needle. You ask her to focus on this image and you guide her in repeating the tapping on the same acupoints. When she completes the tapping sequence, you ask her to rate her fear level again, and she reports that she does not feel any fear. Her SUDS rating is 0. You then ask her to imagine receiving a flu shot in full detail. She does this imaginal exercise without any fear. You review with her the tapping sequence she just used and advise her that she can do this as a self-treatment any time she needs to and that she can use it to help her overcome any fear or limiting beliefs that she encounters in her life. You can tell her in full confidence that because she reached a 0 in this brief treatment, the likelihood is great that she will have little or no fear when she receives her flu shot. You send her over to your nurse, who administers the flu shot. The patient has no adverse reactions. It took you 10 minutes to help this patient.

> The SUDS rating stands for Subjective Units of Distress and is measured from 0 to 10, with 10 being the maximum amount of subjective feelings of distress and unrest.

CASE STUDY 2: BLOATING, WEIGHT GAIN, AND ANXIETY

A 47-year-old woman comes to see you. Her presenting complaints include bloating, 10-pound weight gain over the past 6 months, and anxiety. During the evaluation, you learn that her last child left for college, she faces insecurity at work due to restructuring, and her husband's mother, who lives out of town, had a stroke 8 months ago. You note that this patient has suffered from anxiety in the past and has taken anxiolytics, but did this only briefly because she prefers natural approaches. You discuss the stresses in her life with her and inform her that her body is giving her important messages that her life is out of balance. Because she prefers natural approaches, you introduce the Four Energy Gates practice to her and emphasize the importance of regular daily practice at home. You share with her that you have been doing them as well and noticed improvements in your mood and general well-being. You show her the exercises and give her a home self-practice handout. She agrees to return to the office in 1 month. After 1 week, your nurse follows up with the patient, and the patient says that she has been practicing 4 out of 7 days but that she feels noticeably calmer. When she returns after 1 month, she says that she continues to have concerns about her job security and her mother-in-law's care, but that the bloating has gone away and she is much calmer. She said that she showed her husband the practice and that he is doing it with good results as well.

These two examples show how both focused energy psychology (EP) methods (case report 1) and more global EP wellness methods (case report 2) can be used by physicians, nurse practitioners, and other health care professionals in their offices to introduce patients to effective self-help practices (Box 103.1).

BOX 103.1	Overview of Energy Psychology

1. Uses meridian, chakra, or biofield interventions to treat the symptom
2. Provides rapid, gentle, nonretraumatizing treatment for a wide range of emotional and psychological conditions.
3. Does not require deep emotional processing of the problem.
4. Activates hope because long-standing problems can often be helped.
5. Is easily taught as a self-help method.

WHAT IS ENERGY PSYCHOLOGY?

EP is a family of integrative approaches to psychotherapy, self-improvement, and wellness rooted in mind-body healing traditions that are up to 5000 years old. EP methods blend the bioenergetic insights of these traditions with the best of contemporary psychological practice. EP practitioners combine cognitive interventions (including focused awareness and mindfulness, imaginal exposure of disturbing memories, and cognitive reframing) simultaneously with the activation of one or more of the human bioenergy systems such as meridians, chakras, and biofields. EP is a part of the broader integration of the profound shifts in science as the implications of relativity and quantum theory are applied to healing practices.[1] Along with this is a recognition in health care of the role of consciousness, intention, and energy in wellness and healing.[2] With roots that link to ancient Chinese medicine and acupuncture, including qigong self-healing practices, EP is a bridge that connects this ancient healing wisdom to modern therapeutic practice and research as well as leads modern practitioners to directly explore these ancient practices themselves.

EP emerged in the early 1980s as part of a search for more effective treatments for posttraumatic stress disorder (PTSD) and phobias. It is also an outgrowth of the continuing convergence of medical and healing systems of the West and the East. This convergence broke into public awareness in 1971 when *New York Times* journalist James Reston wrote about his experience of acupuncture successfully treating his postsurgical pain. This occurred while he was in China prior to President Nixon's historic visit.

At the time of this writing, many EP treatment modalities are in use in the United States and are increasingly being used throughout the world. Examples of popular modalities include the Emotional Freedom Techniques (EFT), Thought Field Therapy (TFT), Tapas Acupressure Technique (TAT), Energy Diagnostic and Treatment Methods (EDxTMs), Advanced Integrative Therapy (AIT), and Heart Assisted Therapy (HAT), with EFT being the most commonly used method. They are being used by a range of professionals and lay people. Psychologists, social workers, and other mental health practitioners—along with physicians, nurses, chiropractors, life coaches, educators, sports performance experts, yoga teachers, and lay people, among other groups—are integrating EP methods into their work (see Chapter 116).

By the mid-1990s in the United States, awareness of EP's effectiveness as a rapid and comprehensive trauma treatment spread. Therapists who were already familiar with other effective trauma therapies, such as exposure therapies and eye movement desensitization and reprocessing (EMDR),[3] began to embrace EP because of the positive results they found in the treatment of recalcitrant trauma patients. In their practices, they observed that patients typically experienced rapid and robust relief from trauma symptoms, with significant symptom improvement evident typically after only a couple of sessions.

In the field, trauma-relief teams used EP interventions to help people who were traumatized as a result of both natural and manmade disasters, including survivors of the Newtown school shootings, the attacks of 9/11, the Indonesian tsunami, earthquakes in Guatemala and Pakistan, Hurricane Katrina in New Orleans, the war in Serbia and Bosnia, and the genocide in Rwanda. Because EP can be quickly taught to indigenous relief workers who are not mental health professionals, treatments can be locally administered while relying on only a few trained outside professionals. This method of treatment delivery was used successfully in Guatemala and Indonesia as well as in Rwanda. EP is showing great promise as an effective treatment for PTSD among U.S. military veterans. Similar to other traumatized populations, EP treatment of veterans led to the resolution of chronic disabling symptoms, such as nightmares, flashbacks, hypervigilance, and emotional numbness. As an empowerment strategy, patients were taught how to use EP for symptom maintenance and as an effective generalized self-help method.

Significantly, EP treatment is gentle and does not retraumatize the patient. A holistic therapy, EP treatment typically leads to rapid and simultaneous positive changes in emotions, mind, body, and overall well-being. In general clinical practice, well-trained EP practitioners can help people rapidly recover from a broad range of problems, including panic attacks, phobias, and generalized anxiety; traumatic reactions including PTSD; persistent negative emotional states such as sadness, grief, and anger; and blocks to creative expression and peak performance. EP approaches can be helpful adjuncts to more severe problems such as major depression, bipolar disorder, and personality disorders, including borderline personality disorder.

Despite these promising results, EP has faced significant professional opposition. To support practitioners and to promote EP generally, in 1999, the Association for Comprehensive Energy Psychology (ACEP) was founded (see Key Web Resources). ACEP, a nonprofit international professional organization, which is headquartered in the United States, promotes the education, research, and professional practice of EP. In addition, ACEP is a leader in addressing the ethics and scope of practice issues associated with EP. ACEP offers education and certification in EP. Recognizing that EP methods have an important role in mental health settings, in the broader health care arena, and in all areas in which people are working to help others advance themselves and overcome problems (e.g., education, corrections, coaching, and sports performance), ACEP developed advanced training programs for both mental health professionals and allied health practitioners.

In 2012, as a result of ACEP's efforts, the American Psychological Association (APA) made the historic decision to approve ACEP as a continuing education (CE) provider for psychologists. Both the clinical applications of EP and research into EP have been growing since.

WHAT IS THE EVIDENCE FOR ENERGY PSYCHOLOGY?

The APA decision was based on the fact that research had established a threshold, evidence-based foundation for EP. Studies demonstrated that EP is an effective treatment for anxiety, specifically for certain phobias (e.g., insects and small animals[4] and public speaking anxiety,[5] along with other common fear states).

A good overview of the evidence-based support for EP can be found in Feinstein's 2012 article in the *Review of General Psychology*.[6]

EP's efficacy as a trauma treatment has been shown in clinical field research. In the case of Rwanda, in 2006, members of the Trauma Relief Committee of the Association for Thought Field Therapy Foundation worked with children at the El Shadai orphanage. Children there who had witnessed the murder of their parents and other family members during the Rwandan genocide were profoundly traumatized. The therapists worked with 50 children aged 13–18 years. These children suffered typical PTSD symptoms including flashbacks, nightmares, bedwetting, depression, withdrawal, isolation, difficulty concentrating, and aggression. The children's level of PTSD was evaluated using standardized tests. Their average scores exceeded the cutoffs for a diagnosis of PTSD, as outlined in the fourth edition of the *Diagnostic and Statistical Manual of Mental Disorders*. These 50 children were treated with three TFT sessions lasting 20 minutes each. After the TFT sessions were administered, most of the children experienced an immediate decrease in the frequency and intensity of flashbacks and other symptoms. The clinical improvement was matched by improvement in the children's test scores. At the conclusion of the three sessions, the tests were readministered, and the children's scores were found to be no longer in the PTSD range. These improvements continued to hold a year later when the children were retested.[6,7]

EP methods show great promise in the treatment of returning veterans. In a randomized controlled trial of EP in combat veterans, 49 veterans had scores higher than the PTSD cutoff. After six treatment sessions, 42 of these veterans had scores that were no longer in the PTSD range. These gains were maintained at the 6-month follow-up.[8]

The near instantaneous calming of severe emotional reactions that can occur with EP treatment suggests that EP treatment affects trauma-associated brain systems. Indeed, research suggests that EP treatment produces rapid changes in the brain. As an example, Diepold and Goldstein compared a patient's quantitative electroencephalography pattern before and after a single TFT session. The pattern was abnormal when the subject brought to mind a specific personal trauma, but it was normal when the subject thought about a neutral event. Following a single TFT treatment, no abnormalities were observed in either the traumatic or neutral condition. These positive changes in brain wave patterns remained at 18-month follow-up.[7]

Evidence is growing to support the clinical findings that EP treatments can ameliorate physical problems, including headache and pain. Bougea et al. showed that EFT can reduce the pain associated with tension-type headaches.[9,10]

Church has summarized research to date indicating that clinical EFT is an effective treatment for psychological and many physiological conditions.[11]

> Energy psychology, although a shift from the conventional Western medical belief, appears to be an easy to practice, low-cost with low-harm intervention that can empower patients to recruit internal resources that can resolve stressful emotions. Results have been shown to be sustained over time.

HOW DOES ENERGY PSYCHOLOGY WORK?

The debate on how EP modalities work is lively. Kathleen Hui's work[12] at Harvard University demonstrated that stimulating acupoints can lead to modulation of the limbic system. Some investigators, such as Ruden,[13] argue that the clinical results seen in EP treatment can be explained by extending current neuroscience understanding of neuroplasticity in the brain. Porges' polyvagal theory has been used as a model for understanding trauma and the efficacy of EP.[14,15] Feinstein argued that EP is an accelerated exposure therapy. In other words, the somatic component of EP treatments, by stimulating the meridian system, accesses a much more rapid information processing system that turns off the body's alarm response and leads to repatterning of negative memory patterns (in the amygdala and hippocampus, respectively). Presumably, Feinstein's argument could be expanded to include EP methods (e.g., HAT, TAT, and AIT) that are somatically focused but do not employ percussive tapping on acupuncture points.

Roger Callahan,[16] the developer of TFT, proposed an informational and energetic model suggesting that stimulating meridian points helps to collapse perturbations in the patient's thought field. These energetic perturbations are presumed to be caused by some initial upsetting or traumatic incident. The notion of the existence of a thought field, which is a field of information fundamentally energetic and not localized in brain tissue, appears to be supported by Rupert Sheldrake's work on morphic resonance.[17] In addition, studies on mind effects at a distance offer further support for the possibility that our mind extends beyond the brain.[18] These latter energy- and consciousness-based explanations may better fit actual clinical experience because many clinicians report positive EP clinical outcomes by activating body energy centers without touching the body or through intention only. Larry Dossey[19] argued that the evidence for nonlocal mind is compelling, and this nonmechanistic view points toward new possibilities for healing. At the same time, it echoes ancient ideas about human interconnectedness.[20] EP, like qigong, by focusing on meridians, consciousness, and energy may be helping us rediscover hidden healing capacities that were long overlooked in the Western scientific paradigm.[21]

HOW DO I GET STARTED?

Because EP approaches can be used for self-help, one of the best ways to learn about EP is to begin by trying it out yourself. A basic tenet of EP treatment (similar to acupuncture) is that symptoms occur when we are in a state of energetic imbalance or disharmony. So, a good starting point for self-treatment is a comprehensive energy balancing practice.

A good option is the Four Energy Gates (Fig. 103.1 within the Patient Handout). According to Master Nan Lu, daily practice of these qigong energy exercises drawn from traditional Chinese medicine can promote overall wellness and contribute to the improvement of emotional and physical symptoms.[22]

To work on a personal issue, follow these four basic steps: begin with a basic balancing practice (the Four Energy Gates), identify the problem, perform an energy clearing or balancing exercise (e.g., the EFT tapping sequence), and evaluate the results and repeat if necessary (Box 103.2).

For example, let us say that you have an important speaking event coming up and you are experiencing apprehensions about presenting. As the day of the event approaches, you notice that you are avoiding preparing for the talk; you have an unsettled feeling in your belly when you think about it; when you respond to your colleagues' questions about it, your voice trembles; and you worry that you will embarrass yourself. Of course, these anxieties are common, but you feel your fears are excessive. You decide that you are going to help yourself overcome this problem by using an EP approach. You have already noted the behavioral (avoidance), physical (distress in your belly and shaky voice), emotional (anxiety), and cognitive (worry about embarrassment) components of your anxious reaction. Considering these symptoms, you identify your worry that you will embarrass yourself as the most salient aspect. You establish that your SUDS rating when you think about these worries is a 9. If you choose the more comprehensive of the self-treatment protocols, you would begin with the Four Energy Gates practice. This takes approximately 15–20 minutes. The acupuncture points used in the Four Energy Gates improve the flow and distribution of your body's qi. The first three open up the energy flow to the head, the heart, and the kidneys, respectively. The last one helps to integrate and harmonize the qi flow in the body. Many times, just doing the Four Energy Gates can lead to a significant improvement in the problem (a brief video of the Four Energy Gates can be found here: http://taoofhealing.com/patient-care/self-care/).

If, after completing the Four Energy Gates, your anxiety persists (you still feel distress when you think about embarrassing yourself when you give the speech) and your SUDS rating is not 0, you can proceed to treat your worry of embarrassing yourself by using this EFT protocol (Fig. 103.2 within the Patient Handout):

1. While tapping firmly and steadily on the side of the hand (sh on the chart), say out loud:
2. "Even though I have this worry that I'll embarrass myself, I deeply love and accept myself." Another version you can use is this: "Even though I have this worry that I'll embarrass myself, I'm attracting love and compassion into my heart." Repeat these statements three times.
3. Next, tap approximately seven to nine times on each of these acupoints while repeating at each point this phrase, which serves to keep you attuned to the problem: "this worry." Again, steady and firm tapping works best.
4. Move from one point to the next until you have tapped on all seven points:
5. Eyebrow: eb
6. Side of the eye: oe
7. Under the eye: e
8. Under the nose: un
9. Under the lower lip: ul
10. Under the collarbone: c
11. Under the arm: ua

(Note: You can tap on all the points on the chart, but usually tapping on these seven points is sufficient. Also, do your best to tap on the location shown in the chart. If you are not sure whether you are doing it correctly, do your best and continue with the procedure.)

After you have tapped on these points, stop and reevaluate the intensity of the problem. What is the SUDS rating now? How much distress remains? To what extent are you able to imagine yourself in the situation and be free from worry and distress? If any upset remains, repeat these steps. However, this time adjust the first statement to this: "Even though I still have some of this worry, I deeply love and accept myself." The reminder phrase could be "the remaining worry" or "still have some worry." Complete the tapping sequence and reevaluate. Sometimes, you need to shift the focus of the treatment to a different facet or aspect of the problem, say from the worry of embarrassment to the queasy feeling in your belly. By doing this, usually the problem significantly subsides or disappears after a few rounds of tapping. In some instances, more persistence is required. If you do not experience immediate improvement, keep at it.

Usually, when your SUDS rating reaches 0 and you have no distress when you imagine experiencing the situation, the likelihood is high that you will be able to go through the actual event with little or no distress. However, because the tapping is easy to do, you can always use it as a self-help booster whenever you feel the need. You should test out the treatment as much as possible to be sure that you are completely free of the negative reactions. As you start to notice improvements, push yourself to imagine the target situation at its worst to see whether you experience any distress. If you do, repeat the tapping, targeting those specific reactions.

Patient Handout: Energy Psychology Self-Care Patient Handout

Use the 4 Energy Gates (Figure 103-1) for daily self-care. Also, use this practice when dealing with an emotional, personal, or physical problem that is not passing on its own. You can do one or more of the 4 Energy Gates throughout the day, whenever you need a pick-me-up. *(Remember to consult with your physician if you have any serious health concerns.)*

Use the tapping method (Figure 103-2) to address a particular distressing emotional or personal issue.

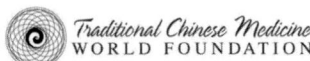

Traditional Chinese Medicine
WORLD FOUNDATION

The Four Energy Healing Gates: Universal Pathways to Health

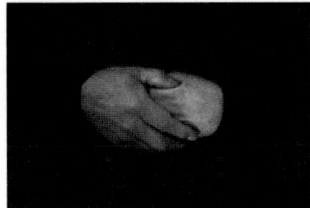

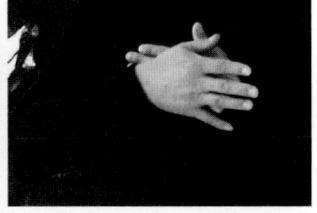

On the web between the thumb and index finger: With firm pressure, make small circles for 4 to 5 minutes. Note: the outside, active hand supports and protects.

On the center line of the body between the breasts: Place one palm over the other, and using light pressure only, circle in a clockwise direction at least 200 times (can also be done counter-clockwise).

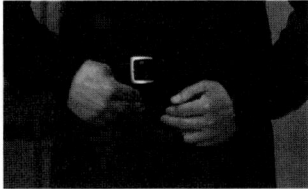

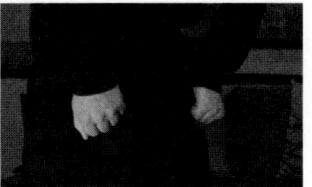

Just to each side of the center line, four fingers below the navel: Tap this area with two fingers of each hand for 4 to 5 minutes.

In the center "dimple" of the main muscle of the buttocks: Keeping arms, shoulders and hips relaxed, hold a loose fist and alternately punch this area for 4 to 5 minutes.

Traditional Chinese Medicine World Foundation
34 West 27th St, Site 1212, New York, NY 10001
212-274-1079 • fax: 212-274-9879 • www.tcmconference.org

Fig 103-1. Energy Psychology Meridian Tapping Protocol
From: Traditional Chinese Medicine World Foundation. http://www.tcmworld.org/_downloads/FourEnergyGates_FullPage.pdf
Accessed June 20, 2011.

1. Identify the problem that is blocking you. Is it primarily an emotional, cognitive, or behavioral issue? Is it physical (e.g., shoulder pain)? Rate it from 0–10 (10 is the most distress).

2. Then while tapping firmly and steadily on the side of the hand (sh on the chart) say outloud (to yourself):
*"Even though I have this **[insert your problem]**, I deeply love and accept myself."* Or, use this:
*"Even though I have this **[insert your problem]**, I attract love and compassion into my heart."*
Repeat 3 times.

3. Next, tap steadily and firmly about 7–9 times on each of the following acupoints while saying at least once at each point a brief reminder of the issue you are working on. (See Fig. 103-2.)
         Eyebrow – eb
         Side of the eye – oe
         Under the eye – e
         Under the nose – un
         Under the lower lip – ul
         Under the collarbone – c
         Under the arm – ua
(Note: You can tap on all of the points on the chart, but usually tapping on these 7 points is sufficient. Also, do your best to tap on the location shown in the chart. If you are not sure if you are doing it correctly, do your best and continue with the procedure.)

FIG. 103.1 ■

BOX 103.2	Steps for Energy Psychology Self-Treatment

1. Begin with a balancing practice (Four Energy Gates).
2. Identify the issue (cognitive, emotional, and behavioral aspects).
3. Hold the problem in mind while doing the Emotional Freedom Techniques tapping sequence.
4. Evaluate the results and repeat, if necessary.

For a shortcut, do only steps 2–4.

HOW DO I GET TRAINED?

EP appears simple, and for many issues it can be. Using EP clinically to treat a diverse clinical population with a range of problems requires advanced training, however. Furthermore, knowledge of various ways of working energetically allows you to individualize treatment. EP training for professionals is becoming more rigorous. ACEP sponsors several training programs, and you can also go to the websites of other methods to discover ways to learn and become certified in those approaches (see the Key Web Resources).

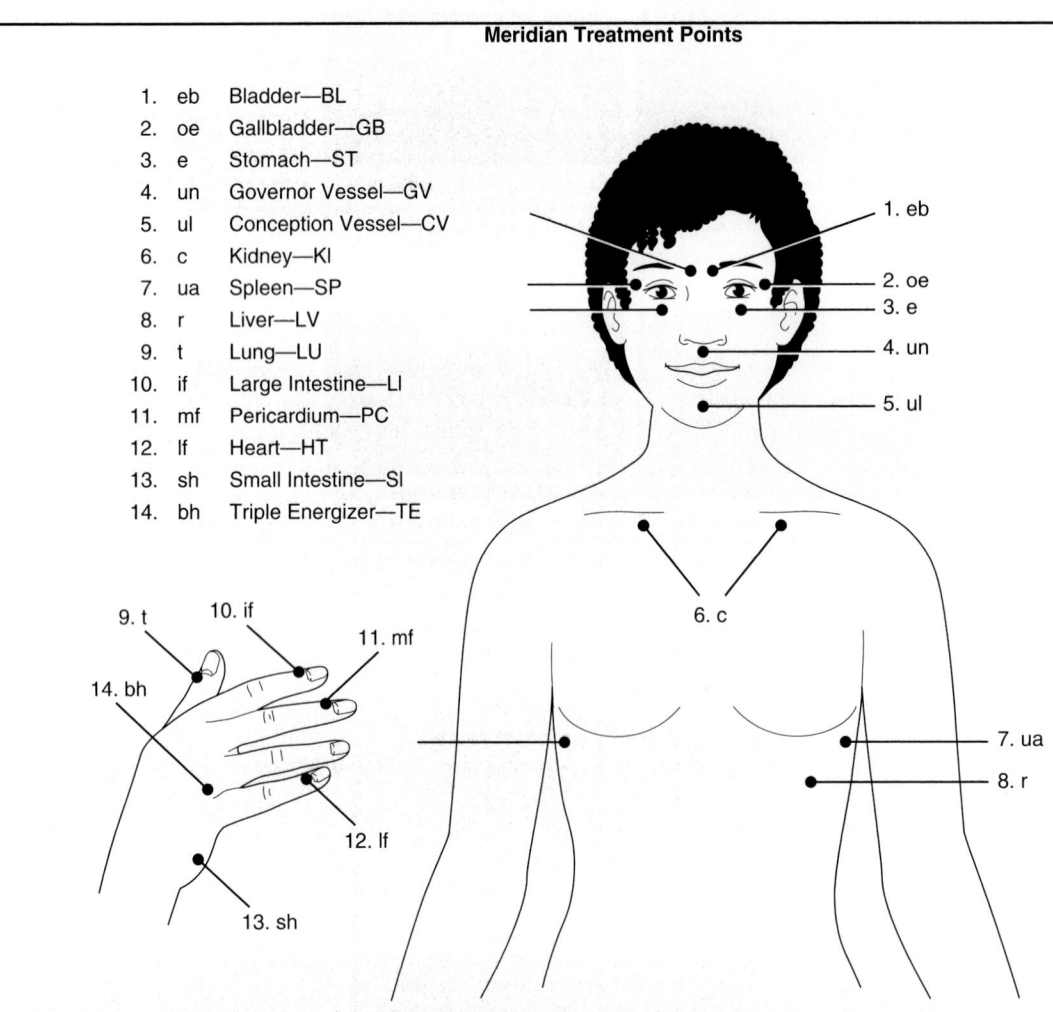

Meridian Treatment Points

1.	eb	Bladder—BL
2.	oe	Gallbladder—GB
3.	e	Stomach—ST
4.	un	Governor Vessel—GV
5.	ul	Conception Vessel—CV
6.	c	Kidney—KI
7.	ua	Spleen—SP
8.	r	Liver—LV
9.	t	Lung—LU
10.	if	Large Intestine—LI
11.	mf	Pericardium—PC
12.	lf	Heart—HT
13.	sh	Small Intestine—SI
14.	bh	Triple Energizer—TE

Figure 103-2. Energy tapping protocol.

(List continues from Fig. 103.1)

4. Reevaluate the problem. How is it now? Repeat steps 2 and 3 if the problem still bothers you. Target the aspect of the problem that it is most distressing. For example, it may have started as a physical discomfort and has become more clearly emotional. Be persistent and repeat as necessary.

5. Usually, when your SUDS reaches 0, and you have no distress when you imagine experiencing the situation, the high likelihood is that you will be able to go through the actual event with little or no distress. However, because the tapping is easy to do, you can always use it as a self-help booster whenever you feel the need. Note: it is important to test out the treatment as much as possible to be sure that you are completely free of the negative reactions. As you start to notice improvements, push yourself to imagine the target situation at its worst to see whether you experience any distress. If you do, repeat the tapping targeting those specific reactions.

FIG. 103.2 ■

IMPORTANCE OF PERSONAL PRACTICE AND DEVELOPMENT

As you use EP methods more frequently, an important shift occurs. You internalize your experience that entrenched and difficult-to-treat problems can often be transformed quickly. Contrary to the generally held idea that you must work through the deep psychological roots of problems, you can reliably facilitate deep and enduring personal change by addressing the energetic foundations of problems.

In all energy work, indeed in all healing, the practitioner's personal development is critical. Caring, compassion, and technical skill are essential to the healing encounter and so is the internal energetic level of the practitioner. Practitioners should establish a personal practice that can increase their energy level. For example, performing the Four Energy Gates everyday gradually improves your internal energy and helps you to be more effective. Other examples could include a regular meditation practice, doing yoga, or taking daily walks in nature. Time devoted to your personal practice has many visible and invisible benefits.

As with any healing-oriented practice, work on yourself first by grounding and balancing your own energy. This can be done in various ways, including the Four Energy Gates technique, meditation, breath work, and others.

ENERGY PSYCHOLOGY AS A FIRST-LINE TREATMENT

Patients come to see their doctors and health care practitioners to seek treatment for disturbing symptoms. That many of these symptoms are not based on any significant pathology is well known. Often, these symptoms are somatic messages related to ongoing stress and disharmony in the patient's life. Having EP as part of your tool set will enable you to alleviate your patients' symptoms by helping them deal with the underlying stress that is at the root of their distress. An added benefit is that by offering EP treatment, you can help patients leave your office feeling better. In addition, they will have an effective, inexpensive, and safe self-help tool that they will be able to use forever.

Key Web Resources

This link provides a brief demonstration of each of the Four Energy Gates.	http://taoofhealing.com/patient-care/self-care/
Association for Comprehensive Energy Psychology: The Association for Comprehensive Energy Psychology is an international nonprofit professional organization whose goals are to promote the education, training, research, and ethical practice of comprehensive energy psychology.	http://www.energypsych.org
EFT Universe: This website contains many articles and case examples of the application of The Emotional Freedom Techniques (EFT).	http://www.eftuniverse.com
A short video showing the before and after results of EFT treatment of four severely traumatized veterans. Very intense.	http://www.innersource.net/ep/component/content/article/60.html
TATLife: This is the home site for the Tapas Acupressure Technique.	http://www.tatlife.com
Energy Psychology: This is the website for Dr. Fred Gallo, who is credited with coining the term energy psychology and who wrote the first textbook on it *(Energy Psychology)*. He has developed numerous methods, including Energy Diagnosis and Treatment Methods (EDxTM).	http://www.energypsych.com
Innersource: This is Dr. David Feinstein's and Donna Eden's website, which includes links to Dr. Feinstein's articles, as well as information about Donna Eden's energy medicine workshops and trainings.	http://www.innersource.net/ep/
Traditional Chinese Medicine World Foundation: This website describes the many programs offered by Master Nan Lu. Energy psychology has direct links to traditional Chinese medicine. Master Lu's programs and training are a natural way to deepen your grasp and appreciation of the healing principles behind energy psychology.	http://www.tcmworld.org

---

REFERENCES

References are available online at **ExpertConsult.com**.

SECTION III

BIOCHEMICAL

SECTION OUTLINE

104 PRESCRIBING BOTANICALS

105 PRESCRIBING PROBIOTICS

106 DETOXIFICATION

107 CHELATION THERAPY

108 INTEGRATIVE STRATEGIES FOR PLANETARY HEALTH

CHAPTER 104

PRESCRIBING BOTANICALS

Paula Gardiner, MD, MPH • Amanda C. Filippelli, MSN, MPH, RN, APRN • Tieraona Low Dog, MD

A careful examination of the evidence regarding the safety and efficacy of herbal medicines should guide the clinician as they partner with their patients in creating optimal health care.

OVERVIEW

In 2012, 33.2% percent of the American population used some form of complementary and alternative medicine (CAM), with 17.7% percent of the population using non-vitamin, nonmineral dietary supplements.[1] During 2012, whole-food supplements had approximately $1.1 billion in sales.[2] This was more than 10% annual growth. It is clear that many of our patients are regularly using herbs and dietary supplements.

WHO USES HERBS?

Rates of herbal product use vary by age, gender, race, and ethnicity. Substantial numbers of all patient groups report using herbs and dietary supplements, particularly women and people with chronic or recurrent illnesses who also receive care from conventional health care professionals. In adult national studies, there are many conditions where herb use has been commonly reported for relief of gastrointestinal conditions, memory improvement, cardiovascular health, and cancer symptom improvement.[3-6] Herbal medicine has also been used in pediatric populations for common conditions, including mental health disorders, headaches, eczema, and asthma.[7-10]

WHAT ELSE ARE THEY TAKING?

Approximately one-third of all adults in the United States might be taking an over-the-counter medication and herb or a prescription medication and herb concurrently.[11] Different patient populations are at high risk for drug/herb interactions; these include human immunodeficiency virus (HIV)-positive patients, chronically ill patients, cancer patients, and elderly Medicare patients.[12-14]

There is no universally accepted guideline for managing a patient's prescription medication and herbal medicine in the outpatient or inpatient setting.[11] However, the Joint Commission Accreditation of Healthcare Organization requires that dietary supplements (herbs, vitamins, and minerals) conform to the same hospital standards as prescription medications.[15]

Despite the documented high prevalence of patient use of herbal products, fewer than half of patients who use herbs typically discuss it with their clinician.[16,17] Therefore, it is critical to have an approach to discussing herb with patients.

TALKING ABOUT HERBS WITH PATIENTS

Health care providers must be able to talk with patients about a wide variety of treatment options, including those that fall outside what the health care provider learned in formal training. Because use of herbs has the potential for both benefit and harm, it is important that providers approach the topic of herb usage in an open and non-judgmental way. Many cultures have a rich history of using botanical medicines; indeed, herbal medicine is the most common form of traditional medicine in the world. Because such a wide variety of herbal practices and products are available in the United States, generalizations are difficult. Nevertheless, by asking a few open-ended questions, the clinician should be able to assess the patient's beliefs and cultural practices regarding his/her use of herbal medicines. Examples of such questions are as follows:

- When you were growing up, did you or your family ever use any medicinal plants or herbal remedies to improve your health or treat an illness?
- If I were to walk around your house and look for containers of herbs, vitamins, or dietary supplements, what would I find?
- How do you use herbs or herbal remedies in your home?
- Are you taking any herbs or herbal medicines now? If so, what are you trying to treat, and do you think the herbs are working?

Using herbs in practice is a holistic process. Besides the patient's cultural and social background, it is important for the clinician to take into account what symptoms the patient has, any chronic or acute illness, prescribed medications the patient is taking, and any nonprescribed medications as well as to judge how adherent the patient will be to the regimen the clinician recommends.

EFFICACY

How does the clinician know whether an herb actually works for a patient's condition? Is there strong historical evidence? Is there a biologically plausible mechanism of action based on in vitro or animal research? Has the herb undergone controlled clinical trials? And if so, which type of product was studied and at what dose? These are important questions to ask when trying to determine efficacy. First, here is a summary of the strengths and weaknesses of different types of evidence used to assess the efficacy of botanical medicines.

In vitro studies, objective measurements using isolated tissue or cell culture, are a well-accepted first step for understanding the physiological and/or pharmacological activity of a particular substance. Animal studies are often used in pharmacological studies because they permit control over a number of variables and can help explain potential mechanisms of action. The strengths of in vitro and animal studies are that they:
- Allow control over a number of variables
- Generate and test hypotheses for mechanism of action
- Help determine safety at varying doses and duration
They do have limitations, which are as follows:
- Results may not accurately predict physiological effects in humans.
- Parenteral administration may give differing results from oral administration.
- Study of isolated constituents may not reflect use of the whole plant.
- Ethical issues surround the use of animals in medical research.

A long history of use is an important source of information regarding the safe and effective use of plant medicines. These historical data are almost exclusively based on observational data, and even today, a clinician's observations remain an important tool for assessing efficacy and adverse effects in the office. One strength of observational data is that they can provide useful insight when a therapy has been used by multiple cultures, over time, for similar purposes. Also, the astute clinician may detect a therapeutic effect, or an adverse effect, that is not well known or recognized. An important limitation is that there is a risk of bias if the observers are not studying a defined cohort of patients.

Nonrandomized and nonblinded, or uncontrolled, studies are a valuable method for generating hypotheses and assisting in the identification of adverse events, although they are best regarded as yielding "supportive" evidence. Strengths of uncontrolled studies are that they are:
- Valuable for generating hypotheses
- Useful for identifying adverse events
The limitation is that the presence of multiple uncontrolled variables increases risk of bias in the results.

Outcome research generally involves a cohort of patients with the same diagnosis (e.g., diabetes, heart disease) that relates their clinical and health outcomes (e.g., death, events, improvement) to the care that they received (e.g., physical therapy, medication). The strengths of outcomes research is that it:
- Reflects more closely the actual day-to-day practice of clinical medicine
- Is well suited for whole-system approaches (e.g., traditional Chinese medicine, Ayurveda, naturopathy)

A challenge in prescribing botanicals is the variation that is naturally found within any growing plant. Where is the active ingredient...the root, stem, leaves, or flowers? What type of soil was it grown in? What was the growing season like? A good botanical is like a good wine.

The limitation is that it is difficult to establish efficacy for any particular aspect of treatment.

It has the following strengths:
- It provides safeguards against numerous forms of bias.
- The model is applicable for the study of many botanical interventions.

Limitations of randomized, double-blind trials are as follows:
- The average randomly allocated patient may not adequately reflect the clinical subgroups seen in clinical medicine.
- This model may not be applicable for answering some clinical questions, such as individualization of therapy.
- The lack of a randomized controlled trial (RCT) is often interpreted as lack of efficacy; this is a problem in botanical medicine in which treatments may have been used for centuries but lack current gold standard evidence.

In addition to clearly understanding the limitations of different research methods, the clinician must understand exactly what type of product is actually being tested. The complex nature of botanicals (e.g., the variations in constituents between species, plant parts, and preparation) makes it essential that authors of research articles clearly provide an adequate description of the product used in the clinical trial. Descriptions should include identification (Latin binomial and authority), plant part (root, leaf, seed, etc.), and type of preparation (tea, tincture, extract, oil, etc.).

Tincture and extract description should include the identity of the solvent and the ratio of solvent to plant material. If the preparation is standardized to a chemical constituent, that information should also be included. Precise and clear dose and dosage form should be provided.[18] These are critically important issues to consider when conducting and publishing research on botanical medicines. Thus it is important for us to ask the question "Is the product that my patient is taking for her particular condition similar to what was clinically tested?" In 2006, the Consolidated Standards of Reporting Trials (CONSORT) developed guidelines in reporting clinical trials of herbal medicine in the peer-reviewed literature, which has been adapted by many journals.[19,20] There is a growing need for more clinical trials examining herbal medicine.

An increasing number of systematic reviews and meta-analyses are now available for busy clinicians to evaluate the evidence of efficacy for a number of botanicals, including echinacea (*Echinacea* spp.),[21] garlic (*Allium sativum* L.),[22] kava (*Piper methysticum* G. Forster),[23] ginkgo (*Ginkgo biloba* L.),[24,25] horse chestnut (*Aesculus hippocastanum* L.),[26] saw palmetto (*Serenoa repens* W. Bartram),[27] and St. John's wort (*Hypericum perforatum* L.).[28] While recognizing the value of meta-analyses in the medical literature, it is important to point out one potential problem with this approach in the field of herbal medicine—the "pooling" of different products to reach a specific conclusion about a particular plant. For example, a review of garlic pooled results from clinical trials using raw garlic, aged garlic extracts, dehydrated garlic, and garlic oil macerates to reach a specific conclusion regarding the benefit of garlic for cardiovascular health.[29] When one evaluates these products from an analytical perspective, it is clear that there are marked chemical differences between them, making any general conclusion about the efficacy of garlic (or lack thereof) questionable.

And finally, we must consider what level of evidence of efficacy is acceptable to support the use of a medicinal plant by our patient. This must take into consideration the relative safety of the product, the medical condition being treated, and the personal beliefs and preferences of the patient.

Before moving on to safety, it is important to consider the use of herbal products in pediatric populations. While herbs are used by children for a variety of reasons, there is a great need for more research on the use of herbs in pediatric populations.

SAFETY CONSIDERATIONS

As with any drug or chemically active constituent, whether an herb is toxic depends on its dose, form of product, what it is taken with, and the underlying condition of the patient. Overall, most herbs commonly used in the United States have a relatively good safety profile, and the incidences of herbal adverse events are low. More than 1500 dietary supplement-related regulatory alerts from the Food and Drug Administration (FDA), MedWatch, and Health Canada websites were identified from 2005 to 2013.[30] In general, many case reports are of poor quality and are anecdotal in nature, and frequently, the adverse effects are caused not by the supplements themselves, but rather by adulteration or contamination of these products.[31]

Modern use of an herbal product may not reflect the use of herbal preparations in traditional medicine. For example, an excellent safety record of a traditional oral preparation may well have limited relevance to use of the same herb in a concentrated product at a high dose. Moreover, herbs that are apparently safe under normal conditions may be more hazardous in specific conditions (e.g., pregnancy, impairment of renal or liver function), under special circumstances (e.g., during the perioperative period), or when combined with certain conventional drugs.

> Adverse effects of botanicals commonly arise not from the supplement itself but from contaminants within it.

When one is considering the safety of botanicals, it is important to look at the framework for regulating the sale of dietary supplements in the United States. The Dietary Supplement and Health Education Act (DSHEA), which was enacted in 1994, has had a profound influence on how herbal products are sold and marketed to the consumer. To discuss herbal products with patients, clinicians must understand this act.[32] The following points are important:
- DSHEA allows dietary ingredients that were in the market before 1994 to be marketed without prior approval

of their efficacy and safety by the FDA. Herbs that were brought to market in the United States after 1994 must submit a notification to the FDA. If it wasn't present in the food supply, the manufacturer must document why they believe it to be safe when used under the conditions suggested on the label.
- The manufacturer of an herbal product is responsible for the truthfulness of claims made on the label and must have evidence that the claims are supported; nevertheless, DSHEA neither provides a standard for the evidence needed nor requires submission of the evidence to the FDA.
- Manufacturers are permitted to claim that the product affects the structure or function of the body, as long as (1) there is no claim of effectiveness for the prevention or treatment of a specific disease and (2) a disclaimer appears on the container informing the user that the FDA has not evaluated the product for any claim.
- The manufacturer is responsible for controlling quality and safety of the product, but if a concern about safety arises, the burden of proof lies not with the manufacturer but with the FDA, which has to prove that the product is unsafe.

The FDA has released good manufacturing practices (GMPs) for herbal products. GMPs set standards for purity, strength, and potency of the supplements to reflect what is stated on the label.[33]

Even if clinicians are able to identify an herbal product that shows strong efficacy, the concern about the safety of herbal products often overshadows our discussions with patients. These concerns include contamination with other products, such as heavy metals, pesticides, microorganisms, or misidentified herbal ingredients, and adulteration with a prescription drug.[31] The quality of plant material varies considerably depending on where it is cultivated or gathered, the times and methods of harvest and drying, and environmental conditions such as climate and soil type. There may be considerable variation in the composition of an herbal product among manufacturers, as well as discrepancies between label information and actual content. Clinicians should be cognizant of potential adverse events from food or drug interactions. For instance, there is sufficient evidence from interaction studies and case reports to demonstrate that St. John's wort (*H. perforatum* L.) induces the cytochrome P450 (CYP) 3A4 enzyme system and the P-glycoprotein drug transporter in a clinically relevant manner, reducing the efficacy of comedications.[34,35]

In December of 2006, the Dietary Supplement and Nonprescription Drug Consumer Protection Act was passed. It requires the reporting of a serious adverse event as a result of a dietary supplement and labeling of the manufacturer's address and phone number. The manufacturer is required to forward information on serious adverse events to the FDA within 15 days. The health care professional can also report a drug/herb interaction or an adverse effect to MedWatch, a program administered by the FDA. Another excellent resource is to contact your local poison control centers; the new nationwide toll-free number for poison control is 800-222-1222. There is also a need for better reporting of adverse events in children following herb use[36].

CHOOSING A BRAND OR PRODUCT: A QUESTION OF QUALITY

Once the clinician has determined that an herb is efficacious and safe for a particular patient, he or she must advise the patient on choosing high-quality products. The quality of an herbal preparation partly determines its efficacy and safety. Even with DSHEA, loopholes in the regulatory system have allowed poor-quality products to be introduced into the marketplace. The FDA is addressing some of the problems associated with manufacturing herbal products with its new GMPs.[33] Nonprofit and for-profit organizations have taken on the task of certifying manufacturers who are following GMPs and testing to see that what is on a label is in the bottle (Table 104.1). It is critical to guide patients toward purchasing the best-quality herbal product; high quality generally translates to better safety and efficacy.

DOSING

Once the correct herb has been chosen for the correct patient's diagnosis, the clinician confronts confusing questions of dosing. Where is the dosing information on the label of the bottle? How much herb should the patient take and for how long? Is the dose different for a child?

There are many ways for patients to prepare and use "herbal medicines" (Table 104.2). A traditional herbalist will individualize every treatment protocol on the basis of the patient's unique situation, often using more than one herb or type of preparation. However, tailoring the herbal treatment for the patient can be difficult for the conventional provider in this age of uncertainty regarding the safety of all herbal products. Traditionally, most herbalists administered crude herbs in the form of teas, decoctions, tinctures, poultices, or compresses. These preparations are relatively inexpensive and easy to use. We encourage our patients to get involved by developing self-care routines (e.g., cooking with herbs, making a cup of tea, taking an herbal bath). The majority of commercial herbal products are sold in solid dosage forms, such as tablets and capsules, although teas, tinctures,

TABLE 104.1 **Information on Testing Dietary Supplement and Herbal Products**

Organization	What to Look for on the Label	Web Address
NSF is a nonprofit public health organization. NSF's certification service includes product testing, Good Manufacturing Practices (GMP) inspections, ongoing monitoring, and use of the NSF Mark.	**NSF** NSF	http://www.nsfconsumer.org/food/dietary_supplements.asp
The United States Pharmacopeia (USP)—testing for contamination, adulteration, and good manufacturing processes. USP also examines products for pharmacological properties.	**USP**	http://www.usp.org/usp-verification-services/usp-verified-dietary-supplements
Consumer Labs evaluates commercially available dietary supplement products for composition, potency, purity, bioavailability, and consistency of products.	**CL** ConsumerLab.com	http://www.consumerlab.com/
U.S. government—GRAS "GRAS" is an acronym for the phrase **G**enerally **R**ecognized **A**s **S**afe. Under sections 201(s) and 409 of the Federal Food, Drug, and Cosmetic Act (the Act), any substance that is intentionally added to food is a food additive, that is subject to premarket review and approval by FDA, unless the substance is generally recognized, among qualified experts, as having been adequately shown to be safe under the conditions of its intended use, or unless the use of the substance is otherwise excluded from the definition of a food additive.	GRAS	http://www.fda.gov/food/ingredientspackaginglabeling/gras/default.htm
Health Canada In Canada dietary supplements are regulated by the government in a natural health products category insuring safety and efficacy of these products. This link includes all dietary supplements that are licensed for sale in Canada.		http://www.hc-sc.gc.ca/

and liquid extracts remain popular. Teas (water extracts) have a long history of use but are often limited by taste and rapid spoilage (they have to be made fresh). Hydro-ethanolic extracts, such as tinctures and fluid extracts, are more concentrated and easier to administer, although the alcohol content can be a problem for some patients.

A growing number of herbal preparations are now standardized to a specific constituent, or group of compounds, helping to ensure batch-to-batch consistency of the product. The standardizing compound may or may not be one of the "active" ingredients in the product. Most clinical trials are conducted on standardized products.

The type of herbal preparation a clinician chooses to use depends on a variety of considerations, including the patient, whether the medical problem is acute or chronic, personal preferences, and medicinal properties of the herb. For example, many people find valerian tea unpleasant tasting; recommending a tincture or capsule may improve the chance that the patient will adhere to therapy. Chamomile tea is quite appropriate for people of all ages. If using garlic for cardiovascular health, the patient could simply add garlic to the daily diet or choose a standardized extract.

For dose, the clinician can start by looking at the clinical trials on the product studied, the dose used, and side effects reported. The majority of herbal clinical trials have been conducted on standardized extracts in solid dosage forms (capsules and tablets). There are also excellent resources about correct dosages on the Internet (Table 104.3). The clinician should nevertheless be aware that products in the marketplace vary widely in dose and may not accurately represent either what was historically used or the dose typically seen in clinical trials.

We recommend asking patients to bring to the office all their dietary supplement bottles, teas, tinctures, and so on. This can be a fruitful exercise in starting an open discussion, teaching the patient how to read supplement labels, and catching potential drug–herb interactions and adverse effects. Table 104.4 contains explanations of the elements of a label on a botanical product bottle.

TABLE 104.2 **Preparation of Herbal Products**

- Balm or salve—A soothing lipid-based topical preparation containing beeswax, vegetable, or mineral oil.
- Bath—Herbal preparation placed in a soaking bath; transdermal absorption extremely limited and mostly relevant to herbs with high volatile oil content. Herbal baths can be useful for skin irritation or enjoyed simply for their pleasant aroma.
- Decoction—An extraction of the soluble compounds from hard plant material (e.g., bark or roots) in boiling water. Herbs are generally simmered for at least 10 minutes.
- Essential oil—Volatile oils extracted from a plant, often through distillation. Essential oils are often many times more potent that the plant itself, which also means an increased risk of potentially adverse effects when used internally. Some popular essential oils include eucalyptus, peppermint, and tea tree oil.
- Fluid extract—A hydroethanol solution with the strength of one part solvent to one part herb (more concentrated than a tincture; alcohol content can vary).
- Glycerite—An herbal compound infused in a solution of glycerin (no alcohol).
- Infusion—An extraction of soluble compounds from fresh or dried flowers, leaves, or seeds in hot water. Infusions are generally steeped for a minimum of 5–10 minutes (a tea).
- Maceration—An herbal infusion made with cold or room temperature water.
- Pills, capsules, or tablets—These may contain the whole herb (or particular plant part such as leaf, root, or seed) or the dried extract of a herb.
- Poultice—An herbal preparation wrapped in cloth and applied to the skin.
- Powders—An herbal preparation applied in a powder form (e.g., talc).
- Syrup—Herbs infused in a syrup product.
- Tincture—A hydroethanolic solution of active plant constituents with a strength of greater than one part herb per one part solvent (alcoholic content can vary).
- Tonic—A preparation used to invigorate and restore the body, generally taken on a daily basis (e.g., nettles).

CONCLUSION

In conclusion, the clinician should remember to:[37]
- Ask all patients about botanicals and the supplements they use. (Offer examples of types of products meant in the question.)
- Record the responses in the patient's record so that anyone consulting the patient can check for possible safety concerns such as herb–drug interactions.
- Advise patients about the safety and effectiveness of the products that they are using or considering using.
- If unable to answer all the patient's questions about some botanicals, the clinician should be prepared to refer the patient to evidence-based sources of information (see Table 104.4).
- The clinician who uncovers a possible adverse effect should report it to MedWatch, as previously discussed.

TABLE 104.3 **Evidence-Based Resources for Dietary Supplements**

Subscription Services	
Dynamed: Reference tool powered by Ebscohost with summaries for more than 3200 topics. There is a mobile application available as well ($395/year for physician subscription).	http://www.dynamed.com/home/
Natural Medicines: You can search by supplement or commercial product name. Also includes information about pregnancy and lactation, as well as adverse events (inquire for pricing).	https://naturalmedicines.therapeuticresearch.com/
HerbMed: HerbMed is an herbal database that provides scientific data underlying the use of herbs for health. HerbMedPro, an enhanced version of HerbMed, is available for subscription, licensing, and data streaming. The public site has 20 herbs; HerbMedPro has an additional 233 herbs and continuous updating (individual subscriber $45.00/year).	www.herbmed.org

Continued

TABLE 104.3   Evidence-Based Resources for Dietary Supplements—cont'd

Nonsubscription Services

The National Center for Complementary and Alternative Medicine (NCCAM): NCCAM is the Federal Government's lead agency for scientific research on CAM. *Herbs at a Glance*, a series of 42 patient information sheets, are listed at http://nccam.nih.gov/health/herbsataglance.htm	http://nccam.nih.gov/
NIH Office of Dietary Supplements: Provides overview of vitamins, minerals, and dietary supplements with two levels of information—Health Professional and QuickFacts.	http://ods.od.nih.gov/
Dietary Supplement Labels Database: Dietary Supplement Labels Database offers information about label ingredients, enabling users to compare label ingredients in different brands. Each dietary supplement has additional links to other government created HDS resources such as Medline, Clinical Trials.gov, and NCCAM.	http://www.dsld.nlm.nih.gov/dsld/
MedlinePlus—Dietary Supplements—For Free: This consumer health database from the National Library of Medicine offers extensive information on dietary supplements. http://www.nlm.nih.gov/medlineplus/druginformation.html	http://medlineplus.gov
American Botanical Council: This nonprofit organization has helpful information and continuing medical education resources.	http://www.herbalgram.org
Health Canada: The Canadian government regulates natural health products in Canada licensing products with proof of safety and efficacy. This is a very helpful site—it lists products licensed in Canada and has helpful monographs.	http://www.hc-sc.gc.ca

TABLE 104.4   Interpreting Product Labels

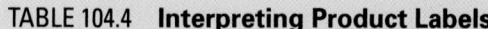

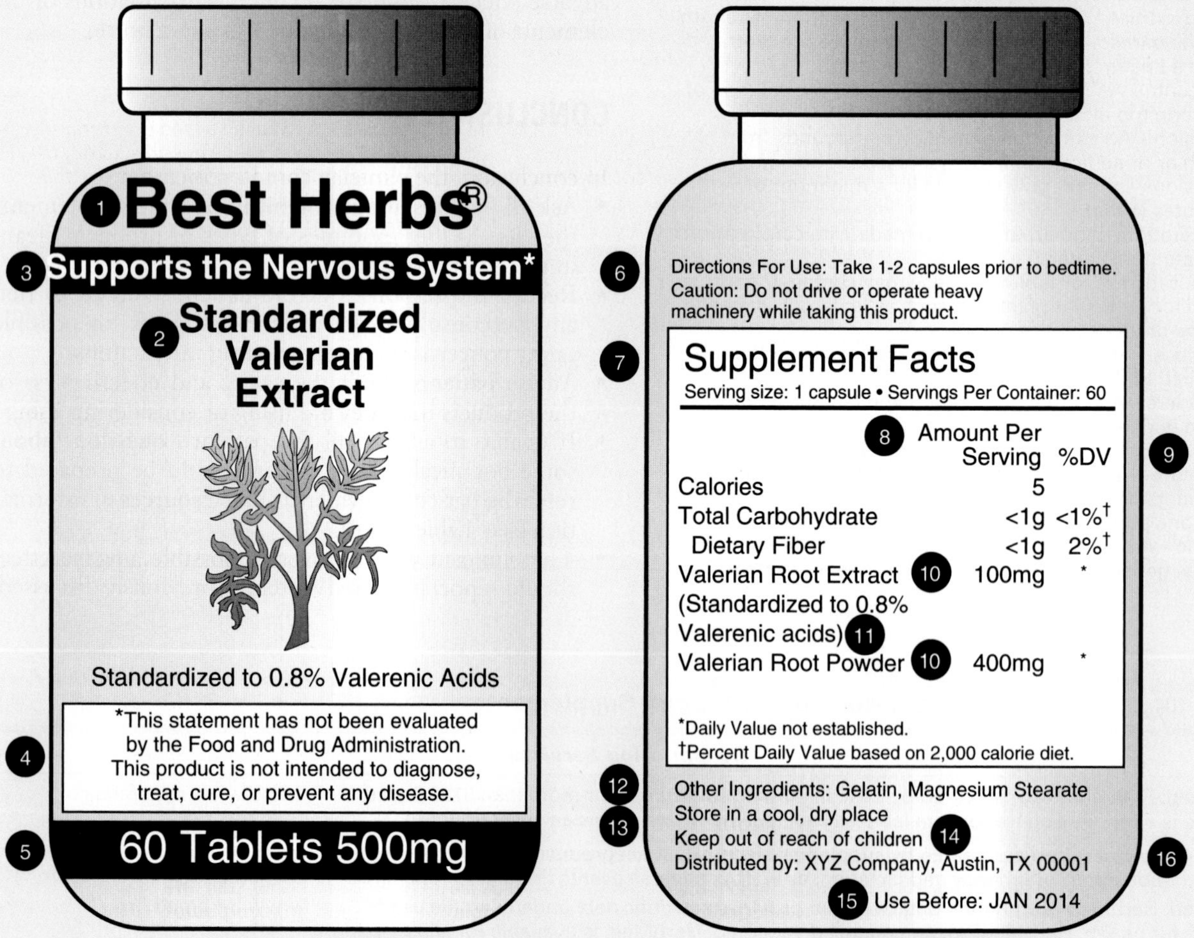

❶Best Herbs®

❸ **Supports the Nervous System***

❷ **Standardized Valerian Extract**

Standardized to 0.8% Valerenic Acids

❹ *This statement has not been evaluated by the Food and Drug Administration. This product is not intended to diagnose, treat, cure, or prevent any disease.

❺ **60 Tablets 500mg**

❻ Directions For Use: Take 1-2 capsules prior to bedtime. Caution: Do not drive or operate heavy machinery while taking this product.

❼ **Supplement Facts**

Serving size: 1 capsule • Servings Per Container: 60

	❽ Amount Per Serving	%DV ❾
Calories	5	
Total Carbohydrate	<1g	<1%†
Dietary Fiber	<1g	2%†
Valerian Root Extract ❿	100mg	*
(Standardized to 0.8% Valerenic acids) ⓫		
Valerian Root Powder ❿	400mg	*

*Daily Value not established.
†Percent Daily Value based on 2,000 calorie diet.

⓬ Other Ingredients: Gelatin, Magnesium Stearate
⓭ Store in a cool, dry place
Keep out of reach of children ⓮
Distributed by: XYZ Company, Austin, TX 00001 ⓰

⓯ Use Before: JAN 2014

TABLE 104.4 **Interpreting Product Labels—cont'd**

1. Brand name
2. Product/herb name
3. Herbal products and other "dietary supplements" may make "statements of nutritional support," often referred to as "structure/function claims," as long as they are truthful and not misleading, are documentable by scientific data, and do not claim to diagnose, cure, treat, or prevent any disease and carry a disclaimer on the product label to this effect. The disclaimer must also note that FDA has not evaluated the claim. The product manufacturer must also notify the FDA of the structure/function claim within 30 days of bringing the product to market. According to current FDA regulations, examples of acceptable structure/function claims include "supports the immune system" and "supports a healthy heart," while claims such as "helps treat the common cold" and "helps prevent heart disease" are considered unacceptable because these are considered drug claims. Thus "helps maintain urinary tract health" is acceptable, while "helps prevent urinary tract infections" is not.
4. A structure/function claim requires this disclaimer when it appears on the label of a dietary supplement as well as in any brochures or advertising. The disclaimer must be in bold type and in a box.
5. Number of tablets, capsules, and net weight of each in package.
6. Directions for use and cautions.

Items 7–10 are part of the "Supplement Facts Panel"

7. ᵃ "Serving Size" is the suggested number of tablets, capsules, softgels, tea bags, liquid extract, or tincture to take at one time.
8. ᵃ "Amount per Serving" first indicates the nutrients present in the herb and then specifies the quantity. The following items must be declared if in excess of what can legally be declared as zero: calories, fat, carbohydrates, sodium, and protein. In addition, the following nutrients must also be declared if present in quantities exceeding what can legally be declared as zero: vitamins A, C, D, E, K, B1, B2, B3, B6, B12, folic acid, biotin, calcium, iron, phosphorus, iodine, magnesium, zinc, selenium, copper, manganese, chromium, molybdenum, chloride, and potassium. Most herbal products contain negligible amounts of these nutrients.
9. ᵃ "Percent Daily Value" (%DV) indicates the percentage of daily intake provided by the herb. An asterisk under the "Percent Daily Value" heading indicates that a Daily Value is not established for that dietary ingredient.
10. ᵃ Herbs should be designated by their standardized common names as listed in the book *Herbs of Commerce*, published in 1992 by the American Herbal Products Association. If the common name is not listed in *Herbs of Commerce*, then the common name must be followed by the herb's Latin name. The plant part must be listed for each herb. The amount in milligrams of each herb must be listed unless the herbs are grouped as a proprietary blend—then only the total amount of the blend need be listed. For herbal extracts, the following information must be disclosed:
    a. the ratio of the weight of the starting material to the volume of the solvent (even for dried extracts where the solvent has been removed, the solvent used to extract the herb must be listed)
    b. whether the starting material is fresh or dry
    c. the concentration of the botanical in the solvent
11. Standardization. If a product is chemically standardized, the product label may list the component used to measure standardization (e.g., ginsenosides in Asian ginseng, valerenic acids in valerian) and the level to which the product is standardized (e.g., 4% ginsenosides). Therefore, if a product contained 100 mg of Asian ginseng extract per capsule and the extract was standardized to 4% ginsenosides, one capsule would contain 4 mg of ginsenosides. In most, but not all, cases, the component used to measure standardization is bioactive, although the standardization component may not be responsible for the intended primary activity of the herbal supplement, other active compounds may be responsible. Products can also be standardized to "marker compounds" for purposes of quality control. Those markers may or may not be active.
12. A list of all other ingredients, in decreasing order by weight, must appear outside the Supplement Facts box. In herb formulas containing multiple herbal ingredients, the herbs must be listed in descending order of predominance.
13. The proper location for storage of herbal products is typically labeled as a cool, dry place.
14. All herbal products and other dietary supplements should be kept out of the reach of children.
15. The herb should be used before the expiration date for maximum potency and effectiveness. Expiration dates are often arbitrarily established by the manufacturer, regardless of the ingredients and their relative stability. Such dates are routinely set at two years from the date of manufacture of the finished dietary supplement, although this period may be longer or shorter depending on the manufacturer's policies, stability testing, dosage form, and other variables.
16. The product must list the manufacturer or distributor's name, city, state, and zip code.

ᵃAdapted with permission from the table "Interpreting Product Labels" in Blumenthal M, Hall T, Goldberg A, et al., eds. *The ABC Clinical Guide to Herbs.* Austin, TX: American Botanical Council; 2003:24. Go to www.herbalgram.org for more information on ABC's additional resources and continuing medical education for health care providers.

REFERENCES

References are available online at ExpertConsult.com.

CHAPTER 105

PRESCRIBING PROBIOTICS

Jonathan Takahashi, MD, MPH • J. Adam Rindfleisch, MPhil, MD

WHY PROBIOTICS?

The Gut Microbiome in Health and Disease

The quantity of microbes in our bodies number approximately 100 trillion cells, ten times more than the number of human cells; the collective genome of these organisms is 100 times larger than our own.[1] Most of these bacteria reside in the intestinal tract, with an estimated 70% in the colon alone.[2] *Metagenomics* is the study of all DNA from a given environment, which for humans includes the DNA from the host and the *microbiota*, a term that refers to the totality of microorganisms that coexist with the host or in a specified part of the host's body, such as the gastrointestinal (GI) tract.[3,4] Recent metagenomic studies have revealed that each individual harbors 160 or more bacterial species from a consortium of about 1150 prevalent species.[5] Given that more than 90% of our "superorganism" is actually microbial rather than human, technological advances in molecular biology have fueled a virtual explosion of research in the quest to better understand the role of the microbiome in physiology, health, and disease.

Scientific interest in the symbiotic relationships between humans and certain microbes is not new, beginning soon after Louis Pasteur and Robert Koch established the idea that microorganisms were responsible for infectious diseases. In 1907, Nobel laureate Ilya Metchnikov postulated that lactic acid bacteria (LAB), such as those consumed in fermented foods, contributed to longevity by replacing pathogenic microbes such as *Clostridia* with beneficial, nonpathogenic microbes. The diet he promoted included milk fermented with what he called "Bulgarian bacillus."[6] Scientific research progressed during the 20th century, but it was only with technological advances in molecular biology and genomics during the latter part of the century that a more detailed understanding of human–microbial symbiosis started to emerge. Recently, the National Institute of Health (NIH)-sponsored Human Microbiome Project (2008–2012) utilized samples from 18 locations, ranging from the nares to the vagina and gut, from nearly 5000 healthy individuals to create an initial characterization of the normal microbiota in healthy adults in a Western population.[5] Our understanding of how the microbiota is intricately entwined with human physiology continues to evolve with each passing year as research brings new discoveries.

As the home for the vast majority of the human microbiota, the GI tract has been the main focus of recent research. While popular understanding views the GI tract as a simple, closed tube through which food and waste products pass, science continues to uncover how it merits its nickname as "our second brain." Gut–microbial interactions have been shown to play a key role in the following physiological processes:

- *Intestinal barrier function.* The extent to which the epithelial barrier allows bacterial translocation into the bloodstream, what is commonly referred to as the "leakiness" of the gut, is affected by the microbiota itself, which regulate the production of desmosomes and tight junctions.[4] The integrity of the intestinal barrier is important in defending against pathogens and also in decreasing circulatory proinflammatory lipopolysaccharides (LPS) that are implicated in a number of chronic inflammatory diseases.[2,4,7,8]

- *Immune regulation.* The mucosal immune system must strike a fine balance between tolerance of beneficial microbes and reaction to potentially pathogenic microbes. The mucus layer changes its composition and thickness in response to microbial stimulation, and maturation of the extensive gut-associated lymphoid tissue (GALT), including Peyer's patches, depends on microbial colonization. Furthermore, specific species drive the differentiation of immune cell subsets, particularly T cell responses, as well as the production of immune mediators such as IgA, which have a range of downstream effects.[4]

- *Metabolism and adiposity.* Facilitation of nutrient absorption is one of the core functions of the intestinal tract, but the microbiota affect not only local but also systemic metabolism. The exact details continue to be elucidated by research, but the complex interplay between the ingested food, bile acids, mucus layer, and microbiota modulates the release of hormones such as glucose-dependent insulinotropic polypeptide, glucagon-like peptide, and lipoprotein lipase inhibitors. Short-chain fatty acids (SCFAs) produced by bacterial fermentation are thought to be key mediators in these processes.[4,8]

- *Brain and behavior effects.* The gut possesses its own enteric nervous system (ENS), which is in constant communication with the central nervous system (CNS) through conduits such as the vagus nerve, and there is clear evidence of bidirectional communication in the physiological stress response. Animal models have begun to reveal how microbes directly produce or stimulate the production of signaling molecules, such as norepinephrine, GABA receptor ligands, and serotonin, even directly influencing behaviors, such as anxiety. This "microbiome–gut–brain neuroendocrine axis" is the subject of ongoing investigation.[4,9,10]

- *Tissue and organ homeostasis.* Evidence from mouse models shows a role for molecular signaling from intestinal microbes in intestinal tissue repair as well as the potential contribution to osteoporosis through influence on bone remodeling. Some studies have associated certain microbial species with the development of colon cancer, possibly through inflammatory mechanisms.[4]

The term *dysbiosis* signifies "an imbalance in the structure and/or function of the microbiota that leads to disruption of host–microorganism homeostasis."[4,7] A familiar example of dysbiosis is *Clostridium difficile* infection, which most commonly occurs after repeated antibiotic or broad-spectrum antibiotic administration. *C. difficile* colitis represents an example of severe imbalance between commensal organism and the pathogenic *C. difficile*, creating levels of inflammation that can even precipitate severe sepsis.[7]

There is growing evidence for the potential role of dysbiosis in noncommunicable chronic diseases that comprise a substantial and growing portion of the global disease burden. A unifying hypothesis for many of these diseases is chronic inflammation, which gut microbes modulate at the local and systemic level, as previously noted. Studies in animal models and correlative studies in humans suggest a possible role for dysbiosis in inflammatory bowel disease,[7] atopic and allergic diseases,[7] obesity,[7,8,11,12] type 2 diabetes and metabolic syndrome,[3,7,8,11,13,14] atherosclerosis,[15,16] and autoimmune diseases.[17,18] It should be noted that studies in humans to date are largely correlative, and further research will be vital in determining causality.

HOW THE HUMAN MICROBIOTA IS ESTABLISHED AND ALTERED

Every person's microbiota begins to be established even before birth. One of the largest influences on the establishment of the infant's microbiota appears to be whether or not the baby is delivered vaginally, with concomitant exposure to the mother's vaginal and gut flora.[19] Perinatal factors found to be associated with differences in the diversity and specific composition of the infant gut microbiota include:[20]

- Maternal exposures such as stress, antibiotic use, smoking
- Length of gestation (term vs. preterm)
- Mode of delivery (cesarean vs. vaginal)
- Nourishment (breastmilk vs. formula)
- Antibiotic administration
- Surrounding environment (e.g., sanitation, urban vs. rural, geographic factors)
- Caregiving structure (e.g., extended family involvement)
- Ethnicity and cultural practices

The composition and diversity of the intestinal microbiota of the breastfed infant is different from that of the formula-fed infant, including greater numbers of beneficial bacteria such as *Bifidobacterium* with breastfeeding.[21,22] In particular, higher concentrations of potentially beneficial *Bifidobacteria* are found in the gut when babies are breast fed, as are fewer potential pathogens.[23] Evidence demonstrates an enteromammary pathway for bacterial

transfer in addition to the substantial provision of prebiotics in breastmilk.[24-26] The establishment of healthy gut microbiota is postulated as one of the possible mechanisms through which breastfeeding decreases the rates of numerous chronic diseases, ranging from allergic diseases to obesity[20] (Fig. 105.1).

> Colonization of the gut with healthy flora can be listed as another benefit of breastfeeding.

A 2013 study of healthy volunteers examining the stability of the human microbiota over time found that in a given individual, an average of 60% of strains remained after 5 years.[27] There was a significant concordance between family members, supporting the idea that the early environment shapes the composition of the lifelong microbiota.[27] The findings of this study, along with results from animal models, hint at a possible, although unproven, role for the early-life microbiota in genetic imprinting, or epigenetics, which has been found to be increasingly important in health and disease.[4] At the same time, a 2012 study showed the most significant similarity between cohabiting mothers and fathers and their children, even if they were genetically unrelated.[28] Furthermore, the 2013 study found a significant change in the microbiota after a subset of four subjects consumed a monotonous low-calorie diet for a portion of the study protocol.[27] This corresponds with results of animal studies demonstrating later-life malleability of the microbiota and potential contributions to disease through dysbiosis.[4,27]

WHAT ARE PROBIOTICS, PREBIOTICS, AND SYNBIOTICS? (TABLE 105.1)

Since the 1980s, tremendous interest has developed regarding the ways the ecosystem of the gut may be altered, not only to decrease pathogen numbers but also to promote overall health by correcting dysbiosis and supporting homeostasis. Many different foods and supplements that contain microbes—namely, species of bacteria or yeasts—are now available over the counter. These products are widely known as *probiotics*, a hybrid word created by combining the Latin *pro-* ("for") with the Greek adjective *-biotic* ("life").[29] The first use of the word in the scientific literature may have been by Kollath in 1953 to describe supplements that help restore health in patients suffering a form of malnutrition resulting from eating too much highly refined food.[29] For all the commercial and scientific attention these supplements currently receive, only in the 1990s did the word *probiotic* enter both medical and general lexicons on a regular basis.

In 2002, the Food and Agriculture Organization of the United Nations clearly defined probiotics as "live microorganisms which, when administered in adequate amounts, confer health benefits upon the host."[30] The International Scientific Association for Probiotics and

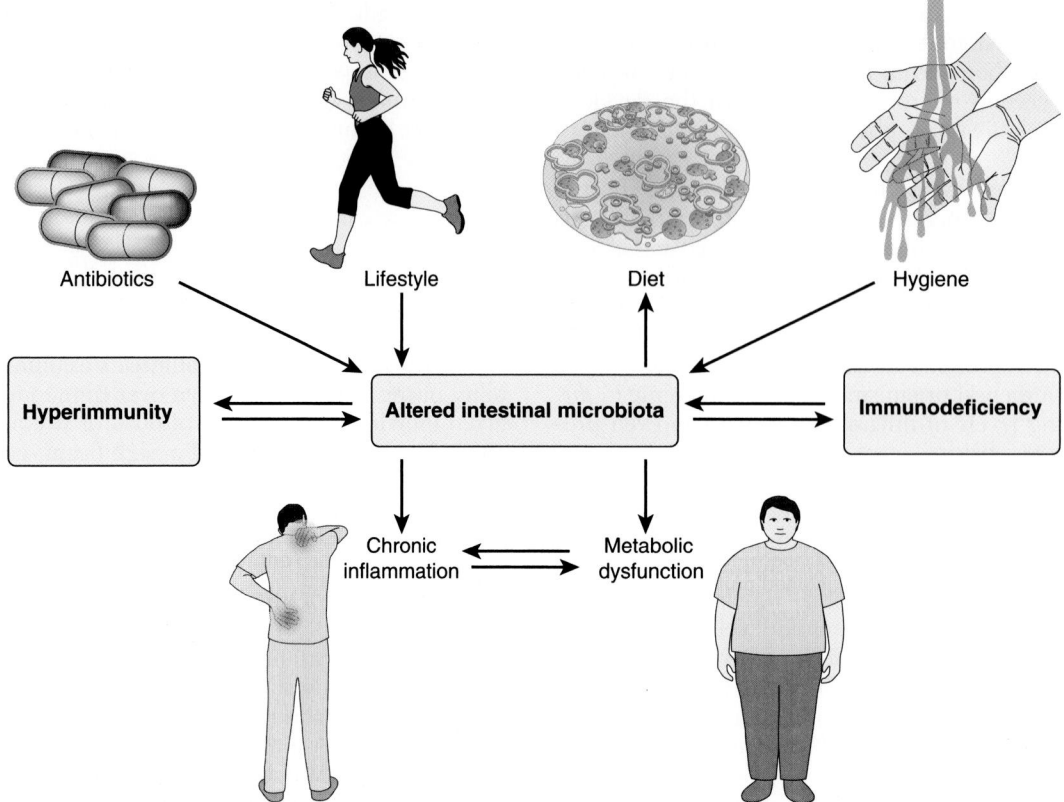

FIG. 105.1 ■ Some of the factors that can shape the composition of the intestinal microbiota and effects of dysbiosis on chronic disease. Environmental factors such as lifestyle, diet, hygiene, and use of antibiotics can impact the gut microbiota. The immune system also impacts the gut microbiota, while a state of dysbiosis alters levels of immune mediators, inducing both chronic inflammation and metabolic dysfunction. (Adapted from Sommer F, Bäckhed F. The gut microbiota--masters of host development and physiology. *Nat Rev Microbiol.* 2013;11(4):227-238.)

TABLE 105.1	**Basic Definitions for Probiotics, Prebiotics, and Synbiotics**
Probiotics	Live microorganisms that confer a health benefit on the host when administered in adequate amounts
Prebiotics	Selectively fermented ingredients that result in specific changes in the composition and/or activity of the gastrointestinal microbiota thus conferring health benefit(s) upon host
Synbiotics	Products that contain both probiotics and prebiotics

Adapted from: Guarner F, Khan AG, Garisch J, et al. World Gastroenterology Organisation Global Guidelines: probiotics and prebiotics October 2011. *J Clin Gastroenterol.* 2012;46(6):468-481.

Prebiotics released a consensus statement in 2014 that supported continued use of this definition and also created the following subcategories of probiotics:[31]

1. Probiotic in a health food or supplement without a health claim (member of a species or specific microbe generally considered safe and supported by evidence that it is "generally beneficial")
2. Probiotic in a health food or supplement with a specific health claim (defined strain with proof of delivery and viability at end of shelf life, with robust clinical evidence of efficacy)

3. Probiotic drug (similar to #2, but also meeting regulatory standards for drugs)

To fulfill these requirements, a useful probiotic should have certain properties: (1) survival to the target organ (e.g., be resistant to both gastric and bile acids), (2) interaction with host systems, (3) antipathogenic/prohealth actions, (4) safety, and (5) amenability to manufacturing.[32]

The most commonly available probiotics today include bacteria from the genus *Lactobacillus* (e.g., *Lactobacillus acidophilus)* and *Bifidobacterium* (e.g., *Bifidobacterium bifidum*) as well as the yeast *Saccharomyces boulardii* (to be distinguished from *Saccharomyces cerevisiae*, used in baking and brewing). Strains of *Streptococcus* and *Enterobacteriaceae* and other genera are less commonly included.

> The most commonly used probiotic species belong to the genera *Lactobacillus* and *Bifidobacterium. S. boulardii*, a probiotic yeast, is also increasingly utilized.

Michel Cohendy, a colleague of Metchnikov working in the early 20th century, carried out further investigations with "the Bulgarian bacillus" (now known as *Lactobacillus delbrueckii* subsp. *bulgaricus*) that led to a product called "Le Ferment" sold by the Pasteur Institute of Paris. However, it was Leo Rettger et al. at Yale University who demonstrated that *Lactobacillus bulgaricus* did not survive gastric passage to the small intestine, calling into question which strains Cohendy may have actually been studying. In 1921, they proposed *L. acidophilus* as a better therapeutic candidate based on its ability to survive gastric passage and transform the intestinal flora with lactose and dextrin supplementation.[6]

Henry Tissier, also of the Pasteur Institute, first isolated *B. bifidum* from the feces of a breastfed infant in 1906. He suggested that this bacterium could be administered to infants with diarrhea to displace pathogenic bacteria.[33,34]

During a cholera outbreak in Indochina in 1920, the French microbiologist Henri Boulard noticed that people drinking a special tea made from the outer skin of lychee and mangosteens seemed to be more protected from the disease. He succeeded in isolating the responsible yeast and named it *S. boulardii*.[33]

Escherichia coli Nissle 1917 (the last part of the name is the subspecies designation) is notable in that it is a non–lactic acid–producing bacterium (non-LAB). This specific strain was discovered by Alfred Nissle in the feces of World War I soldiers who were resistant to salmonellosis and shigellosis, and is more widely used in Europe than in the United States.[32]

Prebiotics

Prebiotics are nutrients that selectively stimulate the growth and activity of one or more colonic microorganisms that act to promote the health and wellbeing of the host.[35] Prebiotics consist mostly of nonstarch polysaccharides and oligosaccharides poorly digested by human enzymes, which have traditionally been used to add fiber to foods without adding bulk.[34] However, since not all dietary carbohydrates may be true prebiotics, Gibson et al. have proposed a specific set of criteria, which are as follows:[36]
1. Resistance to gastric acidity, hydrolysis by mammalian enzymes, and GI absorption
2. Fermentation by intestinal microflora
3. Selective stimulation of the growth and/or activity of intestinal bacteria associated with health and wellbeing
According to the criteria of Gibson et al., only a select few substances have accumulated sufficient research evidence to definitively declare their prebiotic activity. These include the following:
- Inulin-type fructans: inulin, oligofructose, fructooligosaccharides
- Galactooligosaccharides
- Lactulose
- Human milk oligosaccharides

Other molecules that are promising, but have less evidence to date, include isomaltooligosaccharides, lactosucrose, xylooligosaccharides, soya bean oligosaccharides, and glucooligosaccharides.[34,36-38]

Inulin and oligofructose occur naturally in many food sources, including garlic, onions, leeks, asparagus, chicory, bananas, wheat, oats, soybeans, and artichokes.[35]

Although not as extensive as the research on probiotics, there is a growing body of evidence supporting the ability of prebiotics to facilitate significant shifts in the gut ecosystem, for example, away from potentially pathogenic strains toward *Bifidobacterium*,[35] and to potentially offer benefit for conditions such *C. difficile* infection,[39] traveler's diarrhea,[40] allergic disease,[41] and irritable bowel syndrome.[42] In addition, prebiotics can help increase the effective absorption of dietary calcium.[43,44] Much of the ongoing basic research focuses on obesity and the metabolic syndrome. Prebiotics may also have a direct beneficial effect through the action of short-chain fatty acids (SCFAs) produced through fermentation, which modulate intestinal permeability and can decrease circulating inflammatory mediators such as bacterial lipopolysaccharides (LPS).[45]

Synbiotics

Synbiotics are products that contain both prebiotic and probiotic ingredients. The theory is that consuming both at once, instead of just the probiotic alone, may enhance microbe survival and lead to greater positive effects on the beneficial microbes already established in the intestines. Although most studies have focused on probiotics, research on synbiotics is growing. An extensive review of the clinical evidence for synbiotics is beyond the scope of this chapter, but summaries can be found in published reviews.[46]

HOW DO PROBIOTICS WORK? POTENTIAL MECHANISMS

Probiotics are postulated to exert a beneficial effect through numerous mechanisms, many of which may be specific to individual species. Probiotic mechanisms of action relate directly to the basic physiology of the gut–microbial relationships. One central mechanism for probiotics is the restoration of a more normal balance of intestinal flora after some disruptive event that contributes to dysbiosis. Although few studies have included an evaluation of both the restoration of normal microbiota and disease treatment efficacy, a synthesis of the literature for eight common disease indications revealed that many of the probiotics shown to have a restorative effect on intestinal flora, particularly *S. boulardii* and *L. acidophilus*, were also shown be effective in clinical randomized controlled trials (RCTs).[47]

Some of the key mechanisms of action of probiotics, as described in the literature, are summarized in Table 105.2 and Fig. 105.2.

WHAT ARE THE CLINICAL INDICATIONS FOR PREBIOTICS AND PROBIOTICS?

Potential benefits from probiotic therapy are strain specific. A list of many of the conditions that have been studied is shown in Table 105.3.

TABLE 105.2   Summary of Biological Effects and Mechanisms of Action of Probiotics

Immunological effects	• Reduce secretion of proinflammatory cytokines • Increase secretion of antiinflammatory cytokines • Activate local macrophages to increase antigen presentation to B lymphocytes and increase secretory IgA production • Induction of T regulatory lymphocytes • Promote hyporesponsiveness to food antigens
Antimicrobial effects	• Compete for nutrients with pathogens • Compete for adhesion with pathogens • Inhibit translocation • Alter local environment (e.g., decrease pH) to inhibit pathogens • Produce bacteriocins to inhibit pathogens • Modify pathogen-derived toxins • Provide "decoy binding sites" for pathogens
Enhancement of mucosal barrier	• Stimulate epithelial mucin production • Strengthen epithelial barrier, e.g., via tight junction function and alteration of surface proteins
Other effects	• Scavenge superoxide radicals • Produce short-chain fatty acids (SCFAs), which have multiple downstream effects

Modified from references 32,34,46, 48.

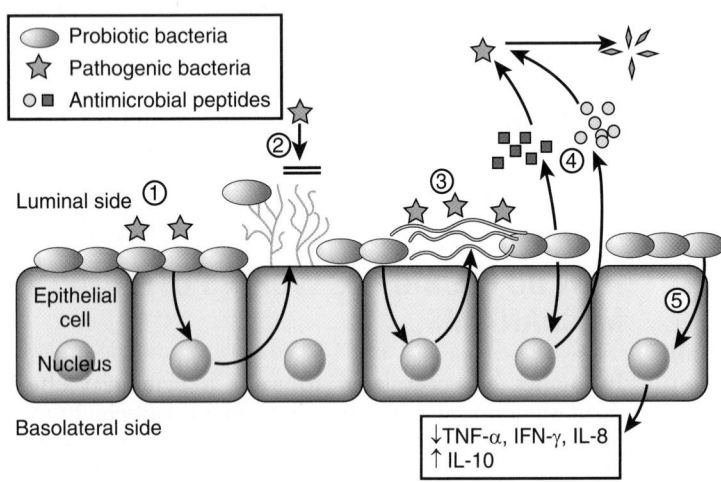

FIG. 105.2 ■ Schematic summary of some of the mechanisms of action of probiotics in the bowel. Probiotics can alter pathogenic bacterial adherence to the bowel wall through (1) a physical barrier, (2) an altered epithelial surface glycosylation pattern, and (3) increased mucin production. Other modes of action include (4) secretion of antimicrobial peptides and (5) modulation of the immune system and altered gene expression. *IFN*, interferon; *IL*, interleukin; *TNF*, tumor necrosis factor. (Redrawn from Borowiec AM, Fedorak RN. The role of probiotics in management of irritable bowel syndrome. *Curr Gastroenterol Rep.* 2007;9(5):393-400.)

TABLE 105.3   Potential Therapeutic Applications for Probiotics

Conditions for which there is moderate to strong level of evidence for benefit	Prevention of necrotizing enterocolitis in preterm infants[49-51] Prevention of upper respiratory infections (URIs) in preschool-age children[52-56] Primary prevention of *Clostridium difficile*-associated diarrhea[57,58] Treatment of acute viral infectious diarrhea[59] Prevention of traveler's diarrhea[60] Prevention of antibiotic-associated diarrhea (children)[61] Irritable bowel syndrome (IBS)[62,63] *Helicobacter pylori* treatment enhancement[64-66]
Conditions for which there is limited evidence for benefit	Bacterial vaginosis (oral and intravaginal)[67,68] Prevention of URIs in adults[52] Prevention of gestational diabetes[69,70] Allergic rhinitis[71] Prevention and treatment of atopic dermatitis (infants)[72-76] Prevention of eczema (infants/children)[77] Infant growth (especially in human immunodeficiency-1 infection)[78,79] Ulcerative colitis (induction or maintenance of remission)[46,80-82] Prevention of ventilator-associated pneumonia[83,84] Cystic fibrosis[85-89]

TABLE 105.3   Potential Therapeutic Applications for Probiotics—cont'd

Conditions for which there is conflicting, inconclusive, or insufficient evidence	Hepatic encephalopathy[90-92] Secondary prevention of *C. difficile*-associated diarrhea[58] Treatment of *C. difficile*-associated diarrhea (together with antibiotics)[93] Prevention of antibiotic-associated diarrhea (adults)[94,95] Persistent diarrhea (children)[96] Functional constipation[97,98] Prevention and treatment of atopic dermatitis[72,74,99] Prevention of chemotherapy- and radiation-induced enteritis/diarrhea[100] Treatment of radiation-induced enteritis[100] Hypertension[101] Hyperlipidemia[102,103] Type 2 diabetes[14,104] Crohn's disease (induction or maintenance of remission)[46,80,105] Pouchitis[46,80] Oral health (e.g., caries, periodontal disease)[106,107] Infant colic[108-110] Prophylaxis of UTIs in infants with vesicoureteral reflux (VUR)[111] Lactose intolerance[112] Autism[113] Nonalcoholic fatty liver disease[114] Prevention of acute otitis media[115] Acute pancreatitis[116,117] Prevention of preterm labor[118] Improving outcomes for malnourished individuals[119] Weight loss[120] Rheumatoid arthritis[121-123] Diverticular disease[124] Chronic fatigue syndrome[125]
Conditions for which there is evidence suggesting lack of benefit	Prevention of food hypersensitivity (infants/children)[41] Prevention of allergic rhinitis (infants/children)[41] Prevention of asthma (infants/children)[41,74]

The methodology for the categorization of clinical evidence was adapted from criteria utilized by the American Academy of Family Physicians (SORT criteria), Oxford Centre for Evidence-based Medicine (Levels of Evidence), and DynaMed (Levels of Evidence), including number, type, and quality of published clinical trials including potential for bias, statistical and clinical significance, and homogeneity of results. This review was based largely on published systematic reviews and meta-analyses.

PRESCRIBING PROBIOTICS: WHICH ONES, WHAT DOSE, AND HOW SHOULD THEY BE TAKEN?

One of the principal challenges in evaluating the clinical efficacy of probiotics is the range of species, dosages, preparations, and treatment duration used in the intervention arm of different clinical trials. These features of the research literature can inhibit meaningful meta-analysis, placing importance instead on the systematic review of multiple, well-conducted trials. Since, from a rigorous scientific standpoint, therapeutic benefits ascribed to probiotic therapy are strain and dose specific, recommending a specific treatment plan to patients can seem daunting. The ideal scenario would be to prescribe exactly the same product used in a given clinical trial; however, considering the very real limitations in cost and availability for many products, a reasonable approach would be to choose probiotic products that are merely as similar as possible. While probiotics are not subject to the same testing requirements as pharmaceuticals, there are some parallels in the use of generic drugs, which claim to have the same active ingredients but do not carry the same requirement for proof of therapeutic efficacy as their brand-name counterparts.[126]

In general, dosages given for prebiotics and probiotics range widely, anywhere from 1 million to 20 billion colony-forming units (CFUs) or more, but recommendations tend toward 1–10 billion CFUs for infants and 10–20 billion CFUs for older children and adults. Probiotics must be administered consistently to ensure a sufficient population and effect on the intestinal microbiota over time.[47] Available data regarding the minimum duration of therapy for various clinical conditions are limited, however.

Table 105.4 lists some of the indications for which probiotics have been shown to be most effective, with examples of the probiotic regimens used in clinical trials.

Recommendations for how to take probiotics can vary and are largely based on expert opinion, but clinical trial protocols can be informative. Some experts recommend taking probiotics on an empty stomach, but the protocols for many trials, particularly in children, often have had patients take probiotics with meals to increase treatment adherence. When taken during a course of antibiotic therapy, probiotics should be started as soon as possible; clinical trials typically have had patients take probiotics only during antibiotic therapy, but since research has suggested that it may take several weeks for the intestinal flora to recover after antibiotic therapy, it is a reasonable recommendation to take probiotics for several days to weeks longer.[143]

Treatment with probiotics is typically well tolerated. Probiotics come in capsules that can be swallowed whole, opened and mixed into drinks or soft foods, in sachets and

TABLE 105.4 **Examples of Probiotic Regimens for Clinical Indications That Have at Least Moderate Evidence of Benefit (see Clinical Evidence Table 105.3)**

Indication	Probiotic Species, Dose (Colony-Forming Units)
Prevention of necrotizing enterocolitis (NEC) in very low birth weight (VLBW)/preterm infants[50,51]	*Lactobacillus acidophilus* + *Bifidobacterium bifidum* 0.056–6 × 10^7 to 0^9 in one or two divided doses per day[51]
Irritable bowel syndrome (IBS)[62,63]	*Lactobacillus rhamnosus GG*, 3 × 10^9 twice daily for 8 wks[63,127] *Lactobacillus plantarum*, 10 × 10^10 daily for 4 wks[62,128] *B. bifidum*, 1 × 10^9 daily[62,129]
Helicobacter pylori treatment enhancement[64-66]	*Saccharomyces boulardii*, 3 × 10^10 three times daily for 4 wks (starting with triple therapy)[65,130] *Lactobacillus gasseri*, ≥ 10^9 twice daily for 4 wks (3 wks before and 1 wk after triple therapy)[65,131] *L. acidophilus*, 5 × 10^6 + *Streptococcus faecalis* 2.5 × 10^6 + *Bacillus subtilis*, 5 × 10^3 daily (for 2 wks before or for 2 wks after triple therapy)[65,132] Kefir, 250 mL daily (*Lactobacillus* + *Bifidobacterium*) for 2 wks (concurrent with triple therapy)[65,133] *L. acidophilus*, 5 × 10^9 three times daily for 10 days (concurrent with and 3 days after triple therapy)[65,134]
Prevention of upper respiratory infections (URIs) in preschool-age children[52-56]	*L. acidophilus*, 10^10 + *Bifidobacterium lactis*, 10^10 twice daily[53] *L. rhamnosus*, GG 10^9 daily[54] *Lactobacillus paracasei*, 10^8 + *Streptococcus thermophilus* 10^7 + *Lactobacillus bulgaricus*, 10^7 (DanActive) daily[56]
Primary prevention of *Clostridium difficile*-associated diarrhea[57,58]	*L. acidophilus* + *Lactobacillus casei*, 10^11 (total) daily for duration of antibiotic treatment then for 5 additional days[57,58,135] *L. acidophilus* + *B. bifidum* 2 × 10^10 (total) within 36 hours of antibiotics then for 20 days[57,136] *L. casei* 1.9 × 10^10 + *L. bulgaricus* 1.9 × 10^10 + *S. thermophilus* 1.8 × 10^9 (DanActive) twice daily for length of course of antibiotics and then for 1 wk[57,137]
Treatment of acute viral infectious diarrhea[59]	*L. rhamnosus*, GG 2 × 10^10 twice daily (for 7 days or duration of symptoms)[59,138] *S. boulardii*, 4 × 10^10 twice daily[59,139]
Prevention of traveler's diarrhea[60]	*S. boulardii*, 2 × 10^10 daily[60,140] (for 5 days before leaving and then throughout trip)
Prevention of antibiotic-associated diarrhea (children)[61]	*S. boulardii*, 250 mg twice daily for duration of antibiotic treatment[61,141] *L. rhamnosus GG*, 1 × 10^10 daily for duration of antibiotic treatment[61,142]

Examples are drawn from the clinical trials that demonstrated more positive results with greater statistical significance.

powder form, and in fermented milk beverages. If effective, treatment can likely continue indefinitely, although it should be noted that long-term safety data are lacking, and precautions do exist (see later in this chapter).

Refrigeration is recommended for products that have been heat dried because they are more likely to die with temperature extremes. Lyophilized preparations (as noted on the bottle) do not need refrigeration and tend to have good long-term survival. Brand choice is important. One study of 14 commercial probiotics sold in the United States found that 93% were incorrectly labeled, nearly 36% did not list strains on the label at all, and nearly 60% had contaminants. Another study that tested 58 products from around the world found that only 38% contained the dose stated on the label and 29% did not contain strains listed on the label.[144,145]

How may one select a reliable probiotic brand? Consider the following:
- Use products from companies that have sponsored probiotics research.
- Consider using www.consumerlab.com (subscription required). The laboratory tests different brands of supplements to verify whether each contains what is claimed on the label.
- Make certain that products have a Good Manufacturing Practice (GMP) seal.

- Ensure that the product specifies which species it contains and in what quantities.

Although many companies manufacture probiotic cocktails (mixtures of several different species), care should be taken to ensure that the specific species known to have clinical efficacy are present in sufficient quantity. For example, different *Bifidobacteria* tolerate different pH levels and vary in terms of fecal recovery rates after they have been consumed.[146]

Examples of some commercially available probiotics that have been utilized in research trials are listed in Table 105.5.

DO NATURAL FOOD SOURCES PROVIDE PROBIOTICS?

Natural food sources can provide probiotics, but not without a few caveats. European, African, and Asian consumers have long been exposed to probiotics found in fermented foods such as yogurt, buttermilk, sauerkraut, kefir, and kimchi. There is a growing body of basic science and clinical research on fermented foods made with LAB, such as kefir, and it appears likely that some of these foods may provide health benefit via their probiotic

TABLE 105.5 **Examples of Some Commercially Available Probiotics That Have Been Utilized in Research Trials**

Probiotic Strain(s)	Brand Name(s)	Producer
Bifidobacterium infantis 35624	Align	Procter & Gamble
Bifidobacterium animalis subsp. *lactis* DN-173010	Activia	Dannon
Lactobacillus casei DN-114001	Actimel, DanActive	Dannon
Lactobacillus rhamnosus GG (ATC 53013)	Culturelle	Amerifit
Lactobacillus casei subsp. *Shirota*	Yakult	Yakult
Lactobacillus acidophilus Lb	Lacteol	Aptalis
Saccharomyces boulardii CNCM I-745 (lyo)	Florastor	Biocodex
L. acidophilus CL 1285 + *L. casei* Lbc80r + *L. rhamnosus* CLR2	Bio K+	BioK+ Intnl
Bifidobacterium breve, Bifidobacterium longum, B. infantis, L. acidophilus, L. plantarum, L. casei, L. bulgaricus, Streptococcus thermophilus	VSL#3	Sigma-Tau

Adapted from McFarland L V. From yaks to yogurt: the history, development, and current use of probiotics. *Clin Infect Dis.* 2015;60(suppl 2): S85-S90 and Garner F, Khan AG, Garisch J, et al. World gastroenterology organisation global guidelines: probiotics and prebiotics october 2011. *J Clin Gastroenterol.* 2012;46(6):468-481.

potential.[133,147-149] However, the organisms typically found within these foods are often not the same microbes for which significant supportive research data regarding health benefits exist. Similar to "prescription" probiotics used in research studies, the potential benefit of a probiotic food for a given clinical indication should be considered strain specific and based on available research, when possible.

In evaluating the potential of a food to provide either specific or general health benefits from probiotic ingredients, consider the following:

- Is the product pasteurized? Yogurt may be "made with live cultures," but pasteurization kills beneficial as well as harmful organisms. A probiotic dairy product must have bacteria added back after pasteurization.
- Is it clear which strains are present in a given food, and whether they are known to have probiotic potential or not?
- Do the "live cultures" in a specific product include species that will survive acidic pH? Yogurts frequently emphasize *L. delbrueckii* subspecies *bulgaricus* and *Streptococcus thermophilus*, two organisms that may not survive passage through gastric acid and bile to colonize the gut mucosa.
- Typically, frozen foods do not contain live cultures, so foods such as frozen yogurt likely do not constitute a good probiotic source. However, work is progressing in the development of probiotic ice creams, which may be able to deliver adequate amounts of *Lactobacillus casei* and *Lactobacillus rhamnosus*.[150]

HOW SAFE ARE PROBIOTICS?

Across numerous systematic reviews, probiotics appear to be extremely safe.* A 2011 Agency for Healthcare Research and Quality (AHRQ) review of RCT data noted that the existing data do not show evidence of increased risk, but "the current literature is not well

equipped to answer questions on the safety of probiotics in intervention studies with confidence."[153] A commentary on this report suggested that, were the AHRQ to attempt to answer the question, "Are apples safe?" it would have come to the same conclusion and argued that in the absence of drug-like toxicology and safety data, the AHRQ results are encouraging.[155] Most safety concerns raised are linked to case reports only, and when compared with commonly used pharmaceuticals (including antibiotics), probiotics and prebiotics fare much better in terms of adverse effects. Among the most commonly reported adverse effects attributable to probiotics are flatulence and bloating.[156]

Case reports of *Lactobacillus* bacteremia, with complications such as endocarditis and liver abscess, do exist.[154,157,158] The mechanism in some cases is thought to be due to bacterial translocation; many case reports have involved immunocompromised people, such as cancer patients receiving chemotherapy or patients with diabetes.[158] The occurrence of bacteremia with *Lactobacillus* is thought to be extremely rare, and there is research to suggest that probiotics may have little effect on its incidence.[154] An observational study in Finland during the 1990s, when *L. rhamnosus* GG consumption increased widely across Finland, showed no increase in the incidence of Lactobacillus-positive blood cultures.[159] There have been rare infectious complications documented with *S. boulardii* in nonimmunocompromised patients who were nonetheless ill.[160,161] Most case reports of fungemia with *S. boulardii* have been in patients with severe comorbidities and/or central venous catheters.[33,153] Nonetheless, in studies focusing on patients with diagnoses such as human immunodeficiency virus (HIV) infection and cancer, as well as elderly adults and premature infants, overall, there has been a very low rate of adverse effects attributable to the probiotic intervention.[152,153]

Perhaps the most well-known instance of an adverse outcome occurring in a trial involving probiotics was the 2008 Dutch Probiotic Prophylaxis in Patients with Predicted Severe Acute Pancreatitis (PROPATRIA) trial

*33,34,41,50,52,57,59,61,67,69,71,81,82,96,99,108,111,119,151-154

in patients with severe acute pancreatitis, which found increased mortality in the intervention group, possibly be due to an increased risk of bowel ischemia.[162] There has been considerable discussion, both by the original study authors as well as others, regarding the possible mechanisms for the higher mortality rate with probiotic treatment as well as issues with the trial design that could have contributed to this high rate.[119,163,164] Following the PROPATRIA trial, the U.S. Food and Drug Administration (FDA) responded by making the restrictions on probiotics used in clinical trials more similar to those on pharmaceutical drugs.[164] Based on the currently available research showing a possible increased risk of mortality, patients with severe, acute pancreatitis should not be given probiotic-supplemented enteral nutrition.

Caution is advised regarding the use of probiotics in the following patient populations:

- Immunocompromised patients.[152,154] The FDA specifically recommends caution for patients taking antirejection medication after stem cell or solid organ transplant, injectable immunosuppressive drugs for autoimmune disease, or corticosteroids (greater than 0.5 mg/kg of body weight prednisone or its equivalent) or those receiving chemotherapy or radiation treatment
- Patients with indwelling medical devices such as central venous catheters[152,164]
- Severe acute pancreatitis[152,164]
- Critically ill patients in general, such as those with organ failure[152,164]
- Patients with valve abnormality or replacement, history of endocarditis[154]
- Premature infants in certain categories.[51,152] The weight of evidence showing benefit for prevention of necrotizing enterocolitis (NEC) has recently shifted the discussion toward whether it would be ethical *not* to administer probiotics to infants at high risk of NEC. However, citing a lack of evidence in specific, particularly vulnerable populations, caution is advised for infants who are extremely low birth weight (ELBW), clinically unstable, and/or have GI, cardiac, or genetic abnormalities.[51]
- Patients with previous bowel surgery and short-gut syndrome and neonates (less than 6 months of age); caution is advised specific to strains that can produce D(−)-lactate.[152,154]
- Patients with lactose hypersensitivity and yeast allergy. Some authorities recommend that *Lactobacillus* preparations be avoided in persons with hypersensitivity to

lactose or milk, and yeasts should not be used in anyone with a yeast allergy. *Bifidobacteria* have no listed contraindications because they are generally considered nonpathogenic and nontoxigenic.[156]
- Patients who are pregnant. A 2009 review examining safety during pregnancy found no adverse effect on gestational age, growth, or cesarean section rate for *Lactobacillus and Bifidobacterium*, and there were no reports of fetal malformation. There was no evidence available for *Saccharomyces*. Due to the limited data availability, the investigators cautioned that further research is needed before definitive conclusions can be made regarding the safety of probiotics in pregnancy, and the FDA recommends caution in pregnant patients.[165,154]
- The use of *Enterobacter* species is controversial, given the potential risk of pathogenicity compared with other species.

> As a general rule, most good-quality probiotics are quite safe with low risk of side effects, but caution must be observed in patients who are immunocompromised, have indwelling medical equipment, or are critically ill and/or have organ failure.

Based on the available data showing a lack of observed adverse effects or negative impacts on growth, a 2011 review concluded that prebiotics and probiotics are safe to use in infant formula, although they are not recommended for routine supplementation and are indicated only for specific conditions.[166]

CONCLUSION

Scientific research in metagenomics and bioinformatics continues to discover more ways in which our lives as human beings are intimately tied to the trillions of microbes that we each harbor. Together with a nutritious, antiinflammatory diet, probiotics are one potential way in which we may influence host–gut–microbiotia interactions and support health and treat disease. Ongoing basic research on mechanisms of action and high-quality clinical trials, along with consistent manufacturing and regulatory standards, will help clinicians and patients make best use of this promising field of therapy.

Key Web Resources

Natural Medicines	https://naturalmedicines.therapeuticresearch.com/
Consumerlab.com	https://www.consumerlab.com
University of Wisconsin Integrative Medicine Patient Handout	http://www.fammed.wisc.edu/sites/default/files/webfm-uploads/documents/outreach/im/handout_probiotics_patient.pdf
American Gastroenterological Association	http://www.gastro.org/info_for_patients/2013/6/6/probiotics
International Scientific Association for Probiotics and Prebiotics	http://www.isapp.net
Food Insight	http://www.foodinsight.org

REFERENCES

References are available online at ExpertConsult.com.

CHAPTER 106

DETOXIFICATION

Luke Fortney, MD, FAAFP · Rian Podein, MD · Michael Hernke, PhD

WHAT IS DETOXIFICATION AND WHY DO IT?

Detoxification, as reviewed here, is the constellation of physiological and psychological processes through which the body identifies, neutralizes, and eliminates toxic substances, metabolic byproducts, habits, and patterns. Alcohol and other narcotic withdrawal therapies are serious medical conditions requiring close supervision and are not discussed here.

For an increasing number of people living in a more polluted and stressful world, body systems can become overburdened and strained by various contaminants that may lead to health problems.[1] In general, these toxins can be identified within the following general categories:[2]

- *Antinutrients* such as high-fructose corn syrup, trans fats, caffeine, alcohol, and processed foods
- *Internal metabolic toxins* such as nitrogen, carbon dioxide, bile, urea, free radicals, and stool
- *Medications* used improperly, inappropriately, or too often
- *Heavy metals* such as mercury, arsenic, lead, cadmium, tin, and aluminum
- *Chemicals* such as pesticides, herbicides, cleaning products, solvents, and glues
- *Allergens* such as food, mold, dust, pollen, and chemicals
- *Infectious organisms* such as bacteria, viruses, yeast, and parasites

Further, the following social, emotional, and spiritual challenges affect health and well-being:[3,4]

- *Stress*, such as lack of personal time, too much work, excessive worry, too little rest, and financial strain
- *Unhealthy mental states*, such as addictions, overeating, and destructive mental patterns
- *Ambient distractions*, such as pervasive noises, smells, lights, and images
- *Overstimulation* from advertisements, radio, computers, television, smart phones, and pagers
- *Lack of spiritual connection*, a loss of meaning and purpose
- *Isolation*, the lack of social support and community
- *Nature deprivation*, being disconnected from natural environments[5]
- *Negative emotions* and persistent self-defeating thoughts, such as anger, fear, guilt, and hopelessness

Although too infrequently acknowledged, the body and mind already possess the capacity to handle these challenges. This process of maintaining biological and mental balance is called *homeostasis*. The major systems that work together synchronously to maintain health and balance include the following:

- Liver and gallbladder (Figs. 106.1–106.3)
- Kidneys
- Gastrointestinal system
- Skin
- Lungs
- Lymphatic and circulatory systems
- Mind and brain

Symptoms that may reflect an overtaxed or dysfunctional detoxification system are often vague and nonspecific, but when seen in constellation, they suggest a problem with the body's ability to restore itself. When potentially serious medical conditions have been ruled out by a reasonable medical workup, symptoms that may be attributed to a detoxification problem with the body often include the following:[1,6,7]

- Fatigue with sleep disruption and brain-fog
- Mood disturbance, especially depression, anxiety, fear, and anger
- Muscle aches and joint pain
- Sinus congestion, dark circles under the eyes, and postnasal drip
- Headaches with neck and shoulder pain
- Bloating and flatulence
- Irritable bowel, foul-smelling stools, and dark urine
- Weight changes and loss of muscle tone
- Heartburn, recurrent colds, and persistent infections
- Infertility and low libido
- Premature aging and weakness
- Fluid retention and excess weight
- Rashes and canker sores
- Bad breath and adverse body odor

Although conclusive scientific data supporting detoxification therapies are largely lacking, the question for a patient suffering from any of these symptoms remains this: *"What can I do to feel better?"* Unfortunately, many gimmicky, expensive, unnecessary, and potentially harmful products and programs exist, and dubious practitioners may exaggerate their claims. In general, patients should avoid dramatic, expensive, and extreme approaches in favor of reasonable, safe, and health-promoting lifestyle changes that empower patients and avoid dependency and unrealistic expectations. The five basic components of any detoxification program should include the following:

- Daily physical activity, such as yoga and walking (preferably in natural "outdoor" environments when possible)[5]
- Regular sweating, through physical activity, use of a sauna or steam room, or a hot-room yoga class
- Healthy nutrition, rich in organic fruits and vegetables and filtered water (see Figs. 106.1–106.3)
- Self-reflection, such as any contemplative practice (e.g., meditation), journaling, and breathing-focused relaxation techniques

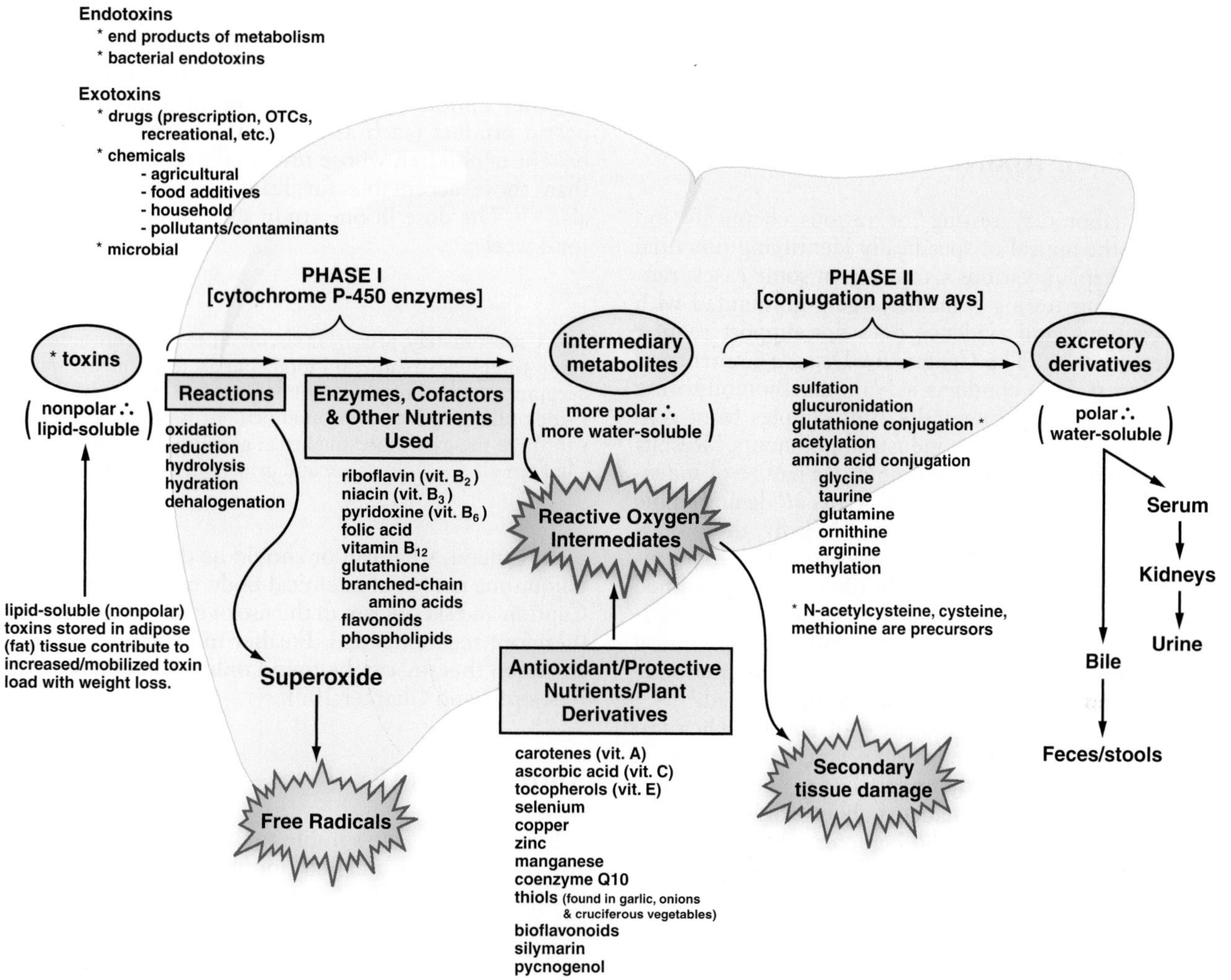

Endotoxins
* end products of metabolism
* bacterial endotoxins
Exotoxins
* drugs (prescription, OTCs, recreational, etc.)
* chemicals
- agricultural
- food additives
- household
- pollutants/contaminants
* microbial
PHASE I
[cytochrome P-450 enzymes]
* toxins
nonpolar ∴ lipid-soluble
Reactions
oxidation
reduction
hydrolysis
hydration
dehalogenation
Enzymes, Cofactors & Other Nutrients Used
riboflavin (vit. B2)
niacin (vit. B3)
pyridoxine (vit. B6)
folic acid
vitamin B12
glutathione
branched-chain amino acids
flavonoids
phospholipids
lipid-soluble (nonpolar) toxins stored in adipose (fat) tissue contribute to increased/mobilized toxin load with weight loss.
Superoxide
Free Radicals
intermediary metabolites
more polar ∴ more water-soluble
Reactive Oxygen Intermediates
Antioxidant/Protective Nutrients/Plant Derivatives
carotenes (vit. A)
ascorbic acid (vit. C)
tocopherols (vit. E)
selenium
copper
zinc
manganese
coenzyme Q10
thiols (found in garlic, onions & cruciferous vegetables)
bioflavonoids
silymarin
pycnogenol
PHASE II
[conjugation pathw ays]
sulfation
glucuronidation
glutathione conjugation *
acetylation
amino acid conjugation
glycine
taurine
glutamine
ornithine
arginine
methylation
* N-acetylcysteine, cysteine, methionine are precursors
Secondary tissue damage
excretory derivatives
polar ∴ water-soluble
Serum
Kidneys
Urine
Bile
Feces/stools

FIG. 106.1 ■ Liver detoxification: over-the-counter (OTC) drugs.

Phase 1 Detoxification
Alcohol
Environmental Toxins
Drugs
P-450 System
–
~100 Enzymes
Free Radicals
Neutralized Toxin
Fat Soluble
Antioxidants
(Glutathione)
Cleared

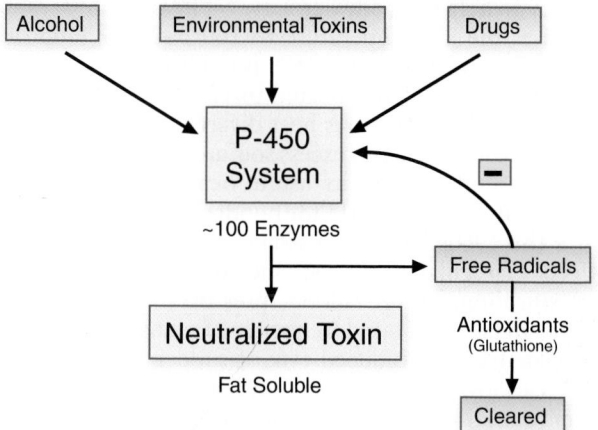

FIG. 106.2 ■ Phase 1 detoxification: cytochrome P-450.

Phase 2 Detoxification
Conjugation
Neutralized Toxin
Fat Soluble
Phase II System
Required Nutrients
Glutathione
Glutathione, B6
Amino Acid
Glycine
Methylation
SAMe
Sulfation
Cysteine, methionine
Acetylation
molybdenum, Acetyl CoA
Glucuronidation
Glucuronic Acid
Toxin Prepared for Excretion
Water Soluble
Bile/Intestines
Urine/Kidneys

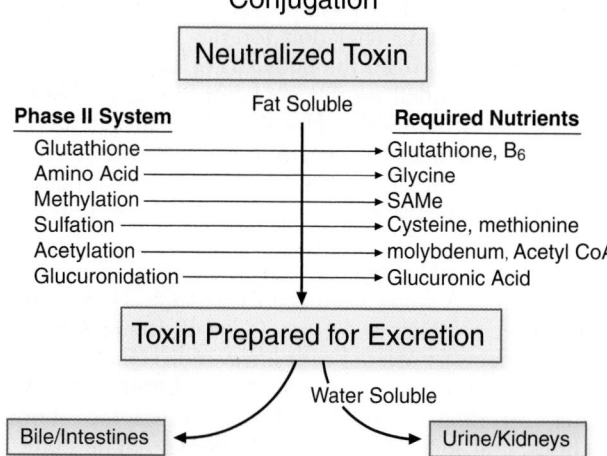

FIG. 106.3 ■ Phase 2 detoxification: *CoA*, coenzyme A; *SAMe*, *S*-adenosylmethionine. (From Bland JS, Costarella L, Levin B, et al. Environment and toxicity. In: *Clinical nutrition: a functional approach.* Gig Harbor, WA: Institute for Functional Medicine; 1999:261.)

- Manual therapies, such as massage and acupuncture
- Regular supportive social time with friends, family, and community[8]

TESTING FOR TOXINS

Although laboratory testing for various chemicals and toxins has the appeal of specifically identifying potential culprits to explain various symptoms in some cases, random screening testing remains largely unfounded with few exceptions, and evidence does not support regular or widespread use. The Centers for Disease Control and Prevention (CDC) conducts a National Biomonitoring Program that tests urine and serum samples from representative populations for industrial pollutants.[9] Results continue to demonstrate the ubiquitous nature of industrial pollutants, or body burdens, across *all* demographic groups regardless of health status.[10-13] Sadly, these findings indicate the widespread presence of societal chemicals and suggest that chemical body burden can be presumed for any presenting patient.[14-19] Given the expense, variable quality, questionable validity, and unclear clinical significance of the majority of specific pollutant body burdens, routine testing is not recommended.[13,20,21] Moreover, the health significance of specific chemical exposures—at what levels, during which times, and at what frequency—is poorly understood.[22] Indiscriminate and unfounded causal statements about exposure, harm, and treatment efficacy should be approached cautiously and skeptically. Therefore the focus should be on reducing the amount of toxicity in our living environments (see Chapter 108).

CHELATION THERAPY

Using safe and effective methods to prevent disease, treat symptoms, and achieve homeostasis is the primary goal of a good detoxification regimen. Appropriate, well-placed skepticism and concern exists over many detoxification therapies, including chelation for the removal of various heavy metals from the body.[23] For example, a common but unfounded use for chelation therapy is autism spectrum disorder (ASD). However, a Cochrane Review found no evidence that chelation therapy was effective. The review went on to caution against its use because the risks of adverse effects far outweigh any potential benefits.[24]

The safety of widespread chelation therapy remains questionable. A study from the Emergency Department at Emory University in Atlanta, Georgia, found common adverse effects associated with intravenous chelation that included diaphoresis, hypotension, tachycardia, leukopenia, thrombocytopenia, electrocardiographic abnormalities, and increased serum creatinine.[25] The clinical significance of chelation therapy is also uncertain. A Cochrane Review concluded that, at present, evidence of the effectiveness or ineffectiveness of chelation therapy in improving clinical outcomes of patients with atherosclerotic cardiovascular disease is insufficient.[26] However, the CDC did recommend that the calcium disodium edetate ($CaNa_2EDTA$) challenge test be considered for children who have blood lead levels of 1.21–2.12 mcmol/L (25–44 mcg/dL) to determine whether chelation is indicated.[27] Another option could include use of a modified citrus pectin product (such as Pectasol), which may also have benefit in children whose test results reveal levels higher than those acceptable for lead and other heavy metals.[28-32] The dose in one study was 5 g three times daily for 4 weeks.

> Unfortunately, pectin is a viscous fiber that is not absorbed into the bloodstream, and food sources (e.g., citrus, apples, legumes, and cabbage) do not help chelate heavy metals outside of the gut. However, modified citrus pectin is absorbed through the gastrointestinal tract and appears to reduce this burden via renal clearance and urinary elimination.

In general, what can or should be done to address the ubiquitous nature of chemical body burden is uncertain. Caution and skepticism in the use of chelation therapy are therefore recommended. Further information regarding chelation therapy can be found online (see the Key Web Resources and Chapter 107).

SAUNA THERAPY

The body stores fat-soluble toxins such as pesticides in adipose tissue (also called lipophilic persistent organic pollutants, or POPs). One well-known example are the flame retardants polybrominated diphenyl ethers (PBDEs); some of the highest levels of these compounds throughout the world have been found in the breasts of lactating American women.[33] These compounds were banned in Europe due to their association with reproductive, neurodevelopmental, and thyroid toxicities.[33]

Taking a relaxing sauna or steam bath is an effective therapy to help the body detoxify.[34] The traditional sauna increases the air temperature to 160°F–200°F (approximately 70°C–90°C), with 25% humidity compared with a steam room, which is heated to 120°F–130°F at 100% humidity. The exogenous heat diverts blood to the skin, where sweating releases excess sodium, nitrogen, and toxins.[35-37] In addition to its use in Scandinavia and many cultures around the world for hundreds of years, research since the 1960s has demonstrated the health-promoting effects of regular sauna use, including stress reduction, detoxification, lower blood pressure, and decreased pain.[38] In fact, increased frequency of sauna use is actually associated with a reduced risk of sudden cardiac death, fatal cardiovascular disease, and all-cause mortality.[39] Sauna cessation is advised for men attempting to conceive with their partners as heat-based therapies temporarily impair sperm count and motility.[40]

Although sauna use is safe for most people of all ages, caution should be used in people who have undergone recent surgery; have unstable cardiovascular conditions such as recent myocardial infarction or cerebrovascular accident; or have multiple sclerosis, acute lung infections, or pregnancy complications.[41] Even people with known heart disease can partake in sauna therapy. The greatest risk for all uses is hypotension and syncope, particularly if alcohol is used during sauna use (which is *not* recommended).[39]

Some evidence indicates that a lower-temperature infrared sauna may offer similar health benefits. Lower-temperature infrared saunas are typically heated to 120°F and are a good option for those who cannot tolerate the higher temperatures of a traditional sauna or steam room (e.g., individuals with multiple sclerosis). For further reading on the many health effects of sauna therapy, please refer to an excellent book entitled, *The Holistic Handbook of Sauna Therapy*, by Nenah Sylver.[42]

EXERCISE

Reasonable and safe approaches to body burden detoxification include increasing awareness and adherence to healthy lifestyle behaviors such as regular physical activity, healthy nutrition, stress reduction, mind-body practices, spiritual connection, and avoidance of harmful behaviors such as smoking. Exercise has been shown to enhance adipose tissue circulation and therefore increases the release of stored toxins.[43] Cardiovascular exercise also supports detoxification through sweating. Starting with gentle, but regular, forms of exercise, such as walking or bicycling for 30 minutes or more per day, is best. Ideally, a person should set a goal of vigorous movement of any kind for 60 minutes or more on a daily basis. Hot room yoga is particularly beneficial for detoxification, but any and all forms of movement are encouraged.

NUTRITION

Nutrition is arguably the first and most important step in promoting health and supporting the body's efforts to remove harmful substances. What a person avoids eating is equally important as what is included in a healthy diet. By avoiding artificial additives and unhealthy fats, reducing excess calories (including less salt, saturated fats, and sugars), and adhering to a diverse whole food organic diet, a person will be better able to support the body's detoxification process, in large part, by avoiding overeating and ingestion of environmental pollutants[44-46] (see Chapter 88).

While annually millions of people worldwide take part in various forms of detoxification, little is mentioned about the role of the gut microbial microbiota. One study evaluated the effects of several 3-day dietary detox regimens and found that they do indeed change the microbial community, with some of them increasing a genus of bacteria thought to help prevent obesity and diabetes.[47] However, with return to their prior standard American diet, the gut microbial changes returned to their pre-detox state at approximately 10 days. These findings are consistent with those of a prior research study that showed that dietary changes can rapidly and reproducibly alter the human gut microbiota but that short-term

TABLE 106.1	The Environmental Working Group's List of the "Dirty Dozen" (Foods Highest in Pesticides Used) and the "Clean 15" (Foods Lowest in Pesticides Used)
Dirty Dozen (Better to Buy Organic)	**Clean 15 (Less Important to Buy Organic)**
1. Celery	1. Onions
2. Peaches	2. Avocado
3. Strawberries	3. Sweet corn
4. Apples	4. Pineapple
5. Blueberries	5. Mangoes
6. Nectarines	6. Sweet peas
7. Bell peppers	7. Asparagus
8. Spinach	8. Kiwi
9. Cherries	9. Cabbage
10. Kale and collard greens	10. Eggplant
11. Potatoes	11. Cantaloupe
12. Grapes (imported)	12. Watermelon
	13. Grapefruit
	14. Sweet potato
	15. Honeydew melon

Data from the Environmental Working Group: http://www.ewg.org.

detox programs may be most effective as a jumpstart to an ongoing dietary lifestyle modification that supports an optimal gut microbiome[48] as well as the many health benefits associated with probiotic supplementation for various medical conditions.[49]

Safe and Environmentally Friendly Fish and Seafood Choices

Consuming fish and seafood a few times per week has many benefits;[50] however, concerns exist about contaminants that may affect our health and the environmental impact of fishing practices. Resources that can be used to help guide safe fish and environmentally sustainable seafood choices are provided in the Key Web Resources.

Pesticides in Produce

When deciding whether to invest in organic produce, it can be helpful to understand which conventional fruits and vegetables are highest and lowest in pesticide content. The Environmental Working Group publishes a helpful guide that lists the "Dirty Dozen" (foods highest in pesticides) and the "Clean 15" (foods lowest in pesticides), as shown in Table 106.1 (see also the Key Web Resources).

Fasting

Occasional and sensible fasting may be helpful as well. Several variations of fasting exist, some involve drinking only water or juices or other nonsolid foods. During fasting, the main source of energy used by the body comes from hydrolyzing fatty acids from triglycerides stored in adipose tissue.[51-54] Because many toxins are sequestered in adipose tissue, fasting may be helpful in eliminating these toxins from the body. Initially, a person may feel worse during a fast because of this mobilization process. Resting and drinking plenty of fluids are therefore helpful during a fast.

MANUAL THERAPIES

Manual therapies such as massage may be helpful to mobilize and eliminate toxins from the body by mobilizing the lymphatic system, among other possible benefits. Together with exercise and sauna therapy, massage can greatly enhance the ability of the lymphatic, cardiopulmonary, and hepatorenal circulatory systems to eliminate toxins. For example, massage has been shown to reduce excessive fluid volume by 65% in patients with lymphedema.[55,56] Other forms of body work such as acupuncture may be helpful as well, in part, by increasing the relaxation response as well as treating qi stagnation and myofascial restrictions.

Mind-Body Connection

Finally, any detoxification review or program that ignores the mind-body connection is remiss. Stress is arguably the most significant toxin confronting patients on a daily

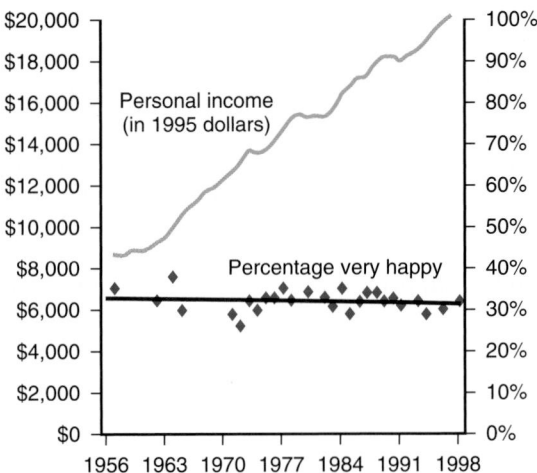

FIG. 106.4 ■ U.S. Department of Commerce, Bureau of the Census.

and long-term basis. As measures of happiness decline in the United States (Fig. 106.4), various mind-body syndromes such as fibromyalgia, migraine, chronic fatigue, irritable bowel, multiple chemical sensitivity, and others continue to affect more people.[57,58] Unfortunately, support and awareness are lacking for mind-body interventions that cultivate understanding, behavior changes, insight, and accountability for patients and health care workers.[59] Various chapters in this text offer helpful tools to support a healthy mind and emotions.

Key Web Resources

University of Wisconsin Department of Family Medicine: This website provides a regularly updated, self-guided 7-day detoxification plan.	http://www.fammed.wisc.edu/integrative/modules
Environmental Working Group: This group offers excellent resources regarding information on harmful toxins in the environment with recommendations on how to avoid them, including information on toxins in fish and pesticides in produce.	http://www.ewg.org http://www.ewg.org/safefishlist
Environmental Defense Fund seafood selector: This organization offers ratings of the best (least contamination) and worst (most contamination) for seafood consumption, as well as a pocket guide for selecting seafood.	http://www.edf.org/page.cfm?tagID=1521
Centers for Disease Control chemical exposure report: This report details the health effects of human exposure to environmental chemicals.	http://www.cdc.gov/exposurereport/
Doctor's Data, Inc.: This laboratory offers toxicology testing, as well as drinking water analysis. It also contains information on chelation therapy.	http://www.doctorsdata.com
Bioneers: This organization offers advice on sustainable living that supports wider social and ecological health.	http://www.bioneers.org
National Center for Complementary and Alternative Medicine: This National Institutes of Health website provides information on many topics, including chelation therapy.	http://www.nccam.nih.gov

Detoxification Program

Patient Handout: Seven Day Detoxification Program

Many detoxification programs are available, but caution is advised before doing one. Very often symptoms are a signal from the body that something is out of balance and needs to be addressed. However, before adding any treatments, it is often the case that something should be removed as the first step to healing (eg smoking cessation for coughing). This program is about jump-starting a healthy lifestyle, which is far more important than any short-term detox. Most importantly, be flexible and adapt this program to your specific needs. The following plan (found online at www.fammed.wisc.edu/integrative/modules) offers a general outline for a self-guided detox program.

Getting Started
• This regimen is not intended to be an exhaustive resource, nor is it a test of will and endurance. It is designed to be a safe, gentle, useful, empowering, and accessible health guide that takes into account personal variability. Adaptations should be made as necessary. However, this process does require planning and preparation, so read through it and make preparations ahead of time.
• In addition to physiologic approaches, this plan equally emphasizes mind-body approaches that can aid the relaxation response and unravel negative and unconscious mental patterns that often result in pain and discomfort.
• The most important part of going through a detox program is to first ask why you are doing it. Being clear about your intentions helps avoid inflated expectations and disappointment. Write-down the reason for going through a detox in your own words.
• The five basic ingredients of this detox regimen are self-reflection, exercise, sauna, nutrition, and manual therapy. The program offered here is designed to support and enhance your body's inherent ability to heal and be well. It is intended for most people with few exceptions.
• The program has a strong emphasis on using organic, sustainable, local, responsible, gentle, natural, whole, and balanced ingredients that honor the global and spiritual aspect of health.

Precautions and Expectations
• **Healing crises** can occur during a detox. Common temporary symptoms can include general malaise, fatigue, headache, lightheadedness, diarrhea, cramps, bloating, body-aches, mood-changes, and generalized weakness. These symptoms are often caused by a combination of factors including the mobilization of toxins, low blood sugar, low fluids, electrolyte imbalance, withdrawal from habitual substances (such as alcohol, caffeine, sugar, nicotine), and even changes in your daily routine.
• Most often the best approach is to continue with the detox. However, you may need to stop or alter the detox if you experience ongoing or worsening symptoms.
• **Dehydration** is unnecessary during a detox. Make sure that you drink a lot of fluids.
• **Address your particular needs** as you go along, such as more frequent snacks, larger meals, increase protein and healthy fats, less physical work, more rest, and less striving in general.
• Continued use of **prescription medications** is advised and should be monitored by a physician. If needed, use "over-the-counter" medications sparingly for relief of headaches or other symptoms.
• **Communicate with your health care provider** about any concerns that arise during the detox as needed.
In the end, you will likely find that you feel better, have more energy, are healthier, and may require less medication.
Below are three examples of different detoxification programs to consider. You can choose the one that best matches your needs and lifestyle. They progress from simple (#1) to more involved (#3).

Version #1 (short) for 5 or more days:
* Eat only fruits and vegetables in any combination, amount, and preparation using healthy oils and spices as needed.
* Drink plenty of filtered water, juice, tea, and broth.
* Move and exercise the body in any variety, intensity, and duration everyday.
* Keep a daily journal and practice any form of self-reflection everyday (eg meditation). Use the "Mind/Body Awareness Writing Exercises" workbook at www.fammed.wisc.edu/integrative/modules as a guide for journaling.

Version #2 (simplified) for 7 or more days (extend days 6 and 7 to a full 10 days if desired):
* **Days 1 and 2:** Eliminate meat, eggs, dairy, wheat, alcohol, caffeine, chocolate, and refined sugars. Eat only organic vegan foods in any arrangement, preparation, and amount using cooking oils and seasonings.
* **Day 3:** Further eliminate all grains, nuts, beans, and legumes. Eat only fruits and vegetables in any combination, amount, and preparation using oils and spices as needed.
* **Day 4:** If possible avoid eating any solid food. Drink plenty of water, broth, juice, and tea. Rest during this day.
* **Day 5:** (same as Day 3)
* **Days 6 and 7 (and optional extended days 8-10):** (same as Days 1 and 2)
* Throughout the detox, keep a daily journal and practice any form of self-reflection everyday (eg meditation). Use the "Mind/Body Awareness Writing Exercises" workbook at www.fammed.wisc.edu/integrative/modules as a guide for journaling.

Version #3 (advanced) with added supplements and probiotic bowel regimen:
Days 1 and 2: For the entire detox week, eliminate all meat (e.g., fish, beef, pork, lamb, poultry), refined sugars (white/brown sugar and especially high-fructose syrup), and especially artificial sweeteners such as *saccharine, aspartame, and Splenda* (natural sweeteners such as honey, maple syrup, molasses, Stevia, and erythritol, are okay to use in small amounts). Also avoid alcohol, tobacco, caffeine, cigarettes, chocolate, and recreational drugs for the entire week. It is advised to avoid dairy, wheat, and eggs during the detox week as well (instead try soy/almond/rice milk, soy cheese, soy yogurt, stanol/sterol spreads). Cooking should be guided by healthy recipes for soups, steaming, sautéing, and baking etc based on your preferences.

Keep a daily journal and practice any form of self-reflection everyday (eg meditation). Use the "Mind/Body Awareness Writing Exercises" workbook at www.fammed.wisc.edu/integrative/modules as a guide for journaling.
Encouraged foods for days 1 and 2 include fresh/frozen/dried vegetables, fruit, and mushrooms (maitake, shiitake, oyster, and/or enoki, etc). Healthy grains are also recommended for days 1 and 2 (brown/wild rice, quinoa, buckwheat, oatmeal, millet etc), as well as seeds, nuts, legumes, and flaxseed.
Other suggestions for days 1 & 2 include the following:
Cold-pressed organic extra virgin olive oil as guided by "detox appropriate" recipes.
Spices and healthy seasonings as needed based on your preferences.
Drink 8–10 glasses of filtered water, including "vitalizing beverage," "detox broth," smoothies, and diluted juices.
Drink tea throughout the day, such as peppermint, decaf green, chamomile, licorice, ginger, rooibos, and digestive tea.
For snacks eat mixed nuts, dried and fresh fruit, vegetables, and detox broth (see Table ***).
Consider using the optional herbs and supplements at recommended dosages.
Consider 15–30 minutes of sauna or steam-room therapy.
Consider 30–60 minutes of light exercise such as walking, running, biking, skiing, jump rope, stretching, yoga, pilates.
Practice any variety of self-reflection, including meditation and breathing exercises. Journaling is encouraged.

Day 3: For day 3 also <u>eliminate</u> grains, nuts, seeds, legumes, beans, and mushrooms.
Eat only fruit and vegetables fresh/frozen/dried in any combination and amount using detox appropriate recipes.
Just like days 1 & 2 the following items are suggested:
> Olive oil
> Spices and seasonings
> Filtered water, tea, vitalizing-beverage, detox broth, smoothies, and diluted juice
> Optional herbs and supplements at recommended dosages
> Sauna or steam-room heat therapy
> Light exercise
> Journaling, self-reflection/meditation

A new suggestion for today is to add a session of <u>massage therapy</u> to help mobilize toxins and stimulate the lymphatic circulation.

Day 4 (Modified Fasting): <u>Eliminate all solid food</u> (i.e., using only water, tea, juices, and broth with adaptations as needed). <u>Pay attention to the needs of your body!</u> *Sensitive, ill, weak, and thin people should avoid or modify this day of fasting if needed, such as drinking more juice and broth as needed.*
> Other suggestions for this day include:
> Rest and relaxation—<u>avoid</u> exercise and sauna today. Do minimal or no work today.
> Stop all previous supplements for today.
> Drink plenty of fluids and keep up with bowel and bladder losses (tea with honey, vitalizing beverage, diluted fruit/vegetable juice, and detox broth).
> Use journaling, self-reflection, or meditation.

A new suggestion for today only is to add an optional bowel cleansing regimen:
> Take 500–1000 mg of activated charcoal capsules (or bentonite clay)—toxin binders for the gut—by mouth three times per day with water.
> Drink 300 mL of **magnesium citrate** (typically one bottle) in the morning as a laxative for bowel elimination.
> Use 1 saline **Probiotic Fleet Enema** in the afternoon or evening (See Table *** below for instructions).

Day 5 (Same as Day 3 except for added Energy Work session): For day 5, <u>add back</u> fruit and vegetables in any combination, preparation, and amount using detox appropriate recipes. Again, encouraged foods include fresh/frozen/dried vegetables and fruit (*but <u>no</u> mushrooms, grains, seeds, beans, legumes, or nuts for this day*). Just like day 3, the following items are suggested:
> Olive oil
> Spices and seasonings
> Filtered water, tea, vitalizing-beverage, detox broth, smoothies, and diluted juice
> Optional herbs and supplements re-started at recommended dosages
> Sauna or steam room therapy
> Light exercise
> Journaling, and self-reflection, or meditation

A new suggestion for today is to add a session of <u>Energy Work</u> such as acupuncture, Reiki, Healing Touch etc to help balance your newly cleansed system.

Days 6 and 7 (Same as Days 1 and 2, extend for days 8-10 if desired): In addition to fruits and vegetables, <u>add back</u> mushrooms, beans, legumes, seeds, nuts, and healthy grains (same as Days 1 & 2 above).
The following suggestions continue to be encouraged:
> Olive oil
> Spices and seasonings
> Filtered water, tea, vitalizing-beverage, detox broth, smoothies, and diluted juice
> Optional herbs and supplements at recommended dosages
> Sauna or steam room heat therapy
> Light exercise
> Journaling, self-reflection, or meditation

Detox Recipes and Supplements

Detox broth recipe:
Use fresh organic ingredients if possible. This is an excellent aid for fasting on Day 4. Ingredients can vary depending on availability.
1 large soup pot or kettle
1 strainer
1 large bowl or container for straining the soup
3–4 quarts of filtered water (fill pot after all ingredients are in)
1 large chopped onion (white or yellow)
3–5 small bunches of various chopped greens (kale, parsley, cilantro, chard, or dandelion)
2 stalks of sliced celery
1 cup of fresh or dried seaweed (nori, dulse, wakame, kelp, or kombu)
1/2 small-medium head of chopped cabbage (any variety)
2 peeled carrots
2 stalks of peeled burdock root
1 large peeled daikon root
1 cup of squash (any variety) chopped into cubes
3 chopped root vegetables (turnip, parsnip, or rutabaga

2–3 cups fresh/dried mushrooms (maitake, shiitake, oyster, or enoki)
Add all ingredients to the large pot at once and bring to a low boil for 40–60 minutes (add water to fill). Strain the stock to remove the solid material (keep the liquid broth and dispose the left over solid parts). Salt to taste. Store in the original soup pot or a tightly sealed
container for use all week. Keep the remaining broth cooled in the refrigerator, and reheat for use. Enjoy as a sipping broth throughout the detox week, especially during the day of fasting on day 4.

Smoothie recipe with optional supplements:
Use organic ingredients when possible. This makes about 1 liter which is divided into 4 servings, or 2 days worth, a glass in the AM and PM.
About 2 tablespoons (20 mL) of organic cold pressed extra virgin olive oil
1/2 avocado

About 4 tablespoons (20 g) of **whey protein powder** *(optional)*
About 4 tablespoons (20 g) of **modified citrus pectin** *(Pectasol, optional)*
1/2 cup of orange juice (or 100% organic juice of choice)
1/2 cup of vanilla flavored soy milk, rice milk, or almond milk
About 4 tablespoons (40 g) of flaxseed (or psyllium)
8–10 ice cubes (or 1/2 cup of filtered water)
1 organic banana (sliced)
1 organic apple or pear with peel (sliced)
1/2 cup organic frozen or fresh blueberries (and/or seasonal berries of choice)
Place ingredients in a blender and grind up until smooth, adding more water as needed. Store remaining mix in the refrigerator. *Be creative; this can be varied according to taste and availability of various fruit.* Enjoy 1 tall glass twice a day with or between meals.

Digestive tea recipe:
1/2 teaspoon (t) of whole fennel seeds
1/2 t of whole coriander seeds
1/2 t of whole cumin seeds
Add seeds to about one quart boiling water. Let the seeds steep for about 10 minutes. Enjoy after meals throughout the detox week. Other recommended teas include ginger, licorice, peppermint, chamomile, rooibos, and decaf green teas.

Vitalizing beverage:
This is an excellent aid for fasting on day 4.
1–2 tablespoons fresh lemon and/or lime juice (about 1/2 crushed or squeezed lemon/lime)
1–2 tablespoons of real maple syrup
1/10 teaspoon cayenne pepper (a small pinch)
Purified, spring, or mineral water (carbonated water can also be used)
In a tall glass combine the juice, syrup, and cayenne. Fill the glass with water and stir well. Add crushed ice as desired. Enjoy throughout the detox, especially during fasting on day 4. Diluted fruit juice of any variety (1/2 real juice and 1/2 water) is also recommended.

Optional supplements list for advanced detox regimen:
- **Hydrolyzed whey protein powder 10 g powder** two times per day mixed in smoothies or juice. Whey protein contains bonded cysteine that increases glutathione, a potent antioxidant, immune modulator, and detoxifier.
- **Pectasol powder** *(modified citrus pectin-MCP,* **NOT pectin fiber)** 10 g powder two times per day mixed in smoothies. MCP is absorbed in the gut and chelates heavy metals in the body that flow to the kidneys and liver where they are eliminated. It may be easier to find online.
- **Milk thistle crude extract capsules** 500–1000 mg three times per day with meals. This is a safe and beneficial herb used for 7 days for liver support.
- **Dandelion root capsules,** 500–1000 mg three times per day with meals. This is a safe and beneficial herb for kidney and gallbladder support. It may increase urination.
- **Multivitamin tablet,** one daily with a meal.
- **Turmeric capsules,** 500–1000 mg three times per day with meals. This is a safe and beneficial herb used for 7 days for inflammation and gut support.
- **Probiotics,** one capsule three times per day. This is a safe and beneficial supplement used for 7-10 days to colonize the gut with healthy supportive bacteria.
- **Fish Oil omega-3 essential fatty acids,** 1000 mg total of EPA and DHA daily in liquid or capsule form. Vegetarian options include 2 tablespoons (T) daily of ground flaxseed or flax oil mixed in with smoothies. This supplement is used to reduce inflammation in the body.
- **Extra virgin, cold-pressed, organic olive oil,** 2 tablespoons in smoothies twice a day (and used in any amount in food for cooking). This healthy oil is rich in essential fatty acids.
- **DAY OF FASTING ONLY: Activated charcoal or bentonite clay capsules,** 500–1000 mg three times per day to bind gut toxins, but only taken during fasting. Always take 1-2 hours before or after anything else by mouth.

Probiotic fleet enema regimen (this is should be done after a bowel movement)
  What you'll need:
    * Over-the-counter <u>saline</u> Fleet Enema (4.5 oz, or 133 mL).
    * Unscrew the Fleet enema cap to access the saline solution.
    * Dissolve 2 probiotic capsules from 3 different probiotic brands/varieties and pour in the contents into the fleet enema solution (each of the 3 different probiotic brands should include a bacterial strain that is <u>different</u> from the other 2 brands for variety).
    * Laying on your LEFT side, insert the probiotic enema rectally, and squeeze the bottle firmly, and then remove.
    * Suggested body poses for use immediately after (rest in each pose for 20-30 seconds): LEFT side, BACK (bridge pose), RIGHT side, child-pose, hands-&-knees, then stand up.
    * Hold the enema as long as you can.

From University of Wisconsin Integrative Medicine, *"Detoxification" Patient Handouts, <u>www.fammed.wisc.edu/integrative/modules</u>*

Patient Handout Detoxification Program. (From University of Wisconsin Integrative Medicine, *"Detoxification" Patient Handouts,* www.fammed.wisc.edu/integrative/modules.)

ACKNOWLEDGMENT

Special thanks to Mandy Fortney for reviewing, testing, and improving this detox program.

REFERENCES

References are available online at ExpertConsult.com.

CHAPTER 107

CHELATION THERAPY

Jeanne A. Drisko, MD

INTRODUCTION

The word chelation has its roots in the late 19th and early 20th centuries with European and American chemical discoveries.[1,2] The word itself is derived from the Greek *CHELE* that means pincher with reference to grabbing by the claws of a crab or lobster. As such, it was recognized that certain types of chemicals could effectively grab and bind metals and minerals, and thus the term chelation arose to describe the incorporation of a metal ion into a heterocyclic ring structure. The understanding of binding and removing of heavy metals in human systems led to therapeutic applications, and this occurred as early as World War II when chelation was introduced as an antidote for arsenic-based poisonous gas exposure.[3–5] Chelation, as a treatment for heavy metal intoxication, has enjoyed robust basic science and clinical research through the years and is the mainstay in conventional toxicology as a resource for documented acute heavy metal poisoning.[4,6–9] Integrative medicine practitioners have also embraced chelation therapy for acute and chronic heavy metal poisoning, although the practice is not always supported by conventional toxicologists.[2,10,11] However, within rigorous guidelines and with accurate laboratory testing, chelation therapy can be an effective tool in the integrative medicine armamentarium for symptomatic patients with positive biological markers for heavy metal toxicity.

There are many types of chelators with wide-ranging chemical structures and differing affinities for metals and minerals that can be obtained from naturally occurring food sources as well as pharmaceutical compounds. Biological systems in both plants and animals are replete with metal-binding proteins such as metallothioneins.[12] These potent chelators of heavy metals are central to the natural response of biological systems to toxic chemicals. Because natural chelators are found ubiquitously, foods have been suggested as ways to reduce absorption or reabsorption of heavy metals found in the gastrointestinal (GI) tract and to support natural detoxification pathways.

Examples of food-based natural chelators include dietary fibers, sulfur-containing foods such as garlic and onions, amino acids, and pectins from fruit.

Chelation as an applied clinical therapeutic intervention usually involves pharmaceutically derived compounds. Some representative types are highlighted later. It is important to understand that the term *chelation* is a general, nonspecific term that defines a chemical equilibrium reaction between a charged metal ion and complexing agent, characterized by the formation of bonds between the two. The metal is said to be chelated, and the complexing agent is the chelator, whether it is from a plant-derived source or an administered pharmaceutical agent.

HISTORY OF CHELATION USES

Heavy Metal Chelation

Biologically based metals/minerals can be used to restore the normal healthy physiology of the body, and this beneficial effect can be accomplished by direct administration of essential metals, such as iron, in deficient states. In addition, toxic metals or minerals found in excess can be chelated and removed.[4] Interested readers looking for more detailed chemical explanations regarding chelation therapy should review several of the following references.[6,7]

Ethylenediaminetetraacetic acid (EDTA) was first used during the 1930s in the German textile industry as a chelating agent to remove calcium during dye processing. In the 1940s, Martin Rubin, PhD, along with chemist Frederick Bersworth discovered the biological effects of EDTA on calcium homeostasis, leading to its laboratory use as an anticoagulant.[13] Rubin subsequently gained approval from the Food and Drug Administration (FDA) for EDTA use in humans with lead poisoning (CaEDTA) and hypercalcemia (disodium EDTA). Norman E. Clarke, Sr. and Albert Boyle separately published case reports that showed improvement in cardiovascular status in patients who received disodium EDTA for lead poisoning.[14,2] Conventional toxicologists continued to administer and study EDTA for its FDA-approved uses of lead toxicity and hypercalcemia. It was during this time that the use of EDTA took divergent paths.

2,3-Dimercaptosuccinic acid (DMSA) was developed in the 1960s from an older chelator, British antilewisite or BAL, that had fallen out of favor because of its highly toxic profile.[4,15] Applied clinically in 1981, DMSA was proposed for use in cases of arsenic poisoning.[16,17] Throughout the 1980s and beyond, the toxicology and basic science literature reported DMSA to be effective in treating a broader range of toxic heavy metals such as lead, arsenic, and mercury.[3,17,18] In the 1980s, Aposhian suggested that oral chelation could replace intravenous (IV) chelation in the future.[3,15] Continued ongoing use of DMSA to the present confirms it proposed place as an effective oral chelator.

In 1972, Russian researchers published the first reports of a dithiol compound, 2,3-dimercaptopropane-1-sulfonate (DMPS), suggesting benefit in improving clinical outcomes in atherosclerotic vascular disease.[4,17,19] With follow-up reports confirming these benefits, DMPS was also found to be beneficial for treatment of hypertension and age-related cognitive decline. Soon, it was discovered that DMPS was found to be particularly efficient at chelating mercury, and this was related to its sulfhydryl chemistry. Its chelating ability was postulated to be the mechanism of improvement in chronic disorders. DMPS is parenterally and orally administered and has enjoyed wide use; however, at this writing, it is not approved for any use in the United States by the FDA.[20]

DMPS is considered to be an experimental drug, and although not approved by the FDA as a drug on formulary, it is allowed as a bulk item to be compounded by compounding pharmacists.

Over ensuing decades, studies continued using DMSA and DMPS with ongoing encouraging outcomes in patients with proven heavy metal toxicity. In 1994, a pharmacokinetic study in patients with lead toxicity showed that DMSA appeared to enter into unhealthy red blood cells at greater rates than that into healthy red blood cells.[21] In 1996, a DMPS pharmacokinetic study found that heavy metals were not redistributed to the brain in an animal model.[6] The numbers of research studies continue to show the utility and safety of oral DMSA and DMPS chelation for removal of heavy metals.[4,18–20,22]

It was during the decade of the 1960s that other types of injectable and oral chelators began to be studied and used for mineral and metal overload. Notably, deferoxamine (DFO) was reported in 1964 to be effective in chelation of iron overload.[23–25] In the following decades after its introduction, DFO gained further credence as an oral chelator of iron and was demonstrated to have significant improvements in cardiovascular function when there was biopsy-proven cardiac iron.[24] Iron chelation remains well accepted.

Cardiovascular Disease

Chelation as a therapy for cardiovascular disease began garnering attention in the 1950s with early anecdotal medical reports of patients, while receiving IV EDTA therapy for lead toxicity, demonstrated reversal of calcified atherosclerotic plaques and reduction in complaints of angina.[14] Endrate, manufactured by Abbott, was the trade name assigned to one form of EDTA with variations of its chemical structure attributed to other trade names. It is this type of intravenously administered chelator that has become synonymous with the practice of chelation therapy for cardiovascular disease and that draws the heat and light of scrutiny. The literature of that time is replete with numerous articles that include case reports, small clinical trials, mechanistic studies, observational studies, and anecdotal reports of benefit

when used in patients with atherosclerotic vascular disease.[2,26,27] However, EDTA chelation for atherosclerotic vascular disease was dealt a blow in 1963 when data published from a study of 10 male patients were combined with another trial of 81 patients.[28] The authors recommended that EDTA chelation therapy be discontinued for atherosclerotic vascular disease because of disappointing results. Of note, across the 2 years of the study, the authors infused EDTA chelation therapy at a dose of 3 grams across 2.5–3 hours in 2000 consecutive infusions without a reported untoward adverse effect. It is not in the best interest of this review to debate the merits or problems with the referenced report of Meltzer et al., but it should be sufficient to say that as a result of the publication, the practice of EDTA chelation as a therapy for atherosclerotic vascular disease was driven underground and continued to be practiced only by alternative medicine physicians. During the intervening years to the present years, rigorous conventional research continued supporting the use of IV EDTA for acute lead toxicity in children and adults.[3,4,22,29–31,32,33]

In 2002, the Cochrane Collaboration published a review of chelation therapy for atherosclerotic vascular disease.[26] At that writing, the report concluded that there were no trials on the effectiveness of chelation therapy for coronary or cerebrovascular disease. The majority of trials had been focused on peripheral vascular disease, specifically investigating EDTA chelation as a treatment for intermittent claudication. The report encouraged randomized trials to be conducted in coronary and cerebrovascular disease to determine if there was an effect. Indeed, a follow-up randomized trial was conducted in 84 participants with known ischemic heart disease and angina, and the trial concluded that there was no evidence to support a beneficial effect of EDTA chelation therapy in this cohort.[34] But, the trial was acknowledged to be underpowered, and the placebo infusions contained IV vitamin C that could not be excluded from having a beneficial effect.[35]

THE TRIAL TO ASSESS CHELATION THERAPY

In 2002, the National Center for Complementary and Alternative Medicine at the National Institutes of Health in partnership with the National Heart, Lung, and Blood Institute funded the largest randomized controlled trial, the Trial to Assess Chelation Therapy (TACT).[36] TACT was the largest multicenter study that assessed EDTA chelation in a randomized placebo–controlled fashion and enrolled 1708 participants with a history of prior myocardial infarction to either the arm to receive 40 infusions of an EDTA chelation solution or the arm receiving a placebo solution[36,37] (Fig. 107.1). It is beyond the scope of this review to discuss the use of low-dose versus high-dose oral multivitamin regimens in the TACT trial.[38] Lamas et al. reported at the conclusion of TACT that the IV chelation regimen with disodium EDTA, compared with placebo, reduced the risk for adverse cardiovascular outcomes, many of which were revascularization procedures.

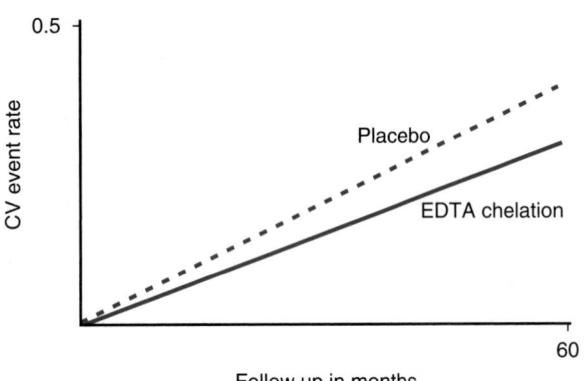

FIG. 107.1 ■ Incidence of cardiovascular events in those with a prior myocardial infarction treated with placebo versus ethylenediaminetetraacetic acid (EDTA) chelation with a 60-month follow-up. (Adapted and modified from Lamas GA, Goertz C, Boineau R, et al. Effect of disodium EDTA chelation regimen on cardiovascular events in patients with previous myocardial infarction: the TACT randomized trial. *JAMA* 2013;309:1241–1250.)

The TACT trial did show a statistically significant effect in decreasing all-cause mortality in the treatment arm in this cohort.[37] A follow-up paper on TACT findings showed a highly significant benefit of EDTA chelation therapy in type 2 diabetic patients.[39] It is important to highlight the fact that the EDTA-based infusion regimen included not only disodium EDTA but also magnesium, procaine hydrochloride, heparin, 7 g of injectable vitamin C, potassium chloride, sodium bicarbonate, pantothenic acid, thiamine, and pyridoxine, all delivered in sterile water.[36,37] The TACT trial was not designed to tease out the effect of each of these components or their contribution to the outcome, nor was it designed to determine a plausible mechanism of action. It was designed, however, to mimic the real-world administration of EDTA chelation therapy as practiced by integrative medicine practitioners. Further trials will be needed to answer these questions and to replicate the TACT findings. As the TACT investigators cautioned, the findings were not sufficient to support the routine use of chelation therapy for the treatment of patients who have had a myocardial infarction.[37] The history of EDTA chelation therapy for cardiovascular disease is certainly at a crossroads and not at a dead end.

CLINICAL USE OF CHELATION THERAPY

Background

Biologically based metals and minerals serve as central components of normal healthy physiology, but when in excess or deficient, serious adverse manifestations may result. In contrast, heavy metals such as mercury, lead, arsenic, and cadmium are found ubiquitously yet have no beneficial role in human biological systems.[40] Recently, gadolinium exposure has been brought into question as a source of heavy metal toxicity that may occur with routine medical imaging.[41] The effects of acute as well as long-term exposure to heavy metals are well known to contribute to human chronic disease burden.[4,31,40,42–49]

For these reasons, chelation of heavy metals is well supported by the scientific literature.*

Heavy metal intoxication induces reactive oxygen species and subsequent depletion of antioxidant cell defenses.[4,43,50,55,56] The generation of reactive oxygen species from heavy metal exposure in biological systems includes such things as superoxide, singlet oxygen, peroxynitrite, hydroxyl radical, and others. The generation of reactive oxygen species and the subsequent cascade of oxidative damage in biological systems initiate reactions resulting in lipid peroxidation, protein oxidation, and damage to DNA and RNA.[5] Oxidative stress can be partially implicated as a mechanism of metal toxicity, and a resultant strategy to increase the antioxidant capacity of affected tissues could enhance its long-term effective treatment. As a point, in fact, acute metal intoxication in experimental systems has been shown to increase antioxidant defense enzymes like superoxide dismutase, catalase, glutathione peroxidase, and others.[4] With the depletion of critical antioxidants such as glutathione and resultant oxidative stress with time and chronic exposure, there is mitochondrial dysfunction, DNA damage, and mutagenesis. This has been shown to lead to abnormal signal transcription, apoptosis, and cell proliferation that have potential for carcinogenesis[57,58] Treatment with supplementation of antioxidant nutraceuticals to augment the cells' antioxidant defenses could reduce the toxic metal interaction with the biological system.[4] Although this appears to be an attractive idea, the usefulness of antioxidants in conjunction with chelation therapy has not been extensively investigated.

In addition to oxidative damage, several mechanisms have been proposed to explain how heavy metals induce toxicity, yet none of these mechanisms has been explicitly defined. Besides the well-described increased oxidative stress, heavy metals are known to alter multiple cellular pathways such as inhibition of DNA repair, alterations in DNA methylation, decreased immune response, and eventual genotoxicity and carcinogenicity.[57] As a carcinogen, there has been increasing evidence that heavy metal exposure promotes carcinogenicity through epigenetic binding of the DNA rather than classic mutations.[50] Although these mechanisms are in the beginning stages of exploration, what it is known is the final alterations result in nervous system dysfunction, immune dysregulation, organ system damage, mitochondrial dysfunction, cardiovascular disease, and endocrine disruption.[1,4]

Toxicity from metal overload or heavy metals can be treated with chelation therapy. Chelation therapy complexes the metal and allows removal of the excess or toxic metal from the system and aids in reducing chronic effects. Although there are a variety of metal chelators approved by the FDA for metal chelation, the identification of the ideal chelator has not been realized. Most of the current chelators have the disadvantage of adverse effects, nonspecific binding, and/or administration difficulties. Currently, with the amount of heavy metal exposure increasing throughout the world, it is imperative to develop better tolerated and more effective chelation compounds and determine if combination therapies of various chelation agents along with antioxidants, vitamins, and minerals might augment

*1,3,4,19,22,50–54

successful outcomes. Better outcomes may be identified and advanced strategies could be developed and tested through large clinical trials.

> Chelators mobilize heavy metals from stores that may be bound in soft tissue or bone, but mobilization does not guarantee excretion and elimination.[19] If the chelation approach is aggressive and reaches beyond what the patient is able to eliminate, then redistribution may occur back into soft tissues and bone with ongoing toxic effects. If the patient is not adequately prepared with good nutrition, a baseline assessment of micronutrients, and repletion of deficiencies prior to chelation, then redistribution may occur.

It is also helpful to evaluate detoxification pathways by genetic screening to determine if there are polymorphisms in key pathways that need support, such as glutathione and methylation. Assuring a healthy terrain prior to chelation avoids health consequences. Approaching chelation of the patient gently and slowly to assess for reactions is wise. Follow-up frequent assessment of critical micronutrients, such as calcium, magnesium, selenium, and zinc, is essential to support what might be lost during the chelation process.[3,4,17] Conservative approaches are rarely wrong. Finally, if there are GI tract abnormalities that result in malabsorption, then oral chelators may be poorly absorbed, and as a result, less available systemically.[10,19,59] If there is an emergent need for chelation prior to GI healing, then it may be necessary to bypass the intestine in favor of using IV chelators.

TREATMENT OF HEAVY METAL INTOXICATION

Testing for Heavy Metal Intoxication

Blood and urine tests are routinely performed by a classically trained toxicologist to search for acute exposures to heavy metals.[1,9,60] This type of testing is valuable for documenting current acute poisoning as seen in industrial exposures, but it is of limited value in assessing the total body burden from chronic exposures. Blood, urine, and hair analyses for heavy metals are poor surrogates for heavy metal body burden from chronic exposures.[10,19,59] Conventional labs that offer testing for heavy metals provide reference ranges for each based on internal standards from their own clientele and are constantly updated with time. Until recently, these labs had no national data points to utilize when setting internal reference ranges. The Centers for Disease Control (CDC) has accumulated a significant database analyzing United States residents and determining the average burden of toxic compounds. These reports are available online (http://www.cdc.gov.exposurereport/). It is from the wealth of these data that more accurate ranges for blood and urine levels are available to evaluate heavy metal burden from acute exposures. Of interest, the findings in the CDC report are from individuals who provided random samples throughout the day without having taken a heavy metal–mobilizing agent or chelator. The reported values are a reflection of the heavy metals present in the blood or urine, which are related to current dietary or environmental exposures and not chronic body stores. Because of the collection method, only a small portion of these ranges are reflective of chronic exposure, with heavy metal buildup bound in soft and/or hard tissues, and therefore are not available in the circulation. It is generally recommended that a nonchelator-challenged collection of urine or blood be obtained as a baseline assessment. This is to determine if there is an acute exposure that needs to be removed and addressed such as in the case of mercury where there is ongoing contaminated fish consumption. If one would directly undergo a chelator-challenged urine collection without the baseline nonchallenged assessment, potential acute ongoing exposure might be overlooked while the patient is treated for chronic exposure with chelation therapy.[10,19,59] It goes without stating that the clinician needs to take an accurate heavy metal exposure history from the patient prior to any type of testing.

> It should be emphasized that no standards or reference ranges are currently in place to support a clinician in evaluating a chelation postprovoked urine heavy metal test. There are no available data to define reference ranges for postchelation challenge urine collection from any of the myriad of chelators used.

There are currently no accepted standards of use for a single chelating agent or proper dosage of any chelating agent to make sense of reference ranges. In addition, not all chelating agents bind all of the heavy metals with efficiency. For example, if a DMSA chelation challenge is given prior to urine collection to assess for mercury, cadmium will be removed at a much lower rate because it has reduced affinity for and is poorly mobilized by DMSA. If there is significant cadmium body burden, this may be poorly evaluated in this setting and improperly treated across the long course.[61] While the postchallenge urine collection is standard among integrative medicine practitioners of chelation, using a prechelation challenge test would augment information that cannot be obtained otherwise. Restated, random samples collected where a chelating agent is not administered are excellent for showing current and acute exposures to heavy metals, whereas urine collection obtained after a chelating agent is given is a reflection of the chronic exposure and total body burden. Clinical information can assist in selecting the correct chelating agent to be administered not only for testing but also possibly for treatment (Table 107.1).

> It is generally recommended that a nonchelator-challenged collection of urine or blood be obtained as a baseline assessment. This determines if there is an acute exposure that needs to be removed and addressed such as in the case of mercury where there is ongoing contaminated fish consumption. If one would go directly to a chelator-challenged urine collection without the baseline nonchallenged assessment, potential acute ongoing exposure might be overlooked while the patient is treated for chronic exposure with chelation therapy.

TABLE 107.1 **Review of Chelating Agents**

Agent	Indications	Route of Administration	Precautions	Notes
EDTA	Lead, and to a much lesser extent, mercury and cadmium	Intravenous administration	Monitor zinc, calcium, iron, and copper levels during chelation; can be nephrotoxic if administered too frequently and rapidly; disodium EDTA is lethal if given by rapid IV push secondary to rapid loss of calcium; limited distribution in biological systems in intracellular space	Pharmaceutical preparation for IV administration; oral and transmucosal agents available OTC but with very limited absorption
DMSA	Lead, mercury, arsenic, antimony, cadmium, others	Oral administration	Limited distribution in biological systems in intracellular space; monitor zinc, copper, and sodium levels during chelation	Pharmaceutical preparation; least toxic of FDA-approved drugs for chelation; various heavy metals have different affinities with some binding stronger and others with less attraction
DMPS	Mercury	Intravenous, transmucosal, and oral administration	Not FDA approved	Is available by compounding; limited chelation of lead and arsenic
Deferoxamine	Iron, and rarely used for aluminum	Subcutaneous, intramuscular, and intravenous administration	Not FDA approved for aluminum toxicity	Pharmaceutical preparation
Deferasirox	Iron	Oral administration	Increased risk for death	Pharmaceutical preparation
Citrus pectin	Postulated arsenic, lead, mercury, cadmium, and strontium	Oral administration	Slow and mild chelation process not suitable for acute severe toxicity; does not appear to reduce essential minerals like zinc and calcium with time	Nutraceutical; appears safe in children
Blue-green algae (spirulina and chlorella)	Postulated arsenic, mercury, cadmium, aluminum, lead	Oral administration	May contain toxins and heavy metals from the way they are harvested; interacts with Coumadin by naturally occurring vitamin K in the product	Nutraceutical
Zeolite	Postulated lead, iron, and cadmium	Oral administration	May bind zinc and manganese; very limited human research	Nutraceutical

DMPS, 2,3-dimercaptopropane-1-sulfonate; *DMSA*, 2,3-dimercaptosuccinic acid; *EDTA*, ethylenediaminetetraacetic acid; *FDA*, Food and Drug Administration; *OTC*, over-the-counter.

PHARMACOLOGICAL APPROACHES

DMPS

DMPS is given orally, intravenously, and transmucosally. DMPS, when administered orally, is approximately 39% absorbed from the GI tract.[19] Pharmacokinetic studies have shown that solutions are stable, rapidly converted to the disulfide form, and excreted largely by the kidneys. It is mainly distributed in the extracellular space but may enter the cell by specific transport mechanisms to aid in chelation and removal of mercury.[4] Currently, DMPS is not considered an appropriate chelator for lead toxicity and has only limited applicability in arsenic toxicity. But, it is reported to be very effective for elimination of mercury.[3,4,20] DMPS has a long history of use in Russia and Germany and is sold as an over-the-counter oral agent because of its demonstrated safety.[3,17] There are reports of minor adverse effects of GI discomfort, skin reactions, mild neutropenia, and elevated liver enzymes.

DMSA

Oral administration of DMSA is possible because of its hydrophilic nature that results in absorption from the GI tract.[4,17,19] It is worth noting that in patients with associated intestinal dysbiosis, DMSA may have limited gut absorption.[19] Oral absorption is approximately 25% of the total dose, and most of the DMSA found circulating is protein-bound; 95% to albumin, and only a small percent is present as the free drug. DMSA is extensively metabolized in humans with approximately 25% excreted in the urine and the remainder excreted in the feces.[17] It has proven to be the least toxic but has a significant drawback in that it lacks the ability to cross cellular membranes and is distributed in the extracellular fluids only.[4,62] DMSA mobilizes lead from soft tissues without redistribution to the brain in contrast with EDTA, which has been demonstrated to do so.[15] However, there may be initial mercury redistribution to the brain that appears to subside as therapy is continued.[15] Because important minerals are also mobilized, bound, and excreted, blood levels of zinc, copper, and sodium should be monitored. This is compared with EDTA, where there is increased urinary excretion of zinc and copper, as well as iron and calcium. Although DMSA it is known to be a safe agent when used in correct clinical settings, there have been reports of GI upsets, skin reactions, mild neutropenia, and elevated liver enzymes.[4] A rare side effect reported is mucocutaneous eruptions and toxic epidermal necrosis that resolves when DMSA is discontinued.[19]

EDTA

EDTA is poorly absorbed from the GI tract (<5%) and, as a consequence, should only be administered by a parenteral route.[4] It is primarily distributed in extracellular fluids, which limit its capacity to chelate intracellular metals. EDTA is also known to redistribute lead to the brain and should not be used to assess for lead mobilization in children.[4] EDTA can be obtained as disodium EDTA or calcium disodium EDTA with different applications of use. The FDA archived a report from 2013 entitled, "Questions and Answers on Edetate Disodium (marketed as Endrate and generic products."[63] EDTA is used to refer to two similar but separate drugs with differing indications of use. The first drug is calcium disodium EDTA (Versinate), and the second drug is disodium EDTA (Endrate). The confusion lies in the common name of EDTA for both drugs; however, there are two very separate indications of use for each. Calcium disodium EDTA is approved by the FDA for use in lead poisoning and has been the mainstay of treatment for childhood lead poisoning since the 1950s.[4] The second drug, disodium EDTA, is approved for use in patients with rhythm disorders from drug intoxication such as digitalis where there is hypercalcemia. Calcium disodium EDTA, Versinate, will not deplete calcium if given rapidly, while disodium EDTA will remove calcium through renal excretion in a life-threatening fashion if administered rapidly. In fact, erroneous administration of a bolus infusion of disodium EDTA for lead poisoning, when calcium disodium EDTA was meant to be administered, resulted in the death of a child.[64] Between 1971 and 2007, there were 11 deaths associated with the use of EDTA infusions. Nine of these deaths were attributed to disodium EDTA specifically, while two of the deaths only refer to EDTA as the causative agent. In fact, in five of the deaths, there was confusion when ordering the drug that resulted in the adverse outcome. There have been no deaths reported from administering calcium disodium EDTA. Risks associated with IV EDTA chelation have been reported to be renal failure, arrhythmia, tetany, hypocalcemia, hypotension, and prolongation of bleeding time, among others.[4,34]

Cardiovascular

The above being said, TACT was the largest randomized clinical trial evaluating disodium EDTA in 1708 patients postmyocardial infarction.[36,37]

TACT found that disodium EDTA infusions, when given according to protocol and not administered as a rapid bolus, were very safe. For practitioners of EDTA chelation therapy, full assessment includes basic laboratory testing including analysis of renal function, mineral status, and close monitoring of vital signs. Safety concerns are real, and the administration of IV EDTA chelation for whatever reason should be done by a trained medical professional in an environment conducive to full assessment of potential problems and the ability to respond immediately to problems if they should occur.

NATURAL PRODUCTS

Over-the-Counter Chelators

It is not uncommon to find EDTA capsules for oral administration advertised to the public on the Internet.[65] While it is well known that this is a powerful chelating agent when given intravenously, oral use of EDTA has not been validated. Pharmacokinetic studies of oral EDTA have not been undertaken. It is well documented that EDTA is only marginally absorbed from the GI tract.[4,19] A case report of a single patient exposed to lead showed that there was a 36-fold mobilization following each IV EDTA chelation but only a three-fold increase in blood excretion with oral EDTA.[59] Certainly, further evaluation is warranted.

The FDA became aware of an increase in the number of oral chelation products offered for sale over the Internet, and these products claimed to treat and prevent disease by cleansing the body of heavy metals and toxic chemicals.[65] The majority of these products contained EDTA and DMSA. Although they were marketed as dietary supplements, they were claiming to treat and prevent disease, and as a result of the language, the FDA designated them as drugs. As such, these products need to be approved by the FDA to be legally marketed. According to the report, the concern for these available chelating products was first and foremost that they targeted vulnerable populations. The objectionable language in the claims was related to treating and preventing disease without specific clinical trial evidence for benefit from any of the products. Products containing EDTA have never been shown to provide any benefit for heavy metal chelation when administered orally or as a suppository. There was also reported a misleading reference to the CDC's recommendation for EDTA chelation therapy for lead poisoning, giving the false impression that the use of an oral EDTA product was approved and/or sanctioned by the CDC.[65] The FDA division of Health Fraud and Consumer Outreach Branch enforced action against several of the websites forcing removal of the products and their claims, although there continue to be a plethora of these types of websites. Caveat emptor.

Antioxidants and Sulfhydryl Compounds

Antioxidants with sulfhydryl chemistry could double as free radical scavengers as well as chelating agents, although clinical trial evidence is only just building.[5,43,44,49,50,67] Examples include N-acetyl cysteine (NAC), taurine, alpha lipoic acid, melatonin, and other natural agents. As antioxidants, these products have the capacity to enhance cellular antioxidant defenses by regenerating endogenous glutathione, vitamin C, and vitamin E. These important natural products have the potential to remove heavy metals from biological systems, quench free radicals, regenerate antioxidants, and excrete the heavy metals without redistribution in the biological system.[5,68] In addition to their role as agents modifying metal toxicity, antioxidants could potentially act as complementary chelating agents or adjuvants that increase the efficacy of a known chelator. Combination therapies with chelators and antioxidants such as glutathione, NAC, lipoic acid, melatonin, and vitamin C, along with supportive therapies such as zinc, copper, vitamins, and sulfhydryl amino acids like methionine have been proposed as adjunctive therapies.[5] The endogenous thiol-containing molecules, glutathione, cysteine, homocysteine, metallothionein, and albumin, all contain sulfur groups that readily bind heavy metals. The higher the thiol concentration is in the biological system, the more it is able to protect against accumulation of heavy metals. Although certainly a plausible mechanism of action could be proposed for the addition of these agents to chelation, no supportive clinical research has been undertaken. Of note, in an animal system exposed to mercury vapor then given a chelating agent with antioxidants or antioxidants alone, glutathione, alpha lipoic acid, and vitamin C administered without a chelating agent were insufficient for reducing mercury content in the brain or kidney.[69]

N-Acetyl Cysteine

NAC has been reported to be a chelator of toxic metals as well as a precursor for glutathione synthesis.[19,43] Pharmacokinetic studies show rapid absorption after oral administration, and because it is a component of glutathione, NAC actively forms glutathione during first-pass metabolism through the liver.[70] The sulfhydryl component of the structure is responsible for the metabolic activity. Of interest, NAC appears to have chelating ability in acute heavy metal poisoning and in fact has been shown to be more effective than EDTA or DMSA by increasing urinary excretion of lead and chromium.[71] An animal study combining NAC with DMSA reduced arsenic-related oxidative stress.[72] One review went so far as to state that NAC is an excellent choice as an antioxidant and could be safely combined with other drugs and chelators to improve outcomes (Table 107.2).[5]

Glutathione

Reduced glutathione is found in high concentrations in cellular systems and plays a major role in detoxification of

TABLE 107.2 Supplements to Support Chelation

Supplement	Dosing	Precautions	Mechanism of Action	Notes
N-acetyl cysteine (NAC)	Oral with doses beginning at 300 mg and as high as 600 mg three times/day (will not cover inhaled dosing or recommendations for other maladies)	Considered likely safe; hypothesized to reduce clotting; may potentiate the effects of nitroglycerin therapy	Important in the production of glutathione; as an antioxidant, can regenerate vitamins C and E; chelates through sulfhydryl chemistry	Not enough human trial data to suggest a significant chelating effect, although early evidence suggests an effect in lead and chromium toxicity
Alpha lipoic acid	Oral with doses beginning at 300 mg and up to 600 mg three times/day	May lower blood sugar in certain individuals; may lower thiamine stores; may interfere with thyroid medication; may redistribute lead and mercury in human systems	As an antioxidant, can regenerate vitamins C and E; chelates through sulfhydryl chemistry; aids in regeneration of glutathione	Not enough human trial evidence to recommend as a chelator
Flavonoids	Oral dosing through food and supplementation as extracts of tea, berries, grapes, etc.	May negatively impact cytochrome P450 enzymes; high doses inhibit platelet aggregation; may bind nonheme iron; may decrease absorption of vitamin C from the intestine	Antioxidant and anti-inflammatory properties; modulates signaling pathways; direct chelating properties through its chemical structure	Common components of the human diet and found ubiquitously in nature; insufficient human trial evidence for recommendation as a chelator
Taurine	Oral with doses beginning at 500 mg and up to 9000 mg/day in divided doses	Generally considered safe; may interact with lithium to reduce levels	Critical in bile production and therefore assists in hepatic clearance; important in phase II detoxification; may chelate through sulfhydryl chemistry; considered an antioxidant	Insufficient human clinical trial evidence as a chelating agent

TABLE 107.2 Supplements to Support Chelation—cont'd

Supplement	Dosing	Precautions	Mechanism of Action	Notes
Selenium	Oral with doses generally recommended at 200–400 mcg (required daily amount is around 50 mcg)	May interfere with glucose control in some diabetics; may be highly toxic if high doses above 400 mcg are taken for a prolonged period	Important functions in selenocysteine enzymes and selenoproteins; important for glutathione function and antioxidant balance; changes metabolism of arsenic	Evidence suggests a use in arsenic toxicity
Glutathione	Oral dosing of 500 mg and upward reported to be safe; intravenous dosing beginning at 400 mg with some reports up to 12,000 mg/infusion without reported significant adverse events; (will not address inhaled dosing and uses)	Oral dosing may be better absorbed in the liposomal form; best to begin with lower doses of intravenous glutathione and slowly increase dosing; no serious adverse events noted and is generally considered safe	Important antioxidant; chelates through sulfhydryl chemistry	Insufficient clinical trial evidence to recommend glutathione as a chelator, although evidence shows it carries mercury and reduces its toxicity; does not appear to become a prooxidant at high intravenous doses

various electrophilic compounds.[5] Deficiency of glutathione puts the cell at risk for oxidative damage. Besides its antioxidant defense and free radical scavenging, glutathione regenerates important antioxidants such as vitamins C and E. Glutathione maintains the redox state of critical protein sulfhydryl groups that are necessary for DNA repair. Besides neutralization of free radicals, glutathione also is suggested to chelate transition metals, thereby reducing their toxic ability.[5] Glutathione is known to be both a carrier of mercury as well as an antioxidant with specific roles in protecting the body from mercury toxicity. Glutathione targets and binds methylmercury, preventing it from binding to other cellular proteins, which results in organ damage. Glutathione also prevents mercury from entering the intracellular environment and becoming an intracellular toxin. It has been suggested that IV glutathione combined with EDTA chelation significantly increases cadmium excretion.[5,73] It was also found that renal protection was augmented. However, this was conducted in a single patient, albeit in a controlled fashion. This suggests that glutathione could provide additional chelation in the proper setting, but needs verification in clinical trials.[73] Oral glutathione administration is not recommended unless it is delivered in a form that protects it from digestion such as liposomal. IV glutathione can bypass the GI tract and is an important physiological chelator as well as antioxidant.[19] Both oral liposomal and IV glutathione have good safety profiles.[74,75]

Glutathione is poorly absorbed orally. If prescribed orally, recommend a product that is liposomal, which protects it against digestion.

Flavonoids

Flavonoids or bioflavonoids are phytochemicals well known to be antioxidants and widely available as dietary supplements. These are found throughout nature as components of seeds, fruits, flowers, vegetables, and beverages. Flavonoids enjoy a reputation as regulators of physiological processes including inflammation, thrombosis, immune reaction, antitumor properties, and vasodilatation.[76] Because of their interesting ring structure, flavonoids may act to sequester heavy metals apart from their antioxidant function and seem to have a synergy between free radical scavenging and formation of metal complexes.[77–79]

Taurine

Two sulfur-containing amino acids, taurine and methionine, have been proposed as adjuncts in removing heavy metals during chelation because of their sulfhydryl chemistry. They appear to have a role in decreasing oxidative stress.[19,80–82] Taurine, when coadministered with DMSA, helped to further reduce the total body burden of arsenic and lead.[19] Taurine is found ubiquitously throughout mammalian tissues and is known to act as a powerful antioxidant.[80,81,83] Taurine is able to form unstable metal complexes with transition metals based on its electrophilic nature.[5] Taurine is a remarkable thiol-containing amino acid and has been shown to maintain calcium homeostasis, bile acid conjugation, neuromodulation, stabilization of membranes, and has scavenging capabilities.[5,80] Part of its ability to protect the cell membranes is related to regulating the enzyme phospholipid methyltransferase, which regulates the activity of phosphatidylethanolamine and phosphatidylcholine critical to cell membrane structure.[82]

Alpha Lipoic Acid

Alpha lipoic acid is characterized as a particularly efficient antioxidant with the capacity to regenerate endogenous antioxidants such as glutathione, vitamin C, and vitamin E with potential therapeutic properties in the treatment of metal-induced oxidative stress.[84–86] Because of its dual lipophilic and hydrophilic nature, it is readily absorbed by the gut and crosses cellular and blood–brain membranes.

It has also been shown to decrease lipid peroxidation in the brain and peripheral nervous tissue when given orally in an animal model.[84] Alpha lipoic acid has been shown to increase both intra- and extracellular levels of glutathione in human systems. Increases in glutathione levels are felt to be related to lipoic acid's antioxidant capabilities.[43,85] Another very important attribute is its metal-chelating activity.[84,85] It is known to be readily absorbed into the intracellular environment and can form complexes with metals that were previously found to be bound to other sulfhydryl-containing proteins. Alpha lipoic acid crosses the blood–brain barrier where it readily binds with lead and mercury. It should be cautioned, however, that it may redistribute metals.[19] Metal ions known to be chelated by alpha lipoic acid include copper, zinc, lead, mercury, and iron. Alpha lipoic acid has been administered both orally and by an IV route without reports of significant toxicity.[5] It is a safe product and has been administered up to 1200 mg intravenously in humans without toxicity and orally in daily divided doses of 1800 mg with negligible reported adverse effects. However, studies have largely been conducted in animals and further human clinical trials need to be done.

Mineral Support

Concomitant administration of selenium, magnesium, zinc, and calcium with chelation therapy has an effect on blood biochemistry and oxidative stress. Selenium was the most effective in reducing arsenic-induced inhibition of blood delta-aminolevulinic acid dehydratase (ALAD) activity and liver oxidative stress.[87] Calcium and magnesium also showed favorable effects on hematological and other biochemical parameters. Because selenium was the most effective, it was recommended to be added to chelation therapy to achieve the best protective effects against arsenic poisoning in humans.[87] Selenium as an important essential element that should be evaluated in the face of heavy metal intoxication. It is capable of forming an insoluble compound with mercury, which may be transported through biological membranes. It is important to remember that selenium depletion in the face of mercury exposure will also deplete selenoenzymes.[19] Zinc and selenium have also been shown to exert protective effects against mercury toxicity, most likely mediated by induction of the metal binding proteins metallothionein and selenoprotein-P.[88] It is critical to follow mineral levels during chelation therapy as depletion may occur.

Modified Citrus Pectin

Modified citrus pectin (MCP) is an over-the-counter nutritional supplement derived from the inner peel white pulp of citrus fruit.[89–91] MCP has a complex polysaccharide structure, and as such, is soluble with the principal component being D-galacturonic acid. Unmodified pectin is nondigestible because the polysaccharides are cross-linked in long polymers. MCP is composed of citrus pectin that has been broken down into shorter chains, and this is accomplished by using enzyme and pH modifications. The shorter structure and lower molecular weight are required for the pectin to be absorbed out of the GI

tract and into the bloodstream during digestion. It has been proposed that MCP is able to bind heavy metals and eliminate them without eliminating essential biological minerals.[91] One postulated mechanism of action of heavy metal binding by MCP appears to be related to passive binding with decreased absorption of heavy metals in the GI tract. This appears to be through bile trapping of heavy metals in intrahepatic circulation with reduced reabsorption of the heavy metals in the gut. Another postulated mechanism of binding is that MCP is absorbed into the bloodstream with subsequent direct chelation of heavy metals and elimination of the metal-pectin complex in the urine.[91] It should be cautioned that no human trials of significance including pharmacokinetic studies have been completed, although case reports are available and there does seem to be a promise of effect. In several uncontrolled human studies, MCP was shown to result in excretion of cadmium, mercury, arsenic, and lead.[91] There is a need for a gentle, safe heavy metal chelating agent, especially for children in areas with endemic chronic heavy metal exposure. MCP appears to be a safe and effective chelating agent that has been shown to lower levels of heavy metals in children, although the trial was small and uncontrolled with questions of conflict of interest on the part of the investigators.[90,92] MCP can be given safely to children in divided doses throughout the day for extended periods of time without apparent adverse events.[90]

> Modified citrus pectin is a safe chelator that can be used in children with lead toxicity.

Algae

Blue-green algae, such as the *Spirulina* and *Chlorella* species, are unicellular organisms and commercially distributed as organic algae dietary supplements.[19,93–95] These species have been proposed for use in chronic disorders including heavy metal toxicity.[91,96–98] Unfortunately, robust controlled clinical trial evidence is lacking and human use is inferred from industrial applications in polluted water and toxic site cleanup. Some limited human trials show improved oxygen consumption and aerobic endurance when chlorella is used orally.[98] It is proposed that alginates passively bind to heavy metals, sequester them, and subsequently excrete these toxins via normal excretory processes. In areas of endemic arsenic poisoning with high incidences of resultant immunotoxicity and oxidative stress, blue-green algae have been proposed as a safe and cheap chelator.[96,99] But, only animal studies of arsenic toxicity have been conducted demonstrating downregulation of immunotoxicity with improved oxygenation after arsenic exposure.[100] In cadmium-exposed rats, chlorella appeared to protect against cadmium-induced liver toxicity.[96] In addition, it was also reported that there were lesser hepatic concentrations of cadmium when chlorella was administered. An uncontrolled prospective study was conducted in 34 human subjects, 17 at high risk for heavy metal exposure and 17 healthy.[94] It appears as if there is preferential binding of heavy metals compared with essential minerals. A proposed mechanism of action for preferential binding of heavy metals appears to be related to the "egg box" structure of the molecule resulting in a high affinity of binding of heavy metals when compared with essential minerals.[89] It was reported that chlorella intake resulted in reductions in body fat percentage, serum total cholesterol, and fasting glucose levels. Gene analysis identified changes in signal transduction molecules, metabolic enzymes, receptors, transporters, and cytokines, particularly in fat metabolism and insulin signaling pathways.[94] However, it is cautioned that arsenic can be found in naturally occurring dietary supplements such as algae because of its inherent chelating ability and the ubiquitous distribution of arsenic in the Earth's crust.[101,102] It is also reported that there is an accumulation of other toxic byproducts such as microcystins in naturally derived algae supplements, and naturally occurring increased levels of vitamin K may result in a drug interaction with Coumadin. An interesting case report in the psychiatric literature describes an adult female with onset of psychosis with no predisposing factors after the ingestion of chlorella.[103] Withdrawal of the chlorella supplement resulted in disappearance of the psychotic symptoms, and when the patient resumed the supplement, the symptoms recurred. The psychiatrist caring for this patient cautioned against the use of the supplement because of unknown adulterants, toxic impurities, or from the effect of the algae itself. Because of the potential for toxicity or adverse events, algae species should not be recommended for regular consumption until further human research is conducted and safety assured.

Zeolites

Zeolites naturally occur and are composed of aluminum complexed with silicate-containing minerals. Most of the commonly found natural zeolites are formed by changes that occur in volcanic rocks when in contact with fresh- or seawater.[104] There is a three-dimensional structure with the aluminum ion occupying the center surrounded by four oxygen atoms, and the complex lattice has a negative charge. This allows the complex to bind with certain cations such as lead, cadmium, zinc, and manganese. The most common use of zeolites is industrial for removal of heavy metals during purification in water management.[104,105] Zeolites are routinely used in water management systems and for animal feed purification. Animal studies have been conducted to evaluate the ability of zeolites to remove heavy metals from biological systems and have been shown to be effective. Although used in integrative health regimens for detoxification, no formal human clinical trials have been conducted using zeolites.[58,105] Oral zeolite is commercially available as a dietary supplement. The author compared a pre- and postzeolite flush test with IV EDTA and DMPS.[58] In this single case report, the author noted that zeolite failed to enhance the excretion of lead, noting that it was ineffective in this particular patient.

SUMMARY

The role of chelation therapy for heavy metal intoxication is well established and supported in the scientific literature. Classically trained toxicologists usually address the effects of acute metal toxicity and treat with chelation therapy when certain rigid testing parameters are followed. Assessment approaches used by integrative practitioners of chelation are less rigid, including the use of provoked urine evaluation, which is not approved of in classic toxicology. The use of FDA-approved chelators such as EDTA and DMSA are used by both groups. However, some practitioners promote off-label use of EDTA for cardiovascular disease and routinely use the non-FDA approved chelator DMPS. Although classically trained toxicologists and integrative practitioner chelationists have been at odds, there appears to be some meeting in the middle because of the recent results of the TACT trial that investigated EDTA for cardiovascular disease and the growing realization of worsening heavy metal exposures around the world and the need for safe, effective, and inexpensive chelators. Only further research will be able to address the unanswered questions.

Case Study

The patient is a 59-year-old male with long-standing metabolic syndrome with dyslipidemia, hypertension, truncal obesity, and borderline elevated glucose and having stent placement in coronary vessels 3 years prior. The patient also had a diagnosis of prostate cancer 2 years prior but is currently without evidence of disease. There was a history of long-standing irritable bowel syndrome with predominant constipation.

The patient visited the University of Kansas Medical Center, KU Integrative Medicine clinic to discover a better approach for his chronic disorders through diet and lifestyle interventions. Laboratory assessment revealed the need for micronutrient replacement based on results of laboratory testing, and he was referred to the KU Integrative Medicine clinic dietitian for the management of his poor-quality diet and food hypersensitivity.

In the course of the patient's workup, it was discovered that he had been a lifelong hunter and had been taught as a young man to reload his shotgun shells with pellets. As a result, he had significant long-term exposure to lead and antimony. Other toxic exposures elicited were related to multiple amalgam fillings, many of which were placed in early adolescence and had not been replaced in the ensuing years in spite of fractures and deterioration. The patient had also been exposed to second-hand tobacco smoke in his childhood but did not smoke himself.

Continued

Case Study—cont'd

HEAVY METAL TESTING

An unprovoked urine collection was obtained for heavy metal analysis, which showed significantly elevated levels of lead, uranium, nickel, and cadmium. Antimony and mercury levels were elevated but were not outside the reference range. Subsequently, DMSA was administered, and a urine sample was collected 6 hours postchelator administration. This showed markedly elevated lead and mercury levels with elevated antimony, cadmium, nickel, and thallium levels. There was no evidence of uranium in the second sample postchelator.

CHELATION THERAPY

The patient was placed on a chelation schedule with DMSA, with frequent laboratory testing for minerals such as zinc that may be removed during chelation and ongoing periodic checks of excreted heavy metals. The patient was supplemented with a mineral complex to support any deficiencies that might occur while undergoing DMSA chelation. He also received micronutrients that he was found to be deficient in at the outset, and those were also followed by serial laboratory testing to ensure adequacy. In addition, it was imperative that he drank plenty of water to flush the excreted chelator–heavy metal complexes through the kidneys and to encourage daily bowel movements for elimination of heavy metal complexes via the bowel. Renal function remained normal.

CHELATION SUPPORT

Other supportive nutritional supplements included green tea extract for bioflavonoids, oral liposomal glutathione, oral vitamin C, whole-foods diet with plenty of cruciferous vegetables, juicing, and cilantro/chlorella supplements. He was also encouraged to add forms of lymphatic drainage with rebounding on a mini trampoline, skin brushing, and infrared sauna.

OUTCOME

Over time, the very high lead and mercury levels began to clear with some increase in cadmium and antimony levels, related to the decreasing competition for binding by DMSA. The patient chose highly filtered water, and uranium did not reappear with time. DMSA chelation was terminated when the last challenged urine collection was found to have only negligible amounts of heavy metals. This occurred during a 6-month period.

With dietary changes and weight loss, micronutrient support, and chelation therapy, the metabolic syndrome cleared with normalization of blood pressure, dyslipidemia, and borderline elevated glucose level. His irritable bowel syndrome was no longer a problem. The patient's therapy was a multipronged approach that resulted in the overall improvements, but the chelation was important because of the well-known cardiovascular adverse effects from heavy metals that would result in ongoing untoward effects if not addressed.

CASE DISCUSSION

This case is instructive for several reasons. First of all, uranium was present in the initial unchallenged sample but not evident after DMSA was given. This tells us that there was an acute exposure of uranium, and this most likely occurred from a water source, as it can be fairly ubiquitous in drinking water. There are two explanations for why it was not present in the postchallenge urine. Either the patient was not exposed to the water source during the follow-up and hence no acute ongoing uranium exposure; or more likely, DMSA, because of its very strong affinity for lead and mercury and low affinity for uranium, preferentially bound the lead and mercury. With the very high levels of lead and mercury in the postchelation sample, the chelator was saturated with heavy metals and unlikely to bind the uranium because of the lower affinity. In any event, the patient was counseled about checking his water source for uranium. Another important point is the initial unchallenged urine collection chelates and excretes heavy metals that are only available from the bloodstream and not from body stores. This may occur when there is turnover of bone with a release of lead, or it may occur when there is breakdown of amalgam dental work with releases of mercury and tin into the circulation. Another consideration is that heavy metals may come from acute exposure such as from food, tobacco use, hobbies, and/or work exposures. Careful patient questioning about diet and lifestyle habits is imperative.

Key Web Resources

American College for Advancement in Medicine (ACAM): This is the oldest physician membership organization for those who practice integrative/alternative medicine. The ACAM has been in the forefront of teaching chelation therapy for heavy metal toxicity.

http://www.acam.org/

American Academy of Environmental Medicine (AAEM): The AAEM is well known for their approach to patient care in the face of toxic environmental exposures, including heavy metal toxicity. They educate physicians about detoxification and chelation therapy.

https://www.aaemonline.org/

International College of Integrative Medicine (ICIM): The ICIM is a physician membership organization composed of chelationists who have been successful in educating how chelation affects cardiovascular disease.

http://www.icimed.com/

REFERENCES

References are available online at ExpertConsult.com.

CHAPTER 108

INTEGRATIVE STRATEGIES FOR PLANETARY HEALTH

Nancy L. Sudak, MD, ABIHM • James Harvie, PEng

Awareness of the ecological impact of modern human activities necessitates urgent action on the part of society. Integrative holistic practitioners intuitively utilize an expansive ecological, or whole-system, model of health. At the individual level, an ecological model embraces the interplay of psychosocial, spiritual, environmental, and other factors in the support and promotion of individual health and well-being. A systems worldview also supports the understanding and interplay of social determinants and diseases. One cannot separate human health from the health of communities and the planet. Holistic integrative practitioners, who are uniquely oriented toward an expansive ecological worldview, are ideal educators for patients and colleagues about the steps that can be taken to mitigate ecological health impacts and advocate for policies and practices that promote health and well-being at individual, community, and planetary levels.

This chapter provides a practical overview of some of the major issues eroding global ecological services and of preventive strategies through the lens of climate change, food system, and toxic chemicals. Although acute toxicity is problematic, this chapter focuses on the chronic toxicity. The chapter does not address the myriad of established environmentally related occupational exposures, and it assumes an everyday workplace that is not dissimilar from our homes with respect to the use of products, technologies, and consumption of foods and water. The important social health impact of our current materials economy is similarly beyond the scope of this chapter.

A SYSTEMS APPROACH

Human populations are tied to ecological functions, and from a wellness perspective, differentiating between human and environmental effects is not logical. What food we grow, and how we grow it, has consequences with respect to nutrition, greenhouse gas emissions, water and air quality, and socioeconomic health.[1] A 2015 Institutes of Medicine report concluded that the food system can be conceptualized as a complex, adaptive system and found that systemic approaches that take full account of social, economic, ecological, and evolutionary factors and processes will be required to meet challenges to the U.S. food system in the 21st century.[2]

Similarly, the toxic, persistent cycle demonstrates the potential for distant releases to cause local exposures and the role of prevention at the local level in promoting global restoration. Fig. 108.1 helps illustrate that when we pour something undesired down the drain, our action

has multiple unseen effects, and although a burden may have been relieved on the home front, another burden occurs elsewhere. A systems approach incorporates the whole. By shifting focus from the parts to the whole, we can better grasp that we are not immune from externalized social and environmental impacts on the products and materials we use, as ultimately they are all connected to individual health.

THE PRECAUTIONARY PRINCIPLE

An important concept that has evolved from the study of environmental health is the precautionary principle, a decision-making tool used if an activity raises the threat of harm, but the cause and effect are not definite. The precautionary principle proposes that the burden of proof that an activity or product is *not* harmful should fall on the purveyors of a potentially harmful activity. This principle embodies the Hippocratic premise, "First do no harm," and is gaining widespread acceptance because it eliminates the barrier of uncertainty to allow for protective action. Rather than asking how much toxic damage is acceptable in a baby or an ecosystem, a precautionary approach asks how much exposure can be avoided.[3] For example, although we know that many industrial chemicals have adverse health effects and that our body burdens are striking, we may not fully understand whether safe threshold limits exist or have the benefit of studies that demonstrate synergism among various chemical combinations. It is also reasonable to consider the biochemical diversity among detoxification mechanisms in human beings[4] and to acknowledge that what may be tolerated in one individual may have a devastating health impact on another. When consequences are not known with certainty, but are judged from available evidence to pose a significant risk, avoidance is the most prudent course of action.

> The precautionary principle proposes that the burden of proof that an activity or product is not harmful should fall on the purveyors of a potentially harmful activity. When consequences are not known with certainty, but are judged from available evidence to pose a significant risk, avoidance is the most prudent course of action.

The burden of scientific proof has become an obstruction to protecting health and the environment because many people will be irreversibly sickened during the

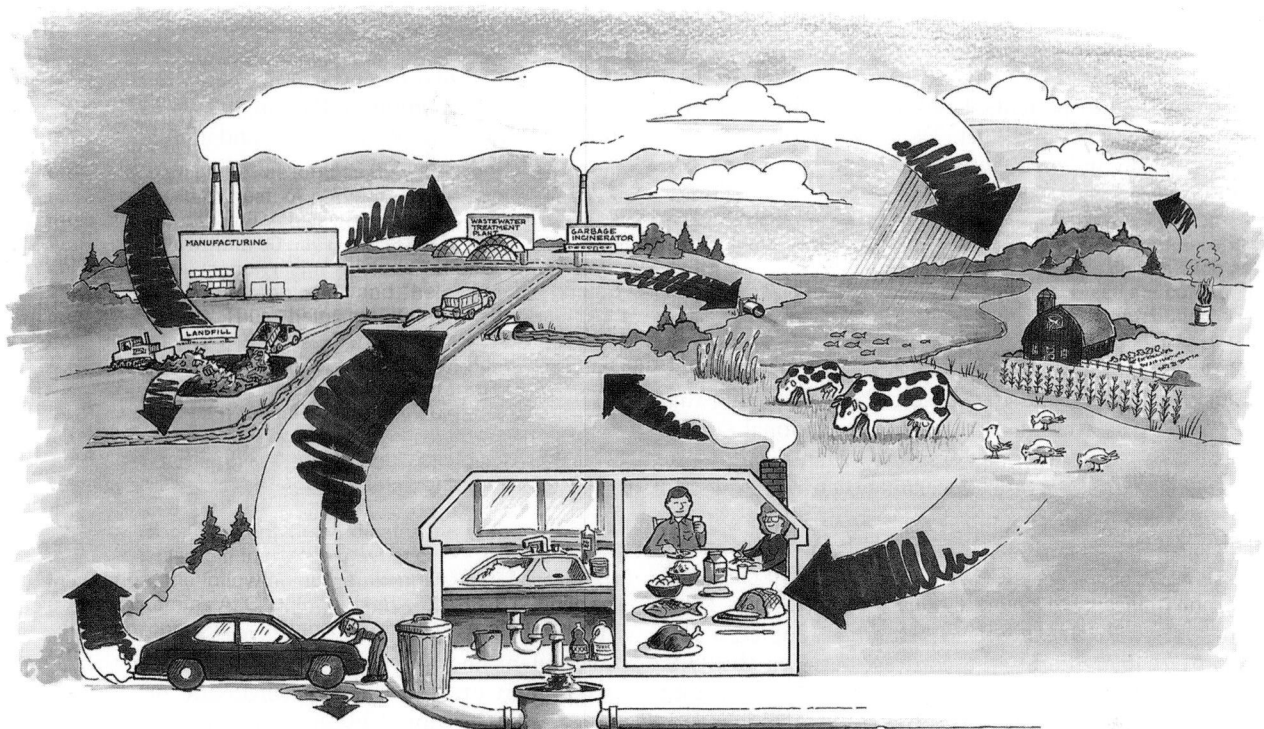

FIG. 108.1 ■ Toxic persistent cycle. (From Western Lake Superior Sanitary District. *Safe solutions to toxic problems: a guide to eliminating persistent toxic substances from the Lake Superior Basin.* Duluth, MN: Western Lake Superior Sanitary District; 2007. http://www.wlssd.com/Safe_Solutions_Toxic_Problems.pdf.)

lengthy process required to prove that a substance is harmful. In fact, under current regulatory practice, proponents of harmful activities are served by investment in research that prolongs uncertainty. Many smokers died of lung cancer before cause and effect were definitively established between cigarette smoking and lung cancer. Application of the precautionary principle has become a critical component of environmental agreements throughout the world because it proactively combines scientific rigor from all current available evidence with the primary concern of protecting public health and serves as an effective evidence-informed tool. When human health and environmental health are at stake, protective action is the most ethical course of action, even when it precedes unequivocal scientific certainty. The challenge is that application of the precautionary approach is still limited in scope. The following two examples demonstrate the importance of these considerations.

Nanotechnology

Nanomaterials are engineered particles made to have extremely small dimensions to take advantage of unique physical and chemical properties that exist at the nanoscale. As a result of their unique size, the physical and chemical properties of nanomaterials differ from those of their larger-scale particles, and they may act unpredictably and in ways that are currently not understood. For example, evidence indicates that nanomaterials can pass through skin and blood–brain barriers[5] and exhibit a host of negative health impacts.[6-9] Scientific bodies have recommended that nanomaterials be treated and regulated as

new chemicals[10] and that the precautionary principle be applied.[11] Nonetheless, hundreds of consumer products and food additives in the marketplace contain nanomaterials. These products are typically undisclosed and untested for their impacts on human and environmental health.

Genetically Engineered Foods

Genetically engineered (GE) foods were first introduced to the marketplace in 1994 when producers in the United States brought out the Flavr Savr tomato. In 1996, GE soy became the first GE crop to be widely grown. GE technologies incorporate genetic material into the food supply to produce foods that would not otherwise occur in nature. Up to 70% of packaged foods in the U.S. supermarkets may contain ingredients from GE corn,[12] soy, canola,[13] or sugar.[14] In 2009, GE beets were introduced to the U.S. market. U.S. residents have therefore been consuming GE foods without the benefit of adequate studies to ensure that these foods will have no adverse impacts on human or animal health or on the environment. Health concerns associated with GE foods include both potential human and ecological impacts. These include allergies,[15] antibiotic resistance,[16-23] food toxicity,[24-28] threats to nontarget species by contamination,[29-32] and gene dispersal.[33-39] Moreover, GE crop use promotes the increased use and toxicity of pesticides.[40-43]

In 1992, the U.S. Food and Drug Administration (FDA) declared that GM crops are generally regarded as safe (GRAS) and therefore do not require any safety evaluations or labeling of genetically modified organisms (GMOs).[44] Problematically, technology stewardship agreements state that the purchase of genetically modified seeds from patent owners (such as Monsanto) for purposes of research is explicitly prohibited unless that research is approved by the technology proponents. Leading researchers released a statement concluding that "as a result of restricted access, no truly independent research can be legally conducted on many critical questions regarding the technology, its performance, its management implications,...and its interactions with insect biology."[45] We continue to face a paucity of studies specifically designed to assess the potential for health effects from GE foods or feed.[46] In 2005, a Parliamentary Assembly of the Council of Europe noted the health and safety issues around GE crops and the lack of studies assessing these threats by stating that "the health risks to humans (allergies, nutritional effects, etc.) so far have hardly been examined...[and] there is as yet no reliable information concerning their medium- and long-term environmental effects."[47] Scientists have stated that the scarcity and contradictory nature of the scientific evidence published to date prevents conclusive claims of safety, or of lack of safety, of GMOs.[48]

In 2011, the Parliamentary Assembly adopted a resolution[49] that highlights the contrast between the U.S. approach to GMOs, which assumes safety without research, and the European approach, which hinges on the precautionary principle. Moreover, the resolution recommended that member countries "take the necessary steps to label products containing GMOs or derived from animals fed with GMOs" and "that the European Union guarantee the right of its member states to decide whether or not to cultivate genetically modified plants and, if such cultivations exist, to establish GMO-free zones." In 2009, a leading U.S. Catholic health system introduced a policy aimed at preferentially purchasing GE-free foods.[50] By 2011, the American Academy of Environmental Medicine (AAEM),[51] the American Nurses Association, the Illinois Public Health Association,[52] and the American Public Health Association[53] endorsed resolutions calling, in part, for the labeling of GMO foods. Specifically, the AAEM stated, "with the precautionary principle in mind, because GM foods have not been properly tested for human consumption and because there is ample evidence of probable harm, the AAEM asks, in part, that physicians educate their patients, the medical community, and the public to avoid GM foods when possible and provide educational materials concerning GM foods and health risks."[51] As of mid-2015, the European Union, Japan, Russia, and China were among the 64 nations worldwide that required GMO foods to be labeled. The European Union has also banned the cultivation of GMO crops altogether, with only minor exceptions. Vermont, Connecticut, and Maine have already passed labeling laws and, as of 2013, more than 70 labeling bills or ballot initiatives were introduced across 30 states.[54]

PRESSING ECOLOGICAL PROBLEMS IN TODAY'S WORLD: THREE EXAMPLES

Exploring ecological health can feel daunting when we begin to comprehend the profound impact of modern life on the planet and its inhabitants. Remaining ignorant with respect to ecological issues or adopting a mindset that an individual has little power to influence the solution is not uncommon. Patients have questions about these issues and look for answers and understanding about how to process these concerns, become empowered, and feel hopeful. Health care practitioners have an important opportunity to engage populations in an understanding of a systems model of health. Clinicians can help them link harm to the planet and harm to themselves and offer health-promoting strategies. The following three interrelated examples are critically important to understand as we engage with our patients and the broader community.

Chemical Exposures and Associated Policies

Since 2000, studies conducted by the U.S. Centers for Disease Control and Prevention (CDC)[55] have documented the scale of our toxic body burden, as measured in human blood and urine. Many toxic chemicals have also been identified in umbilical cord blood, thereby demonstrating in utero exposure. Epigenetic programming is commonly disrupted by environmental exposures, particularly during sensitive windows of development.[56-58] Some well-known human endocrine disruptors include diethylstilbestrol (DES), dioxin, polychlorinated biphenyls (PCBs), dichlorodiphenyl trichloroethane (DDT) and other pesticides, bisphenol A (BPA), and phthalates. Unlike some chemicals, these disruptors have no threshold of toxicity, and their effects do not correlate linearly with the magnitude of exposure; thus miniscule exposures can result in dramatic impacts on function. A newly recognized class of compounds called *obesogens* interferes with the body's adipose tissue biology, endocrine hormone systems, or central hypothalamic-pituitary-adrenal axis. Obesogens are implicated in derailing the homeostatic mechanisms important to weight control.[59-61] Organizations including the World Health Organization (WHO) and the Endocrine Society recognize that industrial chemicals provide a significant risk to public health.[62,63] Substances for use outside of the food and drug industries may be introduced into the marketplace without assessment for toxicity. Thus the burden of harm is on consumers, rather than on product manufacturers. Of the more than 80,000 chemicals in use today, approximately 5000 are used pervasively. At the heart of many of the issues associated with toxic chemicals is the Toxic Substances Control Act of 1976 (TSCA), which was created with the intent to identify and regulate dangerous chemicals. A 2009 report by the U.S. Government Accountability Office (GAO) included the TSCA on its "High-Risk" areas of government needing immediate reform. The GAO concluded that the Environmental Protection Agency (EPA) "does not have sufficient chemical assessment information to determine whether it should establish controls to limit public exposure to many chemicals that may pose substantial health risks."[64]

No animal or individual experiences one toxin at a time, but toxicity studies are conducted individually. Although chemical mixtures represent a huge unknown area in toxicology, chemicals interact with one another to produce effects that may be inhibitory, additive, or synergistic.[65] The American Medical Association advocates for a comprehensive chemicals policy in line with current scientific knowledge and the training of medical students, physicians, and other health professionals about the human health effects of toxic chemical exposures.[66]

Food and Water Concerns

Since the early 20th century, we have radically altered the way we produce and distribute food. The industrialization of our food system is fundamentally affecting the health of individuals and the planet. Not only are the foods we promote misaligned with dietary guidelines but also methods of their production and distribution, divorced from natural ecological processes, are promoting increased antibiotic-resistant bacteria, poisoned air and water, foodborne pathogens, pollinator impacts,[67] and collapsing rural communities.

The impact of pesticides on pollinators is worth highlighting. Bees pollinate approximately 75% of the fruits, nuts, and vegetables grown in the United States.[68] We are currently experiencing a growing problem with bee colony collapse; worldwide, the population of honeybees used as pollinators has been declining precipitously. A report released from the Public Library of Science[69] identified a "remarkably high level" of 98 pesticides/metabolites in bee pollen. No single cause of bee colony collapse has been conclusively proven, but chemical contamination and pathogens are leading theories.[70,71]

> Bees pollinate 75% of food produce in the United States. Bee colony collapse threatens this food supply and may be associated with pesticides because high levels of pesticide metabolites are found in bee pollen.

Because poor nutrition is a risk factor for four of the six leading causes of death in the United States (i.e., heart disease, stroke, diabetes, and cancer), the public health, medical, nursing, and hospital communities have recognized the need to address the food system by promoting nutritious foods from sustainable food systems[72-75] (Boxes 108.1 and 108.2). A United Nations report, endorsed by 57 countries, has called for support of agroecology and local, sustainable economic food models if we are to support ecological services and health communities and reduce hunger.[76,77]

Like food, water is essential for life and good health. The water crisis is the foremost global risk on the basis of the impact to society as a measure of devastation.[78] According to the United Nations, around 700 million people in 43 countries currently suffer from water scarcity. By 2025, 1.8 billion people will be living in countries or regions with absolute water scarcity and two-thirds of the world's population could be living under water-stressed conditions. With the existing climate change scenario, almost half of the world's population will be living in areas of high water stress by 2030, including between 75 million and 250 million people in Africa.[79]

BOX 108.1   Key Principles of Chemical Policy

KEY PRINCIPLES OF A HEALTH-ORIENTED CHEMICALS POLICY

- Immediately initiate action on the worst chemicals. Persistent bioaccumulative toxins are uniquely hazardous.
- Request for basic information for all chemicals. Manufacturers should be required to provide basic information on the health hazards associated with their chemicals, how they are used, and the ways that the public or workers could be exposed.
- Protect the most vulnerable.
- Hold industry responsible for demonstrating chemical safety.
- Promote safer alternatives.
- Ensure the right to know.

Adapted from the Safer Chemicals, Healthy Families Coalition: www.saferchemicals.org.

BOX 108.2   Sustainable or Healthy Food System Characteristics

- Proximate (obtained close to home)
- Healthy, as part of a balanced diet
- Fairly traded
- Nonexploitive
- Environmentally beneficial
- Accessible and affordable
- Meeting animal welfare standards
- Socially inclusive
- Encouraging knowledge of food and food culture

Although most of the U.S. population has access to fresh, treated water, increasing concerns are associated with contaminated water[80-82] and with water scarcity resulting from drought or resource depletion as agriculture, industry, and households become increasingly affected by climate change. In the United States, 40 of 50 state water managers expect water shortages in some portion of their states under average conditions by 2023.[83] Adding to the complexity is the role of water privatization in which water companies are purchasing aquifers, water supplies, and watersheds that had previously been held in the common domain.

Climate Change

According to the Intergovernmental Panel on Climate Change, warming of the climate system is now unequivocal, and evidence from all continents and most oceans shows that many natural systems are being affected by regional climate changes, particularly temperature increases.[84] The direct and indirect impacts on human health are staggering and include asthma, loss of life, a range of infectious disease vectors, respiratory diseases, allergies, and childhood development problems.[85-87] In 2003, more than 35,000 people died in Europe as a result of heat stress. Clearly, the health care system will be required to carry a significant burden in treating climate-related health care costs. Approximately 25% of global emissions leading to climate change are attributable to

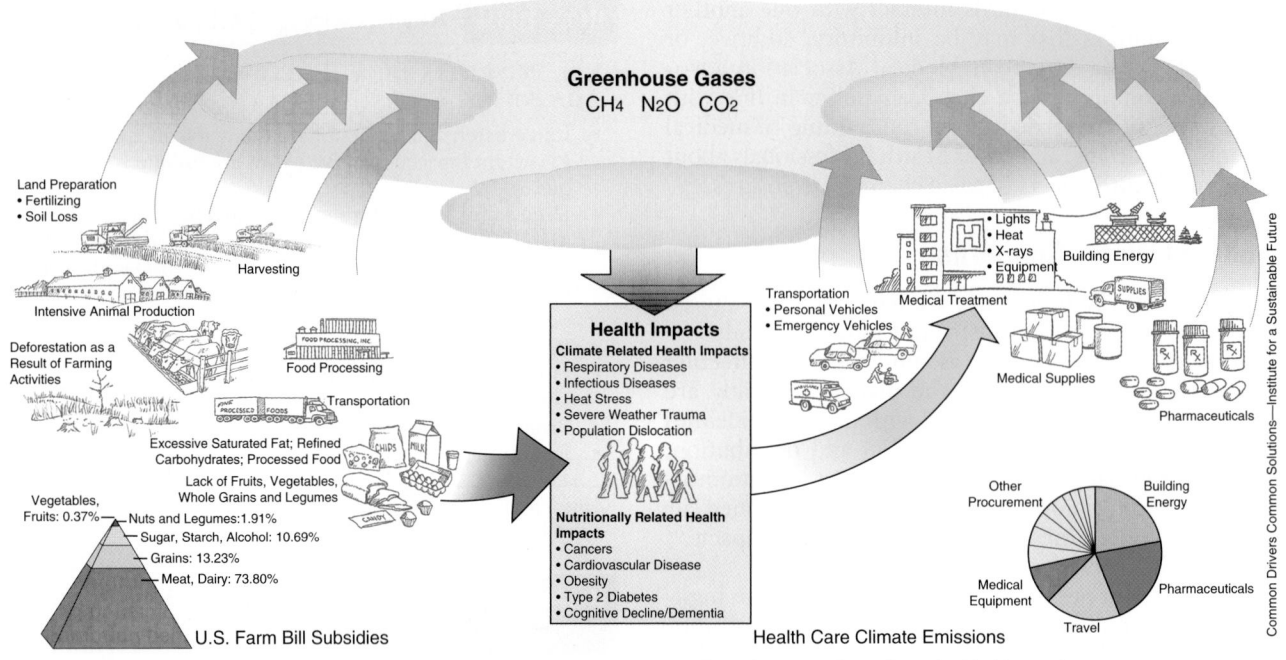

FIG. 108.2 ■ Common drivers common solutions. (From Institute for a Sustainable Future.)

agricultural activities, including land use changes such as deforestation.[88] Without greater efforts to reduce our emissions, these could increase an additional 30% by 2050.[89] We must recognize that health care itself has a sizable greenhouse gas footprint. The National Health System (NHS) of the United Kingdom is a global health care climate mitigation leader through its comprehensive assessment of climate footprint and the development of a climate mitigation and adaptation strategy.[90] The 2004 NHS greenhouse gas footprint was calculated as representing 3% of the total UK greenhouse gas footprint. In a similar, albeit less comprehensive analysis, investigators estimated that the U.S. health care greenhouse gas emissions in 2007 represented 8% of the total U.S. emissons.[91] Consistent with the UK calculations, prescription drugs represented a significant contribution to the U.S. health care footprint: 14% of the total health care greenhouse gas emissions.[91]

Because pharmaceutical interventions are used extensively for nutrition-related diseases, such as stroke, heart disease, and diabetes, and given that our food system is a significant climate emissions contributor, we suggest that a dietary-focused primary prevention strategy would have health and climate benefits. See Fig. 108.2 for an illustration of the role of our food and health systems in climate mitigation.[93] Research indicates that we must increase the resilience of our social and ecological systems considerably to cope with future climate change and other components of global change.[94]

PERSONAL AND PLANETARY HEALTH IN EVERYDAY LIFE

Besides specific occupations and their own unique set of environmental exposures, relative commonality exists in the nature of the foods we eat, water we drink, and products we use on our bodies and in our homes. Moreover, because white collar employment now comprises approximately 50% of the workplace, from an environmental health perspective, our workplaces may be almost indistinguishable from our homes.

Household Products

Many people are unaware of the magnitude of toxic exposure they receive through ordinary household products. Nearly every type of common household cleaner, deodorizer, drain clog substance, and laundry product has been identified as having some toxic properties.[95] Health effects associated with indoor cleaners include cancer, reproductive disorders, and respiratory or skin damage. Cleaning chemicals eventually enter the environment and may have deleterious effects, such as depletion of the ozone layer, diminution of drinking water quality, and accumulation in aquatic life. Some of the less safe chemicals are persistent and remain in the environment for many years or even indefinitely. Many cleaning chemicals are considered hazardous owing to their flammability, corrosivity, or toxicity, and they present safety and cost concerns in their handling, storage, and disposal.[96-98]

Almost all home cleaning products can be effectively replaced by common household ingredients. Recipes for specific uses are abundant on the Internet and available in most public libraries. Typical suggested alternative ingredients are vinegar, baking soda, corn starch, salt, borax (toxic if ingested), lemon juice, olive oil, essential oils, mild liquid nondetergent soaps, reusable nonimpregnated steel wool, and nonchlorine and nonsodium hypochlorite scouring powder. For people less interested in making their own products, many "green" cleaning products are available in the marketplace.[99] Environmentally preferable products have been designated by the Green

Seal Standard for Industrial and Institutional Cleaners (GS-37).[100] Patients should be informed that the safety of a product is not guaranteed even when products are found on the shelves of their trusted stores. Learning to avoid toxic substances does require concern, the ability to read labels, and some scientific literacy. Physicians can help patients by compiling recipes for effective nontoxic cleaning solutions or lists of preferred commercial home cleaners. Hosting demonstrations and lectures in the clinic or hospital settings also send an important message of public health to patients.

> To make a nontoxic home cleaning product, fill a jar with citrus peels (orange, lime, or lemon) and pour undiluted white vinegar over them. Close the lid, and let sit for 2 weeks. Then, strain out the remaining fluid to use as a natural cleaner. Can dilute with water to wash windows or use full strength for washing surfaces and floors.

Because of the toxic persistent cycle, discarding toxic household products can be complicated. As a rule, these substances should not be poured down the drain, flushed down the toilet, or thrown in the trash. Because many common household products are considered hazardous waste, local environmental agencies, university extension services, or public works departments should be contacted for instructions on proper disposal. Some waste facilities have specialized departments that accept and properly manage toxic substances.

Personal Care Products

Most consumers would be surprised to learn that the government does not require health studies or premarket testing for cosmetics and other personal care products. Personal care products include soaps, hair dyes, body lotions, perfumes, cosmetics, deodorants, fragrances, and other similar products. Teenage girls use an average of 17 personal care products per day (compared with adult women, who use an average of 12 products per day).[101]

Serious health effects associated with personal care products include carcinogenicity and reproductive or developmental toxicity. Personal care products are associated with phthalate exposure in children; phthalates are increasingly implicated for serious endocrine-disrupting impacts.[102] Manufacturers are currently reformulating products in Europe to comply with an amendment to the European Union's Cosmetics Directive to ban the use of chemicals that are known or strongly suspected of causing cancer, mutation, or birth defects, but this effort was voluntary within the United States as of 2014. Patients should be counseled to reduce their use of personal care products and avoid products with heavy fragrance, aerosols, and dark hair dyes (which may contain lead acetate). Use of milder soaps and avoidance of nail polish, hairspray, and other phthalate-containing substances (known endocrine disruptors) should be encouraged. Despite the apparent confidence they engender in consumers, commonly used antibacterial soaps are harmful to our ecological system and provide no added protection to household

consumers. Triclosan is a bactericide used in a growing number of consumer products, including antibacterial soaps, toothpaste, shampoos, lotions, and deodorants. Even at low levels, it is acutely toxic to some aquatic organisms, particularly certain algae species, and has been detected in surface waters.[17,103,104] Triclocarban and tricarban are good examples of avoidable toxic substances with pervasive impacts and little to no consumer benefit. Triclosan is problematic for its persistence, its activity as an endocrine disruptor, and its potential to promote antibiotic-resistant organisms. In 2014, the State of Minnesota declared a phase-out of the use of triclosan in consumer products after 2017. As a protective measure to the people and aquatic species exposed, an informed consumer may simply learn to avoid the purchase and use of antibacterial (or antimicrobial) personal care products such as soaps, gels, cleansers, toothpaste, cosmetics, or other "antibacterial" or "antimicrobial" items such as cutting boards, towels, shoes, clothing, and bedding.

Cellular and Cordless Phones

In 1900, our experience of electromagnetic radiation was limited to natural sources. Since 1950, however, we have become increasingly reliant on electric technologies involving various electromagnetic frequencies. Accordingly, concern about health hazards (most notably cancer) has escalated. Conflicting results have emerged with respect to health risks and electromagnetic radiation exposure through microwaves, computers, and televisions. An oft-cited study released in April 2007 revealed an increased risk of ipsilateral acoustic neuroma and high-grade glioma in long-term users (more than 10 years) of cell phones.[105] These same concerns have also been generated by cordless phones.[106] A large subsequent study performed in 2010 by the Interphone Study Group concluded that there is no increased risk of cancer in long-term cell phone users. However, this study has been criticized for design flaws generated by selection bias, exposure bias, and age-range bias.[107,108] In 2011, the WHO issued a press release stating that the International Agency for Research on Cancer, and the WHO classified radiofrequency electromagnetic fields as possibly carcinogenic to humans, on the basis of an increased risk for glioma associated with wireless phone use.[109] Since that time, further evidence has mounted to substantiate concerns of carcinogenic risk posed by cell phones for both acoustic neuroma and glioma relative to area of exposure from cell phone use, and have urged a precautionary approach, especially where children are concerned.[110-112] A newer concern based on compelling case reports is the risk of multifocal invasive breast carcinoma in young women who store their cell phones in their bras.[113]

On the basis of the foregoing studies and the pervasive nature of cell phone and cordless phone use, the Environmental Health Trust has issued practical recommendations regarding cell phone and cordless phone use, including the following:

- Do not hold a cell phone directly up to your head. Use a headset or speakerphone when using the device, or a nonmetal case that has been independently tested to reduce radiation up to 90%.

- Pregnant women should keep cell phones away from their abdomen and men who wish to become fathers should not keep these phones on while in their pocket.
- Do not allow children to play with or use your cell phone. Older children should use a headset or speakerphone when talking on a cell phone.
- Do not text and drive and only use specially adapted antennas when using mobile phones in cars to avoid absorbing maximum power as the phone moves from one cell system to another. When buying a new car, pay attention that the car has a built-in antenna that reduces your direct exposure.
- Turn off your wireless router at night to minimize exposure to radiation.
- Eat green vegetables and get a good night's sleep in a dark room to enhance natural repair of DNA that may have been damaged by radiation.

As wireless usage escalates, it is anticipated that further evidence of harm will continue to emerge. Cities and countries outside of the United States have accordingly adopted proactive policies to curtail exposures, especially in children.

Household Pesticides

The use of pesticides is widespread, and homeowners use substantially more per acre than does the agriculture sector. House dust typically contains concentrations of pesticides and other endocrine-disrupting compounds of magnitudes higher than outdoor air.[114,115] In a Nonoccupational Pesticide Exposure Study, a cross section of homes was found to contain pesticide residues, including those of substances banned years earlier.[116]

By their very nature, pesticides tend to show a high degree of toxicity because they are designed to kill certain organisms and thus create some risk of harm. Within this context, pesticide use has raised serious concerns not only of potential effects on human health but also about impacts on wildlife and sensitive ecosystems. Often, pesticide applications prove counterproductive because they kill beneficial species such as natural enemies of pests and increase the chances of development of resistance to pesticides among pests. Furthermore, many end users have poor knowledge of the risks associated with the use of pesticides, including the essential role of the correct application and the necessary precautions. Even farmers who are well aware of the harmful effects of pesticides are sometimes unable to translate this awareness into their practices.[117]

The Ontario College of Family Physicians completed an extensive literature review of pesticides and determined that "Exposure to all the commonly used pesticides...has shown positive associations with adverse health effects. The literature does not support the concept that some pesticides are safer than others; it simply points to different health effects with different latency periods for the different classes."[118] The College urged a focus on reducing exposure to all pesticides rather than targeting specific pesticides or classes. The investigators encouraged family doctors to learn about high-risk groups (women of childbearing age, occupationally exposed patients, children) and teach methods of reducing pesticide exposures.

Physicians are ideally suited to bring these issues to the grounds of hospitals, schools, and government facilities and suggest safer, yet effective, alternatives for landscaping and lawn care. Finally, the College suggested that physicians convey health concerns to politicians who make regulatory decisions about pesticide use and public health. As of 2010, every province and territory in Canada has pesticide-related legislation in place to protect its citizens from unnecessary exposure.

Various reduction strategies exist through the application of integrated pest management (IPM), an approach to pest management that focuses on preventing and managing pest problems through nontoxic methods by using a hierarchy of strategies, with chemical controls as a last resort. Homeowners who use a pest control or lawn maintenance company should clearly communicate an IPM plan to the contractor. Many contractors now employ IPM, but homeowners are encouraged to request a thorough explanation of individual company IPM policies.

Furnishings

That furnishings of the typical U.S. home contain toxins is not intuitively obvious. However, substances such as wrinkle-resistant fabrics, permanent press sheets, curtains, and clothing, as well as modern furniture made from pressed composite wood, contain and emit formaldehyde and other substances. Carpeting is usually made of synthetic fibers that have been treated with pesticides, fungicides, and adhesives. Many office carpets emit a chemical called *4-phenylcyclohexene*, an additive to the latex backing used in more commercial and home carpets, which is thought to be one of the chemicals responsible for "sick" office buildings.[119] Modern furniture also contains a significant amount of plastics and foam, which are highly flammable petroleum-based products requiring chemical flame retardants (polybrominated diphenyl ethers [PBDEs]). This is a topic of growing concern in environmental health. Perfluorinated compounds (PFCs), associated with fabric protectors and stain guards, constitute another type of persistent bioaccumulative toxin (PBT) of increasing concern. Vinyl (polyvinylchloride [PVC]) plastic coverings contain phthalates and release dioxin and furans during manufacture and breakdown.

Patients, let alone design professionals, may have trouble discerning the differences among various product components. As a general rule, products constructed from solid wood, metal, and natural fibers such as cotton and wool tend to be safe alternatives.

Meat, Poultry, and Seafood

Confined (or Concentrated) Animal Feedlot Operations (CAFOs) epitomize the extreme of our industrialized food system. These operations confine large quantities of livestock to a closed area where all food and water inputs are carefully controlled. CAFOs are defined as more than 1000 beef cattle, 2500 hogs, or 100,000 broiler hens; they generate an estimated 575 billion pounds of manure annually.[120] The largest 2% of U.S. livestock farms now produces 40% of all animals in the United States.[121] In 2002, half of all hogs in the United States were raised on large-scale farms that managed more than 5000 hogs.[122] Five companies control roughly 60% of chicken processing, while four companies control more than 80% of the U.S. beef packing.[123] Although not exclusive to CAFOs, many different feed additives are provided, including growth hormones, antibiotics in feed and water, and arsenic. Public health and medical associations have called for a moratorium on CAFO construction because of concerns that include runoff, community impacts, air quality, worker health and safety, and issues of antibiotic resistance,[124,126] notwithstanding issues of cruelty to animals.

The Food and Agriculture Organization identified meat production alone as responsible for 18% of global greenhouse gas emissions.[127] The wide variety of public health and infectious diseases has called attention to increasing concerns with antibiotic resistance.[128-132] The CDC noted that 90,000 patients died as a result of hospital-acquired infections, and more than 70% of the bacteria that caused hospital-acquired infections were resistant to at least one of the drugs most commonly used to treat them. Investigators estimated that more than 70% of all antibiotics consumed in the United States are used as feed additives for poultry, swine, and beef cattle for nontherapeutic purposes.[133] The strong consensus is that agricultural antibiotic use contributes to antibiotic resistance in humans, and more than 300 organizations, including the American Medical Association, have advised that restrictions on agricultural use of antibiotics are necessary.[134] Yet according to a 2014 FDA report, the total quantity of antibiotics that are known to be important in human medicine and are sold or distributed for use in food-producing animals jumped by 16% between 2009 and 2012.[135] Investigators have recommended that health professionals become aware of these trends as they promote healthier sustainable diets.[136] The 2015 Dietary Guidelines Advisory Committee stated that "Linking health, dietary guidance, and the environment will promote human health and the sustainability of natural resources and ensure current and long-term food security."[137] Meatless Mondays is a global movement of participating individuals, hospitals, schools, worksites, and restaurants around the world working to minimize the ecological footprint of meat production by eliminating meat from the diet on Mondays. Institutions and homeowners are utilizing independent third-party certified food labels, such as organic, certified humane, and fair trade, to support sustainable food procurement.[138]

Although fish is a good source of protein and omega-3 fatty acids, some species should be avoided because of PBT content. Mercury is the PBT most commonly associated with fish contamination; others are PBDEs, dioxin, furans, and PCBs. Mercury is bound to the protein component and cannot be removed. Most other PBTs accumulate in fat, which should be removed. Most fish advisories are based on federal guidelines developed to protect the average 160-lb man; patients should be advised to recognize this fact. Patients who catch and eat their own fish should be advised to become familiar with local fish consumption advisories, which are typically developed for specific inland lakes. Many fish stocks are in serious decline as a result of overfishing. In addition, evidence indicates that salmon produced from the aquaculture industry has higher levels of PCBs than does wild-caught fish.[139,140] Similar to industrialized food production, ecological health issues associated with aquaculture are varied including genetic manipulation, fish waste, forage fish, and antibiotic use.[141] Many websites have developed "fish calculators" that allow users to determine "allowable" fish intake based on individualized weight, age, and sex, while others have developed easy-to-use fish consumption guides, which list fish choices that are of concern with respect to both overfishing and contamination.[142,143]

Organic Food Considerations

Conscientious health care practitioners are well aware of the challenges involved in encouraging patients to consume healthy foods. Warning patients about food contaminants adds a layer of complexity to the discussion. However, the issue of contaminated food is particularly relevant during vulnerable periods of life and should not be overlooked. This information can be introduced in the clinic setting and followed up with handouts, community presentations, and resource lists for patients (see the Key Web Resources). Practitioners need not feel the burden of expressing every pertinent aspect of this problem to the patient. They should enlist the expertise of community professionals.

Growing children consume far more food and water per body weight than adults, and their biological detoxification mechanisms are not fully developed. As a result of these differences and the qualities of foods eaten in high amounts by typical children, a child experiences a substantial burden of pesticide exposure in the first decade.[144] Consequently, elimination of pesticide residues is a sensible precautionary strategy. Although families may have budgetary challenges that do not allow for a complete transition to an organic diet, avoidance of the most contaminated foods is a useful approach (Table 108.1). The Environmental Work Group Shoppers Guide to Pesticides in Produce[145] is a regularly updated list of produce that has been found to be highest in tested pesticide residues and are best to avoid when substitutes are available. The Pesticide Action Network's *What's On*

TABLE 108.1	Foods With High Pesticide Content
Apples	
Bell peppers	
Celery	
Cherries	
Imported grapes	
Nectarines	
Peaches	
Pears	
Potatoes	
Red raspberries	
Spinach	
Strawberries	

My Food app is another helpful app that helps consumers identify which pesticides they might be exposed to, along with toxicological data.[146]

Drinking Water

According to the EPA, the United States has one of the safest water supplies in the world.[147] We are fortunate that public regulation of drinking water has provided a public health benefit, but this relativistic assessment does not address potential exposure to unregulated contaminants found in the drinking water supplies or the relative safety of existing standards. The EPA has drinking water regulations for more than 90 contaminants. The Safe Drinking Water Act set up a process for identification of new contaminants that may require regulation in the future.

The EPA must periodically release a Contaminant Candidate List (CCL).[148] The contaminants on the list are known or anticipated to occur in public water systems. However, they are currently unregulated by existing national primary drinking water regulations. The most current list, published in 2011, contains many different industrial chemicals such as perchlorate (used in the manufacture of rocket fuel) and toluene, as well as a long list of pesticides, and even the pharmaceutical hormone estrogen. As of April, 2015, the EPA was accepting comments on a revised CCL.[149] The water supply for approximately 15% of the U.S. population derives from sources separate from public supplies, such as wells, cisterns, and springs.[150] These sources are unregulated and require the homeowner to test the water for safety.

Many patients interested in a precautionary approach install water filters or treatment systems. Numerous systems are commercially available. Ideal water filtration devices are certified to remove specified contaminants. The National Sanitary Foundation International, an independent standard-setting organization, certifies water treatment systems.[151] Water filtration is especially advisable for patients who have private wells in proximity to industrial sites, landfills, combined annual feedlot operations, contaminated soils, or agricultural areas as surface waters are recognized to be contaminated with pharmaceuticals and other contaminants.[152,153]

Patients may be under the misguided impression that bottled water is purer than tap water. A 1999 report, however, found that some bottled water contained bacterial contaminants and that several brands contained synthetic organic chemicals or inorganic contaminants.[154] The report also noted that bottled water regulations have gaping holes, and both state and federal bottled water regulatory programs are severely underfunded. Bottled water costs up to 10,000 times more than tap water (notwithstanding the energy use and pollution costs associated with transport across the country). Bottled water produces up to 1.5 million tons of plastic waste per year. In 2006, the U.S. population consumed more than 30 billion bottles of water, of which more than 80% went to a landfill or were incinerated. Plastic bottles are one of largest sources of marine debris, 70% of which is plastic.[155] Water is essential to human life and an inherent right, but access to affordable, safe, and sustainable water is becoming increasingly difficult around the world. By supporting and promoting publicly owned water infrastructures, the health care community can provide the moral voice for the right to affordable, safe, and sustainable drinking water. Drinking water concerns represent a challenging issue that jeopardizes our planetary health.

CONCLUSION

Rachel Carson was one of the first scientists to raise an alarm about the unconditional belief in "better living through chemistry" and reminded us of humans' intimate relationship with the environment. Clearly, many modern chemicals provide humans with products that are extraordinarily effective and convenient. We must realize, however, that despite the short-term benefits, these products have a host of recognized long-term impacts that have been either purposely or inadvertently ignored. This lesson parallels what we have learned about our unfettered use of energy and the industrialization of our food system. We are reminded that we are part of a system with intricate feedback loops, and as we interfere with these relationships, we may create unintended consequences. These relationships suggest the necessity for an important global shift in our consciousness from the one that has been oriented toward an efficient, linear, Western scientific model to the one with a greater appreciation of an interconnected resilient systems model.

An important approach forward draws from the research on the "commons" by Nobel Prize economist Elinor Ostrom.[156] The commons represent a broad array of "resources" or gifts of nature, many of which are essential human needs such as seed, water, or fisheries. She drew on examples from around the world to show how local communities have worked together to craft, monitor, enforce, and revise rules to limit their behavior and keep their resources available for the long term. From her work, she articulated a set of shared rules, or commons management principles, which, because of their demonstrated success, has spurred thinking and global application. These principles such as transparency and democratic decision making, localized boundaries or "sense of place," and inclusivity are consistent with many of the fundamental tenets of democratic societies. At their core is an acknowledgment of the importance of a system that provides a means to have an equal say in decision-making and the right to health and well-being.

As integrative providers, this thinking is not new. We have recognized the value of pharmaceutical interventions, but we have worked first to explore primary prevention interventions and naturally sustainable treatment options. We acknowledge patients as primary to decision making. Reports by the United Nations Millennium Assessment, the Intergovernmental Panel on Climate Change, and global governmental scientific bodies add a layer of urgency to holistic thinking and provide clarity that human activities are affecting ecological systems. Our action today is imperative and requires an approach that moves from a model of disease treatment to one of ecological prevention (Box 108.3).

BOX 108.3   Key Advocacy Strategies

DEVELOP AND ADOPT AN ECOLOGICAL HEALTH MISSION STATEMENT AND PLAN

Work with your clinic or institution to develop or tailor an existing ecological health mission statement and plan. Use the plan meaningfully to guide purchasing and other practices.

MODEL BEHAVIOR IN HOME AND PRACTICE

Adopt policies and practices within your clinic and institution consistent with your ecological health mission. As products and services become obsolete, change to those that are more ecologically benign (see Key Web Resources).

EDUCATE

Provide resources and information to patients and colleagues within the clinic or institution as hard copies or on the website.

MEET WITH YOUR HOSPITAL CEO

Numerous hospitals and clinics are adopting ecologically sustainable practices and policies. One clinician's voice is an important support for new or existing "green" or environmental teams; many clinicians' voices add potency to the message.

MEET WITH ELECTED OFFICIALS

Elected officials and their staff are interested in meeting with constituents to hear their views. A physician's voice brings considerable moral authority. Most visitors are paid lobbyists representing industry and corporations, not typically the voice of community and health. Call and make appointments, and if that is not possible, speak to senior staff. Elected officials are busy; stay on point to keep your message relevant and concise. Ask for their specific position, and try to gain a commitment. Follow up with a letter, and keep the ball rolling.

OFFER YOUR VOICE TO A COMMUNITY ORGANIZATION

Most community-based organizations have limited resources and welcome occasional help. Offer to write an article for their newsletter, be a spokesperson at media events, or meet with them and an elected official.

SHARE YOUR VIEWS WITH MEDIA

Although media are changing, sharing your views on issues with the public is important. We need more health advocates. Letters to the editor and opinion editorials are widely read and shared. Call your newspaper to learn about word length and other submission guidelines.

HOST COMMUNITY EVENTS: BOOK SIGNING, MOVIE VIEWING

Many ecological health multimedia resources are available. Host a community movie viewing or book reading and help integrate an ecological health message.

CONDUCT GRAND ROUNDS

Grand rounds are an important way to bring the latest science to your colleagues.

PREVENTION PRESCRIPTION

- Substitute nontoxic alternatives for chemical pesticides for home and garden.
- Choose organically grown, locally raised produce and animal products.
- Prefer third-party food ecolabels (http://www.greenerchoices.org/eco-labels/).
- Eat low on the food chain.
- Select "green cleaners."
- Purchase bath and beauty products that are free of phthalates and other toxic compounds.
- Purchase furniture and building materials that are produced from simple components (wood, metal, cotton materials).
- Avoid polyvinylchloride (vinyl) products and polystyrene and plastic containers made of polycarbonate, respectively designated as recycle numbers 3, 6, and 7 on these plastic containers.[157]
- Purchase "green" computers and home electronics with a priority for those that may be returned to the manufacturer for recycling at the end of the product's life.
- Avoid polytetrafluoroethylene (Teflon) and stain-treatment products.
- Avoid antimicrobial products.
- Prefer metal, ceramic, or glass containers, especially for hot and acidic foods.
- Conserve energy and consume less.

Key Web Resources

The Collaborative on Health and the Environment listserve, webinars, and ebook *Story of Health*	http://www.healthandenvironment.org
Academy of Integrative Health and Medicine	http://www.aihm.org
Consumers Reports Greener Choices Ecolabels	http://www.greenerchoices.org/eco-labels/
Green Guide for Health Care (offers tools for creating healthy, healing environments)	http://www.gghc.org
Pesticide Action Network pesticide guide *(What's on My Food)*	http://www.whatsonmyfood.org
Pesticide Action Network physician network	http://www.panna.org/healthnetwork
Safer Chemicals Safer Families	http://www.saferchemicals.org
Monterey Bay Aquarium Seafood Watch	http://www.montereybayaquarium.org/cr/seafoodwatch.aspx
Environmental Health Trust	http://www.ehtrust.org
Health Care Without Harm: The Campaign for Environmentally Responsible Health Care	http://www.noharm.org
Our Stolen Future (database with focus on endocrine disruption)	http://www.ourstolenfuture.org
Science and Environmental Health Network	http://www.sehn.org
Physicians for Social Responsibility	http://www.psr.org
Environmental Working Group: Environmentally Preferable Purchasing Guides and Databases	http://www.ewg.org
Campaign for Safe Cosmetics	http://www.safecosmetics.org
The Story of Stuff (includes videos on the negative effects of overconsumption)	http://www.storyofstuff.org
Council of Canadians: Water	https://canadians.org/water

REFERENCES

References are available online at ExpertConsult.com.

SECTION IV

BIOMECHANICAL

SECTION OUTLINE

109 STRAIN/COUNTERSTRAIN

110 ACUPUNCTURE FOR HEADACHE

111 ACUPUNCTURE FOR NAUSEA AND VOMITING

112 PROLOTHERAPY FOR CHRONIC MUSCULOSKELETAL PAIN

113 NASAL IRRIGATION FOR UPPER RESPIRATORY CONDITIONS

CHAPTER 109

STRAIN/COUNTERSTRAIN

Harmon Myers, DO[†] • Julia Jernberg, MD

HISTORY AND THEORY OF COUNTERSTRAIN THERAPY

In the 1950s, Lawrence Jones, an osteopathic physician in rural Oregon, discovered a novel, highly effective, low-risk form of manipulation that, six decades later, has become an internationally taught technique. In an attempt to ameliorate a farmer's severe back pain, Dr. Jones noted that the passive positioning of this index patient into a position of comfort and holding of that position resulted in the complete resolution of the patient's back pain. Jones followed up this serendipitous discovery with the meticulous cataloging of hundreds of points that could be relieved by precisely positioning the patient.[1] The position needed to treat the patient's pain effectively could be determined by finding specific points of disease that Jones termed "tender points." Tender points were areas that, when palpated, caused the patient to experience discomfort at that site and felt more taut to the examiner or were of a firmer consistency than the surrounding tissue. Jones believed that the cause—and subsequently the treatment—centered on the pathological features of agonist and antagonist muscles of specific joints.

Jones (and subsequent theorists) ascribed the pathological features of a tender point and the associated pain to the inappropriate and ceaseless firing of muscle proprioceptors and nociceptors that were, as a result, constantly "turned on" without any relaxation. Jones termed his treatment of the pain associated with these tender points, "strain-counterstrain" because he hypothesized that a rapid attempt to return a strained agonist muscle back to its neutral position would excessively accelerate the lengthening of the antagonist muscle. Because the antagonist was short while the agonist was stretched out (the strain), the proprioceptors within the shortened antagonist were hypervigilant for signs of stretch (i.e., the "gain" was increased to enhance the sensitivity to subsequent stretch). Thus when the antagonist was rapidly lengthened (the counterstrain) as the agonist raced back to its neutral position, the antagonist's highly attuned proprioceptors could "see" the prompt lengthening as a signal that the antagonist was being stretched beyond neutral, even though it was not actually longer than its neutral length. This false sensation that the antagonist was being stretched led to chronic overfiring of the antagonist's proprioceptors. Because the muscle was signaling "stretch" when it was not actually lengthened, it had no opportunity to turn down the neural discharge. The muscle therefore continually tried to shorten (i.e., was chronically constricted) in its attempt to alleviate the false sensation of stretch (Fig. 109.1).

Counterstrain is simply the shortening of specific muscles that are in spasm. It is a safe and effective therapy for common myofascial trigger points. Compared to other manual techniques it is relatively easy to learn but takes practice.

Strain-counterstrain, Jones reasoned, was effective because it enabled the cessation of the inappropriate firing of the proprioceptors in the antagonist muscle. If the muscle were shortened while it was not contracted, the perpetual firing that relayed the false sensation of stretch could be shut down and the proprioceptors could be "reset" with the normal length of the muscle as the baseline. Thus Jones' therapy is based on the *passive* shortening of the afflicted muscle into an optimum relaxed position that allows the afferent nerve impulses to dampen. As a result, the muscle can escape from signals to contract on a long-term basis.

While Jones was beginning to appreciate the therapeutic potential of strain-counterstrain manipulations, Janet Travell, MD, John F. Kennedy's physician, was embarking on what was to become an exhaustive study of myofascial trigger points and their pain referral patterns. Travell's trigger points were similar to Jones' tender points—in that they were nodular, taut areas in muscle that were tender to palpation. Travell noted that trigger points could refer pain to areas beyond the region of the trigger point, and she extensively mapped out both mundane and unexpected referred sites. For instance, Travell noted that a trigger point in the soleus muscle in the leg could cause pain in the leg, the sacral area and, surprisingly, the jaw. Travell's therapy of the trigger points differed markedly from Jones' counterstrain manipulations. Travell's preferred method of treating trigger points was to topically anesthetize the skin using a cold spray and then to stretch out the muscle containing the trigger point. In addition, injection into a trigger point was also noted to relieve the associated pain (Box 109.1).

Harmon Myers, DO, was an early student and a subsequent teacher of Jones' technique. Myers synthesized the joint-centered tender points and manipulations of Jones with Travell's myofascial referral patterns of pain stemming from muscular trigger points. Myers realized that Jones' tender points and counterstrain treatment positions actually were locating and shortening Travell's myofascial trigger points and associated muscles. In counterstrain, the passively and optimally shortened position (held for 90 seconds) allowed the inappropriate firing of the proprioceptors located in the muscle containing Travell's trigger point to abate. When the chronically contracted muscle finally relaxed, Travell's trigger point palpably dissolved and the myofascial pattern of pain ceased.

[†] Deceased

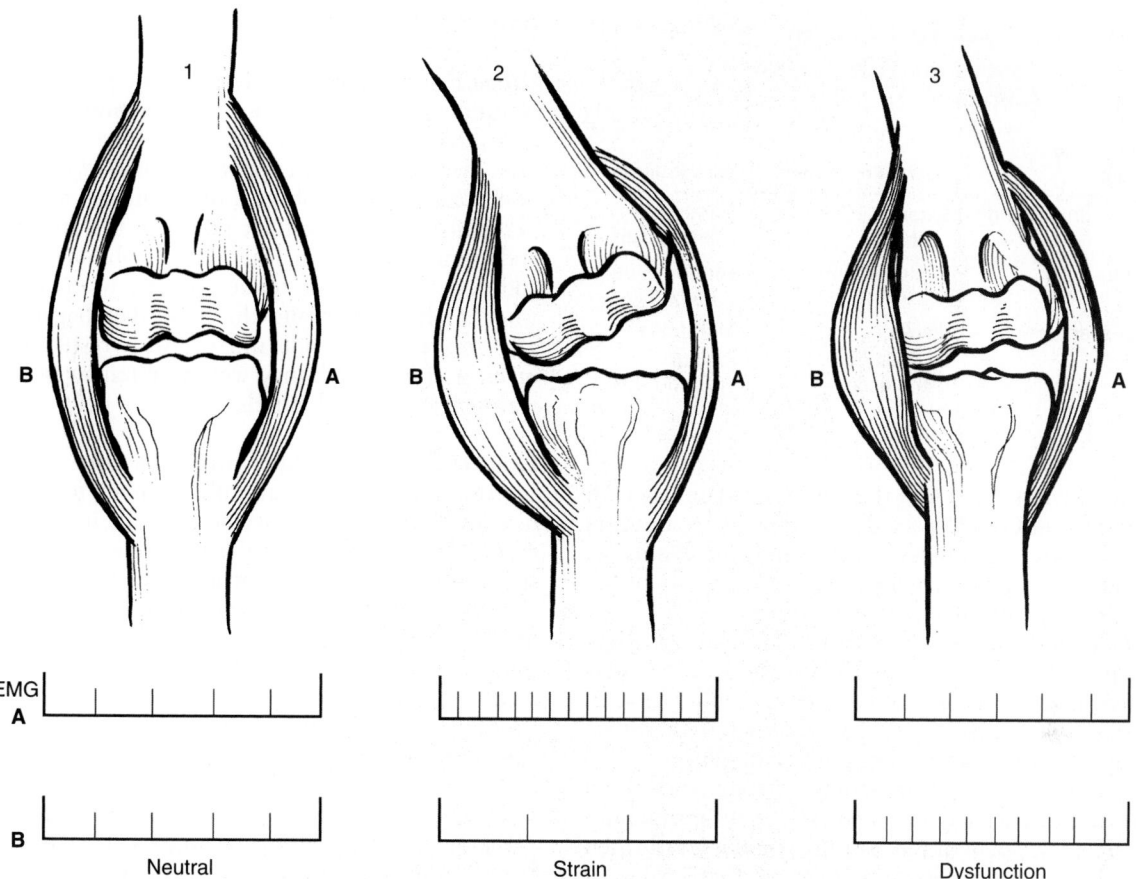

FIG. 109.1 ■ Jones' neuromuscular model. EMG, electromyography. (From D'Ambrogio KJ, Roth GB. *Positional release therapy: assessment and treatment of musculoskeletal dysfunction.* St. Louis: Mosby; 1997; modified from Jones LH. *Strain and counterstrain.* Newark, OH: American Academy of Osteopathy; 1981.)

BOX 109.1	Pathophysiology of a Tender Point

Awareness of tender points in the myofascial system dates back to the Chinese Tang Dynasty (AD 618) when these areas were called Ah Shi points. Descriptions of these points in Western medicine have included terms such as trigger points, fibrositis, muscle callus, chronic myositis, and muscular nodules. The underlying mechanisms of pain and inflammation appear to share common origins. Tender points result from the following three mechanisms:

- A proprioceptive neural response to acute muscular strain that registers the rate of stretch of the muscle spindle fibers
- A nociceptive neural response to visceral disease, muscle strain, or injury that persists because of a lack of response to treatment
- An autonomic–somatic neural response to increased tone of the sympathetic nervous system that can result from anxiety and pain

Within the area of the tender point, proinflammatory and vasoconstrictive chemical mediators, including histamine, prostaglandins, bradykinin, products of anaerobic metabolism, and potassium, accumulate. These mediators team with an influx of calcium ions and lead to chronic hyperstimulation of the associated muscle, thereby causing a neurological reflex arc that further exacerbates and "tightens" the painful muscle. The underlying trigger of this phenomenon can be an acute injury, repetitive strain, imbalance of muscle use, visceral disease, or chronic stress and tension.

Often, complete symptom resolution was obtained with just a few counterstrain sessions. This was true not only for muscular pain but also for other symptoms noted by Travell or Jones. Not uncommonly, patients with complaints of dizziness (sternocleidomastoid muscle), cough (pretracheal fascia and sternocleidomastoid muscle), gastric reflux, and bowel symptoms (rectus abdominis, external abdominal oblique, and longissimus thoracis muscles) dramatically improved with the application of Jones' positioning integrated with Travell's myofascial patterns of pain.

The seemingly remarkable efficacy of this therapy, when administered in a finite number of sessions, along with the relatively benign nature of the treatment led to its appeal among patients and therapists alike. Without further provocation, a few sessions of counterstrain can be quite effective, even for long-standing pain problems.

PRACTICAL APPLICATIONS OF COUNTERSTRAIN THERAPY

Evaluating the Patient for Therapy

To determine whether a patient might be helped by counterstrain, the practitioner must know the myofascial pain referral patterns as well as the associated visceral and

TABLE 109.1	**Myofascial Pain Patterns Associated With Common Ailments**	
Headache and Neck Pain	**Bowel Problems**	**Back Pain**
Sternocleidomastoid	External abdominal oblique	Quadratus lumborum
Trapezius	Rectus abdominis	Longissimus thoracis
Levator scapulae	Iliacus	Multifidus
	Longissimus thoracis	Rectus abdominis

History and Examination

Clues From History. Determine the probable initial or continuing source of pain or dysfunction. This can lead to a directed search for related myofascial referral. For example, a patient with upper back pain who has a history of chronic gastroesophageal reflux disease would prompt evaluation of upper tender points in the anterior rectus abdominis and external abdominal oblique muscles, in addition to posterior tender points, whereas a patient who has headaches and dizziness that began after she ran into a truck's side mirror, with resultant forceful turning of her head, may well have tender points in the sternocleidomastoid muscle.

Exacerbating and Alleviating Factors. Assess what positions the patient naturally assumes to alleviate the discomfort and what movements make it worse. Realize that shortening of the culprit muscle lessens pain and stretching of that muscle worsens it. In addition, active use of an afflicted muscle worsens the pain. For example, low back pain that worsens with lumbar extension could implicate the anterior abdominal muscles, whereas pain in the knee on rising from a sitting position would prompt an examination of the groin for a tender point in the rectus femoris muscle.

Feel the Tender Point. Attentively "listen" to the patient's muscles with your fingers as you search for tender points. Closing your eyes and directing your full attention to the symphony of textures that your fingers encounter will markedly enhance your ability to appreciate tender points.

Treatment Logistics

Once the tender points have been discerned, treatment consists of *shortening* the affected muscles while they are in a *relaxed* state. This passively shortened position enables the constantly firing proprioceptors and nociceptors to sense that continual stretching is no longer occurring; thus they can finally turn down their signal intensity to a normal level. For this to happen, the treatment position must be precisely determined so that the muscle is optimally shortened. A solid knowledge of anatomy helps the counterstrain practitioner envision the correct position, and the palpable softening of the previously taut tender point confirms the optimum treatment position. Subjective input from the patient is also very helpful in finding the correct position. Palpation of the tender point initially elicits a painful sensation in the patient. However, when the patient is perfectly positioned for optimal shortening of the muscle, he or she will experience at least 70% improvement in the level of pain with palpation of the tender point. Often, complete amelioration of the pain with palpation at the tender point coincides with ideal muscle shortening, and the patient is incredulous that the palpating finger is still on the same tender point (as it should be throughout the treatment and after returning the patient to neutral position while the practitioner checks periodically for the texture and the subjective sensitivity of the tender point). Especially when

autonomic symptoms. Once the clinician is familiar with the referral patterns, especially for the more common muscles, a search for tender points within those muscles can ascertain whether counterstrain is likely to be an effective therapy for that particular patient.

To help guide the search for culprit muscles, ask yourself what muscles are stretched when the pain worsens and then look for tender points within those muscles. If a patient complains of back pain and enters the office hunched over (back in flexion), an examination of the anterior muscles (rectus abdominis, external abdominal oblique, and iliacus) may very well yield significant tender points. The back pain in this patient would worsen when the patient is standing straight because of stretching of the anterior (abdominal) thoracic and lumbar muscles.

Myofascial pain is not limited solely to the somatic realm. Multiple examples of muscular pain stemming from the stomach and intestines exist, and ample evidence indicates neural feedback between the viscera and the muscles and vice versa. A thorough understanding of the somatovisceral relationships, followed by subsequent treatment of identified muscular disorders, can prove invaluable in patients who have failed to attain relief by pharmaceutical and other conventional methods (e.g., for gastroesophageal reflux disease, inflammatory bowel disease, irritable bowel syndrome, and the associated back pain).

Some ailments associated with the more common myofascial pain patterns are listed in Table 109.1. More detailed lists can be found in the references.[1-3] Successful treatment of muscle disorders implicated in myofascial pain referral patterns can frequently spare patients unnecessary consumption of pain medications, sometimes prevent surgery (e.g., appendectomy for a tender point in the right lower external abdominal oblique muscle), and, of course, often provide pain relief.

Even if you should decide to refer patients elsewhere for treatment instead of endeavoring to treat them yourself, you must appreciate the contributions of myofascial patterns of pain. A clinician who is adept—or at least competent—in diagnosing myofascial contributions to pain and other dysfunctions will cultivate appreciative patients.

Counterstrain is also referred to as Positional Release Therapy.

a practitioner is first learning counterstrain, the patient's subjective input regarding tenderness from firm palpation of the tender point can be very helpful in guiding his or her proper positioning.

The final test for the efficacy of that position is to check for the disappearance of the tender point on returning the patient to a neutral position. Because the practitioner's finger remains on the tender point during the entire treatment, it is possible to reevaluate the consistency and sensitivity of the tender point after holding the optimum position for 90 seconds. If the maneuver is done correctly, the posttreatment tender point should no longer be tender (or should be at least 70% improved) and should no longer feel taut or ropey in the neutral position.

During counterstrain treatments, the patient is moved into and out of positions very slowly so as not to reset the inappropriate receptor firing with any rapid stretching. The optimal position must be held for 90 seconds to effectively turn off the inappropriately firing neurons. Counterstrain should not be painful, and the patient should not experience any discomfort (except the occasional gentle stretching sensation in muscles opposite to those being shortened). The patient must be instructed to alert the practitioner if any pain or discomfort is experienced, and the practitioner should adjust the position accordingly to ensure that the position is comfortable.

Precautions

Although this technique can be powerfully beneficial, a few potential warnings are in order. Occasionally, the patient will feel sore or have flulike symptoms for 24–48 hours after a treatment, as the inflammatory mediators and byproducts of anaerobic metabolism are released into the circulatory system. This phase typically does not last more than 48 hours, and the patient is usually markedly improved thereafter. A more serious caveat of treatment applies to patients with severe posttraumatic stress disorder (PTSD). Relief of chronic and debilitating pain may destabilize the psychological state of a tenuous patient with PTSD who has come to rely on pain as a distraction from mental trauma. Other than these precautions, if a patient is treated in a position of comfort, counterstrain can be an astonishingly effective, yet reassuringly benign, manual therapy to incorporate in your arsenal.

General Guidelines

Treat Referral Points First

Before you attempt to treat the tender points at the site of pain, search for the important and common myofascial pain referral areas and treat those first. If a patient has a headache, first examine and treat the neck referral muscles (sternocleidomastoid, trapezius, and levator scapulae) before you begin to treat any tender points in the head itself. Approximately half the time, abolition of tender points in these referral muscles alone will resolve the head pain. Similarly, if a patient has sacral or buttock

pain, you must evaluate and alleviate any tender points in the quadratus lumborum or longissimus thoracis muscles that refer pain to this area before trying to remedy any points in the piriformis or gluteus muscles themselves. If you fail to remove disorders in the offending *referral* muscles before addressing the tender points within the area itself, therapy will often be ineffective because the major culprit of the pain—anatomically removed from the site of the discomfort—will continue to cause symptoms until it is treated.

Order of Treatment

Once you have located the tender points, treat the most severe or the middle of a chain of tender points first. Sometimes, this approach can "turn off" adjacent or milder tender points.

Be Slow and Gentle

Move the patient into and out of position very slowly and gently. Ask the patient to tell you if he or she has any discomfort beyond the mild stretching of muscles on the side opposite the one being treated.

Listen to Your Fingers and the Patient

As you strive to position the patient so that the afflicted muscle is at its shortest length, the palpable softening of the texture of the tender point combined with the patient's subjective assessment of the resolution of the discomfort noted during application of pressure to the tender point will guide you to the optimal position.

Hold

Hold the position for 90 seconds. This is how long it takes to reset the inappropriately firing nerves. If pain is long standing, you may need to hold the position for a minute or two more. Use the sensation that the tender point is dissolving to know when the patient can be returned to neutral position.

Check Response

Keep your fingers on the tender point during treatment, and occasionally check back to make sure the tender point is soft and painless. When you return the patient to neutral position after treating that particular muscle, recheck the tender point. It should be at least 70% improved for lasting therapeutic efficacy.

Variations in Position

Although each particular muscle has general guidelines to direct you to the correct position, each patient will differ in the extent needed to achieve ideal resolution of the tender point. Often, younger, more limber patients need more flexing, bending, or rotating, whereas older, stiffer patients experience complete tender point and pain relief with much less dramatic contortion of the body.

Anterior tender points tend to be treated in flexion, whereas posterior tender points tend to be treated in extension. The more lateral tender points tend to need more side-bending or rotation, whereas the more midline tender points tend to evoke more flexion or extension in their resolution.

Comfort Is Paramount

Always treat the patient while he or she is in a position of comfort. Counterstrain is an inherently low-risk therapy as long as the patient is comfortable during treatment. Obviously, extreme extension of the cervical spine (rarely used in counterstrain) should be undertaken with a degree of caution in the older adults or in young women and others more prone to vertebral artery issues.

Sequelae

Inform the patient that he or she may feel sore or have flulike symptoms for 24–48 hours after treatment. Most ailments need three or fewer treatments to resolve. If the pain persists beyond three sessions, the source of pain needs to be reevaluated.

EXAMPLES OF THE TECHNIQUE

This section contains illustrations of referral patterns, tender points, and treatment positions for several muscle groups that are commonly involved in pain. This discussion provides just a short sample, and the reader should refer to referenced resources or continuing medical education for more information.[2,3]

Headache, a common and frequently debilitating complaint, aptly illustrates the need for a clinician to be familiar with the myofascial pain patterns and also provides an example of the ease and efficacy of using counterstrain in clinical practice. Many headaches are associated with tender points in three noncranial muscles: the sternocleidomastoid, trapezius, and levator scapulae. These tender points are relatively easy to locate, and the positions of treatment can be readily learned. Because the neck is not extended, the risk of vertebral artery dissection is not a concern. Thus this is a rewarding set of muscles on which to learn the counterstrain technique. Consider checking to see whether these muscles are implicated in patients with migraines, stress headaches, or other head or neck pain complaints.

Trapezius Muscle

The trapezius muscle, an expansive muscle in the upper back, can have various trigger point locations. The trapezius muscle can refer pain from the posterior neck into the head and sometimes causes discomfort in the frontal sinus area. The two most common tender points (medial and lateral) that refer pain to the head and neck are found by pinching the uppermost area between the shoulder and the neck and are depicted by the Xs in Fig. 109.2A.

Tender Points

- Tender points are located in the fibers of the upper part of the muscle at the junction of the neck and shoulder and are found by pinching the muscle between finger and thumb.
- Medial point: The medial point is found in the webbing at the junction of the neck and thorax (a gentle version of the *Star Trek* "Vulcan death grip").
- Lateral point: The lateral point is found 1 or 2 cm more lateral than the medial point as you pinch out toward the shoulder.

Referral Pattern

- Medial point: Pain can be located at the angle of the jaw, behind the eye, and through the temporal region into the lateral neck.
- Lateral point: Pain is found in the suboccipital area through the posterior neck (see Fig. 109.2B).

Treatment Position

With patient lying on back:
- Medial points: Side-bend the patient's cervical spine toward the side of pain so the ear is moved toward the shoulder.
- Lateral points: Flex the patient's shoulders so that the arms are approximately 150–170 degrees overhead (so that the humerus is through the plane of the eyes), as shown in Fig. 109.2C, and apply steady, gentle cephalic traction (in effect, moving the scapular attachments closer to the vertebral origins of the muscle).

Levator Scapulae Muscle

Chronic contraction within the levator scapulae muscle can be a frequent source of pain in the shoulders and the posterior neck, with radiation of pain into the occipital area. This condition is seen in people with tension and anxiety (chronic shoulder shrug), those who work extensively with a keyboard, or those who regularly hold a telephone between the ear and the shoulder. A hint that the levator scapulae is in need of treatment comes when a patient holds his or her contralateral hand over the area between the shoulder and neck and rubs the upper back with his or her fingers.

- Tender point: This point is located at the superomedial border of the scapula between the scapula and the nape of the neck (Fig. 109.3A). Slide your fingers medially over the scapular spine and move laterally to medially. When the spine of the scapula ends, hook your fingers up and onto the superior medial border of the scapula and press posterior to anterior and medial to lateral against the medial edge of the scapula.
- Referral pattern: Pain is felt in the posterior neck through the shoulder, with referral pain in the occipital area (see Fig. 109.3B).
- Treatment position: With the patient supine, side-bend the neck toward the side of the tender point. Flex the patient's shoulder to approximately 30–45 degrees with the elbow flexed. Abduct the shoulder slightly

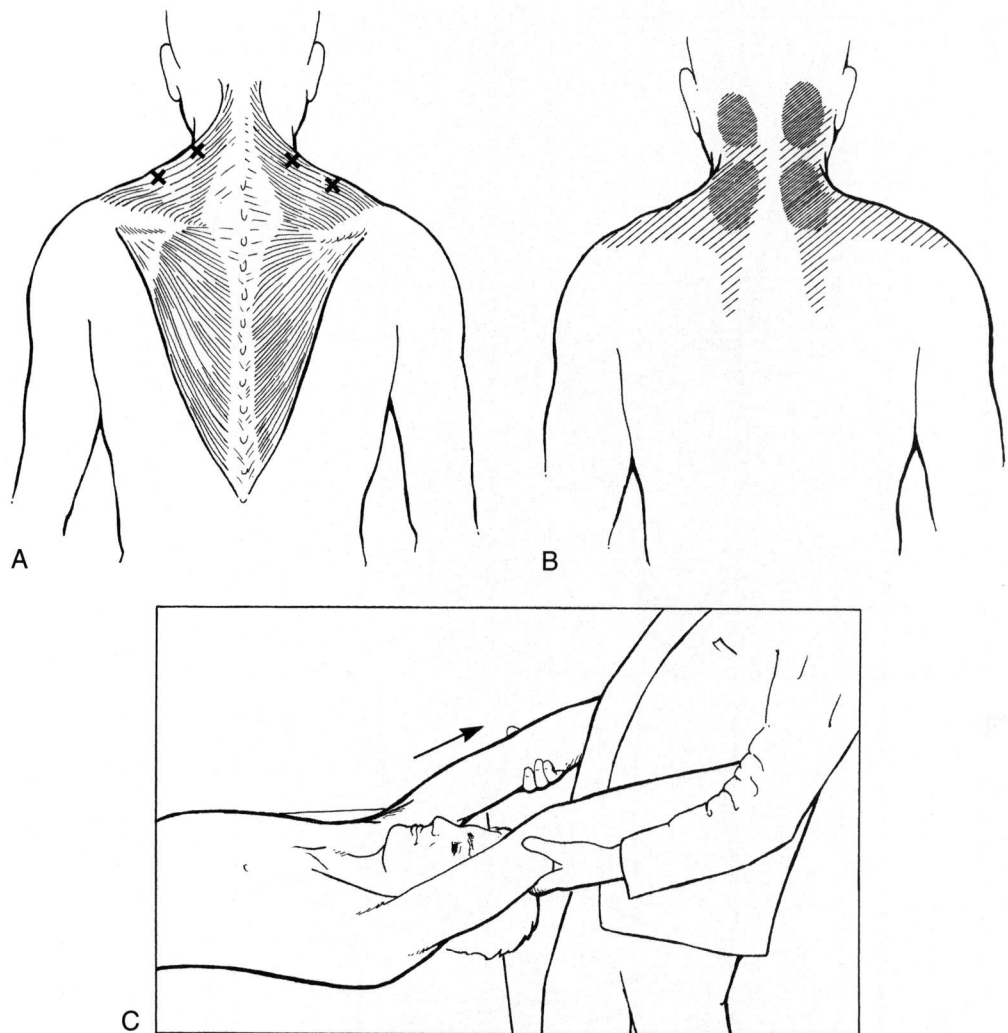

FIG. 109.2 ▪ The counterstrain technique applied to the trapezius muscle. See text for details. A, Tender points. B, Pain referral pattern. C, Treatment position for lateral trapezius points.

and apply a cephalic force through the shaft of the humerus to elevate the scapula. It feels as though you are shoving the shoulder toward the ear (see Fig. 109.3C).

Sternocleidomastoid Muscle

This muscle is a myofascial culprit often implicated in headache, ear pain, or sinus symptoms. Additionally, the sternal branch attachment can be associated with dry cough, whereas disorders of the clavicular belly of the muscle can be associated with postural dizziness and a sense of imbalance. Generally, patients do not actually complain of any discomfort in the anterior neck, and thus awareness of Travell's myofascial patterns of pain can be important in resolving the many headaches and other symptoms originating from dysfunction in the sternocleidomastoid muscle.

- Tender point: This is located anywhere in the body of either the sternal or the clavicular division of the muscle (or the sternal attachment in the case of cough). Pinch the belly of the muscle with your thumb and index finger to help find the tender point. Obviously, care should be taken to avoid carotid massage (Fig. 109.4A).

- Referral pattern: Pain is referred to the suboccipital, frontal, maxillary, or other areas of the head. Further symptoms stemming from the sternocleidomastoid muscle include ear, eye, or temporomandibular joint symptoms; dizziness or imbalance; and dry cough (see Fig. 109.4B).
- Treatment position: With the patient supine, support the head as you gently but markedly flex the neck, rotate the head away from the tender point, and sidebend it toward the tender point. Imagine coaxing the patient's ear toward either the sternum (for the sternal branch) or the clavicular insertion (for the clavicular branch). Sometimes, using a pillow helps the patient relax enough to soften the sternocleidomastoid muscle while the patient's head is elevated off the table (see Fig. 109.4C).

Piriformis Muscle

The sciatic nerve and the piriformis muscle are in close proximity (Fig. 109.5). In fact, in 5% of the population, the nerve runs through or over the muscle, thus making irritation of the nerve much more likely when the muscle

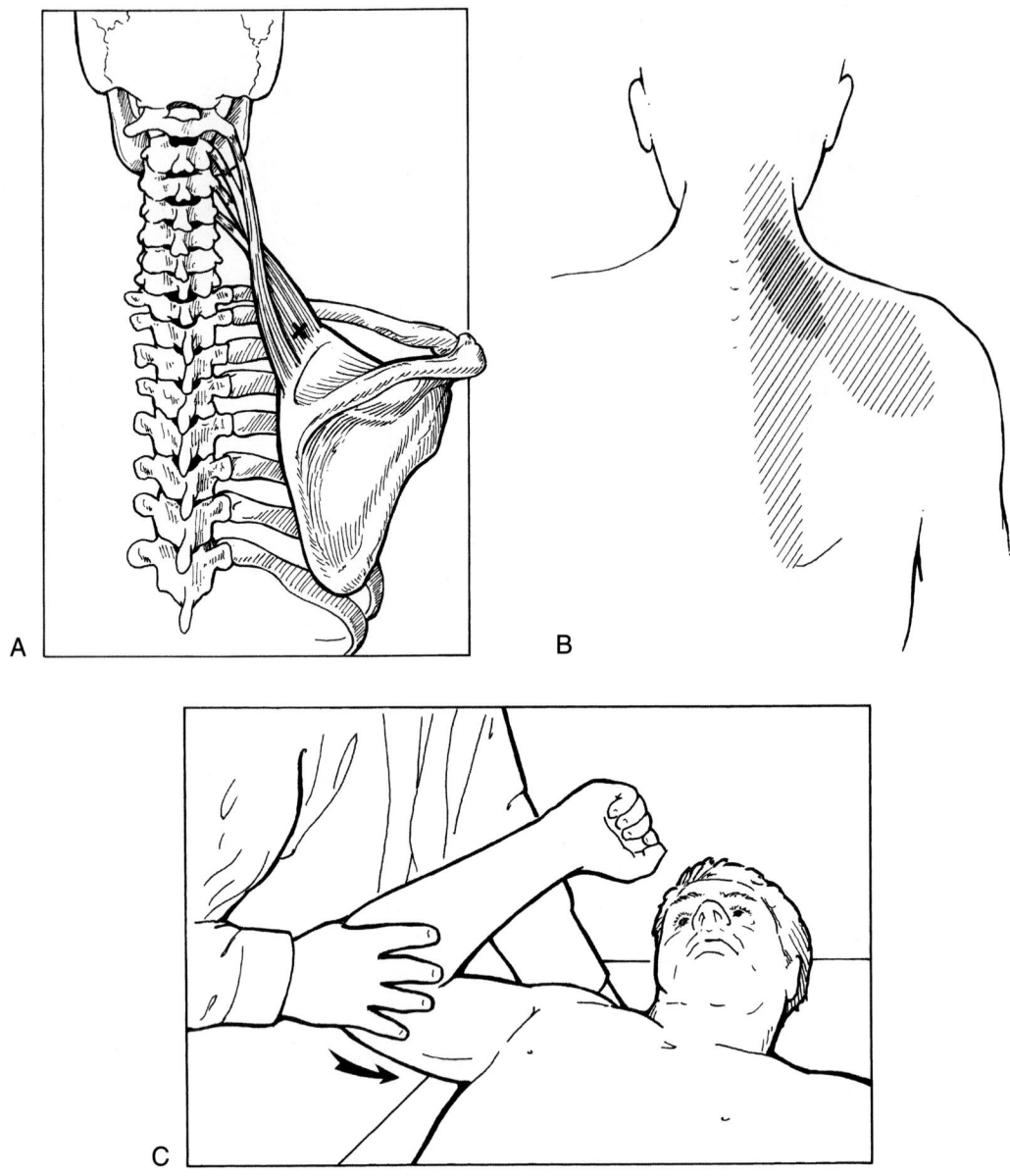

FIG. 109.3 ▇ The manipulation technique applied to the levator scapulae muscle. See text for details. A, Tender point. B, Pain referral pattern. C, Treatment position.

is inflamed. This condition, called piriformis syndrome, is a common cause of buttock pain with radiation of pain down the back of the thigh. Before treating the piriformis muscle, be sure to assess for and treat any tender points in the quadratus lumborum and longissimus thoracis muscles because both these muscles can radiate to the sacral or buttocks area. The rectus abdominis and external abdominal oblique muscles can also be involved anteriorly.

- Tender point: This point is located within the piriformis muscle, which is 3 inches medial and slightly cephalad to the greater trochanter. Tender points can occur anywhere within muscle, which runs between the midsacrum and the greater trochanter of the proximal femur (see Fig. 109.5A).
- Referral pattern: Pain may occur in the buttock and the back of the thigh (see Fig. 109.5B).
- Treatment position: The patient is prone. The therapist sits on the same side as the tender point. The patient's

leg on the tender point side is suspended off the table, with the patient's anterior ankle resting on the therapist's thigh. Flex the patient's hip 120–130 degrees, adduct the hip to tolerance, and slightly rotate the hip internally by gently pulling outward on the foot (see Fig. 109.5C).

BENEFITS

The counterstrain technique is beneficial for the following reasons:

- It often provides immediate relief of discomfort. The benefits are frequently long lasting or even permanent, and they can usually be achieved in a few sessions.
- It readily and efficiently helps the body regain normal function and range of motion that may have been severely and chronically limited by a remote injury that led to continual myofascial dysfunction.

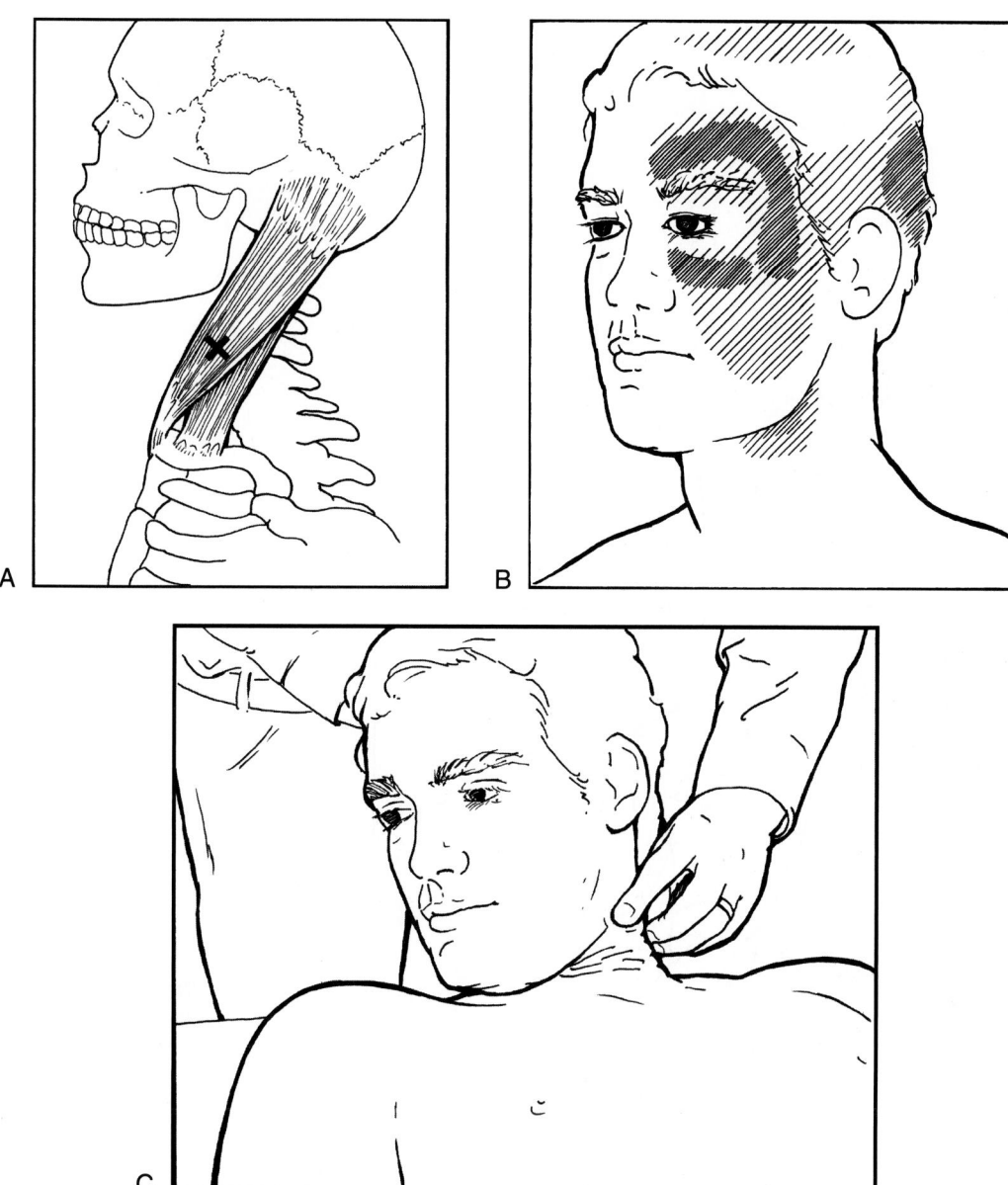

FIG. 109.4 ■ The manipulation technique applied to the sternocleidomastoid muscle. See text for details. A, Tender point. B, Pain referral pattern. C, Treatment position.

- Not only is it comfortable for the patient to experience, but also counterstrain can be highly rewarding for the practitioner to perform. Counterstrain is easy to learn (especially using Myers' method of combining Travell's myofascial trigger point and Jones' positioning) and not difficult to master at an advanced level.
- It enables you to touch the patient and thereby increase a sense of caring and rapport in a time when technology is creating barriers between practitioner and patient.
- In addition to treating pure somatic pain, counterstrain can help relieve visceral symptoms and the associated somatic pain resulting from somatovisceral or viscerosomatic neural feedback loops.
- It uses a position of comfort, with almost negligible inherent risk to the patient.
- The acquisition of this technique can be readily accomplished by most medical practitioners who have a fundamental medical or anatomical knowledge base.

LIMITATIONS

The limitations of counterstrain therapy are as follows:
- Although pain relief is usually permanent, in some cases pain can recur. Recurrence is more likely when the initial source of injury is not adequately addressed.
- A somewhat localized technique such as this may not be the most effective approach for treating a patient with diffuse and disseminated tender points (e.g., fibromyalgia). In addition, it may not be as rewarding when treating someone with frequent or continuous recurrent reinjury (e.g., as seen in untreated Crohn's disease or gastroesophageal reflux disease in which the visceral problem restimulates the somatic disorder).

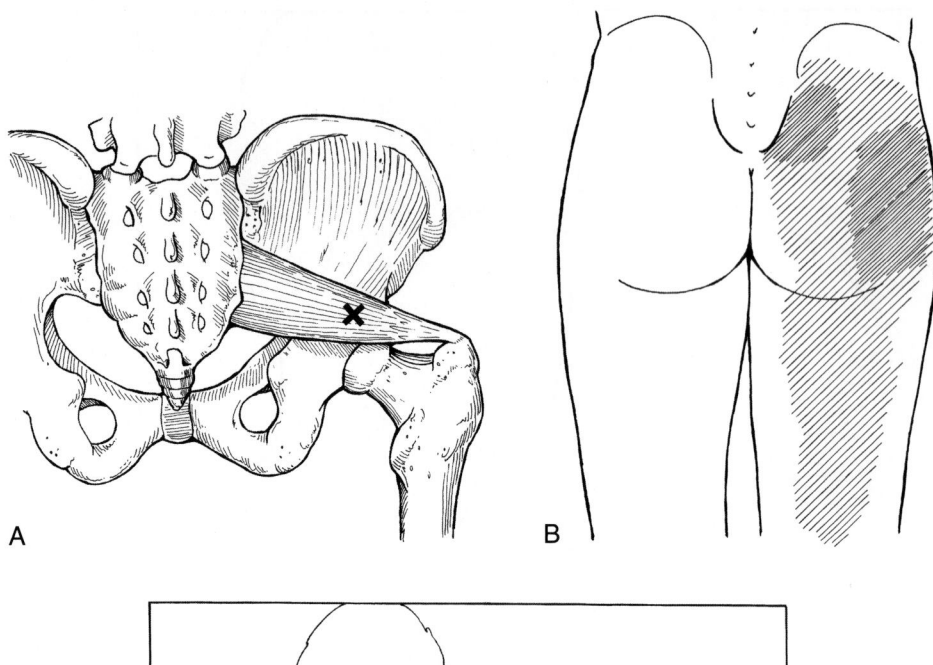

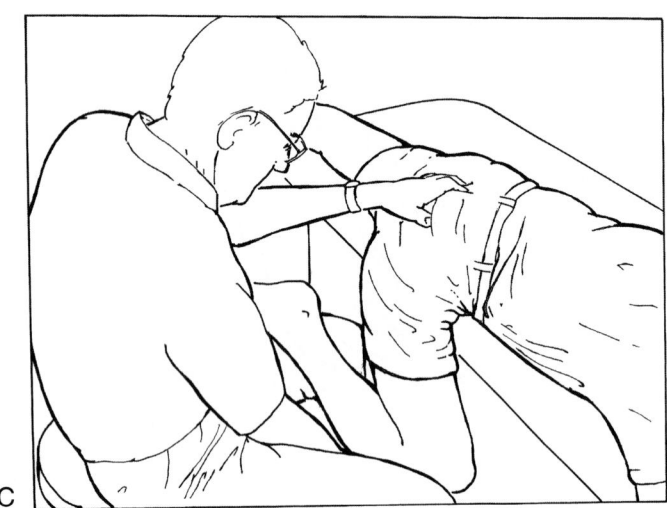

FIG. 109.5 ■ The manipulation technique applied to the piriformis muscle. See text for details. A, Tender point. B, Pain referral pattern. C, Treatment position.

- The technique is conceptually easy to learn, but it takes practice to become thoroughly adept at it. The practitioner should start by becoming familiar with the common and important muscle groups and then progress from there.
- When able, one should begin the counterstrain technique by practicing on children because their limited soft tissue mass allows for easy identification of tender

points and their small frames enable ready maneuverability into treatment positions.
- If psychological problems are not addressed, a patient who "needs" somatic pain to maintain equilibrium can become destabilized. Close coordination with a mental health professional is recommended in patients with a history of severe psychological issues or with significant PTSD before attempts are made to relieve the somatic pain.

Key Web Resources

American Academy of Osteopathy: Many courses in manual medicine, including counterstrain, are offered annually.

http://www.academyofosteopathy.org/

Jones Institute: This organization coordinates counterstrain workshops in the United States and internationally.

http://www.jiscs.com/Article.aspx?a=0

Tucson Osteopathic Medical Foundation: This group offers hands-on classes in strain/counterstrain, taught by Myers twice a year.

http://www.tomf.org

Key Educational Texts

Travell J, Simons D. *Travell and Simons' Myofascial Pain and Dysfunction: The Trigger Point Manual.* Philadelphia: Williams & Wilkins; 2008.

Travell and Simons' two-volume text documenting the myofascial pain and dysfunction referral patterns encompasses an amazingly thorough life's work, replete with interesting observations of common and unique myopathic associations.

Travell J, Simons D. *Travell and Simons' Trigger Point Flip Charts.* Baltimore: Williams & Wilkins; 1996.

This useful trigger point flip chart is based on Travell's work.

Myers H. *Clinical Application of Counterstrain.* Tucson: Osteopathic Press; 2012.

Myers' counterstrain manual combines Travell's findings with Jones' work to provide a succinct, visual, and hands-on approach to learning and applying counterstrain.

Speicher T. *Clinical Guide to Positional Release Therapy.* Human Kinetics, 2016.

Manual for clinicians that also includes access to 60 videos showing the most common therapeutic positions.

REFERENCES

References are available online at **ExpertConsult.com.**

CHAPTER 110

ACUPUNCTURE FOR HEADACHE

Aaron J. Michelfelder, MD

OVERVIEW

Acupuncture is the technique of piercing the skin with needles at specific points on the body to treat or prevent various conditions. Acupuncture has been used for thousands of years by practitioners in many different cultures and societies around the world. Because acupuncture has become more popular, physicians should have at least a basic working knowledge of the technique. The best physicians use all their knowledge of integrative medicine to provide the most comprehensive care available to patients.

Acupuncture points are not random. They are palpable and often correspond to depressions in muscles or bones or to neural foramina. An acupuncture point usually has its own neurovascular bundle, which distinguishes it from the surrounding tissue, and is sometimes quite tender to palpation. In traditional Chinese medicine (TCM), these points connect to energy (qi) channels, called *meridians*, within the body. Fourteen principal meridians (6 bilateral [12 in total] and 2 central) are recognized, typically named after organs of the body: kidney (KI), heart (HT), small intestine (SI), bladder (BL), liver (LV), master of the heart (MH) also called pericardium or (P), triple heater (TH), gallbladder (GB), spleen (SP), lung (LU), large intestine (LI), stomach (ST), conception vessel (CV), and governor vessel (GV).

MECHANISM OF ACTION

The exact mechanism of action of acupuncture is unclear. However, significant evidence indicates that acupuncture effects changes in the muscles where the needle is inserted, changes starting at nerves near the needle and passing all the way up to the higher cortex, and changes in circulating and local hormones, cytokines, neurotransmitters, and other body chemicals.[1]

SAFETY OF ACUPUNCTURE

Because of the use of sterile needles to pierce unsterilized skin, serious adverse reactions to acupuncture are very rare. A systematic review of the world literature on prospective studies of the safety of acupuncture revealed that in nine trials involving tens of thousands of treatments, pneumothorax was the only life-threatening complication, and it occurred twice; infections did not occur at all.[2] A prospective survey of 34,000 treatments by traditional acupuncturists in the United Kingdom found no serious adverse events.[3] In the largest prospective trial to date, involving 97,733 patients and more than 760,000 treatments performed by 7050 physicians in Germany, pneumothorax was found to occur twice, and one occurrence each of exacerbation of depression, acute hypertensive crisis, vasovagal reaction, and asthma attack with hypertension and angina was observed.[4] The most commonly reported reactions were needling pain in 3.28%, hematoma in 3.19%, bleeding in 1.38%, and orthostasis in 0.46% of patients. Overall, nonserious adverse events were reported to occur in 7.1% of patients.[4]

TRAINING IN ACUPUNCTURE

Laws concerning the practice of acupuncture are defined by each state. Practitioners include the following: licensed acupuncturists, who have completed at least 3 years of training at a college of Oriental medicine; chiropractors, who receive variable amounts of training in chiropractic school but may have additional training after chiropractic school; and physicians and dentists who have completed acupuncture training courses outside their regular professional training. For physicians to practice acupuncture, some states require no training at all, others require 200 hours, and some mandate 300 hours of acupuncture training. Board certification is available to physicians through the American Board of Medical Acupuncture. Details on physician training and licensure can be found on the website of the American Academy of Medical Acupuncture (see the Key Web Resources).

TECHNIQUES

Technique for Acupressure

Acupressure is essentially massage, but with the purpose of stimulating an acupuncture point for a desired effect. Acupressure can also be used to relax trigger points, as well as other areas of spasm within muscles that may or may not be acupuncture points.

The technique is to find the point or area to be stimulated as follows:
1. With your index finger or thumb, start superficially and apply just enough pressure to move the skin.
2. Move the finger or thumb in gentle, slow circles.
3. With every few circles, apply more and more pressure until you feel the muscle fibers beginning to relax beneath your fingers. If you are stimulating an area without a muscle, such as over the supraorbital foramen, just keep applying slow, steady, downward, circular pressure over the foramen.

4. With the stimulation of an acupuncture point, the patient should eventually feel a dull, aching sensation. Stimulation of the point should last at least several minutes, past which the patient feels this aching sensation. You may have to apply acupressure intermittently, such as for a few minutes, several times an hour.

This technique is a good one to teach patients to perform on themselves for problems such as sinus headaches and pressure.

Technique for Acupuncture

Acupuncture needles come in all sizes, ranging from very thin (approximately 40 gauge) to much thicker (up to 20 gauge). An acupuncture needle comes with a very sharp point and has a plastic or wrapped metal handle. Because acupuncture needles are not hollow like phlebotomy needles, they are believed to separate tissue more than to cut it (Fig. 110.1).

1. After the desired acupuncture point is found, palpation of the point is important to prepare the body for the needle (Fig. 110.2).

2. A very small needle may need an introducer, which is included with most needles. The introducer is a plastic tube, which is a few millimeters shorter than the needle. Place the introducer on top of the acupuncture point, and then, drop the needle into the introducer (Figs. 110.3 and 110.4). The handle of the needle will protrude a few millimeters from the top of the introducer.

3. Holding the introducer between the thumb and third finger of your dominant hand, tap the needle into the skin using your index finger (Figs. 110.5 and 110.6). With practice, the right amount of force needed to pierce the skin is simple to recognize.

4. After the initial tap of the needle into the skin, carefully remove the introducer. Then, the needle may be pushed in deeper and angled to the desired location. Typically, the needle enters the body of a muscle, but the depth depends on the acupuncture point. A point on the back of the neck may be 2–3 cm deep, but a point on the forehead may only be a few millimeters deep.

Inserting the needles without the plastic introducer requires some training and supervision and is beyond the scope of this chapter.

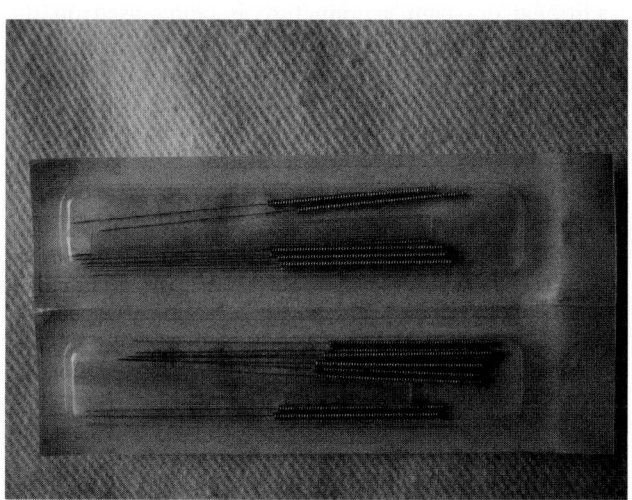

FIG. 110.1 ■ Package of acupuncture needles.

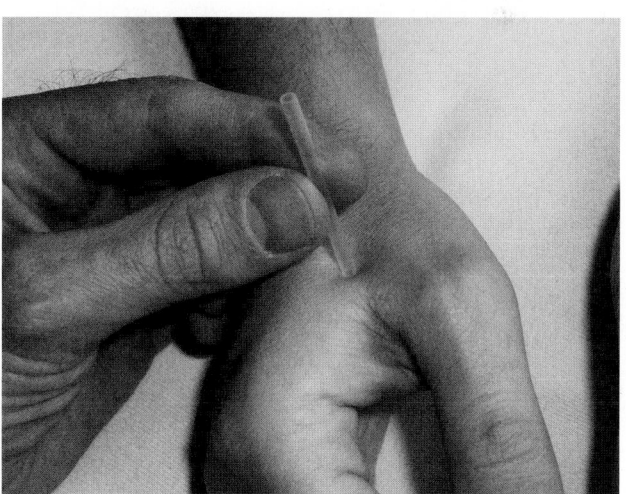

FIG. 110.3 ■ Positioning the introducer.

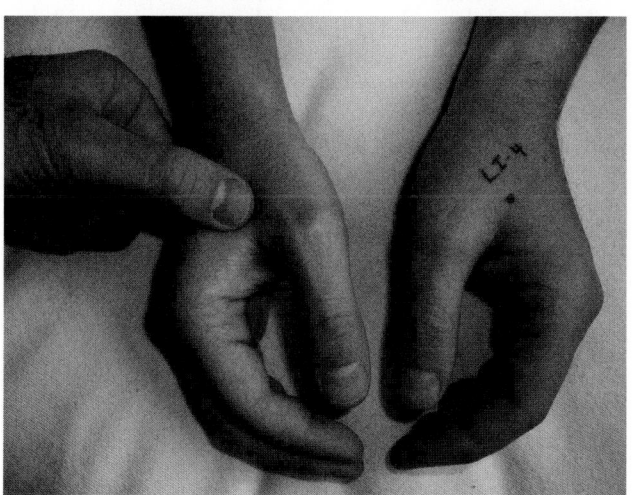

FIG. 110.2 ■ Palpation.

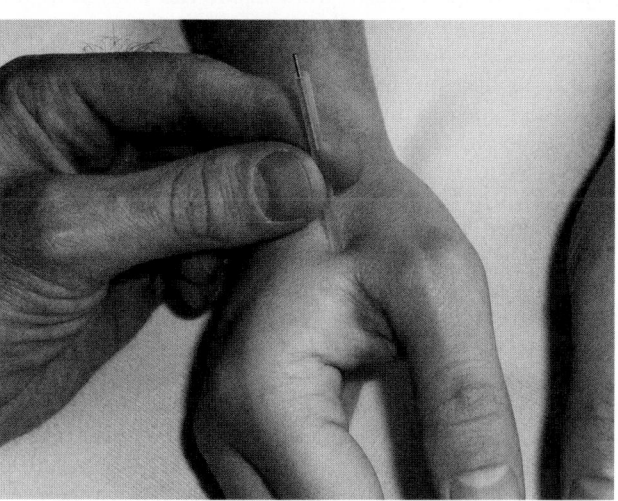

FIG. 110.4 ■ Needle in introducer.

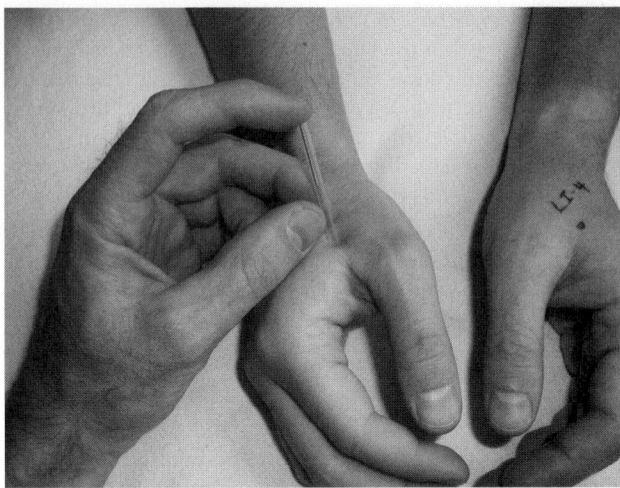

FIG. 110.5 ■ Tapping needle into place.

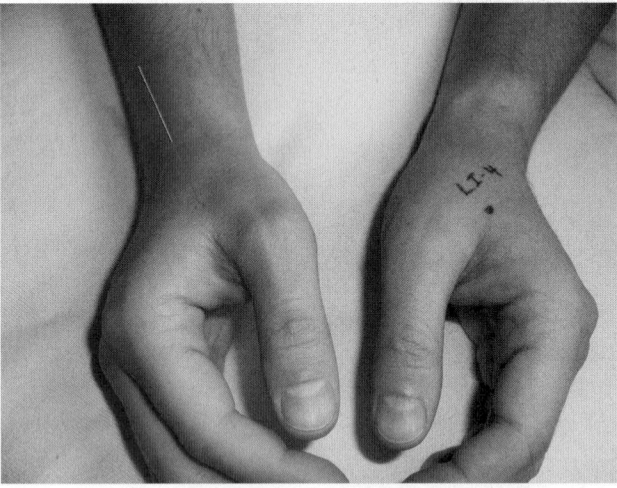

FIG. 110.6 ■ Needle in place.

Once a needle has been inserted, it can either be stimulated or left alone. If it is left alone, the coiled handle and temperature difference between the needle tip in the body and the needle handle at room temperature will cause electrons to move from inside the body into the needle. Inserting a needle and then leaving it alone is called *needle in dispersion*. The needle becomes a capacitor removing electrons from the body. In TCM, this action is believed to be calming, cooling, and depleting.

To add electrons to the body, the needle can be stimulated by a back-and-forth twirling action, which the acupuncturist achieves by rotating the needle approximately 180 degrees, alternating clockwise and counterclockwise. The needle can also be stimulated by warming with something like Chinese moxa, an herb pressed into an incense-like stick that, when lit, smolders and emits a steady stream of heat. Electrical stimulators are very popular and may be connected to the needles in a circuit to add electron flow from one needle to another. This is the process for percutaneous electrical nerve stimulation (PENS), the acupuncture version of transcutaneous electrical nerve stimulation (TENS). Lasers can also be used to stimulate acupuncture points with or without needles.

Both acupuncture and acupressure can be used to stimulate acupuncture points. Patients can be taught to perform their own acupressure, thus empowering them to help themselves.

EVIDENCE FOR ACUPUNCTURE IN HEADACHE

The allopathic tradition of the randomized placebo-controlled clinical trial is very difficult to apply to acupuncture. Defining placebo acupuncture is challenging because many people argue that any needle piercing the skin is acupuncture. Many studies use no acupuncture as the control intervention, or they use sham acupuncture, which usually means inserting needles into places that are not acupuncture points. Some studies have tried to use acupressure as the control. In any case, many studies have been unsuccessful in blinding patients or the clinicians regarding whether they had acupuncture, and the acupuncturist is certainly not blinded regarding whether traditional or sham acupuncture is being used on the patient. Many studies also use protocols whereby every patient receives the same treatment. Most acupuncturists individualize the acupuncture treatment to each patient and modify treatments based on response to earlier treatments.

To put acupuncture studies into context, the U.S. Food and Drug Administration requires only two studies of a drug to show that the drug is better than placebo before the agent can be approved. A drug could show neutral results in many studies, but as long as two studies have positive results, the drug can be approved for use. Possibly because of the difficulties in experimental design, many studies of acupuncture have had positive results and many have had neutral results.

In 1999, Melchart et al.[5] performed a review of 22 randomized controlled trials of acupuncture for headache involving 1042 patients from European countries. These reviewers concluded that the trials tended to be small and had methodological problems; however, the evidence suggested a role for acupuncture in headache treatment.[5] In a well-designed trial reported in 2004, Vickers et al.[6] studied acupuncture in 401 patients with chronic headaches in the United Kingdom. Subjects underwent either acupuncture treatments once a week for 3 months or no acupuncture. Over 1 year, the decrease in headache score was 34% in treatment group versus 16% in the control group. In addition, the treatment group was found to have 20 fewer days of headache per year, 15% less medication use, 25% fewer visits to the general practitioner, and 15% fewer days off work. Wonderling et al.,[7] examining the cost effectiveness of acupuncture for headaches in the United Kingdom, found that acupuncture improved health-related quality of life at a small additional cost and was relatively cost effective.

Two Cochrane Collaboration reviews of acupuncture performed meta-analyses of available acupuncture trials for headache. The first meta-analysis of acupuncture trials included 22 studies with a total of 4419 patients in whom acupuncture was used for migraine prophylaxis. The reviewers concluded that "these studies suggest that acupuncture is at least as effective as, and possibly more effective than, prophylactic drug treatment and has fewer side effects." They recommended acupuncture as a treatment option for patients with migraines.[8] The second meta-analysis concerned acupuncture for tension headaches and included 11 trials with a total of 2317 participants. The reviewers found that patients had a statistically significant reduction in the number, frequency, and intensity of tension headaches over 3 months, but none had studied effects beyond 3 months. The reviewers concluded that "acupuncture could be a valuable nonpharmacological tool in patients with frequent episodic or chronic tension-type headaches."[9]

Yang et al. compared acupuncture to topiramate for chronic migraine prophylaxis and found that the acupuncture group had a larger decrease in moderate to severe headache days, and adverse events occurred in 6% of the acupuncture group compared with 66% of the topiramate group.[10] Additionally, several studies have shown acupuncture to be cost effective when compared with the cost of medications and days or work lost.[11,12] A recent review of all available evidence for acupuncture in migraine prevention concluded that "acupuncture seems to be at least as effective as conventional drug therapy for migraine and is safe, long lasting, and cost effective."[13]

> The latest evidence shows that acupuncture is helpful in treating headaches.

SELECTING ACUPUNCTURE AND ACUPRESSURE POINTS

Selection of acupuncture or acupressure points for the treatment of headaches should proceed as follows:
1. Start with general relaxation or calming points.
2. Release trigger points in the posterior cervical region.
3. Depending on the type of headache, use local points.

General Relaxation and Calming Points

Governor Vessel 20

The GV20 point is located at the top of the head, over the sagittal suture, which is created by the closure of the posterior fontanelle. Often, a bony ridge is present at this point. Visually, GV20 can be found by tracing an imaginary line from the ear lobes up through the middle of the top of the ears (the helix) and up to the midline. The point where that line crosses the sagittal suture (midline) is the GV20 point. Acupressure can be applied to this point, or a needle can be inserted here and left in dispersion (Fig. 110.7).

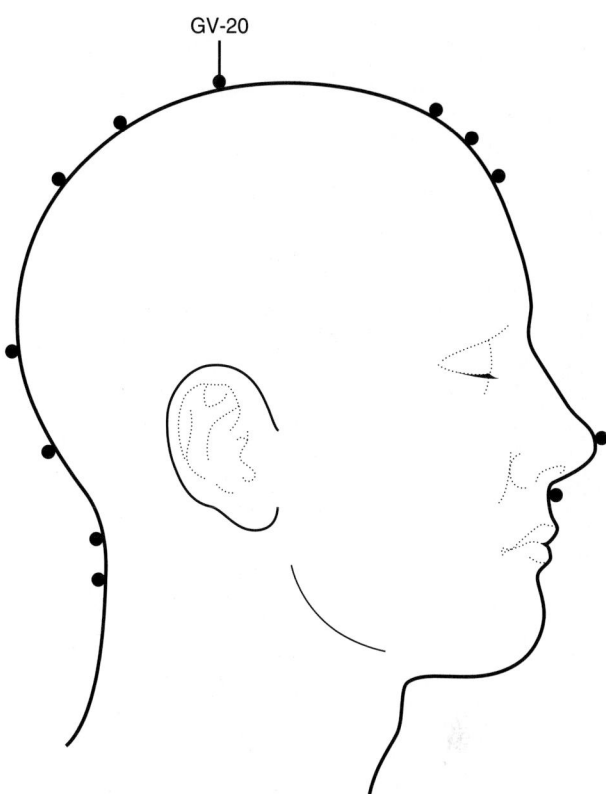

FIG. 110.7 ■ The governor vessel 20 *(GV20)* acupuncture point.

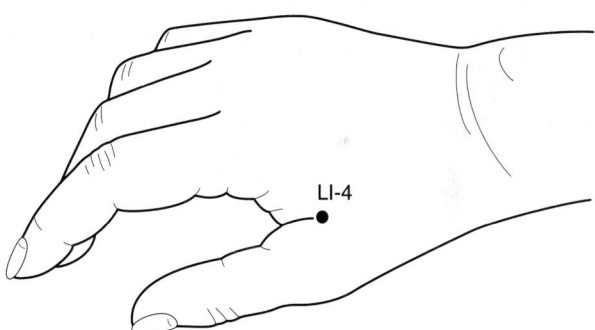

FIG. 110.8 ■ The large intestine 4 *(LI4)* acupuncture point.

Large Intestine 4

The LI4 point is located in the body of the first interosseus muscle in the hand, between the first and second metacarpal bones. This point is usually tender, and patients can easily perform acupressure to this point bilaterally on themselves (Fig. 110.8).

Trigger Points in the Cervical Region

People with headaches tend to have stiff posterior cervical muscles. Massage, heat, chiropractic and osteopathic manipulation, acupressure, trigger point injections, and acupuncture can all help release the muscle spasm.

Gallbladder 20

The GB20 point is located at the base of the skull, posteriorly, between the insertions of the sternocleidomastoid

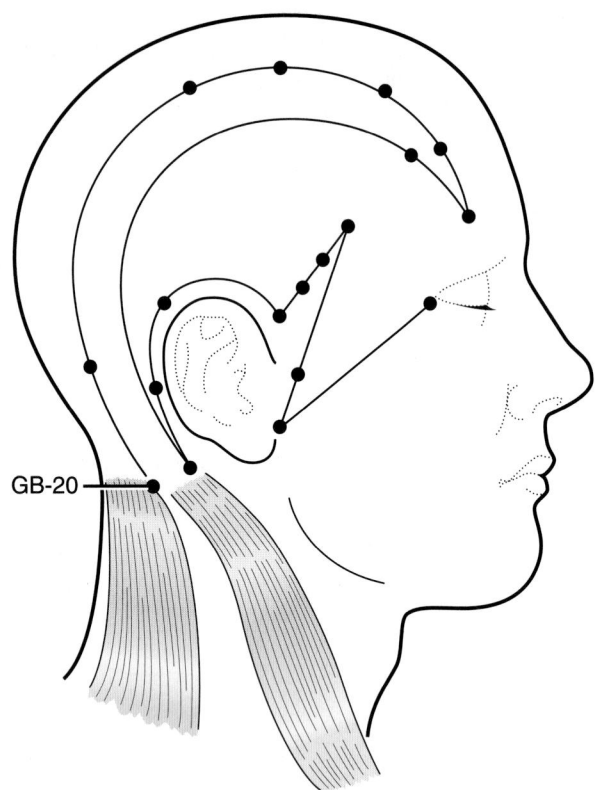

FIG. 110.9 ■ The gallbladder 20 *(GB20)* acupuncture point.

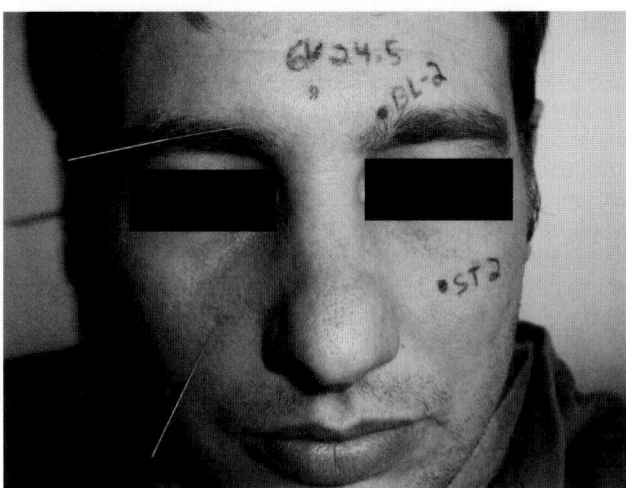

FIG. 110.10 ■ Acupuncture points governor vessel 24.5 *(GV24.5)*, bladder 2 *(BL2)*, and stomach 2 *(ST2)*.

and the trapezius muscles. Start by placing the thumb and index finger of one hand on the mastoid processes and then slide them posteriorly. Your fingertips will "fall into" two depressions at the base of the skull. Superiorly, you will feel the skull. On the either side of your fingers, you will feel the sternocleidomastoid or trapezius muscles (Fig. 110.9).

> Palpate all the muscles of the posterior neck from the base of the skull down to the shoulders. Any tender points or areas of spasm should be addressed with massage, acupuncture, or acupressure.

Local Points

Frontal Headaches

For frontal headaches, including sinus, tension, and migraine, the GV24.5 may be used. This point is located on the glabella between the eyebrows (Fig. 110.10).

Sinus Headaches

- Bladder 2: The BL2 point is located at the frontal notch, just medial to the supraorbital foramen (see Fig. 110.10). Insert the needle from above.
- Stomach 2: The ST2 point is located lateral to the nose in a depression where the infraorbital foramen is found. Needle this point starting laterally, aim toward the medial canthus of the eye, and insert the needle subcutaneously (see Fig. 110.10).

Tension Headaches

- Temporal muscle tender points: Palpate the muscles of the scalp carefully, and perform acupressure or acupuncture at any tender areas or regions of spasm found, especially in the temporal region.

Migraines and Cluster Headaches

Migraines and cluster headaches are complicated to treat with acupuncture. Follow the same principles of general relaxation points, then cervical points, and then GV24.5. After these procedures, search for any tender points on the scalp. If needling tender points on the scalp does not provide satisfactory relief, a more systemic approach with acupuncture may be more successful. Such an in-depth approach is beyond the scope of this chapter.

DURING AN ACUPUNCTURE TREATMENT

Needles stay in place for approximately 30 minutes. Patients should be relaxing in a comfortable room with the lights low and perhaps some calming music in the background. Distractions should be minimized.

Remove acupuncture needles as follows:
1. Place one finger on the skin next to the needle.
2. While holding your finger in place, use the other hand to gently pull the needle out.
3. Sometimes a drop of blood may be released. Applying pressure is not necessary; simply dab the blood away with sterile gauze.

POSTTREATMENT HOME PROGRAM

Patients are instructed to moderate their activity for 24 hours after a treatment. They should avoid very hot or very cold foods or liquids, consumption of alcohol, sexual activity, and other physically demanding activities. They should also drink plenty of water and get adequate sleep.

Patients can continue to perform acupressure on themselves starting 24 hours after the treatment. A good approach is to stimulate GV20, LI4, and local neck and head points twice a day or as needed.

Ideally, acupuncture is integrated into a regimen of headache trigger avoidance, healthful diet, exercise, and stress reduction as well as possible medication therapy. Acupressure is a great way to empower patients to take control of their own symptoms.

WHAT TO LOOK FOR IN AN ACUPUNCTURIST

A physician acupuncturist should have completed training in one of the programs approved by the American Board of Medical Acupuncture. Board certification in medical acupuncture identifies individuals who have completed at least 200 hours of training, passed a board examination, practiced at least 2 years, and performed at least 500 acupuncture treatments.

A nonphysician acupuncturist should be licensed. The letters "L.Ac." should follow a licensed acupuncturist's name. In addition, the National Certification Commission for Acupuncture and Oriental Medicine has a database of certified acupuncturists (see the Key Web Resources).

CONCLUSION

- Training for physicians to learn acupuncture is available through several continuing medical education programs.
- Acupuncture is useful for treating headaches, and patients can be taught acupressure to empower them to take control of their own health.

- In treating headaches: (1) start with general relaxation points (GV20, LI4), (2) release trigger points in the posterior cervical region (GB20 and any tender points), and (3) depending on the type of headache, use local points.
- For referral, look for a physician acupuncturist, licensed acupuncturist, or chiropractor with documented training and, ideally, certification in acupuncture.

Key Web Resources

American Academy of Medical Acupuncture: The main certifying group of physician acupuncturists	http://www.medicalacupuncture.org/
National Certification Commission for Acupuncture and Oriental Medicine (NCCAOM): Certifying group maintaining a database of certified acupuncturists	http://www.nccaom.org
National Center for Complementary and Alternative Medicine (NCCAM): Part of the National Institutes of Health	http://nccam.nih.gov
Acumedico: A list of acupuncture sites with illustrations	http://www.acumedico.com/acupoints.htm
Acupuncture Today: Acupuncture news source with information on clinicians and acupuncture research	http://www.acupuncture-today.com/mpacms/at/home.php

REFERENCES

References are available online at ExpertConsult.com.

CHAPTER 111

ACUPUNCTURE FOR NAUSEA AND VOMITING

Aaron J. Michelfelder, MD

OVERVIEW

For an overview of acupuncture, its mechanism of action, its safety, and training as well as techniques for performing acupuncture and acupressure, please see Chapter 110.

Extensive data are available concerning the use of acupuncture and acupressure for nausea and vomiting, especially with regard to the following causes or types of these conditions:

- Postoperative status
- Chemotherapy
- Pregnancy
- Motion sickness

POSTOPERATIVE NAUSEA AND VOMITING

In 1997, the National Institutes of Health (NIH) convened a panel of nonadvocate scientists to assess the current evidence concerning acupuncture and its efficacy. At that time, the panel concluded that clear evidence indicated that acupuncture was effective for adult postoperative and chemotherapy-induced nausea and vomiting.[1] Since then, six studies have also demonstrated its efficacy in preventing postoperative nausea and vomiting in children.[2-4] A 2004 Cochrane Review of 26 trials involving 3347 children and adults showed that in comparison with controls, acupuncture, with and without electrical stimulation, and acupressure were effective in decreasing the incidence of postoperative nausea and vomiting.[5] When compared, acupuncture and acupressure were equivalent to antiemetic drugs in preventing vomiting but were actually better in preventing nausea.[5] A Cochrane meta-analysis including 40 trials with a total of 4858 participants looked specifically at stimulation of the wrist acupuncture point pericardium 6 (PC6) for preventing postoperative nausea and vomiting.[6] The reviewers found that acupuncture and acupressure at the PC6 acupoint significantly reduced the risk of postoperative nausea and vomiting when compared with sham in both children and adults. The reviewers also found that PC6 stimulation was equivalent to antiemetic drugs.[6] Another meta-analysis of 21 studies from 1996 to 2009 showed that acupuncture reduced nausea but not vomiting when compared with antiemetic prophylaxis alone.[7]

CHEMOTHERAPY-INDUCED NAUSEA AND VOMITING

As previously stated, the 1997 NIH Acupuncture Consensus Panel concluded that acupuncture was effective for chemotherapy-induced nausea and vomiting. Dundee and Yang[8] found that acupressure was effective for decreasing nausea in hospitalized patients but worked much better when the acupressure bands were stimulated every hour. In an attempt to make this effect stronger, these investigators performed acupuncture with electrical stimulation in 105 patients, all of whom had had nausea and/or vomiting after an earlier chemotherapy treatment. This treatment prevented nausea and/or vomiting in 66% of patients and only 6% did not have any benefit from the acupuncture.[8] A meta-analysis of 11 studies including 1247 patients found that self-administered acupressure prevented chemotherapy-induced nausea and vomiting, and electroacupuncture also had a positive effect.[9] The reviewers concluded that these studies suggested a biological effect of acupuncture in preventing and treating chemotherapy-induced nausea and vomiting.[9]

PREGNANCY-RELATED NAUSEA AND VOMITING

The data for the use of acupuncture in pregnancy-related nausea and vomiting are equivocal.[10] A Cochrane Review of available studies found limited evidence to support the use of wrist and ear acupressure or acustimulation to treat pregnancy-related nausea and vomiting and cited the need for higher-quality, more focused studies in this area.[11]

MOTION SICKNESS

Several devices, including those for acupressure and electrical stimulation, have been approved by the U.S. Food and Drug Administration for the prevention of motion sickness. Hu et al.[12] reported that acupressure reduced the symptoms of motion sickness and decreased abnormal gastric myoelectric activity and tachyarrhythmia. However, Miller and Muth,[13] who tested two available acupressure and acustimulation bands for the prevention

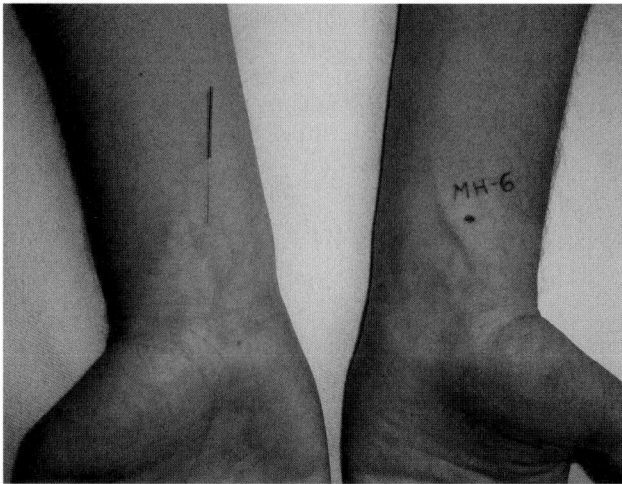

FIG. 111.1 ■ The master of the heart (*MH6;* also called pericardium 6 [PC6 or P6]) acupuncture point.

of motion sickness, found that the devices delayed the onset of, but did not prevent, the sickness.[10]

> Acupuncture and acupressure are effective for postoperative and chemotherapy-induced nausea and vomiting, but data are equivocal for pregnancy-induced nausea and vomiting as well as for motion sickness. Acupuncture, with or without electrical stimulation, and acupressure appear to be equivalent to antiemetic drugs for the prevention of nausea and vomiting.

ACUPUNCTURE POINTS FOR NAUSEA AND VOMITING

Naming of acupuncture points and techniques for performing acupuncture and acupressure is discussed in Chapter 110.

Three main points are relevant to this discussion: (1) master of the heart 6, also called PC 6 (MH6, PC6, or P6), (2) stomach 36 (ST36), and (3) liver 3 (LV3).

Master of the Heart 6

MH6 is located on the anterior surface of the wrist, approximately three fingerbreadths proximal to the distal wrist crease. It lies between the tendons of the flexor carpi radialis and palmaris longus muscles. Because the median nerve can be very superficial, insert the needle only a few millimeters under the skin, starting proximally, and direct it very superficially toward the hand. Warn the patient that if he or she feels a shooting or shock-like sensation into the hand, it is nothing harmful, and slightly withdraw without removing the needle tip from the skin and then redirect the needle more superficially (Fig. 111.1).

Stomach 36

ST36 is a depression in the anterolateral aspect of the shin, between the tibialis anterior and extensor digitorum longus muscles. You can find this point by placing your thumb on the anterior border of the tibia and sliding superiorly. Where the tibia starts to fan out near the patella (tibial tuberosity), allow your thumb to travel laterally until it

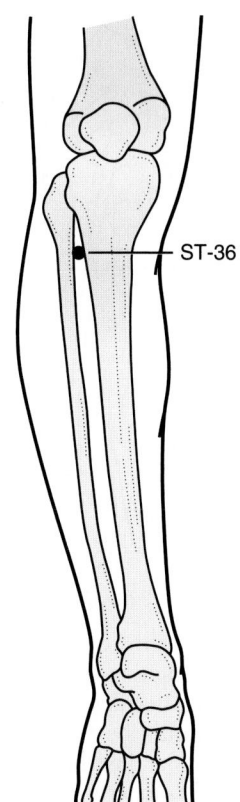

FIG. 111.2 ■ The stomach 36 *(ST36)* acupuncture point.

encounters a depression approximately six fingerbreadths below the patella and one fingerbreadth lateral to the tibial tuberosity. The needle is inserted perpendicular to the skin, approximately 1–2 cm deep, and is stimulated with clockwise and counterclockwise twisting (Fig. 111.2).

Liver 3

LV3, also a very important point for the treatment of nausea and vomiting, is located on the dorsum of the foot between the first and second metatarsal bones. If you place a finger between the first and second toes and slide it up the foot between the first two metatarsal bones, LV3 is the last place where you can access the underlying muscle between those two bones. The needle is directed toward the tip of the calcaneus and is inserted to a depth of approximately 1 cm (Fig. 111.3).

Practical Use of These Points

To prevent nausea, stimulate the MH6 point, either with acupressure (using a finger, a commercially available acupressure band, or an acustimulator) or acupuncture. To treat nausea and vomiting, start with MH6 and then add ST36 with stimulation and LV3 in dispersion (see Chapter 110 for the distinction between stimulation and dispersion).

DURING AN ACUPUNCTURE TREATMENT

For the prevention of nausea, needles should be placed at least 30 minutes before the antiemetic effect is needed

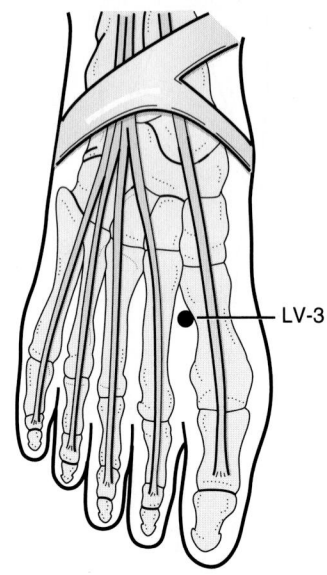

FIG. 111.3 ■ The liver 3 *(LV3)* acupuncture point.

and continued for as long as required. For the treatment of nausea and vomiting, needles should stay in for as long as needed. Patients should be relaxing in a comfortable room with the lights low and perhaps some calming music in the background. Distractions should be minimized.

Remove acupuncture needles as follows:
1. Place one finger on the skin next to the needle.
2. While holding your finger in place, use the other hand to pull the needle out gently.
3. Sometimes a drop of blood may be released. Applying pressure is not necessary; simply dab the blood away with sterile gauze.

POSTTREATMENT HOME PROGRAM

Patients are instructed to moderate their activity for 24 hours after a treatment. They should avoid very hot or very cold foods and liquids, consumption of alcohol, sexual activity, and other physically demanding activities. They should also drink plenty of water and get adequate sleep.

Patients can continue to perform acupressure on themselves whenever needed. Acupressure is a great way to empower patients to take control of their own symptoms.

WHAT TO LOOK FOR IN AN ACUPUNCTURIST

A physician acupuncturist should have completed training in one of the programs approved by the American Board of Medical Acupuncture. Board certification in medical acupuncture identifies individuals who have completed at least 200 hours of training, passed a board examination, practiced for at least 2 years, and performed at least 500 acupuncture treatments.

A nonphysician acupuncturist should be licensed. The letters "L.Ac." should follow a licensed acupuncturist's name. In addition, the National Certification Commission for Acupuncture and Oriental Medicine has a database of certified acupuncturists (see the Key Web Resources).

CONCLUSION

- Acupuncture has been shown to be effective for the prevention and treatment of postoperative and chemotherapy-induced nausea and vomiting. Acupuncture may be helpful for the prevention of pregnancy-induced nausea and vomiting as well as motion sickness.
- For the prevention of nausea, stimulate the MH6 point with acupuncture, acupressure, or electrical stimulation.
- To treat nausea and vomiting, use MH6, but also add ST36 with stimulation (clockwise and counterclockwise twisting action) and LV3 in dispersion (needle left alone).
- For more information about learning acupuncture, visit the American Academy of Medical Acupuncture Web site (see the Key Web Resources).

Key Web Resources	
American Academy of Medical Acupuncture: The main certifying group of physician acupuncturists	http://www.medicalacupuncture.org/
American Board of Medical Acupuncture: The certifying board for physicians. Includes requirements to sit for the board exam.	http://www.dabma.org/requirements.asp
Acumedico: A list of acupuncture sites with illustrations	http://www.acumedico.com/acupoints.htm
National Certification Commission for Acupuncture and Oriental Medicine (NCCAOM): Certifying group maintaining a database of certified acupuncturists	http://www.nccaom.org
Acupuncture Today: Acupuncture news source with information on clinicians and acupuncture research	http://www.acupuncturetoday.com/mpacms/at/home.php
Sea-Band: A commercial product that stimulates PC6 for nausea and vomiting	http://www.sea-band.com/
Mayo Clinic: YouTube video on acupuncture for nausea	http://www.youtube.com/watch?v=XWdDMrS8WIA

REFERENCES

References are available online at ExpertConsult.com.

CHAPTER 112

PROLOTHERAPY FOR CHRONIC MUSCULOSKELETAL PAIN

David Rabago, MD • Bobby Nourani, DO • Michael J. Weber, MD

INTRODUCTION AND HISTORY

Prolotherapy is an injection-based therapy for chronic musculoskeletal pain conditions.[1] Originally termed "sclerotherapy" because of the early use of scar-forming sclerosants or procedures, prolotherapy has been used in a form recognizable to contemporary medical practitioners for at least 80 years; the earliest report appeared in the peer-reviewed allopathic literature in 1937 for temporomandibular joint syndrome.[2] Modern applications and contemporary injection techniques were formalized by George Hackett, a general surgeon in the United States, based on clinical experience.[3] "Sclerotherapy" was replaced by "prolotherapy'" (from "proliferant therapy") based on the observation that newer injectants did not cause scar formation, rather ligamentous tissue sometimes exhibited a larger cross-sectional area after prolotherapy injection in animal models.[3] Because of the purported effects of prolotherapy on degenerative tissue, including revitalization and reorganization, it has also been categorized as a "regenerative" injection therapy by some researchers.[4]

> The term prolotherapy has evolved from sclerotherapy and some now refer to this as "regenerative" injection therapy. Prolo = proliferant.

The popularity of prolotherapy appears to be increasing among patients and physicians; however, data on the prevalence of its use are limited. The current number of medical providers who offer prolotherapy is not known but is likely several hundred in the United States based on attendance at continuing medical education (CME) conferences and physician listings on relevant websites.

WHAT IS PROLOTHERAPY?

Prolotherapy commonly consists of several injection sessions conducted every 2–6 weeks over the course of several months. Hypertonic dextrose is the most common injectant; this chapter will refer to the basic science and clinical effects of prolotherapy using dextrose injection. During an individual prolotherapy session, a dextrose solution is injected at sites of tender ligament and tendon attachments and in adjacent joint spaces.[5] Injected solutions are hypothesized to cause local irritation, with subsequent inflammation and anabolic tissue healing,[6,7] improving joint stability, biomechanics, function, and ultimately, decreasing pain.[3,8] A pain control mechanism at the tissue level is not well elucidated; however, it is likely multifactorial, involving effects in multiple tissue types and plane, and associated with both the physical injection procedure and biological effects of the injectant.

BASIC SCIENCE

Animal model studies suggest an injectant-specific biological effect and have focused on inflammation and ligamentous size and strength. Dextrose has been reported to produce a local inflammatory response in a rat knee ligament model.[9] Injured medial collateral rat ligaments that were injected with dextrose had a significantly larger cross-sectional area than both noninjured and injured saline–injected controls.[10] In a rabbit model, flexor retinaculum tissue showed greater strength (load absorption) and tissue thickness than in saline-injected controls.[11] More recent evidence has suggested that dextrose has a pain-specific sensorineural mechanism associated with neuroinflammation, currently understood to play a role in osteoarthritic pain.[12-14] Clinically, dextrose may reduce pain via a sensorineural mechanism in patients with stable knee cartilage volume.[15] Patients with Achilles tendinopathy who received dextrose prolotherapy injections that targeted sensory nerves and exercise reported improvement compared with exercise alone ($P = .007$).[16] Both reports suggest that injected dextrose acts on relevant chronic pain receptors to reduce neurogenic inflammation and decrease subsequent pain; however, these are preliminary reports, and the specific mechanism is unknown.

In addition to treatment of weakened ligaments and tendons and intraarticular joint space, recent attention has been given to the healing of fascia as a potential contributing mechanism in prolotherapy.[17] Fascia, the network of connective tissue found throughout the body, surrounds muscles, nerves, and organs, creating a complex support apparatus for structure and form, and a mode of transmission for tension forces. Growing evidence suggests that fascial integrity is essential to the proper function of the organism as a whole. Repetitive motion injuries such as tendinopathy and other traumatic injury disrupt fascial integrity; damage is reported to play a role in chronic pain, myofascial disorders, trigger points, and fibrotic scar formation.[18-21] A solution with proliferant properties, such as dextrose, injected into dysfunctional fascial layers may have a number of potential effects, including reorganization of collagen, improved fascial glide between layers, decreased tension between neuromuscular structures, and overall decreased burden of compensatory patterns, all of which could improve function and thereby reduce pain.

CLINICAL RESEARCH

Throughout the twentieth century, practitioners of prolotherapy reported clinical findings. As prolotherapy is primarily practiced and taught outside of academia, the scientific literature is clinically focused and contains few randomized clinical trials (RCTs). A systematic review of prolotherapy for all indications found 42 published reports from 1937–2005.[1] Thirty-six were case reports or case series and reported positive findings in patients with chronic, painful musculoskeletal conditions refractory to then-current best care. Methodological strength varied widely and was generally consistent with publication date. Older reports document injectants and methods no longer used. While these pragmatic studies often lacked control groups and randomization, their strength lies in the assessment of prolotherapy in clinical settings experienced by patients and included the clinician's ability to select the patient and to individually tailor the injection protocol. Most of the participants assessed were treated for low back pain (LBP). However, other indications included in these early studies included knee osteoarthritis (OA), shoulder dislocation, neck strain, costochondritis, lateral epicondylosis, and fibromyalgia.[1]

The publication rate and methodological quality of studies assessing prolotherapy for clinical indications have increased since the mid-1980s (Fig. 112.1).

Prolotherapy has been best assessed for three distinct sets of conditions: OA, tendinopathy, and LBP. Each is a cause of significant pain and disability and is often refractory to best-practice therapies. Finding new effective therapies for these conditions can have an impact on both individual patient care and overall public health. The following section gives a brief description of studies assessing prolotherapy in these clinical indications, and the level of evidence associated with each condition (Table 112.1).

Osteoarthritis

Prolotherapy has been assessed as a treatment for finger and knee OA. In early studies by Reeves et al., participants with symptomatic finger or knee OA were randomized to either prolotherapy with 10% dextrose and lidocaine or control injections with lidocaine and bacteriostatic water on the basis of clinical and radiological criteria.[22,23] Intervention participants in the finger OA trial reported significantly improved "pain with movement" and "flexion range" scores compared with control participants. Intervention participants in the knee OA trial, assessed using a 0–100 visual analog scale (VAS) and compared with control participants, reported significant improvements in pain at rest, walking, and while using stairs. Provocative

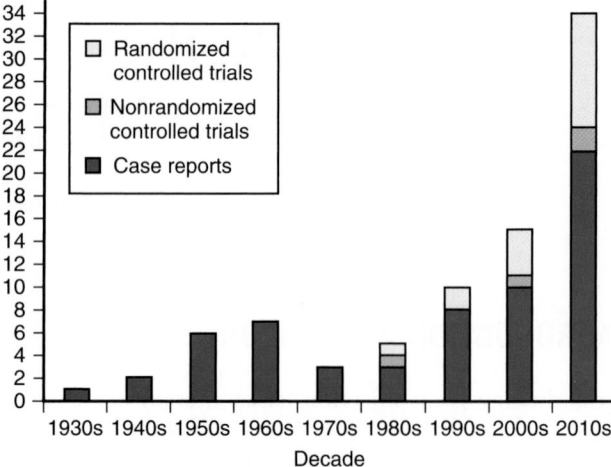

PROLOTHERAPY RESEARCH PUBLICATIONS BY DECADE

FIG. 112.1 ■ The number of published clinical studies on prolotherapy since 1937.

findings in both studies included improved radiological features of OA on plain radiographs, including decreased joint space narrowing and osteophyte grade in the finger study, and increased patellofemoral cartilage thickness in the knee study. While these techniques are limited in their ability to quantify such variables, they suggest the need for further study.

Building on the work of Reeves et al., two groups conducted more rigorous trials of prolotherapy for knee OA, an essential element of which has been the use of the validated Western Ontario McMaster University Osteoarthritis Index (WOMAC, 0–100 points) scale, the recommended self-reported outcome in knee OA research. The WOMAC features subscales of pain, stiffness, and function; the minimal clinical important difference (MCID) on the WOMAC for knee OA is approximately 12 points.[24,25]

Rabago et al. conducted an open-label pilot study that assessed prolotherapy in participants with mild-to-severe knee OA. Methodological elements, effect size of prolotherapy on the WOMAC, and overall feasibility of a more rigorous study were established.[26] Participants reported a 15.9 ± 2.5-point improvement in aggregate WOMAC scores, which were balanced between the three subscales. Shortly thereafter, Dumais et al. corroborated these findings in a crossover study in which participants who received physical therapy and prolotherapy were compared with those who received physical therapy alone.[27] At 16 weeks, prolotherapy was added to the physical therapy group, and the change on the aggregate WOMAC scale, attributed to prolotherapy alone, was 11.9 points.

These studies set the stage for an RCT by Rabago et al. that compared prolotherapy with at-home exercise and blinded saline injection. In this multiply blinded, rigorously reported study, prolotherapy participants reported significantly improved scores compared with both control groups at 9, 24, and 52 weeks, culminating in a 15.3-point improvement on the WOMAC scale, nearly twice that of the controls.[28] These are the most robust data favoring prolotherapy and suggest

TABLE 112.1 **Strength of Evidence for Prolotherapy as a Treatment for Chronic Musculoskeletal Conditions: Osteoarthritis (OA), Tendinopathy, and Low Back Pain Using the Strength of Recommendation Taxonomy (SORT) Criteria**[57]

Key Clinical Recommendation on Prolotherapy	Evidence Rating	Reference(s)
Hand and finger OA: may be effective based on one RCT of modest quality	B	22
Knee osteoarthritis: effective for knee OA based on two strong RCTs; moderately strong methodological quality	A	23,26-29
Lateral epicondylosis: likely effective based on strong positive data in small RCTs	A	34,35,37
Achilles tendinopathy: may be effective based on a high-quality prospective case series and pilot-level RCT	B	16,39
Hip adductor: may be effective based on a high-quality prospective case series	B	58
Plantar fasciitis: may be effective based on a high-quality prospective case series	B	59
Patellar: may be effective based on a high-quality prospective case series	B	60
Osgood-Schlatter disease: may be effective based on one high-quality RCT	B	38
Nonspecific LBP: may be effective; conflicting results in several RCTs	C	40-43
Coccygodynia: may be effective based on a prospective case series	B	47
Sacroiliac joint dysfunction: may be effective in patients with documented failure of load transfer (disability) at the sacroiliac joint based on a prospective case series	B	46
Degenerative disk disease	B	49

that prolotherapy, performed by a trained operator, results in safe, substantial, and sustained improvement on knee-specific quality-of-life indicators. A subsequent open-label prospective study followed participants for an average of 2.5 years and reported continued improvement of an average of 20.9 ± 2.8 points.[29] Consistent with clinical observation, approximately 80% of participants had improved status compared with their baseline status; 20% worsened, consistent with the natural history of knee OA. No study has identified baseline predictive markers of success with prolotherapy. A recent systematic review and meta-analysis reported that prolotherapy resulted in significant, clinically important improvement of knee OA without adverse events and concurred with these findings.[30]

Compared with home exercise and blinded saline injection therapy for osteoarthritis of the knee, prolotherapy resulted in significantly improved pain, stiffness, and function, almost twice that of the controls, with 80% of participants having improvement.[28]

Tendinopathies

Several studies support the use of prolotherapy for chronic, painful overuse tendon conditions formerly called "tendonitis," which are now more correctly termed "tendinosis" or "tendinopathy" to reflect existing, underlying pathophysiology.[31] Tendinopathies are discussed as a group because the current understanding of overuse tendinopathies identifies them as sharing a primarily noninflammatory etiology, association with repetitive motion overuse injury, and painful

degenerative tissue. The purported mechanism of prolotherapy is well matched to the current understanding of overuse tendinopathy, and it has been assessed as a treatment for five tendon disorders: lateral epicondylosis, hip adductor, Achilles, plantar, patellar, and Osgood-Schlatter tendinopathies.

Lateral Epicondylosis ("Tennis Elbow")

While many nonsurgical therapies have been tested for lateral epicondylosis (LE) refractory to conservative measures, none have been shown to be uniformly effective in the long term.[32-34] Three pilot-level RCTs suggest that prolotherapy is effective for LE. In a two-arm study comparing prolotherapy with masked-allocation saline injections, Scarpone et al. assessed 20 adults (10 per group) with at least 6 months of severe painful LE refractory to rest, nonsteroidal antiinflammatory medications (NSAIDs), and corticosteroid injections.[35] Prolotherapy participants reported, on a 0–10 point VAS, significantly decreased resting pain scores at 8 and 16 weeks, from 5.1 ± 0.8 points at baseline to 0.5 ± 0.4 at 16 weeks, versus from 4.5 ± 1.7 to 3.5 ± 1.5 points in controls. Prolotherapy participants also showed significantly improved isometric strength compared with controls, and grip strength compared to baseline status. These clinical improvements seen in prolotherapy subjects were maintained at 52 weeks. These data were corroborated by Rabago et al., who conducted a pilot study of size using the Patient-Rated Tennis Elbow Evaluation, a validated primary outcome.[36] Both studies suggest efficacy but are limited by the small sample size. Data from both studies were used to establish methods for an ongoing, more definitive study.[37] A third small RCT compared prolotherapy with corticosteroid injections. At 6 months, participants in both groups reported substantial improvement, but methodological issues, including a small sample size, precluded conclusions in favor of either therapy.[38]

Achilles Tendinopathy

Maxwell et al. conducted a well-designed case series (N = 36) to assess whether prolotherapy injected under ultrasound guidance would decrease pain and change ultrasound-based parameters of tendon thickness, hypoechogenicity, and neovascularity.[39] At 52 weeks, participants reported improvement in VAS-assessed pain severity by 88%, 84%, and 78% during rest, "usual" activity, and sport, respectively. Tendon thickness decreased significantly; however, other ultrasound-based criteria were not correlated with self-reported outcomes, suggesting that a causal relationship between ultrasound-imaged tissue characteristics and the degree of clinical improvement remains unclear. Prolotherapy has been assessed in multidisciplinary tendinopathy care. Participants in an Achilles tendinopathy study responded earlier and with improved cost-effectiveness when physiotherapy and prolotherapy were combined compared with either treatment alone.[16]

Osgood-Schlatter Disease

This tendinopathy of the patellar tendon at the tibial tubercle is common in children ages 9–17 years old engaged in kicking sports. While it has been historically understood as a self-limited condition that resolves with growth, the condition can become chronic, and morbidity associated with pain and loss of sport is substantial. Topol et al. assessed dextrose prolotherapy using the benchmark criterion "return to asymptomatic sport" and the 0- to 7-point Nirschl Pain Phase Scale (NPPS).[40] Prolotherapy was compared with blinded saline injections and usual care at 3 months; participants in the saline group were offered prolotherapy, and all participants were followed for 1 year. At 3 months, participant athletes receiving dextrose injections reported asymptomatic sport more frequently than knees treated with control injections ($P <$ .01) or usual care ($P <$ .001). At 1 year, asymptomatic sport remained more common in dextrose-treated knees than in injection control ($P =$ .024) or usual care ($P <$ .0001) knees. NPPS score changes between groups at 1 year were consistent with these relationships.

Low Back Pain

Generalized LBP. Four RCTs evaluated prolotherapy for generalized, nonsurgical LBP; three used a nondextrose agent known as phenol–glycerin–glucose (P2G) as the injectant,[41-43] and the fourth used dextrose and is discussed here.[44] Each study used a protocol involving injections to the ligamentous attachments of the L4-S1 spinous processes, sacrum, and ilium. While outcome measures varied, a common measure was the percentage of participants reporting greater than 50% improvement in pain/disability scores at 6 months.

Study participants in a trial by Yelland et al.,[44] the largest and most methodologically rigorous of the LBP

RCTs, were randomized to one of four intervention groups: dextrose and physical therapy, dextrose and "normal activity," saline injections and physical therapy, or saline injections and "normal activity." By 12 months, participants in each group reported improved pain (26%–44%) and disability (30%–44%) scores; a majority of participants (55%) reported that improvements in both pain and disability had been worth the effort of undergoing the intervention, and the percentage of subjects who reached at least 50% pain reduction ranged from 36% to 46%. Changes in outcome scores favored dextrose participants, but not by statistically significant margins, suggesting the study was underpowered.

Interpretation of the LBP RCT data is challenging and methodological problems with each trial have been noted,[45] including the use of a nonstandard, minimal injection protocol in the trial of Yelland et al., which may have rendered the intervention less effective than the conventional protocol, which features more injections and more injectant. While a recent systematic review[46] found insufficient evidence to recommend prolotherapy for nonspecific LBP, the clinical trial data offer generally promising, early investigational results and suggest the need for well-designed, sufficiently powered research. In the context of anecdotal clinical success and the promising aspects of initial RCTs for nonspecific LBP, researchers have begun to assess prolotherapy in patients with more narrowly focused diagnoses of LBP and loss of function in an effort to determine which underlying pathology may be most responsive to prolotherapy. Cusi et al. assessed 25 participants with symptomatic sacroiliac joint dysfunction refractory to 6 months or more of physical therapy and with documented failure of load transfer (disability) at the sacroiliac joint.[47] Compared with baseline, pain and disability scores on three multidimensional outcome measures were significantly improved at the 26-month follow-up in excess of the MCID. Khan et al. assessed 37 subjects with refractory coccygodynia.[48] Average pain scores dramatically improved from 8.5 to 2.5 points at 2 months, far in excess of the reported MCID for chronic pain.[49] In an especially novel study, Miller et al. assessed prolotherapy for leg pain in patients who had moderate-to-severe degenerative disk disease diagnosed by computed tomography,[50] who failed physical therapy, and who had substantial but temporary pain relief with two fluoroscopically guided epidural steroid injections. After an average of 3.5 sessions of biweekly, fluoroscopically guided injections to the relevant disk space with 25% dextrose with bupivacaine, 43% of responders showed a significant, sustained treatment response of a 71% improvement in pain score. VAS scores for responders were 8.9 ± 1.4, 2.5 ± 2.0, and 2.6 ± 2.2 points at baseline, 2, and 18 months, respectively. While these three recent studies of prolotherapy for "specific" LBP were uncontrolled, they suggest the need for future RCTs with more focused clinical indications of axial pain and disability.

These studies in OA, tendinopathy, and LBP suggest that prolotherapy is an appropriate therapy for patients refractory to conservative care with these conditions, and set the stage for further research involving functional radiological and biomarker assessments in addition to dissemination and implementation research including cost-effectiveness.

CONTRAINDICATIONS

Absolute contraindications to prolotherapy with dextrose are few; they include acute skin or joint infection, active rheumatological flare, allergy to corn or topical analgesics, and use of immunosuppressive medications. Relative contraindications include acute gouty arthritis, acute fracture, and bleeding disorders or use of anticoagulants.

COMMON SIDE EFFECTS

The main risk for prolotherapy is pain and mild bleeding or bruising as an outcome of needle trauma. Patients may report pain, tissue "fullness," and occasional numbness at the injection site at the time of injections. These are typically self-limited. Anecdotally reported postinjection pain during the first 72 hours after injections is relatively common; clinical trials have reported that approximately 10% of participants experience such flares.[28] They are typically self-limited and respond well to acetaminophen (500–650 mg every 4 hours as needed). Rarely, postinjection pain may require treatment with opioid medication. NSAIDs are not routinely used after the procedure. Most patients with pain flares experience diminution of pain within 5–7 days after injections; regular activities can be resumed at this time.

ADVERSE EVENTS

While prolotherapy has been reported as safe in clinical trials, the injection in ligaments, tendons, and joints raises safety concerns. Theoretical risks include lightheadedness, allergic reaction, infection, or neurological (nerve) damage. Injections should be performed using universal precautions, and the patient should be prone if possible. Dextrose is extremely safe; it is approved by the Food and Drug Administration (FDA) for intravenous treatment of hypoglycemia and for caloric supplementation.[51] A small number of significant prolotherapy-related complications have been reported associated with perispinal injections. They employed very concentrated solutions, which are no longer conventionally used, and included five cases of neurological impairment from spinal cord irritation[52-54] and one death in 1959 following prolotherapy with zinc sulfate for LBP.[52] In a survey of 95 clinicians using prolotherapy, there were 29 reports of pneumothoraces after prolotherapy for back and neck pain, two of which required hospitalization for a chest tube, and 14 cases of allergic reactions, none of which were classified as serious.[55] A more recent assessment survey of practicing prolotherapists concluded that adverse events were no more common in prolotherapy than in other spinal injection procedures.[56] No serious side effects or adverse events were reported for prolotherapy when used for peripheral joint indications.[56]

PRACTICAL CONSIDERATIONS

Prolotherapy is not governed by any general oversight body, and the procedures are not typically part of medical school or residency curricula. Safe practice of prolotherapy requires specialized training. Differences in technique exist between practitioners depending on the training venue. In the United States, prolotherapy is taught via peer learning and in conference, workshop, and formal CME settings. Prolotherapy is typically performed by MDs or DOs who have underwent such training. Performing prolotherapy for patients is best done in consultation with physicians who are experienced with these procedures. Two organizations, the Hackett Hemwall Patterson Foundation and the American Association of Orthopaedic Medicine, provide a majority of the formal coursework and training in the United States. Physicians interested in learning more about prolotherapy have access to a variety of resources (see the Key Web Resources). A growing number of fellowships in sports and rehabilitation medicine also provide training. The University of Wisconsin Prolotherapy Education and Research Lab (UW PEARL; http://www.fammed.wisc.edu/prolotherapy/) provides an academic portal for those interested in prolotherapy.

A CASE EXAMPLE: LATERAL EPICONDYLOSIS

A 48-year-old construction worker presents to the author's clinic with 5 months of lateral elbow pain consistent with LE. The symptoms have not responded to conservative therapy.

During a consultation for treatment of tennis elbow with prolotherapy, the physician confirms the diagnosis and reviews prior treatments including trials of medication, physical medicine, and other conservative approaches. A physical exam is performed and includes all lateral elbow soft tissue–supporting structures. If the patient appears to be a good candidate for prolotherapy, the risks and benefits of prolotherapy are discussed, as well as alternative treatments. If there is no contraindication and the patient desires to proceed, we offer a trial of dextrose prolotherapy.

We ask that patients stop all NSAIDs and other anti-inflammatory medications for 2 weeks prior to treatment. The day before and of treatment, we suggest that patients drink plenty of water and eat a light meal 1–2 hours prior to treatment and take acetaminophen or other non-NSAID–containing prescribed pain medication.

On the day of the procedure, a 15% dextrose solution is prepared in a 10-mL syringe using 2 mL of 1% lidocaine without epinephrine, 3 mL of 50% dextrose, and 5 mL of bacteriostatic 0.9% sodium chloride solution for extraarticular injections. For intraarticular injections, in a 5-mL syringe, a 25% dextrose solution is prepared using 2.5 mL of 1% lidocaine without epinephrine and 2.5 mL of 50% dextrose.

The patient is positioned supine with the elbow flexed at 90 degrees with the forearm in pronation and resting

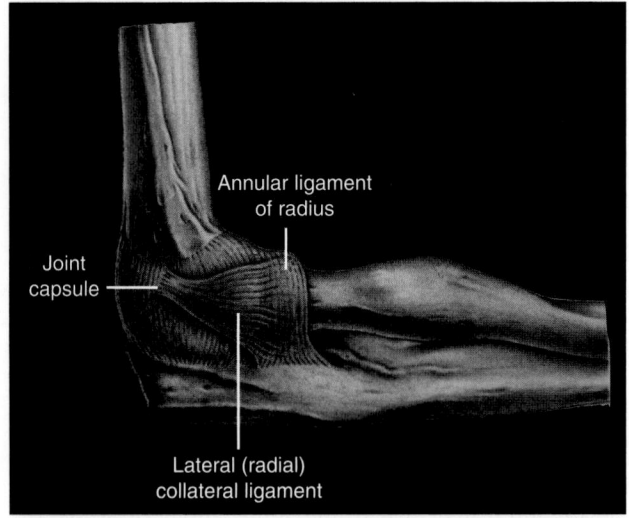

FIG. 112.2 ■ Lateral view. Capsular ligaments of the elbow.

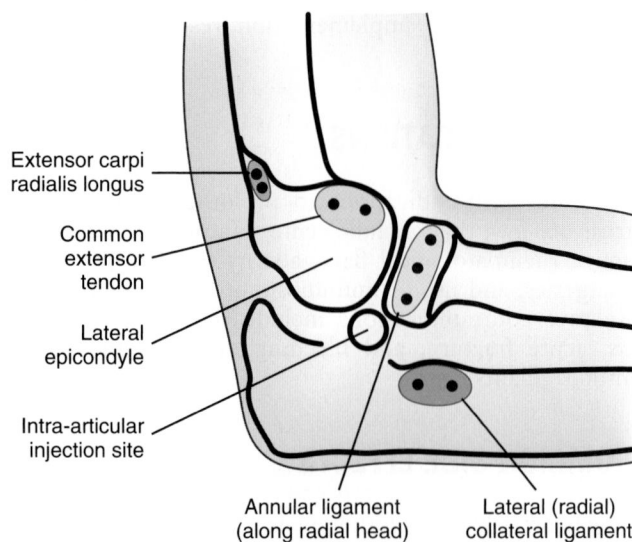

FIG. 112.4 ■ Prolotherapy tender points. Structure identification.

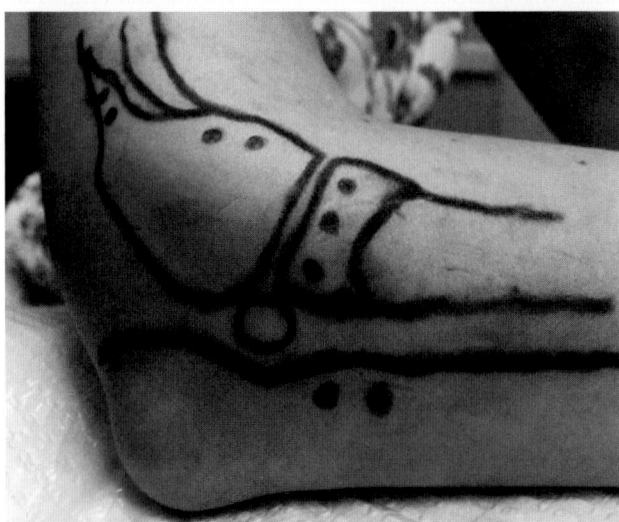

FIG. 112.3 ■ Topical anatomy, lateral elbow. Commonly treated prolotherapy tender points.

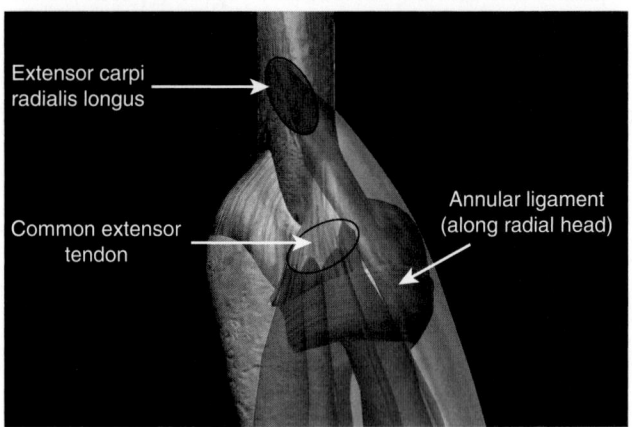

FIG. 112.5 ■ Anteroposterior (AP) view. Elbow anatomy.

on his or her abdomen. The lateral elbow is cleaned with 70% denatured alcohol. Using an surgical marking pen or other appropriate marker, the bony and soft-tissue anatomy are outlined, including the lateral epicondyle, common extensor tendon, attachment of the extensor carpi radialis longus, annular ligament along the radial head, lateral (radial) collateral ligament, and the site of intraarticular injection (Figs. 112.2–112.5). Next, the areas tender to palpation are marked with attention to the radial nerve. The marked area is then cleaned with a solution of chlorhexidine gluconate and allowed to dry. With a 30-G, 0.5-inch needle on a 5-mL syringe, anesthetic skin wheals with 1% lidocaine without epinephrine are placed at areas of tenderness prior to dextrose injection.

For the intraarticular injection, we use a 27-G × 1 ¼″ needle and inject 2–3 mL of the 25% dextrose solution. For extraarticular injections, we use a 27-G × 1 ¼″ needle and inject 0.5–2 mL of the 15% dextrose solution on bone in a peppering fashion. Care is taken to avoid injection through skin markings. Injections are most often placed using a "needle touching bone" peppering technique at the attachments of the common extensor tendon and the annular ligament using a total of 2–3 mL of solution.

Patients typically notice a marked reduction in pain immediately after treatment. After the local anesthetic wears off, patients often notice an increase in stiffness and pain lasting 1–3 days. Pain relief and improved function typically occur 2–6 weeks after treatment. In the post-treatment period, we advise that the patient uses acetaminophen for pain and avoids all NSAIDs for 4 weeks. Heat may be used for soreness; ice is avoided for the first 1–2 weeks as not to inhibit the proliferative response; patients may gradually increase activity to normal levels over the course of approximately 3 days with avoidance of strenuous activities for 1–2 weeks.

Prolotherapy treatments are spaced 3–6 weeks apart. Though some patients see resolution of pain after one treatment, we generally anticipate 3–5 treatments for clinically significant reductions in pain and function. At each visit, an interval history is obtained and physical exam is performed. If the patient does not report improvement after three prolotherapy sessions, alternative interventions are pursued.

INSURANCE COVERAGE

Some third-party payers cover prolotherapy for the indications discussed, but most patients pay out of pocket. Referrals are made in a similar manner to those for more conventional procedures. An initial consultation, including a relevant history and physical, is performed by the prolotherapist to determine if the patient is a candidate for prolotherapy.

Note: Portions of this chapter have appeared in two prior publications: Rabago D, Slattengren A, Zgierska A. Prolotherapy in primary care practice. *Primary Care: Clinics in Office Practice.* 2010;37:69–80; and Rabago D, Patterson JJ, Baumgartner JJ. Prolotherapy: a CAM therapy for chronic musculoskeletal pain. In: Lennard TA, ed. *Pain Procedures in Clinical Practice.* 3rd ed. Elsevier Saunders; 2011:113–130.

Key Web Resources	
"The Anatomy, Diagnosis, and Treatment of Chronic Myofascial Pain with Prolotherapy": Continuing medical education (CME) on the basics of prolotherapy. This 3.5-day conference is offered through the University of Wisconsin School of Medicine and Public Health. All clinical and research aspects of prolotherapy are covered.	http://www.ocpd.wisc.edu/Course_Catalog/
Hackett Hemwall Foundation List of Prolotherapists: The Hackett Hemwall Patterson Foundation is a nonprofit medical foundation whose mission is to provide high-quality treatment of musculoskeletal problems to underserved people around the world. Physicians listed on the site have completed the Foundation's high-volume CME experience in prolotherapy.	http://hacketthemwall.org/List_of_Prolotherapists.html
Commercial Prolotherapy Physician Listing: This site lists physicians by state who perform prolotherapy. It includes contact information and a short biography and prolotherapy credentials. Physicians pay to list themselves on this site.	http://www.getprolo.com
American Association of Orthopaedic Medicine: The American Association of Orthopaedic Medicine is a nonprofit organization that provides information and educational programs on comprehensive nonsurgical musculoskeletal treatment including prolotherapy. This searchable site lists AAOM members who perform prolotherapy.	http://www.aaomed.org
University of Wisconsin Prolotherapy Education and Research Lab (UW PEARL): The UW PEARL is a university-based collaboration between primary care and specialty clinicians to further education and research on prolotherapy.	http://www.fammed.wisc.edu/prolotherapy/

REFERENCES

References are available online at ExpertConsult.com.

CHAPTER 113

NASAL IRRIGATION FOR UPPER RESPIRATORY CONDITIONS

David Rabago, MD • Supriya Hayer, MD • Aleksandra Zgierska, MD, PhD

Nasal irrigation (NI) is an adjunctive therapy for upper respiratory conditions. The most common form of the procedure bathes the nasal cavity with saline (SNI) delivered as a spray or liquid. SNI originated thousands of years ago in the Ayurvedic medical tradition of India.[1] In the West, several administration devices, indications, and solution types for NI were described in the *Lancet* in 1902.[2] The current prevalence of SNI use is not known; however, its popularity has increased over time in the context of studies reporting positive effects in several upper respiratory conditions and due to publicity in news and popular media outlets, including the Oprah Winfrey Show (May 2007) and National Public Radio.[3] The most common method of liquid SNI uses the so-called "neti pot" and has the advantage of gravity-based administration. Other ways to deliver saline to the nasal cavity include hand-operated squeeze bottle and electrically or battery-powered products. SNI recommendation by physicians is common; in a survey of 330 family physicians, 87% reported recommending SNI to their patients for one or more conditions.[4]

THE SCIENCE

The exact mechanism of SNI action is not known. SNI may improve the nasal mucosa's immune response to infectious agents, inflammatory mediators, and irritants through several reported physiologic effects, including the direct cleansing of irrigation,[5-7] the removal of inflammatory mediators,[8,9] and improved mucociliary function, demonstrated by increased ciliary beat frequency.[10,11] Chronic sinus symptoms (lasting longer than 12 weeks) is the most common indication for SNI.[4] Based on positive results in clinical and functional outcomes, the Cochrane Collaboration concluded that SNI is an appropriate adjunctive therapy for the symptoms of chronic rhinosinusitis (CRS).[12-15] Users of liquid SNI also reported significantly decreased antibiotic and nasal spray use.[12] Clinical results have been corroborated for liquid, but not for nasal spray, SNI.[15] Data for the prevention or treatment of other indications, including irritant rhinitis,[16,17] viral upper respiratory tract infection (URI),[18-20] allergic rhinitis,[21-23] and postoperative care for endoscopic sinus surgery,[24] is positive, although less rigorous. Nasal irrigation has been recommended by content experts for mild to moderate rhinitis of pregnancy,[25] acute rhinosinusitis,[26] sinonasal sarcoid,[27] and Wegener's granulomatosis[28] (Table 113.1).

TECHNIQUE VARIATIONS

SNI can be performed using positive pressure (spray or squirt bottle) or "gravity-based" pressure (a vessel with a nasal spout) devices (Fig. 113.1 in the patient handout). Each is available over the counter. Saline is instilled in one nostril and allowed to drain out of the other. While liquid and spray saline have both been assessed, liquid NI is reported to be substantially more effective than spray for chronic sinus symptoms[15] and allergic rhinitis.[9,21] Uniform recommendations regarding liquid saline versus spray and other use-related variables are less evidence-based for other indications. Ideal salinity of SNI for any given condition is not known; 0.9%–3% saline solutions have been most often used. Optimal pH and temperature are likewise not known, although saline mixed with clean water at room temperature has been most often used in clinical trials. Each may be patient specific[22] and has been reported as safe within the ranges used in the cited studies. In the United States, after two cases of tapwater contamination by *Naegleria fowleri*, which may have been associated with SNI use, and fatal infections in two patients in Louisiana,[39] the U.S. Food and Drug Administration (FDA) issued guidelines recommending the use of distilled, sterile, or boiled-then-cooled water for irrigation (FDA Consumer Update, 2012).

Gravity liquid irrigation using a neti pot appears to be more effective than nasal spray irrigation for reducing antibiotic use in patients with recurring sinus infections.

IRRIGANT VARIATIONS

In addition to saline, other irrigants have also been studied and evaluated to determine their efficacy. One such irrigant, xylitol, is a naturally occurring nonabsorbable sugar. Although it has a shorter clinical history, nasal irrigation with xylitol (XNI) has also been reported to be effective in alleviating symptoms associated with CRS.[40] Fluticasone is a corticosteroid that effectively manages CRS symptoms.[29] Traditionally used as a spray, recent studies using fluticasone as an irrigant have shown greater improvement in CRS symptoms.[41] While irrigation with saline is considered as standard care for many upper respiratory conditions, both xylitol and corticosteroid irrigants are not.

TABLE 113.1 Recommended Indications for Saline Nasal Irrigation Among Adults

Key Clinical Recommendation	Evidence Rating	Reference
Nasal irrigation is effective adjunctive treatment for symptoms of chronic rhinosinusitis.	A	1, 14, 15, 22, 29, 43
Nasal irrigation may be effective adjunctive treatment for symptoms of several other conditions based on limited trial evidence: Irritant rhinitis/congestion, allergic rhinitis, viral upper respiratory congestion, postoperative care for endoscopic sinus surgery.	B	16-24, 30-35
Nasal irrigation has been recommended by content experts for mild to moderate rhinitis of pregnancy, acute rhinosinusitis, sinonasal sarcoid, and Wegener's granulomatosis.	C	25-28, 36-38

A, consistent, good-quality patient-oriented evidence; B, inconsistent or limited-quality patient-oriented evidence; C, consensus, disease-oriented evidence, usual practice, expert opinion, or case series.

PEDIATRIC USE

NI has also been shown to be effective in pediatric CRS as a first-line treatment as well as for recurring nasal symptoms. Generally, once daily NI over a 6-week period has been shown to be most effective, leading to symptom resolution while minimizing need for sinus surgery.[37,41,42]

RECOMMENDED DOSE FOR TREATMENT AND PREVENTION

The effective dose of SNI for the treatment of chronic sinus symptoms in randomized controlled settings has been reported to be once[12] or twice[15] daily. Long-term use is less well known, but SNI use by subjects with chronic sinus symptoms in one study stabilized at approximately three times a week for the prevention of symptoms.[43] Recommendations for acute rhinosinusitis, URI, and rhinitis are more difficult to make. Nasal irrigation once daily or spray saline up to three times daily has been reported to be safe.[20,44]

SAFETY

SNI appears safe within the aforementioned water quality recommendations. No study evaluating SNI has reported any adverse events. Nasal irrigation is associated with frequent, minor side effects that are self-limited or resolve with practice or adjustment of the procedure.[12,15,22,45] Minor side effects include a sense of discomfort and nervousness with the first use of liquid SNI.[22] Side effects noted by less than 10% of SNI users included self-limited ear fullness, stinging of the nasal mucosa, and epistaxis (rare)[12,15,45] that were ameliorated by technique modification and salinity adjustment[22] and did not cause discontinuation of SNI by subjects.[12,15]

PRACTICAL USE OF SNI

SNI has been identified as "an important component in the management of most sinonasal conditions and is effective and underutilized."[46] Most interested patients with appropriate conditions would be considered as candidates for a trial of SNI. Examples of inappropriate patients include those with the potential to leak saline to unwanted tissue planes or spaces (e.g., incompletely healed facial trauma), neurological or musculoskeletal problems that could facilitate aspiration, or patients who otherwise cannot perform the procedure. SNI is considered safe, appropriate adjunctive treatment for symptoms associated with CRS. SNI may also be an effective adjunctive treatment for mild-to-moderate viral URIs, allergic rhinitis, and rhinitis of pregnancy. SNI has not been evaluated for acute rhinosinusitis.

Portions of this chapter have appeared in two prior publications: Rabago D, Zgierska A, Mundt M, et al. Efficacy of daily hypertonic saline nasal irrigation among patients with sinusitis: A randomized controlled trial. *J Fam Pract.* 2002;51(12):1049-1055; and Rabago D, Zgierska A. Saline nasal irrigation for upper respiratory conditions. *American Fam Physician* 2009;80(10): 21-22, 1117-1119.

Key Web Resources

Further information, including detailed patient handouts with instructions for making and adjusting salt water using bulk ingredients (in English and Spanish), instructional videos and links, scientific reports, and a radio story by National Public Radio (NPR) can be found at this link.

http://www.fammed. wisc.edu/research/ past-projects/nasal-irrigation

Be sure to use clean, filtered water for nasal irrigation.

Patient Handout: Using Saline Nasal Irrigation for Upper Respiratory Conditions

Chronic sinus symptoms (nasal congestion, runny nose or post nasal drip) are very common and have several potential causes and treatments. Saline nasal irrigation is a therapy you can do at home in addition to your current care plan for sinus symptoms. This technique improves symptoms by rinsing the area behind the nose with salt water. This handout describes how to perform SNI using a nasal cup, also known as a "neti pot".
What you will need: A nasal cup, distilled water and pre-packaged salt are commercially available at many pharmacies.

There are 3 steps to saline nasal irrigation.

Step 1: Mix the solution
- If you are using a pre-packaged salt, simply prepare the salt water as indicated on the packaging using lukewarm distilled or sterile water and put 4 fluid ounces (100 mL) in the nasal cup. If you plan to mix your own salt water using bulk ingredients, please see the website below for detailed instructions.

Step 2: Position the nasal cup (Please see pictures)
- Lean over a sink so you are looking directly into the basin.
- Rotate your head slightly and gently insert the spout of the nasal irrigation pot into the upper nostril so that it forms a comfortable seal. Do not press the spout against the "middle", or septum, of the nose.

Step 3: Irrigate the nose
- *Breathing through your mouth,* raise the nasal irrigation pot so that the solution enters the upper nostril. The solution will soon drain from the lower nostril.
- When the nasal pot is empty, gently exhale through both nostrils to clear them of excess solution and mucus. Gently blow your nose into a tissue.
- Repeat the procedure for the other nostril.

Nasal cup care: Mix new solution when you plan to irrigate your nose, discard extra salt water immediately. Wash nasal pot after irrigation.
Troubleshooting: You may notice some drainage of salt water up to 30 minutes after nasal irrigation; this is normal. Many users of nasal irrigation carry tissues. If stinging or burning occur, try decreasing the salt content by half; you may also adjust the temperature of the water slightly. Do not use very hot or very cold water. Nasal irrigation can also be done in the shower.
Want more information? A more detailed patient handout (including a version in Spanish), instructions for making and adjusting salt water using bulk ingredients, instructional videos and links, scientific reports and a radio story by National Public Radio (NPR) are at:
http://www.fammed.wisc.edu/research/past-projects/nasal-irrigation

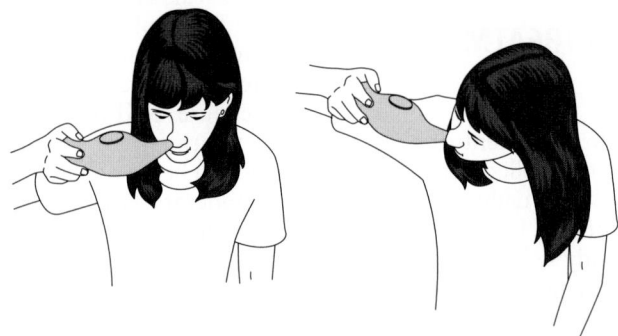

FIG. 113.1 ■ A common nasal irrigation technique using a nasal cup or neti pot. Liquid saline is instilled in one nostril and allowed to drain out the other.[12] (From Rabago D, Zgierska A, Mundt M, et al. Efficacy of daily hypertonic saline nasal irrigation among patients with sinusitis: a randomized controlled trial. *J Fam Pract*. 2002;51:1049-1055.) Redrawn from University of Wisconsin Department of Family Medicine : *Nasal irrigation instructions*. <http://www.fammed.wisc.edu/research/past-projects/nasal-irrigation>; Accessed 15.02.12.

REFERENCES

References are available online at ExpertConsult.com.

SECTION V

BIOENERGETICS

SECTION OUTLINE

114 INTEGRATING SPIRITUAL ASSESSMENT AND CARE

115 THERAPEUTIC HOMEOPATHY

116 BIOFIELD THERAPIES

CHAPTER 114

INTEGRATING SPIRITUAL ASSESSMENT AND CARE

Gregory A. Plotnikoff, MD, MTS • Daniel Wolpert, MDiv, MA •
Douglas E. Dandurand, PhD, MDiv, MA, MAS

Spiritual and religious practices such as prayer represent the most prevalent complementary therapies in the United States. In recent years, more than twice as many U.S. adults have reported preferring prayer over herbal medicines for health and healing.[1] In recent decades, nearly 80% of U.S. adults reported that religion, to a large extent, helps patients and families cope with illness.[2] Nearly 75% of the public have reported that praying for someone else can help cure his or her illness; furthermore, 56% of adults have stated that faith has helped them recover from illness, injury, or disease.[3] Whole-person medical care, by definition, integrates the spiritual dimensions of the patient and his or her family.

Spirituality may or may not involve formal religion. Over the past 40 years, the religious landscape in the United States has changed dramatically. The percentage of people who identify with no religion has risen to more than 20% of the population.[4] Within the Christian tradition, church attendance and participation has dramatically declined. The phrase "spiritual but not religious" has gained enormous traction and popularity within the culture. Furthermore, practices such as meditation, yoga, and other traditional spiritual disciplines have gained popularity, as have New Age spirituality, pagan spirituality, and earth-based spirituality, among others. At the other end of the religious spectrum, fundamentalism has also seen a rise in popularity, particularly in certain parts of the country. Given these changes, it is helpful for clinicians to understand their spiritual and religious context as well as the meanings of some of these terms.

Spirituality and religion are means by which human beings relate to all that which is "Other" than themselves: the rest of the natural world, other people, and even their internal unfamiliar states. Although there are many different rubrics used to define these terms (Table 114.1), religion is generally an organized collective set of practices, dogmas, and rules that describe or talk about our relationship to the greater universe, whereas spirituality tends to define a set of practices that help us to relate directly to that greater universe. Thus a person may attend many religious services that are about God yet also may have no sense that they are relating directly to God. On the other hand, persons who meditate regularly may feel that they have a rich relationship with God and may also define themselves as not being religious. These sometimes subtle, but significant, differences can have important ramifications for a person when he or she is ill or facing a life crisis.

In clinical settings, both spiritual support as well as spiritual distress demand professional attention. Spiritual beliefs are frequently important in medical decisions.[5] Spiritual well-being is closely linked to successful coping,[6] faster recovery,[7] and higher quality of life.[8] Many patients may want help with meaning, hope, or overcoming fears[9]; unmet spiritual needs, spiritual pain, or unresolved spiritual struggles are associated with despair,[10] increased mortality,[11] poorer outcomes from posttraumatic stress disorder (PTSD),[12] and unnecessarily increased use of health care resources.[13] The latter point is crucial for both primary and subspecialty care as this challenges every clinician to expand his or her differential diagnosis to consider patients requiring frequent appointments for ambiguous or nonspecific symptoms (see Fig. 114.1). Compared to patients with less physical or psychological problems, patients who report more concerns are likely to also have more spiritual concerns and greater distress related to these concerns. Patients with such distress often have abuse histories, including the possibility of spiritual abuse. They often carry a diagnosis of major depression and generalized anxiety disorders.[14] The clinically relevant point is that to address physical or psychological distress, a consideration of the patient's spiritual context can help the clinician identify rational, nonpharmacological responses. Although more data is needed, several randomized controlled trials suggest that spiritual practices and interventions determine treatment choices in a number of clinical situations such as anxiety,[15] cancer,[16] or addiction.[17]

American adults consistently report that it is good for doctors to talk to patients about spirituality.[18,19] In 2004, 83% percent of 921 primary care patients surveyed in Ohio reported that they wanted physicians to ask about spiritual beliefs in certain circumstances such as serious illness or the loss of loved ones.[20] In response to the accumulating data on the importance of spirituality and health, even the Joint Commission for the Accreditation of Healthcare Organizations (JCAHO) now requires that patient spirituality be addressed as a part of routine inpatient care.[21] However, despite patient interest and needs, a nation-wide survey of 1,732,562 patients reported very low ratings of satisfaction with the emotional and spiritual aspects of care received.[22]

Integrative clinicians should be prepared to inquire and engage patients in discussions on spirituality. Ignoring the patient's source of meaning, purpose, richness, and direction places the clinician at a risk of providing inefficient, ineffective, and unsatisfactory care.[23] The challenge is to identify the best means for addressing a patient's spiritual concern.

Multiple mnemonics exist to guide clinicians in their interviews with patients. These include FICA,[24]

TABLE 114.1 Three Dimensions of Spirituality: Head, Heart, and Hand

Cognitive	Experiential	Behavioral
Beliefs	Love, compassion, altruism, forgiveness	Duties: daily behavior, moral obligations
Values	Connection, relationship with: self, others, community, environment, nature, the transcendent	Choices: life choices, medical choices
Ideals	Inner energy, strength, resilience	Specific practices: prayer, meditation, yoga, chanting, rituals, diet, nature walks, etc.
Meaning	Inner peace, comfort, support	Participation in religious community
Purpose	Hope	
Truth	Faith (trust)	
Wisdom	Transcendence	
Faith (belief)		

From Anandarajah G. The 3 H and BMSEST models for spirituality in multicultural whole-person medicine. *Ann Fam Med.* 2008;6:448-458.

HOPE,[25] and SPIRIT,[26] which are outlined in Table 114.2. These mnemonics highlight content and provide questions that may lead to important insights into care for the patient and his or her family. However, even before an intake interview, a new patient intake form can honor religious or spiritual concerns. At the Penny George Institute for Health and Healing, we have woven these three helpful questions into the intake form.

1. We recognize that it is often difficult to discuss distressing experiences. As you feel comfortable, please describe any traumatic situations you may have experienced (e.g., abuse, loss of a loved one, divorce, separation, or fire).
2. Of the many forms of stress that individuals can experience (environmental, physical, emotional/spiritual, pharmaceutical, or dietary), are there any in particular that affect your life? Please describe.
3. Please describe your spiritual history, including information about your current practices or routines.

In the context of an intentionally holistic intake form, these questions are perceived as nonthreatening. Each question allows the patient to choose how much information to share. The clinician can review responses before meeting the patient. This previsit review is time efficient and allows the clinician to consider appropriate integration of spiritual assessment and care when creating a customized action plan for the patient. To support this clinical competency, this chapter identifies five practical goals for every clinician. Addressing of these five goals results in three practical outcomes: (1) improved diagnostic accuracy, (2) appropriately focused and directed resources, and (3) a strengthened therapeutic alliance.

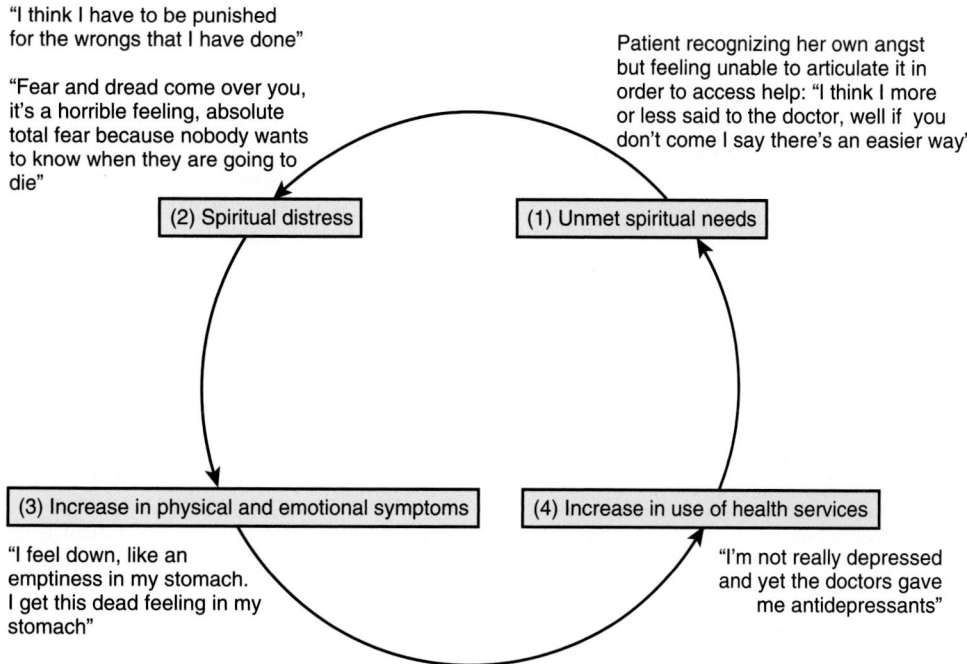

FIG. 114.1 ■ **Unmet spiritual need cycle may result in an increased demand and service use.**
(Redrawn from Grant L, Murray SA, Sheikh A. Spiritual dimensions of dying in pluralist societies. *BMJ.* 2010;341:c4859.)

THE FIVE CLINICAL GOALS OF SPIRITUAL ASSESSMENT AND CARE

Clinical Goal One: Anticipate the Presence of Religious and Spiritual Concerns in Both Adult and Pediatric Care

Spiritual and religious concerns in clinical care range from rituals or practices, such as prayer, to complex crises, such as despair. Every illness is a potential spiritual crisis and also may have, in part or in whole, a spiritual cause. This is true for the patient and his or her family as well as for the care team. These crises can be found in both acute and chronic care settings but may most easily be seen with end-of-life care; common spiritual/religious concerns at that time include the following:

- Not being forgiven by God
- Not reconciling with others
- Dying alone or cutoff from God
- Not having a blessing from a family member or clergy person
- Wondering whether anyone will miss you or remember you over time[27]

TABLE 114.2 **Spiritual Assessment Tools**

FICA—Pulchaski

F: Faith or belief—What is your faith or belief?
I: Importance and influence—Is it important in your life? How?
C: Community—Are you part of a religious community?
A: Awareness and addressing—What would you want me as your physician to be aware of? How would you like me to address these issues in your care?

HOPE—Anandarajah

H: Hope—What are your sources of hope, meaning, strength, peace, love, and connectedness?
O: Organization—Do you consider yourself a part of an organized religion?
P: Personal spirituality and practices—What aspects of your spirituality or spiritual practices do you find most helpful?
E: Effects—How do your beliefs affect the kind of medical care you would like me to provide?

SPIRIT—Maugans

S: Spiritual belief system—What is your formal religious affiliation?
P: Personal spirituality—Describe the beliefs and practices of your religion or spiritual system that you personally accept/do not accept.
I: Integration within a spiritual community—Do you belong to a spiritual or religious group or community? What importance does this group have for you?
R: Ritualized practices and restrictions—Are there specific practices that you carry out as a part of your religion/ spirituality (e.g., prayer and meditation)? What significance do these practices or restrictions have to you?
I: Implications for medical care—What aspects of your religion/spirituality would you like me to keep in mind as I care for you?
T: Terminal events planning—As we plan for your care near the end of life, how does your faith impact on your decisions?

Spiritual concerns can arise at any time in life. To recognize religious and spiritual concerns in others, one should be able to recognize them in oneself. Whole-person health care means proactively engaging in spiritual life as opposed to waiting for a crisis to enlighten that awareness. Hence, all clinicians are challenged to develop self-awareness of their own spiritual history and perspectives.[28] In clinical care, the goal is to not to react to one's own spiritual needs or beliefs, but to acknowledge and bracket them and then respond to the patient's spiritual concerns. This capacity to respond to the patient rather than to one's own emotional needs is termed being present.

Both culture and spirituality can be implicit and unconscious. Both patients and clinicians can be blind to the effects of their own perspective in clinical interviewing and decision making. For this reason, health care professionals should begin by conducting cultural and spiritual assessments of themselves before performing them on patients. The most effective interviewing allows the patient's deeply held implicit and unconscious beliefs to be understood, acknowledged, and affirmed by the clinician. The clinical challenge is to create a safe and conducive setting where spiritual concerns can be recognized and shared.

> One hallmark of spirituality in clinical care is deep listening. The challenge is for health care professionals to step out of their role as answer givers and into their role as listeners. When we listen deeply to our patients, we honor them and their experience. We thus encourage them to listen deeply to themselves.

When patients believe that they will not be judged and that someone will listen and not try to fix, dismiss, or deny their concerns, they will often freely share their most private concerns. The sense of being heard is itself frequently therapeutic.

From an ethical viewpoint, clinicians should maintain respect for their patients' beliefs and recognize patients' vulnerability to their own attitudes. No practitioner should impose his or her own religious, or antireligious, beliefs on patients.[29,30] All practitioners need to recognize that their answers are their answers only.

This is particularly relevant within the field of integrative medicine at this point in its development. For a number of reasons, integrative medicine tends to identify with non-Judeo–Christian spiritualities and practices. Statues of Buddha, pictures of the Tao, and symbols of other non-Western religions regularly adorn integrative medicine clinics. In certain areas of the country, these icons may represent the views of the majority of patients, but in many areas, they do not. Recognizing this bias and understanding that all religions have sources for deep spiritual healing are in the best interests of patients.

To invite the patient to share his or her spiritual and religious concerns does not require specifically religious or spiritual questions. Good open-ended questions include the following:

- How else do you hurt?

- Serious illness can affect lives in many unexpected ways. How has this illness affected your life?
- What do you miss the most or fear the most as a result of this illness?
- What are some of the things you wish you could talk about? Is there anyone you wish you could talk to?
- What's most important to you right now?

The answers to such questions frequently reflect the patient's spiritual values and worldview in addition to identifying important connections that have been disrupted. At the same time, clinicians should not be afraid to directly address religious beliefs, practices, and issues.

Clinical Goal Two: Comprehend How Patients Want Their Religious and/or Spiritual Beliefs and Community to Be Seen as Resources for Strength and Recovery

Faith and related religious worldviews sometimes are considered medically relevant only when they obstruct the implementation of scientifically sound biomedical care.[31] However, this attitude is profoundly naïve. Every religion and cultural tradition has teachings, practices, and rituals that facilitate spiritual healing.[32]

> The challenge is not to seek omnicultural and spiritual competency but to develop a humility that allows patients to teach about what is important to them.

Patients often display many clues that can be keys to the beginning of a conversation. For example, "Mrs. Xiong, I see that you have white and red strings tied around your wrist. Could you please teach me about their importance to you?" Such questioning would lead the health care professional into a deeper understanding of the patient's worldview and sources of strength. Such questioning would also prevent profound patient harm by accidental cutting and removal of sacred objects to make way for an intravenous (IV) line placement or other biomedical intervention.

Three related open-ended questions include the following:

- As your doctor, what do you most want me to know about you as a (religious or spiritual) person?
- In the past, from where have you drawn the strength to cope with difficult situations?
- How can I be most helpful to you regarding your spiritual concerns and practices?

The principal guideline in any such questioning is to listen to understand rather than to express agreement or disagreement.

Clinical Goal Three: Understand Better Your Patients' Subjective Experiences and Subjective Understanding of (Ultimate) Reality

Every effective health care professional is broadly familiar with the religious worldviews of the cultural groups within their patient population. Patients and their families can teach about the specifics. This is important because there is a significant danger in extrapolating the truth for one patient of one cultural group and making it the truth for all such patients. This constitutes practice by stereotype (e.g., this patient is Hmong; therefore...). The challenge is to understand what *this* illness means for *this* patient.[33]

The consideration of seven concepts and questions by clinicians can help generate clinically relevant questions and guide understanding among them. These include, how does this patient (and/or family) understand:

1. Ultimate health?
2. Affliction and suffering?
3. The different parts of a person (e.g., location of the soul, meaning in this life and the next)?
4. The patient's illness/sickness or disease (i.e., is there a nonscientific diagnosis such as loss of soul)?
5. Necessary interventions or forms of care (e.g., specific foods, rituals, herbs)?
6. Who is seen as qualified to address the different parts that need healing?
7. Efficacy or healing?

Given the frequently implicit and unconscious nature of the answers to these questions, these seven questions should be seen only as prompts or guides. Health care professionals should ask themselves if they could answer these questions for their patients on the basis of their interview(s). Doing so directs interviewing toward the clinically relevant meaning of the illness to the patient. The response to an open-ended question such as "What do you fear most about surgery?" can lead to a dialogue that may help answer these questions. Should this reveal a spiritual concern that cannot be addressed medically, further questioning may help identify the interventions that are needed and professionals who should perform them.

Clinical Goal Four: Determine What Impact, Positive or Negative, Your Patients' Spiritual Orientation Has on Their Health Problems and Perceived Needs

Although spirituality is frequently seen in a positive light, there is, of course, a shadow side. The *Diagnostic and Statistical Manual* (DSM-5) includes an axis IV concern—a religious or spiritual problem.[34,35] Examples cited include distressing experiences that involve loss or questioning of faith, problems associated with conversion to a new faith, or questioning of other spiritual values that may not necessarily be related to an organized church or religious institution.

When patients are asked about their sources of support, it is possible that what worked previously is not perceived to be working at present. Spiritual distress is often exacerbated when a patient's understanding of his or her spiritual life and spiritual support conflicts with the religious beliefs of his or her faith tradition. For example, if the Source of Life (God) is feared or understood as punishing, the person in distress has nowhere to turn and thus is at high risk for panic and despair. This often surfaces among patients after hearing the diagnosis of a life-threatening or life-changing illness.

In such cases, traditional spiritual sources of support, such as teachings, practices, and rituals, may paradoxically be barriers to spiritual well-being. For this reason, health care professionals are at a risk of creating a sense of shame or guilt by denying, dismissing, or silencing doubts or theological challenges. Examples of valid spiritual suffering include the following:

Spiritual Alienation
  "Where is God now when I need Him the most?"
  "Why isn't He listening?"
Spiritual Anxiety
  "Will I ever be forgiven?"
  "Am I going to die a horrible death?"
Spiritual Guilt
  "I deserve this."
  "I am being punished by God."
  "I didn't pray hard enough."
Spiritual Anger
  "I'm mad at God."
  "I blame God for this."
  "I hate God."
Spiritual Loss
  "I feel empty."
  "I don't care anymore."
Spiritual Despair
  "There's no way God could ever care for me."
  "I'm just a corpse waiting to happen."[16]

When spirituality is understood as including connections with one's self, others, nature, and God or a higher power, spiritual suffering can be seen as resulting from the loss of such connections—betrayal by one's body, loss of social roles, dependence on technology, and theological doubt or loss of faith. Healing, therefore, is the process of resolving such broken connections and recovering one's wholeness. The focus of healing is the human experience of illness and its associated suffering. Healing can occur in any dimension: physical, emotional, social, and spiritual. Healing as the resolution of brokenness may or may not include curing a disease. One can cure a heart attack but not heal the broken heart. Healing is never quick or easy.

Frequently, when patients are diagnosed with a life-threatening or life-changing illness, they turn toward their God and pray for healing. Healing, in its truest sense of making whole, means personal (spiritual) growth and development through embracing the illness (or any other presenting issue) and discovering God as a source of love in it.

"Healing" and "cure" are terms and intentions that, for many, if not most, are used interchangeably and synonymously. Therefore, when one prays for healing, one might more truly be praying for cure. This lack of distinction between healing and curing is crucial for clinicians to understand because it addresses the patient's understanding of his or her relationship to God or Source of Life. If a person prays for cure—and cure is not always a possibility—that person sets him or herself up for an experience of disconnect with God, experiencing their God as an abandoning one. This experience needs to be considered in the differential diagnosis of spiritual distress or despair.

Spiritual healing begins with the recognition and acknowledgment of spiritual pain. For this reason, the American Academy of Hospice and Palliative Medicine's mnemonic

---

TABLE 114.3 **Spiritual Suffering Response Mnemonic**

LET GO—American Academy of Hospice and Palliative Medicine
L—Listen to the patient's story.
E—Encourage the search for meaning.
T—Tell of your concern and acknowledge the pain of loss.
G—Generate hope whenever possible.
O—Own your own limitations, seek competence, and refer when appropriate.

LET GO can be quite helpful (Table 114.3).[36] The challenge here is to respond not as an expert with the answer(s) but as a fellow human being also struggling to make sense of tragedy. Listening, acknowledging, and validating are means of connecting at a deep level and are the most profound means of strengthening the therapeutic alliance. This connection between clinician and patient is the foundation for healing. Without this connection, without first listening comfortably to the patient at a deep level, referral of patients to those with expertise in pastoral care and counseling may be perceived as abandonment by patients.

Generating hope whenever possible does not mean creating fake scenarios or deceiving patients. It means identifying what is important to the patient and working to achieve that. What constitutes hope and its shadow side, despair, keeps changing throughout the course of an illness. For this reason, first asking and then acting to address what is most important for the patient today (or for a given time period) is an important, concrete, and constructive means of addressing hope.

> As with any medical referral, pastoral experts are available for assistance in understanding complex or difficult cases. Referrals can enhance the quality of care, and, frequently, the patient's quality of life.

Clinical Goal Five: Determine Appropriate Referrals to Chaplains, Clergy, or Traditional Healers for Spiritual Care

Many spiritual concerns are addressed as a variation on the questions "Why? Why me? Why now?" Clearly, multiple members of the health care team can recognize the many varieties of such spiritual concerns in clinical settings. However, even if time allows, these are not the questions that should be answered by health care professionals. To do so is to risk harming patients. For every such question, the best answers are found rather than given. The health care professional's role is to help give voice to such questions and to support the patient's search for answers.

Today, there is no need for any member of the health care team to be a self-sufficient virtuoso. This is especially true when Clinical Pastoral Education (CPE)–trained chaplains are available in hospital settings. Chaplains offer well-tuned skills in listening for and responding to spiritual concerns in acute care settings. Furthermore, they can help identify when a spiritual guide (director) or a culture's spiritual healer (e.g., priest, pipe holder, or shaman) may be the most appropriate professional for a patient's spiritual concerns.

Professionally trained spiritual directors (guides) serve in outpatient settings. This allows the spiritual director to enter a long-term or more expansive relationship with the patient. Spiritual direction is emphatically not about giving preformed or formulaic answers. Spiritual directors are trained in the art of meeting the person where he or she is experiencing life. Spiritual direction ideally addresses integration of the *all* of life without judgment.

Spiritual direction is a method of healing conversation that allows people to listen deeply within their spiritual life as they understand it. For some, this means a sacred time to become more whole or aware. For others, it means deepening their relationship with God. Spiritual direction is not dependent on religion and can occur independently of one's religious beliefs, including not having any religious beliefs. Spiritual direction helps clients to attend to the spirit "part" of who they are, to see the longer arch and journey of their life, and to connect with their innate health and wisdom. Spiritual direction supports healing because we humans are most healthy when our body, mind, and spirit are balanced and nonanxious.

Spiritual direction can be especially helpful for people who:

• feel stuck in their lives and have a general sense of "disease" that they cannot get beyond or alleviate.
• have been suffering for many years with medical and/or psychological difficulties and do not yet see the deeper patterns and threads of both their suffering and potential for health.
• have been suffering from illnesses that may have spiritual abuse or exposure to very negative church or theological messages as their root cause.
• understand or realize that their difficulties would be helped by a deeper relationship with God/Higher Power.
• feel burdened by a difficult diagnosis or a challenging chronic illness in themselves or a loved one.

Both inpatient and outpatient care plans should identify a patient's spiritual resources, spiritual needs, and preferred spiritual care provider. Truly integrative medicine requires that a relationship be built between the clinician and available chaplain and spiritual direction services, leading to the establishment of a network of local consultants and patient- or family-preferred spiritual care providers who can offer assistance.

THERAPEUTIC REVIEW

There are three practical outcomes of integration of spiritual assessment and care into clinical settings: (1) improved diagnostic accuracy, (2) appropriately focused and directed resources, and (3) a strengthened therapeutic alliance. To achieve these outcomes, clinicians should consider integrating these eight summary points:

1. Intake questions and mnemonics exist to guide the inclusion of spirituality in clinical care. Expand the social history.
2. Spiritual needs can arise at any time or place. Anticipate them.
3. Spiritual healing begins with recognition and acknowledgment of spiritual pain. Listen intentionally.
4. Spirituality is about questions, not answers. Help voice the questions.
5. The best answers are found rather than given. Support the search.
6. Care plans should include patients' spiritual needs, resources, and preferred spiritual care providers. Identify them.
7. Every religious tradition has teachings, practices, and rituals that are potential resources of strength and recovery. Integrate these into the care plan, as appropriate.
8. Every illness is a potential spiritual crisis. Refer to pastoral care specialists (chaplains, clergy, and spiritual directors) for assistance.

Key Web Resources

Duke University Center for Spirituality, Theology and Health: The Center is focused on conducting research; training others to conduct research; and field-building activities related to religion, spirituality, and health.

http://www.spiritualityandhealth.duke.edu/

The George Washington Institute for Spirituality and Health: (GWish) is working toward a more compassionate system of health care by restoring the heart and humanity of medicine through research, education, and policy work focused on bringing increased attention to the spiritual needs of patients, families, and health care professionals.

http://www.gwish.org/

HealthCare Chaplaincy: The multifaith HealthCare Chaplaincy is a national leader in the research, education, and practice of spirit-centered palliative care, which helps people with life-altering illness to live well and live fully.

http://www.healthcarechaplaincy.org

REFERENCES

References are available online at ExpertConsult.com.

CHAPTER 115

THERAPEUTIC HOMEOPATHY

Paul E. Bergquist, MD

WHY HOMEOPATHY?

"When I was a medical student I felt sure that any one of us would have been ashamed to be caught looking into a homeopathic book by a professor. We had to sneer at homeopathy by word of command. Such was the school opinion then, and I imagine similar [sentiments]…exist in the medical schools today."[1]

So spoke William James, philosopher and physician, in 1898, when he made a plea to the Massachusetts legislature to support homeopathy. Medical practitioners today are no less skeptical about homeopathy than they were a century ago. Homeopathy is just as implausible, irrational, and misunderstood today as it was then.

How is it possible that homeopathic remedies containing infinitesimal amounts of active substances can cure illness? Proponents of homeopathy believe that the use of microdoses stimulates human defense and homeostatic self-regulatory mechanisms to resolve illness. Cure is possible in many acute and chronic diseases, some of which have little or no chance of cure in regular medicine. Despite a relative lack of scientific data to support its theory, homeopathy has been used safely and effectively by millions of people worldwide for more than 2 centuries.

WHAT IS HOMEOPATHY?

Homeopathy is derived from the Greek words for "like" and "suffering." The guiding principle "likes cure likes" has its origins in ancient Egyptian medicine, as well as in Hippocratic medicine of the ancient Greeks; however, the practice of homeopathy was codified by Samuel Hahnemann, a 17th-century German medical doctor. Disillusioned with the medical practices of those days, which included bloodletting, purging, cathartics, and cupping, Hahnemann decided to experiment with medicinal substances on himself.

He started with quinine, an herbal medicine known at that time to cure malaria:

"I took by way of experiment…four drams of good China (quinine). My feet, fingers, at first became cold; I grew languid and drowsy; then my heart began to palpitate, and my pulse grew hard and small; intolerable anxiety, trembling, prostration throughout all my limbs; then pulsation, in the head, redness of my cheeks, thirst, and, in short, all those symptoms which are ordinarily characteristic of

intermittent fever, make their appearance. This paroxysm lasted two or three hours each time, and recurred if I repeated this dose, not otherwise; I discontinued it and was in good health again."[2]

This was the first proving of a homeopathic medicine and led Hahnemann to formulate the Law of Similars, which states that a remedy can cure a disease if it produces similar symptoms in a healthy person. Hahnemann also found that symptoms of poisoning by a drug were often the same as those of the disease cured by the drug. Hahnemann and his followers went on to prove hundreds of plant, mineral, animal and disease substances. These symptoms were cataloged in homeopathic materia medicas, which today include more than 2000 remedies. Each remedy has a full profile of mental, emotional, and physical pathological symptoms. Homeopathic remedies are compiled in the Homoeopathic Pharmacopoeia of the United States, which is recognized by the U.S. Food and Drug Administration.

HOW ARE HOMEOPATHIC REMEDIES PREPARED?

Because many remedies are toxic in their crude form, Hahnemann attenuated the remedies by serial dilution and succussion, a process whereby the solution is struck on a pad a given number of times between dilutions. This process eliminated almost all the side effects of the crude substance. A 12 C potency, for example, is prepared by diluting 1 drop of the crude tincture in 99 drops of an alcohol–water solution, succussing it, and then taking a drop of that diluted solution and diluting it in another 99 drops of alcohol–water solution; this process is repeated 12 times to reach the 12 C, or 12 centesimal, potency. The decimal (X or D) potencies are diluted on a 1:9 scale and considered less potent. Beyond a 12 C or 24X dilution, the Avogadro's rule designates that not a single molecule of the original substance should remain in the solution. Paradoxically, however, in clinical practice, the higher the number of dilutions and successions, the more potent the remedy. French scientists Jacques Benveniste et al.[3] were able to demonstrate mast cell degranulation using a homeopathic dilution of immunoglobulin E antibodies in a laboratory setting, where even at very high dilutions, not a single molecule of immunoglobulin E remained in the solution. Because of its implausibility, their study, published in the scientific journal *Nature*, was rejected by the scientific community. However, the study

TABLE 115.1 Common Homeopathic Potencies

Common Potencies	Serial Cycles (of Dilution and Succussion)	Usual Dosing Method
6X	1:10 dilution 6 cycles	3–5 pellets every 5 min–every hour for acute illness
12X	1:10 dilution 12 cycles	3–5 pellets every 15 min–every 2 h for acute illness
30X	1:10 dilution 30 cycles	3–5 pellets every 1–8 h for subacute illness
6 C	1:100 dilution 6 cycles	3–5 pellets every 5 min–every hour for acute illness
12 C	1:100 dilution 12 cycles	3–5 pellets four times daily in acute case or 5 pellets daily in chronic case
30 C	1:100 dilution 30 cycles	3–5 pellets three times daily in acute case, or daily for 10 days in subacute case
200 C	1:100 dilution 200 cycles	5 pellets every hour or daily in very acute case, 10 pellets once in chronic case
1 M	1:100 dilution 1000 cycles	5 pellets every hour in severe acute case, 10 pellets once in chronic case
10 M	1:100 dilution 10,000 cycles	5 pellets every hour in severe acute case, 10 pellets once in chronic case
50 M	1:100 dilution 50,000 cycles	5 pellets daily in severe acute case, 10 pellets once in chronic case
CM	1:100 dilution 100,000 cycles	5 pellets daily in severe acute case, 10 pellets once in chronic case

was repeated 10 years later in a rigorous pan-European trial published in 1999. Again, the investigators demonstrated statistically significant results showing activity of hyperdilute solutions.[4]

Table 115.1 lists the common homeopathic potencies and their usual dosing methods.

HOW DO HOMEOPATHIC REMEDIES WORK?

The exact mechanism by which homeopathic remedies work is unknown. The clinical success of homeopathy is often attributed to the placebo effect. Reilly and Taylor

et al.[5-8] conducted four double-blind, placebo-controlled trials of homeopathy in the treatment of allergies and found that homeopathy was significantly more effective than placebo. These researchers concluded that either homeopathy works or the clinical trial method itself was flawed. Since 1980, more than 190 controlled and 115 randomized trials of data were reported, the results of which again suggest that homeopathy is more than a placebo-based approach.[9-14]

Transfer of bioelectrical wave signatures from medicinal substances to water in hyperdilute solutions has been posited as a possible mechanism of the action of homeopathic remedies.[15] French virologist and Nobel Laureate Luc Montagnier and his coworkers[16] published a study showing that dilute solutions containing the DNA of pathogenic bacteria and viruses (including human immunodeficiency virus [HIV]) "could emit low-frequency radio waves" that induced surrounding water molecules to become arranged into nanostructures.[17] Once induced, these water molecules could then also emit radio waves. These investigators suggested that water could retain these properties even after the original DNA-containing solutions were ultradiluted to the point where no molecules of the original DNA remained (much like a diluted and potentized homeopathic remedy).[16]

HOW ARE HOMEOPATHIC MEDICINES PRESCRIBED?

When the body is threatened by harmful external forces, such as trauma, toxins, bacteria, and viruses, it produces symptoms such as fever, cough, and pain. These symptoms often reflect certain innate purposes: to inactivate bacteria or viruses, to carry off irritating byproducts of diseases, and to force the individual to rest and recuperate. Although these symptoms may be uncomfortable for the patient, they represent a healthy reaction of the body's defense mechanisms. They are also the only true guides to individual manifestations of the disease.

The homeopath, recognizing the individual as body, mind, and spirit, takes an extensive history of all physical, mental, and emotional symptoms. The location, quality, severity, frequency, and time of aggravation of symptoms are discovered. Underlying causes such as trauma, bereavement, change of job, abuse, and physiological change (pregnancy, teething, menarche, and menopause) are important. Amelioration or aggravation of symptoms, fears and phobias, food cravings and aversions, sex drive, and energy level are all considered. Body habitus, physiognomy, mannerisms, behavior, and psychological symptoms are examined. The homeopath is especially interested in unusual or strange, rare, and peculiar symptoms.

The homeopath builds a complete picture of the pathological features of a person in the course of taking the history and then attempts to find a remedy that most closely matches the whole picture of symptoms. In an acute case, acute symptoms are primarily

BOX 115.1	Examples of Materia Medicas

- Allen JT. *Encyclopedia of Materia Medica.* New York: Boericke & Tafel; 1879 [reprint: New Delhi: B. Jain Publishing; 1988].
- Boericke W. *Materia Medica Pocket Guide and Reference Works.* New Delhi: B. Jain Publishing; 2004 [reprint].
- Encyclopedia Homeopathica and Reference Works (www.wholehealthnow.com/homeopathy_software/index.html): example of a computer program that contains hundreds of materia medicas from the past to the present, with programs designed to access the symptoms and remedies from the entire homeopathic database.
- Hahnemann S. *Materia Medica Pura* (contains original proving symptoms). New Delhi: B. Jain Publishing; 2002 [reprint].
- Morrison R. *Desktop Guide.* Nevada City, CA: Hahnemann Clinic Publishing; 1993.
- Phatak SR. *Concise Materia Medica.* New Delhi: B. Jain Publishing; 1999.
- Vermeulen F. *Concordant Materia Medica.* Haarlem, The Netherlands: Merlijn; 1994.

BOX 115.2	Examples of Repertories

Homeopathic repertories are books that help guide the most appropriate remedy.
- Kent JT. *Kent's Repertory.* Calcutta (Kolkata): Sett Dey; 1974.
- Radar (www.wholehealthnow.com/homeopathy_software/index.html): a computer program that contains multiple repertories and helps the homeopath choose remedies.
- Schroyens F. *Synthesis 9.1.* London: Homeopathic Book Publishers; 2002.
- Van Zandvoort R. *Complete Repertory.* Leidschendam, The Netherlands: Institute for Research in Homeopathic Information and Symptomatology; 1998.

taken into account. In a chronic case, in what is often called *constitutional prescribing*, all symptoms, past and present, may help the homeopath find the right remedy.

The process of finding the correct remedy can be the most challenging aspect of the clinical practice of homeopathy. A homeopathic repertory of symptoms and the homeopathic materia medica are the two essential references for practicing homeopaths (Boxes 115.1 and 115.2). After the most important symptoms are elicited, a repertory of symptoms is consulted to see which remedies address all or most of the important symptoms in the case. Those remedies are studied more closely in one or more of the materia medicas, which are encyclopedias of remedy characteristics and symptoms. The remedy that appears to match the pathological features and essential nature of the case most accurately is given to the patient. Several remedies may match the case closely enough to stimulate the natural homeostatic mechanisms of the body to move toward cure. If the remedy chosen is not a close match to the case, it will do nothing for the symptoms.

BOX 115.3	Small Sample of Reputable Homeopathic Pharmacies

- Boericke & Tafel, Inc.: 2381 Circadian Way, Santa Rosa, CA 95407; telephone: 707-571-8202; fax: 707-571-8237; www.boerickeandtafel.com
- Boiron-Bornemann, Inc.: Box 449, 6 Campus Avenue, Building A, Newtown Square, PA, 19073; telephone: 800-BLU-TUBE
- Hahnemann Laboratories, Inc.: San Rafael, CA 94901; telephone: 888-4-ARNICA; fax, 415-451-6981; www.hahnemannlabs.com
- Helios Homeopathic Pharmacy: 97 Camden Road, Tunbridge Wells, Kent, TN1 2QR, United Kingdom; telephone 01892-537 254; www.helios.co.uk
- Homeopathic Educational Services: 2124 Kittredge Street, Berkeley, CA 94704; telephone: 510-649-0294; fax: 510-649-1955; www.homeopathic.com
- Standard Homeopathic Company: Box 61067; 204-210 West 131st Street, Los Angeles, CA 90061; telephone: 800-624-9659
- Washington Homeopathic Products: 260 Hawvermale Way, Berkeley Springs, WV 25411; telephone 800-336-1695

Remedy Prescription

In acute illnesses, the remedy is usually given in lower potencies, such as 12 C or 30 C, three to five pellets by mouth every 5–60 minutes. If the remedy does not help the symptoms after four or five doses, a different remedy should be chosen. In less acute illnesses, the remedy can be given three or four times a day for 1–2 days. If no improvement is noted, a different remedy is chosen. Once improvement is noted, the remedy is given only when symptoms recur. In chronic illnesses, a higher potency, such as 200 C, is used once at the beginning of a treatment. Symptoms are monitored over the next 1–2 months. If improvement is followed by relapse, the remedy is repeated once. If no improvement is noted, a different remedy is chosen. A patient who is taking other medications may need a daily dose of a lower potency (e.g., 12 C) after the initial 200 C to counter the interfering effects of the other medications.

AGGRAVATION AND ANTIDOTE

Aggravation of a patient's existing symptoms can occasionally occur when a chronic problem is treated using a homeopathic remedy. This is particularly true for skin problems and diseases or disorders that have been treated with steroids. Usually, the aggravating symptoms resolve within 5–10 days, and the resolution should be followed by gradual improvement beyond the initial baseline condition if the correct remedy has been chosen.

If a patient experiences improvement of chronic symptoms and then has a sudden relapse after trauma, surgery, dental trauma, emotional grief, or severe illness or after initiating coffee, camphor, chamomile, steroids, or other regular allopathic medications, the remedy effects are said to be *antidoted*. These influences or substances do not always antidote the effects of a remedy.

Box 115.3 contains a list of several reputable homeopathic pharmacies.

TABLE 115.2 Remedies for Teething

Remedy[a]	Indication	Better from/in	Worse from/in
Calcarea carbonica	Constipation, delayed teething, milk intolerance	Heat	Cold, wet, dairy products
Chamomile	Irritability, screaming, capriciousness	Being carried, rocked hard, car ride	Night, heat, being held still
Pulsatilla	Weepiness, whining	Gentle rocking, being held	Overheated, stuffy room
Nux vomica	Irritability, burping, gas	Nap, evening	Morning

[a]All doses 12 C–30 C; three pellets given every hour as needed in the cheek. If no improvement is seen after four to five doses, choose another remedy.

TABLE 115.3 Remedies for Colic

Remedy[a]	Indication	Better from/in	Worse from/in
Chamomile	Irritability, being cross	Being carried, being rocked hard	Open air, night
Calcarea carbonica	Sweaty head, plumpness	Dry, warm	Cold, wet
Colocynthis	Doubling up, distended abdomen	Firm pressure, heat, bending legs up	Anger, eating, drinking

[a]All doses 12 C–30 C; three pellets given every hour as needed in the cheek. If no improvement is seen after four to five doses, choose another remedy.

FOR WHICH CONDITIONS CAN HOMEOPATHIC TREATMENTS BE USED?

Many conditions, chronic and acute, can be effectively treated with a homeopathic approach. These include pediatric problems, such as recurrent otitis media,[18-21] pharyngitis, attention-deficit hyperactivity disorder,[22] enuresis,[23] constipation, diarrhea,[24] asthma, allergic rhinitis, eczema,[6,25,26] juvenile arthritis, chronic bronchitis, and recurrent pneumonia. Adult problems well treated by homeopathy include anxiety,[27] bruising and ecchymosis from trauma and surgery,[28-30] poisonings,[31] anemia,[32] acquired immunodeficiency syndrome/HIV infection,[33,34] insomnia,[35,36] vertigo,[37] tinnitus,[38] depression,[27,39,40] bipolar disorder, headaches,[41] gastroesophageal reflux disease, colitis, Sjögren's syndrome,[42] rheumatoid arthritis,[43,44] heart disease,[45] multiple sclerosis (management and arrest of progression), diabetic polyneuropathy,[46] perimenopausal symptoms,[47,48] fibromyalgia,[49,50] chronic fatigue syndrome,[51] infertility,[52] dysmenorrhea,[53,54] postoperative ileus,[55] chronic or recurrent urinary tract infection, trigeminal neuralgia,[56] psoriasis,[57] numerous other dermatological conditions,[58,59] influenza,[60,61] snoring,[62] and chronic cough. Traditionally, homeopathy has been used effectively for the treatment of epidemics; during cholera and severe influenza epidemics, homeopathy was significantly more effective than any of the allopathic approaches to management.

In a study funded by the Cuban government, Bracho et al.[63] created a homeopathic preparation of four strains of *Leptospira* and administered it to 2.3 million people at high risk during an epidemic of leptospirosis in Cuba. A significant decrease in the disease incidence was observed in the intervention regions. No decrease was noted in the regions where no remedy was administered. The epidemic was controlled, and the incidence of leptospirosis fell below the usual levels.[63]

Classical homeopaths use constitutional prescribing for chronic diseases and complicated cases. Although most health care practitioners will choose not to prescribe constitutionally, homeopathy may be used in a cookbook fashion to achieve results in many acute illnesses and some chronic illnesses. Tables 115.2 through 115.5 list some of the commonly used remedies for various problems.[64]

Otitis Media

Acute and chronic recurrent otitis media responds well to homeopathic remedies.[20] Acute otitis media often improves without treatment over 3–5 days. Antibiotics can often be avoided, and the appropriate homeopathic remedy sometimes speeds healing and prevents recurrence (Table 115.6).

Sinusitis

Several remedies are appropriate for acute sinusitis[65] (Table 115.7). Chronic or recurrent sinusitis can be treated by referral to a classical homeopath for constitutional treatment.

Allergies, Asthma, and Atopic Eczema

Allergic rhinitis, asthma, and atopic eczema can be cured over several years using a constitutional homeopathic approach. Referral of a patient with such a problem to a trained homeopath is recommended. Asthma and eczema symptoms are not always easily palliated, and a constitutional homeopathic approach, with or without steroid and bronchodilator inhalers and minimal use of steroid creams, is recommended. Allergic rhinitis symptoms can also be alleviated in a palliative manner.[8] Table 115.8 lists some of the more common remedies for palliation of these problems.[66,67]

TABLE 115.4 **Remedies for Severe Brain Injury and Mild Traumatic Brain Injury**[a]

Severe acute head trauma[b]	Arnica	10 M–100 M (CM)	5 pellets (oral/axilla/buccal mucosa) every 15 min in the first 12–24 h, then every day for 10–30 days Decrease frequency of dose as patient improves Continue through rehabilitation
Chronic effects of head trauma (posttraumatic brain injury)	Suggest constitutional homeopathic therapy (e.g., Arnica, Calcarea Carbonica, Cicuta, Helleborus, Natrum Sulphuricum, Opium Silica)	200 C–1 M	5 pellets once; repeated as necessary if improvement is followed by relapse

[a]Homeopathic remedies have been used for acute severe concussion and intracranial hemorrhage as adjunctive therapy to neurosurgical approaches and in posttraumatic brain injury for speeding rehabilitation.[58]
[b]Homeopathic treatment would be an adjunctive therapy to a hospital intensive care unit protocol for treatment of head injury.

TABLE 115.5 **Remedies for Acute Injury and Emergencies**

Indications	Remedy	Potency	Dose
Shock	Arnica	200 C or up to 50 M	5 pellets PO every 5 min, every day
Shock with fear	Aconite	200 C or up to 50 M	5 pellets PO every 5 min, every day
Head injury	Arnica	200 C or up to 50 M	As mentioned earlier; the more severe the trauma, the more frequently repeated and the higher the potency
Blow to spine or whiplash	Hypericum	200 C or up to 50 M	5 pellets PO every 5 min, every day
Trauma with bleeding, bruising, contusion, laceration	Arnica Hypericum	30 C or up to 200 C 30 C or up to 200 C	As mentioned earlier; remedies may be given concurrently
Eye injury	Aconite	30 C–200 C	Five pellets PO every 5 min, every day
Black eye	Ledum	30 C–200 C	As mentioned earlier
Cut nerves, crush injuries	Hypericum, Arnica	30 C–200 C	As mentioned earlier; may be given concurrently
Fractures	Arnica, Symphytum, Ledum	200 C	5 pellets of each daily for 10–14 days
Puncture wounds	Ledum	30 C–200 C	5 pellets PO every 5 min, every day, depending on the severity
Bites, bee stings	Apis, Ledum	As mentioned earlier	As mentioned earlier
Muscle, ligament, and joint sprains and strains	Arnica, Ruta	30 C–200 C	5 pellets PO three times daily for 10–14 days
Chronic sprains or strains	Rhus toxicodendron	30 C or 200 C	5 pellets daily for 7–10 days or 10 pellets one dose once
Burns	Calendula	Topical oil, lotion	Apply to burn
First degree	Urtica urens	30 C	5 pellets PO every 5 min prn
	Causticum	30 C	5 pellets PO every 5 min prn
Second degree	Urtica urens	30 C–200 C	5 pellets PO every 5 min prn
	Hypericum	30 C–200 C, topical	Tincture dilute 1:3 in water
Third degree	Cantharis, Hypericum	30 C–200 C	5 pellets PO every 5 min prn
Sunburn	Belladonna	30 C	5 pellets PO every 5 min prn
Heatstroke: hot, red, dry	Antimonium Crudum, Belladonna	30 C–200 C	5 pellets every 15 min prn
Throbbing headache	Glonoine	30 C–200 C	As mentioned earlier
Electrical burns	Phosphorus	30 C–200 C	5 pellets PO three times daily prn
Epistaxis	Phosphorus	30 C–200 C	5 pellets PO every 5 min prn
Blood, fluid loss	China Officinalis	30 C–200 C	As mentioned earlier
Dental extraction with blood loss	Phosphorus	30 C–200 C	As mentioned earlier
Syncope, collapse	Carbo Vegetabilis	30 C–200 C	5 pellets PO every 5 min prn
Food poisoning	Arsenicum Album	30 C	5 pellets PO every 5 min prn
Mucus, vomiting	Ipecac	30 C	5 pellets PO every 5 min prn

PO, Orally; *prn,* as needed.

TABLE 115.6 Remedies for Otitis Media

Remedy[a]	Indications	Better from/in	Worse from/in
Aconite	Sudden onset, high fever, restlessness, being hot, dry, thirsty, or fearful	Open air, rest	Night, warm room, noise, cold wind, teething, touch
Belladonna	Red face, being hot, right ear, throbbing pains, high fever	Sitting up, wrapping up in warm room	Light, getting head wet or cold, teething, 3 a.m.–3 p.m.
Calcarea Carbonica	Thick discharge from ear, decreased hearing	Warmth, dryness, lying, massage	Cold, wet, exertion, teething, milk
Chamomile	Being cross, screaming in pain, pushing people away	Being carried rapidly, warm weather	Wind, 10 p.m.–10 a.m., teething, cold, being looked at
Ferrum Phosphoricum	Early stages, gradual onset, pallor	Cold applications, touch, cold drinks	Night, motion, noise, right side, warm drinks
Hepar Sulphuris	Great sensitivity to pain, fits of screaming	Warmth, warm applications	Hating to be examined, cold, drafts of air
Lachesis	Rare, extreme pain, left ear, pharyngitis	Open air, discharge, loosening clothes	After birth of sibling/jealousy, wind, tight clothes
Mercurius Vivus	Sickly child status, precociousness, foul discharge, salivation at night, pus in ears	Rest, morning	Night, warmth of bed, being too hot or too cold, being held
Pulsatilla	Weepiness, sensitivity, thick yellow discharge, left ear	Wanting to be held, carried, or comforted; open air, lying on painful side	Twilight, after eating, warm stuffy room, left side, fat-rich food
Silica	Constipation, being chilly, ruptured eardrum with watery or cheesy discharge, sweaty feet	Rest (fatiguing easily), warmth, covering up	Milk, teething, cold air, night, combing hair, touch

[a]All remedies are 12 C or 30 C; three pellets are given every 5 min–every hour as needed until better. If no improvement is seen after four to five doses, choose another remedy.

TABLE 115.7 Remedies for Sinusitis

Remedy[a]	Indications[b]	Better from/in	Worse from/in
Arsenicum album	Burning nasal discharge, restlessness, anxiety	Warm drinks, hot applications, food, lying head up	Midnight or after, cold, exertion, ice, draft, tobacco
Hepar Sulphuris	Pain at root of nose, sensitivity, irritability, stuffy nose, later stage	Warmth, wrapping up, eating	Cold draft of air, touch, lying on painful side
Hydrastis	Thick, yellow discharge from posterior nares, nose sores, bloody crusts	Pressure, warm wraps, dry weather, rest	Inhaling cold air, night, open air, motion
Kali Bichromicum	Most common sinus remedy, pain in maxillae and bridge of nose, thick stringy discharge, stuffy nose	Heat, pressure, motion	Cold, damp air, undressing, 2–3 a.m., alcohol, after sleep
Mercurius Vivus	Raw nostrils, ulcers, bloody discharge, hurried, bad breath	Moderate temperatures, rest, morning	Night, extremes of temperature, heat, drafts, lying on right side
Natrum Muriaticum	Fluent white nasal discharge, violent sneezing	Rest, open air, lying on right side, massage	Heat of sun, morning, emotions, exertion, consolation, touch
Nux Vomica	Snuffling, stuffiness, impatience, anger, feeling chilly, sneezing on waking	Rest, allowing discharge freely, hot drinks, evenings	Uncovering, coffee, alcohol, drugs, morning, overeating, pressure of clothes
Pulsatilla	Ripe cold with yellow mucus, loss of smell, weepiness, clinginess	Gentle exercise, open air, weeping, massage	Warm and stuffy room, beds, rich fatty food, time before or during menses
Silicea	Dry nose crusts, sensitive nasal bones	Warmth, warm wraps, summer, wet weather	Cold air, noise, light, confrontation, talking, mental exertion

[a]All remedies are three pellets, 12 C or 30 C, given every 2–4 h as needed until better.
[b]If no improvement is seen after four to five doses, choose another remedy.

TABLE 115.8 **Remedies for Allergic Rhinitis**

Remedy[a]	Indications[b]	Better from/in	Worse from/in
Allium Cepa	Bland eye tearing, sneezing, excoriating nasal discharge	Open air, cold room, cold water, motion	Warm room, wet feet, evening, spring, damp weather
Arsenicum Album	Burning eye and nasal discharge, thin mucus, feeling chilly, restlessness	Heat, hot applications, hot drinks, motion, lying with head elevated	Midnight or after, sight or smell of food, cold drinks, alcohol
Arundo	Itching inside nose, palate, or ear canals; salivation with runny nose	Desire for sour foods, drinking	Urination
Arum Triphyllum	Raw sores in nostrils, excoriating discharge, stuffy nose, mouth breathing	Warmth	Talking; overuse of voice; cold, wet wind
Euphrasia	Profuse burning tears, bland nasal discharge, eyes filled with tears, red eyes	Winking, wiping eyes, dark, open air, coffee	Night, lying down, wind, sunlight, warmth, indoors
Galphimia Glauca[13]	Sneezing, hives, cold sores, skin allergy, eyelid edema		Weather changes
Natrum Muriaticum	Watery white nasal discharge, cold sores, sneezing, cracked lip, headache	Fresh air, cool bath, thirst, sweating, skipping meals	Heat, sun, light, 9–11 a.m., time after menses, warm room, consolation, grief, loss
Nux Vomica	Violent sneezing in spells, daytime runny nose with nighttime stuffiness	Indoors, warmth, hot drinks	Outside, cold air, drafts, coffee, stimulants, alcohol, overwork
Sabadilla	Sneezing in spells, exhaustion, tickling in nose, red burning eyelids, dry mouth	Warmth, warm drinks, open air, eating	Cold air, cold drinks, odors (especially flowers), sneezing
Wyethia	Tremendous itching of upper palate, dry mouth	Clucking palate, swallowing saliva	Afternoon, eating, exercise, motion
Homeopathic combination remedies	Many over-the-counter preparations available; can be used for generic rhinitis symptoms		
House dust mite remedy[b]	Used if dust mite allergy is known		

[a]All remedies are three pellets, 12 C–30 C, every 2–4 h as needed until better.
[b]Data from Lewith GT, Watkins AD, Hyland ME, et al. Use of ultramolecular potencies of allergen to treat asthmatic people allergic to house dust mite: double blind randomized controlled clinical trial. BMJ. 2002;324:520–523.

Chronic Cough

For cough that persists after all other causes—such as infection, asthma, allergies, neoplasms, chronic obstructive pulmonary disease, and gastroesophageal reflux disease—have been ruled out and empirical therapy has failed, the homeopath can prescribe Ignatia 200 C once or Ignatia 30 C daily for 7 days. If emotional trauma or loss precedes the cough, this remedy is especially indicated.

Cancer

Homeopathic remedies are used in cancer to stimulate the immune system and for palliation of symptoms.[68-70] They can also be used to reduce the side effects of cancer treatment.

Calendula 30 C or Fluoric acid 30 C at a dose of five pellets every 4 hours daily or calendula ointment applied two times a day after radiation treatment has been found to be highly effective for prevention of grade 2 or higher acute dermatitis in patients with breast cancer.[71] Radiation-induced itching in such patients can also be treated using several other remedies, including Causticum, Ignatia, Kali bichromicum, Psorinum, Rhus toxicodendron, and Gamma ray.[72]

Radium bromatum 30 C, five pellets once or three times daily, can be used against other side effects of

radiation therapy, such as Lhermitte sign, nonhealing burns or ulcers, postradiation pain and myalgias, fatigue, and other skin problems.

Gastrointestinal Disorders

Table 115.9 lists common remedies for gastrointestinal disorders.[24,73]

Obstetrics

Homeopathic remedies are well suited to pregnancy. The remedies have no side effects and can be safely prescribed for various prenatal difficulties, including miscarriage, morning sickness, heartburn, headaches, constipation, induction and management of labor,[74] and preeclampsia, as well as postpartum problems such as hemorrhage,[75] mastitis, depression, and newborn nursing difficulties[76] (Table 115.10).

CONCLUSION

Homeopathy is a safe and effective tool that can be integrated into a practicing clinician's armamentarium as either a first-line therapy or an adjunctive treatment. It is relatively free of adverse side effects, enhances the body's ability to

TABLE 115.9 Remedies for Acute Gastrointestinal Disorders

Remedy[a]	Indications[b]	Better from/in	Worse from/in
Arsenicum Album	Diarrhea, vomiting, thirst for small sips, cramping, blood in stool or emesis	Heat, warm drinks, lying with head up, company, rest	Eating, spoiled food, cold drinks, spicy food, right side, cold
Cantharis	Burning stool, burning pains, blood in stools or emesis	Belching, flatus, warmth, rest, rubbing	Drinking liquids, coffee
Croton Tiglium	Gushing watery diarrhea, vesicular rash, loud gurgling, sloshing intestines	Time after sleep, gentle rubbing	Drinking or eating least amount, touch, motion, summer, washing
Carbo Vegetabilis	Feeling chilly, indigestion, gas, bloating, belching	Belching, fanning, cold, bending over double	Eating, evening, lying down, wine, warmth, rich food
China	Gas that will not come up or down, belching that gives no relief, indigestion	Bending double, hard pressure, open air, warmth	Light touch, night, eating, drafts, every other day
Colocynthis	Vomiting, diarrhea, with severe cramps, doubling up with pain	Warmth, pressure, rest, after stool	Anger, indignation, drafts, taking cold
Gelsemium	Green or white diarrhea, heaviness of limbs and eyelids, tremor	Motion, profuse urination, bending forward, sweating	10 a.m., anticipation, thinking of ailment, emotion, shock, humid weather
Ipecac	Continuous nausea and vomiting, increased salivation	Rest, open air, pressure, cold drinks, motion	Food smells, vomiting, warmth of room, overeating
Lycopodium	Indigestion, bloating, rumbling gas, heartburn, craving for sweets	After midnight, warm food and drink, uncovering, getting cool	Lying on right side, 4–8 a.m., cold drinks, warm room, pressure of clothes
Nux Vomica	Constipation, vomiting, nausea	Evening, nap, warmth, wrapping head, hot drinks	Overindulgence, morning, spicy food, stimulants, narcotics, cold open air
Phosphorus	Vomiting, hematemesis, thirst for cold water	Cold, eating, sleep, cold food and water, dark	Warm food and drink, touch, evening, light, wind, odors, emotion
Podophyllum	Painless gushing diarrhea, colic, flatus, offensive odor	Massage over liver, lying on abdomen	Morning, teething, hot weather, eating, drinking, milk
Pulsatilla	Indigestion, heartburn, weepiness	Open air, motion, cold applications	Rich fatty food, time after eating, warm room
Sulfur	Constipation, diarrhea, burning anus with itching, large hard stools	Open air, lying on right side, dry heat, walking, drawing up limbs	Bathing, standing, warmth of bed, being overheated, suppressed symptoms

[a]All remedies are three pellets, 12 C–30 C, every 2–4 h as needed until better.
[b]Data from Jacobs J, Jonas WB, Jimenez-Perez M, Crothers D. Homeopathy for childhood diarrhea: combined and meta-analysis from three randomized, controlled clinical trials. *Pediatr Infect Dis J.* 2003;22:229–234.

TABLE 115.10 Remedies for Obstetrics

Indication	Remedy	Potency	Dose
Induction of labor	Caulophyllum with Blue Cohosh tincture or capsules	30 C–200 C, one dropperful or one capsule alternating with Caulophyllum every 2 h	5 pellets every 2 h for five doses Repeat next day if no labor If no labor after 2 days, wait for several days before repeating
Turning a breech baby	Pulsatilla	30 C–CM	5 pellets one dose
Weak, exhausted labor, rigid os, poor contractions	Gelsemium	30 C	5 pellets every 5–10 min for four doses
Ineffectual labor, lack of dilation, no progress	Caulophyllum	30 C	5 pellets every 5–10 min for four doses
Arrested labor with shooting pains and cramps in thighs	Cimicifuga	30 C	5 pellets every 5–10 min for four doses
Back labor, occiput posterior position	Kali Carbonicum	30 C	5 pellets every 5–10 min for four doses
Fainting, desire for cool air, labor with poor progress, weepiness	Pulsatilla	30 C	5 pellets every 5–10 min for four doses
Fear, anxiety during labor	Aconite	30 C	5 pellets every 5–10 min as needed
Retained placenta	Cantharis, Sepia	30 C	5 pellets every 5–10 min for two doses of one remedy If no results, try the other remedy

Continued

TABLE 115.10 **Remedies for Obstetrics—cont'd**

Indication	Remedy	Potency	Dose
Completion of a miscarriage	Cimicifuga	200 C–1 M	5 pellets once, with tinctures
	Take with tinctures of Blue and Black Cohosh	1 dropperful of each	Orally every 2–4 h until bleeding slows and tissue passes

restore balance, is curative in some diseases that would otherwise only be managed or palliated, speeds healing in adjunctive approaches, and is inexpensive. Homeopathy has survived the ultimate test of any medical therapy—the test of time in the field of clinical practice. Perhaps elucidation of an underlying mechanism of action that can be understood in scientific terms will impart a more prominent role to homeopathy in clinical practice in the future.

Key Web Resources

American Institute of Homeopathy (AIH): This is the principal professional organization of licensed medical practitioners who are practicing homeopaths. The Institute publishes a quarterly journal for practitioner members.	http://www.homeopathyusa.org
National Center for Homeopathy (NCH): This national organization of lay and professional homeopaths is one of the primary homeopathic associations in the United States. It is dedicated to providing information on postgraduate training in homeopathy and dissemination of homeopathic educational materials and resources.	http://www.nationalcenterforhomeopathy.org
Homeopathic Educational Services: Homeopathic Educational Services is a retail outlet for homeopathic books, tapes, remedies, software, and educational materials. This site also includes the *Homeopathic Family Medicine eBook*, by Dana Ullman, MPH, a review of homeopathic treatment for numerous clinical problems with associated footnoted references.	http://www.homeopathic.com
Whole Health Now homeopathy software: This computer program contains repertories and materia medica designed to help match a remedy to specific symptoms from the entire homeopathic database.	http://www.wholehealthnow.com/homeopathy_software/index.html

Key Resources for Further Study

Coulter H. *Divided Legacy.* Washington, DC: McGrath; 1973.	A comprehensive history of homeopathy.
Dean ME. *The Trials of Homeopathy.* York, UK: University of York; 2001.	A review of all the clinical research conducted on homeopathy from the early 1800s.
Herscu P. *The Homeopathic Treatment of Children.* Berkeley, CA: North Atlantic Books; 1991.	A review of some of the most often used remedies for a variety of common pediatric illnesses.
Morrison R. *Desktop Companion to Physical Pathology.* Nevada City, CA: Hahnemann Clinic Publishing; 1998.	A concise desk reference written for physicians to aid in remedy selection for a group of common disorders.
Panos M, Heimlich J. *Homeopathic Medicine at Home: Natural Remedies for Everyday Ailments and Minor Injuries.* Los Angeles: Jeremy P. Tarcher; 1990.	A resource for patients and practitioners in choosing remedies for common acute ailments at home.
Perko S. *Homeopathy for the Modern Pregnant Woman and Her Infant.* Berkeley, CA: Benchmark Homeopathic; 1997.	A practical guide for using homeopathy in obstetrics and neonatal care.
Ramakrishnan AU, Coulter C. *A Homeopathic Approach to Cancer.* St. Louis: Quality Medical; 2001.	A homeopathic adjunctive approach to the treatment of cancer.
Sankaran R. *Soul of Remedies.* Mumbai: Homeopathic Medicals; 1997.	A description of the constitutional nature of a selected group of remedies by an experienced homeopath.
Ullman D. *Homeopathic Family Medicine* eBook. Homeopathic Educational Services: www.homeopathic.com; 2015	A review of homeopathic treatment for a wide variety of clinical problems with associated footnoted references.

REFERENCES

References are available online at ExpertConsult.com.

CHAPTER 116

BIOFIELD THERAPIES

J. Adam Rindfleisch, MPhil, MD

We are not just surrounded by energy and vibration; we *are* energy and vibration. One of the best-known of all physics equations, e = mc², points to a link between energy and matter. Matter is mostly composed of space that contains (or perhaps gives rise to) a smattering of subatomic particles/waves that influence one another through mysterious forces of attraction and repulsion. The nature of the interconnections of energy, physical reality, and consciousness is one of the great mysteries of our times. Quantum physics offers some tantalizing hints about these relationships, but we still have a great deal to learn.

How do these concepts of physics—vibrations, fields, and energy—inform healing? Dozens, if not hundreds, of different cultures and traditions have terms referring to life energy, which includes vital forces that are closely linked to consciousness and animate everything that is alive. Terms used to name this force include chi, prana, pneuma, fohat, mana, and orgone. Throughout human history, people from different cultures and civilizations spanning the globe have suggested that it is possible to both perceive and manipulate this life force. In fact, what we refer to as our "conventional medicine" is something of a historical and geographical anomaly in the grander scheme. The term "biofield therapy" was coined in a 1992 National Institutes of Health (NIH) report,[1] but energy medicine therapies are not new; they have been practiced for millennia. It is important that integrative clinicians be familiar with them.

This chapter reviews key concepts of energy medicine and describes some of the most commonly used biofield therapies. Key research findings related to these healing approaches are summarized here and ways for clinicians to work collaboratively with energy medicine practitioners are suggested. The final section describes exercises you can try yourself.

One caveat: Energy medicine is perhaps one of the most mysterious and controversial of all forms of therapy. An energy medicine practitioner once stated that as an African American, homosexual woman who practices reiki, she has been unpleasantly surprised to find that the most discrimination she has encountered in her adult life has not been linked to race, sexual orientation, or being a female, but rather to her energy medicine practice. Even for some of the most objective scientists, the topic of energy medicine strikes a highly emotional chord. A 1998 volume of JAMA went so far as to conclude that findings from a child's school science project (which investigated one Therapeutic Touch (TT) practitioner's ability to sense the presence of the child's hands) offered "unrefuted evidence that the claims of TT are groundless and that further professional use is unjustified."[2]

As integrative medicine providers explore the use of these therapies, the concept of "scope of practice" takes on a new meaning. At some point, every integrative provider has to determine his or her stance regarding the validity and utility of these approaches. Patients will most certainly inquire about them. Whatever you decide about how biofield therapies fit (or do not fit) into your practice, you should be able to discuss them knowledgeably with your patients.

A second caveat: A textbook chapter can offer only a taste of this varied and complex array of therapies. Trying to understand energy medicine solely by reading about it is akin to trying to grasp Beethoven's work by reading his biography instead of listening to his compositions or getting a sense of Van Gogh's *Starry Night* without being able to look at it. In other words, you are strongly encouraged to learn and explore through direct experience!

> Truly learning about human energetic therapies requires one to experience them firsthand.

DEFINING ENERGY MEDICINE

The National Center for Complementary and Alternative Medicine, now the National Center for Complementary and Integrative Health (NCCIH), originally classified human energetic therapies as one of five main categories of complementary medicine.[3] They further classified them based on whether the energy being manipulated by practitioners was measurable ("veritable") as opposed to subtle ("putative"). Because of political pressures, the NCCIH has scaled back on its support to biofield research or coverage of energy medicine in its web materials. Because there is some debate on whether certain types of subtle energy can be measured, the distinction between veritable and putative may not be as helpful. In a well-done 2015 review of clinical studies of energy medicine featured in a themed edition of *Global Advances in Health and Medicine*, biofield therapies were defined as "noninvasive, practitioner-mediated therapies that explicitly work with the biofield of both the practitioner and client to stimulate a healing response in the client."[4] The biofield was defined in the same article as "endogenously generated fields, which may play a significant role in information transfer processes that contribute to an individual's state of mental, emotional, physical, and spiritual well-being."

According to 2002–12 data from the Centers for Disease Control, a consistent 0.5% of the U.S. population had used some form of energy medicine in the past year.[3] The 2012 National Health Interview Survey found that more than 3.7 million U.S. adults have visited an energy medicine practitioner at some point and 1.5 million reported receiving a biofield therapy in the past year.[5] Surveys may underestimate the use of energy medicine because practitioners of other modalities, such as massage therapists, chiropractors, and naturopathic doctors, commonly blend energy medicine into their practices without labeling what they are doing as energy medicine per se. Research is limited on the use of energy medicine in hospitals, but a 2005 study reported that more than 50 U.S. hospitals and clinics formally offered energy medicine.[6]

Many different schools, or styles, of human energetic therapies exist, especially if one includes the various shamanic techniques that have arisen in many of the world's indigenous cultures. *The Encyclopedia of Energy Medicine* identifies nearly 50 popular approaches used in the United States.[7]

Although various approaches to energy medicine may work with different aspects, or parts, of the energy field or may enlist different techniques for manipulating or maneuvering energy, most share some common aspects, including the following:[8]

- They assume the presence of an energetic anatomy or pattern that has an influence on health. Examples include the chakra system, the aura, and the meridian system used in acupuncture. Some schools of thought propose the existence of several different layers, or levels, of the energy body, each with unique characteristics. Because the chakra system is intrinsic to most techniques and is often referenced by integrative medicine practitioners, it is described in more detail in Table 116.1.
- Patterns in the energy body may precede or cause physical problems. They may also be linked to emotional, mental, social, or spiritual issues.
- Most energy practitioners enlist one or more methods of perceiving the energy field. For example, some practitioners claim to see it, some feel it through touch, some enlist the use of pendulums or other dowsing techniques to assess it, and some report being guided by intuition or direct knowing. Many enlist the assistance of "helper" energies in their work.
- Many healers have experienced a health crisis (taken the healer's journey) themselves that precipitated their foray into energy healing.
- Energy is said to respond to intention. Practitioners may manipulate energy through any number of means, which may include healing rituals, hands-on techniques, visualization exercises, or nonlocal (distant) healing practices.

Table 116.2 lists various forms of human energetic therapies, with key websites for each.

> Although styles and forms of biofield therapies are myriad, many of them share common elements.

TABLE 116.1 The Chakras

Chakra Name(s)[a]	Location in the Body	Color	Associated Issues
First (root)	Base of spine	Red	Physical health and security, materialism, body awareness
Second	Lower abdomen, just below umbilicus	Orange	Emotions, especially toward oneself, reproduction, creativity (in some traditions)
Third	Solar plexus (just below xyphoid)	Yellow	Mental well-being, logic, will, sense of control
Fourth	Heart area, but in midline rather than to the left	Green (sometimes rose)	Connections to others, relationships, forgiveness, compassion
Fifth	Throat	Blue (sometimes turquoise)	Self-expression, creative pursuits, speaking one's truth
Sixth (third eye)	Center of forehead	Indigo or violet	Vision, perception, intuition, dreams
Seventh (crown)	Top and center of scalp	Purple or white	Spirituality, connection with a higher power, unity
Eighth and higher	Vary greatly among traditions; some describe an eighth chakra 6–12 inches over the seventh chakra and a ninth chakra 6–12 inches below the feet	Varies (the one below the feet is said to be brown)	Variable; eighth chakra sometimes described as a point where the boundaries of an individual begin to disappear; in some traditions, linked to the collective consciousness or past lives; ninth chakra may be tied to grounding, connection with the earth

For more information on how energetic anatomy is conceptualized in different traditions, see the various websites listed in Table 116.2.
[a]Names, numbers of chakras, and locations vary among different traditions. In Indian traditions, each chakra from 1 to 7 has an associated sound (lam, vam, ram, yam, ham, am, and om, respectively), as well as a musical key (the first starts with C and the others follow up the scale). Each chakra is linked to different glands as well; this often guides how energy medicine practitioners work with different conditions. In some traditions, the glands are, from chakras 1 to 7, the adrenals, gonads, pancreas, thymus, thyroid, pituitary, and pineal, respectively. Some traditions ascribe adrenals to the third and some link the prostate to the first.

TABLE 116.2 Energy Healing Modalities: Descriptions and Key Websites[a]

Energy Modality	Description and Related Website[a]
Acupuncture and acupressure	Needles are inserted into points said to be located along different meridians, or energy channels, within the body. In electroacupuncture, electricity is passed through the needles. http://www.yinyanghouse.com/. Look at the "Theory" section on the website.
Barbara Brennan School of Healing	This approach focuses on energy healing according to detailed descriptions of energy anatomy and flow. Many schools of healing are based on the experiences or techniques of a specific individual, and this is one example. http://www.barbarabrennan.com/
Crystal therapy and gem therapy	Minerals are used to influence the energy field. Different stones are believed to have specific vibrational properties. http://www.livescience.com/40347-crystal-healing.html
Emotional freedom techniques and thought field therapy	These methods were created by Gary Craig and Roger Callahan, respectively. Tapping of various meridian points is said to release stored negative emotional energy. http://www.emofree.com/ and http://www.rogercallahan.com/index.php (highly commercial)
Energy psychology	Offered by mental health professionals who combine various forms of psychotherapy with energy medicine approaches. http://www.energypsych.org
Eye movement desensitization and reprocessing (EMDR)	Rapid alternation of eye movements from left to right and tapping of specific groups of points on the body are used in various patterns to release energy-based problems. http://www.emdr.com/
Flower essences	Various flower extracts are said to influence people according to the nature or energy of the extracts' plants of origin, http://www.bachcentre.com/. See the remedies section.
Healing touch	Developed in the 1980s by Janet Mentgen, RN, this method is based on principles used in therapeutic touch and other such techniques. Extensive instruction and training are required for certification. See the "Research/Integrative Health" section. http://www.healingtouchinternational.org/
Homeopathy	Created by Samuel Hahnemann in 1796, this approach uses highly diluted solutions said to hold the vibrational principle of a given remedy, which is carefully tailored after a detailed evaluation of a person's symptoms. http://www.homeopathic.org/
Jin shin jyutsu	Developed by Jiru Murai in the early 1900s and brought to the West by Mary Burmeister in the 1960s, this method focuses on the use of 26 safety energy locks to unlock energy flow. http://www.jsjinc.net/
Johrei	Founded by Mokichi Okada, who envisioned a "paradise on earth" brought about through energetic detoxification and adherence to seven key principles. Does not involve direct physical touch. http://www.johreifoundation.org
Matrix energetics	This system of "consciousness technology" was created by Richard Bartlett, DC, ND. It holds that anyone can be a healer through manipulating the matrix of information that is the foundation on which a person's reality is built. http://www.matrixenergetics.com/
Polarity therapy	Based on the work of Randolph Stone, this approach combines diet, exercise, and other techniques to optimize the health of the energy field. http://www.polaritytherapy.org/
Pranic healing	Systematized by Choa Kok Sui and tied to Arhatic yoga, this method involves visualizing colors and directing them through different techniques. http://www.pranichealing.org/
Qigong	This technique enlists various precise body movements to alter one's capacity to store and manipulate qi, or energy. http://www.qigonginstitute.org/main_page/main_page.php
Quantum-touch	In this system created by Richard Gordon, energy is directed through intention, breathwork, and other techniques, with a strong focus on musculoskeletal issues, among others. http://www.quantumtouch.com/
Reflexology	Certain parts of the feet, believed to be correlated with various body parts, are massaged or treated with essential oils. http://www.reflexology-usa.org/
Reiki	This technique originated in Japan with Mikao Usui. Trainees are given attunements said to allow them to pass universal healing energy through them to others. Many different schools exist. http://www.reiki.org
Shamanic healing	This modality is often classed as spiritual, rather than energetic. The healer intuitively determines the source of a health problem and enlists rituals, helpful spirits, journeys to the spirit world, or other techniques to bring about healing. Hundreds of shamanic traditions exist. https://www.shamanism.com
Therapeutic touch	This technique was developed in the 1970s by Dolores Krieger, a nurse, and Dora Kunz. Gentle touch is used to influence the biofield. http://www.therapeutictouch.org/
Zero balancing	Created by Fritz Smith, MD, in the 1970s, this method holds that gentle touch and traction can balance energy at a "zero point," a place where the energetic and physical bodies are aligned. http://www.zerobalancing.com

[a]Table based, in part, on data from Rindfleisch JA. Biofield therapies: energy medicine and primary care. *Prim Care*. 2010;27:165–179. This list is by no means comprehensive. For instance, prayer and spiritual healing are also classified by some investigators as human energetic therapies. All websites accessed 12.15.15.

ENERGY MEDICINE RESEARCH

Through technology, we routinely perceive and manipulate various forms of energy. Our smartphones and televisions can pick up precise frequencies from among thousands that bounce through the atmosphere. Western medicine relies on energetic properties of the body to obtain electrocardiograms (ECGs), electroencephalograms (EEGs), magnetic resonance imaging (MRI) scans, computed tomography (CT) scans, x-ray studies, and many other tests. All these devices are powered by electricity, another form of energy.

> Research has shown that human energetic therapies can positively influence outcomes in numerous circumstances, but much remains to be learned about the mechanism of action, the differences among different energy modalities in their effect, and the best ways to integrate these approaches into other types of healing practices.

We are aware that energy fields of different individuals interact. When people are near one another, each one's EEG patterns can reflect in the others; to use the quantum physics term, their patterns entrain.[9] A 1994 study reported that, for some pairs of people who knew each other and had a certain degree of rapport, one person's brain seemed to instantaneously relay information to another's over a distance.[10] This was the case even when the people were in different rooms and one of those rooms was an electromagnetically impenetrable (Faraday) chamber. Investigators reported that flashing lights viewed by one subject influenced the EEG for the ophthalmic region of the brain of his or her partner in the sealed room.[9] This study was heavily criticized, but a 2004 study reported similar findings.[10]

What is the status of energy medicine research? The current body of research on human energetic therapies is relatively small but steadily growing, and some fascinating discoveries have been made.

The following three important suppositions related to energetic therapies need to be validated for energy medicine to be considered plausible from a scientific standpoint:
1. Subtle energy exists, and it has scientifically validated mechanisms of action through which it influences biological systems.
2. People can perceive and manipulate this energy.
3. Manipulating this energy has clinically important, beneficial effects on health.

Fascinating studies have explored suppositions 1 and 2, with remarkable results that raise more questions than they answer. Quantum biology, biophoton emissions studies, macroscopic quantum effects, and an array of novel measurement devices have offered insights into the mechanism of action of energy therapies.[11,12] Other research indicates that test subjects can influence random number generators and gather information about distant, unseen objects or events that will occur in the near future better than what would be predicted by chance alone.[9,13]

As for the supposition 3 that energy therapies have clinically meaningful effects, the body of research is slowly growing. For instance, a study conducted in Hawaii found that 11 energy practitioners were able to alter brain activity on functional MRI scans. They were asked to select someone with whom they felt a close connection, and then, once they were separated from their partners by hundreds of miles, they were asked to send "distant intentionality" at random 2-minute intervals. The recipients were blinded to the timing of these transmissions. Functional MRI findings indicated that activity levels in several areas of the brains of the recipients changed precisely at the time the healers were sending their intentions ($p = .0000127$).[14]

A 2014 review was unable to pinpoint any specific physiological changes in biofield therapists, such as alterations in biomarker levels in their blood, related to being in a "healing state."[15]

Table 116.3 summarizes some of the key clinical studies of the effectiveness of human energetic therapies focusing primarily on meta-analyses and systematic reviews.[4,16-43] The most commonly studied therapies are healing touch, reiki, and therapeutic touch.

GUIDELINES FOR MAKING AN ENERGY MEDICINE REFERRAL

The keys to making an appropriate referral to an energy medicine practitioner are in many ways similar to those when one refers to any sort of nonbiomedical or "complementary," practitioner:
1. Know the practice and the practitioner. This not only includes knowing in general about the nature of the modality practiced but also means being aware of the practitioner's qualifications and training. How willing is the practitioner to work collaboratively with Western medicine practitioners? Both innate talent and the amount of experience influence a given healer's effectiveness.[8] The best way to get to know providers is to experience their practice as a client.
2. Know when to refer. Many energy medicine practitioners suggest that any patient-related concern is "fair game" when someone is referred for energy work. However, keep in mind that not all providers work according to the Western medicine diagnostic categories. Trust your instincts as the referral provider. According to many practitioners, biofield therapies are especially worthy of consideration for the following:
- People with generally heightened sensitivity. These people are often uncomfortable with crowds; highly intuitive; finely attuned to the feelings of others; or very sensitive to foods, medications, or environmental pathogens.
- People with a history of severe emotional traumas
- People with pain (physical or otherwise)
- People with fatigue or a sense that they can never "keep their energy in." This can include those who are constantly giving to or supporting others and not taking time for their own needs.

TABLE 116.3	Summary of Key Systematic Reviews, Meta-Analyses, and Randomized Controlled Trials Relating to the Clinical Efficacy of Human Energetic Therapies
Focus of Studies	**Findings**
General Reviews	• A 2015 review reported that more than 30 trials have now been done focusing on energy medicine and pain.[4] Although energy medicine seems to decrease pain intensity, the review noted that therapeutic effects are less clear when certain pain measurement instruments are used. The same review noted that more than 15 studies of biofield therapies for cancer exist, mostly focused on the treatment of adjunctive symptoms.[4] Results were most favorable where depression and fatigue were concerned, but only a few studies found benefit. A 2011 review concluded that energy medicine had no benefit in the treatment of pain based on the findings of 6 quantitative and 2 qualitative studies,[16] and a 2014 review came to the same conclusions.[17] • A 2015 review of 30 palliative care-related studies published from 2008–13 concluded research "supports the use of biofield therapies in relieving pain, improving QOL and well-being, and reducing psychological symptoms of stress."[18] • A 2015 review of biofield therapy studies that focused on *nonhuman* subjects (plants and cell cultures) found that biofield therapies led to a significant improvement in well-being relative to controls.[19] • A 2010 systematic review of 67 studies concluded that biofield therapies "…are promising complementary interventions for reducing pain intensity in numerous populations, reducing anxiety for hospitalized populations, and reducing agitated behaviors in dementia, beyond what may be expected from standard treatment or nonspecific effects. Effects on long-term clinical outcomes are less clear, and more systematic research is needed."[20] • A 2008 Cochrane Review evaluated findings for 1153 patients in 5 healing touch, 15 therapeutic touch, and 5 reiki trials to determine whether touch therapies were helpful for pain. Pain was reduced by an average of 0.83 points on the 10-point pain rating scale, with a 95% confidence interval of –1.16 to –0.5. The investigators concluded that "touch therapies may have a modest effect on pain relief."[21] • A 2003 research survey reviewed 2200 published reports related to spiritual healing, energy, medicine, and the effects of mental intention. Findings were summarized as follows:[22,23] • 75% of 130 studies on the link between religious/spiritual practices and health showed positive findings, but the overall study quality was poor. Nearly all the research was observational. • 11 out of 19 trials of energy healing involving 1122 people reported positive effects (Cohen's D effect of 0.6). Overall research quality was judged as fair (Jadad score, 3–4 out of 5). Most trials involved Therapeutic Touch.
Healing Touch	• A 2011 systematic review of 5 out of 332 reviewed studies concluded that "Though the studies support the potential clinical effectiveness of Healing Touch in improving health-related quality of life in chronic disease management, more studies are required given that even the studies included with high-quality scores had limitations."[24] • A trial conducted in 2011 found that a combination of Healing Touch and guided imagery reduced PTSD symptoms in a group of 123 returning active duty military personnel.[25] • A 2004 review concluded that although 30 available studies of Healing Touch did not allow for generalized conclusions, the technique holds promise.[26] • A 2010 pilot study found that Healing Touch lowered stress and improved heart rate variability in 9 pediatric oncology patients.[27] • Vitality, pain, and physical functioning was improved in a group of 78 women with gynecological cancers who were undergoing radiation therapy.[28] • Healing Touch decreased anxiety and length of stay in patients recovering from coronary bypass surgery, but it led to no change in pain medication or antiemetic use or atrial fibrillation incidence.[29]
Reiki	• A 2015 Cochrane review found that there was insufficient evidence to confirm whether or not Reiki is beneficial in people above the age of 16 years with anxiety or depression.[30] • A 2014 review compiled effect sizes from 12 articles that met criteria and concluded that Reiki has beneficial effects in pain and anxiety.[31] • A 2011 randomized controlled trial found that reiki had a significant positive effect on the mood of anxious or depressed students that lasted for 5 weeks.[32] • A 2009 review that included 12 studies found that 9 of them reported significant therapeutic effects of Reiki, but 11 of the 12 studies were ranked as poor quality based on the Jadad score.[33] • A 2010 study conducted in a Yale University cardiology ward found that heart rate variability and positive emotional status improved markedly with the provision of Reiki to patients, as compared with patients in the control group or those who listened to meditative music.[34] • Review of study data through 2007 concluded that the benefit of Reiki "remains unproven."[35] • A review by Vitale in 2007 held that the Reiki literature includes one of four studies with significant findings for stress and depression, one study with significant findings for acute pain, and one of three studies that showed benefit for chronic pain.[36]
Therapeutic Touch	• A 2014 Cochrane Review found therapeutic touch not helpful for acute wound healing.[37] A 2010 study found that therapeutic touch improved pain and fatigue in a study of 90 patients undergoing chemotherapy.[38] • A 2010 study of 21 postoperative patients found that therapeutic touch significantly decreased pain, cortisol, and natural killer cell levels.[39] • A 2007 Cochrane Review did not find any good-quality studies to assess the general effect of therapeutic touch on anxiety.[40] • A 2008 review concluded that therapeutic touch does reduce pain and anxiety in patients with cancer.[41] • Therapeutic touch was found to decrease behavioral symptoms in people with dementia.[42] In a subsequent study of a group of 64 residential patients, this technique was found to decrease restlessness and cortisol variability significantly.[43]

- Those who seem "starved for energy." This group includes those patients who leave a provider completely drained at the end of a visit.
- Anyone who lacks focus or seems "ungrounded."
- Patients suffering from an array of nonspecific or unrelated complaints or whose symptoms cannot be easily explained from a biomedical perspective
- Patients whose chief complaints have something of a supernatural or paranormal bent. Again, the integrative providers' belief system will guide how they approach such concerns.
3. Be aware of safety concerns. Energy medicine has a very low risk of negative effects or outcomes, although one must use caution about relying on human energetic therapies to the exclusion of conventional, potentially lifesaving interventions, especially during life-threatening emergencies or when dealing with severe physical trauma. In addition, patients with psychosis may not do well with energetic approaches.

> The use of energy medicine can be considered to maintain health or to treat practically any condition, with minimal adverse effects. Caution is recommended for use in people with a history of psychosis or when it could lead to a delay in potentially life-saving allopathic interventions.

4. Obtain feedback from the recipients of the care. Are people getting better after you refer them? Is healing occurring?

INCORPORATING ENERGY MEDICINE APPROACHES INTO ONE'S OWN PRACTICE

As with any approach to healing, practitioners must find appropriate mentorship when adopting new techniques. However, energy medicine is an approach that can be attempted by anyone. Many practitioners teach the family members or friends of an ill person techniques that they can practice with their loved ones themselves.

> The exercises in this chapter are starting points. As you gain experience, create your own, tailoring to the needs of your specific practice. Explore and have fun!

As you experiment with these exercises, keep in mind that a health care provider should not "take on" the energy of others nor is it appropriate for him or her to feel that personal energy is lost during energy work with another person. Always ask for permission before doing one of these exercises with someone. Be sure to allow the recipient of the practice to have sufficient time to recover afterward; some people move into a trancelike state as they work with these techniques. Persons familiar with interactive guided imagery and mindfulness practices will note that many energy exercises contain elements of both.

The following four practices can be readily incorporated into a patient encounter:
1. Sensing the biofield
2. Grounding
3. Charging up your energy
4. Setting appropriate boundaries
5. Draining away a symptom

Sensing the Biofield

According to energy medicine practitioners, the biofield may be perceived in a variety of ways. While it is not clear whether people who claim to see energy actually experience their visuals due to photons striking their retinas or kinesthetic people sense an actual vibration or temperature change that triggers their sense of touch, it is nevertheless common for people to report that they interpret their awareness of energy medicine through one or more senses or through emotions and feelings. That said, some people report that they have a "direct knowing" of information that does not come through one of their five senses.
- With light levels low, face your partner while they sit in front of a monochromatic background. Look past them to a focal point a few feet behind them. Note any senses, especially in your peripheral vision, of light distortions (blurriness), colors, or sparks.
- Next, tune into your sense of hearing. As you face your partner, do you notice any sounds, hear words or music, or pick up on any other auditory imagery?
- Take your partner's hands in yours. What do you notice through your sense of touch? People who sense energy through touch often report temperature changes, vibrations, or tingling.
- Bring your attention to your heart area. What do you notice as you focus on your emotions? What is your partner feeling, or what feelings arise for you?
- Take time to share your impressions with your partner. Trade places, and have them do the same for you.

Grounding

This exercise can be used when people seem overly distracted by their emotions or too much "in their head," thinking about an issue but not remaining aware in other ways. Grounding can be helpful for bringing someone into the present moment or into a more enhanced awareness of their physical state. It is also good for people who tend to go off on tangents in conversation. This exercise can be useful for providers before, between, or following encounters with patients. Caution: Some people cope with pain or suffering by not being grounded; this exercise may be stressful to them.
- Remove your footwear as able. Socks are permissible.
- Sit up or lie straight. If possible, the soles of your feet should be kept in contact with the floor.
- Keep your legs and arms uncrossed, if possible.
- After a few slow, deep breaths, bring all your attention to the soles of the feet. Imagine the breath moving in and out through them. Continue until this feels comfortable. If you feel any resistance, simply note it and continue to breathe.

- Feel, visualize, or imagine the outward breath that the feet are extending into the ground like the roots of the tree, slowly spreading through the soil. Sense how these roots add stability and a sense of connection with the earth.
- With each inward breath, feel, visualize, or imagine energy flowing into the feet through those roots, the way that nutrients and water flow into a tree. Let the energy move into the body up through the feet and to wherever it is needed.
- Continue this exercise for at least 20 breaths.
- It may be helpful to follow this exercise with an overall body scan, in which a person is asked to tune in sequentially, without judging or analyzing, to various parts of the body. (e.g., "Focus on your left toes…then your left foot…then the ankle…knee…thigh")

Charging Up Your Energy

Many variations of this exercise exist. It can be done by anyone who is feeling fatigued or weary as well as by someone intending to share energy with another person. The best approach always is to maintain your own energy level and allow additional energy to flow through to others without ever feeling that you are losing your own energy in the process.

- In a place that feels safe, assume a comfortable position and close your eyes. You may find it helpful to place your hands on your lap, with the palms facing upward.
- Bring your awareness to the breath, and take several deep breaths.
- When you inhale, begin by imagining white light moving in through the soles of the feet and up through the body to the heart.
- After the flow from the feet to the heart can be perceived, do the same with the top of the head, and imagine white light moving in, down through the center of the head, neck, and chest, to the heart.
- Continue this process, and allow the heart to fill and overflow with the white light. Thinking about whatever fills your heart with the strongest sense of joy, compassion, love, or enthusiasm is often helpful.
- Once the heart feels full, it should remain so through the rest of the exercise. Repeat the previous steps if the heart does not continue to feel full.
- As the heart overflows, send the white light (or, if preferred, the feeling of love or compassion) from the heart and down the arms into the hands. This energy is ready to be shared with another part of your own body by placing the palms over wherever extra energy is desired. It may also be shared with another person, with permission.

Setting Appropriate Boundaries

This exercise is especially helpful to people who feel overwhelmed by the energy, emotions, or simply the physical presence of others. It may be useful for people with fibromyalgia, whose senses are heightened to a point of causing dysfunction, or for people with chronic fatigue, whose energy seems to leak out of them in a way they cannot control. This practice may also be useful for people who feel as though others are somehow draining their energy. It can help a person feel less defensive or adversarial.

- Ideally, this exercise should be done at a time and place where you feel safe enough to close your eyes.
- Take a moment to tune in to how you feel, right now. Do you feel drained? Tired? Overwhelmed? Where in the body do you have these feelings? Where do you feel vulnerable?
- After several deep breaths, imagine yourself surrounded by a clear, bright, white, force field. This force field surrounds you like a protective bubble that allows in only what you choose and deflects anything that is unnecessary or harmful away from you.
- Strengthen the force field in any places where you feel vulnerable.
- If desired, you can choose to maintain the knowledge of whatever bounces off the force field; understand that you can do this without it affecting you emotionally or energetically.
- Imagine white light radiating from a point at the exact center of the bubble of force that clears out anything that does not belong inside the bubble.
- Enhance the force field further by using additional imagery, sounds, or feelings that you associate with strength and well-being. Pause after adding each extra layer, and focus on the breath.
- With practice, a person can rapidly move through this exercise before entering an uncomfortable environment or facing a challenging interpersonal encounter. This exercise can also be good to be use on first awakening or when retiring for the night.

Draining Away a Symptom

Healing touch and other human energetic therapies often use this technique in various forms. This exercise can be helpful when a symptom can be localized to a specific area of the body. For example, a pain drain can be used for headaches or joint pain. Practitioners can also ask those experiencing emotional pain about where in the body they feel it the most.

- Close your eyes and focus on the part of the body where you feel the pain, discomfort, or imbalance most strongly.
- Describe what you notice there. Does it have a color? Is it an image? A memory? What sound do you hear when you tune into this area? What is the temperature of this area, and how does it feel compared with the rest of your body?
- Take some time to focus your awareness on the discomfort. This can be distressing, given that we may spend time trying to avoid, ignore, or control our symptoms. Just observe. Stay as neutral as possible.
- Now, focus on how the area should be. At its healthiest, how does it look, sound, and feel? Take time to develop a strong sense of this. Again, stay objective.
- With each exhalation, envision the symptom—all that you noticed about it—being exhaled. Some people let it leave with the breath, and others release it into the ground through the bottoms of their feet. Some

people release it in the form of emotions that arise. For others, it just seems to fade away.

- With each inhalation, breathe in your sense of how the part of your body receiving your attention can feel at its healthiest, at its most whole. Draw in the imagery related to health that you generated for this location. This can come in with the breath, through the top of the head, through the bottoms of the feet, or in any other way that seems appropriate.

As a provider present with someone doing this exercise, you can often enhance the experience by placing your hand on or near the part of the patient's body that is receiving attention. If it seems appropriate, you may envision sending what is required through yourself. Use the steps outlined in the grounding exercise to ensure that you are not giving your own energy, but rather letting it flow into and through you, as though you are an antenna. Similarly, if you, the provider, feel comfortable doing so, you may feel or see the symptom being released from the person being healed into your hands. If this occurs, simply intend that whatever is released be deflected away from both the patient and you into the ground.

> If you choose to try energy medicine exercises with those who seek your care, feel free to experiment. Shape these or other exercises as you find appropriate, and develop some of your own.

If you find the foregoing exercises helpful, you may want to consider some of the following resources, which offer other useful exercises and ways of conceptualizing human energetic therapies:

- Brennan BA. *Hands of Light: A Guide to Healing Through the Human Energy Field.* New York: Bantam Dell; 1993.
- Brennan BA. *Light Emerging: The Journey of Personal Healing.* New York: Bantam Dell; 1993.
- Bruyere RL. *Wheels of Light: Chakras, Auras, and the Healing Energy of the Body.* New York: Fireside; 1994.
- Dale C. *The Subtle Body: An Encyclopedia of Your Energetic Anatomy.* Boulder, CO: Sounds True; 2009.
- Dale C. *The Subtle Body Practice Manual: A Comprehensive Guide to Energy Healing.* Boulder, CO: Sounds True; 2013.
- Eden D. *Energy Medicine for Women: Aligning Your Body's Energies to Boost Your Health and Vitality.* New York: Tarcher Penguin; 2008.
- Eden D. *Energy Medicine: Balancing Your Body's Energies for Optimal Health, Joy, and Vitality.* New York: Tarcher Penguin; 2008.
- Gordon R. *Quantum Touch: The Power to Heal.* 3rd ed. Berkeley, CA: North Atlantic Books; 2006.
- Ingerman S. *Shamanic Journeying: A Beginner's Guide.* Boulder, CO: Sounds True; 2008.
- Myss CM. *Anatomy of the Spirit: The Seven Stages of Power and Healing.* New York: Random House; 1996.
- Weil A, Chiasson AM. *Self-Healing with Energy Medicine (Self Healing CD Series).* Boulder, CO: Sounds True; 2009.

Key Web Resources[a]

International Society for the Study of Subtle Energies and Energy Medicine: Group devoted to the study of energy medicine that publishes a newsletter and hosts annual conferences focused on energy medicine	http://www.issseem.org/
Alternative Medicine Foundation resource guide on energy work: Provides descriptions, links, and introductory readings for a number of different energy medicine modalities.	http://amfoundation.org/energywork.htm
Institute of Noetic Sciences: Group dedicated to the study of consciousness and energetic, founded by astronaut Edgar Mitchell	http://www.noetic.org/

[a]See also the websites listed in Table 116.2.

REFERENCES

References are available online at ExpertConsult.com.

SECTION VI

OTHER

SECTION OUTLINE

117 CREATING A GREENER CLINIC

118 INTEGRATIVE MEDICINE FOR THE UNDERSERVED

CHAPTER 117

CREATING A GREENER CLINIC: THE IMPACT OF GLOBAL WARMING ON HEALTH

Rian Podein, MD • Michael Hernke, PhD

Global warming and climate change are transforming ecosystems on an extraordinary scale and at an extraordinary pace, resulting in what some consider to be the greatest public health disaster facing us today.[1,2] The etiology of climate change has been identified and reported by the Intergovernmental Panel on Climate Change, concluding with strong evidence that most of the global warming that has occurred during the past 50 years is attributable to human activities and specifically to the consumption of fossil fuels, producing carbon dioxide and other greenhouse gases (GHGs).[3] Because of the familiarity and predominance of carbon dioxide among the GHGs, it is often used as a representative, or surrogate, for estimating, monitoring, and reporting GHG emissions. Reporting of carbon dioxide emissions can be expressed as the specific carbon dioxide quantity (e.g., tons per year) if this is the only GHG emission measured. When other GHG emissions are taken into account, the result may be expressed in terms of the global warming potential (GWP). GWP is a measure of how much a given mass of GHG is estimated to contribute to global warming relative to the same mass of carbon dioxide over a given time, facilitating measurements in units of carbon dioxide equivalents.[4] All sectors of society, including health care, contribute to the increasing accumulation of atmospheric GHG. In many countries, the health care sector is responsible for consuming significant amounts of goods and services and is an important contributor to gross domestic products. In general, the more a health care system consumes, the greater the amount of carbon emissions associated with the consumption and thus greater the size of its carbon footprint. Carbon emission estimates have been completed for the United States and the National Health System (NHS) in England. The U.S. health care system emits more than 434 million tons of carbon dioxide annually, which represents 7% of the total annual U.S. carbon emissions; the NHS England carbon emissions amount to a total of 18 million tons per year, which represents 3.2% of total carbon emissions in England.[5,6]

GHG emissions are represented by the quantity of emitted carbon dioxide measured in tons. Global warming potential incorporates all gases and is a measure of how much a given mass of GHG is estimated to contribute to global warming relative to the same mass of carbon dioxide over time.

The public health consequences of GHG accumulation and climate change are already present, and future projections are alarming. The direct effects of climate change on human health have been reported through a multitude of pathways, including temperature-related illnesses and deaths, extreme weather, air pollution, allergic diseases, infectious diseases, malnutrition, and displaced populations.[7] The global burden of disease morbidity and mortality attributable to the human-caused portion of climate change is significant, with approximately 5 million disability-adjusted life years per year and more than 150,000 lives annually, with projections to more than double by 2030.[8]

Whereas the health care sector can play a key role in helping societies adapt to the effects of climate change and the risk it poses to human health, the role of mitigation has more recently emerged. This was demonstrated by a World Health Organization mandate for member states to develop "programs for health systems that will contribute to reducing their own GHG emissions."[9] Individual, organizational, and national motivations for reducing GHG emissions may vary, but health care practitioners and health care organizations must be motivated to do no harm, and it is therefore incumbent on us to reduce, with the goal to eliminate, the carbon footprint of medicine and health care.

The U.S. health care system emits more than 434 million tons of carbon dioxide annually, which represents 7% of the total annual U.S. carbon emissions. The NHS England carbon emissions amount to a total of 18 million tons per year, which represents 3.2% of the total carbon emissions in England.

A PRIMER ON LIFE CYCLE ASSESSMENT

Quantification of the carbon emissions of a health system, hospital, or clinic is important to approximate the overall impact toward climate change, to identify strategies for carbon reduction, and to clarify the potential value of mitigation efforts. Life cycle assessment (LCA) is a technique that can be used for this process. LCA evaluates the environmental impacts precipitated by a product or a

Improving the Environmental Profile of Health Care

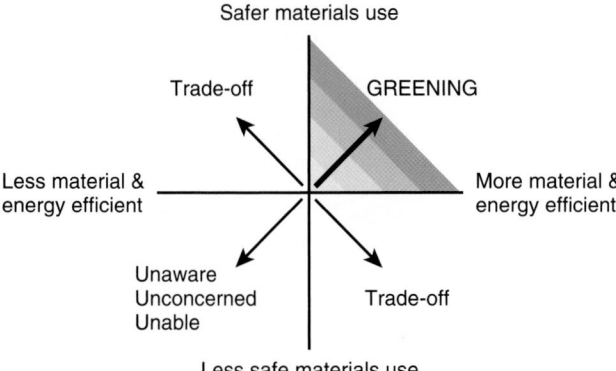

FIG. 117.1 ■ Improving the environmental profile of health care. (Hernke MT. Customer-focus across the lifecycle. Presented at: *10th International Greening of Industry Network Conference: Corporate Social Responsibility—Governance for Sustainability*; June 23-26, 2002; Göteborg, Sweden.)

service (i.e., health care) from sourcing materials through end of life. LCA is composed of three stages:
1. Identify and quantify environmental loads—energy and materials usage, emissions, and waste.
2. Assess and evaluate potential environmental impacts associated with the loads.
3. Assess the opportunities for improvement.

LCA considers all processes over the life cycle—extraction and processing, manufacturing, transport and distribution, use, reuse, maintenance, recycling, and final disposal.[10,11]

A product life cycle can be seen as a linear progression that starts with the extraction of raw materials, such as ore and oil, which are processed into basic materials, such as aluminum and plastics. Finished materials then compose parts and components, such as a car body, which along with other components are assembled into final products. A life cycle also includes the use phase and the end-of-life activities, such as disassembly and recycling. Transportation and distribution between life cycle phases are also considered.

Activities across a life cycle require material and energy resources and generate wastes and emissions, including GHG. LCA gathers information about the quantity of these resources and wastes produced at each life cycle stage. Thus, the effect of manufacturing an automobile would include not only the impacts at the final assembly facility but also the impact from mining metal ores; making electronic parts, windows, and parts that are needed to build the car; and of course, the emissions precipitated from driving.

LCA provides a fairly complete picture within the scope of investigation of a product's or service's known environmental impacts. It lets you see which parts of a product or facility life cycle most negatively affect the environment and thus helps prioritize improvements or select alternative products and services to achieve safer and more efficient energy and materials use (Fig. 117.1). LCA approaches alone do not provide a vision of health care in a sustainable society, a task for which broader science-based principles are useful and have been described elsewhere.[12]

The U.S. and England health sector carbon footprint estimates, mentioned previously, were calculated using the LCA technique. Their findings identified not only the total GHG emissions but also that the three greatest areas of carbon emissions within health care can be attributed to building energy use, pharmaceuticals, and travel, each of which accounted for about 22% of emissions in the England study (Fig. 117.2).[6] In the United States, building energy use and prescription drugs accounted for about 20% and 15% of emissions, respectively; emissions attributable to travel were not considered.[5,13]

Energy Use

Energy use to heat, cool, and power medical facilities is highly intensive and expensive, and it is one of the largest contributors to health care sector's carbon footprint using nonrenewable fossil energy sources. Fortunately, this area offers many opportunities for improving efficiency.

A variety of calculator tools use energy consumption information to enable health care facilities to estimate their GHG (including carbon dioxide) emissions, to compare energy use with similar buildings nationwide, to estimate the health impacts and medical costs due to power plant emissions from the consumed energy, and to obtain third-party recognition and verification for energy consumption benchmarks (see Key Web Resources).

Energy consumption and carbon tracking tools can help people and organizations monitor efforts to reduce energy consumption and resultant carbon emissions. Major targets for energy use mitigation include conserving energy, making operations more energy efficient, and purchasing renewable energy or installing renewable energy infrastructure (Box 117.1).

New health care facilities can reduce their energy use and subsequent carbon emissions by incorporating energy efficiency and renewable energy into their design and construction. To facilitate this goal, the U.S. Green Building Council has created the Leadership in Energy and Environmental Design (LEED) program for the health care industry, a best practices guide for more sustainable building design, construction, and operations.[14] LEED is a certification system providing third-party verification that a building was designed and built with a focus on energy savings, water efficiency, carbon dioxide emissions reduction, improved indoor environmental quality, and stewardship of resources and sensitivity to their impacts.

LEED is perhaps the most well-known green building standard but certainly not the only one worth considering. Retzlaff[15] and Haapio and Viitaniemi[16] reviewed LEED and other green building standards to help users understand their substantial differences and merits with respect to various sustainability dimensions, such as the relative emphasis on energy use and indoor air quality, and other facility goals, such as community or civic use.

When health care facilities, organizations, and national systems reduce their energy use or increase the contribution of renewable energies, cobenefits in addition to carbon reduction and climate change mitigation are realized through direct public health benefits and economic savings. For example, the health effects due to pollution from fossil fuel emissions, especially from coal combustion,

Top Three Sources of Carbon Emissions in Health Care

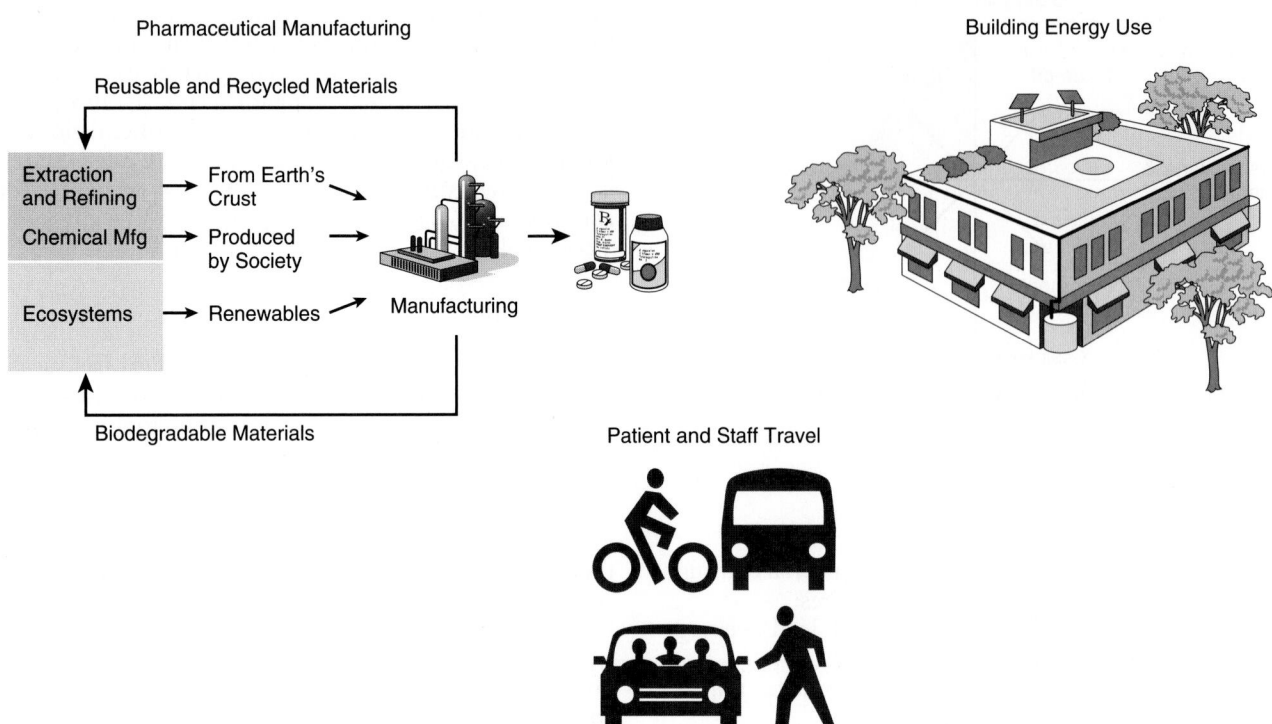

FIG. 117.2 ■ The three greatest areas of carbon emissions within health care.

include cardiovascular disease, cancer, stroke, and respiratory disease as well as asthma and delayed neurological development in children.[17-19] In addition, the cost of fossil fuels is bound to increase over time as supply decreases, thereby positioning energy conservation, efficiency, and alternative energy measures to provide for long-term financial benefits.

Health systems have been encouraged to respond to the challenge of climate change by addressing their own energy consumption and to lead by example: "The health sector is one of the most trusted and respected sections of the society, and it is also one of the largest employer and consumer of energy. This presents both a responsibility and an opportunity to be an 'early mover' to achieve climate-neutrality in its own operations and to demonstrate that this can go hand-in-hand with improved effectiveness and cost savings."[20]

Pharmaceuticals

Pharmaceutical medications are also one of the largest contributors to the health care's carbon footprint; most of such emissions result directly from the energy used in pharmaceutical production in the manufacturing plants.[6] There has been a steady increase in the demand for pharmaceutical interventions and the use of prescription medications within modern medicine. Annual global spending on medicines is expected to reach nearly $1.2 trillion in 2016, with the United States, the single largest market, accounting for 31% of total spending.[21]

If health care continues to increase its reliance on and use of pharmaceutical medications, its contribution to the carbon footprint will also continue to increase in addition

to significant public health and ecological consequences. Medication-related errors at all points of care, including prescription of medications, dispensing by pharmacists, and unintentional nonadherence on the part of patients, are a major contributor to avoidable patient morbidity, mortality, and cost.[22] Ecologically, pharmaceutical medications are being excreted and discarded into the environment at a rate faster than they can degrade, causing them to accumulate in waterways and drinking water. The majority of waterways tested in the United States now show traces of common medications such as acetaminophen, hormones, blood pressure medicine, codeine, and antibiotics, with mounting concerns regarding their deleterious effects on aquatic organisms.[23] Strikingly, a vast array of these pharmaceuticals, including antibiotics, anticonvulsants, mood stabilizers, and sex hormones, have found their way into the drinking water supplies throughout the United States.[24] Because of multiple concerns, including ongoing pharmaceutical use in large amounts, environmental accumulation, resistance of some pharmaceutical parent compounds or active metabolites to biodegradation, newer drugs with poorly understood modes of biochemical actions, potential for ecological harm, and potential for unknown subtle effects from long-term exposures to low concentrations of bioactive compounds, pharmaceuticals have been named by the Environmental Protection Agency as one of the top five "emerging" contaminants affecting human and ecological health.[25]

Integrative medicine, with its incorporation of nonpharmaceutical complementary and alternative medicine interventions, is a proven approach that can reduce health care's reliance on pharmaceuticals.[26,27] Compared

---

BOX 117.1   **Energy Operations: Opportunity for Action**

MAKE BUILDING OPERATIONS MORE ENERGY EFFICIENT

Dedicate personnel and programs to energy conservation, establish baseline energy consumption, install retrofits and institute operational changes, and track progress. Projects may range from minor improvements to capital projects that target a facility's major energy-using systems. Hospitals may bring in an energy use reduction consultant, while Group Purchasing Organizations (GPOs) may make available a contract for energy use reduction consulting. Sample strategies:

- Switch incandescent light bulbs for compact fluorescents and light-emitting diodes (LEDs); install solar parking-lot lighting.
- Install occupancy sensor switches in offices and other intermittent use areas.
- Upgrade at least one major piece of mechanical infrastructure equipment (e.g., boiler, chiller, hot water heater) with the most energy efficient available technology.
- Turn down thermostats slightly (a small lowering, one to two degrees, of temperature can have a big impact).

INSTALL ON-SITE RENEWABLE ENERGY CAPABILITY

Solar photovoltaic panels can generate a portion of your facility's required electricity or power a solar thermal hot water heating system. Installing a combined heat and power (CHP) facility on-site can also reduce greenhouse gas emissions and reduce expenses on energy. CHP systems generate power and heat from a single fuel source, significantly increasing energy efficiency. See the EPA's Combined Heat and Power Partnership.

PURCHASE ENERGY EFFICIENT PRODUCTS

Where Energy Star–qualified or Federal Energy Management Program–designated products are available, hospitals should buy only these products. Group Purchasing Organizations (GPOs) should make these products available on contract. See http://www.eere.energy.gov/femp/pdfs/eep_productfactsheet.pdf for a list of eligible products.

REDUCE "STANDBY" ENERGY USE

Computers and other electronic equipment use energy even when they are turned off or on standby. It is estimated that standby power consumption is responsible for 1% of the world's carbon dioxide emissions. When possible, plug a computer and related devices into a power strip, then turn off the strip when the equipment is not in use—power strips do not draw power. Another energy-saving tool is a software system that manages the power usage of networked systems.

BUY GREEN POWER

Offset 50% or 100% of your power use by purchasing electricity generated renewably.

From Addressing Climate Change in the Health Care Setting. Opportunities for Action. Practice Greenhealth and Health Care Without Harm, 2009.

---

with pharmaceutical interventions alone, an integrative medicine approach often holds the potential to be as effective or even better, to be less expensive, and to pose limited or even positive side effects. One such example is the treatment and prevention of migraine headaches. Acupuncture has demonstrated benefit for the acute treatment of migraine headaches and could therefore be considered in association with or instead of pharmaceuticals.[28] For migraine headache prophylaxis, acupuncture is at least as effective as or possibly more effective than pharmaceutical drug treatment, has fewer adverse effects, and can be cost effective.[28-30] In addition, another nonpharmaceutical intervention, biofeedback, has been shown to be equally efficacious compared with the commonly used pharmaceutical propranolol for migraine headache prevention.[31]

Efforts within the practice of medicine and health care to facilitate pharmaceutical reductions are crucial for the goal of reducing carbon emissions and for providing optimal quality patient care. A couple of areas warrant an increased focus for change. First, providers, organizations, and health systems would benefit by addressing the great imbalance of resources currently provided for disease treatment and away from wellness promotion and disease prevention. The benefits of addressing this issue would reduce the need for pharmaceutical and nonpharmaceutical interventions alike. Second, support for the education of health professional students and providers regarding the role of an integrative medicine approach is already under way, with an increasing presence of complementary and alternative medicine electives in medical schools, integrative medicine curriculum within medical residency programs, integrative medicine fellowships, and continuing medical education programs, all of which will contribute to an increasing base of providers who will have the knowledge and training to consider nonpharmacological interventions when appropriate.

Procurement and Transportation

Other noteworthy areas for carbon mitigation efforts within health care include food procurement and on-road transportation. According to the National Academy of Sciences, outside of direct energy use, these have been identified as the two biggest lifestyle factors when it comes to the net contribution to climate change.[32]

Environmentally preferable purchasing (EPP) is the act of purchasing products and services whose environmental impacts have been considered and found to be less damaging to the environment and human health compared with competing products or services that serve the same purpose. Although EPP can be used for all products and services, one emerging example within health care is the purchase of more local, healthy, and sustainable foods. Most foods travel an average of 1500 miles from "farm to plate," with significant GHG emissions as a result of transportation and fossil fuel use.[33] More locally produced foods reduce the "food miles" of a product, with a resultant reduction in the amount of carbon and GHG emissions. In addition, there are the cobenefits of reduced air and water pollution associated with long-distance transport. More specifically, one of the leading contributors to the food system climate change is recognized to be meat consumption and production, responsible for nearly one-fifth of the total global GHG emissions.[34] Some health care organizations have acted by significantly reducing their meat offerings. Notably, the British NHS has instituted vegetarian menus and reduced meat offerings in all of the nation's public hospitals to reduce its carbon footprint.[35] Inspired by the Meatless Monday project, a nonprofit initiative in association with the Johns Hopkins Bloomberg School of Public Health, numerous health care organizations within the United States have endorsed a voluntary 1-day per week meatless menu (to learn more, visit www.meatlessmonday.com). The United Nations climate chief has validated the utility of these efforts, stating that having a meat-free day every week is the biggest single contribution people could make to curbing climate change in their personal lives.[36]

> People should have one meat-free day a week if they want to make a personal and effective sacrifice that would help tackle climate change.
> Rajendra Pachauri, Chair of the United Nations Intergovernmental Panel on Climate Change (originally published in The Guardian, September 7, 2008.)

Supporting more sustainable food procurement products, including reduced meat consumption, provides health care organizations an opportunity to model healthy eating patterns for patients, reduces carbon and GHG emissions, and offers health benefits too. The regular consumption of meat products increases the risk of chronic diseases, especially some of the leading causes of death, such as cardiovascular disease, stroke, diabetes, and some cancers.

Road transportation in the form of staff and patients driving automobiles plays a significant role in health care's carbon footprint. Health care organizations have the opportunity to encourage staff and patients to shift from sedentary automobile travel to a more active and healthy travel, such as walking, cycling, and public transport. In addition to reducing carbon and GHG emissions, these more active transportation methods provide exercise, reduce fatal accidents, increase social contact, and reduce air pollution.[37]

Consideration should be given to senior-level creation of an active travel plan for the organization, incentives for staff and patients for active travel, establishment of monitoring metrics, routine review of organizational travel needs and alternatives (e.g., teleconferencing), and moving health care delivery closer to the home. Efforts to reduce carbon emissions, including those related to transportation, have the potential to save money, benefit population health, and reduce health inequalities. In fact, many efforts that improve health also contribute to more sustainable development and vice versa. This may be illustrated as a virtuous cycle, a condition in which a favorable circumstance or result gives rise to another that subsequently supports the first, as demonstrated for transportation (Fig. 117.3).

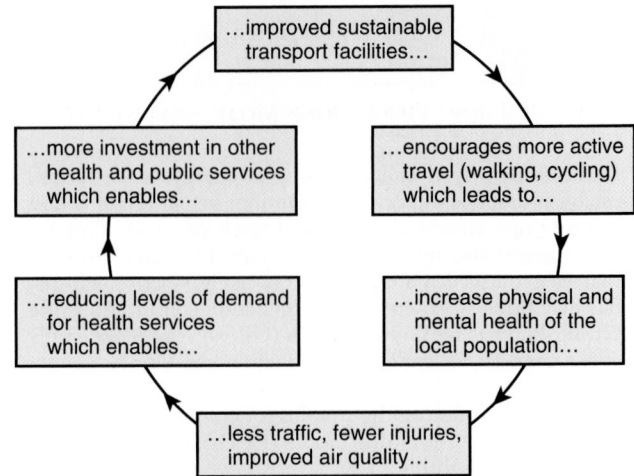

FIG. 117.3 ■ Virtuous cycle for transportation. (From *Saving carbon, improving health*. NHS Carbon Reduction Strategy for England, January 2009.)

CONCLUSION

In 1987, the United Nations published a report that provided guiding principles for sustainable development.

> Sustainable development is development that meets the needs of the present without compromising the ability of future generations to meet their own needs.
> World Commission on Environment and Development (originally published in Our Common Future. New York: Oxford University Press; 1987.)

The more recent Millennium Ecosystem Assessment, an extensive assessment of the consequences of ecosystem change for human well-being, has highlighted our global unsustainability according to this principle, concluding that human actions are depleting the Earth's natural capital, putting such strain on the environment that the ability of the planet's ecosystems to sustain future generations can no longer be taken for granted.[38] Reducing carbon and GHG emissions is a critical component in mitigating the consequences of global climate change and for moving toward a more sustainable society. The common mission of health care professionals and their institutions to facilitate health and to reduce suffering along with good societal standing positions them well to model carbon reduction practices. To transition toward a reduced carbon medical practice and health care system, we may look to prior successes, such as addressing global health interdependence by promoting peace and nuclear disarmament and antismoking advocacy. With climate change, the stakes are high for global catastrophes, as they are with nuclear weapons. In addition, the scientific evidence supports the risks of exposure to secondhand smoke, and the evidence for global warming and climate change is unequivocal that secondhand carbon is harmful too.

Key Web Resources

Practice Greenhealth (membership organization for health care institutions): Energy Impact Calculator: Calculates carbon dioxide emissions on the basis of the amount of energy consumed by the building; estimates health impacts and medical costs due to power plant emissions

http://practicegreenhealth.org/tools-resources/energy-impact-calculator

Energy Star (a joint program of the U.S. Environmental Protection Agency and the U.S. Department of Energy): Portfolio Manager: Calculates greenhouse gas emissions (including carbon dioxide, methane, and nitrous oxide) on the basis of the amount of energy consumed by the building; allows comparison of energy use to similar buildings nationwide; potential to earn Energy Star recognition

http://www.energystar.gov/index.cfm?c=healthcare.bus_healthcare

World Resources Institute and World Business Council for Sustainable Development (a joint project of a global business association and an environmental think tank): Greenhouse Gas Protocol: Provides a comprehensive accounting framework and extensive suite of tools and guidance for emissions accounting for standards and programs around the world, including tools for "office-based and service sector organizations," suitable for health care

http://www.ghgprotocol.org/

Climate Registry (a membership organization for North American organizations): Climate Registry Information System (CRIS): Online tool for greenhouse gas calculation, reporting, and third-party verification; emissions can be estimated on the basis of sources and fuel type or directly reported

http://www.theclimateregistry.org/

REFERENCES

References are available online at ExpertConsult.com.

CHAPTER 118

INTEGRATIVE MEDICINE FOR THE UNDERSERVED

Richard McKinney, MD • Jeffrey Geller, MD

INTRODUCTION

Integrative medicine most often involves provision of high-cost one-on-one consultation. Delivery models now exist that allow dramatic cost reduction, making the challenge of providing this care to underserved populations less daunting. Linked and group visits support financial sustainability even in today's revenue-based health care systems. As the shift toward capitated payment and improved health outcomes continues, other models will become highly valued, particularly for the many issues not well addressed by conventional medicine. Characteristics of integrative medicine make it especially effective in working with the underserved, a group largely living in poverty. It should also be noted that nearly a third of the poor are already using complementary medicine, typically without any real guidance.[1] The time seems right to bring integrative medicine to the underserved! In this chapter we will address the following:

1. Discuss factors suggesting how to approach this population
2. Provide specific examples of low-cost, effective integrative approaches
3. Discuss the challenges inherent in providing these services
4. Share current delivery models that meet those challenges
5. Briefly address the issues of provider self-care versus burnout

HEALTH INEQUITIES

A long list of chronic illnesses disproportionately affect the poor, with the incidence of chronic pain, mental illness, coronary disease, diabetes, and toxin exposure each between one and a half to eight times their incidence in the general population.[2-4] As the focus of conventional medicine has moved excessively toward surgeries and pharmaceuticals, it leaves integrative medicine with much to offer to patients with chronic illness. Many of these health issues resist conventional care, at least as it is most often delivered today, yet respond robustly to integrative approaches, and many of these can be provided at low cost. Many of the interventions described in other chapters are inexpensive and capable of producing real and sustainable relief or healing. See Table 118.3 for a detailed listing.

Chronic pain, one of the most common reasons people of all backgrounds seek integrative care, provides a dramatic example of this. The evidence for the association of higher rates of chronic pain with a lower socioeconomic status (SES) is robust. This population is more likely to develop chronic pain, to be more disabled by it, and to experience a more serious impact of it on their lives. Individuals with a lower SES who are experiencing chronic pain are more disabled and distressed, even when controlling for confounding variables.[5] Ironically, expensive interventions, such as surgery, procedures, and medications, are covered in insurance plans despite little evidence of cost efficacy.[6-8] Meanwhile, less-expensive, effective integrative medicine strategies, such as acupuncture, massage, tai chi, osteopathic adjustment, chiropractic treatment, herbal, and behavioral interventions, are not covered in insurance and therefore are rarely available to this group.

SOCIAL DETERMINANTS OF HEALTH (SDH)

Integrative health has long considered the whole person—body, mind, and spirit—and has worked to encourage fundamental changes in behavior that support health. Caring effectively for patients with limited resources and working to improve the health of the most vulnerable population demands even more efforts. It is clear that health starts in our neighborhoods and communities and not in our clinics. Beyond that, it is not only the decisions all of us make in our daily lives that determine our health but also the environment in which we live, work, and play and the gifts or limitations that the environment provides us with on a daily basis. This collection of issues is referred to as the SDH, which the World Health Organization describes as follows:

These circumstances are shaped by the distribution of money, power, and resources at global, national, and local levels. The social determinants of health are mostly responsible for health inequities—the unfair and avoidable differences in health status seen within and between countries.

The SDH include a wide array of influences, ranging from the availability of resources to meeting daily needs (e.g., food insecurity and affordable housing), accessibility of health care, educational and economic opportunities, community safety versus exposure to violence, quality of education and availability of job training, and social norms and culture. They principally revolve around policies and mores, often implicitly race related, that enforce social inequity. The disproportionate disease burden of the economically disadvantaged is largely a consequence of the SDH, serving as stark examples of how the social determinants promote disease, impede health, and make our jobs more difficult. Most simply put, being poor is an independent risk factor for excess mortality.[9] See Key Web Resources in the following text for the link to the federal Healthy People 2020 program to address SDH. For many of us, these issues demand our involvement outside of the exam room and beyond the work we do every day.

If we consider **health inequities**—the unfair and avoidable differences in health status and disease burden between social classes—a societal disease, then the **social determinants of health** represent the pathophysiology, or perhaps the pathosociology, causing them.

The External Environment of Poverty: Those with a lower SES comprise a complex population whose members experience significant barriers in accessing effective health care and substantial challenges in making healthy changes in lifestyle choices. The social and physical environment of poverty is such that compared with the more affluent, many of our patients live in a very different world. Adler and Newman have described that individuals most affected by poverty are often primarily focused on the survival needs of shelter, safety, and food.[10] The limited time, energy, and resources available for attention to health, esteem, and social connectedness are only a few of the many reasons they experience greater stress and more frequent depression. Substandard housing results in greater exposure to toxins in an environment that may require nearly constant vigilance and impede restful sleep. Increased exposure to violence and difficulty in finding safe spaces for exercise and play contribute to social isolation and to more sedentary lifestyles. Limited access to nutritious food lowers the consumption of fiber, fresh fruits, and vegetables.[10] Collectively, these issues result in such major differences in health among people living in communities only a few miles apart that Jason Coburn, writing for the *RWJF Human Capital Blog*, suggests that a person's zip code is a better predictor of life expectancy than a full genetic analysis, quoting differences of more than 13 years in life expectancy for neighborhoods only a few miles apart from one another.[11] Reduced family and community coherence often produces a surprising degree of social isolation in the poorest of the poor.[10] The estimated impact of this single factor on mortality "ranges between 1.9 to almost 5 times greater than those with better social connections."[10]

Although some of these issues do involve choice, it would be a mistake to consider them simply "lifestyle choices." Behaviors such as cigarette use, high-fat diets, and lack of exercise "are shaped and constrained by social and physical environments linked to SES."[12] Focusing on health behavior is potentially problematic because it can risk "blaming the victim" if the behavior is viewed in this fashion. In addition, health promotion efforts that are not targeted at the poor are likely to increase SES disparities because they are used more readily by those with more resources to act on the information. Changes in rates of smoking, which fell far more quickly among the more educated following the surgeon general's report on smoking, were a dramatic example of health promotion efforts resulting in the current SES gradient in smoking.[10] Awareness of these concerns suggests more attention to the promotion of universal access to the resources needed to engage in health-promoting behavior.[10]

The Internal Environment of Poverty: It is not surprising that the sum of these external environment issues creates huge differences in what might be termed the internal environment—the amalgamation of personal beliefs; attitudes; interpretations; the stories one tells oneself; and the balance of stress, calm, and distress. By affecting lifestyle choices, stress impacts health both directly and indirectly. Even as each of these factors contribute to increased stress in the lives of those with lower SES, our patients are often simultaneously dealing with economic strain, poor paying and insecure employment in jobs with little sense of control, and neighborhoods rife with drug dealing and violence.[13,14]

Christine Bonathan, a clinical and research psychologist with the UK National Health Service, has conservatively described the consequences of such an internal environment: "Social threats raise anxiety and stress, and the consequences of perhaps feeling socially inferior, living in a less socially cohesive neighborhood with a more imminent sense of threat combined with poorer education, and resulting poorer job opportunities are likely to interact with the psychological factors known to increase the risk of negative health outcomes."[5] It is likely that individuals raised in such an environment may frequently self-identify as victims of their upbringing. Those with a victim mentality are generally reluctant to believe that their own decisions can truly improve their health and happiness. Integrative approaches may help these individuals shift their personal narrative from a victim to that of a hero's journey, having survived such a terrible childhood with remarkable positive traits like generosity or compassion or integrity. It is the authors' experience that such a shift may help patients come to believe in their abilities to actually improve both their situation and health. Our counsel can then find fertile soil.

The Importance of Preventive Care: People living in poverty likely have dramatically less support should they lose work or need care for an injury. An effective emphasis on prevention is likely to yield greater benefits for this population. Early detection of poor lifestyle factors, such as stress, sleep loss, poor diet, and decreased exercise, should be taken seriously and addressed as often as possible, taking care to relate them to the patient's own values. Early detection allows more time to plan and implement meaningful changes.

WHY INTEGRATIVE CARE IS ESPECIALLY VALUABLE WITH THE UNDERSERVED

As a group, integrative practitioners spend more time than conventional providers learning about their patients and patient perspectives on the issues they present with. This practice and perspective help them relate to their patients differently. They typically do a better job of meeting the patient where they are at and more commonly seek out and deal with the root causes of issues. In doing so, a wider range of approaches is employed and the least toxic, suitable option is chosen whenever possible. Integrative providers are often more skilled at facilitating and nurturing behavior change and at helping patients deal with conflicting values and ambivalent feelings to succeed in making real changes in lifestyle choices. Because lifestyle is the source of so many chronic diseases and small changes in lifestyle can produce such big changes in health, we can excel at caring for chronic conditions.

Although there are substantial challenges in providing care to this population, the authors' experience in working with the most vulnerable include pleasant surprises as well. We have more frequently encountered "beginner's mind" among the poor than in other consumers of integrative care, with this attitude including a more open willingness to genuinely try out our suggestions. Lifestyle changes are difficult challenges for all of us; this seems especially true for the poor, to whom these suggestions from well-meaning and usually more affluent providers appear to come from a different world. We have found that the same individuals very often listen quite well to their peers. Peer-to-peer learning is inherent to group visits, often making them a more effective agent of change than care delivered one on one. Huge degrees of social isolation and loneliness are often found among the poorest of the poor[15] and can be directly reduced by participation in group programs.[16]

FACILITATING BEHAVIORAL CHANGE

It is recognized that many behaviors that may be adaptive for immediate survival may not be best for long-term health. Behavior change must be approached both carefully and sensitively. For example, working the midnight shift may be the only way a person can support their family, but it causes unhealthy behaviors: eating at irregular hours, loss of sleep, and isolation from other family members who keep a more normal schedule. It is often only through relationship, empathy, and consistent communication and understanding that a willingness to change behavior (i.e., get a new job) can actually emerge. Even then, a longer process is required to consider long-term goals (i.e., training for a new job) while simultaneously addressing short-term health and financial issues. This may necessitate several years of working with the same patient. It most often requires the development of insight, an awareness of the resources available to the patient, and the collaborative consideration of slow, consistent, positive steps rather than large or sudden changes.

Assessing patient priorities is a crucial part of understanding their circumstances and behavior. Securing housing, finding a job, or caring for family may far surpass their focus on preventive health or even the treatment of symptomatic issues. Supporting a person just by listening and building a relationship may sometimes be the most important service that can be offered (see Chapter 4).

PROVIDER CHARACTERISTICS FOR HEALING THE UNDERSERVED

Additional characteristics of style and attitude help determine provider's effectiveness, whether integrative or conventional. The desire to meet the patient where they are at and to understand their perspective provides an important beginning. Active listening with compassion and respect combined with a genuine effort toward acceptance without judgment is also important. Honoring patient autonomy by providing friendly, compassionate, and collaborative care is a clear statement of respect. Because individuals from vulnerable populations are not often offered this respect, they respond better than most once they recognize that it is sincere. Looking for and addressing root causes of difficulties with a strategy based on hope and strength is essential. "Addressing self-confidence and other emotional triggers that affect change and support the client's ability to embrace and sustain positive change"[17] then goes far (see Chapter 3).

Most of us are able to achieve and maintain these attitudes more easily when working with clients who are more like ourselves. The same characteristics may require greater attention on our part when working with patients from quite different backgrounds. More often than not, these efforts are ultimately uniquely productive. The ability to motivate patients to change is largely related to provider style and the ability to create and maintain collaborative relationships.[17]

The techniques of **motivational interviewing** have proven especially valuable with the economically disadvantaged, likely *because they are not often treated collaboratively in a respectful fashion*. They respond well when they encounter a provider who listens well and treats them as partners. "The paradox of change" is often quoted as a maxim of this work—"When people feels accepted for who they are and what they do, no matter how unhealthy, it allows them the freedom to consider the change rather than the need to defend against it"[18] (see Chapter 101).

Motivational interviewing has proven to be a powerful method of patient-centered communication that strengthens motivation for change and reduces resistance by exploring and helping to resolve ambivalence. Sign up for a training program near you at http://www.motivationalinterviewing. org/.

AFFORDABLE APPROACHES AND SUSTAINABLE PROGRAMS

Every community has different strengths and weaknesses. It is wise to take the time to identify what resources already exist in the community. A sample listing can be seen in Table 118.2. Be aware that an increasing number of unconventional practitioners are devoting substantial time and energies to the care of the disadvantaged. Many may be happy to collaborate and extend service options.

A general program might include a number of approaches. Appropriate selection always requires attention to affordability and sustainability. Tables 118.1 and 118.4 offer some ideas that may be helpful toward reaching a cost-effective practice. In keeping with the form and function of this book, an organized guide to low-cost services by the type of intervention is provided.

EXAMPLES OF AFFORDABLE SERVICES BY INTERVENTION TYPE

Biochemical

We already know that many of the poor are already using supplements, vitamins, and botanicals and doing so without guidance.[1] It is helpful to discuss the patient's budget *before* making recommendations and to limit recommended products to two or three, or a total that is affordable to the patient. Some botanicals, supplements, and vitamins are now covered by health insurance, making them more affordable to those with insurance (e.g., vitamin D, magnesium, niacin, B12, folate, fish oil, and probiotics). Other botanicals, pharmaceuticals, and supplements may need to be purchased out of pocket. Cumin, ginger, cinnamon, and similar salutogenic herbs are usually available at local groceries, as are teas, such as mint, chamomile, and ginger, which when wisely

TABLE 118.1	Low-Cost Alternative Treatments for Common Health Conditions
General	Homeopathy: symptom specific
Probiotics	Substituting red star yeast for *Saccharomyces boulardii*
Diet/Nutrition	Healthier foods, more veggies, antiinflammatory, food sources of probiotic and prebiotic (fish oil)
Lifestyle changes	Motivational interviewing approach to ambivalence/resistance
Arthritis	Substituting Knox gelatin for glucosamine, tai chi or other exercise, warm compress, acupressure points near affected joint, and antiinflammatory diet.
ENT	Sinusitis: saline lavage, steam with oil of eucalyptus for sinusitis, *acupressure points*
DERM	Shingles: capsaicin topical cream
	Dermatitis: aloe vera, consumption of oolong tea
	Small, localized infections: honey (sterile), garlic paste
	Fungal infections: topical tea tree oil
Endocrine	Diabetes: dietary changes, increased exercise, sleep, hygiene, and gymnema
Cardiological	Hypertension: garlic, sour milk, soft music, sleep, and hygiene
Lifestyle changes	Motivational interviewing, group medical visits
GI	Upper GI tract: DGL, Swedish bitters, arugula, chamomile, peppermint teas
GERD	Elevating head of the bed, liquid calcium or Cal-Mag, trial of lemon juice or cider vinegar 30 minutes prior to meals.
Nausea	Fresh ginger tea, chamomile tea, peppermint tea for some; use of sea bands or other pressure at acupressure point
Bloating	Fennel, anise, or caraway seeds
Indigestion	Swedish bitters, use of sour foods such as arugula as substitutes for bitters; fennel tea or seeds
IBS, diarrhea predom or mixed	Peppermint oil in enteric coated capsules 0.2 mL or 200 mg
	Ginger rhizome/ground ginger for constipation dominant IBS
Constipation	Gastrocolic reflex, ground flax seeds, bran or high-fiber diet, power pudding (applesauce, stewed prunes, and bran in equal parts; 2–4 tbsp. daily)
Diarrhea, symptom control	Strong tea (green tea being the best, oolong tea second best, and black tea the last)
Gynecology	Bacterial vaginosis and urinary tract infection (UTI) prevention: probiotics
	Bacterial vaginosis or candida vaginitis: boric acid
UTI prevention	Cranberry, D-mannose
Pelvic floor dysfunction:	Yoga, osteopathic manual medicine
Urinary incontinence	Yoga
Neurological	

Continued

TABLE 118.1 Low-Cost Alternative Treatments for Common Health Conditions—cont'd

Migraine	Magnesium, riboflavin; biofeedback with hand warming
Psychological	Anxiety: EFT, support, exercise taught in group settings, Inositol, skullcap, passionflower, chamomile, kava tea, avoiding caffeine
Depression	St. John's wort, fish oil, nutrition, exercise, and group visits (support)
Insomnia	Teas including valerian, chamomile, lemon balm, skullcap, lavender, and melatonin
Toxin reduction	
Household cleaning	White vinegar; mix 1 tsp liquid soap, 1 tsp borax or baking soda, dash of white vinegar or lemon juice in 1 qt water
Window cleaner	¼ cup white vinegar in 1 qt warm water; use squeegee for best results
Oven cleaner	Baking soda, soap and water used with a copper scrubber

DERM, dermatological; *DGL*, deglycyrrhizinated licorice; *EFT*, emotional freedom techniques; *ENT*, ear, nose, and throat; *GERD*, gastroesophageal reflux disease; *GI*, gastrointestinal; *Gyn*, gynecological; *IBS*, irritable bowel syndrome; *liq*, liquid; *Mg*, magnesium; *tbsp*, tablespoon; *tsp*, teaspoon; *qt*, quart.

TABLE 118.2 Identifying Available Resources in Your Community or Practice

Promotion of programs to

Improve access to better quality food

Teach consumers how to prepare healthy food & save money

Creating partnerships with local groups geared toward health

Space at YMCA, church

Sharing programs with a meditation center or food pantry

Food bank with unsold produce from local farmers market

Community gardens where patients can participate

Discounted membership at a local Y or gym

Sliding-scale services at schools training integrative health practitioners

Wild-crafting classes

Collaborating with other health practitioners working within community

There is generally less competition and more collaboration in this setting.

Working with a local bodega to carry specific nutraceuticals, foods, vitamins, spices, etc., at a reduced cost—may benefit the business by bringing local health-conscious consumers into their store.

TABLE 118.3 Mind-Body Modalities for the Underserved

Used in either short individual visits or group visits

Journaling (gratitude, diet survey, etc.)

Breathing techniques (4-7-8 method, alternate nostril, etc.)

Brief meditation techniques (soft music, short scripts, etc.)

Mindfulness techniques (body scan, etc.)

Appropriate for group visits or longer individual visits

Guided imagery

Massage

Hypnosis

Meditation

Yoga

Laughter as medicine groups

Tai chi

Qigong

chosen may provide therapeutic benefit. Food recommendations are often more practical than supplements, and providing vitamins in the form of fresh or frozen vegetables through food can be more effective, acceptable, and sustainable than separate purchases. When supplements or vitamins are needed, less expensive substitutions may be of benefit. An inexpensive chain-store brand multivitamin is almost always a better choice than no vitamin, and several eBusinesses offer substantial savings on better quality items. **Cost-saving substitutions** can also make supplement use more affordable. Examples include gelatin for glucosamine, live-culture yogurt or yeast as a probiotic, sunlight for vitamin D, frozen broccoli or spinach for folate, and Red Star yeast for *Saccharomyces boulardii*.

Biomechanical

Acupuncture, massage, and osteopathy are not often practiced in underserved communities. Because most of this work is out-of-pocket expense to the patient, group visits (shared experience) or linked visit (physician supported) approaches are usually the most sustainable. In addition, some options may be covered by insurance. For example, a physical therapist or osteopath in a hospital may provide osteopathic manual medicine and massage as part of their care, and most insurers cover limited chiropractic services with insurance copayment.

Bioenergetic

Many nurses and clinicians are trained in reiki, acupressure, and healing touch. They, or other community practitioners, may be delighted to find a setting where they can provide these services. Group visits lend themselves to these forms of healing, allowing a nonclinician healer to participate as well.

TABLE 118.4	Ideas for Group Program Activities

Stress Reduction
Prompting awareness: Realization you are not alone
Group programs focused on stress reduction
    Support: friendship/validation of feelings
    Laughter: sharing common experiences
Breathing exercises

Nutrition/Food as Medicine
    Health-center–sponsored farmers markets

Demonstration Cooking and Tastings
Community Gardens
Integrative medicine delivered in group sessions
    Meditation
    Yoga
    Qigong
    Massage
    Acupuncture
    Hypnosis

Condition-Specific Education
Activities incorporated into group sessions
    Exercise: walking/dance/aerobics/strength training
    Art: singing/painting/drawing/collage
    Writing: poetry/children's books/journaling
One-on-one integrative medicine consultations: short visits
    working with the patient to develop a plan

Mind-Body Therapy

These are some of the most used therapies for the underserved as they can be adapted easily to address issues of stress. Those which do not require props are generally more practical and more easily utilized than others. Organized groups can meet regularly at a park to practice tai chi, qigong, yoga, or to work cooperatively in a community garden. Breathing, meditative, or mindful techniques can be simply imparted in just minutes and incorporated into a variety of other activities. If there are local meditation-focused organizations, they may have much to offer. Each are discussed in other chapters of this book.

Lifestyle

Lifestyle choices are most limited by the decreased number of healthy options, safety, and resources in a poor community. Group visits and linked visit models can offer exercise, yoga, or other classes that can become part of a participant's daily life while addressing loneliness, depression, and stress. Many organized groups meet for shared meals, activities, or daily walking.

CHARACTERISTICS OF SUCCESSFUL INTEGRATIVE PROGRAMS FOR THE UNDERSERVED

Finding ways to sustainably deliver integrative care to economically disadvantaged clients involves a number of challenges. Programs need to be accessible, efficient, inexpensive, and demonstrate more rapid efficacy. The meeting location should ideally be convenient to the population being served and perhaps close to mass transit stops. Clinical problems to be addressed should be selected carefully. Programs focused on issues that cause both substantial human suffering and a heavy financial cost to the health care system will be viewed more favorably. Approaches with a better evidence of effectiveness are more likely to produce the impressive results necessary to gain support from both patients and clinicians. Rapid efficacy deserves particular attention, especially for new and less mature programs. Providing services with rapid pay-off helps build support for other slower-acting efforts that may ultimately be of great importance. Efficient programs serve more people quickly and lower overhead, allowing sustainability through the production of revenue. Cultural competence and humility is required throughout—ideas on what is healthy and healing vary.

AN EXAMPLE OF A SUSTAINABLE ALTERNATIVE MEDICINE HOSPITAL PRACTICE

When introducing services provided on-site by licensed acupuncturists at the San Francisco General Hospital, reasoning from these characteristics led us to select chronic pain as our focus. Due to limited capacity, only those dealing with chronic pain for less than 6 years were chosen for the pilot, expecting that results would be more robust and more rapid among this group than among those with a 15- or 20-year history. Because licensed acupuncturists (LAcs) are still unable to produce revenue in the safety net system, linked visits with a doctor provided limited revenue. A research effort was organized simultaneously that focused on the acceptability of this service by the patients and on changes in their quality of life and ability to function in daily life. We are also collecting stories because these personal anecdotes are particularly valuable in building support. The pilot is now underway. In the future, we hope to also assess the effect on the frequency of physician and emergency department visits and ideally on the total cost of care for participating individuals to build a convincing case for the business model. We specifically chose to collect data expected to demonstrate both clinical and cost effectiveness as a method of securing support for future programs.

EXAMPLE OF GROUP VISIT AT A FEDERALLY QUALIFIED COMMUNITY HEALTH CENTER

At the Greater Lawrence Family Health Center in Lawrence, Massachusetts, it was discovered that group medical visits are especially well-suited for vulnerable communities, providing both economic and clinical advantages. These groups use an empowerment model designed to reduce loneliness, which also produces improvements in health outcomes.[16,19] By maximizing **group delivery** of appropriate services and deemphasizing one-on-one visits, productivity was maintained as new integrative services were offered. A single licensed clinician, when paired with a medical assistant trained to help run groups and an instructor, would interact with 8–40 patients simultaneously and bill for many of them. Such programs allowed us to offer longer visits and improved access to health care and thus increased provider productivity. They simultaneously provided the patient with experiences of stress reduction, social connection, and peer-to-peer learning. We ultimately have been able to offer 50 group visits each week with yoga, exercise, meditation, functional medicine, art, games, cooking, and other activities to treat the many chronic illnesses, including heart disease, addiction, childhood obesity, diabetes, and chronic pain, in our community.

ACHIEVING BUY-IN FROM ADMINISTRATION

Although we now have sufficient data demonstrating both the clinical and cost effectiveness of *selected* integrative approaches,[20] "selling" a new program to a health system decision maker often remains an uphill battle. Although clinic and hospital administrators share the same concerns, different issues tend to dominate. A healthy bottom line for financial operations is a necessity for continued operations to serve the mission of the organization. Because clinic administrators are typically dealing with smaller budgets, program changes are proportionately larger, so their first concern is typically financial. The greater time required for one-on-one integrative health visits is not usually accompanied by any increase in revenue. Incorporating group programs, with a realistic billing model, may allow much greater success. Hospital administrators, dealing with a much larger budget, are often more concerned about liability, but in each case, you'll want to be prepared to address costs and revenues. Other vital concerns beyond finance and liability are competence, confidentiality, accountability, and professionalism; each must be addressed directly. Although grant and philanthropic support may be required for start-up costs, care should be exercised while using them for operational expenses—the money eventually runs out. It is vitally important to create financially sustainable programs either by creating revenue or by adding significant value to your organization.

Producing Revenue While Including Noncovered Services

Despite the aim of the Affordable Care Act (ACA), alternative and many preventative services still lack coverage by most insurers in most states. In today's environment, we principally recognize two models for creating revenue.

The Linked Visit

The linked visit provides a brief but meaningful encounter with a conventional provider regarding a billable diagnosis. This visit is then linked to a visit with an alternative provider who can provide appropriate services for the same diagnosis at no additional charge. The conventional provider goes on to see other patients in an efficient manner. These shorter conventional visits result in higher productivity and revenue than usual for that one provider. The difference can be used to provide a modest revenue stream that allows costs to be offset or possibly met.

> **Group medical visits and linked medical visits** can be a financially sustainable way to provide a wider array of integrative care. These practices target the SDH by reducing stress, loneliness, and depression and promoting healthy behaviors while increasing hope and nurturing a spirit of empowerment.

The Group Visit

The group visit provides a longer and more efficient encounter as 8–40 participants can be seen simultaneously. It is becoming a predominant delivery model for alternative treatment experiences (Table 118.4).[21] The longer duration of group visits allows more thorough participant education about alternative therapies (see Table 118.3). Shared appointments and group medical visits seem the most promising approaches to build financial sustainability for alternative services, with one-on-one visits continuing but substantially minimized. This allows for coordinated interprofessional programs, with the team-based care extending the reach of the most highly paid and costly professionals. Costs per individual are minimized despite the longer sessions that are the heart of the program. Surprises come from the more open-minded attitude the groups promote among participants and from the magic of peer-to-peer learning. Hearing confirmation from a member of your own community that an approach you've never before heard of may be effective is very different than hearing it from a strangely dressed and privileged physician, who is clearly from a different planet. Behavioral or lifestyle changes can be more strongly supported in groups than in other settings. The other bonus of group work, particularly in the open model of empowered groups, is the dramatic way in which groups can foster community, sense of belonging, and friendships.[21-24] In this setting, most patients ultimately prefer to minimize their one-on-one time with the doctor, fearing that they will miss something in the group session going on simultaneously.

The group experience can result in higher access to health care, stress reduction, emotional support, and sharing of best practices between peers. These are all highly efficient pathways to health. Most effective group sessions have a check-in period, an educational experience, and an activity portion that is relevant to the particular group. Beginning each session with an unhurried check-in round builds community. Allowing at least an hour for education or demonstrations provides time for peer-to-peer discussion. Don't forget to add music—nearly every group is helped by it. Groups do best when they are consistently scheduled, are in an easily accessible location, are covered by insurance, provide value to the attendees, and actively solicit guidance from group participants.

Most group meetings last at least an hour, and groups can meet monthly, bimonthly, weekly, or biweekly. Some have a drop-in format, whereas others have prescribed attendees and meeting criteria. Groups can be used as therapy for patients with heart disease, diabetes, chronic pain (fibromyalgia, headaches, and back pain), pregnancy, addiction (smoking and heroin), obesity (adults, children, and families), developmental delay, and high utilization of services. Many of our patients suffer with depression, loneliness, social isolation, posttraumatic stress, anxiety, and social stressors. Services offered in groups can address these issues, both physical and psychosocial, by offering a variety of services: acupuncture, hypnosis, meditation, yoga, qigong, dance, yoga, aerobics, strength training, low-impact exercise, exercise of different levels, support, art, writing, demo cooking and tastings, shared meals, planned outings and trips, community gardens, and condition-specific education and training sessions.

Provider Burnout and Self-Care

The underserved and their caregivers both need unique types of support, and the provider's self-care is a crucial issue deserving explicit attention. The need for services far exceeds supply, and burnout ultimately makes services even less available. Adopting the mindset of a well-paced runner is essential—this is not a sprint but a marathon. A proactively chosen mix of more and less generously reimbursed services, perhaps in a mix of integrative and conventional care, may allow maximized professional satisfaction while maintaining personal balance. We will accomplish far more by pacing ourselves to stay involved with a disadvantaged client or community for a longer time, providing consistent care, rather than by burning ourselves out by taking on huge amounts each month. Change takes time.

Taking care of your own needs is vital. Working in an underserved community requires patience and creativity as we strive to overcome the barriers to health that our patients encounter. Creativity most often requires a place of freedom in the mind that allows us to make connections that otherwise may be missed. It takes time to develop different perspectives and to continue the journey of learning as a healer.

> The challenge of providing integrative care to vulnerable populations is huge, so are the rewards. It is a marathon and not a sprint. Good self-care is essential for all—providers and staff.

OUTSIDE THE EXAM ROOM: ACTIVISM

Whether the ACA is ever fully implemented or not, the swing toward capitated payments seems destined to continue. At some point, additional services will likely cease to add incremental income. These changes will increasingly dictate the use of cost-effective ways to promote population health, with a focus on cost savings.[26] Advancing patients' health, improving their experience of care, and saving money—the triple aim—will then be paramount, and the time even more ripe for the approaches that we have discussed, among others. Now is the time to help generate the data to support such a shift. When the time comes, changes will include substantial analysis of our health systems. It is up to us to collect and provide the data that the decision makers will need and use to choose health options wisely.

For many of us, the issues related to the SDH, health equity, and appropriateness of care for the most vulnerable demand our political involvement outside of the exam room. Affecting the SDH is a major challenge but also an area where we can make a difference, most effectively by working with the community. Some movement toward reimbursement of alternative therapies has already begun nationally. The Joint Commission now recommends that organizations provide nonpharmacological therapies as first-line treatment for pain and chronic pain for accreditation and names these nonpharmacological approaches to include osteopathy, acupuncture, and mind-body therapies.[25] By supporting organizations working toward these ends, we can stay informed, help our organizations be prepared, and serve as leaders in the field.

Key Web Resources	
Pt handouts, clinician guidelines, teaching aides. IM4US also hosts an annual meeting in August of each year that focuses on Integrative Medicine for the Underserved.	http://www.IM4US.org
Information regarding the social determinants	http://www.healthypeople.gov/2020/topics-objectives/topic/social-determinants-health
Training and resources for motivational interviewing	http://www.motivationalinterviewing.org/
Clinician learning modules, patient information handouts	http://www.fammed.wisc.edu/integrative
Scientific research on Integrative Care	http://nccih.nih.gov (previously NCCAM)
Herbs at a Glance, patient info sheets on more than 50 herbs	http://nccam.nih.gov/health/herbsataglance.htm
Dietary Supplements Labels Database	http://www.dsld.nlm.nih.gov

REFERENCES

References are available online at ExpertConsult.com.

INDEX

A

Abatacept (Orencia), in rheumatoid arthritis, 498

Abdominal pain, in pediatrics, 457–465.e2
acupuncture in, 463
behavior modification in, 460
bioenergetic therapy in, 463
biofeedback in, 464
biomechanical therapy in, 463
botanicals in, 460–462
breathing exercises in, 464
chamomile in, 460–461, 461b
cyproheptadine in, 463, 463b
dietary fiber in, 459–460, 460t, 460b
food elimination in, 460
ginger in, 461, 461b
guided imagery in, 464
healing touch in, 463
histamine-2 (H2) receptor antagonists in, 462–463
hypnosis in, 464
integrative therapy for, 459–465
lemon balm in, 462, 462b
massage in, 463
mind-body therapy in, 463–465
nutrition in, 459–460
osteopathic manipulative therapy in, 463
pathophysiology of, 457–459, 457b, 458f, 459b
peppermint in, 461, 461b
pharmaceuticals in, 462–463
prevention prescription of, 464b
probiotics in, 462, 462b
progressive muscle relaxation in, 464
proton pump inhibitors in, 462–463
psychotherapy in, 464–465
red flags in, 459
Reiki in, 463
Rome III criteria for, 459
slippery elm in, 462, 462b
supplements in, 462
surgery in, 463
therapeutic review on, 464b–465b
traditional Chinese medicine (TCM) in, 463t
web resources on, 465t

Ablation therapy, in arrhythmias, 284

Abortion, therapeutic, in nausea and vomiting, in pregnancy, 547, 547f

Abreactive ego state therapy, for posttraumatic stress disorder, 89

Absorption, on hormone imbalance, 579–580

Acamprosate, in alcoholism, 819

Acanthopanax senticosus. See Siberian ginseng

Acetaminophen, 153
in carpal tunnel syndrome, 698, 698b
in low back pain, 671
in neck pain, 684t
in osteoarthritis, 646

N-Acetylcysteine, 1010, 1010t–1011t
in Alzheimer disease, 102, 102b
in chronic kidney disease, 414, 414b
in HIV disease, 184, 184b
in homocysteine lowering, 402–403
in inflammatory bowel disease, 506
in Parkinson's disease, 146, 146b
in polycystic ovary syndrome, 364, 364b

Acetyl-L-carnitine
in Alzheimer disease, 101–102, 102b
in chronic fatigue syndrome, 486, 486b
in insulin resistance, 331, 331b
in metabolic syndrome, 331, 331b
in peripheral neuropathy, 126

Achilles tendinopathy, prolotherapy for, 1050

Acid-base balance, in osteoporosis, 370

Acid-base issues, osteoporosis and, 371

Acid-suppressing drugs, in peptic ulcer disease, 446, 446b

Acitretin, in psoriasis, 734, 734b

Acne rosacea, 765–769
botanicals in, 766–767
diet in, 767
emotional stress and, 759
erythematotelangiectatic, 765, 766t
ocular, 765, 766t
papulopustular, 765, 766t
pathophysiology of, 759, 760f
phymatous, 765, 765f, 766t
therapeutic review for, 770b
web resources on, 770t

Acne vulgaris, 759, 767b
azelaic acid in, 763b, 764
benzoyl peroxide in, 762b, 763
botanicals in, 761–762
brewer's yeast in, 761, 761b
diet in, 760
emotional stress and, 759–760
green tea in, 762, 762b
hormonal treatment and, 764, 764b
hygiene in, 759
isotretinoin in, 764b, 765
laser and light therapy in, 765
pathophysiology of, 759, 760f
retinoids in, topical, 763, 763b
salicylic acid in, 763, 763b
supplements in, 760–761
surgery in, 765
tea tree oil in, 762, 762b
therapeutic review for, 767b
therapies to consider for, 765
turmeric in, 762–763, 762b
vitamin A in, 761–762, 761b
web resources on, 770t
zinc in, 761, 761b

Acquired immunodeficiency syndrome (AIDS). *See* Human immunodeficiency virus (HIV) disease

Action, in healing encounter, 22

Acupressure
in dysmenorrhea, 574–575, 575f, 575b
in headache, 1038–1039
in labor pain management, 529, 529f, 529b
in nausea and vomiting in pregnancy, 544, 544b, 545f

Acupuncture
in arrhythmias, 281
auricular, 822, 822f
in autism spectrum disorder, 71
in cholelithiasis, 455
in chronic fatigue syndrome, 490–491
in chronic kidney disease, 419
in chronic prostatitis/chronic pelvic pain syndrome, 620, 620b
in depression, 41
in dysmenorrhea, 574
in energy psychology, 972
in epicondylosis, 708–709, 709b
in fertility, 523
in fibromyalgia, 478
in gout, 692
in headache. *See* Headache, acupuncture for
in heart failure, 250
in herpes simplex virus infection, 194–195
in HIV disease, 188
in inflammatory bowel disease, 514
in irritable bowel syndrome, 430
in labor pain management, 528–529, 528f, 529b
in low back pain, 672–673
in lung cancer, 787
in Lyme disease, 226, 226b
in menopausal symptoms, 554–555, 555b
in migraine, 115–116
in nausea and vomiting, 1044–1046.e1, 1045f–1046f, 1045b
in neck pain, 680, 680b
in osteoarthritis, 644, 644b
in palliative care, 814
in Parkinson's disease, 147, 150b–151b
in pediatric abdominal pain, 463
in peptic ulcer disease, 447
in peripheral neuropathy, 123, 123b
in polycystic ovarian syndrome, 365–366
in postdates pregnancy, 538, 538t
in posttraumatic stress disorder, 90, 92b
in premenstrual syndrome, 566
in psoriasis, 736, 736b
in rheumatoid arthritis, 498
specific and nonspecific variables of, 16, 16f, 17t
in substance abuse, 821–822, 822f, 822b
in tension-type headache, 118

Acupuncture *(Continued)*
in urinary tract infection, 215–216
in urolithiasis, 612, 612b
in uterine fibroids, 589

S-Adenosylmethionine (SAMe), 396
in chronic hepatitis, 203–204
in depression, 38–39, 38f
in fibromyalgia, 479, 479b
in osteoarthritis, 645–646, 645b

Adiponectin, 334, 334b

Adrenal fatigue, 404–409.e1
adrenal glandulars in, 407–408
ashwagandha in, 406, 406b
bioenergetic interventions in, 408
biofeedback in, 408
botanicals in, 406–407
breathing practices in, 408
dehydroepiandrosterone (DHEA) in, 407
diagnosing, 404–405, 405b
integrative therapy for, 406–409, 406b
L-carnitine in, 407, 407b
licorice in, 406, 406b
lifestyle interventions in, 406
mind-body interventions in, 408
natural stress response in, 404, 405f, 406t
nutrition in, 406
Panax ginseng in, 407, 407b
prevention prescription of, 408b
progressive muscle relaxation in, 408
reiki in, 408
Rhodiola rosea in, 407, 407b
Siberian ginseng in, 407, 407b
supplements in, 407–408
therapeutic review in, 409b
therapies to consider in, 408–409
vitamin B complex in, 407, 407b
vitamin C in, 407, 407b
web resources on, 409t
yoga in, 408

Adrenal gland, in chronic fatigue syndrome, 488

Adrenal glandulars, in adrenal fatigue, 407–408

Agaricus brasiliensis, in peripheral neuropathy, 131

Age/aging
Alzheimer disease and, 97. *See also* Alzheimer disease
cataracts and, 833. *See also* Cataracts
heart rate variability and, 925–926

Age-related macular degeneration, 838–846.e1
alpha-lipoic acid in, 843
amino acids in, 843–844
atrophic, 839f
attitude and, 841
B vitamins in, 843
beta-carotene in, 843
bilberry in, 844
bioflavonoids in, 843
botanicals in, 844–845

Page numbers followed by "*b*" indicate boxes; "*f*" figures; "*t*" tables.

Age-related macular degeneration (Continued)
  breathing in, 840–841
  carotenoids in, 843
  Chinese herbs in, 845, 845b
  cold-water fish in, 842
  copper in, 844
  docosahexaenoic acid in, 844, 844b
  estrogen in, 841
  exercise in, 840
  exudative, 839f
  fruits and vegetables in, 841
  gender in, 839–840
  Ginkgo biloba in, 844
  glutathione in, 842–843
  hats and visors in, 840
  hydration in, 840
  inflammation and, 840
  integrative therapy for, 840–846
  lifestyle interventions in, 840–841
  limiting alcohol intake in, 840
  lutein in, 842–843, 843b
  lutein-containing foods in, 841–842, 842b
  magnesium in, 844
  medication effects in, recognition of, 840, 840b
  milk thistle in, 844, 844b
  minerals in, 844
  multivitamins in, 842
  nutrition in, 841–842, 841b
  pathophysiology of, 838
  pharmaceuticals in, 845
  prevention prescription of, 845b
  risk factors for, 839–840
  sage in, 844
  saturated fats in, 842
  screening of, 838–839, 839f
  selenium in, 844
  sleep in, 841
  smoking and other factors in, 840
  stress management in, 840
  sunglasses in, 840
  sunlight in, 839
  supplements in, 842–844
  therapeutic review in, 845b
  tocopherols in, 843
  vitamin A in, 843
  vitamin C in, 843
  vitamin D in, 843
  web resources in, 846t
  whole body health in, 841
  wine in, 842
  zinc in, 844
AIDS. *See* Human immunodeficiency virus (HIV) disease
Air pollution, 157
  in chronic kidney disease, 418.e2
ALCAT testing, 314
Alcohol use/abuse
  age-related macular degeneration and, 840
  anxiety and, 48
  breast cancer and, 582, 775
  cholelithiasis and, 452
  colorectal cancer prevention and, 803
  depression and, 37
  diabetes mellitus and, 336, 336b
  dysmenorrhea and, 569
  osteoporosis and, 377–378
  peptic ulcer disease and, 443
Alcoholics Anonymous, 824–825, 824b
Alcoholism, 817–828.e2
  abstinence from, 819b
  integrative therapy, 818–828
    acupuncture in, 821–822, 822f, 822b
    Alcoholics Anonymous in, 824–825, 824b
    biofeedback in, 823
    botanicals, 821
    guided imagery in, 823
    homeopathy in, 826–828
    hypnosis in, 823

Alcoholism (Continued)
    meditation in, 823
    mind-body therapies in, 823–824, 823b
    Native American interventions in, 825–826, 825f–826f
    nutrition in, 826
    pharmaceuticals, 818–821, 819t
    spirituality in, 824
    therapeutic review on, 826b–827b
    yoga in, 823–824
  moderate, 819b
  pathophysiology of, 818
  prevention, 826b
  risky/hazardous, 819b
  screening for, 819b
  web resources on, 828t
Aldosterone, in premenstrual syndrome, 560
Aldosterone antagonists, in heart failure, 248
Alendronate, in osteoporosis, 378–379, 379t
Alexander technique, 677
Alfuzosin, for urolithiasis, 613, 613b
Alkalinizers, in urolithiasis, 612
Allergic patient, 300–309.e2
  antihistamines in, 305–306, 306b
  integrative therapy for, 302–309
    immunotherapy, 306–307
    mind-body therapy, 307
    nutrition, 302–303
    other botanicals, 305
    pharmaceuticals, 305–306
    supplements, 303–304
    traditional Chinese medicine, 307–309
  pathophysiology of, 300–302, 301f, 301t–302t, 301b
  prevention prescription for, 308b
  therapeutic review for, 308b
  web resources in, 309t
Allergic rhinitis, therapeutic homeopathy in, 1067, 1070t
"Allergic to everything," 317
Allergy
  food, 310–318.e6, 310b
    in cholelithiasis, 452
    diagnosis of, 311t, 313–314
    differentiating from other food reactions, 316
    epidemic of, 310–312
    IgG4 antibody testing to, 314
    integrative therapy of, 314–318
    medical history of, 313, 313b
    migraine and, 313
    nomenclature of, 310
    pathophysiology of, 310–312
    physical examination of, 313
    prevention prescription of, 318b
    pseudoallergy and, 316
    research validation of, 312–313
    specific adaption of, 312, 312f
    symptoms and conditions may cause or exacerbated by, 311t
    therapeutic review of, 318b
    web resources on, 318t
Allergy elimination diet, in atopic dermatitis, 719
AlliMed, for chronic sinusitis, 161, 161b
Allium sativum. See Garlic
Allopurinol, in gout, 695, 695b
Aloe vera
  in constipation, 469, 469b
  in herpes simplex virus infection, 194, 194b
  in inflammatory bowel disease, 509
  in irritable bowel syndrome, 428–429
  in psoriasis, 730–731
Alpha adrenergic agonists, in rosacea, 770b, 770.e5

Alpha blockers, in chronic prostatitis/chronic pelvic pain syndrome, 617, 617b
Alpha-1 channel blockers, in urolithiasis, 612–613
5-Alpha reductase inhibitors, 631, 634b
Alpha-adrenergic blocking agents, in benign prostatic hyperplasia, 604–605, 605b
Alpha-glucosidase inhibitors, 332
L-Alpha-glycerylphosphorylcholine, for Alzheimer disease, 105
Alpha-lipoic acid, 1010t–1011t, 1011–1012
  in age-related macular degeneration, 843
  in Alzheimer disease, 102, 102b
  in chronic hepatitis, 204
  in diabetes mellitus, 340–341, 341b
  in HIV disease, 183, 183b
  in insulin resistance, 330, 330b
  in metabolic syndrome, 330, 330b
  in migraine, 109t
  in peripheral neuropathy, 127
5-Alpha-reductase inhibition, in benign prostatic hyperplasia, 605, 605b
Alpha-synuclein, in Parkinson's disease, 145
Altered intestinal permeability, autism and, 66–67
Althea officinalis. See Marshmallow
Alzheimer disease, 94–107.e4
  antiinflammatory diet in, 875t
  B vitamins for, 101
  case study in, 95b–97b
  clinical course of, 98
  diagnosis of, 97–98, 98f
  integrative therapy for, 98–107, 98b
    botanicals, 102–103
    hormones, 103
    lifestyle factors in, 98–100
    management of behavioral problems, 104
    mind-body techniques, 100–101, 100b
    supplements, 101–102
    therapies to consider for, 103–107
    vitamins and minerals, 101
  mild cognitive impairment and, 97
  pathophysiology of, 95–98
    chronic exposure to toxins, 95–97
    methylation and homocysteine, 95
  plaques in, 95
  prevention prescription for, 106b
  risk factors of, 96t
  screening for, 97
  tangles in, 95
  therapeutic review on, 106b
  web resources on, 107t
Amantadine, in Parkinson's disease, 148–149, 149b
American ginseng, for vaginal dryness, 597, 597b
Amino acids
  in age-related macular degeneration, 843–844
  in attention-deficit/hyperactivity disorder, 55
  in autism spectrum disorder, 70
  in chronic fatigue syndrome, 489
5-Aminosalicylic acid, in inflammatory bowel disease, 511
Amiodarone, herbal and supplement interactions with, 256t
Amitriptyline, in myofascial pain syndrome, 659, 659b
Amlexanox, in aphthous stomatitis, 749, 749b

Amniotomy, in postdates pregnancy, 539
Amoxapine, in depression, 43
Amoxicillin, 155b
  in Lyme disease, 223b
Amsler grid, in age-related macular degeneration, 838, 839f
Amyloid, in Alzheimer disease, 95
Analgesics
  in common cold, 178
  in fibromyalgia, 481
  in peripheral neuropathy, 130
Ananas comosus. See Pineapple
Androgens. *See* Dihydrotestosterone (DHT); Testosterone
Andrographis, for common cold, 171, 171b
Andrographis paniculata extract, in inflammatory bowel disease, 509
Angelica, in arrhythmias, 283
Angioplasty, in coronary artery disease, 255
Angiotensin receptor blockers (ARBs), in heart failure, 248, 249b
Angiotensin-converting enzyme inhibitors
  in heart failure, 247–248, 249b
  in type 2 diabetes mellitus, 345
Animal-assisted therapy, for Alzheimer disease, 104
Antacids, in peptic ulcer disease, 447, 447b
Anthralin, in psoriasis, 733, 733b
Antiandrogens, in polycystic ovarian syndrome, 367, 367b
Antiangiogenesis factors, in uterine fibroids, 585, 585b
Antibiotic-associated diarrhea (children), prevention of, 992t
Antibiotics
  in acne vulgaris
    oral, 764, 764b
    topical, 763, 763b
  in chronic prostatitis/chronic pelvic pain syndrome, 617, 617b
  in irritable bowel syndrome, 430, 430b
  in Lyme disease
    acute infection of, 222–223, 223b
    chronic persistent symptoms of, 224, 224b
  natural, in chronic sinusitis, 161–162
  in otitis media, 153, 155
  in peptic ulcer disease, 446, 446b
  in rheumatoid arthritis, 496
  in rosacea, 769b, 770.e5
  in urinary tract infection, 215
Anti-*Candida* program, 318
Anticholinergics
  in benign prostatic hyperplasia, 605
  in common cold, 178
  in Parkinson's disease, 149, 149b
Anticoagulant therapies, in coronary artery disease, 255
Anticonvulsants
  in fibromyalgia, 481
  in migraine, 113
  in peripheral neuropathy, 129–130
Antidepressants
  in depression, 41, 42t
  in fibromyalgia, 480
  in irritable bowel syndrome, 430
  in myofascial pain syndrome, 659
  in peripheral neuropathy, 129
Antihistamines
  in allergic patient, 305–306, 306b
  in atopic dermatitis, 721, 721b, 724b
  in common cold, 177–178

Antihistamines *(Continued)*
in nausea and vomiting in
pregnancy, 546, 546b
in urticaria, 742–743, 743b
Antihypertensive agents, 413
Antiinflammatory diet. *See* Diet,
antiinflammatory
Antimicrobial drugs, in inflammatory
bowel disease, 510–511, 511b
Antioxidants. *See also* Vitamin C;
Vitamin E
in chronic fatigue syndrome,
487–488, 488b
dietary, in allergic patient, 303
in HIV disease, 183
inflammation and, 869
in neck pain, 678–679
in rheumatoid arthritis, 495
in type 2 diabetes mellitus, 341
Antiplatelet drugs, herbal and
supplement interactions with,
256t
Antipsychotics, for autism spectrum
disorder, 68
Antipyretics, in common cold, 178
Antiretrovirals, in HIV infection,
181–182, 181t, 182b
Antivirals
in common cold, 178–179, 178b
in herpes simplex virus, 195, 195b
Anxiety, 46–52.e1
in alcoholism treatment, 821
botanicals for, 49–50
comorbid conditions of, 46
definition and diagnostic criteria
for, 46
energy psychology in, 971
integrative therapy for, 47–52
mind-body therapy for, 50
nutrition for, 47–48
in palliative care, 809.e1
Parkinson's disease and, 149
pathophysiology of, 46–47, 46b
pharmaceuticals for, 48–49, 49t
prevention prescription for, 51b
ruling out organic disease in, 47,
47t
supplements for, 48, 49t
therapeutic review on, 51b
therapies to consider for, 50–52
web resources on, 52t
Aphthous stomatitis, 747–752.e1, 747f
amlexanox in, 749, 749b
analgesic agents in, 750
antiinflammatory agents in,
749–750
botanicals in, 749
cautery with silver nitrate in, 751,
752b
chlorhexidine gluconate in, 750,
750b
colchicine in, 750–751, 751b
dexamethasone in, 750, 750b
diet in, 748
etiology of, 748b
German chamomile *(Matricaria
recutita)* in, 749, 749b
glutamine in, 748, 748b
homeopathy in, 749, 749b
honey in, 748
integrative therapy for, 747–752
licorice in, 749, 749b
lifestyle in, 747
mind-body therapy in, 749
mouthwashes in, 750
nutrition in, 747–748, 748b
pathophysiology of, 747
prevention prescription in, 751b
supplements in, 748
systemic pharmaceuticals, 750–751
systemic steroids in, 751, 751b
tetracycline-fluocinolone
acetonide-diphenhydramine
mouthwash, 750, 750b
thalidomide in, 751, 751b

Aphthous stomatitis *(Continued)*
therapeutic review in, 752b
therapies to consider in, 751–752
toothpaste in, 747
traditional Chinese medicine in,
751–752
triamcinolone in, 750, 750b
viscous lidocaine (xylocaine 2%
solution) in, 750, 750b
vitamin B$_{12}$ in, 748, 748b
web resources in, 752t
APOE4 gene, in Alzheimer disease,
97
Apple cider vinegar, 328
Appreciation, 924, 924f–925f
Arachidonic acid, 871f
L-Arginine
in heart failure, 247
in vaginal dryness, 596–597, 597b
Arginine, in herpes simplex infection,
192
Arnica, in carpal tunnel syndrome,
701, 701b
Aromatase inhibitors, 631, 632b, 634b
in breast cancer, 777
Aromatherapy
in depression, 44
in labor pain management, 530
with massage, in dysmenorrhea,
575–577, 576b
in neck pain, 686–688, 687b
in palliative care, 813
Arrhythmias, 276–286.e3
ablation therapy in, 284
acupuncture in, 281
L-carnitine, in, 281
coenzyme Q10 in, 281
copper in, 281
food as, trigger of, 279–280
gastric distention and, 279
integrative therapy in, 279–284
ablation therapy, 284
acupuncture, 281
botanicals, 282–283, 283b
diet, 279–280, 280t, 280b
exercise, 280
lifestyle, 281
mind-body therapy, 281
pharmaceuticals, 280t, 283–284,
284b
supplements, 281–282
magnesium in, 281
omega-3 fatty acids in, 282
pathophysiology of, 276–279
approach to the patient,
278–279, 278t–279t, 279f
types and mechanisms of,
276–278
potassium in, 282
prevention prescription for, 284b
referral to a specialist, 279, 279t
risk-to-benefit ratio in, 284
selenium in, 282
therapeutic review on,
284b–285b
vitamins in, 282
web resources on, 285t
zinc in, 281
Arsenic, inorganic, metabolic
syndrome and, 324
Arsenicum album, in asthma, 297
Art therapy, in palliative care, 814
Arthritis. *See also* Osteoarthritis
antiinflammatory diet in, 875t
psoriatic, 726, 728t
rheumatic. *See* Rheumatoid
arthritis
Arthritis Self-Management Program
(ASMP), 642
Arthroplasty, in osteoarthritis, 648
Arthroscopy, in osteoarthritis, 648
Ascorbic acid. *See* Vitamin C
Ashwagandha
in adrenal fatigue, 406, 406b
in multiple sclerosis, 138

Aspartate, in chronic fatigue
syndrome, 487, 487b
Aspirin
in colorectal cancer prevention,
803
in coronary artery disease, 255
Asthma, 287–299.e2
antiinflammatory diet in, 875t
antiinflammatory medications in,
294–295, 295b
Boswellia in, 291
breathing exercises in, 291
bronchodilators in, 294
chiropractic in, 295–296
Coleus in, 291–292
disclosure in, 296
environment and, 288
exercise in, 289
guided imagery in, 296
herbal mixtures in, 292–293
hypnosis in, 296
integrative therapy for, 288–299
biochemical, 291–293
biomechanical approaches,
295–296
lifestyle, 288–289
mind-body therapy, 291, 296
other therapies to consider,
296–299
supplements, 293–294
journaling in, 296, 938
Ma huang in, 292
massage in, 295
nutrition in, 289
osteopathy in, 295
pathophysiology of, 288
prevention prescription of,
297b–298b
Pycnogenol in, 292
risk factors and triggers of, 288,
289f–290f, 289t
selenium in, 294
therapeutic homeopathy in, 1067
therapeutic review for, 298b
traditional Chinese medicine in,
297
vitamin C in, 293
vitamin D in, 293
vitamin E in, 293
web resources on, 299t
yoga in, 291
Astragalus membranaceus
in chronic hepatitis, 206
in common cold, 172
Atherosclerosis. *See* Coronary artery
disease
Atopic dermatitis (AD), 715–725.e2
allergens, in avoidance of, 718
allergy elimination diet in, 719
antihistamines in, 721, 721b
antimicrobials in, 721, 721b, 724b
bleach baths in, 717–718
botanicals in, 720–721
coal tar in, 721
conventional modalities in, 721
diagnosis of, 716–717, 716b
essential fatty acids in, 719–720,
720b
glycyrrhetinic acid in, 720, 720b
homeopathy in, 723–725
humidity in, 718
hydration in, 717
hydrolyzed formula, in infancy,
718–719
immunization in, 721
immunotherapy in, 721
integrative therapy for, 717, 717f
lifestyle and supportive care for,
717–718
loose-fitting clothing in, 718
mild soap in, 718
mind-body therapy for, 719
moisturizers following bathing
in, 718
nutrition for, 718–725

Atopic dermatitis (AD) *(Continued)*
oolong tea for, 719, 719b
other immunomodulators in, 722
pathophysiology of, 716–717,
716b–717b
pharmaceuticals for, 721–722
prevention prescription in, 723b
probiotics in, 720, 720b
supplements for, 719–720
therapeutic review in, 724b
therapies to consider in, 722–725
topical corticosteroids in, 721–722,
722b
topical immunomodulators in,
722, 722b
traditional Chinese medicine in, 722
traditional Japanese medicine in, 723
ultraviolet light in, 721
vitamins in, 719, 719b
web resources in, 725t
wet dressings in, 718, 718b
Atrial fibrillation, 277, 277b
nonvalvular
NOACs for, 286t
therapeutic review for, 280t
Attention-deficit/hyperactivity
disorder (ADHD), 53–63.e4
biochemical therapies for, 60–63
botanicals and dietary supplements
in, 60
comorbidities of, 53
definitions of, 53
emotional self-regulation in,
57–58, 57t
environment and, 60, 60t
epidemiology of, 53
exercise in, 54, 54b
genetic associations of, 53
integrative therapy for, 54, 54f
lifestyle and, 54–60
magnesium in, 55
mind-body therapies in, 56–57
nutrition in, 55–56, 55t
pathophysiology of, 53
pharmaceuticals in, 60–62
presentation of, 53
prevention prescription for, 62b
safety in, 54
sleep in, 54–55
social relationships and, 58–59
stress management in, 57–58, 57t
therapeutic review on, 62b–63b
therapies for, 62–63
web resources on, 63t
Attitude, in age-related macular
degeneration, 841
Audioanalgesia, in labor pain
management, 530
Auditory integrative training, in
autism spectrum disorder, 71
Autism spectrum disorder (ASD),
64–73.e4
botanicals and herbals in, 70
complementary and alternative
medicine therapies for, 64, 65t
epigenetics of, 64–65, 65b
genetics of, 64–65
integrative therapy for, 66–67
mind-body medicine in, 71–73
neuroimaging findings for, 65–66
pathophysiology of, 64–66
pharmaceuticals in, 67–69
prevention prescription for, 72b
supplements for, 69–70
therapeutic review on, 72b
website resources on, 73t
Autogenic training, 911t–912t
Avocado soybean unsaponifiables
(ASU), in osteoarthritis, 648
Ayurveda
in chronic kidney disease,
419–421, 419b
in fertility, 523
in hypertension, 239
in urolithiasis, 612

Azadirachta indica. See Neem
Azelaic acid
in acne vulgaris, 763b, 764
in rosacea, 768b, 770

B
Back pain. *See also* Low back pain
chronic, 963
Balneo-phototherapy, in psoriasis, 727–728
Barbara Brennan School of Healing, 1075t
Bed noise, in insomnia, 82–83, 84b
Bedroom toxicity, 82b
Behavior modification, in carpal tunnel syndrome, 697–698
Behavioral sleep medicine specialists, for insomnia, 83–85
Benfotiamine. *See also* Vitamin B
in peripheral neuropathy, 127
in type 2 diabetes mellitus, 342, 342b
Benign prostatic hyperplasia (BPH), 600–607.e1
alpha-adrenergic blocking agents in, 604–605
5-alpha-reductase inhibition in, 605
beta-sitosterol in, 602–603, 603b
cholesterol and, 601
flaxseed oil in, 601–602
integrative therapy for, 601–607, 603t
botanicals, 603–604
nutrition, 601–602
pharmaceuticals, 604–605
supplements, 602–603
surgery, 605–607, 605b
omega-3 fatty acids in, 601–602
pathophysiology of, 601, 602f
prevention prescription for, 606b
Pygeum africanum in, 604
rye grass pollen in, 604
saw palmetto in, 603–604
soy in, 601
therapeutic review for, 606b
web resources for, 607t
zinc in, 603
Benzoyl peroxide, in acne vulgaris, 762b, 763
Berberine
in dyslipidemias, 273, 273b
in urinary tract infection, 214
Bereavement, in palliative care, 811
Beta blockers, in heart failure, 248–249, 249b
Beta-carotene, in age-related macular degeneration, 843
Betaine hydrochloride
for homocysteine lowering, 402
in irritable bowel syndrome, 430–431, 431b
Beverages. *See also* Alcohol use/abuse; Caffeine; Coffee
urolithiasis and, 610
Bifidobacterium. See Probiotics
Bilberry, in age-related macular degeneration, 844
Bile acid sequestrants, 332
Bindweed, antiangiogenesis property of, 585
Biochemical therapy
integrative medicine and, 1091–1092
in labor pain management, 530
in otitis media, 153
in postdates pregnancy, 537–538
Bioelectromagnetics, in peripheral neuropathy, 122–123
Bioenergetics. *See also* Energy medicine
in adrenal fatigue, 408
in carpal tunnel syndrome, 704
in dysmenorrhea, 573–575, 576b

Bioenergetics *(Continued)*
in epicondylosis, 708–709, 714b
in erectile dysfunction, 625
in heart failure, 250
integrative medicine and, 1092
in neck pain, 680–681, 687b
in pediatric abdominal pain, 463
in peripheral neuropathy, 123
in postdates pregnancy, 538
Biofeedback
in adrenal fatigue, 408
in attention-deficit/hyperactivity disorder, 58
in constipation, 469
in heart rate variability enhancement, 928–929
in HIV disease, 187–188
in hypertension, 238, 238b
in migraine, 114
in neck pain, 680
in pediatric abdominal pain, 464
in peripheral neuropathy, 122
in posttraumatic stress disorder, 91
in substance abuse, 823
in type 2 diabetes mellitus, 337
in urinary tract infection, 216–217, 216b
Biofield therapies, 1073–1080.e1, 1074b. *See also* Energy medicine
Bioflavonoids
in age-related macular degeneration, 843
in cataract prevention, 836
in gout, 691, 691b
Biomechanical therapy. *See also* specific types, e.g., Counterstrain
in carpal tunnel syndrome, 702–704
in dysmenorrhea, 575, 576b
in epicondylosis, 710–713
in GERD, 437
in heart failure, 249–250, 250b
integrative medicine and, 1092
in myofascial pain syndrome, 655–657
in otitis media, 155–156
in pediatric abdominal pain, 463
in peripheral neuropathy, 130
Biotin
in insulin resistance, 330, 330b
in metabolic syndrome, 330, 330b
in multiple sclerosis, 137–138
in seborrheic dermatitis, 755
Birth control pills, in uterine fibroids, 588, 588b
Bisphenol A (BPA), 633
Bisphosphonates, in osteoporosis, 378–379
Black cohosh
in easing menstrual pain, 573t
in labor pain management, 530
in menopausal symptoms, 555–556, 556b
in postdates pregnancy, 537, 537b
in premenstrual syndrome, 565, 565b
Black haw, in dysmenorrhea, 572, 572b
Black tea extract, for herpes simplex virus, 196
Bladder stones. *See* Urolithiasis
Bleach baths, in atopic dermatitis, 717–718
Blood pressure
high. *See* Hypertension
journaling in, 938
normal, 230, 230t
Blood sugar, glycemic index and, 864f
Blue cohosh, in postdates pregnancy, 537, 537b
Blueberries, 328
Body composition, 888, 888b, 891t
Body mass, fat-free, 888

Body noise, insomnia and, 80, 80b, 84b
Bone
DASH diet effects on, 880
depot medroxyprogesterone acetate effects on, 378
strength, assessing, fracture risk, 370
Bone health
osteoporosis and, 371
substances may be harmful to, 377–378
Bone mineral content (BMC), 887–888
Bone mineral density (BMD), 370, 888. *See also* Osteoporosis
"Bone resorption inhibitory food items" (BRIFI), 371b
Borg scale, 889, 890t
Borrelia burgdorferi, 218
Boswellia
in asthma, 291
in fibromyalgia, 479, 479b
in inflammatory bowel disease, 509
in osteoarthritis, 648–649
Botanicals, 331–332. *See also specific types, e.g.*
in acne vulgaris, 761–762
in adrenal fatigue, 406–407
in age-related macular degeneration, 844–845, 845b
in allergic patient, 305
in Alzheimer disease, 102–103
antiinflammatory, 584–585, 585b
in anxiety, 49–50
in aphthous stomatitis, 749, 752b
in arrhythmias, 282–283, 283b
in asthma, 291–293
in atopic dermatitis, 720–721, 721b, 724b
in benign prostatic hyperplasia, 603–604, 603t
in breast cancer, 778
in carpal tunnel syndrome, 700–701
in cataract prevention, 836
in cholelithiasis, 453–454
in constipation, 469–470
in depression, 39–40
in dysmenorrhea, 571–572, 576b
in fibromyalgia, 479
in GERD, 436
in gout, 692, 695, 696b
in heart failure, 243–246
in hypertension, 236–237, 237b
in hypothyroidism, 355
in inflammatory bowel disease, 514b–515b
in insulin resistance, 331–332
in liver detoxification, 583–584
in low back pain, 672
in menopausal symptoms, 555–556
in metabolic syndrome, 331–332
in migraine, 111–112
to modulate pelvic lymphatic drainage, 584, 584b
in multiple sclerosis, 138–139
in osteoporosis, 376
in otitis media, 154
in palliative care, 808
in Parkinson's disease, 147
in pediatric abdominal pain, 460–462
in peptic ulcer disease, 444–446, 446b
in peripheral neuropathy, 123–126
in postdates pregnancy, 536–537
prescribing, 978–985.e1
animal studies of, 980
brand or product, choosing, 982, 982t
dosing of, 982–983, 983t–985t
efficacy of, 979–981, 980b
product labels on, 984t–985t

Botanicals *(Continued)*
safety considerations in, 981–982, 981b
in vitro studies of, 980
in psoriasis, 730–731
in rosacea, 767–768
in seborrheic dermatitis, 755–756, 756b, 758b
in testosterone deficiency, 633–634
in type 2 diabetes mellitus, 337–340
in urinary tract infection, 213–215
in urolithiasis, 611
in urticaria, 740–742, 745b
in uterine fibroids, 583
Botulinum toxin, in migraine, 113
BPH. *See* Benign prostatic hyperplasia (BPH)
Braak hypothesis, of Parkinson's disease, 144
Brain injury, therapeutic homeopathy in, 1068t
Breast, lumpy, guided imagery in, 932–933, 933b
Breast cancer, 771–784.e7, 780b
alcohol and, 582, 775
botanicals in, 778
Brassica (*Cruciferous*) vegetables in, 777, 777b
conventional treatment in, 778–779
edible (medicinal) mushrooms in, 776, 776b
emotional care in, 778
exercise in, 774–775
fiber in, 775
flax in, 776, 776b
glycemic index and, 865
green tea in, 776, 776b
2-hydroxyestrone/16-hydroxyestrone ratio in, 773, 773b, 774f
integrative medicine in, 773–780, 781t
integrative oncology, recommended reading, 780.e1t
lifestyle in, 773, 773b
localized, chemotherapy in, 779–780
Mediterranean diet in, 775
melatonin in, 778, 778b
metastatic, chemotherapy in, 780
monounsaturated fatty acids in, 776
multivitamins in, 777, 777b
nutrition in, 775–777
pathophysiology of, 772
polyunsaturated fatty acids in, 775, 775b
prevention prescription in, 782b
radiation in, 779
risk factors of, 772–773, 772b, 772.e1t
screening of, 773, 773b
side effects from, integrative management of, 780–784, 780b
soy in, 776, 776b
spiritual care in, 778
sugar in, 775
supplements in, 777–778, 777b
surgical approach in, 779
therapeutic review in, 783b
vitamin D in, 777–778, 778b
web resources in, 783t–784t
whey protein in, 776–777, 777b
Breast stimulation, in postdates pregnancy, 537
Breath exercise, for insomnia, 85b
Breath/breathing, 895b, 917
abdominal, 897, 897b
in age-related macular degeneration, 840–841
airway resistance in, 897–899, 897b

Breath/breathing (Continued)
in asthma, 291
coordination of, with movement, 898–899
in heart rate variability enhancement, 928
internal imagery linked to, 898, 898b
mechanism of, 895, 896f, 896t, 896b
muscle/ body emphasis in, 897, 897b
paced and patterned, 895–897, 897b
in pediatric abdominal pain, 464
practices of, in adrenal fatigue, 408
therapeutic, 895–900
  patient handout for, 900f
  resources for practicing, 899
  web resources for, 899t
thoracic, 897
training, in low back pain, 901, 903f–907f
Brewer's yeast, in acne vulgaris, 761, 761b
Bromelain
in gout, 692, 692b
in inflammatory bowel disease, 509
Bronchodilators, in asthma, 294
Bulk-forming laxatives, in constipation, 471
Bupropion
in alcoholism, 820
in depression, 42t, 43
in obesity, 392
1,4-Butane-disulfonate, in depression, 38–39
Butterbur
in allergic patient, 305, 305b
in migraine, 112, 112b
in urticaria, 741, 741b

C
Caffeine
anxiety and, 47–48
in attention-deficit/hyperactivity disorder, 56
depression and, 37
osteoporosis and, 377
type 2 diabetes mellitus and, 337
Calcipotriene, in psoriasis, 731, 731b
Calcitonin, in osteoporosis, 380
Calcium, 372–373, 372b
in cholelithiasis, 453, 453b
in chronic kidney disease, 418.e1
in colorectal cancer prevention, 802, 802b
deficiency in, and FODMaP diet, 884
dietary reference intakes for, 372t
in inflammatory bowel disease, 505, 505b
in menopausal symptoms, 557–558
in osteoporosis, 372–373
in premenstrual syndrome, 562–563, 563b
in urolithiasis, 611
Calcium carbonate, in HIV disease, 184, 185b
Calcium channel blockers
herbal and supplement interactions with, 256t
in migraine, 113
in urolithiasis, 612
Calcium D glucarate, in uterine fibroids, 586, 586b
Calculi. See Cholelithiasis; Urolithiasis
Calming herbs, in attention-deficit/hyperactivity disorder, 60, 60t
Camellia sinensis. See Green tea
Cancer. See also specific cancers, e.g., Breast cancer
antiinflammatory diet in, 875t
DASH diet effects on, 880
glycemic index and, 865
low back pain and, 663t–664t
therapeutic homeopathy in, 1070

Candex, 164
Candida, eliminating fuel for, 164–166, 166b
Candida Questionnaire and Scoresheet, 158, 159f–160f
Candisol, for chronic sinusitis, 164
Cannabinoids
in multiple sclerosis, 138
in peripheral neuropathy, 125, 125b
Cannabis
in anxiety and depression, in palliative care, 809.e1
in inflammatory bowel disease, 509
in insomnia, 79
in nausea, in palliative care, 809, 809b
in pain, in palliative care, 808, 808b
Capsaicin
in myofascial pain syndrome, 657b
in osteoarthritis, 647
in peripheral neuropathy, 128
in psoriasis, 730, 730b
Carbohydrates
in antiinflammatory diet, 872–873, 873f, 873b
in chronic sinusitis, 165
classification of, 884f
in dyslipidemias, 264, 267
fermentable, irritable bowel syndrome and, 882
urolithiasis and, 610
Carbon dioxide emissions, in health care, 1082–1083, 1084f
Cardiac glycosides (Digoxin), in heart failure, 249
Cardiovascular disease. See also Coronary artery disease; Heart failure; Hypertension
integrative approaches to, 253
prevention, in glycemic index, 865
Caregivers, assisting, in Alzheimer disease, 104
L-Carnitine
in adrenal fatigue, 407, 407b
in arrhythmias, 281
in heart failure, 247
in HIV disease, 184, 184b
in type 2 diabetes mellitus, 342, 342b
Carnosine, in cataract prevention, 835
Carotenoids. See also specific types, e.g., Beta-carotene
in age-related macular degeneration, 842–843
type 2 diabetes mellitus and, 341
Carpal tunnel syndrome, 697–706.e2
acetaminophen in, 698, 698b
arnica in, 701, 701b
behavior modification in, 697–698
bioenergetics in, 704
biomechanical therapy in, 702–704
botanicals in, 700–701
causes of, 698t
clinical manifestations of, 697, 697b
corticosteroids in, 699–700, 700b
diagnosis of, 697, 697b
diuretics in, 699
ergonomic keyboards in, 698
exercise in, 698
ginger in, 700, 700b
integrative therapy for, 697–706
laser acupuncture in, 704
lifestyle in, 697–698
massage therapy in, 702
nonsteroidal antiinflammatory drugs in, 698–699, 699b, 699b
occupations associated with, 698t
osteopathic manipulative treatment in, 702–704, 703f
pathophysiology of, 697
pharmaceuticals in, 698–700

Carpal tunnel syndrome (Continued)
prevention prescription in, 705b
supplements in, 701
surgery in, 704, 704b
therapeutic review in, 705b
therapeutic touch in, 704
therapies to consider in, 704–706
traditional acupuncture in, 704
traditional Chinese medicine in, 704
ultrasound therapy in, 702
vitamin B₆ in, 701, 701b
web resources in, 706t
willow bark in, 700–701, 701b
wrist splinting in, 702
yoga in, 702
Carrageenan, for common cold, 172, 172b
Castor oil
in postdates pregnancy, 535–536
in uterine fibroids, 589
Cataracts, 829–837.e1, 830b
botanicals in, 836
  bioflavonoids, 836
  Cineraria maritima, 836
  turmeric, 836
diagnosis of, 830–831
epidemiology of, 831
integrative therapy for, 831–833
  aging and, 833
  alcohol, 832
  corticosteroids, 832
  exercise, lack of, 832
  overweight, 832
  pharmaceuticals, 832
  smoking, 832
  stress management, 832
  sunglasses, ultraviolet light-blocking, 831
nutrition in, 833–834
  algae-eating fish, 834
  B vitamins, 835
  carnosine, 835
  docosahexaenoic acid, 835, 835b
  hydration, 833–834
  lutein-containing foods, 833
  multivitamins, 835, 835b
  saturated animal fat, avoidance of, 833
  sulfur-containing foods, 834
  vitamin A, 835, 835b
  vitamin C, 833–834, 834b
  vitamin E, 835
pathophysiology of, 830
prevention of, 836b
progression of, 831, 831b
risk factors of, 831, 831b
screening of, 830–831
supplements in, 834–835
  lutein, 834, 834b
  zeaxanthin, 834, 834b
surgery in, 836–837
therapeutic review in, 837b
vision, changes with, 830, 830b
web resources on, 837t
Catechol-O-methyl transferase (COMT) inhibitors, in Parkinson's disease, 148, 148b
Cat's claw, in Lyme disease, 224, 224b
Cauda equina syndrome, 663t–664t
Caulophyllum thalictroides. See Blue cohosh
CDP-choline, 146, 146b
Cefuroxime axetil, in Lyme disease, 223b
Celiac disease, 426
nonceliac gluten sensitivity versus, 316, 316b
prevalence of various clinical and laboratory findings in patients with, 317t
Cellular phones, 1021–1022
Cervical support, in neck pain, 678

Chamomile
in atopic dermatitis, 720
in common cold, 172, 172b
in easing menstrual pain, 573t
in GERD, 435t, 436b
in nausea and vomiting, in pregnancy, 543–544, 544b
in pediatric abdominal pain, 460–461, 461b
Chaste tree/chaste berry
in fertility, 522, 522b
in polycystic ovarian syndrome, 365, 365b
in premenstrual syndrome, 564, 564b
Chelation therapy, 1004–1015.e3
N-acetylcysteine, 1010, 1010t–1011t
algae, 1012–1013
alpha lipoic acid, 1010t–1011t, 1011–1012
antioxidants, 1009–1010
in autism spectrum disorder, 69, 69b
in cardiovascular disease, 1005, 1006f, 1009
case study in, 1013b–1014b
chelating agents, 1008t
clinical use of, 1006–1007
in coronary artery disease, 261–263
in detoxification, 998, 998b
DMPS, 1005b, 1008, 1008t
DMSA, 1008–1009, 1008t
ethylenediaminetetraacetic acid (EDTA), 1004, 1008t, 1009
flavonoids, 1010t–1011t, 1011
heavy metal chelation, 1004–1005
mineral support, 1012
modified citrus pectin (MCP), 1012, 1012b
over-the-counter chelators, 1009
sulfhydryl compounds, 1009–1010
taurine, 1010t–1011t, 1011
Trial to Assess Chelation Therapy (TACT), 1005–1006
web resources on, 1015t
zeolites, 1008t, 1013
Chelators, 1007b
food-based natural, 1004b
over-the-counter, 1009
Chemical neutralization, in liver detoxification, 198–199
Chemotherapy
in colorectal cancer prevention, 804
in lung cancer, 788
nausea and vomiting with, 1044
Cherry, in gout, 692, 692b
Chest radiography, in lung cancer, 786
Chili, in peptic ulcer disease, 445, 445b
Chinese herbs, in age-related macular degeneration, 845, 845b
Chinese medicine. See Traditional Chinese medicine
Chiropractic
in asthma, 295–296
in labor pain management, 527
in migraine, 115
in otitis media, 156
in tension-type headache, 118
Chlorhexidine gluconate, in aphthous stomatitis, 750, 750b
Chloride channel activator, in constipation, 471–472
Chocolate, 874
craving, 587b
Cholelithiasis, 450–456.e2
acupuncture in, 455
alcohol consumption in, 452
botanicals in
  choleretic herbs, 453–454
  gallstone-dissolving herbs, 454
calcium in, 453, 453b

Cholelithiasis (Continued)
cholesterol-lowering medications in, 454
coffee consumption in, 452
dandelion in, 453, 453b
dietary fiber in, 451
estrogen supplementation and, 451t
exercise in, 450
fats in, 451
fenugreek in, 454
food allergy in, 452
globe artichoke in, 453, 453b
healthy weight in, maintenance of, 450
homeopathy in, 455
integrative therapy of, 450–456
laparoscopic cholecystectomy in, 454
lifestyle in, 450
magnesium in, 452–453, 453b
milk thistle in, 453, 453b
nut consumption in, 451
nutrition in, 450–452, 452b
olive oil in, 453
osteopathy in, 455–456
pathophysiology of, 450, 451f
peppermint in, 454, 454b
pharmaceuticals in, 454
piperine in, 455
prevention prescription of, 455b
risk factors for, 450, 451t
stress reduction in, 450
sugar consumption in, 451–452
supplements in, 452–453
surgery in, 454
therapeutic review on, 455b–456b
therapies to consider in, 454–456
turmeric in, 454, 454b
ursodeoxycholic acid in, 454, 454b
vitamin C in, 452, 452b
vitamin E in, 453, 453b
water consumption in, 452
web resources on, 456t
Cholesterol. See also Dyslipidemia; Lipoprotein
benign prostatic hyperplasia and, 601
dietary, 264, 267
Choline, in homocysteine lowering, 402
Chondroitin sulfate
in osteoarthritis, 644–645
prostate cancer and, 798b
Chromium
in HIV disease, 185, 185b
in inflammatory bowel disease, 505
in insulin resistance, 330, 330b
in metabolic syndrome, 330, 330b
in polycystic ovarian syndrome, 364, 364b
in type 2 diabetes mellitus, 340, 340b
Chronic fatigue syndrome, 484–492.e2
acetyl-L-carnitine in, 486, 486b
adrenal support in, 488
botanicals in, 490
coenzyme Q10 in, 486–487, 487b
conventional treatment in, 485
dehydroepiandrosterone (DHEA) in, 488, 488b
diagnosis of, 484–485, 485b
energy medicine in, 490–491
etiology of, 484
exercise in, 486
general considerations in, 485–486
hormonal imbalances in, 488
immune system imbalance in, 488–489
integrative therapy for, 485–492
iron in, 489
mind-body therapy in, 490
multivitamins in, 489
nutrition in, 486

Chronic fatigue syndrome (Continued)
pathophysiology of, 484–485
pharmaceuticals in, 491–492
physical modalities in, 490
prevention prescription of, 491b
ribose (D-ribose) in, 487, 487b
sleep disturbances in, 488
supplements in, 486–490
therapeutic review on, 492b
thyroid in, 488
vitamin B12 in, 489
vitamin D in, 489
web resources on, 492t
Chronic hepatitis, 198–210.e5, 198b
adequate protein intake for, 208
botanicals in, 205–206, 207t
coffee and, 209
common etiologies of, 199t
cruciferous vegetables and, 208
dietary fat intake and, 208
dietary fiber for, 208
enhancing liver detoxification for, 198–199
fruit and, 208
green tea for, 208–209
herbal concoctions and traditional Chinese medicine for, 206
histological hallmarks of, 198
integrative therapy for, 199–208
lifestyle interventions for, 207–208
mind-body therapies for, 206–207
nutrition and, 208–209
pathophysiology of, 198–199, 199t
pharmaceuticals for, 199–202, 200t, 207t
prevention prescription for, 209b
reducing free radicals in, 198
supplements for, 202–205
therapeutic review for, 209b–210b
web resources on, 210t
Chronic kidney disease (CKD), 410–421.e11
N-acetylcysteine (NAC) in, 414, 414b
acupuncture in, 419
adverse drug reactions in, 413
air pollution in, 418.e2
alkalinizing therapy in, 413
antihypertensive agents in, 413
arsenic in, 418.e1
astragalus in, 415
Ayurveda in, 419–421, 419b
calcium in, 418.e1
coenzyme Q10 (CoQ10) in, 414, 414b
cordyceps in, 415–416, 416b
curcumin in, 415
definition of, 411
environmental toxins in, 418
exercise in, 419
flame retardants in, 418.e1
folic acid in, 415
food and cosmetic additives in, 418.e1
heavy metals in, 418.e1
herbal toxicities in, 416
herbals in, 415–418
herbicides in, 418.e1
hyperphosphatemia in, 417
inorganic phosphate additives in, 417, 418b
integrative therapy for, 413–421
lead in, 418.e1
lifestyle modification in, 418–419
ligustrazine in, 416, 416b
magnesium in, 413–414, 414b
management of, conventional approach to, 411–413
meditation in, 419
mercury in, 418.e1
mind-body therapies in, 419
niacin in, 415
nutraceuticals in, 413–415
nutrition in, 416–418, 416b

Chronic kidney disease (CKD) (Continued)
omega-3 fatty acid in, 414
organic solvents in, 418.e1
palmitoylethanolamide (PEA) in, 415
pathophysiology of, 411, 412f
pesticides in, 418.e1
pharmaceuticals in, 413
plastics in, 418.e1
prebiotics in, 414–415
prevention prescription of, 420b
probiotics in, 414–415
prognosis of, 411, 412f
raw nuts in, 418
Rheum officinale in, 416, 416b
risk factors of, 411
short-chain fatty acids in, 415
sleep, low quality of, 419
smoking cessation in, 419
sodium in, restriction, 417
stress in, 419
sugar diets in, 418
supplements in, 413–415
synbiotic in, 414–415
Tai chi in, 419
therapeutic review on, 420b
therapies to consider in, 419–421
traditional Chinese medicine (TCM) in, 419
Tripterygium wilfordii Hook F in, 416, 416b
turmeric in, 415
uric acid-lowering agents in, 413
vitamin B6 in, 415
vitamin B12 in, 415
vitamin D 25-OH in, 414
vitamin K in, 415
water pollution in, 418.e2
web resources on, 421t
weight loss in, 418
yoga in, 419
Chronic musculoskeletal pain, prolotherapy for, 1047–1053. e2, 1049t
adverse events of, 1051
basic science of, 1047–1048
case example of, 1051–1052
clinical research of, 1048–1051, 1048f
common side effects of, 1051
contraindications of, 1051
insurance coverage of, 1053
practical considerations of, 1051
web resources on, 1053t
Chronic prostatitis/chronic pelvic pain syndrome, 616–622.e1
acupuncture in, 620, 620b
alpha blockers in, 617, 617b
antibiotics in, 617, 617b
cannabis in, 620
clinical presentation of, 621–622
cognitive behavioral therapy in, 621
diagnosis of, 616–617, 617t
etiology of, 616
exercise in, 620
integrative therapy for, 617–622
lifestyle in, 617
mind-body therapy in, 621
nutrition in, 617–620, 620b
pathophysiology of, 616, 616b
pharmaceuticals in, 617
physical therapy in, 620
prevention prescription for, 622b
quercetin in, 620
questionnaire for, 618f–619f
risk factors for, 616
rye grass pollen extract in, 620
saw palmetto in, 620
supplements in, 620
therapeutic review for, 622b
treatment, by UPOINT phenotype, 621t
web resources on, 622t

Chronic sinusitis, 157–169.e2, 168b
antiinflammatory and antioxidant vitamins and supplements in, 162–163
detoxification in, 166–167
diet for, 163
emotional factors in, 163
improving indoor air quality for, 163
integrative therapy in, 158–161
mind-body therapy in, 167
nasal hygiene in, 162, 162t
nasal sprays in, 162
natural antibiotics in, 161–162
pathophysiology of, 157–158
prevalence of, 157
respiratory healing program for, 158–161
restoring normal bowel bacterial flora for, 166
risk factors for, 158
sleep for, 163
spirituality and, 167–169, 169b
strengthening immune system against, 166
web resources on, 169t
Chronic suppressive therapy, for herpes simplex virus infection, 195–196, 196b
Chrysanthellum indicum, for rosacea, 759, 769b
Cigarette smoking
cataracts and, 832
cessation of, 820, 820b
osteoporosis and, 377
Parkinson's disease and, 144
Cimicifuga racemosa. See Black cohosh
Cineraria maritima, in cataract prevention, 836
Cinnamon, in type 2 diabetes mellitus, 339–340, 340b
Circadian rhythms, in insomnia, 82–83, 82b–83b
Citalopram, in depression, 42, 42t
Citrullus colocynthis, 339, 339b
Citrus bergamot, in dyslipidemias, 273–274, 274b
Citrus pectin, 1008t
CKBM-A01, in HIV disease, 186
Climate change, 1019–1020, 1082
Climatotherapy, in psoriasis, 727–728
Clomid, for infertility, 523
Clomiphene citrate, in polycystic ovarian syndrome, 367, 367b
Clonidine
herbal and supplement interactions with, 256t
in menopausal symptoms, 554, 554b
Clostridium difficile, in inflammatory bowel disease, 510–511
Coal tar, in atopic dermatitis, 721
Cobalamin, for homocysteine lowering, 401, 401b
Cocaine dependence, 821
Coccinia cordifolia, 337, 337b
Cocoa, in hypertension, 232–233, 233b
Coconut oil, 872
Cod liver oil, in otitis media, 153
Codeine, in low back pain, 671
Coenzyme Q10
in Alzheimer disease, 102, 102b
in arrhythmias, 281
in chronic fatigue syndrome, 486–487, 487b
in chronic kidney disease, 414, 414b
in coronary artery disease, 259–260
in heart failure, 246
in hypertension, 235, 235b
in insulin resistance, 331, 331b
in metabolic syndrome, 331, 331b
in migraine, 111, 111b
in Parkinson's disease, 146

Coffee. *See also* Caffeine
  in cholelithiasis, 452
  insomnia and, 80
  Parkinson's disease and, 144
  rheumatoid arthritis and, 494
Cognitive exercise, in Alzheimer
    disease, 99
Cognitive restructuring, in insomnia,
    81, 81b
Cognitive therapy, mindfulness-
    based, in depression, 40
Cognitive-behavioral therapy
  in chronic fatigue syndrome,
    485b
  in chronic prostatitis/chronic
    pelvic pain syndrome, 621
  in fibromyalgia, 477
  in insomnia, 80, 81b, 84f
  in irritable bowel syndrome,
    429–430, 430b
  in menopausal symptoms, 557
  in migraine, 115
  in posttraumatic stress disorder,
    90b
  in type 2 diabetes mellitus, 337
Colchicine
  in aphthous stomatitis, 750–751,
    751b
  in gout, 693, 693b
Cold therapy, in osteoarthritis, 643
Colesevelam, 332
  in dyslipidemia, 274b–275b
Coleus, in asthma, 291–292
Colic, therapeutic homeopathy in,
    1067t
Colloidal oatmeal, for rosacea, 767b,
    768
Colon hydrotherapy, in chronic
    sinusitis, 166–167
Colorectal cancer, 800–805.e2
  incidence of, 800
  medications in
    aspirin, 803
    NSAIDs, 803
    postmenopausal hormone
      replacement, 803–804
  natural history of, 800
  prevalence of, 800
  prevention of, 800–803, 801t, 804b
    dietary supplements, 802–803
    integrative therapy, 800–802
    physical activity, 803
  risk factors for, 800, 801t
  screening of, 800
  survivorship in, 804–805
  therapeutic review, 805b
  treatment of, 804
    complementary therapies, 804t
  web resources on, 805t
Combinations, in dyslipidemias,
    274–275
Combined heat and power (CHP)
    facility, 1085b
Commiphora mukul. See Guggul
Common cold. *See also* Upper
    respiratory infections
  clinician-patient interaction in, 17
  pathophysiology of, 170
Communication
  in palliative care, 807
  technology and, in integrative
    medicine, 2–3
Compassion training, 21, 22t
Complementary and alternative
    medicine (CAM)
  integrative medicine and, 3, 4f
    avoiding labels, 4
    growth of, in United States, 4,
      4f–5f
Complera, for HIV disease, 182b
Conditioned insomnia, 75b
Confined Animal Feedlot Operations
    (CAFOs), 1022–1023
Conjugated linoleic acids, for
    rheumatoid arthritis, 495

Constipation, 466–473.e2
  abdominal massage in, 469
  aloe in, 469, 469b
  behavioral training in, 469, 469b
  biofeedback in, 469
  botanicals in, 469–470
  bulk-forming laxatives in, 471
  chloride channel activator in,
    471–472
  commercially packaged fiber
    supplements in, 467, 467b,
    468t
  dietary fiber in, 466–467,
    466b–467b
  emollient laxatives in, 471
  fluids in, 467
  food triggers in, 467, 467b
  hypnotherapy in, 469
  integrative therapy for, 466–473
  in irritable bowel syndrome, 882
  medications associated with, 467t
  mind-body therapy in, 469
  nutrition in, 466–467
  osmotic laxatives in, 471, 471b
  in palliative care, 808–809
  perineal self-acupressure in, 470
  pharmaceuticals in, 470–472,
    470t–471t
  physical activity in, 466
  prevention prescription of, 472b
  probiotics in, 467–469
  Rome II criteria for, 467t
  slow-transit, 466
  stimulant laxatives in, 471
  stool softeners in, 471
  supplements in, 467–469
  therapeutic review on, 472b
  therapies to consider in, 473
  traditional Chinese medicine
    (TCM) in, 469
  web resources on, 473t
Constriction device, in erectile
    dysfunction, 625
Cool breeze technique, 918
Copper
  in age-related macular
    degeneration, 844
  in Alzheimer disease, 101
  in arrhythmias, 281
  in osteoporosis, 375
Cordless phones, 1021–1022
Coriolus versicolor, in colorectal cancer
    prevention, 803, 803b
Coronary artery disease, 253–263.e2
  angioplasty in, 255
  anticoagulant therapies in, 255
  chelation therapy in, 261–263
  fiber in, 258–260
  fish in, 254
  fish oil in, 259
  folic acid in, 260
  high density lipoprotein in, 257
  integrative therapy for, 253–257
    exercise, 254–255
    lipid management, 255–257
    nutrition, 253–254
    pharmaceuticals, 255, 256t
  low density lipoprotein in,
    256–257
  Mediterranean diet in, 253–254
  mind/body therapy in, 261, 261b
  niacin in, 258
  nuts in, 254
  other therapies in, 261–263
    chelation therapy, 261–263
    enhanced external
      counterpulsation, 261
  pathophysiology of, 253, 253b
  plaques in, 253
  prevention prescription for, 262b
  red yeast rice in, 258–259
  stanols in, 258
  statin-related myalgias in, 257,
    257b

Coronary artery disease *(Continued)*
  stenting in, 255
  sterols in, 258
  supplements for, 258–261, 258t
  therapeutic prescription on, 262b
  vitamin D in, 260
  vitamin E in, 260
  web resources on, 263t
Corticosteroids
  in carpal tunnel syndrome,
    699–700, 700b, 705b
  cataracts and, 832
  in epicondylosis, 709, 709b
  in multiple sclerosis, 139
  nasal, in allergic patient, 306, 306b
  in nausea and vomiting, in
    pregnancy, 547, 547b
  in rheumatoid arthritis, 495–496,
    496b
  in urticaria, 743, 743b
Corticotropin-releasing hormone,
    910
Cortisol, 100
Cough suppressants, in common
    cold, 178
Counseling. *See also* Motivational
    interviewing
  in attention-deficit/hyperactivity
    disorder, 58
  therapeutic, in obesity, 385
Counterstrain, 1027–1037.e1, 1028b,
    1030b, 1032b
  benefits of, 1034–1035
  educational texts of, 1037t
  general guidelines for, 1031–1032
  history of, 1028–1029
  limitations of, 1035–1037
  order of treatment of, 1031
  patient for, evaluating, 1029–1030,
    1030t
  piriformis muscle, 1033–1034,
    1036f
  practical applications of,
    1029–1032
  precautions for, 1031
  referral points in, 1031
  technique, examples of, 1032–1034
    levator scapulae muscle,
      1032–1033, 1034f
    sternocleidomastoid muscle,
      1033, 1035f
    trapezius muscle, 1032, 1033f
  tender points in, 1029b, 1032,
    1033f–1036f
  theory of, 1028–1029, 1029f
  treatment logistics of, 1030–1031
  web resources on, 1037t
Cowhage. *See Mucuna pruriens*
Cramp bark
  in dysmenorrhea, 572, 572b
  in labor pain management, 530
Cramping. *See* Dysmenorrhea;
    Premenstrual syndrome
Cranberry
  in benign prostatic hyperplasia,
    604, 604b
  in peptic ulcer disease, 445, 445b
  in urinary tract infection, 213–214,
    214b
Craniosacral therapy, in migraine,
    116
Crataegus monogyna. See Hawthorn
Creatine
  in chronic fatigue syndrome, 487,
    487b
  in Parkinson's disease, 147
Crohn's disease, 501
  N-acetylcysteine in, 506
  acupuncture in, 514
  aloe vera in, 509
  5-aminosalicylic acid in, 511
  Boswellia serrata in, 509
  bovine colostrum in, 508–509
  butyrate in, 508
  curcumin in, 509–510

folate in, 504–505
  glucocorticoids in, 511–512
  helminths in, 510–512
  immunosuppressants in, 512, 512b
  malnutrition in, 502
  melatonin in, 507
  mind-body medicine in, 512–514,
    513t
  pathophysiology of, 501, 502f
  prebiotics in, 508b
  probiotics in, 507
  Saccharomyces boulardii in, 507–508
Cromolyn, in allergic patient, 305,
    305b
Cruciferous vegetables
  in chronic hepatitis, 208
  in prostate cancer prevention, 794
Crystal therapy, 1075t
Curcumin
  in chronic kidney disease, 415,
    415b
  in colorectal cancer prevention,
    802–803, 803b
  in dyslipidemias, 273, 273b
  in inflammatory bowel disease,
    509–510
  in lung cancer, 787, 787b
  in multiple sclerosis, 138
  in osteoarthritis, 648
  in Parkinson's disease, 147, 147b
  in peripheral neuropathy,
    123–124, 124f
  in psoriasis, 729, 729b
Cyclobenzaprine
  in fibromyalgia, 480, 480b
  in myofascial pain syndrome, 658,
    658b
Cyclooxygenase (COX)-2 inhibitor
  in colorectal cancer prevention,
    801
  in osteoarthritis, 646
Cyclosporine
  herbal and supplement interactions
    with, 256t
  in psoriasis, 734, 734b
  in urticaria, 743, 743b
Cynara scolymus. See Globe artichoke
Cyproheptadine, in pediatric
    abdominal pain, 463, 463b
Cytidine 5'-diphosphocholine
    (CDP-choline), for Alzheimer
    disease, 105
Cytochrome P-450, 997f
Cytokines, in osteoporosis, 370–371
Cytotoxic chemotherapy, in breast
    cancer, 779

D
Dairy, acne vulgaris and, 760, 760b
Dairy calcium, sources of, 373t
Damaged tendon, histology of, 708f
Damiana, for fertility, 522, 522b
Danazol, in uterine fibroids, 587,
    587b
Dandelion, in cholelithiasis, 453,
    453b
Decoction, in preparation of herbal
    products, 983t
Decongestants, in common cold,
    178
Deep brain stimulation surgery, in
    Parkinson's disease, 149
Deep pelvic massage, in uterine
    fibroids, 589
Deferasirox, 1008t
Deferoxamine, 1008t
Deglycyrrhizinated licorice (DGL),
    in peptic ulcer disease, 444,
    444b
Dehydroepiandrosterone (DHEA),
    630, 633, 633b
  in adrenal fatigue, 407
  in Alzheimer disease, 103, 103b
  in chronic fatigue syndrome, 488,
    488b

Dehydroepiandrosterone (DHEA)
(Continued)
in inflammatory bowel disease, 507
prostate cancer and, 797
in uterine fibroids, 588, 588b
Delirium, in palliative care, 809–810,
810b
Dementia. See Alzheimer disease
Denosumab, 380
Depression, 34–45.e3, 45t
acupuncture for, 41
S-adenosylmethionine in, 38–39,
38f
alcohol and, 37
in alcoholism treatment, 821
antidepressants in, 41
antiinflammatory diet in, 875t
aromatherapy in, 44
botanicals in, 39–40
Botox in, 44–45
caffeine and, 37
diet and, 37
dietary supplements in, 38–39, 42t
electroconvulsive therapy in, 43
estrogen replacement therapy in,
43–44
exercise and, 36
folic acid in, 38
grief and, 811
heart rate variability and, 926
hydroxytryptophan in, 39, 42t
integrative therapy for, 36–37
kindling in, 36
metabolic syndrome and, 328
mind-body therapy in, 40–41, 40b
mindfulness-based cognitive
therapy for, 40
mixed reuptake blockers in, 41–42,
42t
music therapy in, 44
neurotransmitters in, 36
novel treatments for, 44–45
nutrition and, 37–38, 37b
omega-3 fatty acids in, 37–38, 38b
in palliative care, 809.e1
Parkinson's disease and, 149
pathophysiology of, 36
pharmaceuticals in, 41–43, 42t
phototherapy in, 41
placebo in, 14–16
pregnancy-related, 36–37
psilocybin for, 44
psychotherapy in, 40
recurrent, 36
refined sucrose and, 37
in rheumatoid arthritis, 493
selective serotonin reuptake
inhibitors in, 41–42, 42t
sleep deprivation therapy for, 44
St. John's wort in, 39, 39b, 42t
stress and, 36
tai chi for, 40–41
traditional healing techniques
for, 41
transcranial magnetic stimulation
in, 44
vitamin B_6 in, 38
vitamin B_{12} in, 38
vitamin D and, 38
web resources on, 45t
yoga in, 40
Dermatitis
atopic. See Atopic dermatitis
seborrheic. See Seborrheic
dermatitis
Desvenlafaxine, in depression, 42t
Detoxification, 996–1003.e2
chelation therapy for, 998, 998b
for chronic sinusitis, 166–167
definition of, 996–998
exercise for, 999
fasting for, 999–1000
liver, 997f
manual therapies for, 1000–1003,
1001f–1003f

Detoxification (Continued)
mind-body connection in,
1000–1003, 1000f
nutrition for, 999–1000
patient handout on, 1001f–1003f
pesticides in, 999, 999t
phase, 997f
sauna therapy for, 998–999
seafood and, 999
toxin, testing for, 998
web resources on, 1000t
Devil's claw, in low back pain, 672,
672b
Dexamethasone, in aphthous
stomatitis, 750, 750b
DHEA. See Dehydroepiandrosterone
(DHEA)
Dhyana, in yoga, for osteoarthritis,
642
Diabetes, 334
antiinflammatory diet in, 875t
natural history of, 323f
Diabetes agents, in obesity, 384t
Diabetes mellitus, type 2, 334–346.
e3. See also Insulin resistance;
Metabolic syndrome
alpha-lipoic acid in, 340–341,
341b
angiotensin-converting enzyme
inhibitors in, 345
antioxidants in, 341
bariatric surgery in, 345–346
benfotiamine in, 342, 342b
biofeedback in, 337
botanicals in, 337–340
L-carnitine, 342, 342b
chromium in, 340, 340b
cognitive-behavioral therapy in,
337
education in, 337
exenatide in, 344, 344b
exercise in, 335
fenugreek in, 340, 340b
incretins in, 344
insulin in, 344–345
integrative therapy of, 334–346
lifestyle and, 334–335
magnesium in, 341, 341b
metformin in, 343, 343b
mind-body therapy in, 337
nutrition in, 335–336, 336f
omega-3 fatty acids in, 341, 341b
pathophysiology of, 334, 335f
pharmaceuticals in, 343–345
prevention prescription of, 345b
sitagliptin in, 344, 344b
sleep hygiene in, 337
smoking and, 335
specific foods and, 336–337
statins in, 345
sulfonylureas in, 343, 343b
supplements in, 340–343
risks of specific, 343
therapeutic review of, 346b
thiazolidinedione in, 343–344,
344b
vitamin D in, 340
vitamin E in, 341–342
vitamin K in, 342, 342b
web resources on, 346t
Diabetes Prevention Program
(DPP), 335
Diabetic neuropathy. See also
Peripheral neuropathy
bioelectromagnetics for, 122–123
biofeedback for, 122
methylcobalamin for, 127–128
Diacerein, in osteoarthritis,
647–648
Diagnostic and Statistical Manual of
Mental Disorders, Fifth Edition
(DSM- 5), 64, 65t, 1061
"Diaphragmatic breathing," 897
Diclectin, for nausea and vomiting,
in pregnancy, 545, 545b

Diclofenac
in myofascial pain syndrome, 657
in osteoarthritis, 647
Diet. See also Nutrition
in acne rosacea, 760
in acne vulgaris, 760
antiinflammatory, 869–877.e4,
877f
in Alzheimer disease, 875t
in arthritis, 875t
in asthma, 875t
in cancer, 875t
carbohydrates in, 872–873, 873f,
873b
in cardiovascular disease, 875t
chocolate in, 874
in chronic obstructive
pulmonary disease, 875t
cocoa in, 874
components of, 870–874
in dementia, 875t
in depression, 875t
fats in, 870–872, 871f, 871t,
871b
fruits in, 873, 873b
in hypertension, 875t
in Lyme disease, 225
medical conditions with, 874,
875t
in nonalcoholic fatty liver
disease, 875t
in obesity, 875t
in peripheral artery disease, 875t
proteins in, 874
in psoriasis, 728–729, 875t
turmeric in, 874
for urticaria, 740
vegetables in, 873, 873b
web resources on, 876t
wine in, 874
in aphthous stomatitis, 748
in arrhythmias, 279–280, 280t,
280b
in chronic sinusitis, 163
DASH, 232, 878–881.e1
benefit of, 878–879, 879b, 880f
blood pressure reduction with,
878, 878b
bone effects of, 880
for cancer, 880
in cardiovascular health,
879–880
definition of, 878, 879t
foods in, 880–881
slow cognitive decline, 880
web resources on, 881t
depression and, 37
elimination, 847–862.e6, 314–315,
314b–315b, 858b
alternative, 315
in atopic dermatitis, 854t–855t
in attention deficit hyperactivity
disorder (ADHD),
854t–855t
in autistic spectrum disorders,
854t–855t
avoidance phase of (step 2),
853–856, 856b
challenge phase of (step 3), 856
in irritable bowel syndrome
(IBS), 854t–855t
leaky gut syndrome,
pathophysiology of,
849–857, 850t–851t, 852b
long-term planning phase of
(step 4), 856
in migraine, 854t–855t
nonallergic food intolerances,
pathophysiology of, 849,
849b
patient handout for, 859f–862f
points to consider before
prescribing an, 853t
precautions with, 316–317, 317b
prescribing an, 852–856, 852t

Diet (Continued)
in psoriasis, 728
in rheumatoid arthritis (RA),
854t–855t
risk of, 856–857, 857b
in serous otitis media, 854t–855t
web resources on, 858t
FODMaP, 882–885.e1
gluten-free diet, in psoriasis, 728
on hormone imbalance, 579–580
in hypothyroidism, 350–351
low-glycemic index, 865
in blood sugar control, 865
in cardiovascular disease (CVD)
prevention, 865
in diabetes mellitus, 865
in insulin resistance, 327
in metabolic syndrome, 327
Mediterranean, 869–870, 870f,
870t
in colorectal cancer prevention,
802
in coronary artery disease,
253–254, 254b
in dyslipidemias, 271
in hypertension, 231–232
in insulin resistance, 327, 327b
in metabolic syndrome, 327, 327b
pyramid, 387f
in obesity, 384
in osteoporosis prevention, 371
prostate cancer and, 794
in rosacea, 767
in specialized allergen avoidance,
302
Dietary fat, 337
premenstrual syndrome and, 562
Dietary Supplement and Health
Education Act (DSHEA), 981
Dietary Supplement and
Nonprescription Drug
Consumer Protection Act,
981–982
Dietary supplements. See
Supplements
Diferuloylmethane, for multiple
sclerosis, 138
Digestion, on hormone imbalance,
579–580
Digestive/absorptive process, 332
Digitalis, herbal and supplement
interactions with, 256t
Digoxin, in heart failure, 249
Dihydrotestosterone (DHT), 630.
See also Testosterone
Diindolylmethane, stomach-
activated, for uterine fibroids,
581, 584, 584b
2,3-Dimercaptopropane-1-sulfonate
(DMPS), 1005, 1005b, 1008,
1008t
2,3-Dimercaptosuccinic acid (DMSA),
1004, 1008–1009, 1008t
Dimethylglycine (DMG), for autism
spectrum disorder, 70
Dinitrochlorobenzene, for HIV
disease, 189–190, 189b
Dipeptidyl peptidase-4 (DPP-4)
inhibitors, 332
Direct-acting HCV antivirals, 200,
200b, 201t
Disclosure, 937, 939
in asthma, 296
journaling for. See Journaling
Disease-modifying antirheumatic
drugs, for rheumatoid arthritis,
496
Disulfiram, in alcoholism, 819, 820b
Diuretics
in carpal tunnel syndrome, 699
in heart failure, 249
Docosahexaenoic acid. See Omega-3
fatty acids
Dong quai, for easing menstrual
pain, 573t

Dopamine agonists, in Parkinson's disease, 148, 148b
Dopamine antagonists, in nausea and vomiting, in pregnancy, 546, 546b
Dopamine norepinephrine reuptake inhibitor antidepressants, in depression, 42t, 43
Dovonex, in psoriasis, 731, 731b
Doxazosin
  in chronic prostatitis/chronic pelvic pain syndrome, 617b
  in urolithiasis, 613, 613b
Doxycycline, in Lyme disease, 223b
Dream health, in insomnia, 81–82, 82b
Dry saunas, for common cold, 175
Dual-energy x-ray absorptiometry (DEXA), 888
Duloxetine, in depression, 42, 42t
Dutasteride, in prostate cancer prevention, 797
Dysbiosis, 579, 987
Dyslipidemia, 264–275.e5
  carbohydrates in, 264, 267
  dietary cholesterol in, 264, 267
  fats in, 267
  garlic in, 272–273, 273b
  integrative therapy in, 267–275
  mechanisms for treatment of, 266t–267t
  Mediterranean diet in, 271
  nutraceutical supplements in, 268–275, 268f
  nutrition in, 267
  nuts in, 271
  omega-3 fatty acids in, 270–271, 271b
  pathophysiology of, 264
  phytosterols in, 269–270
  plant sterols in, 269–270, 270b
  prevention of, 274b
  red yeast rice in, 269, 269b
  saturated fats in, 264, 267
  soy in, 270, 270b
  testing in, 264–265, 265b, 266f
    expanded lipid, 264b, 275t
  therapeutic review on, 274b–275b
  trans-fats in, 264
  web resources on, 275t
Dysmenorrhea, 569–577.e2
  acupressure in, 574–575, 575f, 575b
  acupuncture in, 574
  aromatherapy with massage in, 575–577, 576b
  bioenergetic therapy in, 573–575
  biomechanical therapy in, 575
  black haw (Viburnum prunifolium) in, 572, 572b
  botanicals in, 571–572
  cramp bark (Viburnum opulus) in, 572, 572b
  exercise in, 569
  fennel (Foeniculum vulgare) in, 571, 571b
  French maritime pine bark extract (Pinus pinaster) in, 571, 571b
  heat therapy in, 573–574, 574b
  hormonal treatments in, 572–573
  integrative therapy for, 569–577
  lifestyle in, 569
  magnesium in, 570, 570t, 570b
  magnet therapy in, 574
  mind-body therapy in, 573
  nonsteroidal antiinflammatory drugs in, 572
  nutrition in, 569–570
  omega-3 fatty acids in, 569–570, 570t, 570b
  other herbs in, 572, 573t
  pathophysiology of, 569
  pharmaceuticals in, 572–573
  prevention prescription in, 576b
  primary, 569

Dysmenorrhea (Continued)
  SCA (saffron, celery seed, anise) in, 571–572, 572b
  secondary, 569
  spinal manipulation therapy in, 575
  substance use in, 569
  supplements in, 570–571
  surgery in, 575
  therapeutic review in, 576t
  therapies to consider in, 575–577
  transcutaneous electrical nerve stimulation in, 574
  vitamin B1 (thiamine) in, 570–571, 570t, 571b
  vitamin B6 (pyridoxine) in, 570, 570t, 570b
  vitamin E in, 570t, 571, 571b
  web resources in, 577t
  willow bark extract (Salix cortex) in, 572, 572b
Dyspnea, in palliative care, 809

E
Ear
  anatomy of, 154f
  infection of. See Otitis media
Ear drops, in otitis media, 154
Earache. See Otitis media
Earthing, in hypertension, 239
Echinacea
  in common cold, 172–173, 173b
  in rheumatoid arthritis, 495b
EchinOsha, in chronic sinusitis, 161, 161b
Ectopic beats, 277, 277b
Eczema. See Atopic dermatitis (AD)
Edible (medicinal) mushrooms, in breast cancer, 776, 776b
Education, Alzheimer disease and, 97
Eicosapentaenoic acid (EPA). See also Omega-3 fatty acids
Elderberry
  in chronic sinusitis, 161
  in common cold, 173
  in herpes simplex virus, 196–197
Electrical stimulation, for peripheral neuropathy, 130
Electrocardiography (ECG), 922–923
Electroconvulsive therapy, in depression, 43
Electronic activity monitors, in cardiorespiratory training, 890
Electrotherapeutic point stimulation (ETPS), in myofascial pain syndrome, 656
Eleutherococcus senticosus. See Siberian ginseng
Elevated homocysteine, 395, 395b
Elimination, in liver detoxification, 199, 199t
Elimination diet. See Diet, elimination
ELISA testing, in Lyme disease, 221
Emesis. See Vomiting
Emollient laxatives, in constipation, 471
Emotional awareness, for pain, 963–970.e2, 963b
Emotional care, in breast cancer, 778
Emotional freedom technique, 1075t
  for posttraumatic stress disorder, 88–89
Emotions, neck pain and, 679
Empathy, 21
Endocrine disruptors, in testosterone deficiency, 633, 633b
End-of-life care, 806–816.e4
End-stage renal disease (ESRD), 411
  febuxostat in, 413
  fiber supplementation for, 415
  prebiotic and synbiotic for, 414–415
Energy, usage in health care sector, 1083–1084, 1085b

Energy medicine, 1073b, 1075t, 1078b
  approaches in, 1078–1080, 1078b
  appropriate boundaries in, 1079
  biofield, sensing of, 1078
  chakras in, 1074t
  charging in, 1079
  definition of, 1073–1074
  draining away a symptom in, 1079–1080, 1080b
  grounding in, 1078–1079
  for multiple sclerosis, 136
  in neck pain, 680
  in palliative care, 813
  referral for, 1076–1078
  research on, 1076, 1076b, 1077t
  web resources on, 1080t
Energy psychology, 971–977.e1, 972b
  in bloating, weight gain, and anxiety, 971
  definition of, 972–973
  evidence for, 973, 973b
  as first-line treatment, 977
  in flu shot fear, 971
  Four Energy Gates in, 974, 975f, 977b
  personal practice and development in, 977, 977b
  for posttraumatic stress disorder, 972
  self-care with, 975f
  steps for, 976b
  web resources on, 977t
Energy tapping protocol, 976f
Enhanced external counterpulsation (EECP), in coronary artery disease, 261
Entacapone, in Parkinson's disease, 148, 148b
Enteral/parenteral feedings, in nausea and vomiting, in pregnancy, 547
Enteric inflammatory triggers, 883f
Enteric nervous system (ENS), 424
Environment, in asthma, 288
Environmental toxicities, diagnosis and treatment of, 418
Enzymes, in uterine fibroids, 585, 585b
Eosinophilia myalgia syndrome, hydroxytryptophan and, 39
Ephedra sinica. See Ma huang
Epicondylosis, 707–714.e1
  acupuncture in, 708–709, 709b
  bioenergetic therapy in, 708–709
  biomechanical medicine in, 710–713
  corticosteroid injections in, 709, 709b
  healing context in, 707–708
  injection therapies in, 709–710, 710b
  integrative therapy for, 707–714
  lateral, 1049–1050
  lifestyle in, 707–708
  mind-body therapy in, 708
  nonsteroidal antiinflammatory drugs in, 709, 709b
  orthoses (braces) in, 713, 713b
  osteopathic manipulation treatment in, 710–713, 713b
  pathophysiology of, 707, 707b
  pharmaceuticals in, 709
  physical therapy in, 710, 710b, 711f–712f
  prevention prescription in, 713b
  psychosocial stress in, 708, 708b
  relative rest in, 708, 708f
  surgery in, 713–714, 713b
  therapeutic review in, 714b
  web resources in, 714t
Epidural steroid injections
  in low back pain, 673
  in neck pain, 683

Epidural steroids
  acupuncture versus, 16
  specific and nonspecific variables of, 16, 16f, 17t
Epigallocatechin gallate. See Green tea
Epworth Sleepiness Scale, for insomnia, 76
Erectile dysfunction, 623–629.e2
  bioenergetics in, 625
  emerging therapies for, 627–629
  evaluation for, 623, 623b, 624t
  integrative therapy for, 623–629
  lifestyle and, 626–627, 627b
  manual therapies for, 625
  medications and, 625t
  mind-body therapy in, 625–626
  nutraceuticals in, 625, 626b
  pathophysiology of, 623
  pharmaceuticals in, 623
  prevention prescription of, 628b
  prostaglandin E₁ injection in, 624
  risk factors for, 625b
  testosterone for, 623–624, 624b
  therapeutic review for, 628b
  vacuum erection or constriction device in, 625
  web resources on, 629t
Ergonomic keyboards, for carpal tunnel syndrome, 698
Ergot alkaloids, in migraine, 114
Erythema migrans, 218, 220f
Escitalopram, in depression, 42, 42t
Essential fatty acids
  in atopic dermatitis, 719–720, 720b
  in neck pain, 678
  in osteoporosis, 373–374
  in rheumatoid arthritis, 495
Essential oils
  for neck pain, 686–688
  in preparation of herbal products, 983t
Estriol, 553, 581
  in vaginal dryness, 597, 597b
Estriol-Lactobacilli combination (Gynoflor) vaginal tablet, 597, 598b
Estrogen. See also Hormone replacement therapy
  in age-related macular degeneration, 841
  in menopausal symptoms, 553, 553b
  metabolism of, 583, 583f
  for multiple sclerosis, 139
  role of, 378
  synthesis and catabolism, pathways of, 774f
  in urinary tract infection, 215
Estrogen dominance, 579–581, 579f, 580t
  diet-related increase in, 582
  diet-related reduction in, 583, 583b
  insulin resistance and, 580
  intestinal dysbiosis and, 579
  liver detoxification and, 580–581
Estrogen replacement therapy. See also Hormone replacement therapy
  in depression, 43–44
Ethylenediaminetetraacetic acid (EDTA), 1008t, 1009
Evening primrose oil
  in peripheral neuropathy, 126
  in postdates pregnancy, 536
  in premenstrual syndrome, 565, 565b
Exenatide, 344, 344b
Exercise
  abdominal curl-up, in low back pain, 903f–907f
  aerobic
    for osteoarthritis, 641
    in Parkinson's disease, 145

Exercise (Continued)
in age-related macular
degeneration, 840
in Alzheimer disease, 98–99
in anxiety, 47, 47b
in arrhythmias, 280
in asthma, 289
in attention-deficit/hyperactivity
disorder, 54
in autism spectrum disorder, 67
in breast cancer, 774–775
breathing, in low back pain, 901,
903f–907f
cardiovascular, 891t
in carpal tunnel syndrome, 698
cat/dog stretch, in low back pain,
903f–907f
in cholelithiasis, 450
in chronic fatigue syndrome, 486
in chronic kidney disease, 419
coordination training, in low back
pain, 902, 903f–907f
in coronary artery disease, 254–255
in depression, 36, 37b
in detoxification, 999
in dysmenorrhea, 569, 576b
in fibromyalgia, 477
flexibility
in low back pain, 901–902
in osteoarthritis, 641–642
gluteus maximus, in low back pain,
903f–907f
gluteus medius, in low back pain,
903f–907f
hamstring, in low back pain,
903f–907f
heart rate in, 926–927
hip flexor stretch, in low back pain,
903f–907f
in hypertension, 234
in hypothyroidism, 350
in insulin resistance, 326
in irritable bowel syndrome, 427
Key Three, 891–893, 892f
in low back pain, 901–907.e1, 669,
903f–907f
web resources on, 902t
in Lyme disease, 225, 225b
in menopausal symptoms, 558
relaxation, 556
in metabolic syndrome, 326
in migraine, 108–110
movement. See Movement
therapies
in multiple sclerosis, 134
in muscle strengthening, in
osteoarthritis, 641
in myofascial pain syndrome,
653–654, 654b
in nausea and vomiting, in
pregnancy, 543
in neck pain, 677–678, 687b
in obesity, 385–386
in ocular disorders, 832
in osteoarthritis, 640–642
in osteoporosis, 376–377, 377b
in Parkinson's disease, 145, 145b,
150b–151b
in peripheral neuropathy, 122
piriformis, in low back pain,
903f–907f
in polycystic ovarian syndrome, 362
in posttraumatic stress disorder,
86–87, 86b, 92b
in pregnancy-related depression,
36–37
in prostate cancer prevention,
794–796
as relaxation technique, 911t–912t
in resistance, in osteoarthritis, 641
in rheumatoid arthritis, 494
standing-on-one-leg, in low back
pain, 903f–907f
strength, in low back pain, 902,
902b, 903f–907f

Exercise (Continued)
in testosterone deficiency, 632
in type 2 diabetes mellitus, 335
in uterine fibroids, 583
for vaginal dryness, 596, 596b
Exercise prescription, 886–894.e1
agility in, 893–894
balance in, 891t, 893–894
basic principles of, 887, 887b
body composition and, 888, 888b
cardiorespiratory training in,
888–890
electronic activity monitors in, 890
fitness, five components of,
887–888
FITT principle for, 888, 889f, 890t
flexibility in, 893
key three strength program in,
891–893, 892f
levels of, 891, 891t
resistance training in, 890–891,
890b
stability in, 893
therapeutic review in, 893b
web resources in, 894t
Extracorporeal shockwave
lithotripsy, for urolithiasis,
613–614, 613f
Eye movement desensitization and
reprocessing (EMDR), 1075t
Eyes
cataract of. See Cataracts
dry, prevention of, 834b
macular degeneration of. See Age-
related macular degeneration
Ezetimibe, in dyslipidemias, 267

F
Facet joint injections
in low back pain, 673
in neck pain, 683
Facilitated positional release, in
osteopathic manipulative
techniques, 678t
Facilitating behavioral change,
integrative medicine and, 1090
Famciclovir, for herpes simplex virus
infection, 195, 196b
Far-infrared sauna, in chronic
sinusitis, 166
Fast foods, 328t
Fasting, 999–1000
intermittent, in Alzheimer disease,
99
Fat, 267
cataracts and, 833
in cholelithiasis, 451
in diet, 870–872, 871f, 871t, 871b.
See also Omega-3 fatty acids
saturated, 264, 267
trans-, 264
trans-fatty acids, 872, 872f
Fat-free body mass (FFB), 888
Fatigue, chronic. See Chronic fatigue
syndrome
Fatty acids. See Omega-3 fatty acids;
Omega-6 fatty acids
Febuxostat, for gout, 695, 695b
Feingold diet, in children with
attention-deficit/hyperactivity
disorder, 56
Feldenkrais, in neck pain, 677
Female infertility, 518
Female reproductive life cycle,
physiology of, 550–553,
551f–552f, 551b
Fennel, in dysmenorrhea, 571, 571b
Fenugreek
in cholelithiasis, 454
in type 2 diabetes mellitus, 340,
340b
Fermentable carbohydrates
(FODMaPs)
in irritable bowel syndrome, 426
reactions to, 316

Fertility, herbal medicine for, 522
Fertility blend, 521–522
Fetal heart tones, 923, 924f
Feverfew
in migraine, 111–112, 111b
in rosacea, 768, 768b
Fiber, 336, 873f
in breast cancer, 775
in chronic kidney disease, 415
in colorectal cancer prevention,
801
in coronary artery disease,
258–260
in DASH diet, 878
dietary
in cholelithiasis, 451
in constipation, 466–467,
466b–467b
in irritable bowel syndrome,
426–427, 427b
in pediatric abdominal pain,
459–460, 460t, 460b
in hypertension, 233
in menopausal symptoms, 557
Fibrates, in dyslipidemia, 267
Fibroids. See Uterine fibroids
Fibromyalgia, 474–483.e2
acupuncture in, 478
analgesics in, 481
anticonvulsants in, 481
antidepressants for, 480
autonomic dysfunction in, 475
bodywork in, 477
Boswellia in, 479, 479b
botanicals in, 479
cannabinoids in, 481
exercise in, 477, 477b
four Rs in, 477–478
ginger in, 479, 479b
homeopathy in, 478
integrative therapy for, 476–481,
476b, 482f
magnesium in, 479b
meditation in, 477
mind-body therapy in, 477–478
nonsteroidal antiinflammatory
drugs (NSAIDs) in, 480–481
nutrition in, 476–477
omega-3 fatty acids in, 478b
pain in, 475, 475b
pathophysiology of, 475–476,
475b, 476f
pharmaceuticals in, 480–481
prevention prescription of, 482b
psychotherapeutic interventions
in, 477–478
S-adenosylmethionine (SAMe) in,
479, 479b
selective serotonin reuptake
inhibitors for, 480, 480b
St. John's wort in, 479, 479b
supplements in, 478–479
temperament and, 475–476
therapeutic review on, 483b
turmeric in, 479, 479b
vitamin D in, 478–479
web resources on, 483t
Finasteride, in prostate cancer
prevention, 797
First-generation H1-receptor
antagonists, dosage of, for
urticaria, 742
Fisetin, for allergic patient, 304, 304b
Fish. See also Omega-3 fatty acids
algae-eating, in cataract, 834
in antiinflammatory diet, 874
in coronary artery disease, 254
type 2 diabetes mellitus and, 341
Fish oil. See also Omega-3 fatty acids;
Omega-6 fatty acids
in Alzheimer disease, 102, 102b
in asthma, 294
in chronic sinusitis, 163
in coronary artery disease, 259,
259b

Fish oi (Continued)
in depression, 42t
in migraine, 111
in peripheral neuropathy, 128
in psoriasis, 729, 729b
in vaginal dryness, 596, 596b
Fitness. See also Exercise
five components of, 887–888
FITT principle, for exercise
programming, 888, 889f
Flame retardants, in chronic kidney
disease, 418.e1
Flavonoids, 1010t–1011t, 1011
Flaxseed
in benign prostatic hyperplasia,
601–602
in breast cancer, 776, 776b
in chronic sinusitis, 165
in dyslipidemia, 271, 271b
in hypertension, 233–234
prostate cancer and, 795
Flexibility, 891t, 893
Flora Balance, for chronic sinusitis,
164
Flower essences, 1075t
Fluconazole, in seborrheic
dermatitis, 757
Fluids
in constipation, 467
extract, in preparation of herbal
products, 983t
in menopausal symptoms, 558
in urinary tract infection, 212
Flutamide, in polycystic ovarian
syndrome, 367
FODMaP diet, 882–885.e1
condition for, 882
high and low, 883t
limitations of, 884–885
meaning of, 882
mechanism of action of, 882
sugars, 882t
therapeutic benefit of, 882b
web resources on, 885t
FODMaP sugars, 882t
Foeniculum vulgare. See Fennel
Folate, 399
in colorectal cancer prevention,
802
in inflammatory bowel disease,
504–505
metabolites, increase in, amount
of, 395–396, 396f
Folic acid
in anxiety, 48
in autism spectrum disorder, 69
in chronic kidney disease, 415
in coronary artery disease, 260, 260b
in depression, 38, 42t
in insulin resistance, 329, 329b
in metabolic syndrome, 329, 329b
Follicle-stimulating hormone (FSH),
578
Food(s). See also Diet; Nutrition
adverse reactions to, 850t–851t
celiac disease and, 850t–851t
cross-allergy and, 850t–851t
elimination diet for. See Diet,
elimination
enzymatic and, 850t–851t
eosinophilic
esophagogastroenteritis,
850t–851t
food allergy, 850t–851t
IgG-related intolerance and,
850t–851t
infectious and, 850t–851t
pharmacological reactions and,
850t–851t
physiological reactions and,
850t–851t
pseudoallergies and, 850t–851t
psychogenic and, 850t–851t
structural and, 850t–851t
toxin mediated and, 850t–851t

Food(s) (Continued)
allergy to, 310–318.e6, 310b, 853t
in adverse food reactions, 850t–851t
atopic dermatitis and, 716
cholelithiasis and, 452
diagnosis of, 311t, 313–314
differentiating from other food reactions, 316
in elimination diet, 853t, 853b
epidemic of, 310–312
IgG4 antibody testing to, 314
integrative therapy of, 314–318
in irritable bowel syndrome, 425–426
medical history of, 313, 313b
migraine and, 313
nomenclature of, 310
pathophysiology of, 310–312
physical examination of, 313
prevention prescription of, 318b
pseudoallergy and, 316
research validation of, 312–313
seborrheic dermatitis and, 757
specific adaption of, 312, 312f
symptoms and conditions may cause or exacerbated by, 311t
therapeutic review of, 318b
web resources on, 318t
avoidance of. See also Diet, elimination
in insulin resistance, 328, 328t
in metabolic syndrome, 328, 328t
challenges, individual, 315
cooking techniques for, 327–328
in DASH diet, 880–881
in detoxification, 999, 999t
elimination, in pediatric abdominal pain, 460
extract testing, 314
fear of, and FODMaP diet, 884
glycemic index in, 864–865
high-GI, 863b
intolerance to. See also Food(s)
in elimination diet, 853t, 853b
lutein-containing, 833
pesticides in, 999, 999t
planetary health and, 1019, 1019b
procurement of, as health care's carbon footprint, 1085
proteins, elimination of, 882–883
sensitivities to. See also Food(s), adverse reactions to
in irritable bowel syndrome, 425–426
sulfur-containing, 834
therapeutic
in insulin resistance, 328
in metabolic syndrome, 328
triggers
of arrhythmias, 279–280
in constipation, 467, 467b
rheumatoid arthritis and, 494
type 2 diabetes mellitus and, 335–336
Forgiveness, 940–944.e1
guidelines for, 941–943, 942f
health effects of, 940–941
nature of, 941, 941b
patient handout on, 944f
trauma and, 941b
web resources on, 943t
Four Energy Gates, in energy psychology, 974, 975f, 977b
Fracture
osteoporotic, 370
spinal, 663t–664t
Free radicals, in chronic hepatitis, 198
French maritime pine bark extract, in dysmenorrhea, 571, 571b
Fructose intolerance, irritable bowel syndrome and, 426, 426b

Fructose malabsorption, in pediatric abdominal pain, 458
Fruit
in age-related macular degeneration, 841
in antiinflammatory diet, 873, 873b
in chronic sinusitis, 165
Fumaric acid, for multiple sclerosis, 140
Functional magnetic resonance imaging, in healing encounter, 22b
Functional somatic syndromes, 221
Fungal sinusitis, 158, 158b
treating yeast overgrowth and, 163–166

G
Gabapentin
in fibromyalgia, 481, 481b
in Lyme disease, 224, 224b
in menopausal symptoms, 554, 554b
in myofascial pain syndrome, 659b
in peripheral neuropathy, 130
Gallbladder "flush," in cholelithiasis, 453
Gallstone disease. See Cholelithiasis
Gamma-linolenic acid (GLA), 373–374
in gout, 691–692, 692b
Garlic
in chronic sinusitis, 161
in colorectal cancer prevention, 801
in common cold, 173, 173b
in dyslipidemias, 272–273, 273b
in hypertension, 236–237, 237b
in urinary tract infection, 212
Gastric distention, arrhythmias and, 279, 280b
Gastroesophageal reflux disease (GERD), 433–438.e1
antianxiety botanicals in, 436
antiinflammatory botanicals in, 435–436
biomechanical therapy in, 437
botanical combinations in, 436
chamomile in, 435t, 436b
demulcent botanicals in, 435, 435t
homeopathy in, 437
integrative therapy for, 434–438
licorice in, 435t, 436, 436b
lifestyle modification in, 434–435
marshmallow in, 435, 435t, 435b
mind-body therapy in, 437
pathophysiology of, 433–434, 434f, 434t
pediatric patient, special consideration for, 434, 434b, 437–438
pharmaceuticals in, 436, 436t, 437b
prevention prescription of, 438b
skullcap in, 435t
slippery elm root bark powder in, 435, 435t, 435b
surgery in, 437
symptoms of, 433
therapeutic review on, 438b
therapies to consider in, 437
traditional Chinese medicine in, 437
valerian in, 435t
web resources on, 438t
Gastrointestinal microbes, in rosacea, 767
Gastrointestinal system
disorders of. See also specific disorders
in hypnosis, 917–918
therapeutic homeopathy in, 1070, 1071t
microflora of, establishment of, 987

Gate control theory, 526
Gem therapy, 1075t
Gender
age-related macular degeneration and, 839–840
cataracts and, 832
General adaptation syndrome, 910f, 910b
Generalized anxiety disorder (GAD). See Anxiety
Genetic factors, in multiple sclerosis, 134
Genetically engineered foods, 1017–1018
Geranium oil, in peripheral neuropathy, 125–126
GERD. See Gastroesophageal reflux disease (GERD)
German chamomile (Matricaria recutita)
in aphthous stomatitis, 749, 749b
for common cold, 172, 172b
Ginger
in carpal tunnel syndrome, 700, 700b
in common cold, 173, 173b
in fibromyalgia, 479, 479b
in irritable bowel syndrome, 428, 428b
in nausea, in palliative care, 809, 809b
in nausea and vomiting, in pregnancy, 543, 543b
in osteoarthritis, 649
in pediatric abdominal pain, 461, 461b
in rheumatoid arthritis, 495, 495b
Ginkgo biloba
in age-related macular degeneration, 844
in Alzheimer disease, 105
in multiple sclerosis, 138
in premenstrual syndrome, 565, 565b
in urticaria, 742, 742b
in vaginal dryness, 597, 597b
Ginseng
in common cold, 173–174, 174b
in insulin resistance, 331, 331b
in metabolic syndrome, 331, 331b
Glatiramer acetate (GA), in multiple sclerosis, 141
Global warming, impact on health, 1081–1087.e2
life cycle assessment (LCA), 1082–1086, 1083f
energy use on, 1083–1084, 1085b
pharmaceuticals on, 1084–1085
procurement on, 1085–1086
transportation on, 1085–1086, 1086f
web resources on, 1087t
Globe artichoke, in cholelithiasis, 453, 453b
Glove anesthesia technique, 918–919
Glucocorticoids
in gout, 693, 693b
in inflammatory bowel syndrome, 511–512
Glucosamine sulfate, in osteoarthritis, 644–645, 645b
Glucose. See also Glycemic index; Glycemic load
blood, 335
inflammation and, 869
Glucose and insulin tolerance test (GITT), 325–326
Glucose transporter 4 (GLUT4), 321
Glutamine
in aphthous stomatitis, 748, 748b
in chronic hepatitis, 204
in inflammatory bowel disease, 506
in peptic ulcer disease, 444, 444b
L-Glutamine, in HIV disease, 184, 184b

Glutathione, 1010–1011, 1010t–1011t, 1011b
in age-related macular degeneration, 842–843
in Alzheimer disease, 102
in chronic hepatitis, 202–203, 203b
in Parkinson's disease, 146, 146b
Gluten sensitivity, irritable bowel syndrome and, 426
Gluten-free diet
casein free diet, for autism spectrum disorder, 67
in psoriasis, 728
Gluteus maximus exercise, in low back pain, 903f–907f
Gluteus medius exercise, in low back pain, 903f–907f
Glycemic control, in colorectal cancer prevention, 801–802
Glycemic index, 335–336, 863, 863f, 863b–864b, 864t, 866t–868t
in blood sugar control, 865
in cancer, 865
in cardiovascular disease (CVD) prevention, 865
in diabetes mellitus, 865
in disease prevention and management, 865
in foods, 864–865
in inflammation, 865
in oxidative stress, 865
Glycemic load, 863–865, 864t, 864b, 866t–868t
in disease prevention and management, 865
Glycerite, in preparation of herbal products, 983t
Glycyrrhetinic acid
in atopic dermatitis, 720, 720b
in psoriasis, 731
Glycyrrhizin. See Licorice
Goldenseal
in common cold, 174
in urinary tract infection, 215
Gonadotropin receptor agonists, in uterine fibroids, 587
Gout, 689–696.e1
ACE inhibitors in, 693–695
acupuncture in, 692
allopurinol in, 695, 695b
bioflavonoids in, 691, 691b
botanicals in, 692
bromelain in, 692, 692b
cherry in, 692, 692b
colchicine in, 693, 693b
diuretics in, 693–695
eicosapentaenoic acid in, 691–692, 692b
gamma-linolenic acid in, 691–692, 692b
glucocorticoids in, 693, 693b
Hibiscus in, 692, 692b
history of, 689–690
ice in, 692–693, 693b
integrative therapy for, 690–696
lifestyle in, 690–691
new clinical significance of, 689–690, 690b
nonsteroidal antiinflammatory drugs in, 693, 693b
nutrition in, 690–691
pathogenesis of, 689–690, 689f
pharmaceuticals in, 693
physical medicine in, 692–693
prevention prescription for, 695b
probenecid in, 695, 695b
pyramid, 690f
quercetin in, 692, 692b
rest in, 693
supplements in, 691–692
therapeutic review for, 696b
therapies to consider in, 695–696
traditional Chinese medicine in, 693

Gout *(Continued)*
vitamin C in, 691, 691b
web resources on, 696t
weight loss in, 690
Graded exercise therapy, for chronic fatigue syndrome, 485b
Grape fruit seed, in chronic sinusitis, 162–163, 162b
Green tea
in acne vulgaris, 762, 762b
in Alzheimer disease, 103
in breast cancer, 776, 776b
in dyslipidemia, 270, 270b
in insulin resistance, 331, 331b
in metabolic syndrome, 331, 331b
in multiple sclerosis, 139
in obesity, 388, 388b
in Parkinson's disease, 147, 147b
prostate cancer and, 795
in rosacea, 768
in uterine fibroids, 583, 583b
Greenhouse gases (GHGs), 1082, 1082b
Grief, 811
Grounding
in energy medicine, 1078–1079
in guided imagery, 934
Group visit, integrative medicine and, 1094–1095
Guggul, in hypothyroidism, 355
Guided imagery, 930–936.e1
applications in medicine, 931
in asthma, 296
case history of, 930–933
for chronic fatigue syndrome, 490
contraindications for, 934–935, 936b
definition of, 930–931
evocative imagery for, 933–934
grounding in, 934
in headaches, 930–931
healing imagery for, 933
in heart rate variability enhancement, 929
indications for, 930, 931b
initiation of, 934
inner advisor for, 933
interactive imagery dialogue for, 933
in lumpy breast, 932–933, 933b
mechanism of action of, 931–933
mental and physical relaxation in, 933
in palliative care, 812
for posttraumatic stress disorder, 88
precautions for, 934–935
recordings for, 936
as relaxation technique, 911t–912t
in research, 931
resources for, 935–936
self-study programs for, 936
sessions for, 934, 935b
in substance abuse, 823
techniques for, 933–934
training for, 935–936
web resources for, 936t
Gut health, optimizing, in Alzheimer disease, 99
Gut-immune barrier, 849–857, 852b
Gynostemma pentaphyllum, 339, 339b

H
Hand clasp test, 915
Hand tracing technique, 919, 919f
Harpagophytum procumbens. See Devil's claw
Hats, in age-related macular degeneration, 840
Hawthorn
in heart failure, 243–246, 246b
in hypertension, 237, 237b
Headache, 108–119.e3
acupressure in, 1038–1039

Headache *(Continued)*
acupuncture for, 1038–1043.e1
cervical region, trigger points in, 1041–1042, 1042b
for cluster headache, 1042
definition of, 1038
evidence for, 1040–1041, 1041b
for frontal headache, 1042, 1042f
GB20 point for, 1041–1042, 1042f
general relaxation and calming points in, 1041
GV20 point for, 1041, 1041f
LI4 point for, 1041, 1041f
local points in, 1042
mechanism of action of, 1038
for migraines, 1042
posttreatment home program after, 1042–1043
safety of, 1038
for sinus headaches, 1042, 1042f
techniques for, 1039–1040, 1039f–1040f, 1040b
for tension headaches, 1042
training in, 1038
treatment, during an, 1042
web resources on, 1043t
guided imagery in, 930–931
hypnosis in, 918
migraine. *See* Migraine
"red flag" symptoms in, 108
tension-type, 117
acupuncture in, 118, 1042.
See also Headache, acupuncture for,
chiropractic for, 118
prevention prescription for, 118b
therapeutic review in, 119b
web resources on, 119t
Healing, 14b, 23b
Healing encounter, 20–26.e1, 26b. *See also* Motivational interviewing
action in, 22
empathy in, 21
five questions to consider in, 24–25, 24f
foundations of, 14–18
insight and intuition in, 21–22, 22f
mindfulness in, 20–22
pause in, 22
practitioner *versus* pill in, 20
presence in, 23, 23f
proceed in, 23, 23b
salutogenesis-oriented, 25–26
self-reflection in, 21, 21f
steps to enhance, 25–26
3 Ps of, 22–23
web resources on, 26t
Healing environments
behavioral, 13–14
business case for, 18–19
in clinical setting, 14, 15t
creating, 12–19.e2
external, 14
genetic expression and, 18, 18f
health teams in, 17, 18t
internal, 12
interpersonal, 12
optimal, 13f, 13t, 19t
practitioner's influence on, 17, 17f
spiritual connection and, 14
value of, 18–19
Healing foods pyramid, 335–336, 336f
Healing touch. *See* Therapeutic/healing touch
Healing-oriented medicine, 7, 7b, 8f
Health
as continuum, 19
definition of, 7
forgiveness and, 940–941
gut microbiome in, 986–987, 988f
healing-oriented medicine and, 7, 7b, 8f

Health care system, twenty-first century simple rules for, 7t
Health teams, 17, 18t
Heart failure, 242–252.e5, 242b, 243t
acupuncture in, 250
angiotensin receptor blockers in, 248
angiotensin-converting enzyme inhibitors in, 247–248
L-arginine in, 247
beta blockers in, 248–249
cardiac glycosides in, 249
carnitine in, 247
coenzyme Q10 in, 246
hawthorn in, 243–246
hydralazine in, 249
integrative therapy for, 243–252, 244f–245f
biomechanical therapy, 249–250
botanicals, 243–246
herbs and supplements, 243
lifestyle, 250–251
mind-body therapy, 250
nutrition, 251–252
pharmaceuticals, 247–249
supplements, 246–247
prevention prescription of, 251b
therapeutic review on, 251b–252b
web resources on, 252t
Heart rate variability (HRV), 922–929.e6
age and, 925–926
background to, 922–923, 922b–923b
basics matter in, 928
biofeedback effects in, 928–929
biofeedback with paced slow breathing in, 927
in cardiovascular health, 926
congestive heart failure and, 924f
deep, slow breathing in, 928
in depression, 926
enhancement of
beginning of, 928–929
recommendations for, 928
steps to, 928
web resources on, 929t
environmental effects on, 926
in exercise, 926–927
factors that improve, 926–927
in frustration to appreciation, 924, 924f–925f
health and, 925–927
measurement of, 923–925, 924f–925f
in meditation, 927
in nutrition, 926
in pharmaceuticals, 926
physiology of, 923–925, 925b
temperature changes and, 927
willpower and, 927, 927b
Heat therapy
in dysmenorrhea, 573–574, 574b
in osteoarthritis, 643
Heavy metal chelation, 1004–1005, 1007b
Heavy metal intoxication, treatment for, 1007, 1007b
Heavy metals, in chronic kidney disease, 418.e1
Helicobacter pylori, 439, 440f
rosacea and, 767
treatment enhancement, 992t
Helminths, in inflammatory bowel disease, 510–512
Helping styles, 954–955. *See also* Motivational interviewing
directing, 954, 956t
following, 954
guiding, 954
Hemoglobin, glycosylated (HbA1c), 326
Hepatitis A vaccination, 202
Hepatitis B vaccination, 202

Hepatitis C virus (HCV), 198
direct-acting antiviral therapy for, 200, 200b, 201t
ribavirin for, 202
Herbal products
information on testing, 982t
preparation of, 983t
Herbal remedies, with nephrotoxic potential, 416, 417t
Herbal toxicities, in chronic kidney disease, 416
Herbalism, 337, 338t
Herbicides, chronic kidney disease and, 418.e1
Herbs. *See also* Botanicals
talking about, 979
uses of, 979
Herpes simplex virus, 191–197.e2
acupuncture in, 194–195
clinical manifestations of, 191, 191b
dietary considerations in, 193t
epidemiology of, 191
integrative therapy for, 192–197
lifestyle and, 192
mind-body therapies for, 195
nutrition and, 192
pharmaceuticals and, 195–196
prevention prescription of, 196b
reactivation, potential triggers of, 192t
supplements and, 192–193
therapeutic review for, 197b
therapies to consider for, 196–197
web resources on, 197t
Heterocyclic antidepressants, 43
Heterocyclic serotonin modulator, for depression, 43
Hibiscus, in gout, 692, 692b
Hip flexor stretch exercise, 903f–907f
Hip fracture prevention studies, 379t
Hippotherapy, for autism spectrum disorder, 71
Histamine-2 (H2) receptor antagonists
dosage of, for urticaria, 742–743
in pediatric abdominal pain, 462–463, 463b
Histamine-releasing foods, 740t
Histamine-rich foods, 740t
Hives. *See* Urticaria
Homeopathy, 1075t
in aphthous stomatitis, 749, 749b, 752b
in asthma, 297
in atopic dermatitis, 723–725
in cholelithiasis, 455
in fibromyalgia, 478
in GERD, 437
in labor pain management, 532
in migraine, 116–117
in nausea and vomiting, in pregnancy, 548
in otitis media, 156
in postdates pregnancy, 536, 536b
in psoriasis, 736–738, 736b
in seborrheic dermatitis, 757
in substance abuse, 826–828
in urticaria, 744–746, 745b
in uterine fibroids, 589–591
Homocysteine, in Alzheimer disease, 95
Homosexual, 938
Honey
in aphthous stomatitis, 748
in common cold, 175, 175b
HOPE, in spiritual assessment tools, 1060t
Hops
in easing menstrual pain, 573t
in insomnia, 79, 79b
Hormonal imbalances, in chronic fatigue syndrome, 488
Hormonal treatment
acne vulgaris and, 764, 764b
in dysmenorrhea, 572–573

Hormone(s)
  in Alzheimer disease, 103
  in multiple sclerosis, 139
  in uterine fibroids, 588
Hormone balance
  estrogen dominance and, 579
  intestinal dysbiosis and, 579
Hormone replacement therapy,
    male. *See also* Testosterone,
    deficiency of
  contraindications of, 635, 635b
Hormone-altering medications,
    prostate cancer and, 797
Hot baths, for common cold, 175,
    175b
Hot flashes, hypnosis for, 918
Hot toddy, in common cold, 176
Household pesticides, 1022
Household products, 1020–1021,
    1021b
Human immunodeficiency virus
    (HIV) disease, 180–190.e2
  N-acetylcysteine in, 184, 184b
  acupuncture in, 188
  biofeedback in, 187–188
  botanicals in, 186–187
  calcium carbonate in, 184, 185b
  L-carnitine in, 184, 184b
  Chinese herbal approaches for,
    186, 186b
  chromium in, 185, 185b
  L-glutamine in, 184, 184b
  herb-supplement-medication
    interactions in, 187
  hypnosis in, 188
  K-PAX Immune Support Formula
    in, 185, 185b, 186t
  α-lipoic acid in, 183, 183b
  massage therapy in, 188
  milk thistle in, 186–187, 187b
  mind-body therapy in, 187–188
  mindfulness and stress reduction
    in, 188
  multivitamins in, 183
  nutrition in, 182–183
  omega-3 polyunsaturated fatty
    acids in, 185, 185b
  pathophysiology of, 180
  pharmaceuticals in, 181–182
  prevention of, 189b
  progressive muscle relaxation in,
    187–188
  red rice yeast extract in, 187,
    187b
  selenium in, 183, 183b
  smoking and, 182
  spirituality in, 188
  therapeutic review on, 190b
  types of, 180b
  vitamin A in, 183, 183b
  vitamin B_{12} in, 183, 183b
  vitamin C in, 183, 183b
  vitamin D in, 184b
  vitamin E in, 183, 183b
  web resources on, 190t
  zinc in, 185, 185b
Human microbiota, 987, 987b
Humidity, in atopic dermatitis,
    718
Humulus lupulus. See Hops
Huperzine A, in Alzheimer disease,
    102–103, 103b
Hydrastis canadensis. See Goldenseal
Hydration. *See also* Fluids
  in age-related macular
    degeneration, 840
  in atopic dermatitis, 717
  in cataract prevention, 833–834
Hydrocortisone, in chronic fatigue
    syndrome, 491
Hydrotherapy, in myofascial pain
    syndrome, 657
Hydroxychloroquine, in rheumatoid
    arthritis, 496, 496b

2-Hydroxyestrone/
    16-hydroxyestrone ratio, in
    Breast cancer, 773, 773b, 774f
5-Hydroxytryptamine receptor
    1B/1D agonists (triptans), for
    migraine, 114
5-Hydroxytryptamine₃ receptor
    agonists, for nausea and
    vomiting, in pregnancy, 546,
    546b
5-Hydroxytryptophan
  in anxiety, 48
  caution for, 48
  precautions for, 48b
Hydroxytryptophan, in depression,
    39, 42t
Hygiene
  in acne rosacea, 759
  in acne vulgaris, 759
  in rosacea, 767–768
Hyperarousal, insomnia and, 76, 76b
Hyperbaric oxygen therapy, in
    autism spectrum disorder, 72
Hypercalciuria, 608
Hypericum perforatum. See St. John's
    wort
Hyperoxaluria, 608
Hypertension, 229–241.e3, 230t,
    230b–231b
  asymptomatic, 230
  Ayurveda in, 238
  botanicals, 236–237, 237b
  cocoa in, 232–233
  coenzyme Q10 in, 235
  DASH diet in, 878–881.e1, 232
  dietary supplements and, 234–236
  exercise and, 234
  fiber in, 233
  garlic in, 236–237
  hawthorn in, 237
  integrative therapy for, 231–239
  lifestyle modification, 231
  Mediterranean diet in, 231–232
  mind-body therapy for, 237–239
  nutrition and, 231–234
  olive oil in, 232
  prevention prescription for, 240b
  qi gong in, 239
  red wine in, 233
  relaxation response in, 237–238
  smoking cessation in, 231
  tai chi in, 239
  therapeutic review on, 240b
  therapies to consider for, 239–241
  traditional Chinese and East Asian
    medicine, 240–241
  transcendental meditation in, 238
  vitamin D in, 235–236
  web resources on, 241t
  weight loss and, 234
Hyperuricemia, 690b. *See also* Gout
Hypnosis
  in asthma, 296
  in herpes simplex virus, 195
  in HIV disease, 188
  in irritable bowel syndrome, 429
  in menopausal symptoms, 557
  in migraine, 115
  in nausea and vomiting, in
    pregnancy, 544–545
  in neck pain, 679
  in palliative care, 812
  in pediatric abdominal pain, 464
  in psoriasis, 735
  as relaxation technique, 911t–912t
  in substance abuse, 823
  in urticaria, 744, 744b
Hypnotherapy, 529
  in constipation, 469
  in labor pain management, 529
  in posttraumatic stress disorder, 89
Hypnotic induction, 921b
Hypocitraturia, 608
Hypoglycemia, in premenstrual
    syndrome, 560

Hypothalamus, in stress, 910
Hypothyroidism, 347–360.e3
  botanicals in, 355
  Brassica vegetable avoidance in,
    350–351, 351b
  in chronic fatigue syndrome, 488
  clinical presentation of, 348
  diet in, 350–351
  endocrine disruptors and,
    348–350
  environmental toxins and,
    348–350
  exercise in, 350
  guggul in, 355
  hypothalamic, 347
  integrative therapy in, 350–360,
    350f, 350b
  iodine deficiency in, 351, 351t,
    351b
  iodine excess in, 352, 352b
  iodine testing in, 352, 352b
  iron in, 354, 354b
  laboratory studies in, 348
  normal thyroid physiology and,
    347
  nutrition in, 350–351
  omega-3 in, 354, 354b
  optimal lab values in, 348, 348b
  pathophysiology of, 347–350
  pharmaceuticals in, 355–358,
    355.e1t
  prevention prescription of, 359b
  primary, 347
  probiotics in, 354–355
  seaweed preparations in, 351t, 355
  secondary, 347
  selenium in, 353, 353t, 353b
  soy in, 351
  stress reduction in, 358
  subclinical, 347–348, 347b
  supplements in, 351–355
  tertiary, 347
  therapeutic review on, 359b–360b
  therapies to consider in, 358–360
  timing of blood collection in, 348
  traditional Chinese medicine in,
    358
  transient, 347
  treatment algorithm, 349f
  treatment targets in, 348, 348b
  vitamin A in, 353, 353b
  vitamin D in, 354, 354b
  web resources on, 360t
  yoga in, 358–360, 358b, 359f
  zinc in, 353–354, 354b
Hypovitaminosis D, 373
Hysterectomy, in fibroids, 578, 588

I

Ibandronate, in osteoporosis,
    378–379, 379t
Ibuprofen, 153, 153b
Ice
  in epicondylosis, 708
  in gout, 692–693, 693b
Ideosensory experience, 915
Imagery. *See* Guided imagery
Immune system
  in chronic fatigue syndrome,
    488–489
  guided imagery effects on, 932b
Immunization, childhood diseases
    and, 721
Immunoglobulin E (IgE), 301b
Immunosuppressants, in
    inflammatory bowel syndrome,
    512, 512b
Immunotherapy
  in allergic patient, 306–307
  sublingual, 307, 307b
  in atopic dermatitis, 721
  in autism spectrum disorder, 69
In vitro fertilization, 523
Incretins, 344
Indian frankincense. *See* Boswellia

Indian ginseng. *See* Ashwagandha
Indigo naturalis extract, in psoriasis,
    730, 730b
Indinavir, St. John's wort interaction
    with, 187b
Indole-3-carbinol (I-3-C), in uterine
    fibroids, 581, 584, 584b
Infection. *See also specific infections*
  Borrelia burgdorferi. See Lyme
    disease
  ear. *See* Otitis media (OM)
  respiratory tract. *See* Upper
    respiratory infections
  spinal, 663t–664t
  urinary tract. *See* Urinary tract
    infection (UTI)
Infertility
  causes of, 518
  conventional medicine for, 523
  environmental chemicals and, 520,
    520b
  in female, 518
  integrative therapy for, 519–525
  lifestyle in, 519–520
  in male, 518
  micronutrients in, 521
  mind-body therapies in, 522–523
  nutrition in, 519, 519b
  physical activity in, 519
  prevention prescription for, 524b
  spirituality and, 519–520
  supplements in, 521–522
  therapeutic review for, 524b
  in vitro fertilization for, 523
Inflammation
  age-related macular degeneration
    and, 840
  antioxidants and, 869
  carbohydrates and, 872–873
  diet and, 869–877.e4. *See also* Diet,
    antiinflammatory
  eicosanoid and, 869
  food and, 869
  gastrointestinal dysbiosis and, 869
  gene expression and, 869
  glucose level and, 869
  glycemic index and, 865
  insulin level and, 869
  in insulin resistance, 321f
  in irritable bowel syndrome,
    423–424
  markers of, 869
  measurement of, 869
  mechanisms of, 869
  in osteoporosis, 370–371
  role of, 370–371, 371b
Inflammatory bowel disease,
    501–516.e8. *See also* Crohn's
    disease; Ulcerative colitis
  acupuncture in, 514
  botanicals in, 514b–515b
  bovine colostrum in, 508–509
  dehydroepiandrosterone in, 507
  helminths in, 510–512
  herbal therapies in, 509–510
  mind-body medicine in, 512–514,
    513t
  nutritional approaches in,
    514b–515b
  pathophysiology of, 501, 502f
  pharmaceuticals in, 510–512
  prebiotics in, 508, 508b
  prevention in, 514b
  probiotics in, 507
  supplements in, 507–509
  surgery in, 512
  synbiotics in, 508
  therapeutic review on, 514b–515b
  web resources on, 516t
Inhaled analgesia, for labor pain
    management, 531–532, 531t
Inhaled hot moist air, for common
    cold, 175–176
Innate immunity, disordered, in
    rosacea, 766–769

Inner advisor, in guided imagery, 933
Innovative health systems, 27–28, 28f, 28t
Inositol, in psoriasis, 730, 730b
D-*chiro*-Inositol (DCI), in polycystic ovarian syndrome, 363–364, 364b
Inositol family, in polycystic ovarian syndrome, 363–364
Insight, in healing encounter, 21–22, 22f
Insomnia, 74–85.e3
    comorbid, 74, 75b
    definitions of, 74
    etiology of, 74–75, 75b
    evaluating, 76–77, 76b
    integrative therapy for, 77–79, 77b
    mind-body therapy for, 80–85
    noise reduction approach for, 80–83
    objective measures for, 76–77, 77f
    pathophysiology of, 75–77, 75b
    pharmaceuticals and substances for, 77, 77b–78b
    primary care intervention for, 83–85, 83b
    self-report scales for, 76
    supplements for, 77–79
    web resources on, 85t
Insulin, 320
    fasting, 326
    glycemic index and, 864f
    inflammation and, 869
    in type 2 diabetes mellitus, 344–345
Insulin receptor, 322
Insulin resistance (IR), 319–333.e5, 324b, 334
    abnormalities associated with, 321t
    acetyl-L-carnitine in, 331, 331b
    alpha lipoic acid in, 330, 330b
    bile acid sequestrants in, 332
    biotin in, 330, 330b
    botanicals in, 331–332
    chromium in, 330, 330b
    coenzyme Q10 (CoQ10) in, 331, 331b
    in colorectal cancer, 802
    comorbidities of, 323t
    criteria for clinical diagnosis of, 321t
    defining, 320
    diagnosis of, 325–326
    environmental toxins and, 323
    estrogen dominance and, 580
    exercise in, 326, 328b
    fiber in, 327
    folic acid in, 329, 329b
    food avoidance in, 328
    ginseng (*Panax ginseng*) in, 331, 331b
    green tea (*Camellia sinensis*) in, 331, 331b
    integrative therapy of, 326–333, 326b
    interrelationship between, 324–325
    lifestyle factors and, 326–327
    low-glycemic index foods in, 327
    magnesium in, 330, 330b
    Mediterranean diet in, 327, 327b
    milk thistle (*Silybum marianum*) in, 331–332, 332b
    mind body, 328
    nutrition in, 327–328
    pathophysiology of, 320–325
    pharmaceuticals in, 332
    in polycystic ovarian syndrome, 363–364
    prevalence of, 320
    prevention prescription of, 333b
    risk factors for, 320
    stress management in, 328, 328b
    summary of, 323f
    supplements in, 328–331

Insulin resistance (IR) (*Continued*)
    surgery in, 332–333
    syndrome of, 320
    therapeutic foods in, 328
    therapeutic review of, 333b
    vitamin B6, 329, 329b
    vitamin B₁₂, 329, 329b
    vitamin C, 329, 329b
    vitamin D, 329, 329b
    vitamin E, 330, 330b
    web resources on, 333t
    weight management in, 326–327, 327b
Insulin sensitizers, 332
    in polycystic ovarian syndrome, 366, 366b
Insulin signaling pathways, 322f
Integrative medicine, 6–9, 7b
    academic center respond and, 3–4, 4f, 4b
    for attention-deficit/hyperactivity disorder, 54, 54f
    board certification in, 6
    in breast cancer, 773–780, 781t
    brief history, 2–6
    change in public interest and, 3, 3f
    changing medical culture and, 4–6, 6b
    for chronic hepatitis, 199–208
    for chronic sinusitis, 158–161
    definition of, 7t
    future of, 9–10
    for HIV disease, 180–190
    for hypertension, 231–239
    increasing value through, 7–8, 8f
    for inflammatory bowel disease, 501–516
    integration, 9
    organizations in, name changes of, 6t
    for palliative care, 811–816
    philosophy of, 1–11.e1
    in postdates pregnancy, 535–541
    prevention in, 9
    in prostate cancer, 793–799
        chemotherapy, 793
        conventional treatments, 793–794
        hormonal therapy, 793
        immunotherapy, 793–794
        observation, 793
        surgery and radiation, 793
    red flags of, 187t
    reducing suffering with, 9, 9f, 9b
    for sinus infections and colds, 161–169
    technology and communication in, 2–3
    therapeutic review for, 10b
    titles in, evolution of, 6f
    for underserved, 1088–1095.e1
        achieving buy-in from administration, 1094–1095
        affordable approaches and sustainable programs, 1091, 1092t
        affordable services by intervention type, 1091–1093
        characteristics of successful integrative programs for, 1093
        facilitating behavioral change, 1090
        group visits at Lawrence family health center, 1093–1094
        health inequities, 1088, 1089b, 1093t
        integrative care, 1090
        outside exam room: activism, 1095
        provider characteristics for healing, 1090
        social determinants of health, 1088–1089

Integrative medicine (*Continued*)
    sustainable alternative medicine hospital practice, 1093
    web resources on, 1095t
    for uterine fibroids, 582–591
    web resources on, 10t–11t
Integrative oncology, 780.e1t
Integrative provider, on discussing forgiveness, 942, 943b
Intensive behavioral therapy, for autism spectrum disorder, 66
Interactive Guided Imagery, 930–936.e1, 935b.
    See also Guided imagery
    in neck pain, 679–680
Interdisciplinary team, in optimal healing environment, 18t
Interferon beta, in multiple sclerosis, 140
Internal optimal healing environments, 12
International Classification of Disease code book, 20b
Interpersonal optimal healing environments, 12
Interviewing. *See* Motivational interviewing
Intolerance, 310–318.e6
    diagnosis of, 311t, 313–314
    integrative therapy of, 314–318
    key web resources on, 318t
    medical history of, 313, 313b
    nomenclature of, 310
    pathophysiology of, 310–312
    physical examination of, 313
    prevention prescription of, 318b
    research validation of, 312–313
    therapeutic review of, 318b
Intravenous immunoglobulin therapy (IVIG), for Alzheimer disease, 106–107
Intravenous micronutrient therapy, in Lyme disease, 225, 225b
Intuition, in healing encounter, 21–22, 22f
Iodine
    deficiency of, 351, 351t, 351b.
        See also Hypothyroidism
    excess, 352, 352b
    loading test, 352
    skin patch test, 352
    testing, 352, 352b
Iodine loading test, 352
Iodine skin patch test, 352
Iodoral tablet, 352, 352b
Iron
    in chronic fatigue syndrome, 489
    in chronic hepatitis, 204
    deficiency of, 354
    in hypothyroidism, 354, 354b
    in inflammatory bowel disease, 505
    in uterine fibroids, 586, 586b
Irrigation. *See* Nasal irrigation/spray
Irritable bowel syndrome, 313, 422–432.e3, 992t
    acupuncture in, 430
    aloe in, 428–429
    antibiotics in, 430, 430b
    antidepressants in, 430
    betaine hydrochloride in, 430–431, 431b
    botanical medicines in, 428–429
    celiac disease and, 426
    cognitive behavioral therapy (CBT) in, 429–430, 430b
    combination herbal therapies in, 429
    diagnosis of, 424–425, 424t
    differential diagnosis of, 425t, 425b
    digestive function in, 423
    enteric nervous system (ENS) in, 423
    exercise in, 427
    fermentable carbohydrates in, 426, 882

Irritable bowel syndrome (*Continued*)
    fiber in, dietary, 426–427, 427b
    FODMaP diet for, 882
    food allergies in, 425–426
    food sensitivities in, 425–426
    fructose intolerance in, 426, 426b
    ginger in, 428, 428b
    gluten sensitivity and, 426
    gut microflora and, 423, 424b
    hypnosis in, 429, 917
    immune dysfunction and, 423–424
    inflammation and, 423–424
    integrative therapy for, 425–432
    intestinal permeability in, 423
    journaling on, 938
    lactose intolerance in, 426, 426b
    mind-body therapies in, 429–430
    nutrition in, 425–427
    oral cromolyn in, 430, 430b
    osteopathic medicine in, 431–432
    Padma Lax in, 429, 429b
    pancreatic enzymes in, 428, 428b
    pathophysiology of, 423–425
    peppermint oil in, 428, 428b
    pharmaceuticals in, 430
    placebo effects in, 430
    prebiotics in, 427–428, 428b
    prevention prescription of, 431b
    probiotics in, 427, 427b
    psychotherapy in, 429–430, 430b
    Rome III criteria for, 424–425, 424t
    sleep hygiene in, 427
    stress management in, 429
    STW-5 in, 429, 429b
    supplements in, 427–428
    symptoms of, reduced by FODMaP diet, 882
    therapeutic review on, 431b
    therapies to consider in, 430–432
    traditional Chinese medicine (TCM) in, 429
    web resources on, 432t
Isometheptene, in migraine, 114
Isosorbide dinitrate, in heart failure, 249
Isotretinoin
    for acne vulgaris, 765
    in rosacea, 769b, 770.e5
Ivermectin, for rosacea, 769b, 770.e5
Ixodes scapularis, 218, 219f

J
Jin shin jyutsu, 1075t
Johre, 1075t
Joint loading, reduction of, for osteoarthritis, 643
Joints
    inflammation of. *See* Rheumatoid arthritis
    normal, 639
Jones' neuromuscular model, 1029f
Journaling, 587
    in asthma, 296
    for health, 937–939.e1
        after stressful event, 937, 938f, 938b
        in asthma, 938
        in blood pressure, 938
        in employment, 938–939
        health and, 939, 939b
        in infectious disease, 938
        in irritable bowel syndrome, 938
        memory function and, 938
        precautions with, 939
        relationship-centered care and, 939
        in rheumatoid arthritis, 938
        web resources on, 939t
        in wound healing, 938
    in neck pain, 679
Justicia paniculata, for common cold, 171, 171b

K

Kava
  in anxiety, 49–50
  caution for, 49–50
  precautions for, 49b
  in premenstrual syndrome, 566
Keratolytics
  in psoriasis, 731, 731b
  in seborrheic dermatitis, 756, 756b
Ketoconazole (Nizoral) cream,
    in seborrheic dermatitis, 756–757,
    757b
Key Three Strength Program,
    891–893, 892f
Kidney stones. *See* Urolithiasis
Kindling, in depression, 36
Kirtan kriya, in Alzheimer disease, 100
Koebner phenomenon, 726b
K-PAX Immune Support Formula,
    in HIV disease, 185, 185b, 186t
Kudzu, in substance abuse, 821, 821b

L

Labor pain
  acupressure in, 529, 529f, 529b
  aromatherapy in, 530
  audioanalgesia in, 530
  bioenergetics in, 528–529
  biofeedback in, 530
  biomechanical therapy in, 527–528
  black cohosh in, 530
  botanicals in, 530
  chiropractic therapy in, 527
  cramp bark in, 530
  doula for, 526
  first-stage of, 526
  gate control theory in, 526
  homeopathy in, 532
  hypnotherapy in, 529
  integrative therapy for, 526–534
  lifestyle and, 527
  local anesthesia in, 532, 532t
  management of, 526–534.e3
  manual therapy in, 527
  massage in, 527–528
  mind-body therapy in, 529–530
  motherwort in, 530
  music in, 530
  opioid analgesia in, 531, 531t
  pharmaceuticals in, 530–532
  physiology of, 526
  prevention prescription of, 533b
  raspberry leaf in, 530
  reflexology in, 532–534
  regional anesthesia in, 532,
    532t–533t
  second stage of, 526
  sedatives in, 532
  sterile water injections in, 528, 528b
  therapeutic review on, 534b
  three stages of, 526
  transcutaneous electrical nerve
    stimulation (TENS) in, 528,
    528b
  water immersion and, 527, 527b
  web resources on, 534t
  yoga in, 529–530
Lactobacillus GG, in inflammatory
    bowel disease, 507
Lactobacillus rhamnosus
  in atopic dermatitis, 720
  in inflammatory bowel disease, 507
Lactose intolerance, irritable bowel
    syndrome and, 426, 426b
Laser bronchoscopy, in lung cancer,
    786
Lateral epicondylosis, 707, 707b,
    708f, 1051–1052, 1052f
  prolotherapy and, 1049–1050
Latera Flora, 164
LDL particle number (LDL-P), 265,
    265f, 265b
Leaky gut, 66–67
Leaky gut syndrome, 849–857,
    850t–851t, 852b

Leflunomide, in rheumatoid arthritis,
    496–498
Leiomyomata. *See* Uterine fibroids
Lemon, for common cold, 174
Lemon balm
  in herpes simplex virus, 194, 194b
  in insomnia, 79, 79b
  in pediatric abdominal pain, 462,
    462b
Leukotriene inhibitors, in urticaria,
    743, 743b
Leuprolide acetate, in uterine
    fibroids, 587, 587b
Levator scapulae muscle,
    counterstrain for, 1032–1033,
    1034f
Levodopa, in Parkinson's disease,
    147–148, 148b
Levothyroxine, 355–356, 355.e1t
Lewy bodies, 144, 144f
Licorice
  in adrenal fatigue, 406, 406b
  in aphthous stomatitis, 749, 749b
  in asthma, 292
  in chronic hepatitis, 205
  in GERD, 435t, 436, 436b
  in polycystic ovarian syndrome,
    365, 365b
  in psoriasis, 731
  in rosacea, 768, 768b
Lidocaine, in myofascial pain
    syndrome, 657, 657b
Life cycle assessment (LCA),
    1082–1086, 1083f
  energy use on, 1083–1084, 1085b
  pharmaceuticals on, 1084–1085
  procurement on, 1085–1086
  transportation on, 1085–1086,
    1086f
Lifestyle. *See also* Diet; Exercise
  in age-related macular
    degeneration, 840–841
  in aphthous stomatitis, 747
  in arrhythmias, 281
  in asthma, 288–289
  in atopic dermatitis, 717–718
  in breast cancer, 773, 773b
  in carpal tunnel syndrome,
    697–698, 705b
  in chronic hepatitis, 207–208
  in dysmenorrhea, 569
  in epicondylosis, 707–708, 714b
  in gout, 690–691, 696b
  in heart failure, 250–251
  in inflammatory bowel disease, 513
  integrative medicine and, 1093
  in migraine, 108–110
  in multiple sclerosis, 134
  in neck pain, 677, 687b
  in peripheral neuropathy, 122
  in postdates pregnancy, 538
Ligustrazine, in chronic kidney
    disease, 416, 416b
Linked visit, integrative medicine
    and, 1094, 1094b
Linolenic acid, 55
Liothyronine, 355.e1t, 357
Lipodystrophy, HIV disease and, 182
Lipoprotein. *See also* Dyslipidemia
  high density, 257
  low density, 256–257
Liraglutide, 344
  in obesity, 391, 391b
Lithium succinate, in seborrheic
    dermatitis, 757
Liver
  detoxification of, 997f
    botanicals for, 583–584
    for chronic hepatitis, 198–199
    estrogen dominance and,
      580–581
  fatty disease, nonalcoholic, 324
  in insulin resistance, 321f
Liver fibrosis, stages of, 199t
Lobelia, in smoking cessation, 821

Local anesthesia, for labor pain
    management, 532, 532t
Localized breast cancer,
    chemotherapy in, 779–780
Long chain polyunsaturated fatty
    acids, for nutritional imbalances,
    in chronic fatigue syndrome,
    489
Long QT interval syndrome, 282
Loose-fitting clothing, in atopic
    dermatitis, 718
Lorcaserin (Belviq), in obesity,
    390–391, 391b
Loving-kindness/compassion
    meditation, for posttraumatic
    stress disorder, 88
Low back extension exercise,
    903f–907f
Low back flexion exercise,
    903f–907f
Low back pain
  acetaminophen in, 671
  acupuncture in, 672–673
  acute, 662
  biomechanical interventions in,
    669–670
  biopsychosocial model of, 663f
  botanicals in, 672
  chronic, 662–675.e3
  devil's claw in, 672, 672b
  education for, 668
  evaluation of, 664
  exercises in, 901–907.e1, 669,
    903f–907f
    breathing and relaxation
      training, 901, 903f–907f
    coordination, 902, 903f–907f
    flexibility training, 901–902
    low back extension, 903f–907f
    low back flexion, 903f–907f
    web resources on, 902t
  fear-avoidance beliefs in, 665
  first-line pharmaceuticals for, 671
  imaging of, 667–668, 668b
  injections in, 673, 673b
  integrative therapy for, 668–675
  lifestyle and, 668, 668t
  massage in, 670
  mind-body therapies in, 670–671
  neuromusculoskeletal (NMS)
    dysfunction and, 663
  nonsteroidal antiinflammatory
    drugs (NSAIDs) in, 671
  nonthrust manual therapy in, 670
  opioids in, 671–672, 672b
  optimal healing environment for,
    15t, 16
  pathophysiology of, 662–664,
    662b, 663t–664t, 663f
  patient history in, 664
  physical examination in, 664–665,
    665t
  prevention prescription of, 674b
  prolotherapy and, 1050–1051
  red flags in, 665, 665t
  second-line pharmaceuticals for,
    671–672
  self-care strategies in, 668–669
  skeletal muscle relaxants for, 671
  spinal manipulation in, 669–670,
    670b
  subgrouping of, 665–667
  supplements in, 672
  surgery in, 673–675
  tai chi in, 671
  therapeutic review on, 674b
  treatment-based classification of,
    666–667, 667f
  tricyclic antidepressants in, 671
  Waddell's nonorganic signs in,
    666f
  web resources on, 675t
  willow bark in, 672, 672b
  yellow flags in, 665, 666t
  yoga for, 671

Low density lipoprotein, in coronary
    artery disease, 256–257
Low-cost alternative treatments,
    for common health conditions,
    1091t–1092t
Lower esophageal sphincter (LES),
    433, 434f
  decreased tone of, 433, 434t. *See
    also* Gastroesophageal reflux
    disease (GERD)
Low-glycemic index foods, 327
Low-glycemic load diet, for acne
    vulgaris, 760–761
Low-level laser therapy
  for myofascial pain syndrome, 655
  for rheumatoid arthritis, 498
L-theanine, for insomnia, 79, 79b
Lubricants, vaginal, 593–595, 594t,
    595b
Lugol solution, 352, 352b
Lumbar radiculopathy, 663t–664t
Lumpy breast, guided imagery in,
    932–933, 933b
Lung cancer, 785–789.e2, 785b,
    788b–789b
  acupuncture in, 787
  chemotherapy in, 788
  chest radiography in, 786
  curcumin in, 787, 787b
  environmental carcinogens and,
    785
  exercise-based pulmonary
    rehabilitation for, 787
  genetics and biomarkers in, 785,
    785b
  integrative therapy of, 786–789
  laser bronchoscopy in, 786
  massage in, 787
  mind-body modalities of, 786–787
  nutrition in, 787, 787b
  pathophysiology of, 785–786
  radiation therapy for, 788
  radiofrequency ablation for, 788,
    788b
  risk factors of, 785
  screening and detection for, 786
  signs and symptoms of, 785
  smoking and, 785, 785b
  smoking cessation for, 787
  spiral computed tomography of,
    786, 786f, 786b
  surgery for, 788
  therapies to consider for, 788–789
  tobacco use and, 785
  traditional treatments for, 787–788
  web resources on, 789t
  yoga for, 787
Lutein
  in age-related macular
    degeneration, 842–843, 843b
  in cataract prevention, 834b
Luteinizing hormone (LH), 578, 630
Lycopene
  in dyslipidemias, 274, 274b
  in prostate cancer prevention, 795
Lyme disease, 218–228.e5
  acute infection of, 222–223
    pharmaceuticals, 222–223
    supplements, 223
  CDC criteria for, 221
  chronic persistent symptoms of,
    223–228
    acupuncture for, 226, 226b
    lifestyle, 225
      massage therapy for, 226, 226b
      mind-body therapy for, 226
      pharmacological, 224
      supplements, 225
  clinical course of, 218–221, 218b,
    220f, 221b
  diagnosis of, 221–222, 222b
  epidemiology of, 218–222, 219f
  exercise in, 225
  gabapentin in, 224
  integrative therapy of, 222

Lyme disease *(Continued)*
  intravenous micronutrient therapy
    in, 225
  medically unexplained symptoms
    of, 218–221
  omega-3 fatty acids in, 225
  prevention prescription for,
    226b–227b, 227f
  probiotics in, 223, 225
  risk reduction in, 222
  stages of, 218
  tai chi in, 226
  therapeutic review on, 228b
  therapies to consider for, 226–228,
    228b
  web resources on, 228t
Lymphatic techniques, in osteopathic
  manipulative techniques, 678t
Lysine, in herpes simplex virus
  infection, 192, 192b

M
Ma huang, in asthma, 292, 292b
Macular degeneration. *See* Age-
  related macular degeneration
Magnesium, 375
  in age-related macular
    degeneration, 844
  in allergic patient, 304, 304b
  in arrhythmias, 281
  in asthma, 293–294
  in attention-deficit/hyperactivity
    disorder, 55
  in autism spectrum disorder, 70
  in cholelithiasis, 452–453, 453b
  in chronic kidney disease,
    413–414, 414b
  in DASH diet, 878
  in dysmenorrhea, 570t, 570b
  in fibromyalgia, 479, 479b
  in hypertension, 236, 236b
  in inflammatory bowel disease, 505
  in insulin resistance, 330, 330b
  in metabolic syndrome, 330, 330b
  in migraine, 110, 110b–112b
  in multiple sclerosis, 137
  in osteoporosis, 375
  in premenstrual syndrome, 563,
    563b
  in type 2 diabetes mellitus, 341,
    341b
  in urolithiasis, 611
  in uterine fibroids, 586–587, 586b
Magnesium-L-threonate, for
  Alzheimer disease, 105
Magnet therapy
  in dysmenorrhea, 574
  in multiple sclerosis, 136
  in osteoarthritis, 649
Magnetic resonance imaging (MRI),
  in lower back pain, 667
Maitake, 776
Malnutrition. *See also* Nutrition
  in inflammatory bowel disease, 502
D-Mannose, in urinary tract
  infection, 213
Mantra meditation, for posttraumatic
  stress disorder, 87
Manual therapy. *See also specific types,*
  e.g.,
  in detoxification, 1000–1003,
    1001f–1003f
  in erectile dysfunction, 625
  in labor pain management, 527
  in myofascial pain syndrome, 655
  in neck pain, 681–683
    chiropractic and physical
      therapy studies in, 682
    gua sha in, 682
    research in, 681
    safety in, 681, 681b
    strain-counterstrain in,
      682–683
    suboccipital release in, 682–683,
      682f, 683b

Marine collagen peptides (gelatin),
  339, 339b
Marshmallow, in GERD, 435, 435t,
  435b
Massage
  in asthma, 295
  in autism spectrum disorder,
    71–72
  in carpal tunnel syndrome, 702
  in chronic fatigue syndrome, 490
  in fibromyalgia, 477
  in HIV disease, 188
  in labor pain management,
    527–528
  in low back pain, 670
  in lung cancer, 787
  in Lyme disease, 226, 226b
  in myofascial pain syndrome, 655
  in osteoarthritis, 643–644
  in palliative care, 813
  in pediatric abdominal pain, 463
Mastic, in peptic ulcer disease, 445,
  445b
Matricaria recutita. See Chamomile
Matrix energetics, 1075t
Meat
  in colorectal cancer prevention,
    801, 801b
  planetary health and, 1022–1023
Medial epicondylosis, 707, 707b,
  708f
Medical foods, for Alzheimer disease,
  105
Medications. *See also*
  Pharmaceuticals
  for Alzheimer disease, 103–104,
    103b, 104t
Meditation, 945–953.e2
  in Alzheimer disease, 100
  in arrhythmias, 281
  in attention-deficit/hyperactivity
    disorder, 57–58
  in chronic kidney disease, 419
  definition of, 945
  in fibromyalgia, 477
  heart rate variability and, 927
  medical benefits of, 945
  mindfulness, 945, 945b–947b,
    948f
    goal of, 945
    in medical practice, 948, 949b
    in psychophysiological
      disorders, 968
    SOLAR or SOL acronym for,
      947b, 946b
    TIES mnemonic, 947b
  movement as, 949–953, 952f
  postures for, 952f
  precautions for, 947b
  in psoriasis, 735
  reason of, 947b, 945, 945b–947b
  as relaxation technique, 911t–912t
  research on, 945–947
  in substance use, 823
  systems in, 950t–951t
  transcendental, in hypertension,
    238
  types of, 948–949, 949b, 950t–951t
  web resources on, 953t
Mediterranean diet. *See* Diet,
  Mediterranean
Melaleuca alternifolia. See Tea tree oil
Melatonin
  in Alzheimer disease, 103, 103b
  in attention-deficit/hyperactivity
    disorder, 57b, 60
  in autism spectrum disorder, 70
  in breast cancer, 778, 778b
  in inflammatory bowel disease, 507
  in insomnia, 78, 78b
  in migraine, 112, 112b
Melissa officinalis. See Lemon balm
Membrane sweeping, in postdates
  pregnancy, 539
Memory, journaling on, 938

Memory loss, 97. *See also*
  Alzheimer disease
Menopause. *See also* Hormone
  replacement therapy
  acupuncture in, 554–555, 555b
  bioenergetic therapy in, 554–555
  black cohosh in, 555–556, 556b
  botanicals in, 555–556
  calcium in, 557–558
  clonidine in, 554, 554b
  cognitive behavior therapy (CBT)
    in, 557
  estrogen in, 553, 553b
  exercise in, 558
    relaxation, 556
  fiber in, 557
  fluids in, 558
  gabapentin in, 554, 554b
  healthy fats in, 557
  hypnosis in, 557
  insomnia and, 80, 80b
  integrative therapy of, 553–559
  mind-body therapy in, 556–557
  mindfulness-based stress reduction
    (MBSR) in, 557
  nonhormonal medication in, 554,
    554f, 554b
  nutrition in, 557–558
  pharmaceuticals in, 553–554
  prevention prescription of, 558b
  progesterone in, 553, 553b
  Rheum rhaponticum in, 556, 556b
  spiritual exploration in, 558–559
  St. John's wort in, 556, 556b
  symptoms in
    managing, 550–559.e1
    nonvasomotor, 552
    vasomotor, 552
  therapeutic review on, 558b
  transition, 552
    well-being in, 552–553
  web resources on, 559t
  yoga in, 555, 555b
Menorrhagia
  botanicals for, 584–585
  with uterine fibroids, 584–585, 588
Menstrual cramps, vitamins B in,
  586b
Menstrual cycle, 578–579
Mentha piperita. See Peppermint
Menthol, in myofascial pain
  syndrome, 657
Menthol-containing products, for
  topical use, 742b
Mercury, in chronic kidney disease,
  418.e1
Mesalamine, in inflammatory bowel
  disease, 511
Metabolic syndrome, 319–333.e5,
  324d
  acetyl-L-carnitine in, 331, 331b
  alpha lipoic acid in, 330, 330b
  benign prostatic hyperplasia and,
    601
  biotin in, 330, 330b
  botanicals, 331–332
  chromium in, 330, 330b
  clinical identification of, 384t
  coenzyme Q10 (CoQ10) in, 331,
    331b
  comorbidities of, 323t
  criteria for clinical diagnosis of,
    321t
  defining, 320
  diagnosis of, 325–326
  environmental toxins and, 323
  estrogen dominance and, 580
  exercise in, 326, 328b
  fiber in, 327
  folic acid in, 329, 329b
  food avoidance in, 328
  ginseng (*Panax ginseng*) in, 331,
    331b
  green tea (*Camellia sinensis*) in,
    331, 331b

Metabolic syndrome *(Continued)*
  integrative therapy of, 326–333,
    326b
  lifestyle factors and, 326–327
  low-glycemic index foods in, 327
  magnesium in, 330, 330b
  Mediterranean diet in, 327, 327b
  milk thistle (*Silybum marianum*) in,
    331–332, 332b
  mind body therapy in, 328
  nutrition in, 327–328
  pathophysiology of, 320–325
  pharmaceuticals in, 332
  prevalence of, 320
  prevention prescription of, 333b
  risk factors for, 320
  stress management in, 328, 328b
  supplements in, 328–331
  surgery in, 332–333
  therapeutic foods in, 328
  therapeutic review of, 333b
  vitamin B6, 329, 329b
  vitamin B₁₂, 329, 329b
  vitamin C, 329, 329b
  vitamin D, 329, 329b
  vitamin E, 330, 330b
  web resources on, 333t
  weight management in, 326–327,
    327b
Metastatic disease, chemotherapy
  in, 780
Metformin, 332
  in obesity, 391, 391b
  in polycystic ovarian syndrome, 366
  in type 2 diabetes mellitus, 343,
    343b
Methadone, for pain, in palliative
  care, 807
Methotrexate
  in psoriasis, 734, 734b
  in rheumatoid arthritis, 496
Methyl B12 injections, for autism
  spectrum disorder, 69–70
Methyl donors, side effects with, 402b
Methylation
  in Alzheimer disease, 95
  for chronic fatigue syndrome, 489
Methylcobalamin. *See* Vitamin B₁₂
Methylenetetrahydrofolate reductase
  (MTHFR)
  dietary and supplemental folates
    in, 399–401, 400f, 400t, 401b
  folate activator and, 395–396, 396f
  health risks associated with, 398
  homocysteine, nutrient needs and,
    395–403.e2
  integrative therapy for, 398–403,
    399b
  mutations and polymorphisms in,
    396–397, 396t
  pathophysiology of, 395–398
  prevention prescription of, 402b
  related homocysteine lowering
    therapies in, 401–403
  testing of, 398, 398b
  therapeutic review on, 403b
  Web resources on, 403t
Methylenetetrahydrofolate reductase
  polymorphisms
  health risks associated with, 398
  testing for, 398, 398b
Methylsulfonylmethane (MSM), in
  osteoarthritis, 646
Methyltestosterone, 635–637, 635b
Metoclopramide, for nausea, in
  palliative care, 808
Metronidazole
  in inflammatory bowel disease, 511b
  in rosacea, 768b, 769
Microbiome
  altered, and FODMaP diet, 884
  osteoporosis and, 371
Migraine, 108
  abortive pharmaceutical therapies
    in, 109t, 113–114

Migraine (Continued)
acupuncture in, 115–116, 1042. See also Headache; acupuncture for
anticonvulsants in, 113
β-blockers in, 113
botanicals in, 111–112
botulinum toxin in, 113
butterbur in, 112, 112b
calcium channel blockers in, 113
chiropractic in, 115
coenzyme Q10 in, 111, 111b
cognitive-behavioral therapy in, 115
craniosacral therapy in, 116
ergot alkaloids in, 114
exercise in, 108–110
feverfew in, 111–112, 111b
fish oil in, 111
homeopathy in, 116–117
hypnosis in, 115
intranasal lidocaine in, 114
isometheptene in, 114
lifestyle in, 108–110
α-lipoic acid in, 109t
magnesium in, 110, 110b–112b
melatonin in, 112, 112b
mind-body techniques in, 109t, 114–115
mindfulness meditation in, 115
neurolinguistic programming in, 109t
nonsteroidal antiinflammatory drugs in, 113–114
nutrition in, 110
omega-3 fatty acids in, 111, 111b
osteopathic manipulation in, 115
pathophysiology of, 108, 108b, 109f
pharmaceuticals in, 109t, 112–114
physical therapy in, 115
prevention of, 109t, 112–113, 116b
relaxation in, 115
riboflavin in, 110–111, 111b
spinal manipulation in, 115
therapeutic review on, 116b–117b
tricyclic antidepressants in, 113
triptans in, 114
valerian in, 112, 112b
web resources on, 119t
Mild cognitive impairment, in Alzheimer disease, 97
Milk thistle
in age-related macular degeneration, 844, 844b
in cholelithiasis, 453, 453b
in chronic hepatitis, 205, 205b
in detoxifying prior to conception, 522
in HIV disease, 186–187, 187b
in insulin resistance, 331–332, 332b
in metabolic syndrome, 331–332, 332b
in psoriasis, 731, 731b
in uterine fibroids, 584, 584b
Mind noise, insomnia and, 80–82, 81b, 84b
Mind-body connection, 376
in detoxification, 1000–1003, 1000f
in osteoporosis, 376
Parkinson's disease and, 149–151, 150b–151b
Mind-body therapy, 389–390
in adrenal fatigue, 408
in allergic patient, 307
in Alzheimer disease, 100–101, 100b
in aphthous stomatitis, 749, 752b
in arrhythmias, 281
in asthma, 291, 296
in atopic dermatitis, 719, 724b
in attention-deficit/hyperactivity disorder, 56–57
in chronic fatigue syndrome, 490

Mind-body therapy (Continued)
in chronic hepatitis, 206–207
in chronic kidney disease, 419
in chronic sinusitis, 167
in constipation, 469
in depression, 40–41, 40b
in dysmenorrhea, 573, 576b
in epicondylosis, 708, 714b
in erectile dysfunction, 625–626
in fibromyalgia, 477–478
in GERD, 437
in heart failure, 250
in HIV disease, 187–188
in hypertension, 237–239
in infertility, 522–523
in inflammatory bowel disease, 512–514, 513t
in insulin resistance, 328
integrative medicine and, 1092t, 1093
in irritable bowel syndrome, 429–430
in labor pain management, 529–530
in low back pain, 670–671
in Lyme disease, 226
in metabolic syndrome, 328
in migraine, 109t, 114–115
in multiple sclerosis, 134–135
in myofascial pain syndrome, 654–655
in neck pain, 679–680, 687b
in obesity, 389–390
in osteoarthritis, 642–643
in palliative care, 812–814
in pediatric abdominal pain, 463–465
in peripheral neuropathy, 122–123
in polycystic ovarian syndrome, 366
in posttraumatic stress disorder, 87–90, 92b
in premenstrual syndrome, 566
prostate cancer and, 796
in psoriasis, 735, 735b
in rheumatoid arthritis, 494
in seborrheic dermatitis, 756
in substance abuse, 823–824, 823b
in testosterone deficiency, 632
in type 2 diabetes mellitus, 337
in urinary tract infection, 216
in urticaria, 744–746, 745b
in uterine fibroids, 587
Mindfulness, 20–22, 337
Mindfulness medical practice, 948, 949b
Mindfulness meditation, 57, 945, 945b–947b, 948f
goal of, 945
in medical practice, 948
in migraine, 115
in multiple sclerosis, 135
in posttraumatic stress disorder, 87
in psychophysiological disorders, 968
SOLAR or SOL acronym for, 947b, 946b
TIES mnemonic for, 947b
Mindfulness-based cognitive therapy, in depression, 40
Mindfulness-based interventions, in inflammatory bowel disease, 513
Mindfulness-based stress reduction, 947
in hypertension, 238
in Lyme disease, 226, 226b
in menopausal symptoms, 557
in palliative care, 812
Minerals
in age-related macular degeneration, 844
in Alzheimer disease, 101
in autism spectrum disorder, 70, 70b

Mirtazapine, in depression, 42t, 43
Misoprostol, in postdates pregnancy, 538, 538b
Mitochondrial hypothesis, 144–145
Mixed reuptake blockers, in depression, 41–42, 42t
Modified citrus pectin (MCP), 1012, 1012b
Moisturizers, in atopic dermatitis, 718
Mold-containing foods, for chronic sinusitis, 165
Monounsaturated fatty acids
in breast cancer, 776
in dyslipidemia, 271, 271b
Motherwort, in labor pain management, 530
Motion sickness, 1044–1045
Motivational interviewing, 954–962.e1, 954b, 957b, 960t, 1090b. See also Healing encounter; Helping styles
change talk in, 958t–960t, 959
with directing helping style, 956t
effectiveness of, 956, 957f
foundation or spirit of, 955–956
helping client access motivation for change in, 960–961
helping style consistent with, 956t
knowing about versus using, 955
skills in, enhancement of, 961–962, 962b
sustain talk in, 957, 958t–961t
web resources on, 962t
Mouthwashes, in aphthous stomatitis, 750
Movement therapies
as meditation, 949–953, 952f
in neck pain, 677–678
for peripheral neuropathy, 122
MTHFR 677C→T Polymorphism (C677T), 396–397, 397t
MTHFR 1298 A→C Polymorphism (A1298C), 397, 397t
Mucuna pruriens, in Parkinson's disease, 147
Multidisciplinary team, in optimal healing environment, 18t
Multiple sclerosis, 133–142.e2
ashwagandha in, 138
diagnosis of, 134, 135f–136f
environmental factors in, 133–134
etiology of, 133–134
exercise in, 134
genetic factors in, 134
glatiramer acetate in, 141
immunological factors in, 133
infectious agents in, 134
integrative therapy for, 134–142
botanicals, 138–139
disease-modifying treatments, 140–141
energy medicine, 136
hormones, 139
lifestyle, 134
mind-body therapy, 134–135
nutrition, 135–136
pharmaceuticals, 139
supplements, 137–138
therapies to consider, 141–142
mindfulness meditation in, 135
natalizumab in, 141
pathophysiology of, 133
prevention prescription for, 141b
psychosocial factors in, 134
sunshine in, 134
testosterone in, 139
therapeutic review on, 141b–142b
web resources on, 142t
Multivitamin. See also specific vitamins
in age-related macular degeneration, 842
in Alzheimer disease, 101, 101b
in autism spectrum disorder, 70
in breast cancer, 777, 777b

Multivitamin (Continued)
in cataract prevention, 835, 835b
in chronic fatigue syndrome, 489
in HIV disease, 183
in insulin resistance, 328–329
in metabolic syndrome, 328–329
prostate cancer and, 796–797
Muscle counterstrain. See Counterstrain
Muscle energy, in osteopathic manipulative techniques, 678t
Muscle relaxants
in low back pain, 671
in myofascial pain syndrome, 658
in neck pain, 684t
Music therapy
in Alzheimer disease, 104
in autism spectrum disorder, 71
in depression, 44
in labor pain management, 530
in palliative care, 812–813
as relaxation technique, 911t–912t
Myalgias, statin-related, 257, 257b
Myofascial pain patterns, 1030, 1030t
Myofascial pain syndrome, 651–661.e2. See also Chronic fatigue syndrome
antidepressants in, 659
bioenergetics in, 660
biomechanical therapy in, 655–657
central biostimulation in, 656–657, 656f
diagnosis of, 651, 651b–652b
diet in, 659
epidemiology of, 651, 651b, 652t
exercise in, 653–654, 654b
hydrotherapy in, 657
integrative therapy for, 652–660, 653f, 654t
low-level laser therapy in, 655
manual therapy in, 655
massage therapy in, 655
mind-body therapy in, 654–655
muscle relaxants in, 658
myofascial release techniques in, 655
nonsteroidal antiinflammatory drugs in, 658, 658b
pathophysiology of, 651–652, 651b, 652t, 653f
peripheral biostimulation in, 655–656, 656f
pharmaceuticals in, 658–659
posture correction in, 655
prevention prescription for, 660b
relaxation and awareness technique in, 654–655, 654b
sleep in, 654
supplements in, 659, 659b
synonyms for, 651b
therapeutic review for, 660b–661b
thermotherapy in, 657
topical therapy in, 657
traditional Chinese medicine in, 660
trigger point needling or injection in, 657–658
web resources on, 661t
Myofascial release, 676
in osteopathic manipulative techniques, 678t
Myolysis techniques, in uterine fibroids, 589
Myomectomy, in uterine fibroids, 589
Myringotomy, in otitis media, 156b

N
NADH (Coenzyme I), for chronic fatigue syndrome, 487, 487b
Nails, psoriasis of, 726
Naltrexone
in alcoholism, 819, 820b
in inflammatory bowel disease, 511
Nanotechnology, 1017

Nasal hygiene, for chronic sinusitis, 162, 162t
Nasal irrigation/spray
  in chronic sinusitis, 162
  in upper respiratory conditions, 1054–1056.e1
    dose for, 1055
    indications for, 1055t
    mechanism of, 1054
    patient handout on, 1056f
    pediatric use of, 1055
    safety of, 1055, 1055b
    technique variations for, 1054, 1054b, 1056f
    web resources on, 1055t
Nasal rescue, in chronic sinusitis, 162, 162b
Nasal saline, for common cold, 176
Natalizumab, in multiple sclerosis, 141
National Institute of Clinical Excellence (NICE), and stimulant medications, for children with ADHD, 61b
Native American Interventions, in alcoholism, 825–826, 825f–826f
Natural Cellular Defense, in chronic sinusitis, 166
Natural procreative technologies (NPT), 523–525
Natural products, for posttraumatic stress disorder, 91–93
Natural stress response, in adrenal fatigue, 404, 405f, 406t
Nausea
  acupuncture in, 1044–1046.e1, 1045b
    LV3 point for, 1045, 1046f
    MH6 point for, 1045, 1045f
    needle removal for, 1046
    posttreatment home program for, 1046
    ST36 point for, 1045, 1045f
    training for, 1046
    web resources on, 1046t
  chemotherapy-induced, 1044
  in palliative care, 808–809
  postoperative, 1044
  in pregnancy, 542–549.e2, 548b
    acupressure in, 544, 544b, 545f
    antihistamines in, 546, 546b
    avoid odors in, 542–543
    bioenergetics in, 544
    chamomile in, 543–544, 544b
    corticosteroids in, 547, 547b
    counseling in, 545
    dopamine antagonists in, 546, 546b
    enteral/parenteral feedings in, 547
    exercise in, 543
    ginger root in, 543, 543b
    homeopathy in, 548
    5-hydroxytryptamine₃ receptor agonists in, 546, 546b
    hypnosis in, 544–545
    increase rest in, 543
    integrative therapy for, 542–549
    intractable, 547
    intravenous fluids in, 547
    lifestyle in, 542–543
    mind-body therapy in, 544–545
    nutrition in, 543
    pathophysiology of, 542
    peppermint leaf for, 544, 544b
    pharmaceuticals in, 546–547
    phenothiazines in, 546, 546b
    psychotherapy in, 545
    supplements in, 545
    therapeutic abortion in, 547, 547f
    therapies to consider in, 548–549
    traditional Chinese medicine in, 548–549, 548b
    vitamin B₆ in, 545
    web resources on, 549t
  pregnancy-related, 1044

Neck pain, 676–688.e4
  acupuncture in, 680, 680b
  Alexander technique in, 677
  antioxidants in, 678–679
  aromatherapy/essential oils in, 686–688
  bioenergetic therapies in, 680–681
  biofeedback in, 680
  cervical support in, 678
  emotions and, 679
  energy medicine modalities in, 680
  essential fatty acids in, 678
  evaluation of, 677b
  exercise and movement in, 677–678
  Feldenkrais in, 677
  gua sha in, 682
  hypnosis in, 679
  injections in, 683
  integrative therapy for, 676–688
  interactive guided imagery in, 679–680
  journaling in, 679
  lifestyle in, 677
  manual therapies in, 681–683
  mind-body therapy in, 679–680
  nutrition in, 678–679
  omega-3 fatty acids in, 685, 685b
  pathophysiology of, 676
  pharmaceuticals in, 683–684, 684t
  phytoantiinflammatory agents in, 685, 685t–686t
  Pilates in, 677
  prevention prescription in, 687b
  relaxation exercises in, 680
  risk factors for, 677b
  saturated fatty acids in, 679, 679b
  strain-counterstrain in, 682–683
  suboccipital release in, 682–683, 682f, 683b
  supplements in, 685
  surgery in, 683
  therapeutic review in, 687b
  web resources for, 688t
  yoga in, 677–678
Necrotizing enterocolitis (NEC), prevention of, 992t
Needles
  in dispersion, 1040
  fear of, 971
Neem, in peptic ulcer disease, 445–446, 446b
Nefazodone, in depression, 43
Neurofeedback, in attention-deficit/ hyperactivity disorder, 58b
Neurolinguistic programming, in migraine, 109t
Neuromuscular stimulation, in myofascial pain syndrome, 655, 656f
Neuroplasticity, hypnosis in, 920–921
Neurotransmitters, in depression, 36
Niacin
  in chronic kidney disease, 415
  in coronary artery disease, 258, 258b
  in dyslipidemia, 268–269, 269b
  in menstrual cramps, 586b
  in vaginal dryness, 597, 597b
Nifedipine, in urolithiasis, 612, 612b
Nitrates, inorganic, in hypertension, 234, 234f
Nitric oxide, in vaginal lubrication, 592, 593t, 598f
Nonalcoholic fatty liver disease, 324
  illustration of molecular events involved in pathogenesis of, 325f
  interrelationship between, 324–325
Nonceliac gluten sensitivity, 313, 426
  celiac disease versus, 316, 316b
  prevalence of various clinical and laboratory findings in patients with, 317t

Noncompliance, 955b
Noncovered services, integrative medicine and, 1094–1095
Nondairy calcium, sources of, 373t
Nonhormonal medication, in menopausal symptoms, 554, 554f, 554b
Noni, in gout, 695
Nonsteroidal antiinflammatory drugs (NSAIDs)
  in carpal tunnel syndrome, 698–699, 699t, 699b
  in colorectal cancer, 803
  in dysmenorrhea, 572
  in epicondylosis, 709, 709b
  in fibromyalgia, 480–481
  in gout, 693, 693b
  in low back pain, 671
  in migraine, 113–114
  in myofascial pain syndrome, 658, 658b
  in neck pain, 684t
  in osteoarthritis, 646
  peptic ulcer disease and, 443
  in prostate cancer prevention, 797–799
  in rheumatoid arthritis, 495
  in uterine fibroids, 588, 588b
Nonvalvular atrial fibrillation
  NOACs for, 286t
  therapeutic review for, 280t
Non-vitamin-mineral supplements, in inflammatory bowel disease, 505–507
Norethindrone acetate, in uterine fibroids, 588, 588b
Normal tendon, histology of, 708f
NT factor energy lipids, for chronic fatigue syndrome, 487, 487b
Number needed to screen (NNS), 800b
Nutraceuticals
  in dyslipidemias, 268–275, 268f
  in erectile dysfunction, 625, 626b, 627t
  in uterine fibroids, 585–587
Nutrition, 318
  in adrenal fatigue, 406
  in age-related macular degeneration, 841–842, 841b, 845b
  in allergic patient, 302–303
  in Alzheimer disease, 99, 100t
  in anxiety, 47–48
  in aphthous stomatitis, 747–748, 747b, 752b
  in asthma, 289, 289b
  in atopic dermatitis, 718–725, 724b
  in attention-deficit/hyperactivity disorder, 55–56, 55t
  in benign prostatic hyperplasia, 601–602
  in breast cancer, 775–777
  in cataract prevention, 833–834
  in cholelithiasis, 450–452, 452b
  in chronic fatigue syndrome, 486
  in chronic kidney disease, 416–418, 416b
  in chronic prostatitis/chronic pelvic pain syndrome, 617–620, 620b
  in colorectal cancer prevention, 800
  in constipation, 466–467
  in coronary artery disease, 253–254, 254b
  in depression, 37–38, 37b
  in detoxification, 999–1000
  in dyslipidemia, 267
  in dysmenorrhea, 569–570, 576b
  in fibromyalgia, 476–477
  in gout, 690–691, 691b, 696b
  in heart failure, 251–252
  in HIV disease, 182–183

Nutrition (Continued)
  in hypertension, 231–234
  in hypothyroidism, 350–351
  infertility and, 519, 519b
  in inflammatory bowel disease, 501, 502f, 503b, 514b–515b
  in insulin resistance, 327–328
  in irritable bowel syndrome, 425–427
  in lung cancer, 787, 787b
  in menopausal symptoms, 557–558
  in metabolic syndrome, 327–328
  in migraine, 110
  in multiple sclerosis, 135–136
  in nausea and vomiting, in pregnancy, 543
  in neck pain, 678–679, 687b
  in obesity, 386–387
  in osteoporosis, 372–376
  in otitis media, 153
  in palliative care, 811
  in Parkinson's disease, 145, 145b, 150b–151b
  in pediatric abdominal pain, 459–460
  in peptic ulcer disease, 440–442, 442b
  for peripheral neuropathy, 122
  in polycystic ovarian syndrome, 363
  in postdates pregnancy, 535
  in premenstrual syndrome, 562, 562t, 562b
  in prostate cancer, 794–795
  in psoriasis, 728–729
  in rheumatoid arthritis, 494–495
  in seborrheic dermatitis, 754–755, 758b
  in substance abuse, 826
  in testosterone deficiency, 631–632
  in type 2 diabetes mellitus, 335–336, 336f
  in urinary tract infection, 212
  in urolithiasis, 609–611, 609t–610t
  in urticaria, 740, 745b
  in uterine fibroids, 582–583
Nuts
  in antiinflammatory diet, 872
  in coronary artery disease, 254
  in dyslipidemias, 271
Nystatin, in seborrheic dermatitis, 757, 757b

O
Oatmeal baths, 727b
Obesity. See also Insulin resistance; Metabolic syndrome
  abdominal pain and, 458
  in breast cancer, 773, 773b
  bupropion in, 392
  cataracts and, 832
  caution for supplements used for weight loss, 389, 389t
  classification of, associated disease and, 383t
  in colorectal cancer prevention, 802
  counseling in, 385
  definition of, 382, 382b
  diet in, 384
  exercise in, 385–386
  green tea in, 388, 388b
  integrative approach to, 382–394.e2
    integrative therapy, 385–394
    pathophysiology of, 382–385
  integrative assessment of, 384–385, 385b
  metformin in, 391, 391b
  mind-body therapy in, 389–390
  morbidity, 382
  nutrition in, 386–387
  omega-3 fatty acids in, 388, 388b
  orlistat in, 391, 391b
  over-the-counter weight loss aids in, 391

Obesity (Continued)
pathogenesis of, 382–383
pharmaceuticals in, 390–391
for combined weight loss and
type II diabetes mellitus,
391–392
phentermine in, 390, 390b
pre-meal water loading, 387–388
prevention prescription of, 393b
related health risk, 382, 383t
supplements in, 388–389
surgery in, 392–394
therapeutic counseling of, 385
therapeutic review on, 393b–394b
topiramate in, 392
vitamin D in, 388, 388b
web resources on, 394t
Obesogens, 1018
Obstetrics. See also Labor pain
therapeutic homeopathy in, 1070,
1071t–1072t
Occupational therapy, in carpal
tunnel syndrome, 702
Oenothera biennis. See Evening
primrose oil
Olive oil, 872
in cholelithiasis, 453
in hypertension, 232
Omega-3 fatty acids
in acne vulgaris, 761, 761b
in allergic patient, 302–303
in Alzheimer disease, 99–100
in anxiety, 48
in arrhythmias, 282, 282b
for attention-deficit/hyperactivity
disorder, 55
in autism spectrum disorder, 70
in benign prostatic hyperplasia,
601–602
in chronic kidney disease, 414
in colorectal cancer prevention,
801
in depression, 37–38, 38b
in dyslipidemias, 270–271, 271b
in dysmenorrhea, 569–570, 570t,
570b
in fibromyalgia, 478, 478b
in HIV disease, 185, 185b
in hypertension, 233, 233b
infertility and, 521, 521b
in inflammation, 871, 871f
in insulin resistance, 331, 331b
in Lyme disease, 225, 225b
in metabolic syndrome, 331,
331b
in migraine, 111, 111b
in neck pain, 685, 685b
in obesity, 388, 388b
in osteoarthritis, 648
in osteoporosis, 373–374
in Parkinson's disease, 145
in peripheral neuropathy, 128
in polycystic ovarian syndrome,
363
in prostate cancer prevention,
797
in psoriasis, 729, 729b
in rheumatoid arthritis, 494
in seborrheic dermatitis, 754,
754b
sources of, 872b
in type 2 diabetes mellitus, 341,
341b
in urolithiasis, 609t, 610–611
in uterine fibroids, 587, 587b
in vaginal dryness, 596, 596b
Omega-6 fatty acids, in
inflammation, 871, 871f
Onions
in type 2 diabetes mellitus, 337
in urinary tract infection, 212
Oolong tea, in atopic dermatitis,
719, 719b
Opiate withdrawal and recovery,
management of, 820

Opioids
in fibromyalgia, 481b
in labor pain management, 531,
531t
in low back pain, 671–672, 672b
in neck pain, 684t
in osteoarthritis, 647
in palliative care, 807
in testosterone deficiency, 632–633
Optimal healing environments,
12–19.e2, 13f, 13t
behavioral, 13–14
business case for, 18–19
in clinical setting, 14, 15t
external, 14
genetic expression and, 18, 18f
health teams in, 17, 18t
internal, 12
interpersonal, 12
practitioner's influence on, 17, 17f
spiritual connection and, 14
value of, 18–19
Oral antifungals, in seborrheic
dermatitis, 757
Oral contraceptives
in multiple sclerosis, 139
in polycystic ovarian syndrome,
366–367, 366b
Oral cromolyn, in irritable bowel
syndrome, 430, 430b
Oral medications, 332
Oregon grape root (Mahonia
aquifolium), in atopic dermatitis,
720
Orlistat (Xenical)
in obesity, 391, 391b
in polycystic ovarian syndrome,
366
Orthotics, in epicondylosis, 713,
713b–714b
Osgood-Schlatter disease, 1050
Osmotic laxatives, in constipation,
471, 471b
Osteoarthritis (OA), 638–650.e3,
640f
acetaminophen in, 646
acupuncture in, 644, 644b
S-adenosylmethionine (SAMe)
in, 645b
antiinflammatory diet in, 640
arthrodesis in, 648
arthroplasty in, 648
arthroscopy in, 648
biological approaches for, 648
Boswellia serrata in, 648–649
capsaicin cream in, 647
chondroitin sulfate in, 644–645
cold therapy in, 643
curcumin in, 648
cyclooxygenase-2 inhibitor in, 646
diacerein in, 647–648
diclofenac in, 647
exercise in, 640–642, 641b
ginger in, 649
group programs for, 642
integrative approaches for, 640–650
intraarticular steroid injections
in, 647
lifestyle and, 640
magnet therapy in, 649
massage in, 643–644
methylsulfonylmethane (MSM)
in, 646
mind-body therapies in, 642–643
nonbiological approaches for, 648
nonopioid analgesics in, 646
nonsteroidal antiinflammatory
drugs in, 646
normal joints and, 639
early changes of, 639
late changes of, 639
omega-3 fatty acids in, 648
opioid analgesics in, 647
osteotomy in, 648
pathophysiology of, 639

Osteoarthritis (OA) (Continued)
pharmaceuticals in, 646
physical modalities in, 643–644
prevention prescription of, 649b
prolotherapy in, 1048–1049, 1049b
reduction of joint loading in, 643
supplements in, 644–646
surgery in, 648
susceptibility to, 640f
tai chi in, 642
telemedicine interventions in, 642
therapeutic review on, 649b–650b
therapeutic touch in, 649–650
topical analgesics in, 647
tramadol in, 646
transcutaneous electrical nerve
stimulation (TENS) in, 643
web resources on, 650t
weight loss in, 640
yoga in, 642
Osteopathy, 678t. See also
Counterstrain
in asthma, 295
in carpal tunnel syndrome,
702–704, 703f, 705b
in cholelithiasis, 455–456
in epicondylosis, 710–713, 713b
in irritable bowel syndrome,
431–432
in labor pain management, 527
in migraine, 115
in neck pain, 682
in otitis media, 155
in pediatric abdominal pain, 463
in peptic ulcer disease, 447–449
Osteopenia, 370
Osteoporosis, 370–381.e5, 381t
acid-base issues in, 371
alcohol effects in, 377–378
bisphosphonates in, 378–379
bone strength, assessing, fracture
risk in, 370
botanicals in, 376
caffeine effects in, 377
calcitonin in, 380
calcium in, 372–373
cigarette smoking effects in, 377
considerations in childhood,
adolescence, and young
adulthood, 376
definition of, 370
epidemiology of, 370–372
essential fatty acids in, 373–374
exercise in, 376–377, 377b
fracture risk in, 370
inflammation in, 370–371
integrative therapy of, 372–381
magnesium in, 375
mind-body connection, 376
nutrition in, 372–376
pathophysiology of, 370–372
pharmaceuticals in, 378–381
to avoid, 380–381
phosphorus effects in, 374
prevention prescription of, 380b
protein in, 374, 374b
role of inflammation, 370–371, 371b
selective estrogen receptor
modulators in, 379–380
sodium effects in, 377
soy in, 375–376, 376b
substances may be harmful to bone
health, 377–378
supplements in, 372–376
teriparatide in, 380
therapeutic review on, 381b
trace minerals in, 375
vitamin A in, 377
vitamin C in, 375, 375b
vitamin D in, 373, 373b
vitamin K in, 374–375, 375b
web resources on, 381t
Osteotomy, in osteoarthritis, 648
Otitis media (OM), 152–156.e1
antibiotics in, 153, 155

Otitis media (OM) (Continued)
chiropractic intervention in, 156
cod liver oil in, 153
herbal extract ear drops in, 154
homeopathy in, 156
integrative therapy for, 153–156
biochemical in, 153, 153b
biomechanical in, 155–156
botanicals in, 154
nutrition in, 153
pharmaceuticals in, 155, 155f,
155b
supplements in, 154
myringotomy in, 156b
osteopathy in, 155
pathophysiology of, 153, 154f
pharmaceuticals in, 155, 155f, 155b
prevention of, 156b
therapeutic homeopathy in, 1067,
1069t
therapeutic review on, 156b
therapies to consider for, 156
tympanostomy tube in, 156
web resources on, 156t
xylitol in, 154, 154b
Over-the-counter (OTC) drugs, in
detoxification, 997f
Overweight
adult classification of being, 383t
classification of, and associated
disease, 383t
definition of, 382, 382b
Oxalobacter formigenes, in urolithiasis,
611–612
Oxidative stress, glycemic index in,
865
Oxytocin, in postdates pregnancy,
539, 539b

P
Paced breathing, 895–897, 896t, 897b
Padma Lax, in irritable bowel
syndrome, 429, 429b
Pain. See also Psychophysiological
disorders
abdominal. See Abdominal pain
back. See Low back pain
emotional awareness for, 963–970.
e2, 963b
in fibromyalgia, 475, 475b
forgiveness and, 941
hypnosis in, 918–919
labor. See Labor pain
myofascial. See Myofascial pain
syndrome
neck. See Neck pain
palliative care and, 807–808, 808b
pathways, 964
psychology of, 964–965, 964b.
See also Psychophysiological
disorders
reality of, 963–964
Pain referral pattern
in levator scapulae muscle, 1034f
in piriformis muscle, 1036f
in sternocleidomastoid muscle,
1035f
in trapezius muscle, 1032, 1033f
Palliative care, 806–816.e4, 806f,
814b–816b
acupuncture in, 814
anxiety in, 809.e1
aromatherapy in, 813
art therapy in, 814
bereavement in, 811
botanicals for, 808
common issues in, 807
communication in, 807
constipation in, 808–809
conventional and alternative
modalities (CAM) in, 806
delirium in, 809–810, 810b
depression in, 809.e1
dyspnea in, 809
energy medicine in, 813

Palliative care *(Continued)*
forgiveness and, 941
guided imagery in, 812
hypnosis in, 812
integrative therapies for, 811–816
life review in, 812
massage in, 813
mind-body therapies in, 812–814
mindfulness-based stress reduction in, 812
movement in, 811–812
music therapy in, 812–813
nausea in, 808–809
nutrition in, 811
pain management in, 807
pathophysiology of, 807
Reiki therapy in, 813–814
reminiscence therapy in, 812
spiritual care in, 810–811, 810t
supplement in, 812
traditional Chinese medicine in, 814
vomiting in, 808–809
web resources in, 816t
Palpitations, 277–278
Panax ginseng. *See* Ginseng
Pancreas, in insulin resistance, 321f
Pancreatic enzymes, in irritable bowel syndrome, 428, 428b
Pancreatic insufficiency, 428, 428b
Pancreatitis, acute, 993–994
Panic disorder. *See* Anxiety
Pantethine, in dyslipidemias, 272, 272b
Parkinson's disease (PD), 143–151.e3
acupuncture in, 147
advanced, 143
alpha-synuclein in, 145
amantadine in, 148–149, 149b
anticholinergic medications in, 149, 149b
Braak hypothesis of, 144
catechol-O-methyl transferase inhibitors in, 148, 148b
clinical signs and symptoms of, 143–144
coenzyme Q10 in, 146
creatine in, 147
curcumin in, 147, 147b
deep brain stimulation surgery in, 149
dopamine agonists in, 148, 148b
early symptoms of, 143
exercise in, 145, 145b, 150b–151b
glutathione in, 146, 146b
green tea in, 147, 147b
integrative therapy for, 145–147
botanicals in, 147
exercise in, 145, 145b
nutrition in, 145, 145b
supplements in, 146–147
levodopa in, 147–148, 148b
Lewy bodies in, 144, 144f
mind-body connection in, 149–151, 150b–151b
mitochondrial hypothesis of, 144–145
motor freezing in, 143
Mucuna pruriens (velvet bean or cowhage) in, 147
N-acetyl cysteine in, 146, 146b
nonmotor symptoms of, 143, 144t
pathophysiology of, 144–145
pharmaceuticals and, 147–149
preclinical symptoms of, 143
prevention prescription in, 149b
rasagiline in, 148, 148b
risk factors for, 143–144
supplements in, 146–147, 150b–151b
surgery in, 149
tai chi in, 145
therapeutic review in, 150b–151b
tremor in, 143
vitamin B$_{6 in}$, 147b
vitamin D in, 146

Parkinson's disease (PD) *(Continued)*
vitamin E in, 146–147
web resources on, 151t
zonisamide in, 149, 149b
Paroxetine, in depression, 42t
Patient expectations, healing encounter and, 25
Patient handout
on detoxification, 1001f–1003f
on forgiveness, 944f
Patient-defined goals, 27, 28t
Patient-driven care, in whole health, 28
Patterned breathing, 895–897, 896t, 897b
Pause
in healing encounter, 22
meditation and, 948
Pediatric patient, GERD in, 434, 434b, 437–438
Pelargonium sidoides. See Umckaloabo
Pelargonium spp. See Geranium oil
Pelvic pain questionnaire, 618f–619f
Peppermint
in cholelithiasis, 454, 454b
in common cold, 174
in irritable bowel syndrome, 428, 428b
in nausea and vomiting, in pregnancy, 544, 544b
in pediatric abdominal pain, 461, 461b
in urticaria, 741–742, 741b
Peptic ulcer disease (PUD), 439–449. e3
acid-suppressing drugs in, 446, 446b
acupuncture in, 447
alcohol avoidance or moderation in, 443
antacids in, 447, 447b
antibiotics in, 446, 446b
botanicals in, 444–446, 446b
cabbage in, 445, 445b
chili in, 445, 445b
cranberry in, 445, 445b
deglycyrrhizinated licorice (DGL) in, 444, 444b
diagnosis of, 440, 441f
glutamine in, 444, 444b
Helicobacter pylori in, 439, 440f
integrative therapy for, 440–449
mastic in, 445, 445b
neem in, 445–446, 446b
nonsteroidal antiinflammatory drugs (NSAIDs) and, 443
nutrition in, 440–442, 442b
osteopathy in, 447–449
pathophysiology of, 439–440, 439b, 440f
pharmaceuticals in, 446–447
physical activity in, 442
polyunsaturated fatty acids (PUFAs) in, 444, 444b
prevention prescription of, 448b
probiotics in, 443, 443b
sleep in, inadequate, 442
stress reduction in, 442, 442f
sucralfate in, 447, 447b
supplements in, 443–444
therapeutic review on, 448b
therapies to consider in, 447–449
tobacco cessation in, 442
traditional Chinese medicine (TCM) in, 447
turmeric in, 444, 444b
vitamin C in, 443, 443b
web resources on, 449t
zinc in, 443–444, 444b
Percutaneous electrical nerve stimulation (PENS), 130, 1040
Percutaneous nephrolithotomy, for urolithiasis, 614–615, 614f
Peripheral biostimulation, in myofascial pain syndrome, 655–656, 656f

Peripheral neuropathy, 120–132.e8
acetyl-L-carnitine in, 126
alpha-lipoic acid in, 127
analgesics in, 130
antidepressants in, 129
B-complex multivitamin in, 128, 128b
bioelectromagnetics in, 122–123
biofeedback in, 122
biomechanical modalities in, 130
electrical stimulation in, 130
evening primrose oil in, 126
exercise in, 122
geranium oil in, 125–126
integrative therapy for, 121–132
biomechanical modalities, 130
botanical medicine, 123–126
lifestyle, 122
mind-body therapy, 122–123
movement therapies, 122
pharmaceuticals, 128–130
supplements, 126–128
surgery, 131
therapies to consider, 131–132
neural blockade in, 130
pathophysiology of, 120–121, 121f
pharmaceutical agents for, 121t
prevention prescription for, 131b
serotonin norepinephrine reuptake inhibitors in, 129
therapeutic review on, 131b–132b
with toxic neuropathy, 121t
tricyclic antidepressants in, 129
web resources on, 132t
Persea americana. See Avocado
Personal care products, 1021
Personal health plan, 31–32
Personalized care, in whole health, 28
Pesticides
in chronic kidney disease, 418.e1
household, 1022
in produce, 999, 999t
Petasites hybridus. See Butterbur
pH, vaginal, 594
Pharmaceuticals. *See also specific pharmaceuticals*
in acne vulgaris, 762
in age-related macular degeneration, 845, 845b
in AIDS, 181–182
in alcoholism, 818–821, 819t, 820b
in allergic patient, 305–306
in anxiety, 48–49, 49t
in aphthous stomatitis, 752b
in arrhythmias, 280t, 283–284, 284b
in asthma, 294–295
in atopic dermatitis, 721–722, 724b
in attention-deficit/hyperactivity disorder, 60–62
in benign prostatic hyperplasia, 603t, 604–605
in carpal tunnel syndrome, 698–700
in cholelithiasis, 454
in constipation, 470–472
in coronary artery disease, 255, 256c
in depression, 41–43, 42t
in dyslipidemias, 274b–275b
in dysmenorrhea, 572–573, 576b
in epicondylosis, 709, 714b
in erectile dysfunction, 623
in fibromyalgia, 480–481
in GERD, 436, 436t, 437b
in gout, 693, 696b
as health care's carbon footprint, 1084–1085
in heart failure, 247–249
in hypothyroidism, 355–358, 355. e1t
in inflammatory bowel disease, 510–512

Pharmaceuticals *(Continued)*
in insulin resistance, 332
in irritable bowel syndrome, 430
in Lyme disease, 222–223
in menopausal symptoms, 553–554
in metabolic syndrome, 332
in migraine, 109t, 112–114
in multiple sclerosis, 139
in myofascial pain syndrome, 658–659
in neck pain, 683–684, 684t, 684b
in obesity, 390–391
in osteoarthritis, 646
in osteoporosis, 378–381
in otitis media, 155, 155f, 155b
in Parkinson's disease, 147–149, 150b–151b
in pediatric abdominal pain, 462–463
in peptic ulcer disease, 446–447
in peripheral neuropathy, 121t, 128–130
in polycystic ovarian syndrome, 366–367
in postdates pregnancy, 538–539
in prostate cancer prevention, 797–799
in psoriasis, 731–733
in rheumatoid arthritis, 495–498
in rosacea, 768, 770.e5
in seborrheic dermatitis, 756–757, 758b
in type 2 diabetes mellitus, 343–345
in urinary tract infection, 215
in urolithiasis, 612–613
in urticaria, 742–744, 745b
in uterine fibroids, 587
Pharmacotherapies, for posttraumatic stress disorder, 90–93, 92b
Phenazopyridine, in urinary tract infection, 215
Phenothiazines, in nausea and vomiting, in pregnancy, 546, 546b
Phentermine, in obesity, 390, 390b
Phobias. *See* Anxiety
Phosphatidylcholine
in Alzheimer disease, 105
in inflammatory bowel disease, 506–507
Phosphodiesterase 4 inhibitor, in psoriasis, 735
Phosphodiesterase inhibitors, for erectile dysfunction, 623, 623b, 626t
Phosphodiesterase-5 (PDE5) inhibitors
in benign prostatic hyperplasia, 605, 605b
in vaginal dryness, 598, 598b
Phosphorus, osteoporosis and, 374
Phototherapy
in depression, 41
in psoriasis, 733–734, 733b
Phthalates, 633
Phyllanthus niruri, in urolithiasis, 611, 611b
Physical activity. *See also* Exercise
in colorectal cancer prevention, 803
in constipation, 466
in peptic ulcer disease, 442
Physical therapy
in carpal tunnel syndrome, 702
in chronic prostatitis/chronic pelvic pain syndrome, 620
in epicondylosis, 710, 710b, 711f–712f, 712b
in gout, 692–693, 696b
in migraine, 115
in neck pain, 677
Physical vascular therapy, for peripheral neuropathy, 122–123
Phytoantiinflammatory agents, in neck pain, 685, 685t–686t

Phytosterols, in dyslipidemias, 269–270

Pilates, in neck pain, 677

Pills, in preparation of herbal products, 983t

Pineapple, in postdates pregnancy, 535

Pinus pinaster. See French maritime pine bark

Piper methysticum. See Kava

Piperine, in cholelithiasis, 455

Piriformis exercise, in low back pain, 903f–907f

Piriformis muscle, counterstrain for, 1033–1034, 1036f

Pistacia lentiscus. See Mastic

Placebo
    common cold and, 177
    in depression, 14–16
    in irritable bowel syndrome, 430

Planetary health
    advocacy strategies for, 1025b
    cellular phone and, 1021–1022
    chemical exposures and associated policies in, 1018–1019
    climate change and, 1019–1020, 1020f
    cordless phone and, 1021–1022
    drinking water and, 1024
    ecological problems in, 1018–1020
    food concerns in, 1019, 1019b
    furnishings and, 1022
    genetically engineered foods and, 1017–1018
    household pesticides and, 1022
    household products and, 1020–1021, 1021b
    integrative strategies for, 1016–1026.e4, 1025b
    meat and, 1022–1023
    nanotechnology and, 1017
    organic food considerations in, 1023–1024, 1023t
    personal care products and, 1021
    personal health and, 1020–1024
    poultry and, 1022–1023
    precautionary principle in, 1016–1018, 1016b
    seafood and, 1022–1023
    systems approach to, 1016, 1017f
    water concerns in, 1019, 1019b
    web resources on, 1026t

Plant stanols, in dyslipidemias, 269–270

Plant sterols, in dyslipidemias, 269–270, 270b–271b

Plaques
    in Alzheimer disease, 95
    in coronary artery disease, 253
    in multiple sclerosis, 134, 135f

Plastics, in chronic kidney disease, 418.e1

Platelet-rich plasma (PRP), in epicondylosis, 709–710, 714b

Polarity therapy, 1075t

Polycystic ovarian syndrome (PCOS), 361–369.e2
    N-acetylcysteine in, 364, 364b
    acupuncture in, 365–366
    antiandrogens in, 367, 367b
    botanicals in, 365
    chaste tree berry *(Vitex Agnus-castus)* in, 365, 365b
    chromium in, 364, 364b
    Cinnamomum cassia in, 365, 365b
    clomiphene citrate in, 367, 367b
    complementary healing approaches, 365–366
    criteria for, 361, 362t
    evaluation of, 361
    hormone modulators in, 366–367
    inositol family in, 363–364
    insulin sensitizers in, 366, 366b
    integrative therapy of, 362–369, 362b

Polycystic ovarian syndrome (PCOS) *(Continued)*
    licorice in, 365, 365b
    lifestyle of, 362
    macronutrients in, 363
    mind-body therapy in, 366
    nutrition in, 363
    omega-3 fatty acids in, 363
    oral contraceptives in, 366–367, 366b
    orlistat in, 366
    pathophysiology of, 361–362
    pharmaceuticals in, 366–367
    phenotypic expression of, 362f
    physical activity in, 362
    prevention prescription of, 368b
    progestins in, 367, 367b
    soy in, 363b
    statins in, 367, 367b
    supplements in, 363–365
    surgery in, 367–369
    theories for, 361
    therapeutic review on, 368b
    vitamin D in, 364, 364b
    web resources on, 369t
    weight management in, 362

Polyol sugars, 883b

Polysomnography, in insomnia, 76–77

Polyunsaturated fatty acids
    in breast cancer, 775, 775b
    in peptic ulcer disease, 444, 444b

Polyvagal theory, heart rate variability and, 923

Pomegranate juice
    in dyslipidemias, 273, 273b
    in prostate cancer, 795

Pomi-T, in prostate cancer prevention, 797

Popular diets, in obesity, 386–387, 387b

Positional release therapy, 1030b

Postdates pregnancy, 535–541.e1
    acupuncture in, 538, 538t
    amniotomy in, 539
    biochemical therapy in, 537–538
    bioenergetics in, 538
    black cohosh in, 537, 537b
    blue cohosh in, 537, 537b
    botanicals in, 536–537
    breast stimulation in, 537
    castor oil in, 535–536
    evening primrose oil in, 536
    homeopathy in, 536, 536b
    integrative therapy in, 535–541
    lifestyle in, 538
    mechanical methods in, 539–541
    membrane sweeping in, 539
    misoprostol in, 538, 538b
    nutrition in, 535
    oxytocin in, 539, 539b
    pathophysiology of, 535
    pharmaceuticals in, 538–539
    pineapple in, 535
    prevention prescription of, 540b
    red raspberry leaf in, 536–537, 537b
    sexual intercourse and, 538
    shiatsu in, 537–538
    supplements in, 535–536
    therapeutic review on, 540b
    transcervical Foley catheter or Cook catheter insertion in, 539–541, 539f
    vaginal prostaglandins in, 539, 539b
    web resources on, 541t

Posttraumatic stress disorder (PTSD), 86–93.e3. *See also* Anxiety
    acupuncture in, 90, 92b
    definition of, 86
    diagnostic criteria of, 86
    emotional freedom technique in, 88–89
    energy psychology in, 972
    exercise in, 86–87, 86b, 92b
    hypnotherapy in, 89

Posttraumatic stress disorder (PTSD) *(Continued)*
    integrative therapy in, 86–87
    meditation in, 87–88, 87b
    mind-body therapy in, 87–90, 92b
    pharmacotherapies in, 90–93, 92b
    prevention prescription in, 91b–92b
    psychotherapy in, 89–90
    repetitive transcranial magnetic stimulation (rTMS) in, 90
    thought field therapy in, 88–89
    visualization and guided imagery in, 88
    web resources on, 93t
    yoga in, 88

Posture
    correction of, in myofascial pain syndrome, 655
    for meditation, 952f

Potassium
    arrhythmias and, 282
    in DASH diet, 878

Potassium citrate, in urolithiasis, 612, 612b

Poultice, in preparation of herbal products, 983t

Powders, in preparation of herbal products, 983t

Pramipexole, in Parkinson's disease, 148, 148b

Pranic healing, 1075t

Prayer
    in asthma, 296
    as relaxation technique, 911t–912t

Prebiotics, 988t, 988b–989b, 989. *See also* Probiotics
    in chronic kidney disease, 414–415
    dietary source of, 418
    clinical indications for, 989
    in inflammatory bowel disease, 508, 508b
    in irritable bowel syndrome, 427–428, 428b

Preconception counseling and fertility, 517–525.e2, 524b
    preconception multivitamin ingredients and, 521b
    web resources on, 525t

Prediabetes, 320

Pregabalin (Lyrica)
    in fibromyalgia, 481, 481b
    in peripheral neuropathy, 130

Pregnancy. *See* Labor pain
    nausea in. *See* Nausea, in pregnancy
    postdates. *See* Postdates pregnancy
    vomiting in. *See* Vomiting, in pregnancy

Pregnancy-related depression, exercise to prevent, 36–37

Pregnenolone
    in Alzheimer disease, 103, 103b
    in chronic fatigue syndrome, 488, 488b

Pre-meal water loading, in obesity, 387–388

Premenopausal women, vaginal dryness in, 592

Premenstrual syndrome, 560–568.e2
    acupuncture in, 566
    aldosterone in, 560
    black cohosh in, 565b
    botanicals in, 564–566
    calcium in, 562–563, 563b
    chaste tree *(Vitex agnus-castus)* in, 564b
    clinical evaluation of, 561–562
    diet in, 562, 562t, 562b
    endogenous opiates in, 560
    exercise in, 562
    ginkgo *(Ginkgo biloba)* in, 565, 565b
    hormonal influences in, 560
    hypoglycemia in, 560
    integrative therapy for, 562–568
    mind-body therapy in, 566

Premenstrual syndrome *(Continued)*
    nutrition in, 562, 562t, 562b
    pathophysiology of, 560–562, 561t
    pharmaceuticals in, 566–568
    prevention prescription of, 567b
    prolactin in, 560
    prostaglandins in, 560
    psychosocial theory in, 560
    pyridoxine in, 563–564
    selective serotonin reuptake inhibitors in, 566–568
    St. John's wort *(Hypericum perforatum)* in, 565–566, 566b
    supplements in, 562–564
    symptoms of, 560–561, 561t
    therapeutic review on, 567b
    valerian *(Valeriana officinalis)* in, 566b
    vitamin B$_6$ in, 563–564, 564b
    web resources on, 568t

Primary uncomplicated herpes simplex virus infection, pharmaceuticals in, 195

Proactive care, in whole health, 28

Probenecid, in gout, 695, 695b

Probiotics
    in atopic dermatitis, 720, 720b
    in autism spectrum disorder, 66–67
    biological effects, 990t
    in chronic kidney disease, 414–415
    dietary source of, 418
    clinical indications of, 992t
    in common cold, 176
    in constipation, 467–469
    definition of, 986–989, 988t, 988b
    dosage for, 991–992, 992t–993t
    human microbiota, 987, 987b
    indications for, 989
    in inflammatory bowel disease, 507
    in irritable bowel syndrome, 427, 427b
    in Lyme disease, 223, 223b, 225, 225b
    mechanisms of action of, 990t
    natural food sources of, 992–993
    in obesity, 389, 389f
    in otitis media, 154
    pancreatitis in, 993–994
    in pediatric abdominal pain, 462, 462b
    in peptic ulcer disease, 443, 443b
    potential mechanisms of, 989, 990f
    potential therapeutic applications for, 990t–991t
    prescribing, 986–995.e4
    safety, 993–994, 994b
    in seborrheic dermatitis, 755, 755b
    in urinary tract infection, 213, 213b
    web resources on, 995t

Product labels, interpreting, 984t–985t

Progesterone, in menopausal symptoms, 553, 553b

Progesterone-containing intrauterine devices, in uterine fibroids, 588, 588b

Progestins, in polycystic ovarian syndrome, 367, 367b

Progressive muscle relaxation, 911t–912t
    in HIV disease, 187–188
    in pediatric abdominal pain, 464

Prolactin, in premenstrual syndrome, 560

Prolotherapy, 1047b
    in chronic musculoskeletal pain, 1047–1053.e2, 1049t
        adverse events of, 1051
        basic science of, 1047–1048
        case example of, 1051–1052
        clinical research of, 1048–1051, 1048f
        common side effects of, 1051
        contraindications of, 1051

Prolotherapy *(Continued)*
  insurance coverage of, 1053
  practical considerations of, 1051
  web resources on, 1053t
  in epicondylosis, 710, 714b
Promethazine, in nausea, in palliative care, 808–809
Prophylaxis, pre- and postexposure, HIV disease and, 182
Propionibacterium acnes, 759, 760f. *See also* Acne vulgaris
Propolis, in herpes simplex virus, 193–194, 194b
Propranolol, herbal and supplement interactions with, 256t
Prostaglandin E₁ injection, in erectile dysfunction, 624
Prostaglandins, premenstrual syndrome and, 560
Prostate cancer, 790–799.e2
  acupuncture in, 796
  chondroitin sulfate and, 798b
  diagnosis and staging of, 791–792, 791t–792t
  diet and, 794
  green tea in, 795
  integrative therapy for, 793–799
    conventional treatments, 793–794
  lifestyle therapy and, 794–796, 794b, 796b
  mind-body medicine in, 796
  multivitamins and, 796–797
  pomegranate juice in, 795
  prevention of, 797–799, 798b
    cruciferous vegetables in, 794
    dutasteride in, 797
    exercise in, 794
    finasteride in, 797
    lycopene in, 795
    NSAIDs in, 797–799
    selenium in, 796
    soy protein in, 794–795
    vitamin D, 796
    vitamin E, 796
  recurrence of, 797
  risk factors of, 790, 790b
  screening for, 790–791, 791b
  smoking and, 794
  soy protein and, 794–795
  supplements and, 797
  therapeutic review on, 798b
  web resources on, 799t
Prostate gland, cancer of. *See* Prostate cancer
Prostate-specific antigen (PSA), 790, 792t
Protein
  in chronic sinusitis, 165
  in diet, 874
  in osteoporosis, 374, 374b
  in urolithiasis, 610
Proton pump inhibitors
  in GERD, 436, 436t, 437t
  in pediatric abdominal pain, 462–463
Provider burnout, integrative medicine and, 1095, 1095b
Prunus africana, in benign prostatic hyperplasia, 604
Pseudoallergy, 316
Psoralen and ultraviolet A light therapy, 734, 734.e1, 734.e1b
Psoriasis, 726–738.e2
  acitretin in, 734, 734b
  acupuncture in, 736, 736b
  aloe vera in, 730–731
  anthralin in, 733, 733b
  antiinflammatory diet in, 728–729
  apremilast in, 735
  arthritis with, 726, 728t
  balneo-phototherapy in, 727–728
  biological immune response modifiers in, 735
  botanicals in, 730–731
  calcipotriene in, 731, 731b

Psoriasis *(Continued)*
  capsaicin in, 730, 730b
  climatotherapy in, 727–728
  clinical background of, 726, 727f
  curcumin in, 729b
  cyclosporine in, 734, 734b
  environmental factors in, 726
  glycyrrhetinic acid in, 731
  homeopathy in, 736–738, 736b
  hypnosis in, 735
  indigo naturalis extract in, 730, 730b
  inositol in, 730, 730b
  keratolytics in, 731, 731b
  licorice in, 731
  meditation in, 735
  methotrexate in, 734, 734b
  milk thistle in, 731, 731b
  mind-body therapy in, 735, 735b
  of nails, 726
  nutrition in, 728–729
  omega-3 fatty acids in, 729b
  pathophysiology of, 726
  pharmaceuticals in, 731–733
  phototherapy of, 733–734, 733b
  prevention prescription, 736b
  Silybum marianum in, 731, 731b
  skin care in, 726–728
  steroids in, 731, 731b, 732t–733t
  subtypes of, 727t
  supplements in, 729–730
  tar in, 733, 733b
  tazarotene in, 731–733, 733b
  therapeutic review, 737b
  traditional Chinese medicine in, 735–736
  ultraviolet A and psoralen therapy in, 734.e1, 734.e1b
  ultraviolet B therapy in, 733, 733b
  web resources in, 738t
  zinc in, 729–730, 730b
Psychophysiological disorders, 965, 965b
  diagnosis of, 965–968, 966t
  diagnostic interview in, 966–968, 967t
  neurology of, 964f
  personality traits in, 965, 965t
  research support in, 968
  therapeutic program for, 968–969, 968t, 969b
  treatment approach for, 968–969
  trigger in, 968–969, 969b
  web resources on, 970t
Psychosocial stress, for epicondylosis, 708, 708b
Psychotherapy
  in anxiety, 50
  in depression, 40
  in irritable bowel syndrome, 429–430, 430b
  in nausea and vomiting, in pregnancy, 545
  in optimal healing environment, 17
  in pediatric abdominal pain, 464–465
  in posttraumatic stress disorder, 89–90
Psyllium, in idiopathic constipation, 467
Purines, in urolithiasis, 611
PUVA, in psoriasis, 734, 734.e1, 734.e1b
Pycnogenol
  in allergic patient, 303–304, 304f, 304b
  in asthma, 292
  in testosterone deficiency, 634, 634b
Pygeum africanum, in benign prostatic hyperplasia, 604, 604b
Pyridoxine. *See* Vitamin B₆

Q
Qigong, 911t–912t, 1075t
  in autism spectrum disorder, 71–72
  in chronic fatigue syndrome, 491
  in hypertension, 239
Quantum-touch therapy, 1075t
Quassia amara, in rosacea, 770.e5
Quercetin, 832
  in allergic patient, 303, 303b
  in chronic prostatitis/chronic pelvic pain syndrome, 620, 620b
  in gout, 692, 692b
  in testosterone deficiency, 633–634, 634b
  in urticaria, 741, 741b

R
Radiation therapy
  in breast cancer, 779
  in colorectal cancer prevention, 804
  in lung cancer, 788
Radiofrequency ablation, for lung cancer, 788, 788b
Range of motion, in osteoarthritis, 641–642
Rasagiline, in Parkinson's disease, 148, 148b
Raspberry leaf
  in labor pain management, 530, 530b
  in postdates pregnancy, 536–537, 537b
Rechallenge diets, elimination and, in clinical practice, 315–316
Recombinant biologics, for rheumatoid arthritis, 498
Recurrent uncomplicated herpes simplex virus infection, pharmaceuticals for, 195–196
Red flags
  in headache, 108
  in low back pain, 665, 665t
Red wine, in hypertension, 233
Red yeast rice
  in coronary artery disease, 258–259
  in dyslipidemias, 269, 269b
  in HIV disease, 187, 187b
Referral
  for arrhythmias, 279, 279t
  for cataracts, 831
  for energy medicine, 1076–1078
  for hypnosis, 921
Refined starchy foods, 328t
Reflexology, 1075t
  in labor pain management, 532–534
Regional anesthesia, for labor pain management, 532, 532t–533t
Reiki therapy, 1075t, 1077t
  in adrenal fatigue, 408
  in Alzheimer disease, 104
  in palliative care, 813–814
  in pediatric abdominal pain, 463
Relationship-centered care, 8–9, 939
Relative rest, for epicondylosis, 708, 708f
Relaxation techniques, 908–913.e1, 911t–912t. *See also* Mind-body therapy
  active participation in, 912
  for anxiety, 50
  duration and frequency of practice of, 912
  essentials of, 912
  in herpes simplex virus, 195
  in hypertension, 237–238
  in inflammatory bowel disease, 513–514
  in insomnia, 81
  in migraine, 115
  mindset in, 912
  in myofascial pain syndrome, 654–655

Relaxation techniques *(Continued)*
  in neck pain, 680
  in posttraumatic stress disorder, 88
  prescribing, 912–913, 913t
  stress and, 910–912, 910f
  web resources on, 913t
Religion, 1058, 1059t
Reminiscence therapy, in palliative care, 812
Repetitive strain, in neck pain, 678
Repetitive transcranial magnetic stimulation (rTMS), for posttraumatic stress disorder, 90
Resistance training, 890–891, 890b
Respiratory healing program, for chronic sinusitis, 158–161
  components of, 161
Rest, in gout, 693
Resveratrol/grape seed extract
  in dyslipidemias, 273, 273b
  in testosterone deficiency, 634, 634b
Retinoids, topical, in acne vulgaris, 763, 763b
Rheumatoid arthritis, 313, 493–500.e1
  acupuncture in, 498
  antibiotics in, 496
  antioxidants in, 495
  botanicals in, 495
  coffee and, 495
  conjugated linoleic acids in, 495
  corticosteroids in, 495–496, 496b
  diagnosis of, 493, 494f
  disease-modifying antirheumatic drugs in, 496
  essential fatty acids in, 495
  exercise in, 494
  food triggers in, 494
  ginger for, 495, 495b
  hydroxychloroquine in, 496, 496b
  integrative therapy for, 494–500
  journaling in, 938
  leflunomide in, 496–498
  low-level laser therapy in, 498
  methotrexate in, 496
  mind-body therapy in, 494
  nonsteroidal antiinflammatory drugs in, 495
  nutrition in, 494–495
  omega-3 fatty acids in, 494
  omega-9 fatty acids in, 494
  pathophysiology of, 493
  pharmaceuticals in, 495–498
  physical and occupational therapy in, 494
  prevention prescription of, 499b
  recombinant biologics in, 498
  sulfasalazine in, 496, 496b
  supplements in, 495
  surgery in, 498
  therapeutic review on, 499b–500b
  tobacco use and, 495
  treatment algorithm for, 497f
  turmeric in, 495, 495b
  web resources on, 500t
Rhodiola, in arrhythmias, 283
Rhubarb, in herpes simplex virus infection, 196
Ribavirin, in HCV, 202
Riboflavin
  for homocysteine lowering, 402, 402b
  for migraine, 110–111, 111b
D-Ribose, in chronic fatigue syndrome, 487, 487b
Risedronate, in osteoporosis, 378–379, 379t
Roman chamomile (*Chamaemelum nobile*), for common cold, 172, 172b
Ropinirole, in Parkinson's disease, 148, 148b
Rosacea, 765
  abnormal barrier function in, 766
  antibiotics in, 769b, 770.e5

Rosacea *(Continued)*
botanicals in, 767–768
Chrysanthellum indicum in, 759, 769b
classification of, 759–764, 765t, 767
colloidal oatmeal in, 767b
diet in, 767
disordered innate immunity in, 766–769
feverfew in, 768, 768b
genetics of, 766
green tea in, 768
hygiene for, 767–768
introduction/epidemiology of, 766
isotretinoin in, 769b, 770.e5
laser and light therapy, surgery in, 769
licorice extract in, 768, 768b
microbes in, 767
neurovascular dysregulation in, 766
pathophysiology of, 766
pharmaceuticals in, 768, 770.e5
Quassia amara for, 770.e5
therapeutic review on, 770.e5b
UV radiation in, 766–767
Rotenone, 144
Rotigotine, 148, 148b
Rubus. See Raspberry leaf
Rye grass pollen
in benign prostatic hyperplasia, 604, 604b
in chronic prostatitis/chronic pelvic pain syndrome, 620, 620b

S
Saccharomyces boulardii, in inflammatory bowel disease, 507–508
Saccharomyces cerevisiae, in acne vulgaris, 761, 761b
Safety
in headache acupuncture, 1038
in nasal irrigation, 1055, 1055b
in prescribing botanicals, 981–982, 981b
on probiotics, 993–994, 994b
Saffron
in depression, 40, 42t
in dysmenorrhea, 571–572, 572b
Sage
in age-related macular degeneration, 844
in herpes simplex virus infection, 196
Salacia reticulate, 339, 339b
Salai guggal. *See* Boswellia
Salicylic acid, in acne vulgaris, 763, 763b
Saline nasal irrigation
dose for, 1055
indications for, 1055t
mechanism of, 1054
patient handout on, 1056f
pediatric use of, 1055
safety of, 1055, 1055b
technique variations for, 1054, 1054b, 1056f
web resources for, 1055t
Salix cortex. See Willow bark
Salutogenesis, 20b
Salutogenesis-oriented healing encounter, 25–26
Salutogenesis-oriented sessions, 25–26
Salve, in preparation of herbal products, 983t
Sambucus. See Elderberry
SAMe. *See* S-Adenosylmethionine (SAMe)
Sanctuary, sense of, in insomnia, 83, 83b

Sangre de Grado, in herpes simplex virus, 194, 194b
Sarsaparilla, in urticaria, 741, 741b
Saturated fats
in age-related macular degeneration, 842
decrease, in neck pain, 679
Sauna therapy, for detoxification, 998–999
Saw palmetto
in benign prostatic hyperplasia, 603–604, 604b
in testosterone deficiency, 634, 634b
SCA (saffron, celery seed, anise), in dysmenorrhea, 571–572, 572b
Schisandra
in chronic hepatitis, 206
in detoxifying prior to conception, 522
Screening
alcoholism, 819b
breast cancer, 773, 773b
cataracts, 830–831
colorectal cancer prevention, 800
prostate cancer, 790–791, 791b
Sea buckthorn oil, for vaginal dryness, 597, 597b
Seafood
detoxification and, 999
planetary health and, 1022–1023
Seaweed preparations, in hypothyroidism, 351t, 355
Seborrheic dermatitis (SD), 753–758.e1
botanicals in, 755–756, 756b
energy-based treatments in, 757–758
fluconazole in, 757
food allergy in, 757
homeopathy in, 757
integrative therapy for, 754–758, 754b
keratolytic treatments in, 756, 756b
ketoconazole in, 757
lithium succinate in, 757
mind-body therapy in, 756
nutrition in, 754–755
nystatin in, 757, 757b
omega-3 essential fatty acids in, 754, 754b
oral antifungals in, 757
other creams in, 756–757, 757b
pathophysiology of, 753–754, 753b
pharmaceuticals in, 756–757
prevention prescription in, 758b
probiotics in, 755, 755b
shampoos in, 756, 756b
supplements in, 755
therapeutic review in, 758b
therapies to consider in, 757–758
topical corticosteroids in, 756, 756b
topical nicotinamide (vitamin B3) in, 755, 755b
vitamins in, 755, 755b
web resources in, 758t
yeast elimination in, 754–755
Secale cereale. See Rye grass pollen
Second-generation H1-receptor antagonists, dosage of, for urticaria, 742
Secretin, 69
Sedatives, in labor pain management, 532
Selective estrogen receptor modulators, 379–380
in osteoporosis, 379–380
Selective norepinephrine reuptake inhibitors (SNRIs), in menopausal symptoms, 554
Selective serotonin reuptake inhibitors (SSRI)
in autism spectrum disorder, 68

Selective serotonin reuptake inhibitors (SSRI) *(Continued)*
in depression, 41–42, 42t
in fibromyalgia, 480, 480b
in menopausal symptoms, 554
in premenstrual syndrome, 566–568
Selenium, 1010t–1011t
in age-related macular degeneration, 844
in Alzheimer disease, 101
arrhythmias and, 282
in asthma, 294
in chronic hepatitis, 203
in HIV disease, 183, 183b
in hypothyroidism, 353, 353t, 353b
in inflammatory bowel disease, 505
in polycystic ovarian syndrome, 364–365, 365b
in prostate cancer prevention, 796
in uterine fibroids, 586, 586b
Self-care
integrative medicine and, 1095, 1095b
in low back pain, 668–669
Self-hypnosis techniques, 915b
breathing/breath technique for, 917
debriefing for, 920
education about, 914–915, 920
eye fixation and closure technique for, 916–917
in gastrointestinal disorders, 917–918
hand clasp test for, 915
in headache, 918
for hot flashes, 918
ideosensory experience test for, 915
neuroplasticity in, 920–921
in pain, 918–919
patient encouragement in, 920–921
re-alerting in, 920
referral for, 921
relaxation staircase image in, 916
strategies for, 917
in surgical outcomes, 919–920
talent for, 915
thumb-and-finger technique in, 916
trance induction in, 915–917
in warts, 919, 919f
web resources on, 921t
Self-reflection. *See also* Meditation
in healing encounter, 21, 21f
Self-report scales, for insomnia, 76
Self-treatment, energy psychology for, 976b
Sensitization, 300–301, 301f
Serenoa repens. See Saw palmetto
Serotonin norepinephrine reuptake inhibitors. *See also* Selective serotonin reuptake inhibitors (SSRI)
in depression, 42t
in fibromyalgia, 480, 480b
in peripheral neuropathy, 129
Serotonin reuptake inhibitors (SRI), in autism spectrum disorder, 68
Sertraline, in depression, 42t
Sesame, in dyslipidemias, 272, 272b
Sexual intercourse, postdates pregnancy and, 538
Sexual lubricant safety, 593–594
Sexual lubricant safety, 593–594
Shamanic healing, 1075t
Shampoos, in seborrheic dermatitis, 756, 756b, 758b
Shatavari
for easing menstrual pain, 573t
for fertility, 522, 522b
Shiatsu, in postdates pregnancy, 537–538
SHINE protocol, for chronic fatigue syndrome, 485–486, 486b

Siberian ginseng
in adrenal fatigue, 407, 407b
in arrhythmias, 283
Sigmoidoscopy, in colorectal cancer prevention, 800
Sildenafil, in vaginal dryness, 598, 598b
Silver nitrate, cautery with, in aphthous stomatitis, 751
Silver spray, ionic, for chronic sinusitis, 162, 162b
Silybum marianum. See Milk thistle
Silymarin, 339, 339b
in HIV disease, 186, 187b
Simple sugars, depression and, 37
Sinus survival spray, in chronic sinusitis, 162, 162t, 162b
Sinusitis
chronic, 157–169.e2, 168b
antiinflammatory and antioxidant vitamins and supplements for, 162–163
detoxification for, 166–167
diet for, 163
emotional factors in, 163
improving indoor air quality for, 163
integrative therapy for, 158–161
mind-body therapy for, 167
nasal hygiene for, 162, 162t
nasal sprays for, 162
natural antibiotics for, 161–162
pathophysiology of, 157–158
prevalence of, 157
respiratory healing program for, 158–161
restoring normal bowel bacterial flora for, 166
risk factors for, 158
sleep for, 163
spirituality and, 167–169, 169b
strengthening immune system against, 166
common cold and, 157–158
symptoms and diagnosis of, 157–158
therapeutic homeopathy in, 1067, 1069t
Sitagliptin, 344, 344b
Skin, microbes, in rosacea, 767
Skullcap, in GERD, 435t
Sleep
in age-related macular degeneration, 841
in Alzheimer disease, 101
chronic fatigue syndrome in, 488
in chronic sinusitis, 163
dysfunctional thoughts about, 81b
inadequate, in peptic ulcer disease, 442
lack of, cataracts and, 833
low quality of, in chronic kidney disease, 419
in myofascial pain syndrome, 654
promotion of, for insomnia, 77, 77b
stages of, 77f
Sleep deprivation therapy, for depression, 44
Sleep efficiency, 75b
Sleep environment, for insomnia, 82, 82b
Sleep hygiene, 337
in insomnia, 81
in irritable bowel syndrome, 427
in type 2 diabetes mellitus, 337
Sleep restriction therapies, in insomnia, 81
Slippery elm
in GERD, 435, 435t, 435b
in pediatric abdominal pain, 462, 462b
Small intestinal bacterial overgrowth, and rosacea, 767

Smoking, 377
  in age-related macular
    degeneration, 840
  cessation
    in addressing peptic ulcer
      disease, 442
    in chronic kidney disease, 419
    in hypertension, 231
    lung cancer and, 787
    for multiple sclerosis, 134, 134b
    in colorectal cancer prevention, 803
  diabetes mellitus and, 335
  in HIV disease, 182
  lung cancer and, 785, 785b
  prostate cancer and, 794
Social relationship, in attention-
  deficit/hyperactivity disorder,
  58–59, 58t
Sodium, 377
  osteoporosis and, 377
  restriction, in chronic kidney
    disease, 417
  in urolithiasis, 610
Sodium sulfacetamide, for rosacea,
  768b, 770.e1
Sodium-glucose cotransporter 2
  inhibitors, 344, 344b
Sodium-glucose transporter-2
  (SGLT-2) inhibitors, 332
Soft tissue techniques, in osteopathic
  manipulative techniques, 678t
SOLAR or SOL acronym, for
  meditation, 947b, 946b
Solar photovoltaic panels, 1085b
Sorbitol pathway, 833f
Soy
  in benign prostatic hyperplasia, 601
  in breast cancer, 776, 776b
  in colorectal cancer prevention, 801
  in dyslipidemias, 270, 270b
  in hypothyroidism, 351
  in osteoporosis, 375–376, 376b
  in polycystic ovarian syndrome,
    363, 363b
  prostate cancer prevention and,
    794–795
Space, healing encounter and, 25
Specialized allergen avoidance diets,
  for allergic patient, 302
Specific Carbohydrate Diet (SCD),
  for irritable bowel syndrome,
  426
Spinal canal stenosis, 663t–664t
Spinal manipulation
  in dysmenorrhea, 575
  in low back pain, 669–670
  in migraine, 115
Spiral computed tomography, of
  lung cancer, 786, 786f, 786b
SPIRIT, in spiritual assessment tools,
  1060t
Spiritual assessment, 1057–1063.e1
  five clinical goals of, 1060–1063
    appropriate referrals,
      1062–1063
    health problems and perceived
      needs, 1061–1062, 1062b
    patients' subjective
      experiences and subjective
      understanding of (ultimate)
      reality, 1061
    religious and spiritual concerns
      in both adult and pediatric
      care, 1060–1061, 1060b
    resources for strength and
      recovery, 1061, 1061b
    therapeutic review in, 1063b
    tools for, 1060t, 1060b
    web resources on, 1063t
Spiritual care, 1057–1063.e1
  in breast cancer, 778
  five clinical goals of, 1060–1063
    appropriate referrals, 1062–1063
    health problems and perceived
      needs, 1061–1062, 1062b

Spiritual care (Continued)
    patients' subjective
      experiences and subjective
      understanding of (ultimate)
      reality, 1061
    religious and spiritual concerns
      in both adult and pediatric
      care, 1060–1061, 1060b
    resources for strength and
      recovery, 1061, 1061b
  in palliative care, 810–811, 810t
  therapeutic review in, 1063b
  web resources on, 1063t
Spiritual need cycle, 1059f
Spiritual suffering response
  mnemonic, 1062t
Spirituality, 1058. See also
    Spiritual care
  in Alzheimer disease, 104–105
  chronic sinusitis and, 167–169, 169b
  in HIV disease, 188
  in substance abuse, 824
  three dimensions of, 1059t
Spironolactone, in polycystic ovarian
  syndrome, 367, 367b
Spondyloarthropathy, 663t–664t
Springing, in osteopathic
  manipulative techniques, 678t
St. John's wort
  in anxiety and depression, in
    palliative care, 809.e1, 809.
    e1b
  in depression, 39, 39b, 42t
  in fibromyalgia, 479, 479b
  indinavir interaction with, 187b
  in menopausal symptoms, 556, 556b
  in premenstrual syndrome,
    565–566, 566b
Stability, 893
Stages of Reproductive Aging
  Workshop (STRAW), 550, 551f
Staircase trance technique, 916
Standing-on-one-leg exercise, in low
  back pain, 903f–907f
Stanols, in coronary artery disease,
  258
Statin-related myalgias, 257, 257b
Statins
  in dyslipidemias, 274
  herbal and supplement interactions
    with, 256t
  in polycystic ovarian syndrome,
    367, 367b
  in type 2 diabetes mellitus, 345
Steam inhaler, for chronic sinusitis,
  162
Stenting, in coronary artery disease,
  255
Sterile water injections, in labor pain
  management, 528, 528b
Sternocleidomastoid muscle,
  counterstrain for, 1033, 1035f
Steroid hormones, in obesity, 384t
Steroid injection, for carpal tunnel
  syndrome, 705b
Steroids, in psoriasis, 731, 731b,
  732t–733t
Sterols
  in coronary artery disease, 258
  in dyslipidemias, 269–270, 270b
Still technique, in osteopathic
  manipulative techniques, 678t
Stimulant laxatives, in constipation,
  471
Stimulants
  for attention-deficit/hyperactivity
    disorder, 61, 61t
  for autism spectrum disorder, 67–68
Stimulus control therapy, in
  insomnia, 81, 81b
Stinging nettle
  in allergic patient, 305, 305b
  in urticaria, 741, 741b
Stones. See Cholelithiasis;
    Urolithiasis

Stool softeners, in constipation, 471
Strain-counterstrain, 682–683
  in osteopathic manipulative
    techniques, 678t
Strength training, 891t
Stress. See also Stress management
  chronic, in Alzheimer disease, 100
  in chronic kidney disease, 419
  in depression, 36
  disclosure in, 937. See also
    Journaling
  emotional
    acne rosacea and, 759–760
    acne vulgaris and, 759–760
  GERD and, 433
  increased levels of, Parkinson's
    disease and, 149
  inflammatory bowel disease and,
    512–513
  multiple sclerosis and, 134b
  relaxation for. See Relaxation
    techniques
Stress management. See also
    Journaling; Meditation
  in age-related macular
    degeneration, 840
  in attention-deficit/hyperactivity
    disorder, 57, 57t
  in cataract prevention, 832
  in HIV disease, 187
  in insulin resistance, 328, 328b
  in irritable bowel syndrome, 429
  in metabolic syndrome, 328,
    328b
Stress reduction
  in cholelithiasis, 450
  in peptic ulcer disease, 442, 442f
STW-5, in irritable bowel syndrome,
  429, 429b
Subjective units of distress, 971b
Sublingual immunotherapy, for
  allergic patient, 307, 307b
Suboccipital release, for neck pain,
  682–683, 682f, 683b
Substance abuse, 817–828.e2
  acupuncture in, 821–822, 822f,
    822b
  Alcoholics Anonymous in,
    824–825, 824b
  biofeedback in, 823
  botanicals in, 821
  guided imagery in, 823
  homeopathy in, 826–828
  hypnosis in, 823
  integrative therapy for, 818–828
  meditation in, 823
  mind-body therapies in, 823–824,
    823b
  Native American interventions in,
    825–826, 825f–826f
  nutrition in, 826
  pharmaceuticals, 818–821, 819t
  spirituality in, 824
  therapeutic review, 826b–827b
  web resources on, 828t
  yoga in, 823–824
Sucralfate, in peptic ulcer disease,
  447, 447b
Suffering, reduction of, 9, 9f, 9b
Sugar sweetened beverages, 328t
Sugars
  in breast cancer, 775
  in cholelithiasis, 451–452
  in chronic kidney disease, 418
  elimination of, 882–883
  fermentable, 882
  FODMaP, 882t
  simple, depression and, 37
Sulfasalazine, in rheumatoid arthritis,
  496, 496b
Sulfonylureas, 343, 343b
Sunglasses
  in age-related macular
    degeneration, 840
  in cataract prevention, 831

Sunlight
  in age-related macular
    degeneration, 839
  in multiple sclerosis, 134
Supplements
  in acne vulgaris, 760–761
  in adrenal fatigue, 407–408
  in age-related macular
    degeneration, 842–844, 845b
  in allergic patient, 303–304
  in Alzheimer disease, 101–102
  in anxiety, 48, 49t
  in aphthous stomatitis, 748, 752b
  in arrhythmias, 281–282
  in asthma, 293–294
  in atopic dermatitis, 719–720,
    724b
  in benign prostatic hyperplasia,
    602–603, 603t
  in breast cancer, 777–778, 777b
  in carpal tunnel syndrome, 701
  in cataracts, 834–835
  in cholelithiasis, 452–453
  in chronic fatigue syndrome,
    486–490
  in chronic prostatitis/chronic
    pelvic pain syndrome, 620
  in colorectal cancer prevention,
    802–803
  in constipation, 467–469
  in coronary artery disease,
    258–261, 258t
  dietary
    for depression, 38–39, 42t
    evidence-based resources for,
      983t
    information on testing, 982t
  in dysmenorrhea, 570–571, 576b
  fertility and, 521–522
  in fibromyalgia, 478–479
  for gout, 691–692, 695–696,
    696b
  in heart failure, 246–247
  in HIV disease, 183–185
  in hypothyroidism, 351–355
  in inflammatory bowel disease,
    507–509
  in irritable bowel syndrome,
    427–428
  in low back pain, 672
  in Lyme disease
    acute infection of, 223
    chronic persistent symptoms
      of, 225
  in metabolic syndrome, 328–331
  in multiple sclerosis, 137–138
  in myofascial pain syndrome, 659,
    659b
  in neck pain, 685, 687b
  in obesity, 388–389
  in osteoarthritis, 644–646
  in osteoporosis, 372–376
  in otitis media, 154
  in Parkinson's disease, 146–147,
    150b–151b
  in pediatric abdominal pain, 462
  in peptic ulcer disease, 443–444
  in peripheral neuropathy,
    126–128
  in polycystic ovarian syndrome,
    363–365
  in postdates pregnancy, 535–536
  prostate cancer and, 797
  in psoriasis, 729–730
  in rheumatoid arthritis, 495
  in seborrheic dermatitis, 755, 758b
  in testosterone deficiency, 633
  in type 2 diabetes mellitus,
    340–343
  in urinary tract infection, 213
  in urolithiasis, 611
  for urticaria, 745b
Support, healing encounter and, 25
Supportive care, in atopic dermatitis,
  717–718

Surgery
  in benign prostatic hyperplasia, 605–607, 605b
  in breast cancer, 779
  in carpal tunnel syndrome, 704, 704b–705b
  in cataract prevention, 836–837
  in cholelithiasis, 454
  in colorectal cancer prevention, 804
  in dysmenorrhea, 575
  in epicondylosis, 713–714, 713b–714b
  in GERD, 437
  hypnosis for, 919–920
  in inflammatory bowel disease, 512
  in insulin resistance, 332–333
  in low back pain, 673–675
  in metabolic syndrome, 332–333
  in neck pain, 683
  in obesity, 392–394
  in osteoarthritis, 648
  in otitis media, 156
  in pediatric abdominal pain, 463
  in peripheral neuropathy, 131
  in polycystic ovarian syndrome, 367–369
  in rheumatoid arthritis, 498
  in urolithiasis, 613–615
  in uterine fibroids, 578, 588–589
Swallowing, 433, 434f
Sympathomimetic effects, supplements with, 392t
Synbiotics, 988t, 988b, 989. See also Probiotics
  in chronic kidney disease, 414–415
  in inflammatory bowel disease, 508
Syrup, in preparation of herbal products, 983t
Systemic enzymes, in uterine fibroids, 585, 585b
Systemic exertion intolerance disease (SEID), 485b
Systemic steroids, in aphthous stomatitis, 751, 751b

T
Tablets, in preparation of herbal products, 983t
Tachyarrhythmia, 276, 277f
Tai chi, 911t–912t
  in Alzheimer disease, 99
  in chronic kidney disease, 419
  in depression, 40–41
  in hypertension, 239
  in Lyme disease, 226, 226b
  in osteoarthritis, 642–643
  in Parkinson's disease, 145
  in peripheral neuropathy, 122
Tamsulosin, in urolithiasis, 613, 613b
Tanacetum parthenium. See Feverfew
Tangles, in Alzheimer disease, 95
Tar, in psoriasis, 733, 733b
Taraxacum officinalis. See Dandelion
Target behavior, 957
Taurine, 1010t–1011t, 1011
Tazarotene, in psoriasis, 731–733, 733b
Tea, 376. See also Caffeine; Green tea.
Tea tree oil, in acne vulgaris, 762, 762b
Teething, therapeutic homeopathy in, 1067t
Telemedicine interventions, in osteoarthritis, 642
Tender points, 1028. See also Counterstrain
  in levator scapulae muscle, 1034f
  pathophysiology of, 1029b
  in piriformis muscle, 1036f
  in sternocleidomastoid muscle, 1035f
  in trapezius muscle, 1032, 1033f
Tendinopathy(ies), 707, 1049
  prolotherapy and, 1049–1050

TENS. *See* Transcutaneous electrical nerve stimulation (TENS)
Tension-type headache, 117
Terazosin, in chronic prostatitis/chronic pelvic pain syndrome, 617b
Teriparatide, in osteoporosis, 379t, 380
Testosterone
  creams, 635, 635b
  cypionate injections, 635, 635b
  decrease in, 601
  deficiency of, 630–637.e1
    bisphenol A exposure and, 633
    botanicals in, 633–634
    endocrine disruptors in, 633, 633b
    exercise in, 632
    integrative therapy for, 631–637
    laboratory testing in, 635, 635b
    maca in, 634, 634b
    mind-body therapy in, 632
    nutrition in, 631–632
    opioids in, 632–633
    pathophysiology of, 630–631
    pharmaceuticals in, 634–637
    phthalate exposure and, 633
    prevention prescription for, 636b
    Pycnogenol in, 634, 634b
    quercetin in, 633–634, 634b
    resveratrol/grape seed extract in, 634, 634b
    saw palmetto in, 634, 634b
    signs and symptoms of, 632b
    supplements in, 633
    therapeutic review for, 636b
    toxins in, 632–633
    web resources for, 637t
    zinc in, 633, 633b
  in erectile dysfunction, 623–624, 624b
  gels and patches, 635, 635b
  in multiple sclerosis, 139
  production of, 630, 631f–632f
  prostate cancer and, 793
  replacement of, 635b
Tetracycline-fluocinolone acetonide-diphenhydramine mouthwash, in aphthous stomatitis, 750, 750b
Thalidomide, in aphthous stomatitis, 751, 751b
Theobroma cacao. See Cocoa
Therapeutic breathing, 895–900
  as relaxation technique, 911t–912t
Therapeutic homeopathy, 1064–1072.e2
  in acute injury and emergencies, 1068t
  aggravation with, 1066b
  in allergic rhinitis, 1067, 1070t
  antidote with, 1066b
  in asthma, 1067
  in atopic eczema, 1067
  in cancer, 1070
  in chronic cough, 1070
  in colic, 1067t
  definition of, 1064
  in gastrointestinal disorders, 1070, 1071t
  key resources on, 1072t
  in obstetrics, 1070, 1071t–1072t
  in otitis media, 1067, 1069t
  preparations for, 1064–1065, 1065t
  prescription for, 1065–1066, 1066b
    remedy, 1066, 1066b
  rationale for, 1064
  in severe brain injury and mild traumatic brain injury, 1068t
  in sinusitis, 1067, 1069t
  in teething, 1067t
  use of, 1067–1070, 1067t–1068t
  web resources on, 1072t

Therapeutic/healing touch, 1075t, 1077t
  in carpal tunnel syndrome, 704
  in osteoarthritis, 649–650
Thermotherapy, in myofascial pain syndrome, 657
Thiamine. *See* Vitamin B1
Thiazide diuretics, in urolithiasis, 613
Thiazolidinedione, 366
  in type 2 diabetes mellitus, 343–344, 344b
Thiol-based antioxidants, for multiple sclerosis, 137
Thioctic acid. *See* Alpha-lipoic acid
Thought field therapy, 1075t
  in posttraumatic stress disorder, 88–89
Thumb-and-finger technique, 916
Thyroid hormone
  dose, excessive, 356
  replacement therapy
    approach to, 355–356, 355.e1t, 356b
    inadequate response to, 356–357
    indications for, 349f
    LT4 + LT3 combination therapy, 357–358, 357b–358b
Thyroid-stimulating hormone, 347
Thyroxine (T4), 347
Tick bite. *See also* Lyme disease.
  prevention of, 226b–227b
TIES mnemonic, 947b
Time, healing encounter and, 25
Tincture
  in preparation of herbal products, 983t
  in uterine fibroids, 584, 584b
Tobacco cessation, in peptic ulcer disease, 442
Tobacco use
  in dysmenorrhea, 569
  elimination of, and rheumatoid arthritis, 495
  lung cancer and, 785
Tocopherols, in age-related macular degeneration, 843
Tocotrienols
  in dyslipidemias, 272, 272b
  in peripheral neuropathy, 131–132
Tolcapone, in Parkinson's disease, 148, 148b
Tonic, in preparation of herbal products, 983t
Toothpaste, in aphthous stomatitis, 747
Topical analgesics, for osteoarthritis, 647
Topical anesthetic agents, for herpes simplex virus infection, 195
Topical corticosteroids
  in atopic dermatitis, 721–722, 722b, 724b
  in seborrheic dermatitis, 756, 756b
Topical immunomodulators, for atopic dermatitis, 722, 722b, 724b
Topical nicotinamide (vitamin B3), in seborrheic dermatitis, 755, 755b
Topiramate
  in alcoholism, 820, 820t
  in obesity, 392
Total allergic load, 317
Total testosterone (TT), 630, 630b
Touch. *See* Therapeutic/healing touch
Touchi (soy), 339, 339b
Toxic neuropathy, peripheral neuropathy with, 121t
Toxic persistent cycle, 1016, 1017f
Toxin(s)
  in detoxification, 996
  metabolic syndrome and, 323
  testing for, 998
Trace minerals, in osteoporosis, 375

Traditional acupuncture, for carpal tunnel syndrome, 704, 705b
Traditional Chinese medicine. *See also* Acupuncture
  in allergic patient, 307–309
  in aphthous stomatitis, 751–752
  in asthma, 297
  in atopic dermatitis, 722
  in carpal tunnel syndrome, 704
  in chronic fatigue syndrome, 491
  in chronic hepatitis, 206
  in chronic kidney disease, 419
  in constipation, 469
  in GERD, 437
  in gout, 693, 693b
  in hypothyroidism, 358
  in infertility, 523
  in inflammatory bowel disease, 514–516
  in irritable bowel syndrome, 429
  in multiple sclerosis, 141
  in myofascial pain syndrome, 660
  in nausea and vomiting, in pregnancy, 548–549, 548b
  in pediatric abdominal pain, 463
  in peptic ulcer disease, 447
  in psoriasis, 735–736, 736b
  in urolithiasis, 612
  in urticaria, 744, 745b
Traditional Japanese medicine (Kampo), for atopic dermatitis, 723
Training
  cardiorespiratory, 888–890, 890t
  resistance, 890–891, 890b
  strength, 891t
Tramadol
  in fibromyalgia, 481, 481b
  in osteoarthritis, 646
Trametes, in colorectal cancer prevention, 803, 803b
Trance, 914–917. *See also* Hypnosis
  debriefing after, 920
  re-alerting after, 920
Tranexamic acid, in uterine fibroids, 588, 588b
Transcendental meditation, in hypertension, 238
Transcervical Foley catheter or Cook catheter insertion, in postdates pregnancy, 539–541, 539f
Transcranial magnetic stimulation
  in autism spectrum disorder, 71
  in depression, 44
Transcutaneous electrical nerve stimulation (TENS), 130, 1040
  in dysmenorrhea, 574
  in labor pain management, 528, 528b
  in myofascial pain syndrome, 655
  in osteoarthritis, 643
Transdisciplinary team, in optimal healing environment, 18t
Trans-fatty acids, 872, 872f
Transportation
  as health care's carbon footprint, 1085–1086
  virtuous cycle for, 1086f
Transurethral incision of the prostate (TUIP), in benign prostatic hyperplasia, 606
Transurethral microwave thermotherapy (TUMT), in benign prostatic hyperplasia, 605
Transurethral needle ablation (TUNA), in benign prostatic hyperplasia, 605
Transurethral resection of the prostate (TURP), in benign prostatic hyperplasia, 605–606
Trapezius muscle, counterstrain for, 1032, 1033f
Trauma, forgiveness and, 941b
Traveler's diarrhea, prevention of, 992t

Trazodone
  in depression, 43
  in fibromyalgia, 480, 480b
Tremor, in Parkinson disease, 143
Trial to Assess Chelation Therapy
    (TACT), 1005–1006
Triamcinolone, in aphthous
    stomatitis, 750, 750b
Trichloroethylene (TCE), 144
Tricyclic antidepressants
  in depression, 43
  in fibromyalgia, 480, 480b
  in low back pain, 671
  in migraine, 113
  in neck pain, 684t
  in peripheral neuropathy, 129
Trigger points, in myofascial pain
    syndrome, 651b
  biostimulation of, 656f
Triglyceride-to-HDL cholesterol
    ratio (TG:HDL-C), 326
Trigonella foenum graecum. See
    Fenugreek
Triiodothyronine (T3), 347
Trimethoprim-sulfamethoxazole,
    for chronic prostatitis/chronic
    pelvic pain syndrome, 617b
Trimethylglycine, for autism
    spectrum disorder, 70
Triptans, in migraine, 114
Tripterygium wilfordii Hook F, in
    chronic kidney disease, 416,
    416b
Triticum aestivum, in inflammatory
    bowel disease, 510
Tumor necrosis factor-α blockade,
    512
Turmeric
  in acne vulgaris, 762–763, 762b
  in Alzheimer disease, 103
  in antiinflammatory diet, 874
  in cataract prevention, 836
  in cholelithiasis, 454, 454b
  in chronic kidney disease, 415,
    415b
  in fibromyalgia, 479, 479b
  in inflammatory bowel disease,
    509–510
  in peptic ulcer disease, 444, 444b
  in rheumatoid arthritis, 495,
    495b
Twelve-Step Programs, 824–825,
    824b
Tympanostomy tube, 156
Type 2 diabetes mellitus, 334
  in obesity, 391–392
  pathophysiology of, 335f
  three major pathogenic defects,
    321f

U

Ubiquinone. *See* Coenzyme Q10
Ulcerative colitis
  N-acetylcysteine in, 506
  acupuncture in, 514
  aloe vera in, 509
  5-aminosalicylic acid in, 511
  Boswellia serrata in, 509
  bovine colostrum in, 508–509
  butyrate in, 508
  curcumin in, 509–510
  folate in, 504–505
  glucocorticoids in, 511–512
  helminths in, 510–512
  immunosuppressants in, 512,
    512b
  malnutrition in, 502
  melatonin, 507
  mind-body medicine, 512–514,
    513t
  pathophysiology, 501, 502f
  prebiotics, 508b
  probiotics, 507
  Saccharomyces boulardii, 507–508
  synbiotics, 508

Ulmus fulva. See Slippery elm
UltraInflamX-360, for chronic
    sinusitis, 166
Ultrasound therapy, in carpal tunnel
    syndrome, 702, 705b
Ultraviolet A and psoralen therapy,
    in psoriasis, 734.e1, 734.e1b
Ultraviolet B therapy, in psoriasis,
    733, 733b
Ultraviolet light, in atopic dermatitis,
    721
Ultraviolet radiation, in psoriasis,
    727
Umckaloabo, for common cold,
    174–175, 175b
Uncaria tomentosa. See Cat's claw
United States Pharmacopeia (USP),
    700
  verified brands, 700t
University of Michigan integrative
    medicine health foods pyramid,
    336f
Upper respiratory infections
  prevention of, 992t
  viral, 170–179.e7, 178b–179b
    botanicals in, 171–175
    integrative therapies for,
      171–179
    mind body therapy in, 177
    pathophysiology of, 170–171,
      170b
    pharmaceuticals and
      conventional cold products
      in, 177–179
    psychosocial influences of, 171,
      171b
    vitamins, minerals, and home
      remedies in, 175–177
    web resources on, 179t
Ureteroscopy, in urolithiasis, 614,
    614f
Uric acid-lowering agents, in chronic
    kidney disease, 413
Urinary tract infection (UTI),
    211–217.e2
  acupuncture in, 215–216
  antibiotics in, 215
  behavioral changes in, 215
  berberine in, 214
  biofeedback in, 216–217
  bladder irritants in, 212
  clinical presentation of, 211
  cranberry in, 213–214
  D-mannose in, 213
  fluids in, 212
  goldenseal in, 215
  integrative therapies for, 212–217
    botanicals, 213–215
    nutrition, 212
    other therapies to consider,
      215–217
    pharmaceuticals, 215
    supplements, 213
  pathophysiology and epidemiology
    of, 211–212
  phenazopyridine in, 215
  prevention prescription for, 216b
  probiotics in, 213
  risk factors for, 211–212, 212t
  therapeutic review on, 216b
  vitamin C in, 213
  web resources on, 217t
Urolithiasis, 608–615.e1, 609f
  acupuncture in, 612, 612b
  alfuzosin in, 613, 613b
  alkalinizers in, 612
  allopurinol in, 613, 613b
  alpha-1 channel blockers in,
    612–613
  Ayurvedic medicine in, 612
  beverages in, 610
  botanicals in, 611
  calcium in, 611
  calcium-channel blockers in, 612
  carbohydrates in, 610

Urolithiasis *(Continued)*
  chlorthalidone in, 613, 613b
  citrate in, 608, 608b, 609t
  doxazosin in, 613, 613b
  extracorporeal shockwave
    lithotripsy in, 613–614, 613f
  herbals in, 612
  hydrochlorothiazide in, 613
  magnesium in, 611
  nifedipine in, 612, 612b
  nutrition in, 609–611, 609t–610t
  omega-3 fatty acids in, 609t,
    610–611
  oxalate in, 611
  pathophysiology of, 608–609
  percutaneous nephrolithotomy in,
    614–615, 614f
  pharmaceuticals in, 612–613
  potassium citrate in, 612, 612b
  prevention prescription of, 614b
  probiotics in, 611–612
  protein in, 610
  purines in, 611
  sodium bicarbonate in, 612, 612b
  sodium in, 610
  supplements in, 611
  surgery in, 613–615
  tamsulosin in, 613, 613b
  therapeutic review on, 615b
  traditional Chinese medicine in,
    612
  ureteroscopy in, 614, 614f
  vitamin C in, 611
  vitamin D in, 611
  water in, 610
  web resources on, 615t
  weight and, 609–610
  xanthine inhibitors in, 613
  zinc in, 611
Ursodeoxycholic acid, in
    cholelithiasis, 454, 454b
Urtica dioica. See Stinging nettle
Urticaria, 739–746.e2
  antihistamines in, 742–743, 743b
  antiinflammatory diet in, 740
  botanicals in, 740–742
  butterbur in, 741, 741b
  corticosteroids in, 743, 743b
  cyclosporine in, 743, 743b
  dietary limitations in, 740
  general principles of, 740
  Ginkgo biloba in, 742, 742b
  homeopathy in, 744–746, 745b
  hypnosis in, 744, 744b
  integrative therapy for, 740–746
  leukotriene inhibitors in, 743,
    743b
  mind-body techniques in,
    744–746
  nutrition in, 740
  omalizumab (xolair) in, 744, 744b
  pathophysiology of, 739–740
  peppermint in, 741–742, 741b
  pharmaceuticals in, 742–744
  prevention prescription in, 745b
  quercetin in, 741, 741b
  sarsaparilla in, 741, 741b
  stinging nettle in, 741, 741b
  therapeutic review in, 745b
  traditional Chinese medicine in,
    744
  valerian root in, 742, 742b
  web resources in, 746t
Uterine artery embolization, in
    uterine fibroids, 589
Uterine fibroids, 578–591.e2
  acupuncture in, 589
  antiangiogenesis factors in, 585,
    585b
  birth control pills in, 588, 588b
  botanicals in, 583
  calcium D glucarate in, 586,
    586b
  castor oil packs in, 589
  danazol in, 587, 587b

Uterine fibroids *(Continued)*
  deep pelvic massage in, 589
  dehydroepiandrosterone in, 588,
    588b
  diindolylmethane for, 581, 584,
    584b
  dysbiosis and, 579
  epigallocatechin gallate in, 583,
    583b
  estrogen dominance and, 579–581,
    579f, 580t
  etiology of, 578
  evaluation for, 582, 582t
  exercise in, 583
  gonadotropin receptor agonists
    in, 587
  green tea in, 583, 583b
  homeopathy in, 589–591
  hormones in, 588
  indole-3-carbinol (I-3-C) for, 581,
    584, 584b
  integrative therapy for, 582–591
  iron in, 586, 586b
  leuprolide acetate in, 587, 587b
  lifestyle in, 583
  magnesium in, 586–587, 586b
  malignant potential of, 581–582,
    582t
  menorrhagia with, 584–585, 588
  mind-body therapy in, 587
  norethindrone acetate in, 588,
    588b
  NSAIDs in, 588, 588b
  nutraceuticals in, 585–587
  nutrition and, 582–583
  omega-3 fatty acids in, 587, 587b
  pathophysiology of, 578–582
  pharmaceuticals in, 587
  prevalence of, 578
  prevention prescription in, 589b
  progesterone-containing
    intrauterine devices in, 588,
    588b
  selenium in, 586, 586b
  surgical treatment for, 588–589
  systemic enzymes in, 585, 585b
  therapeutic review in, 590b
  tranexamic acid in, 588, 588b
  vitamin C in, 585, 585b
  vitamin D and, 578–579, 586,
    586b
  web resources in, 591t
  zinc in, 586–587, 586b
UV radiation, and rosacea,
    766–767
Uva ursi, in urinary tract infection,
    214

V

Vaccinium oxycoccos. See Cranberry
Vaginal dryness, 592–599.e2
  behavioral therapy in, 595–596
  botanicals in, 597
  description and prevalence of,
    592
  exercise in, 596, 596b
  integrative therapy for, 593–599,
    598b
  Mediterranean diet in, 596, 596b
  nutrition in, 596
  pharmaceuticals in, 597–599
  risk factors for, 592, 592t
  therapeutic review on, 599b
  topical vaginal lubricants in,
    593–595
  vaginal renewal program for, 595,
    595b
  vibrating wand massage in, 596
  vitamins and supplements in,
    596–597
  web resources on, 599t
Vaginal epithelium, pathophysiology
    of, 593
Vaginal lubrication, physiology of,
    592–593, 593b

Vaginal penetration, for vaginal dryness, 595, 595b
Vaginal pH, 594
Vaginal prostaglandins, in postdates pregnancy, 539, 539b
Vaginal renewal program, 595, 595b
Valacyclovir, 195, 196b
Valerian
  in anxiety, 50, 50b
  in GERD, 435t
  in insomnia, 78–79, 79b
  in migraine, 112, 112b
  in premenstrual syndrome, 566, 566b
  in urticaria, 742, 742b
Valeriana officinalis. See Valerian
Vascular disease, optimizing, in Alzheimer disease, 99
Vasomotor symptoms, in menopause, 552
  management of, 553
Vegan diets, osteoporosis and, 371–372
Vegetables
  in age-related macular degeneration, 841
  in antiinflammatory diet, 873, 873b
  in cataract prevention, 833
  in chronic sinusitis, 164
Vegetarian, osteoporosis and, 371–372
Velvet bean. *See Mucuna pruriens*
Venlafaxine, in depression, 42, 42t
Vertebral fracture prevention studies, 379t
Vibrating wand massage, in vaginal dryness, 596
Viburnum opulus. See Cramp bark
Viburnum prunifolium. See Black haw
Visceral hyperalgesia, pathogenesis of, 458f, 458b
Viscous lidocaine (Xylocaine 2% solution), in aphthous stomatitis, 750, 750b
Visors, in age-related macular degeneration, 840
Visualization, for posttraumatic stress disorder, 88
Vitamin A, 377
  in acne vulgaris, 761–762, 761b
  in age-related macular degeneration, 843
  in cataract prevention, 835, 835b
  deficiency of, 353
  in HIV disease, 183, 183b
  in hypothyroidism, 353, 353b
  in inflammatory bowel disease, 503–504
  in osteoporosis, 377
Vitamin B
  in adrenal fatigue, 407, 407b
  in age-related macular degeneration, 843
  in anxiety, 48
  in cataract prevention, 835
  in menstrual cramps, 586b
  for peripheral neuropathy, 127–128
  in uterine fibroids, 585–586, 585b
Vitamin B1
  in dysmenorrhea, 570–571, 570t, 571b
  in peripheral neuropathy, 127
Vitamin B2. *See also* Riboflavin
  in migraine, 110–111
Vitamin B3, 268–269
  in seborrheic dermatitis, 755, 755b
Vitamin B6
  in autism spectrum disorder, 70
  in carpal tunnel syndrome, 701, 701b
  in chronic kidney disease, 415
  in colorectal cancer prevention, 802, 802b

Vitamin B6 *(Continued)*
  in depression, 38
  in dysmenorrhea, 570, 570t, 570b
  in homocysteine lowering, 402, 402b
  in insulin resistance, 329, 329b
  in metabolic syndrome, 329, 329b
  in nausea and vomiting, in pregnancy, 545
  in Parkinson's disease, 147b
  in premenstrual syndrome, 563–564, 564b
Vitamin B12. *See also* Cobalamin
  in Alzheimer disease, 101, 101b
  in aphthous stomatitis, 748, 748b
  in chronic fatigue syndrome, 489
  in chronic kidney disease, 415
  in depression, 38
  in HIV disease, 183, 183b
  in inflammatory bowel disease, 504
  in insulin resistance, 329, 329b
  in metabolic syndrome, 329, 329b
  in multiple sclerosis, 137
  in peripheral neuropathy, 127–128
Vitamin C
  in adrenal fatigue, 407, 407b
  in age-related macular degeneration, 843
  in Alzheimer disease, 101
  in asthma, 293
  in cataract prevention, 833–834, 834b
  in cholelithiasis, 452, 452b
  in chronic hepatitis, 203
  in chronic sinusitis, 162
  in common cold, 176–177
  in fertility, 522, 522b
  in gout, 691, 691b
  in herpes simplex virus infection, 192, 192b
  in HIV disease, 183, 183b
  in inflammatory bowel disease, 504
  in insulin resistance, 329, 329b
  in metabolic syndrome, 329, 329b
  in osteoporosis, 375, 375b
  in peptic ulcer disease, 443, 443b
  in urinary tract infection, 213
  in urolithiasis, 611
  in uterine fibroids, 585, 585b
Vitamin D
  in age-related macular degeneration, 843
  in Alzheimer disease, 101
  in asthma, 293
  in breast cancer, 777–778, 778b
  in chronic fatigue syndrome, 489
  in colorectal cancer prevention, 802, 802b
  in common cold, 177
  in coronary artery disease, 260
  deficiency, uterine fibroids and, 578–579
  in depression, 38
  dietary reference intakes for, 372t
  in fibromyalgia, 478–479, 479b
  in HIV disease, 184, 184b
  in hypertension, 235–236
  in inflammatory bowel disease, 504
  in insulin resistance, 329, 329b
  in metabolic syndrome, 329, 329b
  in multiple sclerosis, 137
  in obesity, 388, 388b
  in osteoporosis, 373, 373b
  in otitis media, 154, 154b
  in Parkinson's disease, 146
  deficiency of, 146
  in polycystic ovarian syndrome, 364, 364b
  in prostate cancer prevention, 796
  in psoriasis, 729–730, 729b
  in type 2 diabetes mellitus, 340
  in urolithiasis, 611
  in uterine fibroids, 586, 586b
Vitamin D 25-OH, in chronic kidney disease, 414

Vitamin D3
  in chronic sinusitis, 162–163
  in vaginal dryness, 596, 596b
Vitamin E
  in Alzheimer disease, 101
  in asthma, 293
  in cataract prevention, 835
  in cholelithiasis, 453, 453b
  in chronic hepatitis, 203
  in coronary artery disease, 260, 260b
  in dysmenorrhea, 570t, 571, 571b
  in HIV disease, 183, 183b
  in inflammatory bowel disease, 504
  in insulin resistance, 330, 330b
  in metabolic syndrome, 330, 330b
  in Parkinson's disease, 146–147
  in prostate cancer prevention, 796
  in type 2 diabetes mellitus, 341–342
Vitamin K
  in chronic kidney disease, 415
  in inflammatory bowel disease, 504
  in osteoporosis, 374–375, 375b
  in type 2 diabetes mellitus, 342, 342b
Vitamin K1, in osteoporosis, 375b
Vitamin K2, in osteoporosis, 374
Vitamin-mineral supplements, in inflammatory bowel disease, 503–505
Vitamins
  in arrhythmias, 282
  in atopic dermatitis, 719, 719b
  in attention-deficit/hyperactivity disorder, 55
  in seborrheic dermatitis, 755, 755b
Vitex agnus-castus. See Chaste tree/chaste berry
Voiding, dysfunctional, 216, 216b
Vomiting
  acupuncture in, 1044–1046.e1, 1045b
    LV3 point for, 1045, 1046f
    MH6 point for, 1045, 1045f
    needle removal for, 1046
    posttreatment home program for, 1046
    ST36 point for, 1045, 1045f
    training in, 1046
    web resources on, 1046t
  chemotherapy-induced, 1044
  in palliative care, 808–809
  postoperative, 1044
  in pregnancy, 542–549.e2, 548b
    acupressure in, 544, 544b, 545f
    antihistamines in, 546, 546b
    avoid odors in, 542–543
    bioenergetics in, 544
    chamomile in, 543–544, 544b
    corticosteroids in, 547, 547b
    counseling in, 545
    dopamine antagonists in, 546, 546b
    enteral/parenteral feedings in, 547
    exercise in, 543
    ginger root in, 543, 543b
    homeopathy in, 548
    5-hydroxytryptamine3 receptor agonists in, 546, 546b
    hypnosis in, 544–545
    increase rest in, 543
    integrative therapy for, 542–549
    intractable, 547
    intravenous fluids in, 547
    lifestyle in, 542–543
    mind-body therapy in, 544–545
    nutrition in, 543
    pathophysiology of, 542
    peppermint leaf in, 544, 544b
    pharmaceuticals in, 546–547
    phenothiazines in, 546, 546b
    psychotherapy in, 545
    supplements in, 545

Vomiting *(Continued)*
    therapeutic abortion in, 547, 547f
    therapies to consider in, 548–549
    traditional Chinese medicine in, 548–549, 548b
    vitamin B6 in, 545
    web resources on, 549t
  pregnancy-related, 1044
VSL#3, in inflammatory bowel disease, 507

W
Walk to a Healthy Future, 889–890
Warfarin
  in coronary artery disease, 255
  herbal and supplement interactions with, 256t
Warts, hypnosis in, 919, 919f
Water. *See also* Fluids
  in cholelithiasis, 452
  in chronic sinusitis, 166
  drinking, planetary health and, 1024
  in urolithiasis, 610
Water immersion, in labor pain management, 527, 527b
Water pollution, in chronic kidney disease, 418.e2
Weight gain
  energy psychology in, 971
  medications associated with, 384t
Weight loss
  caution for supplements used for, 389, 389t
  in chronic kidney disease, 418
  in gout, 690
  in hypertension, 234
  pharmaceuticals for combined, 391–392
  in psoriasis, 728–729
Weight loss medications, PCOS and, 366, 366b
Weight loss program, common, 386–387, 387b
Weight management.
  See also Obesity
  in insulin resistance, 326–327, 327b
  in metabolic syndrome, 326–327, 327b
  osteoarthritis and, 640
  in polycystic ovarian syndrome, 362
Western blot testing, in Lyme disease, 221
Wet dressings, in atopic dermatitis, 718, 718b
Wheat grass juice, in inflammatory bowel disease, 510
Whole body health, in age-related macular degeneration, 841
Whole grains, in coronary artery disease, 254, 254b
Whole health process, 27–33.e1, 33t
  case scenario in, 31b
  Circle of Health in, 28, 29f
  four-step process for health planning in, 32
  innovative health systems for, 27–28, 28f, 28t
  patient-defined goals in, 27, 28t
  personal health plan in, 31–32
  three questions in, 28–31, 29f–30f
  value of, 32–33
  value over volume in, 27
Willow bark
  in carpal tunnel syndrome, 700–701, 701b
  in dysmenorrhea, 572, 572b
  in low back pain, 672, 672b
Wine, 874
  in age-related macular degeneration, 842

Withania somnifera, for multiple sclerosis, 138
Wolff-Parkinson-White syndrome, 279f
Wormwood, in inflammatory bowel disease, 510
Worry, stress physiology and, 931–932, 932b
Wound healing, journaling on, 938
Wrist splinting, in carpal tunnel syndrome, 702

X
Xanthine inhibitors, in urolithiasis, 613
Xenoestrogens, 581
Xilei-san (XLS), in inflammatory bowel disease, 510
Xylitol, in otitis media, 154, 154b

Y
Yangweishu, for ulcer healing, 447
Yeast elimination, in seborrheic dermatitis, 754–755

Yeast overgrowth, reducing, 163–164
Yin chiao, for chronic sinusitis, 161, 161b
Yoga
in adrenal fatigue, 408
in Alzheimer disease, 99
in asthma, 291
in autism spectrum disorder, 71
in carpal tunnel syndrome, 702, 705b
in chronic kidney disease, 419
in depression, 40
in hypertension, 238–239
in hypothyroidism, 358–360, 358b, 359f
in labor pain management, 529–530
in low back pain, 671
in lung cancer, 787
in menopausal symptoms, 555, 555b
in multiple sclerosis, 135
in neck pain, 677–678
in osteoarthritis, 642

Yoga *(Continued)*
in peripheral neuropathy, 122
in posttraumatic stress disorder, 88
as relaxation technique, 911t–912t
in substance abuse, 823–824

Z
Zeaxanthin, in cataract prevention, 834, 834b
Zeitgebers, 82
Zeolites, 1008t, 1013
Zero balancing, 1075t
Zinc
in acne vulgaris, 761, 761b
in age-related macular degeneration, 844
in Alzheimer disease, 101
in arrhythmias, 281
in attention-deficit/hyperactivity disorder, 55
in benign prostatic hyperplasia, 603, 603b
in chronic hepatitis, 204
in common cold, 177, 177b

Zinc *(Continued)*
deficiency of, 353
in herpes simplex virus, 193, 193b
in HIV disease, 185, 185b
in hypothyroidism, 353–354, 354b
in inflammatory bowel disease, 505
in insulin resistance, 330, 330b
in metabolic syndrome, 330, 330b
in osteoporosis, 375
in peptic ulcer disease, 443–444, 444b
in psoriasis, 729–730, 730b
in testosterone deficiency, 633, 633b
in uterine fibroids, 586–587, 586b
Zingiber officinale. See Ginger
Zoledronic acid, 379
Zonisamide, in Parkinson's disease, 149, 149b